Principles and Practice of
Geriatric Psychiatry

Principles and Practice of
Geriatric Psychiatry

Third Edition

Edited by

Mohammed T. Abou-Saleh

St George's Hospital Medical School, London, UK

Cornelius Katona

University College London, London, UK

Anand Kumar

University of Illinois, Illinois, USA

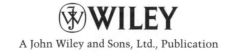

A John Wiley and Sons, Ltd., Publication

Library of Congress Cataloging-in-Publication Data

Principles and practice of geriatric psychiatry / [edited by] Mohammed T. Abou-Saleh, Cornelius Katona, Anand Kumar. –3rd ed.
       p. ; cm.
   Includes bibliographical references and index.
   ISBN 978-0-470-74723-0 (cloth)
   I. Abou-Saleh, Mohammed T. II. Katona, C. L. E. (Cornelius L. E.), 1954- III. Kumar, Anand, 1956-
   [DNLM: 1. Mental Disorders–diagnosis. 2. Aged. 3. Aging–physiology. 4. Aging–psychology.
   5. Mental Disorders–therapy. WT 150]
   Geriatric psychiatry.
   618.97′689–dc22

                                                                                2010025369

A catalogue record for this book is available from the British Library.

This book is published in the following electronic formats: ePDF 9780470669594; Wiley Online Library 9780470669600

Set in 9/11 Times by Laserwords Private Limited, Chennai, India
Printed and bound in Singapore by Markono Print Media Pte Ltd.

First Impression 2011

Dedication

Dedicated to our wives and families

Associate Editors

Contents

Contributors

Charlene S. Aaron University of Iowa College of Nursing, 101 Nursing Building, 50 Newton Road, Iowa City, IA 52242-1121, USA

Melanie Abas Institute of Psychiatry, Kings College London, Box P060, De Crespigny Park, London SE5 8AF, UK

Mohammed T. Abou-Saleh Division of Mental Health, St George's, University of London, Cranmer Terrace, London SW17 0RE, UK

Marc E. Agronin University of Miami Miller School of Medicine, and Medical Director for Mental Health and Clinical Research, Miami Jewish Health Systems, Miami, FL 33137, USA

Howard Aizenstein University of Pittsburgh School of Medicine, Pittsburgh, USA

Olusola Ajilore Department of Psychiatry, University of Illinois-Chicago, 5841 S. Maryland Ave, Chicago, IL 60637, USA

David N. Anderson Mersey Care NHS Trust, Older People's Mental Health Services, Sir Douglas Crawford Unit, Mossley Hill Hospital, Liverpool L18 8BU, UK

David N. Anderson Mersey Care NHS Trust, Older People's Mental Health Services, Sir Douglas Crawford Unit, Mossley Hill Hospital, Liverpool L18 8BU, UK

Toni C. Antonucci Institute for Social Research, University of Michigan, 426 Thompson Street, Ann Arbor, MI 48106-1248, USA

Carolina Aponte Urdaneta Duke University Medical Center, Room 3059 Yellow Zone, 200 Trent Dr, Durham, NC 27710 2, USA

Liana G. Apostolova Department of Neurology, UCLA David Geffen School of Medicine, Los Angeles, CA 90095, USA

Brian S. Appleby Division of Geriatric Psychiatry and Neuropsychiatry, The Johns Hopkins Hospital, Baltimore, MD 21287, USA

Tom Arie University of Nottingham, Ageing and Disability Research Unit, The Medical School, Queen's Medical Centre, Nottingham NG7 2UH, UK

Kunle Ashaye Hertfordshire Partnership NHS Trust, Mental Health Unit, Lister Hospital, Coreys Mill Lane, Stevenage, Hertfordshire SG1 4AB, UK

Stefanie Auer MAS Alzheimerhilfe, Bad Ischl, Austria

Olusegun Baiyewu Department of Psychiatry, College of Medicine, University of Ibadan, Nigeria

Robert Baldwin Manchester Mental Health & Social Care Trust, Edale House, Manchester Royal Infirmary, Manchester M13 9BX, UK

Clive Ballard Wolfson Centre for Age Related Diseases, King's College London, Guy's Campus, London SE1 1UL, UK

Sube Banerjee Institute of Psychiatry, King's College London, 16 De Crespigny Park, London, SE5 8AF, UK

Stephen J. Bartels Department of Psychiatry, Dartmouth Centers for Health and Aging Dartmouth Medical School, Hanover, NH 03755-1404, USA

Aartjan T. F. Beekman VU Medical Center and GGZ in Geest, A.J. Ernststraat 887, Amsterdam 1081 HL, and EMGO Institute for Health and Care Research, VU University and VU University Medical Center, Amsterdam, The Netherlands

Jean Beh King's College London, London SE1 1UL, UK

Lynn M. Bekris Departments of Medicine, Neurology and Psychiatry and Behavioral Sciences, University of Washington School of Medicine, Seattle, WA 98195, USA

Susan Mary Benbow Centre for Ageing and Mental Health, Staffordshire University, Stafford ST18 0AD, UK

German E. Berrios Department of Psychiatry, Addenbrooke's Hospital, Cambridge University Hospitals NHS Foundation Trust, Cambridge CB2 0QQ, UK

John L. Beyer Duke University Medical Center, Room 3059 Yellow Zone, 200 Trent Dr, Durham, NC 27710 2, USA

Ashok J. Bharucha University of Miami Miller School of Medicine, Miami, Florida, 33136 USA

David Bienenfeld Department of Psychiatry, Wright State University Boonshoft School of Medicine, Dayton, OH 3640, USA

Thomas D. Bird Geriatrics Research Service, Veterans Affairs Puget Sound Health Care System, Seattle, WA 98108, USA

Douglas Blackwood Division of Psychiatry, University of Edinburgh, The Royal Edinburgh Hospital, Edinburgh, EH10 5HF, UK

Dan G. Blazer Duke University School of Medicine, Duke University Medical Center, Durham, NC 27710, USA

Mats Bogren Department of Clinical Sciences, Psychiatry, The Lundby Study, Lund University Hospital, SE-221 85 Lund, Sweden

Susan Y. Bookheimer Center for Cognitive Neurosciences, Semel Institute for Neuroscience and Human Behavior, David Geffen School of Medicine at UCLA, Los Angeles, CA 90095, USA

Walter Pierre Bouman Mental Health Services for Older People, University Hospital, Nottingham NG7 2UH, UK

Ann Bowling Department of Primary Care and Population Health, University College London, London WC1E 6BT, UK

Carol Brayne – Chapter 48 Department *of* Public Health & Primary Care, Institute of Public Health, Robinson Way, Cambridge CB2 2SR, UK

John C. S. Breitner GRECC, VA Puget Sound Health Care System, Division of Geriatric Psychiatry, University of Washington School of Medicine, Seattle, WA 98108, USA

Dawn Brooker University of Worcester Association for Dementia Studies, Institute of Health and Society, University of Worcester, Henwick Grove Campus, Worcester WR2 6AJ, UK.

Kathleen C. Buckwalter University of Iowa College of Nursing, 101 Nursing Building, 50 Newton Road, Iowa City, IA 52242-1121, USA

Rob Butler Suffolk Mental Health Partnership NHS Trust, St Clement's Hospital, Foxhall Road, Ipswich, Suffolk IP3 8LS, UK

Ashley Cain Department of Psychiatry, University of California – San Diego, MC 0680, 9500 Gilman Drive, La Jolla, CA 92093-0680, USA

Veronica Cardenas Department of Psychiatry, University of California – San Diego, MC 0680, 9500 Gilman Drive, La Jolla, CA 92093-0680, USA

Ruoling Chen Centre for Health and Social Care Improvement, School of Health and Wellbeing, University of Wolverhampton, Wulfruna Street, Wolverhampton, WV1 1LY, UK

Nicolas Cherbuin Centre for Mental Health Research, Australian National University, 63 Eggleston Road, Canberra, ACT 0200, Australia

Carolyn Chew-Graham Primary Care Research Group, School of Community Based Medicine, University of Manchester, 5th Floor Williamson Building, Oxford Road, Manchester M13 9PL, UK

Ramilgan Chitramohan Birmingham and Solihull Mental Health Foundation Trust, Heartlands Hospital, Birmingham B9 5SS, UK

Helen Chiu Department of Psychiatry, Faculty of Medicine, The Chinese University of Hong Kong, Shatin, New Territories, Hong Kong

Linda Clare School of Psychology, Bangor University, Bangor, Gwynedd LL57 2AS, UK

Brian Clarke Department of Clinical Gerontology, King's College Hospital, Denmark Hill, London, SE5 9RS, UK

Mary Coats Department of Neurology, Washington University in St Louis, 660 S. Euclid Avenue, CB 8111, St. Louis, MO 63110, USA

Jiska Cohen-Mansfield George Washington University Medical Center and School of Public Health, Washington DC 20037, USA Tel Aviv University Herczeg Institute on Aging and Sackler Faculty of Medicine, Tel-Aviv, Israel

Peter Connelly Murray Royal Hospital, Perth PH2 7BH, UK

J. E. Cooper Department of Psychiatry and Behavioural Science, Medical Research Foundation Building, Level 3 Rear, 50 Murray Street, Perth, WA 6000, Australia

John R. M. Copeland University of Liverpool, Department of Psychiatry, Section of Old Age Psychiatry, St Catherine's Hospital, Birkenhead, Wirral, CH42 0LQ, UK

Monica Crugel Oxleas NHS Foundation Trust, Memorial Hospital, Shooters Hill, London, SE18 3RZ, UK

Pim Cuijpers VU University Amsterdam, Van der Boechorststraat 1, Amsterdam 1081 BT, and EMGO Institute for Health and Care Research, VU University and VU University Medical Center, Amsterdam, The Netherlands

Hugo de Waal East of England Postgraduate School of Psychiatry, Fulbourne, Cambridge CB21 5XB, UK

Colin Depp Department of Psychiatry, University of California – San Diego, MC 0680, 9500 Gilman Drive, La Jolla, CA 92093-0680, USA

Davangere P. Devanand College of Physicians and Surgeons, Columbia University, and Division of Geriatric Psychiatry, New York State Psychiatric Institute, New York, NY 10032, USA

Markus Donix Center for Cognitive Neurosciences, Semel Institute for Neuroscience and Human Behavior, David Geffen School of Medicine at UCLA, Los Angeles, CA 90095, USA

Brian Draper School of Psychiatry, University of NSW, Sydney, NSW 2052, Australia

Stephen B. Dunnett School of Biosciences, Cardiff University, Museum Avenue Box 911, Cardiff, CF10 3US, UK

Linda Ercoli Department of Psychiatry and Biobehavioral Sciences, Geriatric Psychiatry Division, Semel Institute for Neuroscience and Human Behavior, David Geffen School of Medicine at UCLA, 760 Westwood Plaza, Suite 37-440, Los Angeles, CA 90024, USA

Mavis Evans Elderly Mental Health Directorate, Wirral and West Cheshire Community NHS Trust, Clatter bridge Hospital, Bebington, Wirral L63 4JY, UK

Lisa T. Eyler University of California, San Diego, 9500 Gilman Drive, # 9151-B, La Jolla, CA 92093, USA

Waleed Fawzi Oxleas NHS Foundation Trust, Memorial Hospital, Shooters Hill, London, SE18 3RZ, UK

Steven Ferris Aging and Dementia Clinical Research Center, New York University Langone Medical Center, Center of Excellence on Aging, New York, NY 10016, USA

Cynthia D. Fields Department of Psychiatry and Behavioral Sciences, Johns Hopkins School of Medicine, Baltimore, MD 21287, USA

Jonathan Folstein Vanderbilt Universit, Nashville, Tennessee, USA

Marshal Folstein University of Miami Miller School of Medicine, Nashville, USA

Susan Folstein University of Miami Miller School of Medicine, Nashville, USA

Brent Forester Harvard Medical School, McLean Hospital, 115 Mill Street, Belmont, MA 02478, USA

Hans Förstl Klinik und Poliklinik für Psychiatrie und Psychotherapie, Klinikum rechts der Isar, Technische Universität München, Ismaninger Str. 22, 81675 München, Germany

Chris Fox Folkestone Health Centre, 15-25 Dover Road, Folkestone, Kent CT20 1JY, UK

Paul T. Francis King's College London, Wolfson Centre for Age-Related Diseases, Guy's Campus, London SE1 1UL, UK

Emile Franssen Aging and Dementia Clinical Research Center, New York University Langone Medical Center, Center of Excellence on Aging, New York, NY 10016, USA

D. Gallagher-Thompson Department of Psychiatry & Behavioral Sciences, Stanford University School of Medicine, 401 Quarry Road, Stanford, CA 94305-5717, USA

Mary Ganguli Western Psychiatric Institute and Clinic, 3811 O'Hara St. Pittsburgh, PA 15213, USA

V. Gardner Department of Psychiatry and Behavioral Sciences, Duke University Medical Center, Durham, NC 3950, USA

Serge Gauthier McGill Center for Studies in Aging, Douglas Hospital, Montreal, Quebec H4H 1R2, Canada

J P Gibbons Department of Psychiatry and Behavioral Sciences, Center for the Study of Aging and Human Development, Duke University Medical Center, Room 3521 Blue Zone Duke Clinics, Box 3003, Durham, NC 27710, USA

Ben Green Department of Psychiatry, University of Liverpool 147, UK

Faith M. Gunning Institute of Geriatric Psychiatry, Department of Psychiatry, Weill Cornell Medical College, 21 Bloomingdale Road, White Plains, NY 10605, USA

Jeffrey T. Guptill Duke University School of Medicine, Duke University Medical Center, Durham, NC 27710, USA

David Gwyn Seymour Medicine for the Elderly, University of Aberdeen, Aberdeen, AB24 3EN, UK

Scott M. Hayes Joseph and Kathleen Bryan Alzheimer's Disease Research Center, Department of Psychiatry. Duke University, Durham, NC 27705, USA

C. Michael Hendricks Department of Psychiatry, Wright State University, Boonshoft School of Medicine, OH 3640, USA

Adriana P. Hermida Fuquay Center for Late Life Depression, Emory University School of Medicine, Atlanta, GA 30329-5120, USA

N. Herrmann Sunnybrook Health Sciences Centre, Toronto, Ontario, M4N 3M5, Canada

Claire Hilton Mental Health Service for Older Adults, Central and North West London NHS Foundation Trust, Bentley House, Harrow HA3 5QX, UK

John V. Hindle School of Medical Sciences, University of Bangor, Llandudno Hospital, Llandudno, Conwy, LL30 1LB, UK

Juanita Hoe Department of Mental Health Sciences, University College London, London W1W 7EJ, UK

Allan House School of Healthcare, University of Leeds, Leeds LS2 9JT, UK

Julian C. Hughes Northumbria Healthcare NHS Foundation Trust and Institute for Ageing and Health, Newcastle University, Newcastle Upon Tyne, NE1 7RU UK

Celia F. Hybels Department of Psychiatry and Behavioral Sciences, Center for the Study of Aging and Human Development, Duke University Medical Center, Room 1505 Blue Zone Duke Clinics, Box 3003, Durham, NC 27710, USA

Thomas Idiculla Mental Health Services Evaluation Dept, McLean Hospital, 115 Mill St, Belmont, MA 02478, USA

James S. Jackson Institute for Social Research, University of Michigan, Ann Arbor 48502, USA

S. H. D. Jackson Department of Clinical Gerontology, King's College Hospital, Denmark Hill, London, SE5 9RS, UK

A. Jablensky Department of Psychiatry and Behavioural Science, Medical Research Foundation Building, Level 3 Rear, 50 Murray Street, Perth, WA 6000, Australia

Imran A. Jamil Aging and Dementia Clinical Research Center, New York University Langone Medical Center, Center of Excellence on Aging, New York, NY 10016, USA

Dilip V. Jeste University of California, San Diego, 9500 Gilman Drive, # 0664, La Jolla, CA 92093, USA

David Jolley Personal Social Services Research Unit, Manchester University, Manchester M13 9PL, UK

Rob Jones Mental Health Services for Older People Directorate and Nottingham University Section of Old Age Psychiatry, Queen's Medical Centre, Nottingham NG7 2UH, UK

Anthony Francis Jorm ORYGEN Research Centre, Department of Psychiatry, University of Melbourne, Parkville, Victoria 3052, Australia

Eileen M. Joyce UCL Institute of Neurology, Queen Square, London WC1N 3BG, UK

Andrea June University of Colorado at Colorado Springs, Colorado Springs, CO 80918, USA

Barbara Kamholz Department of Psychiatry, Duke University, Durham, NC 27708, USA

Jason Karlawish University of Pennsylvania Institute on Aging, Philadelphia, PA 19104, USA

Robert J. Kastenbaum Arizona State University at Tempe, Tempe, AZ 85287, USA

Cornelius Katona Department of Mental Health Sciences, University College London, Charles Bell House, 7-73 Riding House Street, London WIW 7EJ, UK

Sharjeel Khan Aging and Dementia Clinical Research Center, New York University Langone Medical Center, Center of Excellence on Aging, New York, NY 10016, USA

Zunera Khan King's College London, London SE1 1UL, UK

Jeanne Kim Memory and Aging Research Center, Geriatric Psychiatry Division, Semel Institute for Neuroscience and Human Behavior, David Geffen School of Medicine at UCLA, 760 Westwood Plaza, Suite 88-201, Los Angeles, CA 90024, USA

Susan Kim Geriatric Psychiatry Research Program, McLean Hospital, 115 Mill Street, Belmont, MA 02478, USA

Paul D. Kirwin Associate Professor of Psychiatry, Geriatric Psychiatry Fellowship Director, Yale University School of Medicine, VA CT Healthcare System

Eran Klein The Johns Hopkins Berman Institute of Bioethics, Baltimore, MD 21201, USA

Alan Kluger Aging and Dementia Clinical Research Center, New York University Langone Medical Center, Center of Excellence on Aging, New York, NY 10016, USA

Anthony Klugman Old Age Psychiatry, South London and Maudsley NHS Foundation Trust, Bethlem Royal Hospital, Monks Orchard Road, Beckenham, Kent, BR3 3BX, UK

Robert Kohn The Warren Alpert Medical School of Brown University, Miriam Hospital, 164 Summit Ave, Fain Building Suite 2B, Providence, RI 02906, USA

Maritha J. Kotze Department of Pathology, Faculty of Health Sciences, Stellenbosch University, Tygerberg, 7505, Cape Town, South Africa

Peter Knapp School of Healthcare, University of Leeds, Leeds LS2 9JT, UK

Anand Kumar Department of Psychiatry, University of Illinois-Chicago, 912 South Wood Street, Chicago, IL 60637, USA

Yookyung Kwon Stanford Geriatric Education Center, 1215 Welch Road, Stanford, CA 94304-5403, USA

Helen H. Kyomen McLean Hospital, 115 Mill Street, Belmont, MA, 02478, USA

Iain Lang Peninsula Medical School, University of Exeter, Plymouth, PL6 8BU, UK

Nicole M. Lanouette University of California, San Diego, 9500 Gilman Drive, # 0664, La Jolla, CA 92093, USA

Maria I. Lapid Mayo Clinic College of Medicine, Mayo Clinic Rochester, Rochester, MN 55905, USA

Helen Lavretsky Departments of Psychiatry and Biobehavioral Sciences, Semel Institute for Neuroscience and Human Behavior, David Geffen School of Medicine at UCLA, Los Angeles, CA 90095, USA

Vanessa Lawrence Institute of Psychiatry, King's College London, 16 De Crespigny Park, London, SE5 8AF, UK

Orly Lazarov Department of Anatomy and Cell Biology, College of Medicine, The University of Illinois at Chicago, Chicago, IL 60612, USA

Barry D. Lebowitz University of California, San Diego School of Medicine, 9500 Gilman Drive, La Jolla, CA 92093, USA

Susan W. Lehmann Department of Psychiatry and Behavioral Sciences, The Johns Hopkins University School of Medicine, 600 North Wolfe Street, Meyer 279, Baltimore, MD 21287-7279, USA

Alex D. Leow Department of Psychiatry, University of Illinois at Chicago, Chicago, IL 60637, USA

James Lindesay Department of Health Sciences, University of Leicester, Leicester LE5 4PW, UK

Benjamin Liptzin Department of Psychiatry, Baystate Medical Center, 759 Chestnut Street, Springfield, MA, 01199, USA

Gill Livingston Department of Mental Health Sciences, University College London, London W1W 7EJ, UK

Constantine G. Lyketsos The Johns Hopkins Bayview Medical Center 5300 Alpha Commons Drive Alpha Commons Building, 4th Floor, Baltimore, MD 21224, USA

David Aaron Maroof Department of Psychiatry and Behavioral Sciences, The Johns Hopkins University School of Medicine, 600 North Wolfe Street, Meyer 218, Baltimore, MD 21287-7218, USA

Renee Marquett Department of Psychiatry & Behavioral Sciences, Stanford University School of Medicine, 401 Quarry Road, Stanford, CA 94305-5717, USA

Meghan A. Marty University of Colorado at Colorado Springs, Colorado Springs, CO 80918, USA

E. Wayne Massey Duke University School of Medicine, Duke University Medical Center, Durham, NC 27710, USA

Fiona E. Matthews MRC Biostatistics Unit, Institute of Public Health, Cambridge, CB2 2SR, UK

Cecilia Mattisson Department of Clinical Sciences, Psychiatry, The Lundby Study, Lund University Hospital, SE-221 85 Lund, Sweden

Donna D. McAlpine School of Public Health, University of Minnesota, Minneapolis, MN 55455, USA

William M. McDonald Fuquay Center for Late Life Depression, Emory University School of Medicine, Atlanta, GA 30329-5120, USA

Bernadette McGuinness Centre for Public Health, School of Medicine, Dentistry and Biomedical Sciences, The Queen's University of Belfast, Belfast BT9 7BL, UK

I. G. McKeith Department of Old Age Psychiatry, Institute for Health of the Elderly, Wolfson Research Centre, Newcastle General Hospital, Newcastle upon Tyne NE4 6BE, UK

David Mechanic Institute for Health, Health Care Policy and Aging Research, Rutgers, the State University of New Jersey, New Brunswick, NJ 08901, USA

David Melzer Peninsula College of Medicine & Dentistry, Universities of Exeter and Plymouth, John Bull Building, Plymouth, PL6 8BU, UK

Mario F. Mendez Departments of Neurology and Psychiatry, VA Greater Los Angeles Healthcare System and David Geffen School of Medicine at UCLA, Los Angeles, CA 90095, USA

David A. Merrill Department of Psychiatry and Biobehavioral Sciences, David Geffen School of Medicine at UCLA and VA Greater Los Angeles Healthcare System

Sujatha Merve Chasefarm Hospital, Enfield EN2 8JL, UK

Catherine Messinger University of Iowa College of Nursing, 101 Nursing Building, 50 Newton Road, Iowa City, IA 52242-1121, USA

Karen Miller Aging and Memory Research Center, Geriatric Psychiatry Division, Semel Institute for Neuroscience and Human Behavior, David Geffen School of Medicine at UCLA, 760 Westwood Plaza, Suite 88-201, Los Angeles, CA 90024, USA

Alisoun Milne School of Social Policy, Sociology and Social Research, University of Kent, Canterbury, Kent CT2 7LZ, UK

Gary S. Moak University of Massachusetts Medical School, Worcester, MA and Medical Director, Moak Center for Healthy Aging, 18 Lyman Street, Suite 285 Westborough, MA 01581, USA

Victor Molinari University of South Florida, Tampa, FL 33620, USA

Isabel Monteiro Aging and Dementia Clinical Research Center, New York University Langone Medical Center, Center of Excellence on Aging, New York, NY 10016, USA

John C. Morris Department of Neurology, Washington University School of Medicine, 660 S. Euclid Avenue, St. Louis, MO 63110, USA

Pat Mottram Evidence Based Practice Centre, Department of Psychiatry, University of Liverpool 147, UK

Cynthia A. Munro Department of Psychiatry and Behavioral Sciences, The Johns Hopkins University School of Medicine, 600 North Wolfe Street, Meyer 218, Baltimore, MD 21287-7218, USA

Declan G. M. Murphy Department of Forensic and Neurodevelopmental Sciences, Institute of Psychiatry at the Maudsley, King's College London WC2R 2LS, UK

Joanna Murray Institute of Psychiatry, King's College London, 16 De Crespigny Park, London, SE5 8AF, UK

Asim Naeem Division of Mental Health (Psychiatry of Disability), Level 6 – Hunter Wing, St George's University of London, Cranmer Terrace, London, SW17 0RE, UK

Per Nettelbladt Department of Clinical Sciences, Psychiatry, The Lundby Study, Lund University Hospital, SE-221 85 Lund, Sweden

Ruth O'Hara Department of Psychiatry and Behavioral Sciences, Stanford University School of Medicine, Stanford University, Stanford, CA 94305, USA

VA Sierra-Pacific Mental Illness Research Education and Clinical Center, Palo Alto, USA

John O'Hare Centre for Public Health, School of Medicine, Dentistry and Biomedical Sciences, The Queen's University of Belfast, Belfast BT9 7BL, UK

Esther Oh Johns Hopkins School of Medicine and Johns Hopkins Bayview, Baltimore, MD 21224, USA

Martin Orrell Department of Mental Health Sciences, 48 Riding House Street, University College London, London W1W 7EY, UK

Dana Scherr Parchi The Child and Family Institute at St. Luke's and Roosevelt Hospitals, New York, NY 10025, USA

Laura Parisi Clinica Neurologica University Campus Bio-Medico, Rome, Italy

A. Peter Passmore Centre for Public Health, School of Medicine, Dentistry and Biomedical Sciences, The Queen's University of Belfast, Belfast BT9 7BL, UK

Vikram Patel London School of Hygiene and Tropical Medicine (UK) and Sangath (India); Sangath Centre, 841/1 Alto Porvorim, Goa 403521, India

Thomas L. Patterson Department of Psychiatry, University of California – San Diego, MC 0680, 9500 Gilman Drive, La Jolla, CA 92093-0680, USA

Ian Peate School of Nursing and Midwifery, Thames Valley University, London W5 5RF, UK

Renee Pepin University of Colorado at Colorado Springs, Colorado Springs, CO 80918, USA

Robert Perneczky Klinik und Poliklinik für Psychiatrie und Psychotherapie, Klinikum rechts der Isar, Technische Universität München, Ismaninger Str. 22, 81675 München, Germany

Richard Perry Department of Neurosciences, Imperial College and Imperial College Healthcare NHS Trust, Charing Cross Hospital, Fulham Place Road, London, W6 8RF, UK

Adolf Pfefferbaum Neuroscience Program, SRI International, 333 Ravenswood Ave., Menlo Park, CA 94025, USA

Michael Philpot Mental Health of Older Adults, South London and Maudsley NHS Foundation Trust, Maudsley Hospital, London SE5 8AZ, UK

Ben Pickard Strathclyde Institute of Pharmacy and Biomedical Sciences (SIPBS), University of Strathclyde, The John Arbuthnott Building, 27 Taylor Street, Glasgow, G4 0NR, UK

Felix C.V. Potocnik Department of Psychiatry, Faculty of Health Sciences, Stellenbosch University, Tygerberg, 7505, Cape Town, South Africa

Bevin Powers VA Sierra-Pacific Mental Illness Research Education and Clinical Center, Veterans Administration Health Care System, Palo Alto, CA 94304, USA

Department of Psychiatry and Behavioral Sciences, Stanford University School of Medicine, USA

Aparna Prasanna Wolverhampton Primary Care Trust, Penn Hospital, Wolverhampton WV4 5HN, UK

Neil Prentice Murray Royal Hospital, Perth PH2 7BH, UK

Martin Prince Centre for Global Mental Health, Department of Health Service and Population Research, Institute of Psychiatry, King's College London, 16 De Crespigny Park, London, SE5 8AF, UK

Patrick Rabbitt Age and Cognitive Performance Research Centre, University of Manchester, Oxford Road, Mancehster M13 9PL, UK

Peter V. Rabins Department of Psychiatry and Behavioral Sciences, Johns Hopkins School of Medicine, Baltimore, MD 21287, USA

Oyepeju Raji Division of Mental Health (Psychiatry of Disability), Level 6 – Hunter Wing, St George's University of London, Cranmer Terrace, London, SW17 0RE, UK

Barry Reisberg New York University Langone Medical Center, Center of Excellence on Aging, New York, NY 10016, USA

Kenneth Rockwood Division of Geriatric Medicine, Dalhousie University, 1421–5955 Veterans' Memorial Lane, Halifax, NS, B3H 2E1, Canada

Joanne Rodda Department of Mental Health Sciences, University College London, WC1E 6BT, UK

Heather R. Romero Joseph and Kathleen Bryan Alzheimer's Disease Research Center, Department of Psychiatry. Duke University, Durham, NC 27705, USA

Steven P. Roose College of Physicians and Surgeons, Columbia University, and Division of Geriatric Psychiatry, New York State Psychiatric Institute, New York, NY 10032, USA

Paolo Maria Rossini Clinica Neurologica University Campus Bio-Medico, Rome, Italy

Teresa A. Rummans Mayo Clinic College of Medicine, Mayo Clinic Rochester, Rochester, MN 55905, USA

Marwan Sabbagh Cleo Ruberts Center, Banner-Sun Health Research Institute, Sun City, AZ 85351, USA

Sahlgrenska Academy at the University of Gothenburg, Gothenburg, Sweden

Sunita Sahu Oxleas NHS Foundation Trust, Memorial Hospital, Shooters Hill, London, SE18 3RZ, UK

M. Sajatovic Case Western Reserve University School of Medicine and University Hospitals Case Medical Center, Cleveland, OH, 44106, USA

Oludamilola Salami Johns Hopkins School of Medicine and Johns Hopkins Bayview, Baltimore, MD 21224, USA

George M. Savva Department of Public Health and Primary Care, University of Cambridge, Institute of Public Health, Cambridge CB2 0SR, UK

Stephen M. Scheinthal New Jersey Institute for Successful Aging, University of Medicine and Dentistry of New Jersey – School of Osteopathic Medicine, Stratford, NJ 08084, USA

Martin M. Schmidt Division of Mental Health, St George's University of London, London SW17 0RE, UK

Jerome J. Schulte Department of Psychiatry, Wright State University, Boonshoft School of Medicine, OH 3640, USA

Daniel L. Segal University of Colorado at Colorado Springs, Colorado Springs, CO 80918, USA

Sati Sembhi Suffolk Mental Health Partnership NHS Trust, St Clement's Hospital, Foxhall Road, Ipswich, Suffolk IP3 8LS, UK

Andrew Moore Severn Department of Anaesthesia, Royal Lancaster Infirmary, Lancaster LA1 4RP, UK

K.S. Shaji Department of Psychiatry, Government Medical College, Thrissur, Kerala 680596, India

Bart Sheehan Health Sciences Research Institute, Medical School Building, Warwick Medical School, Coventry CV4 7AL, UK

Melanie B. Shulman Aging and Dementia Clinical Research Center, New York University Langone Medical Center, Center of Excellence on Aging, New York, NY 10016, USA

K.I. Shulman Sunnybrook Health Sciences Centre, Toronto, Ontario, M4N 3M5, Canada

Marcus Simmgen Thomas Addison Unit, St George's Hospital NHS Trust, Blackshaw Road, Tooting, London SW17 0QT, UK

Ingmar Skoog Institute of Neuroscience and Physiology, Unit of Neuropsychiatric Epidemiology, Sahlgrenska Academy at the University of Gothenburg, Gothenburg, Sweden

Gary W. Small Department of Psychiatry and Biobehavioral Sciences, Semel Institute for Neuroscience and Human Behavior, David Geffen School of Medicine at UCLA, Los Angeles, CA 90095, USA

Gary W. Small Parlow-Solomon

Filip Smit Professor of Public Mental Health Trimbos Institute (Netherlands Institute of Mental Health and Addiction) and EMGO Institute of Health and Health Care Research, VU University Medical Centre. PO Box 725, Utrecht 3500 AS, The Netherlands

B. Joy Snider 660 S. Euclid Avenue, CB 8111, Department of Neurology, Washington University in St Louis, St. Louis, MO 63110, USA

Christian Sorg Klinik und Poliklinik für Psychiatrie und Psychotherapie, Klinikum rechts der Isar, Technische Universität München, Ismaninger Str. 22, 81675 München, Germany

Reisa A. Sperling Memory Disorders Unit, Brigham and Women's Hospital, Alzheimer's Disease Research Center and Gerontology Research Unit, Massachusetts General Hospital, Department of Neurology and Psychiatry, Harvard Medical School, Boston, MA 02215, USA

D. C. Steffens Department of Psychiatry and Behavioral Sciences, Duke University Medical Center, Durham, NC 3702, USA

Dan J. Stein Department of Psychiatry and Mental Health, University of Cape Town, Cape Town, South Africa

Elliott M. Stein Jewish Home of San Francisco, 302 Silver Avenue San Francisco, CA 94112, USA and Department of Psychiatry, University of Miami School of Medicine, Miami, FL 33136, USA

Max L. Stek Department of Psychiatry, VUmc Medical Centre and GGZinGeest, AJ Ernst street 887, 1081HL Amsterdam, The Netherlands

Martin Steinberg Johns Hopkins Bayview Medical Center, 5300 Alpha Commons Drive, Baltimore, MD 21224, USA

Robert Stewart King's College London (Institute of Psychiatry), De Crespigny Park, London SE5 8AF, UK

Mary Ellen Stolder University of Iowa College of Nursing, 101 Nursing Building, 50 Newton Road, Iowa City, IA 52242-1121, USA

David L. Sultzer Department of Psychiatry and Biobehavioral Sciences, David Geffen School of Medicine at UCLA and VA Greater Los Angeles Healthcare System 11301 Wilshire Blvd. Los Angeles, CA 90073, USA

Edith V. Sullivan Department of Psychiatry and Behavioral Sciences, Stanford University School of Medicine, 401 Quarry Rd., Stanford, CA 94305, USA

Cindy Tam Department of Psychiatry, The Chinese University of Hong Kong, Shantin, New Territories, Hong Kong

Giles MY Tan Department of Forensic and Neurodevelopmental Sciences, Institute of Psychiatry at the Maudsley, King's College London WC2R 2LS, UK

Rawan Tarawneh Department of Neurology, Washington University in St Louis, 660 S. Euclid Avenue, CB 8111, St. Louis, MO 63110, USA

John-Paul Taylor Department of Old Age Psychiatry, Institute for Health of the Elderly, Wolfson Research Centre, Newcastle General Hospital, Newcastle upon Tyne NE4 6BE, UK

Alexander M. Thomson Department of Elderly Care, Salford Royal Hospitals NHS Foundation Trust, Stott La, Salford M68HD, UK

Dolores Gallagher-Thompson Department of Psychiatry & Behavioral Sciences, Stanford University School of Medicine, 401 Quarry Road, Stanford, CA 94305-5717, USA

Paul M. Thompson Department of Neurology, UCLA David Geffen School of Medicine, Los Angeles, CA 90095, USA

Stephen Todd Centre for Public Health, School of Medicine, Dentistry and Biomedical Sciences, The Queen's University of Belfast, Belfast BT9 7BL, UK

Carol Torossian Aging and Dementia Clinical Research Center, New York University Langone Medical Center, Center of Excellence on Aging, New York, NY 10016, USA

Adrian Treloar Oxleas NHS Foundation Trust, Memorial Hospital, Shooters Hill, London, SE18 3RZ, UK

JoAnn T. Tschanz Department of Psychology and Center for Epidemiologic Studies, Utah State University, Logan, UT 84322, USA

Joshua Tsoh Associate Consultant in Psychiatry, Prince of Wales Hospital, Shatin, New Territories, Hong Kong

Debby Tsuang Geriatric Research, Education, and Clinical Center and Mental Illness Research, Education, and Clinical Center, Veterans Affairs Puget Sound Health Care System, Seattle, WA 98108, USA

H. W. J. van Marwijk Department of General Practice, VUmc Medical Centre and GGZinGeest, AJ Ernst street 887, 1081HL Amsterdam, The Netherlands

Susan J. van Rensburg Division of Chemical Pathology, National Health Laboratory Service, Sandringham, Cape Town, South Africa

Vijay Venkatraman University of Pittsburgh School of Medicine, Pittsburgh, USA

Martin J. Vernon Department of Elderly Medicine, Burton House, Withington Hospital, Nell LAne, West Didsbury, Manchester M20 8LR, UK

Ottavio V. Vitolo Memory Disorders Unit, Brigham and Women's Hospital, Massachusetts General Hospital, Department of Psychiatry, Harvard Medical School, Boston, MA 02215, USA

Zuzana Walker Department of Mental Health Sciences, St Margaret's Hospital, Epping, Essex, CM16 6TN UK

John P. Wattis Professor of Old Age Psychiatry, Centre for Health and Social Care Research, University of Huddersfield, Queensgate, Huddersfield HD1 3DH, UK

Jerzy Wegiel New York State Institute for Basic Research in Developmental Disabilities, Staten Island, New York 10306, USA

Kathleen A. Welsh-Bohmer Joseph and Kathleen Bryan Alzheimer's Disease Research Center, Department of Psychiatry. Duke University, Durham, NC 27705, USA

Eric Wexler Division of Geriatric Psychiatry and Center for Neurobehavioral Genetics, David Geffen School of Medicine at UCLA, Los Angeles, CA 90095, USA

Kirsten M. Wilkins Assistant Professor of Psychiatry, University of Oklahoma College of Medicine-Tulsa, Tulsa, OK

David G. Wilkinson Moorgreen Hospital, Botley Road, West End, Southampton SO30 3JB, UK

Philip Wilkinson Department of Psychiatry, University of Oxford, Warneford Hospital, Old Road, Headington, Oxford OX3 7JX, UK

Kenneth C. M. Wilson St Catherine's Hospital, Church Road, Birkenhead, Wirral L42 OLQ, UK

Anders Wimo KI Alzheimer's Disease Research Center, Department of Neurobiology, Care Sciences and Society, Karolinska institutet, Stockholm, Sweden

Philip Wong Johns Hopkins School of Medicine and Johns Hopkins Bayview, Baltimore, MD 21224, USA

Matthew R. Woodward Geriatric Psychiatry Research Program, McLean Hospital, Belmont, MA 02478, USA

Graeme A. Yorston St Andrew's Hospital, Northampton NN1 5DG, UK

Chang-En-Yu Geriatric Research, Education, and Clinical Center and Mental Illness Research, Education, and Clinical Center, Veterans Affairs Puget Sound Health Care System, Seattle, WA 98108, USA

Natalie M. Zahr Department of Psychiatry and Behavioral Sciences, Stanford University School of Medicine, 401 Quarry Rd., Stanford, CA 94305, USA

L. McKenzie Zeiss University of California, Irvine, CA 92697-2800, USA

Richard A. Zweig Ferkauf Graduate School of Yeshiva University, Bronx, NY 10461, USA

Preface

It has been eight years since the second edition of *Principles and Practice of Geriatric Psychiatry* was published. During this time there has been substantial progress in the science and practice of geriatric psychiatry. This third edition attempts to capture these advances and provide an up-to-date summary for trainees and practitioners.

Two of the Editors of the previous editions, John R M Copeland and Dan G Blazer, decided to withdraw and two new Editors (one from the UK and one from the US) have been recruited. We wish first of all to express our grateful thanks to John and Dan for their remarkable stewardship over the production of the two previous editions. We would also like to acknowledge the invaluable contribution of the six Associate Editors in bringing this third edition to completion.

The previous edition received good reviews as well as some helpful criticisms. We therefore decided to maintain the textbook's overall scope, structure, headings, list of contents and international authorship. The majority of the textbook's chapters have been updated by the original authors. We have, however, recruited several new authors who are internationally recognized experts in their fields and commissioned substantial completely new material.

We believe that the value and the strengths of this textbook rest in its comprehensive coverage of the basic and clinical sciences of normal and abnormal ageing, of the full range of psychiatric disorders in the elderly, and of the organization of psychogeriatric services in the UK and the US as well as chapters on prevention, training and education.

We hope that this third edition is well received by its readers and that it proves to be a useful and readable way for them to update their knowledge of the science and practice of geriatric psychiatry.

Mohammed T Abou-Saleh
Cornelius L E Katona
Anand Kumar

Preface to Second Edition

The editors were very gratified that the first edition of this textbook was generally well received and that a second edition has been called for. It is now seven years since the original book appeared, and there have been many more advances in the subject. In spite of new sections and some wholesale rewriting, it has been possible once again, to contain the information in one volume. Very sadly some of our original contributors have died. New authors have replaced them while others have been added in an endeavour to keep the text authoritative and up-to-date. The helpful criticisms of the first edition have been carefully considered in the preparation of this one. Having so many distinguished authors with such a breadth of interest, while greatly enhancing the book, has led to a long gestation period, but we believe that it has been worthwhile. Much of the original format has been retained in order to continue to stimulate lively debate and exchange of views. If the book contributes to the growing strength of Geriatric Psychiatry internationally, it will have done its work.

John R. M. Copeland
Mohammed T. Abou-Saleh
Dan G. Blazer

Preface to First Edition

The discipline of the psychiatry of old age has moved rapidly in recent years and the number of practitioners has expanded worldwide. An authoritative text is required which draws on the knowledge of these experts and which reflects both new scientific advances and innovations in service development.

In a comparatively new subject many of the issues are still contentious and on some of these we have tried to provide the opportunity for the expression of different points of view. Readers are asked to judge the issues for themselves from the evidence set out.

Here and there short, special articles have been commissioned which present research findings in more detail and describe new aspects of care.

They are intended to enliven the text and their choice has been dependent on timing and opportunity.

We have also tried to give a "feel" for what is happening in developing countries and the scope of the problems experienced by local practitioners.

Even a book of this size can never be complete and no doubt gaps in the coverage of subjects will be identified. We would be glad to have them pointed out. The more comprehensive a book aims to be the longer it takes to come to publication and in a fast-moving area of knowledge this can be a problem. Many of our authors have been kind enough to update their contributions at a late stage, which we hope has overcome this difficulty to some extent.

In the early stages of the development of a subject there is insufficient corpus of knowledge to assemble in book form. This situation has changed dramatically for geriatric psychiatry in recent years. We hope that the knowledge gathered here from our distinguished international panel of authors bears this out.

John R. M. Copeland
Mohammed T. Abou-Saleh
Dan G. Blazer

Part A

Historical Background

A Conceptual History in the Nineteenth Century

German E. Berrios

Department of Psychiatry, Addenbrooke's Hospital, Cambridge, UK

The history of geriatric psychiatry can be written from two viewpoints. The 'externalist' approach focuses on the social and political variables that have controlled attitudes towards abnormal behaviour in old age, and on the professionalization of those charged with the care of the mentally infirm elderly. The 'internalist' approach – to be followed in this chapter – concentrates on the origin of the scientific language of psychogeriatrics. An adequate historical account should include information on theories of ageing, both physical and mental, brain sclerosis and the formation of a viable concept of mental illness. On the first rubric much research has been done[1-9]; far less work exists on the other two. On psychogeriatric care before the nineteenth century[10,11] there is very little: this may simply reflect a historical reality.

VIEWS ON AGEING BEFORE THE NINETEENTH CENTURY

Like most other aspects of human life, ageing has also been portrayed in terms of metaphors. Classical views, following the nature–nurture controversy, conceived of ageing as resulting from either internal instructions or from the buffeting of foreign factors[4,8].

The 'wear and tear' view happened to be popular during the early nineteenth century, the period on which this chapter will concentrate. It was based, as it had always been, on the ageless observation that all natural objects, whether animate or not, are subject to the ravages of time. Surprisingly enough, the 'wear and tear' view has not always generated an understanding attitude. In fact, across times and cultures great ambiguity has existed in regard to the treatment of old folk. Fortunately, a realistic acceptance seems to have predominated although there is plenty of evidence of hostility. The Hebrew tradition, and indeed its Christian offshoot, encouraged much reverence towards the wisdom and value of old age. But even in societies that have made great play of this view, veneration has been reserved for those in positions of power or influence[12]. Little is known about attitudes towards elderly women or old men in humbler stations[11].

So, it can be concluded that, all in all, a view seems to have predominated that ageing was undesirable and that the identification of wear factors was important to devising ways of prolonging life[5,13].

A second ambiguity can be detected in these earlier writings. It concerns the extent to which the ageing process necessarily involves the human mind. While it was a palpable fact that all human frames decayed, not everyone accepted that this had necessarily to affect the soul or mind. Extant descriptions of the psychological changes brought about by old age suggest that people were aware that the mind also underwent a decline. However, theory and religion encouraged the view that the spirit could or did escape wear and tear, and that human beings grew ever more wise and useful, thanks to the accumulation of experience and knowledge. This belief must have been available in all those societies that felt the need to create adequate spaces for all manner of intellectual and/or sociopolitical gerontocracies[2]. Some seem even to have separated chronological age and functional age in order to justify such concessions. From the point of view of the history of psychogeriatrics, it would be useful to know to what extent this belief was undermined by the occasional case of dementia among those elderly in positions of power[1]. Historical evidence seems to show that these situations were neither more nor less perturbing than mental illness occurring at other periods of life. Indeed, fail-safe devices seem to have been available in these societies to cope with the upheavals created by such occurrences.

Men like Buffon, Darwin and Goethe reshaped ideas on ageing during the eighteenth century. Buffon[14] wrote: 'All changes and dies in Nature. As soon as it reaches its point of perfection it begins to decay. At first this is subtle and it takes years for one to realise that major changes have in fact taken place' (p. 106). Buffon put this down to an 'ossification' process similar to that affecting trees: 'this cause of death is common to animals and vegetables. Oaks die as their core becomes so hard that they can no longer feed. They trap humidity, and this eventually makes them rot away' (p. 111).

Erasmus Darwin's views resulted from the application of yet another metaphor, namely that ageing results from a breakdown of 'communication' between man and his environment[15]. Darwin suggested that such breakdown followed a loss of irritability (a property of nerve fibres) and a decreased response to sensation:

> It seems our bodies by long habit cease to obey the stimulus of the aliment, which support us ... three causes may conspire to render our nerves less excitable: 1. If a stimulus be greater than natural, it produces too great an exertion of the stimulated organ, and in consequence exhausts the spirit of animation; and the moving organ ceases to act, even though the stimulus is continued. 2. If excitations weaker than natural be applied, so as not to excite the organ into action, they may be gradually increased, without exciting the organ into action, which will thus acquire a habit of disobedience to the stimulus. 3. When irritative motions continue to be produced in consequence of stimulus, but are not succeeded by sensation. (p. 365)

Principles and Practice of Geriatric Psychiatry, 3rd edn. Edited by Mohammed T. Abou-Saleh, Cornelius Katona and Anand Kumar
© 2011 John Wiley & Sons, Ltd

VIEWS ON AGEING DURING THE NINETEENTH CENTURY

In 1807 Sir John Sinclair[16] published a major compendium on ageing and longevity, which included references to most pre-nineteenth century sources. It was, in a way, the last grand glance to the past. Soon afterwards work started by those who, like Léon Rostan (1791–1866), based their claims on empirical findings. Rostan, one of the most original members of the Paris school, published in 1819 his *Recherches sur le Ramollissement du Cerveau*[17], where the view commenced that vascular disorders might be as important as parenchymal ones in brain ageing. Even more important was his uncompromising anti-vitalistic position enshrined in the claim that all diseases were related to pathological changes in specific organs[18,19].

During the 1850s Reveillé-Parise[3] saw his task as writing on 'the history of ageing, that is, mapping the imprint of time on the human body, whether on its organs or on its spiritual essence' (p. v). In regard to ageing itself he wrote: 'the cause of ageing is a gradual increase in the work of decomposition . . . but how does it happen? What are the laws that control the degradation that affects the organization and mind of man?' (p. 13). Reveillé-Parise dismissed the toxic view defended by the Italian writer Michel Lévy[20] according to which there was a gradual accumulation of calcium phosphates that led to petrification, to an 'anticipation of the grave'. This view, he stated, had no empirical foundation and was based on a generalization from localized findings. Reveillé-Parise supported the view that ageing results from a negative balance between composition and elimination, which equally affected the cardiovascular, respiratory and reproductive organs.

Finally, the views should be mentioned of J. M. Charcot, who in 1868 offered a series of 24 lectures on the diseases affecting the elderly[21]. Charcot dedicated Lecture 1 to the 'general characters of senile pathology'; he started by saying that all books on geriatrics up to his time had 'a particularly literary or philosophical turn [and had been] more or less ingenious paraphrases of the famous treatise De Senectute' (p. 25). He praised Rostan for his views on asthma and brain softening in the elderly, and predictably also mentioned Cruveilhier, Hourman and Dechambre, Durand-Fardel and Prus. He criticized Canstatt and other German physicians because in their work, 'imagination holds an immense place at the expense of impartial and positive observation' (p. 26). Charcot's own contribution was based on the general principle that 'changes of texture impressed on the organism by old age sometimes become so marked, that the physiological and pathological states seem to merge into one another by insensible transitions, and cannot be clearly distinguished' (p. 27).

THE DEVELOPMENT OF THE NOTION OF BRAIN SCLEROSIS

When in 1833 Lobstein[22] described the basic pathology of arteriosclerosis, he did not imagine that it would, during the second half of the century, become the mechanism of 'senility' par excellence[14,23,24]. Motor and sensory deficits, vertigo, delusions, hallucinations and volitional, cognitive and affective disorder were all attributed to the effect of arteriosclerosis[25,26]. They related to the brain via a two-stage speculative pathophysiology: parenchymal and/or vascular disorders could affect the brain, and the distribution of the lesions could be diffused or focal. Vascular changes included acute ischaemia (on which clinical observation was adequate)[27,28]

and chronic ischaemia, invented as a separate syndrome by extrapolating from the symptoms and signs observed during the acute states[24]. The role of arteriosclerosis as a causal and prognostic factor in relation to the involutional psychoses was challenged early in the twentieth century[29] but this paper remained unnoticed. Hence, some of the old notions, such as that of 'arteriosclerotic dementia', remained active well into the 1960s[30].

Alienists during the same period, however, were already able to distinguish between states where a putative chronic and diffuse reduction in blood supply had taken place from focalized damage, i.e. what they called 'multifocal arteriosclerotic dementia' and was equivalent to what is currently called multi-infarct dementia[24,31,32].

NINETEENTH CENTURY VIEWS ON MENTAL DECAY IN THE ELDERLY

It is against this background that the history of the language and concepts dedicated to understanding mental disorders in the elderly must be understood. In addition to these neurobiological frameworks, a psychological theory that explained the manner of the decline was required. Such a psychopathology was provided by the heuristic combination of associationism, faculty psychology[33], and statistics[34] that characterized the early and middle parts of the nineteenth century.

Yet another perspective, originating in clinical observation, was added during the 1830s. It led to the realization that, in addition to the well-known forms of mental disorder, the elderly might exhibit specific forms of deterioration, and that these could be related to recognizable brain changes. There is only space in this chapter to deal with two examples: one typifying a 'specific' disorder of old age, namely the history of chronic cognitive failure or dementia; the other illustrating the effect of a general mental disorder (melancholia) on the elderly.

THE FORMATION OF THE CONCEPT OF SENILE DEMENTIA

The history of the word and concept of dementia before the nineteenth century has been touched upon elsewhere[35]. Suffice it to say here that, at the beginning of the nineteenth century, 'dementia' had a 'legal' and a 'medical' meaning and referred to most acquired states of intellectual dysfunction that resulted in serious psychosocial incompetence. Neither age of acquisition nor reversibility was part of its definition. These two dimensions were only incorporated during the nineteenth century and completely changed the semantic territory of the dementia concept.

Anecdotal observation of cases of senile dementia abound both in the fictional literature and in historical documents[36], but the concept of 'senile dementia', as it is currently understood, only took shape during the latter part of the nineteenth century. Indeed, it could not have been otherwise, as the neurobiological and clinical language that made it possible only became available during this period[37,38]. But even after the nosological status of senile dementia had become clearer, there were many who, like Rauzier[39], felt able to state: 'it may appear either as a primary state or follow most of the mental disorders affecting the elderly' (p. 615). Following Rogues de Fursac[40], Adrien Pic – the author of one of the most influential geriatric manuals during this period[41] – defined senile dementia as: 'a state of intellectual decline, whether or not accompanied by delusions, that results from brain lesions associated with ageing' (pp. 364–365). It was against this background that the concept of Alzheimer's disease, which became the prototype for all senile dementias, was created during the first decade of the twentieth century[37]. Recent work has shown that its 'discovery' was controlled by ideological forces well beyond what could be described as 'scientific'[37,42]. These forces also introduced unwarranted clinical strictures, such as the exclusion of non-cognitive symptoms[43,44] and false age boundaries, which took many years to disappear.

THE FORMATION OF THE CONCEPT OF INVOLUTIONAL MELANCHOLIA

The concept of 'senile or involutional psychoses', which featured so prominently in Kraepelin's early classification, included presenile delusional insanity, senile dementia, late catatonia and involutional melancholia[45,46]. The reasons that led Kraepelin to separate this group were mostly theoretical, to wit, that they appeared during a period of life when 'sclerotic' changes were beginning to occur; the same factor accounted for their bad prognosis[46].

The general history of melancholia and depression has been analysed elsewhere[47-49]. Suffice it to say here that by the 1860s depression was considered to be an independent syndrome resulting from a primary disorder of affect. This meant that hallucinations, delusions and cognitive impairment were secondary to the pathological feelings. This conviction was particularly strong towards the end of the century, when emotional mechanisms became popular in the explanation of most forms of mental disorder[50]. By the end of the century the metaphor of depression as a form of 'reduction' or 'loss' had become firmly established. No better example can be found than the fact that up to 1893 (fourth edition) Kraepelin felt obliged to classify all forms of agitated depression as mania![51]

KRAEPELIN AND INVOLUTIONAL MELANCHOLIA

Much of the current confusion on the meaning of involutional melancholia can be explained if attention is given to the circumstances of its historical development (for a full analysis of this process and list of references, see Berrios[52]). The conventional story[53-56] is that up to the seventh edition of his textbook Kraepelin considered involutional melancholia as a separate disease, and that when confronted by the evidence collected by Dreyfus[57], he decided to include it, in the eighth edition, under the general heading of manic depressive insanity. Indeed, this account was first offered by Kraepelin himself (see Dreyfus, p. 169).

The story is, however, more complex and it is unlikely that the findings of Dreyfus alone caused Kraepelin's change of heart. For example, Thalbitzer[58] claimed that his own work had also been influential (p. 41). In the eighth edition Kraepelin abandoned not only involutional melancholia but the entire group of 'senile psychoses'. A recent statistical analysis of Dreyfus's old series has also shown that his conclusion that the natural history of involutional melancholia was no different from that of depression affecting younger subjects was wrong[51].

CONCLUSIONS

This short chapter, providing a historical vignette on the origin of the language of old age psychiatry, suggests that it was born during the nineteenth century from three conceptual sources: theories of ageing, neurobiological hypotheses concerning brain sclerosis, and the realization that specific forms of mental disorder might affect the elderly. Two clinical illustrations were provided, one pertaining to the origins of the concept of senile dementia, and the other to the notion of involutional melancholia.

REFERENCES

1. Huber J-P, Gourin P. Le vieillard dément dans l'Antiquité classique. *Psychiatr Fr* 1987; **13**: 12–18.
2. Minois G. *Histoire de la Vieillesse. De l'Antiquité à la Renaissance*. Paris: Fayard, 1987.
3. Reveillé-Parise JH. *Traité de la Vieillesse*. Paris: Baillière, 1853.
4. Grmek MD. *On Ageing and Old Age*. The Hague: W Junk, 1958.
5. Legrand MA. *La Longévité à Travers les Âges*. Paris: Flammarion, 1911.
6. Freeman JJ. *Aging. Its History and Literature*. New York: Human Sciences Press, 1979.
7. Kotsovsky D. Le problème de la vieillesse dans son développement historique. *Riv Biol* 1931; **13**: 99–111.
8. Grant RL. Concepts of aging: an historical review. *Persp Biol Med* 1963; **6**: 443–78.
9. Bastai P, Dogliotti GC. *Physiopathologie de la Vieillesse*. Paris: Masson, 1938.
10. Robinson DR. The evolution of geriatric psychiatry. *Med Hist* 1972; **16**: 184–93.
11. Kastenbaum R, Ross B. Historical perspectives on care. In Howells J (ed.), *Modern Perspectives in the Psychiatry of Old Age*. Edinburgh: Churchill Livingstone, 1975, 421–49.
12. Cicero. *De Senectute, De Amicitia, De Divinatione*, trans. Falconer WA. London: Loeb, 1923.
13. Gruman GJ. A history of ideas about the prolongation of life. *Trans Am Phil Soc* 1966; **56**: 1–97.
14. Buffon M le Comte, Georges-Louis Leclerc. *Histoire Naturelle de l'Homme, de la Vieillesse et de la Mort*, vol. 4: *Histoire Naturelle de l'Homme*. Paris: De L'imprimerie Royale, 1774.
15. Darwin E. *Zoonomia; or, the Laws of Organic Life*, 2 vols. London: Johnson, 1794–1796.
16. Sinclair Sir J. *The Code of Health and Longevity*. Edinburgh: Constable, 1807.
17. Rostan LL. *Recherches sur le Ramollissement du Cerveau*. Paris: Bechet, 1819 and 1823.
18. Rostan LL. Jusqu à quel point l'anatomie pathologique peut-elle éclairer la thé rapeutique des maladies. Thèse de concours. Paris: Moessard, 1833.
19. Chereau A. Rostan. In Dechambre A, Lereboullet L (eds), *Dictionnaire Encyclopédique des Sciences Médicales*, vol. 84. Paris: Masson, 1877, 238–40.
20. Lévy M. *Traité d'hygiène Publique et Priveé*. Paris: Baillière 1850.
21. Charcot JM. *Clinical Lectures on Senile and Chronic Diseases*, trans. Tuke WS. London: The New Sydenham Society, 1981.
22. Lobstein JG. *Traité de Anatomie Pathologique*, vol. 2. Paris: Baillière, 1838.
23. Demange E. *Étude Clinique et Anatomopathologique de la Vieillesse*. Paris: Ducost, 1886.
24. Potain C. Cerveau (Pathologie). In Dechambre A, Lereboullet L (eds), *Dictionnaire Encyclopédique des Sciences Médicales*, vol. 14. Paris: Masson, 1873, 214–345.
25. Marie A. *Démence*. Paris: Doin, 1906.
26. Albrecht T. Manischdepressiven Irresein und Arteriosklerose. *Allg Z Psychiatr* 1906; **63**: 402–47.

27. Schiller F. Concepts of stroke before and after Virchow. *Med Hist* 1970; **14**: 115–31.
28. Fields WS, Lamak NA. *A History of Stroke*. New York: Oxford University Press, 1989.
29. Walton GL. Arteriosclerosis probably not an important factor in the etiology and prognosis of involution psychoses. *Boston Med Surg J* 1912; **167**: 834–6.
30. Weitbrecht HJ. *Psychiatrie im Crundriss*. Berlin: Springer, 1968.
31. Ball B, Chambard E. Démence. In Dechambre A, Lereboullet L (eds), *Dictionnaire Encyclopédique des Sciences Médicales*, vol. 26. Paris: Masson, 1882, 559–635.
32. Spielmeyer W. *Die Psychosen des Rückbildungs und Creisenalters*. Leipzig: Deuticke, 1912.
33. Berrios GE. Historical background to abnormal psychology. In Miller E, Cooper PJ (eds), *Adult Abnormal Psychology*. Edinburgh: Churchill Livingstone, 1988, 26–51.
34. Birren JE. A brief history of the psychology of ageing. *Gerontologist* 1961; **1**: 69–77.
35. Berrios GE. Dementia during the seventeenth and eighteenth centuries: a conceptual history. *Psychol Med* 1987; **17**: 829–37.
36. Torack RM. The early history of senile dementia. In Reisberg B (ed.), *Alzheimer's Disease*. New York: Free Press, 1983, 23–8.
37. Berrios GE. Alzheimer's disease: a conceptual history. *Int J Geriatr Psych* 1990; **5**: 355–65.
38. Schwalbe J. Dementia senilis. In *Lehrbuch der Greisenkrankheiten*. Stuttgart: Enke, 1909, 479–89.
39. Rauzier G. *Traité des Maladies des Vieillards*. Paris: Baillière, 1909.
40. Rogues de Fursac J. *Manual de Psiquiatría*, trans. of 5th French edn by Peset J. Valencia: Editorial Pubul, 1921.
41. Pic A. *Précis des Maladies des Vieillards*. Paris: Doin, 1912.
42. Dillman R. *Alzheimer's Disease. The Concept of Disease and the Construction of Medical Knowledge*. Amsterdam: Thesis Publishers, 1990.
43. Berrios GE. Non-cognitive symptoms and the diagnosis of dementia. Historical and clinical aspects. *Br J Psychiat* 1989; **154**(suppl 4): 11–16.
44. Berrios GE. Memory and the cognitive paradigm of dementia during the 19th century: a conceptual history. In Murray RM, Turner TH (eds), *Lectures on the History of Psychiatry*. London: Gaskell, 1990, 194–211.
45. Cabaleiro Goas M. Los sindromes psicóticos de la presenilidad. *Actas Luso Esp Neurol Psiquiatr* 1955; **14**: 17–26.
46. Cabaleiro Goas M. Psicosis preseniles no orgánicocerebrales y su prevención. In *Proceedings of I Congreso Nacional de Geronto-Psiquiatría preventiva. Xl Reunión de la Sociedad Española de Psiquiatría*. Madrid: Liade, 1974, 117–42.
47. Berrios GE. Melancholia and depression during the 19th century: a conceptual history. *Br J Psychiatry* 1988; **153**: 298–304.
48. Berrios GE. Depressive and manic states during the 19th century. In Georgotas A, Cancro R (eds), *Depression and Mania*. New York: Elsevier, 1988, 13–25.
49. Berrios GE. The history of the affective disorders. In Paykel ES (ed.), *Handbook of Affective Disorders*, 2nd edn. Edinburgh: Churchill Livingstone, 1992, 43–56.
50. Berrios GE. The psychopathology of affectivity: conceptual and historical aspects. *Psychol Med* 1985; **15**: 745–58.
51. Kraepelin E. *Psychiatrie*, 4th edn. Leipzig: Meixner, 1893.
52. Berrios GE. Affective symptoms in old age: a conceptual history. *Int J Geriatr Psychiatry* 1991; **6**: 337–46.
53. Sérieux P. Review of Dreyfus's Melancholie. *L'Encéphale* 1907; **2**: 456–8.
54. Post F. *The Clinical Psychiatry of Late Life*. Oxford: Pergamon, 1965.
55. Kendell RE. *The Classification of Depressive Illness*. Oxford: Oxford University Press, 1968.
56. Jackson SW. *Melancholia and Depression. From Hippocratic Times to Modern Times*. New Haven, CT: Yale University Press, 1985.
57. Dreyfus GL. *Die Melancholie. Ein Zustandsbild des manischdepressiven Irreseins*. Jena: Gustav Fischer, 1907.
58. Thalbitzer S. *Emotions and Insanity*. London: Kegan Paul, Trench, Trubner, 1926.

The Development of Old Age Psychiatry in the UK

Claire Hilton[1] and Tom Arie[2]

[1]Central and North West London NHS Foundation Trust, Harrow, UK
[2]University of Nottingham, Ageing and Disability Research Unit, Nottingham, UK

Old age psychiatry in Britain was born in the 1960s and 1970s, and came of age at its recognition by the government as a distinct specialty in 1989.[i] Yet the need for it had been recognized as far back as the 1940s. Why was the gestation so long, and how has it developed in the last twenty years since its recognition? What can we learn from this history?

THE EARLIEST DAYS

The likelihood that older people would become major users of psychiatric services was identified during the Second World War. Increasing longevity meant there were more, and even older, old people. Falling birth rates increased the proportion of old people and since more women were in employment it was harder for them to take on traditional caring roles. Some of the more frail older people were cared for in 'chronic sick' and mental hospitals, which might be needed for war casualties.

Until the 1940s mental and physical ill health in old age had been considered largely irremediable. In the 1940s Marjory Warren, the pioneering geriatrician, demonstrated the scope for rehabilitating old people[1], psychiatrist Felix Post wrote on psychiatric differential diagnosis and multidisciplinary approaches to treatment[2], and Willi Mayer-Gross described how severely depressed old people could improve with electroconvulsive therapy (ECT)[3][ii]. Despite the evidence of successful treatment, older people were not given priority in health policy. In 1942 the Beveridge Report laid the foundations of the 'welfare state' and a National Health Service (NHS). However, it stated, 'It is dangerous to be in any way lavish to old age, until adequate provision has been assured for all other vital needs'[4].

After the war, at the instigation of Professor Aubrey Lewis, a psychiatric 'geriatric unit' was opened at the Bethlem Hospital in South London, part of the Bethlem-Maudsley postgraduate psychiatric teaching hospital (see Chapter 03). This unit was for functionally ill patients regarded as treatable. Patients with dementia, especially those requiring long stay care, were excluded, in part because of

opposition from academic psychiatrists who did not see their care as being worthy of study and investigation.

We shall touch on matters relating to these early influences, since all run throughout the development of the specialty. In addition, each generation rediscovers the demography of ageing as if it were a new phenomenon. Yet unlike, say, trends in fertility, or in transportation, which cannot be predicted with certainty, we always know the size of prospective populations of older people and the epidemiology of the crucial illnesses[5]. Repeatedly, the government has laid plans and failed adequately to implement or fund them, and then has 'discovered' afresh the scale of need. In 1950 we hear, 'It is recognised that the present conditions of financial stringency limit opportunities for action at this time'[6]. In 2001, a national service 'framework' for older people had no allocated new funding for mental health[7], whereas a parallel framework for mental health for younger people was substantially funded[8].

Another initiative in 2007 to improve access to psychological therapies has followed an economic model and has been targeted towards getting unemployed younger people into work, although this may well be changing to become more inclusive across all ages[9]. A contrast exists even within Britain: since 2002, Scotland provides both free personal and nursing care, if deemed appropriate after assessment, while England and Wales do not.

WORKING WITH GERIATRICIANS

Working with geriatricians is crucial in view of the multiple and interlinked disorders of old people, yet at times this has been erratic. Although active treatment, both physical and mental, was being advocated by the 1940s, geriatrics developed much earlier than psychogeriatrics. This was in part because many early geriatricians saw themselves as holistic practitioners for older people, therefore requesting little psychiatric assistance. The advocacy of Lord Amulree, a civil servant and geriatrician, and the other founders of geriatrics drew the successes of rehabilitation, including emptying hospital beds, to the attention of the government[10]. Such a phenomenon did not occur in old age psychiatry until around 1970 when new local services, such as that established at Goodmayes Hospital in 1969[11], were drawn to the attention of the Department of Health and Social Security[12]: only then it was recognized that a modern approach could reduce bed occupancy, improve outcomes and save money. Until the 1970s old age psychiatry in the UK was

---

[i]Originally called 'psychogeriatrics', 'old age psychiatry' is now more commonly used. However, the former is retained in some contexts, e.g. journal titles such as *International Psychogeriatrics*. The Royal College of Psychiatrists has a Faculty of the Psychiatry of Old Age, while many clinical departments refer to themselves as 'Mental Health Services' for older people or older adults.
[ii]Before antidepressants, ECT was the only effective physical treatment.

Principles and Practice of Geriatric Psychiatry, 3rd edn. Edited by Mohammed T. Abou-Saleh, Cornelius Katona and Anand Kumar
© 2011 John Wiley & Sons, Ltd

characterized by research in clinical treatment, nosology, pathology and epidemiology, with only small pockets of local service innovation.

In 1970 there were 200 geriatric medicine consultants[13] but only a handful of psychogeriatricians[14,15]. By 2006 there were 700 psychogeriatricians[16]. Where enthusiastic geriatricians and psychiatrists existed in a particular locality they collaborated. In addition, collaboration between the Royal College of Psychiatrists and the British Geriatrics Society[17] since the 1970s has led to the development of guidelines for good practice and working collaboratively[18]. Moving services away from isolated mental and 'chronic sick' hospitals and their coming together in district general hospitals has given better access to each other's services. Sometimes this facilitated joint working, but formal joint services were rare. In 1977, a department of Health Care of the Elderly, comprising both medicine and psychiatry working together, along with other relevant disciplines and professions was set up in Nottingham. There was an orthopaedic-geriatric unit, a stroke unit and a continence service, and joint research, along with extensive teaching of medical students and postgraduate trainees of relevant disciplines, and of overseas workers[19–21].

'Memory clinics' are another development, now widespread, with their roots in both psychogeriatric and geriatric practice in the mid-1980s[22]. More recent developments include psychiatric liaison services for patients with acute physical illness in district general hospitals[23]. Jointly run 'intermediate care' or 'convalescent' rehabilitation units for confused older people, especially those recovering from both delirium and physical illness, are also new. Geriatricians and psychiatrists still have much to learn from each other, and 'seamless' services remain the ideal. 'Guidelines for collaboration' have recently been updated[24].

WORKING WITH PSYCHIATRISTS CARING FOR YOUNGER PEOPLE

Before the establishment of the specialty, mentally ill old people requiring secondary care were the responsibility of general psychiatrists, but they rarely showed interest in actually working with them, especially those with dementia. However, some of the pioneering psychogeriatric services, such as Sam Robinson's in Dumfries (1958)[25], or Brice Pitt's at Claybury, Essex (1966)[26], emerged in part due to the far sightedness and encouragement of general psychiatrists who were medical superintendents of mental hospitals. Despite such early developments, it took until 1989 for the Royal College of Psychiatrists and the government to agree officially to the creation of the new specialty of old age psychiatry. Until then, lack of recognition meant that it had often been impossible to extract from official statistics adequate data on older people's use of services, and hence to establish the scale of need for services and for training.

Competition for resources is inevitable, so long as resources are limited. The low status of the aged, the perceived needs of people of working age, and the common misperception that young severely mentally ill people are frequently dangerous have generally resulted in funding for services for younger people disproportionately exceeding that for older people.

A CENTRAL BODY FOR COORDINATING DEVELOPMENT

A powerful national focus for securing improved recognition and better resources has been the flourishing Faculty of the Psychiatry of Old Age at the Royal College of Psychiatrists (since 1988), and its predecessor bodies (from 1973). It has, among other things, encouraged research, innovation, multidisciplinary working, and links with voluntary and statutory organizations and with the government, and has taken an interest in architecture and design for elderly confused people[27]. A first series of newsletters in the 1980s served as a constructive means of communication among clinicians. A second series since 1996, available online since 2000 (www.rcpsych.ac.uk/college/faculties/oldage/newsletter.aspx), often expresses thoughtful comment related to current clinical and policy dilemmas. Faculty meetings have remained a source of debate, education, inspiration and problem solving. The Faculty's website is a mine of information (www.rcpsych.ac.uk/college/faculties/oldage.aspx).

RESEARCH AND ACADEMIC DEVELOPMENT

Research on older people's mental health has flourished and has helped the development of evidence-based practice. Sir Martin Roth in the 1950s defined the major diagnostic categories in older people[28], rather as Emil Kraepelin had done 50 years earlier for younger people. Felix Post undertook follow-up studies of treatment of depression and psychotic disorders. Nick Corsellis[29] followed by Bernard Tomlinson, Martin Roth[30] and Elaine and Robert Perry unpicked the neurochemical and neuropathological features of Alzheimer's disease[31]. Early research by Raymond Levy into lecithin and later tacrine was a forerunner of today's evidence-based antidementia drugs[32].

Difficulty in obtaining funding for research has been characteristic[15]. But the growth of the neurosciences, along with the influence of bodies such as the Alzheimer's Society, has enhanced the scale of funding for research into the dementias, and has attracted able workers.

Research has also grown through the development of academic departments of old age psychiatry. The first old age psychiatrist to be appointed professor became head of the joint department of Health Care of the Elderly in Nottingham in 1977. The first professor of old age psychiatry, at Guy's Hospital, London, was appointed in 1983. The *International Journal of Geriatric Psychiatry* was started in 1986. In 1989 there were half a dozen professorial departments[33]; now most medical schools have an academic presence for old age psychiatry, and many NHS consultants are involved in teaching medical students and postgraduates. Many other departments in universities are now conducting relevant research, and there are further thriving journals.

TEACHING AND TRAINING

Biographical information reveals that many colleagues did not envisage becoming old age psychiatrists, but were *inspired* by others to do so; they saw and experienced what could be done to help old people. Such effective teaching is crucial[15].

Sharing our knowledge with other specialties and disciplines can change the way colleagues respond to elderly mentally ill people – in primary care, in management, in palliative care, social services, learning disability services, voluntary organizations, Citizens Advice Bureaux, and within the multidisciplinary teams within which we work. Other groups that have sought teaching include architects, designers, lawyers and the police.

Structured training for old age psychiatrists has also evolved over the years. The earliest psychogeriatricians in the 1960s and 1970s had little or no specific training. Six months' experience in old age psychiatry is considered valuable for trainees in psychiatry and in general practice. Specialized training for career old age psychiatrists is during the last three years of a six-year psychiatry training scheme. There is a competency-based curriculum[34], and at least two years (full-time equivalent) old age psychiatry in recognized training posts are usually required.

CLINICAL INNOVATION

The demise of the vast Victorian mental hospitals, the coming of community care, more liberal mental health legislation and new effective psychopharmacology have all helped to shape the progress of psychiatry since the 1950s. The psychogeriatricians have consistently fought to prevent older people being left behind younger people in new developments. Important classic texts of innovation in old age psychiatry such as *In the Service of Old Age* by Tony Whitehead (1971)[35] deserve particular mention, as do the reports in the 1960s and 1970s of abuses in the unfashionable sectors of care. The Ely Hospital Report (1969)[36] was also instrumental in bringing about the Hospital (later Health) Advisory Service (HAS), which advised on the neglected areas of the health service. The HAS was a valuable ally of the early old age psychiatrists, encouraging and spreading good practice. Its first director became an old age psychiatrist upon demitting office[37]

Home assessment and support by consultants and other team members was the norm: in some services this is still the usual first point of contact. Initial assessment at home was introduced in the 1960s, in order to evaluate, in the light of knowledge of the home setting, who could be helped without hospital admission, or who might need a medical or a surgical bed rather than psychiatric help. Often the entire management of the patient could be undertaken in the patient's home. Home assessment and treatment is valued by patients, carers and staff, and it helps to build a close working relationship with the local community, and is popular with medical students.

The importance of support for carers of people with dementia has long been recognized. Respite admissions[38], social services day care, help with personal care at home and the Admiral Nurse service established in 1994 (www.fordementia.org.uk/admiral.htm) are important in delivering such support.

Psychotherapy, including family therapy with old people and their adult children, dates from the 1960s[39] but is still not widespread, despite pockets of enthusiasm[40]. In a very few places psychiatric intensive care units, in particular providing care for elderly men with dementia and disruptive behaviours, have evolved, such older people being excluded from similar services for younger people[41]. Elsewhere, intensive home treatment teams are appearing for even those with severe mental illness such as would traditionally require admission.

Old age psychiatry day hospitals date from the 1950s onwards. They were often a substitute for long stay care for people with chronic mental illness living at home or with their family. More recently they have developed to offer assessment, treatment, rehabilitation and support such as might be beyond the capacity of a social care day centre. They enable some with particularly disruptive behaviours unmanageable by a social care day centre to remain in the community[42].

More recently as 'ethnic minority' populations have aged, understanding cultural and religious customs and attitudes to mental illness and ageing has become important in many local communities.

Other disciplines have developed in parallel to old age psychiatry. The British Psychological Society, for example, established a special

Table 2.1 Core features of a service in 2009

Core features are likely to include:
Community: assessment, diagnosis, treatment, rehabilitation
Inpatients: acute assessment and continuing care
Day hospital
Memory service
Support for carers
Liaison service to geriatric, medical and surgical wards
Other:
    planning
    teaching
    research
    liaison with related professions and organizations
    advocacy for patients
    advice on medico-legal matters, e.g. mental capacity

interest group for psychologists working with older people in 1980 (www.psige.org/index.php).

Without evaluated creativity, we would not have the rich array of services that, despite constraints of limited funding, serve our patients, their relatives and carers. But by no means every service for older people yet has all the components described above (see Table 2.1).

LONG STAY CARE

Up to the 1980s, most long stay care for dementia, along with that of aged people with chronic psychosis, took place in hospitals. Local authority residential homes were intended to care for frail old people, but with the passage of time they too increasingly became facilities for demented people, but lacking nursing skills and facilities appropriate to their residents' needs. During the Thatcher era of the 1980s, long stay care in hospitals was replaced by care in commercial, or, less often, charitable homes. Surveillance of standards in multiple dispersed units became very difficult. Third party inspection and definition of 'minimum standards' was instituted by the Blair government[43]. Education and training of care home staff, long virtually absent, is now becoming more prevalent. But 'scandals' in the care of old people continue, and although they often achieve publicity, they generally evoke less indignation and less remedial action than similar scandals in child care. Fortunately, architects and designers often now devote special skills to the needs of old people.

THE FUTURE

Old age psychiatrists, like workers in other health specialties, practise within the context of the structure and culture of society. At the time of writing we enter a recession, with uncertainty about the future, but with ever more evidence of the effectiveness of our interventions.

There are more government initiatives. The *National Dementia Strategy*, emphasizes raising awareness, early diagnosis and intervention, and improving quality of care in dementia, and is welcome on that account. However, the government's initial financial backing for the strategy amounts to less than 1% of the total annual cost of dementia care. It is hard to believe that this will make any significant impact. In addition it states, 'Decisions on funding for subsequent years will only be made once we have had the opportunity to consider the results from the initial demonstrator sites and evaluation work. There is no expectation therefore that all areas will necessarily be able to implement the Strategy within five years'[44]. This resonates with previous policies advocating good practice, which are neither mandatory nor adequately funded.

A new Mental Capacity Act seeks to provide a statutory framework to protect vulnerable people who are not able to make their own decisions[45]. There is also new legislation relating to 'deprivation of liberty', significantly affecting people with dementia who lack capacity to decide on their place of care, to determine whether and how they can be confined to a care home or hospital in their best interests. The new Equality Bill should prevent discrimination in services on the basis of chronological age[46]. However, it also carries the paradoxical risk that a separate service for old people may be regarded as discriminatory. Challenges to our special services have long arisen from this viewpoint, and we must continue to show that special services for an inherently low status and thus usually neglected group make for better care, and to point to the reasons why.

Legal and medical changes, and changes in society, will raise new questions, but the 1970s adage for an old age psychiatrist will continue to be 'occasional militancy... to gain for the elderly a fair share of scant resources, to put them to best use, to make do with too little while wheeling, dealing, and fighting for more'[47].

REFERENCES

1. Warren M. Care of chronic sick. *Br Med J* 1943; **ii**: 822–3.
2. Post F. Some problems arising from a study of mental patients over the age of 60 years. *J Ment Sci* 1944; **90**: 554–65.
3. Mayer-Gross W. Electric convulsion treatment in patients over 60. *J Ment Sci* 1945; **91**: 101–3.
4. Beveridge W. *Social Insurance and Allied Services* (Cmnd 6404). London: HMSO, 1942.
5. Kay DWK, Beamish P, Roth M. Old age mental disorders in Newcastle upon Tyne, Part 1: A study of prevalence. *Br J Psychiatry* 1964; **110**: 146–58.
6. Ministry of Health. Care of the Aged Suffering from Mental Infirmity, report HMC (50) 25. Typescript in King's Fund Library, London, 1950.
7. Department of Health. *National Service Framework for Older People*, 2001. At www.dh.gov.uk/en/publicationsandstatistics /publications/publicationspolicyandguidance/DH_4003066, accessed 9 Jan 2010.
8. Department of Health. *National Service Framework for Mental Health*, 2001. At www.dh.gov.uk/en/Publicationsandstatistics /Publications/PublicationsPolicyAndGuidance/DH_4009598, accessed 9 Jan 2010.
9. Department of Health. *Commissioning IAPT for the Whole Community: Improving Access to Psychological Therapies*, 2008. At www.dh.gov.uk/en/Publicationsandstatistics/Publications/DH_0 _90011, accessed 9 Jan 2010.
10. Exton-Smith AN. Obituary: Lord Amulree. *Br Med J* 1984; **288**: 156.
11. Arie T. The first year of the Goodmayes psychiatric service for old people. *Lancet* 1970; **ii**: 1179–82.
12. Fry J. The Keppel Club (1952–74): lessons from the past for the future. *Br Med J* 1991; **303**: 1596–8.
13. Brocklehurst JC. *The Geriatric Day Hospital*. London: King Edward's Hospital Fund for London, 1970.
14. Arie T, Jolley D. Psychogeriatrics. In Freeman H. (ed.), *A Century of Psychiatry*. London: Mosby-Wolfe, 1999, 260–65.
15. Hilton C (ed.). *The Development of Old Age Psychiatry from the 1960s until 1989*, Guthrie Trust Witness Seminar, Centre for the History of Medicine, University of Glasgow, 9 May 2008. At www.gla.ac.uk/media/media_107314_en.pdf, accessed 9 Jan 2010.
16. Royal College of Psychiatrists. *Workforce Figures for Psychiatrists*. London: Royal College of Psychiatrists, 2006. At www.rcpsych.ac.uk/PDF/Results%20for%20the%202006%20 Census%20(2).pdf, accessed 9 Jan 2010.
17. British Geriatrics Society Cerebral Ageing and Mental Health Special Interest Group. At www.bgs.org.uk/Special%20Interest/ cerebral_ageing.htm, accessed 9 Jan 2010.
18. British Geriatrics Society and Royal College of Psychiatrists. Joint report on matters relating to the care of psycho-geriatric patients. *Br J Psychiatry* 1973; **123**: News and Notes 2–3.
19. Arie T. Combined geriatrics and psychogeriatrics: a new model. *Geriatr Med* 1990; April: 24–7.
20. Arie T. Education in the care of the elderly. *Bull N Y Acad Med* 1985; **61**(6): 492–500.
21. Bendall MJ. The interface between geriatrics and psychogeriatrics. *Curr Med Lit Geriatr* 1988; **1**(1): 2–7.
22. Van der Cammen TJM, Simpson JM, Fraser RM, Preker AS, Exton-Smith AN. The memory clinic: a new approach to the detection of dementia. *Br J Psychiatry* 1987; **150**: 359–64.
23. Working Group for Liaison Mental Health Services for Older People, Faculty of Old Age Psychiatry. *Who Cares Wins*. London: Royal College of Psychiatrists, 2005. At www.bgs.org.uk/PDF Downloads/WhoCaresWins.pdf, accessed 9 Jan 2010.
24. British Geriatrics Society. *Guidelines for Collaboration between Physicians of Geriatric Medicine and Psychiatrists of Old Age*, BGS Best Practice Guide 3.4, 2007. At www.bgs.org.uk/Publications/Compendium/compend_3-4.htm, accessed 9 Jan 2010.
25. Robinson RA. The organisation of a diagnostic and treatment unit for the aged in a mental hospital. In *Psychiatric Disorders in the Aged*, report on the World Psychiatric Association Symposium. Manchester: Geigy, 1965, 186–205.
26. Pitt B, interviewed for *Oral History of Geriatrics as a Medical Specialty*, National Sound Archive, 1991. At http://cadensa.bl.uk/uhtbin/cgisirsi/BLMW1dvUMJ/10190012/9 (summary), accessed 9 Jan 2010.
27. Kemp M. Accommodation for elderly patients with severe dementia, minutes, Group for the Psychiatry of Old Age, Royal College of Psychiatrists 28 Mar 1974 (13), 13 June 1974 (4).
28. Roth M. The natural history of mental disorders in old age. *J Ment Sci* 1955; **101**: 281–301.
29. Corsellis JAN. *Mental Illness and the Ageing Brain*, Maudsley Monograph 9. London: Oxford University Press, 1962.
30. Roth M, Tomlinson BE, Blessed G. The relationship between qualitative measures of dementia and degenerative change in cerebral grey matter of elderly subjects. *Proc R Soc Med* 1967; **60**: 254–60.
31. Perry EK, Perry RH, Blessed G, Tomlinson B. Necropsy evidence of central cholinergic deficits in senile dementia. *Lancet* 1977; **i**: 189.
32. Eagger SA, Levy R, Sahakian BJ. Tacrine in Alzheimer's disease. *Lancet* 1991; **337**: 989–92.

33. Arie T. Martin Roth and the 'Psychogeriatricians'. In Davison K, Kerr A. (eds), *Contemporary Themes in Psychiatry: A Tribute to Sir Martin Roth*. London: Gaskell, 1989, 231–8.

34. Royal College of Psychiatrists. *A Competency Based Curriculum for Specialist Training in Psychiatry: Specialist Module in Old Age Psychiatry*, 2009. At www.rcpsych.ac.uk/PDF/Old_Age _Feb09.pdf, accessed 9 Jan 2010.

35. Whitehead T. *In the Service of Old Age: The Welfare of Psychogeriatric Patients*. Harmondsworth: Penguin, 1970.

36. DHSS. *Report of the Committee of Inquiry into Allegations of Ill-treatment of Patients and other Irregularities at the Ely Hospital, Cardiff* (Cmnd 3975). London: HMSO, 1969.

37. Baker AA. Why psychogeriatrics? *Lancet* 1974; **i**: 795–6.

38. De Largy J. Six weeks in, 6 weeks out. A geriatric hospital scheme for rehabilitating the aged and relieving their relatives. *Lancet* 1957; **i**: 418–19.

39. Colwell C, Post F. The parent–child relationship in the treatment of elderly psychiatric patients. *Ment Health (Lond)* 1964; **23**: 7–9.

40. Benbow SM, Marriott A. Family therapy with elderly people. *Adv Psychiatr Treat* 1997; **3**: 138–45.

41. Department of Health. *Mental Health Policy Implementation Guide: National Minimum Standards for General Adult Services in Psychiatric Intensive Care Units (PICU) and Low Secure Environments*, 2002. At www.dh.gov.uk/en/Publicationsandstatistics /Publications/PublicationsPolicyAndGuidance/DH_4010439, accessed 9 Jan 2010.

42. Arie T. Day care in geriatric psychiatry 1978. *Age Ageing* 1979; **8**(suppl): 87–91.

43. Department of Health. *Fit for the Future? National Required Standards for Residential and Nursing Homes for Older People* (Consultation Document), 1999. At www.dh.gov.uk/en/ Publicationsandstatistics/Publications/PublicationsPolicyAnd-Guidance/DH_4009506, accessed 9 Jan 2010.

44. Department of Health. *Living Well with Dementia: A National Dementia Strategy*, 2009. At www.dh.gov.uk/en/socialcare /deliveringadultsocialcare/olderpeople/nationaldementiastrategy /index.htm, accessed 9 Jan 2010.

45. Office of Public Sector Information. *Mental Capacity Act 2005*, 2005. At www.opsi.gov.uk/ACTS/acts2005/ukpga_20050009 _en_1, accessed 9 Jan 2010.

46. Office of Public Sector Information. *Equality Act 2006*, 2006. At www.opsi.gov.uk/acts/acts2006/pdf/ukpga_20060003_en.pdf, accessed 9 Jan 2010.

47. Anon. Group into section? Minutes, Group for the Psychiatry of Old Age, Royal College of Psychiatrists, 1977 (typescript).

Commentary on 'In the Beginning' by Felix Post

Claire Hilton

Central and North West London NHS Foundation Trust, Harrow, UK

INTRODUCTION

Felix Post was probably the first dedicated old-age psychiatrist anywhere in the world. 'In the Beginning' is his autobiographical account of the earliest days of old-age psychiatry in Britain. Such accounts are valuable primary sources for understanding the development of the specialty. We are now reaching a point in time when our earliest pioneers like Felix Post (1913–2001) and Martin Roth (1917–2006) have died. It is important that we remember the contributions of our teachers from the past who have set the foundations for our specialty, just as Phillipe Pinel, Emil Kraepelin, Sigmund Freud and many others are celebrated for their contributions to the mental well-being of mainly younger people.

This short chapter by Felix Post has been described as 'pure Felix'. It characteristically reveals his humility and modesty, and his praise of others, attributing little achievement to himself. A brief biographical note and commentary are therefore warranted to set it in context.

'IN THE BEGINNING' BY THE LATE FELIX POST

In 1943, after a year's early training as one of the war-time refugees of the Maudsley Hospital, Professor Aubrey Lewis passed me on to Professor D.K. Henderson and the Royal Edinburgh Hospital for Nervous and Mental Diseases, where I initially worked in the private department. During one of his rounds, Henderson said to me: 'Post, do you see all these old people here? Why don't you write 'em up?' This I obediently did, and my article appeared in the *Journal of Mental Science*[i]. The article started by demonstrating that the admission rate of patients over 60 to the Royal Edinburgh Hospital had risen between 1901 and 1941 more steeply than the proportion of this age group in the Scottish population. Interestingly, at this early date, I had found no difficulties in the differential diagnosis of my colleagues' and my own patients. There were 22 senile, arteriosclerotic and presenile dementia patients, 20 manic–depressive patients, 25 patients suffering from involutional or senile melancholia and 51 patients with schizophrenia. Assuming that the functional psychoses were the concern of general psychiatry, the rest of the paper dealt with the dementias and with an attempt to link the type associated with delusions and hallucinations to earlier personality characteristics. I noted that a high proportion of dementia admissions had been precipitated by terminal confusional states, and that of 111 patients admitted over the preceding four years with organic psychoses, only

23 were still occupying beds. I made the false prediction that in the future the main burden of the hospital services would be represented by the chronicity and survival of melancholic and paranoid patients. I did not anticipate that electroconvulsive therapy (ECT) and antidepressive drugs, while producing lasting recoveries in only 25% of cases, would make at least temporary discharge from inpatient care possible in most cases.

Aubrey Lewis was more farsighted. He had published, with a psychiatric social worker[ii] a paper describing the psychiatric and social features of the patients in the Tooting Bec Hospital for Senile Dementia, London, UK, and in 1946 predicted, in the *Journal of Mental Science*[iii] that ageing and senility would become a major problem of psychiatry.

After army service, I consulted Lewis about possible positions and he recommended me for the post of assistant physician at the Maudsley Hospital. I flattered myself that in me Lewis had seen a future brilliant psychiatrist, but was soon to be disillusioned. Even before the Bethlem Royal and Maudsley Hospitals were united in 1948, Lewis had conceived the idea of using some of the Bethlem beds to establish a unit for patients over the age of 60. After a heated discussion with the Bethlem matron, Lewis obtained agreement for the admission of senile patients to a hospital which, like the Maudsley, had previously admitted only patients thought to be recoverable. Uncovering his batteries, he asked me to take on the development of this Geriatric Unit. Once again, I obeyed (to say without enthusiasm would be an understatement) and, right up to my retirement, I continued also to run a unit and outpatient clinic for younger adults.

A report in the *Bethlem Maudsley Gazette*[iv] demonstrated that both the Bethlem staff and I had 'caught fire'. The article started with a tribute to Professor Aubrey Lewis and his almost revolutionary idea of including experience in geriatric psychiatry within postgraduate training. The article went on to describe how patients over 60 had gradually infiltrated the Bethlem wards to emerge as a unit for 26 women and 20 men. The two wards were staffed by the same number of senior and junior nurses as the other adult wards, with two trainee psychiatrists changing every six months to other departments. There was one psychiatric social worker, later usually assisted by a trainee. The occupational therapy department had collaborated with the nursing staff to devise and carry out a daily occupational programme as well as socializing activities. The psychiatric social worker ran a weekly afternoon of handicrafts, tea and talk near the Maudsley, where throughout my tenure I conducted a weekly follow-up and

Principles and Practice of Geriatric Psychiatry, 3rd edn. Edited by Mohammed T. Abou-Saleh, Cornelius Katona and Anand Kumar
© 2011 John Wiley & Sons, Ltd

supportive clinic. The first year during which the unit had been in full swing was 1952, and it was recorded that during that year there had been 3.00 admissions to each geriatric bed compared to 3.74 admissions to each general psychiatric place. Patients who had been dementing, but whose home care was no longer possible had been excluded from admission, though not rigidly, as well as patients with recurring illnesses that had been adequately treated at the Bethlem-Maudsley or other hospitals. Of 133 patients, nine died, only four had to be transferred to their regional mental hospitals, seven were resettled in homes for the elderly, while 113 could be returned to family care. One year after discharge, information was successfully obtained about 121 of 124 cases. Seven patients had died, including one suicide of a woman who had discharged herself. Thirty ex-patients had to be readmitted to our or other hospitals, 35 were still outside hospital but by no means symptom-free, but 45 patients would be classified as recovered. These relatively favourable results were due to 89 patients having suffered from affective illnesses: 24 had symptoms associated with brain damage, 10 were mainly paranoid and 10 were regarded as having psychoneurosis. In spite of 4–6 weeks of conservative management 52 patients had to be given ECT. I concluded the article by pointing to research needs and by opining that with 30–40% of patients admitted to British mental hospitals being over the age of 60, training in the special problems of this age group was essential for all entrants to general psychiatry.

The history of the beginning would be incomplete without a brief account of further developments. My little textbook (rightly out of print) and publications on the long-term outcome of affective, para-phrenic and schizo-affective illnesses were largely my own work, but many of the junior psychiatrists made contributions and they and clinical psychologists, as well as social workers, instigated their own researches. Many later made a name for themselves, and some became leading psychogeriatricians. Among them were Tom Arie, the late L.K. Hemsi, David Jolley, Robin Jacoby, David Kay, Kenneth Shulman and, last but certainly not least, Raymond Levy. After the Bethlem-Maudsley had accepted a district commitment and the admission of involuntary (sectioned) patients, Raymond Levy and my successor, Klaus Bergmann (not a Bethlem trainee), managed to move the Geriatric Unit to the Maudsley, so much closer to the patients' family homes. Raymond Levy succeeded in establishing an Academic Department of Old Age Psychiatry, which has continued to conduct research into the dementias of late life, that most important subject, previously neglected on account of admission restrictions before the hospital abandoned its ivory tower to accept a district commitment. With similar developments elsewhere, psychogeriatrics became a world movement, and Sir Aubrey Lewis would be pleased.

REFERENCES

i. Post F. Some problems arising from a study of mental patients over the age of sixty years. J Ment Sci 1944; **90**: 554–65.

ii. Lewis AJ, Goldschmidt H. Social causes of admission to a mental hospital for the aged. Sociol Rev 1943; **365**: 86–98.

iii. Lewis AJ. Ageing and senility: a major problem of psychiatry. J Ment Sci 1946; **92**: 150–70.

iv. Post F. Geriatric unit (a report on progress made, with special reference to 1952). Bethlem Maudsley Hosp Gaz 1955; **1**: 270–71.

COMMENTARY

Felix was a refugee from Nazi Germany[1]. He enrolled at St Bartholomew's Hospital in 1934, qualifying in 1939. He entered medicine in an era when it was widely assumed that older mentally ill people were 'senile' and therefore nothing could be done for them.

Felix refers to his 1944 paper[2]. He commented on his 'false prediction' for older people requiring long-stay care in hospital, that those with chronic functional illnesses would numerically exceed those with organic illnesses. However, he did not emphasize the real significance of his paper, his observations that 'Old age alone does not produce mental illness', that appropriate diagnoses can be made, and that a multidisciplinary approach is important in treating older people. The possibility of differential diagnosis from a hopeless mass of mental symptoms in old age was not widely recognized until Martin Roth's classic paper in 1955[3]. Felix was a decade ahead. His conclusions were radical. Felix's paper caught the attention of Professor Aubrey Lewis (1900–1975); he referred to it in his own landmark paper[4]; they shared a common, new and challenging belief that something *could* be done to treat elderly mentally ill people.

Lewis had three contemporaries writing constructively on mental illness in older people. Two were relatively senior refugee psychiatrists: Willi Mayer-Gross[5] and Erwin Stengel[6]. The third, Felix, was earmarked by Lewis for a clinical role with older people. However, Felix had no intentions of becoming a psychiatrist, let alone one working with older people. But he was aware that refugee doctors were having difficulty in securing senior appointments, especially in traditional elitist teaching hospitals. Lewis offered him a post in 1947 at the Maudsley Hospital, London, a psychiatric teaching hospital. Henceforth, he regarded himself as owing Lewis a huge debt, and thus when Lewis asked him to be consultant on the new Geriatric Unit he could not refuse. Felix's ambivalence to working there stemmed from the prevailing belief that nothing could be done therapeutically to help the old and mentally ill[7], despite his own published work.

Lewis's objective was to make the Bethlem-Maudsley Hospital a great centre of postgraduate psychiatric teaching and research, of which mental illness of older people would be part[8]. Once established, the Geriatric Unit for functionally ill old people was sufficient for the teaching purposes envisaged by Lewis. With this objective fulfilled, Lewis and his colleagues offered Felix no further support for developing additional services for older people. 'In the Beginning' rightly attributes the founding of the Geriatric Unit to Lewis, but it would be inaccurate to attribute any further developments to him. The rest should be Felix's accolade.

Felix also modestly reported the outcome of treatment of his first inpatients in 1952 as 'relatively favourable'[9]. However, his results could perhaps better be described as 'spectacular'. This is for two reasons. First, at that time most mentally ill old people requiring mental hospital admission would have been admitted to long-stay wards without any assessment, let alone treatment, for their apparent all encompassing label of 'senility'. The expectation of any recovery was extremely low. Second, the only effective therapeutic tools were electroconvulsive therapy (ECT) and psychotherapeutic approaches; antidepressants, antipsychotics and mood stabilizers were yet to be introduced. Sadly, however, this outcome study was published in a journal with only a small circulation; had it been published in a more widely read journal it might have had a greater impact. For Felix himself, however, such results began to produce a sense of 'therapeutic optimism'[10].

Felix also referred to 'my little textbook (rightly out of print)'. This is a valid statement, but fails to reflect on the importance of the 'little textbook', *The Clinical Psychiatry of Late Life*[11]. It was the first book of its kind to emphasize an evidence-based approach to actively treating older mentally ill people. Highly readable, its philosophy remains at the foundations of good clinical practice today. It ends with the words:

> Sometimes, we may effect cures; frequently, we may be able to ameliorate the patient's condition; we shall always endeavour to give him and his family sympathetic support... *Quelquefois guérir; soulager souvent; consoler toujours.*

Why, one may ask, did so many of Felix's junior doctors go on to become leading psychogeriatricians? It was not chance, but likely to be related to his inspiring and enthusiastic teaching. Felix's personal career experience, moving from ambivalence to optimism to conveying his enthusiasm to others raises another contemporary lesson: we need to engage our medical students and junior staff and let them experience what can be done in order that they may carry with them the knowledge and ideals of the specialty, and possibly enter the field themselves. Felix's widespread influence lay largely in his clinical acumen, his meticulousness, his wisdom and his teaching skills[12].

Felix's autobiographical sketch ends with the words 'psychogeriatrics became a world movement, and Sir Aubrey Lewis would be pleased'. Lewis would undoubtedly have revelled in such lasting recognition, and hopefully the more unassuming Felix Post would also be pleased to have his legacy remembered.

REFERENCES

1. Hilton C. Felix Post (1913–2001) pioneer in the psychiatry of old age. *J Med Biog* 2007; **15**: 31–36.
2. Post F. Some problems arising from a study of mental patients over the age of 60 years. *J Ment Sci* 1944; **90**: 554–65.
3. Roth M. The natural history of mental disorders in old age. *J Ment Sci* 1955; **101**: 281–301
4. Lewis AJ. Ageing and senility: a major problem of psychiatry. *J Ment Sci* 1946; **92**: 150–70.
5. Mayer-Gross W. Electric convulsion treatment in patients over 60. *J Ment Sci* 1945; **91**: 101–103.
6. Stengel E. A study on the symptomatology and differential diagnosis of Alzheimer's disease and Pick's disease. *J Ment Sci* 1943; **89**: 1–20.
7. Post F. Interviewed by Professor Margot Jefferys for *Oral History of Geriatrics as a Medical Specialty* 1991: National Sound Archive F3264–F3265.
8. Lewis AJ. The education of psychiatrists. *Lancet* 1947; **ii**: 79–83.
9. Post F. Geriatric unit. *Bethlem Maudsley Hosp Gaz* 1955; **1**: 270–71
10. Post F. Tape recording in possession of Julian Post. Unknown interviewer c. 1996.
11. Post F. *The Clinical Psychiatry of Late Life*. London: Pergamon Press, 1965.
12. Arie T. Remembering Felix Post. *Psychiatr Bull* 2002; **26**: 199–200.

Part B

Normal and Abnormal Ageing

Changes in the Macrostructure and Microstructure of the Ageing Brain

Natalie M. Zahr[1], Adolf Pfefferbaum[2] and Edith V. Sullivan[1]

[1]Department of Psychiatry and Behavioral Sciences, Stanford University School of Medicine, CA, USA
[2]Neuroscience Program, SRI International, Menlo Park, CA, USA

MACROSTRUCTURAL CHANGES IN NORMAL AGEING DETECTED WITH CONVENTIONAL MRI

Conventional brain structural magnetic resonance imaging (MRI) produces images of protons, with contributions primarily from water and some from fat. Tissue contrast is possible because of the fundamental differences in water content in the primary tissues of the brain: white matter consists of about 70% water, grey matter 80% and cerebrospinal fluid (CSF) 99%. Tissue contrast also depends on differences in the degree to which water is bound and differences in the local environment. By judicious choice of imaging acquisition parameters that yield high conspicuity between grey and white matter (e.g. Figure 4.1a), segmentation of brain tissue is possible. Segmentation provides the basis for volumetric and morphological quantification of brain structure[1,2]. In addition to manual delineation of specific structures, methods for quantitative survey of the brain include voxel-based morphometry, as is widely used with spatial parametric mapping (SPM)[3,4], parcellation[2,5] and deformation morphometry[6-8]. The achievement of quantitative analysis was an essential step for rendering MR images useful in the quest for reliable identification of age-related macrostructural change.

In vivo structural MRI reveals age-related increases in the volume of CSF-filled spaces primarily at the expense of cortical grey matter (cross-sectional[9-14], longitudinal[15-19]).

Despite evidence for widespread thinning of the cerebral cortex as a feature of normal ageing[16,20,21], specific grey matter structures of the brain exhibit differential patterns of ageing. A preponderance of data indicates an excessive vulnerability of the frontal lobes, and in particular the prefrontal cortex, as documented cross-sectionally[22-23]. Other grey matter structures demonstrating cross-sectional decline in volume with age include, but are not limited to, segments of the temporal[20,25] and parietal cortices[20], thalamus[12,26], and cerebellum[11,21,27]. Longitudinal studies, although less frequently reported, support cross-sectional results by revealing disproportionate effects of age on frontal grey matter regions[15,17,28], entorhinal[28,29], temporal[17,28], parietal[17] cortices, and cerebellum[21]. Some[30], but not all[27,31] MRI studies of subcortical structures report little shrinkage of basal ganglia structures. Similarly, although some reports are equivocal[16,28,32], it is generally accepted that hippocampal volume shrinks little with age[20,33,34]. That hippocampal volume shrinkage is not a reliable marker of healthy ageing makes it a robust marker of age-related diseases affecting this structure, notably, Alzheimer's disease.

The relevance of structural MRI findings to age-related decline in function is underscored by correlations with selective behaviours. For example, smaller prefrontal volume predicts poorer performance on the Wisconsin Card Sorting test[35] and other tasks involving inhibitory control[36,37]. Deficits in the working memory that occur in normal ageing correlate with frontal system volume[38], whereas episodic memory deficits that occur in Alzheimer's disease correlate with medial temporal lobe/hippocampal volume[39-41]. Such findings support a double dissociation between normal ageing and Alzheimer's disease: frontal brain volume reductions and executive dysfunction mark normal ageing, whereas volume reductions in the medial temporal lobe/hippocampus and the corresponding memory deficits indicate Alzheimer's pathology[20,42,43].

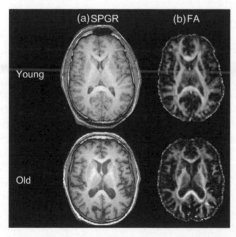

Figure 4.1 (a) Structural magnetic resonance imaging (spoiled gradient recalled, SPGR), and (b) diffusion tensor imaging (fractional anisotropy, FA) images from a young (32 year old) and an elderly (73 year old) male volunteer. SPGR images exemplify those that yield conspicuity between grey and white matter permitting brain tissue segmentation. Fractional anisotropy images facilitate fibre tracking

Principles and Practice of Geriatric Psychiatry, 3rd edn. Edited by Mohammed T. Abou-Saleh, Cornelius Katona and Anand Kumar

MICROSTRUCTURAL CHANGES IN NORMAL AGEING DETECTED WITH DTI

Whole-brain white matter volume shrinkage is small, estimated at no more than 2% per decade[27] (but see [31,44]). Yet postmortem investigations, in contrast to macrostructural approaches, have provided fruitful leads to age-related changes in white matter by revealing microstructural white matter compromise[45] including degradation of microtubules, myelin and axons[46-48]. *In vivo*, white matter microstructure is detectable with DTI, which has successfully revealed evidence of regional white matter disruption in normal ageing even in regions appearing normal on bulk volume imaging.

Quantification of DTI Data

Water molecules in the brain are in constant Brownian motion. Although movement of water protons affects conventional structural imaging to some degree, DTI allows quantification of this microscopic movement *within* each voxel, providing a depiction of local water molecular movement in terms of the preferred orientation of the motion. Along a white matter fibre, the path of a water molecule is constrained and this movement is called 'anisotropic', because diffusion along the long axis of a fibre (axial diffusion) is greater than diffusion across the fibre (radial diffusion[49]). Conversely, regions with few or no constraints imposed by physical boundaries such as CSF in the ventricles allow water movement to be random in every direction; this is therefore 'isotropic'. Disruption of white matter microstructure detectable with DTI can reflect compromise of cytoskeletal structure, myelin or axon density[50,51].

DTI quantification requires computation of a tensor, a mathematical description of a three-dimensional ellipsoid depicting the magnitude and orientation of diffusion in individual voxels. The tensor is associated three eigenvalues, with three corresponding orientational vectors (eigenvectors, $\lambda_1, \lambda_2, \lambda_3$), describing the diffusion ellipsoid by its major axes. The eigenvalue average, or trace, reflects the magnitude of diffusion, referred to as mean diffusivity or the apparent diffusion coefficient. The extent to which one eigenvalue, λ_1, dominates the other two, λ_2 and λ_3, determines the degree of anisotropy, that is, the degree of orientational preference within a voxel, typically measured as fractional anisotropy, ranging between 0 and 1 on a normalized scale (Figure 4.1b[52]). The largest eigenvalue, λ_1, is the longitudinal or axial diffusivity, λ_L, and reflects axonal integrity, whereas λ_2 and λ_3 quantify transverse or radial diffusivity, $\lambda_T = (\lambda_2 + \lambda_3)/2$, and reflect myelin integrity[49,53]. For both clinical and research studies, most DTI data sets are reduced to an anisotropy image and a diffusivity image. (For more information about DTI, see[54].)

Regional Quantification of DTI Data

A variety of approaches have been developed for quantification of DTI data; each has strengths and weaknesses that should be considered when critically evaluating published reports. Approaches for regional quantification of the DTI metrics of anisotropy and diffusivity include manually placing small, geometric samples (cubes, ovals, circles) onto selective white matter bundles, manually identifying anatomically based regions of interest (ROI, e.g. midsagittal corpus callosum), application of whole-brain analysis using SPM or other voxel-based morphometric methods, or tract-based spatial statistics (TBSS[55]). Geometric ROIs have the advantage of yielding rarefied samples of white matter with minimal effects from partial voluming (i.e. inclusion of grey matter, CSF or both) but the potential disadvantage of under-representing the condition of the full extent of the fibre system under study. Manual identification of the entire fibre tract has the advantage of providing an anatomically based sample of the target fibre with the possibility of examining subdivisions for regional variation; a disadvantage can be its susceptibility to partial voluming artefact because of the extended region sampled[56]. Voxel-based morphometry is attractive because it provides an automated, whole-brain survey of fractional anisotropy or diffusivity, but more often than not, has the under-appreciated cost of inadequate registration[6]. Such misregistration can disproportionately bias results and conclusions drawn from data, especially of the elderly[57], who have dilated CSF-filled spaces invading targeted white matter samples[58]. TBSS is another survey approach that does not actually track fibres but is used to quantify the whole-brain fractional anisotropy skeleton[59].

AGEING EFFECTS ON DTI METRICS

With advancing age and senescence, a consensus maintains a decline in fractional anisotropy in brain white matter[56,60-65] (but see [66,67]). Furthermore, consistent evidence supports an anterior–posterior gradient of fractional anisotropy decline with age[57,58,60,61,65,68-74] that has been confirmed in a monkey model of ageing[75]. TBSS likewise substantiates an anterior–posterior gradient, namely by identifying lower fractional anisotropy values in the frontal, parietal and temporal lobes, corpus callosum (particularly the genu and body) and the internal capsule[76].

In complement to white matter fractional anisotropy decline in ageing, diffusivity in white matter increases[58,65,67,77-80]. As with fractional anisotropy, profile analysis reveals that the primary locus of the age effect is in anterior white matter[80]. This pattern of age-related decline of fractional anisotropy and increase in diffusivity mirrors postmortem observations with predominant age-related findings in anterior white matter systems[45,81].

QUANTITATIVE FIBRE TRACKING IN AGEING

The degree to which the diffusion orientation of a voxel is similar to its neighbours, or in other words, coherence of diffusivity measures between voxels[82,83], serves the conceptual basis for quantitative fibre tracking[55,84-87]. Connectivity and coherence between different brain regions on vector and fibre tracking maps is readily apparent on visual inspection[88]. Methods for quantitative analysis of structural connectivity of white matter include fibre-tract trajectories[89-91] and maps of the degree of 'alignment' among neighbouring vectors, on a voxel-to-voxel basis, resulting in a measure of intervoxel coherence[82]. Advantages of quantitative fibre tracking over focal ROI analysis include the ability to measure the entire extent of a fibre tract and to characterize its integrity along its full extent.

Quantitative fibre tracking confirms focal DTI measures of an anterior-to-posterior pattern of disruption of white matter integrity[92,93] as, for example, the elderly have lower fractional anisotropy and higher diffusivity than the young in anterior but not posterior sectors of the fibres coursing through the corpus callosum (Figure 4.2)[94-96]. Recent work also supports a superior–inferior gradient of ageing effects on white matter (Figure 4.3)[97-99], whereas pontocerebellar and cerebellar hemisphere white matter tracts are relatively preserved[97].

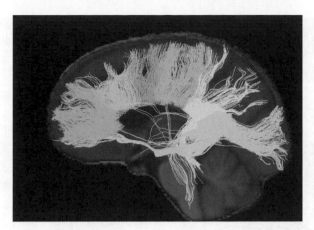

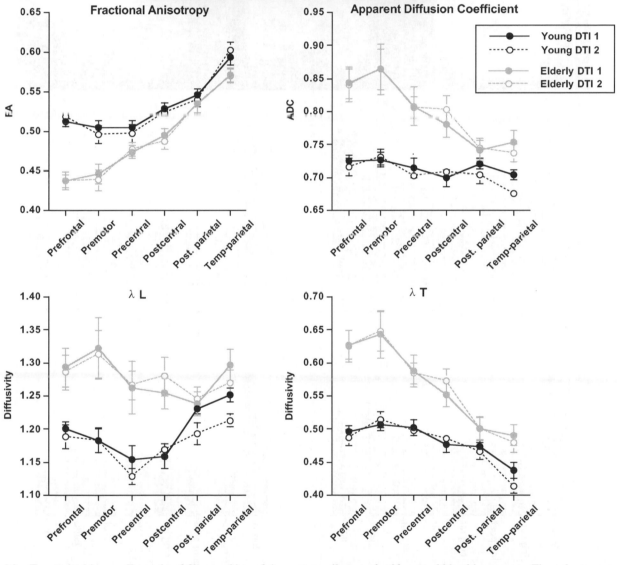

Figure 4.2   Top sagittal image: Example of fibre tracking of the corpus callosum of a 23-year-old healthy woman. The colours represent six different fibre bundles based on previously described divisions[148] identified with fibre tracking based on diffusion tensor imaging (DTI)-derived fractional anisotropy. From anterior (far left) to posterior (far right), the bundles are deemed prefrontal, premotor, precentral, postcentral, posterior parietal, and temporal-occipital. Bottom data figures: Mean $\pm$ SE of the six callosal sectors for the young and elderly groups at MRI sessions two years apart of the four principal metrics of DTI: fractional anisotropy, apparent diffusion coefficient (ADC), λ_1 and λ_t. The elderly group had lower fractional anisotropy and higher diffusivity than the young group at both scanning sessions, and the group differences were greatest in anterior sectors. Reproduced with permission from Sullivan *et al.*[105]

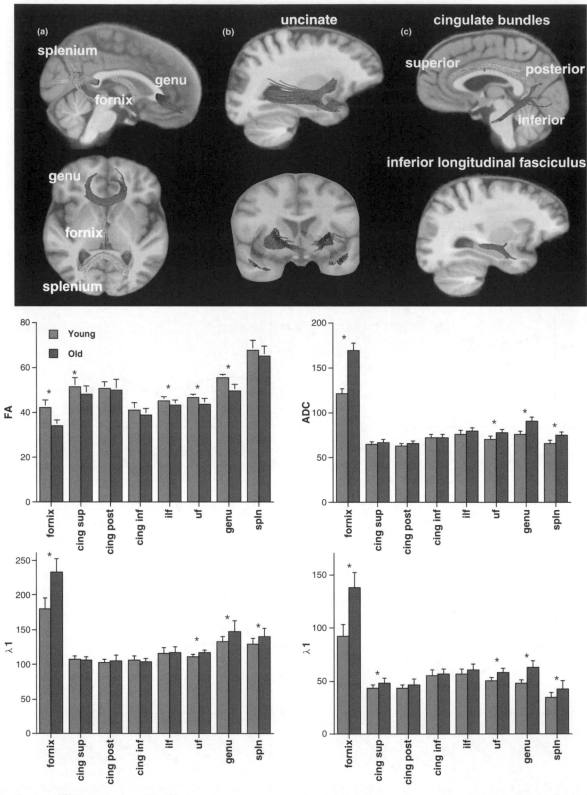

Figure 4.3 Images: Fibre tracts were identified on the group-average fractional anisotropy image in common space. (a) Sagittal (top) and axial (bottom) views of the genu, splenium and fornix. (b) Sagittal (top) and coronal (bottom) views of the uncinate fasciculus. (c) Sagittal (top) view of the cingulum (superior, posterior, inferior) and inferior longitudinal fasciculus (bottom). Bar graphs: Mean $\pm$ SD for fractional anisotropy, apparent diffusion coefficient (ADC), λ_1 and λ_t for young (grey) and elderly (white) subjects for each fibre bundle. *$P \leq 0.05\,t$-test. Modified from Zahr *et al*.[99]

LONGITUDINAL STUDIES OF AGEING BRAIN MICROSTRUCTURE

Longitudinal studies of normal, healthy men and women across the adult age range document normative age-related, DTI-detectable changes in brain white matter that are requisite for interpreting DTI data from individuals with neuropsychiatric disorders and other conditions affecting the brain. However, longitudinal studies have their own problems with respect to measurement reliability within and across research centres, selective attrition, and hardware and software system modifications and drift[100]. For example, a study of five normal adults imaged five times each resulted in 5% across-subject variation and a mean variation of 2.3 ± 1.2 SD% in diffusivity[78]. Another study measured the reliability of global and regional fractional anisotropy and diffusivity measurements in ten healthy young adults, imaged three times on two different 1.5-T scanners made by the same manufacturer[101]. When reliability was measured on a voxel-by-voxel basis or on a slice-by-slice basis, fractional anisotropy and diffusivity values were equivalently and significantly higher within than across scanners. In addition to reliability of a common measurement approach, substantial differences can arise when different analysis schemes are applied to the same data set[102].

Longitudinal DTI studies of healthy ageing are only now emerging. The few studies reporting longitudinal results in normal ageing do so secondarily, in that the target study groups were individuals with neurological conditions, including head injury[103] and amyotrophic lateral sclerosis[104]; in neither control group were age-related declines in fractional anisotropy or increases in diffusivity detected. One small prospective study followed eight young and eight elderly individuals over two years[105] but found no evidence of change in any of the six sectors of the corpus callosum examined; instead, the measurement was highly reliable across the interval (see Figure 4.2).

BRAIN WHITE MATTER STRUCTURE–FUNCTION RELATIONSHIPS

The functional ramifications of the DTI metrics have been regularly verified with observations of correlations between regionally specific low fractional anisotropy or high diffusivity and poor cognitive[61,62,71–73,106,107] or motor[68] test performance in humans and also a monkey model of ageing[75]. Lower whole-brain fractional anisotropy and higher mean diffusivity correlated with working memory performance[106,108]. The alternating finger-tapping task, a test of interhemispheric information transfer, revealed a relationship between splenium and parietal pericallosal white matter fractional anisotropy and finger-tapping output that was selective to the alternating condition, requiring interhemispheric motor coordination, and not unimanual conditions, free of transcallosal information exchange[68]. Task switching[61,109] and lower scores on tests of executive functions[63,109] correlated with low fractional anisotropy and greater diffusivity in anterior brain regions; lower verbal fluency scores correlated with lower fractional anisotropy in central samples of white matter[61].

Functional correlates of regional fibre tracking are also emerging. Correlations between fibre tracking quantification and the Stroop color-word reading were noted[94]. A large, multifactorial battery of neuropsychological tests reduced to three factor scores revealed that problem solving and working memory factor scores correlated with indices of callosal genu and fornix integrity, whereas the motor factor score correlated with a widespread set of fibre systems, likely reflecting the multiple brain loci required to execute the tasks, which included speed, dexterity and choice reaction time (Figure 4.4)[99].

LIMITATIONS OF DTI

DTI studies indicate widely varying fractional anisotropy across brain regions, with lower anisotropy and higher in diffusivity in older than younger healthy adults, that is prominent in the anterior supratentorial white matter but minimal to none in posterior cortical and corticospinal tracts. A caveat to this generalization is that selective deletion of uniformly orientated white matter fibres from a tissue sample of crossing fibres, as can occur with Wallerian degeneration, can cause abnormally high anisotropy[110]. Therefore, interpretation of fractional anisotropy results requires guidance by knowledge of the underlying regional architecture, especially white matter[111] and supplemented with non-human primate studies, affording the opportunity for *in vivo* examination and postmortem verification of imaging results (cf.[88]).

Furthermore, the diameters of axons, for example in the corpus callosum ranging from 0.4 to 5 μm, with most less than 1 μm, means that a cross-section of the genu of the human corpus callosum contains approximately 400 000 fibres per mm^2 and a single DTI voxel using relatively high resolution ($2 \times 2 \times 2$ mm^3) for current standards could contain 1.6 million fibres in a cross-section[112]. Consequently, caution must be used when interpreting the anatomical meaning of observations made with radiological measures, which are coarse on the size scale of the underlying fibres.

Finally, the diffusion-weighted signal can also be influenced by iron accumulation with age, and the resulting effect is different among deep grey matter structures and white matter and needs to be considered, especially when using DTI to characterize structures known to accumulate iron (*in vivo*[113], postmortem[114]) or in conditions, such as stroke, that produce high ferritin deposition (cf.[115]).

OTHER STRUCTURAL MAGNETIC RESONANCE OBSERVATIONS IN AGEING

Convergent postmortem[114] and *in vivo* data indicate that deep grey matter brain structures accumulate ferritin at different rates throughout adult ageing[113,116,117]. Abnormal iron accumulation has been reported in neurological conditions involving the basal ganglia, including Parkinson's disease, multiple sclerosis and Huntington's disease (reviewed in: [113,118–122]), and suggests that iron burden contributes to age- and disease-related functional decline[123,124].

Iron can be measured *in vivo* with MR imaging because of iron's effect on signal intensity, causing signal darkening on T2* and T2-weighted images that is greater with increasing magnetic field strength. By estimating the transverse relaxivity increase across field strengths, the MR field-dependent relaxivity increase (FDRI) can be calculated[113,125,126]. For example, acquisition of spin-echo data with a constant TR and multiple echoes at 1.5-T and 3.0-T allows the computation of R2 (the inverse of T2) at each field strength with the difference between R2s divided by the field strength difference producing FDRI in units of s^{-1}/T (Figure 4.5a).

In addition to affecting relaxivity, local iron influences MR gradient-echo image phase, which forms the basis for another method for iron quantification, susceptibility-weighted imaging (SWI) (Figure 4.5b)[127]. The paramagnetic properties of tissue ferritin cause local field inhomogeneity that can also be quantified by examining the phase of the computed spins. The ferromagnetic

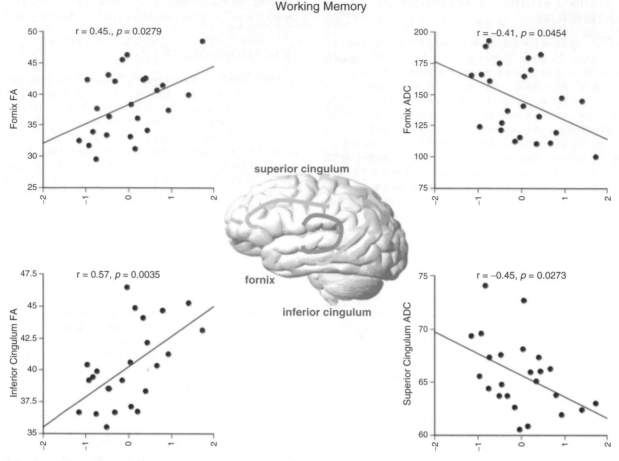

Figure 4.4 Correlations (Spearman rank and Bonferroni corrected) between a working memory domain isolated using principal component analysis and diffusion tensor imaging (DTI) metrics (fractional anisotropy and apparent diffusion coefficient) by tract. Modified from Zahr et al.[99]

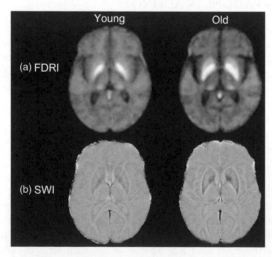

Figure 4.5 Group averages for 11 younger (mean= 24 years old, 5 men, 6 women) and 12 older (mean= 74 years old, 6 men, 6 women) participants for (a) field-dependent relaxivity increase (FDRI) and (b) susceptibility-weighted imaging (SWI) techniques for measuring brain iron. Greater iron concentration yields higher (brighter) FDRI signal but lower (darker) SWI signal. Modified from Pfefferbaum et al.[126]

property of iron causes protons to accrue more negative phase in iron-rich tissue. At optimal acquisition parameters, the more iron in a voxel, the lower will be the measured phase[127].

FDRI and SWI document increasing iron deposition with age in deep brain structures such as the caudate and putamen, globus pallidus, red nucleus, substantia nigra and thalamus[113,119,126,128]. In a recent comparison study between FDRI and SWI, both methods detected high globus pallidus iron concentration independent of age and significantly greater iron in putamen with advancing age[126].

Further senescent changes in brain tissue composition and emblematic of tissue degradation are the increases in presence and volume of white matter hyperintensities (WMHIs) (e.g. [129–131]), typically visible in T2-weighted and fluid-attenuated inversion recovery (FLAIR, Figure 4.6) images. WMHIs are associated, for example, with hypertension, stroke, traumatic brain injury and respiratory dysfunction[132–134]. The current controversy regarding WMHIs aetiology is whether a common pathophysiological mechanism underlies the formation of periventricular and deep white matter lesions[134–136]. It is thought that demyelination or ependymal lining damage commonly occurs periventricularly, whereas rarefication of myelin or cavitations from fibre loss, concomitant of ischaemic damage or arteriosclerosis, commonly occurs in deep white matter[130]. Depending on the location of WMHIs, different types of functional decline can ensue[136,137].

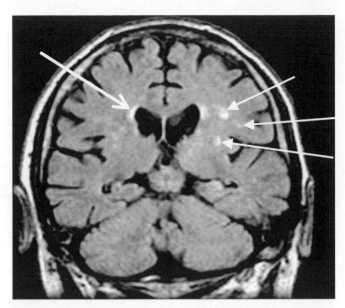

Figure 4.6 Coronal image from a healthy elderly adult volunteer (72 years old) displaying white matter hyperintensities in deep (closed arrows) and periventricular (open arrow) regions of the brain

CONCLUSION

The twentieth century has seen a dramatic increase in life expectancy in developed countries. Estimates from the Health and Retirement Study, sponsored by the US National Institute on Ageing, indicate that ~10% of individuals aged 70 and older in the United States suffer moderate to severe cognitive impairment that rises to ~20% by age 85 years[138]. Therefore, expanding longevity coupled with declining CNS function will dictate the need for continued development of clinically practical and sensitive imaging modalities to assist in the differential diagnosis of age-related diseases.

Advances in neuroradiology have contributed to the neuroscience of normal ageing and to characterizing morphological and tissue changes that occur in the brain with age. Among these is the identification of previously underappreciated occurrence of decline in white matter integrity. The *in vivo* interrogation of the brain has also highlighted the dramatic, involutional brain tissue shrinkage and replacement with CSF, less apparent at the autopsy table as the brain collapses in on itself when removed from the skull[139].

Finally, a principal aim of this paper was to emphasize neuroradiological concomitants of apparent normal ageing, thereby providing an essential context in which to interpret radiological evidence for neurodegenerative diseases and other conditions of brain insult. Careful history taking and clinical description of presumed healthy men and women have proved essential in identifying factors that underlie departure from normality[28] or are categorized as 'normal variants'[140]. Factors increasing in prevalence with age and affecting brain tissue and potentially function include hypertension[141], cerebrovascular disease[135,142], and iron deposition[113]. DTI can be more sensitive than conventional MRI for detection of subtle and perhaps prodromal changes in tissue that occur with age (cf. [126,143,144]), including those characteristic of stroke[145–147]. Use and quantification of tractography may also enable monitoring white matter fibre regrowth[148] following trauma, disease or recovery from alcohol and drug dependence and to test models of white matter recovery in normal ageing, trauma and disease.

ACKNOWLEDGEMENTS

This work was supported by NIH grants AG017919, AA017168, and AA005965.

REFERENCES

1. Lim KO, Pfefferbaum A. Segmentation of MR brain images into cerebrospinal fluid spaces, white and gray matter. *J Comput Assist Tomogr* 1989; **13**: 588–93.
2. Makris N, Meyer JW, Bates JF, Yeterian EH, Kennedy DN, Caviness VS. MRI-based topographic parcellation of human cerebral white matter and nuclei. II. Rationale and applications with systematics of cerebral connectivity. *Neuroimage* 1999; **9**: 18–45.
3. Frackowiak RSJ, Zeki S, Poline JB, Friston KJ. A critique of a new analysis proposed for functional neuroimaging. *Eur J Neurosci* 1996; **8**: 2229–31.
4. Ashburner J, Friston K. Voxel-based morphometry – The methods. *Neuroimage* 2000; **11**: 805–21.
5. Tzourio-Mazoyer N, Landeau B, Papathanassiou D *et al.* Automated anatomical labeling of activations in SPM using a macroscopic anatomical parcellation of the MNI MRI single-subject brain. *Neuroimage* 2002; **15**: 273–89.
6. Rohlfing T, Sullivan EV, Pfefferbaum A. Deformation-based brain morphometry to track the course of alcoholism: Differences between intra-subject and inter-subject analysis. *Psychiatry Res NeuroImaging* 2006; **146**: 157–70.
7. Studholme C, Cardenas V, Maudsley A, Weiner M. An intensity consistent filtering approach to the analysis of deformation tensor derived maps of brain shape. *Neuroimage* 2003; **19**: 1638–49.
8. Lepore N, Brun C, Pennec X *et al.* Mean template for tensor-based morphometry using deformation tensors. *Med Image Comput Comput Assist Interv Int Conf Med Image Comput Comput Assist Interv* 2007; **10**: 826–33.
9. Pfefferbaum A, Mathalon DH, Sullivan EV, Rawles JM, Zipursky RB, Lim KO. A quantitative magnetic resonance imaging study of changes in brain morphology from infancy to late adulthood. *Arch Neurol* 1994; **51**: 874–87.
10. Raz N, Gunning FM, Head D *et al.* Selective ageing of the human cerebral cortex observed *in vivo*: Differential vulnerability of the prefrontal gray matter. *Cereb Cortex* 1997; **7**: 268–82.
11. Sullivan EV, Deshmukh A, Desmond JE, Lim KO, Pfefferbaum A. Cerebellar volume decline in normal ageing, alcoholism, and Korsakoff's syndrome: relation to ataxia. *Neuropsychology* 2000; **14**: 341–52.
12. Sullivan EV, Rosenbloom MJ, Serventi KL, Pfefferbaum A. Effects of age and sex on volumes of the thalamus, pons, and cortex. *Neurobiol Aging* 2004; **25**: 185–92.
13. Courchesne E, Chisum HJ, Townsend J *et al.* Normal brain development and ageing: quantitative analysis at *in vivo* MR imaging in healthy volunteers. *Radiology* 2000; **216**: 672–82.
14. Taki Y, Kinomura S, Sato K *et al.* Both global gray matter volume and regional gray matter volume negatively correlate with lifetime alcohol intake in non-alcohol-dependent Japanese men: a volumetric analysis and a voxel-based morphometry. *Alcohol Clin Exp Res* 2006; **30**: 1045–50.

15. Pfefferbaum A, Sullivan EV, Rosenbloom MJ, Mathalon DH, Lim KO. A controlled study of cortical gray matter and ventricular changes in alcoholic men over a five year interval. *Arch Gen Psychiatry* 1998; **55**: 905–12.
16. Liu RS, Lemieux L, Bell GS *et al*. A longitudinal study of brain morphometrics using quantitative magnetic resonance imaging and difference image analysis. *Neuroimage* 2003; **20**: 22–33.
17. Resnick SM, Pham DL, Kraut MA, Zonderman AB, Davatzikos C. Longitudinal magnetic resonance imaging studies of older adults: a shrinking brain. *J Neurosci* 2003; **23**: 3295–301.
18. Raz N, Rodrigue KM, Kennedy KM, Acker JD. Vascular health and longitudinal changes in brain and cognition in middle-aged and older adults. *Neuropsychology* 2007; **21**: 149–57.
19. Fotenos AF, Mintun MA, Snyder AZ, Morris JC, Buckner RL. Brain volume decline in ageing: evidence for a relation between socioeconomic status, preclinical Alzheimer disease, and reserve. *Arch Neurol* 2008; **65**: 113–20.
20. Fjell AM, Westlye LT, Amlien I *et al*. High consistency of regional cortical thinning in aging across multiple samples. *Cereb Cortex* 2009; **19**: 2001–12.
21. Tang Y, Whitman GT, Lopez I, Baloh RW. Brain volume changes on longitudinal magnetic resonance imaging in normal older people. *J Neuroimaging* 2001; **11**: 393–400.
22. Salat DH, Buckner RL, Snyder AZ *et al*. Thinning of the cerebral cortex in ageing. *Cereb Cortex* 2004; **14**: 721–30.
23. Taki Y, Goto R, Evans A *et al*. Voxel-based morphometry of human brain with age and cerebrovascular risk factors. *Neurobiol Aging* 2004; **25**: 455–63.
24. Brickman AM, Habeck C, Zarahn E, Flynn J, Stern Y. Structural MRI covariance patterns associated with normal ageing and neuropsychological functioning. *Neurobiol Aging* 2007; **28**: 284–95.
25. Raz N, Gunning-Dixon F, Head D, Rodrigue K, Williamson A, Acker J. Aging, sexual dimorphism, and hemispheric asymmetry of the cerebral cortex: replicability of regional differences in volume. *Neurobiol Aging* 2004; **25**: 377–96.
26. Van Der Werf YD, Tisserand DJ, Visser PJ *et al*. Thalamic volume predicts performance on tests of cognitive speed and decreases in healthy ageing. A magnetic resonance imaging-based volumetric analysis. *Brain Res Cogn Brain Res* 2001; **11**: 377–85.
27. Walhovd KB, Fjell AM, Reinvang I *et al*. Effects of age on volumes of cortex, white matter and subcortical structures. *Neurobiol Aging* 2005; **26**: 1261–70; discussion 75–78.
28. Raz N, Lindenberger U, Rodrigue KM *et al*. Regional brain changes in ageing healthy adults: General trends, individual differences, and modifiers. *Cereb Cortex* 2005; **15**: 1676–89.
29. Rodrigue KM, Raz N. Shrinkage of the entorhinal cortex over five years predicts memory performance in healthy adults. *J Neurosci* 2004; **24**: 956–63.
30. Sullivan EV, Deshmukh A, de Rosa E, Rosenbloom MJ, Pfefferbaum A. Striatal and forebrain nuclei volumes: Contribution to motor function and working memory deficits in alcoholism. *Biol Psychiatry* 2005; **57**: 768–76.
31. Jernigan TL, Archibald SL, Fennema-Notestine C *et al*. Effects of age on tissues and regions of the cerebrum and cerebellum. *Neurobiol Aging* 2001; **22**: 581–94.
32. Scahill RI, Frost C, Jenkins R, Whitwell JL, Rossor MN, Fox NC. A longitudinal study of brain volume changes in normal ageing using serial registered magnetic resonance imaging. *Arch Neurol* 2003; **60**: 989–94.
33. Sullivan EV, Pfefferbaum A, Swan GE, Carmelli D. Heritability of hippocampal size in elderly twin men: Equivalent influence from genes and environment. *Hippocampus* 2001; **11**: 754–62.
34. Sullivan EV, Marsh L, Pfefferbaum A. Preservation of hippocampal volume through adulthood in healthy men and women. *Neurobiol Aging* 2005; **26**: 1093–98.
35. Gunning-Dixon FM, Raz N. Neuroanatomical correlates of selected executive functions in middle-aged and older adults: a prospective MRI study. *Neuropsychologia* 2003; **41**: 1929–41.
36. Head D, Rodrigue KM, Kennedy KM, Raz N. Neuroanatomical and cognitive mediators of age-related differences in episodic memory. *Neuropsychology* 2008; **22**: 491–507.
37. Elderkin-Thompson V, Ballmaier M, Hellemann G, Pham D, Kumar A. Executive function and MRI prefrontal volumes among healthy older adults. *Neuropsychology* 2008; **22**: 626–37.
38. Sullivan EV, Marsh L, Mathalon DH, Lim KO, Pfefferbaum A. Age-related decline in MRI volumes of temporal lobe gray matter but not hippocampus. *Neurobiol Aging* 1995; **16**: 591–606.
39. Raz N, Gunning-Dixon FM, Head D, Dupuis JH, Acker JD. Neuroanatomical correlates of cognitive ageing: evidence from structural magnetic resonance imaging. *Neuropsychology* 1998; **12**: 95–114.
40. Head D, Snyder AZ, Girton LE, Morris JC, Buckner RL. Frontal-hippocampal double dissociation between normal ageing and Alzheimer's disease. *Cereb Cortex* 2005; **15**: 732–39.
41. Cahn DA, Sullivan EV, Shear PK *et al*. Structural MRI correlates of recognition memory in Alzheimer's disease. *J Int Neuropsychol Soc* 1998; **4**: 106–14.
42. Jack CR, Jr., Shiung MM, Weigand SD *et al*. Brain atrophy rates predict subsequent clinical conversion in normal elderly and amnestic MCI. *Neurology* 2005; **65**: 1227–31.
43. Hedden T, Gabrieli JD. Healthy and pathological processes in adult development: new evidence from neuroimaging of the ageing brain. *Curr Opin Neurol* 2005; **18**: 740–47.
44. Miller AKH, Alston RL, Corsellis JAN. Variations with age in the volumes of grey and white matter in the cerebral hemispheres of man: measurements with an image analyzer. *Neuropathol Appl Neurobiol* 1980; **6**: 119–32.
45. Kemper TL. Neuroanatomical and neuropathological changes during ageing and dementia. In Albert ML, Knoefel JE (eds), *Clinical Neurology of Aging*, 2nd edn. New York: Oxford University Press, 1994, 3–67.
46. Meier-Ruge W, Ulrich J, Bruhlmann M, Meier E. Age-related white matter atrophy in the human brain. *Ann N Y Acad Sci* 1992; **673**: 260–69.
47. Aboitiz F, Rodriguez E, Olivares R, Zaidel E. Age-related changes in fibre composition of the human corpus callosum: sex differences. *Neuroreport* 1996; **7**: 1761–64.
48. Marner L, Nyengaard JR, Tang Y, Pakkenberg B. Marked loss of myelinated nerve fibers in the human brain with age. *J Comp Neurol*. 2003; **462**: 144–52.
49. Song SK, Sun SW, Ramsbottom MJ, Chang C, Russell J, Cross AH. Dysmyelination revealed through MRI as increased radial (but unchanged axial) diffusion of water. *Neuroimage* 2002; **17**: 1429–36.
50. Spielman D, Butts K, de Crespigny A, Moseley M. Diffusion-weighted imaging of clinical stroke. *Int J Neuroradiol* 1996; **1**: 44–55.

51. Basser PJ, Pierpaoli C. Microstructural and physiological features of tissues elucidated by quantitative diffusion tensor MRI. *J Magn Reson B* 1996; **111**: 209–19.

52. Pierpaoli C, Basser PJ. Towards a quantitative assessment of diffusion anisotropy. *Magn Reson Med* 1996; **36**: 893–906.

53. Sun SW, Liang HF, Le TQ, Armstrong RC, Cross AH, Song SK. Differential sensitivity of *in vivo* and ex vivo diffusion tensor imaging to evolving optic nerve injury in mice with retinal ischemia. *NeuroImage* 2006; **32**: 1195–204.

54. Jones DK. Fundamentals of diffusion MR imaging. In Gillard J, Waldman AD, Barker P (eds), *Clinical MR Neuroimaging*. Cambridge: Cambridge University Press, 2005.

55. Smith SM, Johansen-Berg H, Jenkinson M *et al.* Acquisition and voxelwise analysis of multi-subject diffusion data with tract-based spatial statistics. *Nat Protoc* 2007; **2**: 499–503.

56. Abe O, Aoki S, Hayashi N *et al.* Normal ageing in the central nervous system: quantitative MR diffusion-tensor analysis. *Neurobiol Aging* 2002; **23**: 433–41.

57. Bhagat YA, Beaulieu C. Diffusion anisotropy in subcortical white matter and cortical gray matter: changes with ageing and the role of CSF-suppression. *J Magn Reson Imaging* 2004; **20**: 216–27.

58. Pfefferbaum A, Sullivan EV. Increased brain white matter diffusivity in normal adult ageing: Relationship to anisotropy and partial voluming. *Magn Reson Med* 2003; **49**: 953–61.

59. Yeh PH, SImson K, Durazzo TC, Gazdzinski S, Meyerhoff D. Tract-based spatial statistics (TBSS) of diffusion tensor imaging data in alcohol dependence: Abnormalities of the motivational neurocircuitry. *Psychiatry Res* 2009; **173**: 22–30.

60. Pfefferbaum A, Sullivan EV, Hedehus M, Lim KO, Adalsteinsson E, Moseley M. Age-related decline in brain white matter anisotropy measured with spatially corrected echo-planar diffusion tensor imaging. *Magn Reson Med* 2000; **44**: 259–68.

61. O'Sullivan M, Jones D, Summers P, Morris R, Williams S, Markus H. Evidence for cortical 'disconnection" as a mechanism of age-related cognitive decline. *Neurology* 2001; **57**: 632–38.

62. Stebbins G, Carrillo MD, Medina D *et al.* Frontal white matter integrity in ageing and its relation to reasoning performance: a diffusion tensor imaging study (abs 456.3). *Soc Neurosci Abstr* 2001; **27**: 1204–.

63. Madden DJ, Whiting WL, Huettel SA, White LE, MacFall JR, Provenzale JM. Diffusion tensor imaging of adult age differences in cerebral white matter: relation to response time. *Neuroimage* 2004; **21**: 1174–81.

64. Salat DH, Tuch DS, Greve DN *et al.* Age-related alterations in white matter microstructure measured by diffusion tensor imaging. *Neurobiol Aging* 2005; **26**: 1215–27.

65. Head D, Buckner RL, Shimony JS *et al.* Differential vulnerability of anterior white matter in nondemented ageing with minimal acceleration in dementia of the Alzheimer type: Evidence from diffusion tensor imaging. *Cereb Cortex* 2004; **14**: 410–23.

66. Chepuri NB, Yen YF, Burdette JH, Li H, Moody DM, Maldjian JA. Diffusion anisotropy in the corpus callosum. *Am J Neuroradiol* 2002; **23**: 803–808.

67. Helenius J, Soinne L, Perkio J *et al.* Diffusion-weighted MR imaging in normal human brains in various age groups. *Am J Neuroradiol* 2002; **23**: 194–99.

68. Sullivan EV, Adalsteinsson E, Hedehus M *et al.* Equivalent disruption of regional white matter microstructure in ageing healthy men and women. *Neuroreport*. 2001; **12**: 99–104.

69. Salat DH, Tuch DS, Hevelone ND *et al.* Age-related changes in prefrontal white matter measured by diffusion tensor imaging. *Ann N Y Acad Sci* 2005; **1064**: 37–49.

70. Takahashi T, Murata T, Omori M *et al.* Quantitative evaluation of age-related white matter microstructural changes on MRI by multifractal analysis. *J Neurol Sci* 2004; **225**: 33–37.

71. Grieve SM, Williams LM, Paul RH, Clark CR, Gordon E. Cognitive ageing, executive function, and fractional anisotropy: a diffusion tensor MR imaging study. *AJNR Am J Neuroradiol* 2007; **28**: 226–35.

72. Bucur B, Madden DJ, Spaniol J *et al.* Age-related slowing of memory retrieval: Contributions of perceptual speed and cerebral white matter integrity. *Neurobiol Aging* 2008; **29**: 1070–79.

73. Madden DJ, Spaniol J, Whiting WL *et al.* Adult age differences in the functional neuroanatomy of visual attention: a combined fMRI and DTI study. *Neurobiol Aging* 2007; **28**: 459–76.

74. Yoon B, Shim YS, Lee KS, Shon YM, Yang DW. Region-specific changes of cerebral white matter during normal ageing: a diffusion tensor analysis. *Arch Gerontol Geriatr* 2008; **47**: 129–38.

75. Makris N, Papadimitrioua GM, van der Kouwe A *et al.* Frontal connections and cognitive changes in normal ageing rhesus monkeys: A DTI study. *Neurobiol Aging* 2007; **28**: 1556–67.

76. Damoiseaux JS, Smith SM, Witter MP *et al.* White matter tract integrity in ageing and Alzheimer's disease. *Hum Brain Mapp* 2009; **30**: 1051–59.

77. Chen ZG, Li TQ, Hindmarsh T. Diffusion tensor trace mapping in normal adult brain using single-shot EPI technique. A methodological study of the ageing brain. *Acta Radiol* 2001; **42**: 447–58.

78. Naganawa S, Sato K, Katagiri T, Mimura T, Ishigaki T. Regional ADC values of the normal brain: differences due to age, gender, and laterality. *Eur Radiol* 2003; **13**: 6–11.

79. Engelter ST, Provenzale JM, Petrella JR, DeLong DM, MacFall JR. The effect of ageing on the apparent diffusion coefficient of normal-appearing white matter. *Am J Roentgenol* 2000; **175**: 425–30.

80. Pfefferbaum A, Adalsteinsson E, Sullivan EV. Frontal circuitry degradation marks healthy adult ageing: Evidence from diffusion tensor imaging. *Neuroimage* 2005; **26**: 891–99.

81. Peters A, Sethares C. Aging and the myelinated fibers in prefrontal cortex and corpus callosum of the monkey. *J Comp Neurol* 2002; **442**: 277–91.

82. Pfefferbaum A, Sullivan EV, Hedehus M, Adalsteinsson E, Lim KO, Moseley M. *In Vivo* detection and functional correlates of white matter microstructural disruption in chronic alcoholism. *Alcohol Clin Exp Res* 2000; **24**: 1214–21.

83. Jones D, Simmons A, Williams S, Horsfield M. Non-invasive assessment of axonal fiber connectivity in the human brain via diffusion tensor MRI. *Magn Reson Med* 1999; **42**: 37–41.

84. Gerig G, Corouge I, Vachet C, Krishnan KR, MacFall JR. Quantitative analysis of diffusion properties of white matter fiber tracts: a validation study. Paper presented at the 13th Proceedings of the International Society for Magnetic Resonance in Medicine, 2005, Miami, FL.

85. Fillard P, Gerig G. Analysis tool for diffusion tensor MRI. In *Proceedings of Medical Image Computing and Computer-assisted Intervention, Lecture Notes in Computer Science*. Saint-Malo, France: Springer, 2003.

86. Le Bihan D. The 'wet mind': water and functional neuroimaging. *Phys Med Biol* 2007; **52**: R57–90.

87. Mori S, Wakana S, Nagae-Poetscher LM, Van Zijl PMC. *An Atlas of Human White Matter*. Amsterdam: Elsevier, 2005.

88. Schmahmann JD, Pandya DN, Wang R *et al*. Association fibre pathways of the brain: parallel observations from diffusion spectrum imaging and autoradiography. *Brain* 2007; **130**: 630–53.

89. Masutani Y, Aoki S, Abe O, Hayashi N, Otomo K. MR diffusion tensor imaging: recent advance and new techniques for diffusion tensor visualization. *Eur J Radiol* 2003; **46**: 53–66.

90. Basser PJ, Pierpaoli C. A simplified method to measure the diffusion tensor from seven MR images. *Magn Reson Med* 1998; **39**: 928–34.

91. Mori S, van Zijl PC. Fiber tracking: principles and strategies – a technical review. *NMR Biomed* 2002; **15**: 468–80.

92. Davis SW, Dennis NA, Buchler NG, White LE, Madden DJ, Cabeza R. Assessing the effects of age on long white matter tracts using diffusion tensor tractography. *NeuroImage* 2009; **46**: 530–41.

93. Falangola MF, Jensen JH, Babb JS *et al*. Age-related non-Gaussian diffusion patterns in the prefrontal brain. *J Magn Reson Imaging* 2008; **28**: 1345–50.

94. Sullivan EV, Adalsteinsson E, Pfefferbaum A. Selective age-related degradation of anterior callosal fiber bundles quantified *in vivo* with fiber tracking. *Cereb Cortex* 2006; **16**: 1030–29.

95. Pfefferbaum A, Rosenbloom MJ, Adalsteinsson E, Sullivan EV. Diffusion tensor imaging with quantitative fibre tracking in HIV infection and alcoholism comorbidity: Synergistic white matter damage. *Brain* 2007; **130**: 48–64.

96. Hasan KM, Ewing-Cobbs L, Kramer LA, Fletcher JM, Narayana PA. Diffusion tensor quantification of the macrostructure and microstructure of human midsagittal corpus callosum across the lifespan. *NMR Biomed* 2008; **21**: 1094–101.

97. Sullivan EV, Rohlfing T, Pfefferbaum A. Quantitative fiber tracking of lateral and interhemispheric white matter systems in normal ageing: Relations to timed performance. *Neurobiol Aging* 2010; **31**: 464–81.

98. Stadlbauer A, Salomonowitz E, Strunk G, Hammen T, Ganslandt O. Age-related degradation in the central nervous system: assessment with diffusion-tensor imaging and quantitative fiber tracking. *Radiology* 2008; **247**: 179–88.

99. Zahr NM, Rohlfing T, Pfefferbaum A, Sullivan EV. Problem solving, working memory, and motor correlates of association and commissural fiber bundles in normal ageing: a quantitative fiber tracking study. *NeuroImage* 2009; **44**: 1050–62.

100. Birren JE, Schaie KW. *Handbook of the Psychology of Aging*, 5th edn. San Diego: Academic Press, 2001.

101. Pfefferbaum A, Adalsteinsson E, Sullivan EV. Replicability of diffusion tensor imaging measurements of fractional anisotropy and trace in brain. *J Magn Reson Imaging* 2003; **18**: 427–33.

102. Jones DK, Symms MR, Cercignani M, Howard RJ. The effect of filter size on VBM analyses of DT-MRI data. *Neuroimage* 2005; **26**: 546–54.

103. Sidaros A, Engberg AW, Sidaros K *et al*. Diffusion tensor imaging during recovery from severe traumatic brain injury and relation to clinical outcome: a longitudinal study. *Brain* 2008; **131**: 559–72.

104. Blain CR, Williams VC, Johnston C *et al*. A longitudinal study of diffusion tensor MRI in ALS. *Amyotroph Lateral Scler* 2007; **8**: 1–8.

105. Sullivan EV, Rohlfing T, Pfefferbaum A. Longitudinal study of callosal microstructure in the normal adult ageing brain using quantitative DTI fiber tracking. *Dev Neuropsychol* 2008 (in press).

106. Charlton R, Landau S, Schiavone F *et al*. A structural equation modeling investigation of age-related variance in executive function and DTI measured white matter damage. *Neurobiol Aging* 2008; **29**: 1547–55.

107. Shenkin SD, Bastin ME, MacGillivray TJ, Deary IJ, Starr JM, Wardlaw JM. Childhood and current cognitive function in healthy 80-year-olds: a DT-MRI study. *Neuroreport* 2003; **14**: 345–49.

108. Charlton RA, Barrick TR, McIntyre DJ *et al*. White matter damage on diffusion tensor imaging correlates with age-related cognitive decline. *Neurology* 2006; **66**: 217–22.

109. Kennedy KM, Raz N. Aging white matter and cognition: differential effects of regional variations in diffusion properties on memory, executive functions, and speed. *Neuropsychologia* 2009; **47**: 916–27.

110. Pierpaoli C, Barnett A, Pajevic S *et al*. Water diffusion changes in Wallerian degeneration and their dependence on white matter architecture. *Neuroimage* 2001; **13**: 1174–85.

111. Virta A, Barnett A, Pierpaoli C. Visualizing and characterizing white matter fiber structure and architecture in the human pyramidal tract using diffusion tensor MR. *Magn Reson Imaging* 1999; **17**: 1121–33.

112. Aboitiz F, Scheibel A, Fisher R, Zaidel E. Fiber composition of the human corpus callosum. *Brain Res* 1992; **598**: 143–53.

113. Bartzokis G, Tishler TA, Lu PH *et al*. Brain ferritin iron may influence age- and gender-related risks of neurodegeneration. *Neurobiol Aging* 2007; **28**: 414–23.

114. Hallgren B, Sourander P. The effect of age on the non-haemin iron in the human brain. *J Neurochem* 1958; **3**: 41–51.

115. Herve D, Molko N, Pappata S *et al*. Longitudinal thalamic diffusion changes after middle cerebral artery infarcts. *J Neurol Neurosurg Psychiatry* 2005; **76**: 200–205.

116. Bartzokis G, Mintz J, Sultzer D *et al*. *In Vivo* MR evaluation of age-related increases in brain iron. *Am J Neuroradiol* 1994; **15**: 1129–38.

117. Bizzi A, Brooks RA, Brunetti A *et al*. Role of iron and ferritin in MR imaging of the brain: a study in primates at different field strengths. *Radiology* 1990; **177**: 59–65.

118. Brass SD, Chen NK, Mulkern RV, Bakshi R. Magnetic resonance imaging of iron deposition in neurological disorders. *Top Magn Reson Imaging* 2006; **17**: 31–40.

119. Haacke EM, Mittal S, Wu Z, Neelavalli J, Cheng YC. Susceptibility-weighted imaging: technical aspects and clinical applications, part 1. *AJNR Am J Neuroradiol* 2009; **30**: 19–30.

120. Wallis LI, Paley MN, Graham JM *et al*. MRI assessment of basal ganglia iron deposition in Parkinson's disease. *J Magn Reson Imaging* 2008; **28**: 1061–67.

121. Griffiths PD, Crossman AR. Distribution of iron in the basal ganglia and neocortex in postmortem tissue in Parkinson's disease and Alzheimer's disease. *Dementia (Basel, Switzerland)* 1993; **4**: 61–65.

122. Schenck JF, Zimmerman EA, Li Z *et al*. High-field magnetic resonance imaging of brain iron in Alzheimer disease. *Top Magn Reson Imaging* 2006; **17**: 41–50.

123. Bartzokis G, Lu PH, Tingus K *et al*. Lifespan trajectory of myelin integrity and maximum motor speed. *Neurobiol Aging* 2009 (in press).

124. Sullivan EV, Adalsteinsson E, Rohlfing T, Pfefferbaum A. Relevance of iron deposition in deep gray matter brain structures to cognitive and motor performance in healthy elderly men and women: exploratory findings. *Brain Imaging Behav* 2009 (in press).

125. Bartzokis G, Aravagiri M, Oldendorf WH, Mintz J, Marder SR. Field dependent transverse relaxation rate increase may be a specific measure of tissue iron stores. *Magn Resonance Med* 1993; **29**: 459–64.

126. Pfefferbaum A, Adalsteinsson E, Rohlfing T, Sullivan EV. MRI estimates of brain iron concentration in normal ageing: Comparison of field-dependent (FDRI) and phase (SWI) methods. *NeuroImage* 2009; **47**: 493–500.

127. Haacke EM, Xu Y, Cheng YC, Reichenbach JR. Susceptibility weighted imaging (SWI). *Magn Reson Med* 2004; **52**: 612–18.

128. Harder SL, Hopp KM, Ward H, Neglio H, Gitlin J, Kido D. Mineralization of the deep gray matter with age: a retrospective review with susceptibility-weighted MR imaging. *AJNR Am J Neuroradiol* 2008; **29**: 176–83.

129. Malloy P, Correia S, Stebbins G, Laidlaw DH. Neuroimaging of white matter in ageing and dementia. *Clin Neuropsychol* 2007; **21**: 73–109.

130. Fazekas F, Kleinert R, Offenbacher H *et al*. Pathologic correlates of incidental MRI white matter signal hyperintensities. *Neurology* 1993; **43**: 1683–89.

131. Cahn DA, Malloy PF, Salloway S *et al*. Subcortical hyperintensities on MRI and activities of daily living in geriatric depression. *J Neuropsychiatry Clin Neurosci* 1996; **8**: 404–11.

132. Liao D, Cooper L, Cai J *et al*. The prevalence and severity of white matter lesions, their relationship with age, ethnicity, gender, and cardiovascular disease risk factors: the ARIC Study. *Neuroepidemiology* 1997; **16**: 149–62.

133. Kuller LH, Longstreth WT, Jr., Arnold AM, Bernick C, Bryan RN, Beauchamp NJ, Jr. White matter hyperintensity on cranial magnetic resonance imaging: a predictor of stroke. *Stroke* 2004; **35**: 1821–25.

134. Holland CM, Smith EE, Csapo I *et al*. Spatial distribution of white-matter hyperintensities in Alzheimer disease, cerebral amyloid angiopathy, and healthy ageing. *Stroke* 2008; **39**: 1127–33.

135. DeCarli C, Fletcher E, Ramey V, Harvey D, Jagust WJ. Anatomical mapping of white matter hyperintensities (WMH): exploring the relationships between periventricular WMH, deep WMH, and total WMH burden. *Stroke* 2005; **36**: 50–55.

136. Kim KW, MacFall JR, Payne ME. Classification of white matter lesions on magnetic resonance imaging in elderly persons. *Biol Psychiatry* 2008; **64**: 273–80.

137. Kochunov P, Ramage AE, Lancaster JL *et al*. Loss of cerebral white matter structural integrity tracks the gray matter metabolic decline in normal ageing. *NeuroImage* 2009; **45**: 17–28.

138. National Institute on Aging. *Growing Older in America: The Health & Retirement Study*, 2009. At www.nia.nih.gov/NR/exeres/C80ADCEA-DE6E-4EF0-8D75-FD32AAE9BE6A.html, accessed Feb 2010.

139. Pfefferbaum A, Sullivan EV, Adalsteinsson E, Garrick T, Harper C. Postmortem MR imaging of formalin-fixed human brain. *Neuroimage* 2004; **21**: 1585–95.

140. DeCarli C, Massaro J, Harvey D *et al*. Measures of brain morphology and infarction in the Framingham heart study: establishing what is normal. *Neurobiol Aging* 2005; **26**: 491–510.

141. Brickman AM, Schupf N, Manly JJ *et al*. Brain morphology in older African Americans, Caribbean Hispanics, and whites from northern Manhattan. *Arch Neurol* 2008; **65**: 1053–61.

142. Nordahl CW, Ranganath C, Yonelinas AP, Decarli C, Fletcher E, Jagust WJ. White matter changes compromise prefrontal cortex function in healthy elderly individuals. *J Cogn Neurosci* 2006; **18**: 418–29.

143. Tullberg M, Fletcher E, DeCarli C *et al*. White matter lesions impair frontal lobe function regardless of their location. *Neurology* 2004; **63**: 246–53.

144. O'Brien JT, Erkinjuntti T, Reisberg B *et al*. Vascular cognitive impairment. *Lancet Neurol* 2003; **2**: 89–98.

145. Moseley ME, Kucharczyk J, Mintorovitch J *et al*. Diffusion-weighted MR imaging of acute stroke: correlation with T2-weighted and magnetic susceptibility-enhanced MR imaging in cats. *Am J Neuroradiol* 1990; **11**: 423–29.

146. Moseley ME, Mintorovitch J, Cohen Y *et al*. Early detection of ischemic injury: comparison of spectroscopy, diffusion-, T2-, and magnetic susceptibility-weighted MRI in cats. *Acta Neurochir Suppl* 1990; **51**: 207–209.

147. Peters A, Sethares C. Is there remyelination during ageing of the primate central nervous system? *J Comp Neurol* 2003; **460**: 238–54.

148. Pandya DN, Seltzer B. The topography of commissural fibers. In Lepore F, Ptito M, Jasper HH (eds), *Two Hemispheres – One Brain: Functions of the Corpus Callosum*. New York: Alan R. Liss, 1986, 47–74.

Functional Imaging of the Ageing Brain

Robert Perneczky, Christian Sorg and Hans Förstl

*Department of Psychiatry and Psychotherapy, Klinikum rechts der Isar,
Technische Universität München, München, Germany*

INTRODUCTION

Modern imaging techniques such as functional magnetic resonance imaging (fMRI), positron emission tomography (PET) and single photon emission tomography (SPECT) provide the groundwork to test mechanistic hypotheses derived from basic neuroscience studies in healthy individuals and patients with neurological and psychiatric disorders. Apart from these scientific applications, functional imaging studies can also provide important diagnostic information in the field of geriatric psychiatry. Therefore, functional imaging scans are recommended by diagnostic guidelines to resolve certain differential diagnostic issues[1], and costs are also reimbursed for these special cases in selected countries (e.g. Medicare Coverage Criteria for FDG-PET for Alzheimer's disease, http://nps.cardinal.com/nps/PETFoundations/documents/PETADCovFinal.pdf). In addition to its benefits for the diagnosis and differential diagnosis of neurological and psychiatric disorders, functional brain imaging has also been shown to increase the confidence of experts in their clinical diagnosis. For example, Foster et al.[2] reported that visual rating of ^{18}F-fluoro-2-deoxy-glucose (FDG) PET scans after a short training period was more reliable and accurate in distinguishing Alzheimer's disease from frontotemporal dementia (FTD) than clinical assessment on its own. This was particularly true when the raters were uncertain with their clinical diagnosis. Hence, FDG PET is able to add important diagnostic information that appropriately improves diagnostic confidence.

Biomarkers including functional imaging are also gaining importance for the evaluation and monitoring of treatment effects. Modern, sensitive techniques are able to detect subtle brain functional changes resulting from therapeutic interventions, even if the therapeutic effect is not immediately mirrored by clinical improvement. This could lead to the identification of treatment responders in very early treatment phases[3] or before the actual treatment period has even started. Furthermore, for some potentially preventive treatments to have their greatest impact, patients need to be identified at the presymptomatic stage. This means that individuals with an increased risk for a certain disease, but who do not yet show any clinical signs, need to be identified. Persons at risk for Alzheimer's disease, for example, can already be identified on the basis of brain metabolic deficits in their FDG PET scans before first symptoms, such as forgetfulness, appear[4].

This chapter provides an overview of a selection of functional imaging techniques and brain functional changes associated with ageing, some prevalent neurodegenerative and psychiatric disorders, and those due to treatment. Important clinical aspects and future research perspectives will be discussed.

FUNCTIONAL IMAGING TECHNIQUES

Functional neuroimaging is broadly defined as techniques that provide measures of brain activity. Commonly used techniques are electroencephalography (EEG), magnetoencephalography (MEG), PET, SPECT and fMRI. Here we focus on PET and fMRI, which primarily aim at the regional mapping of mental processes. These techniques measure metabolic and haemodynamic brain processes closely linked with neuronal activity. PET and fMRI allow both the detection of regional activity changes in response to experimentally presented stimuli or cognitive tasks and the detection of synchronous co-activity changes across brain regions in response on stimuli or during rest. In this section we review the biological basis of functional neuroimaging signals, then we describe the physics of PET and fMRI signals, and finally we discuss two basic principles underlying functional neuroimaging data analysis: functional specialization and functional integration.

Behaviourally evoked changes in blood flow are at the heart of functional neuroimaging[5]. Blood flow changes reflect metabolic changes, which in turn reflect changes in neuronal activity. From a metabolic point of view neuronal activity is dominated by transmitter recycling. Eighty per cent of brain energy is used for glutamate recycling. Central to glutamate recycling are aerobic glycolysis and oxidative phosphorylation. These activity-dependent processes with their main substrates H_2O, O_2 and glucose provide the basis for[15] O-H_2O-PET, FDG PET, and blood oxygen level-dependent (BOLD) fMRI.

Oxygen-15 and fluorine-18 are isotopes with short half-lives that are introduced into the body incorporated into H_2O and glucose. As the tracers decay, emitted gamma rays are detected by the PET scanner and used for image construction. The spatial resolution is about 1.5 cm and the temporal resolution is about 60 s; both values strongly influence the experimental design of neurocognitive paradigms. The fundamental signal for BOLD fMRI comes from hydrogen atoms mainly bonded to H_2O within the brain. In the presence of a static magnetic field, these hydrogen atoms absorb energy that is applied at a characteristic radio frequency. After radiofrequency excitation,

Principles and Practice of Geriatric Psychiatry, 3rd edn. Edited by Mohammed T. Abou-Saleh, Cornelius Katona and Anand Kumar

hydrogen atoms emit energy at the same radiofrequency until they gradually return to their equilibrium state (resonance phenomenon). The MRI scanner measures the emitted radiofrequency energy. The measured radiofrequency signal decays over time, influenced by distinct factors, including the presence of inhomogeneities in the magnetic field. BOLD fMRI techniques are designed to measure primarily changes of inhomogeneity within a small volume of tissue that result from changes in blood oxygenation. Deoxy- and oxyhaemoglobin ($Hb\text{-}CO_2$, $Hb\text{-}O_2$) have different magnetic properties; $Hb\text{-}CO_2$ is paramagnetic and introduces an inhomogeneity into the nearby magnetic field, whereas $Hb\text{-}O_2$ is weakly diamagnetic with little effect. Hence, an increase in the concentration of $Hb\text{-}CO_2$ causes a decrease in image intensity, and a decrease in $Hb\text{-}CO_2$ causes an increase in image intensity (BOLD effect). The spatial resolution of BOLD fMRI is about 0.5 cm and temporal resolution about 1–4 seconds.

There are two key topics in the analysis of functional imaging data, reflecting the long-standing debate in neuroscience about functional specialization versus functional integration in the brain[6]. The first is brain 'mapping', where three-dimensional images of neuronal activation are generated showing which parts of the brain respond to a given sensory stimulus or cognitive task. This is also known as the study of functional specialization and generally proceeds using some form of statistical parametric mapping (SPM) based on a voxel-wise analysis. A classic example here is the identification of human V4 and V5, the areas specialized for the processing of colour and motion. The second topic is 'functional integration', where models are used to analyse how different brain areas interact. A classic example is the use of models to find increased connectivity between dorsal and ventral visual streams after subjects learn object–place associations. A large number of statistical techniques are used to detect interregional connectivity (e.g. independent component analysis, support vector machine, dynamic causal modelling).

AGE-RELATED FUNCTIONAL CHANGES

Brain Functional Decline

'Normal ageing' is associated with numerous biological deteriorations in the human body, which also include brain functional changes. However, 'normal ageing' is a rather fuzzy concept and it is sometimes difficult to separate age-related and disease-related brain changes. All the same, with age the brain undergoes both structural and functional changes that underlie subjective complaints. The pre-frontal cortex shows the most prominent functional deterioration in most studies, whereas other regions including the anterior hippocampus, the thalamus and the posterior cingulate cortex are affected to a much lesser extent[7]. These results support the theory that the first areas to emerge phylo- and ontogenetically are the most resistant to age effects and the last to emerge are the most vulnerable. Furthermore, the relative functional preservation of brain structures during 'normal ageing' that are affected early in Alzheimer's disease, such as the hippocampus and the posterior cingulate cortex[8], seems to mark the parting of the ways between ageing and brain disease. This is also supported by the finding that cognitively normal elderly individuals with a pathological brain metabolic pattern are more likely to experience memory decline[9] and are at elevated risk of developing symptoms of Alzheimer's disease[10]. Also in line with these findings, Alzheimer's disease-like brain functional patterns are also found in cognitively normal elderly individuals with an increased genetic risk for Alzheimer's disease (i.e. carriers of the

apolipoprotein E allele $\varepsilon4$ (*APOE4*)[11]). Alzheimer's disease-like changes are already present at even younger ages in pre-symptomatic individuals from families with known early-onset autosomal dominant Alzheimer's disease-carrying mutations in the *PRESENILIN1* gene[12]. Interestingly, a maternal history of Alzheimer's disease also predisposes cognitively normal individuals to progressive metabolic deficits in Alzheimer's disease-vulnerable brain regions, which may be related to a higher risk of developing the disease[4]. Although the exact causes of these abnormalities are not yet known, these results suggest the involvement of maternally inherited predisposition to brain metabolic failure, possibly connected to mitochondrial DNA. The facts that mitochondrial DNA is entirely maternally inherited in humans, and diseases associated with mitochondrial DNA mutations often present as sporadic disorders, support this hypothesis.

Adaptation and Compensation

Age- and disease-related changes are not only associated with functional deterioration but also with counteractive measures. Accessory neural networks are activated to solve increasingly difficult tasks (adaptation). Similar mechanisms are deployed if a task cannot be solved by the usual means because of damage to the brain regions normally involved due to age-related changes or neurodegeneration (compensation)[13]. To offset brain functional deterioration, networks and cognitive patterns less susceptible to interference are activated; furthermore, additional networks not involved in young healthy individuals for the same task are recruited. These activity adjustments are exemplified by two well-described phenomena. The PASA (posterior-anterior shift in aging) phenomenon describes one possible reaction of the human brain to age-associated cognitive impairment. An increased activation of pre-frontal areas in conjunction with a decreased activation of occipital areas is found for the same cognitive paradigm in elderly individuals compared to healthy young persons. The degree of this activity shift is positively associated with task performance[14]. The HAROLD (hemispheric asymmetry reduction in older adults) phenomenon, on the other hand, delineates a reduction of hemispheric asymmetry in elderly individuals[15]; compared to young individuals, elderly persons tend to activate additional contralateral and to deactivate ipsilateral brain regions for the same cognitive task. Again, task performance positively correlates with the degree of the activity change. Taken together, PASA and HAROLD are good examples of the three possible mechanisms of cerebral activity changes associated with efficient information processing during ageing: (i) increased activation of brain regions already involved at the same task difficulty level in young individuals; (ii) activation of additional networks in other brain regions; (iii) more efficient deactivation of interfering networks.

FUNCTIONAL CHANGES IN NEURODEGENERATIVE DISORDERS

Neurodegenerative disorders are associated with distinct brain functional patterns. These patterns help to separate different disorders and to identify patients at oligosymptomatic stages.

Mild Cognitive Impairment and Alzheimer's Disease

In Alzheimer's disease functional brain damage is typically found in the hippocampus, and the pre-frontal, temporoparietal and posterior cingulate association cortices[8,16]. The hippocampus and the posterior cingulate cortex seem to be affected in very early disease stages; metabolic deterioration of these two regions is already present in patients with mild cognitive impairment (MCI)[17,18]. Furthermore, an FDG PET suggestive of Alzheimer's disease in patients with MCI is a strong predictor for progression to dementia, especially in the presence of other risk factors such as an *APOE ε4* allele[19]. The degree of posterior cingulate cortex hypometabolism is also positively correlated with clinical disease severity in MCI[20]. However, several studies show that there is no linear association between brain damage and clinical symptoms, and that individual characteristics related to cognitive reserve modify the association between neurodegenerative damage and clinical signs[21-23]. Therefore, clinical symptoms tend to be less severe in individuals with higher estimated cognitive reserve than would be predicted by the amount of their brain damage.

Frontotemporal Lobar Degenerations

The clinical syndromes FTD, semantic dementia (SD) and non-fluent progressive aphasia (NFPA) have distinct morphological and functional imaging correlates. Furthermore, associations between specific clinical symptoms and focal functional brain pathology can be established. For example, metabolic reductions in brain regions related to micturition can be found in patients with FTD who suffer from urinary incontinence in contrast to those patients who do not experience this distressing symptom[24].

In FTD, bi-hemispheric functional brain pathology, which predominantly affects the pre-frontal cortex, the anterior cingulate cortex, the caudate nucleus and the insula, is already present in early clinical stages[25]. As the disease progresses, the functional pathology crosses the boundaries of the pre-frontal cortex and spreads to temporal and parietal regions[26]. Davies *et al.*[27] recently reported a group of patients with FTD without any structural brain changes that seem to have a better prognosis. However, brain functional alterations and the clinical relevance of this finding have yet to be explored. It is interesting to note that the degree of functional brain pathology is also influenced by genetic characteristics[28] and cognitive reserve[29,30]. In SD, initially asymmetric, in most cases left-sided, functional lesions of the temporal cortex, more specifically the temporal pole, are found[25]. It was recently shown in a follow-up study that the metabolic deficit only worsened in the anterior cingulate cortex after 15 months; this limited worsening was, however, associated with a considerable clinical decline[31]. In NFPA, the asymmetric functional deficit is predominantly located in the left temporal and insular cortex, the caudate nuclei and the thalami[32-34]. However, right hemispheric functional pathology was reported in left-handed patients[35] (Figure 5.1).

Lewy Body-Associated Disorders

Parkinson's disease dementia (PDD) and dementia with Lewy bodies (DLB) probably both belong to a spectrum of Lewy body-associated disorders. This notion is supported by a similar pattern of functional cerebral pathology, which includes brain regions also affected in Alzheimer's disease, such as the pre-frontal, temporoparietal and posterior cingulate cortex, and additional areas in the visual association cortex[36,37]. In a direct comparison, patients with DLB had a significant metabolic reduction in the anterior cingulate cortex compared with patients with PDD[36]. Associations between focal metabolic deficits and typical neuropsychiatric symptoms were reported, for example between right pre-frontal metabolism and delusions[38], and metabolism in visual association areas and visual hallucinations[39,40]. Furthermore, the impairment of daily activities was also linked to focal functional brain pathology[41,42].

FUNCTIONAL CHANGES IN PSYCHIATRIC DISORDERS

Next we review some studies in major depression and in schizophrenia using fMRI and FDG PET. Since explicit neuroimaging studies exploring the effect of age on major depression and schizophrenia are rare, we focus here on some recent imaging studies in major depression and schizophrenia, providing some new insights in disease mechanisms and demonstrating the potential of neuroimaging techniques for a better understanding of disease-related symptoms by altered brain processes. For both disorders changes in the default mode network (DMN) will be of special interest. The DMN comprises the medial pre-frontal cortex, the posterior cingulate cortex, and the lateral parietal cortex (for review see[43]). Areas of the DMN show elevated metabolism at rest, they are functionally connected by synchronized co-activity at rest and they consistently deactivate across a wide range of attention demanding, goal-directed behaviours; since DMN activation is related to self-referential functions such as remembering the past, planning the future or perspective taking of the mental state of others, deactivations during goal-directed behaviour are suggested as an attenuation of self-referential processes in order to improve goal-oriented attention[43].

The first finding pointing at a potential role of the DMN in major depression was reported by Greicius and colleagues[44]; the authors observed increased synchronized co-activity of the medial pre-frontal cortex within the DMN in major depression during rest. Examining the relevance of this result, Sheline *et al.*[45] found that in major depression medial pre-frontal regions of the DMN exhibited failure to deactivate during both looking at negative stimuli and appraising them. Patients with major depression and healthy controls were instructed to look at pictures inducing negative emotions in a passive mode and to appraise them actively (making a negative picture positive by depersonalizing it such that it does not pertain to the viewer or that the picture is not real). For the passive viewing and the active regulating condition patients and controls demonstrated reduced activations compared to the baseline state (i.e. deactivations) in the DMN. However, compared with controls, depressed patients' deactivations were less distinctive in several areas of the DMN, notably in the medial pre-frontal cortex. This result suggests that patients with major depression might have problems in reducing self-referential processes both during emotion-related activity and also during subsequent emotion regulation.

In a similar design to that of Sheline *et al.* Grimm and colleagues[46] found that the degree of deactivation failure correlated with the severity of depressive symptoms and reported hopelessness. These results together point at the prominent role of the DMN in major depression: the DMN seems to be critically involved in some key deficits of major depression such as emotion regulation or increased self-focused cognitions.

Several recent studies have revealed substantial changes within the DMN of patients with schizophrenia. Garrity and colleagues[47] found reduced synchronized co-activity within superior parts of the posterior cingulate cortex and the precuneus and increased co-activity within the inferior posterior cingulate cortex and the

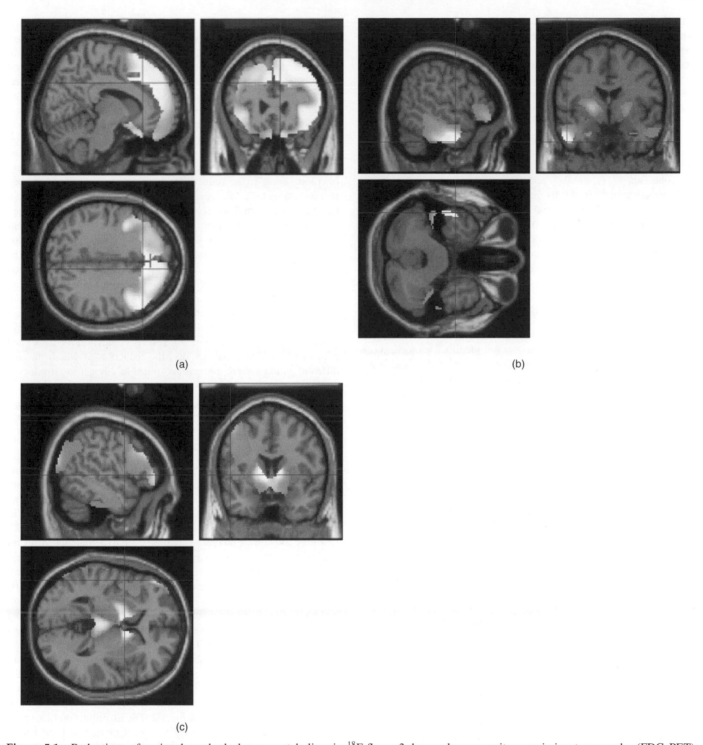

(a)

(b)

(c)

Figure 5.1 Reductions of regional cerebral glucose metabolism in ^{18}F-fluoro-2-deoxy-glucose positron emission tomography (FDG PET) studies of patients with (a) frontotemporal dementia, (b) semantic dementia and (c) progressive non-fluent aphasia compared with healthy control subjects (sagittal, axial, and coronal slices; areas with reduced metabolism are displayed in colour). *A full colour version of this figure appears in the colour plate section*

medial pre-frontal cortex in patients with schizophrenia during an auditory oddball attention task. In particular, increases in co-activity (i.e. functional hyperconnectivity) were correlated with positive symptoms. Looking at a potential relation between hyperconnectivity within the frontal DMN and already known hyperactivation of areas within and outside of the DMN in schizophrenia, Whitfield-Gabrieli et al.[48] instructed patients with early schizophrenia, first-degree relatives of patients with schizophrenia, and healthy control subjects to perform a working memory task during fMRI. They found gradually reduced deactivations of the medial pre-frontal cortex across patients with schizophrenia, relatives of patients and controls with deactivations correlating with the cognitive performance. In the patient group deactivations were related to the severity of positive symptoms. Both patients and relatives hyper-activated in the dorsolateral pre-frontal cortex. With regard to functional connectivity, synchronized co-activity of the medial pre-frontal cortex during rest was highest in patients and lowest in controls. This hyperconnectivity of the medial pre-frontal cortex was related to both the hyperactivity of the dorsolateral pre-frontal cortex and the deactivation of the medial pre-frontal cortex, indicating an association between hyperactivation and hyperconnectivity in schizophrenia.

Hyperactivation of the DMN may blur the boundary between internal, self-focus-based thinking and external world-focus-based perceptions. Since many symptoms of schizophrenia involve an increased sense of self-relevance in the world or a smearing of internal reflection and external perception, hyperactivity and hyperconnectivity of the DMN may contribute to these critical symptoms of schizophrenia.

TREATMENT EFFECTS ON BRAIN FUNCTION

Including functional neuroimaging in clinical trials and clinical treatment monitoring procedures may identify neurochemical and anatomic differences between treatment responders and non-responders. These differences may serve as biomarkers for the prediction of treatment response and provide valuable information for treatment development by identifying mechanisms of treatment resistance.

Treatment Effects in Dementia

In Alzheimer's disease, cholinergic treatment with donepezil was associated with a stabilized regional cerebral blood flow in treatment responders, whereas blood flow declined in non-responders in a study by Nobili et al.[49]. Similar treatment effects of donepezil were also shown in patients with cognitive impairment after traumatic brain injury[50]. The binding of donepezil to acetylcholinesterase can also be directly measured in vivo with PET, allowing quantitative analyses of acetylcholinesterase and direct investigation of the pharmacokinetics of donepezil in the human brain[51]. Okamura et al.[52] reported that up to 60% of acetylcholinesterase donepezil-binding sites were occupied after the oral application of 5 mg donepezil. Cholinergic treatment with galantamine also caused sustained inhibition of acetylcholinesterase activity in patients with Alzheimer's disease; this effect was associated with attentional rather than memory improvement[53]. Brain functional changes were also demonstrated for drugs targeting transmitter systems other than the cholinergic system. Fellgiebel et al.[54], for example, reported clinical and brain metabolic improvements in a patient with FTD under treatment with aripiprazole, a newer antipsychotic with partial agonistic properties at serotonin 5-HT$_{1A}$ and dopamine D$_2$ receptors, and partial antagonism at serotonin 5-HT$_2$ receptors. This study also suggests that common functional imaging techniques can be used to provide neurobiological evidence for the clinical effects of different psychotropic drugs.

Treatment Effects in Geriatric Depression

Most studies on antidepressant interventions in unipolar depression, including antidepressant drugs[3], total sleep deprivation[55],

psychotherapy[56] and electroconvulsive therapy[57], focus on mid-life individuals. The available data in geriatric depression are limited. Nobler et al.[58] reported that after treatment with nortriptyline or sertraline, the study group as a whole did not show any blood flow changes; furthermore, there were no global blood flow differences between treatment responders and non-responders. However, the blood flow pattern differed significantly between treatment responders and non-responders: responders showed regional blood flow reductions in the pre-frontal and anterior temporal cortices. Brain metabolic reductions in the anterior cingulate cortex and the amygdalae were observed under chronic citalopram treatment by Liotta et al.[59]; the reductions were greater in responders than in non-responders. Wu et al.[60] showed that improvement under treatment with sertraline and after sleep deprivation was associated with a metabolic decrease in the orbitofrontal cortex, whereas clinical worsening was related to a metabolic increase in the dorsolateral pre-frontal cortex. Early metabolic decreases of the right cingulate gyrus after total sleep deprivation in combination with sertraline treatment were furthermore associated with clinical improvement[61]. However, these synergistic effects of antidepressant drug and sleep deprivation could not be replicated in a randomized, placebo-controlled study by the same group[62]. Taken together these results suggest that the state of severe depression is associated with increased functional activity, the reduction of which through different antidepressant therapies is linked to clinical improvement.

CLINICAL APPLICATION AND FUTURE PERSPECTIVES

Functional Neuroimaging in Clinical Practice

Structural imaging of the brain is an integral diagnostic procedure in psychiatry. It can provide indispensable information on possible organic aetiologies of psychiatric disorders, sometimes with immediate therapeutic consequences; furthermore, structural imaging can also support the clinical diagnosis in geriatric psychiatry, such as in the case of marked mediotemporal atrophy in Alzheimer's disease[63]. However, functional imaging techniques are experiencing increased popularity in the search for more sensitive and specific biomarkers for distinct psychiatric disorders. For a limited number of indications, functional imaging studies are already recommended by diagnostic guidelines. These indications include the assessment of regional cerebral blood flow or metabolism by means of PET or SPECT imaging for the differentiation of Alzheimer's disease and other neurodegenerative dementias such as FTD. Functional imaging should, however, never replace structural imaging; functional imaging should rather be used to provide complementary information in uncertain clinical cases. The added clinical value of functional imaging in several psychiatric and neurological disorders, including major depression and schizophrenia, is still to be determined. The identification of responders and non-responders in early treatment phases or even before starting a treatment would be especially desirable. Furthermore, novel imaging procedures such as resting state fMRI (rs-fMRI) could not only help to clarify the brain functional basis of neurodegenerative and psychiatric disorders but also serve as non-invasive biomarkers for the diagnosis and differential diagnosis in geriatric psychiatry[64].

Future Perspectives

Representing a new tool of functional neuroimaging research with some potential for reaching clinical relevance in psychiatric disorders, rs-fMRI focuses on changes of functional interactions between

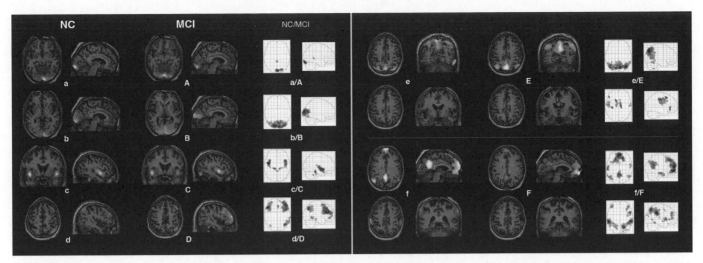

Figure 5.2 Brain networks characterized by synchronized co-activity during rest in normal controls (NC) and patients with mild cognitive impairment (MCI) detected by 4 min of resting state functional magnetic resonance imaging (fMRI). Brain networks correspond with networks found during characteristic cognitive task conditions such as seeing or attending. Selectively in both networks of part f/F patients had reduced co-activity compared with controls: the default mode network and an attention network

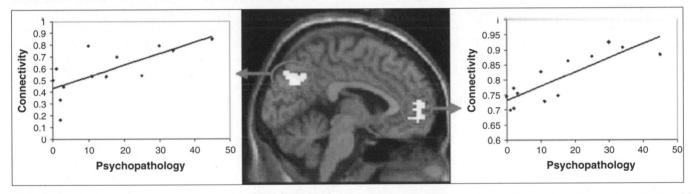

Figure 5.3 The functional connectivity at rest within the default mode network (DMN) correlates with psychopathology in patients with schizophrenia. Psychopathology reflects positive symptoms (composite Scale for the Assessment of Positive Symptoms (SAPS) score of positive symptoms); connectivity reflects whole brain functional connectivity with seed in the medial pre-frontal cortex. Adapted with permission from data published in Whitfield-Gabrieli et al.[48]

brain areas. Since it is performed at rest, rs-fMRI only needs minimal compliance of patients during imaging, making it appropriate for clinical purposes. Because it focuses on interactions between brain areas, rs-fMRI detects functional changes characteristic of several psychiatric disorders (Figures 5.2 and 5.3)[65].

In addition to this new brain mapping tool, several other new approaches aim at the integration of distinct structural and functional imaging parameters. Of particular note, machine learning-related methods such as support vector machines and various clustering procedures have been used. The basic idea of these approaches is to identify distinct patterns that are specific for a set of patients[66]. However, further research is warranted to explore the real potential of these newer methods.

REFERENCES

1. Knopman DS, DeKosky ST, Cummings JL *et al*. Practice parameter: diagnosis of dementia (an evidence-based review). Report of the Quality Standards Subcommittee of the American Academy of Neurology. *Neurology* 2001; **56**: 1143–53.

2. Foster NL, Heidebrink JL, Clark CM *et al*. FDG-PET improves accuracy in distinguishing frontotemporal dementia and Alzheimer's disease. *Brain* 2007; **130**: 2616–35.

3. Brockmann H, Zobel A, Joe A *et al*. The value of HMPAO SPECT in predicting treatment response to citalopram in patients with major depression. *Psychiatry Res* 2009; **173**: 107–12.

4. Mosconi L, Mistur R, Switalski R *et al*. Declining brain glucose metabolism in normal individuals with a maternal history of Alzheimer disease. *Neurology* 2009; **72**: 513–20.

5. Raichle ME, Mintun M. Brain work and brain imaging. *Annu Rev Neurosci* 2006; **29**: 449–76.

6. Cohen J, Tong F. Neuroscience. The face of controversy. *Science* 2001; **293**: 2405–407.

7. Kalpouzos G, Chetelat G, Baron JC *et al*. Voxel-based mapping of brain gray matter volume and glucose metabolism profiles in normal ageing. *Neurobiol Aging* 2009; **30**: 112–24.

8. Mosconi L, Tsui WH, Herholz K *et al*. Multicenter standardized 18F-FDG PET diagnosis of mild cognitive impairment, Alzheimer's disease, and other dementias. *J Nucl Med* 2008; **49**: 390–98.

9. Caselli RJ, Chen K, Lee W *et al.* Correlating cerebral hypometabolism with future memory decline in subsequent converters to amnestic pre-mild cognitive impairment. *Arch Neurol* 2008; **65**: 1231–36.

10. Mosconi L, Mistur R, Switalski R *et al.* FDG-PET changes in brain glucose metabolism from normal cognition to pathologically verified Alzheimer's disease. *Eur J Nucl Med Mol Imaging* 2009; **36**: 811–22.

11. Rimajova M, Lenzo NP, Wu JS *et al.* Fluoro-2-deoxy-D-glucose (FDG)-PET in APOEepsilon4 carriers in the Australian population. *J Alzheimers Dis* 2008; **13**: 137–46.

12. Mosconi L, Sorbi S, de Leon MJ *et al.* Hypometabolism exceeds atrophy in presymptomatic early-onset familial Alzheimer's disease. *J Nucl Med* 2006; **47**: 1778–86.

13. Stern Y, Habeck C, Moeller J *et al.* Brain networks associated with cognitive reserve in healthy young and old adults. *Cereb Cortex* 2005; **15**: 394–402.

14. Davis SW, Dennis NA, Daselaar SM *et al.* Que PASA? The posterior-anterior shift in ageing. *Cereb Cortex* 2008; **18**: 1201–209.

15. Cabeza R Hemispheric asymmetry reduction in older adults: the HAROLD model. *Psychol Aging* 2002; **17**: 85–100.

16. Herholz K, Salmon E, Perani D *et al.* Discrimination between Alzheimer dementia and controls by automated analysis of multicenter FDG PET. *Neuroimage* 2002; **17**: 302–16.

17. Mosconi L, Tsui WH, de Santi S *et al.* Reduced hippocampal metabolism in MCI and AD: automated FDG-PET image analysis. *Neurology* 2005; **64**: 1860–67.

18. Minoshima S, Giordani B, Berent S *et al.* Metabolic reduction in the posterior cingulate cortex in very early Alzheimer's disease. *Ann Neurol* 1997; **42**: 85–94.

19. Drzezga A, Grimmer T, Riemenschneider M *et al.* Prediction of individual clinical outcome in MCI by means of genetic assessment and[18]F-FDG PET. *J Nucl Med* 2005; **46**: 1625–32.

20. Perneczky R, Hartmann J, Grimmer T *et al.* Cerebral metabolic correlates of the clinical dementia rating scale in mild cognitive impairment. *J Geriatr Psychiatry Neurol* 2007; **20**: 84–88.

21. Perneczky R, Drzezga A, Diehl-Schmid J *et al.* Schooling mediates brain reserve in Alzheimer's disease: findings of fluorodeoxy-glucose-positron emission tomography. *J Neurol Neurosurg Psychiatry* 2006; **77**: 1060–63.

22. Scarmeas N, Zarahn E, Anderson KE *et al.* Association of life activities with cerebral blood flow in Alzheimer disease: implications for the cognitive reserve hypothesis. *Arch Neurol* 2003; **60**: 359–65.

23. Perneczky R, Wagenpfeil S, Lunetta K *et al.* Education attenuates the effect of medial temporal lobe atrophy on cognitive function in Alzheimer's disease: the MIRAGE study. *J Alzheimers Dis* 2009; **17**: 855–962.

24. Perneczky R. Therapie der frontotemporalen Demenz. *Z Psychiatr Psychol Psychother* 2007; **56**: 47–49.

25. Diehl J, Grimmer T, Drzezga A *et al.* Cerebral metabolic patterns at early stages of frontotemporal dementia and semantic dementia. A PET study. *Neurobiol Aging* 2004; **25**: 1051–56.

26. Diehl-Schmid J, Grimmer T, Drzezga A *et al.* Decline of cerebral glucose metabolism in frontotemporal dementia: a longitudinal 18F-FDG-PET-study. *Neurobiol Aging* 2007; **28**: 42–50.

27. Davies RR, Kipps CM, Mitchell J *et al.* Progression in frontotemporal dementia: identifying a benign behavioral variant by magnetic resonance imaging. *Arch Neurol* 2006; **63**: 1627–31.

28. Laws SM, Perneczky R, Drzezga A *et al.* () Association of the tau haplotype h2 with age at onset and functional alterations of glucose utilization in frontotemporal dementia. *Am J Psychiatry* 2007; **164**: 1577–84.

29. Perneczky R, Diehl-Schmid J, Drzezga A *et al.* Brain reserve capacity in frontotemporal dementia: a voxel-based[18] F-FDG PET study. *Eur J Nucl Med Mol Imaging* 2007; **34**: 1082–87.

30. Borroni B, Premi E, Agosti C *et al.* Revisiting brain reserve hypothesis in frontotemporal dementia: evidence from a brain perfusion study. *Dement Geriatr Cogn Disord* 2009; **28**: 130–35.

31. Diehl-Schmid J, Grimmer T, Drzezga A *et al.* Longitudinal changes of cerebral glucose metabolism in semantic dementia. *Dement Geriatr Cogn Disord* 2006; **22**: 346–51.

32. Nestor PJ, Balan K, Cheow HK *et al.* Nuclear imaging can predict pathologic diagnosis in progressive nonfluent aphasia. *Neurology* 2007; **68**: 238–39.

33. Nestor PJ, Graham NL, Fryer TD *et al.* Progressive non-fluent aphasia is associated with hypometabolism centred on the left anterior insula. *Brain* 2003; **126**: 2406–18.

34. Perneczky R, Diehl-Schmid J, Pohl C *et al.* Non-fluent progressive aphasia: Cerebral metabolic patterns and brain reserve. *Brain Res* 2007; **1133**: 178–85.

35. Drzezga A, Grimmer T, Siebner H *et al.* Prominent hypometabolism of the right temporoparietal and frontal cortex in two left-handed patients with primary progressive aphasia. *J Neurol* 2002; **249**: 1263–67.

36. Yong SW, Yoon JK, An YS *et al.* A comparison of cerebral glucose metabolism in Parkinson's disease, Parkinson's disease dementia and dementia with Lewy bodies. *Eur J Neurol* 2007; **14**: 1357–62.

37. Minoshima S, Foster NL, Sima AA *et al.* Alzheimer's disease versus dementia with Lewy bodies: cerebral metabolic distinction with autopsy confirmation. *Ann Neurol* 2001; **50**: 358–65.

38. Perneczky R, Drzezga A, Boecker H *et al.* Right prefrontal hypometabolism predicts delusions in dementia with Lewy bodies. *Neurobiol Aging* 2008; **30**: 1420–29.

39. Boecker H, Ceballos-Baumann AO, Volk D *et al.* Metabolic alterations in patients with Parkinson disease and visual hallucinations. *Arch Neurol* 2007; **64**: 984–88.

40. Perneczky R, Drzezga A, Boecker H *et al.* Cerebral metabolic dysfunction in patients with dementia with Lewy bodies and visual hallucinations. *Dement Geriatr Cogn Disord* 2008; **25**: 531–38.

41. Perneczky R, Drzezga A, Boecker H *et al.* Activities of daily living, cerebral glucose metabolism, and cognitive reserve in Lewy body and Parkinson's disease. *Dement Geriatr Cogn Disord* 2008; **26**: 475–81.

42. Perneczky R, Haussermann P, Drzezga A *et al.* Fluoro-deoxy-glucose positron emission tomography correlates of impaired activities of daily living in dementia with Lewy bodies: implications for cognitive reserve. *Am J Geriatr Psychiatry* 2009; **17**: 188–95.

43. Buckner R, Andrews-Hanna J, Schacter D. The brain's default network: anatomy, function, and relevance to disease. *Ann N Y Acad Sci* 2008; **1124**: 1–38.

44. Greicius M, Flores B, Menon V *et al.* Resting-state functional connectivity in major depression: abnormally increased contributions from subgenual cingulate cortex and thalamus. *Biol Psychiatry* 2007; **62**: 429–37.

45. Sheline Y, Barch D, Price J *et al*. The default mode network and self-referential processes in depression. *Proc Natl Acad Sci USA* 2009; **106**: 1942–47.

46. Grimm S, Boesinger P, Beck J *et al*. Altered negative BOLD responses in the default-mode network during emotion processing in depressed subjects. *Neuropsychopharmacology* 2009; **34**: 932–43.

47. Garrity A, Pearlson G, McKiernan K *et al*. Aberrant 'default mode' functional connectivity in schizophrenia. *Am J Psychiatry* 2007; **164**: 450–57.

48. Whitfield-Gabrieli S, Thermenos H, Milanovic S *et al*. Hyperactivity and hyperconnectivity of the default mode network in schozophrenia and in first-degree relatives of persons with schizophrenia. *Proc Natl Acad Sci USA* 2009; **106**: 1279–84.

49. Nobili F, Koulibaly M, Vitali P *et al*. Brain perfusion follow-up in Alzheimer's patients during treatment with acetylcholinesterase inhibitors. *J Nucl Med* 2002; **43**: 983–90.

50. Kim YW, Kim DY, Shin JC *et al*. The changes of cortical metabolism associated with the clinical response to donepezil therapy in traumatic brain injury. *Clin Neuropharmacol* 2009; **32**: 63–68.

51. Hiraoka K, Okamura N, Funaki Y *et al*. Quantitative analysis of donepezil binding to acetylcholinesterase using positron emission tomography and [5-(11)C-methoxy]donepezil. *Neuroimage* 2009; **46**: 616–23.

52. Okamura N, Funaki Y, Tashiro M *et al*. In vivo visualization of donepezil binding in the brain of patients with Alzheimer's disease. *Br J Clin Pharmacol* 2008; **65**: 472–79.

53. Kadir A, Darreh-Shori T, Almkvist O *et al*. PET imaging of the in vivo brain acetylcholinesterase activity and nicotine binding in galantamine-treated patients with AD. *Neurobiol Aging* 2008; **29**: 1204–17.

54. Fellgiebel A, Muller MJ, Hiemke C *et al*. Clinical improvement in a case of frontotemporal dementia under aripiprazole treatment corresponds to partial recovery of disturbed frontal glucose metabolism. *World J Biol Psychiatry* 2007; **8**: 123–26.

55. Gillin JC, Buchsbaum M, Wu J *et al*. Sleep deprivation as a model experimental antidepressant treatment: findings from functional brain imaging. *Depress Anxiety* 2001; **14**: 37–49.

56. Brody AL, Saxena S, Stoessel P *et al*. Regional brain metabolic changes in patients with major depression treated with either paroxetine or interpersonal therapy: preliminary findings. *Arch Gen Psychiatry* 2001; **58**: 631–40.

57. Henry ME, Schmidt ME, Matochik JA *et al*. The effects of ECT on brain glucose: a pilot FDG PET study. *J ECT* 2001; **17**: 33–40.

58. Nobler MS, Roose SP, Prohovnik I *et al*. Regional cerebral blood flow in mood disorders, V.: Effects of antidepressant medication in late-life depression. *Am J Geriatr Psychiatry* 2000; **8**: 289–96.

59. Liotti M, Mayberg HS, Brannan SK *et al*. Differential limbic–cortical correlates of sadness and anxiety in healthy subjects: implications for affective disorders. *Biol Psychiatry* 2000; **48**: 30–42.

60. Wu JC, Gillin JC, Buchsbaum MS *et al*. Sleep deprivation PET correlations of Hamilton symptom improvement ratings with changes in relative glucose metabolism in patients with depression. *J Affect Disord* 2008; **107**: 181–86.

61. Smith GS, Reynolds CF, 3rd, Houck PR *et al*. Glucose metabolic response to total sleep deprivation, recovery sleep, and acute antidepressant treatment as functional neuroanatomic correlates of treatment outcome in geriatric depression. *Am J Geriatr Psychiatry* 2002; **10**: 561–67.

62. Smith GS, Reynolds CF, 3rd, Houck PR *et al*. Cerebral glucose metabolic response to combined total sleep deprivation and antidepressant treatment in geriatric depression: a randomized, placebo-controlled study. *Psychiatry Res* 2009; **171**: 1–9.

63. Jack CR, Jr., Dickson DW, Parisi JE *et al*. Antemortem MRI findings correlate with hippocampal neuropathology in typical ageing and dementia. *Neurology* 2002; **58**: 750–57.

64. Sorg C, Riedl V, Perneczky R, Kurz A, Wohlschläger AM. Impact of Alzheimer's disease on the functional connectivity of spontaneous brain activity. *Curr Alzheimer Res* 2009; **6**: 541–53.

65. Sorg C, Riedl V, Muhlau M *et al*. Selective changes of resting-state networks in individuals at risk for Alzheimer's disease. *Proc Natl Acad Sci USA* 2007; **104**: 18760–65.

66. Schmidt J, Hapfelmeier A, Mueller M *et al*. Interpreting PET scans by structured patient data: a data mining case study in dementia research. *KAIS* 2009; 23 Jul 2009 (epub).

Neurophysiology of the Ageing Brain

Paolo Maria Rossini and Laura Parisi

Clinica Neurologica University Campus Bio-Medico, Rome, Italy

INTRODUCTION

The few individuals who reach very old age are called 'longevity outliers'. This particular group represents the fastest growing age group worldwide. For instance, the number of centenarians increases steadily in the US population and their numbers are expected to grow to more than 400 000 in the next 30 years[1].

Awareness of age-related diseases such as dementia has prompted considerable interest in the study of the ageing human brain to trace a clear boundary between physiological and pathological ageing, to carry out primary prevention on populations at high risk of developing dementia, to achieve secondary prevention and to apply eventual disease-modifying therapy to at-risk subjects. Results from these types of studies could be used to plan political and public health interventions. Recent investigations have prompted advancement in biochemical, structural, functional and neurophysiological fields.

Ageing is a physiological dynamic process due to a specific property of the central nervous system (CNS) known as neuronal plasticity. The concept of 'plasticity' applied to neurobiology typically denotes the *potential for change* in addition to the mechanisms of self-repair and/or of reorganization of neural connections. Neural plasticity underlies learning as well as endogenous brain function repair[2], including synaptic efficacy and *synaptic redundancy*; on this basis the functional status and distribution of a network depends on the balance between neural excitation and inhibition, with some areas appearing silent or 'masked' by a mechanism of active tonic inhibition, the latter being prone to alteration or removal, causing a rapid change of the functional network, a process termed 'unmasking'[3]. Additional mechanisms include *long-term potentiation* (LTP) and *long-term depression* (LTD), which contribute to the functional strengthening or weakening of existing synapses by which information is stored in the CNS. LTP has been regarded as the prototypic mechanism of modified synaptic efficacy, and it can differently occur via modification of the input to a postsynaptic cell, the concomitant synchronous input to the synapse from another cell, or postsynaptic depolarization. LTD stems from Na^+ or Ca^{2+} channels at least for short-term changes, while LTP-like mechanisms include glutamate-dependent NMDA receptor activation for long-term changes, a process that can be antagonized by GABA inhibition[4]. Another plasticity-related process is neuronal sprouting and formation of new synapses influenced by local neurotransmitter, neurotrophic factors and synaptic protein synthesis[5]. In particular, dendrites and related spines with synaptic connections undergo continuous remodelling most likely also modulated by interaction with neighbouring astrocytes[4].

Postmortem examinations show that brain ageing is characterized by the formation of neurofibrillary tangles and senile plaques in both cognitively intact individuals and patients with dementia, namely Alzheimer's disease[1]. The ubiquitous presence of these lesions and the steady increase of the prevalence of dementia up to 85 years have strongly supported a continuum between normal and pathological brain ageing.

Ageing is a physiological process that occurs asynchronously in different areas of the brain, its rate being also dependent on the style of life. The differential age-related changes produced in several regions of the brain in the anatomy of neurons, volume tissue, density and dynamics of several neurotransmitters give support to this suggestion[6].

From a macroscopic point of view, brain ageing becomes evident by atrophy. In 1955 Brody estimated that the neuronal loss was about 40%. In 1986 Braak and Braak specified that during the ageing, especially pyramidal cells of frontal lobes die. Some studies suggest that the *primum movens* is a functional and then a structural modification of synapses[7]. It is followed by a modification of the dendritic tree and then by the neuronal death, today known as *aposklesis*. Particularly, the hippocampus seems to be one of the most vulnerable structures in brain ageing.

Functional modifications precede the structural ones, so it is hoped that by integrating structural techniques with the functional ones it will be possible to better investigate brain ageing. Moreover, modern neurophysiological techniques (transcranial magnetic stimulation, TMS; electroencephalography, EEG; magnetoencephalography, MEG; event-related potentials, EPRs) could be helpful for this purpose, being of low cost and non-invasive[8]. Modern techniques of functional neurophysiological imaging allow investigation with high accuracy of the cortico-cortical 'connectivity' that is the base for synchronization and functional binding. These phenomena allow neuronal populations, even at a distance, to contribute to a specific task or to process a specific input working together only for a few milliseconds. Analysis of EEG and MEG signals and TMS techniques gives us worthwhile information about that.

TRANSCRANIAL MAGNETIC STIMULATION

TMS is a brief and intense magnetic field, created by a strong electric current circulating within a coil resting on the scalp; it penetrates human tissue painlessly and, if the current amplitude, duration and direction are appropriate, it induces in the brain (or in spinal roots, or in nerves) electric currents that can depolarize neurons or their axons. TMS can demonstrate causal relationships between the stimulated area and behaviour. It can be used to interfere with the neuronal activity underlying sensory processing, motor planning or execution, attention and visual processing or awareness, different forms of declarative and non-declarative memory, reasoning, mathematics, language and consciousness. This temporary disruptive effect of TMS on cortical function is often referred to as a 'virtual lesion' and is likely to occur because the stimulus transiently synchronizes the activity of a large proportion of neurons under the coil, thus inducing a long-lasting, generalized inhibitory postsynaptic potential that reduces cortical activity for the next 50 to 200 milliseconds, depending on stimulus intensity and duration. Moreover, repetitive TMS (rTMS) can produce changes – outlasting the period of stimulation – in cortical excitability[9].

rTMS studies are increasing knowledge about correlation between anatomic structures and their functions. For example, they showed that dorsolateral prefrontal cortex (DLPCF) is implicated in working memory and in verbal episodic memory tasks.

Lesions of frontal lobes cause a reduction of learning and memory abilities but they do not cause the same memory loss as bilateral hippocampal lesions do. So, it has been demonstrated that prefrontal cortex (PFC) is involved in episodic memory tasks and that during encoding or retrieval, there are different areas of PFC that are activated with different *patterns*. It has been demonstrated that left PFC is involved in encoding processes; instead right PFC is involved in retrieval processes. This theory is known as hemispherical encoding retrieval asymmetry (HERA)[9-11]. Nowadays, it is known that the HERA model is not so absolute but that there could be variations due to the nature of the presented stimuli, the strategies of memorization used and the grade of difficulty of the task. Recently, positron emission tomography (PET) and functional magnetic resonance imaging (fMRI) studies have demonstrated that PFC activity tends to be less asymmetric in older than in younger adults (hemispheric asymmetry reduction in old adults, HAROLD). This change may help counteract age-related neurocognitive decline (compensation hypothesis) or it may reflect an age-related difficulty in recruiting specialized neural mechanisms (dedifferentiation hypothesis)[12,13]. Functional neuroimaging techniques could not be used to study whether the loss of asymmetry during ageing reflects compensatory mechanisms or dedifferentiation processes; in fact, they show only the activation of a specific area during a task, but this activation could be related to the performance of the task without being the cause. Instead, this issue was addressed by using rTMS to assess causal relationships between performance and stimulated brain regions. Rossi *et al.* studied the effects of rTMS applied to the left or right DLPFC simultaneously with the presentation of memoranda on visuo-spatial recognition memory task, in a population of healthy subjects divided into two classes by age (<45 and >50 years). In the younger subjects, rTMS of the right DLPFC interfered with retrieval more than left DLPFC stimulation. The asymmetry of the effect progressively vanished with ageing, as indicated by bilateral interference effects on recognition performance. Conversely, the predominance of left DLPFC effect during encoding was not abolished in the older subjects, thereby indicating its causal role

for encoding along the life span. Findings with rTMS suggest that the bilateral engagement of the DLPFC has a compensatory role on episodic memory performance across the age span[13].

CORTICAL EXCITABILITY

Physiological ageing is associated with more complex activations of the motor system to compensate for the reduced skill in motor performance[14,15]. Therefore, TMS variables can provide useful clues to investigate causally subclinical changes of cortical excitability at the motor cortex level. Unfortunately, studies do not show converging findings, probably as a result of technical and experimental differences among them[13,16-18]. Apart from assessing cortical excitability, TMS can be used to measure intracortical facilitatory and inhibitory mechanisms resulting from the balance among neurotransmitters, and dynamic synaptic adaptations to progressive neuronal loss. Motor threshold is generally reduced in Alzheimer's disease compared to healthy age-matched controls and is similarly reduced in subcortical ischaemic vascular dementia[16,19,20], even if several reports have not found reduction of motor thresholds[21,22], with one study noting increased rather than decreased motor thresholds in Alzheimer's disease[23]. Global cortical hyperexcitability while the brain is 'at rest' in Alzheimer's disease is a consistent result[22], which seems to occur independently of GABAergic and cholinergic cortico-cortical mechanism dysfunction as reduced motor thresholds and intracortical inhibition (ICI) and short-latency afferent inhibition (SAI) are uncorrelated. Since TMS does not provide specific pathophysiological information but is sensitive to the 'global weight' of several neurotransmitters as well as subcortical and cortical motor inputs, interpretation of cortical hyperexcitability in Alzheimer's disease is not yet possible.

The majority of these TMS results indicate that the cortex of Alzheimer's disease patients is hyperexcitable, and that such hyperexcitability may offer clues for the differential diagnosis from other dementias in which the cholinergic deficit is not predominant. An intriguing issue that can be addressed by TMS is the study of cortical reorganization of the motor output in Alzheimer's disease. Indeed, motor cortex physiological organization is early involved in Alzheimer's disease, despite the lack of clinically evident motor deficits, which only appear later[24]. This observation is not surprising considering that the motor cortex, through muscarinic receptors and cholinergic terminals, receives a major input from the nucleus basalis of Meynert[25]. Mapping of motor output in mild Alzheimer's disease patients asymptomatic for motor deficits has demonstrated frontal and medial shift of the cortical motor maps for hand muscles. In healthy controls the centre of gravity of motor cortical output is coincident with the site of maximal excitability (hot spot[26]), whereas in Alzheimer's disease patients it shifts towards frontal and medial regions in the absence of changes in the hot spot[22]. An altered synaptic plasticity in Alzheimer's disease also has been demonstrated by applying brief trains of high-frequency rTMS to motor cortex and recording motor-evoked potentials (MEPs) from the contralateral hand muscles. This procedure can induce a progressive increase in MEP size in normal age-matched controls, but it produces opposite changes in Alzheimer's disease. This finding was interpreted as an altered short-term synaptic enhancement in excitatory circuits of the motor cortex. Additional assessment of these findings will be required by evaluating Alzheimer's disease patients after different pharmacological treatments (e.g. cholinergic versus drugs acting on NMDA glutamate receptors).

In summary, TMS assays of cortical disinhibition in Alzheimer's disease as a dysfunction of a single neurotransmitter in a single neural circuit or as the net effect of a complex involvement of more than one neurotransmitter system in several brain areas likely reflects a single facet of a pathological mosaic. A lasting preclinical condition under the attack of pro-degenerative agents could produce the Alzheimer's disease brain as alternative strategies of functioning belonging to the brain reserve even for the execution of simple motor tasks[15,22]. The emerging evidence indicates that the 'stressed synapses' may acquire a different function both in terms of effects and of utilized neurotransmitter and may be strongly dependent on the sampling time of the tested patients[27].

rTMS could be useful to improve cognitive performance in healthy subjects or in patients with mild cognitive impairment (MCI). These effects include selective shortening of picture naming[28] and action naming without changing verbal reaction times for naming objects[29], improving subjects' speed at finding the solution to a reasoning puzzle[30], and improving performance on a choice reaction task[31]. It can be hypothesized that rTMS – by shifting the level of cortical excitability – might allow either more or less access (by interfering, for example, with the functioning of local inhibitory circuits) to brain networks relevant to the experimental task. These effects might vary depending on the timing of the TMS stimulation and on the hierarchical role of the brain area stimulated within the whole functional network underpinning the function under investigation.

These findings reflect the potential of rTMS to recruit compensatory networks that underlie the memory-encoding process and suggest that rTMS is capable of transient and positive rehabilitative influences on brain function[9,32].

EEG/MEG RHYTHMS

Advanced EEG analysis techniques together with analysis of MEG signals contribute to the investigation of brain ageing. Among EEG analysis techniques, the most worthy are the surface Laplacian transformation or coherence analysis of EEG, which can illustrate changes in specific oscillatory frequencies over time and can provide quantitative measurements of individual rhythm[33]. Moreover, the low resolution electromagnetic topography algorithm (LORETA) technique computes three-dimensional linear solutions from multi-channel input to localize generators *in* the brain from the EEG field distribution on the scalp by employing a three-shell spherical head model of the scalp, skull and brain compartments[34]. LORETA solutions consist of voxel z-current density values that are used to predict EEG spectral power density at scalp electrodes. A normalization method yields current density at each voxel for the power density averaged across all frequencies (0.5–45 Hz) and voxels of the brain volume.

Instead, MEG is a non-invasive technique that permits spatial identification of neuronal activation from spontaneous cerebral or external stimulus presentation. MEG signal characteristics are not influenced by extracerebral tissue layers (i.e. meninges, skull, scalp, muscles). MEG signals originate from current flow of tangential dipoles in cortical gyri and sulci[35,36]. The signals reflect the spatial and temporal production of a dipolar source modelled as an equivalent current dipole (ECD). This method provides three-dimensional localization of dipolar field distributions over the scalp with time resolution of milliseconds. Hence, MEG signals can directly estimate the number of active neural pools and provide accurate measures of the intracellular currents in a limited shallow brain region below the recording sensor without influence from volume conduction.

Resting EEG changes across physiological ageing, with gradual changes in spectral power profile indicating a pronounced amplitude decrease of alpha (8–13 Hz) and a global 'slowing' of the background EEG, with increases in power and topographic location in the slower delta (2–4 Hz) and theta (4–8 Hz) frequency ranges[37–39]. Ageing effects on parieto-occipital alpha rhythms reflect the activity of dominant oscillatory neural network modulated by thalamo-cortical and cortico-cortical interactions facilitating/inhibiting the transmission of sensorimotor information and the retrieval of semantic information from cortical storage[40,41]. Low-frequency alpha is primarily related to the subject's global attentive readiness, whereas high-frequency alpha reflects the oscillation of neural systems for the elaboration of sensorimotor or semantic information[39]. Over the course of age, alpha power decreases combined with changes in cholinergic basal forebrain system and in the excitatory activity in the cholinergic brainstem pathway[42]. Despite the relative consensus on alpha decrease, there is no general agreement on the modulation of delta and theta activity in brain ageing[43].

Resting EEG changes in pathological brain ageing. When compared to healthy normal elderly (Nold) subjects, Alzheimer's disease patients exhibit high power for delta and theta and low power for posterior alpha (8–12 Hz) and/or beta (13–30 Hz) frequencies[44–47]. EEG abnormalities were associated with altered regional blood flow/metabolism and with impaired global cognitive function as evaluated by Mini-Mental State Examination (MMSE)[48,49].

MEG also has provided contributions to the understanding of the cortical rhythms in pathological ageing. Parieto-temporal delta and theta sources enhanced in power in Alzheimer's disease compared to Nold subjects in association with hippocampal atrophy[50]. Furthermore, Alzheimer's disease subjects demonstrated a decrease of alpha sources in parieto-occipital region possibly compensated by an increase of temporal alpha sources[51]. Finally, cortical theta and alpha rhythms as revealed by MEG have discriminated the severity level of Alzheimer's disease and distinguished it from Lewy body dementia.

EEG power *per se* does not capture one of the main features of Alzheimer's disease, namely the impairment of functional neural connectivity. It has been reported that Alzheimer's disease patients present an abnormal linear coupling of EEG rhythms among cortical regions, as revealed by spectral EEG coherence[52–56], suggesting a linear temporal synchronicity of coupled EEG rhythms from simultaneously engaged neural sources. Such findings imply that functional coupling of cortical rhythms is modulated by cholinergic systems, and that a decrease of cortical EEG coherence may be a fine-grained marker of Alzheimer's disease, since it is characterized by defective basal forebrain cholinergic inputs to cortex and hippocampus[57]. Most EEG studies of Alzheimer's disease have reported a prominent decrease of alpha band coherence[52,54–56,58–60]. This result also has been found to be associated with ApoE genetic risk, which is hypothesized to be mediated by cholinergic deficit[52]. However, delta and theta band coherence changes in Alzheimer's disease are not homogeneous, as some studies demonstrate a decrease of slow-band EEG coherence, whereas others find an increase[56,61].

MCI subjects present an intermediate magnitude of low-frequency alpha (8–10.5 Hz) activity from parietal, occipital and limbic areas, compared to mild Alzheimer's disease and normal elderly[62]. Increase of slow EEG power coupled with a decrease in alpha activity is linked to cognitive performance decline in MCI patients compared to Nold. More importantly, the magnitude of these sources is correlated negatively with MMSE scores across subjects of the three groups, suggesting that EEG evidence of alpha power decrease in MCI compared to normal subjects is related to behavioural cognition[60,63–65].

The relative decrement of posterior low-frequency alpha sources in MCI may be related to an initial selective impairment of the cholinergic basal forebrain, which could induce a sustained increase of the excitatory activity in the cholinergic brainstem pathway[42]. As a consequence, the increased excitability of thalamo-cortical connections would desynchronize the resting alpha rhythms and enhance the cortical excitability as seen in Alzheimer's disease. Hence, changes of low-frequency alpha power in MCI and mild Alzheimer's disease suggest a progressive impairment of the thalamo-cortical and cortico-cortical systems that govern visual attention. This hypothesis is consistent with clinical findings of increasing deficits of visuospatial abilities in MCI and mild Alzheimer's disease. Similarly, limbic sources imply a progressive impairment of thalamo-cortical and cortico-cortical systems regulating attention tone for memory functions.

Quantitative EEG is able to predict with a good approximation MCI progression to Alzheimer's disease in a short run; this was demonstrated by Rossini et al.[66], who investigated whether combined analysis of EEG power and coherence provides early and reliable discrimination of MCI subjects who will convert to Alzheimer's disease after a relatively brief follow-up.

EEG and MEG rhythms can change over time in relation to a specific event. Event-related desynchronization (ERD) and event-related synchronization (ERS) of EEG or MEG rhythms describe neuroelectric events preceding and following a task execution[39]. ERD/ERS is defined as reduction/increase in EEG power during event (sensory, motor, cognitive) when compared to baseline at a certain frequency band. Alpha band hyper-reactivity in Alzheimer's disease as indexed by increased alpha ERD suggests an abnormal increase of the cortical excitation or disinhibition even during simple cognitive demands. Such findings agree with previous functional neuroimaging studies on memory, which demonstrated a stronger allocation of cortical resources in Alzheimer's disease when compared to Nold subjects[66,67]. In addition, they are consonant with other findings of abnormal central rhythms when processing sensory stimuli or performing voluntary movements and with hyper-reactivity of Alzheimer's disease primary motor cortex as revealed by TMS[15,68].

Artificial neural networks (ANNs) are a useful tool in early diagnosing of dementia; they elaborate in an innovative way EEG signals. Starting from a standard EEG recorded with the international 10–20 system, it is a low cost and non-invasive procedure, it is widespread and it does not require highly qualified staff at the moment of recording. It has been shown that a correct automatic classification of MCI and Alzheimer's disease subjects can be obtained extracting spatial information content of the resting EEG voltage by ANNs with an accuracy greater than 92%[69]. Moreover, the classification of the individual Nold and MCI subjects, with this tool, could reach a sensitivity of 95.87% and a specificity of 91.06% (93.46% accuracy)[70,71]. ANNs could be a worthy tool to improve screening of high-risk population one day.

CONCLUSION

Doubtless the only approach to trace a narrow line between physiological and pathological ageing is integrating genetic, biological, structural and functional variables. The latter change early, so measurement of functional variables could be helpful for early diagnosis. Neurophysiological tools that are low cost, non-invasive and widespread could be useful for large-scale screening and follow-up of populations at high risk of developing dementia. One of the most exciting challenges is to improve them.

REFERENCES

1. Imhof A, Kövari E, von Gunten A et al. Morphological substrates of cognitive decline in nonagenarians and centenarians: a new paradigm? J Neurol Sci 2007; **257**: 72–9.
2. Rossini PM, Rossi S, Babiloni C, Polich J. Clinical neurophysiology of aging brain: from normal aging to neurodegeneration. Prog Neurobiol 2007; **83**(6): 375–400.
3. Jacobs KM, Donoghue JP. Reshaping the cortical motor map by unmasking latent intracortical connections. Science 1991; **251**: 944–7.
4. Ziemann U, Hallett M, Cohen LG. Mechanisms of deafferentation induced plasticity in human motor cortex. J Neurosci 1998; **18**, 7000–7007.
5. Lisman J, Spruston N. Postsynaptic depolarization requirements for LTP and LTD: a critique of spike timing-dependent plasticity. Nat Neurosci 2005; **8**: 839–41.
6. Mora F, Segovia G, del Arco, A. Aging, plasticity and environmental enrichment: structural changes and neurotransmitter dynamics in several areas of the brain. Brain Res Rev 2007; **55**: 78–88.
7. Braak H, Braak E. Staging of Alzheimer's disease-related neurofibrillary changes. Neurobiol Aging 1995; **16**; 271–8, discussion 278–84.
8. Rossini PM, Caltagirone C, Castriota Scanderberg A et al. Hand motor cortical area reorganization in stroke: a study with fMRI, MEG and TCS maps. Neuroreport 1998; **9**(9): 2141–6.
9. Rossini PM, Rossi S. Transcranial magnetic stimulation: diagnostic, therapeutic, and research potential. Neurology 2007; **68**: 484–8.
10. Hallett M. Transcranial magnetic stimulation and the human brain. Nature 2000; **406**: 147–50.
11. Walsh V, Cowey A. Transcranial magnetic stimulation and cognitive neuroscience. Nat Rev Neurosci 2000; **1**: 73–9.
12. Babiloni C, Ferri R, Binetti G et al. Fronto-parietal coupling of brain rhythms in mild cognitive impairment: a multicentric EEG study. Brain Res Bull 2006; **69**(1): 63–73.
13. Rossi S, Miniussi C, Pasqualetti P et al. Age-related functional changes of prefrontal cortex in long-term memory. A repetitive transcranial magnetic stimulation (rTMS) study. J Neurosci 2004; **24**. 7939–44.
14. Ward NS, Frackowiack RS. Age-related changes in the neural correlates of motor performance. Brain 2003; **126**: 873–88.
15. Babiloni C, Babiloni F, Carducci F et al. Movement-related electroencephalographic reactivity in Alzheimer disease. Neuroimage 2000; **12**(2): 139–46.
16. Pepin JL, Bogacz D, De Pasqua V, Delwaide PJ. Motor cortex inhibition is not impaired in patients with Alzheimer's disease: evidence from paired transcranial magnetic stimulation. J Neurol Sci 1999; **170**: 119–23.
17. Oliviero A, Profice P, Tonali PA et al. Effects of aging on motor cortex excitability. Neurosci Res 2006; **55**: 74–7.
18. Rossini PM, Desiato MT, Caramia MD. Age-related changes of motor evoked potentials in healthy humans: non-invasive evaluation of central and peripheral motor tract excitability and conductivity. Brain Res 1992; **593**: 14–19.
19. De Carvalho M, de Mendoza A, Miranda P, Garcia C, De Lourdes M. Magnetic stimulation in Alzheimer's disease. J Neurol 1997; **244**: 304–7.

20. Di Lazzaro V, Pilato F, Dileone M et al. In vivo cholinergic circuit evaluation in frontotemporal and Alzheimer dementias. Neurology 2006; 66: 1111–13.

21. Liepert J, Bar KJ, Meske U, Weiller C. Motor cortex disinhibition in Alzheimer's disease. Clin Neurophysiol 2001; 112: 1436–41.

22. Ferreri F, Pauri F, Pasqualetti P et al. Motor cortex excitability in Alzheimer's disease: a transcranial magnetic stimulation study. Ann Neurol 2003; 53: 102–8.

23. Perretti A, Grossi D, Fragassi N et al. Evaluation of the motor cortex by magnetic stimulation in patients with Alzheimer disease. J Neurol Sci 1996; 135: 31–7.

24. Suva D, Favre I, Kraftsik R et al. Primary motor cortex involvement in Alzheimer disease. J Neuropathol Exp Neurol 1999; 58: 1125–34.

25. Selden NR, Gitelman DR, Salamon-Muruyama N et al. Trajectories of cholinergic pathways within the cerebral hemispheres of the human brain. Brain 1998; 121: 2249–57.

26. Cicinelli P, Traversa A, Bassi A et al. Interhemispheric differences of hand muscle representation in human motor cortex. Muscle Nerve 1997; 20: 535–42.

27. Armstrong DM, Sheffield R, Mishizen-Eberz AJ et al. Plasticity of glutamate and GABAA receptors in the hippocampus of patients with Alzheimer's disease. Cell Mol Neurobiol 2003; 23: 491–505.

28. Mottaghy FM, Hungs M, Brügmann M et al. Facilitation of picture naming after repetitive transcranial magnetic stimulation. Neurology 1999; 53: 1806–12.

29. Cappa SF, Sandrini M, Rossini PM, Sosta K, Miniussi C. The role of left frontal lobe in action naming: rTMS evidence. Neurology 2002; 59: 720–23.

30. Boroojerdi B, Phipps M, Kopylev L et al. Enhancing analogic reasoning with rTMS over the left prefrontal cortex. Neurology 2001; 56: 526–8.

31. Evers S, Böckermann I, Nyhuis PW. The impact of transcranial magnetic stimulation on cognitive processing: an event-related potential study. Neuroreport 2001; 12: 2915–18.

32. Rossi S, Rossini PM. TMS in cognitive plasticity and the potential for rehabilitation. Trends Cogn Sci 2004; 8: 273–9.

33. Babiloni F, Carducci F, Cincotti F et al. Linear inverse source estimate of combined EEG and MEG data related to voluntary movements. Hum Brain Mapp 2001; 14(4): 197–209.

34. Pascual-Marqui RD, Lehmann D, Koenig T et al. Low resolution brain electromagnetic tomography (LORETA) functional imaging in acute, neurolepticnaive, first-episode, productive schizophrenia. Psychiatry Res 1999; 90(3): 169–79.

35. Hari R, Lounasmaa OV. Recording and interpretation of cerebral magnetic fields. Science 1989; 244(4903): 432–6.

36. Romani GL, Williamson SJ, Kaufman L. Tonotopic organization of the human auditory cortex. Science 1982; 216(4552): 1339–40.

37. Dujardin K, Bourriez JL, Guieu JD. Event-related desynchronization (ERD) patterns during memory processes: effects of aging and task difficulty. Electroencephalogr Clin Neurophysiol 1995; 96(2): 169–82.

38. Klass DW, Brenner RP. Electroencephalography of the elderly. J Clin Neurophysiol 1995; 12(2): 116–31.

39. Klimesch W. EEG alpha and theta oscillations reflect cognitive and memory performance: a review and analysis. Brain Res Brain Res Rev 1999; 29(2–3): 169–95.

40. Steriade M, Llinas RR. The functional states of the thalamus and the associated neuronal interplay. Physiol Rev 1988; 68(3): 649–742.

41. Pfurtscheller G, Lopez da Silva F. Event-related EEG/MEG synchronization and desynchronization: basic principles. Clin Neurophysiol 1999; 110: 1842–57.

42. Sarter M, Bruno JP. Cortical acetylcholine, reality distortion, schizophrenia, and Lewy Body Dementia: too much or too little cortical acetylcholine? Brain Cogn 1998; 38(3): 297–316.

43. Hartikainen P, Soininen H, Partanen J, Helkala EL, Riekkinen P. Aging and spectral analysis of EEG in normal subjects: a link to memory and CSF AChE. Acta Neurol Scand 1992; 86(2): 148–55.

44. Dierks T, Jelic V, Pascual-Marqui RD et al. Spatial pattern of cerebral glucose metabolism (PET) correlates with localization of intracerebral EEG-generators in Alzheimer's disease. Clin Neurophysiol 2000; 111(10): 1817–24.

45. Ponomareva NV, Selesneva ND, Jarikov GA. EEG alterations in subjects at high familial risk for Alzheimer's disease. Neuropsychobiology 2003; 48(3): 152–9.

46. Babiloni C, Binetti G, Cassetta E et al. Mapping distributed sources of cortical rhythms in mild Alzheimer's disease: a multicentric EEG study. Neuroimage 2004; 22(1): 57–67.

47. Prichep LS. Use of normative databases and statistical methods in demonstrating clinical utility of QEEG: importance and cautions. Clin EEG Neurosci 2005; 36(2): 82–7.

48. Sloan EP, Fenton GW, Kennedy NS, MacLennan JM. Electroencephalography and single photon emission computed tomography in dementia: a comparative study. Psychol Med 1995; 25(3): 631–8.

49. Rodriguez G, Nobili F, Copello F et al. 99mTc-HMPAO regional cerebral blood flow and quantitative electroencephalography in Alzheimer's disease: a correlative study. J Nucl Med 1999; 40(4): 522–9.

50. Fernandez A, Arrazola J, Maestu F et al. Correlations of hippocampal atrophy and focal low-frequency magnetic activity in Alzheimer disease: volumetric MR imaging-magnetoencephalographic study. AJNR Am J Neuroradiol 2003; 24(3): 481–7.

51. Osipova D, Ahveninen J, Jensen O, Ylikoski A, Pekkonen E. Altered generation of spontaneous oscillations in Alzheimer's disease. Neuroimage 2005; 27(4): 835–41.

52. Jelic V, Julin P, Shigeta M et al. Apolipoprotein E epsilon4 allele decreases functional connectivity in Alzheimer's disease as measured by EEG coherence. J Neurol Neurosurg Psychiatr 1997; 63(1): 59–65.

53. Locatelli T, Cursi M, Liberati D, Franceschi M, Comi G. EEG coherence in Alzheimer's disease. Electroencephalogr Clin Neurophysiol 1998; 106(3): 229–37.

54. Wada Y, Nanbu Y, Koshino Y, Yamaguchi N, Hashimoto T. Reduced interhemispheric EEG coherence in Alzheimer disease: analysis during rest and photic stimulation. Alzheimer Dis Assoc Disord 1998; 12(3): 175–81.

55. Knott V, Mohr E, Mahoney C, Ilivitsky V. Electroencephalographic coherence in Alzheimer's disease: comparisons with a control group and population norms. J Geriatr Psychiatry Neurol 2000; 13(1): 1–8.

56. Adler G, Brassen S, Jajcevic A. EEG coherence in Alzheimer's dementia. J Neural Transm 2003; 110(9): 1051–8.

57. Stam CJ, Jones BF, Manshanden I *et al*. Magnetoencephalographic evaluation of resting-state functional connectivity in Alzheimer's disease. *Neuroimage* 2006; **32**(3): 1335–44.

58. Leuchter AF, Newton TF, Cook IA *et al*. Changes in brain functional connectivity in Alzheimer-type and multi-infarct dementia. *Brain* 1992; **115**(5): 1543–61.

59. Cook IA, Leuchter AF. Synaptic dysfunction in Alzheimer's disease: clinical assessment using quantitative EEG. *Behav Brain Res* 1996; **78**(1): 15–23.

60. Jelic V, Johansson SE, Almkvist O *et al*. Quantitative electroencephalography in mild cognitive impairment: longitudinal changes and possible prediction of Alzheimer's disease. *Neurobiol Aging* 2000; **21**(4): 533–40.

61. Brunovsky M, Matousek M, Edman A, Cervena K, Krajca V. Objective assessment of the degree of dementia by means of EEG. *Neuropsychobiology* 2003; **48**(1): 19–26.

62. Babiloni C, Binetti G, Cassetta E *et al*. Sources of cortical rhythms change as a function of cognitive impairment in pathological aging: a multicenter study. *Clin Neurophysiol* 2006; **117**(2): 252–68.

63. Grunwald M, Busse F, Hensel A *et al*. Correlation between cortical theta activity and hippocampal volumes in health, mild cognitive impairment, and mild dementia. *J Clin Neurophysiol* 2001; **18**(2): 178–84.

64. Kwak YT. Quantitative EEG findings in different stages of Alzheimer's disease. *J Clin Neurophysiol* 2006; **23**(5): 456–61.

65. Rossini PM, Del Percio C, Pasqualetti P *et al*. Conversion from mild cognitive impairment to Alzheimer's disease is predicted by sources and coherence of brain electroencephalography rhythms. *Neuroscience* 2006; **143**(3): 793–803.

66. Grady CL, Furey ML, Pietrini P, Horwitz B, Rapoport SI. Altered brain functional connectivity and impaired short-term memory in Alzheimer's disease. *Brain* 2001; **124**(4): 739–56.

67. Grossman M, Koenig P, Glosser G *et al*. Neural basis for semantic memory difficulty in Alzheimer's disease: an fMRI study. *Brain* 2003; **126**(2): 292–311.

68. Babiloni C, Miniussi C, Moretti DV *et al*. Cortical networks generating movement-related EEG rhythms in Alzheimer's disease: an EEG coherence study. *Behav Neurosci* 2004; **118**(4): 698–706.

69. Rossini PM, Buscema M, Capriotti M *et al*. Is it possible to automatically distinguish resting EEG data of normal elderly vs. mild cognitive impairment subjects with high degree of accuracy? *Clin Neurophysiol* 2008; **119**(7): 1534–45.

70. Buscema M, Capriotti M, Bergami F *et al*. The implicit function as squashing time model: a novel parallel nonlinear EEG analysis technique distinguishing mild cognitive impairment and Alzheimer's disease subjects with high degree of accuracy. *Comput Intell Neurosci* 2007; 35021.

71. Buscema M, Rossini P, Babiloni C, Grossi E. The IFAST model, a novel parallel nonlinear EEG analysis technique, distinguishes mild cognitive impairment and Alzheimer's disease patients with high degree of accuracy. *Artif Intell Med* 2007; **40**(2): 127–41.

7

Potential Regeneration of the Ageing Brain

Stephen B. Dunnett

School of Biosciences, Cardiff University, UK

The brain does not spontaneously regenerate. As long ago as 1928, Cajal recorded that 'once development was ended, the founts of growth and regeneration of axons and dendrites dried up irrevocably. In adult centres ... everything may die, nothing may be regenerated'[1]. Although it remains the case that the damaged mammalian central nervous system (CNS) does not in general generate new nerve cells in response to disease or injury, the intervening 70 years have identified a considerable plasticity of axons to remodel nerve connections and a limited degree of neurogenesis that opens new opportunities for promoting regeneration and repair in the damaged, diseased or ageing nervous system (see Figure 7.1).

ADAPTIVE PLASTICITY

Even if lost cells are not replaced, spared neurons and fibres retain a considerable degree of plasticity to adapt to lost connections by adaptive biochemical compensation both at the presynaptic level – for example by changes in cell firing, transmitter synthesis, release and reuptake – and postsynaptically, by changes in receptor density, receptor sensitivity and post-synaptic signalling (Figure 7.1C)[2,3].

COLLATERAL SPROUTING

The first clear evidence that Cajal's dictum was overly pessimistic in relation to the mammalian CNS came from the demonstration that if a septal cell loses some of its normal axonal inputs then other afferent axons can sprout into the vacated spaces to form new synaptic connections with the target cell[4]. If the new inputs are from a different source they are by and large not functional. However, collateral sprouting of spared fibres of the same systems do appear to be able to sustain functional recovery in a number of model circuits of the brain (Figure 7.1D)[3,5,6].

REGENERATIVE SPROUTING

A major problem for extensive axonal reorganization in the adult brain is that although axons can undergo a degree of local sprouting, they do not typically retain the developmental capacity for long-distance growth through the CNS to distant targets (Figure 7.1E)[3,7]. Long-distance growth of axons can nevertheless be promoted by providing an alternative substrate for growth such as Schwann cells from the peripheral nervous system (PNS) which can be used to bridge a gap caused by a lesion cutting a pathway, or be implanted as a track along which new axons can grow (Figure 7.1H)[8].

NEURAL TRANSPLANTATION

When essential populations of neurones are lost they may be replaced by transplantation. The techniques are now well established for transplantation of embryonic cells derived from the CNS into the brain of adult or aged experimental animals (Figure 7.1G), and such grafts have been demonstrated to survive, repopulate areas of denervation, replace deficient innervations, and restore lost functions in a wide variety of model systems[9,10]. There is now compelling clinical evidence that such grafts can provide a substantial alleviation of symptoms in Parkinson's disease[11], and clinical trials are now underway in Huntington's disease, spinal cord injury and stroke[12-14]. It remains a matter of speculation whether neuronal transplantation can alleviate the more diffuse and widespread degeneration associated with ageing and the dementias.

TROPHIC SUPPORT

Neuronal connections are dependent upon trophic support from their targets, and neurodegenerative diseases of ageing may in part be attributable to a decline in growth factor support[15]. Thus, an alternative approach to prevention of progressive neurodegeneration, and to induction and guidance of regenerative axon growth, is to apply or replace identified trophic factors explicitly. For example, dopaminergic neurones, which decline in several neurodegenerative diseases of ageing, are dependent upon trophic factors (including brain-derived neurotrophic factor (BDNF) and glial cell-derived neurotrophic factor (GDNF)) for trophic support. Chronic infusion of GDNF into the striatum or midbrain can inhibit progressive lesion and age-related atrophy of midbrain dopamine neurons and block the functional decline in motor abilities (Figure 7.1F) both in experimental animals[16] and in man[17]. A similar strategy involving chronic central infusions of nerve growth factor (NGF) has been attempted in a pilot experiment in Alzheimer's disease with only modest success[18]. A major issue to be resolved is how to deliver large trophic factor molecules – which do not cross the blood–brain barrier – to defined targets in the brain; the most powerful experimental techniques to date involve either implantation of cells that are engineered to secrete the particular trophic factor molecule (Figure 7.1G)[19] or direct *in vivo* gene transfer (Figure 7.1F)[20,21].

Principles and Practice of Geriatric Psychiatry, 3rd edn. Edited by Mohammed T. Abou-Saleh, Cornelius Katona and Anand Kumar
© 2011 John Wiley & Sons, Ltd

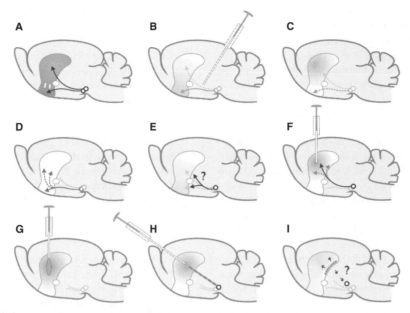

Figure 7.1 Schematic illustration of examples of regeneration and repair in the nigrostriatal system of rats **A**. Normal dopaminergic projections to the striatum arising from dopamine neurons in the ventral mesencephalon. **B**. Toxin 6 OHDA injections into the nigrostriatal pathway deplete striatal dopamine, typically more extensively in the dorsal neostriatum than in the ventral striatum. **C**. Compensatory adaptation of striatal receptors and biochemical turnover from residual spared. **D**. Compensatory collateral sprouting of ventral afferents following complete lesions of dorsal striatum. **E**. Long-distance regenerative axon growth from ventral mesencephalon typically is not a feature of nigrostriatal damage. **F**. Chronic delivery of growth factors such as GDNF by infusion or *in vivo* gene transfer can protect damaged axons and promote axon regeneration within the neostriatum. **G**. Implantation of ventral mesencephalic cells can restore dopaminergic innervation of the denervated striatum. **H**. Implantation of bridge grafts, e.g. of GDNF-secreting glial cells, can provide a substrate for long-distance axon regrowth from the ventral mesencephalon. **I**. Although adult neuron stem cells in the subventricular zone can provide functional cell replacement in dentate gyrus and olfactory bulb, evidence for a similar capacity for cell replacement in the striatum or ventral mesencephalon is weak

ADULT NEUROGENESIS

It was believed until recently that all neurones of the mature nervous system are born in early development so that once lost they are not replaced. It is now clear that there exists in the adult human brain a small population of resting 'neuronal stem cells' with the capacity both to undergo further cell division and to differentiate into both neurones and glia[22]. This opens the hope that such cells may be recruited for repair, either by isolation, expansion and differentiation into defined neuronal cell types *in vitro*, and reimplantation, or by finding the means to induce their spontaneous division, migration to areas of cell loss, and local differentiation into appropriate neuronal phenotype to replace lost target cells *in vivo* (Figure 7.1I). However, claims that endogenous adult stem cells can underlie recovery of function in the adult brain remain largely unsubstantiated, and substantial technical and theoretical problems remain in translating such procedures into applications for repair in human ageing.

CONCLUSION

Although the repair of neuronal damage associated with neurodegenerative disease and normal ageing remains experimental, rapid advances are being made in the techniques for inhibiting degeneration, promoting regenerative growth and replacing lost populations of cells. The pessimism that has for long surrounded the poor prognosis of brain damage in ageing and disease is being transformed to an optimism that these novel experimental approaches may find direct clinical application in the neurodegenerative diseases of ageing. Nevertheless, formidable technical problems still need to be overcome to transform theoretical prospects into practical therapies.

REFERENCES

1. Cajal SRy. *Degeneration and Regeneration of the Nervous System*. Oxford: Oxford University Press, 1928.
2. Zigmond MJ. Do compensatory processes underlie the preclinical phase of neurodegenerative disease? Insights from an animal model of Parkinsonism ? *Neurobiol Dis* 1997; **4**(3–4): 247–53.
3. Navarro X. Neural plasticity after nerve injury and regeneration. *Int Rev Neurobiol* 2009; **87**: 483–505.
4. Raisman G. Neuronal plasticity in the septal nuclei of the adult brain. *Brain Res* 1969; **14**: 25–48.
5. Bohn MC, Cupit L, Marciano F, Gash DM. Adrenal grafts enhance recovery of striatal dopaminergic fibers. *Science* 1987; **237**: 913–16.
6. Buonomano DV, Merzenich MM. Cortical plasticity: from synapses to maps. *Ann Rev Neurosci* 1998; **21**: 149–86.
7. Fawcett JW. Factors responsible for the failure of structural repair in the central nervous system. In Hunter AJ, Clark M (eds), *Neurodegeneration*. New York: Academic Press, 1992, 81–96.
8. Wilby M, Sinclair SR, Muir EM, Zietlow R, Adcock KH, Horellou P *et al*. A GDNF-secreting clone of the Schwann cell line SCTM41 enhances survival and fibre outgrowth from embryonic

nigral neurones grafted to the striatum and the lesioned substantia nigra. *J Neurosci* 1999; **19**(6): 2301–12.

9. Barker RA, Dunnett SB. *Neural Repair, Transplantation and Rehabilitation*. Hove: Psychology Press, 1999.

10. Dunnett SB, Björklund A. Transplantation of dopamine neurons: extent and mechanisms of functional recovery in rodent models of Parkinson's disease. In Iversen LL, Iversen SD, Dunnett SB, Björklund A (eds), *Dopamine Handbook*. New York: Oxford University Press, 2010, 454–77.

11. Lindvall O. Clinical experiences with dopamine neuron replacement in Parkinson's disease: what is the future ? In Iversen LL, Iversen SD, Dunnett SB, Björklund A (eds), New York: Oxford University Press, 2010, 478–88.

12. Falci S, Holtz A, Åkesson E, Azizi M, Ertzgaard P, Hultling C *et al.* Obliteration of a posttraumatic spinal cord cyst with solid human embryonic spinal cord grafts: first clinical attempt. *J Neurotrauma* 1997; **14**(11): 875–84.

13. Kondziolka D, Wechsler L, Goldstein S, Meltzer C, Thulborn KR, Gebel J *et al.* Transplantation of cultured human neuronal cells for patients with stroke. *Neurology* 2000; **55**(4): 565–9.

14. Bachoud-Lévi AC, Gaura V, Brugières P, Lefaucheur JP, Boissé MF, Maison P *et al.* Persistent benefit of foetal neural transplants in patients with Huntington's disease six years after surgery. *Lancet Neurol* 2006; **5**(4): 303–9.

15. Hefti F. Is Alzheimer's disease caused by a lack of nerve growth factor? *Ann Neurol* 1983; **13**: 109–10.

16. Sauer H, Rosenblad C, Björklund A. Glial cell line-derived neurotrophic factor but not transforming growth factor b3 prevents delayed degeneration of nigral dopaminergic neurons following striatal 6-hydroxydopamine lesion. *Proc Natl Acad Sci USA* 1995; **92**(19): 8935–9.

17. Gill SS, Patel NK, Hotton GR, O'Sullivan K, McCarter R, Bunnage M *et al.* Direct brain infusion of glial cell line-derived nmeurotrophic factor (GDNF) in Parkinson's disease. *Nat Med* 2003; **9**(5): 589–95.

18. Seiger Å, Nordberg A, von Holst H, Bäckman L, Ebendal T, Alafuzoff I *et al.* Intracranial infusion of purified nerve growth factor to an Alzheimer patient: the first attempt of a possible future treatment strategy. *Behav Brain Res* 1993; **57**: 255–61.

19. Nakao N, Yokote H, Nakai K, Itakura T. Promotion of survival and regeneration of nigral dopamine neurons in a rat model of Parkinson's disease after implantation of embryonal carcinoma-derived neurons genetically engineered to produce glial cell line-derived neurotrophic factor. *J Neurosurg* 2000; **92**(4): 659–70.

20. Martinez-Serrano A, Fischer W, Söderström S, Ebendal T, Björklund A. Long-term functional recovery from age-induced spatial memory impairments by nerve growth factor gene transfer to the rat basal forebrain. *Proc Natl Acad Sci USA* 1996; **93**(13): 6355–60.

21. Kirik D, Rosenblad C, Björklund A. Preservation of a functional nigrostriatal dopamine pathway by GDNF in the intrastriatal 6-OHDA lesion model depends on the site of administration of the trophic factor. *Eur J Neurosci* 2000; **12**(11): 3871–82.

22. Eriksson PS, Perfilieva E, Björk-Eriksson T, Alborn AM, Nordborg C, Peterson DA *et al.* Neurogenesis in the adult human hippocampus. *Nat Med* 1998; **4**(11): 1313–17.

8

Neuroendocrinology of Ageing

Marcus Simmgen

Thomas Addison Unit, St George's Hospital NHS Trust, Blackshaw Road, Tooting, London, UK

INTRODUCTION

The subject of neuroendocrinology is the interface between the nervous and endocrine systems within the brain. Their structural and functional interaction is bi-directional; that is, neuronal activity modulates endocrine secretion and, in turn, hormones influence brain function. Both neurons and endocrine cells transmit signals to distinct target cells by releasing a chemical mediator that is recognized by specific receptors. There is overlap, as some secreted substances serve as both neurotransmitter and hormone, for example arginine vasopressin (AVP, also called antidiuretic hormone, ADH) or vasoactive intestinal peptide (VIP). Virtually all neurotransmitting systems are involved in the neuroendocrine interaction, and jointly they regulate metabolic homeostasis, growth, development and reproductive function and they influence behaviour, learning, emotional and mental state.

Within the brain, the anatomical sites of closest interaction between the two systems are the hypothalamic-pituitary unit and the pineal gland. Peripherally, endocrine secretion is controlled either by direct innervation through autonomic secretomotor fibres or, indirectly, through the regulation of blood flow.

The endocrine effects on the CNS are widespread: the limbic system structures of hippocampus, amygdala, hypothalamus and cingulate gyrus, as well as the pre-frontal cortex and various other parts of the brain, are responsive to endocrine signals that may alter their morphology or functional behaviour.

The neuroendocrine interface is also linked closely to the body's immunological responses, and the increasingly complex interactions have been described as a neuroendocrine-immune network. Significant immunological changes occur during the ageing process, in part as a consequence of these interactions; however, these aspects are beyond the scope of this chapter.

As in other regions of the brain, the number and function of certain hypothalamic neurons and neuroendocrine cells declines during senescence, while other cell populations remain intact or even hypertrophy[1,2]. Circadian rhythms of secretion undergo a phase shift or become less pronounced and increasingly irregular[3]. Some endocrine axes undergo a significant physiological decline in their activity as a consequence of altered central regulation, loss of peripheral endocrine secretory capacity, tissue responsiveness or post-receptor signalling changes. While the menopause is an established life event for women, the effects of the gradual decline of male sex hormone levels (sometimes termed 'andropause'), of adrenal androgen production ('adrenopause') and of growth hormone ('somatopause') on healthy ageing are still the subjects of ongoing debate and research. In senescence, there are changes in body composition, loss of muscle strength, reduction in endurance and frequently a decline in cognitive, emotional and psychological function. Various hormonal changes contribute to these developments, and the chapter is arranged by endocrine axis and peripheral hormone. A brief overview of its physiology and CNS-related regulation is followed by a description of the changes occurring during senescence, and the implications for the ageing person.

ADENOHYPOPHYSIS

The anterior, glandular lobe of the pituitary gland is derived from pharyngeal ectoderm rather than from neuroectoderm. It achieves a close functional relationship with its regulatory neurons through the capillary portal circulation that exists between the median eminence of the hypothalamus and the adenohypophysis. Releasing and inhibiting hormones thus reach the anterior pituitary gland to exert control over its secretion of hormones with a tropism for the peripheral endocrine glands. All anterior pituitary hormones are released in a pulsatile manner. While they provide feedback inhibition at hypothalamic neurons (short loop), the peripheral hormones exert negative feedback at pituitary and hypothalamic level to ensure stable plasma levels (long loop). The pituitary generally reduces in size during senescence[4].

Somatopause

Growth hormone is synthesized by the somatotroph cell population of the anterior pituitary gland and released in pulsatile bursts with a peak after the onset of sleep. Two hormones are known to stimulate growth hormone synthesis and secretion: growth hormone-releasing hormone (GHRH) and ghrelin, both of which are produced in the hypothalamic arcuate nucleus. The former acts via its cognate GHRH receptor (GHRHR), and the latter via the growth hormone secretagogue receptor (GHSR). In addition, a range of other factors exert control over growth hormone release; such as metabolic substrates, physiological stimuli (sleep, exercise or stress) and certain neurotransmitters. Somatostatin, a hormone produced in the hypothalamic anterior paraventricular nucleus (PVN) inhibits growth hormone release, and the overall output effectively reflects an integration of all these stimuli.

Under the influence of growth hormone, primarily the liver produces insulin-like growth factor 1 (IGF-1), which mediates many of the effects of growth hormone on target tissues. Metabolic effects of growth hormone are: increased muscle mass and strength, reduced fat mass, increased bone density and improved cholesterol levels[5].

Growth hormone levels peak in adolescence and decline by 14% each decade, a process that is further accelerated in postmenopausal women. The amplitude of nocturnal growth hormone pulses falls and may disappear[6]. Since physiological ageing is associated with an increase in body fat and a reduction in muscle mass, as well as with a fall in bone density, there are similarities with adult growth hormone deficiency, and the term 'somatopause' has been used for this. A trial of supplementary growth hormone in a cohort of ageing men showed significant improvement in these parameters[7]. After 12 months of administration, however, side effects of carpal tunnel syndrome, gynaecomastia and hyperglycaemia became evident[8]. A meta-analysis concluded that, while growth hormone replacement was beneficial in growth hormone deficiency, supplementation in an otherwise healthy elderly person showed no evidence for improvements in maximal oxygen consumption, bone mineral density, lipid levels and fasting glucose and insulin levels. There was no suggestion that growth hormone prolonged life. Since there is also a theoretical risk of increased neoplastic disease, there are no grounds to advocate growth hormone supplementation in healthy ageing[5].

As an alternative, small molecules have been developed to act at the GHSR as a long-acting oral ghrelin analogue[9]. One trial was reported after one year to have achieved enhanced growth hormone pulsatility, restored IGF-1 values to juvenile levels, increased fat-free body mass and marginally lowered LDL-cholesterol. Observed side effects were a mild increase in fasted glucose, insulin resistance, cortisol levels and a weight gain of 2.7 kg vs. 0.8 kg in the placebo group[10]. Another compound improved lean body mass and functional strength, balance and coordination. Side effects were deterioration in parameters of insulin resistance, fatigue and insomnia[11]. Neither drug has reached the market.

Prolactin

Prolactin is structurally related to growth hormone, and its secretory regulation is unusual in that the pituitary lactotroph cells are under tonic inhibition by dopamine-producing hypothalamic neurons. Circulating prolactin levels comprise of a combination of basal and pulsatile release[12]. Prolactin levels rise in response to sleep to peak in the early hours[13], and secretion is increased by stress and other stimuli. In men and non-pregnant women, prolactin concentrations gradually decline with advancing age. Frequent nocturnal sampling showed this to be a result of falling basal prolactin secretion that is associated with a reduced lactotroph cell mass or responsiveness, and also to be due to a reduction in hypothalamic stimuli for pulsatile bursts[14]. In ageing rats, the circadian rhythm of prolactin secretion loses the ability to adapt to changes in the light–dark cycle[15].

In a large observational study of a cohort of middle-aged men (52 ± 12.9 years) attending for sexual dysfunction, the lowest quartile of prolactin concentrations was associated with increased risk for metabolic syndrome, atherogenic erectile dysfunction, premature ejaculation and anxiety. There also is evidence for immune-modulating properties of prolactin since, in mice, prolactin deficiency caused impaired lymphocyte function by reducing cytokine-induced macrophage activation[16]. However, the clinical relevance of reduced prolactin levels in senescence is unclear and no trials of replacement therapy in ageing humans have been conducted.

Menopause

The female cycle is under complex regulation by luteinizing hormone (LH) and follicle-stimulating hormone (FSH), which are produced by the gonadotroph cell population of the anterior pituitary gland. Both are released in pulsatile fashion under control by hypothalamic gonadotrophin-releasing hormone (GnRH). In addition to the daily high-frequency pulsatility, their secretion is cyclical over the period of a lunar month. Complex feed-forward and feedback regulation between the hypothalamus, the pituitary gonadotroph cells and the ovary leads to the menstrual cycle during a woman's fertile years. Oestrogen is produced mainly in the granulosa cells of the developing ovarian follicle from an androgenic precursor and is the main female sex steroid hormone.

Follicular depletion, however, is not the sole reason for the menopause. Studies in rats demonstrated that prior to any cycle irregularities there was an early decline in GnRH-neuron response and a consequently reduced LH surge in response to oestrogen around the time of ovulation. Thus the functional loss begins centrally at the level of hypothalamus and pituitary which, together with the changes at ovarian level, leads to the menopause[17].

With the loss of follicular activity, which usually occurs around the mid-sixth decade of life, a rapid fall of oestrogen levels ensues and FSH and LH levels rise due to absence of feedback inhibition. Consequences of a lack of oestrogen are manifold: Atrophy of oestrogen-responsive tissues, rapid loss of bone mass, adverse changes to the lipid profile with increased atherogenic risk, depressive mood swings, lack of concentration, anxiety and loss of libido. Vasomotor symptoms of hot flashes not only impair quality of life, but also represent altered blood vessel physiology that is associated with increased cardiovascular risk[18]. Since the reduction in oestrogen leads to a narrowing of the 'thermoneutral' zone of temperature regulation in the hypothalamus, small changes in core body temperature can trigger symptoms[19].

Oestrogen-containing hormone replacement therapy (HRT) can ameliorate vasogenic menopausal symptoms and delay biochemical changes. To avoid a concomitant excess risk of cardiovascular events, HRT should be taken early[20] and for a limited period only to minimize the additional hazard of thromboembolism and breast cancer[21]. Contrary to expectations, HRT in elderly women did not preserve cognitive ability but was associated with an increased risk of dementia and global cognitive decline that correlated with a reduction in hippocampal, frontal lobe and total brain volumes[22]. It should be noted, however, that some of the noted CNS effects might be (i) specific to the hormone molecule used in the quoted studies, (ii) related to the late timing of HRT, and (iii) due to elevated levels of LH itself, rather than related to oestrogen deficiency[23].

Andropause

Testosterone, the predominant male sex steroid hormone, is produced by testicular Leydig cells under the influence of LH and FSH. As in women, both gonadotrophins are released in pulses from the anterior pituitary gland under GnRH control. Testosterone levels in men follow a diurnal rhythm with peak concentrations occurring in the morning. At puberty, bioavailable testosterone levels begin to rise; they peak around the third decade of life and gradually fall thereafter at an annual rate of 1.3%[24]. Circulating testosterone binds to sex-hormone-binding globulin (SHBG) and, with less avidity, to albumin. Thus the availability of free testosterone reduces as SHBG levels rise with age by 1.2% per annum. Leydig cell attrition, reduced steroid synthetic activity and a lower responsiveness to LH are the main testicular factors contributing to this decline[25]. The circadian variation in testosterone also declines with age. The term 'andropause' has hence come into use as a male equivalent to the menopause, even though the decline in sex hormone levels is gradual in men compared to the relatively sudden reduction in women.

Reduced testosterone availability exerts major metabolic effects on metabolism and thus lowers muscle mass and strength, raises body fat content and negatively affects bone health, libido and reproductive function, as well as mood and cognition[26]. As in menopausal women, the elevation of LH has been implicated in the pathophysiology of Alzheimer's disease in men, as low testosterone concentrations were correlated with increased amyloid-beta protein levels[27]. While a significant proportion of ageing males over the age of 65 years have reduced levels of testosterone, there was wide variability within a large cohort of community-dwelling men and serum concentrations were a poor indicator of symptoms[28,29]. A recent consensus statement therefore emphasized the need for correlation of clinical symptoms with testosterone levels, the lack of cardiovascular and bone fracture outcome data and the need for surveillance for prostate carcinoma, among others, in case of replacement therapy[30].

Thyroid Axis

The hormones thyroxine (or tetra-iodo-thyronine, T4) and tri-iodo-thyronine (T3) are synthesized and secreted by thyroid follicular cells. Only a small proportion of T4 is converted to T3 prior to its release from the thyroid; almost all of the remainder undergoes mono-deiodination in peripheral tissues. T3 has greater biological activity than T4 and a shorter half-life. Plasma levels of both hormones are regulated by thyroid-stimulating hormone (TSH, also called thyrotrophin) that is released by the thyrotroph cells of the anterior pituitary gland, which in turn are under hypothalamic thyrotrophin-releasing hormone (TRH) control.

Virtually all tissues possess receptors for the thyroid hormones, through which the latter regulate the basal metabolic rate, tissue function, protein, fat and carbohydrate metabolism, as well as influence mental function and psychological well-being. The prevalence of thyroid autoantibodies significantly increases with age and, if primary thyroid dysfunction is present (subclinical or overt hypo- or hyperthyroidism), cognitive function is almost invariably affected[31]. Such conditions clearly merit thyroid hormone replacement or suppressive therapy, respectively. In primary hypothyroidism, the pituitary thyrotroph cells appear to lose their responsiveness to low thyroid hormone levels, as the TSH response was significantly reduced at ages over 80 years[32].

In a large, thyroid disease-free population, however, senescence *per se* led only to a minor increase in TSH levels, which remained well within the normal range[33].

Adrenocortical Axis

The hypothalamic–pituitary–adrenal (HPA) axis is central to the adaptive stress response that follows an initial, catecholamine-mediated 'fight-or-flight' reaction. Cortisol is released from the adrenal cortex following stimulation by adrenocorticotropic hormone (ACTH, also called corticotrophin), which is produced by the corticotroph cell population of the anterior pituitary gland. Corticotrophin-releasing hormone (CRH), from hypothalamic neurons residing in the PVN, regulates ACTH secretion in a diurnal pattern.

Cortisol is the main glucocorticoid in humans. It induces insulin resistance and raises blood glucose levels, causes protein and bone catabolism and an elevation in blood pressure. It also dampens the immune response. While a short-term stress response is necessary to deal with the challenges to the body's homeostasis, this reaction must itself be regulated. The hippocampus expresses glucocorticoid receptors and exerts inhibitory control over HPA axis activation, thus limiting the stress response[36]. The physiological day-to-day stress adaptation has been termed 'allostasis'[34], with its regulatory failure leading to an 'allostatic load'[35]. The hippocampus expresses glucocorticoid receptors and exerts inhibitory control over HPA axis activation, thus limiting the stress response[36].

The adrenal capacity for cortisol production is not affected by ageing, although its circadian rhythm is blunted and basal activity increased[37]. However, with advancing age the negative-feedback sensitivity reduces at hippocampal level and the HPA axis activity increases[3]. In both sexes, mean cortisol levels increased by 20–50% between the ages of 20 and 80 years[38]. Magnetic resonance imaging showed that the volumes of hippocampus and anterior cingulated gyrus were inversely correlated with baseline ACTH levels, and that older subjects demonstrated a slower decrease in ACTH in response to an infusion of cortisol than younger volunteers[39]. The stress-induced remodelling of the hippocampus and the resulting rise in glucocorticoid levels thus increases the allostatic load, with negative results for a range of metabolic parameters and the immune system that is associated with ageing[40].

Furthermore, the hippocampus and related limbic structures of the amygdala and pre-frontal cortex are of key importance for learning and memory function, including emotional learning and processing. Persistent elevation of glucocorticoid levels is involved in the emotional memory disturbances found in depression and posttraumatic stress disorder[41].

Adrenopause

Dehydroepiandrosterone (DHEA) and its sulfate ester (DHEAS) are abundant androgenic steroid molecules that serve as precursor molecules for other androgens and oestrogen. DHEA is produced by the adrenal cortex and also serves as a neurosteroid[42]. ACTH regulates its secretion and, in contrast to cortisol and aldosterone, DHEA levels physiologically decline with ageing from the third decade onwards by around 2% annually[43,44]. At the age of 80 years, DHEA concentrations are approximately 20% of those of younger controls[45].

Observational studies have associated low DHEA levels with cardiovascular disease, low bone density, type 2 diabetes, low mood and Alzheimer's disease. However, no causal relationship has been established[46].

DHEA replacement therapy is the focus of research for its potential anti-ageing properties in otherwise healthy older subjects. So far, however, no firm therapeutic indication has emerged[43,47].

NEUROHYPOPHYSIS

The posterior, neural lobe of the pituitary gland contains axonal projections of neurons from the supraoptic (SON) and paraventricular (PVN) hypothalamic nuclei. Axoplasmic flow transports arginine-vasopressin (AVP) and oxytocin to the neurohypophysis for storage.

The nuclei receive cholinergic and noradrenergic innervation and hormone secretion is triggered by a rise in plasma osmolality, reduction in circulating fluid volume, nausea, pain or emotional stress. While the AVP receptor V2 is mainly expressed in the kidney, V1a and V1b receptors are widely distributed within the brain[48].

Arginine-Vasopressin

AVP is central to the maintenance of fluid and osmolality homeostasis throughout life. Basal AVP levels in men were higher in older subjects and showed less responsiveness to fluctuations in osmolality compared to young volunteers. Reduced satiation to water consumption after induction of thirst by infusion of hypertonic saline was demonstrated by altered blood flow in the anterior mid-cingulate cortex on positron emission tomography[49]. The renal tubules become less responsive to AVP in ageing humans and rodents. In the rat, the reduced urine-concentrating ability was found to be due to a down-regulation of the V2 receptor, while AVP levels remained normal[50].

In addition to its function in fluid homeostasis, abnormal plasma AVP levels have been implicated in a range of mental disorders. Elevated concentrations of AVP have been noted in depression, posttraumatic stress disorder, acute schizophrenia and other mental illness[48]. In depressed patients with Alzheimer's disease, however, the content of AVP and oxytocin mRNA in SON and PVN was unchanged compared to controls, and there was no correlation with depression[51]. In rodent models and (confirmed in part) in humans, AVP has also been determined to modify memory and social behaviour such as aggression and affiliation[52].

Oxytocin

Oxytocin plays no significant physiological role in senescence. Basal levels and the response to hypoglycaemia-induced stress remained comparable in older compared to young men[53].

PINEAL GLAND

The pineal gland is situated within the roof of the third ventricle above the Sylvian aqueduct. In fish and amphibians the equivalent structure is light sensitive, whereas in humans the pineal gland receives input from the hypothalamic suprachiasmatic nucleus (SCN) that, in turn, is connected to the retina via non-visual photosensitive pathways. The SCN functions as the master clock for circadian rhythmic activity, which is further entrained by external zeitgebers.

Melatonin

The pineal gland synthesizes and secretes melatonin predominantly during periods of darkness and thus conveys a biological diurnal rhythm as well as an annual seasonal rhythm to the body.

While daytime melatonin production remains virtually unchanged throughout life, nocturnal secretion of melatonin peaks in early childhood and thereafter continuously declines with age. After the age of 60 years, peak peripheral night-time melatonin concentrations fall to 40 pg/ml, compared to 160 pg/ml at the age of 10 years. Background daytime levels are in the order of 30 pg/ml[54].

The SCN and the hypothalamus express a high density of MT1 receptors, allowing for chronobiological feedback to the central clock. In senescence, the circadian rhythm becomes weaker, sleep disturbances more common and there is an associated increasingly irregular diurnal melatonin secretion. The reduced number and density of MT1 receptor-expressing neurons that was found in the SCN of older subjects compared to young controls can, in part, explain this. In the last stages of Alzheimer's disease the prevalence of these neurons was further reduced[55].

Melatonin has non-sedative sleep-inducing properties, and trials of prolonged-release melatonin administration to patients with insomnia aged 55 years and older have shown to improve sleep quality, morning alertness and psychomotor performance. The supplement was administered for three weeks and no withdrawal or rebound symptoms were observed[56,57].

CONCLUSION

Complex neuroendocrinological changes occur during the healthy ageing process at hypothalamic, hypophyseal and target endocrine tissue level. There is increasing evidence that altered neuronal function with irregularities in biological rhythm and decreased secretory responsiveness leads to the significant reduction in availability of several peripheral hormones[3]. Declining levels of sex steroids, growth hormone, adrenal androgens and melatonin secretion contribute to significant adverse changes in body composition and endurance, cardiovascular risk profile, bone strength, sexual physiology, circadian rhythms, cognition and emotional and psychological well-being. Attempts at restoring youthfulness through the replacement of physiologically declining hormones have so far concentrated on time-limited, perimenopausal therapy with low-dose oestrogen. However, promising molecules to improve the growth hormone axis and the melatonin -mediated sleep–wake cycle are being tested. As senescence is a multifactorial process in which other morbidities and drug therapy frequently play a major part, any neuroendocrine changes should naturally not be viewed in isolation. Furthermore, whether a physiological change in life is perceived as being pathological and warranting treatment must be considered within the individual's social, environmental and lifestyle context. An optimistic outlook has the potential to prolong life considerably[58].

REFERENCES

1. Hofman MA. Lifespan changes in the human hypothalamus. *Exp Gerontol* 1997; **32**(4-5): 559–75
2. Zhou JN, Swaab DF. Activation and degeneration during aging: a morphometric study of the human hypothalamus. *Microsc Res Tech* 1999; **44**(1): 36–48.
3. Smith RG, Betancourt L, Sun Y. Molecular endocrinology and physiology of the aging central nervous system. *Endocr Rev* 2005; **26**(2): 203–50.
4. Melmed S. Mechanisms for pituitary tumorigenesis: the plastic pituitary. *J Clin Invest* 2003; **112**(11): 1603–18.
5. Liu H, Bravata DM, Olkin I *et al*. Systematic review: the safety and efficacy of growth hormone in the healthy elderly. *Ann Intern Med* 2007; **146**(2): 104–15.
6. Sherlock M, Toogood AA. Aging and the growth hormone/insulin like growth factor-I axis. *Pituitary* 2007; **10**(2): 189–203.
7. Rudman D, Feller AG, Nagraj HS *et al*. Effects of human growth hormone in men over 60 years old. *N Engl J Med* 1990; **323**(1): 1–6.

8. Cohn L, Feller AG, Draper MW, Rudman IW, Rudman D. Carpal tunnel syndrome and gynaecomastia during growth hormone treatment of elderly men with low circulating IGF-I concentrations. *Clin Endocrinol (Oxf)* 1993; **39**(4): 417–25.

9. Smith RG. Development of growth hormone secretagogues. *Endocr Rev* 2005; **26**(3): 346–60.

10. Nass R, Pezzoli SS, Oliveri MC *et al.* Effects of an oral ghrelin mimetic on body composition and clinical outcomes in healthy older adults: a randomized trial. *Ann Intern Med* 2008; **149**(9): 601–11.

11. White HK, Petrie CD, Landschulz W *et al.* Effects of an oral growth hormone secretagogue in older adults. *J Clin Endocrinol Metab* 2009; **94**(4): 1198–206.

12. Veldhuis JD, Iranmanesh A, Johnson ML, Lizarralde G. Twenty-four-hour rhythms in plasma concentrations of adenohypophyseal hormones are generated by distinct amplitude and/or frequency modulation of underlying pituitary secretory bursts. *J Clin Endocrinol Metab* 1990; **71**(6): 1616–23.

13. Sassin JF, Frantz AG, Kapen S, Weitzman ED. The nocturnal rise of human prolactin is dependent on sleep. *J Clin Endocrinol Metab* 1973; **37**(3): 436–40.

14. Iranmanesh A, Mulligan T, Veldhuis JD. Mechanisms subserving the physiological nocturnal relative hypoprolactinemia of healthy older men: dual decline in prolactin secretory burst mass and basal release with preservation of pulse duration, frequency, and interpulse interval – a General Clinical Research Center study. *J Clin Endocrinol Metab* 1999; **84**(3): 1083–90.

15. Lewy H, Ashkenazi IE, Touitou Y. Prolactin rhythms-oscillators' response to photoperiodic cues is age and circadian time dependent. *Neurobiol Aging* 2005; **26**(1): 125–33.

16. Bernton EW, Meltzer MS, Holaday JW. Suppression of macrophage activation and T-lymphocyte function in hypoprolactinemic mice. *Science* 1988; **239**(4838): 401–4.

17. Downs JL, Wise PM. The role of the brain in female reproductive aging. *Mol Cell Endocrinol* 2009; **299**(1): 32–8.

18. Thurston RC, Sutton-Tyrrell K, Everson-Rose SA, Hess R, Matthews KA. Hot flashes and subclinical cardiovascular disease: findings from the Study of Women's Health Across the Nation Heart Study. *Circulation* 2008; **118**(12): 1234–40.

19. Freedman RR. Pathophysiology and treatment of menopausal hot flashes. *Semin Reprod Med* 2005; **23**(2): 117–25.

20. Rossouw JE, Prentice RL, Manson JE *et al.* Postmenopausal hormone therapy and risk of cardiovascular disease by age and years since menopause. *JAMA* 2007; **297**(13): 1465–77.

21. Chen WY. Exogenous and endogenous hormones and breast cancer. *Best Pract Res Clin Endocrinol Metab* 2008; **22**(4): 573–85.

22. Coker LH, Espeland MA, Rapp SR *et al.* Postmenopausal hormone therapy and cognitive outcomes: The Women's Health Initiative Memory Study (WHIMS). *J Steroid Biochem Mol Biol* 2010, in print.

23. Webber KM, Perry G, Smith MA, Casadesus G. The contribution of luteinizing hormone to Alzheimer disease pathogenesis. *Clin Med Res* 2007; **5**(3): 177–83.

24. Kaufman JM, Vermeulen A. The decline of androgen levels in elderly men and its clinical and therapeutic implications. *Endocr Rev* 2005; **26**(6): 833–76.

25. Wu FC, Tajar A, Pye SR *et al.* Hypothalamic-pituitary-testicular axis disruptions in older men are differentially linked to age and modifiable risk factors: the European Male Aging Study. *J Clin Endocrinol Metab* 2008; **93**(7): 2737–45.

26. Veldhuis JD. Aging and hormones of the hypothalamo-pituitary axis: gonadotropic axis in men and somatotropic axes in men and women. *Ageing Res Rev* 2008; **7**(3): 189–208.

27. Verdile G, Yeap BB, Clarnette RM *et al.* Luteinizing hormone levels are positively correlated with plasma amyloid-beta protein levels in elderly men. *J Alzheimers Dis* 2008; **14**(2): 201–8.

28. Orwoll E, Lambert LC, Marshall LM *et al.* Testosterone and estradiol among older men. *J Clin Endocrinol Metab* 2006; **91**(4): 1336–44.

29. Araujo AB, Esche GR, Kupelian V *et al.* Prevalence of symptomatic androgen deficiency in men. *J Clin Endocrinol Metab* 2007; **92**(11): 4241–7.

30. Wang C, Nieschlag E, Swerdloff R *et al.* Investigation, treatment and monitoring of late-onset hypogonadism in males: ISA, ISSAM, EAU, EAA and ASA recommendations. *Eur J Endocrinol* 2008; **159**(5): 507–14.

31. Bégin ME, Langlois MF, Lorrain D, Cunnane SC. Thyroid function and cognition during aging. *Curr Gerontol Geriatr Res* 2008 (e-journal); Article ID 474868. DOI:10.1155/2008/474868.

32. Carlé A, Laurberg P, Pedersen IB *et al.* Age modifies the pituitary TSH response to thyroid failure. *Thyroid* 2007; **17**(2): 139–44.

33. Hollowell JG, Staehling NW, Flanders WD *et al.* Serum TSH, T(4), and thyroid antibodies in the United States population (1988 to 1994): National Health and Nutrition Examination Survey (NHANES III). *J Clin Endocrinol Metab* 2002; **87**(2): 489–99.

34. Sterling P, Eyer J. Allostasis: a new paradigm to explain arousal pathology. In Fisher S, Reason J (eds), *Handbook of Life Stress, Cognition and Health*. New York: John Wiley & Sons, Inc., 1988, 629–49.

35. McEwen BS. Physiology and neurobiology of stress and adaptation: central role of the brain. *Physiol Rev* 2007; **87**(3): 873–904.

36. Sapolsky RM, Krey LC, McEwen BS. Glucocorticoid-sensitive hippocampal neurons are involved in terminating the adrenocortical stress response. *Proc Natl Acad Sci U S A* 1984; **81**(19): 6174–7.

37. Deuschle M, Gotthardt U, Schweiger U *et al.* With aging in humans the activity of the hypothalamus-pituitary-adrenal system increases and its diurnal amplitude flattens. *Life Sci* 1997; **61**(22): 2239–46.

38. Van Cauter E, Leproult R, Kupfer DJ. Effects of gender and age on the levels and circadian rhythmicity of plasma cortisol. *J Clin Endocrinol Metab* 1996; **81**(7): 2468–73.

39. Wolf OT, Convit A, de Leon MJ, Caraos C, Qadri SF. Basal hypothalamo-pituitary-adrenal axis activity and corticotropin feedback in young and older men: relationships to magnetic resonance imaging-derived hippocampus and cingulate gyrus volumes. *Neuroendocrinology* 2002; **75**(4): 241–9.

40. Bauer ME, Jeckel CM, Luz C. The role of stress factors during aging of the immune system. *Ann N Y Acad Sci* 2009; **1153**: 139–52.

41. Wolf OT. The influence of stress hormones on emotional memory: relevance for psychopathology. *Acta Psychol (Amst)* 2008; **127**(3): 513–31.

42. Aldred S, Mecocci P. Decreased dehydroepiandrosterone (DHEA) and dehydroepiandrosterone sulfate (DHEAS) concentrations in plasma of Alzheimer's disease (AD) patients. *Arch Gerontol Geriatr* 2010, in press.

43. Arlt W. Dehydroepiandrosterone and ageing. *Best Pract Res Clin Endocrinol Metab* 2004; **18**(3): 363–80.

44. Orentreich N, Brind JL, Rizer RL, Vogelman JH. Age changes and sex differences in serum dehydroepiandrosterone sulfate concentrations throughout adulthood. *J Clin Endocrinol Metab* 1984; **59**(3): 551–5.

45. Vermeulen A. Dehydroepiandrosterone sulfate and aging. *Ann N Y Acad Sci* 1995; **774**: 121–7.

46. Chahal HS, Drake WM. The endocrine system and ageing. *J Pathol* 2007; **211**(2): 173–80.

47. Allolio B, Arlt W. DHEA treatment: myth or reality? *Trends Endocrinol Metab* 2002; **13**(7): 288–94.

48. Egashira N, Mishima K, Iwasaki K, Oishi R, Fujiwara M. New topics in vasopressin receptors and approach to novel drugs: role of the vasopressin receptor in psychological and cognitive functions. *J Pharmacol Sci* 2009; **109**(1): 44–9.

49. Farrell MJ, Zamarripa F, Shade R *et al.* Effect of aging on regional cerebral blood flow responses associated with osmotic thirst and its satiation by water drinking: a PET study. *Proc Natl Acad Sci U S A* 2008; **105**(1): 382–7.

50. Tian Y, Serino R, Verbalis JG. Downregulation of renal vasopressin V2 receptor and aquaporin-2 expression parallels age-associated defects in urine concentration. *Am J Physiol Renal Physiol* 2004; **287**(4): F797–805.

51. Meynen G, Unmehopa UA, Hofman MA, Swaab DF, Hoogendijk WJ. Hypothalamic vasopressin and oxytocin mRNA expression in relation to depressive state in Alzheimer's disease: a difference with major depressive disorder. *J Neuroendocrinol* 2009; **21**(8): 722–9.

52. Caldwell HK, Lee HJ, Macbeth AH, Young WS 3rd. Vasopressin: behavioral roles of an "original" neuropeptide. *Prog Neurobiol* 2008; **84**(1): 1–24.

53. Chiodera P, Volpi R, Capretti L *et al.* Oxytocin response to challenging stimuli in elderly men. *Regul Pept* 1994; **51**(2): 169–76.

54. Karasek M. Does melatonin play a role in aging processes? *J Physiol Pharmacol* 2007; **58** (Suppl 6): 105–13.

55. Wu YH, Zhou JN, Van Heerikhuize J, Jockers R, Swaab DF. Decreased MT1 melatonin receptor expression in the suprachiasmatic nucleus in aging and Alzheimer's disease. *Neurobiol Aging* 2007; **28**(8): 1239–47.

56. Luthringer R, Muzet M, Zisapel N, Staner L. The effect of prolonged-release melatonin on sleep measures and psychomotor performance in elderly patients with insomnia. *Int Clin Psychopharmacol* 2009; **24**(5): 239–49.

57. Lemoine P, Nir T, Laudon M, Zisapel N. Prolonged-release melatonin improves sleep quality and morning alertness in insomnia patients aged 55 years and older and has no withdrawal effects. *J Sleep Res* 2007; **16**(4): 372–80.

58. Levy BR, Slade MD, Kunkel SR, Kasl SV. Longevity increased by positive self-perceptions of aging. *J Pers Soc Psychol* 2002; **83**(2): 261–70.

9

Genetic Aspects of Ageing

Ben Pickard[1] and Douglas Blackwood[2]

[1]*Strathclyde Institute of Pharmacy and Biomedical Sciences (SIPBS), University of Strathclyde, UK*
[2]*Division of Psychiatry, University of Edinburgh, UK*

INTRODUCTION: LIVING LONGER VERSUS CHEATING DEATH

That there may be specific biological processes determining life span is an intriguing concept, and one which has attracted interest from both the academic and commercial sectors. Such interest has often focused on the simple numerical indicator of life span but this can often be at odds with the clinical perspective that centres on quality of life for the elderly. In this chapter we will review the latest findings and current ideas in the fields studying the biological process of ageing, its evolutionary underpinning and the genetic factors intertwined with environmental exposure that determine our life span. There is also a semantic issue of whether a discussion of ageing should include factors contributing to longevity if they merely afford protection against the dominant degenerative disorders or serious illnesses of the elderly or only concentrate on mechanisms that actively delay the ageing process[1]. Plainly, these two aspects of ageing are inextricably linked but from a research point of view, and in the context of genetic models, only the latter offers fundamental insights into the process.

AGEING GENETICS, HERITABILITY AND EVOLUTIONARY INFLUENCES

Danish epidemiological studies have reported that the heritability of human longevity is approximately 25%[2,3]: a figure similar to that for lower organisms. Thus there exists scope for the genetic dissection of the phenotype and a substrate for the processes of evolution to act on[4]. In its purest form, evolution requires that advantageous genetic variation is favoured and increases its frequency in the population through the process of natural selection. This is mediated through its ability to increase a carrier individual organism's 'fitness' and thus its ability to reproduce at a greater than average level. It can be appreciated that this raises fundamental conceptual issues in the context of the genetics of longevity. Female reproductive fitness, in particular, occupies only a proportion of the modern human life span and so it could be hypothesized that gene variants influencing life span in the age range from 55–85 years would be under minimal selection compared to those dictating survival within the 15–45-year age range. It has also been argued that, for some species, individuals living beyond reproductive age are counterproductive to species survival – they are a drain on limited resources and thus compete with actively reproducing individuals. Selection pressure for a

biologically programmed 'cap' on life span might avoid this conflict. A second argument against a clear genetic contribution to human longevity would be the vast period of human existence on Earth for which 45 years was 'old age'. In the case of humans, long life spans are a modern phenomenon – average life expectancy dropped in the transition from 'hunter-gatherer' (Mesolithic Stone Age) to agrarian (Neolithic Stone Age) lifestyles[5] and did not significantly exceed the median life span of approximately 30–35 years until recent centuries. The implications are that not only does a long life harm fellow members of one's species, it also has no evolutionary outlet in the form of increased reproductive fitness. The genetics of ageing is left evolutionarily 'rudderless' in these circumstances.

However, two hypotheses offer an alternative view, supporting an evolutionarily 'visible' role for ageing. Firstly, the adoption of agriculture inevitably led to community living and increased social complexity. These social organization developments might be manifest in the altruistic role of the elderly in supporting the community – perhaps through leadership, childcare or other division of labour favourable for group survival. The impact of cultural effects (a form of environment) on ageing can never be entirely separated from genetics in the study of ageing in particular and will be covered in more detail below. Secondly, and perhaps more biologically tractable, is the argument that the genetic variants altering later life survival also play a role in earlier life fitness and are thus relevant to reproductive potential.

Finally, it is also worth considering the corollary of the sudden upturn in life span in recent human history – it has exposed humans to the consequences of genotypes that were never previously expressed for so long. For example, gene variants increasing susceptibility to Alzheimer's disease might be the result of random mutational drift or positive selection for their benefit in the young, but it is only now that they have been exposed to the environment of the ageing brain and consequently deemed pathological.

AGEING BIOLOGY: CLUES FROM HUMAN SYNDROMES

The fact that well-characterized human disorders of premature ageing (progeria) exist suggests that there are real biological processes at work, and ones which are tractable to genetics research. Individuals with progeroid disorders present with a spectrum of phenotypes which closely resemble natural ageing but these occur in young adulthood or even childhood. A multitude of mutations in two particular genes, *WRN* and *LMNA*, account for the majority of these cases. Werner syndrome (WS) is perhaps the best studied of these and is caused by mutations in the *WRN* gene which encodes a helicase/exonuclease protein that functions during the critical processes of active nuclear DNA functioning such as replication, recombination and repair – when potentially pathological errors can be introduced into our DNA. Thus, the consequences to genomic integrity in WS patients are an accelerated version of those hypothesized to occur in normal individuals as a result of a lifetime of environmental exposure and mutation accumulation. The phenotypes are similar too, ranging from osteoporosis, cataracts, type II diabetes, atherosclerosis and cancers (particularly mesenchymal sarcomas) such that WS patients tend to die in their 50s as a result of complications arising from these conditions. Interestingly, the phenotypic spectrum of WS doesn't seem to include the neurodegenerative conditions such as Alzheimer's disease. It is tempting to speculate that these particular disorders are due to the accumulation of protein aggregates (plaques and tangles), i.e., protein attrition rather than genomic DNA attrition.

Mutations in the lamin A gene, *LMNA*, encoding a nuclear intermediate filament protein involved in the packaging of nuclear chromatin, cause 'atypical' WS, or in extreme cases involving a particular *LMNA* splice mutation, the severe and very early-onset Hutchinson–Gilford progeria syndrome (HGPS). A number of other rare progeroid syndromes exist and, of these, Cockayne syndrome type 1 (CS) is the only other one discussed here. This is caused by mutations in the transcription-coupled nucleotide excision repair genes, *CSA* and *CSB*, which also contribute to the cell's battle against genomic damage.

The genes emerging from these human conditions unequivocally point to the maintenance of genomic integrity as a vital process in ageing, involving the concerted action of several different systems to achieve it. Mutations in these systems seem to result in either progerias or cancer syndromes, or occasionally both (e.g. WS). It has been suggested that these alternative outcomes result from the specific responses to DNA damage initiated by the various systems: repair, apoptosis or senescence[6].

AGEING BIOLOGY: CLUES FROM LOWER ORGANISMS

The validity of certain mouse models of ageing has sometimes been questioned for the very reasons discussed previously – distinguishing genuine progeroid features from a numerically shorter life span due to pathological state[7]. Therefore, the presence of features such as kyphosis, as an indicator of an osteoporotic state, stereotypical fat deposition and atrophy of the epidermis are often employed as benchmarks of true ageing models. The progeroid conditions in humans point towards accumulating DNA damage as a mechanism of ageing and the increased life span of mice over-expressing the antioxidizing protein thioredoxin seems to confirm the importance of this process. However, other transgenic mouse models with modulated life spans suggest that additional contributory mechanisms are at play. Historically, it has been suggested that cellular, organ and organismal ageing are affected by the rate of cell proliferation and apoptosis. This has manifest itself in such concepts as the Hayflick limit[8] whereby oxygen levels encountered and cell divisions undergone are recorded by each cell using the gradual shortening of the telomere sequences located at the ends of chromosomes as an internal clock. At a defined telomere threshold length the cell enters a state of protective

self-induced senescence, thus reducing the potential for DNA damage to be manifest as oncogenic cellular changes.

Indeed, a number of mouse mutations linked with altered life span involve proteins that can be classified as regulators of mitosis and cellular proliferation (e.g. p53, Brca1 and p21[WAF1]) and these have been reviewed elsewhere[9]. Alternatively, other mouse models centre on the signalling pathways modulating and modulated by growth hormone, insulin and insulin-like growth factor such as the Ames dwarf and Laron mouse strains. Mice deficient for the *Klotho* gene product, encoding a hormone that inhibits the action of the insulin/IGF-1 pathway, show a progeria phenotype whereas *Klotho* over-expressing mice are longer lived. Finally, *SIRT1*, a member of the sirtuin class of genes, downregulates the production of insulin and IGF-1 thus promoting increased life span. These mouse models, particularly the dwarf strains, and other observations point to a correlation between longevity and body size within a species. It has been reported that shorter humans have on average a greater life span – this is even despite the observation that taller individuals are generally protected against atherosclerosis. The speculation is that body size is closely related to 'cellularity', or the number of divisions during the growth process. This in turn is a reflection of the proliferative potential of an individual's cells as discussed above. The correlation is clearly not a simple one as those with progeroid syndromes are often of short stature. Moreover, the role of the growth hormone/insulin pathway in aspects of cell proliferation, growth, DNA repair and caloric intake (discussed below) means that these processes are all interconnected at some level in their contribution to the rate of ageing.

Naturally, many mouse strains deficient in aspects of genomic repair have been generated given the seeming importance of this process in ageing. One intriguing and counterintuitive result comes from the study of *Csb*, *Xpa* and *Ercc1* mouse mutants and combinations thereof. These mice show definitive progeroid symptoms but also display a downregulation of the insulin/IGF-1 signalling pathway. Normally, such downregulation is protective and life prolonging as discussed in detail below, but in these instances it appears to be an innate compensatory mechanism responding to increased levels of genome instability.

It may be the case that ageing is such a fundamental property of life or the environmental insults so similar that organisms from across all taxa have adopted the same molecular machinery to counter it. In this way there are a growing number of studies which seek to address human ageing through the study of yeast, nematode worm and fruit fly in addition to the mouse. McCarroll *et al.* pursued this approach to the genetics of ageing by employing cross-species profiling of gene expression changes correlated with age[10]. What they observed was a shared set of age-responsive gene expression changes between the nematode *C. elegans* and the fruit fly *D. melanogaster*. Genes involved in oxidative metabolism (such as respiratory chain proteins, ATP synthase and citric acid cycle proteins) and active molecular transport were significantly reduced with age. However, the timing of these changes suggested that this was part of an active programme rather than solely a response to environmental attrition. For instance, in both species, experimentally reducing oxidative stress had the greatest effect on life-span extension during early adulthood. Conversely, modulating the insulin/IGF-1 system had a more pronounced effect on life span in the middle-aged organism. We can interpret these findings to mean that the body has set in place metabolic strategies to pre-empt and minimize the damage associated with ageing. As the authors suggest, a greater appreciation of human health-affecting behaviour in early adulthood might yield benefits in later life.

The same laboratory pursued the role of the *insulin/IGF-1* and *daf-2* (insulin/IGF-1 receptor) pathway that was already known to affect life span in *C. elegans*[11]. Using mutant strains and RNAi methodologies, they showed through microarray screens that the FOXO transcription factor *daf-16* is required to mediate this signalling pathway: *daf-2* deficiency releases *daf-16* from repression and allows it to activate its downstream target genes. Interestingly, the insulin/IGF-1 signalling system has close parallels in mammals – a mammalian orthologue of *daf-16* exists, *FOXO3A*, that is regulated by the IGF-1 pathway effector and ageing gene, p66[SHC]. In the *C. elegans* experiment, sets of *daf-16* upregulated and downregulated genes were identified in longer living mutant strains. In the former group, the genes encoding for stress response and antioxidant genes such as *superoxide dismutase 3* and a *metallothionein* gene were identified together with lipid hormone metabolism and antimicrobial genes. In mammals, *FOXO3A* seems to additionally upregulate components of the genome maintenance pathway. In the latter, downregulated, group of genes were examples of metabolic genes, ubiquitination genes and genes of the vitellogenin structural egg yolk protein group. In the light of the earlier discussion regarding whether longevity is the result of active life extension or avoidance of death, it is interesting to see examples of both mechanisms (antioxidant/metabolic inhibition vs. antimicrobial) represented in the gene lists.

REACTIVE OXYGEN SPECIES, CELLULAR DAMAGE AND GENETICS

The damage to DNA and other cell macromolecules is caused by the reactive oxygen species (ROS) produced as a result of the energy-generating oxidative phosphorylation occurring within the mitochondria in each of our cells[12] – a small proportion of the oxygen consumed in this process is released as reactive superoxide species. Because mitochondria themselves possess a genome (encoding some of the components of the oxidative phosphorylation machinery) located near the source of the ROS, it has been suggested that it is very likely to be subject to high levels of damage (mutation accumulation) as the organism ages. Mitochondrial mutations would potentially cause feed-forward degeneration: a reduction in oxidative phosphorylation efficiency causing an increase in ROS production and, therefore, further propensity for cellular damage. Ageing not only results in the accumulation of mutations in the mitochondrial genome but it also permits the mutated genomes to accumulate within each cell (each cell has anywhere between 10s and 100s of mitochondrial genomes). At some point, a threshold will be crossed where the accumulating mitochondrial deficits impinge on cell function – and it can be appreciated that if such cells are part of the proliferating stem cell niche then either the dissemination of the deficit could be accelerated within a tissue or the proliferation process inhibited by the reduction in oxidative phosphorylation leading to a decrease in tissue regeneration[13]. It is now well documented that multiple organ systems are compromised by mitochondrial failure[14]. Perhaps due to their high energy demands, the central and peripheral nervous systems appear particularly susceptible to mitochondrial dysfunction which manifests itself in the form of neuropathies and dementia. Nevertheless, pathologies of the heart, lungs, musculature, pancreas and thymus have also been linked to mitochondrial failure in humans. Two studies have shown particularly clear age-dependent accumulation of definitively pathological mitochondrial mutations in the substantia nigra – a region of the brain implicated in the aetiology of Parkinson's disease in the elderly. The causal link with illness is not straightforward, however, as the mutation prevalence appears to be equal in aged individuals with or without Parkinson's disease[15,16]. Mitochondria, like nuclei, have dedicated mechanisms for repairing damaged DNA and thus mouse models have been generated that lack one of the repair proteins encoded by the *Polg1* gene. These mice have greatly increased levels of mitochondrial mutations and show a decreased life span associated with typical ageing phenotypes such as osteoporosis and weight loss[17,18].

A GENE–ENVIRONMENT INTERACTION BETWEEN CALORIC INTAKE RESTRICTION AND LONGEVITY

A longstanding direction for ageing research is based on the observation that a reduction in caloric intake results in not only an increase in life span but also an increase in general health including a reduction in illnesses of old age[19]. These studies seem to hold true across a wide range of species from yeast, *C. elegans* and *D. melanogaster* through to mouse and monkey. In terms of reproductive fitness, however, dietary restriction actually reduces fecundity. This suggests that variants leading to reduction in food uptake or slowed metabolism are unlikely to be favoured by genetic selection processes as they will be outcompeted by variants promoting an 'eat fast–die young' strategy that produces greater numbers of offspring

Dietary restriction seems to exert its effect on life span through a number of mechanisms. These can be essentially divided into two classes: those that alter intracellular pathways governing metabolism and survival and those that counteract the production of the harmful reactive oxygen species that are a byproduct of the oxidative phosphorylation pathway[20].

As detailed earlier, metabolic control through the insulin and insulin-like growth factor pathway is implicated in ageing and this is highlighted by its role in the response to dietary restriction. In times of freely available nutrition, insulin signalling results in the phosphorylation and subsequent degradation of Forkhead transcription factors (*daf-16* in *C. elegans* and *FOXO3A* in mammals). However, when food is limited, these transcription factors are able to enter the nucleus where they activate a set of genes which are thought to mediate a change in organismal strategy geared towards survival or even hibernation-like states. New insights from *C. elegans* are rapidly filling in the gaps at the 'top' part of the pathway translating caloric restriction into longevity. The *eat-2* gene encodes a nicotinic acetylcholine receptor subunit which is involved in the innervation of musculature required for eating. Mutants for this gene mimic the dietary restriction phenotype of increased longevity because of mechanical difficulties in eating. This reduced ageing phenotype is absent, however, in the presence of a second mutation in *wwp-1*, which breaks the link between dietary restriction, altered metabolism and life extension. The *wwp-1* and *ubc-18* genes encode interacting E3 and E2 subunits, respectively, of a ubiquitin ligase complex that targets other proteins for destruction. Current research suggests that components of the TOR pathway (a sensor of amino acid nutrition) and PHA-4 protein (FOXA, a transcription factor that overlaps functionality with daf-16/FOXO) may be such targets, ultimately leading to the activation of the life-prolonging metabolic state[21]. TOR signalling has received considerable interest recently because a large-scale study of dietary supplements affecting ageing in mice showed that a TOR inhibitor, rapamycin, significantly extended life span[22] even when administered to aged mice. Rapamycin, already used as a cancer treatment, has immunosuppressant activity meaning that it is unlikely to be used as the first anti-ageing therapy.

However, direct suppression of the pathways targeted by TOR (translation of mRNAs into protein and the breakdown and recycling of cellular components through the process of autophagy) might provide more specific and less harmful therapeutic options.

Two principal conclusions can be made by the reader of longevity research literature. Firstly, the various pathways described above exhibit significant cross-talk at several levels. This cooperation is required to ensure detection and integration of all relevant nutritional/environmental signals and to coordinate responses across metabolic, cell cycle and genomic repair systems. Secondly, this is perhaps the clearest example of gene–environment interaction. It will be interesting to see how quickly this research moves from 'bench to bedside', either in the form of proactive and preventative health education policies or in the search for drug therapies mimicking the beneficial effects of dietary restriction.

Finally, we may speculate on the efficiencies of evolution such that the biological processes used by unicellular organisms to withstand primordial boom-and-bust conditions have been molecularly conserved but now reworked as homeostatic mechanisms impacting on cellular proliferation, fecundity and, ultimately, life span.

REFERENCES

1. Bostock CV, Soiza RL, Whalley LJ. Genetic determinants of ageing processes and diseases in later life. *Maturitas* 2009; **62**: 225–9.
2. Herskind AM, McGue M, Iachine IA, Holm N, Sorensen TI, Harvald B *et al*. Untangling genetic influences on smoking, body mass index and longevity: a multivariate study of 2464 Danish twins followed for 28 years. *Hum Genet* 1996; **98**: 467–75.
3. McGue M, Vaupel JW, Holm N, Harvald B. Longevity is moderately heritable in a sample of Danish twins born 1870–1880. *J Gerontol* 1993; **48**: B237–44.
4. Olshansky SJ. From Michelangelo to Darwin: the evolution of human longevity. *Isr Med Assoc J* 2003; **5**: 316–18.
5. Richards MP. A brief review of the archaeological evidence for Palaeolithic and Neolithic subsistence. *Eur J Clin Nutr* 2002; **56**: 16.
6. Garinis GA, van der Horst GT, Vijg J, Hoeijmakers JH. DNA damage and ageing: new-age ideas for an age-old problem. *Nat Cell Biol* 2008; **10**: 1241–7.
7. Hasty P, Vijg J. Accelerating aging by mouse reverse genetics: a rational approach to understanding longevity. *Aging Cell* 2004; **3**: 55–65.
8. Hayflick L. The limited *in vitro* lifetime of human diploid cell strains. *Exp Cell Res* 1965; **37**: 614–36.
9. de Magalhaes JP, Faragher RG. Cell divisions and mammalian aging: integrative biology insights from genes that regulate longevity. *Bioessays* 2008; **30**: 567–78.
10. McCarroll SA, Murphy CT, Zou S, Pletcher SD, Chin CS, Jan YN *et al*. Comparing genomic expression patterns across species identifies shared transcriptional profile in aging. *Nat Genet* 2004; **36**: 197–204.
11. Murphy CT, McCarroll SA, Bargmann CI, Fraser A, Kamath RS, Ahringer J *et al*. Genes that act downstream of DAF-16 to influence the life span of *Caenorhabditis elegans*. *Nature* 2003; **424**: 277–83.
12. Linnane AW, Marzuki S, Ozawa T, Tanaka M. Mitochondrial DNA mutations as an important contributor to ageing and degenerative diseases. *Lancet* 1989; **1**: 642–5.
13. Taylor RW, Barron MJ, Borthwick GM, Gospel A, Chinnery PF, Samuels DC *et al*. Mitochondrial DNA mutations in human colonic crypt stem cells. *J Clin Invest* 2003; **112**: 1351–60.
14. Reeve AK, Krishnan KJ, Turnbull D. Mitochondrial DNA mutations in disease, aging, and neurodegeneration. *Ann N Y Acad Sci* 2008; **1147**: 21–9.
15. Bender A, Krishnan KJ, Morris CM, Taylor GA, Reeve AK, Perry RH *et al*. High levels of mitochondrial DNA deletions in substantia nigra neurons in aging and Parkinson disease. *Nat Genet* 2006; **38**: 515–7.
16. Kraytsberg Y, Kudryavtseva E, McKee AC, Geula C, Kowall NW, Khrapko K. Mitochondrial DNA deletions are abundant and cause functional impairment in aged human substantia nigra neurons. *Nat Genet* 2006; **38**: 518–20.
17. Kujoth GC, Hiona A, Pugh TD, Someya S, Panzer K, Wohlgemuth SE *et al*. Mitochondrial DNA mutations, oxidative stress, and apoptosis in mammalian aging. *Science* 2005; **309**: 481–4.
18. Trifunovic A, Wredenberg A, Falkenberg M, Spelbrink JN, Rovio AT, Bruder CE *et al*. Premature ageing in mice expressing defective mitochondrial DNA polymerase. *Nature* 2004; **429**: 417–23.
19. McCay CM, Crowell MF, Maynard LA. The effect of retarded growth upon the length of life span and upon the ultimate body size. *Nutrition* 1989; **5**: 155–71; discussion 72.
20. Mair W, Dillin A. Aging and survival: the genetics of life span extension by dietary restriction. *Annu Rev Biochem* 2008; **77**: 727–54.
21. Carrano AC, Liu Z, Dillin A, Hunter T. A conserved ubiquitination pathway determines longevity in response to diet restriction. *Nature* 2009; **460**: 396–9.
22. Harrison DE, Strong R, Sharp ZD, Nelson JF, Astle CM, Flurkey K *et al*. Rapamycin fed late in life extends life span in genetically heterogeneous mice. *Nature* 2009; **460**: 392–5.

10

The Clinical Pharmacology of Ageing

Brian Clarke and S. H. D. Jackson

Department of Clinical Gerontology, Kings College Hospital, London, UK

INTRODUCTION

The proportion of the world's population over the age of 60 years doubled in the last century and will increase two- to threefold in the first century of this millennium[1]. This population has a higher prevalence of chronic illnesses including cardiovascular diseases, cancers, osteoporosis, diabetes, Parkinson's disease, dementia and many other conditions. An increasing body of research is adding further prescribing indications for diseases that occur in the elderly population. This, along with the increasing size of the population, means that the numbers of prescriptions for elderly patients are increasing. Depending on the age group between 60% and 80% of elderly people are taking medication and between 20% and 30% of these patients are taking at least three drugs[2]. It is also estimated that although those over 75 years account for 14% of the population, they receive 33% of medication prescribed[3].

An appreciation of the physiology of the ageing process and how it affects an individual's response to, and handling of, drugs (and drug combinations) is essential to ensure safe prescribing for this vulnerable population[4]. The ageing process can be described as the consequences of the sum of local effects at the cellular and molecular level. A feature of cellular ageing is the disruption of regulatory processes between cells and organs with consequent failure to maintain homeostasis. There is also time-related loss of functional units (the smallest structures still capable of performing the specific physiological activity characteristic to the organ involved) such as nephrons and neurons[5]. These age-related physiological changes affect all organ systems in the body, they significantly affect how the ageing body handles and responds to pharmacological agents and hence need to be considered when prescribing. Chronic illness in older age and related organ dysfunction can compound these ageing-associated changes.

In this chapter we describe the age-associated changes in physiology and consequent changes in pharmacokinetics and pharmacodynamics and their implications for prescribing in elderly patients.

PHARMACOKINETICS AND THE AGEING PROCESS

Pharmacokinetics is the description of how the body handles drugs after administration. It incorporates the liberation, absorption, distribution, metabolism and excretion of drugs and their metabolites. These processes may be affected by the physiological changes associated with ageing resulting in changes in the pharmacokinetics of drugs.

Absorption

Following administration, a number of factors affect a drug's entry into the circulation. These include properties such as particle size, molecular weight, charge, solubility and pK_a (the pH at which 50% remains in an un-ionized, lipid-soluble state). Most drugs are weak acids or bases and are present in solution as both ionized and non-ionized species. Non-ionized drugs are lipid soluble and diffuse easily across the cell membrane. Following liberation some absorption may take place in the stomach, depending on the pK_a of the drug and the pH of the stomach. Gastric acid secretion decreases with normal ageing, confounded by the widespread use of proton pump inhibitors and, to a lesser extent, H2 receptor antagonists, as well as eradication of *Helicobacter pylori*[5]. Drugs requiring an acidic environment to become ionized will be affected most (e.g. iron compounds). However, for most drugs the large surface area of the small bowel makes it the main site of drug absorption. With ageing, although many drugs show no change in absorption, there is slightly reduced small bowel absorption of some substances (including iron, calcium and sugar). There is slower colonic transit time with age, and an associated decrease in peristalsis, largely due a loss of neurons involved in control of the gastrointestinal tract[1]. Passive intestinal permeability is probably unchanged in old age for most substances. However, active transport of other agents such as vitamin B12 is impaired. The effects of these age-related changes would influence primarily those drugs with low permeability and low solubility, e.g. cephalexin. Agents such as benzodiazepines and lithium are readily absorbed. Some agents such as neuroleptics can be esterified with long-chain fatty acids to yield depot formulations that are only slowly absorbed from the site of peripheral injection, e.g. flupentixol where the elimination half-life ($t_{1/2}z$) can be prolonged from 6 hours to 36 hours by use of an intramuscular depot preparation.

Distribution

The volume of distribution (V), also known as apparent volume of distribution, is a pharmacological term used to quantify the distribution of a medication between plasma and the rest of the body after oral or parenteral dosing. It is defined as the volume in which the amount of drug would need to be uniformly distributed to produce a given plasma concentration. Put another way it refers to the fluid volume that would be required to contain all of the drug in the body at the same concentration as that in the blood or plasma. A drug

Principles and Practice of Geriatric Psychiatry, 3rd edn. Edited by Mohammed T. Abou-Saleh, Cornelius Katona and Anand Kumar

with a high V (e.g. morphine -300 litres) implies extensive distribution outside the blood or plasma to other tissues such as fat or muscle. The V is dependent on lipophilicity and the ability of the drug to bind to plasma proteins such as albumin (acidic drugs) and $\alpha 1$-acid glycoprotein (basic drugs) thus holding drug in the blood compartment and reducing V[6,7].

An initial phase of distribution reflects cardiac output and regional blood flow, to well-perfused organs (heart, liver, kidney and brain). A second phase, involving a larger fraction of the body mass, to muscle, skin, viscera and fat can take several minutes to hours to reach steady state. Drugs accumulating in a given tissue, such as fat, may serve as a reservoir that prolongs drug action in that same tissue or at a distant site[7].

With ageing there is a decrease in lean body weight, muscle mass and body water and an increase in body fat per kg of body weight. As a result, lipid-soluble drugs such as benzodiazepines, morphine, neuroleptics and amitriptyline have an increased V due to the higher proportion of body fat. With ageing the higher V for such lipid-soluble drugs, (along with reduced clearance) will result in prolonged elimination half-life and hence drug effects. For water-soluble drugs, V will fall hence higher concentrations will be reached after initial administration. Loading doses of water-soluble drugs should, therefore, be reduced in elderly patients unless the drug also binds to muscle such as digoxin when the muscle mass would be a relevant consideration.

Protein Binding

Many drugs are protein bound to a varying degree. Bound drugs are inactive. An unbound drug is free to mediate its effect. The binding is usually reversible. Most acidic drugs (diazepam, phenytoin, warfarin) bind to albumin. Basic drugs such as lidocaine and tricyclic antidepressants bind to $\alpha 1$-acid glycoprotein. With healthy ageing there is no substantial change in plasma proteins, however, intercurrent illness can result in a drop in albumin and an increase in $\alpha 1$-acid glycoprotein (an acute phase protein)[5]. Chronic disease tends to accelerate the age-related decline in serum albumin. This can produce clinically significant increases in the free fraction of very heavily protein-bound drugs such as ibuprofen (99.5% bound)[5]. Other highly protein-bound drugs include benzodiazepines (>90%) and many antipsychotics (>90%). Lithium, however, is not protein bound and is excreted unchanged rather than being metabolized.

Clearance – Hepatic

Hepatic metabolism of drugs is dependent on the ability of the liver to extract drugs from the blood passing through the organ. Lipophilic drugs are metabolized into more hydrophilic compounds to facilitate elimination, particularly through the urine. However, in some cases metabolites are biologically active or even toxic. Thus risperidone is metabolized to an active metabolite (9-OH risperidone) which has a $t_{1/2}z$ of 22 hours versus the parent drug $t_{1/2}z$ of 4 hours. Similarly, diazepam is metabolized to an active metabolite (desmethyl diazepam) and amitriptyline is metabolized to nortriptyline. Both active metabolites have a longer $t_{1/2}z$ than the respective parent drugs. In the liver, phase I metabolism introduces a functional group onto the parent compound, generally resulting in loss of pharmacological activity. Phase I reactions are located primarily on the endoplasmic reticulum and are performed largely through the cytochrome P450 system of enzymes. This family of enzymes

oxidize, hydroxylate or hydrolyse the drug substrate[6,7]. Several studies have shown an age-related decline in the clearance of drugs by phase I metabolism, probably reflecting a reduced hepatic mass (and, for high clearance drugs, blood flow), as enzyme activity is preserved[5]. Induction or increased synthesis of the cytochrome P450 enzymes induced by drugs, such as phenytoin, isoniazid, glucocorticoids and alcohol, may decrease the bioavailability of parent drug compounds.

Inhibition of drug biotransformation enzymes, commonly by depletion of necessary co-factors, results in elevated levels of parent drugs. This can lead to increased pharmacological effects and an increased incidence of drug-induced toxicity. Inhibition of different isoforms of cytochrome P450 enzymes can be seen with erythromycin and ketoconazole (CYP450 3A4); SSRIs (CYP450 2D6). For two of these enzymes, CYP4502D6 and CYP4502C19, genetic polymorphisms exist that lead to poorly functioning enzymes causing individuals to be poor metabolizers. Thus when prescribing drugs metabolized by these enzymes where the therapeutic window is narrow, prescribing should be on the basis the patient is a poor metabolizer. For example when prescribing haloperidol starting doses should be those appropriate to poor CYP2D6 metabolizers.

Many pharmacokinetic drug interactions occur at the level of hepatic metabolism. For example the inhibition of clozapine and chlorpromazine metabolism by cimetidine.

Phase II reactions are conjugations. They are performed in the cytosolic compartment. Glucuronidation is the most important of the conjugation reactions. The increased water solubility of the glucuronide conjugates promotes their elimination in the urine or bile. Examples of drugs metabolized this way are benzodiazepines and morphine. The two main metabolites of morphine are morphine-3-glucuronide and the active metabolite morphine-6-glucuronide. Although they are formed in the liver they are excreted renally and hence accumulate in chronic kidney disease. Much less effort has been directed at the investigation of the effects of ageing on the conjugative mechanisms. In general, however, studies have not reported a major effect of ageing on the pathways of conjugation.

Clearance – Renal

Excretion of drugs and metabolites in the urine involves three processes: glomerular filtration; active tubular secretion; and passive tubular reabsorption. With ageing, renal mass decreases, as does glomerular filtration rate (GFR). There is also a reduced ability to concentrate urine and a reduced thirst during water deprivation.

GFR decreases at an average rate of 1 ml/min/year after middle age, and is often considered the most important pharmacokinetic change in older age. A normal GFR in a young adult is 120 ml/min depending on body size. Reduction in GFR with age affects the clearance of many drugs such as water-soluble antibiotics, diuretics and lithium and some non-steroidal anti-inflammatory drugs. Declining renal function cannot be quantified by measuring serum creatinine alone as creatinine production is a reflection of muscle mass, which declines with age. Clinically significant reduced renal function may be present with a serum creatinine still within the normal range. GFR can be calculated using several equations. The Cockroft–Gault (CG) equation uses age, weight, gender and serum creatinine[8]:

$$GFR (ml/min) = 1.23 \times \frac{(140 - age)(years) \times weight(kg) \times (0.85 \text{ if female})}{Creatinine\ (\mu mol/L)}$$

The Renal National Service Framework recommends that all laboratories report a formula-based estimation of GFR when serum creatinine is requested in adults[8]. The Modification of Diet in Renal Disease (MDRD) study equation (based on serum creatinine, age, gender and ethnic group) is widely used. The MDRD formula has the advantage of not requiring a weight, and can therefore be issued by the laboratory at the same time as a creatinine result is reported, however, it takes no account of muscle mass other than via age. Cockroft and Gault estimates tend to be lower than MDRD estimates. The adjustment of drug dosing in becomes particularly relevant where drugs are substantially or entirely excreted by the kidney. Routine pre-prescribing estimation of GFR is an essential adjunct to good prescribing in this vulnerable group. Given that the MDRD estimated GFR is now routinely provided this is the method of choice.

Where there is a narrow therapeutic index, significant toxicity can occur if doses are not adjusted downwards to account for renal impairment and subsequent reduced excretion. Examples include lithium, aminoglycosides and digoxin. Lithium toxicity is manifest as neuromuscular excitability, coarse tremors, fasicular twitching, motor agitation, delirium, nausea and even seizures if severely toxic. It is the most dialysable toxin known due to its low molecular weight. Indications to dialyse include high lithium concentrations (>4 mEq/L), or a concentration >2.5 mEq/L in a markedly symptomatic patient.

The presence of causes of chronic kidney disease such as hypertension and diabetes will potentiate the age-associated decline in renal function. It is especially important to review regularly drug therapy in frail older patients who may have, along with other known cardiovascular morbidities, undetected significant renal dysfunction.

Elimination Half-Life

The elimination half-life ($t_{1/2}z$) is the time it takes for the plasma concentration to be reduced by 50% during the elimination phase. This is distinct from the absorption half-life ($t_{1/2abs}$) or distribution half-life ($t_{1/2\,1}$). It is a function of both volume of distribution and clearance, where clearance is the nominal volume of blood that is cleared of drug per unit time:

$$t_{1/2}z = V/Cl$$

where $t_{1/2}z$ = elimination half-life; V = volume of distribution; Cl = clearance

The $t_{1/2}z$ provides a good indication of the time required to achieve steady state after a drug is started, and also an estimate of the time required to remove a drug from the body, and of appropriate dosing intervals. It takes approximately five half-lives to reach steady state during chronic dosing and a similar time to remove the drug when dosing is stopped. Thus for amiodarone with a $t_{1/2}z$ in excess of two months in elderly patients, it would take at least 10 months to reach steady state or to remove the drug from the body. For lipid-soluble drugs, the elimination half-life increases with age, due to both reduced clearance and increased V[6,7]. For water-soluble drugs such as lithium the reduced volume of distribution partially offsets the effect of reduced clearance on $t_{1/2}z$.

Renal tubular interactions are a common cause of pharmacokinetic drug interactions. For example renal tubular reabsorption of lithium is increased by thiazide and loop diuretics. This leads to reduced clearance of lithium and hence rising concentrations. Thus therapeutic drug monitoring can help manage such interactions unlike pharmacodynamic interactions (see below).

Bioavailability and First-Pass Metabolism

Bioavailability is a term used to describe the fractional extent to which an unchanged drug reaches the systemic circulation from its original site of administration. This takes into account the absorption, hepatic metabolism and biliary excretion of a drug that may occur before an oral drug reaches the systemic circulation.

Drugs that undergo substantial first-pass metabolism in the liver are avidly extracted from the blood during passage through the presystemic circulation (gut wall and liver), reducing their bioavailability. Ageing is associated with a reduction in first-pass metabolism, probably due to a 20–30% reduction in liver volume with age and a concomitant reduction in liver blood flow. As a result the bioavailability of drugs that undergo extensive first–pass metabolism, such as chlormethiazole, propranolol and labetalol can be significantly increased[5].

Pharmacodynamics

Pharmacodynamics can be defined as the study of the biochemical and physiological effects of drugs and their mechanisms of action. This includes therapeutic effects and unwanted effects. The effect of ageing may result in increased or decreased effect of a given drug concentration, when compared to the effect of the same concentration in a younger patient. These changes in sensitivity occur independently of any changes in pharmacokinetics that may also exist. Drugs exert their effect by binding selectively to target molecules within the body, these are usually proteins, but are also other macromolecules. The main drug targets are receptors, enzymes, ion channels, transporters (carriers) and DNA. An agonist drug uses a receptor site to activate or enhance a cellular response to that specific receptor. Benzodiazepines, for example, act as agonists at GABAa receptors. A drug that binds to a receptor target but is unable to elicit a maximal tissue response, in effect demonstrating less intrinsic activity or efficacy, is termed a partial agonist. Buspirone is an example of a partial agonist at $5\text{-}HT_{1A}$ receptors, providing anxioselective effects without inducing extra-pyramidal side effects. The antipsychotic aripiprazole acts as a partial agonist at dopamine D2 receptors.

An antagonist binds to a target site and inhibits the action of an endogenous agonist at that site. Mirtazapine is an antagonist at presynaptic α_1-adrenergic, $5\text{-}HT_2$ and $5\text{-}HT_3$ receptors. Most antagonists are competitive, in that they bind reversibly to a site and the effect of the antagonist may be overcome by raising the concentration of the agonist, as an example, many antipsychotics competitively antagonize dopamine receptors.

Other mechanisms of antagonism include irreversible competitive antagonism, whereby raising the concentration of endogenous agonists does not overcome the antagonist's effect: selegiline, for example, irreversibly inhibits monoamine oxidase-B. Non-competitive antagonist drugs do not block receptors, but block the signal transduction process initiated by receptor activation. Pharmacokinetic antagonism reduces free concentration of a drug by reducing its absorption or by accelerating its elimination. A chemical antagonist combines with the drug to neutralize its effect, e.g. protamine sulphate neutralizes the action of heparin[6,7].

Receptor activity and expression changes with ageing and the effect of age on drug sensitivities will vary depending on the drug studied. This makes generalizations difficult. However, there is evidence of reduced β-adrenoreceptor function in advancing age, reducing the elderly patients response to propanolol (β-adrenoceptor antagonist) and salbutamol (β2-adrenoceptor agonist). The responsiveness of α-adrenoceptors on the other hand is preserved with advancing age.

The ageing cardiovascular system also has reduced aortic and large artery elasticity and compliance, leading to higher systolic blood pressure, increased impedance to left ventricular ejection, with resultant tendency towards left ventricular hypertrophy. There is also a reduction in intrinsic heart rate and a reduction in baroreceptor sensitivity.

Orthostatic intolerance increases, as the response to posture change is blunted, leading to increased postural sway and propensity to falls[5,9]. This can of course be exacerbated by the concomitant use of anti-hypertensives and vasodilating drugs, and by drugs that may cause this as a side effect such as the α-blocker, tamsulosin.

In the brain, cholinergic function decreases with age, thermoregulation is also impaired, especially in frail individuals. There is also reduced shivering and vasoconstriction responses to hypothermia. Frail elderly patients are particularly prone to the adverse effects of neuroleptics, including delirium (anticholinergic effect), extrapyramidal symptoms (D_2 blockade), arrhythmias (prolongation of QT) and postural hypotension (α_1 blockade).

Of significant concern to elderly patients is the increased risk of death and cerebral ischaemia or stroke among those receiving treatment for psychosis or behavioural manifestations of dementia[10]. On the basis of 17 placebo-controlled trials of new neuroleptics, involving 5106 patients with dementia-related psychosis, the US FDA reported a 1.6- to 1.7-fold increase in the risk of death associated with all atypical antipsychotics[11]. The relative risk of stroke or transient ischaemic attack with risperidone is reported as high as 3.3 in this group versus controls[13]. It is, however, the only neuroleptic to have a marketing authorization for short-term use in the management of persistent aggression in patients with moderate to severe Alzheimer's disease.

There is increased sensitivity to the central nervous system effects of benzodiazepines, sedation being induced at much lower concentrations with advancing age. In addition these drugs are associated with an increase in postural sway and consequently falls. Table 10.1 lists some of the more common drug-specific pharmacodynamic changes that are seen with ageing along with some examples where ageing has no effect[5].

Pharmacodynamic drug interactions are those where drug A changes the effect of drug B without affecting its pharmacokinetics. Examples include the potentiation of the effects of lithium by calcium channel blockers, the lowering of seizure threshold by tricyclics and lithium reducing the effect of anticonvulsants.

ADVERSE DRUG REACTIONS

Approximately 5–10% of hospital admissions are related to managing drug-toxicity effects. Adverse drug reactions (ADRs) are common in elderly patients – it has been estimated that ADRs are the fourth to sixth leading cause of death. When adverse reactions occur in elderly patients, they are more likely to be severe and are less likely to be reported or recognized[1]. ADRs can be described as dose related, in that they are predictable based on the drug's pharmacological properties. Alternatively they may be idiosyncratic and not predictable on the basis of the pharmacological properties of the drug. These are often of an unknown mechanism and more likely to be more serious than dose-related ADRs (e.g. anaphylaxis)[1,13]. Recent data suggest that half of all disability or premature deaths from medication-related problems are preventable through prescribing vigilance and monitoring[3].

The presence of multiple drug treatments has been identified as an important factor associated with ADRs – the more medication the greater the chance of an ADR. However, ageing can be associated with an increased risk of adverse effects due to changes in pharmacodynamics independent of pharmacokinetics and multiple drug prescriptions. Non-steroidal anti-inflammatory drug (NSAID)-induced adverse events such as gastrointestinal haemorrhage and perforation increase with age, as does NSAID antagonism of antihypertensive therapy.

POLYPHARMACY VERSUS APPROPRIATE PRESCRIBING

The art of prescribing for the elderly patient is a balance between the conflicting demands of research evidence, practical considerations and patients' wishes. Polypharmacy can be defined as the concurrent use of multiple drugs (variously defined as the use of five or more drugs). It is no longer a useful term as it fails to encompass the omission of treatments for which there are clinical indications. Appropriate prescribing has been used to describe various aspects of medicines such as formulation and packaging, but should also be used to cover overuse, underuse and misuse of treatments. This term therefore describes not only the omission of medicines not indicated but also the use those that are indicated[14]. The National Service

Table 10.1 Selected pharmacodynamic changes with ageing

Drug	Pharmacodynamic effect	Age-related change in sensitivity
Adenosine	Heart-rate response	⇔
Diazepam	Sedation, postural sway	⇑
Diltiazem	Acute and chronic anti-hypertensive effect	⇑
Diphenhydramine	Postural sway	⇔
Enalapril	ACE inhibition	⇔
Furosemide	Peak diuretic response	⇓
Heparin	Anticoagulant effect	⇔
Morphine	Analgesic effect, respiratory depression	⇑
Temazepam	Postural sway	⇑
Warfarin	Anticoagulant effect	⇑

⇔ = no significant change; ⇑ = increase; ⇓ = decrease

Table 10.2 Causes of suboptimal drug prescribing

Clinical skills
* Inadequate clinical assessment leading to incorrect diagnosis
* Failure to obtain history of or document previous adverse drug reactions
* Failure to record current medication including over-the-counter medication
* Failure to monitor response to treatment
* Failure to recognize potentially serious drug interactions
* Failure to recognize subtle adverse drug reactions
* Failure to review repeat medication
* Failure to take account of altered pharmacokinetics and pharmacodynamics
* Simple error

Source: Modified from the Royal College of Physicians[16]

Table 10.3 Prescription checklist

* What are the patient's views?
* What is the diagnosis (or diagnoses) you are treating?
* What is the main aim of treatment?
* What are the treatment possibilities in this patient? (non-pharmacological potential?)
* How are your preferred drug and its metabolites (if active) cleared?
* Will other disease states affect your choice?
* Will physiological states (e.g. ageing) affect your choice?
* Could one drug treat more than one problem?
* What is the best route and dosage?
* When will you dose titrate?
* What will its duration be?
* What are the potential adverse effects?
* What potential drug interactions are relevant?
* Would discontinuing another drug help?
* What information should you discuss with the patient?

Framework for Older People highlights the need for appropriate prescribing[15]. Optimizing prescribing includes developing an awareness of the causes of suboptimal prescribing (Table 10.2) and the use of a prescription checklist to aid decisions (Table 10.3). Certain drugs should be actively avoided in elderly patients including: long-acting oral hypoglycemics as they present a high risk of hypoglycemia; long-acting benzodiazepines due to an increased risk of falls and disorientation; and non-selective anticholinergics as they can impair cognition and have significant peripheral anticholinergic side effects.

CONCLUSIONS

The ageing process is characterized by functional changes in all organ systems and results in reduced homeostatic capacity. These changes affect the pharmacokinetics and pharmacodynamics of many drugs commonly used in this age group. The high prevalence of co-morbidities and consequent high number of concomitant prescribed drugs are major factors in the development of ADRs. The reduced functional reserve associated with ageing is also responsible for an increased vulnerability to the effects of prescribed drugs and ADRs. A knowledge and appreciation of these processes, and their consequences, is necessary to ensure appropriate and safe prescribing in this age group.

REFERENCES

1. McLean AJ, Couteur DG. Aging biology and geriatric pharmacology. *Pharmacol Rev* 2004; **56**: 163–84.
2. Jackson SHD. Clinical trials in elderly patients. In Venitz J, Sittner W (eds), *Appropriate Dose Selection: How to Optimize Clinical Drug Development*. New York: Springer, 101–9, 2007.
3. Jackson SHD, Donnelly T. Therapeutics. In Rai, GS, Mulley, GP (eds), *Elderly Medicine: A Training Guide*, 2nd edn. London: Churchill Livingstone, 2007.
4. Swift CG. The clinical pharmacology of ageing. *Br J Clin Pharmacol* 2003; **56**: 249–53.
5. Jackson SHD, Mangoni AA. Age-related changes in pharmacokinetics and pharmacodynamics: basic principles and practical applications. *Br J Clin Pharmacol* 2003; **57**: 6–14.
6. Brunton LL, Lazo JS, Parker KL. *Goodman Gilman's Pharmacological Basis of Therapeutics*, 11th edn. London: McGraw-Hill, 2006.
7. Rang HP, Dale MM, Ritter JM, Flower R. *Rang & Dales Pharmacology*, 6th edn. London: Churchill Livingstone, 2007.
8. Lamb EJ, Webb MC, O'Riordan SE. Using the modification of diet in renal disease (MDRD) and Cockroft–Gault equations to estimate glomerular filtration rate (GFR) in older people. *Age Ageing* 2007; **36**, 689–92.
9. Moore A, Mangoni AA, Lyons D, Jackson SHD. The cardiovascular system in the ageing patient. *Br J Clin Pharmacol* 2003; **56**: 254–60.
10. Gardner DM, Baldessarini RJ, Waraich P. Modern antipsychotic drugs: a critical overview. *CMAJ* 2005; **172**: 1703–11.
11. Rockville (MD). FDA issues public health advisory for antipsychotic drugs used for treatment of behavioral disorders in elderly patients *[FDA Talk Paper] US Food and Drug Administration*,. 2005. At www.fda.gov/bbs/topics/ANSWERS/2005/ANS01350.html.
12. Summary of clinical trial data on cerebrovascular adverse events (CVAEs) in randomized clinical trials of risperidone conducted in patients with dementia. London: Medicines and Healthcare Products Regulatory Agency, 2004.
13. Routledge PA, O'Mahony MS, Woodhouse KW. Adverse drug reactions in elderly patients. *Br J Clin Pharmacol* 2003; **57**: 121–6.
14. Jackson SHD, Mangoni AA, Batty GM. Optimization of drug prescribing. *Br J Clin Pharmacol* 2003; **57**: 231–6.
15. UK Department of Health. *National Service Framework for Older People*. London: Department of Health, 2001.
16. Royal College of Physicians. *Medications for Older People*. London: Royal College of Physicians, 1997.

11

Cognitive Gerontology

Patrick Rabbitt

Neurocognitive Development Unit, School of Psychology, University of Western Australia, Australia

'Cognitive gerontology' is the study of changes in mental abilities and behaviour in old age and so also of changes in the brain and central nervous system that cause them. It developed alongside the rapid growth in academic psychology during the 1950s, promoted by the respect, and the access to funding that investigators, who then termed themselves 'human experimental psychologists', had gained by work on military applications during World War II. Leading figures of that decade were James Birren in the USA and Alan Welford in the UK. Welford was trained in applied experimental psychology and in ergonomics by Sir Frederick Bartlett. His book, *Ageing and Human Skill* (1958), summarizes his research with gifted colleagues in the Cambridge UK Nuffield Unit[1]. This was funded to discover how the contributions of older workers to the post-war economy might be optimized by appropriate training, systems and equipment. Present sensitivity to the imminent demands of ageing populations makes these key aims of current cognitive gerontology. Birren, was convinced by his work with the distinguished psychophysicist, 'Smitty' Stevens that the study of perceptual systems and response times must be the most direct way to use behavioural evidence to deduce changes in the central nervous system. He greatly broadened this view when he became director of the Section on Aging in the National Institutes of Health in Bethesda, MD, where his congenial personality facilitated collaborations that confronted him with medical, biological, epidemiological, demographical and social concomitants of old age. His friend Nathan Shock had begun at Baltimore the first, longest and most thorough longitudinal study of physiological, medical social and psychological changes in a large sample of older people[2]. From Shock's experience Birren learned to appreciate the separate and interacting effects of these factors in contributing to the enormous variability between individual trajectories of ageing – points missed by colleagues with backgrounds solely in 'mainstream' psychology who, because neurophysiological data was then unobtainable, typically borrowed from 'mainstream cognitive psychology' experimental paradigms originally designed to test functional models of mental abilities in young adults. The study of age changes in mental abilities potentially offered a timely challenge to the models then current in mainstream cognitive psychology which, at that time, represented unrealistic 'steady-state' systems that described neither individual differences nor processes of change within them. This challenge was not met until the late 1990s, when unanticipated results from brain imaging and electrophysiology began to bring into question models that had been derived solely from behavioural evidence. These new opportunities now allow us more sensibly to address some of the basic questions for cognitive gerontology: Why do cognitive changes occur? Arc thcy inexorable or can we delay them? What, precisely, are the changes that occur in the brain and central nervous system and how do these affect mental abilities and behaviour? When do changes first begin and how fast do they proceed? Do all individuals age at the same rate or do some age earlier and faster than others? Do all cognitive abilities change at the same or at different rates? Do individuals experience similar or different patterns of changes in their abilities? How does ageing affect our everyday cognitive competence and what can we do to mitigate its effects?

Physiologists had long recognized that because changes in the brain, body and central nervous system occur at markedly different rates in different species and individuals it is not useful to index ageing only by calendar time. They tried to derive algorithms to quantify progress of 'biological ageing' from a variety of different markers of the progress of physiological change[3]. These algorithms are interesting in actuarial and epidemiological contexts, but have proved less fruitful than study of associations between changes in specific biological subsystems, such as are involved in vision, hearing, touch and motor control and concomitant changes in mental abilities. Sensory changes evidently affect cognitive abilities because losses of visual acuity contrast sensitivity and colour vision[4], hearing, especially in higher frequencies, tactile sensitivity, smell and taste all degrade the information that we need to perceive and interpret objects and events[5] and losses of fine motor control impair our ability to respond rapidly and appropriately to our environments[6]. However in addition to these direct effects of information degradation, sensory changes also have other 'knock-on' entrained effects because the additional effort necessary to resolve degraded sense data draws on the limited pool of information-processing resources necessary to interpret and remember what we have seen or heard[7,8]. Because the time courses of sensory changes correlate robustly with those of declines in mental abilities such as intelligence, decision speed and memory, amounts of sensory losses are very effective biological markers for the extents of cognitive changes[9,10]. A logical problem in interpreting such associations between changes is key to many issues in ageing studies: because all physiological, neurophysiological and cognitive changes occur over the same periods of time between their progress are inevitable but may be as functionally uninformative as between independent clocks running at different rates. Imaging of brains *in vivo* now resolves this issue, showing that most of the shared variance between sensory and cognitive changes is accounted for by concomitant gross changes in brain volume and blood flow[11] and prevalence of white matter lesions[12].

A further question is what are the basic functional causes of these interdependent changes in general physiology and neurophysiology? Whether, for example, they are the burden of damage from pathologies and accidents that accumulates throughout the lifespan or whether some other processes, distinct from the effects of the sum of all pathologies and acquired physiological damage, that acts on all biological systems, though possibly at different rates, that is possibly genetically programmed, and so can be loosely described as 'biological ageing'. Like most apparent dichotomies in the 'nature/nurture' debate, this is misleading because both endogenous and exogenous factors operate jointly and strongly interact. There is good evidence for a 'medical model' of ageing based on the premise that, even after differences in their calendar ages have been taken into account, the pathologies and 'negative biological life events' that individuals have experienced account for a large proportion of the variance in mental abilities between them. Exceptionally healthy older men retain greater ability than those with poorer health[13]. Mental changes accelerate as death approaches[14] and some terminal pathologies, such as diabetes and infections, are associated with faster 'terminal decline' in cognitive abilities than others[15]. Thus, even apart from the incidence of particular neuropathologies such as dementias and cerebrovascular accidents that directly affect brain integrity, a substantial proportion of age-related decline in mental abilities is driven by a variety of pathologies that affect cerebrovasuclar sufficiency and brain metabolism. It would be useful to have quantitative estimates of exactly how much of that proportion of variance in mental abilities between older individuals, that is associated with differences in their calendar ages, can be accounted for by experience of particular pathologies. Though exact quantitative data are not yet available it seems no longer useful to argue whether cognitive changes are brought about 'mainly' by inexorable processes of endogenous 'normal ageing' or 'mainly' by pathologies and accidents. New technologies such as brain imaging, transient magnetic stimulation and cortical evoked potentials will soon tell us to what extent the amounts and patterns of central nervous system changes differ between individuals, what pathologies, genetic factors or life events may produce faster changes or different patterns and precisely how brain changes affect different mental abilities.

'Cognitive gerontology' is now a science in transition between a legacy of models to interpret a rich archive of behavioural observations and to gain an increasingly better understanding of the relationships of changes in abilities to the ageing brain and central nervous system that reveals these models to be inadequate – as indeed their proposers knew that they would as better neurophysiological evidence accumulated.

Discussion of the behavioural legacy may begin with Jim Birren's conviction that measurements of response times are an exceptionally good tool to investigate age-related cognitive change[16,17]. This idea had been reinforced by Joseph Brinley's discovery that exact estimates of average decision times for groups of older adults can be closely estimated by multiplying those of young adults by a simple constant[18]. John Cerella verified this for reported data from 108 different tasks on which older and younger groups had been compared[19]. Tim Salthouse greatly extended the implications of these findings by a further discovery that age-related variance in response times can also account for most of the age-related variance in errors on tests of verbal memory in which decision times are not constrained[20,21].

He argued from this that 'general slowing' of the cognitive system not only reflects, but also is the main functional driver of losses in all or most other mental abilities, so that behaviourally measured changes in performance on all, or most, cognitive tasks can be related to changes in a single, very simply measured, index of task performance. This idea became central to discussions for the next 20 years. This was a very powerful theory, but also became uncomfortable because it seemed to leave nothing further to investigate.

Investigators attempted various escapes. Some argued that 'general slowing theory' confused levels of description because behaviourally measured performance indices, such as response times, are distinct logical entities from psychometric statistical constructs such as 'general fluid intelligence' or 'information processing speed' that are computed on the basis of shared variance between performances on different tasks, and that both these entities are distinct from 'neurophysiological system characteristics': the many and various properties of neurones and their mutual interactions that determine their efficiency. Others re-evaluated the implications of the simple linear scaling suggested by 'Brinley plots'[22].

Other investigators beyond discussions of simple relationships between task complexity and averages of decision times to propose sophisticated models to account differences between distributions of response times produced by older and younger adults[23,24]. A third escape from the constraints on discussion imposed by 'general slowing theory' derived from observations that neuronal changes occur earlier and are greater in the frontal and prefrontal and temporal cortex than in other parts of the brain[25]. This makes it plausible that tasks derived from diagnostic tests for frontal damage, such as inhibition of irrelevant information in perception, planning, 'working' memory or task alternatives, may be especially sensitive to increasing age. Considered across all published studies in which no neurophysiological information is available, have been unclear. This is probably because while it is increasingly apparent that the range and variety of patterns of brain ageing differ widely between individuals behavioural comparisons have been made on small samples often of 20 persons or fewer who have not been selected on imaging data. Nevertheless more sophisticated mathematical analyses do suggest that some differences in distributions of reaction times and errors consistent with the frontal ageing hypothesis can be found, even on relatively small and unselected samples.

The frequency of elderly individuals' complaints of memory inefficiency is second only to that of their complaints about arthritic[26]. Nevertheless subjective reports of memory problems seem to be associated more with current levels of depression than with objective performance. Models for age-related declines in memory efficiency have been influenced by evidence of 'general slowing'. Craik and Lockhart showed that because the longer people are allowed to inspect and process words the better they can subsequently recall and recognize them, consequently age impairments can, at least partly, be attributed to reduced 'depth of processing' caused by slowing of information processing[27]. There is also support for the idea that impairment may be specific to some aspects of memory tasks rather than general to all. Craik and Byrd report that age impairs the ability to select critical information to be remembered[28]. However, discussions of age-related memory losses have been less constrained by the 'general slowing' hypothesis because most investigators have been more concerned with the nature of our memory representations of events and information than with the speed with which these can be established and retrieved. Consequently, a large literature discusses whether old age makes it more difficult to encode and recall some kinds of information rather than others. Differences are reported between verbal and spatial information, for faces, for proper names, for hymn tunes, and for the sources and context of correctly recalled material. There are also 'natural history' experiments comparing age-differences reports of vividness, detail and accuracy of so-called 'flashbulb memories' of striking public or private events (e.g. see[29]). Another critical distinction is between memory for information that has been acquired, used and so rehearsed over many years and memory for more recently learned material (e.g. see[30]). Conceptually related to this distinction between memory for recall of recent and distant information, for more and less frequently rehearsed material and for more and less emotionally charged and striking information are investigations of the numbers of memories that elderly people can retrieve of events from different periods of their lives[31]. Most studies find a scarcity of quantity, but not necessarily of the vividness of memories from childhood. This contrasts with a 'reminiscence bump' of memories relating to adolescence and young adulthood, with a marked decline in memories for the very recent past[31]. One explanation is that the greater efficiency of the central nervous system in youth makes memories of earlier experiences more detailed and durable. Another is that events experienced in youth are, at least when they are experienced, novel, possibly also more exciting and are likely to have been more frequently recalled in subsequent years than the probably more often repeated, and possibly more banal, experiences of late middle age and senescence. Consistent with this idea are findings that, irrespective of the ages of individuals when they experienced them, particularly eventful historical periods such as World War II are especially numerous and vivid, and of course also more often provide material for reminiscence.

This distinction between the ability to recall and to use information and skills acquired over a long lifetime and continually updated by practice and the ability to remember new information and events and to learn new lessons from them is a key issue that differentiates between the study of abilities in old age and in youth. It is best defined in the work of John Horn who distinguished between what he termed 'fluid abilities' that are early impaired by age and 'crystallized' abilities' that show relatively little decline[32]. Fluid abilities are indexed by scores on tests of general intelligence and of the ability to acquire and recall new information and 'crystallized' abilities are indexed by tests of acquired, and subsequently continuously practised, material such as vocabulary and social skills.

Memory studies have also been influenced by the hypothesis that because ageing affects the frontal and temporal lobes of the brain earlier and more severely than other areas, so the selection of relevant from irrelevant information held in memory must be more sensitive to age than other abilities (e.g. see[33]). Also associated with the frontal and temporal lobes are the abilities, collectively termed 'prospective memory', to use past information to anticipate what is likely to happen next, to plan how to cope with anticipated events and to retain these plans until they can be appropriately implemented[34]. A key insight has been that, in old age, the efficiency of prospective memory, as indeed other kinds of memory, depends on the availability of environmental information to support recall.

Studies of cognitive ageing use two methodologies: cross-sectional comparisons between groups of different ages and longitudinal studies in which the same groups are repeatedly assessed. These can very profitably be combined by analyses including both kinds of comparisons[35] (see Baltes, 1968). A pervasive difficulty for both is inadvertent selection of participants. Elderly individuals who volunteer for demanding studies are atypically able and well members of their generations and are usually also better educated, more likely to have practised intellectually demanding professions and are usually

also not socioeconomically disadvantaged. Representation of ethnic minorities is also questionable. In more arduous longitudinal studies self-selection of volunteers not only biases initial recruitment but also brings about selective attrition because less healthy and so least able participants withdraw or die leaving a progressively elite group of survivors. So, in longitudinal studies, true rates of cognitive change will be miscomputed unless the incidence of these deaths and dropouts is taken into consideration[14]. Another difficulty for longitudinal studies of mental abilities is that if participants are repeatedly given the same, or similar, tests even at intervals of many years, they show significant practice effects. This also leads to potential miscomputations of trajectories of change, more particularly because older and less able individuals, and those who approach dropout or death, experience less improvement from practice than the younger, more intelligent and more healthy. Anstey, Hofer and Luszcz illustrate how some of these issues can be dealt with in an exploration of both cross-sectional and longitudinal examinations of the ways in which correlations between sensory and cognitive variables change over time[9].

It is becoming questionable whether very large and prolonged longitudinal studies that collect only behavioural data on cognitive change, with additional data on health and demographics, are the most resource-effective way of learning how and why age affects mental abilities. The rapid development of non-invasive brain imaging means that we can now detect changes in the brain and central nervous system over periods measured in months rather than decades that can be related to cotemporaneous patterns of cognitive changes within individuals. Thus, even with small samples we can study variability in idiosyncratic patterns of brain changes and correspondingly patterned changes in cognition[36]. Raz et al. provide excellent general discussions of how such studies can be carried out and what they can tell us[37]. An explosion of studies of relationships between changes in specific brain locations and in particular aspects of cognitive performance includes age differences in the functional neuroanatomy of verbal recognition memory[38], the functional neuroanatomy of age related changes in visual attention[39], changes in entorhinal cortex and losses of memory function, age-related differences in working memory using real-time fMRI, differences in brain activity associated with age-related changes in memory function and brain changes associated with changes in motor performance.

These relationships between changes in specific brain locations and in specific abilities proceed against a background of global changes affecting all parts of the brain such as increasing prevalence and distribution of white-matter lesions, losses in brain volume and declines in cerebral blood flow that all appear to be associated with declines in information processing rate[11,12]. This complicates interpretation of cognitive effects of localized brain changes that may be masked or blurred by these global changes that affect all systems, but to different degrees. This may partially explain apparent contradictions between the results of the many studies using behavioural evidence alone to test the sensible hypothesis that earlier and faster 'ageing' of the prefrontal cortex must result in correspondingly more marked age decrements in abilities such as working memory, planning, attention and executive functions. For example most of the adapted behavioural clinical diagnostic tests for frontal damage tests used to test this hypothesis are scored in terms of the relative speed with which decisions can be made. Since we know that gross brain changes such as white-matter lesion incidence specifically impair processing speed, scores on so-called 'frontal' tasks must evidently reflect some complex combination of local and global effects. It is therefore unsurprising that comparisons between small groups of 30 or fewer individuals for whom information on brain status is not available should only sometimes find evidence for the 'frontal ageing' hypothesis.

With these cautions, 'cognitive gerontology' is now becoming an exciting science in which a rich body of behavioural data and growing sophistication in understanding brain changes is rapidly transforming our understanding of how and why our mental abilities change, why all of us do not change at the same speed or in the same ways and, hopefully, suggest what we may do about this.

REFERENCES

1. Welford AT. *Ageing and Human Skill*. Oxford: Oxford University Press, 1958.
2. Shock NW, Greulich RC, Andres R, Arenberg D, Costa PT, Lakatta EG, Tobin JD. *Normal Human Aging. The Baltimore Longitudinal Study of Aging*. NIH Publ. No 84-2450. Washington, DC: US Government Printing Office, 1984.
3. Borkan GA, Norris AH. Biological age in adulthood. Comparison of active and inactive US males. *Hum Biol* 1980; **52**: 787–802.
4. Faubert J. Visual perception and aging. *Can J Exp Psych* 2000; **56**: 164–75.
5. Corso J. *Aging, Sensory Systems and Perception*. New York. Praeger, 1981.
6. Goodpaster BH, Park SW, Harris TB, Kritchevsky SB, Nevitt M, Schwartz AV *et al*. The loss of skeletal muscle strength, mass, and quality in older adults: the health, aging and body composition study. *J Gerontol Med Sci* 2006; **61A**: 1059–64.
7. Dickenson CM, Rabbitt PMA. Simulated visual impairment: effects on text comprehension and reading speed. *Clin Vision Sci* 1991; **6**: 301–8.
8. van Boxtel MPJ, van Beijsterveldt CEM, Houx PJL, Acteunis JC, Metsemakers JFM, Jolles J. Mild hearing impairment can reduce verbal memory performance in a healthy adult population. *J Clin Exp Neuropsychol* 2000; **22**: 147–54.
9. Anstey KJ, Hofer SM, Luszcz MA. A latent growth curve analysis of late-life sensory and cognitive function over 8 years: evidence for specific and common factors underlying change. *Psychol Aging* 2003; **18**: 714–26.
10. Lindenberger U, Scherer H, Baltes B. The strong connection between sensory and cognitive performance in old age: not due to sensory acuity reductions operating during cognitive assessment. *Psychol Aging* 2001; **16**: 196–205.
11. Rabbitt P, Mogape O, Scott M, Lowe C, Thacker N, Pendleton N *et al*. Effects of global atrophy, white matter lesions and cerebral blood flow on age-related changes in speed, memory, intelligence, vocabulary, and frontal function. *Neuropsychol* 2007; **21**: 684–95.
12. Deary IJ, Leaper SA, Murray AD, Staff RT, Whalley LJ. Cerebral white matter abnormalities and lifetime cognitive change: a 67 year follow up of the Scottish Mental Survey 1932. *Psychol Aging* 2003; **18**: 140–8.
13. Houx PJ, Vreeling FW, Jolles J. Rigorous health screening reduces age effects on a memory scanning task. *Brain Cogn* 1991; **15**: 246–60.
14. Rabbitt P, Lunn M & Wong D. Understanding terminal decline in cognition and risk of death: Methodological and theoretical implications of practice and dropout effects. *European Psychologist* 2006; **11**: 164–171.
15. Small BL, Fratiglione L, vonStrauss E & Backman L. Terminal Decline and Cognitive Performance in Very Old Age: Does Cause of Death Matter? *Psychology and Aging* 2003; **18**: 193–202.
16. Birren JE. The significance of age-changes in speed of perception and psychomotor skills. In Anderson JE (ed.), *Psychological Aspects of Aging*. Washington, DC: American Psychological Association, 1956.
17. Birren JE. Tutorial review of changes in choice response time with advancing age. In Baumeister H (ed.), *Bayer Symposium No 6*. Bonn: Springer-Verlag, 1979, 232–47.
18. Brinley JE. Cognitive sets, speed and accuracy of performance in the elderly. In Welford AT, Birren JE (eds), *Behavior, Aging and the Nervous System*. Springfield, IL: Charles Thomas, 1965.
19. Cerella J. Information processing rates in the elderly. *Psychol Bull* 1985; **98**(1): 67–83.
20. Salthouse TA. *A Theory of Cognitive Aging*. Amsterdam: Elsevier Science, 1985.
21. Salthouse TA. The processing-speed theory of adult age differences in cognition. *Psychol Rev* 1996; **103**(3): 403–28.
22. Myerson J, Hale S, Wagstaff D, Poon L & Smith G. The information-loss model: A mathematical theory of age-related cognitive slowing. *Psychological Review* 1990; **97**(4): 475–87.
23. Ratcliff D, Spieler D, McKoon G. Explicitly modeling the effects of aging on response time. *Psychonom Bull Rev* 2000; **7**(1): 1–25.
24. Verhaeghen P, Cerella J. Everything we know about aging and response times: a meta-analytic integration. In Hofer SM, Alwin DF (eds), *The Handbook of Cognitive Aging: Interdisciplinary Perspectives*. Thousand Oaks: Sage, 2008, 134–50.
25. West RL. An application of prefrontal cortex function theory to cognitive aging. *Psychol Bull* 1996; **120**(2): 272–92.
26. Guttman JM. The elderly at home and in retirement housing: a comparative study of health problems, functional difficulties and support service needs. In Marshall VW (ed.), *Aging in Canada: Social Perspectives*. Ontario: Fitzhugh & Whiteside, Don Mills, 1980, 232–59.
27. Craik FIM, Lockhart RS. Levels of processing: a framework for memory research. *J Verb Learn Verb Behave* 1972; **11**: 671–84.
28. Craik FM, Byrd TD. Aging and cognitive deficits: the role of attentional resources. *Aging Cogn Proc* 1982; 191–211.
29. Cohen G, Conway MA, Maylor EA. Flashbulb memories in older adults. *Psychol Aging* 1994; **9**(3): 454–63.
30. Charness N, Kelley CL, Bosman EA, Mottram M. Word processing training and retraining: effects of adult age, experience and interface. *Psychol Aging* 2001; **16**(1): 110–27.
31. Fitzgerald JM, Lawrence R. Autobiographical memory across the life-span. *J Gerontol B* 1984; **39**: 692–8.
32. Horn, J. The theory of fluid and crystallized intelligence in relation to concepts of cognitive psychology and aging in adulthood. In Craik FM, Trehub S (eds), *Aging and Cognition Processes*. New York: Plenum Press, 1982, 237–78.
33. Zacks RT, Hasher L. Directed ignoring: inhibitory regulation of working memory. In Dagenbach D, Carr TH (eds), *Inhibitory Mechanisms in Attention, Memory, and Language*. New York: Academic Press, 1994, 241–64.
34. McDaniel A, Einstein G, Stout S, Morgan R. Aging and maintaining intentions over delays: do it or lose it. *Psychol Aging* 2003; **18**(4): 823–35.

35. Baltes PB. Longitudinal and cross-sectional sequences in the study of age and generation effects. *Human Development* 1968; **11**: 145–171.

36. Grady CL. Functional brain imaging and age-related changes in cognition. *Biol Psychol* 2000; **54**(1–3): 259–81.

37. Raz N, Lindenberger U, Rodrigue KM, Kennedy HM, Head D, Williamson A *et al*. Regional brain changes in aging healthy adults: general trends, individual differences and modifiers. *Cerebral Cortex* 2005; **15**: 1676–89.

38. Madden DJ, Turkington TG, Provenzale JM, Denny LL, Hawk TC, Gottlob LR, Coleman RE. Adult age differences in the functional neuroanatomy of verbal recognition memory. *Hum Brain Mapping* 1999; **7**: 115–35.

39. Madden DJ, Spaniol J, Whiting WL, Bucur B, Provenzale JM, Cabeza R *et al*. Adult age differences in the functional neuroanatomy of visual attention. A combined fMRI and DTI study. *Neurobiol Aging* 2007; **3**: 459–76.

12

Chronological and Functional Ageing

David Melzer and Iain Lang

Peninsula Medical School, University of Exeter, UK

INTRODUCTION

Ageing is a surprisingly difficult process to define or measure. In a superficial sense it is everything that happens to an individual over time but, for geriatricians and gerontologists, notions of ageing are tied to physiological deterioration and increasing vulnerability to diseases absent in the young. This notion of ageing is synonymous with 'senescence' and is defined[1] as progressive deterioration during adult life that underlies an increasing vulnerability to challenges and a decreased chance of survival.

The relationship between chronological and functional age has implications for ageing research and public policy. In this chapter we describe more meaningful ways of thinking about human ageing than through the proxy of elapsed time, or chronological ageing.

THE PLASTICITY OF AGEING

Ageing is widely seen as the result of lifelong accumulation of random molecular damage[2]. Damage results in declining function at many levels[3], including in mitochondrial function, DNA transcription (through unrepaired somatic DNA mutations) and in the ability of cells to divide and repair tissues. The balance between damage and repair mechanisms determines the amount of unrepaired damage, which manifests as ageing at the cellular and organism level. Secondary responses to damage can then occur, including chronic inflammation, hypothesized as a major element in human ageing[4].

Ageing processes are surprisingly plastic and variable. This is evident at all levels from the molecular to the societal and global population levels. The most dramatic demonstration of the plasticity of ageing is the finding that hundreds of mutant genes (mainly knockouts) can produce radical life extensions in model organisms[5]. In addition to affecting stress responses and telomeres, endocrine signalling has also emerged as particularly important in these models. In general, the impact of 'longevity' gene manipulation on lifespan becomes progressively smaller on moving up the evolutionary ladder[6] and relevance to human ageing is speculative.

In addition to genetic manipulation, caloric restriction in laboratory settings also increases lifespan when compared to unlimited feeding[7,8]. In humans, obesity is a risk for mortality and functioning in older people[9] but whether there are benefits in radically reducing caloric intakes below those required for maintaining a healthy weight is unclear.

The variability of ageing in humans is apparent both in single organs and in the longevity and functioning of individuals. Analyses of the Baltimore Longitudinal Study of Ageing have shown marked heterogeneity in the rates of decline in function of different organ systems: for example, mean maximum work rate and renal blood flow generally decline far faster than measures of nerve conduction[10]. More surprising, individuals show great heterogeneity in patterns of impairment of individual systems, with little indication of typical patterns. In human population studies, it is usual to find people functioning at a higher level than others aged 20 or 30 years younger.

One potential means of identifying an individual's 'true' age is through identifying biomarkers of ageing. The concept of biomarkers of ageing is appealing because it implies biological measures can reflect the rate of ageing and that successful interventions on the ageing process may affect these markers. The American Federation for Aging Research proposed that a biomarker of ageing must[11]:

- predict the rate of ageing – i.e. it should be a better predictor of lifespan than chronological age;
- monitor a basic process that underlies the ageing process, not the effects of disease;
- be testable repeatedly without harming the person;
- be valid in humans and in laboratory animals.

Markers showing potential include telomere length[12] and p16^{INK4a} expression[13].

The search for biomarkers of ageing assumes there is an underlying biological state of ageing that can be summed up as a single number but counterarguments regard ageing as a complex, uncoordinated phenomenon that cannot be encapsulated so simply[14]. Despite much research effort, most gerontologists accept that no biomarkers of ageing have yet been validated[11,15].

FUNCTIONAL HEALTH STATUS

A key aspect of functional ageing or functional health status assesses functioning at the level of the whole older person. Functional health status is related to chronological age, disease and need for care, and understanding the functional aspects of ageing is an important part of geriatric medicine. In the medical model of disease, the clinician gathers symptoms and signs, makes a diagnosis and bases the therapeutic approach on this diagnosis. Complementing this

Principles and Practice of Geriatric Psychiatry, 3rd edn. Edited by Mohammed T. Abou-Saleh, Cornelius Katona and Anand Kumar
© 2011 John Wiley & Sons, Ltd

disease-orientated approach, functional assessment provides an understanding of the impact and consequences of the older person's disease or diseases, giving information on level of independence and prognosis, as well as health care, rehabilitation and social needs.

Since a major impact on functional health comes from disease, a framework that represents the relationship between disease and disability is valuable in developing the concept of functional ageing. The World Health Organization (WHO) originally proposed a theoretical pathway progressing from disease to impairment to disability to handicap[16]. An alternative pathway, proposed by Nagi[17] and utilized by the US Institute of Medicine[18], progresses from diseases and conditions to impairment to functional limitation to disability. An effort to operationalize this latter pathway defines 'impairment' as dysfunction and structural abnormalities in specific body systems, 'functional limitation' as restriction in basic physical and mental actions such as ambulating, grasping, and stepping up, and 'disability' as difficulty in doing activities in daily life such as personal care, household management, job and hobbies[19]. The importance of identifying external factors that needlessly cause disablement outside the individual is a major theme in the more recent WHO classification systems[20].

Means of assessing and reporting functional health status include the following.

Self-Reported Functioning

Physical functioning shows a downwards trend with age and is often assessed through self-report of the ability to perform specific tasks, including self-care activities such as bathing and dressing (activities of daily living), and activities necessary to maintain independence in the community, such as shopping and food preparation (instrumental activities of daily living)[21–24]. A concern with self-reported functioning is that different individuals and groups may have different thresholds for reporting difficulty or inability to carry out activities[25].

Performance Measures

Performance measures of functioning, in which the individual is asked to carry out standardized tasks, offer a way of benchmarking function and comparing over time or across populations[26]. Self-reported functional status may differ from measured function for a variety of reasons, including differences in the domains measured. Assessing both allows us to combine an objective measure of poor performance with an indication of how much everyday function is affected[27]. Tests of physical function are used in clinical assessments of older people[28,29] and can help identify individuals with pre-clinical limitations who are at increased risk of developing disabilities[30,31]. One established measure is the short physical performance battery, including measures of gait speed, chair stands and tandem balance tests: this score has been widely used in clinical settings for the assessment of mobility limitations[32]. Other approaches include these measures plus muscle strength and respiratory function[33].

Frailty

Frailty, generally taken to mean multisystem impairment and a high level of vulnerability, has been defined in two ways: as a phenotype; and as a score of age-related deficits or 'frailty index'. The phenotypic approach defines frailty as a clinical syndrome in relation to five criteria: unintentional weight loss (10 lbs or more in the preceding year); self-reported exhaustion; weakness (grip strength); slow walking speed; and low physical activity[34]. Using these criteria, individuals are defined as either frail (three or more criteria present) or not frail (fewer than three criteria). The frailty index approach sums the number of age-associated deficits experienced by an individual, including symptoms, signs, diseases and disabilities[35] (Rockwood 2007). The resulting score provides an indication of the likelihood that frailty is present, and the index demonstrates characteristic changes with age. Each of these operationalizations of frailty has been validated in multiple populations. Although the two approaches overlap there are substantial differences between them[36] and it has been suggested each represents a different form of frailty and a different trajectory of age-related loss of function[37].

Cognitive Function

Age-related functional decline has cognitive as well as physical aspects. These often occur together, and they share some risk[38] as well as protective[39] factors. The care burden associated with dementia, on both a societal[40] and a household level[41] level, is large. There are major public health concerns about the impact on health and social care services of growing numbers of older people with declining cognitive function and dementia[42]. Among the challenges of dealing with this growing problem is the shortage of effective treatments for dementia, and attention has been drawn to identifying individuals with mild cognitive impairment – that is, those who are not demented but have a memory impairment beyond that expected for age and education[43]. Cognitive function and dementia are covered in more details in Part IV of this book.

Factors Affecting Functional Health Status

The prevalence of disability in activities of daily living (ADL) in the non-institutionalized population rises steeply with increasing age and is higher in women than men at the older ages[44] – see Figure 12.1.

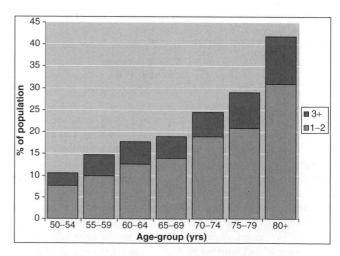

Figure 12.1 Percentage of community-living respondents reporting one to two, and three or more disabilities in activities of daily living. Activities include dressing, walking across a room, getting in and out of bed, eating and using the toilet
Source: Data from the English Longitudinal Study of Ageing (Steel *et al.*, 2004)

The prevalence of ADL disabilities in institutional settings is generally very high. It is important to keep in mind that, although chronological age is strongly related to disability prevalence, many other factors, particularly socioeconomic status, have large impacts on disability that are independent of age[45,46]. Large differences in functional health status exist between groups, with those in less privileged social positions having higher rates of incidence and prevalence of disability, in both developed[47] and emerging countries[48].

Cognitive impairment is a major contributor to functional disability[49,50], as are depressive symptoms[51,52]. A number of potentially modifiable behaviours are associated with physical function or functional decline in later life. These include obesity[53], smoking[54] and low levels of physical activity[55]. The onset of functional disability often occurs relatively early in life: recent studies have identified that up to one in five adults aged 50–64 experiences some problems with walking a quarter of a mile[56,57].

LONG-TERM TRENDS IN FUNCTIONAL HEALTH STATUS AND POLICY IMPLICATIONS

An important issue connected to functional ageing is the relationship between length of life and time spent in a disabled state. Life expectancy increased substantially through the 20th century. One consequence of reduced early-life mortality may be that more people survive to ages where they suffer from chronic diseases, leading to increased prevalence of long-term disability and loss of independence. Increases in life expectancy which bring longer periods of life with impaired function are undesirable both for individuals and for societies and a major goal of gerontology is increasing longevity without increasing the number of years spent in the disabled or dependent state.

An important concept in relation to evaluating the consequences of worldwide population ageing is 'active life expectancy' or 'disability-free life expectancy'[58]. Active life expectancy is defined as the average number of years an individual at a given age will survive and remain in the active, or non-disabled, state. Most analyses of active life expectancy define disability in relation to activities of daily living, with active life expectancy calculated using life-table techniques that consider transitions from the active, non-disabled state to a disabled state or death. The original analysis of active life expectancy considered the transitions to both death and disability as irreversible[58] but recent studies have shown a substantial proportion of disabled persons returns, at least temporarily, to the non-disabled state[59].

Compression of Morbidity

A related theory is 'compression of morbidity'[60], the idea that the burden of lifetime illness may be compressed into a shorter period prior to death. Fries argued that in all species the maximum lifespan is fixed, human beings are quickly approaching this limit, and with a stable life expectancy any postponement of disease and disability would result in a compression of morbidity. He stated the compression of morbidity was inevitable and predicted a decrease in the period people could expect to spend with severe disease and disability. The relationship over time between life expectancy and active life expectancy can be used to assess the occurrence of a compression of morbidity. Three possible scenarios for population morbidity in women are illustrated schematically in Figure 12.2. The total length of the bars in this figure represents life expectancy for Non-Hispanic black U.S. females projected by the Census Bureau for 2050. The

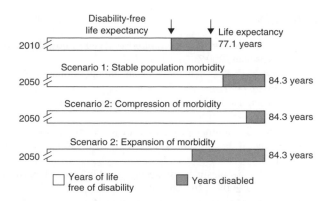

Figure 12.2 Scenarios for change in average burden of population disability level: compression of morbidity and alternatives

length of the unshaded segments of the bars represents active or disability-free life expectancy, and the shaded areas of the bars represent the average number of years in the disabled state. In scenario 1, the onset of disability has been postponed the same number of years as life expectancy has increased, and the number of years spent in the disabled state is unchanged from 2010. In scenario 2, there has been a compression of morbidity. Finally, in scenario 3, although disability-free life expectancy in 2050 has increased compared with 2010, it has not kept pace with increases in life expectancy and there is an expansion of population morbidity.

Active life expectancy is not always easy to assess and debates persist about whether compression of morbidity is taking place. However, trends in disability can be estimated in other ways. It is possible to estimate disability prevalence, which is not equivalent to disabled life expectancy but reflects a cross-sectional picture of the proportion of the population that is disabled. Much attention has been focused on examining longitudinal trends in disability by analysing annual estimates of disability prevalence. In the US, it appeared that in the 1970s the prevalence of age-related disability was rising but in the 1980s rates declined[61–63] and this trend seems to have continued. A number of studies have reported ongoing year-on-year improvements in the health of the older population[61,64–66] and reports from other countries, including New Zealand[67] and England[68] suggest similar patterns of decline in age-related disability may also be occurring there.

Possible causes of these declines in disability prevalence include environmental changes making daily tasks easier[19], more intensive use of assistive devices[69] and other social changes, including attitudes to being active in old age. In addition, the proportion of older people who have little education (a potent risk factor for disability) has declined[63,70]. There is evidence of declining prevalence of some medical conditions in old age, especially cardiovascular disease, and health risk avoidance and improved diagnostic and therapeutic techniques will also have contributed[71].

The future burden of morbidity and disability in the older population is of great concern to those involved in planning, financing and delivering health care and social services. If current rates of disabling diseases such as Alzheimer's disease and hip fracture remain unchanged, the numbers of older people with these diseases will increase substantially during this century[72]. Understanding the factors that affect functional ageing is critical to reducing the burden of disability and compressing morbidity. Effective interventions are needed to prevent the onset and mitigate the consequences of diseases and conditions that lead to much disability in later life.

REFERENCES

1. Masaro EA. *Handbook of the Biology of Ageing*, 6th edn. Amsterdam: Elsevier, 2006.
2. Kirkwood TB. A systematic look at an old problem. *Nature* 2008; **451**: 644–7.
3. Vijg J, Campisi J. Puzzles, promises and a cure for ageing. *Nature* 2008; **454**: 1065–71.
4. Franceschi C. Inflammageing as a major characteristic of old people: can it be prevented or cured? *Nutr Rev* 2007; **65**: S173–6.
5. Kenyon C. The plasticity of ageing: insights from long-lived mutants. *Cell* 2005; **120**: 449–60.
6. Kuningas M, Mooijaart SP, Van Heemst D, Zwaan BJ, Slagboom PE, Westendorp RG. Genes encoding longevity: from model organisms to humans. *Ageing Cell* 2008; **7**: 270–80.
7. Hursting SD, Lavigne JA, Berrigan D, Perkins SN, Barrett JC. Calorie restriction, ageing, and cancer prevention: mechanisms of action and applicability to humans. *Annu Rev Med* 2003; **54**: 131–52.
8. Masoro EJ. Overview of caloric restriction and ageing. *Mech Ageing Dev* 2005; **126**: 913–22.
9. Lang IA, Llewellyn DJ, Alexander K, Melzer D. Obesity, physical function, and mortality in older adults. *J Am Geriatr Soc* 2008; **56**: 1474–8.
10. Arking R. *The Biology of Ageing*, 2nd edn. Sunderland, MA: Sinauer, 1998.
11. Johnson TE. Recent results: biomarkers of ageing. *Exp Gerontol* 2006; **41**: 1243–6.
12. Von Zglinicki T, Martin-Ruiz CM. Telomeres as biomarkers for ageing and age-related diseases. *Curr Mol Med* 2005; **5**: 197–203.
13. Krishnamurthy J, Torrice C, Ramsey MR, Kovalev GI, Al-Regaiey K, Su, L, Sharpless NE. Ink4a/Arf expression is a biomarker of ageing. *J Clin Invest* 2004; **114**: 1299–307.
14. Costa PT, McCrae RR. Design and analysis of ageing studies. In Masoro EJ (ed.), *Handbook of Physiology, Section 11: Ageing*. New York: Oxford University Press, 1995.
15. Butler RN, Sprott R, Warner H, Bland J, Feuers R, Forster M *et al*. Biomarkers of ageing: from primitive organisms to humans. *J Gerontol A Biol Sci Med Sci* 2004; **59**: 560–7.
16. World Health Organization. *International Classification of Impairments, Disabilities, and Handicaps*. Geneva: World Health Organization, 1980.
17. Nagi SZ. An epidemiology of disability among adults in the United States. *Milbank Mem Fund Q Health Soc* 1976; **54**: 439–67.
18. US Institute of Medicine. Committee on a National Agenda for Prevention of Disabilities. *Disability in America: Toward a National Agenda for Prevention*. Washington, DC: Institute of Medicine, 1991.
19. Verbrugge LM, Jette AM. The disablement process. *Soc Sci Med* 1994; **38**: 1–14.
20. World Health Organization. *International Classification of Functioning, Disability and Health*. Geneva: World Health Organization, 2001.
21. Branch LG, Meyers AR. Assessing physical function in the elderly. *Clin Geriatr Med* 1987; **3**: 29–51.
22. Applegate WB, Blass JP, Williams TF. Instruments for the functional assessment of older patients. *N Engl J Med* 1990; **322**: 1207–14.
23. Guralnik JM (ed.). *Assessing Physical Function in Older Populations*. New York: Oxford University Press, 1991.
24. Lawton MP, Brody EM. Assessment of older people: self-maintaining and instrumental activities of daily living. *Gerontologist* 1969; **9**: 179–86.
25. Melzer D, Lan TY, Tom BDM, Deeg DJH, Guralnik JM. Variation in thresholds for reporting mobility disability between national population subgroups and studies. *J Gerontol A Biol Sci Med Sci* 2004; **59**: 1295.
26. Guralnik JM, Branch LG, Cummings SR, Curb JD. Physical performance measures in ageing research. *J Gerontol* 1989; **44**: M141–6.
27. Reuben DB, Seeman TE, Keeler E, Hayes RP, Bowman L, Sewall A *et al*. Refining the categorization of physical functional status: the added value of combining self-reported and performance-based measures. *J Gerontol A Biol Sci Med Sci* 2004; **59**: 1056–61.
28. Guralnik JM, Ferrucci L. Assessing the building blocks of function: utilizing measures of functional limitation. *Am J Prev Med* 2003; **25**: 112–21.
29. Studenski S, Perera S, Wallace D, Chandler JM, Duncan PW, Rooney E *et al*. Physical performance measures in the clinical setting. *J Am Geriatr Soc* 2003; 51: 314–22.
30. Cesari M, Kritchevsky SB, Penninx BW, Nicklas BJ, Simonsick EM, Newman AB *et al*. Prognostic value of usual gait speed in well-functioning older people – results from the Health, Ageing and Body Composition Study. *J Am Geriatr Soc* 2005; **53**: 1675–80.
31. Melzer D, Gardener E, Lang IA, Williams B, Guralnik JM. Measured physical performance. In Banks J, Lessof C, Nazroo J (eds), *Retirement, Health and Relationships of the Older Population in England: The 2004 English Longitudinal Study Of Ageing (Wave 2)*. London: Institute for Fiscal Studies, 2006, 165–78.
32. Studenski S, Perera S, Wallace D, Chandler JM, Duncan PW, Rooney E *et al*. Physical performance measures in the clinical setting. *J Am Geriat Soc* 2003; **51**: 314–22.
33. Lan TY, Melzer D, Tom BD, Guralnik JM. Performance tests and disability: developing an objective index of mobility-related limitation in older populations. *J Gerontol A Biol Sci Med Sci* 2002; **57**: M294.
34. Fried LP, Tangen CM, Walston J, Newman AB, Hirsch C, Gottdiener J *et al*. Frailty in older adults: evidence for a phenotype. *J Gerontol A Biol Sci Med Sci* 2001; **56**: M146–56.
35. Rockwood K, Mitnitski A. Frailty in relation to the accumulation of deficits. *J Gerontol A Biol Sci Med Sci* 2007; **62**: 722–7.
36. Hubbard RE, O'Mahony MS, Woodhouse KW. Characterising frailty in the clinical setting – a comparison of different approaches. *Age Ageing* 2009; **38**: 115–19.
37. Cigolle CT, Ofstedal MB, Tian Z, Blaum CS. Comparing models of frailty: the Health and Retirement Study. *J Am Geriatr Soc* 2009; **57**: 830–9.
38. Llewellyn DJ, Lang IA, Xie J, Huppert FA, Melzer D, Langa KM. Framingham stroke risk profile and poor cognitive function: a population-based study. *BMC Neurol* 2008; **8**: 12.
39. Williamson JD, Espeland M, Kritchevsky SB, Newman AB, King AC, Pahor M *et al*. Changes in cognitive function in a randomized trial of physical activity: results of the lifestyle interventions and independence for elders pilot study. *J Gerontol A Biol Sci Med Sci* 2009; **64**: 688–94.
40. Schneider EL, Guralnik JM. The ageing of America. Impact on health care costs. *JAMA* 1990; **263**: 2335–40.

41. Dunkin JJ, Anderson-Hanley C. Dementia caregiver burden: a review of the literature and guidelines for assessment and intervention. *Neurology* 1998; **51**: S53–60; discussion S65–7.

42. Ferri CP, Prince M, Brayne C, Brodaty H, Fratiglioni L, Ganguli M *et al*. Global prevalence of dementia: a Delphi consensus study. *Lancet* 2005; **366**: 2112–7.

43. Petersen RC, Smith GE, Waring SC, Ivnik RJ, Tangalos EG, Kokmen E. Mild cognitive impairment: clinical characterization and outcome. *Arch Neurol* 1999; **56**: 303–8.

44. Steel N, Huppert FA, McWilliams B, Melzer D, Marmot M, Banks J *et al*. Physical and cognitive function. *Health, Wealth and Lifestyles of the Older Population in England: The 2002 English Longitudinal Study of Ageing*. London: Insitute of Fiscal Studies, 2004.

45. Stuck AE, Walthert JM, Nikolaus T, Bula CJ, Hohmann C, Beck JC. Risk factors for functional status decline in community-living elderly people: a systematic literature review. *Soc Sci Med* 1999; **48**: 445–69.

46. Lang IA, Llewellyn DJ, Langa KM, Wallace RB, Huppert FA, Melzer D. Neighborhood deprivation, individual socioeconomic status, and cognitive function in older people: analyses from the English Longitudinal Study of Ageing. *J Am Geriatr Soc* 2008; **56**: 191–8.

47. Melzer D, Izmirlian G, Leveille SG, Guralnik JM. Educational differences in the prevalence of mobility disability in old age: the dynamics of incidence, mortality, and recovery. *J Gerontol B Psychol Sci Soc Sci* 2001; **56**: S294.

48. Parahyba MI, Stevens K, Henley W, Lang IA, Melzer D. Reductions in disability prevalence among the highest income groups of older Brazilians. *Am J Public Health* 2009; **99**: 81–6.

49. Melzer D, McWilliams B, Brayne C, Johnson T, Bond J. Profile of disability in elderly people: estimates from a longitudinal population study. *BMJ* 1999; **318**: 1108.

50. McGuire LC, Ford ES, Ajani UA. Cognitive functioning as a predictor of functional disability in later life. *Am J Geriatric Psych* 2006; **14**: 36–42.

51. Ormel J, Rijsdijk FV, Sullivan M, Van Sonderen E, Kempen GI. Temporal and reciprocal relationship between IADL/ADL disability and depressive symptoms in late life. *J Gerontol B Psychol Sci Soc Sci* 2002; **57**: P338–47.

52. Berkman LF, Berkman CS, Kasl S, Freeman DH, Leo L, Ostfeld AM *et al*. Depressive symptoms in relation to physical health and functioning in the elderly. *Am J Epidemiol* 1986; 124: 372–88.

53. Angleman SB, Harris TB, Melzer D. The role of waist circumference in predicting disability in periretirement age adults. *Int J Obes (Lond)* 2006; **30**: 364.

54. Vita AJ, Terry RB, Hubert HB, Fries JF. Ageing, health risks, and cumulative disability. *N Engl J Med* 1998; **338**: 1035–41.

55. Lang IA, Guralnik JM, Melzer D. Physical activity in middle-aged adults reduces risks of functional impairment independent of its effect on weight. *J Am Geriatr Soc* 2007; **55**: 1836–41.

56. Gardener EA, Huppert FA, Guralnik JM, Melzer D. Middle-aged and mobility-limited: prevalence of disability and symptom attributions in a national survey. *J Gen Intern Med* 2006; **21**: 1091.

57. Mottram S, Peat G, Thomas E, Wilkie R, Croft P. Patterns of pain and mobility limitation in older people: cross-sectional findings from a population survey of 18,497 adults aged 50 years and over. *Qual Life Res* 2008; **17**: 529–39.

58. Katz S, Branch LG, Branson MH, Papsidero JA, Beck JC, Greer DS. Active life expectancy. *N Engl J Med* 1983; **309**: 1218–24.

59. Hardy SE, Dubin JA, Holford TR, Gill TM. Transitions between states of disability and independence among older persons. *Am J Epidemiol* 2005; **161**: 575–84.

60. Fries JF. Aging, natural death, and the compression of morbidity. *N Engl J Med* 1980; **303**: 130–5.

61. Manton KG, Stallard E, Corder LS. The dynamics of dimensions of age-related disability 1982 to 1994 in the U.S. elderly population. *J Gerontol A Biol Sci Med Sci* 1998; **53**: B59–70.

62. Crimmins EM, Saito Y, Reynolds SL. Further evidence on recent trends in the prevalence and incidence of disability among older Americans from two sources: the LSOA and the NHIS. *J Gerontol B Psychol Sci Soc Sci* 1997; **52**: S59–71.

63. Freedman VA, Martin LG. Understanding trends in functional limitations among older Americans. *Am J Public Health* 1998; **88**: 1457–62.

64. Freedman VA, Crimmins E, Schoeni RF, Spillman BC, Aykan H, Kramarow, E *et al*. Resolving inconsistencies in trends in old age disability: report from a technical working group. *Demography* 2004; **41**: 417–41.

65. Manton KG, Corder L, Stallard E. Chronic disability trends in elderly United States populations: 1982–1994. *Proc Natl Acad Sci USA* 1997; **94**: 2593–8.

66. Kramarow E, Lubitz J, Lentzner H, Gorina Y. Trends in the health of older Americans, 1970–2005. *Health Aff (Millwood)* 2007; **26**: 1417–25.

67. Graham P, Blakely T, Davis P, Sporle A, Pearce N. Compression, expansion, or dynamic equilibrium? The evolution of health expectancy in New Zealand. *J Epidemiol Community Health* 2004; **8**: 659–66.

68. Jagger C, Matthews R, Matthews F, Robinson T, Robine JM, Brayne C. The burden of diseases on disability-free life expectancy in later life. *J Gerontol A Biol Sci Med Sci* 2007; **62**: 408–14.

69. Manton KG, Corder L, Stallard E. Changes in the use of personal assistance and special equipment from 1982 to 1989: results from the 1982 and 1989 NLTCS. *Gerontologist* 1993; **33**: 168–76.

70. Singer BH, Manton KG. The effects of health changes on projections of health service needs for the elderly population of the United States. *Proc Natl Acad Sci USA* 1998; **95**: 15618–22.

71. Schoeni RF, Freedman VA Martin LG. Why is late-life disability declining? *Milbank Q* 2008; **86**: 47–89.

72. Jagger C, Matthews R, Lindesay J, Robinson T, Croft P, Brayne C. The effect of dementia trends and treatments on longevity and disability: a simulation model based on the MRC Cognitive Function and Ageing Study (MRC CFAS). *Age Ageing* 2009; **38**: 319–25; discussion 251.

13

Successful Ageing

Ann Bowling

Department of Primary Care and Population Health, University College London, UK

BACKGROUND

Population ageing and increases in life expectancy in the developed world have led to international interest in how to age 'successfully'. But there is no interdisciplinary agreement on what successful ageing is. The literature reveals that conceptual definitions and measurement of successful ageing vary both within and between disciplines; there is little interdisciplinary cross-referencing. Biomedical models emphasize physical and mental functioning as successful ageing, while sociopsychological models focus on social functioning, life satisfaction and psychological resources. Older people themselves adopt multifaceted definitions of successful ageing[1,2]. Moreover, research shows that older people consider themselves to have aged successfully, but classifications based on traditional, narrower domain models do not[1-3]. This suggests that a model of successful ageing needs to be multidimensional, cut across disciplines, and incorporate a lay perspective for social significance. Moreover, there is overlap, and lack of clarity, in the literature between concepts of successful ageing, active ageing and quality of life. Analysis of overlap between lay perceptions of these concepts in surveys using comparable methods showed that lay perceptions of active ageing emphasized striving to *maintain* health, functioning, and wider well-being (e.g. exercising the body and/or mind in order to maintain health and functioning), while lay definitions of successful ageing and quality of life focused on the existence of a state, rather than the striving for its achievement (e.g. the having health and ability *per se*[4]). This distinction is consistent with the literature on active ageing, which portrays quality of life, and also having 'successfully *aged*', as the end points, although 'successful *ageing*' can also be viewed as a dynamic process.

An earlier interdisciplinary systematic review of the literature by this author[1,3] found that the most common definitions of successful ageing were based on theories of social functioning, life satisfaction, psychological resources and biomedical approaches. A small body of literature focused on lay views. The distinction between concepts as either predictor or constituent variables was not always clear. The survey with the highest citations for successful ageing was the MacArthur Foundation studies of successful ageing[5-7], which are based on a biomedical model, broadened to include active engagement with life.

SOCIAL FUNCTIONING

Social functioning has been conceptualized and measured in many different ways, including social engagement, social roles, participation and activity, social contacts and exchanges, and/or positive social relationships. The main theoretical approaches relating to successful ageing and social functioning are disengagement, activity and continuity theories, although each suffers from limitations, and all are now outdated (see Bearon for critique[8]).

LIFE SATISFACTION

A smaller number of authors included life satisfaction, well-being or their elements in their conceptual and empirical definitions of successful ageing. Components of life satisfaction include zest, resolution, fortitude, relationships between desired and achieved goals, self-concept and mood, including happiness[9-11]. Havighurst[11] (p. 305) stated, 'a person is aging successfully if he feels satisfied with his past and present life', thus arguing that life satisfaction is an attribute of successful ageing, although others have argued that it is a condition for its achievement. Feelings of well-being were an outcome indicator of successful ageing in the Berlin Aging Study[12]. There is lack of consistency about the status of life satisfaction, in particular, as an indicator or constituent variable.

PSYCHOLOGICAL RESOURCES

Few investigators have included psychological resources as their study definition of successful ageing, and again it was not always clear whether the concepts used were predictor or constituent variables. Psychological models include possession of the resources of personal growth, creativity, self-efficacy, autonomy, independence, effective coping strategies, sense of purpose, self-acceptance and self-worth. These models have been criticized for their emphasis on autonomy, thus marginalizing frail older people[13].

Baltes and colleagues[14] developed a strong theoretical model based on the need to employ compensatory strategies when facing the dynamic between challenges and depleting reserves: selective optimization with compensation (SOC). With this model, it is proposed that individuals can contribute to their own successful ageing: when *selected* activities can no longer be performed, strategies are needed to find new ones, and to maximize reserves. There is some supportive evidence from the Berlin Aging Study that people who use these strategies have better well-being than others[12].

Ryff's theoretical model of successful ageing emphasizes a life course approach, and holds that a developmental focus is required[15,16]. She argues that successful ageing includes 'positive or ideal functioning' and is related to development over the life course. Fisher[17] also emphasized adaptability and coping, and defined successful ageing as an ability to continue to grow and learn by using past experiences to cope with present circumstances and set goals for development.

BIOMEDICAL THEORIES

Biomedical or decline theories generally define successful ageing as the optimization of life expectancy, while minimizing physical and mental deterioration. The MacArthur Foundation in the USA commissioned a major study of successful ageing led by Rowe, which comprised a three-site longitudinal study of adults living in the community aged 70–79 in 1988. It was rooted in Rowe and Kahn's[5–7] model of successful ageing as absence, or avoidance of, disease and risk factors; maintenance of physical and cognitive functioning; and active engagement with life (with others and in productive activities). They made the distinction between 'usual ageing', which describes normal decline in physical, social and cognitive functioning with age, and 'successful ageing', in which physiological and cognitive functional loss is minimized, there is active engagement with life, and capabilities even enhanced. This only partly recognizes heterogeneity among older people, and criticisms of Rowe and Kahn's model include its narrowness, neglect of life course dynamics, failure to address adaptation to disease, and neglect of those who are incapacitated who cannot age successfully by the criteria used. A small number of studies have used elements of both biomedical and psychosocial approaches.

LAY VIEWS OF SUCCESSFUL AGEING

Lay views are important to investigate in order to ensure that models of successful ageing have social significance, and to minimize the danger that definitions reflect mainstream cultural expectations and norms for the behaviour of older people. Without social significance, policy initiatives to enhance successful ageing are likely to fail.

The systematic review of the literature, and empirical research by this author, illustrated that lay people view this concept multidimensionally, and included the following elements in their definitions: physical health and functioning; mental and cognitive health; psychological well-being and life satisfaction, including happiness; social functioning – relationships, support, activities and productivity; psychological resources, including personality, personal growth, accomplishments, sense of purpose, physical appearance, self-acceptance, coping, positive outlook, sense of humour; spirituality; lifestyles; neighbourhood; financial circumstances and security. It is also perceived as a dynamic concept. Von Faber *et al.*[18] reported, from the Leiden longitudinal study of people aged 85+, that older people defined successful ageing as a process of adaptation rather than as a state of being, supporting psychological rather than biomedical models. Thus, investigations of older people's views of successful ageing

have indicated that they are far more multifaceted than existing models, crossing the boundaries between the physical, psychological and social self. Moreover, research shows that, overall, many older people consider themselves to have aged successfully while biomedical classifications do not categorize them so. Strawbridge *et al.*[19] compared self-ratings of successful ageing among their sample members aged 65–69 from the longitudinal Alameda County Study with Rowe and Kahn's three-factor model. They reported that, while half the sample could be categorized as having aged successfully with their own self-ratings, only 19% could be so categorized with Rowe and Kahn's model. Bowling's further national survey of people aged 50+ living at home in Britain, asked people what they understood by the term successful ageing, then to rate the extent to which they had aged successfully[2]. Two-thirds of respondents defined successful ageing in terms of having good health and functioning; almost half defined it psychologically. Others defined it mainly in relation to social roles and activities, social relationships, neighbourhood and local community. About four in ten (39%) respondents rated themselves as ageing successfully 'Very well', and a further 37% as 'Well', as opposed to 'All right', 'Not well' or 'Not very well' (see Figure 13.1).

There were positive correlations between self-rated ageing successfully and good self-rated health, no reported longstanding illness, and good quality of life. There were no statistically significant associations with age. The main reasons people gave for their self-ratings of successful ageing included their physical and mental functioning, followed by psychological well-being, social relationships and financial circumstances[1,2]. Also, while over a quarter indicated that they felt defiant about ageing when asked how they thought ageing would affect them, about 40% mentioned worse health and/or functioning, about a fifth thought they would be limited in their lives, and about 10% each mentioned worsening mental health and dependency (see Figure 13.2).

In a further study, Bowling and Iliffe[20] constructed and tested alternate biomedical, social, psychological and multifaceted lay-based models of successful ageing in a national population survey of people

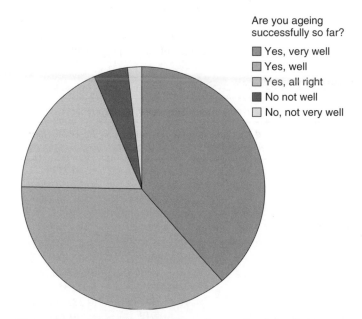

Figure 13.1 Self-rated successful ageing: national population sample aged 50+ in Britain. Data from the *English Longitudinal Study of Ageing* (Steel *et al.*, 2004)

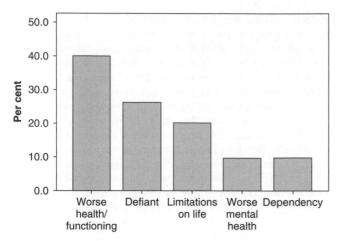

Figure 13.2 How do you think getting older will affect you? (Most common responses shown)

aged 65+ living at home in Britain. Respondents classified as successfully aged with the multifaceted lay model, compared to those classified as not successfully aged, had over five times the odds of rating their quality of life as good rather than not good. The comparable odds ratios from the other, single domain models, while significant, were considerably lower.

Table 13.1 shows the associations between pairs of successful ageing themes mentioned by respondents. While the table shows several instances where mention of one definition was associated with reduced odds of mentioning another, it also indicates the multidimensionality of lay definitions. Respondents who defined successful ageing in terms of health had almost twice the odds, compared to those who did not, of also defining it in terms of finances. Respondents who mentioned social activity had almost twice the odds of mentioning social relationships (and vice versa), possibly reflecting the perceived need for companionship to undertake social activities (e.g. to accompany one on outings). Those mentioning social relations also had over twice the odds of mentioning finances, compared to those who did not. Similarly, respondents who mentioned finances had almost twice the odds of mentioning health and twice the odds of mentioning social relationships (and vice versa). And respondents who defined successful ageing in terms of neighbourhood factors had almost twice the odds of also mentioning financial circumstances. The importance of these results is the demonstration that successful ageing is not perceived narrowly by lay people, in contrast to most theoretical models. It also illustrates the interaction between domains of life, e.g. social relationships may be needed for people to participate in social activities (to accompany people), and people see having both health and money as important for successful ageing.

CONCLUSION

In conclusion, most authors in this field have made unwarranted conceptual leaps and assumed, often, that they have addressed 'successful' ageing with their chosen outcome indicators, with relatively few attempts at theoretical or conceptual justification. Rowe and Kahn's three-factor biomedical model (including social elements) of successful ageing is the most popular and widely used in biomedical research, even outside the MacArthur studies of successful ageing[5-7]. In contrast, lay models of successful ageing are more multidimensional, and, in particular, include more psychosocial elements. Also, to be realistic, the concept needs to be broadened, and to be seen on a continuum, rather than categorized dichotomously in terms of successful or unsuccessful. Also, given the inconsistency with which variables are used as either predictor or constituent variables in the study of successful ageing, advances could be made by grounding the term in older people's definitions, and building on multidimensional theoretical approaches.

Thus a definition of successful ageing would include longevity, physical, cognitive, psychological and social health and functioning, including effective coping, living circumstances (finances, neighbourhood) and overall life satisfaction. Precursors of effective coping strategies are likely to be possession of resources such as SOC, as hypothesized by Freund and Baltes (1998)[12]. Using this approach, the different models are complementary to each other, and successful ageing is not only about maintaining good health and functioning, but it is also about coping and remaining in control of one's life over the life-course, with the aim of achieving dynamically a status

Table 13.1 Logistic regression: associations (odds ratios; CI, confidence intervals) between successful ageing theme pairs ($n = 854$)[a]

Themes (mentioned 1 versus not mentioned 0 = referent) (y):

Themes (mentioned 1 vs. not mentioned 0 = referent) (x):	Health Exp b (95% CI)	Psychological Exp b (95% CI)	Social activity Exp b (95% CI)	Finances Exp b (95% CI)	Social relations Exp b (95% CI)	Neighbourhood Exp b (95% CI)
Health	–	0.713* (0.529–0.960)	0.725** (0.534–0.983)	1.915*** (1.355–2.706)	0.581*** (0.417–0.810)	0.903 (0.551–1.480)
Psychological	0.712** (0.528–0.959)	–	0.643** (0.478–0.866)	0.546*** (0.398–0.748)	0.539*** (0.387–0.751)	0.744 (0.460–1.204)
Social activity	0.725* (0.534–0.983)	0.639** (0.475–0.862)	–	0.703* (0.504–0.981)	1.842*** (1.330–2.551)	0.980 (0.602–1.597)
Finances	1.903***	0.543*** (0.396–0.745)	0.694* (0.498–0.968)	–	2.001*** (1.417–2.825)	1.981** (1.221–3.215)
Social relations	0.576*** (0.413–0.803)	0.535*** (0.385–0.745)	1.839*** (1.327–2.547)	2.004*** (1.421–2.826)	–	1.000 (0.594–1.684)
Neighbourhood	0.912 (0.555–1.500)	0.755 (0.467–1.221)	0.965NS (0.591–1.575)	1.990** (1.231–3.217)	1.008 (0.599–1.697)	–

[a] Fully adjusted for age, sex and socioeconomic status; *$p < 0.05$; **$p < 0.01$; ***$p < 0.001$; NS not significant at 0.05 level.

of having successfully aged. Then the question of whether, and the extent to which, successful ageing is achievable can be addressed. Also, clinicians involved in the care of older people need to balance a *dis-ease* with a health and psychosocial perspective of older age, in order to enhance mutual understandings about desired treatment goals.

REFERENCES

1. Bowling A, Dieppe P. What is successful ageing and who should define it? *Br Med J* 2005; **331**: 1548–51.

2. Bowling A. Successful ageing from older people's perspectives. Results from a British survey of ageing. *Eur J Ageing* 2006; **3**: 123–36.

3. Bowling A. Aspirations for older age in the 21st century: what is successful ageing? *Int J Aging Hum Dev* 2007; **64**: 263–97. [Italian translation at www.geragogia.net.]

4. Bowling A. Enhancing later life: how older people perceive active ageing. *Ageing Ment Health* 2008; **12**: 293–301.

5. Rowe JW, Kahn RL. Human aging: usual and successful. *Science* 1987; **237**: 143–9.

6. Rowe JW, Kahn RL. Successful aging. *Gerontologist* 1997; **37**: 433–40.

7. Rowe JW, Kahn RL. *Successful Aging*. New York: Pantheon.

8. Bearon LB. Successful aging: what does the 'good life' look like? *Forum Fam Consum Issues* (North Carolina State University) 1996; **1**: 1–6.

9. Neugarten BL, Havighurst RJ, Tobin SS. The measurement of life satisfaction. *J Gerontol* 1961; **16**, 134–143.

10. Vaillant GE. Avoiding negative life outcomes: evidence from a forty five year study. In Baltes PB, Baltes MM (eds), *Successful Aging: Perspectives from the Social Sciences*. New York: Cambridge University Press, 1990.

11. Havighurst RJ. Successful aging. In Williams RH, Tibbits C, Donahue W (eds), *Processes of Aging*. New York: Atherton Press, 1963.

12. Freund AM, Baltes PB. Selection, optimisation, and compensation as strategies of life management: correlations with subjective indicators of successful aging. *Psychol Aging* 1998; **13**: 531–43.

13. Nolan M. Successful aging: keeping the 'person' in person-centred care. *Br J Nurs* 2001; **10**: 450–54.

14. Baltes PM, Baltes MM (eds). *Successful Aging: Perspectives from the Social Sciences*. New York: Cambridge University Press.

15. Ryff CD. Successful aging: a developmental approach. *Gerontologist* 1982; **22**: 209–14.

16. Ryff CD. Beyond Ponce de Leon and life satisfaction: New directions in quest of successful aging. *Int J Behav Dev* 1989; **12**: 35–55.

17. Fisher BJ. Successful aging: life satisfaction and generativity in later life. *Int J Aging Hum Dev* 1995; **41**: 239–50.

18. Von Faber M, Bootsma-van der Wiel A, van Excel E *et al.* Successful aging in the oldest old: who can be characterized as successfully aged? *Arch Intern Med* 2001; **161**: 2694–700.

19. Strawbridge WJ, Wallhagen MI, Cohen RD. Successful aging and well-being: self-rated compared with Rowe and Kahn. *Gerontologist* 2002; **42**: 727–33.

20. Bowling A, Iliffe S. Which model of successful ageing should be used in epidemiological surveys? Baseline findings from a British survey of ageing. *Age Ageing* 2006; **35**: 607–14.

14

Sexuality, Non-Traditional Relationships and Mental Health in Older People

Ian Peate

School of Nursing and Midwifery, Thames Valley University, London, UK

INTRODUCTION

Despite an ageing population, little is known or understood about the sexual behaviours and sexual function of older people in society. Individuals (including the older person) manage their sexuality and sexual identity in a number of ways. Assumptions concerning ageing and intimacy in later life are now being challenged. Specific issues concerning sexuality and ageing will be discussed. In a minority of cases clinicians will be working more and more with older people who are involved in non-traditional relationships – a non-heterosexual context. Issues may arise for clinicians and older people concerning sexual identity. Many of those working with the older person will have had little training or education regarding non-heterosexual relationships and the older person. This chapter will emphasize the need to respect the fact that the expression of sexuality in older age is an important aspect of an individual's being, as well as remembering that for some older people coming to terms with their sexuality may bring with it psychological distress. The chapter addresses the mental health of the older lesbian, gay and bisexual (LGB) person; issues concerning transgender and gender dysphoria will not be addressed here. A brief discussion concerning HIV and the older population has been included.

SEXUALITY AND AGEING

Sexuality according to Ginsberg *et al.*[1] is an activity of daily living that is important for a number of older people. Despite this, Edwards[2] notes that within health care systems the sexual needs of the older person are often unrecognized and unmet, often as a result of negative attitudes and beliefs towards sexuality, sex and sexual desires. Many believe that these complex concepts can only be likened to youthfulness. Other factors can impinge on the individual's ability to express freely their sexuality, for example, environmental (structure) constraints in long term care facilities may hinder an older person being able to express their sexual needs[3]. Some common barriers to enjoying sex as a person ages are health problems or lack of a partner as opposed to lack of desire. Little research has been carried out with respect to stereotypical ideas about sex and ageing.

Healthy people are often sexually active people and this has an impact on the quality of an individual's life, therefore to deny an elderly person the option of being sexually active may result in dysfunction and distress. Among older adults there is an internal drive or need for sexual fulfilment[4].

As people age the frequency in which they engage in sexual activity declines. Nevertheless, a substantial number of men and women engage in vaginal intercourse, fellatio, cunnilingus and masturbation, and some people remain sexually active in their eighties and nineties. The limited data that has been analysed demonstrates that there are some men and women who maintain sexual and intimate relationships and desires throughout their lives[4].

Illness can seriously impede sexual activity but there is a dearth of literature regarding how illness impacts on the sexual activity of the older person. Altered pathophysiological changes often associated with the ageing process impact on sexual response in men and women, and most of the changes have a negative bearing on the person, both physically and psychologically.

The loss of a partner as a person ages is common (particularly in older women). Problems associated with the sex act may be a precursor to problems related to an underlying illness such as diabetes mellitus, a genitourinary tract infection or cancer[5]. There are a number of age-related changes in the vasculature and smooth muscle tissues involved in the erectile process as well as increased sensitivity to inhibitory signals in the smooth muscle[6,7]. There are physiological changes that are associated with the menopause (these are complex); for example, a reduction in vaginal lubrication in response to a decrease in oestrogen levels. Attitudinal responses by society to postmenopausal women and their sexuality may also lead to an increase in vulnerability to depression.

Sexual problems for men can include difficulty in achieving or maintaining an erection, lack of interest in sex, climaxing too quickly, anxiety about performance and an inability to climax. For elderly women bothersome problems include lack of interest in sex, difficulty with lubrication, an inability to climax, disliking sex and pain – often felt at the vagina during entry[4].

If problems associated with sexual activity are not treated or are left undiagnosed this may lead to depression or social withdrawal. There are also a number of medications that can result in sexual dysfunction that patients need to take for an ongoing physical or psychiatric illness. The result of sexual problems arising from the taking of prescribed medications may induce the person to stop taking them in an attempt to reduce the negative side effects related to them.

Principles and Practice of Geriatric Psychiatry, 3rd edn. Edited by Mohammed T. Abou-Saleh, Cornelius Katona and Anand Kumar
© 2011 John Wiley & Sons, Ltd

Bancroft *et al.*[8] emphasize the effect of relationship factors and mental health (particularly with regard to women) as being more important predictors of sexual well-being than the physiological factors of sexual arousal and response. For a number of women (tentatively, this could also be said for some men) being in a relationship, the quality of that relationship and a partner's sexual problems are more important than their sexual responsiveness. Bancroft *et al.*[8] considered only heterosexual women in his study; further research is needed to consider the impact of relationships versus sexual responsiveness in the LGB population. Kellett[9] suggests that counselling may allow a couple who are experiencing sexual problems to express their fears and inhibitions, with the therapist educating the couple about the normal changes that accompany ageing.

ISSUES OF CONSENT AND COGNITIVE IMPAIRMENT

The law demands that both parties engaging in sexual relations must consent; this is equally true for the older person, who may have issues associated with cognitive impairment such as dementia. Sexual abuse is a criminal offence. Free will and capacity are germane to informed consent. It may be difficult to ascertain if a person who is cognitively impaired has the capacity to consent to sexual relationships and as such this renders that person vulnerable. There are several potential ethical and legal issues that may arise as a result of this (Mental Capacity Act, 2005). Assuming that a person with dementia cannot make decisions and consent to intimate relationships or that they are unable to comprehend the consequences of decisions associated with consent, sex is unacceptable.

Dementia leads to a variety of changes in people's lives and one area that receives little attention is in respect to sexual relationships. Dementia in the older person is common, as is drug-induced confusional state; these issues are discussed elsewhere in this text. In drug-induced confusional state, a review of current medication is needed. A feature of dementia is the development of several cognitive deficits that include memory impairment. These cognitive deficits can be so severe that they can cause impairment in social functioning, including the ability to consent freely to engage in sexual activity with another person. The deficits may also predispose the person to inappropriate sexual behaviour.

Dementia can impact on the individual's feelings, desires and needs; sexual behaviour and their ability to express intimacy can change. The clinician should explain to the person and others that these changes are not a reflection on any individual and that it is possible to express intimacy in other ways if their chosen way has changed. People with dementia can experience sudden changes associated with their ability to express their sexuality. A range of behaviours can occur depending on what aspect of the brain is affected; sexual interest may diminish or conversely it may increase; there may also be a change in the level of inhibition.

Usually, sex for many people is a private affair; dementia has the potential to bring many private activities out into the open, revealing many private intimate thoughts, feelings and sexually charged actions; for example, inappropriate touching of self and others, undressing and using sexually loaded language. While these actions may be embarrassing for others, they can also be confusing and distressing for the older person with dementia.

What may appear to be inappropriate sexual behaviour may have a number of diverse causes. The causes can be identified by analysis of antecedents, behaviours and consequences, thus providing the clinician with information that will inform the most appropriate intervention if needed. Staff may need training in respect to the management of inappropriate sexual behaviours and the most appropriate ways to help the individual, families and other staff.

MENTAL HEALTH OF LESBIAN, GAY AND BISEXUAL PEOPLE

Older LGB people may experience mental health distress for a number of reasons unconnected with their sexuality, as is the case with older heterosexual people. There are, however, a variety of social factors that may have an impact on the lives of the older LGB person and hence their mental health. There are some personal and social characteristics that may further exacerbate mental distress, for example, ethnicity and disability.

Little is known about the mental health of the LGB population in the UK and even less is known about the LGB older population. Evidence that has been collected suggests that anxiety, depression, self-harm and suicidal feelings are more common among the LGB population when compared with the heterosexual population[10]. There are also higher rates of drug and alcohol misuse among LGB people. The LGB population has been found to have the highest levels of mental distress. The data cited here refers to the LGB population as a whole in the UK and not specifically the older LGB population; nevertheless, as with all populations, LGB people will age and become older LGB people and some of these findings may well reflect those of the older LGBs. The reasons underpinning these findings are complex and as yet not fully understood. Warner *et al.*[10] note that poor mental health in the LGB population has often been linked to experiences of homophobia, discrimination and bullying. Older people are not immune to the effects of homophobic discrimination and bullying by society generally and by those who provide and plan health care.

HOMOPHOBIA AND HETEROSEXISM

Homophobia could be defined as the unreasonable hatred, prejudice and fear of LGB people. Extreme forms of homophobic behaviour can manifest as bullying and physical attacks. Heterosexism – where a society or community is conditioned to expect everyone to live and behave as heterosexual people do – can have a subtle impact on a person's self-esteem and self-image. There are a number of instances where homophobic and heterosexist behaviours exist in the provision of health care with the outcome being detrimental to the health and well-being of the older LGB person.

Institutional homophobia relies on the promotion of heterosexuality as the norm and when health services are provided where policy provision has neglected to take account of the needs of LGB people. In these instances an individual's sexuality has been seen as inferior to the dominant hegemony – the heterosexual. The health service, legal system and police force all have histories of institutionalized homophobia. There are a number of organizations that work with older LGB people who neglect to take into account the reality that not all service users are heterosexual. Some residential care homes and sheltered housing are often mixed sex and are usually set up in such a way that service provision is directed towards heterosexuals, neglecting or refusing to accept that some of their clientele may be lesbian, gay or bisexual.

Homophobia can have an impact in a number of ways. Being lesbian, gay or bisexual is not in itself a mental health problem; however, coping with the consequences of homophobia can have damaging effects on the health and well-being of an LGB person.

Warner *et al.*[10] have demonstrated a possible correlation between levels of homophobia and mental ill health among LGB people. Levels of anxiety, self-harm and depression among participants in this study were higher than average among the LGB participants. Homophobic experiences include damage to property, physical attack and bullying.

OLDER LESBIAN, GAY AND BISEXUAL PEOPLE

There is often little value in using rigid categories when describing who is old or older as these terms can include a number of different generations. There is the potential when using such descriptions that the person (or people) being described may be disempowered and as such the term should be used with caution and tact.

For the majority of older LGB people, living their life predominantly in the twentieth century may have meant that being open about their sexuality would have resulted in oppression and abuse within the mental health services[11] as well as from society. There may be a number of reasons why this occurred; for example, mental health services then reflected the homophobia of the wider society. The Local Government Act (1998) made it illegal for teachers to sanction homosexuality in schools and described gay family relationships as false; this Act was repealed in 2003. Homophobia was also given legitimacy within psychiatry and psychology; theories of mental health pathologised homosexuality. Homosexuality was seen as the cause and effect of a mental illness or even as a mental illness itself. Damaging aversion therapies were often used regularly during the 1960s and 1970s to try to 'cure' homosexuality. Homosexuality was not officially struck off the UK government's list of psychiatric disorders until 1993.

Change is on the horizon and a number of legislative modifications have occurred to combat institutional homophobia in the UK. LGBs are now legally protected from discrimination associated with their sexual orientation from providers of goods and services; this also includes those who provide mental health services. There are some problems that remain. Some people who use mental health services and counselling or psychotherapy services are still being discriminated against with regards to their sexuality, and in some cases this is further exacerbated because of their age. The key factor for such discrimination is associated with lack of awareness among clinicians and due in part to ignorance as opposed to malevolence. A systematic review has been undertaken by the British Association for Counselling and Psychotherapy into the experiences of LGB people who have received counselling or psychotherapy services[12]. Gaps in knowledge have been identified as well as revealing negative attitudes among some therapists. The review recommends that these gaps should be addressed in the training and education of therapists.

Caution must always be taken with reviews of mental health services and the needs of the LGB population, as the results may under-represent the actual number of LGB people taking part in or being included in studies or reviews. There are some people who may be reluctant to disclose their sexuality and there may also be some discomfort and embarrassment on the part of the researcher in asking questions concerning sexuality and the older LGB person.

As well as being lesbian, gay or bisexual, other characteristics such as age, ethnicity or disability can complicate or exacerbate an LGB person's experience of mental illness. Attempts in the past to cure some older LGB people may have left these people with feelings of guilt accompanied with emotional damage. There may be a number of older people who have never acknowledged to themselves or others that they are lesbian, gay or bisexual.

Negative societal attitudes towards sexuality in older age can also have detrimental effects on a person's health and well-being. Older people are often seen as unattractive and socially uninteresting. The 'gay scene' is generally geared towards meeting the needs of the younger LGB population. Lack of social opportunities can deny older LGB people the chance to meet other older LGB people; social isolation may ensue. Harmful societal attitudes can impact on communication between the physician and the patient. The outcome may be an unwillingness of patients and physicians to initiate discussion concerning sex.

HIV INFECTION IN OLDER POPULATION

HIV infection in the older population has until recently in the main been ignored. Much of the published data regarding immunologic and clinical responses to highly active antiretroviral treatment (HAART) are associated with younger cohorts. The reasons why older people have for the most part been ignored are varied, and could include the risk of age related co-morbidity associated with clinical trials.

With increased life expectancy and the success of HAART accompanied by an enhanced length of survival as a result of the improvement of the immunodeficiency caused by HIV infection, the number of older people with HIV is likely to continue to increase. As a result of this, clinical trials (research) that are age specific, taking into account the needs of the older person (i.e. considering co-morbidity and potential drug interactions) are required in relation to the impact of HIV on this population, including therapeutic and clinical outcomes.

CONCLUSION

There are a number of older people who are sexually active although little is known about their sexual activities, behaviours and attitudes. Sexual problems are widespread among the older sexually active population; these problems are rarely discussed with clinicians. A number of older people may become sexually inactive because of a variety of sexual problems – these may be physiological in origin or as a result of their sexuality and societal reactions.

For some older people heterosexual and LGB sex may play an important part in their relationships and well-being; there are also some who do not see this aspect of their lives as crucial. There may be some older people who would benefit from the input of clinicians who are willing to broach what is sometimes seen as the embarrassing and taboo subject of sexuality and the older person.

Evidence suggests that being able to express one's sexuality is positively correlated with good physical and mental health. Allowing the older person to express their sexuality will enhance their health and well-being in a number of ways. For this to happen clinicians must encourage the older person to discuss the issues that concern them. However, for this to take place the clinician must first feel comfortable with their sexuality and challenge any stereotypes they may have that concern the older person's sexuality.

REFERENCES

1. Ginsberg TB, Pomerantz SC, Kramer-Feeley V. Sexuality in older adults: behaviours and preferences. *Age Ageing* 2005; **34**(5): 475–80.
2. Edwards DJ. Sex and intimacy in the nursing home. *Nurs Homes Long Term Care Manag* 2003; **52**(2): 18–21.

3. Bouman WP, Arcelus J, Benbow SM. Nottingham Study of Sexuality and Ageing (NoSSA I): Attitudes regarding sexuality and older people. A review of the literature. *Sex Relatsh Ther* 2006; **21**(2): 149–61.

4. Lindau ST, Schumm LP, Laumann EO *et al*. A study of sexuality and health among older adults in the United States. *N Engl J Med* 2007; **357**(8): 762–74.

5. Rosen RC, Wing R, Schneider S, Gendrano N. Epidemiology of erectile dysfunction: the role of medical comorbidities and lifestyle factors. *Urol Clin North Am* 2005; **32**: 403–17.

6. Bancroft JHJ. Sex and ageing. *N Engl J Med* 2007; **357**(8): 820–22.

7. Schiavi RC. *Aging and Male Sexuality*. Cambridge: Cambridge University Press, 1999.

8. Bancroft JHJ, Loftus J, Long JS. Distress about sex: a national survey of women in heterosexual relationships. *Arch Sex Behav* 2003; **32**: 193–208.

9. Kellett JM. Sexual disorders. In Copeland JRM, Abou-Saleh MT, Blazer DG (eds), *Principles and Practice of Geriatric Psychiatry*, 2nd edn. Chichester: John Wiley & Sons, 2002.

10. Warner J, McKeown E, Griffin M, Johnson K, Ramsay A. Rates predictors of mental illness in gay men and lesbians and bisexual men and women. *Br J Psychiatry* 2004; **85**(6): 479–85.

11. Sayce L. *Breaking the Link between Homosexuality and Mental Illness: An Unfinished History*. London: Mind.

12. King M, Semlyen J, Killapsy H, Nazareth I, Osborn D. *A Systematic Review of Research on Counselling and Psychotherapy for Lesbian, Gay, Bisexual and Transgender People*. London: British Association for Counselling and Psychotherapy, 2007.

15

The Care Home Experience

Alisoun Milne

School of Social Policy, Sociology and Social Research, University of Kent, Canterbury, UK

INTRODUCTION

This chapter aims to highlight the key dimensions of the evidence base exploring the experience of living in a care home, with a particular focus on dementia. Despite the extent of recent policy and practice attention paid to care homes in both the UK and the US, surprisingly little is known about residents' lived experience. Research is only now beginning to take account of the perspective of users with dementia and is embarking on the not inconsiderable task of developing tools and methodologies that can meaningfully capture their voices[1]. By way of introduction, the broader context within which the care home experience is located is provided before moving onto the chapter's core focus. Although much of the evidence presented is drawn from UK research, key messages are equally applicable to the US and mainland Europe.

Background

In the United Kingdom about 5% of the total population aged over 65 lives in care homes. This is comparable with other European countries, the figure being slightly higher in Scandinavia[2]. In the United States 4.2% of the 65 and over population live in nursing homes[3]. In terms of absolute numbers, in 2007 420 000 people lived in care homes in the UK while in the US over 1.8 million people lived in nursing homes. It is important to note that US figures do not include 'assisted living facilities' whereas UK figures incorporate care homes that do *not* provide nursing care[i] as well as those that do.

Care homes' residents tend to be very elderly and frail; multiple physical problems and/or co-morbidity with mental disorders are common[4]. Typically, UK residents are aged over 80 years, are female, have previously lived alone, are on a low income and have multiple disabilities. In a recent UK study of 16 000 residents, over half had dementia, stroke or other neurodegenerative disease, 78% had at least one form of mental impairment, 71% were incontinent and 76% needed help with mobility or were immobile[5]; 27% were immobile, confused *and* incontinent. It is estimated that over two thirds of people living in *all* UK care homes have dementia, most often in the advanced stage, and about a third of all care home

places are registered to provide specialist dementia care[6]. In the US it is estimated that 23–42% of residential community/assisted living residents have moderate or severe dementia. Many residents with dementia experience behavioural problems such as activity disturbances (agitation), aggression and psychosis; reported prevalence of these so-called 'challenging behaviours' can be as high as 90%[7].

In addition, an estimated 50% of all care home residents have depressive disorders that would warrant intervention[8]. Depression in care home populations is associated with functional impairment (e.g. sensory loss, incontinence, loss of mobility), physical health problems (notably pain, dysphasia and heart disease), and social problems such as loneliness[9]. Due to the complexity of assessing the extent of depression among people with dementia and the limited evidence base, it has been suggested that depression in care home residents is often either under- or misdiagnosed[10]. Anxiety symptoms are also relatively common; they are particularly associated with depression and stroke[11].

Living with Dementia in a Care Home

Despite the predominance of older people with dementia in care homes, research that draws on the experience of this group of residents has only recently emerged. In part, this reflects the liminal status of people with dementia inside, and outside, the 'care system', as well as the genuine complexity of collecting data from people whose cognitive capacity and communication skills may be limited[12]. It is notable that an accumulating body of evidence offers valuable insights into the subjective experience of living with early stage dementia. It is also increasingly accepted that people in the middle to late stages of dementia retain the capacity for emotional expression and many can reliably express preferences[13]. As improving long term care for people with dementia is now a key policy priority in both the UK and US, the continuing marginalization of this pivotal perspective in both the practice and research arenas can no longer be justified[14].

Currently, there are two main sources of evidence about 'the care home experience'. One draws on practice-based work whose core aim is that of improving care. 'Dementia care mapping' (DCM) is the most prominent example of this type of work; its influence also extends into the realms of research and inspection (see below)[1]. The second source is drawn from research that has attempted to capture the nature and dimensions of care home life 'from the inside' and/or through the eyes of carers[15]. Predominantly this material is

---

[i]The term 'care home' covers any establishment providing accommodation with personal or nursing care. There are broadly two types of care home: homes that provide nursing care (nursing homes) and homes that provide personal care and support (residential homes).

gathered from observational or questionnaire-based studies, which provide valuable insights and include evidence about the experience of the person with dementia; work that focuses specifically on the subjective experience of users is a new addition to the research portfolio[16].

These two areas of activity combine around the concepts of quality of life and quality of care, both pivotal to the experience of living with dementia in a care home. As quality indicators used by the Commission for Social Care Inspection[ii,iii] (CSCI) move to focus more on 'outcomes of care', taking account of the perspective of the person with dementia becomes increasingly important[17]. A brief review of research findings about quality of life in care homes for people with dementia and 'what is important' to residents will be offered before turning to evidence about their lived experiences.

Quality of Life and Quality of Care

Assessing quality of life among care home residents is a difficult task; it is a complex construct, which is variously measured and evaluated. A number of scales do exist, several of which have been specifically developed for people with dementia; these include the Quality of Life in Alzheimer's Disease (QoL AD)[18] scale, the DEMQOL[19] and the DQol[20]. A persistent challenge in evaluating quality of life is that there are often differences between the ratings of staff, carers and residents. This appears to be a consequence of a difference in emphasis: a recent study found that residents' quality of life scores were most affected by the presence of depression and anxiety, whereas staff ratings were associated with dependency and behaviour problems[21]. A full picture of quality of life may thus require a combination of measures, incorporating the observations of all three groups[22].

Despite the difficulties associated with measurement, evidence to date suggests that quality of life in care homes is largely determined by the existence of mental health problems and subjective well-being[11]. Systematic assessment of residents' needs, and consideration of whether or not they have been met, has been suggested as a means of improving quality of life. The Camberwell Assessment of Need for the Elderly has been used towards this end[23].

Limited consensus also exists in relation to the linked concept of quality of care. First – as with quality of life – there are multiple perspectives to be accommodated. Second, the components of 'care' include those elements that are provided within the home as well as those offered by external sources, such as medical care. Third, good quality care depends on a range of micro level (satisfied staff) and macro level (financial stability of the provider) factors and their interaction; this make its assessment complex and multifaceted. An important contribution to this field has been the development of DCM, an observational approach where items recording residents' activity can be combined to calculate a care index score[24] (see Chapter 30 for details on DCM). Given the limitations of all approaches to gathering information about quality of life and quality of care, an approach that accommodates multiple methods is recommended, rather than relying on a single source of evidence[25].

As might be expected, evidence about the quality of care in homes is mixed. Some of the variation between studies results from methodological differences. For example, studies adopting a 'checklist' approach tend to reach more positive conclusions than those using direct observations[26]. There is more robust evidence in relationship to those issues that impact negatively on user quality of life. These include prescribing patterns and covert administration of medication, physical restraint, electronic tagging and abuse[27].

In terms of therapeutic care practice, a recent survey undertaken by the Alzheimer's Society[28] of 4 084 family carers, and care home workers and managers found that people with dementia are not always afforded dignity and respect. 'Dementia' had become a label that subsumes all other needs and submerges the person's characteristics; this tendency undermines the delivery of individualized care and encourages a task-oriented approach. Lack of activity and stimulation were also highlighted, particularly for people with severe dementia. As the availability of activities and opportunities for occupation is a major determinant of quality of life affecting depression, physical function and behavioural symptoms, this is a primary concern.

A 2007 CSCI[17] inspection of care homes for people with dementia echoes a number of these themes. Although the inspectors found some excellent examples of one-to-one attention and care offered with warmth, understanding and tolerance, impersonal assistance was widely in evidence. The report noted that quality of staff communication with residents – both verbal and non-verbal – had a significant impact on well-being. Positive communication that is warm and friendly results in the person with dementia feeling happy and relaxed. Conversely, negative or neutral communication – interactions that are impersonal or task focused – leave residents feeling distressed and withdrawn. It is thus evident from this and other CSCI inspections that residents with dementia do not always receive person-centred care – care which is delivered in ways that promote independence and which draw on the individual's life course and experiences. It is to the role of experience in extending understanding of the person with dementia's life in a care home that we now turn.

Evaluating the Experiences of the Person with Dementia

Structured observational methods developed specifically for evidencing quality in long term care settings have a sustained history. They provide an opportunity to include the perspective of the person with dementia by collecting data on their experiences in communal areas, how they spend their time, and how they are treated. The most widely used dementia-specific observational tool is DCM. Kitwood, who developed the early prototype of DCM, described it as 'a serious attempt to take the standpoint of the person with dementia, using a combination of empathy and observational skill' (p. 4)[29]. DCM requires training to employ but even with a standardized training programme the inter-rater reliability of practitioners is not high; those who use DCM for research purposes can achieve good reliability[22]. A linked example of an observational tool is the Short Observation Framework for Inspection (SOFI). This draws heavily on DCM and involves structured observation of a sample of five residents in a communal area and over an extended lunch period[17]. As part of an overall inspection, SOFI adds observational depth and detail.

More recently video and digital recordings have also been used in care settings[30]. They can provide fine-grained analysis enabling in-depth observation to occur. Video evidence can be particularly valuable when working with people with very advanced dementia whose speech on first listening seems meaningless, but on repeated replay shows clear attempts at communication[31].

[ii]The CSCI has responsibility for monitoring standards in care homes. In April 2009, the CSCI was replaced by the Care Quality Commission.

[iii]Regulatory bodies are established in each UK country to apply and monitor care standards: in England, it is the Care Quality Commission; in Wales, the Care Standards Inspectorate; and in Scotland, the Care Commission.

The extent to which selfhood or identity is preserved in people with dementia has been a key focus of observational studies[32]. Results suggest that although the self is affected by dementia, manifestations of selfhood persist even in late stages of the illness along with the capacity to develop positive relationships[33]. Questionnaire-based studies have also begun to address this issue, concluding that aspects of identity, as with selfhood, are retained by people with advanced dementia[34]. Research also identifies recurrent issues of loss, communication difficulties, frustration and sadness among residents along with lack of meaningful occupation. Minimal levels of well-being are widely noted in many studies of care homes; these are particularly pronounced for people with the greatest dependency needs[35].

Very recently attempts to explore the subjective experiences of people with advanced dementia in long term care have been made. A seminal study by Clare et al.[16] provides an interpretive phenomenological account of the subjective, psychological experience of living with moderate to severe dementia in a care home. The thematic account highlights four interrelated experiences (see Table 15.1). Daily experience was shaped by the losses resulting from dementia for most residents and was characterized, to a considerable degree, by distressing thoughts and feelings. The psychological impact of 'being in the home' was associated with a sense of uncertainty, lack of control and limited self-determination. These feelings were compounded by multiple experiences of loss – lost abilities, lost memories, and lost identity – which resulted, for some, in feelings of worthlessness. Fear of 'being alone' or 'being lost' was also a dominant experience. However, through their accounts the residents emerged as 'agents actively seeking to cope with their situation' (p. 718). Many found ways to contribute and focused on the positive aspects of home life, including being part of supportive relationships. Such relationships appeared to be pivotal to maintaining a sense of well-being; their absence contributed to feelings of distress and alienation[36]. Although participants displayed many constructive ways to cope, the effects of changes resulting from dementia, coupled with the context of institutional care, placed severe limitations on their expression of personal agency. Consequently, some residents experienced frustration, anger and boredom, especially around minimal activity and daily occupation[37]. Lack of freedom and independence was experienced by some residents as 'restrictive' and communal living could give rise to considerable confusion. If we are serious about addressing current deficits in care home provision, understanding the subjective experience of people with dementia is a fundamental dimension of enhancing practice and thereby improving both quality of life for users and quality of care. The implications of this shift in emphasis are the focus of the final section.

IMPLICATIONS FOR PRACTICE: ENHANCING QUALITY OF LIFE IN CARE HOMES

Much of the evidence reviewed above identifies an overarching need to embed person-centred values into care planning and delivery in care home settings. The pivotal role of developing meaningful relationships and an emphasis on effective communication appear to be the twin routes to enhancing well-being in residents with dementia[38]. There is a related need to address a number of practical and therapeutic deficits. Extending levels of engagement for people with dementia by offering meaningful activities is a prominent example; supporting the continued expression of personal agency and autonomy is a secondary challenge[39]. Managing the difficult and often negative emotions that many residents experience is also important; this depends on the establishment of genuine staff–resident relationships and the capacity of staff to respond sensitively and on an individual basis to need. Supporting role identity is another element of good care; this depends on staff engaging with residents' life course and promoting opportunities for residents to have a continued social role. Being aware of the challenges of living a semi-public life in an institutional setting is an additional facet; this includes working with residents to deal with difficult relationships and providing opportunities for privacy[16].

As noted above, evidence suggests that preservation of self and identity is possible even in those with advanced dementia. The maintenance of previous relationships with friends and relatives is key to providing biographical continuity. Moving into a care home tends to disrupt existing relationships, which may impact negatively on users' sense of self, a process compounded by loss of independence[40]. In this context the relevance of care that is truly person centred becomes clear and understanding what matters to an individual, including his or her wishes, is critical. Story-telling and biographical work can help to develop relationships between staff and residents; this not only increases the likelihood of the resident being seen and valued as an individual[41] but also helps to maintain their cultural and ethnic identity.

Recognition of residents' emotional and social needs – in addition to their physical needs – is crucial to achieving person-centred care. Spending time engaging people with dementia 'in conversation' can also provide a powerful counterweight to the often task-oriented exchanges between residents and staff. It has been suggested that relationships are the key to maintaining well-being in people with dementia and that effective communication – the by-product of a good relationship – undergirds good quality dementia care[42]. Some commentators even argue that caring for a person with advanced dementia is *essentially* about finding ways to communicate even when these may be unfamiliar. Meaningful interactions require the development of a set of core skills among staff: attentiveness, active listening, observation of non-verbal signs, and the use of personal objects to support communication[43]. Staff can also enhance effective communication by ensuring that they face a resident when speaking, have light upon them rather than behind them, using gestures that are consistent with what they are saying, and presenting information simply and slowly[44]. A part of this process is also supporting the 'coping strategies' the user has developed to manage the difficulties he or she encounters in the home.

For many care staff, being able to effect meaningful communication with residents is a crucial component of job satisfaction; lack

Table 15.1 Key themes from the study of Clare et al.[16]

Nothing's right: isolation, alienation, lack of choice, lack of control, fear, worthlessness

I'll manage: making the best of things, valuing contacts and friendships, finding ways of continuing to be useful, being accepted as you are, having a friend in the home, having links with relatives/family, acknowledgement of getting older

I still am somebody: part of coping, affirming one's sense of identity, managing well despite limitations

It drives me mad: frustration and anger at the situation, confined, wanting more independence, boredom, lack of activity, annoying behaviour of other residents, uncertainty, fear, irritation

of opportunity to build personal attachments is a strong predictor of staff burnout[45]. This evidence suggests that enhancing communication skills – a widely noted practice deficit – needs to be a distinctive focus of dementia care training and that care homes need to find ways to ensure staff have the time and expertise to build up and sustain interactions with residents. It is important to recognize that providing care that takes residents' emotional experiences and wishes seriously, facilitates choice and provides a sense of security and reassurance is both time consuming and intensive[46].

A number of key characteristics mark out those care homes that successfully promote and sustain good quality care: clear leadership, a positive ethos, and staff training and support to enhance communication skills and promote retention[47]. A recent project – the 'Enriched Opportunities Programme' – offered a multilevel approach to enhancing the quality of care in three care homes for people with dementia: it included a strong emphasis on leadership and dementia expertise, a trained care team with empathy for residents, and a programme of care and activity developed to meet the needs of individuals. It evidenced that by adopting a coherent focused approach that takes full account of the experiences of residents, care practice and the overall culture of care can be significantly improved[48].

CONCLUSION

People with dementia living in care homes face enormous challenges. In addition to declining cognitive powers, users have to cope with a new and often unpredictable environment. They may also be cared for by people who know very little about them and who are, encouraged by an over-reliance on 'procedures', to focus on their physical safety rather than their emotional well-being. Additionally, frailty, communication difficulties and dependency on others often means that their needs are overlooked and their voices marginalized. Understanding more about the experience of living with dementia in a care home is a critical contribution to improving both quality of life and quality of care. Prioritizing relationships and communication, the establishment of genuine staff–resident attachment, managing distressing emotions, and ensuring that care is individually planned and delivered are key dimensions of practice that place the user experience at its core. Intimate biographical knowledge about the user and their life history, and bolstering the user's abilities, sense of self and identity are key aspects of providing person-centred care. The provision of tailored day activities and recognition of the stresses communal life can cause are also important issues highlighted by research. Excellence in dementia care begins with an understanding of what it is like to live with the illness *throughout* its trajectory[49]. As there is no doubt that residential care is, and will continue to be, one of the dominant types of provision for people with advanced dementia in the developed world, increased emphasis on research that explores the user experience and practice that foregrounds it, is a central component of effective and positive practice in care home settings.

REFERENCES

1. Brooker D. Quality: the perspective of the person with dementia. In Downs M, Bowers B (eds), *Excellence in Dementia Care: Research into Practice*. Open University Press, Milton Keynes, 2008, 476–91.
2. Organisation for Economic Co-operation and Development. *Long-Term Care for Older People*. Paris: OECD, 2005.
3. Zimmerman S, Gruber-Baldini AL, Sloane PD *et al*. Assisted living and nursing homes: apples and oranges? *Gerontologist* 2003; **45**: 105–17.
4. Alzheimer's Society *Dementia UK*. London: Alzheimer's Society, 2007.
5. Bowman C, Whistler J, Ellerby M. A national census of care home residents. *Age Ageing* 2004; **33**: 561–6.
6. Matthews FE, Dening TR. Prevalence of dementia in institutional care. *Lancet* 2002; **360**: 225–6.
7. Brodaty H, Draper B, Saab D *et al*. Psychosis, depression and behavioural disturbances in Sydney nursing home residents: prevalence and predictors. *Int J Geriatr Psychiatry* 2001; **16**: 504–12.
8. Dening T, Milne A. Mental health in care homes for older people. In Jacoby R, Oppenheimer C, Dening T, Thomas A (eds), *The Oxford Textbook of Old Age Psychiatry*. Oxford: Oxford University Press, 2001.
9. Jones RN, Marcantonio ER, Rabinowitz T. Prevalence and correlates of recognized depression in US nursing homes. *J Am Geriatr Soc* 2003; **51**: 1404–9.
10. Evers MM, Samuels SC, Lantz M *et al*. The prevalence, diagnosis and treatment of depression in dementia patients in chronic care facilities in the last six months of life. *Int J Geriatr Psychiatry* 2002; **17**: 464–72.
11. Smallbrugge M, Pot AM, Jongenelis L *et al*. The impact of depression and anxiety on well being, disability and use of health care services in nursing home patients. *Int J Geriatr Psychiatry* 2006; **21**: 325–32.
12. Dening T, Milne A. Depression and mental health in care homes for older people. *Qual Ageing* 2009; **10**(2): 40–46.
13. Phinney A. Toward understanding subjective experiences of dementia. In Downs M, Bowers B (eds), *Excellence in Dementia Care: Research into Practice*. Milton Keynes: Open University Press, 2008, 35–51.
14. Department of Health. *National Dementia Strategy*. London: Department of Health, 2008.
15. Nolan M, Lundh U, Grant G, Keady J. *Partnerships in Family Care*. Milton Keynes: Open University Press, 2003.
16. Clare L, Rowlands J, Bruce E *et al*. The experience of living with dementia in residential care: an interpretive phenomenological analysis. *Gerontologist* 2008; **48**(6): 711–20.
17. Commission for Social Care Inspection. *See Me, Not Just the Dementia: Understanding People's Experience of Living in a Care Home*. London: CSCI, 2008.
18. Hoe J, Katona C, Roch B *et al*. Use of the QOL-AD for measuring quality of life in people with severe dementia – the LASER-AD study. *Age Ageing* 2005; **34**: 130–35.
19. Smith SC, Lamping DL, Banerjee S *et al*. Measurement of health related quality of life for people with dementia: development of a new instrument (DEMQOL) and an evaluation of current methodology. *Health Technol Assess* 2005; **9**(10): 1–93, iii–iv.
20. Brod M, Stewart AL, Sands L, Watson P. Conceptualisation and measurement of quality of life in dementia: the dementia quality of life instrument (DQoL). *Gerontologist* 1999; **39**(1): 25–35.
21. Hoe J, Hancock G, Livingston G *et al*. Quality of life of people with dementia in residential care homes. *Br J Psychiatry* 1999; **188**: 460–64.
22. Sloane PD, Zimmerman S, Williams CS *et al*. Evaluating the quality of life of long-term care residents with dementia. *Gerontologist* 2005; **45**(special issue 1): 37–49.

23. Orrell M, Hancock G. *CANE: Camberwell Assessment of Need for the Elderly*. London: Gaskell, 2004.

24. Brooker D. *Person-Centred Dementia Care: Making Services Better*, Bradford Dementia Group Good Practice Guides. London: Jessica Kingsley, 2007.

25. Innes A, Kelly F. Evaluating long stay care settings: reflections on the process with particular reference to DCM. In Innes A, McCabe L (eds), *Evaluation in Dementia Care*. London: Jessica Kingsley, 2007.

26. Ballard C, Fossey J, Chithramohan R *et al*. Quality of care in private sector and NHS facilities for people with dementia: cross-sectional study. *Br Med J* 2001; **323**: 426–7.

27. Help the Aged and National Care Home Research and Development Forum. *My Home Life: Quality of Life in Care Homes*. London: Help the Aged, 2006.

28. Alzheimer's Society. *Home from Home*. London: Alzheimer's Society, 2007.

29. Kitwood T. *Dementia Reconsidered: The Person Comes First*. Milton Keynes: Open University Press, 1997.

30. Cook A. Using video observation to include the experiences of people with dementia in research. In Wilkinson H (ed.), *The Perspectives of People with Dementia: Research Methods and Motivations*. London: Jessica Kingsley, 2002.

31. Killick J, Allan K. The Good Sunset Project: making contact with those close to death. *J Dement Care* 2006; **14**(1): 22–4.

32. Hubbard G, Tester S, Downs M. Meaningful social interactions between older people in institutional care settings. *Ageing Soc* 2003; **23**: 99–114.

33. Williams CL, Tappen RM. Can we create a therapeutic relationship with nursing home residents in the later stages of Alzheimer's disease? *Journal of Psychosocial Nursing* 1999; **37**: 28–35.

34. Cohen-Mansfield J, Golander H, Arnheim G. Self-identity in older persons suffering from dementia: preliminary results. *Soc Sci Med* 2000; **51**: 381–94.

35. Hubbard G, Cook A, Tester S, Downs M. (2002) Beyond words: older people with dementia using and interpreting nonverbal behaviour. *J Aging Stud* 2002; **16**: 155–67.

36. Surr CA. Preservation of self in people with dementia living in residential care: a socio-biographical approach. *Soc Sci Med* 2006; **62**: 1720–30.

37. Train GH, Nurock SA, Mandela M *et al*. A qualitative study of the experiences of long-term care for residents with dementia, their relatives and staff. *Aging Ment Health* 2005; **9**: 119–28.

38. Fossey J, James I. *Evidence Based Approaches to Improving Dementia Care in Care Homes*. London: Alzheimer's Society, 2008.

39. Cohen-Mansfield J, Parpura-Gill A, Golander H. Utilization of self-identity roles for designing interventions for persons with dementia. *J Gerontol B Psychol Sci Soc Sci* 2006; **61**(4): P202–12.

40. Brown-Wilson C, Cook G, Forte D. The use of narrative in developing relationships in care homes. In Froggatt K, Davies S, Meyer, J (eds), *Understanding Care Homes: A Research and Development Perspective*. London: Jessica Kingsley, 2009, 70–90.

41. Brooker D. Person centred care. In Jacoby R, Oppenheimer C, Dening T, Thomas A (eds), *The Oxford Textbook of Old Age Psychiatry*. Oxford: Oxford University Press, 2008.

42. Robinson J, Banks P. *Care Services Enquiry: The Business of Caring*. London: King's Fund, 2005.

43. Allan K, Killick, J. Communication and relationships: an inclusive social world. In Downs M, Bowers B (eds), *Excellence in Dementia Care: Research into Practice*. Milton Keynes: Open University Press, 2008, 212–29.

44. Adams T. From person-centred to relationship-centred care. *Generations Rev* 2005; **15**: 4–7.

45. Moyle W, Skinner J, Rowe G, Gork C. Views of job satisfaction and dissatisfaction in Australian long-term care. *J Clin Nurs* 2003; **12**(2): 168–76.

46. Davies S, Nolan M. Attending to relationships in dementia care. In Downs M, Bowers B (eds), *Excellence in Dementia Care: Research into Practice*. Milton Keynes: Open University Press, 2008, 438–54.

47. Commission for Social Care Inspection. *The State of Social Care in England 2006–07*. London: CSCI, 2008.

48. Fossey J. Care homes. In Downs M, Bowers B (eds), *Excellence in Dementia Care: Research into Practice*. Milton Keynes: Open University Press, 2008, 336–58.

49. Phinney A. Toward understanding subjective experiences of dementia. In Downs M, Bowers B (eds), *Excellence in Dementia Care: Research into Practice*. Milton Keynes, Open University Press, 2008, 35–51.

16

Ageing: International Statistical Trends and Prospects

Fiona E. Matthews[1] and George M. Savva[2]

[1]MRC Biostatistics Unit, Institute of Public Health, Cambridge, UK
[2]Department of Public Health and Primary Care, Institute of Public Health, Cambridge, UK

INTRODUCTION

The term 'ageing' is a generalized complex terminology that can address a number of concepts, including aspects such as the demography of the whole population or trends within specific age groups (such as births or the older population). But the term 'ageing' is also a generic term for the older population and factors associated with it. Within this chapter we aim to investigate some of these factors and show how the population of the world has changed, how historical changes will affect health in the next decades, how our estimates of population change are challenged by diseases and treatments and what can we currently say about the health of the older population.

TRENDS IN POPULATION SIZE

The historic, current and future population demography demonstrates historic and interesting changes. Over the course of the last 50 years and in the next 50 years there has been and will be a fundamental shift in the distribution of the human population. Different areas of the world display different demographic shift patterns; for example the shifts in the United Kingdom and United States show patterns that are different from those seen in China and India[1]. Nevertheless, all countries are experiencing population ageing.

Figure 16.1 shows the demographic changes across different regions of the world. China and India have not only had a large change in the distribution of the population, they have also increased dramatically in size. The shift in this distribution means that the proportion of the population that is already considered 'older' varies greatly by country. Current estimates of the proportion of the population aged 60 years and over are shown in Figure 16.2. Although the relative distribution shifts from Europe and North America in 1950 towards Asia by 2050 (Table 16.1) there are large numbers in the older population throughout the whole world.

Despite these differing demographic patterns already 64% of the older population (aged 60 and over) live in developing countries and by 2050 nearly 80% of those aged 60 and above will live in developing countries[2]. This definition, however, includes only Europe, North America, Japan, Australia and New Zealand within the developed countries – a pattern that may not reflect true differences[3].

Table 16.1 Percentage distributions of those aged 65 and older by region, 1950–2050

Region	1950	1975	2000	2025	2050
World	100	100	100	100	100
More developed regions	49.0	48.7	40.7	31.5	21.7
Less developed regions	51.0	51.3	59.3	68.5	78.3
Africa	5.5	5.4	6.2	6.8	9.4
Europe	34.4	33.5	25.6	17.8	12.1
Asia	43.9	43.6	51.6	57.9	62.1
North America	10.8	10.8	9.3	8.7	6.4
Latin America and the Caribbean	4.7	6.0	6.7	8.1	9.4
Oceania	0.7	0.7	0.7	0.7	0.6

TRENDS IN FERTILITY

Trends in fertility affect the composition of the older population many years later. While this ensures that surprises are not often encountered in the description of the older population it also means that demographic influences are less immediate at solving the challenges predicted. The decisions made on childbirth both between the two World Wars and after the Second World War are now shaping the composition of the older population. The generation of children to the 'baby boomers' in the 1960s are now reaching middle age and the size of this demographic bubble can be clearly seen in the population pyramids (Figure 16.1). Many European countries have for a number of years been below the reproductive factor (2.1 births per woman[2]). This rate of replacement of the younger population will again shift the relative balance of the population in terms of young and old. In this case there is a double impact, as the baby boomers reach old age with a lack of grandchildren to replace the status quo of the pyramid. This will create, at least for the next 50 years, an ageing society. The current fertility decisions of the early adults are not suggesting that this imbalance will refocus. In fact the decisions to delay or reduce childbirth across the whole of the developed population (and wider in many cases) mean that the majority of countries are now below the 2.1 factor.

Principles and Practice of Geriatric Psychiatry, 3rd edn. Edited by Mohammed T. Abou-Saleh, Cornelius Katona and Anand Kumar

In the less developed regions where infant mortality is still high, despite advances resulting from the Millennium Development Goals (UN Millennium Goal 4), the fertility rate is still relatively high but is reducing dramatically. The developing countries are still experiencing an ageing population, but in a more historically understood way, although many unknowns remain[4]. A recent UN report states that fertility levels are unlikely to rise again to the historic highs and therefore the expression of population ageing is irreversible[5]. However future population size is sensitive to small but sustained deviations from the replacement level[5].

The patterns of fertility affect not only the absolute level of the future middle-aged and older population but they also have a direct impact on the life of the older population at the individual level. The number of available carers within a population is almost universally linked to the extended family support. As this family structure shifts so will the life of the older person[6]. An international comparative survey on the older population undertaken in 1996 showed that the proportion of the older population aged 60 and over living in three-generation households was 29–43% in Asian countries compared with 2% for European and North American countries[7]. If this structure is mimicked with the changing demographic then it will impact enormously on policy.

TRENDS IN LIFE EXPECTANCY AND HEALTHY LIFE EXPECTANCY ACROSS THE AGE RANGE

There has been a steady and consistent increase in life expectancy at birth across all continents and in both males and females (Figure 16.3). However, the major issue in the statistical trends in healthy life expectancy is whether with the extension of longer life there is also an extension of healthy life (i.e. the total remaining life that can be expected to be free of disability). Three patterns of

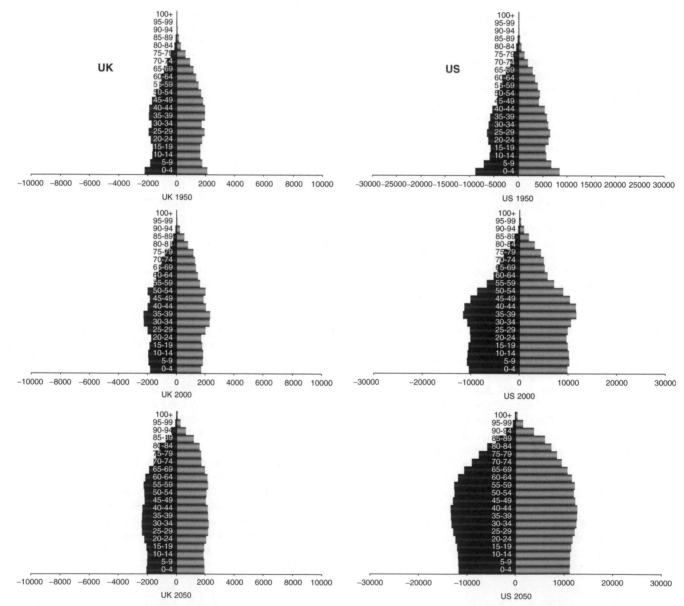

Figure 16.1 Population pyramids and changing distribution. Bars refer to the size of the population (in thousands) of men (left) and women (right) in each age group

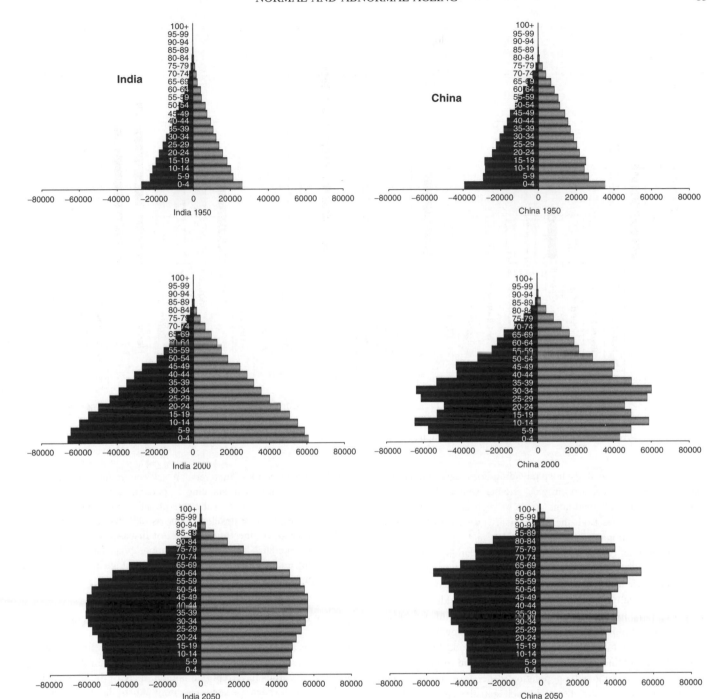

Figure 16.1 (*continued*)

population change in healthy life expectancy have been proposed, an expansion of morbidity[8], a compression of morbidity[9] or dynamic equilibrium[10]. Expansion of morbidity would imply longer life expectancy but at the same time longer life expectancy in ill-health, compression of morbidity would imply that the life extension is predominantly from the healthy life and dynamic equilibrium implies that severity may change, but the burden remains constant. Evidence to date suggests that all three scenarios can occur in different populations at different times.

MEASURING THE CHANGING HEALTH STATUS OF THE OLDER POPULATION

Assessing the compression or expansion of morbidity relies on being able to measure the health status of the older population. Complementary insights regarding the changing health of the older population can be gained from several major sources, each with their own merits and drawbacks. In developed countries routinely gathered statistics such as census data and birth and death certification may be used and these provide reliable information on demographic changes. Routine

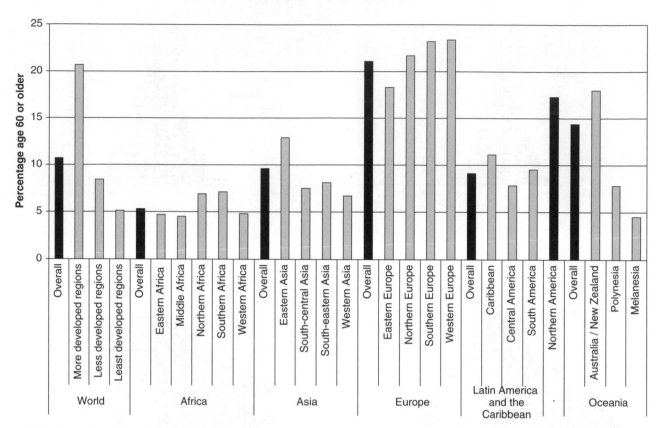

Figure 16.2   Proportion of the older population by country

medical databases, such as hospital admissions data, prescription records or disease registers provide another source. However the reporting of medical conditions to these registers may be biased by various processes. Both the mechanisms by which older people come to the attention of health care providers and reporting practices change with time, particularly in the older population, as a result of changing awareness, attitude and perception of health both by older people and their health care providers. Reporting practices can also vary geographically. Psychiatric conditions in the older population are particularly likely to be under-reported, and death certificates often do not mention major diseases such as dementia despite it being present or a major contributing factor to the death of an older person. Using routine data to record the health and in particular the psychiatric health of the older population is therefore unreliable. Furthermore in many areas of the world such statistics are not collected routinely.

To overcome some of these methodological difficulties, epidemiological studies are conducted. These typically involve recruitment of a cohort who are chosen to be as representative of the population as possible, and these are then subjected to a standardized assessment of their health. Repeating standardized assessments in the same cohort over time leads to a longitudinal study in which changes in the health of the population can be examined. Longitudinal epidemiological studies of health are not without their difficulties. Biases in selection and drop-out are possible and must be examined carefully. Epidemiological studies often have limited applicability outside the populations in which they are conducted, and compared with routine statistics they are limited by their size in terms of detecting small changes. Studies that rely on self-report may still be influenced by changing understanding or perceptions of health[11], or by cross-cultural differences in the interpretation of questions, and so questionnaires must be designed to be as objective as possible.

Projections about the future burden of disease in the older population are generated by combining demographic data on the likely future numbers of older people with epidemiological data regarding disease prevalence and the impact of disease.

TRENDS IN GLOBAL HEALTHY LIFE EXPECTANCY

The international patterns of disability and healthy life expectancy are not consistent with different patterns seen within different populations. Countries have reported both an increase in the prevalence of disability (Sweden[12]), rates stagnating (Australia[13]), or decreasing (United States[14], France[15], Finland[16], Japan[17]) and different evolutions reported for subgroups (men and women in Spain[18] and Denmark[19]) or for mild rather than severe disability (Netherlands[20]). Trends in disability rates are not sufficient, however, as changes in the age distribution of the population need to be combined with the changes in the disability rates to see the full population, and hence conflicting results with another study from Australia found evidence of a compression of morbidity[21]. A recent European comparison has shown that there are still large variations across Europe, and that these inequalities may be becoming larger, particularly between Eastern and Western Europe, and that healthy life expectancy may show more variations than life expectancy[22].

In the developing world there is currently little evidence to investigate whether there is a compression of morbidity or an

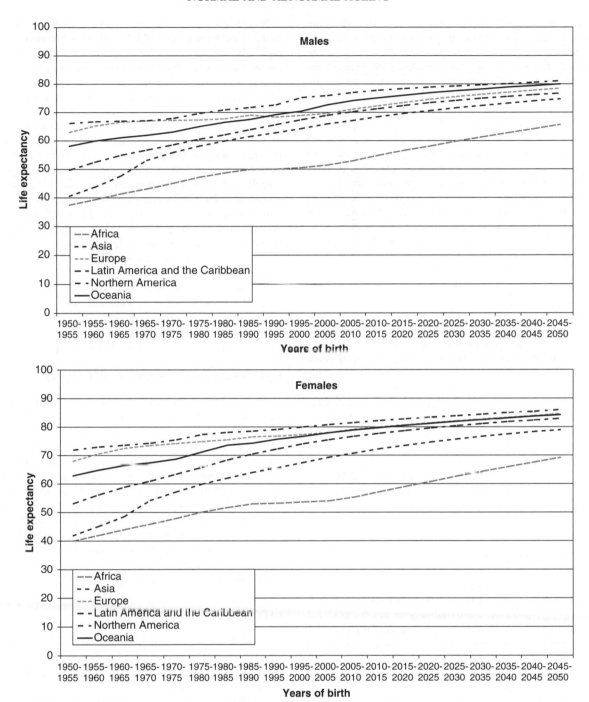

Figure 16.3 Life expectancy at birth across world regions. From Population Division of the Department of Economic and Social Affairs of the United Nations Secretariat[1].

expansion[23]. These countries are at the early stages of the chronic disease growth, though it is becoming an increasing problem. The challenge for a healthy older population across the entire world is one of a focus on lifelong health, not just health in mid to late life[24]. This sort of focus is long term and often overlooked within a resource scarce environment.

It is also possible that these different balances will fluctuate in different populations at different times and may well be modified by intervention strategies and changes to national care policies.

CHANGES IN MARKERS OF HEALTH

As well as varying across cultures, whether the health of the older population is improving or worsening also depends on which measures of health are considered[25,26]. Most studies of changes of health in the older population focus on changes in the levels of disabilities, since this is one of the major determinants of poor quality of life, the inability to live independently and the need for long-term care. Many such studies have shown improvements between cohorts with time. However, the level of disability of an individual is determined both by their underlying health conditions leading to functional impairment and by their environment. Changes in levels of disability may therefore be caused by changes in lifelong exposure to risk factors affecting the prevalence of diseases, the changes in the impairments caused by diseases when they occur, and by changes in technology and the environment. Changes in the prevalence of health conditions may reflect both changes in incidence and in survival with that condition.

The evidence regarding age-specific trends in disability in the older population is mixed. Some evidence of an improvement has been seen in the prevalence of mild disability, while the level of more severe disabilities has remained constant or has worsened slightly. In contrast, most comparisons of health conditions in the older population have shown an increase in major disease prevalence and co-morbidity as well as in objective measures of specific functional limitations[12,27,28]. Consistent improvements in survival with diseases such as heart disease and stroke have not been offset by reductions in their incidence, leading to an increase in prevalence. On the other hand, disability among stroke survivors and those with heart disease has decreased.

Although much of the increase in human life expectancy in the past century has been caused by a reduction in infant mortality, life expectancy of the older population is also increasing. This will lead to changes of the population structure within the older population, particularly in an increase in the numbers of the oldest old compared with the younger old[29]. The oldest old are an emerging population group in terms of research and information on changes in their health and demographic characteristics are only beginning to become available. The oldest old have high rates of physical and cognitive impairment and are likely to live in institutions[30]. A recent report highlighted changes in the demographic and socioeconomic characteristics of the oldest old population in England and Wales[31], revealing an increase in the numbers of the oldest old living alone and as well as an increase in health care resource utilization. More research is needed on the oldest old.

CHANGES IN MENTAL HEALTH

Mental health is increasingly recognized as a significant independent contributor to the burden of disease and as a mediator of aetiological factors for other diseases[32], and maintaining healthy brains in later life is now a research priority[33]. Mental health issues such as schizophrenia and depression affect the whole population, and in the older population dementia and cognitive decline are of specific importance. Mental health in early and midlife is a strong predictor of mental health in old age.

Little reliable evidence is available regarding trends in the prevalence of psychiatric conditions in the older population. A comparison of two studies with similar methodology carried out 10 years apart showed a significant increase in major depression diagnoses in all sociodemographic groups[34].

The effect of changes in age structure of the global population on the number of people with dementia was estimated by a Delphi consensus study, which combined all the available evidence regarding dementia prevalence and future population trends[35]. The number of people aged over 60 with dementia in Europe and North America is likely to have increased by 50% from 2001 numbers by 2020 and will have doubled or trebled by 2040. The numbers with dementia in East Asia and Africa are expected to increase by four times in this time period. There are projected to be 81.1 million people worldwide with dementia in 2040 compared with 24.3 million in 2001, with 70% living in the developing world. However these estimates are based on limited information; while reliable estimates for dementia prevalence are available in the developed world, direct estimates are not available in many areas, although cross-cultural studies that have been undertaken suggest that patterns may be different and further information on global dementia epidemiology is urgently being sought.

Changing incidence and survival with dementia and changes to the disability associated with dementia will affects its impact in the ageing population, and these trends will depend on changing prevalence of risk factors as well as interventions and management. The age-specific incidence of dementia and cognitive impairment has been suggested to have decreased slightly, possibly due to the effects of improved health-related lifestyle and education[36], while the increase in survival from stroke, might suggest an increasing prevalence[37]. Social networks and intellectual stimulation are increasingly recognized as being important determinants of health and mental health in the older population. Models estimating the impact that changes in dementia trends and treatments will have on the future disability burden illustrate the uncertainty in predictions and highlight the need for treatments that will alleviate that burden[38].

FUTURE PROSPECTS AND DIRECTIONS

International trends in ageing are difficult to predict, though recent publications have attempted to investigate not only the population shift[5], but also the trends in disability and health[38]. However it is not just the population shift that requires careful consideration, other factors including changes in food, water, housing, education, early and midlife health and behaviour and the physical and biological environment will all affect our future health prospects[39]. Trends seen across the world raise a number of concerns for the future of the ageing population, foremost of which are the increase in the burden of disease and dependency. Interdisciplinary research across the whole world and in all populations is required in both the ageing process of an individual and the effects of an ageing population, in order to understand and meet the challenges now and in the years ahead[40].

REFERENCES

1. Population Division of the Department of Economic and Social Affairs of the United Nations Secretariat, *World Population Prospects: The 2008 Revision*, 2009. At http://esa.un.org/unpp, accessed 26 Mar 2009.
2. United Nations. *World Population Prospects 2006*. At www.un.org/esa/population/publications/wpp2006/wpp2006.htm, accessed Mar 2009.
3. Kinsella K, Velkoff V, US Census Bureau. *An Aging World*. Washington, DC: US Government Printing Office, 2001.
4. Morgan S. Is low fertility a twenty-first-century demographic crisis? *Demography* 2003; **40**: 589–603.
5. United Nations. *World Population Ageing*, 2007. At www.un.org/esa/population/publications/WPA2007/wpp2007.htm, accessed Mar 2009.
6. Ogawa N. Ageing trends and policy responses in the ESCAP region. In *Population and Development: Selected Issues*. Asian Population Studies Series No, 161. New York: United Nations, 2003, 89–127.

7. Management and Coordination Agency. *Brief Summary of the Fourth International Comparative Survey of the Elderly*. Tokyo: Gyosei Printing Company, 1997.

8. Gruenberg EM. The failures of success. *Milbank Mem Fund Q Health Soc* 1977; **55**: 3–24.

9. Fries J. Aging, natural death, and the compression of morbidity. *N Engl J Med* 1980; **303**: 130–35.

10. Manton KG. Changing concepts of morbidity and mortality in the elderly population. *Milbank Mem Fund Q Health Soc* 1982; **60**: 183–244.

11. Wolf DA, Hunt K, Knickman J. Perspectives on the recent decline in disability at older ages. *Milbank Q* 2005; **83**: 365–95.

12. Parker MG, Ahacic K, Thorslund M. Health changes among Swedish Oldest old: prevalence rates from 1992 and 2002 show increasing health problems. *J Gerontol A Biol Sci Med Sci* 2005; **60**: 1351–55.

13. Davis E, Beer J, Gligora C, Thorn A. Accounting for change in disability and severe restriction, 1981–1998. Australian Bureau of Statistics Working Paper 2001.

14. Freedman VA, Martin LG, Schoeni RF. Recent trends in disability and functioning among older adults in the United States: a systematic review. *JAMA* 2002; **288**: 3137–46.

15. Robine J, Mormiche P, Sermet C. Examination of the causes and mechanisms of the increase in disability-free life expectancy. *J Aging Health* 1998; **10**: 171–91.

16. Aijänseppä S, Notkola I, Tijhuis M, van Staveren W, Kromhout D, Nissinen A. Physical functioning in elderly Europeans: 10 year changes in the north and south: the HALE project. *J Epidemiol Community Health* 2005; **59**: 413–19.

17. Schoeni RF, Liang J, Bennett J, Sugisawa H, Fukaya T, Kobayashi E. Trends in old-age functioning and disability in Japan, 1993–2002. *Popul Stud (Camb)* 2006; **60**: 39–53.

18. Sauvaget C, Tsuji I, Haan M, Hisamichi S. Trends in dementia-free life expectancy among elderly members of a large health maintenance organization. *Int J Epidemiol* 1999; **28**: 1110–18.

19. Brønnum-Hansen H. Trends in health expectancy in Denmark, 1987–1994. *Dan Med Bull* 1998; **45**: 217–21.

20. Perenboom RJM, Van Herten LM, Boshuizen HC, Van Den Bos GAM. Trends in disability-free life expectancy. *Disabil Rehabil* 2004; **26**: 377–86.

21. Doblhammer G, Kytir J. Compression or expansion of morbidity? Trends in healthy-life expectancy in the elderly Austrian population between 1978 and 1998. *Soc Sci Med* 2001; **52**: 385–91.

22. Jagger C, Gillies C, Moscone F *et al*. Inequalities in healthy life years in the 25 countries of the European Union in 2005: a cross-national meta-regression analysis. *Lancet* 2008; **372**: 2124–31.

23. Kalache A, Keller I. The greying world: a challenge for the twenty-first century. *Sci Prog* 2000; **83**: 33–54.

24. Kalache A, Aboderin I, Hoskins I. Compression of morbidity and active ageing: key priorities for public health policy in the 21st century. *Bull World Health Org* 2002; **80**: 243–44.

25. Parker MG, Thorslund M. Health trends in the elderly population: getting better and getting worse. *Gerontologist* 2007; **47**: 150–58.

26. Crimmins EM. *Trends in the Health of the Elderly*, 2004. At: http://arjournals.annualreviews.org/doi/full/10.1146/annurev .publhealth.25.102802.124401?cookieSet=1, accessed Mar 2009.

27. Jagger C, Matthews R, Matthews F *et al*., the Medical Research Council Cognitive Function and Ageing Study (MRC-CFAS). Cohort differences in disease and disability in the young-old: findings from the MRC Cognitive Function and Ageing Study (MRC-CFAS). *BMC Public Health* 2007; **7**: 156.

28. Perenboom RJM, van Herten LM, Boshuizen HC, van den Bos GAM. Life expectancy without chronic morbidity: trends in gender and socioeconomic disparities. *Public Health Rep* 2005; **120**: 46–54.

29. Robine J, Michel J, Herrmann FR. Who will care for the oldest people in our ageing society? *BMJ* 2007; **334**: 570–71.

30. Xie J, Matthews FE, Jagger C, Bond J, Brayne C. The oldest old in England and Wales: a descriptive analysis based on the MRC Cognitive Function and Ageing Study. *Age Ageing* 2008; **37**: 396–402.

31. Tomassini C. The oldest old in Great Britain: change over the last 20 years. *Population Trends (Lond)* 2006, 12332.

32. Prince M, Patel V, Saxena S, Maj M, Maselko J, Phillips MR, Rahman A. No health without mental health. *Lancet* 2007; **370**: 859–77.

33. Brayne C. The elephant in the room – healthy brains in later life, epidemiology and public health. *Nat Rev Neurosci* 2007; **8**: 233–39.

34. Compton WM, Conway KP, Stinson FS, Grant BF. Changes in the prevalence of major depression and comorbid substance use disorders in the United States between 1991–1992 and 2001–2002. *Am J Psychiatry* 2006; **163**: 2141–47.

35. Ferri CP, Prince M, Brayne C *et al*. Global prevalence of dementia: a Delphi consensus study. *Lancet* 2005; **366**: 2112–17.

36. Llewellyn D, Matthews F. Increasing levels of semantic verbal fluency in elderly English adults. *Neuropsychol Dev Cogn B Aging Neuropsychol Cogn* 2009; 1–13.

37. Ukraintseva S, Sloan F, Arbeev K, Yashin A. Increasing rates of dementia at time of declining mortality from stroke. *Stroke* 2006; **37**: 1155–59.

38. Jagger C, Matthews R, Lindesay J, Robinson T, Croft P, Brayne C. The effect of dementia trends and treatments on longevity and disability: a simulation model based on the MRC Cognitive Function and Ageing Study (MRC CFAS). *Age Ageing* 2009; afp016.

39. Cohen J. Human population: the next half century. *Science* 2003; **302**: 1172–75.

40. Franco O, Kirkwood T, Powell J, Catt M, Goodwin J, Ordovas J, van der OF. Ten commandments for the future of ageing research in the UK: a vision for action. *BMC Geriatr* 2007; 710.

17

Economics of Ageing and Mental Health

Anders Wimo

KI Alzheimer's Disease Research Center, Department of Neurobiology, Care Sciences and Society, Karolinska institutet, Stockholm, Sweden

INTRODUCTION

The greying of the world and the high prevalence of mental disorders have highlighted the vulnerability of the social and health-care systems. Based on demographic forecasts, almost apocalyptic scenarios have been presented. The number of people 65 years and older will increase from about 500 million people in 2010 to about 1 billion in 2030. The diseases of the elderly and mental disorders are in general chronic, resource demanding, more or less incurable and long lasting (decades). These disorders also involve many sectors of the society; not only the health-care sector but also to a greater extent social services and informal carers, and they cause a substantial loss of well-being and life-years worldwide[1]. If we also add a financial crisis in the many public care systems we must consider fundamental issues such as economic burden, cost effectiveness of treatments, priority settings, equity, how to organize, finance and distribute care in any health economics analysis.

Health economics is the application of economic theory to health care[2]. There are, however, several methodological issues in this field, which also link to fundamental health economics questions. Some basics in health economics must also be considered. The main focus in this chapter is on dementia and similar disorders, but the principles are applicable to any mental or chronic disorder and so we have also included examples from other mental conditions.

PERSPECTIVE

A health economics analysis can be seen from different viewpoints such as a societal perspective or specific cost-bearers (e.g. county councils, municipalities, insurance companies)[3]. A societal perspective is preferable and should include all relevant costs (that is both direct costs within the health sector and indirect costs due to production losses and costs of informal care) and outcomes. Depending on the selected viewpoint, the outcome of the analysis may vary.

RESOURCE UTILIZATION AND COSTING

A key issue in all economics is the cost concept. The opportunity cost, which most economists recommend using in descriptive studies and economical evaluations, is the value of a resource in its best alternative use[2]. Care resources are more or less always scarce and the use of a resource in one specific way will result in some lost benefit because resources were not allocated to another option[4].

Ideally, opportunity costs should be based on market prices, which in health care are not always easy to identify. For example, for an informal caregiver, who because of the care-cost demands is not working, the opportunity cost is the value of the forgone work that could have been done.

Costs can be divided into direct medical costs, direct non-medical costs and indirect costs. In a simplified approach, direct costs refer to the value of resources used and indirect costs to resources lost. Direct medical costs refer to resources used in the medical care system, such as costs of hospital care, drugs and visits to clinics. Direct non-medical costs are those outside the medical care system, such as costs for formal community care and transports. Depending on how care is organized, costs of long-term care and home care can be regarded as a medical or non-medical direct cost.

Indirect costs are costs due to production losses (such as sick leave, early pension, impaired productivity) or mortality. Costs of informal care (see below) is a complicated issue in itself[5,6], and are often classified as indirect costs, but this is not always obvious.

The costing process usually consists of two phases: first the use of resources is measured in terms of physical units (e.g. days in hospital, hours of home support) during a specified period of time; secondly, this resource utilization is calculated into costs. For economic studies of dementia, we have developed a process called resource utilization in dementia (RUD) (Table 17.1)[11]. Because the organization of dementia care varies between countries, the process must be adapted to the particular national situation. This process also includes linguistic adaption, because the meaning and the costs of care concepts (such as 'institutional care') may vary between countries even if the basic language is similar, e.g. if English is spoken in the UK and South Africa, it does not necessarily mean that the interpretation of care concepts is the same. In multinational trials, it is recommended that the aggregation of results from different countries is in physical units and not in costs.

TYPES OF STUDIES

Several approaches can be used in health economics analyses (see Table 17.2)[7]. With the cost description (CD) approach, the costs of a single treatment are described without outcomes/effect measures

Table 17.1 Components of a resource utilization in dementia (RUD) plan[38]

Patient	Caregiver
Accommodation/long-term care	Informal care time (for patient)
(Work status)	Work status
Respite care	(Respite care)
Hospital care	Hospital care
Outclinic visits	Outclinic visits
Social service	Social service
Home nursing care	Home nursing care
Day care	Day care
Drug use	Drug use

Table 17.2 Different types of health economics studies

CD	Cost description
CA	Cost analysis
CMA	Cost minimization analysis
CEA	Cost effectiveness analysis
CBA	Cost benefit analysis
CUA	Cost utility analysis
CCA	Cost consequence analysis
COI	Cost of illness

and without making any comparisons with alternative treatments. In a cost analysis (CA), the costs of different treatments/therapies are compared, but there are no outcomes/effects included in the analysis. A complete health economics analysis should include both measurements of costs and outcomes and comparisons between different treatment alternatives. This is often expressed as a ratio: the the incremental cost-effectiveness ratio (ICER)

$$\Delta C / \Delta E = (C_A - C_B)/((E_{AT1} - E_{AT0}) - (E_{BT1} - E_{BT0}))$$

where C = costs, E = outcomes/effects, A,B = treatments, T0,T1 = time for assessments.

There are, however, other approaches such as net benefit analyses (net monetary benefits and net health benefits)[7]. Irrespective of approach, a willingness-to-pay level (for a specific outcome) is crucial.

In a cost minimization analysis (CMA) there is evidence that the effects/outcomes are similar between the treatment options and thus the analysis is focused on identifying the therapy with the lowest cost. The difference between CA and CMA is that in a CA there is no data about effects/outcomes.

In a cost-effectiveness analysis (CEA), the effect is expressed as a non-monetary quantified unit such as the cost per death or nursing home admission averted. Other outcomes may be functional measures such as activities in daily living (ADL) capacity, severity states of disease and cognition (e.g. scoring on different scales). In a cost benefit analysis (CBA), costs and outcomes are described in the same unit (usually monetary). Early CBA analyses had a simple human capital approach, while the modern theory of CBA is complex and includes willingness-to-pay approaches such as contingent valuation[8,9]. In a cost utility analysis (CUA), the effect is expressed in terms of utilities, such as quality of life. In CUA, the concept of quality adjusted

life years (QALY) is frequently used (as well as other similar measures such as disability adjusted life years (DALY) and healthy years equivalents (HYE)).

In a cost consequence analysis (CCA), cost and outcomes are analysed and presented separately and there is no direct mathematical connection between these two measures.

Cost of illness (COI) studies are descriptive (such as the costs of illness of dementia in Sweden in SEK 50 billion/year). Two approaches can be used: the prevalence method and the incidence method. With the prevalence approach the costs include for all cases for a specified time period, most often one year, including those already suffering from dementia and for new cases occurring during the period in question[10,11]. With the incidence approach the costs for new cases during e.g. one year are estimated, here both the annual costs and future (discounted) costs are included. The choice of approach depends on the purpose of the study: if the aim is to illustrate the economic consequences of interventions, the incidence approach is preferable. If the idea is to estimate the economic burden during a defined year the prevalence approach is the best option.

Another issue in COI studies is whether to use a top-down or a bottom-up approach. In top-down analysis, the total costs for a specific resource (e.g. health-care costs) are distributed over different diseases. Such studies often rely on data from national registers or similar. The bottom-up method starts from a defined sub-population (often from a local area) with for example dementia and registers all cost of illness related to the disease, followed by an extrapolation to the total dementia population. The problem here is compensating for co-morbidity and net costs may be difficult to estimate. It is also important to specify the included cost categories (e.g. cost of informal care). COI studies can be expressed as costs per case and year or as total costs in a specific country/region. Examples of COI studies of mental disorders are seen in Table 17.3. The cost figures highlight the great variation in cost estimates and the importance of identifying the included cost categories.

INFORMAL CARE

Family members and friends or others close to people with mental disorders are heavily involved in their care. Their situation is of great interest from two aspects. First, mental disorders have consequences for the carers themselves. In this sense, their situation is often very stressing (it can be described in terms of burden, coping, but also in terms of morbidity and mortality).

Secondly, in their role as informal carers they are producers of unpaid care. This production of care is a very important part of the costs of mental disorders from a societal perspective. Costing of informal care is complicated and controversial. There are two frequently used methods: the replacement cost approach and the opportunity cost approach, both of which have drawbacks when applied to mental disorders. The replacement cost approach means that if informal care has not been provided, professional staff must be hired on a 1:1 ratio (e.g. one hour of informal care corresponds to one hour of professional care).

In our opinion, informal care should be valued by its opportunity cost, which for a person of working age, is a production loss, but regarding leisure time and contributions by retired persons or persons with no position on the labour market, it is more complicated and there is no given answer.

In most cases, the replacement cost approach results in higher costs of informal care than the opportunity cost approach.

Table 17.3 Examples of COI studies of mental disorders

Country/ Region	Disorder	Costs (billion US$ 2006)	Annual costs per patient (US$ 2006)	Cost categories included	Source
World	Dementia	326.8	11 138	D, IC	(42)
EU27	Dementia	195.6	26 761	D, IC	(43)
UK	Dementia	34.7	47 847	D, IND, IC	(44)
Sweden	Dementia	7.4	52 095	D, IND, IC	(45)
Europe	Depression	138.5	5 016	D, IND	(46)
Sweden	Depression	4.8	NA	D, IND	(47)
Europe	Psychosis/schizophrenia	46.2	10 011	DC	(48)
UK (London)	Schizophrenia	NA	11 981	DC	(49)
Spain (Santander)	Schizophrenia	NA	2 365	DC	(49)

D = Directs costs; IND = Indirect costs; IC = Costs of informal care
Currency conversions by PPPs (purchase power parities), time transformations by national price index of health
Sources: see[39-41].

Table 17.4 Randomized controlled trials with empirical economic data on pharmacological interventions in Alzheimer's disease

Drug	Disorder	Country	Duration	Results (US$ 2006)	Reference
Donepezil	Alzheimer's disease	Nordic	1 year	1 228 (ns)	(50)
Donepezil	Alzheimer's disease	Canada France, Australia	6 months	320 (ns)	(51)
Donepezil	Alzheimer's disease	UK	60 weeks	−907 (ns)	(52)
Memantine	Alzheimer's disease	USA	6 months	7 946 (p < 0.05)	(53)
Risperidone (r), olanzapine (o) and quetiapine (q)	Alzheimer's disease	USA	9 months	(per month)2002, ITT 193(r),−9(o), −199 (q) Overall p = 0.02 (placebo lower)	(54)

BOOTSTRAPPING

Cost data are often skewed (large variation in resource utilization and costs and lots of zero values), making traditional statistical analyses questionable. To compensate for these problems, bootstrapping is frequently used. By resampling from the original database, a new database is created. After each drawing from the original database to the new database, the drawn case is returned to the original database. There are many ways of bootstrapping but in general the new database has the same number of cases as the original sample. After repeating the resampling process several times (e.g. 100–10 000 times, using statistical software), statistical analyses, such as calculating confidence intervals, can be performed, assuming a better representativeness compared to the original reference population[12]. Confidence intervals are often more narrow with bootstrapping than without.

OUTCOME MEASURES

A health economics analysis is incomplete if there is no outcome/effectiveness measure related to the costs (mostly as a cost-effectiveness ratio). In mental disorders or diseases of the elderly, the choice of effectiveness measure is not obvious. The priority discussions may be between different treatments of a particular disease, but also between treatments of different diseases (e.g. schizophrenia and stroke). In the first situation, diagnosis-specific outcomes may be used (e.g. depression scales in depression,

cognition in dementia), but in the latter case, generic outcomes are necessary. Also when diagnosis-specific outcomes are used, there may be interpretation problems – what is the societal value of an incremental cost of X US$ for a one-point reduction in a depression scale?

Health-related quality of life (HRQoL) is often suggested as the most relevant outcome measure in chronic disorders (such as mental diseases). HRQoL instruments consist of several dimensions (e.g. ADL, social interaction, cognition, perception, pain, anxiety, economic status) and they can be diagnosis-specific or generic[13]. A specific problem in dementia and other mental disorders is that the subjective dimension may be difficult to measure. Thus, proxies (mostly caregivers) are often used[14]. Indirect measurement per se, with proxies is, however, not necessarily a problem – the US Panel for cost effectiveness recommended that the general public should value health states[15]. However, if the proxy is a family member, the answers may more or less reflect the situation and interests of the proxy and not the patient's viewpoint.

Examples of instruments used in dementia are the dementia quality of life instrument (DQoL)[16] and quality of life – Alzheimer's disease (QoLAD)[17,18]. The quality of life assessment schedule (QoLAS) is an instrument that has been used in neuropsychiatric disorders[19-21]. Since these instruments are not preference based[15,22], they are less appropriate for cost utility analysis.

Generic HRQoL scales provide opportunities to make comparisons with other diseases. There are also two types of generic scales.

Table 17.5 Economic evaluations with bootstrapping approaches

Intervention	Disorder	Country	Design	Study length	Outcome	Cost difference (US$ 200€*)	ICER in base option (US$ 2006)	Sensitivity analysis or similar	References
Case management	Dementia	Netherlands	RCT + bootstrapping	6 months	Successful treatment	$246*	4 315/unit	95% vs. WTP of 34 000€	(55)
Case management	Dementia	Netherlands	RCT + bootstrapping	3 months	Successful treatment	$2 247*	Dominance (94% probability)	99% vs. WTP of €2000 per 'successful treatment'	(56)
Psychotherapy of 55+	Depression	Netherlands	RCT + bootstrapping	12 months	Recovery, QALYs	$798	ICER 366 921/ recovery Intervention not cost effective	Bootstrapping: 17% more effective, less expensive. 35% more effective, more expensive. 37% less effective, more expensive. 11% less effective, less expensive	(57)

Table 17.6 Examples of economic evaluations with modelling approaches

Intervention	Disorder	Country	Design	Model length	Outcome	Cost difference (US$ 2006)	ICER in base option	Sensitivity analysis or similar	Reference
Donepezil	Alzheimer's disease	USA	Markov model	2 years	QALYs	92	Dominance	<0 to 529 566 (all scenarios)	(58)
Rivastigmine	Alzheimer's disease	Canada	Survival model	2 years	QALYs	438	Dominance	NA	(59)
Galantamine	Alzheimer's disease	UK	AHEAD model	10 years	QALYs	−817	14 755	9 861–29 585	(60)
Memantine	Alzheimer's disease	Sweden	Markov model	5 years	QALYs	13 454	Dominance	<0 in all scenarios	(61)

Examples of indexes or profiles are the sickness impact profile[23], the short form 36 (SF-36)[24] and shorter versions; SF-20 and SF-12.

Regarding caregivers, burden scales, such as the burden interview[25], can in some sense be used as indicators of QoL, but the interplay between patient characteristics, caregiver QoL and burden is complex[26].

Other types of generic scales are used to calculate quality adjusted life years (QALY)[27]. These include the health utilities index (HUI)[22,28], the EuroQoL/EQ-5D[29] and the index of well-being/quality of well-being scale (QWBS)[30].

The QALY concept reflects both quantity of life and quality of life[22,31] and is expressed as figures between 0 (death) and 1 (perfect health); it is widely used in CUA. The use of QALYs is under debate, particularly regarding the elderly[32]. Chronic, incurable, progressive disorders may be disfavoured when compared with e.g. surgical treatment such as cataract or hip replacement surgery.

Postponing institutional (long-term) care has sometimes been defined as an advantageous effect of interventions, making itself a potential outcome. However, this approach can be questioned for several reasons. The concept of institution is not homogeneous[33]. There are also situations where institutional care is a better alternative that insufficient care 'at home'. If postponing nursing home care is successful, there will also probably be a shift from formal care in an institution to formal home care but, which is more notable, also to an increased period of informal care. The latter shift may cause consequences on the caregiver's private situation, and also from a societal cost perspective.

MODELLING

Dementia and other mental disorders most often last for many years. The economic literature in this field with empirical data from interventions is often based on short periods of time. Such studies are shown in Tables 17.4 and 17.5 (Table 17.5 with bootstrapping approaches). The longest study period in these studies is 60 weeks. Since for practical reasons is difficult to perform interventions studies lasting for several years, there is a great interest in using different approaches of modelling to catch the long-term effects[34]. In an economic model, results from a short empirical core period are extrapolated to a longer period. Inputs from several sources, e.g. efficacy, costing and progression, are used. Various applications of Markov models[35] are frequently used, but several other approaches are at hand. In a review, Cohen and Neumann identified 13 types of models regarding Alzheimer's disease[36].

Discounting of costs (and perhaps outcomes) with rates between 3–5% is recommended[15]. Examples of different modelling approaches are given in Table 17.6. Notable is that most models tend to indicate cost effectiveness. One reason is that the models are based on a positive efficacy effect of the active treatment and a relation between disease progression and costs. Factors that neutralize are the costs of the treatment itself (e.g. not only the drug but also diagnostics and laboratory tests that follow treatment), effects on mortality and costs of side effects.

Models are controversial: the results are highly dependent on the assumptions. Long-term effects, such as exhaustion of carers and staff, which do not occur in the early stages of a disease, and symptoms which do have not a linear progressive course, such as behavioural and psychological symptoms in dementia (BPSDs)[37], are difficult to model. A model is also linked, implicitly or explicitly, to a specific organization of care. Although we regard modelling as an essential part of health economics, many drug authorities and clinical researchers are often sceptical about models; they regard such studies as not being 'empirical'.

PHARMACOECONOMICS AND PROGRAMMES

Even if the literature on health economics is sparse, there is a great deal concerning health economic evaluations of drug treatment. Other clinical interventions (here referred to as 'programmes') such as day care, caregiver support, psychotherapy, case management, housing programmes are common in the clinical reality, but sparse in the health economics literature of dementia and other mental disorders. There are several reasons for this. A drug intervention is rather easy to define and operationalize, while concepts such as 'day care' are more vague. Furthermore, it is difficult to include a sufficient number of study objects in an evaluation of a programme, resulting in poor statistical power. The basic field conditions (e.g. care structure, staff situation) at one study centre may differ considerably from another, making the intervention itself (e.g. day care) difficult to differentiate between different sites. In this sense a pill is much easier to define. The costs of a programme may also be very high if a lot of staff is involved and the economical strength of the sponsors is often weaker than the resources of drug companies.

CONCLUSION

Due to the enormous socioeconomic impact of chronic disorders of the elderly (such as dementia and other mental disorders), it is obvious that there is a great need to obtain information about 'value for money'. Many clinicians take a position that it is unethical to discuss cost effectiveness of diseases that affect weak patient groups. Our position is the opposite: it is unethical NOT to discuss cost effectiveness of the treatment and management of these disorders. Care for these patients demands great investment and if we have no idea of what we get for the money, there is a great risk for a waste of money and resources. This is indeed unethical.

REFERENCES

1. Prince M, Patel V, Saxena S, Maj M, Maselko J, Phillips MR et al. No health without mental health. *Lancet* 2007; **370**(9590): 859–77.

2. Drummond MF, O'Brien B, Stoddart GL, Torrance GW. *Methods for the Economic Evaluation of Health Care Programmes*. Oxford: Oxford University Press, 1997.

3. Winblad B, Hill S, Beermann B, Post SG, Wimo A. Issues in the economic evaluation of treatment for dementia. Position paper from the International Working Group on Harmonization of Dementia Drug Guidelines. *Alzheimer Dis Assoc Disord* 1997; **11**(Suppl 3): 39–45.

4. Donaldson C, Mugford M, Vale L. *Evidence-Based Health Economics*. London: BMJ Books, 2002.

5. van den Berg B, Brouwer WB, Koopmanschap MA. Economic valuation of informal care. An overview of methods and applications. *Eur J Health Econ* 2004; **5**(1): 36–45.

6. Jonsson L. Pharmacoeconomics of cholineesterase inhibitors in the treatment of Alzheimer's disease. *Pharmacoeconomics* 2003; **21**: 1025–37.

7. Drummond MF, Sculper MJ, Torrance GW, O'Brien BJ, Stoddart GL. *Methods for the Economic Evaluation of Health Care Programmes*, 3rd ed. Oxford: Oxford University Press, 2004.

8. Johannesson M, Johansson PO, Jonsson B. Economic evaluation of drug therapy: a review of the contingent valuation method. *Pharmacoeconomics* 1992; **1**(5): 325–37.

9. Johannesson M, Weinstein MC. Designing and conducting cost-benefit analyses. In Spilker B (ed.), *Quality of Life and Pharmacoeconomics in Clinical Trials*, 2nd edn. Philadelphia: Lippincott-Raven, 1996.

10. Rice DP, Hodgson TA, Kopstein AN. The economic costs of illness: a replication and update. *Health Financing Rev* 1985; **7**: 61–80.

11. Lindgren B. *Costs of Illness in Sweden 1964–1975*. Lund: Liber, 1981.

12. Cameron CA, Trivedi PK. *Microeconometrics using Stata*. College Station: Stata Press, 2009.

13. Walker MD, Salek SS, Bayer AJ. A review of quality of life in Alzheimer's disease. Part 1: Issues in assessing disease impact. *Pharmacoeconomics* 1998; **14**(5): 499–530.

14. Stewart A, Brod M. Measuring health related quality of life in older and demented people. In Spilker B (ed), *Quality of Life and Pharmacoeconomics in Clinical Trials*. Philadelphia: Lippincott-Raven, 1996, 819–30.

15. Siegel JE, Torrance GW, Russell LB, Luce BR, Weinstein MC, Gold MR. Guidelines for pharmacoeconomic studies. Recommendations from the panel on cost effectiveness in health and medicine. Panel on cost Effectiveness in Health and Medicine. *Pharmacoeconomics* 1997; **11**(2): 159–68.

16. Brod M, Stewart AL, Sands L, Walton P. Conceptualization and measurement of quality of life in dementia: the dementia quality of life instrument (DQoL). *Gerontologist* 1999; **39**(1): 25–35.

17. Logsdon RG, Gibbons LE, McCurry SM, Teri L. Assessing quality of life in older adults with cognitive impairment. *Psychosom Med* 2002; **64**(3): 510–19.

18. Selai C, Vaughan A, Harvey RJ, Logsdon R. Using the QOL-AD in the UK. *Int J Geriatr Psychiatry* 2001; **16**(5): 537–8.

19. Jonsson L, Jonsson B, Wimo A, Whitehouse P, Winblad B. Second International Pharmacoeconomic Conference on Alzheimer's Disease. *Alzheimer Dis Assoc Disord* 2000; **14**(3): 137–40.

20. Elstner K, Selai CE, Trimble MR, Robertson MM. Quality of Life (QOL) of patients with Gilles de la Tourette's syndrome. *Acta Psychiatr Scand* 2001; **103**(1): 52–9.

21. Selai CE, Elstner K, Trimble MR. Quality of life pre and post epilepsy surgery. *Epilepsy Res* 2000; **38**(1): 67–74.

22. Torrance GW, Feeny DH, Furlong WJ, Barr RD, Zhang Y, Wang Q. Multiattribute utility function for a comprehensive health status classification system. Health Utilities Index Mark 2. *Med Care* 1996; **34**(7): 702–22.

23. Bergner M, Bobbitt RA, Carter WB, Gilson BS. The Sickness Impact Profile: development and final revision of a health status measure. *Med Care* 1981; **19**(8): 787–805.

24. Ware JE, Jr, Sherbourne CD. The MOS 36-item short-form health survey (SF-36). I. Conceptual framework and item selection. *Med Care* 1992; 30(6): 473–83.

25. Zarit SH, Reever KE, Bach-Peterson J. Relatives of the impaired elderly: correlates of feelings of burden. *Gerontologist* 1980; **20**(6): 649–55.

26. Deeken JF, Taylor KL, Mangan P, Yabroff KR, Ingham JM. Care for the caregivers: a review of self-report instruments developed to measure the burden, needs, and quality of life of informal caregivers. *J Pain Symptom Manage* 2003; **26**(4): 922–53.

27. Torrance GW. Preferences for health outcomes and cost-utility analysis. *Am J Manag Care* 1997; **3**: S8–20.

28. Neumann PJ, Sandberg EA, Araki SS, Kuntz KM, Feeny D, Weinstein MC. A comparison of HUI2 and HUI3 utility scores in Alzheimer's disease. *Med Decis Making* 2000; 20(4): 413–22.

29. Coucill W, Bryan S, Bentham P, Buckley A, Laight A. EQ-5D in patients with dementia: an investigation of inter-rater agreement. *Med Care* 2001; **39**(8): 760–71.

30. Kerner DN, Patterson TL, Grant I, Kaplan RM. Validity of the Quality of Well-Being Scale for patients with Alzheimer's disease. *J Aging Health* 1998; **10**(1): 44–61.

31. Torrance G. Designing and conducting cost-utility analysis. In Spilker B (ed.), *Quality of Life and Pharmacoeconomics in Clinical Trials*. Philadelphia: Lippincott-Raven, 1996, 1105–21.

32. Tsuchiya A, Dolan P, Shaw R. Measuring people's preferences regarding ageism in health: some methodological issues and some fresh evidence. *Soc Sci Med* 2003; **57**(4): 687–96.

33. Jacobzone S, Cambois E, Chaplain E, Robine J. *Long Term Care Services to Older People. A Perspective on Future Trends: The Impact of an Improved Health of Older Persons*. Paris: OECD, 1998.

34. Buxton MJ, Drummond MF, Van Hout BA, Prince RL, Sheldon TA, Szucs T et al. Modelling in economic evaluation: an unavoidable fact of life. *Health Econ* 1997; **6**(3): 217–27.

35. Sonnenberg FA, Leventhal EA. Modeling disease progression with Markov models. In Wimo A, Jonsson B, Karlsson G, Winblad B (eds), *Health Economics of Dementia*. Chichester: Wiley, 1998, 171–96.

36. Cohen JT, Neumann PJ. Decision analytic models for Alzheimer's disease: state of the art and future directions. *Alzheimers Dement* 2008; **4**(3): 212–22.

37. Ferris SH, Mittelman MS. Behavioral treatment of Alzheimer's disease. *Int Psychogeriatr* 1996; **8**(Suppl 1): 87–90.

38. Wimo A, Wetterholm AL, Mastey V, Winblad B. Evaluation of the resource utilization and caregiver time in anti-dementia drug trials – a quantitative battery. In Wimo A, Jonsson B, Karlsson G, Winblad B (eds), *Health Economics of Dementia*. Chichester: Wiley, 465–99.

39. Eurostat, 2009. At http://nui.epp.eurostat.ec.europa.eu/nui/show.do?dataset=prc_hicp_aind&lang=en.

40. ECB Statistical Data Warehouse, 2009 At http://sdw.ecb.europa.eu/browseTable.do?DATASET=0&CURRENCY=USD&node=2018794&SERIES_KEY=120.EXR.A.USD.EUR.SP00.A.

41. Data and Statistics, IMF, 2009 At http://www.imf.org/external/data.htm.

42. Wimo A, Jönsson L, Winblad B. An estimate of the total worldwide societal costs of dementia in 2005. *Alzheimers Dement* 2007; **3**: 81–91.

43. Wimo A, Jönsson L, Gustavsson A. The cost of illness and burden of dementia in Europe. In Europe A (ed.), *Dementia in Europe Yearbook 2008*. Luxembourg: Alzheimer Europe, 2008, 67–71.

44. Knapp M, Prince M. *Dementia UK*. London: Alzheimer's Society, 2007.

45. Wimo A, Johansson L, Jönsson L. *Demenssjukdomarnas samhällskostnader och antalet dementa i Sverige 2005* [The societal costs of dementia and the number of demented in Sweden 2005] (in Swedish). Stockholm: Socialstyrelsen, 2007.

46. Sobocki PA, Jönsson B, Wittchen HU, Olesen J. Cost of disorders of the brain in Europe. *Euro J Neurology* 2005; **12**(Suppl 1): 1–27.

47. Sobocki P, Lekander I, Borgstrom F, Strom O, Runeson B. The economic burden of depression in Sweden from 1997 to 2005. *Eur Psychiatry* 2007; **22**(3): 146–52.

48. Andlin-Sobocki P, Rossler W. Cost of psychotic disorders in Europe. *Eur J Neurol* 2005; **12**(Suppl 1): 74–7.

49. Knapp M, Chisholm D, Leese M, Amaddeo F, Tansella M, Schene A *et al*. Comparing patterns and costs of schizophrenia care in five European countries: the EPSILON study. European Psychiatric Services: Inputs Linked to Outcome Domains and Needs. *Acta Psychiatr Scand* 2002; **105**(1): 42–54.

50. Wimo A, Winblad B, Engedal K, Soininen H, Verhey F, Waldemar G *et al*. An economic evaluation of donepezil in mild to moderate Alzheimer's disease: results of a 1-year, double-blind, randomized trial. *Dement Geriatr Cogn Disord* 2003; **15**(1): 44–54.

51. Feldman H, Gauthier S, Hecker J, Vellas B, Hux M, Xu Y *et al*. Economic evaluation of donepezil in moderate to severe Alzheimer disease. *Neurology* 2004; **63**(4): 644–50.

52. Courtney C, Farrell D, Gray R, Hills R, Lynch L, Sellwood E *et al*. Long-term donepezil treatment in 565 patients with Alzheimer's disease (AD2000): randomised double-blind trial. *Lancet* 2004; **363**(9427): 2105–15.

53. Wimo A, Winblad B, Stöffler A, Wirth Y, Möbius HJ. Resource utilization and cost analysis of memantine in patients with moderate to severe Alzheimer's disease. *Pharmacoeconomics* 2003; **21**(5): 327–40.

54. Rosenheck RA, Leslie DL, Sindelar JL, Miller EA, Tariot PN, Dagerman KS *et al*. Cost-benefit analysis of second-generation antipsychotics and placebo in a randomized trial of the treatment of psychosis and aggression in Alzheimer disease. *Arch Gen Psychiatry* 2007; **64**(11): 1259–68.

55. Melis RJ, Adang E, Teerenstra S, Van Eijken MI, Wimo A, Achterberg T *et al*. Multidimensional geriatric assessment: back to the future cost-effectiveness of a multidisciplinary intervention model for community-dwelling frail older people. *J Gerontol A Biol Sci Med Sci* 2008; **63**(3): 275–82.

56. Graff MJ, Adang EM, Vernooij-Dassen MJ, Dekker J, Jonsson L, Thijssen M *et al*. Community occupational therapy for older patients with dementia and their care givers: cost effectiveness study. *BMJ* 2008; **336**(7636): 134–8.

57. Bosmans JE, Van Schaik DJ, Heymans MW, Van Marwijk HW, Van Hout HP, de Bruijne MC. Cost-effectiveness of interpersonal psychotherapy for elderly primary care patients with major depression. *Int J Technol Assess Health Care* 2007; **23**(4): 480–7.

58. Neumann PJ, Hermann RC, Kuntz KM, Araki SS, Duff SB, Leon J *et al*. Cost-effectiveness of donepezil in the treatment of mild or moderate Alzheimer's disease. *Neurology* 1999; **52**(6): 1138–45.

59. Hauber AB, Gnanasakthy A, Mauskopf JA. Savings in the cost of caring for patients with Alzheimer's disease in Canada: an analysis of treatment with rivastigmine. *Clin Ther* 2000; **22**(4): 439–51.

60. Ward A, Caro JJ, Getsios D, Ishak K, O'Brien J, Bullock R. Assessment of health economics in Alzheimer's disease (AHEAD): treatment with galantamine in the UK. *Int J Geriatr Psychiatry* 2003; **18**(8): 740–7.

61. Jonsson L. Cost-effectiveness of memantine for moderate to severe Alzheimer's disease in Sweden. *Am J Geriatr Pharmacother* 2005; **3**(2): 77–86.

18

The Influence of Social Factors on Mental Health

Donna D. McAlpine[1] and David Mechanic[2]

[1] School of Public Health, University of Minnesota, Minneapolis, USA
[2] Institute for Health, Health Care Policy and Aging Research, Rutgers University, New Brunswick, USA

Social factors have an enormous influence on the life course, affecting development and socialization; the relative influence of family and peers; opportunities for education, work, recreation, social participation and patterns of social integration; and independence as one reaches the later years of life. They also influence the availability of various health providers and health care settings if one seeks medical care. It is not surprising, therefore, that almost every aspect of mental health and well-being is influenced by social factors[1].

Understanding the social context of mental illness requires appreciating how social factors may be causally related to either the first-onset or re-occurrence of mental illness, and, in turn, how individuals' social circumstances are shaped by having a mental health problem early in life. Moreover, at all stages of the life course, social context and social policies help explain variation in response to symptoms, treatment patterns and outcomes.

A life course perspective acknowledges that individuals carry into their later years all their prior experiences that influence health status as they age. Such a perspective also directs attention to cohort and historical differences in life circumstances and the experience of health and illness. With the rapidity of social change, persons living a normal life span are required to modify their expectations and behaviour on many occasions if they are to adapt successfully to shifting social conditions. Transformations in technology, sexuality, fertility, family and work life, household structure and many other aspects of life also make it inevitable that different age cohorts will have diverse life experiences and thus, different experiences of health and illness.

Epidemiological studies indicate that ageing is not associated with greater risk of experiencing a mental disorder. Moreover, among community residents, the lifetime prevalence of disorders such as depression appears to be lower among older persons compared to their younger counterparts[2]. This finding may be due to methodological difficulties inherent in asking persons to recall their first onset of disorder, the omission of elders living in institutional settings from these studies, age differences in willingness to acknowledge feelings, or the fact that persons with mental disorder die earlier than those without such disorders. Given recall and selective reporting problems, the reliability and validity of lifetime estimates of mental illness can be seriously questioned. But the finding may also in part be suggestive of an important cohort difference; younger cohorts may be at greater risk of some mental disorders such as depression[2]. If these findings are supported by further evidence, and these conditions are not self-limited, we might expect that as younger cohorts age, the prevalence and societal burden of mental illness among older persons may increase.

The discussion that follows focuses more on severe mental illness than on levels of psychological distress or emotional well-being. The distinction between major mental illness and emotional distress is not always clear. The boundaries between what constitutes elevated symptoms of distress and what constitutes clinical disorder are porous and do not always reflect clinical reality. While the risk of experiencing a clinical disorder may not increase with ageing, there is evidence that depressive symptoms or psychological distress do increase in older age[3]. Mirowsky and Ross suggest the approximation of a U-shaped pattern with high depressed mood in late adolescence and young adulthood, lower levels in the middle years, and highest levels at old age[4]. Many studies deal with symptoms that do not reach the threshold of disorder but such symptoms can still have devastating effects on functioning and quality of life, and are a major source of disability, surpassing in impact many serious chronic diseases[5].

Overwhelmingly, research indicates that mental illnesses are neither randomly distributed nor solely the result of one's genetic heritage. But, investigating the social causes of mental illness is not inconsistent with the potential causal role of biology or genetics. Severe mental illnesses such as major depression, bipolar conditions and schizophrenia result from complex, but poorly understood, interactions between biological vulnerabilities and psychological and social influences. Adverse social and developmental factors may increase susceptibility to serious mental illness, or may trigger illness among vulnerable persons. There is increasing interest in gene–environment interactions and the role of early abuse and stress interacting with genetic vulnerabilities[6].

There is a large body of research documenting that social characteristics and position are associated with the prevalence and incidence of mental disorder. Generally, the research indicates being female, unmarried or from a disadvantaged social class increases risk for experiencing mental health problems. Much debate continues on the relative role of social selection and social causation in influencing these patterns. While the impact of these factors among the elderly has been less well studied, it appears that similar patterns characterize later life[7].

Explanations for the social patterning of mental disorder have explored both social causation and social selection. The search for the

Principles and Practice of Geriatric Psychiatry, 3rd edn. Edited by Mohammed T. Abou-Saleh, Cornelius Katona and Anand Kumar
© 2011 John Wiley & Sons, Ltd

social causes or contributors to these disorders has been dominated by the stress paradigm that largely focuses on depressive symptoms. Childhood abuse, stressful events and chronic strains, poor coping resources, lack of intimate and instrumental relations and low self-efficacy have all been found to be associated with the occurrence of depressive symptoms and to a lesser extent major depression. Experiences very early in life such as death of a parent, and physical or sexual abuse during childhood may be related to onset of depressive disorders well into adulthood[8]. Prenatal and nutritional deficiencies may play a role in neurodevelopmental processes and possibly conditions such as schizophrenia[9,10]. Research among the elderly supports the significance of the stress process for understanding the occurrence of depressive disorders in later life[7].

Research has also emphasized the importance of social support, both as a buffer to life stress and its absence directly contributing to the onset of depressive symptoms or disorder. However, social support remains a vague concept, having varying operational definitions ranging from marital status, network size and instrumental support, to the subjective qualities of relationships such as intimacy[11]. While not conclusive, the research suggests that lack of emotional support is most strongly associated with risk of major depression and most strongly buffers the potential deleterious effects of life stress[12]. Contrary to popular impressions, research indicates that individuals are able to maintain supportive relationships as they age; emotional support appears relatively stable across old age, while instrumental support appears to increase[13]. However, as people reach old age, lifetime networks become depleted as friends and intimates die. Support when significantly diminished may increase vulnerability to mental distress.

There is growing attention to the role of religion or spirituality as causally related to health outcomes, including mental disorder[14,15]. Results from many studies indicate that persons who are more involved in religious activities such as going to church report less psychological distress and lower rates of depressive disorder than those who are not involved in such activities[15]. Religion may be particularly important for the elderly and for specific cultural groups such as African Americans[16]. The pathways through which religiosity affects mental health remain unclear. One plausible hypothesis is that the emotional support and instrumental assistance that might result from religious involvement contribute directly to better health as well as help one cope with the difficulties of life. Research in this area continues to confront difficult selection bias, in that persons in better health may be more able and inclined toward religious participation and that persons drawn to various religious practices may be different in their personalities, attitudes and behaviours than those with lesser or no participation[17,18].

While it remains difficult to control for selection effects when trying to untangle the causal roles of social factors, it seems clear that social causation more powerfully explains social patterns of less severe disorders such as depression and is less significant in explaining psychotic disorders such as schizophrenia[19].

Understanding the importance of social selection requires taking a life course perspective that highlights the importance of social or health experiences for understanding the occurrence and consequences of mental disorder among the elderly. People bring into later life all the experiences related to family, friends, stressful life events and strains, employment and socioeconomic status that they have accumulated over their lives. All of these experiences influence how we are sorted or selected into various circumstances as we age. The early onset of mental disorder is one such experience. Having a severe mental disorder early in life increases the likelihood of remaining unmarried, especially for men, and increases the risk

of divorce and separation among those who do marry[20]. Thus many people with severe mental illness will enter their later years without the benefits of a partner to provide emotional and instrumental support. Early onset also shapes later opportunities for education, employment and earnings[21,22]. Even if symptoms remit later in life, it is difficult to overcome these early experiences, and persons with early onset of mental disorder are more likely to find themselves living with significant economic disadvantages in later life.

Selection effects are particularly important for understanding the social correlates of severe and persistent disorders such as schizophrenia. Scant research suggests that social factors cause schizophrenia, although early work in the area found that stress acts as a trigger affecting the occurrence and timing of episodes[23]. A significant body of work on 'expressed emotion' indicates how modification of interactions can prevent and/or reduce episodes[24]. Experiences subsequent to the onset of schizophrenia importantly shape one's life course. The weight of the evidence supports the view that the impairment associated with schizophrenia prevents upward mobility comparable to one's age cohort and loss of social position because of difficulties completing one's education and maintaining employment[19,25]. Older persons with schizophrenia often carry these deficits they acquired when they were younger.

It is clear that those persons who had their first onset of major mental illness early in life bring into their later years life histories likely to be characterized by significant periods of disorder and disruption. But, they also may bring an array of skills and coping strategies, acquired through dealing with illness over many years, and such adaptive skills may help mitigate the potential negative impact of illness during later life. Research indicates, for example, that having a sense of meaning in life, especially a sense of purpose, buffers the effects of traumatic events early in life on symptoms of depression in old age[26].

For the majority of older people who have a mental health disorder, it will be a recurrence or continuation of a condition that first occurred much earlier in life. By some estimates, 95% of all cases of major depression have first onset before age 65[2]. For the majority of persons with depression, age of onset is early in life and seems to be causally related to social factors such as socioeconomic status, exposure to stressful life events and chronic strains, limited coping resources, and deficient social support. Re-occurrence of depression when one is older is commonly associated with similar social factors. In contrast, for the minority of persons who experience first onset of depression in later life, health status may play a larger role. Some research suggests that first-onset of depression in later life is more driven by the experience of health problems than psychosocial circumstances[27]. Similar findings have been observed for first onset of bipolar disorder in later life[28].

Like depression, most persons with psychotic disorders such as schizophrenia have onset early in life. The prevalence and aetiology of late-onset psychoses remain unclear, although there is a growing literature devoted to the topic. It has been suggested that there may be two types of late-onset psychoses: schizophrenia that occurs first after the age of 40, and schizophrenia-like psychotic disorder that first occurs after the age of 60[29]. Both types of disorders are rare and few social factors seem to be associated with risk. One notable exception is gender; the bulk of research suggests that women are at greater risk for late-onset schizophrenia[29], although the reasons for this increased risk are not well understood.

It is also clear that social factors matter a great deal for understanding responses to symptoms of mental illness, treatment patterns and outcomes. Processes of help-seeking are influenced by broad social beliefs about the nature and what should be treated, characteristics of the individual and the social context in which mental illness occurs, and the organization of services and their physical, social and economic accessibility[1]. Members of varying age cohorts have been socialized differently in relation to the recognition of symptoms, appropriate sources of help and social stigma of seeking help from particular types of providers. Selection from the community to varying types of service providers is a two-stage process, which depends on general factors affecting the inclination to seek assistance, and other factors more specific to choice among alternative practitioners. Recent evidence suggests that older persons with a mental disorder are less likely to receive care than their younger counterparts[30] and are more likely to seek care in the general medical care sector than in the specialty mental health sector.

Treatment for mental disorders in older age is shaped by other social factors. Women are more likely to receive care than are men[31]. Economic disadvantage is also a substantial barrier to access to health services and prescription medications in settings without adequate health insurance coverage[32]. While treatment of depression among older persons has increased dramatically in recent years, there remain significant ethnic and socioeconomic status disparities[33].

Differences in patterns of treatment may reflect variation in help seeking behaviours and differences in response to symptoms by health professionals. Older persons with mental disorder are less likely than their younger counterparts with the same disorder to perceive a need for mental health care[34]. Many may normalize the symptoms of depression as part of normal ageing[35] or perceive such symptoms as less important compared to competing physical and social problems[36].

Interpreting symptoms as indicative of mental illness is also complicated by common use of drugs to treat physical illnesses during this stage of life. Prescription and non-prescription drug use is high in elderly populations because of the prevalence of physical illnesses and dementia. The inappropriate use of pharmaceuticals among elderly persons is also common and includes physicians over-prescribing to older patients, self-medication and drug interactions[37]. Drug sensitivity changes with age-related changes in individuals' capacity to absorb and metabolize drugs; therefore dosages effective in young patients may be ineffective or excessively high for older patients. Antipsychotics are commonly used 'off-label' to treat older persons with dementia, but there is current controversy about such treatment practices because they appear to increase risk of mortality[38].

Social factors such as socioeconomic status put persons with mental illness at risk for a number of negative outcomes not directly associated with the illness. Inadequate housing or homelessness remain significant problems for persons with mental illnesses and compromise efforts to provide meaningful services, yet we know little about these issues in older populations[39].

Ageing brings more positive outcomes for persons with schizophrenia than might be expected based on research focused on younger persons and clinical samples who remain in treatment for long periods. Research indicates that with ageing, the positive symptoms of schizophrenia abate or remain in remission for longer periods, and that for a significant minority of persons complete remission is possible[40]. Longitudinal studies of persons with schizophrenia observe much heterogeneity in its long-term course, with many patients having long remissions, late course improvements and complete remissions[41,42]. Most make adequate adjustments to living in the community although social isolation and limited quality of life are common[1,43]. The impact of family on the course of schizophrenia has received the most research attention, although this research is focused on younger persons. This research suggests that a highly involved critical orientation contributes to relapse[24]. Other research suggests that maternal warmth and praise is associated with better quality of life outcomes among middle-aged persons with schizophrenia[44].

Social policies also influence the types of institutions where elderly people receive care. In the 1950s and 1960s, the organization of services in the United States and many Western nations meant that many persons with mental disorders ended up in psychiatric hospitals and nursing homes, and many elderly persons with mental illnesses had spent much of their lives in such institutions. In the United States large scale deinstitutionalization was only possible with the expansion of welfare programmes that provided subsistence and payment for alternative residential care for mentally ill patients in the community.

Current cohorts of elderly persons with major mental illnesses confront a much different landscape of services than their predecessors. Among those seeking help, most will be seen in primary care, not specialty mental health care[34]. Assessing depression within the constellation of physical concomitants that might be attributed to a variety of other conditions poses diagnostic challenges to the general physician. It is not surprising, therefore, that depression among older persons often goes undiagnosed[45]. This problem may be even more pronounced for African American patients[46].

There has been much recent effort to integrate mental health services into primary medical care. Large-scale multifaceted interventions bringing mental health care into primary care settings have been found to be effective in reducing symptoms and improving quality of life for persons with depression, while also being cost effective. These interventions are intensive, typically including enhanced screening to improve the identification of cases of depression, patient and provider education, case managers responsible for tracking patient outcomes and adherence to treatment, and the availability of a psychiatrist for consultations. However, even at their best, these interventions show how difficult it is address the needs of the elderly with depression. In the most widely replicated model, IMPACT, for example, only about one quarter of patients in the intervention (compared to less than 10% in usual care) achieved remission at 12 months[17].

While most of the research on how social factors impact the occurrence of mental illness or the response to symptoms of mental illness is based on community samples, nursing homes remain the social environment where many elderly persons find themselves. In some sense, the traditional nursing home echoes the conditions of the long term psychiatric hospitals that characterized care for the mentally ill in the past. Typically admissions to nursing homes occur when individuals are incapable of caring for themselves, when their physical and psychiatric problems create unmanageable burdens for their caretakers, or when community caretakers are no longer available. Admission is often triggered by such events as a loss of function following trauma, such as hip fractures, confusion and wandering, and incontinence. Traditional nursing homes, like the traditional long-term mental hospital, contribute to an institutional syndrome resulting from vulnerabilities of patients as they respond to decreased social participation, sensory deprivation, loss of efficacy and control over daily life decisions, institutionalization, routinization and the like. There is persuasive evidence that efforts to keep patients involved and participating in valued activities help for both mental and physical function. Many nursing homes fail to give these social aspects of life adequate attention, and patients spend much of their time in isolation and uninvolved. Moreover, historically, there has been evidence that psychotropic drugs were being over-prescribed in nursing homes to control patients and ease staff workloads. Recent evidence suggests that these practices have been reduced as the result of legislation in the late 1980s in the United States[48].

Nursing care may be the best treatment context for some patients who are seriously incapacitated and require a broad range of services difficult to provide in the home or in other community settings, but most impaired elderly benefit from settings that are more successful in sustaining self-efficacy and social engagement. Recent developments in the nursing home industry suggest that such settings are possible; for example, the Green House model emphasizes small residential (family-like) housing, privacy, independence and control over activities of daily life as much as clinical status allows[49]. Early results indicate that functioning and quality of life, including emotional well-being, are more positive for individuals in such types of homes compared to traditional nursing home settings[50].

Demographic shifts mean that the social patterning of mental illness in later life and our responses to it may be very different with future cohorts of older persons than what we see today. The United States and many other nations are facing an ageing population, with the number of older persons with mental illness more prevalent. The capacity for any society to cope with mental illness depends on the organization of kinship groups and households, and the existing social institutions in a society. The growing prevalence of divorce, single-person households, small families, high female participation in the workforce, geographic mobility and other trends make it difficult to put increasing reliance on informal social networks for caretaking. Developing alternative structures that are financially viable and humane constitutes a growing challenge.

REFERENCES

1. Mechanic D. *Mental Health and Social Policy: Beyond Managed Care*, 5th edn. Boston, MA: Allyn & Bacon, 2008.
2. Kessler RC, Berglund P, Demler O *et al*. Lifetime prevalence and age-of-onset distributions of DSM-IV disorders in the National Comorbidity Survey Replication. *Arch Gen Psychiatry* 2005; **62**: 593–602.
3. Mirowsky J, Ross CE. Age and depression. *J Health Soc Behav* 1992; **33**: 187–205.
4. Mirowsky J, Ross CE. Well-being across the life course. In Horwitz AV, Scheid TL (eds), *A Handbook for the Study of Mental Health: Social Contexts, Theories, and Systems*. Cambridge: Cambridge University Press, 1999, 328–47.
5. Wells KB, Sturm R, Sherbourne CD, Meredith LS. *Caring for Depression*. Cambridge, MA: Harvard University Press, 1996.
6. Brown GW, Harris TO. Depression and the serotonin transporter 5-HTTLPR polymorphism: a review and a hypothesis concerning gene–environment interaction. *J Affect Disord* 2008; **111**: 1–12.
7. Cairney J, Krause N. The social distribution of psychological distress and depression in older adults. *J Aging Health* 2005; **17**: 807–35.
8. Kessler RC, Davis CG, Kendler KS. Childhood adversity and adult psychiatric disorder in the US National Comorbidity Survey. *Psychol Med* 1997; **27**: 1101–19.
9. St Clair D, Xu M, Wang P *et al*. Rates of adult schizophrenia following prenatal exposure to the Chinese famine of 1959–61. *JAMA* 2005; **294**: 557–62.
10. Susser E, Hoek HW, Brown A. Neurodevelopmental disorders after prenatal famine: the story of the Dutch famine study. *Am J Epidemiol* 1998; **147**: 213–16.
11. Thoits PA. Conceptual, methodological and theoretical problems in studying social support as a buffer against life stress. *J Health Soc Behav* 1982; **23**: 145–59.
12. Blazer DG, Hybels CF. Origins of depression in later life. *Psychol Med* 2005; **35**: 1241–52.
13. Shaw BA, Krause N, Liang J, Bennett J. Tracking changes in social relations throughout late life. *J Gerontol B Psychol Sci Soc Sci* 2007; **62**: S90–99.
14. Idler EL, Kasl SV. Religion among disabled and non-disabled persons II: Attendance at religious services as a predictor of the course of disability. *J Gerontol B Psychol Sci Soc Sci* 1997; **52**: S306–16.
15. Moreira-Almeida A, Neto FL, Koenig HG. Religiousness and mental health: a review. *Rev Bras Psiquiatr* 2006; **28**: 242–50.
16. Chatters LM, Bullard KM, Taylor RJ *et al*. Religious participation and DSM-IV disorders among older African Americans: findings from the National Survey of American Life. *Am J Geriatr Psychiatry* 2008; **16**: 957–65.
17. Idler EL. Religion and aging. In Binstock RH, George LK (eds), *Handbook of Aging and the Social Sciences*, 6th edn. San Diego, CA: Elsevier, 2006, 277–300.
18. Idler EL. Health and religion. In Cockerham W (ed.), *The New Blackwell Companion to Medical Sociology*. Oxford: Blackwell, 2010, 133–158.
19. Dohrenwend BP, Levav I, Shrout PE *et al*. Socioeconomic status and psychiatric disorders: the causation–selection issue. *Science* 1992; **255**: 946–52.
20. Kessler RC, Walters EE, Forthofer MS. The social consequences of psychiatric disorders, III: Probability of marital stability. *Am J Psychiatry* 1998; **155**: 1092–6.
21. Breslau J, Lane M, Sampson N *et al*. Mental disorders and subsequent educational attainment in a US national sample. *J Psychiatr Res* 2008; **42**: 708–16.
22. Kessler RC, Heeringa S, Lakoma MD *et al*. Individual and societal effects of mental disorders on earnings in the United States: results from the National Comorbidity Survey Replication. *Am J Psychiatry* 2008; **165**: 703–11.
23. Brown GW, Birley JL. Crises and life changes and the onset of schizophrenia. *J Health Soc Behav* 1968; **9**: 203–14.
24. Leff J, Vaughn C. *Expressed Emotion in Families*. New York: Guilford, 1985.
25. Mechanic D. *Medical Sociology*, 2nd edn. New York: Free Press, 1978.
26. Krause N. Evaluating the stress-buffering function of meaning in life among older people. *J Aging Health* 2007; **19**: 792–812.
27. Sneed JR, Kasen S, Cohen P. Early-life risk factors for late-onset depression. *Int J Geriatr Psychiatry* 2007; **22**: 663–7.
28. Hays JC, Krishnan KR, George LK *et al*. Age of first onset of bipolar disorder: demographic, family history, and psychosocial correlates. *Depress Anxiety* 1998; **7**: 76–82.
29. Howard R, Rabins PV, Seeman MV *et al*. Late-onset schizophrenia and very-late-onset schizophrenia-like psychosis: an international consensus. *Am J Psychiatry* 2000; **157**: 172–8.
30. Wang PS, Lane M, Olfson M *et al*. Twelve-month use of mental health services in the United States: results from the National

Comorbidity Survey Replication. *Arch Gen Psychiatry* 2005; **62**: 629–40.

31. Ojeda VD, McGuire TG. Gender and racial/ethnic differences in use of outpatient mental health and substance use services by depressed adults. *Psychiatr Q* 2006; **77**: 211–22.

32. Berk ML, Schur CL, Cantor JC. Ability to obtain health care: recent estimates from the Robert Wood Johnson Foundation National Access to Care Survey. *Health Affairs* 1995; **14**: 139–46.

33. Crystal S, Sambamoorthi U, Walkup JT *et al.* Diagnosis and treatment of depression in the elderly Medicare population: predictors, disparities, and trends. *J Am Geriatr Soc* 2003; **51**: 1718–28.

34. Klap R, Unroe K, Unützer J. Caring for mental illness in the United States: a focus on older adults. *Am J Geriatr Psychiatry* 2003; **11**: 517–24.

35. Sarkisian CA, Lee-Henderson MH, Mangione CM. Do depressed older adults who attribute depression to 'old age' believe it is important to seek care? *J Gen Intern Med* 2003; **18**: 1001–5.

36. Proctor EK, Hasche L, Morrow-Howell N *et al.* Perceptions about competing psychosocial problems and treatment priorities among older adults with depression. *Psychiatr Serv* 2008; **59**: 670–75.

37. Lipton HL, Lee PR. *Drugs and the Elderly: Clinical, Social, and Policy Perspectives*. Stanford, CA: Stanford University Press, 1988.

38. Jeste DV, Blazer D, Casey D *et al.* ACNP White Paper: update on use of antipsychotic drugs in elderly persons with dementia. *Neuropsychopharmacology* 2008; **33**: 957–70.

39. Cohen CI. Aging and homelessness. *Gerontologist* 1999; **39**: 5–14.

40. Cohen CI (ed.). *Schizophrenia into Later Life: Treatment, Research and Policy*. Arlington, VA: American Psychiatric Publishing, 2003.

41. Davidson L, McGlashan TH. The varied outcomes of schizophrenia. *Can J Psychiatry* 1997; **42**: 34–43.

42. Harding CM, Zubin J, Strauss JS. Chronicity in schizophrenia: fact, partial fact, or artifact? *Hosp Community Psychiatry* 1987; **38**: 477–86.

43. Mechanic D. Organization of care and quality of life of persons with serious and persistent mental illness. In Katschnig H, Freeman H, Sartorius N (eds.), *Quality of Life in Mental Disorders*, 2nd edn. New York: Wiley Interscience, 2006, 309–19.

44. Greenberg JS, Knudsen KJ, Aschbrenner KA. Prosocial family processes and the quality of life of persons with schizophrenia. *Psychiatr Serv* 2006; **57**: 1771–7.

45. Unützer J. Clinical practice. Late-life depression. *N Eng J Med* 2007; **357**: 2269–76.

46. Gallo JJ, Bogner HR, Morales KH *et al.* Patient ethnicity and the identification and active management of depression in late life. *Arch Intern Med* 2005; **165**: 1962–8.

47. Hunkeler EM, Katon W, Tang L *et al.* Long term outcomes from the IMPACT randomised trial for depressed elderly patients in primary care. *Br Med J* 2006; **332**: 259–63.

48. Hughes CM, Lapane KL. Administrative initiatives for reducing inappropriate prescribing of psychotropic drugs in nursing homes: how successful have they been? *Drugs Aging* 2005; **22**: 339–31.

49. Rabig J, Thomas W, Kane RA *et al.* Radical redesign of nursing homes: applying the green house concept in Tupelo, Mississippi. *Gerontologist* 2006; **46**: 533–9.

50. Kane RA, Lum TY, Cutler LJ *et al.* Resident outcomes in small-house nursing homes: a longitudinal evaluation of the initial green house program. *J Am Geriatr Soc* 2007; **55**: 832–9.

Part C

Diagnosis and Assessment

19

Classification of Dementia and other Cognitive Disorders in ICD-10 and DSM-IV

A. Jablensky and J.E. Cooper

Department of Psychiatry and Behavioural Science, Medical Research Foundation Building, Perth, Australia

The classification of mental disorders in the Tenth Revision of the International Classification of Diseases (ICD-10) includes a revised content that reflects the most important advances in research and clinical practice at the time of its conception. It is presented in different versions for different types of professional users. The differences are, however, in degrees of detail, and the versions are compatible with each other since they are all derived from the same basic document, the 'Clinical Descriptions and Diagnostic Guidelines'[1].

THE USES OF ICD-10

ICD-10 has necessarily retained its historical purpose of facilitating the recording of national and international statistics of morbidity and mortality, but has the added values of also being designed as a uniquely international aide to clinical work, teaching, and research. It achieves these objectives by means of an updated list of diagnostic rubrics, a set of glossary-type definitions of disorders, and additional explicit diagnostic criteria. The latter have been developed in two versions: (a) clinical diagnostic guidelines for routine use, allowing sufficient flexibility and discretion in the application of "clinical judgement" in the hospital ward or the out-patient clinic; and (b) diagnostic criteria for research (ICD-10-DCR) providing stringent decision-making rules to increase the specificity of diagnostic classification and thus ensure a high level of sample homogeneity for the purposes of clinical, biological and other research[2].

As a result of a great deal of collaboration between the advisers to the World Health Organisation and the several Task Forces that assembled DSM-IV on behalf of the American Psychiatric Association during the last few years of the preparation of both the classifications, there are very few important differences between them. Since the same body of internationally published research experience and literature was available to both sets of experts during the processes of development, those differences that remain are mainly differences of opinion rather than of fact. Some differences reflect the need for ICD-10 to accommodate a much broader base of international experience and opinions than a national classification. In the development of ICD-10, experts from many different cultures and languages were involved from the earliest stages.

As in ICD-9, Chapter V deals with "Mental and Behavioural Disorders", and is intended for the recording of the clinical syndromes as presented and experienced by the patient. If a specific underlying cause of the disorder is known (or highly probable), additional codes should also be used from other chapters of ICD-10, such as Chapter I; Infectious and parasitic diseases, Chapter II; Neoplasms, or Chapter VI; Diseases of the Nervous System.

DEMENTIA IN ICD-10

In ICD-10, the dementias are embedded in the section on organic and symptomatic mental disorders (codes F00-F09) which contains the following major rubrics:

- Dementia in Alzheimer's disease.
- Vascular dementia.
- Dementia in diseases classified elsewhere.
- Unspecified dementia.
- Organic amnestic syndrome, other than induced by alcohol and drugs.
- Delirium, other than induced by alcohol and drugs.
- Other mental disorders due to brain damage and dysfunction and to physical disease.
- Personality and behavioural disorders due to brain disease, damage and dysfunction
- Unspecified organic or symptomatic mental disorder.

In contrast to ICD-9, the distinction between psychotic and non-psychotic illnesses is of no taxonomic consequence in ICD-10, where disorders of different psychopathological expression are grouped together on the basis of established or presumed common aetiology. In the particular instance of section F0, in which the dementing disorders are included, the underlying classificatory characteristic of "organic" is defined in the sense that "the syndrome so classified can be attributed to an independently diagnosable cerebral or systemic disease or disorder". The subsidiary term "symptomatic" is not used in the titles of individual disorders but it is included in the overall title of the block F00 – F09. This is because it is widely used in many countries to indicate those organic mental disorders in which cerebral involvement is secondary to a systemic extra-cerebral disease or disorder. In other words, 'symptomatic' in this context is a subdivision of the wider term 'organic'.

Principles and Practice of Geriatric Psychiatry, 3rd edn. Edited by Mohammed T. Abou-Saleh, Cornelius Katona and Anand Kumar
© 2011 John Wiley & Sons, Ltd

Another feature of ICD-10, as compared to earlier classifications, is the omission of any reference to age as a defining criterion of the disorders accompanied by a cognitive deficit. The terms "senile" and "presenile" are practically absent in the classification, and there is no provision for identifying any mental disorder as necessarily a result of aging. The classification does, however, allow the recording of an unusually early or late onset of the disorder. In other words, the mental disorders occurring in the elderly are no longer considered to belong in a separate category of morbidity. This is very much in line with research conducted in the past three decades which has demonstrated that the relatively high prevalence of mental morbidity in the elderly in Western cultures is related to a wide range of psychosocial factors (e.g. social isolation, cultural uprooting and institutionalization), as well as to physical co- morbidity, but that the aging process itself does not produce nosologically specific forms of disorders.

If section F0 of ICD-10 is used as a diagnostic decision tree, there is a choice of five entry points at the level of clinical syndrome: (i) dementia; (ii) amnesic syndrome; (iii) delirium; (iv) organic quasi-functional disorder (affective, delusional, hallucinatory or other); and (v) personality or behavioural disorder. Once a disorder is identified at this general syndrome level, the next step is defined by the diagnostic guidelines which lead into more specific diagnostic categories. The diagnostic decision rules for dementia illustrate the point.

The syndrome of dementia is defined in ICD-10 by "evidence of a decline in both memory and thinking, which is of a degree sufficient to impair functioning in daily living", in a setting of clear consciousness. For a confident diagnosis to be established, such disturbances should have been present for at least 6 months. Deterioration of emotional control, social behaviour and motivation represent significant additional features but the overriding criterion is the presence of memory, learning and reasoning decline. The ICD-10 DCR (research criteria) add anchor points for a grading of the deficits into mild, moderate and severe, separately for memory and intellectual capacity. The overall grading of the severity of dementia is made on the basis of the function which is more severely impaired.

Once the presence of the syndrome of dementia is established, the diagnostic process branches off into the different clinical varieties of dementia typical of Alzheimer's disease, vascular dementia, and dementia in diseases classified elsewhere (including Pick's disease, Creutzfeldt-Jakob disease, Huntington's disease, Parkinson's disease, HIV disease, and a range of systemic and infectious diseases such as hepatolenticular degeneration, lupus erythematosus, trypanosomiasis, and general paresis). Dementia in Alzheimer's disease is subdivided into Type I (onset after the age of 65) and Type 2 (onset before the age of 65). Although the ICD-10-DCR criteria emphasize the ultimate criterion of the neuropathological examination and the supporting role of brain imaging, they nevertheless allow for a confident clinical diagnosis to be made, if clear evidence of a memory and intellectual performance deterioration has been present for 6 months or more. The ICD-10 criteria for vascular dementia are broader than the corresponding DSM-IV criteria: they include not only multi-infarct (predominantly cortical) vascular dementia, but also the subcortical dementias (Binswanger's encephalopathy being an example), as well as the mixed cortical and subcortical forms.

As regards the diagnosis of delirium, ICD-10 has abandoned the distinction between acute and subacute deliria; the condition is defined as "a unitary syndrome of variable duration and degree of severity ranging from mild to very grave", with an upper limit of 6 months' duration and a subdivision into delirium superimposed on dementia and delirium not superimposed on dementia.

The rubric "other mental disorders due to brain damage and dysfunction and to physical disease" includes disorders with "functional" characteristics (e.g. hallucinosis, catatonia, schizophrenia-like disorder, and mood disorders) which arise in the context of demonstrable organic illness, such as cerebral disease, systemic disorders, and brain dysfunction associated with toxic disorders (other than due to alcohol or drugs). An important, not yet fully validated, addition to this rubric is the "mild cognitive disorder" attributable to physical co-morbidity which is defined as transient but nevertheless involving memory and learning difficulties. However, the requirement that "this diagnosis should be made only in association with a specified ohysical disorder" is in need of revision, since in a proportion of cases this diagnosis may reflect the early, pre-dementia stage of Alzheimer's disease.

Finally, personality and behavioural disorders due to brain disease, damage and dysfunction include familiar conditions such as organic personality disorder (the frontal lobe syndrome but also other lesions to circumscribed areas of the brain), postencephalitic syndrome, post-concussional syndrome, and some new entities, e.g. right hemispheric organic affective disorder (altered ability to express and comprehend emotion without true depression).

In conclusion, two features of ICD-10 should be emphasized. First, as already noted, it does not identify the mental disorders in the elderly as a separate or special category of psychiatric morbidity. In addition to the F0 section listing the organic and symptomatic mental disorders, psychiatric disturbances arising in the elderly population can be classified, according to their presentation and course, in any of the other major sections of ICD-10 (except for F8 and F9, which deal with developmental disorders and behavioural and emotional disorders occurring in childhood and adolescence).

Second, although ICD-10 is not explicitly a multiaxial classification, there are two ways in which multi-axial coding can be achieved if required. The simplest way is to use extra codes from the other chapters of ICD-10 in addition to those in Chapter V; any physical disorders present can be recorded by codes form Chapters I to XIX, and codes from the final two chapters can be used to cover other noteworthy aspects of the clinical picture. These are Chapter XX; External Causes of Morbidity and Mortality (the X and Y codes, covering drugs causing adverse effects in therapeutic use, and injuries and poisoning), and Chapter XXI; Factors Influencing Health Status and Contact With Health Services (the Z codes, which include a variety of social, family and life-style factors). Another and more comprehensive option is to use the special Multi-axial System now available, which was developed by means of an international collaborative study organised by WHO Geneva[3]. This provides three descriptive axes: Axis 1 – Clinical Diagnosis, Axis II – Disablements, and Axis III – Contextual Factors. These Axes are a convenient re-arrangement of the chapters of ICD-10 listed above, with the addition of a brief set of ratings covering physical disabilities.

DEMENTIA AND OTHER COGNITIVE DISORDERS IN DSM-IV

In DSM-IV (and its revised version DSM-IV TR) dementias and other mental disorders associated with brain disease are grouped into a section entitled "Delirium, dementia, and amnestic and other cognitive disorders". In contrast to ICD-10 and the earlier DSM-IIIR, the term "organic" mental disorders is no longer used in DSM-IV, to avoid the implication that "nonorganic" mental disorders do not have a biological basis[14]. While ICD-10 retains a general description of dementia as a syndrome occurring in Alzheimer's disease, cerebrovascular disease and "other conditions primarily or secondarily affecting the brain", the DSM-IV classification lists dementias as specific disorders which "share a common symptom presentation but are differentiated based on etiology". Specific diagnostic criteria are provided for dementia of the Alzheimer's type, vascular dementia, and dementia due to other medical conditions (HIV disease, head trauma, Parkinson's disease, Huntington's disease, Pick's disease and Creutzfeldt-Jakob disease). A separate DSM-IV category, which has no counterpart in ICD-10, is substance-induced persisting dementia, defined as significant cognitive impairment persisting long after the symptoms of substance intoxication or withdrawal have abated. Another difference from ICD-10 involves the category of "dementia due to multiple etiologies", introduced to cover "the common situation in which the dementia has more than one etiology", such as a condition arising as a result of Parkinson's disease with co-occurring long-term substance use. Finally, the DSM-IV section contains residual categories for "dementia not otherwise specified" and "cognitive disorder not otherwise specified", to enable the coding of dementing illnesses or other cognitive dysfunction that do not meet the criteria for any of the specific types, or for which no specific etiology has yet been established.

While the DSM-IV diagnostic criteria and the ICD-10 diagnostic guidelines for delirium essentially agree, there are differences between the two classifications regarding the specific rubrics and their composition. Thus, the ICD-10 heading for the group of delirious disorders is "delirium, not induced by alcohol and other psychoactive substances", with separate coding provisions for delirium not superimposed on dementia, delirium superimposed on dementia, other delirium and delirium unspecified (alcohol or substance use induced delirium is coded in the ICD10 section "Disorders due to psychoactive substance use"). In DSM-IV, both "delirium due to a general medical condition" and substance-induced delirium are coded within the same section, along with "delirium due to multiple etiologies" and "delirium not otherwise specified".

Another difference between ICD-10 and DSM-IV concerns the placement of psychiatric syndromes and personality or behavioural disorders associated with cerebral disease. The ICD-10 section "Delirium, dementia, and amnestic and other cognitive disorders" provides a fairly detailed classification of "organic" hallucinosis, catatonic disorder, delusional disorder, mood and anxiety disorders, personality disorders and specific syndromes, such as postconcussional and postencephalitic syndrome. Notably, the same section contains the category "mild cognitive disorder" and provides diagnostic guidelines for this rubric, while acknowledging that "the boundaries of this category are still to be firmly established". In DSM-IV, "mild neurocognitive disorder" is an inclusion term under "cognitive disorder not otherwise specified", with diagnostic criteria contained in Appendix B "for further study".

Both ICD-10 and DSM-IV have proved to be essential tools for clinicians, epidemiologists, and – perhaps to a lesser degree – for researchers working in the rapidly evolving areas of the neuroscience and genetics of neurocognitive disorders. In a thoughtful commentary and critique of the two classifications, Reisberg[13] noted that in several respects the present diagnostic manuals reflect knowledge that is somewhat dated and fail to incorporate recent advances. Thus, the DSM-IV definition of dementia requires "impairment in memory" as a cardinal and necessary criterion, not acknowledging

that diseases such as vascular dementia and frontotemporal dementia are not characterized by prominent memory impairment, at least in their early stages. The DSM-IV definition mentions disturbance in executive functioning but omits the behavioural and emotional changes, as well as the diminishing capacity to carry out activities of daily living. Importantly, the DSM-IV definition proposes that the diagnosis of Alzheimer's type dementia can only be made by exclusion, i.e. once other etiologies for the dementia have been ruled out. This is at variance with the current international consensus (including the American Geriatric Society) that Alzheimer's disease should be amenable to diagnosis by inclusion, rather than exclusion. Another suggested change is the removal, from both DSM and ICD, of the distinction between early onset (before 65 years of age) and late onset (after 65 years) Alzheimer's disease. Further proposals concern introducing in the future classifications staging procedures for dementia; broadening the definition of Pick's disease to include frontotemporal dementia; and revising the description of dementia in Parkinson's disease and Lewy body dementia.

PROSPECTS FOR THE FUTURE

It is only a few years before the next edition of the international classification, ICD-11 is ready for use, and there are at present plenty of issues worthy of debate. Both terminological and conceptual issues related to the current ICD-10 classification of this group of conditions have been raised since its introduction in the early 1990s. Thus, the term "organic", sitting uneasily within the title of the ICD-10 section, has often been singled out for critique as a legacy of a dualist tradition and a schism between brain-based "neurological" diseases and "functional" psychiatric disorders that is no longer tenable[4,5]. The non-invasive techniques for brain imaging, such as MRI, SPECT and PET-scans, are demonstrating a variety of structural and functional abnormalities in the brains of some (but by no means all) patients with the familiar clinical syndromes, that are also present in substantial proportions of normal subjects. These changes are 'organic' in a general sense of being something physical, but not in the way the term is used in the ICD (that is, to indicate a concurrent and diagnosable physical disorder).

It will probably soon be time to abandon 'organic' as a term to be used in a classification, and to develop new terms and concepts that will make these more subtle differentiations clear. The term "neurocognitive disorders", thought to capture both the concepts of cognitive disturbance and of an altered neural substrate, has been proposed in a recent review of the evidence supporting the grouping of the dementias, amnesic syndromes and deliria into a single classificatory "cluster"[6]. In addition, a critical examination of the very term "dementia" has also found it wanting for three main reasons[7]. First, it is now clear that memory impairment is just one of several cognitive domains that are affected to varying degrees in this group of disorders (other domains include language, attention, executive function, visuospatial ability, speed of information processing and manual dexterity). Secondly, the operational definitions of the diagnostic criteria for dementia in both ICD-10 and DSM-IV are insufficiently specific, leading on occasions to gross discrepancies in the assessment of the prevalence of dementia in population studies[8,9]. Thirdly, in its categorical usage the term is stigmatizing and has connotations of extreme disability and dependence that tend to arouse severe anxiety in patients and family members. As a possible remedy, terms like "vascular cognitive disorder", or "cognitive disorder in Alzheimer's disease" have been proposed.

Complex problems with far-reaching conceptual implications for the classification of this group of disorders arise out of recent advances in their study with the tools of molecular genetics, proteomics and biomarker research. While conditions such as Alzheimer's disease, Huntington's disease, or Creutzfeldt-Jakob disease have been traditionally regarded as being among the few "true" discrete disease entities within the psychiatric classification, owing to the presence of "hallmark" brain lesions, recent evidence challenges seriously this view[10]. Current molecular classifications distinguish between four groups of neurodegenerative diseases: tauopathies (e.g. Alzheimer's disease, Pick's disease, frontotemporal dementia, progressive supranuclear palsy); alpha-synucleinopathies (e.g. Parkinson's disease, dementia with Lewy bodies, multiple system atrophy); neurofilamentopathies (e.g. dementia with neurofilament inclusions); and prion diseases (e.g. Creutzfeldt-Jakob disease, Gerstmann-Sträussler-Scheinker syndrome, fatal familial insomnia). There is, however, increasing evidence of marked individual variability within the groups, as well as extensive overlap across the diseases and syndromes in terms of structure, molecular composition and distribution of brain lesions, raising the question of common aetiological and pathogenetic mechanisms[11,12]. In the presence of both genetic heterogeneity and clinical pleiotropy, the nosological status of the individual disorders becomes less certain that previously assumed. Generally, two positions have been articulated in the recent literature (Armstrong et al. 2005): (i) the benefits of retaining the concept of distinct nosological entities outweighs its limitations; the latter can be constrained by using the existing diagnostic criteria in conjunction with refined molecular and other biomarker analysis; (ii) the traditional disease entities represent points on a continuum of neuropathological change and a clinical spectrum of syndromes rather than diseases.

Whatever form the ICD-11 classification takes, it seems likely that the principle of recording the clinical picture by means of Chapter V and the underlying cerebral or other physical cause by means of other chapters will remain. Research is now providing many, though not entirely consistent, clues about the exact place and the histological and molecular nature of the lesions in the central nervous system that give rise to the clinical syndromes, but the clinical syndromes themselves will not change, and will always need to be reliably recorded.

REFERENCES

1. WHO (1992) *The ICD-10 Classification of Mental and Behavioural Disorders. Clinical Descriptions and Diagnostic Guidelines*. World Health Organization. Geneva

2. WHO (1993) *The ICD-10 Classification of Mental and Behavioural Disorders. Diagnostic Criteria for Research*. World Health Organization. Geneva.

3. WHO (1997) *Multi-axial Presentation of ICD-10 for Use in Adult Psychiatry*. Cambridge: Cambridge University Press.

4. Spitzer RL, First MB, Williams JBW et al. (1992) Now is the time to retire the term "organic mental disorders". *American Journal of Psychiatry* **149**, 240–244.

5. Sachdev P. (1996) A critique of 'organic' and its proposed alternatives. *Australian and New Zealand Journal of Psychiatry* **30**, 165–170.

6. Sachdev P, Andrews G, Hobbs MJ et al. (2009) Neurocognitive disorders: Cluster 1 of the proposed meta-structure for DSM-V and ICD-11. *Psychological Medicine* (in press).

7. Sachdev P. (2000) Is it time to retire the term "dementia"? *Journal of Neuropsychiatry and Clinical Neuroscience* **12**, 276–279.

8. Wetterling T, Kaniz R-D, Borgis K-J. (1996) Comparison of different criteria for vascular dementia (ADDTC, DSM-IV, ICD-10, NINDS-AIREN). *Stroke* **27**, 30–36.

9. Erkinjuntti T, Ostbye T, Steenhuis R et al. (1997) The effect of differential diagnostic criteria on the prevalence of dementia. *New England Journal of Medicine* **337**, 1667–1674.

10. Armstrong RA. (2005) Overlap between neurodegenerative disorders. *Neuropathology* **25**, 111–124.

11. Perl DP, Olanow CW, Calne D. (1998) Alzheimer's disease and Parkinson's disease: distinct entities or extremes of a spectrum of neurodegeneration? *Annals of Neurology* **44**, S19–31.

12. Morris JC. (2000) The nosology of dementia. *Neurologic Clinics* **18**, 773–788.

13. Reisberg B (2006) Diagnostic criteria in dementia: A comparison of current criteria, research challenges, and implications for DSM-V. *Journal of Geriatric Psychiatry and Neurology* **19**, 137–146.

14. American Psychiatric Association (1994) Diagbostic and Statistical Menual of Mental Disorders. Fourth Edition. Washington DC.

20

Taking a Psychiatric History from Elderly Patients

Sunita Sahu and Monica Crugel

Oxleas NHS Foundation Trust, Memorial Hospital, Shooters Hill, London, UK

INTRODUCTION

When taking a psychiatric history from an elderly person, the general guidance on establishing rapport and taking a medical and psychiatric history apply, but there are also a few particularities. The great heterogeneity of this population in terms of general health and frailty, cognitive abilities and the need for support requires the approach to be adjusted in each case. Clinicians may often be enquiring about someone's life lived before 'their time' and can use this as an opportunity to allow the patient to feel empowered – after all the clinician might know better than the patient what their general and mental health problems are at the moment but only he/she is an expert in their own life history. Sometimes, a little more encouragement and verbal and non-verbal cues of friendliness, respect and openness than with an younger adult patient are needed for establishing a good rapport and obtaining the information. For fear of wasting your time or bringing irrelevant issues into discussion, your elderly patient might not tell you part of the story. Also, pre-conceptions about 'normal' ageing might lead to essential symptoms such as acute or chronic pains, low energy, lack of hope, poor sleep, boredom or lack of social interaction not being mentioned by the patient. Attention to non-verbal cues as well as reassurance that you are interested to hear it all and prompting can help complete the picture.

GETTING READY FOR THE INTERVIEW

Before meeting the patient prepare for the interview. Determine the reason for referral and look at the available medical and psychiatric history and current medication. Ask if the patient will be attending alone or accompanied and if special arrangements will be required in the room, for example if the patient is in a wheelchair.

THE INTERVIEW

After introducing yourself, make sure the patient and their companion are comfortable and check if the patient can hear and understand you. If not, can communication be improved with hearing aids or writing things down and/or involvement of interpreter or the sensory team?. Apart from sensory problems, cognitive deficits (short attention span, memory problems) and dysphasia can affect communication and prevent relevant information being obtained from the patient. In these cases an informant is essential for proper assessment. Adjust the pace of dialogue to the patient's needs: too slow for a cognitively intact patient can sound condescending, too fast for people who cannot keep up can be disastrous.

If the patient is accompanied, establish who the companion is and what their role will be during the interview. Are they an informant or will they provide support for the patient? Have they requested the assessment?

The first interview with the patient and the psychiatric history obtained in this session is extremely important as future assessments will refer to it. Thus, details on nature and onset of all previous episodes, triggers and prodromes, risk factors, duration of episodes, medical co-morbidities, interventions (medication, hospitalization, sectioning, psychotherapy, home help, etc.) and their effect, pharmacological history including compliance, quality of recovery and level of functioning when recovered, should be recorded whenever possible. Your knowledge in psychopathology should guide the questions into obtaining relevant information.

To start the interview, allow the patient or/and informant to explain their view of the presenting complaint.

Start with general questions such as 'Have you ever had any problems to do with your mental health?' and 'Have you ever seen your GP or a psychiatrist for these?', then explore each concern in turn. A patient with poor insight into his previous psychiatric problems might acknowledge having been under psychiatrists for a long time but not having had a mental health problem. Conversely, many people suffer from sub-clinical symptoms or even disorders of clinical severity but have never been assessed or had any treatment.

HISTORY OF THE PRESENTING COMPLAINT

The context of symptoms' onset is of great relevance in geriatric psychiatry. Social and medical factors can play a greater role than genetics in some psychiatric disorders with late onset and, without addressing these, the patient might not recover fully.

Consideration of recent losses such as retirement, bereavement, change in social and financial circumstances, social isolation, loss of abilities and increase in dependency etc. must inform therapeutic intervention, thus recording them is important.

Medical conditions as well as medications prescribed for these can be associated with psychiatric disorders: stroke[1] and cancer[2] have a high co-morbidity with depression; organ failure may cause delirium[3]; respiratory problems are frequently associated with anxiety or panic attacks[4]; some antihypertensives can cause depression[5]; cortisone[6] and anti-Parkinsonian drugs may cause psychosis; drugs

Principles and Practice of Geriatric Psychiatry, 3rd edn. Edited by Mohammed T. Abou-Saleh, Cornelius Katona and Anand Kumar
© 2011 John Wiley & Sons, Ltd

with anticholinergic effects can cause or accentuate confusion, to enumerate only some.

Conversely, care must be given to falsely perceived onset of symptoms. A classic example is memory problems starting 'suddenly' after the spouse's death; it is often the case that the patient's memory problems had been more longstanding but not apparent due to spouse's interventions and prompting. Careful questioning of relatives and other informants would probably reveal cognitive problems prior to bereavement. Sometimes the perceived onset is in fact an aggravation of pre-existing symptoms or the moment at which their intensity becomes significant.

An answer such as 'I have always had this problem' requires clarification as to why they presented for assessment now.

The present disorder might have started in a different form, for example psychosis or confusion following a long depressive episode pointing towards a diagnosis of psychotic depression; confusion following a serious illness, surgery or stroke suggesting delirium; depression with previous episode(s) of mania suggesting bipolar disorder; dementia starting with depression, anxiety or psychosis; substance abuse starting with anxiety or depression. A sudden onset of psychiatric symptoms can suggest organic aetiology.

After identifying the presenting complaint, brief questioning about any other problem, be it social, medical or psychiatric, will help complete the picture.

PAST PSYCHIATRIC HISTORY

One approach is to start with the personal history and once you have information about the patient's lifeline and major life events start asking about the psychiatric history. On one hand this reassures the patient that you are assessing them in an holistic way and are not only 'fishing' for symptoms and, on the other hand, it gives you a better view of the previous level of functioning and, if applicable, the impact of the psychiatric problem on their lives. Some patients may prefer to go straight to the problem.

It is not unheard of for serious lifelong psychiatric illnesses to be diagnosed in old age and a thorough psychiatric history is essential to achieve this. People suffering from generalized anxiety disorder, phobias or obsessive compulsive disorders, might never have seen a psychiatrist before. Careful questioning about long-lasting symptoms (e.g., 'Have you always been a worrier?' Have you always avoided travelling in cars/trains/planes?') can reveal a long history of psychopathology. The mood fluctuations in bipolar disorder sometimes accentuate with age and retrospective diagnosis of a sub-clinical lifelong disorder can be made on a thoroughly taken history.

You will need to actively ask about important issues such as mood symptoms, psychotic features, anxiety, sleep and appetite problems, suicidality.

PHARMACOLOGICAL HISTORY

Obtaining an accurate pharmacological history is important as response to previous treatments and their side effects can inform current prescriptions. However, this can be more difficult than with younger adults as elderly patients might not remember the names of drugs they have been taking over the years. Your knowledge of older psychiatric treatments and interventions as well as older indications for certain types of treatments will help put the information into the right context[7]. For example, ECT, lithium, chlorpromazine and haloperidol were the only treatments available for mental illnesses

until the 1950s when imipramine (the first antidepressant) was introduced; although the current use of antipsychotics is mainly for psychosis, low doses of neuroleptics used to be prescribed in the treatment of depression, anxiety and somatic symptoms; ECT, now mainly used for severe depression and catatonia, was frequently used in the treatment of various psychiatric disorders 30–40 years ago; admissions for treatment were more frequent and much longer than nowadays.

Enquiring about the patient's previous compliance with prescribed treatments, as well as the reasons for non-compliance, when this was the case, can reveal important information. Poor compliance can have various causes and most are similar to those in younger adults, for example, the patient is not convinced that trying a treatment would help, is lacking insight into their psychiatric problem, is experiencing side effects or unpleasant effects from the drugs, stops treatment when they feel better, stops after just a few days due to lack of effect etc. In elderly patients, especially those with cognitive deficits, poor compliance can be due to forgetfulness. This is a serious problem in this population with high levels of co-morbidity and chronic conditions and can lead to relapse of physical or mental condition, under- or overdosing, withdrawal syndromes or other adverse drug reactions. There are various ways to address this such as, enhancing the doctor–patient relationship, psychoeducation, technical solutions (e.g. using dossette boxes), intensifying care (e.g. prompting by carer, administration of drugs by a carer, moving to a more supported accommodation) or, at the extreme, stopping some or all medication if none of the options work and there are associated risks[8].

FAMILY HISTORY

There are understandable differences between taking a family history in a younger adult and an elderly patient. In the elderly, usually the parents of the patient would have died a long time ago, possibly at a younger age than one would expect to now, as a result of which there may not be a history of any problems with an onset in old age, for example dementia. Often the condition from which the parent was suffering may not be known, as the diagnosis may not have been given or may not have been known. Siblings, children, grandchildren and great grandchildren would now be part of the family history. Family interactions can be complex and exploring them can shed light on factors associated with the patient's problems. It will be important to note if the patient is involved in looking after any young children in case child protection issues arise. The converse may also be true if the children or grandchildren are involved in caring for the patient and younger adult protection concerns arise.

Any history of mental disorders in the family must be recorded when available, be it in the patient's parents, children or grandchildren. This would represent third-party information and appropriate confidentiality must be maintained. A history of suicide in a first degree family member represents a risk factor for the patient[9].

PERSONAL HISTORY

This would usually be of much greater length than that of a younger patient. Information on developmental milestones might not be available or relevant but educational attainment and work history will be important for assessing the impact of the psychiatric problem on their lives or when interpreting test results for dementia. It is also an important indicator of the premorbid level of intellectual functioning. Your patient might want to tell you about their war experiences which may have left important psychological marks on their lives. Many more significant life events would have taken place such as loss of parents, relatives and friends. Other kinds of losses such as perceived loss of social status due to retirement, loss of earnings and having to live on a meagre pension, are almost always present. They may have to be living at a lower standard than they were accustomed to and poverty is significant among the elderly[10].

Retirement is a stressful life event for some[11]. Circumstances of retirement may have precipitated depression. Symptoms of dementia interfering with their job may have led to early retirement on medical grounds.

Gross inaccuracies in recalling family history, names and birthdays can be a clue of memory problems.

PAST AND PRESENT SOCIAL SITUATION

This is a broad domain that must be explored in detail when assessing elderly patients. Social and medical care often go hand in hand in helping to improve the patient's quality of life and minimize the risks. For example, a social history revealing a patient living alone, unable to care for himself and under a significant risk to health, might be the single most essential information which will change your short-term treatment plan from prescribing a treatment at home to transferring to hospital or other care facility.

It may be helpful to start with the patient describing a typical day. This should yield rich information about their current circumstances, what they can and cannot manage and what help they are getting from family, friends and neighbours, and voluntary or statutory services. It will also reveal the degree of impairment and the risks to the patient and can point towards other available services which the patient would benefit from, for example day centre, sitting service.

Risks that might need immediate attention can be revealed by asking about the patient's participation in activities of daily living (ADLs). Can they attend to personal hygiene, are they able to do the house chores, use the cooker or the telephone, are they safe on the stairs, are they safe outside the house etc.? (see chapter 34).

Try and obtain information on the finances of your patient and most importantly their ability to manage them. It is necessary to enquire about their current pensions (state or private), benefits and savings, and think about any other benefits they might be entitled to. You can always request social services, working in partnership, to do a full financial assessment. If the patient is unable to manage their finances, arrangements for this to be done by someone else must be made. Family and patient may need to be encouraged to make a lasting power of attorney (LPA) for both property and welfare, a will or an advance decision or at least to start thinking about where they want to live in the future, what kind of care would be acceptable to them etc. Information about the patient's religion, values and beliefs must be recorded as this can play a great role in their life and must be taken into account when planning future care.

A driving history would indicate whether the patient is at risk when driving. If there are issues, the patient or you might need to inform the DVLA.

PERSONALITY

While a thorough personality assessment cannot normally be done in a first interview, keeping a careful eye on personality issues right from the beginning can be very useful. We usually take our personality into old age and a history of significant changes from the premorbid personality reported by the informant will sometimes be a clue to a diagnosis of frontal lobe dementia. Knowledge of premorbid personality traits can be helpful in identifying personality change caused by a mental illness. It may also suggest coping strategies which manifest as symptoms.

PSYCHOSEXUAL HISTORY

As in younger adults, this is an area that can be relevant to your patients' relationships and mental health as well as compliance with medication so offer to discuss this with them. Specific problems in the elderly include sexual dysfunction, the loss of sexual partner by death or serious illness and sexual urges in people with dementia living in care homes.

ALCOHOL AND DRUGS HISTORY

Incidence of alcohol misuse in elderly is thought to be lower then in younger adults but a failure to identify patient's presenting with alcoholism might contribute to the lower figures[12]. With the increase in life expectancy it is predicted the actual number of cases with alcohol-related problems will increase in the following years[13].

Presentation with a fall, confusion or medical complications may mask an underlying alcohol problem. Hence enquiring about current or past alcohol and drug use must be a routine part of the assessment. This should include the age when first used, development of the problem, quantity and frequency and presence of dependence syndrome for each substance used. If alcohol abuse has started in old age, the circumstances might reveal underlying loss, bereavement or depression.

In this age group physical or psychiatric complications of alcohol abuse (e.g. cirrhosis, peripheral neuropathy, cognitive impairment) might have already developed and can be found in the context of continuing or past alcohol abuse. Also, effects of previously well-tolerated quantities of alcohol may increase due to changed physiology.

Onset of memory problems can interfere with a person's usual pattern of alcohol use, for example, by precipitating withdrawal in someone with alcohol dependency who forgets how to obtain the alcohol or causing acute intoxication or even dependency in someone with no prior history of abuse, but regular use, who repeatedly drinks his usual non-harmful amount to intoxication levels.

Knowledge of the type of alcohol consumed can suggest strategies of changing the alcohol to one of lower strength and then gradually tapering the amount, effectively detoxifying the patient. One can use alcohol assessment screening tools but these need to be age-specific, as many of the more traditional rating scales lack validity. The Short MAST-G is commonly used, but others such as the Drinking Problems Index and Alcohol-Related Problems Survey, are used in more specialized settings.

Physical complications of alcohol misuse are numerous, but commonly affect the stomach (ulceration), liver (alcoholic hepatitis, progressing to cirrhosis), blood (anaemia), nervous system (peripheral neuropathy – lack of sensation in legs) and can lead to instability and falls related to episodes of intoxication. Falls may lead to head injury and subdural hematoma. Alcohol may also alter the way in which medication is metabolized by the body and can accentuate the side effects of drugs such as opiates (commonly found in prescribed painkillers).

Inadvertent benzodiapine dependence is common in the elderly. Again, this relates to a time when not enough was known about benzodiazepines and they were prescribed for anxiety or depression and continued for long periods resulting in dependence. A thorough history of use of these drugs would provide useful information about past illness.

FORENSIC HISTORY

In elderly presenting for psychiatric assessment a forensic history is very rarely present. The number of elderly offenders has remained stable over the years; however, the number of elderly in prisons has increased sharply[14].

When taking a psychiatric history in a usual community or hospital setting the interviewer may feel that asking about forensic history can offend the patient and is not relevant. However, it is worth exploring and should not be ignored. There is a risk of offending in people with frontal lobe dementia when this is associated with disinhibition, hoarding or obliviousness to social rules. Also, aggressive behaviour in all types of dementia is frequent, especially towards the carer. In Lewy body dementia, vivid hallucinations, hallucinatory behaviour and cognitive fluctuations can sometimes lead to high risk of harm to others. But even when these lead to serious incidents. Police are rarely involved and charges are often not brought.

REFERENCES

1. Gainotti G, Marra C. Determinants and consequences of post-stroke depression. *Curr Opin Neurol* 2002; **15**(1): 85–9.
2. Jillian RS, Wolfgang L, Melanie JP. Depression as a predictor of disease progression and mortality in cancer patients. *Cancer* 2009; **9999**(9999).
3. Ely EW, Siegel MD, Inouye SK. Delirium in the intensive care unit: an under-recognized syndrome of organ dysfunction. *Semin Respir Crit Care Med* 2001; **22**(2): 115–26.
4. Maurer J, Rebbapragada V, Borson S, Goldstein R, Kunik ME, Yohannes AM *et al*. Anxiety and depression in COPD: current understanding, unanswered questions, and research needs. *Chest* 2008; **134**(4 Suppl): 43S–56S.
5. Ried LD, Tueth MJ, Handberg E, Kupfer S, Pepine CJ, the ISG. A study of antihypertensive drugs and depressive symptoms (SADD-Sx) in patients treated with a calcium antagonist versus an atenolol hypertension treatment strategy in the International Verapamil SR-Trandolapril Study (INVEST). *Psychosom Med* 2005; **67**(3): 398–406.
6. Ritchie EA. Toxic psychosis under cortisone and corticotrophin. *J Ment Sci* 1956; **102**(429): 830–7.
7. Moncrieff J. An investigation into the precedents of modern drug treatment in psychiatry. *Hist Psychiatry* 1999; **10**(40): 475–90.
8. van Dulmen S, Sluijs E, van Dijk L, de Ridder D, Heerdink R, Bensing J. Patient adherence to medical treatment: a review of reviews. *BMC Health Serv Res* 2007; **7**: 55.
9. Kim CD, Seguin M, Therrien N, Riopel G, Chawky N, Lesage AD *et al*. Familial aggregation of suicidal behavior: a family study of male suicide completers from the general population. *Am J Psychiatry* 2005; **162**(5): 1017–19.
10. UK elderly fourth poorest in EU BBC News, 2009.
11. Bosse R, Aldwin CM, Levenson MR, Workman-Daniels K. How stressful is retirement? Findings from the Normative Aging Study. *J Gerontol* 1991; **46**(1): P9–14.
12. O'Connell H, Chin A-V, Cunningham C, Lawlor B. Alcohol use disorders in elderly people – redefining an age old problem in old age. *BMJ* 2003; **327**(7416): 664–7.
13. Nina L. Alcohol use amongst community-dwelling elderly people: a review of the literature. J Adv Nurs 1997; **25**(6): 1227–32.
14. Yorston GA, Taylor PJ. Commentary: older offenders – no place to go? *J Am Acad Psychiatry Law* 2006; **34**(3): 333–7.

21

Mental State Examination in the Elderly

Joanne Rodda and Zuzana Walker

Department of Mental Health Sciences, University College London, UK

The Mental State Examination (MSE) provides a snapshot of a patient's symptoms and signs at the time of the interview. The approach to the MSE in older adults is very similar to that in the younger adult population, although there are a number of important considerations. For example, a significant proportion of patients in old age psychiatry services present with cognitive impairment and there are generational differences between older and younger adults. Physical illness can also complicate the MSE; the assessment of mood can be difficult if someone is frail, immobile or in pain, and acute confusion can be mistaken for dementia, psychosis or mania. These and other factors mean that the observable manifestations of mental illness in the elderly often differ from those in younger adults.

APPEARANCE AND BEHAVIOUR

A great deal of information can be gained from simple observation of the patient walking into the room; for example, posture, gait, presence of abnormal movements, level of personal hygiene and appropriateness of attire can immediately direct the clinician towards important areas for further enquiry.

A deterioration in dress presentation may reflect a decline in personal care; clothing can also give clues about disinhibition or dressing dyspraxia. The level of personal hygiene can clearly demonstrate personal neglect although a well-kempt appearance might be maintained by a carer.

The level of general awareness and alertness may be affected by physical illness or drugs, and fluctuations may be associated with delirium[1,2] or dementia with Lewy bodies[3,4]. Too little or too much eye contact might suggest low mood or disinhibition although it may be necessary to make allowances for visual impairment. Similarly, hearing or visual impairment may result in the appearance of distractibility and confusion. Irritability and hostility are sometimes said to be more common in mania in older adults. However, objective evidence from the few studies available suggests that the presentation of mania in older adults is similar to that in their younger counterparts[5,6].

Over-familiarity or disinhibition is suggestive of mania or frontal lobe syndromes and can be a feature of many types of neurodegenerative disorder. An older person may be more reserved in their interactions with others and so a level of familiarity or inhibition that fits into the realms of social acceptability may still represent a change from normal for that individual. Conversely, a gregarious person may always have been that way; information from relatives or carers is therefore often important to determine whether the current presentation represents a change from the patient's usual way of interacting.

Psychomotor changes are often prominent in depression in the elderly[7–9] although bradykinesia and reduced mobility in Parkinson's disease can be difficult to distinguish from psychomotor retardation or apathy. There are a host of motor signs – e.g. dystonic movements, mannerisms and stereotypies – that may occur as a feature of schizophrenia, mania or organic disorder[10,11] or as a result of side effects of medication. Hyperorality and stereotyped, utilization or repetitive behaviours are suggestive of pathology involving the frontal lobes, e.g. frontotemporal dementia[10].

SPEECH

In the elderly, speech can be affected by a number of factors unrelated to mental state, including ill-fitting dentures or oral pathology. An increase or decrease in the rate, quantity and/or volume of speech can be associated with mania and depression, respectively. Pressure of speech is characteristic of mania or frontal lobe involvement. In depression, poverty of speech may occur to a degree that the patient appears to be mute or dysphasic, although such a severe impairment in language is more frequently a result of neurodegenerative or cerebrovascular disease than functional illness. Circumstantiality and tangentiality occur in psychosis and mania, but are often related to dementia in the elderly. Similarly, flight of ideas is characteristic of mania but can also occur in frontal lobe syndromes.

Nominal dysphasia is common in the early stages of Alzheimer's disease when it would normally be associated with at least some degree of memory impairment. Conversely, in primary progressive aphasia (PPA) impairments in language precede deficits in other cognitive domains[12,13]. Language deficits in PPA are predominantly expressive and usually associated with loss of fluency; in semantic dementia there is loss of expressive and receptive vocabulary in the presence of fluent but 'empty' speech[10,14]. Clearly, it is important to ensure that any apparent receptive dysphasia cannot be accounted for by a hearing impairment and that an apparent expressive dysphasia is not in fact the result of dysarthria. Dysphonia is a disorder of phonation due to inability to produce voice sounds using the vocal organs; this is distinct from dysarthria and can occur in Parkinson's disease, stroke and other organic disorders[15] or as a psychogenic phenomenon[16].

Other abnormalities of speech are suggestive of specific disorders. For example, perseverative speech is almost pathognomonic of organic brain disease, particularly involving the frontal lobes. Verbal

Principles and Practice of Geriatric Psychiatry, 3rd edn. Edited by Mohammed T. Abou-Saleh, Cornelius Katona and Anand Kumar
© 2011 John Wiley & Sons, Ltd

stereotypies, mannerisms, echolalia, paraphasia and neologisms also occur in organic (often frontal) syndromes although may also occur in mania and psychosis.

MOOD

Elderly people may be less likely than younger adults to report sadness or dysphoria. This does not appear to be a cohort effect and has been reported in different generations of older adults[17]; whether this will hold true for the current young-old population is not known. The concept of 'depression without sadness' has, however, been criticized by some, who suggest that apathy, withdrawal and loss of vigour can represent a depletion or disengagement syndrome that reflects normal age-related changes[18]. A similar picture may also result from physical illness due to chronic pain, fatigue and disability. Likewise, the bradykinesia and bradyphrenia of Parkinson's disease can lead to difficulties in differentiating depressive from physical symptomatology. Apathy, loss of interest and motivation and even abulia may occur in dementia, particularly in subcortical[19,20] and frontotemporal subtypes[21], and can overlap with or be misinterpreted as depression[22,23]. Changes in mood may be also present in the prodromal stages of dementia, before cognitive deficits are apparent[24]. In established dementia, affective disturbances are common and may present with behavioural changes[25-27].

Given the overlap of symptomatology, it is helpful to pay close attention to the presence of biological features of depression, particularly diurnal mood variation, appetite, early morning waking and anhedonia. Cognitive symptoms of guilt, helplessness and worthlessness are also useful pointers towards a depressive disorder.

Emotional lability can be present in affective disorder and psychosis but can also be a feature of organic syndromes, e.g. cerebrovascular disease[28], Parkinson's disease[29] and other brain pathology[30], and may be confused with depression. Euphoria is a feature of mania and frontal lobe dysfunction, and may be present in other organic disorders.

THOUGHT

Thought Form

As in younger patients, psychotic illness in the elderly can be associated with a broad spectrum of abnormalities of thought form, e.g. circumstantiality, flight of ideas, loosening of associations (from tangentiality through to word salad) and, at the other extreme, thought block. However, apparent thought disorder in the elderly may represent confusion or language disorder as a result of delirium or neurodegenerative illness. Careful attention to the overall picture, including the context of the patient's presentation and simple cognitive testing, can help to clarify the situation.

Thought Content

Delusions are fixed beliefs out of keeping with an individual's social, cultural and religious background, which are based on unsound reasoning and are maintained even in the presence of evidence to the contrary. In the elderly, delusions may form part of a psychotic or affective illness but are also common in delirium and dementia. In delirium, delusions are often fleeting and persecutory. In dementia, delusions of theft are common and often relate to misplacement of objects. Well-formed delusional systems are uncommon in dementia

but do occur. Delusional misidentification is also common in organic disorder[31], e.g. patients with dementia may insist that their spouse or even their own reflection in the mirror is an impostor.

As in young adults, delusions can be sub-classified into several types, e.g. persecutory, grandiose, nihilistic and bizarre delusions, and delusions of jealousy. Autochthonous or primary delusions arise spontaneously and 'out of the blue' while secondary delusions occur as a result of some other experience, e.g. secondary to hallucinations or affective disturbances. Primary delusions in the elderly suggest functional rather than organic disorder. Delusions must be differentiated from overvalued ideas, which are beliefs that may not be unreasonable but are pursued to an unreasonable degree by the patient. Overvalued ideas are often associated with personality disorders.

Obsessions are recurrent and persistent thoughts, images or impulses that the patient tries to but is unable to resist. They may occur in the context of an obsessive disorder but can also be a feature of depression or dementia. Sometimes repeated checking in dementia is related to anxiety and forgetfulness rather than obsessive–compulsive behaviour and can present a diagnostic challenge, particularly in the early stages.

Passivity Phenomena

Thought insertion and withdrawal, thought broadcast and 'made actions' represent a disintegration of boundaries between the self and the outside world and are typical of a functional psychotic disorder rather than dementia or delirium.

PERCEPTION

A hallucination is a perception in the absence of an external stimulus and may occur in any modality (auditory, visual, tactile, olfactory, gustatory, somatic) in the context of psychosis, affective disorder, organic disorder or delirium. Sensory impairment, both visual and auditory, is particularly important in older people and predisposes to hallucinations. Charles Bonnet's syndrome of visual hallucinations in people with visual impairment in the absence of psychiatric or neurological illness is well known. These hallucinations are typically complex, not distressing and are usually associated with a good degree of insight. The most common cause is age-related macular degeneration (see Schadlu et al.[32] for a recent detailed review). Auditory hallucinations (typically of music) occurring in clear consciousness in people with hearing impairment are also common and have been described as an auditory form of Charles Bonnet syndrome[33]. The pathophysiology underlying these experiences may relate to deafferentiation of visual or auditory cortical structures, resulting in hyperexcitability and increased spontaneous activity[34]. Sensory impairment is also an important maintaining factor for hallucinations occurring in the context of schizophrenia or other disorders.

Auditory hallucinations occur in schizophrenia regardless of the age of onset, although in late-onset psychotic illness visual and olfactory hallucinations are also relatively common[35]. It is important to ensure that an acute confusional state or other organic cause is excluded before new-onset hallucinations in the elderly are attributed to functional illness. Visual hallucinations, typically of people or animals, are one of the core features of dementia with Lewy bodies and are often associated with some degree of insight[4].

Illusions are false internal perceptions that result from a combination of imagery and the perception of a real external object. They are common in people with visual impairment as well as in psychotic or organic disorder and are accentuated by affect and poor attention. Sensory distortions are changes in the perceived quality or intensity of a stimulus (e.g. hyperacusis) and are suggestive of organic disorder or drug intoxication. Perceptual abnormalities must be discriminated from visual agnosia, which is the failure to recognize objects despite normal function of the eye.

COGNITION

General observation throughout the interview will provide information about cognition, e.g. the general level of orientation, the presence of confabulation, repetition of questions or statements and the ability to follow the conversation and to remember facts and names. The presence of hearing impairment, anger, irritability, anxiety, depression and psychosis can lead to an underestimation of cognitive ability and it is important to bear these factors in mind. Conversely, older people with marked cognitive impairment can maintain a façade that is convincing enough to mask their deficits in the absence of collateral history or objective cognitive testing, particularly in the context of a high premorbid level of intellectual ability. Memory is relatively well preserved in the early stages of some dementias and in these cases deficits in other cognitive domains may only become apparent on formal testing. Examples include visuo-spatial impairments in dementia with Lewy bodies[4] or deficits in sequencing and executive function in frontotemporal dementia[10].

Relatives' accounts of cognitive function can also be inaccurate, e.g. due to expectations of increasing forgetfulness with ageing, the insidious nature of their relative's decline or difficulties in accepting the change in their loved one and its significance. It is therefore important to include at least some form of objective cognitive testing during even the most basic examination of mental state. The Mini Mental State Examination (MMSE)[36] is the most widely used cognitive screening tool in clinical practice, although it is weighted towards verbal memory and does not include items to assess executive function. Furthermore, individuals with high premorbid intellectual function may score well within the normal range despite marked cognitive and functional decline from previous levels[37].

More detailed brief assessment scales include the Addenbrooke's Cognitive Examination – Revised (ACE-R)[38], Modified Mini Mental State Examination (3MS)[39] and Cognitive Abilities Screening Instrument (CASI)[40], although all take longer to complete than the MMSE[41]. Supplementing the MMSE with other brief tests like letter fluency (FAS)[42] and the clock drawing test[43,44] may be a practical compromise for the initial assessment and to guide the need for more detailed neuropsychological assessment.

INSIGHT

Insight is a fluid and multifaceted phenomenon and has been conceptualized in many ways. The dimensions of insight in psychosis have been summarized as: (i) recognition of the illness, (ii) attribution of the illness to a mental disorder, (iii) awareness of the benefit of treatment, and (iv) awareness of the social consequences of the mental disorder[45]. Insight in dementia is also a complex entity, and both explicit and implicit awareness are worth considering[46]. For example, an individual may deny any problem with their memory but acknowledge that they have performed poorly on a test or need to use memory aids at home to ensure that they remember appointments. It can sometimes be difficult to discriminate between lack of insight and cognitive impairment itself; this is particularly relevant when considering medication compliance.

It has been suggested that some individuals have insight into subtle cognitive deficits before they are apparent on objective testing, and that as these objective cognitive deficits develop, insight progresses in an inverse U-shaped curve so that ultimately there is established dementia with little insight[47]. However, insight in mild cognitive impairment is variable[48] and the significance of subjective memory complaints in the absence of objective cognitive deficits is as yet uncertain.

REFERENCES

1. Burns A, Gallagley A, Byrne J. Delirium. *J Neurol Neurosurg Psychiatry* 2004; **75**(3): 362–7.
2. Taylor D, Lewis S. Delirium. *J Neurol Neurosurg Psychiatry* 1993; **56**(7): 742–51.
3. Ferman TJ, Smith GE, Boeve BF *et al*. DLB fluctuations: specific features that reliably differentiate DLB from AD and normal aging. *Neurology* 2004; **62**(2): 181–7.
4. McKeith IG, Dickson DW, Lowe J *et al*. Diagnosis and management of dementia with Lewy bodies: third report of the DLB Consortium. *Neurology* 2005; **65**(12): 1863–72.
5. Benedetti A, Scarpellini P, Casamassima F *et al*. Bipolar disorder in late life: clinical characteristics in a sample of older adults admitted for manic episode. *Clin Pract Epidemiol Ment Health* 2008; **4**: 22.
6. Broadhead J, Jacoby R. Mania in old age: a first prospective study. *Int J Geriatr Psychiatry* 1990; **5**: 215–22.
7. Brodaty H, Luscombe G, Parker G *et al*. Increased rate of psychosis and psychomotor change in depression with age. *Psychol Med* 1997; **27**(5): 1205–13.
8. Parker G. Classifying depression: should paradigms lost be regained? *Am J Psychiatry* 2000; **157**(8): 1195–1203.
9. Parker G, Roy K, Hadzi-Pavlovic D, Wilhelm K, Mitchell P. The differential impact of age on the phenomenology of melancholia. *Psychol Med* 2001; **31**(7): 1231–6.
10. Neary D, Snowden JS, Gustafson L *et al*. Frontotemporal lobar degeneration: a consensus on clinical diagnostic criteria. *Neurology* 1998; **51**(6): 1546–54.
11. Peralta V, Cuesta MJ. Motor features in psychotic disorders. I. Factor structure and clinical correlates. *Schizophr Res* 2001; **47**(2–3): 107–16.
12. Mesulam MM. Primary progressive aphasia – differentiation from Alzheimer's disease. *Ann Neurol* 1987; **22**(4): 533–4.
13. Rogalski EJ, Mesulam MM. Clinical trajectories and biological features of primary progressive aphasia (PPA). *Curr Alzheimer Res* 2009; **6**(4): 331–6.
14. Hodges JR, Patterson K. Semantic dementia: a unique clinico-pathological syndrome. *Lancet Neurol* 2007; **6**(11): 1004–14.
15. Merati AL, Heman-Ackah YD, Abaza M *et al*. Common movement disorders affecting the larynx: a report from the neurolaryngology committee of the AAO-HNS. *Otolaryngol Head Neck Surg* 2005; **133**(5): 654–65.
16. Seifert E, Kollbrunner J. Stress and distress in non-organic voice disorder. *Swiss Med Wkly* 2005; **135**(27–28): 387–97.
17. Gallo JJ, Rabins PV, Anthony JC. Sadness in older persons: 13-year follow-up of a community sample in Baltimore, Maryland. *Psychol Med* 1999; **29**(2): 341–50.
18. Adams KB. Depressive symptoms, depletion, or developmental change? Withdrawal, apathy, and lack of vigor in the Geriatric Depression Scale. *Gerontologist* 2001; **41**(6): 768–77.

19. Dujardin K, Sockeel P, Devos D *et al*. Characteristics of apathy in Parkinson's disease. *Mov Disord* 2007; **22**(6): 778–84.

20. Moretti R, Torre P, Antonello RM, Cazzato G. Behavioral alterations and vascular dementia *Neurologist* 2006; **12**(1): 43–7.

21. Chow TW, Binns MA, Cummings JL *et al*. Apathy symptom profile and behavioral associations in frontotemporal dementia vs dementia of Alzheimer type. *Arch Neurol* 2009; **66**(7): 888–93.

22. Starkstein SE, Ingram L, Garau ML, Mizrahi R. On the overlap between apathy and depression in dementia. *J Neurol Neurosurg Psychiatry* 2005; **76**(8): 1070–74.

23. Tagariello P, Girardi P, Amore M. Depression and apathy in dementia: same syndrome or different constructs? A critical review. *Arch Gerontol Geriatr* 2009; **49**(2): 246–9.

24. Onyike CU, Sheppard J M, Tschanz JT *et al*. Epidemiology of apathy in older adults: the Cache County Study. *Am J Geriatr Psychiatry* 2007; **15**(5): 365–75.

25. Lyketsos CG, Olin J. Depression in Alzheimer's disease: overview and treatment. *Biol Psychiatry* 2002; **52**(3): 243–52.

26. Olin JT, Schneider LS, Katz IR *et al*. Provisional diagnostic criteria for depression of Alzheimer disease. *Am J Geriatr Psychiatry* 2002; **10**(2): 125–8.

27. Verkaik R, Francke AL, van Meijel B, Ribbe MW, Bensing JM. Comorbid depression in dementia on psychogeriatric nursing home wards: which symptoms are prominent? *Am J Geriatr Psychiatry* 2009; **17**(7): 565–73.

28. O'Brien J. Behavioral symptoms in vascular cognitive impairment and vascular dementia. *Int Psychogeriatr* 2003; **15**(suppl 1): 133–8.

29. Phuong L, Garg S, Duda JE, Stern MB, Weintraub D. Involuntary emotional expression disorder (IEED) in Parkinson's disease. *Parkinsonism Relat Disord* 2009; **15**(7): 511–15.

30. Richter RW. The pathophysiology of emotional lability: many paths to a common destination. *Am J Geriatr Pharmacother* 2005; **3**(suppl A): 9–11.

31. Fleminger S, Burns A. The delusional misidentification syndromes in patients with and without evidence of organic cerebral disorder: a structured review of case reports. *Biol Psychiatry* 1993; **33**(1): 22–32.

32. Schadlu AP, Schadlu R, Shepherd JB, III. Charles Bonnet syndrome: a review. *Curr Opin Ophthalmol* 2009; **20**(3): 219–22.

33. Griffiths TD. Musical hallucinosis in acquired deafness. Phenomenology and brain substrate. *Brain* 2000; **123**(10): 2065–76.

34. Burke W. The neural basis of Charles Bonnet hallucinations: a hypothesis. *J Neurol Neurosurg Psychiatry* 2002; **73**(5): 535–41.

35. Howard R, Rabins PV, Seeman MV, Jeste DV. Late-onset schizophrenia and very-late-onset schizophrenia-like psychosis: an international consensus. The International Late-Onset Schizophrenia Group. *Am J Psychiatry* 2000; **157**(2): 172–8.

36. Folstein MF, Folstein SE, McHugh PR. 'Mini-mental state'. A practical method for grading the cognitive state of patients for the clinician. *J Psychiatr Res* 1975; **12**(3): 189–98.

37. O'Bryant SE, Humphreys JD, Smith GE *et al*. Detecting dementia with the mini-mental state examination in highly educated individuals. *Arch Neurol* 2008; **65**(7): 963–7.

38. Mioshi E, Dawson K, Mitchell J, Arnold R, Hodges JR. The Addenbrooke's Cognitive Examination Revised (ACE-R): a brief cognitive test battery for dementia screening. *Int J Geriatr Psychiatry* 2006; **21**(11): 1078–85.

39. Teng EL, Chui HC. The Modified Mini-Mental State (3MS) examination. *J Clin Psychiatry* 1987; **48**(8): 314–18.

40. Teng EL, Hasegawa K, Homma A *et al*. The Cognitive Abilities Screening Instrument (CASI): a practical test for cross-cultural epidemiological studies of dementia. *Int Psychogeriatr* 1994; **6**(1): 45–58.

41. Cullen B, O'Neill B, Evans JJ, Coen RF, Lawlor BA. A review of screening tests for cognitive impairment. *J Neurol Neurosurg Psychiatry* 2007; **78**(8): 790–99.

42. Benton A. Differential behavioural effects in frontal lobe disease. *Neuropsychologia* 1968; **6**: 53–8.

43. Agrell B, Dehlin O. The clock drawing test. *Age Ageing* 1998; **27**: 399–403.

44. Pinto E, Peters R. Literature review of the clock drawing test as a tool for cognitive screening. *Dement Geriatr Cogn Disord* 2009; **27**(3): 201–13.

45. Amador XF, Strauss DH, Yale SA *et al*. Assessment of insight in psychosis. *Am J Psychiatry* 1993; **150**(6): 873–9.

46. Howorth P, Saper J. The dimensions of insight in people with dementia. *Aging Ment Health* 2003; **7**(2): 113–22.

47. Reisberg B, Gauthier S. Current evidence for subjective cognitive impairment (SCI) as the pre-mild cognitive impairment (MCI) stage of subsequently manifest Alzheimer's disease. *Int Psychogeriatr* 2008; **20**(1): 1–16.

48. Roberts JL, Clare L, Woods RT. Subjective memory complaints and awareness of memory functioning in mild cognitive impairment: a systematic review. *Dement Geriatr Cogn Disord* 2009; **28**(2): 95–109.

22

The Physical Examination: A Guide for Old Age Psychiatrists

Stephen Todd, John O'Hare, Bernadette McGuinness and A. Peter Passmore

Centre for Public Health, School of Medicine, Dentistry and Biomedical Sciences,
The Queen's University of Belfast, Belfast, UK

INTRODUCTION

The medical and psychiatric history obtained from the patient and informant, together with the mental status assessment, provide the majority of the information required in the evaluation of the older person presenting to the old age psychiatrist. However, the physical examination retains a crucial role in the evaluation of the older person for several reasons (Table 22.1).

First, it is an expected component of the consultation by the patient and/or their relative or carer and assists in developing the doctor–patient relationship. Second, a particular physical sign or constellation of signs will increase or decrease the pretest probabilities in the differential diagnosis under consideration following the history. Third, a more rational and focused plan of investigation will be instituted. Fourth, serial examination over time allows the clinician to observe the course of the disease, assess the effectiveness of any treatments commenced, and, if necessary, reconsider the diagnosis in the light of these data. Fifth, on occasions, an adequate history may not be obtainable, for example in delirium. The physical examination therefore assumes greater weight in determining further management until such history becomes available. Finally, co-morbidity is the rule rather than the exception in the older person. Commonly, there will be several aetiologies for a particular presenting complaint. The old age psychiatrist assesses the older person in a variety of settings, including the home, clinic, hospital ward, or institution, and may be the first or only contact that person may have with a clinician. Therefore, the old age psychiatrist should have the skill and ability to perform a brief but thorough physical examination, interpret the findings, plan a logical series of investigations, and determine if referral to a specialist, including other members of the multidisciplinary team, is indicated[1].

Table 22.1 Role of the physical examination in the older person

Expectation by patient and/or relative in consulting a doctor
Provides additional, pertinent information to history obtained
Allows judicious use of investigations and resource
Repeated assessment permits observation of disease course and
    therapeutic effects
Detection of contributory or important co-morbidity

CONSIDERATIONS

A number of differences between older and younger people are reflected in the pattern and presentation of illness (Table 22.2). First, diseases that commonly occur in older people have taken many years, sometimes decades, to develop. Examples of such chronic 'degenerative' diseases are atherosclerosis, cancer, degenerative joint disease, and neurodegenerative disorders, such as Parkinson's and Alzheimer's diseases.

Second, co-morbidity is common and interacts with normal physiological ageing changes of the body to modify presentation of disease. Impairment of physiological homeostatic mechanisms results in reduced capacity to cope with changes in the body (brought about by disease) or in the environment (such as absence of a carer or admission to hospital). Thus, the older person will be more severely affected by an insult that might be relatively minor to a younger adult. These 'reduced reserves' of older age also lead to slower recovery from an acute insult. For example, hospital length of stay is twice that of younger adults. However, even old, seriously ill individuals can recover if given sufficient time and support.

Third, in older people symptoms of disease often are less specific and uninformative, making the task of establishing the diagnosis/diagnoses more challenging for the clinician. This non-specific mode of presentation often takes the form of a 'giant of geriatrics' syndrome – instability (falls); immobility ('off feet' or 'off legs'); incontinence; intellectual impairment (delirium and dementia). However, a thoughtful approach and careful attention during physical examination will frequently direct the choice of investigations and treatment.

Some practical considerations in the conduct of the physical examination should be kept in mind and will reap considerable reward in the information obtained (Table 22.3). Time and patience are necessary virtues of clinician and patient.

Table 22.2 Differences between older and younger people

Background of chronic disease
Impaired homeostasis/physiological changes of ageing
Less specific presentation of disease

Principles and Practice of Geriatric Psychiatry, 3rd edn. Edited by Mohammed T. Abou-Saleh, Cornelius Katona and Anand Kumar
© 2011 John Wiley & Sons, Ltd

Table 22.3 Practice points when examining the older person

Older people may require longer, and need assistance, to:
- Transfer from chair to standing
- Mobilize into the consulting room
- Transfer from chair to examination couch
- Remove items of clothing
- Replace items of clothing

The examination may also be limited by:
- Fatigue
- Frailty
- Pain
- Breathlessness
- Poor hearing or eyesight and missing aids
- Confusion

The student and doctor in training are encouraged to take the time to follow a standard scheme of examination for each body system and to repeat this scheme again and again not in a thoughtless way but with consideration to each point in the scheme, the finding elicited being examined for its significance in light of the other available data. Such an approach will produce a skilled clinician who can not only perform a rapid and seamless physical examination but also detect pertinent physical signs of relevance to the care of the older person.

GENERAL EXAMINATION

During the Interview

Physical examination commences on first meeting the older person, continues during the interview, and concludes with the 'formal' examination. Observation is thus the key initial tool, later to be supplemented, to a greater or lesser degree, by inspection, palpation, percussion and auscultation. Brief mention is made of the carer. Attention to carer demeanour and their relationship with the patient is important. Mental and physical ill health in the carer may adversely impact on the patient.

The general appearance of the clothes, face and hands, including nails, may be the first clue to self-neglect or neglect or abuse from a carer, depression, or functional decline in completion of basic activities of daily living due to underlying disease(s). Body habitus may suggest malnourishment or cachexia.

The handshake allows closer inspection of hands and nails and will also permit observation of tremor, whether resting or action, wasting of the small muscles, joint swelling or stiffness, or loose jewellery, for example, that will assist in directing enquiry and subsequent examination. Ability to transfer, requirement for an aid or an arm, and gait provide information on functional ability and may suggest dysfunction at various levels of the musculoskeletal and neurological systems which will require more detailed scrutiny.

Observation of the face during the interview may reveal the blank appearance of Parkinson's disease or the lack of expression and poor eye contact of depression. Asymmetry in facial appearance may indicate neurological dysfunction, for example due to stroke or Bell's palsy. Less obvious, perhaps, are symmetrical changes in facial appearance, such as the pallor of anaemia, the fat deposition and telangiectasia of Cushing's syndrome, or the proptosis and lid retraction of an overactive thyroid gland.

Abnormal movements may be noted during the interview. In the head and face, titubation, orofacial dyskinesia, facial tics or myoclonus, or fasciculation of the tongue all require explanation. Wincing or grimacing indicates uncontrolled pain, which requires evaluation and alleviation. In the limbs, tremor may again be apparent. The position and posture of the limbs may suggest current or previous musculoskeletal or neurological problems.

Speech will be assessed during the interview and might direct further testing to determine if there are one or more problems affecting comprehension, such as loss of hearing or receptive dysphasia; articulation and pronunciation, such as dysarthria, expressive dysphasia and dysphonia; or content, such as confusional states, delusional or psychotic disorders, or depression. Limitation of speech due to pain or dyspnoea indicates serious cardiovascular and/or respiratory compromise or perhaps profound anaemia.

Examination

The general examination continues from and expands on observations made during the interview. A general 'head to toe' inspection of the patient will take closer note of the hands, face, head and neck, nutritional and hydration status, and the presence of abnormal swellings and masses.

A systematic approach to the hands will inform the examiner on the presence of a multitude of systemic disorders. The nails may be pitted in psoriasis or clubbed in a number of respiratory, cardiac, gastrointestinal and other disorders. The pattern and distribution of swelling and deformity of the small joints may suggest the presence of osteoarthritis, rheumatoid arthritis or psoriatic arthropathy. Abnormal pigmentation of the skin may indicate anaemia if pale or chronic liver disease if jaundiced. Atrophy of the small muscles may be a marker of generalized weight loss and ill health or suggest median nerve entrapment at the wrist if isolated to the thenar eminence.

Closer inspection of the eyes may also suggest anaemia or liver disease if there is pallor of the conjunctiva or jaundice of the sclera, respectively. Aphthous ulceration of the mouth is a marker of ill health. The presence of oral thrush can suggest recent antibiotic therapy, deficient oral hygiene or poorly controlled diabetes mellitus. Poorly fitting dentures can cause trauma. The condition of teeth that are present should be noted. Poor dentition can cause pain and reduction in oral intake.

The neck should be inspected for the presence of masses and the thyroid gland palpated before and while the patient swallows a glass of water. This should prompt general consideration of thyroid status and evidence of over- (warm sweaty hands, tachycardia, particularly atrial fibrillation, or tremor) or under- (cold, hoarseness, bradycardia, 'peaches and cream' complexion) activity. The cervical lymph nodes should be palpated. Localized or generalized enlargement will be confirmed by subsequent palpation of axillary and inguinal chains.

The skin should be exposed, with judicious use of a gown or drape, to assess colouration and pigmentation and characterize contusions, rashes, masses or tumours. Skin turgor in older people is less reliable than in younger adults as an indicator of hydration. Dryness of mucous membranes or axillae and sunken eyes are suggestive of dehydration whereas a moist tongue is evidence against dehydration. Further evaluation of hydration follows in the cardiovascular section.

CARDIOVASCULAR SYSTEM

The patient should be positioned at forty-five degrees with neck and chest exposed. While palpating the radial pulse at the wrist, the examiner should note the rate and rhythm. Atrial fibrillation is the commonest arrhythmia in older people and is a strong risk factor for cerebral infarction. The character of the pulse is better assessed by palpation of the carotid artery. The blood pressure is measured both lying and after standing for two minutes. Falls are common in older patients, particularly in those with dementia. Postural hypotension is indicated by a fall of 20 mmHg or greater on standing for at least one minute.

The face should be inspected briefly with consideration of jaundice or xanthelasma at the eyes and cyanosis of the lips and tongue. In the neck, the right internal jugular vein is inspected for the jugular venous pressure (JVP), noting the vertical height above the sternal notch and the character. The carotid arteries are palpated separately, noting the character.

Inspect the praecordium for scars, deformity, position of the apex beat and pulsations. Palpation for the apex beat should consider the position and character. A laterally displaced apex beat can denote left ventricular dilatation. Tapping, thrusting and heaving beats occur in mitral stenosis, mitral regurgitation and left ventricular hypertrophy, respectively.

Auscultation is done in the area of maximal acoustic advantage for each of the four valves – apex (mitral); lower left sternal edge (tricuspid); second left (pulmonary) and right (aortic) intercostal spaces. The examiner listens separately to each phase of the cardiac cycle. The first and second heart sounds should be identified and considered normal or abnormal in intensity. The presence of added sounds (extra heart sounds or murmurs) is considered, noting location in the cardiac cycle, character and position heard maximally. Added sounds may be accentuated by repositioning the patient – left lateral for mitral stenosis and upright for aortic regurgitation.

With the patient sitting forward, the examiner may inspect and palpate for sacral oedema. The peripheral pulses should be palpated and other evidence of peripheral vascular disease, such as cool dusky skin, loss of hair and prolonged capillary refill, and peripheral oedema sought.

Other signs to consider during later examination are dullness to percussion and reduced breath sounds (pleural effusion), inspiratory crepitations (pulmonary oedema), hepatomegaly (right ventricular failure) and a pulsatile epigastric mass (abdominal aortic aneurysm).

RESPIRATORY SYSTEM

During the general inspection, notice whether the subject is dyspnoeic or using accessory muscles of respiration. In the hands, observe for tar staining, clubbing, anaemia or wasting of small muscles. The respiratory rate should be counted. In the face, unilateral meiosis and ptosis may suggest Horner's syndrome (damage to the sympathetic nervous system). The contents of the sputum pot should be inspected. Listen for the high-pitched inspiratory note of stridor. In the neck, palpate for tracheal position and presence of cervical lymphadenopathy.

Expose the chest completely and place the patient in a seated position. Both front and back of the chest should be examined with the following suggested scheme. First, inspect for scars and deformity and assess the degree and symmetry of expansion on maximal inspiration. Expansion is then assessed by palpation. Next, palpate for tactile vocal fremitus. The position of the apex beat may suggest mediastinal displacement.

Chest percussion compares left side with right side as the examiner progresses down the chest, not forgetting apices and axillae. The percussion note may be dull, for example with pleural effusion or consolidation, or resonant, with pneumothorax or emphysema. Finally, the chest is auscultated. The character of the breath sounds, whether normal or bronchial, and their intensity is noted. The presence, location and timing of added sounds are then considered. Crepitations or crackles may be pan-inspiratory and in the lower zones in pulmonary oedema or end-inspiratory and with either an upper or lower zone location in pulmonary fibrosis. Wheeze is generally expiratory and polyphonic in chronic obstructive pulmonary disease (COPD). Expiration is prolonged in COPD. Asthma is less prevalent than COPD in older people.

GASTROINTESTINAL SYSTEM

The abdomen should be completely exposed and the patient recumbent with one pillow to support the head. On general inspection, the examiner should have appreciated body habitus. In the hands, evidence of chronic liver disease such as clubbing, white nails, palmar erythema or Dupuytren's contracture may be noted. Bruising, scratch marks and spider naevi may be noted on the torso. Jaundice is best appreciated at the sclera. The mouth should be illuminated and inspected for stomatitis, glossitis and ulceration. Parotid enlargement and, in men, gynaecomastia are also pointers to chronic liver disease.

The abdomen should be inspected for scars, masses, bruising, distension, hernia and prominent veins. The examiner should also bend down to inspect from the side as masses may be visible. Abdominal movement on respiration is then noted.

The patient should be asked to indicate the site of pain, if present. On light palpation of all areas of the abdomen, the examiner should observe for evidence of pain, including wincing, grimacing or guarding. Each region should be deeply palpated in turn for masses if no pain is elicited. Continue to palpate specifically for the presence and location of hepatomegaly and splenomegaly. The kidneys may be bimanually palpable. The groins are palpated for adenopathy and hernia. Percussion of the abdomen starts in the midline and works toward the flank. If dullness is noted the examiner should seek to demonstrate if it shifts on repositioning the patient. Auscultate for the presence of bowel sounds and for bruits over the renal areas. The gastrointestinal examination is completed with digital rectal examination.

NEUROLOGICAL SYSTEM

Neurological examination is an essential component of the evaluation of every older person presenting to the old age psychiatrist. An experienced clinician will complete a thorough screening assessment in a few minutes and conduct a detailed follow-up examination as indicated with only minimum further effort. Neurological examination is crucial for several reasons (Table 22.4).

Observation during interview and general examination of tremor or blank facies will direct the examiner towards other evidence of Parkinsonism, whereas a drooping lip or stiff, immobile limb might suggest stroke and a search for asymmetric upper motor neurone deficits. However, it is recommended that a standard scheme is followed to ensure thorough assessment.

Table 22.4 Importance of neurological examination

Diagnostic criteria specify neurological signs[2–4]
Development of signs can mark disease progression
Recognize side effects of psychiatric medications
Ability to localize pathology by pattern of signs

Cranial Nerves

Assessment of olfaction is generally limited to an enquiry regarding the sense of smell.

The eyes are examined 'from out to in'. Visual acuity, corrected with the person's glasses, is assessed in each eye with a Snellen chart. If the top line cannot be read, acuity should be recorded as the best of finger counting, hand movement, or light appreciation. Knowledge of visual acuity is important in cognitive testing. Visual fields are assessed by confrontation to the examiner's (which are assumed to be normal). The examiner should be seated at least one metre from the patient and on the same level. Each eye is tested in turn and, as a minimum, all four quadrants in each eye should be probed. Any deficit detected must be mapped in detail. The presence of visual inattention is assessed by stimulating both fields simultaneously. Extraocular muscle function is assessed by asking the subject to track a moving object through a horizontal and then a vertical arc from the neutral point. The examiner may place a hand on the patient's forehead to prevent movement. In addition to the direction of reduced or absent movement, the presence of diplopia and direction and speed of nystagmus is noted. The pupils are inspected for size, shape and regularity and compared for equality. The direct reaction of the pupil to light and the consensual reaction of its pair are tested with a bright light shone from the temporal side. Reaction of the pupils to accommodation is tested by asking the patient to change focus from the distance to an object placed close to the face. Cataract may be detected by absence of the red reflex. The corneal reflex is elicited using a strand of cotton wool advanced from the temporal side. On fundoscopy, evidence of retinopathy from diabetes mellitus or hypertension and papilloedema from raised intracranial pressure should be sought.

A scheme of examination of lower cranial nerves is described, although it should be noted that this does not follow each nerve in sequence. Thus, the examiner should remain cognisant of what is being tested. A simple command, followed by demonstration of the desired manoeuvre facilitates compliance with motor examination not only of cranial nerves but also the limbs, to be described below.

Instructions to 'raise your eyebrows', 'close your eyes tightly', 'puff/blow out your cheeks', 'show me your teeth' and 'clench your teeth' assess motor function of the facial and trigeminal nerves. The ability to raise the eyebrow in the presence of ipsilateral lower facial palsy indicates upper motor neurone aetiology. Sensation is tested in the dermatome of each of the three branches of the trigeminal nerve by touching forehead, cheek and jaw on each side. The sensation of taste is not routinely assessed clinically.

Several functions should be assessed once the patient is instructed to 'open your mouth'. While the tongue rests in the floor of the mouth fasciculation may be noted. Movement of the uvula to one side on the command 'say ah' indicates a palsy of the contralateral glossopharyngeal nerve. The gag reflex is tested using an orange stick to press on each side of the oropharynx. Finally, the patient is asked to 'stick out your tongue'. A deviated tongue points to the side of the lesion. Assessment of motor function is completed by asking the patient to 'look to the side' (sternomastoid) and 'shrug your shoulders' (trapezius). Hearing is assessed informally by asking the patient to repeat a phrase whispered into each ear in turn.

Primitive reflexes, such as pouting or palmo-mental, may be present in advanced dementia.

Limbs

Tables 22.5 and 22.6 summarize the scheme of neurological examination of the limbs.

Table 22.5 Neurological examination of the upper limbs

Inspection	
• wasting	
• fasciculation	
Tone	
Power	
• pronator drift	
• shoulder abduction	(C5,6)
• elbow flexion	(C5,6)
• elbow extension	(C6,7)
• wrist & finger extension	(C7)
• wrist flexion & grip	(C8)
Coordination	
• finger-nose	
• rapid alternating movements	
Reflexes	
• biceps	(C5,6)
• supinator	(C5,6)
• triceps	(C6,7)
Sensation	
• pin-prick	
• vibration	
• joint position	
• light touch	

Table 22.6 Neurological examination of the lower limbs

Inspection	
• wasting	
• fasciculation	
Tone	
Power	
• hip flexion	(L2,3)
• knee flexion	(L5,S1)
• knee extension	(L3,4)
• ankle dorsi flexion	(L4,5)
• ankle plantar flexion	(S1,2)
Coordination	
• heel-shin	
• foot tapping	
Reflexes	
• knee	(L3,4)
• ankle	(S1,2)
• plantar	
Sensation	
• pin-prick	
• vibration	
• joint position	
• light touch	
Gait	

Upper limbs (Table 22.5)

Assessment of tone may be affected by voluntary or involuntary movement and is often confounded by the instruction to 'relax' or 'let your arm go floppy'. Asking the patient to tap the foot can help. Reduced tone occurs in the early stage following stroke but usually indicates lower motor neurone pathology. The increased tone of longstanding upper motor neurone lesions eventually releases in a 'clasp-knife' pattern. In Parkinsonian syndromes, tremor superimposed on rigidity leads to a 'cog-wheel' pattern. Extrapyramidal signs may be caused by chronic neuroleptic use.

Pronator drift remains a sensitive marker for weakness. One muscle group innervated from each cranial nerve root should be tested (Table 22.5). It is prudent to assess grip strength and function of the hand and fingers. Power is tested in the position of maximal activity and graded on a standard scale, according to age, build and gender. Stroke predominantly affects flexor muscles.

If the deep tendon reflexes are increased, a positive Hoffmann's reflex (flicking the nail of either the second, third or fourth finger will cause a flexion of the thumb) and finger jerk confirm hyperreflexia. Reinforcement, for example by clenching the teeth, may be required if a reflex appears absent. Coordination is assessed by the finger–nose test – assessing for intention tremor and past-pointing – and rapid, alternating hand movements – which may be slow and clumsy in cerebellar and extrapyramidal disorders.

When testing sensation, the distribution of any abnormality should be determined and may be dermatomal (nerve root or spinal cord lesion), involve a single peripheral nerve territory (for example, carpal tunnel syndrome) or the 'glove' loss of a peripheral neuropathy. Testing for sensation may be unrewarding in subjects with dementia.

Lower limbs (Table 22.6)

Tone is assessed during hip rotation and knee flexion. Clonus, a sustained, rhythmical contraction of muscles under sudden stretch, is checked at the knee and ankle and is present with increased tone from an upper motor neurone lesion. Each lumbosacral nerve root is tested for motor and sensory function. Loss of posterior column modalities is often found in normal elderly people.

The plantar reflex (Babinski sign) is elicited by drawing the stimulus along the lateral border of the sole of the foot from posterior to anterior and then medially across the ball of the foot. Spreading of the toes and dorsiflexion (extension) of the great toe due to upper motor neurone pathology must be distinguished from a withdrawal response.

In the heel–shin test the patient is instructed to slide the foot smoothly down the shin from the knee to the ankle and repeat. Rapid, alternating movement is tested by the patient tapping the foot on the ground.

Finally, the gait is observed with the patient walking normally, turning and walking back. Walking heel to toe and performing Romberg's test (the patient stands with the feet together and is asked to close their eyes) assesses cerebellar and posterior column function.

REFERENCES

1. Royal College of Psychiatrists. *A Competency Based Curriculum for Specialist Training in Psychiatry: Specialist Module in Old Age Psychiatry*. London: Royal College of Psychiatrists, 2006.
2. McKhann G, Drachman D, Folstein M et al. Clinical diagnosis of Alzheimer's disease: report of the NINCDS-ADRDA Work Group under the auspices of Department of Health and Human Services Task Force on Alzheimer's Disease. *Neurology* 1984; **34**: 939–44.
3. McKeith IG, Dickson DW, Lowe J et al. Diagnosis and management of dementia with Lewy bodies: third report of the DLB Consortium. *Neurology* 2005; **65**: 1863–72.
4. Roman GC, Tatemichi TK, Erkinjuntti T et al. Vascular dementia: diagnostic criteria for research studies. Report of the NINDS-AIREN International Workshop. *Neurology* 1993; **43**: 250–60.

23

Investigations in Old Age Psychiatry

Sujatha Merve[1] and Robert C. Baldwin[2]

[1]*Chasefarm Hospital, Enfield, UK*
[2]*Manchester Royal Infirmary, Manchester, UK*

INTRODUCTION

This chapter reviews a range of laboratory and imaging investigations with which an old age psychiatrist should be familiar. Physical illness has been shown to be present in 20–80% of psychiatric patient populations surveyed[1]. Physical illness of relevance to the presenting psychiatric symptoms is reportedly in the range 9–46%[1]. Concomitant medical disorder was found in up to 63% of psychiatric patients presenting to an emergency department[2]. However, a retrospective study demonstrated that only 0.8–4.0% of abnormal tests were clinically significant[1] (defined as those that contributed to a diagnosis of a medical disorder not identified by history taking and physical examination and which led to a medical consultation or changed further management). Accordingly, some have argued against using routine batteries of tests[1,2].

The older adult population may be an exception to this, as the chances of a physical illness presenting primarily with psychiatric symptoms is increased. Examples include delirium (infections, metabolic abnormalities, polypharmacy); dementia (thyroid disease, B_{12} deficiency); psychosis (substance withdrawal/toxicity, space occupying lesions in the brain); depression (anaemia, thyroid disease, some drugs, malignancy); mania (stroke, drug side effects); anxiety (thyroid disease, cardiac arrhythmia); and perceptual abnormalities (visual defects, migraine, temporal lobe epilepsy, withdrawal from drugs). Further, mental disorder may contribute to the onset of new physical illness or deterioration in an existing one due to factors such as self-neglect or cognitive difficulties.

Investigations should be guided by findings from history taking, mental state examination and relevant physical examination. Unlike in general medicine, the role of laboratory and other investigations is mainly supportive and to rule out an organic aetiology of psychiatric presentations. However, there are several other reasons for conducting physical investigations in the older patient (Table 23.1).

Ancillary investigations can aid diagnosis, especially in the dementias and in delirium. Many older patients have known physical co-morbidity that requires further evaluation or are at high risk of common morbidities, which can affect management (ischaemic heart disease, anaemia, etc.). Because of self-neglect, those with dementia and depression may suffer under-nutrition and require investigation for this. Last, some psychiatric procedures and medication require pre- and/or post-testing (Figure 23.1).

Investigations may therefore be classified as primary or 'routine' (most patients receive them), secondary (indicated only in patients with certain clinical characteristics) and mandated (patients meeting certain criteria must have them) (Figure 23.1). The limitations of this approach should be recognized. Some tests (e.g. for neurosyphilis, see below) will show abnormal results very rarely but with important clinical implications. Others (e.g. full blood count or plasma viscosity) will often be slightly abnormal and of uncertain significance. A good deal of skill is required to interpret results in relation to a particular patient.

An example of an investigation of immediate relevance to management is a patient with a history of depression now presenting with what appeared to be a recurrence but also with recent confusion and difficulty in walking. On computerized tomography (CT) brain scan he was found to have a glioma. In another instance a patient with dementia deteriorated with poor appetite and weight loss. Investigations revealed anaemia and a markedly raised C-reactive protein, found on further testing to be due to inflammatory bowel disease. Here investigations helped clarify whether it was dementia or co-morbid pathology causing physical deterioration. Sometimes investigations are of uncertain relevance. An example is a patient presenting with late-onset psychosis and who was found to have a sodium of 125 mmol/l due to the syndrome of inappropriate antidiuretic hormone secretion (SIADH; see below) and a raised thyroid stimulating hormone (TSH) level caused by not taking thyroxine for former radio-iodine treated thyrotoxicosis. Optimizing these abnormalities made no obvious difference to her mental state, which improved only after the introduction of an antipsychotic agent. This also illustrates that even when there is an apparently obvious physical cause for an observed mental state, it is often necessary to treat psychiatric co-morbidity as well as optimizing the management of physical disorder.

HAEMATOLOGICAL INVESTIGATIONS

The full blood count (FBC) and differential count help detect various conditions, including anaemia (low haemoglobin, low red cell count, micro/macrocytosis), infections (raised white cell count, neutrophilia), allergies or parasitic infections (eosinophilia), blood malignancies (raised cell count, abnormal cells in blood smear) and effects of drugs on particular cell lines (neutropenia or

Table 23.1 Reasons for conducting investigations in old age psychiatry

To rule out causative organic physical illness

To aid in the diagnosis of some psychiatric conditions (e.g. dementia)

To assess secondary physical effects of the presenting psychiatric disorder

To help assess the impact of known medical co-morbidities

To screen for common co-morbidities not obvious at presentation but likely to affect management

To screen prior to the commencement of some medications and procedures

To monitor drug levels in the blood

To monitor potential side effects of prescribed drugs

agranulocytosis with clozapine). The erythrocyte sedimentation rate (ESR) and C-reactive protein (CRP) are non-specific tests that can point to infection, inflammation, anaemia, malignancy, temporal arteritis and autoimmune conditions. The ESR rises with advancing age and so becomes more difficult to interpret.

The incidence of psychiatric symptoms with B_{12} deficiency has been reported to vary between 4% and 50% depending on the population studied[3]. A correlation between serum cobalamin level and measures of cognitive function has been noted in some studies, although this has been disputed in those aged over 60[4]. Deficiency of folate may be more likely to cause depressive symptoms and a low B_{12} has been linked to psychosis[5]. The true nature and reversibility of a B_{12} deficiency-induced dementia has been debated. In addition,

deficiency of folate has been linked to poorer response to antidepressant treatment[6]. Confirmatory tests for the aetiology of vitamin B_{12} deficiency include gastric parietal cell antibodies, intrinsic factor antibodies and the Schilling test.

BIOCHEMISTRY

Routine biochemistry may detect electrolyte disturbances, dehydration and abnormal organ functioning (kidney, liver). The commonest psychiatric presentation of most of these is delirium. In addition, biochemical investigations are used to monitor the metabolic side effects of antidepressants or antipsychotics (e.g. SIADH and abnormal liver function tests [LFT]) and mood stabilizers (urea and electrolytes and thyroid function with lithium). SIADH is characterized by hyponatraemia (levels below 125 mmol/l are usually symptomatic), low serum osmolality and inappropriately elevated urine osmolality. SIADH can develop early after initiation of drug therapy, especially with selective serotonin re-uptake inhibitors (SSRIs). Increasing age, female gender and medical co-morbidities are risk factors.

Transient asymptomatic rise in LFT is not uncommon during the first few weeks of prescribing psychotropic drugs. Gamma glutamyl transpeptidase (γGT) is elevated in liver disease, pancreatic disease, obesity and enzyme induction by drugs or alcohol, and 52% of alcohol dependent patients have been reported to have high γGT[7]. Due to its low specificity, γGT is not indicated as a screening test for alcohol misuse. More specific is the carbohydrate-deficient transferrin (CDT) enzyme immunoassay.

A random glucose above 11 mmol/l suggests diabetes. Hypoglycaemia can cause delirium and can be seen in depressed diabetic patients who take their medication but neglect to eat.

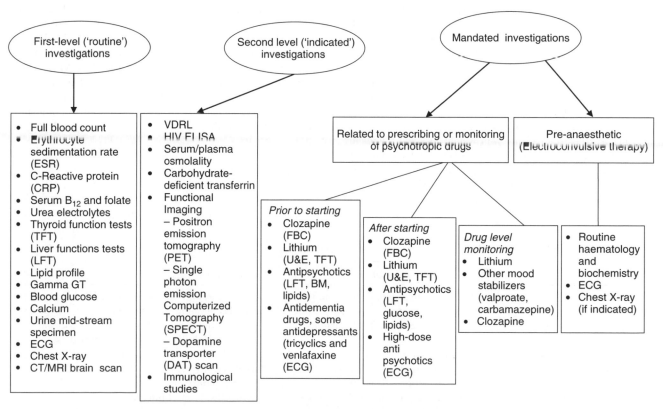

Figure 23.1 Types of investigations in old age psychiatry (see text for meaning of abbreviations)

Thyroid function testing (TFT) should be performed because of the well-known association of depression and hypothyroidism, easily overlooked in the elderly, and because 'apathetic hyperthyroidism' can be mistaken for depression. Patients on lithium should undergo TFT every six months. Raised corrected serum calcium can indicate malignancy (metastasis, multiple myeloma and lung cancer) and these patients may present with depressive symptoms. Iron studies including serum ferritin and total iron binding capacity are performed to help diagnose the type of anaemia (iron deficiency, sideroblastic or anaemia of chronic disease).

Because of the risk of the metabolic syndrome, fasting lipid screening is important in patients receiving antipsychotics. Waist measurement is a simple test of risk for this syndrome and there are international guidelines on waist measurement[8].

MICROBIOLOGY

Mid-stream urine (MSU) assessment is usually carried out to assess patients with confusion. In a sample of 68 patients Gregory *et al.*[2] reported an overall percentage of significant results in 3.1% of their review of general psychiatry patients. Kolman[9], though, studied older patients and found positive test results in 21% of patients. Non-contaminated samples are hard to obtain from patients with delirium or dementia.

RADIOLOGY

The patient's age correlates with the frequency of abnormal findings on chest X-ray[10]. A review of 746 psychiatric admissions[11] identified that the 9% of patients who had a significant X-ray finding also had concomitant physical signs and symptoms. Chest radiology of all patients presenting with psychiatric symptoms is not warranted, and clinical suspicion remains the best yardstick. It should always be performed on patients at risk of conditions like tuberculosis (homeless persons, alcohol/drug misuse and patients with HIV infection) and (ex-) smokers with weight loss.

Chest radiography is usually performed routinely as a pre-anaesthetic screening tool prior to patients receiving ECT (some centres perform it on a mandatory basis on patients aged above 35).

Endoscopy and barium X-ray tests of the gastrointestinal system may be indicated for patients with weight loss and microcytic anaemia. These investigations are sometimes poorly tolerated by psychiatric patients so advances in CT imaging are important. Helical CT scanning of the abdomen with oral contrast, besides being rapid and non-invasive, can identify a range of pathologies of the gut and other structures.

SPECIALIZED BLOOD TESTS

Syphilis

The Venereal Disease Research Laboratory test, commonly known as the VDRL test, is a screening test for syphilis that measures antibodies to the spirochete *Treponema pallidum* in the blood or cerebrospinal fluid (CSF). The newer test analogous to this is the rapid plasma reagin (RPR). *Treponema pallidum* haemagglutination assay and the fluorescent Treponema antibody tests (TPHA/FTA ABS) are highly specific for Treponema antigens and are used at some centres as confirmatory tests, especially of CSF.

Clinically significant results were found in 0.3% (0–0.6%) of psychiatric patients routinely screened[1]. A retrospective study of all inpatients (mean age 74.5) undergoing syphilis screening in a UK hospital[12] revealed that 16 of 423 tests were positive (3.8%). In four of the seven patients who received treatment, syphilis was identified as a likely contributor to the psychiatric presentation. The authors suggested that routine screening of elderly patients was justifiable where an organic aetiology was suspected, especially in dementia. Hilton[13], though, highlighted the importance of considering local epidemiology, risk factors, neurological/neuropsychiatric features and ethics prior to the routine screening of patients. In the guidance on dementia issued by the National Institute for Health and Clinical Excellence (NICE), routine testing for syphilis is not recommended[14].

Immunology

Psychiatric symptoms may be caused by systemic autoimmune diseases such as systemic lupus erythematosus, scleroderma, sarcoidosis, Sjögren syndrome, primary vasculitides and antiphospholipid syndrome. The range of autoimmune antibodies found in the spectrum of conditions include antinuclear antibody (ANA), anti-DNA (single stranded or double stranded), anti-Ro, anti-La, anti-phospholipid antibodies, anti-smooth muscle, rheumatoid factor (RF), anti-neutrophil cytoplasmic antibodies (ANCA) and antibodies to thyroid peroxidase. Table 23.2 illustrates the more common tests in relation to some immunological conditions. Catatonia and some rare encephalopathies are associated with autoimmunity, e.g. anti-NMDAR antibodies[15].

NEUROIMAGING

Focal neurological signs on physical examination or an acute change in the mental status not completely explained by other causes require

Table 23.2 Autoimmune conditions and relevant investigations

Condition	Psychiatric presentation	Relevant tests
Systemic lupus erythematosus	Psychosis, delirium, depression, global cognitive deficits	Anti-nuclear, anti-double stranded DNA, antiphospholipid, anti-neuronal
Hashimoto's thyroiditis	Dementia, delirium, hallucinations	Thyroid antibodies (antithyroid peroxidase and antithyroglobulin), anti-neural antibodies
Sjögren's syndrome	Cognitive dysfunction	Anti-nuclear, rheumatic factor
Polyarteritis nodosa	Delirium, auditory and visual hallucinations, dementia	Raised erythrocyte sedimentation rate (ESR), arterial biopsy
Temporal arteritis and polymyalgia rheumatica	Delirium, depression, hallucinations, cognitive dysfunction	Raised ESR, arterial biopsy

consideration of neuroimaging. Subdural haematoma is easily overlooked in older adults, especially when chronic. Fluctuating confusion, unsteady gait, falls and heavy alcohol use are all clues. Imaging is important if normal pressure hydrocephalus (cognitive impairment, gait disorder, incontinence) is suspected. On magnetic resonance imaging (MRI) the typical 'fluid void' sign may be seen but imaging alone is often not diagnostic.

There are clinical diagnostic rules for assessing which patients with dementia should undergo neuroimaging but they are not precise enough to ensure that patients with potentially reversible lesions are not missed[16]. The cost-effectiveness of routine imaging in patients with suspected dementias has been questioned but with the likelihood of more effective treatments emerging in the future the situation may change. Guidelines concerning the indications for neuroimaging are available from the National Institute for Health and Clinical Excellence[14], the Scottish Intercollegiate Guidelines Network[17] and the American Psychiatric Association (APA)[18]. NICE recommends MRI scanning as the preferred modality to assist early diagnosis and detect subcortical (vascular) white matter changes. The APA recommends neuroimaging in cases with subacute onset (less than one year), symptom onset before age 65, vascular risk factors suggesting a higher likelihood of cerebrovascular contributory factors or a history or neurological examination findings suggesting a possible focal lesion. The usefulness of neuroimaging in late stage disease has not been established[18].

CT is widely available and may be acceptable for anxious/disturbed patients. In one study[19] of 178 CT scans carried out, only 4 cases of potentially reversible neurological conditions were identified and in no case did this knowledge change treatment. On the other hand 32.8% had evidence of ischaemic white matter disease. As CT is not as sensitive as MRI (see below) in detecting this, when unequivocally reported on CT scanning such ischaemic changes ('leukoaraiosis') support a diagnosis of mixed type dementia.

MRI provides more detail of brain structure and function. As the patient must remain motionless in a tunnel for up to 20 minutes, MRI is not suitable for anxious or claustrophobic patients nor for those with metallic implants (pacemakers, aneurysm clips). There are few diagnostic signs relevant to psychiatry with MRI. An exception is the pulvinar sign in variant Creutzfeldt–Jakob disease (CJD), which has been found to be highly accurate and may obviate the need for more invasive testing[20]. More usual is the frequent finding on MRI of white matter hyperintensities, which are commonly interpreted as evidence of small vessel ischaemia but are of uncertain diagnostic significance unless graded as severe.

Positron emission tomography (PET) and single photon emission computed tomography (SPECT) utilize radioactive isotopes to assess brain metabolism (PET) and perfusion (SPECT) and provide information about the functional status of brain tissue. These investigations are discussed in detail elsewhere. Although clinical criteria may be more sensitive than SPECT, the latter is more specific in differentiating different types of dementia[21] and so is recommended to aid in the differential in cases of doubt[17].

Functional imaging of the dopamine transporter to assess the integrity of the nigrostriatal dopaminergic pathways is the basis of the DAT scan. DAT scanning can be helpful in distinguishing drug-induced Parkinsonism from idiopathic Parkinson's disease and in the diagnosis of Lewy body dementia. In the latter, low striatal DAT occurs whereas DAT activity is normal in Alzheimer's[22].

The development of additional imaging tools such as quantitative MRI, functional MRI, investigational PET compounds, and other methods aimed at imaging senile plaques in the brain may help improved diagnosis, early recognition, and more precise assessment of disease progression in the future.

ELECTROCARDIOGRAPHY (ECG)

The main use of ECG in psychiatry is to monitor serious cardiac side effects of psychotropic medication (Table 23.3). It is ordered in at-risk populations, e.g. those with pre-existing cardiac abnormalities or

Table 23.3 Summary of common cardiac effects of psychotropics

ECG parameter	Drug	Effect
Heart rate	Clozapine; drugs with antimuscarinic side effects: TCAs, MAOIs	Sinus tachycardia; clinicians should suspect myocarditis/cardiomyopathy in patients on clozapine if patients have fever or other cardiac symptoms such as persistent tachycardia
Heart rate variability	Clozapine	Reduced variability associated with increased risk of cardiac death
Cardiac conduction	Tricyclic antidepressants	Prolong QRS complex; such changes in a patient with pre-existing conduction defect can cause complete heart block; in toxic doses (overdose) this can prove fatal
	Antipsychotics	Can prolong QTc interval
	Haloperidol in high doses	At-risk patients can develop torsades de pointes and fatal ventricular arrhythmia
	Any intravenous antipsychotic	Some antipsychotics may cause atrial fibrillation, heart block, changes to P and T waves
	Lithium	May affect T waves and rarely cause heart block
Cardiac rhythm	All drugs that have an effect on cardiac conduction	Torsades de pointes, ventricular arrhythmias and sudden cardiac death have all been reported; monitoring mandatory for at-risk population (pre-existing cardiac disease, high-dose antipsychotic use, overdoses especially TCAs and those with metabolic/electrolyte abnormalities)
Cardiac conduction and rhythm	Acetylcholinesterase inhibitors	Can cause bradycardia, atrial arrhythmias; angina, syncope

conduction defects, those on other drugs that have an effect on cardiac conduction (antiarrhythmics), those with or at risk of metabolic abnormalities (anorexia, renal failure) and patients who have taken an overdose. An ECG should be performed prior to the commencement of a tricyclic antidepressant or a cholinesterase inhibitor.

Patients on high-dose antipsychotics are at increased risk of arrhythmias and sudden cardiac death, and hence ECG monitoring in this group of patients is mandatory[23,24]. Lithium can change the morphology of T waves and in rare instances has been associated with heart block (Table 23.3).

ELECTROENCEPHALOGRAPHY (EEG)

The EEG is no longer widely used in assessment of patients in old age psychiatry and has been largely superseded by structural neuroimaging. However, in some cases the EEG can provide valuable additional information, e.g. in differential diagnosis of rapidly progressive dementia, episodic neurological symptoms and signs, or complex presentations with inconsistencies in the clinical picture and investigations.

The EEG in patients with Alzheimer's dementia may show non-specific abnormalities even in the early stages of the disease. In frontotemporal dementia the EEG remains unremarkable until late in the disorder. Although not routinely recommended. The EEG can be highly specific (although not sensitive) in cases of sporadic CJD[17], in which case a lumbar puncture to assess for the presence of protein 14-3-3 may help with the diagnosis. The role of MRI in CJD has been discussed.

Patients with dementia of Lewy body type show a characteristic early slowing of dominant EEG rhythm and 50% show focal delta wave activity in temporal regions[25]. The EEG in patients with vascular dementia is more likely to be normal in the early stages.

Abnormality correlates with the amount of damage in the underlying brain structure, often with focal or asymmetrical changes.

EEG findings of pseudo-periodic sharp wave activity (triphasic) are found in 70% of cases of CJD.

Quantitative EEG (qEEG) uses a computerized programme to statistically analyse EEG recordings and may assist in diagnosis. A literature review[26] suggests that abnormalities in qEEG tend to increase with the severity of the dementia. Studies have reported a moderate to high accuracy of differentiating EEG recordings in normal ageing populations and patients with dementia.

PSYCHOTROPIC DRUG MONITORING

Therapeutic drug monitoring is primarily used for drugs with a narrow therapeutic index or which show high inter-patient pharmacokinetic variability[27]. Drug monitoring is mandatory for some drugs that are toxic in higher concentrations such as lithium. Monitoring can also help confirm treatment adherence. Serum monitoring was useful for tricyclic antidepressants where there was known to be a therapeutic window but with the newer antidepressants, where effective doses are close to starting doses, the need has disappeared.

Most drug levels are measured when they reach steady state concentration; this takes four to five drug half-lives[28]. Also sample collection should be made within 1–2 hours of the recommended time (trough or pre-dose and 12-hour post-dose, as with lithium). Mood stabilizers are one of the most commonly monitored classes of psychotropic drug (Table 23.4), although lithium is the most important because of its narrow therapeutic-to-toxic ratio. Blood levels of valproate and carbamazepine do not necessarily relate to clinical effectiveness.

For clozapine, a number of patient factors have been identified that influence the serum levels. These include the age of the patient,

Table 23.4 Serum monitoring of mood stabilizers

Drug	Investigations prior to prescribing	Side effects	Average daily dosages	Target serum levels
Lithium	Renal function	Polyuria, gastrointestinal upset, tremor, neurological disturbance (toxicity), weight gain, oedema, psoriatic rash		
	Electrolytes ECG Thyroid function Blood glucose (preferably fasting)		400 mg (slow release)	0.6–0.8 mEq/l
Valproate	Liver enzymes	Sedation, nausea, unsteadiness, tremor, weight gain	500–1500 mg	65–90 μg/ml (not definitely established)
	Full blood count ECG (if history or clinical condition suggests)			
Carbamazepine	Liver enzymes	Sedation, ataxia, nystagmus, blurred vision, agranulocytosis, hyponatraemia	400–800 mg	4–12 μg/l (levels for epilepsy)
	Full blood count ECG (if history or clinical condition suggests)			

ethnicity, smoking status and interactions with other drugs. Plasma levels of 350–500 µg/l have been suggested for optimal clinical response. Seizures have been identified to be commoner in patients with levels higher than 1000 µg/l[29]. Some authors have suggested the prophylactic use of valproate to prevent seizures when the plasma levels are >600 µg/l.

OTHER INVESTIGATIONS

Cerebrospinal Fluid Analysis

Lumbar puncture (LP) is generally performed under the care of physicians or neurologists with the main indications being confirmation of CNS infections (bacterial, tubercular, fungal), inflammatory conditions (vasculitis) or malignancy. With the developments in neuroimaging, many of these conditions can be identified on scans. The role of LP in suspected CJD can be diagnostic and has been discussed.

Sleep Studies

Common sleep complaints include insomnia, excessive daytime sleepiness and parasomnias such as REM sleep behaviour disorder (SBD), as seen in dementia with Lewy bodies. Other conditions that may be misdiagnosed as primary psychiatric illnesses include narcolepsy and sleep apnoea syndrome. The latter is increasingly recognized as a cause of or contributory factor to confusional states.

Primarily the assessment of sleep-related disorders relies on clinical evaluation and sleep charts. Polysomnography is available in specialist centres and involves measurement and observation of different stages/components of sleep along with recordings of EEG, electro-oculogram and electromyogram. Sleep apnoea is diagnosed with simultaneous monitoring of respiratory effort and oxygen saturation overnight and is offered by respiratory medicine departments.

Genetic Studies

Genetic screening and prediction of risk raises many ethical dilemmas. However, old age psychiatrists increasingly see younger patients with dementia for whom genetic considerations apply and they should know when to refer to a colleague specializing in psychiatric genetics.

Ethical issues of confidentiality and information sharing pose a great challenge to clinicians and geneticists. The experience may be emotionally challenging to patients and the results may not be conclusive. Issues of 'the right not to know' and implications for the individual's future employment and discrimination in access to insurance policies need to be considered. Some tests can result in stigmatization and unwarranted anxiety among family members. Genetic testing is predictive for only some conditions.

Alzheimer's disease has been associated with mutations in amyloid precursor protein (APP) and presenilin 1 and 2 genes. Frontotemporal dementia studies have suggested mutations in *tau* protein (in some families involving autosomal dominance) and *α-synuclein* has been recognized in Parkinson's disease. Early onset (<65 years) Alzheimer's disease is associated with gene mutations that are transmitted in an autosomal dominant fashion.

While late onset Alzheimer's disease (>65 years) is generally considered to be idiopathic or sporadic, numerous studies have shown increased risk of developing the disease (odds ratio between 3 and 15) in individuals with APO E4 allele on chromosome 19[30].

However, testing for apolipoprotein E4 (*APOE4*) is not recommended for use in the diagnosis of dementia[31]. Commercial kits are available for testing certain genes, for example presenilin 1 (*PSEN1*) on chromosome 14 but careful interpretation is required and should only be undertaken in the context of pre- and post-test counselling[18]. In addition, specific genetic testing is available for Huntington's disease and CADASIL (cerebral autosomal dominant arteriopathy with subcortical infarcts and leukoencephalopathy – Notch 3 gene polymorphisms). Lastly, there is current interest in the glucocerebrosidase gene in Lewy body dementia, which may in the future have implications for genetic testing[32].

LEGAL CONSIDERATIONS

Always record whether the patient consents to undergoing investigations and if they are unable whether it is in their best interests to undergo them. In English law, in an emergency, the Capacity Act (2005) permits reasonable and proportionate force for necessary testing and the Mental Health Act (2007) allows the Responsible Clinician to make arrangements for testing of detained patients where this is of direct relevance to their mental disorder (this includes withdrawing blood for clozapine monitoring). It does not, however, mandate testing of an unrelated condition, e.g. an endoscopy for incidental anaemia. Colleagues responsible for carrying out the investigation must conduct their own assessment of capacity. For example, an endoscopist must be satisfied that the patient understands the procedure and if this is not clear they will often seek the advice of the psychiatrist who has referred the patient. Colleagues undertaking investigations for the psychiatric team should be forewarned if the patient lacks capacity, both for their own safety and because certain tests will be difficult to perform without collaboration of the patient.

Testing of a patient for the good of others without consent is not permitted. The Human Tissue Act (2004) makes this clear. For example, this includes a member of staff who has been bitten by a patient with dementia and who may wish to know the patient's hepatitis and AIDS status. The Capacity Act (2005) may permit testing if it can be demonstrated that such knowledge is in the patient's interest, e.g. if it might lead to less restrictive nursing. Legal advice would still be needed regarding the disclosure of results to a third party.

REFERENCES

1. Anfinson TJ, Kathol RG. Screening laboratory evaluation in psychiatric patients: a review. *Gen Hosp Psychiatry* 1992; **14**: 248–57.
2. Gregory RJ, Nihalani ND, Rodriguez E. Medical screening in the emergency department for psychiatric admissions: a procedural analysis. *Gen Hosp Psychiatry* 2004; **26**: 405–10.
3. Goebels N, Soyka M. Dementia associated with vitamin B12 deficiency: presentation of two cases and review of literature. *J Neuropsychiatry Clin Neurosci* 2000; **12**: 389–94.
4. Ellinson M, Thomas J, Patterson A. A critical evaluation of the relationship between serum B, folate and total homocysteine with cognitive impairment in the elderly. *J Hum Nutr Diet* 2004; **17**(4): 371–83.
5. Hutto BR. Folate and cobalamin in psychiatric illness. *Compr Psychiatry* 1997; **38**(6): 305–14.
6. Mischoulon D, Raab MF. The role of folate in depression and dementia. *J Clin Psychiatry* 2007; **68**(suppl 10): 28–33.

7. Niemela O. Biomarkers in alcoholism. *Clin Chim Acta* 2007; **377**: 39–49.
8. Alberti KGGN, Zimmet P, Shaw J. The metabolic syndrome: new world-wide definition from the International Diabetes Federation Consensus. *Lancet* 2005; **366**: 1059–62.
9. Kolman PB. The value of laboratory investigations of elderly psychiatric patients. *J Clin Psychiatry* 1984; **45**(3): 112–16.
10. Liston EH, Gerner RH, Robertson AG *et al.* Routine thoracic radiography for psychiatric inpatients. *Hosp Community Psychiatry* 1979; **30**: 474–66.
11. Hughes J, Barraclough BM. Value of routine chest radiography of psychiatric patients. *Br Med J* 1980; **281**: 1461–2.
12. Cleare AJ, Jacoby R. Syphilis, neither dead nor buried – a survey of psychogeriatric inpatients. *Int J Geriatr Psychiatry* 1993; **8**: 661–4.
13. Hilton C. General paralysis of the insane and AIDS in old age psychiatry: epidemiology, clinical diagnosis, serology and ethics – the way forward. *Int J Geriatr Psychiatry* 1998; **13**: 875–85.
14. National Institute for Health and Clinical Excellence, and Social Care Institute for Excellence. *Dementia: Supporting People with Dementia and Their Carers in Health and Social Care*, NICE clinical guideline 42. London: NICE/SCIE, 2006.
15. Fink M, Taylor MA. The catatonia syndrome: forgotten but not gone. *Arch Gen Psychiatry* 2009; **66**: 1173–7.
16. Gifford DR, Holloway RG, Vickrey BG. Systematic review of clinical prediction rules for neuroimaging in the evaluation of dementia. *Arch Intern Med* 2000; **160**: 2855–62.
17. Scottish Intercollegiate Guidelines Network (SIGN). *Management of Patients with Dementia*, clinical guideline 86. Edinburgh: SIGN, 2006.
18. American Psychiatric Association. *Practice Guidelines for the Treatment of Psychiatric Disorders Compendium: Alzheimer's Disease and Other Dementias*, 2nd edn. Arlington, VA: APA, 2006.
19. Fielding S. The value of cranial computed tomography in old age psychiatry: a review of the results of 178 scans. *Psychiatr Bull* 2005; **29**: 21–3.
20. Collie DA, Summers DM, Sellar RJ *et al.* Diagnosing variant Creutzfeldt–Jakob disease with the pulvinar sign: MR imaging findings in 86 neuropathologically confirmed cases. *Am J Neuroradiology* 2003; **24**: 1560–69.
21. Talbot PR, Lloyd JL, Snowden JS, Neary D, Testa HJ. A clinical role for ^{99m}Tc-HMPAO SPECT in the investigation of dementia? *Neurol Neurosurg Psychiatry* 1998; **64**: 306–13.
22. McKeith IG, Dickson DW, Lowe J *et al.* Diagnosis and management of dementia with Lewy bodies: third report of the DLB consortium. *Neurology* 2005; **65**(12): 1863–72.
23. O'Brien P, Oyebode F. Psychotropic medication and the heart. *Adv Psychiatr Treat* 2003; **9**: 414–23.
24. Rowland JP, Rigby J, Harper AC *et al.* Cardiovascular monitoring with acetylcholinesterase inhibitors: a clinical protocol. *Adv Psychiatr Treat* 2007; **13**: 178–84.
25. Briel R. EEG findings in dementia with Lewy bodies and Alzheimer's disease. *J Neurol Neurosurg Psychiatry* 1999; **66**: 401–3.
26. Coburn KL, Lauterbach EC, Boutros NN *et al.* The value of quantitative encephalography in clinical psychiatry: a report by the committee on research of the American Neuropsychiatric Association. *J Neuropsychiatry Clin Neurosci* 2006; **18**: 460–500.
27. Hiemke C. Clinical utility of drug measurement and pharmacokinetics – therapeutic drug monitoring in psychiatry. *Eur J Clin Pharmacol* 2008; **64**: 159–66.
28. Taylor D, Paton C, Kerwin R. Plasma level monitoring of psychotropics and anticonvulsants. In *The Maudsley Prescribing Guidelines*, 9th edn. London: Informa Healthcare, 2007, 1–5.
29. Greenwood-Smith C, Lubman DI, Castle DJ. Serum clozapine levels: a review of their clinical utility. *J Psychopharmacol* 2003; **17**(2): 234–8.
30. Bertram L, Tanzi RE. The genetic epidemiology of neurodegenerative disease. *J Clin Invest* 2005; **115**: 1449–57.
31. Knopman DS, DeKosky ST, Cummings JL *et al.* Practice parameter: diagnosis of dementia (an evidence-based review), report of the Quality Standards Subcommittee of the American Academy of Neurology. *Neurology* 2001; **56**; 1143–53.
32. Leverenz JB, Lopez OL, DeKosky ST. The expanding role of genetics in the Lewy body diseases: the glucocerebrosidase gene. *Arch Neurol* 2009; **66**(5): 555–6.

Internet Resources

Dementia guidelines

NICE Dementia Guidelines: www.scie.org.uk/publications/misc/dementia/index.asp; http://guidance.nice.org.uk/CG42/Guidance/doc/English

SIGN dementia guidelines: www.sign.ac.uk/pdf/sign86.pdf

American Psychiatric Association: www.psychiatryonline.com/pracGuide/loadGuidelinePdf.aspx?file=AlzPG101007

American Academy of Neurology: www.aan.com/professionals/practice/pdfs/dementia_guideline.pdf

Neurology (journal): www.neurology.org/cgi/content/full/56/9/1143

Legal and Ethical considerations

Mental Capacity Act (2005): www.opsi.gov.uk/acts/acts2005/ukpga_20050009_en_1

Mental Health Act (2007): www.dh.gov.uk/en/Healthcare/Mentalhealth/index.htm

Human Tissue Act (2004): www.dh.gov.uk/en/Publichealth/Scientificdevelopmentgeneticsandbioethics/Tissue/Tissuegeneralinformation/DH_4102169

24

Bedside Assessment of Cognitive Functioning

Richard Perry

*Department of Neurosciences, Imperial College and Imperial College Healthcare NHS Trust,
Charing Cross Hospital, London, UK*

INTRODUCTION

In the future, clinicians are likely to make ever more use of newer diagnostic techniques such as multimodal MRI imaging, PET imaging and CSF analysis. These ancillary investigations are only helpful in the appropriate clinical context in terms of their ability to discriminate between various diseases and in how their results are interpreted. As always in medicine, this clinical context comes from careful and considered history and examination.

HISTORY TAKING IN COGNITIVE ASSESSMENT

One key aspect of the cognitive history is the necessity of gaining a witness or corroborative account. By their nature, cognitive impairments may include lack of insight and impaired ability to express details of the history as a result of memory, language or other cognitive deficits. It is therefore strongly recommended that a witness history is taken and it is often beneficial to perform this separately from the patient, particularly if personality or behavioural changes are to be exposed.

An in-depth discussion of all aspects of the cognitive history is beyond the scope of this chapter and we have excluded the well-known aspects of past psychiatric history, past medial history, educational and occupational history and social and family history in favour of highlighting some tips specific to cognitive history taking, which although not meant to be foolproof, nevertheless may provide helpful clues to direct the clinician.

Initial Presentation and Impressions

Although not without exception, on the whole, if a spouse, friend or carer is the instigator of the referral, this is more suspicious of an underlying organic brain disorder than patients who self-present. Patients who attend a clinic alone have a much greater chance of having an underlying affective cause of their symptoms than those who are accompanied.

Many patients who are 'brought' to a consultation adopt this role very quickly and defer to their spouse or friend in sitting down and answering questions. A common occurrence is the response to the first greeting or question – when the examiner asks why the patient has come to see them, the patient may immediately turn to their spouse for help or confirmation without actually addressing the question. Anecdotally this reaction seems to have a fairly high specificity for underlying organic brain disease.

Presenting Complaint

It is important to clarify the first symptom that has been noticed by the patient or carer. Patients presenting with moderate stages of dementia may have a multitude of symptoms that overlap between dementia subtypes and often the first symptom can be instructive regarding diagnosis. For example, memory deficits are invariably the earliest feature of Alzheimer's disease whereas behavioural changes are invariably the initial feature of frontotemporal dementia despite both sets of symptoms being present in both conditions as they progress.

It is often difficult for patients or informants to be accurate about the duration of symptoms which are usually underestimated. A little gentle probing can often extend the history from an initial estimate of six months to several years, thereby narrowing the differential diagnosis. It is useful to ask such questions as 'how were they three years ago – were they the same as 20 years ago?'

Behavioural and Personality Changes

To get a clear history of behavioural or personality change, the interviewing of an informant is critical as lack of insight often accompanies such behavioural changes. Major personality change is usually a result of pathology in the limbic, paralimbic and frontal striatal systems. They may be seen in space occupying lesions of the frontal lobe and subcortical dementias but the condition where specific personality changes are virtually diagnostic is frontotemporal dementia.

A simple question such as 'have you noticed any changes in X's behaviour or personality?' is usually a helpful opening gambit. A not uncommon response in frontotemporal dementia is that 'they are not the same person that I married'.

Behaviours to probe for include apathy, passivity and lack of initiation. Indeed some patients are often content to let others discuss less than complimentary changes in their behaviour or personality without need to interject or justify themselves in any way. Disinhibited behaviour can be enquired about in terms of whether the patient has done or said anything that causes embarrassment or is inappropriate, especially in public. Rigidity in behaviour may be evidenced by strict and unnecessary time keeping or eating habits such as always eating the same food at the same time of day. Obsessive and compulsive

Principles and Practice of Geriatric Psychiatry, 3rd edn. Edited by Mohammed T. Abou-Saleh, Cornelius Katona and Anand Kumar
© 2011 John Wiley & Sons, Ltd

behaviour should be questioned and the duration of this ascertained to differentiate from longstanding personality traits. Gradual loss of empathy and blunting of emotional repertoires should be sought and a change in food preferences for sweet things or the development of a catchphrase are both behavioural changes that are virtually pathognomonic of frontotemporal dementia.

Autobiographical History

It is useful to go through details of schooling and major life events in early adulthood, primarily to see if the subject has impaired autobiographical memory. An inability to remember where they went to school, when they were married and where, or what their first job was, is concerning for an organic dementia as these memory abilities are not usually affected in psychiatric disorders.

Medications

Elderly populations may have a multitude of medical and psychiatric co-morbidities and hence multiple medications, many of which may affect cognition. Particular medications to note are opiate-based analgesics such as codeine or tramadol, medications with anticholinergic properties such as tricyclic antidepressants, antispasmodics, anti-emetics, anti-parkinsonian medication, bronchodilators, or anti-arrhythmics.

Activities of Daily Living

Ask about performance at work if appropriate, ability to travel to new locations alone, handling of finances and bank accounts, social events, use of household devices including telephones, TVs etc., preparation of meals, organizing of family events such as trips and holidays. A gradual change of responsibilities from patient to spouse or other carer over several years is revealing.

BEDSIDE COGNITIVE ASSESSMENT

Initial Observations

The bedside cognitive assessment starts with observation of the patient. Watch how the patient enters into the consultation room, paying particular attention to their gait and observe how they sit down in a chair.

The gait abnormality of idiopathic Parkinson's disease is easy to recognize if one is watching for it. Slow and shuffling with short steps, narrow base, stooped posture with decreased arm swing. It is surprising how often this is overlooked. If a diagnosis can be made before the patient has sat down, it is very helpful for the rest of the consultation! The gait of cerebrovascular disease is characterized by the sense that the feet are rooted to the ground with a more wide-based gait, again with small steps. The gait of normal pressure hydrocephalus is usually more wide-based than that of cerebrovascular disease and is unsteady with less adherence of the feet to the floor.

Further useful information can be taken from watching the patient sit in a chair – difficulty in orienting to the chair or sitting on the edge or armrest of a chair by mistake suggests significant apraxia. If a patient falls back heavily into a chair, be on the lookout for additional signs of progressive supranuclear palsy.

Throughout a cognitive assessment it is useful to keep the question in mind of whether one is dealing with a predominantly cortical or subcortical picture of impairment. The cardinal features of

a subcortical cognitive impairment are slowing of thought, response and movement with impaired attention. The major cortical deficits to look out for are language impairment (aphasia), visuospatial impairment and praxis and so the finding of one of these deficits suggests cortical involvement (note the rare exceptions of aphasia from basal ganglia lesions). Memory deficits may be present in both cortical and subcortical syndromes.

Another important question to return to during the consultation is whether the patient has an organic or psychiatric origin to their symptoms. Although it is not always possible to be certain, there are certain clues from both the history and examination that may guide the examiner. Symptoms that are fluctuating or specific to either the home or workplace are suspicious for psychiatric symptoms, as are symptoms that are noticed solely by the patient rather than others. In the examination, psychiatric syndromes may often manifest with impaired memory, executive functions and processing speed deficits but the presence of real language deficits, apraxia or visuospatial function is far more concerning for organic brain disease.

Cognitive Rating Scales

The most widely used screening tool for bedside cognitive assessment is the Mini Mental State Examination (MMSE) which typically takes 8–10 minutes to administer and assesses orientation, memory, language and visuospatial function and is scored out of 30 points. As the MMSE is the subject of a separate chapter (see Chapter 27), it will not be described in detail here, but it is worth considering a few of its major advantages and disadvantages.
Advantages:

- ease of administration;
- wide use helps comparison of scores across patients and testing centres;
- suitable for longitudinal assessment;
- quick.

Disadvantages

- does not assess speed of information processing or executive function;
- minimal assessment of memory;
- ceiling effect in mild cognitive impairment and frontotemporal dementia;
- test–retest reliability (intra-rater) of +/− 3;
- inter-rater reliability suspect on serial 7s and 'world' backwards.

Because of these limitations, which are likely to be inherent in any short screening tool, various adaptations of the MMSE have been devised. The most promising of these is the Addenbrooke's Cognitive Examination (ACE) which includes all of the subtests of the MMSE but is expanded to include more detailed tests that provide scores for each of the five domains of episodic memory, verbal fluency, naming, language and visuospatial function. The latest revised version, the ACE-R, comes on six pages of A4, takes approximately 20 minutes to administer and is scored out of a total of 100. The full ACE-R with administration and scoring guidelines is available on line at http://pn.bmj.com/supplemental.

The memory domain includes a seven-item name-and-address test in which the patient is asked to register a name and address (e.g. Simon Williams, 17 Somerfield Road, Croydon, Surrey) across three learning trials and then recall after a 10-minute delay. There are two tests of verbal fluency. In letter fluency, the patient is asked to produce as many words beginning with 'p' as possible in one minute and in category fluency, as many animals as possible. The naming section is far more sensitive than that on the MMSE and consists of 10 line drawings of low-frequency items.

The authors of the ACE-R have carried out validation studies suggesting two cut-off scores of 88/100 or 82/100 for clinical practice. In the initial publication the upper cut-off score of 88 has a good sensitivity for dementia of 94% and a specificity of 89%[1]. This high sensitivity was reproduced in a later study although specificity was considerably lower with many false positives[2]. The specificity of the ACE for dementia is increased at the lower cut-off score of 82 without a major loss of sensitivity.

Proponents of the ACE have examined its potential to differentiate between dementia subtypes. The initial reports used a ratio of the domain scores of verbal fluency + language/orientation + memory (VLOM ratio) to differentiate between Alzheimer's disease and frontotemporal dementia and found that a ratio >3.2 supports Alzheimer's disease whereas a ratio of <2.2 is in favour of frontotemporal dementia[1]. Follow-up studies have confirmed the ratio of >3.2 as being reasonably sensitive and specific for AD although the sensitivity of a ratio of <2.2 for frontotemporal dementia is probably too low for clinical utility, especially when such studies do not take into account the pre-test probability of a diagnosis[7]. In clinical practice a diagnosis is not based on the ACE alone but in combination with the history, examination findings and imaging investigations.

A more recent study has attempted to use the ACE in conjunction with episodic memory tests such as the Rey Auditory Verbal Memory Test and the CANTAB Paired Associates Learning to identify MCI cases at greatest risk of conversion to Alzheimer's disease[3]. There was reasonable evidence that the combination of a broad screening tool of multiple cognitive domains such as the ACE plus two or more episodic memory tasks was effective in terms of both positive and negative predictive value. Indeed it is likely that this combination, which could be performed in a clinical assessment, is almost as effective as a more formal and extended neuropsychological assessment.

In the author's own practice, the subtests that appear to be the most helpful in adding to the MMSE to aid differential diagnosis are the episodic memory task, the verbal fluency task and the naming task. If the ACE were to be improved upon, it would be to further develop the episodic memory task to a word-list learning task with trials of registration and delayed recall. In clinical practice we are often trying to reliably identify which patients have impaired episodic memory that may be the earliest stages of Alzheimer's disease and the current name-and-address task may be too insensitive to fulfil this role, particularly in patients who have been cognitively high performing. Despite this limitation, the ACE is already becoming more widely used and appears to be an easily administered and helpful tool in the memory clinic.

Assessing Different Cognitive Domains

Orientation to time usually includes an assessment of day, month and year. In general, orientation to time is lost before orientation to space and this is particularly true of Alzheimer's disease. Not knowing the date is not specific and indeed many normal subjects are unaware of the date. Usually when testing date with the MMSE a margin of +/− two days is given. It is notable that disorientation to person in the absence of obtundation of conscious level is suspicious of factitious disorder. The catch is with severely and suddenly aphasic patients who can present to the unwary as confused and even as functional in origin.

Attention can be tested at the bedside with the *serials 7s* or *'world' backwards* of the MMSE or ACE.

Memory. The history informs us about autobiographical memory and further assessment can probe for deficits in episodic, working or semantic memory.

Working memory refers to information that is kept 'online' and in constant rehearsal for periods of up to around 30 seconds. It can be disrupted by interference and memories are not actually laid down for later recall. At the bedside this can be tested by forward and backward digit spans: In *forward-digit span*, a series of numbers, usually starting with three (e.g. 492) is read to the subject evenly at one integer every second who then repeats the numbers back. The digit span is taken as the maximum number of digits repeated back until two successive failures at a string length have occurred. The normal range is 6 +/− 1. *Backward-digit span* is performed in the same way except that the subject is asked to repeat the string of numbers backwards (e.g. examiner reads 947, subject repeats 749). The normal range is 5 +/− 1.

Episodic memory refers to memory for events that have been personally experienced. It has two main components: *anterograde memory* (new learning) and *retrograde memory* (memory for past events). The functional neuroanatomy of episodic memory involves the limbic-diencephalic system and its frontal connections and most importantly the hippocampal complex. Patients with disorders of episodic memory will present with forgetfulness for recent events, have difficulty keeping to the plot of novels or even films, may forget messages and rely on lists and may be repetitive.

Assessment of retrograde memory is predominantly from the history including the autobiographical history (see above) and specific questions related to more recent events such as details of holidays over the last year or two, details of family events such as weddings or Christmas and knowledge of recent major news events.

Anterograde memory can be assessed at the bedside and clinicians often use the memory subtests of the MMSE although the seven-item name-and-address task of the ACE is more sensitive. A patient's previous level of performance should be taken into account and even recall of all seven items may be obtained in those high functioning but in the earliest stages of a degenerative disease.

Semantic memory refers to our memory for facts, word meanings and general knowledge. The neural substrate that appears to be important for semantic memory is the cortical area of the anterior/inferior temporal lobe. Deficits can be apparent from the history by 'empty speech' with circumlocutions. Speech content is diminished and words are replaced with generics such as 'things'. Bedside assessment can be with verbal fluency tests, naming of objects or line drawings, tests of verbal knowledge and reading of regular or irregular words. Verbal fluency, as used in the ACE, can test both phonemic fluency (words beginning with 'p', 'd', 'f' etc.) in a minute or with semantic fluency (e.g. animals, tools, fruits etc.). In conditions characterized by semantic memory impairment there tends to be a discrepancy between semantic and phonemic fluency whereas predominant impairment of phonemic fluency is typical of subcortical syndromes such as cerebrovascular disease, parkinsonism, or depression[4,5]. Tests of semantic knowledge in the verbal domain include questions such as: what colour is grass? where do elephants live? which animal has four legs, a hump and lives in deserts? The ACE language subtests probe for impairment in the reading of irregular words, a difficulty which is often associated with semantic memory impairment. In this context, patients may have difficulty in reading irregular words such as height or yacht and when asked to read 'mint', 'pint' and then 'rint' may read 'rint' as in 'pint'.

If significant and disproportionate semantic impairment is suspected, further assessment of knowledge about famous people or famous faces can be helpful. Right temporal lobe atrophy and involvement of the fusiform gyrus as seen in the right temporal variant of frontotemporal dementia seems to be particularly associated with face recognition and knowledge impairments[6]. This is one of the only uses the author has found for publications such as *celebrity* magazines!

Language. It is important to differentiate actual language disorders (aphasias) from *dysarthria* which refers to the impairment of the mechanical aspects of sound production. From the history, the examiner will be able to gather important information about spoken language such as its degree of fluency, whether there are any articulatory problems, difficulties with word finding, impairment of intonation, rhythm or musicality (*dysprosodia*), or paraphasic errors. When assessing fluency, the most important issue will be whether the person is able to produce language effortlessly or not, regardless of the actual content. Non-fluent speech is effortful and halting with reduced sentence length, agrammatism and impaired prosody where the normal rhythms and undulations of speech are affected. Phonemic paraphasias may be detected where the sounds within words are incorrect, e.g. incollect rather than incorrect. Where the speech deficits are characterized by slow speech, increased pauses between words and distorted sounds but without phonemic problems, the term apraxia of speech may be used. Fluent speech is characterized by lack of effort and normal articulation but with lack of content and circumlocutions. After listening to speech output a simple assessment of comprehension is valuable using simple instructions in a graded manner. It is helpful to start with one-stage commands such as 'close your eyes' before more complicated commands such as 'lift up your left hand and then stick out your tongue' or 'after touching the desk, touch your left ear with your left hand'

Repetition is likewise tested in a graded manner starting with simple words such as 'toaster' before more complicated and polysyllabic words such as 'accordion' or 'catastrophe' and then on to short sentences such as 'The orchestra played and the audience applauded' as in the Cambridge ACE. Watch for phonemic paraphasias as described above and whether these are consistent mistakes.

Naming is tested by asking the patient to name particular objects or line drawings. There is a *frequency effect* in which commonly used words are less affected than uncommon words. For example, patients might be able to name high-frequency objects such as 'pen' and 'watch' (MMSE), but may have problems with more low frequency ones such as 'anchor' or 'barrel'.

Reading and its testing at the bedside is influenced by educational factors which need to be taken into account. An in-depth assessment of reading is not frequently required unless the history and general cognitive screen (e.g. 'close your eyes' from the MMSE) identifies specific problems in this area. The Cambridge ACE is a suitable screening tool as it includes regular and non-regular words which can help determine the presence of a surface dyslexia. This form of dyslexia is typical of semantic memory impairment, possibly because these words require semantic knowledge of the word in order to read it, unlike regular words or non-words which can be read without understanding the meaning of the word.

Like reading, writing may not require a detailed assessment unless there are specific symptoms or a fairly circumscribed language deficit is suspected. In these situations, assessment of written spelling and sometimes writing of individual letters is required.

Calculation. A few simple tests of calculation can be extremely useful in a bedside assessment, especially in the situation of progressive aphasia where the clinician wish to differentiate between a perisylvian or frontal opercular syndrome. This cognitive function is highly susceptible to the person's previous arithmetic ability, which will have to be taken into consideration in order to interpret the findings but a few simple examples of mental arithmetic will usually suffice.

Visuospatial function. These can be easily assessed at the bedside by asking patients to copy simple line drawings such as the intersecting pentagons from the MMSE or the cube or clock face from the ACE. If there is disproportionate visuospatial impairment further analysis should include examination for features of *Balint's syndrome*. Although it often presents in a partial or impure state, it classically has several components, the most striking of which is simultanagnosia, which refers to the inability to widen a visual focus and synthesize a wider scene. Often described as a narrowed spotlight of attention, subjects may report only one part of a scene and ignore the wider picture. This can be picked up at the bedside by dot counting (as in the ACE) or in describing visual scenes from magazine photographs. The other features of Balint's syndrome include optic ataxia, which is the inability to accurately reach for objects in the absence of limb ataxia and optic apraxia or sticky fixation which is the inability to move the eyes to a target. The neural substrates of Balint's syndrome are invariably bilateral damage to the parieto-occipital cortex which may result from watershed infarcts or from neurodegenerative conditions such as the posterior cortical atrophy variant of Alzheimer's disease.

Praxis is typically defined as the inability to perform skilled motor movements in the absence of any deficit of power or sensation. Although usually associated with lesions in the left parietal lobe, apraxia may also be seen after lesions to the right parietal lobe, frontal lobes and subcortical structures in the basal ganglia. The description of many subtypes of apraxia such as ideational or ideomotor apraxia has led to considerable confusion due to the inconsistency with which different terms are used by different investigators but in practice such differentiations rarely help in differential diagnosis. The most important aspect of bedside assessment is to demonstrate impaired praxis, which, like visuospatial impairment, is rarely seen in purely psychiatric disorders. This can usually be achieved by asking the patient to copy a series of hand gestures, e.g. 'hitchhiking sign', or by asking them to mimic the use of objects e.g. 'show me how you brush your teeth' or 'show me how you comb your hair'. The presence of impairment in praxis usually suggests organic cortical dysfunction.

Executive function refers to those higher order cognitive capabilities that are called upon to formulate new plans of action and to select, schedule and monitor appropriate sequences of action. A lot of these functions are mediated by the dorsolateral prefrontal cortex and the subserving fronto-subcortical circuit. However, other aspects of the prefrontal cortex are also involved in some of these functions, such as the inferior frontal areas, in abilities that relate to impulse control and inhibition.

Although best tested with formal neuropsychological measures, some assessment is possible at the bedside. Verbal fluency, as described above and assessed in the ACE, is invariably impaired in dysexecutive syndromes, particularly phonemic or letter fluency. Studies show that 15 items in one minute represents a normal performance. Less than 10 items is definitely abnormal. Marked and particular impairment in letter fluency is a hallmark of subcortical disorders. Another bedside task of executive function is cognitive estimates where a subject is asked to make an educated guess to a question to which they are not expected to know the exact answer. Examples include 'how many people live in London?', 'how fast can a horse run?', or 'how many camels are there in Holland?'. Patients with marked executive impairment tend to give answers that are completely off the mark such as 3000 people living in London. Proverb interpretation, e.g. 'what is the meaning of the phrase 'people in glass houses shouldn't throw stones'?' can be helpful although a patient's age and cultural background may affect their knowledge of such proverbs. A particular aspect of executive function called response inhibition can be tested with the go-no-go test. In this test the examiner asks the subject to place a finger on the desk. The examiner can then tap with their own finger under the desk either once or twice. The subject is instructed to tap once when the examiner taps twice and to tap twice when the examiner taps once. The examiner then begins a series of taps, either once or twice and switches between the two stimuli. Normal subjects pick up the rules to this quickly and can switch without perseverating in their responses.

It is important to remember that executive functions and 'frontal lobe' functions are not synonymous. Executive impairment can manifest from brain injury outside the frontal lobes. A case in point is the cerebellar affective syndrome where cerebellar injuries produce a range of behavioural and neuropsychological deficits very like those seen in frontal lobe syndromes.

The Neurological Examination in Bedside Cognitive Assessment

Specific neurological signs often accompany cognitive and neurobehavioural disorders and although a full discussion of the relevant neurological examination techniques is outside the scope of this chapter, there are some specific systems that should be examined. These should be taken in the context of the observations made of the patient throughout the consultation regarding speed of movement and thought, speech and other motor deficits.

Eye movements. In the context of the bedside cognitive assessment the most important aspects of the eye movements are to look for evidence of cerebellar dysfunction or of supranuclear gaze palsy. Probably the most sensitive measure of dysfunction of the cerebellar system and its connection to the brainstem is the examination of eye movements and nystagmus should be observed for in lateral gaze, upgaze and downgaze. Pursuit movements refer to the smooth tracking of a target from one side to the other and saccadic movements refer to the rapid movement of the eyes from one target to another. All of these eye movements may be affected in cerebellar disease.

Evidence of impairment of supranuclear gaze can be sought by asking the patient to look up to a target and then down while the examiner gently holds the head still. Restriction of upgaze is common with age and is a non-specific marker for extrapyramidal degenerative syndromes. Impairment of downward saccades, particularly slowed downward saccades may support a suspicion of PSP in the right clinical context.

Extrapyramidal signs The cardinal extrapyramidal signs are bradykinesia, rigidity and involuntary movements such as tremor or chorea. Bradykinesia refers to a gradual decrease in speed of movements with repetition and can be elicited in repetitive hand movements or foot tapping. Limb rigidity is suggestive of parkinsonism and axial rigidity, particularly when accompanied by a history of falls and a supranuclear gaze palsy is suggestive of PSP. The tremor of Parkinson's disease is usually, but not always, more prominent at rest and increases with distraction. Lower limb tremor,

particularly unilateral, is very suggestive of Parkinson's disease. Chorea is usually seen as restless flowing involuntary movements, which if mild may just give the impression of a patient being fidgety and should prompt for further exploration of a family history consistent with Huntington's disease and previous psychoactive drug use. Myoclonus refers to intermittent sudden jerks, usually of the limbs and may be stimulus sensitive. Provocation of stimulus sensitive myoclonus may be with a loud clap out of the patient's field of vision. Alternatively upward flicking movements on the underside of fingers of outstretched hands may elicit myoclonic jerks of the same or even contralateral limb. While myoclonus may be present in many neurodegenerative diseases such as Alzheimer's disease, dementia with Lewy bodies and corticobasal degeneration, it is most commonly associated with prion diseases such as Creutzfeldt-Jacob disease, particularly in the presence of a rapidly progressive dementia.

Primitive reflexes. These reflexes are present in newborn babies and tend to disappear with brain maturation. Their re-emergence in adult life suggests disconnection of the fronto-striatal circuits and hence brain pathology. The grasp reflex refers to the involuntary gripping of the examiner's hand when this stimulates the patient's palm. The examiner must tell the patient to let go off the hand. Often attempted withdrawal of the examiner's hand leads to more pronounced grasping. The pout reflex is elicited by putting an orange stick vertically onto the closed lips of the patient and tapping. Other primitive reflexes such as the glabellar tap or palmomental reflex seem to have less discriminatory value.

CONCLUSIONS

As with all aspects of clinical medicine the history is paramount and should be used to guide the clinician to an initial differential diagnosis that can be refined with the examination. While further diagnostic tests are often necessary after bedside assessment, these are most directed and informative if based on a sound clinical assessment.

During this process it is helpful for the clinician to keep in mind a few cardinal questions that can be answered along the way. What were the first presenting symptoms and how long ago did they really start? How is the patient moving and can this help me? Have I got a reliable witness history? Is the presentation psychiatric or organic? Is the pattern cortical or subcortical and what cognitive domains are involved?

By reference back and forth to these questions during the assessment the clinician can interpret the pattern of deficits of a simple cognitive screening tool such as the MMSE or ACE and add refinements to the examination to probe different cognitive functions in more detail. This should lead to a formulation of 'where' the problem lies in terms of the functional neuroanatomy of the brain, which when considered in the light of the onset and progression of the symptoms, can guide towards an accurate differential diagnosis.

REFERENCES

1. Mathuranath PS, Nestor PJ, Berrios GE, Rakowicz W, Hodges JR. A brief cognitive test battery to differentiate Alzheimer's disease and frontotemporal dementia. *Neurology* 2000 December 12; **55**(11): 1613–20.
2. Larner AJ. Addenbrooke's Cognitive Examination (ACE) for the diagnosis and differential diagnosis of dementia. *Clin Neurol Neurosurg* 2007 July; **109**(6): 491–4.

3. Mitchell J, Arnold R, Dawson K, Nestor PJ, Hodges JR. Outcome in subgroups of mild cognitive impairment (MCI) is highly predictable using a simple algorithm. *J Neurol* 2009 September; **256**(9): 1500–9.

4. Steffens DC, Otey E, Alexopoulos GS, Butters MA, Cuthbert B, Ganguli M *et al*. Perspectives on depression, mild cognitive impairment, and cognitive decline. *Arch Gen Psychiatry* 2006 February; **63**(2): 130–8.

5. Potter GG, Steffens DC. Contribution of depression to cognitive impairment and dementia in older adults. *Neurologist* 2007 May; **13**(3): 105–17.

6. Chan D, Anderson V, Pijnenburg Y, Whitwell J, Barnes J, Scahill R *et al*. The clinical profile of right temporal lobe atrophy. *Brain* 2009 May; **132**(Pt 5): 1287–98.

FURTHER READING

Ancelin ML, Artero S, Portet F *et al*. Non-degenerative mild cognitive impairment in elderly people and use of anticholinergic drugs: longitudinal cohort study. *BMJ* 2006; **332**: 455–9.

Bak TH, Mioshi E. A bedside cognitive assessment beyond the MMSE: the Addenbrooke's Cognitive Examination. *Prac Neurol* 2007; **7**, 245–9.

Bonelli RM, Cummings JL. Frontal-subcortical dementias. *Neurologist* 2008; **14**: 100–7.

Hodges JR. *Cognitive Assessment for Clinicians*. Oxford: Oxford University Press, 1994.

Hodges JR, Patterson K. Semantic dementia: a unique clinicopathological syndrome. *Lancet Neurol* 2007; **6**: 1004–14.

Schott JM, Rossor MN. The grasp and other primitive reflexes. *J Neurol Neurosurg Psychiatry* 2003; **74**: 558–60.

25

Neuropsychological Assessment

Linda Clare

School of Psychology, Bangor University, Bangor, Gwynedd, UK

Neuropsychological assessment offers a rigorous method of identifying the presence, extent and severity of cognitive impairments. Brief observation and informal interaction can yield valuable information about a patient's condition, but this level of assessment does not usually provide a sufficient foundation for evaluating the degree or extent of cognitive difficulties, and may mean that subtle or mild difficulties are missed. Therefore, a more systematic approach to assessing patients' cognitive functioning is often needed. Neuropsychological assessment achieves this aim through the use of standardized tests.

THE USE OF STANDARDIZED TESTS

Standardized tests assess aspects of current functioning in a systematic way, providing results that can be compared with normative data[1]. They are developed with the aim of maximizing reliability and validity; that is, they should provide a consistent measure of the construct of interest. Standardized tests are always administered in the same way, following administration procedures set out in the test manual. Thus, the instructions given to each person taking the test, and all the parameters of the test such as the length of time for which stimuli are presented, are identical. These conditions are exactly the same as those used to obtain data from the reference group or normative sample against which the individual's test scores will be compared, ensuring a valid comparison. Norms typically take into account the effects of age, providing stratified norms for different age groups, and adjustment may be made for other demographic factors that affect test performance, such as level of education. It follows that familiarity with the test procedures is essential in order to administer the test appropriately. Similarly, familiarity with the scientific basis and technical properties of the test, as well as the ability to consider the complex range of factors that may impact on test performance, is necessary for accurate interpretation of test results. For this reason, use of many standardized tests is restricted to those professionals who can demonstrate either by virtue of their professional education or as a result of further training that they are specifically trained in test administration and interpretation.

Neuropsychological assessment of older people combines two traditions of standardized testing: psychometric testing and clinical neuropsychological assessment. These two approaches have been described as *population-based* and *deficit-oriented*, respectively[2]. In practice, the two approaches are typically used alongside one another, with an emphasis on considering patterns of scores across a range of tasks.

Psychometric testing assumes that the ability or factor being tested is normally distributed in the general population, and seeks to establish how the individual's scores relate to those found in a representative sample of that population; for example, whether scores are close to the average for the reference group, or whether they are exceptionally high or low, and thus unusual. The classic example of this would be the measurement of IQ. Standardized tests of this kind typically include items across the range of difficulty, such that there will be some easy items that just about everyone should be able to do and some very challenging items that hardly anyone will be able to answer. Some tests identify different starting and finishing points for different age groups so that a range of items of appropriate levels of difficulty is administered, and some tests have rules specifying that the task should be discontinued in the event of incorrect answers being given on a specified number of items, on the basis that further, more difficult items would not be expected to be answered correctly. Therefore, these tests are suitable for individuals across the ability range and provide a challenging test for even those individuals with the highest levels of ability.

Clinical neuropsychological assessment sets out to determine whether there is evidence of impairment in a particular ability, such that the individual's scores are different to what they would have been if illness or injury had not intervened. This may be determined by comparing performance on abilities thought to be affected by the illness or injury with performance in areas thought to remain intact, or may be inferred from a comparison of the individual's scores with scores obtained by a normative sample, taking into account what would be expected on the basis of the individual's background. In the latter case, normative data will typically have been used to identify a cut-off score, signifying that scores more extreme than this value are unlikely to occur within the normal range. Standardized tests based on this approach rest on the assumption that the normal population will generally perform well and that poor scores are indicative of neurological abnormality.

Scores on standardized tests may be expressed in a number of ways. Most frequently, raw scores are typically converted to either a standard score or percentile rank, allowing comparison across subtests and against norms. The standard scores corresponding to given raw scores on a test are calculated on the basis of normative data collected from a large sample, taking into account the distribution of scores in the sample and the mean level of achievement. Where age is likely to affect performance, the standard scores derived from the raw scores are compared to norms for the relevant age group. The

Principles and Practice of Geriatric Psychiatry, 3rd edn. Edited by Mohammed T. Abou-Saleh, Cornelius Katona and Anand Kumar
© 2011 John Wiley & Sons, Ltd

use of percentile ranks serves a similar purpose, indicating whether a score is in the average range or is very infrequent and therefore unusual. Standard scores provide a consistent scale with a defined mean and standard deviation; for example, in the Wechsler Scale of Adult Intelligence (WAIS-III)[3], a scale with a mean of 100 and a standard deviation of 15 is used. Subtest scores are converted to this scale and overall scores are calculated on the same scale. Scores that are two standard deviations above or below the mean are generally considered exceptional, in that they arise very rarely. Scores of 70 (two standard deviations below the mean of 100) or below occur in approximately 5% or fewer of the population. Some tests use a mean of 10 and a standard deviation of 3; in this case, scores of 5 or below occur only in 5% or fewer of the population.

With tests that use population-based norms, the fact that a score is unusual does not in itself indicate that there is an impairment. The observed score may simply reflect the individual's long-standing ability level: the individual may be one of the 5% of the population who score very poorly on the task. Therefore, information about the expected level of performance is needed in order to interpret the results. If the individual's performance is widely discrepant from what would be expected for that individual, this suggests there may be a difficulty or impairment resulting from illness or injury. In practice, expectations about likely performance are usually based on consideration of a number of factors such as the individual's educational and occupational background and level of achievement. For a very high-achieving individual, a score that is in the low average range may reflect a significant decline from previous, superior performance levels. However, in some cases, tests are available that can provide an estimate of expected performance levels. For example, in the English language, the ability to read irregularly-spelled words can be tested with the Wechsler Test of Adult Reading (WTAR)[4] or the National Adult Reading Test (NART)[5]. Since this is considered a 'crystallized' ability, and fairly resistant to many forms of brain injury as well as the very early signs of dementia, scores on this task can be converted to obtain a predicted score on the WAIS-III[3]. If comparing this predicted score with the observed score yields a significant discrepancy, with the observed score lower than the predicted score, this is suggestive of a decline in overall intellectual functioning. Similarly, a comparison might be made between the WAIS IQ score and the Wechsler Memory Scale (WMS-III)[6] score; normative data are available to indicate whether or not a discrepancy in scores is large enough, and unusual enough, to be considered a significant indicator of an impairment in memory relative to what would be expected on the basis of the IQ score.

With deficit-oriented tests, a score that would be unusual in the reference group is generally considered to provide an indication of impairment, given that the poor score cannot be explained by other, contextual factors. The 5th percentile often provides in effect a cut-off for identifying impairment. Scores at or below the 5th percentile in the normal population may be defined as falling into the impaired range. An example of a test using this approach is the Visual Object and Space Perception Battery[7]. For tests using standard scores, as noted above, a score at or below the 5th percentile approximately translates into a score of 70 or below (on the scale with a mean of 100 and standard deviation of 15) or a score of 5 or below (on the scale with a mean of 10 and standard deviation of 3). Some tests use their own classifications, indicating whether a particular score is 'impaired', 'poor', or 'normal'. An example of a test using this approach is the Rivermead Behavioural Memory Test[8]. Some tests reflect tasks that should be achievable by anyone with normal functioning and thus the presence of errors in itself reflects likely impairments; for example, the Behavioural Inattention Test[9] identifies scores as impaired if they are below those of the lowest performing normal controls.

Provision of appropriate test norms is not straightforward, and this is especially the case with older age-groups (for a fuller discussion of this issue, see Busch et al.[2]). Where tests were initially developed for younger adults, norms for older people may be unavailable, or may relate to a restricted age range. They may be based on more limited sample sizes than those for younger age groups, or may have drawn upon a non-representative sample containing only those highly motivated to assist with research. Some measures have only one set of norms available, while other frequently used measures offer numerous sets of norms among which the clinician can select those that are most appropriate for the patient and for the questions being addressed in the assessment. Details of many of these can be found in the compendium compiled by Strauss et al.[10]. Cultural differences may mean that the available norms are not directly appropriate for the individual; for example, an individual who has grown up in a developing country and immigrated to the United Kingdom or United States as an adult will have had different formative and educational experiences from the indigenous population, and thus norms based on a United Kingdom or United States indigenous population may be inappropriate. This in itself does not necessarily preclude the use of the test, but the lack of appropriate norms will place constraints on the interpretation of results. Availability of neuropsychological tests in languages other than English is limited, and use of interpreters during testing is unsatisfactory, especially where these are family members. Translation of tests is a highly skilled and complex task and cultural, as well as linguistic, equivalence must be established. For a fuller discussion of cultural issues in assessment, see the review by Manly[11].

Comparison with test norms provides an indication of the degree to which the observed score would be infrequent or unusual in a healthy population of the same age. In some cases, this is sufficient to clarify the presence of an impairment in a particular area. However, as noted above, the situation is not always clear-cut. Furthermore, individual test scores elicited on a given occasion may be affected by a range of factors. Some of these relate to the individual, for example low mood, anxiety about being tested, physical health problems, pain, drug effects or fatigue. Some relate to the testing environment, for example uncomfortable seating, inadequate lighting or high levels of noise. Other factors relate to the tests used, for example the extent to which they require dexterity or mobility, whether stimuli are in large enough print to be easily visible, and so forth. The extent to which the assessor is able to build rapport with the individual, and respond to any emotional reactions to the assessment, may influence motivation and willingness to engage. Therefore, individual scores must be interpreted in the context of the overall situation. The neuropsychologist's observations of the individual during testing, and comments on the testing situation, will form an important part of the picture when drawing conclusions based on the test results.

The neuropsychological assessment provides a profile of the individual's strengths and difficulties. This profile may be used to contribute to problem identification or diagnosis, to inform decisions about treatment or management, or to monitor change over time. In so doing, information from the neuropsychological assessment must be considered alongside information obtained from other sources[12]. The pattern of scores on neuropsychological tests is only one part of the picture, and needs to be considered alongside the medical history and the results of other tests, for example those that can detect possible physical causes of cognitive impairment, such as heart disease, vitamin deficiency or infection. It is also important to consider information about functional ability. Although cognitive status is related to functional ability[13], performance on cognitive tests does not fully predict functional ability. Therefore a direct assessment of activities of daily living may be advisable. See Little and Doherty[14] and Chapter 34, for a discussion of assessment of functioning, behaviour and daily living skills. An informant perspective is extremely important and should be obtained wherever possible, with the informant interviewed separately in order to obtain a full account. A home visit can provide valuable insights into the person's living situation and social networks.

If results are unclear, they can be seen as providing a baseline, and testing can be repeated after a suitable interval (e.g. one year) to see if there has been any change. However, repeated testing may give rise to practice effects and therefore needs to be undertaken with a degree of caution, and only in those cases where it is really essential. Some tests provide parallel versions of equivalent difficulty which can be used for repeated testing, for example the Rivermead Behavioural Memory Test[8] and the Test of Everyday Attention[15]. The need for repeated assessment is particularly likely to arise in cases where the aim is to differentiate the very early stages of dementia from normal ageing, given the range of factors that can affect test performance on any given occasion. Sometimes the appropriate outcome of a neuropsychological assessment is a decision to re-evaluate after a period of time has elapsed. While there is sometimes pressure to assign a diagnostic category following initial assessment, it is very important for the sake of the individual and family to avoid the risk of a false-positive diagnosis, and in many cases the best approach is to reassess after a period of time has elapsed in order to monitor the presence or absence of change over time, which in itself may be the most significant diagnostic indicator[1].

AIMS AND SCOPE OF NEUROPSYCHOLOGICAL ASSESSMENT

Usually a neuropsychological assessment will be indicated where information about the cognitive profile will assist in answering a specific question or set of questions. Perhaps the most common situation is the need to distinguish between normal ageing, mild cognitive impairment and the early stages of dementia, or to identify whether cognitive difficulties are the result of depression or mental health issues or an indication of early-stage dementia, or to distinguish between different subtypes of dementia or help identify the precise nature of the progressive neurological condition involved (see also Chapters 42 and 62). An assessment might be required in order to identify the presence and nature of cognitive difficulties following a stroke or in the context of other conditions such as Parkinson's disease. In some cases, information from the neuropsychological assessment may be needed to contribute to decisions about ability to continue driving or about the extent to which the individual has capacity to make specific decisions and choices regarding, for example, medical treatment, financial affairs, or where to live.

When conducting neuropsychological assessment with older people, it is important to have a sound knowledge of the profile of cognitive changes arising as a part of normal ageing, including the underlying neuroanatomy, as well as the diagnostic profiles of the range of relevant neurological and psychiatric disorders and their

behavioural presentation in older people, and an understanding of the potential impact on cognition of neurological injury (for a fuller discussion of these issues, see by Potter and Attix[16]). Special considerations arise with regard to particular groups of older people, such as those with lifelong intellectual disability or those with long-term mental illness, where the availability of suitable tests may be limited and change may be especially difficult to detect (e.g.[17]). It is also necessary to be aware of the way in which neuropsychological factors relate to abilities such as driving or to definitions of capacity (for a fuller discussion, see pp. 175–87 in Zarit and Zarit[1]).

While we typically think of cognitive functions as somewhat discrete entities, such as memory, attention or language, in practice these functions are closely interrelated. Changes in one may be mistaken for problems with another; for example an impairment in attention may mean that information is not encoded, giving the appearance of a problem with memory. Furthermore, if the assessment is contributing to a diagnostic process, sampling just one cognitive function will be inadequate; for example, a diagnosis of Alzheimer's disease requires impairment in memory and at least one other cognitive domain. In most cases, it will be necessary to sample a broad range of cognitive functions. Generally it is the pattern of results across domains that is most informative.

The questions that will be asked are first whether there is an overall decline in cognitive functioning, second whether there are impairments in specific domains and processes; and third, if the answer to either of these is affirmative, whether there are any factors other than neurological impairment that could account for the poor performance. Where neurological impairments are identified, this leads to the questions of what the pattern of impairments suggests, what are the implications for the individual's daily life, and for the family where appropriate; and whether intervention is indicated. If there are factors other than neurological impairment that may be affecting performance, such as depression, then these may be treated prior to reassessment. It is also worth noting that some patients may not show any objective impairment, and in such cases it is necessary to consider the reasons for the expressed concern and how best to respond.

In gathering the necessary information, various approaches can be taken. An extensive standard battery of tests can be applied to every individual, or tests can be selected on an individual basis for each new patient. Most commonly, clinicians use a combination of these two methods. A comprehensive selection of tests that covers the essential cognitive functions and is likely to help in answering the most important kinds of questions can be supplemented by the selection of particular tests that are appropriate for the particular questions raised by the individual patient's profile and that make it possible to follow up on particular hypotheses that the clinician may have developed based on the initial test responses. For example, if initial testing suggests an impairment in language, attention or executive function, further tests can be selected to provide a more detailed profile. It is important to tailor the selection of tests to the level of functioning of the individual patient and the aims of the assessment. Thus, an assessment aimed at identifying very subtle difficulties that might constitute the earliest signs of dementia in a 65 year old would require a challenging and extensive set of tasks, while it would be more appropriate to test a patient who showed more obvious signs of impairment, or who was very frail, with a briefer neuropsychological screening battery, perhaps supplemented by one or two brief tasks.

A comprehensive assessment will usually include an evaluation of general intellectual functioning (IQ). The most widely used test for this purpose is the WAIS-III[3]. This includes seven tests of verbal ability (e.g. vocabulary, comprehension, digit span) and seven tests of performance ability (e.g. block design, picture arrangement, matrix reasoning). The full test is lengthy to administer but an overall score can be obtained by administering selected sub-tests or by using the Wechsler Abbreviated Scale of Adult Intelligence[18]. Alongside this, a test that predicts lifelong optimal level of intellectual functioning, such as the WTAR[4], is usually administered. As discussed above, a significant discrepancy between predicted and current IQ would indicate a decline in current functioning. Several specific cognitive domains will also be assessed, typically visuo-spatial perception, language, attention, executive function (the capacity for abstract thinking, planning, problem-solving and inhibition), and memory. For a full discussion of these areas and of the tests that can be used to assess them, see books by Lezak *et al.*[19] and Strauss *et al.*[10].

Memory assessment will usually cover both long-term memory, comprising episodic memory (memory for personally experienced events) and semantic memory (memory for factual information) and working memory. It may also cover prospective memory (ability to remember future intentions) and autobiographical memory. As well as these types of memory, assessment should consider the processes that constitute memory and learning: registration and encoding of information, storage of information and recall of information. Memory should be tested in various ways including recognition, immediate recall and delayed recall, and in various modalities including visual and verbal. Where there has been a discrete injury or insult, such as a closed head injury or stroke, it is useful to consider whether memory difficulties relate to information acquired before the injury (retrograde) or since the injury (anterograde). One of the most widely used memory assessments is the WMS-III[6], which includes 11 subtests providing scores for general memory, working memory, immediate memory, auditory immediate memory, visual immediate memory, auditory delayed memory, auditory reception delayed and visual delayed memory. As with the WAIS-III[3], the WMS-III is a lengthy test and in some cases it may be appropriate to use only a selection of subtests. Many other tests are available to assess specific aspects of memory, for example the Rey-Osterrieth Auditory Verbal Learning Test (RAVLT)[10] or California Verbal Learning Test (CVLT-II)[20]. The Rivermead Behavioural Memory Test[8] focuses on everyday uses of memory, testing memory through the kinds of activities that require memory skills in daily life.

Visual perception can be assessed with subtests from the Visual Object and Space Perception Battery[7], with figure drawing using the Rey-Osterrieth Complex Figure Test[10], or with the clock drawing test[10]. Language is often assessed through tests of naming such as the Boston Naming Test[21] or Graded Naming Test[22]. Attention can be assessed with subtests from the Test of Everyday Attention, and executive function with subtests from the Delis-Kaplan Executive Function System (D-KEFS)[23], which include trail-making and verbal fluency.

As noted above, neuropsychological screening batteries can be employed where patients have obvious impairments or are unable to complete a full assessment. An example of the latter is the Repeatable Battery for the Assessment of Neuropsychological Status (RBANS)[24]. This includes 12 subtests, providing scores in five categories: immediate memory, delayed memory, attention, language and visuo-spatial/constructional ability. The availability of parallel versions of equivalent difficulty is an advantage where repeated testing is indicated. For people with very marked impairments, the Severe Impairment Battery[25] assesses various aspects of cognition using a range of simple tasks.

THE PROCESS OF NEUROPSYCHOLOGICAL ASSESSMENT

The process of conducting a neuropsychological assessment will be influenced by whether the neuropsychologist works as part of a multidisciplinary team or receives referrals as an individual professional. If working as part of a team, information about medical history and factors such as mental state and mood may be available from the psychiatric examination. These areas may therefore require less extensive evaluation as part of the neuropsychological assessment, although some investigation will still usually be made, and standard questionnaires such as the Hospital Anxiety and Depression Scale[26] or Geriatric Depression Scale[27] (see Chapter 29) may be used. The advantage of teamwork lies in drawing together the results of the neuropsychological assessment with the findings from other aspects of the assessment, including for example functional assessments conducted by an occupational therapist.

In planning a neuropsychological assessment, the first consideration will be to ensure that sufficient time is available. A comprehensive assessment may require several hours' contact with the patient and may need to be conducted over more than one visit. Even a brief assessment using a neuropsychological screening battery may take 1.5–2 hours. The neuropsychologist will require sufficient information to select an appropriate set of tests. It is particularly important for the neuropsychologist to be made aware of any factors that would influence the selection of tests, including illiteracy, sensory impairment, restricted mobility and likelihood of fatigue. It is essential that patients are asked to bring with them reading glasses and hearing aids if they use these. Cultural factors should also be considered. In particular, if English is not the patient's first language, this will place constraints on the assessment. Even if the patient speaks very good English, comparison with norms derived from native speakers is unlikely to be appropriate.

On meeting the patient, the neuropsychologist will be concerned to establish a good rapport and ensure that the patient fully understands the nature and aims of the assessment process. At this stage informal discussion can help to elicit the patient's views about his or her difficulties, about the assessment and about the reasons for attending. If an informant is available, the neuropsychologist will want to talk with him or her individually as well as together with the patient. Patients are often anxious about being tested and worried about giving the wrong answers. It can be helpful to explain to them that the tests are designed to challenge everyone, so there is no expectation that anyone would get all the answers right, and the important thing is just to do the best they can. There is no doubt that patients, especially those in the older age groups, often find the neuropsychological assessment a strange process, but there is no need for it to be aversive if the neuropsychologist is able to develop a good rapport and show sufficient sensitivity. Throughout the assessment the neuropsychologist must be attentive to signs of fatigue and to expressions of frustration or distress. The former can be alleviated by suggesting a short break and offering refreshments, while the latter can be addressed by sequencing tasks so that tests which the patient finds difficult are followed by tasks that can be completed more easily. The neuropsychologist will also carefully observe the patient's reactions and behaviour during the session in order to gain an impression of the patient's level of motivation and awareness, and identify any factors that may have affected performance.

Following the assessment, the neuropsychologist will calculate the patient's scores on the various tests administered, a process which can be quite time-consuming, and will usually prepare a concise but comprehensive report detailing the results of the assessment[28]. This will typically contain the following sections: background to the referral and any relevant history, and the reasons for the assessment; outline of the neuropsychologist's observations of the patient's behaviour and responses during testing; details of the tests administered; profile of results for each domain of cognitive functioning assessed; any additional data such as findings from questionnaires assessing mood; summary and recommendations. In the summary and recommendation section, the neuropsychologist will usually comment on the profile of results and what this implies; for example, he or she may comment that the profile is, or is not, consistent with a diagnosis of Alzheimer's disease. This section will also contain any practical recommendations that the neuropsychologist is able to make regarding how to assist or support the patient and family, or improve management of the patient's condition.

The neuropsychologist will generally aim to meet with the patient, and if appropriate the family as well, to provide feedback on the results of the assessment. Feedback should be tailored to the needs and concerns of the patient and family. In the team context this meeting may be jointly arranged with another professional such as the psychiatrist. In some cases it may be necessary to convey unwelcome news such as the diagnosis of dementia. Diagnostic disclosure should be 'patient led' and based on the individual situation[29]. The process should be conducted sensitively and sufficient time should be allowed to ensure that discussion is not rushed and that the patient and family are able to ask questions. A single meeting may not be adequate and it may be advisable to arrange a follow-up discussion. Emphasis should be placed on linking the patient and family with appropriate support networks and on identifying any possible treatment approaches.

Finally, it is important to emphasize that the scope of the neuropsychological assessment is not restricted to assisting in reaching a diagnosis. Ideally, and perhaps particularly so in the case of older people, the knowledge gained about the patient's strengths and difficulties in cognitive functioning as a result of the neuropsychological assessment will form a basis for offering information and advice about managing the patient's condition or informing the development of a treatment plan[30] based on principles of neuropsychological rehabilitation.

REFERENCES

1. Zarit SH, Zarit JM. *Mental Disorders in Older Adults: Fundamentals of Assessment and Treatment*, 2nd edn. New York: Guilford, 2007.

2. Busch RM, Chelune GJ, Suchy Y. Using norms in neuropsychological assessment of the elderly. In Attix DK, Welsh-Bohmer KM (eds), *Geriatric Neuropsychology: Assessment and Intervention*. New York: Guilford, 2006, 133–57.

3. Wechsler D. *Wechsler Adult Intelligence Scale. Third UK edition (WAIS-III)*. London: Harcourt Assessment, 1999.

4. Wechsler D. *Wechsler Test of Adult Reading (WTAR)*. San Antonio, TX: Harcourt Assessment, 2001.

5. Nelson HE, Willison JR. *National Adult Reading Test*, 2nd edn. Windsor: NFER-Nelson, 1991.

6. Wechsler D. *Wechsler Memory Scale. Third UK edition (WMS-III)*. London: Harcourt Assessment, 1999.

7. Warrington E, James M. *Visual Object and Space Perception Battery*. Bury St Edmunds: Thames Valley Test Company, 1991.

8. Wilson BA, Greenfield E, Clare L et al. *Rivermead Behavioural Memory Test. Third Edition. (RBMT-3)*. London: Harcourt Assessment, 2007.

9. Wilson BA, Cockburn J, Halligan P. *Behavioural Inattention Test (BIT)*. Bury St Edmunds: Thames Valley Test Company, 1987.

10. Strauss E, Sherman EMS, Spreen O. *A Compendium of Neuropsychological Tests: Administration, Norms and Commentary*, 3rd edn. New York: Oxford University Press, 2006.

11. Manly J. Cultural issues. In Attix DK, Welsh-Bohmer KM (eds), *Geriatric Neuropsychology: Assessment and Intervention*. New York: Guilford, 2006, 198–222.

12. Clare L. Neuropsychological assessment of the older person. In Woods WT, Clare L (eds), *Handbook of the Clinical Psychology of Ageing*, 2nd edn. Chichester: John Wiley & Sons Ltd, 2007, 363–83.

13. Marson D, Hebert KR. Functional assessment. In Attix DK, Welsh-Bohmer KM (eds), *Geriatric Neuropsychology: Assessment and Intervention*. New York: Guilford, 2006, 158–97.

14. Little A, Doherty D. Assessing functioning, behaviour and need. In Woods RT, Clare L (eds), *Handbook of the Clinical Psychology of Ageing*, 2nd edn. Chichester: John Wiley & Sons Ltd, 2007, 385–414.

15. Robertson IH, Ward T, Ridgeway V, Nimmo-Smith I. *The Test of Everyday Attention*. Bury St Edmunds: Thames Valley Test Company, 1994.

16. Potter G, Attix DK. An integrated model for geriatric neuropsychological assessment. In Attix DK, Welsh-Bohmer KM (eds), *Geriatric Neuropsychology: Assessment and Intervention*. New York: Guilford, 2006, 5–26.

17. Oliver C, Adams D, Kalsy S. Ageing, dementia and people with intellectual disability. In Woods RT, Clare L (eds), *Handbook of the Clinical Psychology of Ageing*, 2nd edn. Chichester: John Wiley & Sons Ltd, 2007, 341–59.

18. Wechsler D. *Wechsler Abbreviated Scale of Adult Intelligence (WASI)*. London: Harcourt Assessment, 1999.

19. Lezak MD, Howieson DB, Loring DW. *Neuropsychological Assessment*, 4th edn. New York: Oxford University Press, 2004.

20. Delis DC, Kaplan E, Cramer JH, Ober BA. *California Verbal Learning Test, second UK edition (CVLT-II)*. London: Harcourt Assessment, 2000.

21. Kaplan E, Goodglass H, Weintraub S. *Boston Naming Test*. Philadelphia: Lea and Febiger, 1983.

22. Warrington E. The Graded Naming Test: a restandardisation. *Neuropsychol Rehabil* 1997; **7**: 143–46.

23. Delis DC, Kaplan E, Kramer JH. *Delis-Kaplan Executive Function System (D-KEFS)*. London: Harcourt Assessment, 2001.

24. Randolph C. *Repeatable Battery for the Assessment of Neuropsychological Status (RBANS-UK)*. London: Harcourt Assessment, 1998.

25. Saxton J, McGonigle KL, Swihart AA, Boller F. *The Severe Impairment Battery*. Bury St Edmunds: Thames Valley Test Company, 1993.

26. Snaith RP, Zigmond AS. *The Hospital Anxiety and Depression Scale*. Windsor: NFER-Nelson, 1994.

27. Yesavage JA, Brink TL, Rose TL *et al*. Development and validation of a geriatric depression screening scale: a preliminary report. *J Psychiatr Res* 1983; **17**: 37–49.

28. Green J. Feedback. In Attix DK, Welsh-Bohmer KM (eds), *Geriatric Neuropsychology: Assessment and Intervention*. New York: Guilford, 2006, 223–36.

29. Bamford C, Lamont S, Eccles M, Robinson L, May C, Bond J. Disclosing a diagnosis of dementia: a systematic review. *Int J Geriatr Psychiatry* 2004; **19**: 151–69.

30. Clare L. *Neuropsychological Rehabilitation and People with Dementia*. Hove: Psychology Press, 2008.

26

Overview of Rating Scales in Old Age Psychiatry

Kenneth C. M. Wilson, Ben Green and Pat Mottram

Department of Psychiatry, University of Liverpool, UK

SOME OF THE ISSUES

The needs which rating scales are expected to fulfil in the psychiatry of old age differ little from those in other age groups. However there are a few issues, which are worth considering.

The rating of behaviour concerned with the ageing process remains a contentious issue and does not play a significant role in driving the development of rating scales designed for this age group. The main influences have been the problems imposed by the measurement of psychiatric symptoms in the context of co-morbidity and the relatively high prevalence of organic cerebral disease experienced by older people. These two issues have informed the development of numerous rating scales for the assessment of cognition and have led to adaptation and subsequent development from many well-recognised rating scales used for the assessment of functional symptoms in younger people. Both significant physical morbidity and cognitive dysfunction will impact on the design as well as the content of the rating scale. Such rating scales need to be brief, allowing for problems in concentration and fatigue. Data may have to be recruited from sources other than the patient. In addition, it is important to emphasise the influence of age related cultural differences. It is usual for the interviewer to be as much as two generations younger than the interviewee. Such a generation gap will carry with it differing expectations, understandings and experiences.

An interesting example of this is that up to one third of older people say that they do not feel depressive mood when many other symptoms point inevitably to the presence of a depressive syndrome. This is unlike the experience of other age groups. It is tempting to introduce the concept of denial when trying to explain this. However, it is just possible that older people understand the term differently or have, throughout their life described the feeling of depression differently; such as feeling 'empty inside'. If a particular rating scale is weighted so as to emphasise the importance of experiencing depressed mood then it may well not address the experiences of a significant proportion of older people with depressive syndrome.

A well-recognised book, devoted to the compilation of rating scales in old age psychiatry lists well over 200 different rating scales[1]. It is well beyond the scope of this brief overview to provide a comprehensive review of each of these instruments. However, as the field of instrumentation expands it is equally important to draw attention to issues relating to the development and selection of these rating scales.

THE DEVELOPMENT OF A RATING SCALE

A number of approaches have been taken in developing rating scales. Good examples are found in scales designed to rate depression; some are developed from 'gold standard' diagnostic criteria. For example, the OARS Depressive scale[2] is derived from depressive symptoms listed by DSM III diagnosis. Other scales have been developed from already existing rating scales. A good example of this is the Carroll Rating Scale (CRS)[3] which was developed from the Hamilton Depression Rating Scale and the Beck Depression Inventory. Being aware of the developmental source of an individual instrument will inform choice in the context of the purpose and population in which the instrument is to be applied. For example, there are significant and important questions relating to the validity of DSM criteria in the diagnosis of depression in people with other disorders such as Parkinson's disease[11]. This generates the obvious question as to whether rating scales derived from these criteria are suitable for, or have been validated in these specific populations. Likewise, those rating scales that have been developed from other rating scales pose the same questions; have the source rating scales been validated in the target populations? Has there been subsequent validation of the specific rating scale in the relevant population? An obvious example is the use of rating scales for rating depression in patients with dementia. Another lies in the problem of rating depression in people with significant physical illness, where some of the physical illness symptoms, such as appetite loss; may be the same as some of those that are rated as depressive symptoms by the scale.

The same issue relates to rating scales designed to rate cognitive symptoms. The Mini Mental State Examination[4] is probably one of the most commonly used cognitive assessment instruments. Its original purpose was to differentiate organic from functional disorders and was designed to quantify change in cognitive state. Despite its popularity, the instrument does have its critics as a screening instrument[5]. There are two important issues worth highlighting in relation to its use. Firstly, the instrument does not and should not be used to allocate a diagnosis. When used in the context of an acute medical ward, it is as likely to pick up cognitive deficit in people with acute confusional states as a consequence of physical illness as it is to identify cognitive problems associated with dementias. Secondly, the instrument fails to assess all cognitive domains, in particular, failing to address specific deficits relating to frontal cortex. This problem is reflected in the adaptation of the instrument over many years of use.

Principles and Practice of Geriatric Psychiatry, 3rd edn. Edited by Mohammed T. Abou-Saleh, Cornelius Katona and Anand Kumar

A good example of this is the development of the ACE-R[12], which was derived from the Mini Mental State Examination but includes a section addressing frontal lobe assessment.

VALIDITY OF AN INSTRUMENT

Many of the above issues fall within the over-all heading of 'validity'. Proving the validity of an instrument is seminal to its development. The concept addresses a number of issues in which the characteristics of the instrument in terms of its performance are addressed within defined populations. Hence, an instrument may be valid in one setting (or in rating symptoms in one type of population) but may not be valid in another. In testing the validity of an instrument; the degree to which it adequately probes the specific issues that are being rated is tested. Its ability to differentiate between people that are known to be dissimilar is tested, and finally, the instrument is examined in terms of the demonstrating that certain explanatory constructs account to some degree for the performance of the test. From a practical point of view it is critical that the choice of an instrument is informed by evidence of validation in populations similar to those that are intended to be interviewed.

Many rating scales have been developed as potential 'case' finding instruments. Usually a rating scale will generate a numerical 'score', often purported to represent severity of a particular set of signs or symptoms. Common examples include the Geriatric Depression Scale.

The scale is not a diagnostic instrument in that it does not exclude conditions, other than depression, which might affect its performance. However it can be used as a screening instrument in that, using a 'cut-off' score it will identify individuals with a degree of symptom severity that correlates with a depression diagnosis. This is done by examining the sensitivity and specificity of the instrument in relationship to an already established instrument or other clinical criteria. In the case of the full, 30-item Geriatric depression Scale; a cut-off score of 11 has been established[6]. However this is further complicated by subsequent developments of the instrument. There now exist shortened versions of 15, 10 and four items, all of which have different 'cut-offs'. It is self-evident that when choosing an instrument the right 'cut-off' score should be used. Many studies fail to report which version of the instrument is used, making comparisons between studies and study replication very difficult.

RELIABILITY OF THE SCALE

Understanding why the instrument was developed in the first place, the subsequent evolution of the instrument and being aware of the populations in which the instrument has proven validity are critical in informing choice of instrument. The 'Reliability' of the instrument must also be considered. This is a technical term referring to a number of concepts.

Firstly; the internal consistency of an instrument refers to the reproducibility of measurement across different items within the rating scale. The 'test-retest reliability' refers to the likelihood of the instrument producing similar ratings when consecutively conducted on the same patient (assuming the condition being measured has not changed in the intervening period).

Secondly; the inter-rater reliability refers to the likelihood of the instrument producing similar results when delivered by two different interviewers simultaneously. Obviously, the interviewer plays an important role in terms of reliability performance. This issue is generally addressed (particularly in the context of research) through training and standardisation. Unfortunately, this is not common practice in clinical settings. The implications of this can be fairly profound in terms of patient care. Again, taking the example of the Mini Mental State Examination; which is recommended in the rating of change in cognition in the context of prescribing anticholinesterase inhibitors in England and Wales. If the instrument is not used in a standardised way then the generated scores will vary; affecting patient care. However, when used appropriately the reliability is fairly good[7]. Another area of potential concern lies in applying those rating scales employing graded or continuous variables in rating individual items. An example of this is the Nursing Home Behaviour problem Scale[10]. This instrument requires a rating of 'never', 'sometimes', 'often', 'usually' and 'always'. Each of these options is associated with a different score. One of the problems facing the rater will lie in the differentiation between these grades. For example, how does one consistently differentiate between' often' and 'usually'? The answer lies in clear instructions/descriptions and standardisation through training of the raters. A good example of a well-established and reliable instrument of this nature is the BECK Depression Inventory[13] (not specifically designed for older people), which rates each item 0–3. Each score has a brief but clear description associated with it, facilitating high levels of reliability. This is one of many self-rating scales.

DIFFERENT METHODS OF DELIVERY

Another typical example of a self-rating scale, specifically designed for older people is the SELF-CARE D rating scale[9]. It is derived from the Comprehensive Assessment and Referral Evaluation Schedule (CARE)[8] and is used to differentiate between people with and without depression in primary care settings. It takes about 15 minutes to complete. The advantages of using self-rating scales have to be balanced by the disadvantages. Experience suggests that the apparent time and resource savings may be offset by the frequent need to help people complete them. Obviously, the patient population must be able to read the questions (if required) and understand the instructions. The BASDEC is a hybrid rating scale, designed to measure depression in institutionalised settings in which patients may be over-heard or embarrassed by answering sensitive questions out loud. Nineteen cards with statements on are presented to the patient and the patient indicates whether each statement is true or false. Each 'True' answer generates a score of '1', 'don't know' generates a score of half a point and 'false' generates a '0' score.

Some scales are specifically designed to capture information about the patient from other sources. The Cornell Scale for Depression in Dementia has been designed to capture information from informants and through observation[14]. The Dysfunctional Behaviour ~Rating Scale[15] was designed for carers to make observations relating to older people with cognitive impairment. In particular cases, data may be gleaned from either the patient or the rater; as is the case in the 'Quantification of physical illness in psychiatric research in the elderly'[16].

TYPES OF INSTRUMENTS

Even though some rating scales have been developed as screening or 'case finding' instruments; these should not be confused with diagnostic instruments that have been specifically designed to enable an allocation of a standardised diagnosis. Such instruments are usually derived from diagnostic systems such as the International Classification of Diseases (ICD) or the Diagnostic and Statistical Manual (DSM criteria). These are usually semi-structured interviews in which a psychiatric syndrome is established. Importantly, they will often include' exclusion criteria' in which specific psycho-syndromes are excluded as part of the process in establishing a diagnosis. For example, the exclusion of cerebro-vascular disease will influence the certainty by which Alzheimer's Disease may be diagnosed.

Rating scales are specifically designed to rate specific variables and can usually be classified by the nature of the variables that they are designed to rate. This overview has already drawn on rating scales designed to measure depression severity, physical illness severity and behavioural problems in people with cognitive disturbance. There are of course, a wide variety of instruments including those designed more specifically for rating aspects of the dementias, quality of life, morale, issues relating to carers and activities of daily living performance. In addition to the Mini Mental State Examination, there are a number of rating scales designed to rate memory and other aspects of cognition. A good example of a practical and innovative instrument is the IQCODE[17], which is used with an informant to quantify cognitive decline over time. These rating scales should not be confused with formal psychometric assessments usually carried out by experienced and trained psychologists.

RATING SCALE SELECTION

In the first instance it is important to establish why and when a rating scale should be used. Staff on acute medical wards often use rating scales for the identification of patients with dementia and may use these to trigger referral for psychiatric assessment. Often enough, the psychiatrist will be referred a patient in an acute or sub-acute confusional state as a consequence of unstable physical illness. This is a classical mistake in that the rating scale is being used as a surrogate diagnostic instrument for dementia as opposed to a screening instrument for cognitive impairment. Inherent to this, is the question 'what is intended to be measured?'. Once the answer to this question has been established then a rating scale developed and designed to measure particular criteria can be selected. The next issue to determine is whether the rating scale is designed to measure the symptoms in populations similar to that in which it the ratings are intended. Determination of this will go some way in establishing the valid use of the rating scale in any particular setting.

The next question worth considering is whether the rating scale is to be used as a screening instrument or to measure change over time. If used as a screening instrument then it is important to determine the appropriate 'cut-off score'. Again this might be specific to a particular population and may need some background literature research. As already mentioned, rating scales can be completed by the individual target patient or carer, by the interviewer or by a third party and by a mixture of agents. The choice will depend on the reasons why a scale is being used and whether or not the person who is subjected to the interview is able to actively contribute towards the rating.

Other considerations relating to choice include; the length of the procedure. In patients with severe illness or short attention span, long interviews may prove problematic. As already indicated, training is required for some rating scales. This is important in terms of validity, reliability and generalisability of the findings. Research protocols in which rating scales are utilised will often include training and subsequent standardisation and inter-rater reliability sessions over the period of data collection. Lastly, the use of many commonly used rating scales are restricted by copyright.

SUMMARY

This brief overview of the use of rating scales in old age psychiatry has attempted to provide a general background to the development of rating scales, drawing on examples of commonly used rating scales in Old Age Psychiatry. The practical implications of validity and reliability of rating scales have been exemplified in the context of selection of rating scales within this age group. As rating scales develop, health expectations increase and resources become more limited, rating scales may offer an apparent, easy alternative to comprehensive psychiatric assessment. It is important to remember; rating scales are refined and specific and if used inappropriately are likely to cause as much harm as they can good.

REFERENCES

1. Burns A, Lawlor B, Craig S 2004, Assessment scales in Old Age Psychiatry. 2nd Ed. Pubs; Martin Dinitz, London.
2. Blazer D. Thediagnosis of depression in the elderly. *Journal of the American Geriatrics Society* 1980, **28**. 52–58.
3. Carroll BJ, Feinberg M, Smouse PE, Rawson SG, Greden JF. The Carroll rating scale for depression1. Development, reliability and valiodation. *British Journal of Psychiatry* 1981; **1238**: 194–200.
4. Folstein MF, Folstein SE, McHugh PR. Mini MnetalStae; a practyical method for grading the cognitive state of patients for the clinician. *Journal of Psychiatric Research* 1975; **12**: 189–198.
5. Anthony J, LeResche L, Niaz U *et al.* Limits of the Mini mental State as a screening test for dementias and delirium among hospital patients. *Psychological Medicine* 1982; **12**: 397–408.
6. Brink T, Yesavage J, Lum O *et al.* Screening tests for Geriatric depression. *Clinical gerontologist* 1982; **1**: 37–43.
7. Tombaugh TN, McIntyre NJ. The Mini Mental State Examination: a comprehensive review. *Journal of the American geriatrics society* 1992; **40**: 922–35.
8. Guralnd B, Kuriansky J, Sharpe L *et al.* The Comprehensive Assessment and Referral Evaluation (CARE) – rationale, development and relaibilty. *International Journal of Ageing in Human development* 1997; **8**: 9–24.
9. Bird AS, macDonald AJD, Mann AH, Philpot MP. Preliminary experience with the SELFCARE-D: a self rating depression questionnaire for the use in elderly, non-institutionalised subjects. *International Journal of geriatric psychiatry* **2**: 31–8.
10. Taylor R, Lichtenstein MJ, Meador KG. The Nursing Home behaviour Problem Scale. *Journal of gerontology* 1992; **47**: M9–16.

11. Weintraub D, Morales KH, Morberg PJ *et al*. Antidepressant studies in Parkinson's Disease: a review and meta-analysis. *Movement Disorders* 2005; **20**: 1161–1169.

12. Mioshi E, Dawson K, Mitchell J *et al*. The Addenbrooke's Cognitive Examination Revised (ACE-R): a brief cognitive test battery for dementia screening. *Int J Geriatr Psychiatry* 2006; **21**: 1078–1085.

13. Beck AT, Ward CH, Mendelson M, Mock J, Erbaugh J. An inventory for measuring depression. *Archives of General Psychiatry* 1961; **4**: 53–63.

14. Alexopoulos GS, Abrams RC, Young RC, Shamoian CA. Cornell Scale for Depression in Dementia. *Biological Psychiatry* 1988; **23**: 271–84.

15. Molloy DW, McILroy WE, Guyatt GH, Lever JA. Validity and reliability of the Dysfunctional Rating Instrument. *ActaPsychiatricaScandinavica* 1991; **84**: 103–6.

16. Burvill PW, Mowry B, Hall WD. Quantification of physical illness in psychiatric research in the elderly. *International Journal of Geriatric Psychiatry* 1990; **5**: 161–170.

17. Jorm A. The informant questionnaire on cognitive decline in the elderly (IQCODE): A review. *International Psychogeriatrics* 2004; **16.3**: 1–19c.

27

The Mini-Mental State Examination*: A Brief Cognitive Assessment

Marshal Folstein[1], Susan Folstein[1] and Jonathan Folstein[2]

[1]*University of Miami Miller School of Medicine, Nashville, USA*
[2]*Vanderbilt University, USA*

The Mini-Mental Status Examination (MMSE) is a scored, 10-minute form of the traditional cognitive mental status examination. The items include orientation to place and time; registration and recall; attention and calculation; language function; and praxis. It is 'mini' because it tests cognitive aspects of mental functions, but excludes mood, abnormal mental experiences, and the form of thinking[1].

It has been standardized with normative values for age and education and is used by physicians and other clinical professionals worldwide to estimate and communicate the presence and severity of cognitive impairment[2,3]. The easily understandable items are useful for helping subjects and caregivers to understand the overall severity of cognitive impairment, as well as particular areas of deficits. For example, caregivers benefit from knowing that the patient can understand a one-stage command: 'put on your socks', but not a three-stage command: 'put on your socks, your shoes, and your pants'.

We highlight several instructions from the manual. First, a single administration given under supervision is adequate for training. Second, subjects should receive an explanation of why they are being tested and how the answers might help in their care or, in the case of research, accomplish the aim of the study. Third, successes should be praised, but errors ignored to avoid inducing emotions that might lower the subject's cognitive capacity. Fourth, fearful subjects can be reassured by early success by beginning with easier items such as naming a pencil and watch. Finally, we recommend that the serial sevens test be given, followed by world-backwards only if the subject refuses to do serial sevens, or refuses to complete one subtraction. The world task is easier than serial sevens and decreases the sensitivity of the test.

A score below 24 detects cognitive impairment in most populations[4] while a score below 27 suggests the need for an evaluation of individuals with greater than a 10th grade education. The MMSE has significant floor and ceiling effects. Many severely impaired patients score zero and the MMSE does not assess superior cognitive capacity.

The MMSE can be used in any population or cultural group; authorized translations are available from the publisher. The distribution of scores in some populations is lower than those established in the United States. This mainly is due to lower education. In the cultures studied to date, the scores are comparable when education is taken into account. The relationship between education and MMSE reflects social class, nutrition, intelligence and other exposures that affect cognition. Low education is also a risk for some diseases that affect cognition. The MMSE score is thus a snapshot of the end result or composite of the many factors that have influenced cognition over the life span: social class, nutrition, intelligence, disease, and other exposures that have occurred throughout life. If the effects of disease and education are controlled, the effect of age on the MMSE is small.

RELIABILITY AND VALIDITY

The MMSE has excellent test–retest and inter-rater reliability. The MMSE accurately reflects the results of psychological tests and structural and functional measures of brain pathology. For example, the MMSE correlates significantly with the Wechsler Adult Intelligence Scale and many other neuropsychological measures of memory, attention, executive function and language. MMSE has been shown to decline on average 3.3 points per year in Alzheimer's disease and correlates with the severity of pathology found at autopsy or by structural and functional imaging[5]. The MMSE score improves in response to treatments such as donepezil for Alzheimer's disease[6].

The score of MMSE is more similar in elderly identical twins than fraternal twins, suggesting a strong genetic component to the score. By these methods, the MMSE is 50% heritable in older adults from several countries, i.e. genetic factors account for about half the variance in scores.

Low MMSE scores occur with dementia, delirium, mental retardation, cortical and subcortical dementia and discrete cognitive disorders such as amnesia, aphasia and executive dysfunction. Hearing-impaired and vision-impaired subjects obtain lower MMSE scores. However, if instructions are written, MMSE can be used with hearing-impaired persons. Vision is required for only two points on MMSE.

Although the MMSE is often low in frontal/subcortical dementia as occurs in Huntington's disease, Parkinson's disease, AIDS

*Disclosure: The Mini-Mental State Examination (MMSE) and all its authorized translations are published by PAR, from which the authors receive royalties. Manuals and forms are available at Mini-Mental.com.

dementia and frontal dementia, MMSE is less sensitive to early frontal/subcortical than to cortical dementia. Because of these limitations, we have recently published a revision of the MMSE (MMSE~2), which includes tests that are more sensitive to subcortical cognitive impairment. Low MMSE scores occur in elderly depressed patients; many depressed patients with cognitive impairment later show cognitive deterioration. The MMSE can be used to track delirium but because the cognitive state in delirium fluctuates, MMSE reliability and sensitivity are difficult to determine. The reliability and validity of the MMSE has not been established for children or for developmental disorders of cognition.

The MMSE score does not provide a diagnosis, pathology or aetiology, which must instead be established from the patient's history, physical examination and laboratory findings. Nor does the MMSE define competency to perform complex social functions, such as giving informed consent or driving an automobile; these functions must be tested directly.

REFERENCES

1. Folstein MF, Folstein SE, McHugh PR. 'Mini-mental state'. A practical method for grading the cognitive state of patients for the clinician. *J Psychiatr Res* 1975; **12**(3): 189–98.

2. Anthony JC, LeResche L, Niaz U, von Korff MR, Folstein MF. Limits of the 'Mini-Mental State' as a screening test for dementia and delirium among hospital patients. *Psychol Med* 1982; **12**(2): 397–408.

3. Crum RM, Anthony JC, Bassett SS, Folstein MF. Population-based norms for the Mini-Mental State Examination by age and educational level. *JAMA* 1993; **269**(18): 2386–91.

4. Tombaugh TN, McIntyre NJ. The Mini-Mental State Examination: a comprehensive review. *J Am Geriatr Soc* 1992; **40**(9): 922–35.

5. Bancher C, Jellinger K, Lassmann H, Fischer P, Leblhuber F. Correlations between mental state and quantitative neuropathology in the Vienna Longitudinal Study on Dementia. *Eur Arch Psychiatry Clin Neurosci* 1996; **246**(3): 137–46.

6. Wallin AK, Andreasen N, Eriksson S. Donepezil in Alzheimer's disease: what to expect after 3 years of treatment in a routine clinical setting. *Dement Geriatr Cogn Disord* 2007; **23**(3): 150–60.

28

The Informant Questionnaire on Cognitive Decline in the Elderly (IQCODE)

Nicolas Cherbuin[1] and Anthony Francis Jorm[2]

[1]Centre for Mental Health Research, Australian National University, Canberra, ACT, Australia
[2]ORYGEN Research Centre, University of Melbourne, Department of Psychiatry, Parkville, Victoria, Australia

INTRODUCTION

Efficient early detection of cognitive decline and dementia is becoming increasingly important. A large number of screening instruments are available, but they vary greatly in their ease of use, psychometric properties and validity in differing cultural contexts, as well as in the presence of co-morbid conditions. In addition, there is a need for cost-effective screening tests which can be administered to large populations across a variety of mediums (orally, paper and pencil, by mail, by telephone, or by computer).

The Informant Questionnaire on Cognitive Decline in the Elderly (IQCODE) is a brief questionnaire for the assessment of change in cognition which shows very good psychometric properties, has been validated across multiple cultural contexts, and which can be used in clinical practice as well as in large-scale epidemiological studies.

The IQODE was developed to assess cognitive decline from a pre-morbid level based on informant reports[1]. The parent instrument was composed of 39 interview questions assessing memory function (acquisition and retrieval) and intelligence (verbal and performance). Informants were asked to rate the magnitude of change over the previous 10 years in these domains. After initial evaluation, the number of items was reduced to 26 which correlated well together and were relatively easy to rate. The questionnaire was formatted for self-completion and named IQCODE. In its present form the IQCODE requires each item to be rated on a 5-point scale from 1, 'much improved' to 5, 'much worse'[2]. The questions are framed in the form: 'Compared to 10 years ago, how is this person at...' (e.g. remembering things about family and friends such as occupations, birthdays, addresses, etc.).

A short version of the IQCODE consisting of 16 items has been developed[2]. It was found to correlate highly (0.98) with the full version and to have equivalent validity against clinical diagnosis. Consequently there is little advantage in using the longer version.

Versions of the IQCODE have been developed and validated in other languages (Chinese, Dutch, Finnish, French, Canadian French, German, Italian, Japanese, Korean, Norwegian, Persian, Polish, Portuguese, Spanish, and Thai) and copies are available for download at cmhr.anu.edu.au/ageing/iqcode.

Other variations on the IQCODE have also been produced, including questionnaires based on shorter[3,4] or more flexible[5] retrospective time frames, as well as short forms in Spanish[6], Chinese[7], Portuguese[8] and in other languages (which to our knowledge have not been validated).

SCORING

Scoring the IQCODE involves summing the items and dividing by the number of items, thus producing a measure ranging from 1 to 5, however, some investigators have preferred adding up all items. Norms have been developed by Jorm and Jacomb[9] for five-year age groups from 70 to 85+ years, but in practice individual researchers have generally chosen to use an absolute cut-off ranging from 3.3–3.6 in community samples to 3.4–4.0 in patient samples. A practical strategy to choose a cut-off is to identify studies (e.g. in Table 28.1) with characteristics most similar to the target population and select their cut-offs.

ADMINISTRATION

The IQCODE is a pen and paper test which takes between 10 and 25 minutes to complete, depending on the form chosen (long/short) and is generally perceived as relatively easy to answer. It can be mailed to informants and could potentially be administered by telephone or by computer (although we are not aware of any validation data with these administration media). The IQCODE can also be used as an alternative screening test when individuals are not able to complete another test such as the Mini-Mental State Examination (MMSE). In a survey of 839 community-based older individuals, Khachaturian et al.[10] found 74 subjects who were unable to complete the 3 MS but the IQCODE could be completed by an informant. Seventy-one of these were subsequently diagnosed with dementia. In addition, Cherbuin et al.[11] reviewed the literature to assess the suitability of dementia screening instruments for self- or informant-assessment, particularly in an electronic format (local computer or web-based). They concluded that the IQCODE was one of three most

Table 28.1 Performance of the Mini-Mental State Examination (MMSE), and the long and short versions of the IQCODE as a screening test for dementia[47-51]

Study	Sample	Diagnostic criteria[a]	Cutoff	N	Age/Age range	Sensitivy	Specificity	ROC curve
MMSE								
Morales et al. (1997)[14]	Urban epidemiological study (Spain)	1	21/22	97	75	0.73	0.78	–
Morales et al. (1997)[14]	Rural epidemiological study (Spain)	1	21/22	160	74	0.83	0.74	–
Callahan et al. (2002)[47]	Epidemiological study (USA)	1	23/24	344	74	0.95	0.87	0.96
Swearer et al. (2002)[51]	Primary care clinic outpatients and independent retirement community residents (USA)	2	23/24	46	80	0.13	1.00	–
Ferrucci et al. (1998)[48]	Geriatric clinic patients (Italy)	2	23/24	104	75	0.97	0.55	–
Heun et al. (1998)[49]	Epidemiological study (Germany)	1, 4	23/24	287	77	0.84	0.99	–
Jorm et al. (1996)[27]	Ex-servicemen (half former prisoners of war) (Australia)	1	23/24	144	73	0.45	0.99	0.81
Knafelc et al. (2003)[52]	Memory clinic patients (Australia)	1	23/24	323	75	0.84	0.73	0.86
Nasreddine et al. (2005)[50]	Memory clinic patients (Canada)	2	25/26	183	75	0.78	1.00	–
Isella et al. (2006)[21]	Cognitively normal volunteers and 45 MCI patients (Spain)	6	28	100	71	0.82	0.73	–
IQCODE (long version)								
Jorm et al. (1991)[18]	Patients seen by a geriatrician (Australia)	3, 4	3.60+	69	80	0.80	0.82	0.87
Jorm et al. (1994)[40]	Epidemiological study (Australia)	1	3.60+	684	70	0.69	0.80	0.77
Law and Wolfson (1995)[36]	Epidemiological study (Canada)	1	3.30+	237	81	0.76	0.96	–
Fuh et al. (1995)[7]	Non-demented community resident and dementia patients (Taiwan)	1	3.40+	399	69	0.89	0.88	0.91
Morales et al. (1997)[14]	Urban epidemiological study (Spain)	1	3.27+	97	75	0.82	0.90	0.89
Morales et al. (1997)[14]	Rural epidemiological study (Spain)	1	3.31+	160	74	0.83	0.83	0.83
Jorm et al. (1996)[27]	Ex-servicemen (half former prisoners of war) (Australia)	3	3.30+	144	73	0.79	0.65	0.77
Mulligan et al. (1996)[37]	Geriatric patients (Switzerland)	1	3.60+	76	82	0.76	0.70	0.86
Del-Ser et al. (1997)[38]	Neurology clinic outpatients (Spain)	1	3.62+	53	69	0.84	0.73	0.81
Flicker et al. (1997)[53]	Memory clinic patients (young, Australia)	1, 5	3.9	299	73	0.74	0.71	–
Flicker et al. (1997)[53]	Memory clinic patients (old, Australia)	1, 5	3.9	78	80	0.79	0.78	–
De Jonghe (1997)[12]	Psychiatric patients (49 with dementia) (Netherlands)	1	3.90+	82	78	0.88	0.79	–
Senanarong et al. (2001)[54]	Community elderly (Thailand)	2	All	87	52–85	–	–	0.93
Lim et al. (2003)[55]	Cognitively normal volunteers and 53 dementia patients (Singapore)	2	3.40+	153	–	0.94	0.94	–
Stratford et al. (2003)[56]	Memory clinic patients (Australia)	4	4.00+	577	73	–	–	0.82
Tang et al. (2003)[15]	Stroke patients (China)	2	3.40+	189	68	0.88	0.75	0.88
Isella et al. (2006)[21]	Cognitively normal volunteers and 45 MCI patients (Spain)	6	3.45	100	71	0.84	0.75	–
IQCODE (short version)								
Jorm (1994)[2]	Epidemiological study (Australia)	1	3.38	684	70+	0.79	0.82	0.85
Jorm et al. (1996)[27]	Ex-servicemen (half former prisoners of war) (Australia)	3	3.38+	144	73	0.75	0.68	0.77
Del-Ser et al. (1997)[38]	Neurology clinic outpatients (Spain)	1	3.88	53	69	0.79	0.73	0.77
Harwood et al. (1997)[57]	Medical inpatients (England)	1	3.44	177	65+	1.00	0.86	–
Knafelc et al. (2003)	Memory clinic patients (Australia)	1	3.60+	323	44–93	0.94	0.47	0.82
Narasimhalu et al. (2007)[58]	Dementia clinic patients and stroke patients (Singapore)	2	3.38+	576	66	0.78	0.86	0.89

[a] 1 = DSM-IIIR dementia; 2 = DSM-IV dementia; 3 = ICD-9; 4 = ICD-10 dementia; 5 = Clinical diagnosis; 6 = Mild cognitive impairment (Petersen 1996 criteria).

promising tools and they recommended further validation studies for these delivery platforms.

PSYCHOMETRIC CHARACTERISTICS

The IQCODE's reliability and validity have been extensively researched. A number of studies have assessed the internal consistency of the scale using Cronbach's alpha. Alpha was found to range between 0.93 and 0.97 across nine studies[1,7,9,12-17] which can be regarded as excellent. The stability of scores over short periods was found to be high, with test–retest reliability showing correlations of 0.96 over three days and 0.75 over one year[9,18].

Other studies have conducted factor analyses to investigate the factor structure of the IQCODE. They all found a large main factor accounting for 42–73% of the variance which is thought to represent 'cognitive decline', while other factors were generally small with the second factor explaining less than 10% of the variance[7,9,13,14,17,19].

VALIDATION AGAINST CLINICAL DIAGNOSIS

Many studies have assessed the validity of the IQCODE against clinical diagnosis. Table 28.1 contrasts measures of sensitivity and specificity of the long and short forms of the IQCODE and the MMSE[11,20] and shows comparable findings for the two tests, confirming that the IQCODE is a valid screen for dementia. However, moderate correlations between the IQCODE and the MMSE in 15 studies ranging from −0.37 to −0.78[20] with a sample size weighted average of −0.58 suggest that these two tests, although largely overlapping, each have some unique variance. As a consequence, a number of studies have investigated whether the concurrent administration and scoring of the IQCODE and the MMSE improves dementia detection. They generally reported somewhat increased sensitivity and/or specificity of the combined tests, but cost-benefits of this combination varied depending on the methodology or the type of sample used[20]. The IQCODE has also been investigated as a predictor of conversion to mild cognitive impairment over three years and was found to be as sensitive as the MMSE for this population (sensitivity 0.82, specificity 0.71 for a cut-off of 3.19)[21].

In addition, the IQCODE has been shown to be a predictor of incident dementia in stroke patients[22] and in non-demented hospital inpatients[23] over 2–3 years follow-up. However, application of the IQCODE to complex clinical populations should be considered carefully, as one study found that the IQCODE and the MMSE were poor at detecting dementia in a sample of first-ever stroke patients[24].

VALIDATION AGAINST NEUROPATHOLOGY AND NEUROIMAGING

Diagnoses of dementia based on post-mortem histological examinations have been compared to pre-mortem IQCODE scores in two studies. Using a cut-off of 3.7 and a neuropathological diagnosis of Alzheimer's disease, Thomas et al.[25] found the IQCODE to have a sensitivity of 73% and a specificity of 75%. While Rockwood et al.[26], with a cut-off of 3.42 and a diagnosis of Alzheimer's disease, vascular or mixed dementia, reported a sensitivity of 97% and a specificity of 33%. Another six studies found associations between neuroimaging measures and the IQCODE. Jorm et al.[27] found significant associations between the IQCODE and the width of the third ventricle ($r = 0.29$), and infarcts in the left ($r = 0.35$)

and right ($r = 0.26$) hemispheres in a community sample of older ex-servicemen. Cordoliani-Mackowiak et al.[28] reported significant correlations between leukoaraiosis ($r = 0.38$) and IQCODE in elderly stroke patients. Henon et al.[29] found significantly higher mean IQCODE measures in individuals with smaller medial temporal lobe measures. And in a diffusion tensor imaging study of stroke patients, Viswanathan et al.[30] detected lower diffusion measures in the non-affected hemisphere, which were interpreted as showing decreased cerebral tissue integrity in those whose pre-morbid cognition was below a cut-off of 3.4 on the IQCODE. High scores on the IQCODE have also been associated with greater cerebral atrophy[31,32].

BIAS AND LIMITATIONS

One complicating issue associated with many cognitive tests is that they can be open to bias when applied to specific sociodemographic, ethnic, language, gender, clinical or cultural groups. For example, scores on the most widely used dementia screening test, the MMSE, have been shown to be affected by gender, age, education, cultural background, language spoken at home, socioeconomic status, occupation and presence of a mood disorder[33,34]. The IQCODE has been shown to be minimally influenced by education[2,7,9,12,35-38] and by proficiency in the language of the country of residence[39]. However, small associations between the IQCODE and anxiety and depression have been reported[14,37,38,40]. They may be due to a direct link between mood disorders and cognitive function or to the fact that the informant may have difficulty differentiating between cognitive decline and depression and anxiety.

In addition, the influence of informant characteristics has also been investigated as possible bias. Jorm et al.[41] found that measures of informant anxiety, depression and their perception of how caring or controlling the subject was perceived to be were more strongly correlated with IQCODE scores than with the MMSE score. This suggests some contamination of the informant's ratings by the respondent's characteristics but these influences appear to be relatively weak and account for less than 6% of the variance in IQCODE scores. In contrast, the length and type of relationship and the age and education of the informant have not been found to be associated with the IQCODE[7,42].

OTHER APPLICATIONS

Although the IQCODE was developed to assess cognitive decline from a premorbid state, it has also been used for other purposes. Priner and colleagues[43] assessed the short form of the IQCODE as a screen for the prediction of postoperative delirium following hip or knee surgery and found that those with a score greater than 3.1 had a more than 12-fold increased risk of delirium. In another study, the premorbid cognitive status of stroke patients was assessed retrospectively with the IQCODE and those with a score greater than 4 were found to be at higher risk of developing epileptic seizures[44] and of dying[45]. Pasquini et al. also investigated the risk of institutionalization in stroke patients[46] and found that those with an IQCODE score greater than 4 at admission had a higher risk of being institutionalized three years later.

Finally, the feasibility of using the IQCODE as a self-report instrument has been investigated by Jensen et al.[16] who administered the questionnaire by mail to 2841 individuals (58.9% of target population) initially recruited during general practice visits. They found that more than 60% reported completing the questionnaire without help and, although responses were not validated against full clinical diagnoses, mean IQCODE scores were higher (3.7 versus 3.3) in patients suspected of having dementia by their GP and the authors commented 'the IQCODE-SR meets the basic requirements of a good measurement'.

CONCLUSION

The IQCODE is a valid screening instrument for dementia and cognitive decline. It is particularly useful in assessing individuals with less proficient language skill, lower education levels or different cultural background or when direct cognitive testing is not possible. Its administration in conjunction with other tests (e.g. MMSE) can improve overall detection rates. Its ease of use and format make it suitable for use in clinical settings as well as in large epidemiological studies.

Acknowledgements

Cherbuin is funded by the National Health and Medical Research Council (NHMRC) Fellowship No. 418020. Jorm was supported by an NHMRC Fellowship

REFERENCES

1. Jorm AF, Korten AE. Assessment of cognitive decline in the elderly by informant interview. *Br J Psychiatry* 1988; **152**: 209–13.
2. Jorm AF. A short form of the Informant Questionnaire on Cognitive Decline in the Elderly (IQCODE): Development and cross-validation. *Psychol Med* 1994; **24**: 145–53.
3. Barba R, Martinez-Espinosa S, Rodriguez-Garcia E, Pondal M, Vivancos J, Del Ser T. Poststroke dementia: clinical features and risk factors. *Stroke* 2000; **31**: 1494–501.
4. Pisani MA, Inouye SK, McNicoll L, Redlich CA. Screening for preexisting cognitive impairment in older intensive care unit patients: use of proxy assessment. *J Am Geriatr Soc* 2003; **51**: 689–93.
5. Patel P, Goldberg D, Moss S. Psychiatric morbidity in older people with moderate and severe learning disability. II: The prevalence study. *Br J Psychiatry* 1993; **163**: 481–91.
6. Morales JM, Gonzalez-Montalvo JI, Bermejo F, Del-Ser T. The screening of mild dementia with a shortened Spanish version of the 'Informant Questionnaire on Cognitive Decline in the Elderly.' *Alzheimer Dis Assoc Disord* 1995; **9**: 105–11.
7. Fuh JL, Teng EL, Lin KN et al. The Informant Questionnaire on Cognitive Decline in the Elderly (IQCODE) as a screening tool for dementia for a predominantly illiterate Chinese population. *Neurology* 1995; **45**: 92–96.
8. Perroco T, Damin AE, Frota NA et al. Short IQCODE as a screening tool for MCI and dementia. *Dement Neuropsychol* 2008; **2**: 300–304.
9. Jorm AF, Jacomb PA. The Informant Questionnaire on Cognitive Decline in the Elderly (IQCODE): socio-demographic correlates, reliability, validity and some norms. *Psychol Med* 1989; **19**: 1015–22.
10. Khachaturian AS, Gallo JJ, Breitner JC. Performance characteristics of a two-stage dementia screen in a population sample. *J Clin Epidemiol* 2000; **53**: 531–40.
11. Cherbuin N, Anstey KJ, Lipnicki DM. Screening for dementia: a review of self- and informant-assessment instruments. *Int Psychogeriatr* 2008; **20**: 431–58.
12. de Jonghe JF. Differentiating between demented and psychiatric patients with the Dutch version of the IQCODE. *Int J Geriatr Psychiatry* 1997; **12**: 462–65.
13. Jorm AF, Scott R, Jacomb PA. Assessment of cognitive decline in dementia by informant questionnaire. *Int J Geriatr Psychiatry* 1989; **4**: 35–39.
14. Morales JM, Bermejo F, Romero M, Del-Ser T. Screening of dementia in community-dwelling elderly through informant report. *Int J Geriatr Psychiatry* 1997; **12**: 808–16.
15. Tang WK, Chan SS, Chiu HF et al. Can IQCODE detect poststroke dementia? *Int J Geriatr Psychiatry* 2003; **18**: 706–10.
16. Jansen AP, Van Hout HP, Nijpels G et al. Self-reports on the IQCODE in Older Adults: A Psychometric Evaluation. *J Geriatr Psychiatry Neurol* 2008; **21**: 83–92.
17. Butt Z. Sensitivity of the informant questionnaire on cognitive decline: an application of item response theory. *Neuropsychol Dev Cogn B Aging Neuropsychol Cogn* 2008; **15**: 642–55.
18. Jorm AF, Scott R, Cullen JS, MacKinnon AJ. Performance of the Informant Questionnaire on Cognitive Decline in the Elderly (IQCODE) as a screening test for dementia. *Psychol Med* 1991; **21**: 785–90.
19. de Jonghe JF, Schmand B, Ooms ME, Ribbe MW. [Abbreviated form of the Information Questionnaire on Cognitive Decline in the Elderly]. *Tijdschr Gerontol Geriatr* 1997; **28**: 224–29.
20. Jorm AF. The Information Questionnaire on Cognitive Decline in the Elderly (IQCODE): a review. *Int Psychogeriatr* 2004; **16**: 275–93.
21. Isella V, Villa L, Russo A, Regazzoni R, Ferrarese C, Appollonio IM. Discriminative and predictive power of an informant report in mild cognitive impairment. *J Neurol Neurosurg Psychiatry* 2006; **77**: 166–71.
22. Henon H, Pasquier F, Durieu I et al. Preexisting dementia in stroke patients. Baseline frequency, associated factors, and outcome. *Stroke* 1997; **28**: 2429–36.
23. Louis B, Harwood D, Hope T, Jacoby R. Can an informant questionnaire be used to predict the development of dementia in medical inpatients? *Int J Geriatr Psychiatry* 1999; **14**: 941–45.
24. Srikanth V, Thrift AG, Fryer JL et al. The validity of brief screening cognitive instruments in the diagnosis of cognitive impairment and dementia after first-ever stroke. *Int Psychogeriatr* 2006; **18**: 295–305.
25. Thomas LD, Gonzales MF, Chamberlain A, Beyreuther K, Master CL, Flicker L. Comparison of clinical state, retrospective informant interview and the neurpathologic diagnosis of Alzheimer's disease. *Int J Geriatr Psychiatry* 1994; **9**: 233–36.
26. Rockwood K, Howard K, Thomas VS et al. Retrospective diagnosis of dementia using an informant interview based on the Brief Cognitive Rating Scale. *Int Psychogeriatr* 1998; **10**: 53–60.
27. Jorm AF, Broe GA, Creasey H et al. Further data on the validity of the Information Questionnaire on Cognitive Decline in the Elderly (IQCODE). *Int J Geriatr Psychiatry* 1996; **11**: 131–39.
28. Cordoliani-Mackowiak MA, Henon H, Pruvo JP, Pasquier F, Leys D. Poststroke dementia: influence of hippocampal atrophy. *Arch Neurol* 2003; **60**: 585–90.
29. Henon H, Pasquier F, Durieu I, Pruvo JP, Leys D. Medial temporal lobe atrophy in stroke patients: relation to pre-existing dementia. *J Neurol Neurosurg Psychiatry* 1998; **65**: 641–47.

30. Viswanathan A, Patel P, Rahman R et al. Tissue microstructural changes are independently associated with cognitive impairment in cerebral amyloid angiopathy. Stroke 2008; 39: 1988–92.

31. Klimkowicz A, Dziedzic T, Polczyk R, Pera J, Slowik A, Szczudlik A. Factors associated with pre-stroke dementia: the Cracow stroke database. J Neurol 2004; 251: 599–603.

32. Mok V, Wong A, Tang WK, Lam WW et al. Determinants of prestroke cognitive impairment in stroke associated with small vessel disease. Dement Geriatr Cogn Disord 2005; 20: 225–30.

33. Tombaugh TN, McIntyre NJ. The Mini-Mental State Examination: a comprehensive review. J Am Geriatr Soc 1992; 40: 922–35.

34. Anderson TM, Sachdev PS, Brodaty H, Trollor JN, Andrews G. Effects of sociodemographic and health variables on Mini-Mental State Exam scores in older Australians. Am J Geriatr Psychiatry 2007; 15: 467–76.

35. Christensen H, Jorm AF. Effect of premorbid intelligence on the Mini-Mental State and IQCODE. Int J Geriatr Psychiatry 1992; 7: 159–60.

36. Law S, Wolfson C. Validation of a French version of an informant-based questionnaire as a screening test for Alzheimer's disease. Br J Psychiatry 1995; 167: 541–44.

37. Mulligan R, Mackinnon A, Jorm AF, Giannakopoulos P, Michel JP. A comparison of alternative methods of screening for dementia in clinical settings. Arch Neurol 1996; 53: 532–36.

38. Del-Ser T, Morales JM, Barquero MS, Canton R, Bermejo F. Application of a Spanish version of the 'Informant Questionnaire on Cognitive Decline in the Elderly' in the clinical assessment of dementia. Alzheimer Dis Assoc Disord 1997; 11: 3–8.

39. Bruce DG, Harrington N, Davis WA, Davis TM. Dementia and its associations in type 2 diabetes mellitus: the Fremantle Diabetes Study. Diabetes Res Clin Pract 2001; 53: 165–72.

40. Jorm AF. A short form of the Informant Questionnaire on Cognitive Decline in the Elderly (IQCODE): development and cross-validation. Psychol Med 1994; 24: 145–53.

41. Jorm AF, Christensen H, Henderson AS, Jacomb PA, Korten AE, Mackinnon A. Informant ratings of cognitive decline of elderly people: relationship to longitudinal change on cognitive tests. Age Ageing 1996; 25: 125–29.

42. Jorm AF, Broe GACH, Sulway MR et al. Further data on the validity of the Informant Questionnaire on Cognitive Decline in the Elderly (IQCODE). Int J Geriatr Psychiatry 1996; 11: 131–39.

43. Priner M, Jourdain M, Bouche G, Merlet-Chicoine I, Chaumier JA, Paccalin M. Usefulness of the short IQCODE for predicting postoperative delirium in elderly patients undergoing hip and knee replacement surgery. Gerontology 2008; 54: 116–19.

44. Cordonnier C, Henon H, Derambure P, Pasquier F, Leys D. Influence of pre-existing dementia on the risk of post-stroke epileptic seizures. J Neurol Neurosurg Psychiatry 2005; 76: 1649–53.

45. Henon H, Durieu I, Lebert F, Pasquier F, Leys D. Influence of prestroke dementia on early and delayed mortality in stroke patients. J Neurol 2003; 250: 10–16.

46. Pasquini M, Leys D, Rousseaux M, Pasquier F, Henon H. Influence of cognitive impairment on the institutionalisation rate 3 years after a stroke. J Neurol Neurosurg Psychiatry 2007; 78: 56–59.

47. Callahan CM, Unverzagt FW, Hui SL, Perkins AJ, Hendrie HC. Six-item screener to identify cognitive impairment among potential subjects for clinical research. Med Care 2002; 40: 771–81.

48. Ferrucci L, Del Lungo I, Guralnik JM et al. Is the telephone interview for cognitive status a valid alternative in persons who cannot be evaluated by the Mini Mental State Examination? Aging (Milano) 1998; 10: 332–38.

49. Heun R, Papassotiropoulos A, Jennssen F. The validity of psychometric instruments for detection of dementia in the elderly general population. Int J Geriatr Psychiatry 1998; 13: 368–80.

50. Nasreddine ZS, Phillips NA, Bedirian V et al. The Montreal Cognitive Assessment, MoCA: a brief screening tool for mild cognitive impairment. J Am Geriatr Soc 2005; 53: 695–99.

51. Swearer JM, Drachman DA, Li L, Kane KJ, Dessureau B, Tabloski P. Screening for dementia in 'real world' settings: The Cognitive Assessment Screening Test: CAST. Clin Neuropsychol 2002; 16: 128–35.

52. Knafelc R, Lo Giudice D, Harrigan S, Cook R, Flicker L, Mackinnon A, Ames D. The combination of cognitive testing and an informant questionnaire in screening for dementia. Age Ageing 2003; 32: 541–47.

53. Flicker L, Logiudice D, Carlin JB, Ames D. The predictive value of dementia screening instruments in clinical populations. Int J Geriatr Psychiatry 1997; 12: 203–209.

54. Senanarong V, Assavisaraporn S, Sivasiriyanonds N et al., The IQCODE: an alternative screening test for dementia for low educated Thai elderly. J Med Assoc Thai 2001; 84: 648–55.

55. Lim HJ, Lim JP, Anthony P, Yeo DH, Sahadevan S. Prevalence of cognitive impairment amongst Singapore's elderly Chinese: a community-based study using the ECAQ and the IQCODE. Int J Geriatr Psychiatry 2003; 18: 142–48.

56. Stratford JA, LoGiudice D, Flicker L, Cook R, Waltrowicz W, Ames D. A memory clinic at a geriatric hospital: a report on 577 patients assessed with the CAMDEX over 9 years. Aust N Z J Psychiatry 2003; 37: 319–26.

57. Harwood DM, Hope T, Jacoby R. Cognitive impairment in medical inpatients. I: Screening for dementia – is history better than mental state? Age Ageing 1997; 26: 31–35.

58. Narasimhalu K, Lee J, Auchus AP, Chen CP. Improving detection of dementia in Asian patients with low education: combining the Mini-Mental State Examination and the Informant Questionnaire on Cognitive Decline in the Elderly. Dement Geriatr Cogn Disord 2008; 25: 17–22.

29

Geriatric Depression Scale

Meghan A. Marty, Renee Pepin, Andrea June and Daniel L. Segal

University of Colorado at Colorado Springs, USA

The Geriatric Depression Scale (GDS) is a popular and well-validated screening measure for depression among older adults. It consists of 30 self-report items and is widely used in research and clinical services. This chapter provides an overview of its development, psychometric properties, alternate forms, and use with special populations.

DEVELOPMENT, ADMINISTRATION AND SCORING

The GDS was developed to address the limited applicability of existing depression scales with older adults[1,2]. One such problem with scales that were developed and validated with younger populations relates to somatic complaints. Though somatic complaints can be a useful indicator of depression in younger samples, it is common for older adults to report somatic problems that can skew the sensitivity and specificity of a screen where older adults are more likely to have false positive depression scores. As such, the GDS does not include many somatic components in the scale and also consists of questions that are appropriate for the ageing population both in content and format. Initially, 100 questions were selected by researchers and clinicians with geriatric experience and administered to both non-depressed and depressed older adults. Of the original 100 items, the 30 items that correlated most highly with the total score were included in the final scale.

The scale was designed so that it could be administered easily in a self-rating format that would not be cumbersome for patients or medical personnel[2]. Most individuals complete the GDS in under 10 minutes. The GDS has a forced-choice response format where individuals are asked to respond *yes* or *no* to each item. However, some patients have problems with the yes/no dichotomy, instead preferring to answer 'sometimes' by either writing it in or by circling the space between the yes and no responses, though neither is a scored answer. It can help if explicit instructions are provided to patients to respond to each item in the way that *best* answers the question. In the initial validation study, the examiner read the items orally and recorded responses for individuals who could not complete the form without assistance. However, later studies found significant differences between mean scores for self-administered and staff-administered modes of presentation, with higher scores reported for self-administered scales[3,4]. There is no significant difference between scores of a card-based administration and verbal administration of the GDS[5].

For each of the 30 GDS items, the depressive response garners 1 point for a maximum total of 30 points. Regarding general cut-offs, total scores ranging from 0 to 9 indicate normal mood; scores ranging from 10 to 19 indicate mild depressive symptoms, and scores ranging from 20 to 30 indicate severe depressive symptoms. The measure is free to use and in the public domain. It can be accessed at www.stanford.edu/~yesavage/GDS.html.

PSYCHOMETRIC PROPERTIES

Reliability

The GDS has been shown to be internally consistent and reliable over time. In the original reliability study, split-half and alpha coefficients were both 0.94[2]. Other studies have demonstrated similar findings with diverse populations, showing alpha and split-half coefficients ranging from 0.80 to 0.99[6-8]. Several studies have examined reliability of scores over time, finding high test–retest correlations between 0.85 and 0.94[2,7-9].

Validity

An important psychometric property of a depression screen is its ability to differentiate between depressed and non-depressed individuals (i.e. criterion validity). The sensitivity of the GDS refers to its ability to correctly identify individuals who are depressed whereas the specificity refers to its ability to correctly identify those individuals who are not depressed. Brink *et al.*[1] found an 84% sensitivity rate and a 95% specificity rate for the GDS among community-dwelling older adults. Several other studies have examined the sensitivity and specificity of the GDS with diverse populations, finding acceptable levels above 80%. These have included medical patients, stroke patients, individuals suffering from dementia, nursing home residents, and psychiatric inpatients (for a thorough review, see Stiles and McGarrahan[10]).

The correlation between the GDS and other screening measures for depression is an indicator of the scale's construct validity. The GDS was initially validated against the Hamilton Rating Scale for Depression[11] (HRS-D) and the Zung Self-Rating Depression Scale[12] (SDS), finding high correlations suggesting that the GDS measures similar constructs as the HRS-D and SDS. Other comparisons with the GDS have also been conducted, including the Beck Depression

Inventory[13] (BDI) and the Center for Epidemiological Studies Depression Scale[14] (CES-D). These comparisons also yielded significant correlations, adding to evidence supporting the construct validity of the GDS[15-18]. Furthermore, the GDS has non-significant correlations with measures of cognition, adding to the empirical evidence that the GDS measures depression and not another construct[19-21].

Dimensionality

Factor studies on the 30 items of the GDS have yielded mixed results. Sheikh et al.[22] proposed a five-factor solution among community-dwelling older adults. Abraham and colleagues[23] proposed a six-factor solution among nursing home residents. These studies contrast the findings from Parmelee et al.[9] and Salamero and Marcos[24], which both found the GDS items to be highly intercorrelated and suggested the scale has only one factor. Based on these results, both advised the GDS should only be interpreted from a single total score.

ALTERNATE FORMS

Brief Forms

Several brief forms of the GDS have been designed for use in settings where time is limited for depression assessment and with frail individuals for whom fatigue and poor concentration are concerns. Sheikh and Yesavage[25] developed a 15-item version of the GDS, commonly referred to as the Short Form (GDS-SF), by taking the 15 items from the original scale that had the highest correlation with depressive symptoms in earlier studies. Findings from their validation study suggested both forms were highly correlated ($r = 0.84$) and effectively differentiated depressed from non-depressed individuals. A subsequent study reported cut-off scores for the GDS-15 as *normal* (0–4), *mild* (5–9) and *moderate to severe* (10–15)[26]. Older adults rated the GDS-15 as an acceptable measure that was not difficult or stressful to complete[27].

Evidence for the validity of the GDS-15 is mixed. Some studies suggest the GDS-15 is not a suitable substitute for the full scale GDS in community-dwelling older adults[26,28] or cognitively impaired individuals[29]. It does appear effective for screening depression in older adults who are cognitively intact and medically ill[29], have affective disorders[30], or who are seen in primary care clinics[27,31]. The GDS-15 was shown to consistently identify depressed individuals in a VA nursing home population[32]. Chiang and colleagues[33] suggest that the GDS-15 may be less effective as a screening tool, but that it could be most effectively used to detect changes in moderate levels of depression.

Hoyl and colleagues[34] developed a five-item GDS for use in a geriatric outpatient population by selecting items from the GDS-15 that had the highest correlation with a clinical diagnosis of depression. Using a score of 2 or greater to indicate possible depression, the GDS-5 had a sensitivity of 97%, specificity of 85%, and alpha coefficient of 0.80. The GDS-5 was found to be as effective as the GDS-15 in an Italian sample of cognitively intact older adults across three settings: a geriatric acute care ward, a geriatric outpatient clinic and a nursing home[35]. In addition, validity of the GDS-5 has been demonstrated for older sedentary adults[36]. Weeks and colleagues[37] compared two versions of four-item GDS measures and the GDS-5 to the GDS-15 in a sample of acute care patients. They found the GDS-5 showed the highest sensitivity (97%), but led to a high number of false positives. The researchers re-ordered the GDS-15 items

into a two-tiered instrument, named the GDS-5/15, so that the full GDS-15 would only be administered to individuals who scored a 2 or greater on the initial GDS-5 items[37].

Many brief forms of the GDS have been compared to a single-item depression screen. For example, D'Ath et al.[27] created three versions of the GDS containing 10 items, 4 items, or 1 item ('Do you feel that your life is empty?'). While the 10-item form performed well using either 2/3 or 3/4 cut-off scores, the 4- and 1-item versions had low sensitivity and specificity. Hoyl et al.[34] found a single-item depression screen ('Do you often feel sad or depressed?') performed significantly worse than the 15- and 5-item GDS, with a sensitivity of 85% and specificity of 65%. Likewise, a comparison of different versions of the GDS in a Dutch population found the diagnostic value of 30-, 15-, 10- and 4-item scales did not differ significantly; however, the 1-item version performed no better than chance[38]. Almeida and Almeida[39] determined the 15- and 10-item scales were good screening instruments for depression in a Brazilian population, but cautioned against using 4- and 1-item forms because of low reliability and failure to show severity of depressive episodes.

Nursing Home Forms

A 12-item GDS was created for use with individuals living in residential care settings, including those with cognitive impairment (GDS-12R)[40]. During administration of the longer GDS in residential care facilities, interviewers found difficulties with a few of the items that appeared irrelevant or ambiguous to residents (e.g. 'Do you prefer staying in rather than going out and doing new things?'). Removal of these items increased internal reliability from 0.76 to 0.81, with no significant difference in internal reliability for those with cognitive impairment. A cut-off score of 4/5 maximized both sensitivity and specificity of the GDS-12R and was suggested for research purposes. A cut-off of 3/4 was suggested for clinical use[40].

Similarly, Jongenelis et al.[41] developed a version of the GDS that would be more user-friendly for nursing home residents. Clinical experts (a psychologist, a physician and a nurse) reviewed and rated the usefulness of the items of the GDS-15, eliminating seven items that were presumed to be offensive or confusing to nursing home residents. The eight-item instrument demonstrated high internal consistency (alpha coefficient of 0.80) with equal sensitivity (96.3%) and greater specificity than the GDS-15 (71.7% versus 63.3%) at a cut-off point of 2/3. They concluded that although the GDS was created for older adults, it was not necessarily designed for frail nursing home residents and alternate versions perform better with this specific population[41].

Collateral Forms

Nitcher et al.[42] created a 30-item Collateral Source Geriatric Depression Scale (CS-GDS) by simply changing the pronouns from *you* to *they* on the original GDS items. Patients with cognitive functioning ranging from normal to moderate dementia and an informant with extensive personal knowledge about the patient completed a self-report version of the GDS-30 and the CS-GDS respectively. Informants reported a higher frequency of symptomatic responses for all symptoms, but both versions were consistent with an independent diagnosis of depression. Correlations between the CS-GDS and the GDS varied by familial relation, ranging from 0.55 for sons to 0.32 for daughters-in-law. A cut-off score of 21 maximized sensitivity and specificity (both at 68%). In addition, the CS-GDS has been shown to maintain adequate reliability and validity when administered via telephone, using a cut-off score of 19[43].

Brown and Schinka[44] developed a 15-item informant version of the GDS (GDSI-15) for use as an adjunctive measure to self-report versions of the GDS or as an independent measure of depression. Cognitively intact older adults and an informant completed a self-report version of the GDS-30 and the 30-item CS-GDS, respectively. Item characteristics for all 30 items of the CS-GDS were examined; the same items used in the original version of the GDS-15 were found to have the best scale characteristics for the shortened informant version. Consistent with findings from the CS-GDS, informant scores were significantly higher than patient scores and had a 0.55 correlation with the self-report GDS-15. A cut-off score of 5 for the GDSI-15 was found to be optimal[44].

USE WITH SPECIAL POPULATIONS

Long-Term Care

The GDS has been shown to be a reliable and valid instrument for identifying depressed nursing home residents[8,45,46]. Abraham et al.[23] demonstrated that the factor structure of the GDS represents six common facets of depression in nursing home residents: life dissatisfaction, dysphoria, hopelessness/decreased self-attitude, rumination/anxiety, social withdrawal/decreased motivation, and decreased cognition.

Compared to a visual analogue scale, which required participants to mark their level of depression on a line, the GDS was better able to predict ratings of depression by a psychologist, particularly with residents with better cognitive functioning[47]. These researchers slightly modified four items of the GDS to be tailored to nursing home residents. Heiser[48] found the GDS was better at detecting depression in nursing home residents than the Minimum Data Set.

Targeting the concern of nursing home residents being too frail to complete a multiple item scale, Jongenelis et al.[49] evaluated the diagnostic accuracy of the GDS (30-, 15-, 12-, 10-, 5-, 4- and 1-item versions) among nursing home residents. Scales with greater than or equal to four items were useful for screening depression, but scales with lower numbers of items had less specificity. That is, scales with 4 items were able to detect major depression, but 10 items were necessary to effectively detect milder depression.

In a similar study, researchers[50] examined various versions of the GDS (30-, 15- and 8-item) and compared them to the Montgomery Asberg Depression Rating Scale (MADRS)[51]. Using the same data set utilized in the study by Jongenelis et al.[41] mentioned previously, not surprisingly, the authors found a similar pattern of results from the various forms of the GDS. They found the GDS was preferable to the MADRS due to the ease of administration; however, the MADRS, a longer instrument, was superior to all GDS versions in detecting depression in nursing home residents.

Cognitive Impairment

Several studies suggest that the accuracy of the GDS decreases as the level of cognitive impairment increases[29,47,52–54]. The majority of these authors (with the exception of Burke et al.[52]) suggest that the GDS can be used with older adults with mild to moderate cognitive impairment. A more preferable type of screen may involve the reporting of a collateral source such as the Cornell Scale for Depression in Dementia[54] (CSDD) or the informant versions of the GDS.

Some authors[54,55] propose shifting the cut-off score (between 4 and 6) when using the GDS with a cognitively impaired individual.

Primary Care

A large study[56] of older adult primary care patients found the GDS to be reliable and valid in this population. A systematic review[57] of nine studies of the GDS in primary care settings found high sensitivity (ranging from 79% to 100%) and adequate specificity (ranging from 67% to 80%). Bijl et al.[31] examined the cut-off score of 5 in primary care patients and reported adequate sensitivity (79%) and specificity (67%). These positive results suggest that use of the GDS provides reliable and accurate depression screening in primary care settings[58].

Oldest-Old Individuals

De Craen et al.[59] examined the sensitivity and specificity of the GDS-15 in adults aged 85 years and older. Results indicated a low cut-off point (2/3) had high sensitivity (100%) and adequate specificity (68%). Findings from another study with adults aged 85 and older demonstrated that the GDS was able to detect increases in depressive symptoms after negative life events such as the loss of a spouse[60]. This suggests that the GDS is an appropriate measure to use for assessing longitudinal changes in older adults. A comparison between the GDS-15 and the General Health Questionaire-12[61] (GHQ-12) in Chinese old-old adults found the GDS-15 had higher reliability and higher sensitivity[62].

Ethnic Groups

The GDS has been evaluated in several different ethnic groups both within and outside of the US, with mixed results. It has shown to be a satisfactory screening tool in Chinese[63], Portuguese[64], Iranian[65] and Japanese American older adults[66]. Results from a study comparing Korean and American older adults indicated the GDS-SF had good reliability with both groups, but the underlying factor structure differed[67]. Costa and colleagues[68] found that reliability was good for the GDS, but it did not perform better than the GHQ-12[61] and neither was an ideal screening tool for Brazilian older adults even with adjustment of cut-off scores.

SUMMARY

Use of the GDS for the screening and detection of depression among older adults is widespread. As with any psychological measure, test performance of the GDS varies depending upon population characteristics (e.g. individuals with different levels of cognitive functioning). Brief forms of the GDS, as well as versions designed for specific populations (e.g. residents in nursing homes), detect depressive symptoms as well as, if not better than, the original GDS. Further research is needed to explore the factor structure of the GDS. The GDS remains a popular and well-validated screening tool for diverse older adult clinical and research settings.

REFERENCES

1. Brink TL, Yesavage JA, Lum O et al. Screening tests for geriatric depression. *Clin Gerontol* 1982; **1**: 37–44.

2. Yesavage JA, Brink TL, Rose TL *et al*. Development and validation of a geriatric depression screening scale: a preliminary report. *J Psychiatr Res* 1983; **17**: 37–49.

3. Cannon BJ, Thaler T, Roos S. Oral versus written administration of the Geriatric Depression Scale. *Aging Ment Health* 2002; **6**: 418–22.

4. O'Neill D, Rice I, Blake P, Walsh JB, Coakley D. The Geriatric Depression Scale: rater-administered or self-administered? *Int J Geriatr Psychiatry* 1992; **7**: 511–15.

5. Brewer L, Connolly R, Smith D, O'Neill D. The Geriatric Depression Scale: feasibility of cardbased-administration. *Ir J Psychol Med* 2002; **19**: 132.

6. Agrell B, Dehlin O. Comparison of six depression rating scales in geriatric stroke patients. *Stroke* 1989; **20**: 1190–94.

7. Brink TL, Curran P, Dorr ML *et al*. Geriatric Depression Scale reliability: order, examiner, and reminiscence effects. *Clin Gerontol* 1985; **3**: 57–60.

8. Lesher EL. Validation of the Geriatric Depression Scale among nursing home residents. *Clin Gerontol* 1986; **4**: 21–8.

9. Parmelee PA, Lawton MP, Katz IR. Psychometric properties of the Geriatric Depression Scale among the institutionalized aged. *J Consult Clin Psychol* 1989; **1**: 331–8.

10. Stiles PG, McGarrahan PF. The Geriatric Depression Scale: a comprehensive review. *J Clin Geropsychol* 1998; **4**: 89–110.

11. Hamilton M. A rating scale for depression. *J Neurol Neurosurg Psychiatry* 1960; **23**: 56–62.

12. Zung WWK. A self-rating depression scale. *Arch Gen Psychiatry* 1965; **12**: 63–70.

13. Beck A, Ward C, Mendelson M, Mock J, Erbaugh J. An inventory for measuring depression. *Arch Gen Psychol* 1961; **4**: 561–71.

14. Radloff LS. The CES-D scale: a self-report depression scale for research in the general population. *Appl Psychol Meas* 1977; **1**: 385–401.

15. Brink TL, Niemeyer L. Assessment of depression in college students: Geriatric Depression Scale versus Center for Epidemiological Studies Depression Scale. *Psychol Rep* 1992; **71**: 163–6.

16. Hickie C, Snowdon J. Depression scales for the elderly: GDS, Gilleard, Zung. *Clin Gerontol* 1987; **6**: 51–3.

17. Hyer L, Blount J. Concurrent and discriminant validities of the Geriatric Depression Scale with older psychiatric patients. *Psychol Rep* 1984; **54**: 611–16.

18. Norris JT, Gallagher DE, Wilson A, Winograd CH. Assessment of depression in geriatric medical outpatients: the validity of two screening measures. *J Am Geriatr Soc* 1987; **35**: 989–95.

19. Feher EP, Larrabee GJ, Cook TH. Factors attenuating the validity of the Geriatric Depression Scale in a dementia population. *J Am Geriatr Soc* 1992; **40**: 906–9.

20. Parmelee P, Katz IR, Lawton MP. The relation of pain to depression among institutionalized aged. *J Gerontol A Biol Sci Med Sci* 1991; **46**: P15–21.

21. Rapp SR, Parisi SA, Walsh DA, Wallace CE. Detecting depression in elderly medical inpatients. *J Consult Clin Psychol* 1988; **56**: 509–13.

22. Sheikh JI, Yesavage JA, Brooks JO, III *et al*. Proposed factor structure of the Geriatric Depression Scale. *Int Psychogeriatr* 1991; **3**: 23–8.

23. Abraham IL, Wofford AB, Lichtenberg PA, Holroyd S. Factor structure of the Geriatric Depression Scale in a cohort of depressed nursing home residents. *Int J Geriatr Psychiatry* 1994; **9**: 611–17.

24. Salamero M, Marcos T. Factor study of the Geriatric Depression Scale. *Acta Psychiatr Scand* 1992; **86**: 283–6.

25. Sheikh JI, Yesavage JA. Geriatric Depression Scale (GDS): recent evidence and development of a shorter version. *Clin Gerontol* 1986; **5**: 165–73.

26. Alden D, Austin C, Sturgeon R. A correlation between the Geriatric Depression Scale long and short forms. *J Gerontol B Psychol Sci Soc Sci* 1989; **44**: 124–5.

27. D'Ath P, Katona P, Mullan E, Evans S, Katona C. Screening, detection and management of depression in elderly primary care attenders. I: The acceptability and performance of the 15 item Geriatric Depression Scale (GDS15) and the development of short versions. *Fam Pract* 1994; **11**: 260–66.

28. Ingram F. The short Geriatric Depression Scale: a comparison with the standard form in independent older adults. *Clin Gerontol* 1996; **16**: 49–56.

29. Burke WJ, Roccaforte WH, Wengel SP. The short form of the Geriatric Depression Scale: a comparison with the 30-item form. *J Geriatr Psychiatry Neurol* 1991; **4**: 173–8.

30. Herrmann N, Mittmann N, Silver IL *et al*. A validation study of the Geriatric Depression Scale short form. *In J Geriatr Psychiatry* 1996; **11**: 457–60.

31. Bijl D, van Marwijk HWJ, Adèr HJ, Beekman ATF, de Haan M. Test-characteristics of the GDS-15 in screening for major depression in elderly patients in general practice. *Clin Gerontol* 2005; **29**: 1–9.

32. Aikman GG, Oehlert ME. Geriatric Depression Scale: long form versus short form. *Clin Gerontol* 200; **22**: 63–70.

33. Chiang KS, Green KE, Cox EO. Rasch analysis of the Geriatric Depression Scale-Short Form. *Gerontologist* 2009; **49**: 262–75.

34. Hoyl MT, Alessi CA, Harker JO *et al*. Development and testing of a five-item version of the Geriatric Depression Scale. *J Am Geriatr Soc* 1999; **47**: 873–8.

35. Rinaldi P, Mecocci P, Benedetti C *et al*. Validation of the five-item Geriatric Depression Scale in elderly subjects in three different settings. *J Am Geriatr Soc* 2003; **51**: 694–8.

36. Marquez DX, McAuley E, Motl RW *et al*. Validation of the Geriatric Depression Scale-5 scores among sedentary older adults. *Educ Psychol Meas* 2006; **66**: 667–5.

37. Weeks SK, McGann PE, Michaels TK, Penninx BWJH. Comparing various short-form Geriatric Depression Scales leads to the GDS-5/15. *J Nurs Scholarsh* 2003; **35**: 133–7.

38. van Marwijk HWJ, Wallace P, de Bock GH *et al*. Evaluation of the feasibility, reliability, and diagnostic value of shortened versions of the Geriatric Depression Scale. *Br J Gen Pract* 1995; **45**: 195–9.

39. Almeida OP, Almeida SA. Short versions of the Geriatric Depression Scale: a study of their validity for the diagnosis of a major depressive episode according to the ICD-10 and DSM-IV. *Int J Geriatr Psychiatry* 1999; **14**: 858–65.

40. Sutcliffe C, Cordingley L, Burns A *et al*. A new version of the Geriatric Depression Scale for nursing and residential home populations: the Geriatric Depression Scale (Residential) (GDS-12R). *Int Psychogeriatr* 2000; **12**: 173–81.

41. Jongenelis K, Gerritsen DL, Pot AM *et al*. Construction and validation of a patient- and user-friendly nursing home version of the Geriatric Depression Scale. *Int J Geriatr Psychiatry* 2007; **22**: 837–42.

42. Nitcher RL, Burke WJ, Roccaforte WH, Wengel SP. A collateral source version of the Geriatric Depression Rating Scale. *Am J Geriatr Psychiatry* 1993; **1**: 143–52.

43. Burke WJ, Rangwani S, Roccaforte WH *et al.* The reliability and validity of the collateral sources version of the Geriatric Depression Rating Scale administered by telephone. *Int J Geriatr Psychiatry* 1997; **12**: 288–94.

44. Brown LM, Schinka JA. Development and initial validation of a 15-item informant version of the Geriatric Depression Scale. *Int J Geriatr Psychiatry* 2005; **20**: 911–18.

45. Gerety MB, Williams JW, Mulrow CD *et al.* Performance of case-finding tools for depression in the nursing home: influence of clinical and functional characteristics and selection of optimal threshold scores. *J Am Geriatr Soc* 1994; **42**: 1103–9.

46. Soon JA, Levine M. Screening for depression in patients in long-term care facilities: a randomized controlled trial of physician response. *J Am Geriatr Soc* 2002; **50**: 1092–9.

47. Snowdon JS, Lane F. Use of Geriatric Depression Scale by nurses. *Aging Ment Health* 1999; **3**: 227–33.

48. Heiser D. Depression identification in the long-term care setting: the GDS vs. the MDS. *Clin Gerontol* 2004; **27**: 3–18

49. Jongenelis K, Pot AM, Eisses AMH *et al.* Diagnostic accuracy of the original 30-item and shortened versions of the Geriatric Depression Scale in nursing home patients. *Int J Geriatr Psychiatry* 2005; **20**: 1067–74.

50. Smalbrugge M, Jongenelis L, Pot AM, Beekman ATF, Eefsting JA. Screening for depression and assessing change in severity of depression. Is the Geriatric Depression Scale (30-, 15- and 8-item versions) useful for both purposes in nursing home patients? *Aging Ment Health* 2008; **2**: 244–8.

51. Montgomery SA, Asberg M. A new depression scale designed to be more sensitive to change. *Br J Psychiatry* 1979; **143**: 382–9.

52. Burke WJ, Houston MJ, Boust SJ, Roccaforte WH. Use of the Geriatric Depression Scale in dementia of the Alzheimer type. *J Am Geriatr Soc* 1989; **37**, 856–60.

53. Debruyne H, Van Buggenhout M, Le Bastard N *et al.* Is the geriatric depression scale a reliable screening tool for depressive symptoms in elderly patients with cognitive impairment? *Int J Geriatr Psychiatry* 2009; **24**: 556–62.

54. Kørner A, Lauritzen L, Abelskov K *et al.* The Geriatric Depression Scale and the Cornell Scale for Depression in Dementia. A validity study. *Nord J Psychiatry* 2006; **60**: 360–64.

55. Schreiner AS, Hayakawa H, Morimoto T, Kakuma T. Screening for late life depression: cut-off scores for the Geriatric Depression Scale and the Cornell Scale for Depression in Dementia among Japanese subjects. *Int J Geriatr Psychiatry* 2003; **18**: 498–505.

56. Friedman B, Heisel MJ, Delavan RL Psychometric properties of the 15-item Geriatric Depression Scale in functionally impaired, cognitively intact, community-dwelling elderly primary care patients. *J Am Geriatr Soc* 2005; **53**: 1570–76.

57. Watson LC, Pignone MP. Screening accuracy for late-life depression in primary care: a systematic review. *J Fam Pract* 2003; **52**: 956–64.

58. Peach J, Koob JJ, Kraus MJ. Psychometric evaluation of the Geriatric Depression Scale (GDS): supporting its use in health care settings. *Clin Gerontol* 2001; **23**: 57–67.

59. de Craen AJM, Heeren TJ, Gussekloo J. Accuracy of the 15-item Geriatric Depression Scale (GDS-15) in a community sample of the oldest old. *Int J Geriatr Psychiatry* 2003; **18**: 63–6.

60. Vinkers, DJ, Gussekloo J, Stek ML, Westendorp RGJ, van der Mast RC. The 15-item Geriatric Depression Scale (GDS-15) detects changes in depressive symptoms after a major negative life event. The Leiden 85-plus study. *Int J Geriatr Psychiatry* 2004; **19**: 80–84.

61. Goldberg DP. *Detection of Psychiatric Illness by Questionnaire.* London: Oxford University Press, 1972.

62. Boey KW, Chiu HFK. Assessing psychological well-being of the old-old: a comparative study of GDS-15 and GHQ-12. *Clin Gerontol* 1998; **19**: 65–75.

63. Boey KW. The use of the GDS-15 among the older adults in Beijing. *Clin Gerontol* 2000; **21**: 49–75.

64. Pocinho MTS, Farate C, Dias CA, Lee TT, Yesavage JA. Clinical and psychometric validation of the Geriatric Depression Scale (GDS) for Portuguese elders. *Clin Gerontol* 2009; **32**: 223–36.

65. Malakouti SK, Fatollahi P, Mirabzadeh A, Salavati M, Zandi T. Reliability, validity, and factor structure of the GDS-15 in Iranian elderly. *Int J Geriatr Psychiatry* 2006; **21**: 588–93.

66. Iwamasa GY, Hilliard KM, Kost CR. The Geriatric Depression Scale and Japanese American older adults. *Clin Gerontol* 1998; **19**: 13–24.

67. Jang Y, Small BJ, Haley WE. Cross-cultural comparability of the Geriatric Depression Scale: comparison between older Koreans and older Americans. *Aging Ment Health* 2001; **5**: 31–7.

68. Costa E, Barreto SM, Uchoa E *et al.* Is the GDS-30 better than the GHQ-12 for screening depression in elderly people in the community? The Bambui health aging study (BHAS). *Int Psychogeriatr* 2006; **18**: 493–503.

30

Dementia Care Mapping

Dawn Brooker

University of Worcester Association for Dementia Studies, Institute of Health and Society, University of Worcester, Worcester, UK

INTRODUCTION

Dementia Care Mapping (DCM)[1,2] is an observational tool that has been used in formal dementia care settings such as hospital wards, care homes and day care facilities since 1991. Its main uses are:

- at an individual clinical level to elucidate situations where an individual is displaying distress behaviours or to improve well being;
- as an instrument of practice development for shifting the culture of care to one that is person-centred rather than task focused;
- as a tool in research to assess quality of care and quality of life.

DCM is grounded in the theoretical perspective of a person-centred approach to dementia care. Person-centred care values all people regardless of age and health status, is individualized, emphasizes the perspective of the person with dementia and stresses the importance of relationships[3]. DCM originated from the pioneering work of the late Professor Tom Kitwood in person-centred approaches to dementia care. In his final book[4] Kitwood described DCM as: 'a serious attempt to take the standpoint of the person with dementia, using a combination of empathy and observational skill' (p. 4).

THE DEVELOPMENT OF DCM

Tom Kitwood and his PhD student Kathy Bredin developed the original tool through ethological observations of many hours in nursing homes, hospital facilities, and day care facilities in the United Kingdom[1]. It was designed primarily as a tool to develop person-centred care practice over time with data being fed back to care teams who could then use it to improve their practice. The original development work is not available in the public domain[5].

DCM has been through a number of changes since its inception. From 1991 to 1997, the first publically available version, DCM 6th edition, was used. This was revised based on feedback from practitioners in the UK resulting in the 7th edition being launched in 1997. The unexpected death of Tom Kitwood in 1998 created a need to have more formalized structures around DCM. The role of strategic lead for DCM was created at the University of Bradford in 2001 which the author fulfilled until 2009. The formal network of DCM trainers and the DCM International Implementation Group had their inaugural meetings in 2001 and 2002 respectively. DCM underwent a further major revision 2002–2004 drawing on the international perspectives. In 2005 DCM 8 was launched. The revised tool (DCM 8) was validated against DCM 7th edition[6].

The DCM tool is only available through undertaking a registered courses delivered by licensed trainers using standardized training methods. Those undertaking the basic DCM training course (3–4 days duration) do not need any formal qualification although the complexity of the method requires reasonable numeracy and literacy skills. DCM is not aligned to a particular discipline. There are a number of different levels of training that have developed over the years to equip users of DCM at a variety of different levels.

DCM training has been available in the UK since 1991. The worldwide spread of DCM has been remarkable. Tom Kitwood taught the first DCM course outside the United Kingdom in the United States in 1998. In the same year, the materials were translated into German and training commenced there. Australia ran its first course in 2001. The Danish translation and the first course in Denmark took place in 2002. Training has been available in Switzerland with support from Germany since 2002. The materials were translated into Japanese and the first basic course took place in Japan in 2003. Translation into Korean occurred a couple of years later. Spanish and Catalan translations were completed in 2009. At the time of going into press the translations into Flemish, Dutch and Italian are being done. Strategic partnerships exist between the University of Bradford and organizations in all these countries to ensure that training in DCM adheres to international quality standards. At time of going into press there are approximately 8000 people trained at basic level worldwide.

The DCM International Implementation Group is an association of all those countries where DCM training is offered or who are preparing to offer training. Its purpose is to consider the training, care practice and research associated with DCM drawing on expertise from around the world and ensuring a common set of quality standards.

DCM has grown in popularity over the years. Many practitioners have used DCM in many different situations and continue to do so. This may be because DCM appears to provide a vehicle for those wishing to systematically move dementia care from primarily a custodial and task-focused model into one that focuses on the well-being of people living with dementia. There are very few other tools that purport to do this or that have been shown to be effective in this endeavour. Whether it has had a sustained impact on practice is difficult to assess. The investment of time and effort in undertaking training and sustaining mapping cycles can be a barrier in practice.

Principles and Practice of Geriatric Psychiatry, 3rd edn. Edited by Mohammed T. Abou-Saleh, Cornelius Katona and Anand Kumar
© 2011 John Wiley & Sons, Ltd

There has been no survey of how many care providers actually use DCM in practice. A survey undertaken some years ago indicated that around 50% of people undertaking the training actually used mapping in practice although many more reported a beneficial impact on their own practice of undertaking the training[7].

THE DCM TOOL

During a DCM evaluation, an observer (mapper) tracks five people with dementia (participants) continuously over a representative time period. Observation takes place in communal areas of care facilities. Guidelines are provided during training about how to observe in a way that does not increase the ill-being of people with dementia. After each 5-minute period (a time frame) two types of codes are used to record what has happened to each individual. The behavioural category code (BCC) describes one of 23 different domains of participant behaviour that has occurred.

Based on behavioural indicators, a judgement is also made of the relative state of affect and engagement experienced by the person with dementia. This is called a mood/engagement value (ME value) and is rated on a scale ranging from -5 (extreme negative state) to $+5$ (extreme positive state. ME values are averaged over the mapping period to arrive at a well- and ill-being score (WIB score). This provides an index of relative well-being for a particular time period for an individual or a group. Being in a state of well-being is defined as experiencing a preponderance of positive over negative experiences and feelings over a period of time. Therefore, for a person with dementia, experiencing relative well-being would relate to experiencing more of the indicators of well-being over a period of time than the indicators of ill-being.

Personal detractions (PDs) and personal enhancers (PEs) are recorded whenever they occur. PDs are staff behaviours that have the potential to undermine the personhood of those with dementia. These are described and coded according to type and severity. PEs are staff behaviours that are thought to enhance personhood. These are described and coded according to type and the degree to which it is thought they enhance personhood.

From published papers on DCM[8] there is consistency of what is reported in DCM data. In long-term care facilities, behaviour codes indicating social interaction, passive watching, and eating and drinking appear as the most frequent codes almost without exception. Codes for walking and sleeping appear as the next most frequently cited. In facilities with lower well-being scores, withdrawn and repetitive behaviours are frequently seen. In facilities with higher well-being scores, creative activity, physical exercise and general leisure activities occur more frequently. Generally, a greater diversity of behaviour and higher well-being scores are reported in day-care facilities. These scores both increase generally during periods of therapeutic activity. Higher levels of personal detractions occur in those facilities with the lowest well-being scores.

LENGTH OF OBSERVATION PERIOD

Most of the published studies here have mapped continuously for 6 hours, although those using DCM for practice-development purposes mapped for longer[9-12]. It also is evident from practice that useful insights can be gained from mapping for just a couple of hours[13]. Mapping an individual at a particular time of day may throw light on the causes and triggers of distress behaviours. Length of maps will depend, in part, on the reason for mapping. Sometimes mapping

is spread over a couple of days. This can have the advantage of sampling a greater amount of variety of staffing situations but some of the continuity may be lost at an individual participant level. For research purposes, a statistically significant correlation between the hour prior to lunch and a 6-hour map on all their key indicators at the group level has been described[14]. It is likely that there would be more variation for individual level data.

Maps above 4 hours' duration have been reported to correlate well with longer maps but that those below 4 hours do not[6]. When comparing maps over time it is important to try to map for the same time period to ensure that the same opportunities are available for activity on both occasions. Mapping over a meal time will increase levels of activity for example. So if on the first occasion of mapping, only one meal time is observed it is important to ensure only one meal time is observed on the second occasion.

WHAT DCM EVALUATES

The DCM tool provides in-depth detail about the following:

- variations in individual and group care facility levels of well-being and ill-being;
- how people with dementia spend their time and how this is linked to relative well- and ill-being; and
- staff behaviour that promotes personhood and staff behaviours that undermine personhood.

DCM tells us about the quality of care as it impacts on the quality of life of those living in dementia care settings. Within Kitwood's writing was the assumption that, for people with dementia, well-being is a direct result of the quality of relationships they enjoy with those around them. The interdependency of the quality of the care environment to the relative quality of life experienced by people with dementia is central to person-centred care practice. In placing DCM in the taxonomy of measures of quality of life and quality of care, DCM attempts to measure elements of both. In its BCCs and WIBs, DCM measures relative well-being, affect, engagement and occupation, which are important elements of quality of life. Through PDs and PEs, DCM records the quality of care practice as it promotes or undermines the personhood of those being mapped.

In terms of concurrent validity with other measures there is some evidence that DCM is related to indicators of quality of care[9,15] and with proxy quality-of-life measures[14,16]. With persons with more advanced dementia it is difficult to ascertain whether there is a correlation between DCM scores and direct quality-of-life interviews. One study[16] did not find a correlation on a subsample with participants with mild cognitive impairment. In a multi-method study[17] it was noted that during interviews, people with dementia rated their quality of life as better than their DCM scores would suggest.

DCM measures something similar to proxy measures and other observation measures. It is somewhat different from other quality-of-life and quality-of-care measures in that it attempts to measure elements of both. In training to use DCM, mappers are explicitly taught to increase their empathy for the viewpoint of the person with dementia and to use this during their coding decisions.

RELIABILITY OF DCM

In research papers it appears that a reasonable agreement between trained mappers can be achieved. Nineteen studies reported inter-rater coding agreements ranging from 0.7 to 1.0, most reporting concordance coefficients of 0.8[8]. Mappers in routine practice are likely not to spend time ensuring that their inter-rater reliability is adequate. When many different mappers are engaged in mapping at different points in time, drifts in coding can have a significant impact on results[18] unless systematic checking is in place to prevent this. There are various ways in which reliability can be achieved in routine mapping[19].

Only one paper has reported on test–retest reliability on the same individuals a week apart[14]. There was satisfactory correlation between +3 and +5 ME values, overall WIB score and type of BCC. To date DCM data has only been published on DCM 7 data.

POPULATIONS THAT DCM IS USED WITH

DCM is used primarily with people with dementia living in long-term care settings. This covers a wide range of cognitive ability and dependence. There is evidence to suggest that level of dependency is correlated with DCM scores, specifically that low WIB scores are associated with high dependency levels[9,16,18]. However, this is not always the case[20,21]. The correlations between low WIB scores and high dependency may of course be related to a third factor of poorer quality of psychosocial care for people with dementia who have high dependency needs. In two studies where DCM was used in a systematic way to improve practice over time, the relationship between dependency and WIB scores disappeared as care quality improved[9,10]. DCM helps to focus care staff to consider the needs of those whose well-being is lowest, who are usually those with the greatest levels of dependency. Accordingly, DCM can help staff to refocus and adapt their care practices to better meet the needs of more dependent clients.

The evidence that dependency level skews DCM results is strong enough to suggest that a measure of dependency should be routinely taken alongside DCM evaluations so that the results can be scrutinized for this relationship.

Although DCM was originally developed in formal care services for people living with dementia, over the years it has also been used in services for people with learning disabilities[22] on general elderly care wards[23] and with people with Huntington's disease[24].

USING DCM TO IMPROVE THE QUALITY OF CARE

DCM lends itself well to improving well-being and quality of life for people with dementia at an individual care-plan level. The analysis of individual maps provides a lot of information about how to optimize an individual's well-being over the day. Small things that engender joy or distress, that are easy to miss as part of general care, become very clear in the process of mapping. This can be built upon to ensure that people have the opportunity to experience well-being more often.

At a group level, for example in the management of a hospital ward or nursing home, DCM can be used to improve the organization of care towards one that is person-centred rather than task-focused. An analysis of key events over the day – such as meal times or activity sessions or handovers – often reveals where changes can be made that will improve levels of well-being of the whole group of service users.

At a management level within care organizations, DCM data can help in decisions around skill mix, training needs and staff development. DCM sheds light on those skills that engender well-being. It can be useful in tailoring training and staff development programmes

around specific examples from the lived experience within an organization.

An advantage of DCM is that it can be used over time to monitor change at all these levels, thus evaluating whether the changes have had an impact. DCM data can be analysed to monitor change over time at an individual resident level and at an organizational level. DCM data can be utilized to good effect in fulfilling a number of reporting requirements for commissioners and inspections.

USING DCM TO CHANGE THE CULTURE OF CARE

In 2001, an international 'think tank' of DCM practitioners came together to review their collective experience on DCM[25]. Their conclusions from practice were that DCM, used within an organizational framework that supported person-centred care, could improve levels of well-being, increase the diversity of occupation, and decrease the incidence of personal detractions. The published developmental evaluations although limited in number supports this assertion both for larger scale quality-assurance initiatives[9,10] and more in-depth developments in single establishments[12,26]. A recent Australian cluster-randomized control trial of DCM demonstrated that DCM improved levels of agitation and that the number of falls decreased in care homes that used DCM[27].

Using DCM to achieve culture change is not an easy or trivial process. It does not provide a quick fix solution. This fact needs to be engaged with by both staff and management teams prior to deciding to use DCM. DCM is unlikely to have a positive impact unless staff have the necessary knowledge and skills base to use the information it generates. Also, as DCM works through helping staff teams reflect on their practice to bring about quality improvements, mechanisms such as supervision, mentoring, governance and quality assurance groups need to be established at an organizational level for DCM to work effectively over a sustained period of time.

Bringing DCM into an organization as a driver for person-centred care practice is a major undertaking. It requires clear strategic and operational planning if there is to be a maximum return on investment. Many organizations spend over a year planning and ensuring they are prepared before embarking on their first DCM evaluation. The British Standards Institute have developed a Publically Accessible Specification[28] to provide health and social care organizations with comprehensive guidance to assist them in this process.

USING DCM IN RESEARCH

The University of Bradford maintains a DCM bibliographic database that contains all known publications on DCM (http://www.bradford.ac.uk/acad/health/dcm). It is updated by the Bradford Dementia Group with annual bibliographic searches on Medline, Cinahl, and Psychinfo using the terms 'DCM' and 'dementia care mapping' as well as personal correspondence from practitioners and researchers.

A review of the published literature on DCM[8] revealed a number of papers of variable quality dating back to 1995 that have used DCM in a research context. These were categorized into the following types:

1. Cross-sectional surveys: Ten papers reported DCM results across a number of different facilities, and the results either compared or pooled. An additional three papers used DCM to investigate the relationship between participants' characteristics and well-being and activity.

2. Evaluations of interventions: In a further ten papers DCM was used to evaluate the impact of various interventions including a number of non-pharmacological therapeutic interventions and a double-blind, placebo-controlled, neuroleptic discontinuation study[29].
3. Practice development evaluations: Six papers investigated the ability of DCM to develop practice over time by means of repeated evaluations.
4. Multi-method evaluations: Three articles reported using DCM as part of a multi-method evaluation of a single facility or service.

DCM was not designed to be a research tool. Careful consideration should be given in deciding whether DCM is fit for purpose given the specific topic under investigation. In terms of cross-sectional surveys, there are tools that may be more suited to this task that do not have the attendant time-consuming problems and specialist training associated with DCM.

DCM seems to be suited to smaller scale within-subjects or group comparison intervention evaluations, given that it appears to demonstrate discrimination on a variety of interventions. In multi-method qualitative designs, DCM appears to enrich the data derived from proxy and service-user interviews and focus groups. DCM provides an opportunity to represent a reflection on what could be the viewpoint of service users who are unable to participate fully in interviews.

What is clear is that BCCs do not measure real-time estimates of different types of behaviour[18]. Because of the rules of coding in DCM, it will underestimate the occurrence of socially passive and withdrawn behaviour compared with data collected with continuous time sampling. Researchers interested in looking at withdrawn and passive behaviour might be better advised to use another tool. It is worthy of note, however, that despite this, three studies[21,30,31] found DCM discriminated between groups on social withdrawal in their evaluations. There are a number of modifications to DCM that might prove useful when using DCM in research[32].

CONCLUSIONS

DCM has a long history and it has changed over time. It has been taken up by practitioners in many countries who wish to improve the quality of care for people with dementia. It can be used on an individual client level or to improve group care. It requires specialist training to use and it takes careful planning to ensure that it is used to good effect. It has been utilized as a research tool for a variety of purposes.

DCM's advantages are that it is standardized, quality controlled, international, responsive to change, multidisciplinary and has an increasing research base. Its disadvantages are that it is resource heavy in terms of its training and administration. DCM holds a unique position in relation to quality of life in dementia care, being both an evaluative instrument and a vehicle for practice development in person-centred dementia care.

REFERENCES

1. Kitwood T, Bredin K. A new approach to the evaluation of dementia care. *J Adv Health Nurs Care* 1992; **1**: 41–60.
2. Brooker D, Surr CA. *Dementia Care Mapping: Principles and Practice*. Bradford: University of Bradford, 2005.
3. Brooker D. What is person-centred care for people with dementia? *Rev Clin Gerontol* 2004; **13**: 215–22.
4. Kitwood T. *Dementia reconsidered: the person comes first*. Buckingham: Open University Press, 1997.
5. Adams T. Kitwood's approach to dementia and dementia care: a critical but appreciative review. *J Adv Nurs* 1996; **23**: 948–53.
6. Brooker D, Surr C. Dementia Care Mapping (DCM): Initial validation of DCM 8 in UK field trials. *Int J Geriatr Psychiatry* 2006; **21**: 1018–25.
7. Surr C, Brooker D. The effects of undertaking a DCM training course on care practice. *Signpost* 2002; **7**: 16–18.
8. Brooker D. Dementia Care Mapping (DCM): a review of the research literature. *The Gerontologist* 2005; **45**: 11–18.
9. Brooker D. Foster N. Banner A. Payne M, Jackson L. The efficacy of Dementia Care Mapping as an audit tool: report of a 3-year British NHS evaluation. *Aging Mental Health* 1998; **2**: 60–70.
10. Martin GW, Younger D. Person-centred care for people with dementia: a quality audit approach. *J Psychiatr Mental Health Nurs* 2001; **8**: 443–48.
11. Williams J, Rees J. The use of 'dementia care mapping' as a method of evaluating care received by patients with dementia: an initiative to improve quality of life. *J Adv Nurs* 1997; **25**, 316–23.
12. Wylie K. Madjar I, Walton J. Dementia Care Mapping: a person-centered approach to improving the quality of care in residential settings. *Geriaction* 2002; **20**: 5–9.
13. Brooker D. Edwards P, Benson S (eds), *DCM: Experience and Insights into Practice*. London: Hawker Publications, 2004.
14. Fossey J, Lee L, Ballard C. Dementia Care Mapping as a research tool for measuring quality of life in care settings: psychometric properties. *Int J Geriatr Psychiatry* 2002; **17**; 1064–70.
15. Bredin K, Kitwood T, Wattis J. Decline in quality of life for patients with severe dementia following a ward merger. *Int J Geriatr Psychiatry* 1995; **10**: 967–73.
16. Edelman P, Fulton BR, Kuhn D. Comparison of dementia-specific quality of life measures in adult day centers. *Home Health Care Serv Q* 2004; **23**: 25–42.
17. Parker J. Education and learning for the evaluation of dementia care: The perceptions of social workers in training. *Educ Ageing* 1999; **14**: 297–314.
18. Thornton A, Hatton C, Tatham A. DCM reconsidered: Exploring the reliability and validity of the observational tool. *Int J Geriatr Psychiatry* 2004; **19**: 718–26.
19. Surr C, Bonde-Nielsen E. Inter-rater reliability in DCM. *J Dement Care*, 2003; **11**: 33–36.
20. Jarrott SE, Bruno K. Intergenerational activities involving persons with dementia: an observational assessment. *Am J Alzheimer's Dis Other Dement* 2003; **18**: 31–37.
21. Gigliotti CM, Jarrott SE, Yorgason J. Harvesting health: effects of three types of horticultural therapy activities for persons with dementia. *Dementia* 2004; **3**: 161–70.
22. Finnamore T, Lord S. The use of Dementia Care Mapping in people with a learning disability and dementia. *J Intellect Disabil* 2007; **11**: 157–65.
23. Woolley RJ, Young JB, Green JR, Brooker DJ. The feasibility of care mapping to improve care for physically ill older people in hospital. *Age Ageing* 2008; **37**: 390–95.
24. Boor A, Knight C. The utility of dementia care mapping within a Huntington's disease service as a quality outcome measure. *Huntington's Dis Assoc Newsl* 2007 (December).

25. Brooker D, Rogers L (eds). *DCM Think Tank Transcripts 2001*. Bradford: University of Bradford, 2001.

26. Lintern T, Woods R, Phair L. Training is not enough to change care practice. *J Dement Care* 2000; **8**: 15–17.

27. Chenoweth L, King MT, Jeon Y *et al*. Caring for Aged Dementia Care Resident Study (CADRES) of person-centred care, dementia-care mapping, and usual care in dementia: a cluster-randomised trial. *Lancet* 2009; **18**: 317–421.

28. British Standards Institute. *PAS 800:2010 Use of Dementia Care Mapping for person-centred care in a care provider organization – Guide*. BSI: London, 2010.

29. Ballard C, Thomas A, Fossey J *et al*. A 3-month, randomised, placebo-controlled, neuroleptic discontinuation study in 100 people with dementia: The Neuropsychiatric Inventory is a predictor of clinical outcome. *J Clin Psychiatry* 2004; **65**: 114–19.

30. Ballard C, O'Brien JT, Reichelt K, Perry E. Aromatherapy as a safe and effective treatment for the management of agitation in severe dementia: The results of a double blind, placebo-controlled trial with Melissa. *J Clin Psychiatry* 2002; **63**: 553–58.

31. Potkins D, Myint P, Bannister C *et al*. Language impairment in dementia: Impact on symptoms and care needs in residential homes. *Int J Geriatr Psychiatry* 2003; **18**: 1002–1006.

32. Sloane P, Brooker D, Cohen L *et al*. Dementia Care Mapping as a research instrument. *Int J Geriatr Psychiatry* 2007; **22**: 580–99.

31

Staging Dementia

Barry Reisberg[1], Imran A. Jamil[1], Sharjeel Khan[1], Isabel Monteiro[1], Carol Torossian[1], Steven Ferris[1],
Marwan Sabbagh[2], Serge Gauthier[3], Stefanie Auer[4], Melanie B. Shulman[1], Alan Kluger[1],
Emile Franssen[1] and Jerzy Wegiel[5]

[1]Aging and Dementia Clinical Research Center, New York University Langone Medical Center,
Center of Excellence on Brain Aging, New York, NY, USA
[2]Cleo Ruberts Center, Banner-Sun Health Research Institute, Sun City, AZ, USA
[3]McGill Center for Studies in Aging, Douglas Hospital, Montreal, Quebec, Canada
[4]MAS Alzheimerhilfe, Bad Ischl, Austria
[5]New York State Institute for Basic Research in Developmental Disabilities, Staten Island, New York, USA

INTRODUCTION AND OVERVIEW OF DEMENTIA STAGING

Dementia is a progressive pathological process extending over a period of many years. Clinicians and scientists have long endeavoured to describe the nature of dementia progression. Such descriptions have generally been encompassed within two broad categories: global staging and more specific staging, sometimes referred to as axial or multi-axial staging. A comparison of the major current dementia staging systems with the most widely used mental status assessment in Alzheimer's disease, the major cause of dementia, is shown in Figure 31.1.

This Figure illustrates some of the major potential advantages of staging. These advantages include: (i) staging can identify premorbid, but potentially manifest conditions which may be associated with the evolution of subsequent dementia, such as subjective cognitive impairment, a condition which is not differentiated with mental status or psychometric tests; (ii) staging can be very useful in identifying subtle predementia states, such as mild cognitive impairment (MCI), wherein mental status assessments and psychometric tests, while frequently altered, are generally within the normal range and, consequently, are not reliable markers[17-19]; and (iii) staging can track the latter 50% of the potential time course of dementias such as Alzheimer's disease (AD), when mental status assessments are virtually invariably at bottom (zero) scores[20]. Furthermore, apart from their utility in portions of dementia where mental status and psychometric assessments are out of range, or insensitive, there are clear data indicating that staging procedures can more accurately and sensitively identify the course of dementia in the portion of the condition which is conventionally charted with mental status assessments. This latter evidence comes from longitudinal investigation of the course of AD[9], pharmacological treatment investigation of AD[21-23], and study of independent psychometric assessments of AD[24]. For example, longitudinal study has demonstrated that the Functional Assessment Staging procedure (FAST)[5] and the Global

Deterioration Scale (GDS)[3] accounted for more than twice the variance in the course of AD over a five-year mean interval, compared to the Mini-Mental State Examination (MMSE)[7,9]. When employed together, the GDS and the FAST staging procedures explained nearly three times the variance in the temporal course of AD compared to the MMSE (i.e. change in measure versus change in time), with the MMSE encompassing only 10% of temporal change variance and the GDS and FAST together encompassing 28% of the temporal change variance[9]. In pharmacological studies, staging procedures have frequently demonstrated sensitivity to effects of the interventions in pivotal studies where mental status assessment has not shown a significant effect. This superiority in the demonstration of pharmacological treatment efficacy for staging procedures over mental status assessment has been seen for both classes of currently approved pharmacotherapeutic agents; that is, for N-methyl-D-aspartate (NMDA) receptor antagonist treatment decreasing glutamate-induced excitotoxicity, and for cholinesterase inhibitor treatment enhancing cholinergic brain functioning. For example, a pivotal, multicentre trial associated with worldwide approvals of memantine treatment for AD found a robust statistically significant effect of the memantine, NMDA receptor antagonist treatment with the FAST staging procedure, but no significant effect was observed with the MMSE evaluation[21]. Similarly, in a pivotal study associated with worldwide approval of the cholinesterase inhibitor, rivastigmine, it was found that low dose treatment (1–4 mg/day) was associated with significant improvement on the GDS staging procedure, but not on the MMSE assessment[22]. Additionally, study of predominantly institutionalized persons with more advanced AD in the latter portion of the MMSE range (i.e. with MMSE scores of 10 or below), with specially designed psychometric procedures for advanced AD patients, have clearly shown that the FAST staging procedures can robustly track progressive change in these more advanced AD patients, in conjunction with special psychometric procedures, whereas the MMSE does not sensitively change in this more severe range[24]. Another potential advantage of staging procedures in comparison with mental status

Principles and Practice of Geriatric Psychiatry, 3rd edn. Edited by Mohammed T. Abou-Saleh, Cornelius Katona and Anand Kumar
© 2011 John Wiley & Sons, Ltd

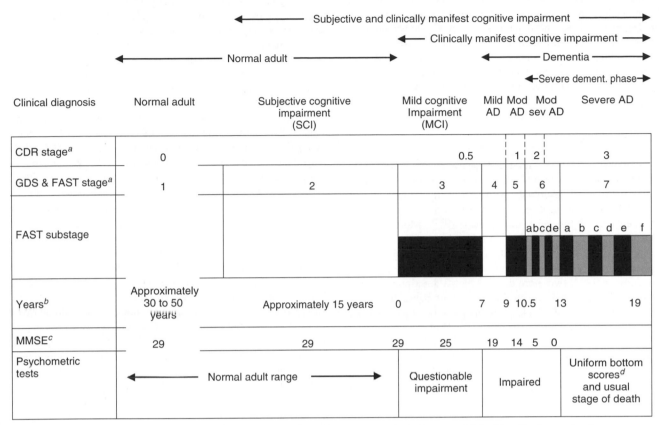

^{a} Stage range comparisons shown between the CDR and GDS/FAST stages are based upon published functioning and self-care descriptors.

^{b} Numerical values represent time in years.

For GDS and FAST stage 1, the temporal values are subsequent to the onset of adult life.

For GDS and FAST stage 2, the temporal value is prior to onset of mild cognitive impairment symptoms.

For GDS and FAST stage 3 and above, the values are subsequent to the onset of mild cognitive impairment symptoms.

In all cases, the temporal values refer to the evolution of Alzheimer's disease pathology.

All temporal estimates are based upon the GDS and FAST scales and were initially published based upon clinical observations in Reisberg, *Geriatrics* 1986; **41**(4): 30–46[8]. These estimates have been supported by subsequent clinical and pathological cross-sectional and longitudinal investigations (e.g. Reisberg *et al.*, *Int Psychogeriatr* 1996; **8**: 291–311[9]; Bobinski *et al.*, *Dementia* 1995; **6**: 205–10[10]; Bobinski *et al.*, *J Neuropathol Exp Neurol* 1997; **56**: 414–20[11]; Kluger *et al.*, *J Geriatr Psychiatry Neurol* 1999; **12**: 168–79[12]; Prichep *et al.*, *Neurobiol Aging*, 2006; **27**: 471–81[13] ; Reisberg and Gauthier, *Int Psychogeriatr* 2008; **20**: 1–16[14]; Wegiel *et al.*, *Acta Neuropathol* 2008; **116**: 391–407[15]; Reisberg *et al.*, *Alzheimers Dement* 2010; **6**(1): 11–24[16]).

The spacing in the figure is approximately proportional to the temporal duration of the respective stages and substages, with the exception of GDS and FAST stage 1, for which the broken lines signify an abbreviated temporal duration spacing for this normal adult condition which lasts approximately 30 to 50 years.

^{c} MMSE scores are approximate mean values from prior published studies.

^{d} For typical adult psychometric tests.

Figure 31.1 Typical time course of normal brain ageing; mild cognitive impairment associated with Alzheimer's disease and the dementia of Alzheimer's disease. AD, Alzheimer's disease; CDR, Clinical Dementia Rating[1,2]; GDS, Global Deterioration Scale[3,4]; FAST, Functional Assessment Staging[5,6]; MMSE, Mini-Mental State Examination[7]; Mod AD, moderate Alzheimer's disease; Mod sev AD, moderately severe Alzheimer's disease. Copyright © 2007, 2009 Barry Reisberg, MD. All rights reserved

or psychometric assessment of AD and other dementias, is in identifying the management concomitants of severity assessments[25,26]. Staging procedures have also been successfully applied postmortem to retrospectively assess the diagnoses (i.e. AD or other non-AD dementia) of a diverse assortment of dementia-related cases available for 'brain banking', but on which no antemortem clinical data were available[27]. Similarly, postmortem retrospective staging procedures have been successful in establishing remarkably robust clinicopathological correlations in longitudinally studied AD cohorts[10,11,15,20].

GLOBAL STAGING

Efforts to globally stage progressive dementia can be traced back at least to the early nineteenth century when the English psychiatrist, James Prichard, described four stages in the progression of dementia: '(1) impairment of recent memory, (2) loss of reason, (3) incomprehension, (4) loss of instinctive action'[28,29]. More recently, the American Psychiatric Association's[30] Diagnostic and Statistical Manual of Mental Disorders, 3rd edition (DSM-III) recognized three broad stages in its definition of primary degenerative dementia[30]. Subsequently, in 1982, two more detailed global descriptions of the progression of dementia were published. One of these, the Clinical Dementia Rating (CDR) scale[1], describes five broad stages from normality to severe dementia. The other, the Global Deterioration Scale (GDS)[3], identifies seven clinically recognizable stages from normality to most severe dementia of the Alzheimer type. A recently published abridged version of the GDS is shown in Table 31.1[31].

Complete versions of the CDR and the GDS scales can be found in the literature (e.g. for the original CDR, references[1,32] and for the CDR 'current version', reference[2]; for the GDS, reference[3], and for the tabular format of the GDS, reference[4]). These two global staging instruments, the GDS and the CDR, are generally compatible except that the GDS is more detailed and specific and identifies two stages which the CDR staging does not.

One of these stages identified by the GDS staging procedure but not by the CDR is a stage in which subjective complaints of cognitive deficit occur in the absence of clinically identifiable symptoms (GDS stage 2). These subjective complaints are now recognized as occurring very commonly in older persons (e.g.[33–35]). Although this stage of subjective complaints continues to be identified only by the GDS staging system, studies have indicated that persons with these complaints are at increased risk for subsequent overt dementia (e.g.[12,16,36–38]). A distinct diagnostic terminology, namely, 'subjective cognitive impairment' (SCI), has recently been suggested for otherwise healthy older persons with these symptoms who are free of overtly manifest symptoms of mild cognitive impairment (MCI) or dementia[14,39]. A recent study, which is apparently the first to systematically examine the prognosis of GDS stage 2, SCI persons, in comparison with persons with no cognitive impairment (NCI, GDS stage 1), from the perspective of the subsequent development of MCI or dementia, has indicated the true morbidity associated with this SCI condition. Over a mean seven-year follow-up, the risk of subsequent decline to MCI or dementia was 4.5-times greater in persons with SCI (GDS stage 2) than in persons who are free of these subjective complaints, after controlling for differences in age and other demographic variables, as well as follow-up time[16]. Physiological differences between otherwise healthy older persons with these subjective complaints of cognitive impairment and similarly aged persons without these symptoms (i.e. between GDS stage 2 and GDS stage 1 subjects) have now been reported for brain metabolism and cortisol levels[40,41]. Longitudinal studies are also presently confirming[13,14] a previously estimated 15-year duration[8] for this GDS stage 2 condition, identifying subjective impairment only, in the evolution of brain ageing and AD pathology.

The GDS staging measure and associated assessments from the GDS staging system also identify a stage, GDS stage 3, for which the terminology mild cognitive impairment (MCI) was originally coined in 1988[42]. This GDS stage 3 is described, in part, as a stage in which: (i) the 'earliest clear-cut deficits' become manifest; (ii) 'objective evidence of memory deficit is obtained only with an intensive interview', and (iii) there is 'decreased performance in demanding employment and social settings'. Many of the early observations with respect to the nature of MCI were made using this GDS stage 3 definition (see[17] for a review), and the GDS 3 definition of MCI remains compatible

Table 31.1 Abridged global deterioration scale

Stage 1: NCI. No subjective memory deficit (no cognitive impairment); no problems with activities of daily living.
Stage 2: SCI. Subjective cognitive impairment (subjective memory and/or other cognitive complaints): observations, sometimes accompanied by complaints, of being forgetful, such as of difficulties with recall of names, and/or of misplacing objects.
Stage 3: MCI. Earliest subtle deficits (mild cognitive impairment): difficulties often noted at work; may have become lost; may have misplaced a valuable object.
Stage 4: Mild dementia. Clear deficits on clinical examination (moderate cognitive impairment): decreased knowledge of personal and/or current events; often difficulties with finances or shopping or meal preparation or travel.
Stage 5: Moderate dementia. Can no longer survive independently in the community without some assistance (moderately severe cognitive impairment): difficulty with recall of some important personal details (e.g. address, names of one or more important schools attended); may require cueing for activities for daily living.
Stage 6: Moderately severe dementia. Largely unable to verbalize recent events in their life (severe cognitive impairment): may forget name of spouse; incontinence develops as this stage progresses; requires increasing assistance with activities for daily living such as dressing and showering. Increased behavioural problems (e.g. agitation) or other personality problems are common.
Stage 7: Severe dementia. Few intelligible words or no verbal abilities (very severe cognitive impairment): the ability to walk is lost as this stage evolves. Later, basic capacities such as the ability to sit up independently, to smile, and to move and/or to hold up the head independently are progressively lost.

2009 abridged version. Original abridged version published in *Canadian Medical Association Journal* 2008; **179**(12): 1281. Modified from Reisberg B, Ferris SH, de Leon MJ *et al*. The global deterioration scale for assessment of primary degenerative dementia. *Am J Psychiatry* 1982; **139**: 1136–9.

with the current international consensus definition of MCI, published by Winblad *et al.* in 2004[19]. The CDR staging methodology identifies a CDR 0.5 stage originally termed 'questionable dementia', which is somewhat broader in scope than the MCI entity, and which encompasses some of early (mild) dementia, as well as the MCI clinical timeframe.

At the other end of the pathological spectrum, the CDR does not identify any stage beyond that in which dementia patients 'require much help with personal care' and are 'often incontinent'. In contrast, the GDS identifies a final seventh GDS stage in which patients are already incontinent and over the course of which language and motor capacities are progressively lost. Importantly, the CDR does not stage or substage the latter portion of the dementia of AD, representing nine or more years of potential life and continuing decline for these patients (see Figure 31.1). This absence of attention to the nature of severe dementia clinical changes in the CDR staging methodology may add to the neglect of persons with more advanced dementia and, in particular, the dementia of Alzheimer's disease. In marked contrast with the CDR, the GDS identifies two stages (GDS stages 6 and 7), corresponding to the CDR 3 stage range. Additionally, the other elements of the GDS staging system, described below, chart this latter portion of the dementia of AD in detail. For example, the FAST scale (described below) identifies eight substages corresponding to the CDR stage 3, 'severe dementia' range.

In addition to the range differences discussed above and differing staging numbers, the CDR scale and the GDS staging scale also have different procedures for scoring. The original CDR versions used a 'sum of boxes' procedure, with means of the sum of boxes in six CDR assessment categories, i.e. (1) Memory, (2) Orientation, (3) Judgement and Problem Solving, (4) Community Affairs, (5) Home and Hobbies, and (6) Personal Care. However, current scoring procedures for the CDR are much more complex and more weighted towards the memory category. The GDS staging procedure simply requires the choice of the most appropriate global stage, based upon cognition and functioning. GDS staging descriptors acknowledge common emotional concomitants of the stages; however these are not employed in the stage selection. The comparisons shown in Figure 31.1 between the CDR and the GDS/FAST staging categories and other assessment procedures are based upon the CDR functioning and self-care descriptions.

In summary, with respect to range, the GDS staging and associated measures from the GDS Staging System, are much more detailed at both ends of the pathological spectrum of brain ageing and progressive dementia than the CDR staging. As discussed, the GDS staging identifies an SCI stage prior to the development of mild cognitive impairment, which the CDR staging does not refer to. Also, the GDS staging procedures are more rigorous in the definition of MCI and the separation of MCI from early dementia. In the severe end of the dementia spectrum, the GDS staging and the associated GDS Staging System, described in greater detail in the next section, are much more detailed than the CDR.

Staging procedures have been shown to be valid and reliable methods for assessing the magnitude of pathology in AD and related dementing conditions. This validity and reliability is illustrated in this brief review for the GDS, the most detailed and explicit staging procedure.

The validity of the GDS has been demonstrated in several ways. Cross-sectional studies have confirmed the consistency of the ordinal sequence and the optimal weighting of the hierarchically sequenced items embodied in the GDS stages in ageing and progressive Alzheimer's disease (AD)[42–45]. Thus, the specific impairments

characteristic of each stage almost always follow the impairments described for the previous stage. Also, the grouping of impairment characteristics within stages appears to be optimal.

For example, naturalistic study has supported the identification of staging phenomena, largely identical to the GDS stages, by independent layperson observers. In this study[44], a 30-item questionnaire derived from the GDS was completed by a relative or caregiver for each of 115 patients with varying degrees of dementia. Principal components analysis was used to combine the items into a single composite scale that more reliably represents distances between the 30 clinical manifestations along the continuum of cognitive decline. In the study it was found that 'the scale scores for the clinical manifestations were observed to cluster into relatively discrete groups, suggesting naturally occurring stages or phases. Objective cluster analysis methods further confirmed the presence of distinct transitions along the cognitive decline continuum.' It was concluded that the 'utility of empirically derived scale values in staging the course of primary degenerative dementia is suggested.'

The relationship between the GDS stages and mental status assessments, other dementia assessments, scores on cognitive tests and other objective tests and *in vivo* assessments of brain change in ageing and progressive dementia have been studied in considerable detail[3,42]. These studies have indicated significant correlations between all of these measures of dementia severity and the GDS stages. However, the strongest relationships have been observed between comprehensive dementia assessments such as the Mini-Mental State Examination (MMSE)[7] and the progression of dementia on the GDS[42]. The GDS also correlates well with independent physical markers of AD progression such as changes in neurological reflexes[46]. Thus the construct validity of the GDS has been well substantiated.

At least six separate studies have examined the reliability of the GDS[47–52]. Reliability coefficients have ranged from 0.82 to 0.97 in these studies using disparate procedures in diverse settings. These studies have indicated that the GDS is at least as reliable as any other instruments upon which clinicians rely, such as the MMSE. In a reliability study in a nursing home setting[51], the GDS was found to be somewhat more reliable than the MMSE. Importantly, GDS staging has also been shown to be a reliable procedure when assessed using a telephone format[52].

Global staging scales such as the GDS have certain important advantages in dementia assessment. First and foremost, these scales are strongly anchored to the clinical symptoms, behaviour and functional changes in progressive degenerative dementia, and particularly those of Alzheimer's disease. Consequently, they discourage misdiagnosis. Unlike many mental status and other dementia test instruments, global stages are relatively stable over time and relatively resistant to practice effects. Equally importantly, global staging instruments are minimally influenced by educational background and socioeconomic status, whereas mental status and similar assessments are strongly influenced by such factors. Also, as previously noted, global staging, and in particular the GDS, covers the entire range of pathology in central nervous system (CNS) ageing and progressive dementia, whereas, for example, mental status assessments and most psychometric tests entirely fail to distinguish GDS stages 1 and 2 (i.e. NCI and SCI). Occasionally, patients may display GDS stage 3 symptomatology (MCI) and still score a perfect 30 on the MMSE. Uncommonly, dementia patients may display GDS stage 4 symptomatology (mild dementia), and still score a perfect 30 on the MMSE. Much more commonly, patients may display the clear-cut dementia symptomatology characteristic of GDS stage 4 and achieve

MMSE scores which are near perfect or within the so-called 'normal' range. At the other end of the pathological spectrum, most patients at GDS stage 6 (moderately severe dementia) achieve only bottom scores on traditional psychometric tests. Over the entire course of the GDS 7 (severe dementia) stage, most patients attain only zero (bottom) scores on the MMSE. The GDS, however, describes a final seventh stage, over the course of which patients may survive for many years.

AXIAL AND MULTI-AXIAL STAGING

The observation that the progression of dementia pathology is accompanied by progressive changes in more specifically defined processes, termed 'axes' has resulted in efforts to stage dementia in terms of those processes. Generally, axial staging has attempted to exploit progressive changes in cognition or functioning, although attempts have also been made to hierarchically stage progressive mood and behavioural changes, progressive motoric changes and progressive neurological changes, as well as other observable concomitants of dementia. These efforts can be traced back more than 40 years to the work of de Ajuriaguerra and associates[53-55]: Swiss investigators who were strongly influenced by Piaget's investigations of the stages of normal infant and childhood development. More recently, Cole and co-workers in Canada employed this approach in their Hierarchic Dementia Scale[56-58]. A similar approach was pursued, apparently independently, by Gottfries and associates in Sweden[59].

The CDR staging has a 'sum of boxes' approach which employs a hierarchical, multi-axial-like procedure[60], or, more recently, a modified, multi-axial-like procedure[2]. Based upon the seven-stage GDS, Reisberg and associates also described axial and multi-axial concomitants of progressive dementia[61,62] in a measure termed the Brief Cognitive Rating Scale (BCRS). Each of the BCRS axes has been enumerated to be optimally concordant with the corresponding GDS stages. Ultimately, the functional component of these BCRS axes resulted in the most detailed hierarchical staging of progressive dementia proposed to date, a 16-stage and substage measure of progressive functional change. This latter assessment is termed Functional Assessment Staging or FAST[5] (Table 31.2).

Like the BCRS axes, the FAST has been enumerated to be optimally concordant, in dementia of the Alzheimer type, with the corresponding GDS stages, discussed above. The FAST can be used as an independent staging measure of the magnitude of dementia pathology, or as part of the GDS Staging System[45]. Advantages of the FAST staging procedure include the following: (i) the FAST is capable of describing the entire course of brain-ageing associated, cognition-based functional changes and subsequent dementia of the Alzheimer type, ordinally (i.e. hierarchically), in unprecedented detail; (ii) the scale can assist in differentiating dementia of the Alzheimer type from other dementia processes[8,65,66]; (iii) the scale can assist in identifying premature and potentially remediable functional changes in AD patients (e.g. premature loss of ambulation due, for example, to the side effects of medication)[8,65,66]; (iv) the scale permits the retrospective as well as prospective examination of the temporal course of AD[10,11]; and (v) the scale is the only current measure which permits the detailed staging of severe AD[20,23,24,43]. A strong relationship between this FAST procedure and comprehensive cognitive assessments such as the MMSE has long been noted[64,67]. However, because the MMSE and other cognitive modalities bottom out prior to the final five to eight FAST substages, complete concurrent validation and examination of the FAST had to await the development of cognitive measures useful in most severe dementia. Such measures were developed towards the end of the twentieth century and do, in fact, evidence strong relationships with the final FAST stages[24]. Subsequent work showed approximately equally strong relationships between this latter portion of the FAST and ostensibly cognition-independent neurological reflex changes[46], as well as hippocampal neuropathological changes in volume[10], cell number[11] and the percentage of remaining hippocampal neurons with neurofibrillary changes[11], with the advance of AD as per the FAST stages and substages (reviewed in[20]). Also, the second layer of the entorhinal cortex is believed to be a very early site of AD pathology. In this layer, a very robust relationship, across the FAST severity spectrum from FAST stage 3 to 7f, with the decrement in neuronal numbers has recently been reported ($r = 0.9$)[15]. The correlations between the advance of AD as measured with the FAST in the latter portion of the course of AD, generally after the MMSE bottom (zero) point, and cognitive, neurological reflex and neuropathological hippocampal measures are generally approximately 0.8–0.9. These diverse relationships are comparable to the correlation between the FAST and the MMSE in the MMSE-sensitive portion of the FAST staging assessment. Because of these properties and others, the FAST has proven to be of widespread utility. For example, in the United States, the FAST staging procedure has been utilized as the Medicare mandated 'gold standard' for hospice admission for more than a decade[68]. Importantly, because of the sensitivity of the FAST staging procedure to the course of AD, not only over the final seventh stage when the MMSE is zero, but also over the course of FAST stage 6, when patients still score on measures such as the MMSE, the FAST measure has shown a significant effect on the course of AD in a pivotal multicentre drug trial, associated with worldwide approvals for memantine as the first medication for advanced AD, whereas the MMSE was not sensitive to change in this study[21]. At the present time, the FAST has been used as an efficacy and/or severity assessment in all pivotal trials associated with United States and European Union approvals of medications for advanced AD (for a review, see[23]).

Apart from the utility of the FAST staging, other elements of the multi-axial BCRS staging procedures have also proven useful in AD assessment. On the BCRS, Axis I assesses concentration; Axis II, recent memory; Axis III, remote memory; Axis IV, orientation; and Axis V, functioning. Axis V of the BCRS was developed and expanded in the process of the creation of the FAST staging procedure. All of these elements of the BCRS, including the FAST, have been utilized as part of the syncretic NYU CIBIC-Plus assessment measure[69]. As part of the NYU CIBIC-Plus, these measures have been used as primary outcome measures in pivotal trials associated with regulatory body (e.g. FDA) approvals of two of the three medications currently approved and marketed for the treatment of AD in the United States (i.e. rivastigmine and memantine) (for a review, see[23]). At the other end of the brain-ageing and AD continuum, the BCRS Axes I to V have been found to add significantly to the GDS global assessment in predicting the risk of decline and the time to decline to MCI or dementia in ostensibly normal subjects with NCI or SCI (GDS stages 1 and 2)[16].

SUMMARY

Behaviourally based brain-ageing and progressive dementia staging procedures can be useful and, frequently, superior to other assessment modalities in identifying potential treatments for AD and related

Table 31.2 Functional Assessment Staging (FAST) and time course of functional loss in normal brain ageing and Alzheimer's disease

FAST stage	Clinical characteristics	Clinical diagnosis	Estimated duration in AD[a]	Mean MMSE[b]
1	No decrement	Normal adult		29–30
2	Subjective deficit in word finding or recalling location of objects	Subjective cognitive impairment	15 years	29
3	Deficits noted in demanding employment settings	Mild cognitive impairment	7 years	24–27
4	Requires assistance in complex tasks, e.g. handling finances, planning dinner party	Mild AD	2 years	19–20
5	Requires assistance in choosing proper attire	Moderate AD	18 months	15
6a	Requires assistance in dressing	Moderately severe AD	5 months	9
b	Requires assistance in bathing properly		5 months	8
c	Requires assistance with mechanics of toileting (such as flushing, wiping)		5 months	5
d	Urinary incontinence		4 months	3
e	Faecal incontinence		10 months	1
7a	Speech ability limited to about a half-dozen words	Severe AD	12 months	0
b	Intelligible vocabulary limited to a single word		18 months	0
c	Ambulatory ability lost		12 months	0
d	Ability to sit up lost		12 months	0
e	Ability to smile lost		18 months	0
f	Ability to hold up or move head independently lost		12 months or longer	

Adapted from Reisberg, 1986[8]. Copyright © 1984 by Barry Reisberg, MD.

[a] In subjects without other complicating illnesses who survive and progress to the subsequent deterioration stage[9–16].

[b] MMSE = Mini-Mental State Examination score (Folstein et al., 1975[7]). Estimates based in part on published data summarized in Reisberg et al., 1989[63] and in Reisberg et al., 1992[64]. It should be noted that the educational level of the subjects in these studies is high (mean ~15.5 years ± ~ 3 years, of formal education). The influence of these educational levels on the mean MMSE scores should be given consideration.

dementias[70–72], as well as in assessing the course and the management needs of the dementia patient, and also in the diagnosis and differential diagnosis of dementing disorders. In providing an overview of the course of dementias such as AD, from the initial to final clinical symptoms, staging is uniquely useful. Staging is also singularly useful in assessment at various specific points in the evolution of dementing processes. Very importantly, staging can uniquely relate to management needs and the general management import of dementing processes.

ACKNOWLEDGEMENT

This work was supported in part by US DHHS grants AG03051 and AG08051 from the National Institute on Aging of the US National Institutes of Health; by grants 90AZ2791, 90AM2552 and 90AR2160 from the US Department of Health and Human Services Administration on Aging; by grant NCRRM01 RR00096 from the General Clinical Research Center Program and by Clinical and Translational Science Institute grant 1UL1RR029893 from the National Center for Disease Research Resources of the US National Institutes of Health; by the Zachary and Elizabeth M. Fisher Center for Alzheimer's Research Foundation; by a grant from Mr. William Silberstein; by the Leonard Litwin Fund for Alzheimer's Disease Research; by the Woodbourne Foundation; and by the Hagedorn Fund.

REFERENCES

1. Hughes CP, Berg L, Danziger WL et al. A new clinical scale for the staging of dementia. Br J Psychiatry 1982; **140**: 566–72.
2. Morris JC. The Clinical Dementia Rating (CDR): current version and scoring rules. Neurology 1993; **43**: 2412–14.
3. Reisberg B, Ferris SH, de Leon MJ et al. The global deterioration scale for assessment of primary degenerative dementia. Am J Psychiatry 1982; **139**: 1136–9.
4. Reisberg B, Ferris SH, de Leon MJ et al. The Global Deterioration Scale (GDS). Psychopharmacol Bull 1988; **24**: 661–3.
5. Reisberg B. Functional assessment staging (FAST). Psychopharmacol Bull 1988; **24**: 653–9.
6. Sclan SG, Reisberg B. Functional assessment staging (FAST) in Alzheimer's disease: reliability, validity and ordinality. Int Psychogeriatr 1992; **4**: 55–69.
7. Folstein MF, Folstein SE, McHugh PR. Mini-mental state: a practical method for grading the cognitive state of patients for the clinician. J Psychiatr Res 1975; **12**: 189–98.
8. Reisberg B. Dementia: a systematic approach to identifying reversible causes. Geriatrics 1986; **41**(4): 30–46.
9. Reisberg B, Ferris SH, Franssen E et al. Mortality and temporal course of probable Alzheimer's disease: a five-year prospective study. Int Psychogeriatr 1996; **8**: 291–311.

10. Bobinski M, Wegiel J, Wisniewski HM *et al.* Atrophy of hippocampal formation subdivisions correlates with stage and duration of Alzheimer disease. *Dementia* 1995; **6**: 205–10.

11. Bobinski M, Wegiel J, Tarnawski M *et al.* Relationships between regional neuronal loss and neurofibrillary changes in the hippocampal formation and duration and severity of Alzheimer disease. *J Neuropathol Exp Neurol* 1997; **56**: 414–20.

12. Kluger A, Ferris SH, Golomb J *et al.* Neuropsychological prediction of decline to dementia in nondemented elderly. *J Geriatr Psychiatry Neurol* 1999; **12**: 168–79.

13. Prichep LS, John ER, Ferris SH *et al.* Prediction of longitudinal cognitive decline in normal elderly using electrophysiological imaging. *Neurobiol Aging* 2006; **27**: 471–81.

14. Reisberg B, Gauthier S. Current evidence for subjective cognitive impairment (SCI) as the pre-mild cognitive impairment (MCI) stage of subsequently manifest Alzheimer's disease. *Int Psychogeriatr* 2008; **20**: 1–16.

15. Weigel J, Dowjat K, Kaczmarski W *et al.* The role of overexpressed DYRK1A protein in the early onset of neurofibrillary degeneration in Down syndrome. *Acta Neuropathol* 2008; **116**: 391–407.

16. Reisberg B, Shulman MB, Torossian C, Ling L, Zhu W. Outcome over seven years of healthy adults with and without subjective cognitive impairment. *Alzheimers Dement* 2010; **6**(1): 11–24.

17. Reisberg B, Ferris SH, Kluger A *et al.* Mild cognitive impairment (MCI): a historical perspective. *Int Psychogeriatr* 2008; **20**: 18–31.

18. Gauthier S, Reisberg B, Zaudig M *et al.* Mild cognitive impairment. *Lancet* 2006; **367**: 1262–70.

19. Winblad B, Palmer K, Kivipelto M *et al.* Mild cognitive impairment – beyond controversies, towards a consensus: report of the International Working Group on Mild Cognitive Impairment. *J Intern Med* 2004; **256**: 240–6.

20. Reisberg B, Wegiel J, Franssen E *et al.* Clinical features of severe dementia: staging. In Burns A, Winblad B (eds), *Severe Dementia*. London: John Wiley & Sons, Ltd, 2006, 83–115.

21. Reisberg B, Doody R, Stöffler A *et al.* Memantine in moderate-to-severe Alzheimer's disease. *N Engl J Med* 2003; **348**: 1333–41.

22. Corey-Bloom J, Anand R, Veach J. A randomised trial evaluating the efficacy and safety of ENA 713 (rivastigmine tartrate), a new acetylcholinesterase inhibitor, in patients with mild to moderately severe Alzheimer's disease. *Int J Geriatr Psychopharmacol* 1998; **1**: 55–65.

23. Reisberg B. Global measures: utility in defining and measuring treatment response in dementia. *Int Psychogeriatr* 2007; **19**: 421–56.

24. Auer SR, Sclan SG, Yaffee RA, Reisberg B. The neglected half of Alzheimer disease: cognitive and functional concomitants of severe dementia. *J Am Geriatr Soc* 1994; **42**: 1266–72.

25. Reisberg B, Kenowsky S, Franssen EH *et al.* President's Report: Towards a science of Alzheimer's disease management: a model based upon current knowledge of retrogenesis. *Int Psychogeriatr* 1999; **11**: 7–23.

26. Reisberg B, Franssen EH, Souren LEM *et al.* Evidence and mechanisms of retrogenesis in Alzheimer's and other dementias: management and treatment import. *Am J Alzheimers Dis Other Demen* 2002; **17**: 202–12.

27. Rockwood K, Howard K, Thomas VS *et al.* Retrospective diagnosis of dementia using an informant interview based on the Brief Cognitive Rating Scale. *Int Psychogeriatr* 1998; **10**, 53–60.

28. Cohen GD. Historical views and evolution of concepts. In Reisberg B (ed.), *Alzheimer's Disease*. New York: Free Press/Macmillan, 1983, 29–33.

29. Prichard JC. *A Treatise on Insanity*. Philadelphia: Haswell, Barrington and Haswell, 1837.

30. American Psychiatric Association. *Diagnostic and Statistical Manual of Mental Disorders*, 3rd edn. Washington, DC: American Psychiatric Association, 1980.

31. Reisberg B. Abridged Global Deterioration Scale. In Hermann N, Gauthier S. Diagnosis and treatment of dementia: 6. Management of severe Alzheimer's disease. *CMAJ* 2008; **179**: 1281.

32. Berg L. Clinical Dementia Rating (CDR). *Psychopharmacol Bull* 1988; **24**: 637–9.

33. Jonker C, Geerlings MI, Schmand B. Are memory complaints predictive for dementia? A review of clinical and population-based studies. *Int J Geriatr Psychiatry* 2000; **15**: 983–91.

34. Wang P-N, Wang S-J, Fuh J-L *et al.* Subjective memory complaint in relation to cognitive performance and depression: a longitudinal study of a rural Chinese population. *J Am Geriatr Soc* 2000; **48**: 295–9.

35. Brucki SMD, Nitrini R. Subjective memory impairment in a rural population with low education in the Amazon rainforest: an exploratory study. *Int Psychogeriatr* 2008; **21**: 164–71.

36. Geerlings MI, Jonker C, Bouter LM *et al.* Association between memory complaints and incident Alzheimer's disease in elderly people with normal baseline cognition. *Am J Psychiatry* 1999; **156**: 531–7.

37. St John P, Montgomery P. Are cognitively intact seniors with subjective memory loss more likely to develop dementia? *Int J Geriatr Psychiatry* 2002; **17**: 814–20.

38. van Oijen M, de Jong F, Hofman A *et al.* Subjective memory complaints, education, and risk of Alzheimer's disease. *Alzheimers Dement* 2007; **3**: 92–7.

39. Reisberg B, Prichep L, Mosconi L *et al.* The pre–mild cognitive impairment, subjective cognitive impairment stage of Alzheimer's disease. *Alzheimers Dement* 2008; **4**: S98–108.

40. Mosconi L, De Santi S, Brys M *et al.* Hypometabolism and altered cerebrospinal fluid markers in normal apolipoprotein E E4 carriers with subjective memory complaints. *Biol Psychiatry* 2008; **63**: 609–18.

41. Wolf OT, Dziobek I, McHugh P *et al.* Subjective memory complaints in aging are associated with elevated cortisol levels. *Neurobiol Aging* 2005; **26**: 1357–63.

42. Reisberg B, Ferris SH, de Leon MJ *et al.* Stage-specific behavioral, cognitive, and in vivo changes in community residing subjects with age-associated memory impairment and primary degenerative dementia of the Alzheimer type. *Drug Dev Res* 1988; **15**: 101–14.

43. Reisberg B, Franssen E, Bobinski M *et al.* Overview of methodologic issues for pharmacologic trials in mild, moderate, and severe Alzheimer's disease. *Int Psychogeriatr* 1996; **8**: 159–93.

44. Overall JE, Scott J, Rhoades HM *et al.* Empirical scaling of the stages of cognitive decline in senile dementia. *J Geriatr Psychiatry Neurol* 1990; **3**(4): 212–20.

45. Reisberg B, Sclan S, Franssen E *et al.* The GDS Staging System: Global Deterioration Scale (GDS), Brief Cognitive Rating Scale (BCRS), Functional Assessment Staging (FAST). In Rush AJ, First Jr MB, Blacker D (eds.), *Handbook of Psychiatric*

Measures, 2nd edn. Washington, DC: American Psychiatric Publishing, 2008, 431–5.

46. Franssen EH, Reisberg B. Neurologic markers of the progression of Alzheimer disease. *Int Psychogeriatr* 1997; **9**(Suppl 1): 297–306.

47. Foster JR, Sclan S, Welkowitz J *et al*. Psychiatric assessment in medical long-term care facilities: reliability of commonly used rating scales. *Int J Geriatr Psychiatry* 1998; **3**: 229–33.

48. Gottlieb GL, Gur RE, Gur RC. Reliability of psychiatric scales in patients with dementia of the Alzheimer type. *Am J Psychiatry* 1988; **45**: 857–9.

49. Reisberg B, Ferris SH, Steinberg G *et al*. Longitudinal study of dementia patients and aged controls: an approach to methodologic issues. In Lawton MP, Herzog AR (eds.), *Special Research Methods for Gerontology*. Amityville, NY: Baywood Publishers, 1989, 195–231.

50. Dura JR, Haywood-Niler E, Kiecolt-Glaser JK. Spousal caregivers of persons with Alzheimer's and Parkinson's disease dementia: a preliminary comparison. *Gerontologist* 1990; **30**: 332–6.

51. Hartmaier SL, Sloan PD, Guess HA *et al*. The MDS Cognition Scale: a valid instrument for identifying and staging nursing home residents with dementia using the Minimum Data Set. *J Am Geriatr Soc* 1994; **42**: 1173–9.

52. Monteiro IM, Boksay I, Auer SR *et al*. The reliability of routine clinical instruments for the assessment of Alzheimer's disease administered by telephone. *J Geriatr Psychiatry Neurol* 1998; **11**: 18–24.

53. de Ajuriaguerra J, Rey Bellet-Muller M, Tissot R. A propos de quelques problèmes posés par le déficit opératoire des vieillards atteints de démence dégénérative en début d'evolution. *Cortex* 1964; **1**: 103–32.

54. de Ajuriaguerra J, Tissot R. Some aspects of psychoneurologic disintegration in senile dementia. In Mueller CH, Ciompi L (eds.) *Senile Dementia*. Bern: Huber, 1968, 69–79.

55. de Ajuriaguerra J, Tissot R. Some aspects of language in various forms of senile dementia: comparisons with language in childhood. In Lennenberg EH, Lennenberg E (eds.) *Foundations of Language Development*, vol. 1. New York: Academic Press, 1975, 323–39.

56. Cole MG, Dastoor D. Development of a dementia rating scale: preliminary communication. *J Clin Exp Gerontol* 1980; **2**: 46–63.

57. Cole MG, Dastoor DP, Koszycki D. The Hierarchic Dementia Scale. *J Clin Exp Gerontol* 1983; **5**: 219–34.

58. Cole MG, Dastoor D. A new hierarchic approach to the measurement of dementia. *Psychosomatics* 1987; **28**: 298–304.

59. Gottfries CG, Brane G, Steen B. A new rating scale for dementia syndromes. *Gerontology* 1982; **28**(suppl): 20–31.

60. Hughes CP, Berg L, Danziger WL *et al*. Clinical dementia rating (CDR) scale. In American Psychiatric Association, Task Force for the Handbook of Psychiatric Measures, *Handbook of Psychiatric Measures*. Washington, DC: American Psychiatric Association, 2000, 446–50.

61. Reisberg B, Schneck MK, Ferris SH *et al*. The Brief Cognitive Rating Scale (BCRS): findings in primary degenerative dementia (PDD). *Psychopharmacol Bull* 1983; **19**: 47–50.

62. Reisberg B, London E, Ferris SH *et al*. The Brief Cognitive Rating Scale: language, motoric, and mood concomitants in primary degenerative dementia. *Psychopharmacol Bull* 1983; **19**: 702–8.

63. Reisberg B, Ferris SH, de Leon MJ *et al*. The stage specific temporal course of Alzheimer's disease: functional and behavioral concomitants based upon cross-sectional and longitudinal observation. In Iqbal K, Wisniewski HM, Winblad B (eds.), *Alzheimer's Disease and Related Disorders: Progress in Clinical and Biological Research*, vol. 317. New York: Alan R. Liss, 1989, 23–41.

64. Reisberg B, Ferris SH, Torossian C *et al*. Pharmacologic treatment of Alzheimer's disease: a methodologic critique based upon current knowledge of symptomatology and relevance for drug trials. *Int Psychogeriatr* 1992; **4**(Suppl 1): 9–42.

65. Reisberg B, Ferris SH, Franssen E. An ordinal functional assessment tool for Alzheimer's-type dementia. *Hosp Community Psychiatry* 1985; **36**: 593–5.

66. Reisberg B, Ferris SH, de Leon MJ. Senile dementia of the Alzheimer type: diagnostic and differential diagnostic features with special reference to functional assessment staging. In Traber J, Gispen WH (eds.), *Senile Dementia of the Alzheimer Type*, vol.2. Berlin: Springer-Verlag, 1985, 18–37.

67. Reisberg B, Ferris SH, Anand R *et al*. Functional staging of dementia of the Alzheimer's type. *Ann N Y Acad Sci* 1984; **435**: 481–3.

68. US Health Care Financing Administration. *Hospice – Determining Terminal Status in Non-Cancer Diagnoses – Dementia, Policy Number: (YPF #163) (Y Med #20), The Medicare News Brief (A Publication for all Medicare Part B Providers)*, Issue no. MNB-98-7, September 1998. Washington, DC: US HCFA. For a current reference see Centers for Medicare and Medicaid Services (CMS), Medicare Coverage Database, LCD for Hospice Alzheimer's Disease and Related Disorders (L16343); www.medicare.gov/coverage/home.asp, searching for ID L16343.

69. Reisberg B, Ferris SH. Clinician's interview–based impression of change-plus. In Kelly C, Newton-Howes G (eds.), *Guide to Assessment Scales in Dementia*. London: Science Press, Ltd, 2004, 9–10, and 21-page scale reproduction.

70. Sabbagh MN, Silverberg N, Bircea S *et al*. Is the functional decline in Parkinson's disease similar to the functional decline of Alzheimer's disease? *Parkinsonism Relat Disord* 2005; **11**: 311–15.

71. Sabbagh MN, Lahti T, Connor DJ *et al*. Functional ability correlates with cognitive impairment in Parkinson's disease and Alzheimer's disease. *Dement Geriatr Cogn Disord* 2007; **24**: 327–34.

72. Paul RH, Cohen RA, Moser DJ. The Global Deterioration Scale: relationships to neuropsychological performance and activities of daily living in patients with vascular dementia. *J Geriatr Psychiatry Neurol* 2002; **15**: 50–4.

32

The Clinical Dementia Rating

Rawan Tarawneh, B. Joy Snider, Mary Coats and John C. Morris

Washington University in St. Louis, St. Louis, MO, USA

INTRODUCTION

The Clinical Dementia Rating (CDR) is an instrument used to assess the presence and severity of dementia of the Alzheimer type (DAT); it may be applicable to other dementias as well. The CDR was developed at Washington University School of Medicine in 1982 and revised in 1993 to improve the distinction between different severity levels.

Determination of the CDR is based on separate semi-structured interviews with the patient and an appropriate informant, such as spouse or adult child, to provide information regarding the patient's current level of cognitive function and daily activity in comparison with previously attained abilities.

DEVELOPMENT OF THE CDR

Measuring dementia severity is useful for research as well as for clinical decision making. Accurate staging of dementia is particularly important in clinical trials, both to select appropriate participants with similar levels of disease severity and to monitor disease progression[1]. The importance of a standardized approach to dementia staging in clinical trials is highlighted by the US Food and Drug Administration's Guidelines for the Clinical Evaluation of Anti-Dementia Drugs: 'the stage and severity of the dementia affecting each subject participating in a clinical trial must be assessed and recorded systematically in a manner that will be readily understood by other workers in the field'[2].

Prior to the introduction of the CDR, most attempts at the clinical staging of dementia were based on psychometric tests and behavioural rating scales. Some early instruments included the Dementia Scale (DS) of Blessed, the Global Deterioration Scale (GDS), the 29-item Blessed Information and Memory Scale (BIMC), and the Short Blessed Test, an abbreviated 6-item version of the BIMC.

The CDR is a 'global' scale that assesses impairment in cognitive ability, including the impact of cognitive changes on everyday functioning; it was designed to be performed independently of psychometric test results. The CDR assesses intra-individual change from the individual's prior cognitive and functional ability. Psychometric testing typically compares individual performance to reference group norms. By comparing functional and cognitive changes to the premorbid (predementia) level of function for that individual, the CDR minimizes effects of confounding factors such as age, educa-

tional level and ethnicity (i.e. the individual serves as his or her own control).

The CDR has been validated in several neuropathological studies of Alzheimer's disease[3]. It has demonstrated strong correlations with other behavioural and functional tests, as well as strong inter-rater correlations, attesting to its validity and reliability. While it may not be suitable for every situation, the CDR has become internationally recognized as a highly reliable diagnostic and severity-ranking scale for dementia, has been cited in over 1000 references (http:/apps.isiknowledge.com) and translated into 60 different languages and dialects (http://alzheimer.wustl.edu-/cdr/PDFs/translation/). Although primarily developed to assess DAT, the addition of language and behaviour domains in the Uniform Data Set version of the CDR (UDS) has allowed its use in the evaluation of other causes of dementia[4].

Online training in the use of the CDR is available at http://alzheimer.wustl.edu/cdr/Application/Step1.htm or by writing to the authors.

OVERVIEW OF THE CDR

The CDR is performed in two components: a semi-structured interview with a collateral source that provides information on the individual's premorbid level of function and any changes that have occurred, and an interview with the individual that includes some objective testing. It is determined by rating cognitive, behavioural and functional changes resulting from cognitive loss in each of six categories: Memory, Orientation, Judgement and problem solving, Community affairs, Home and hobbies, and Personal care (Table 32.1). Each category is scored independently on a 5-point scale of impairment (0 = no impairment, 0.5 = questionable or very mild, 1 = mild, 2 = moderate and 3 = severe impairment); one category, Personal care, does not have a 0.5 impairment level. The CDR scoring table includes descriptive 'anchors' that guide the rater in determining individual domain ratings based on both collateral source report and patient performance. The clinician uses his or her judgement to determine each rating, scoring each as independently as possible. With CDR training, clinicians can successfully distinguish between physical and cognitive causes of functional impairment and assign a CDR that accurately reflects dementia severity even in the presence of impaired physical performance[6].

The global CDR is determined by applying a scoring algorithm (www.biosat.wustl.edu/~adrc/cdrpgm/index.html), where global

---

Principles and Practice of Geriatric Psychiatry, 3rd edn. Edited by Mohammed T. Abou-Saleh, Cornelius Katona and Anand Kumar

Table 32.1 The clinical dementia rating scale

	None 0	*Questionable 0.5*	*Mild 1*	*Moderate 2*	*Severe 3*
Memory	No memory loss or slight Inconsistent forgetfulness	Consistent slight forgetfulness; partial recollection of events; 'benign' forgetfulness	Moderate memory loss: more marked for recent events; defect interferes with everyday activity	Severe memory loss, only highly learned material retrained: new material rapidly lost	Severe memory loss only fragments remain
Orientation	Fully oriented	Fully oriented but with slight difficulty with time relationships	Moderate difficulty with time relationships; oriented for place at examination; may have geographic disorientation elsewhere	Severe difficulty with time relationships; usually disoriented to time, often to place	Oriented to person only
Judgement and problem solving	Solves everyday problems and handles business and financial affairs well; judgement good in relation to past performance	Slight impairment in solving problems, similarities and differences	Moderate difficulty in handling problems, similarities and differences; social judgement usually maintained	Severely impaired in handling problems, similarities and differences; social judgement usually impaired	Unable to make judgements or solve problems
Community affairs	Independent function as usual in job, shopping, volunteer and social groups	Slight impairment in these activities	Unable to function independently at these activities though may still be engaged in some, appears normal to casual inspection	No pretence of independent function home; appears well enough to be taken to functions outside the family home	Appears too ill to be taken to functions outside the family home
Home and hobbies	Life at home, hobbies and intellectual interests well maintained	Life at home, hobbies and intellectual interests slightly impaired	Mild but definite impairment of functions at home; more difficult chores, and complicated hobbies and interests abandoned	Only simple chores preserved; very restricted interests, poorly maintained	No significant function in the home
Personal care	Fully capable of self-care		Needs prompting	Requires assistance in dressing, hygiene and keeping of personal effects	Requires much help with personal care; frequent incontinence

Score only as decline from previous usual level due to cognitive loss, not impairment due to other factors.
Source: Morris, J.C. (1993) The Clinical Dementia Rating (CDR): current version and scoring rules. *Neurology*, **43**, 2412–4.

CDR 0 = no dementia and CDR = 0.5, 1, 2 and 3 for very mild, mild, moderate and severe dementia. The CDR-sum of boxes (CDR-SB) is obtained by summing the scores in the individual categories, so CDR-SB ranges from 0 to 18 ('best' to 'worst' performance)[7]. The CDR-SB offers some advantages: it does not require an algorithm to calculate and can be treated as interval data in statistical analysis whereas the global CDR represents ordinal data. More importantly, the CDR-SB offers a wider range of values and increased precision for tracking changes across time. For example, mild DAT (global CDR 1) spans CDR-SB scores from 3.5 to 10, whereas moderate DAT (global CDR 2) spans 8–15.

CHARACTERISTICS

The CDR has two important properties of a global staging measure: hierarchy and concordance[8]. Hierarchy means that dementia severity is proportional to the CDR score (e.g. global CDR 3 is more severe than global CDR 2). The CDR captures different disease patterns and can identify subgroups of patients through concordance, another important property. In individuals with DAT, most of the six domains are expected to be reasonably concordant with the memory score (e.g. in global CDR 0.5 most domains would have scores of either 0.5 or 0 or 1). Disconcordance between different cognitive domains (e.g. a mix of 0, 2 and 3s) is suggestive of a non-Alzheimer's cause of dementia.

The CDR has demonstrated excellent 'face validity' in that it assesses the influence of cognitive loss on the ability to conduct everyday activities. It provides a standardized and meaningful way to describe clinically relevant changes to patients and their families[8].

The CDR has demonstrated its validity in multiple longitudinal studies with neuropathological confirmation of Alzheimer's disease; both the CDR and CDR-SB have been shown to correlate with the densities of neurofibrillary tangles and senile plaques, particularly in the neocortex[3]. Since the inception and revision of the CDR, the diagnosis of dementia has evolved, with increasing interest in and recognition of milder stages of dementia. The CDR has demonstrated a high degree of sensitivity (91%) in distinguishing individuals with even the mildest stages of dementia from normal individuals in longitudinal studies with neuropathological confirmation of Alzheimer's disease[9].

When administered in a standardized fashion, the CDR has excellent reliability. Inter-rater reliability of the CDR in several single and multicentre clinical trials including both physicians and non-physicians is 80% or greater for overall CDR, and ≥80% for almost all of the individual boxes[10,11].

The stability of the CDR over time was investigated in a 30-year longitudinal study of 1768 patients 63–83 years of age and with CDRs 0, 0.5 or 1 at Washington University[13]. Over time, the participant sample became older, more highly educated, more ethnically diverse, more likely to be female and more likely to have non-Alzheimer's disease dementias. There was a high turnover in the individual clinicians. Despite these changes, the psychometric test scores of individuals with similar CDR ratings did not change significantly over the 30-year period.

DIAGNOSIS AND DETECTION OF EARLY STAGES OF DEMENTIA

In its original form, CDR 0.5 denoted a heterogeneous group with questionable dementia. However, there is a growing body of evidence that many in the CDR 0.5 group are very similar to those with mild DAT in cognitive, behavioural, psychometric performance, longitudinal progression, as well as in neuroimaging and CSF biomarker characteristics.

By relying on intra-individual cognitive decline rather than inter-individual comparison of psychometric performances with arbitrary cut-points for impairment, CDR 0.5 allows the identification of individuals with cognitive impairment that may be too mild to fulfil criteria for mild cognitive impairment. Longitudinal studies have consistently demonstrated that the CDR 0.5 designation, when impairment is believed clinically to be caused by DAT, is followed by progressive cognitive and functional decline over time and by the histopathological changes of Alzheimer's disease at autopsy even when the CDR 0.5 diagnosis is 'pre-mild cognitive impairment'[9].

CDR 0.5 is now considered to characterize 'very mild' rather than 'questionable' dementia. We attempt to diagnose the aetiology of

dementia even when the degree of impairment is very mild (CDR 0.5).

ADAPTATIONS OF THE CDR

The CDR has been adapted to other clinical settings such as nursing homes and chronic care facilities (CDR-CC). A more abbreviated form of the CDR has been included into the Diagnostic and Statistical Manual for the identification of dementia.

The CDR interview can take 45–60 minutes and may be impractical for some clinical and research settings. A software system for administration and automatic scoring of the CDR using a hand-held device platform was recently developed. The platform includes specific algorithms for each scoring domain and the global CDR. The platform increases ease of data collection and management and is transferable to other platforms, allowing its use in both research and clinical settings. The Palm-based CDR has excellent validity, reliability and high correlation with the traditional CDR and is accurate for distinguishing CDR 0 and 0.5, which is probably the most challenging distinction in practice[14].

A brief informant questionnaire, referred to as 'AD8', has been developed in another attempt to avoid the time limitations of the CDR. The AD8 scores responses to eight questions. It offers a practical screening tool for the presence of dementia, with high sensitivity, specificity and face validity. However, in contrast to the CDR, it cannot be used as a staging tool for dementia[15].

POTENTIAL LIMITATIONS OF THE CDR

The CDR is not without limitations, including reliance on clinical judgement and the availability of an observant collateral source, and the length of time required for administration. Although the semi-structured interview format is flexible and can be adapted to different cultures and socioeconomic groups, social, cultural and educational factors may influence some domains of the scale. Therefore, additional validation studies will be needed to establish the validity and reliability of the CDR in ethnic subpopulations[16].

ACKNOWLEDGEMENTS

This chapter was supported by grants from the National Institutes of Aging (NIH/NIA P01AG003991, NIH/NIA P50AG005681).

REFERENCES

1. Perneczky R, Wagenpfeil S, Komossa K, Grimmer T, Diehl J, Kurz A. Mapping scores onto stages: mini-mental state examination and clinical dementia rating. *Am J Geriatr Psychiatry* 2006; **14**: 139–44.
2. Leber P. *Guidelines for the Clinical Evaluation of Antidementia Drugs*. Rockville, MD: US Food and Drug Administration, 1990.
3. Berg L, McKeel DW, Jr., Miller JP *et al*. Clinicopathologic studies in cognitively healthy ageing and Alzheimer's disease: relation of histologic markers to dementia severity, age, sex, and apolipoprotein E genotype. *Arch Neurol* 1998; **55**: 326–35.
4. Morris JC, Weintraub S, Chui HC *et al*. The Uniform Data Set (UDS): clinical and cognitive variables and descriptive data from Alzheimer Disease Centers. *Alzheimer Dis Assoc Disord* 2006; **20**: 210–16.

5. Morris JC. The Clinical Dementia Rating (CDR): current version and scoring rules. *Neurology* 1993; **43**: 2412–14.

6. Shah KR, Carr D, Roe CM, Miller JP, Coats M, Morris JC. Impaired physical performance and the assessment of dementia of the Alzheimer type. *Alzheimer Dis Assoc Disord* 2004; **18**: 112–19.

7. O'Bryant SE, Waring SC, Cullum CM *et al*. Staging dementia using Clinical Dementia Rating Scale Sum of Boxes scores: a Texas Alzheimer's research consortium study. *Arch Neurol* 2008; **65**: 1091–95.

8. Rockwood K, Morris JC. Global staging measures in dementia. In Gauthier S (ed), *Clinical Diagnosis and Management in Alzheimer's Disease*. London: Martin Dunitz, 1996, 141–53.

9. Storandt M, Grant EA, Miller JP, Morris JC. Longitudinal course and neuropathologic outcomes in original vs revised MCI and in pre-MCI. *Neurology* 2006; **67**: 467–73.

10. Morris JC, Ernesto C, Schafer K *et al*. Clinical dementia rating training and reliability in multicenter studies: the Alzheimer's Disease Cooperative Study experience. *Neurology* 1997; **48**: 1508–10.

11. Burke WJ, Miller JP, Rubin EH *et al*. Reliability of the Washington University Clinical Dementia Rating. *Arch Neurol* 1988; **45**: 31–32.

12. McCulla MM, Coats M, Van Fleet N, Duchek J, Grant E, Morris JC. Reliability of clinical nurse specialists in the staging of dementia. *Arch Neurol* 1989; **46**: 1210–11.

13. Williams MM, Roe CM, Morris JC. Stability of the Clinical Dementia Rating 1979–2007. *Arch Neurol* 2009; **66**: 773–77.

14. Galvin JE, Meuser TM, Coats MA, Bakal DA, Morris JC. The 'portable' CDR: translating the Clinical Dementia Rating interview into a PDA format. *Alzheimer Dis Assoc Disord* 2009; **23**: 44–49.

15. Galvin JE, Roe CM, Powlishta KK *et al*. The AD8: a brief informant interview to detect dementia. *Neurology* 2005; **65**: 559–64.

16. Morris JC, Cummings JL. Workshop reports from the third Asia-pacific regional meeting of the international working group on harmonization of dementia drug guidelines. *Alzheimer Dis Assoc Disord* 2006; **20**: 313.

33

GMS-HAS-AGECAT Package and the Global Mental Health Assessment Tool (GMHAT): Epidemiology and Closing the Treatment Gap

John R. M. Copeland

Division of Psychiatry, University of Liverpool, UK

For epidemiological and other studies of mental illness and morbidity in older age it is important to ensure as far as possible that the differences in the levels of cases of illness found between geographical areas and between studies at different points in time are not due to methodological differences and, in particular, the way the diagnoses themselves are made. To overcome this problem, standardized interviews were introduced. The GMS-HAS-AGECAT Package consists of a series of interviews designed to be given to a person for assessing the dementias and depression, with optional sections for minor mental illness. The Geriatric Mental State (GMS) was derived originally from the Present State Examination and the Mental Status Schedule (see the GMS Resource Centre at www.liv.ac.uk/gms). Substantial modifications and additions were incorporated to make it more applicable to older populations and to increase emphasis on organic states. The Package now provides, in addition to the GMS, which is an interview with the subject, the History and Aetiology Schedule (HAS) for an informant, which allows the assessment of onset and course of illness, past history, family history and certain risk factors for dementia, depression and other mental illness.

Standardization of diagnosis is achieved by the Automated Geriatric Examination for Computer Assisted Taxonomy (AGECAT) computer-assisted differential diagnosis based on an extensive decision tree method. The system aggregates the data into scores and allots each subject to levels of 'diagnostic confidence' on each of eight diagnostic syndrome clusters: organic, schizophrenia/paranoid, mania, depression (psychotic and neurotic type) (levels 0–5), obsessional, hypochondriacal, phobic and anxiety neurosis (levels 0–4). Level 3 and above are what would usually be recognized by psychiatrists as cases of illness. The computer then compares these levels with one another to derive a final diagnosis and flags cases where the decision has been difficult. The validity of the AGECAT diagnosis has been assessed against psychiatrists' diagnoses on the same patients. The range of kappa values for the agreement between AGECAT and psychiatrists' diagnoses for organic states is 0.80–0.88 and for depressive states 0.76–0.80. Outcome studies are now providing additional validation. After three years of follow-up, over 83% of AGECAT cases of organic disorder identified in the community study were either dead or still dementing. One third of

depressed cases were also depressed three years later. Postmortem studies have provided some validation of the dementia diagnosis[1].

In the second stage AGECAT uses the data from the HAS to take the diagnosis to a further stage, dividing organic states into acute or chronic, and the latter into the different types of dementia using a standardized form of the Hachinski Ischaemia Score. It also identifies bereavements and flags co-existent immobility, pain, lifelong intellectual function and physical illness.

The GMS can be used by trained lay workers and provides a diagnosis by AGECAT. When used in epidemiological studies it is possible to derive prevalence figures for the full range of psychiatric morbidity using a one-stage design. The measures are therefore economical as well as reliable and valid. The Package does not rely on special psychological tests as these are not applicable across cultures or socioeconomic groups or with populations of varying literacy. The interviews have also been transferred for presentation on laptop computer, which improves accuracy and communication, avoids delays and costs in inputting data, and provides rapid access to results and easy quality control of interviewing techniques.

These measures have been used in a number of projects, including the Medical Research Council (UK) ALPHA study of the incidence of the dementias (Liverpool, UK) and the multicentre MRC Cognitive Function and Ageing Study of six centres in the UK, the EURODEP EC-funded Concerted Action across nine European centres, the ongoing ASIADEP studies in five Asian centres, and the 10/66 Dementia Research Group (www.alz.co.uk), a collective of dementia researchers from the developing world examining the validity of dementia diagnosis in 27 centres in Latin America, Africa, India and South Asia, China and Southeast Asia, as well as forming part of the minimum dataset required by the EURODEM (EC Concerted Action on Epidemiology and Prevention of Dementia). The GMS has been translated and used in 40 different languages. The HAS has been shortened and modified to provide for the criteria of Lewy body dementia, and other recognized dementia classifications[2].

Of particular interest has been the question of how accurately the GMS Package diagnosed dementia among those persons with little or no education, an environment for which it was not initially developed. Findings now suggest that the GMS does tend to over-identify

Principles and Practice of Geriatric Psychiatry, 3rd edn. Edited by Mohammed T. Abou-Saleh, Cornelius Katona and Anand Kumar

organic disorder in low education groups free of dementia. However, overall the GMS appears to have performed well, and with some minor modifications when used in conjunction with the Community Screening Instrument for Dementia (CSI-D) has made an important contribution to one-stage dementia diagnosis for use in the developing world. Ongoing studies have continued to address these issues[3].

A recent development has been aimed at developing a clinical tool for areas of the world where there are no or very few psychiatrists or psychiatrically trained nurses. The Global Mental Health Assessment Tool (GMHAT[4]; see www.gmhat.org) has been developed in two versions. The first is for use as a diagnostic tool in primary care for the identification and treatment of mental illness in both young adult and older populations. Taking only 15 minutes on average and only requiring brief training in its use at high school educational level, it can be employed much as a blood test or an X-ray but much more cheaply and quickly. The second or full version, for secondary care where there is no psychiatrist, is designed to be given by a psychiatric nurse trained briefly in the method. The extensive computerized diagnostic algorithms based on the AGECAT system have been much extended to include mental illnesses encountered in younger age groups as well as those in older people (All-AGECAT) and more extended treatment options. Preliminary trials have begun in the UK, the Netherlands, Ireland, India and Africa. Closing the treatment gap particularly in low and middle income countries is now of growing concern. Achieving a reliable diagnosis and instituting treatment is the vital rate-limiting step on the road to recovery and return to work. In many parts of the world older people need to continue to work to support themselves and their families, especially in countries ravaged by HIV AIDS.

REFERENCES

1. MRC CFAS. Pathological correlates of late-onset dementia in a multicentre, community-based population in England and Wales. *Lancet* 2001; **357**: 169–75.
2. Copeland JR, Prince M, Wilson KC *et al*. The Geriatric Mental State Examination in the 21st century. *Int J Geriatr Psychiatry* 2002; **17**: 729–32.
3. Prince M, Acosta D, Chiu H, Scazufca M, Varghese M, for the 10/66 Dementia Research Group. Dementia diagnosis in developing countries: a cross-cultural validation study. *Lancet* 2003; **361**: 909–17.
4. Sharma VK, Lepping P, Cummins AGP *et al*. The Global Mental Health Assessment Tool – Primary care version (GMHAT/PC) development, reliability and validity. *World Psychiatry* 2004; **3**(2): 115–19.

34

Assessing Life Skills

Colin Depp, Veronica Cardenas, Ashley Cain and Thomas L. Patterson

Department of Psychiatry, University of California – San Diego, USA

INTRODUCTION

Particularly among older adults with mental illnesses, functional impairments play a critical role in clinical decisions, whether in determining a patient's ability to maintain residence in the community or gauging how well interventions aid patients in fulfilling life roles. The goal of mental health interventions is to restore functioning as much as possible, ideally to the individual's premorbid level of functioning, and so it follows that the measurement of functional abilities is of paramount clinical importance. By virtually any measure, the functional impact of psychiatric illness is immense and typically lifelong. Among people with schizophrenia, about two-thirds are unable to perform social roles and fewer than one-third are ever employed[1]. According to the World Health Organization (WHO), depression is among the commonest causes of days of disability, among all diseases, in the developed world[2]. Dementia due to Alzheimer's disease, which is now the sixth-leading cause of death, is also a leading cause of nursing-home placement in older adults[3]. In addition to the personal losses associated with functional impairment, disability associated with late-life mental illness imposes substantial monetary costs on society, such as wages lost by sufferers and their caregivers, the expense of services that compensate for functional deficits and other supportive costs.

Historically, much of the focus in psychiatry has been on quantifying and treating the symptoms of mental illness, with relatively less methodological rigour on the conceptualization and measurement of everyday functioning and skills for daily life. However, recent years have seen a rapid increase in the sophistication of approaches to measure the capacity to perform activities of daily living and in the quantification of 'real-world' outcomes that patients and providers care about. In this chapter, we will review the domains of interest and approaches to assessing daily living skills in older people with psychiatric disorders, provide a model linking the factors that contribute to functional disability and review the measurement modalities and the instruments available to measure functional outcomes in geriatric psychiatric patients.

CONSIDERATIONS IN MEASURING FUNCTIONING

Functional abilities encompass a number of life domains and there is no definitive subset of abilities under the umbrella of functional status nor a 'gold standard' defining functional independence or dependence. As a result, dozens of measures of functioning exist that cover different life domains, with varying theoretical bases and psychometric properties. Recent initiatives, such as the Measurement and Treatment Research to Improve Cognition in Schizophrenia (MATRICS)[4] (sponsored by the National Institute of Mental Health) have attempted to rectify the heterogeneity of functional measurement approaches by validating and recommending a core set of functional assessments. Other NIH initiatives, such as the Patient Reported Outcomes Measurement Information System (PROMIS)[5], are also underway to provide a standard 'toolbox' with which researchers and clinicians can select standardized population-normed instruments to measure functioning with self-report measures.

While the process of identifying a 'core' set of functional measures is ongoing, several important dimensions must be considered in any approach. The conceptualization of functional impairments generally separates what an individual *can* do (capacity) from what an individual *does* do (actual performance). Functional capacity refers to the ability of an individual to perform a task under optimal conditions and that performance can be measured with the observational or performance-based approaches described in the latter portion of this chapter. Actual performance may be discrepant from functional capacity, as real-world performance is affected by motivation, opportunities and environmental barriers.

In addition to the distinction between capacity and actual performance, the functional consequences of an illness can be judged in a number of ways. Functional status can be assessed relative to age-adjusted norms, premorbid ability or a criterion devised by an external entity (e.g. some government agency standard). The normative basis for assessing functioning is important when interpreting scores from instruments that are generic (e.g. the Medical Outcomes Study – Short Form) and meant to be applicable to the broad population. Alternatively, functioning measures can be disease-specific, such as those focusing on severe mental illnesses (e.g. the Independent Living Skills Survey). Although these latter measures may not provide an estimate of functioning relative to healthy older adults, the items may have a lower 'floor' and thus can guide rehabilitation targets in functionally impaired people.

Another way in which functioning can be classified, typically in population-based studies, are preference-weighted approaches. These approaches use population data on preferences for states of health to create indices of disability adjusted life years (DALYs) or quality adjusted life years (QALYs), which can be compared across illnesses or treatments. For example, the Quality of Well-Being Scale uses a preference-weighted approach. Previous use of this instrument

Principles and Practice of Geriatric Psychiatry, 3rd edn. Edited by Mohammed T. Abou-Saleh, Cornelius Katona and Anand Kumar
© 2011 John Wiley & Sons, Ltd

estimates that the 'well years' lost to schizophrenia among middle-aged and older adults are slightly more than that experienced by ambulatory individuals with AIDS[6].

Yet another distinction in assessing functioning involves the source of the information. Not surprisingly, ratings of functioning provided by patients, their family members and their clinicians often show inconsistencies – for example, patients with depression may overestimate their impairment, while patients with diminished insight due to dementia may believe they are fully capable when they are not. Family and clinician judgements of functioning may depend upon the degree to which they are familiar with the individual's functioning in the community. Some indicators of functioning, such as employment status or medication adherence, may be dependent on contextual factors such as availability of social support. Furthermore, daily living skills must be assumed to fluctuate within the individual, based both on the context and on the course of the psychiatric illness and its treatment, such that any point-in-time assessment of functioning may be biased by state-level factors (e.g. mood state, fatigue).

Taking all these considerations together, it is clear that attaining reliable and accurate representations of an individual's level of functioning presents a challenge for clinicians and researchers. The best approach typically utilizes multiple measures of functioning (e.g. performance-based, subjective ratings) in different contexts (e.g. at home and in the clinic).

WHAT ARE THE SKILLS OF DAILY LIVING?

There is no single definition of daily life skills, but the primary functional categories include activities of daily living, social role functioning, decision-making capacity and recovery. The activities of daily living (ADLs) were defined in the 1960s and a decade later they were differentiated from instrumental activities of daily living (IADLs). ADLs include toileting, dressing, transferring and other activities basic to maintaining residence in the community. IADLs are more cognitively complex and involve fine motor movements, including managing medications, using the telephone, arranging transportation, managing money and preparing meals. In the general population, impairment in ADLs and IADLs increases with age, although the overall prevalence of ADL impairment in older people seems to have declined over the past several decades[7]. Change in ADLs often corresponds to change in disease status and not infrequently triggers placement in a care facility. Typically, ADLs and IADLs are rated by an observer or clinician, but self-perceived impairment in functional tasks is also frequently evaluated. Measures of perceived ability to complete functional tasks are embedded in subjective questionnaires (e.g. 'Are you impaired in your ability to walk one mile?') as well as whether a disease impacts functioning (e.g. 'Has your mental health interfered with your social activities?'). Finally, a number of approaches to the measurement of general physical function are used to assess physical fitness in older adults (e.g. grip strength, sit to stand tests), but because these are not specifically tied to daily life skills, we will not describe them here. Interested readers are referred to an excellent review on these physical functioning instruments[8].

Social functioning is another key domain in functional assessment. Actual performance can be measured in regard to an individual's roles in the workplace, in close relationships and in leisure activities. In geriatric populations, particularly after retirement, social roles may be less culturally prescribed than among younger adults, which makes determining the extent of social impairment more challenging. Particularly in schizophrenia as opposed to mood disorders or dementia, social skills may be measured in standardized role-play tasks. These simulate conversations in which the participant's performance is graded. The use of performance-based measures of social functioning is generally restricted to research.

Another context of functional status that clinicians are frequently asked to evaluate in older adults with mental health problems is decision-making capacity, particularly with regard to medical or other major life decisions. The assessment of capacity to make decisions should be specific to the context. For example, it cannot be assumed that impairment in the handling of personal finances signifies impairment in the making of medical decisions, such as the refusal of treatment. Assessing decisional capacity typically includes four components: understanding, appreciation, reasoning and expressing a choice. Understanding describes the extent to which the individual comprehends what is at stake, i.e. probable outcomes, risks and benefits. Appreciation measures how well the individual can relate the decision to his or her own situation, while reasoning measures the quality of the mental process by which the individual arrives at that decision. Finally, expressing a choice concerns whether the individual is capable and/or willing to express a decision. Research in older patients with schizophrenia or bipolar disorder using standardized measures of decisional capacity has indicated that cognitive impairments are the single greatest predictor of impairment in decisional capacity, over and above psychotic or affective symptoms. However, the manner in which the information is conveyed to the patient, particularly whether it is repeated, appears to make a significant difference in whether capacity is achieved. It cannot be assumed that the presence of a psychiatric disorder translates to a lack of capacity.

Finally, recent years have seen an emergence of a more patient-centred concept of functioning that is termed 'recovery'. The precise definition of this term is debated, but a consensus panel formed by the US Substance Abuse and Mental Health Services Administration (SAMHSA) provided the following: 'Mental Health recovery is a journey of healing and transformation enabling a person with a mental health problem to live a meaningful life in a community of his or her choice while striving to achieve his or her full potential'[9]. Although recovery shares a focus with the above domains on functional outcomes, greater emphasis is placed on the patient's sense of self-efficacy and meaning. The measurement of recovery is thus more idiographic than that of the domains just described. How the construction of recovery changes, if at all, across the lifespan of people with mental illnesses has received little research.

WHAT ARE THE INFLUENCES ON DAILY LIVING SKILLS?

Many factors influence functioning and daily living skills, including illness, cultural issues, environmental contexts and age-related changes. In this section, we review the impact of these factors and provide an integrative model that combines them.

Emerging evidence in a variety of psychiatric disorders suggests that cognitive impairments are the greatest contributors to diminished functional status[10,11]. On average, the relative influence of cognitive impairments on functioning probably increases over the course of a long-term illness. This is in part due to declines in the acuity of psychopathological symptoms for people with early-onset mental illnesses[12] and also because cognitive impairments beyond those associated with normal ageing may cross thresholds to create functional impairment. A number of studies have examined the relative impact of cognition on functioning in older patients with mental illness and the general conclusion is that cognitive impairments supersede psychopathologic symptoms in their associations with functional deficits of older adults with schizophrenia, bipolar disorder and depression[13]. Among cognitive abilities, impairment in executive functioning, which includes planning, task switching and other higher order mental abilities, appears to be most influential on functional status. Recent research has suggested that even among older patients with depression or bipolar disorder, both cognitive impairments and functional problems appear to persist between mood episodes.

However, concurrent symptoms do appear to produce disability, particularly in subjective functioning. In addition to cognitive impairments, among older patients with schizophrenia, negative symptoms appear to be more closely associated with functional impairment than are positive symptoms. In mixed-age patients with bipolar disorder, depressive symptoms appear to be more disabling on average than manic symptoms, in part because they are, on average, more frequent and intractable. Another general trend among older adults with severe mental illnesses is that earlier age of onset is associated with greater functional impairment, likely because functional problems have had a longer time to accrue and because patients have a comparatively shorter time in which to establish life roles free of illness. Medical co-morbidities and substance abuse also appear to produce added functional impairment.

Another strong determinant of functional status and one frequently overlooked in assessment, is the patient's environment. The concept of person–environment fit[14] posits that functioning is a product of individual abilities and environmental supports. In this model, the physical and social environment may support or detract from autonomous function. For example, the elimination of high curbs can enable individuals in wheelchairs to function at a level similar to those who are not wheelchair-bound. By contrast, chaotic or novel environments may overwhelm cognitive resources and exacerbate functional deficits in vulnerable older people. Some recently developed interventions for schizophrenia[15] and for dementia[16] emphasize environmental supports to compensate for cognitive deficits and maintain functioning.

Finally, sociocultural influences affect functioning in geriatric patients with psychiatric disorders. Culturally based expectations regarding functioning and mental illness can influence the kinds of daily tasks an older adult can accomplish. For example, older immigrants may have a language barrier or lack the means to acquire resources needed to improve functioning. Moreover, culturally diverse older adults may be accustomed to carrying out daily activities following a different set of steps or using different means from those of the dominant culture. For example, a person may not know how to refill medication by way of telephone as is often done in the United States. The person may also come from a culture with clearly defined gender roles that impede the learning of such tasks as cooking, cleaning or driving a vehicle. Culturally held beliefs about the elderly can also influence daily functioning. For example, family members may feel obligated to do things for ageing relatives to ease their burden, ensure their safety, or to express culturally appropriate reverence. This sense of duty may intensify when a psychiatric illness is involved.

INTEGRATING THE CONTRIBUTORS TO FUNCTIONAL DISABILITY: A MODEL

A number of disablement models have been developed over the past three decades. Most recently, the WHO developed what it termed a revised working disability model. This model clarified certain constructs and operationalized functioning across three levels[17-20]: the body; the person as a whole; and the person in social contexts. While this model is useful, it lacks specificity and fails to consider a host of other factors which may influence functional capacity, such as cognitive deficits, earlier age of onset of illness, the environment in which a person lives and co-morbidities such as substance abuse.

The following conceptual model of functional capacity (see Figure 34.1), which incorporates many of the issues mentioned above, elaborates on the WHO model. Hypothetical paths between concepts are indicated by arrows. An important feature of this model is the role of mediation – i.e. causal links are implied between illness features and disability. Among older adults with

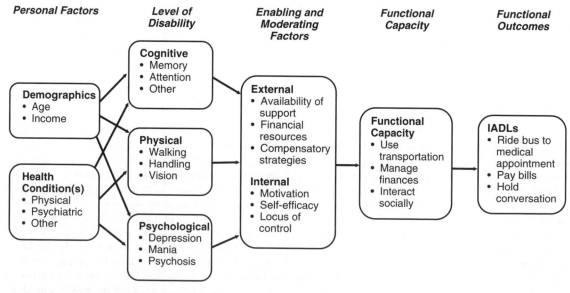

Figure 34.1 Model of functional capacity

schizophrenia, recent evidence shows that the pathway between cognitive abilities and functioning may be mediated by functional capacity. Bowie *et al.*[10] examined the relationships between functional capacity data, scores on the UCSD Performance-Based Skills Assessment (UPSA), case-manager ratings of real-world functioning (covering interpersonal skills, work skills and community activities), neuropsychological test scores and symptom levels, and they constructed a path model showing that neuropsychological performance predicted functional capacity, which in turn predicted all three domains of real-world functioning. Psychiatric symptoms, specifically depression, predicted interpersonal and work skills, while negative symptoms affected interpersonal skills independently of other predictors. However, while real-world adaptive life skills were predicted by neuropsychological performance, symptoms and functional capacity, neuropsychological performance contributed little to the prediction of real-world performance after accounting for functional capacity. This study illustrates how specific paths in our proposed model can be validated with data and the model provides a heuristic by which to organize assessment data in gauging individual functioning.

DESCRIPTIONS OF SPECIFIC MEASURES OF FUNCTIONING

As described in the introduction, many measures of functioning exist with different psychometric properties, formats and content. In considering which measure to use, it is important to recognize that all have limitations in terms of completeness, ceiling and floor effects, sensitivity to change and applicability across multiple patient groups (e.g. inpatients vs. outpatients). Measures for assessing functioning fall into four broad categories: self-reports, informant reports, clinician ratings and observational measures. Below and in Table 34.1 we have selected from among the best validated of these measures and describe the instruments in detail.

Table 34.1 An overview of specific functional instruments

Measure	Time to administer	Domains assessed	Type of administration	Validity, relationship to real-world outcomes
UPSA	30 minutes	Functional capacity: household chores, communication, finance, transportation and planning recreational activities	Performance-based	Predictive of one's ability to live independently in the community
UPSA-Brief	10–15 minutes	Functional capacity: finances and communication	Performance-based	Highly correlated with full UPSA
SSPA	20 minutes	Social skills	Performance-based	Excellent inter-rater reliability, good test–retest reliability; scores correlate with health-related QWB and observed performance on activities of daily living
MMAA	15 minutes	Medication management ability	Performance-based	Significantly related to prescription refill records, performance-based measures of everyday functioning and self-reported quality of life
ILSS-SR	20–30 minutes	Functional living skills (see text for full list)	Self-report	Marginal to good internal consistency, stability and inter-rater reliability; good ability to predict employability
GAF	5–15 minutes	Functional impairment secondary to mental illness	Clinician-rated	Good reliability and a valid measure of psychiatric disturbance in severely mentally ill
SF-36	5–10 minutes	Mental and physical health-related quality of life	Self-report	Good internal reliability and construct validity
QWB-SA	15 minutes	Quality adjusted life years Health-related quality of life	Self-report	Results comparable to interviewer-administered version
SAFE		Adaptive functioning; social-interpersonal, instrumental and life skills functioning	Observational	Good convergent, discriminant and predictive validity
MOSES		Levels of functioning in self-care, levels of organization, depressed and anxious mood, irritability and behavioural withdrawal	Observational	Satisfactory validity against other established measures (Zung depression, Robertson short mental status, Kingston dementia, PAMIE scales)

SELF-REPORT

Generic Measures

SF-36

The Medical Outcomes Study (MOS) 36-item short-form Health Survey (SF-36) is a self-report measure that covers eight different domains: physical functioning, role limitations due to physical health problems, bodily pain, general health perceptions, vitality, social functioning, role limitations due to emotional problems and mental health. These eight subscales are combined to produce two summary scores: the physical and the mental composite score[21]. An even shorter 12-item (SF-12) scale has been developed that can be completed in one or two minutes[22].

QWB

The Quality of Well-Being (QWB) is a preference-based questionnaire that measures health-related quality of life. The original version was administered by an interviewer, but a self-administered version (QWB-SA) was subsequently developed to avoid some of the difficulties associated with interviewer administration. The QWB-SA consists of five sections totalling 56 items that assess acute or chronic symptoms, self-care, mobility, physical functioning and performance of everyday activities. Participants are asked to think about the past three days and indicate if they experienced the symptom or problem on the previous day, two days ago, three days ago, or some combination thereof. The QWB-SA takes approximately 15 minutes to complete[23].

Disease-Specific Measures

ILSS

The Independent Living Skills Survey (ILSS) tests basic functioning in patients with severe and persistent mental illness. There are two versions: informant-rated (ILSS-I) and self-report (ILSS-SR). The ILSS-I consists of 103 items that assess 12 areas of basic community living skills. The ILSS-SR has 70 items that cover 10 different domains: personal hygiene, appearance and care of clothing, care of personal possessions and living space, food preparation, care of personal health and safety, money management, transportation, leisure and recreational activities, job seeking and job maintenance. Participants are asked to indicate by a 'yes' or 'no' response whether they had performed a specific task in the past month. The ILSS-SR takes approximately 20 to 30 minutes to complete[24].

INFORMANT RATINGS

ADL

Some patients, such as in Alzheimer's disease, may not be able to complete a self-report measure. In such cases, an informant provides information on life skills. Typically, the informant is a spouse, an adult child, or a caregiver who spends at least two days a week in direct contact with the patient. The Katz activities of daily living (ADL) index is one of the more widely used informant-rated measures. Caregivers rate the patient's level of dependence on others in six different areas: bathing, dressing, toileting, transferring, continence and feeding. A zero score indicates complete independence, while a three is complete dependence. Slightly more sensitive than the Katz is the Barthel index, which uses 10 different categories. In addition to the six categories used in the Katz, the Barthel index divides toileting into bladder and bowel control and adds walking, stair climbing and grooming. Higher scores are assigned to those with higher levels of independent functioning, for a possible total of 100 points[26].

IADL

The Instrumental Activities of Daily Living Scale (IADL) covers the more complex instrumental activities that are needed to live independently. The IADL evaluates ability to use a telephone, shop, prepare food, keep house, do laundry, use transportation, take medication and manage finances. Typically, women are scored on all eight domains, while for men, food preparation, housekeeping and laundering are sometimes excluded[27].

RIL

Another example of an informant-completed measure is the Record of Independent Living (RIL). The informant rates the patient on the categories of activities, communication and behaviour. Ratings for activities range from 0 (no change when compared to previous competence) to 4 (patient no longer performs this activity) with allowances for 'don't know' or 'not applicable.' Similarly, ratings for communication range from 0 (no difficulty) to 4 (no longer performs this function). The behaviour section consists of a checklist on which the informant indicates whether specific problem behaviours were present before the illness and whether they are currently present[28].

CLINICIAN-RATED

GAF

The Global Assessment of Functioning (GAF) describes a person's overall psychological, social and occupational functioning. It is used as Axis V in the *Diagnostic and Statistical Manual of Mental Disorders*, Fourth Edition and consists of 10 'ranges of function' that total 10 points each, for an overall possible score of 100. A perfect score indicates superior functioning, while a score of less than 10 indicates 'persistent danger of severely hurting self or others, or inability to maintain minimal personal hygiene, or serious suicidal act with clear expectation of death'. The GAF co-mingles functional impairment and psychiatric symptoms and so it is not a 'pure' measure of functioning as is the ILSS[25].

OBSERVATION

SAFE

The Social Adaptive Functioning Evaluation (SAFE) was developed for a geriatric psychiatric inpatient population to evaluate social-interpersonal, instrumental and life-skills functioning. This 17-item scale is scored using observation, caregiver contact and interaction with the subject. These items assess self-care, social competence and adjustment and miscellaneous skills such as impulse control and cooperativeness. Items are rated on a 5-point scale with higher scores reflecting greater impairment. This scale is useful because the patient can be rated regardless of their cooperation or responses[29].

MOSES

The Multidimensional Observation Scale of Elderly Subjects (MOSES) is an observation-based measure that can be completed by nurses or staff at residential facilities. It consists of 40 items that measure five different areas of functioning related to life in a residential facility: self-care, levels of organization, depressed and anxious mood, irritability and behavioural withdrawal. There is also a briefer 24-item version[30-32].

PERFORMANCE-BASED MEASURES

UPSA

The UCSD Performance-Based Skills Assessment (UPSA) uses role-play tasks to examine five areas of everyday functioning including household chores, communication, finance, transportation and planning recreational activities. Patients are asked to plan a trip to the beach, write a cheque, read a bus route map, complete a shopping list and call a doctor to reschedule an appointment. It typically takes about 30 minutes to administer and includes several props such as grocery items, maps and a telephone. The UPSA has shown excellent reliability as well as strong convergent validity and good criterion validity with real-world outcome measures[33]. Also available is the UPSA-Brief, which includes only the communication and finances sections of the original UPSA. The UPSA-Brief and UPSA show high levels of convergence in predicting real-world functional outcomes.

MMAA

The Medication Management Ability Assessment (MMAA) also uses role-playing tasks, specifically focused on assessing a patient's ability to manage a moderately complex prescription medication regimen similar to one an older adult might typically encounter. The interviewer shows the patient four standard prescription pill bottles with mock labels and filled with differently coloured dried beans. The labels read: Parlenol: Take 2 tablets twice a day with food; BRB: Take 1 tablet 3 times per day; Cyclomeovan: Take 2 tablets three times a day on an empty stomach (i.e. at least 1 hour before or 2 hours after a meal); and Linophen: Take 2 tablets 4 times a day. The interviewer then removes the bottles and an hour later the interviewer asks the participant to 'walk' verbally through his or her day, handing the interviewer the appropriate type and number of pills at the appropriate times. Scores are based on the total number of correct responses for a possible total of 25 points. The number of pills over and under the prescribed amount is also scored. The MMAA has excellent test–retest reliability and good construct validity, with scores significantly correlated with two other performance-based measures of functionality[34].

SSPA

The Social Skills Performance Assessment (SSPA) is designed to measure everyday social skills. This performance-based measure consists of two role-playing tasks, each lasting three minutes. In the first task, the interviewer plays a new neighbour and the participant's goal is to initiate an acquaintance with the new neighbour in a 'friendly and informative manner'. In the second task, the participant plays a tenant who must contact his or her landlord (played by the interviewer) to discuss a leak that needs to be repaired immediately. Each scenario is scored from 1 (low) to 5 (high) on various factors including: interest/disinterest, fluency, clarity, focus, affect, grooming, social appropriateness, overall conversation, negotiation ability, submission/persistence and overall argument. The entire measure takes about 20 minutes to administer[35].

SUMMARY

We have described a general approach to assessing life skills in older people with psychiatric disorders, an integrative model linking the determinants of functioning with each other and specific instruments that cover multiple modalities. The best approach to measuring functioning integrates multiple assessments modalities in different contexts and uses both subjective and objective data obtained from the patient, family or other proxy informants and direct observation. The use of instruments validated in geriatric populations, such as the ones we have described, will increase the reliability and interpretability of assessment. As the focus of psychiatric care shifts from symptoms to broader functional outcomes and recovery, expanding the evidence base for functional assessments will become all the more important.

ACKNOWLEDGEMENTS

The authors would like to acknowledge the following sources of funding which supported the writing of this chapter: for Dr Depp, K-award No. MH077225; for Dr Cardenas, training grant No. T32 MH 019934-15 (Jeste, Dilip); and Dr Patterson, R01 MH078737 and the Department of Veteran Affairs.

REFERENCES

1. Jablensky A. Epidemiology of schizophrenia: the global burden of disease and disability. *Eur Arch Psychiatry Clin Neurosci* 2000; **250**: 274.
2. Murray CJ, Lopez AD. Global mortality, disability and the contributions of risk factors. *Lancet* 1997; **349**: 1436–42.
3. 2009 Alzheimer's Disease Facts and Figures. Alzheimer's Association, 2009.
4. Marder SR, Fenton W. Measurement and treatment research to improve cognition in schizophrenia: NIMH MATRICS initiative to support the development of agents for improving cognition in schizophrenia. *Schizophr Res* 2004; **72**: 5.
5. Cella D, Yount S, Rothrock N, Gershon R, Cook K, Reeve B et al. The Patient-Reported Outcomes Measurement Information System (PROMIS): progress of an NIH roadmap cooperative group during its first two years. *Med Care* 2007; **45**: S3–11.
6. Patterson TL, Kaplan RM, Grant I, Semple SJ, Moscona S, Koch WL et al. Quality of well-being in late-life psychosis. *Psychiatry Res* 1996; **63**: 169.
7. Freedman VA, Martin LG, Schoeni RF. Recent Trends in disability and functioning among older adults in the United States: a systematic review. *JAMA* 2002; **288**: 3137–46.
8. Subashan P, Samir HM, Richard CW, Stephanie AS. Meaningful change and responsiveness in common physical performance measures in older adults. *J Am Geriatr Soc* 2006; **54**; 743–9.
9. Administration SAaMHS. National Consensus Statement on Mental Health Recovery. US Department of Health and

Human Services, 2004, updated 22 June 2009. At http://mentalhealth.samhsa.gov/publications/allpubs/sma05-4129/.

10. Bowie CR, Reichenberg A, Patterson TL, Heaton RK, Harvey PD. Determinants of real-world functional performance in schizophrenia subjects: correlations with cognition, functional capacity and symptoms. *Am J Psychiatry* 2006; **163**: 418–25.

11. Twamley EW, Doshi RR, Nayak GV, Palmer BW, Golshan S, Heaton RK *et al*. Generalized cognitive impairments, ability to perform everyday tasks and level of independence in community living situations of older patients with psychosis. *Am J Psychiatry* 2002; **159**: 2013–20.

12. Jeste DV, Twamley EW, Zorrilla LTE, Golshan S, Patterson TL, Palmer BW. Aging and outcome in schizophrenia. *Acta Psychiatr Scand* 2003; **107**: 336–43.

13. Green M. Cognitive impairment and functional outcome in schizophrenia and bipolar disorder. *J Clin Psychiatry* 2006; **67**: 3–8.

14. Teresi JA, Holmes D, Ory MG. The therapeutic design of environments for people with dementia: further reflections and recent findings from the National Institute on Aging Collaborative Studies of Dementia Special Care Units. *Gerontologist* 2000; **40**: 417–21.

15. Velligan DI, Prihoda TJ, Ritch JL, Maples N, Bow-Thomas CC, Dassori A. A randomized single-blind pilot study of compensatory strategies in schizophrenia outpatients. *Schizophr Bull* 2002; **28**: 283–92.

16. Iwarsson S, Wahl H-W, Nygren C, Oswald F, Sixsmith A, Sixsmith J *et al*. Importance of the Home environment for healthy aging: conceptual and methodological background of the European ENABLE-AGE project. *Gerontologist* 2007; **47**: 78–84.

17. Nagi SZ. An Epidemiology of disability among adults in the United States. *The Milbank Memorial Fund Quarterly Health Soc* 1976; **54**: 439.

18. Pope AM, Tarlov AR. *Disability in America: Toward a National Agenda for Prevention*. Washington, DC: National Acadamy Press, 1991.

19. Verbrugge L, Jette A. The disablement process. *Soc Sci Med* 1994; **38**: 1–14.

20. Whiteneck G, Fougeyrollas P, Gerhart K. Elaborating the model of disablement. In Fuhrer M (ed.), *Assessing Medical Rehabilitation Practices: The Promise of Outcome Research*. Baltimore: PH Brooks, 1997, 91–102.

21. Ware JE, Jr, Sherbourne CD. The MOS 36-ltem Short-Form Health Survey (SF-36): I. Conceptual framework and item selection. *Med Care* 1992; **30**: 473–83.

22. Gandek B, Ware JE, Aaronson NK, Apolone G, Bjorner JB, Brazier JE *et al*. Cross-validation of item selection and scoring

for the SF-12 health survey in nine countries: results from the IQOLA project. *J Clin Epidemiol* 1998; **51**: 1171.

23. Kaplan RM, Sieber WJ, Ganiats TG. The quality of well-being scale: Comparison of the interviewer-administered version with a self-administered questionnaire. *Psychol Health* 1997; **12**: 783–91.

24. Wallace CJ, Liberman RP, Tauber R, Wallace J. The Independent Living Skills Survey: a comprehensive measure of the community functioning of severely and persistently mentally ill individuals. *Schizophr Bull* 2000; **26**: 631–58.

25. Jones SH, Thornicroft G, Coffey M, Dunn G. A brief mental health outcome scale-reliability and validity of the Global Assessment of Functioning (GAF). *Br J Psychiatry* 1995; **166**: 654–9.

26. Katz S, Akpom C. A measure of primary sociobiological functions. *Int J Health Serv* 1976; **6**: 493–508.

27. Lawton MP, Brody EM. Assessment of older people: self-maintaining and instrumental activities of daily living. *Gerontologist* 1969; **9**: 179–86.

28. Weintraub S. The record of independent living: an informant-completed measure of activities of daily living and behavior in elderly patients with cognitive impairment. *Am J Alzheimers Dis Other Dement* 1986; **1**: 35–9.

29. Harvey PD, Davidson M, Mueser KT, Parrella M, White L, Powchik P. Social-Adaptive Functioning Evaluation (SAFE): a rating scale for geriatric psychiatric patients. *Schizophr Bull* 1997; **23**: 131–45.

30. Helmes E, Csapo KG, Short J-a. Standardization and Validation of the Multidimensional Observation Scale for Elderly Subjects (MOSES). *J Gerontol* 1987; **42**: 395–405.

31. Pruchno RA, Kleban MH, Resch NL. Psychometric Assessment of the Multidimensional Observation Scale for Elderly Subjects (MOSES). *J Gerontol* 1988; **43**: P164–9.

32. Diehl M, Spore DL, Smyer MA. Measurement Properties of the Short Multidimensional Observation Scale for Elderly Subjects (MOSES. *J Appl Gerontol* 1997; **16**: 403–26.

33. Patterson TL, Goldman S, McKibbin CL, Hughs T, Jeste DV. UCSD Performance-based skills assessment: development of a new measure of everyday functioning for severely mentally ill adults. *Schizophr Bull* 2001; **27**: 235–45.

34. Patterson TL, Lacro J, McKibbin CL, Moscona S, Hughs T, Jeste DV. Medication management ability assessment: results from a performance-based measure in older outpatients with schizophrenia. *J Clin Psychopharmacol* 2002; **22**: 11–19.

35. Patterson TL, Moscona S, McKibbin CL, Davidson K, Jeste DV. Social skills performance assessment among older patients with schizophrenia. *Schizophr Res* 2001; **48**: 351.

35

Quality of Life Measures in Old Age

Juanita Hoe, Martin Orrell and Gill Livingston

Department of Mental Health Sciences, University College London, UK

INTRODUCTION

The maintenance of physical and cognitive functioning and the avoidance of disease are associated with well-being and quality of life (QoL) in old age, as poor health can lead to loss of control, autonomy and independence[1,2]. Traditionally, outcomes of treatment have been evaluated in terms of mortality or symptoms, but a more important outcome measure may be the patient's perspective, as symptoms may improve in one area while overall quality of life decreases because of the negative effects of treatment[3]. The emergence of QoL as a fundamental measure for evaluating and monitoring health outcomes in old age is attributed to the ethical and economic concerns associated with the ageing population and the concomitant increase in chronic illness and disability. Birren and Dieckmann[4] identify three main areas of concern associated with this increase: (i) the impact on health service resources and the potential financial burden anticipated; (ii) the intrusive use of medical technologies; and (iii) the QoL for people in institutions. In chronic illness, people can suffer from both the disability and the treatment[5]. Moreover, treatment can often result in limited gains in terms of survival, or absence of cure, which changes the balance as to acceptable side effects. Aggressive interventions may have therapeutic benefits that are overshadowed by the negative effects, thus leading to reduced QoL overall. Any detrimental impact on QoL needs to be weighed against the advantages offered through treatment[6]. It is the individual's perception that predicts whether they seek help, accept treatment or regard themselves to be well and recovered, and therefore, should be part of any outcome measures[7]. Thus, subjective health measures can be used to help provide a fuller picture of the individual's health state.

THE MEANING OF QoL

The term quality of life is used frequently in everyday life, with most people assuming they know what it means without considering how to define or measure it. In terms of health, QoL has become a popular, broadly used expression that is frequently taken for granted without the meaning being clear. There is debate about the true definition and meaning of QoL, particularly whether ratings should be objective or subjective, what criteria should be used and what is actually being measured, 'the quality of an individual's life, state of life, or the meaning of life in general'[8]. QoL is argued to be less related to basic needs than to individual expectations and experiences of life, which include individual perceptions of well-being, happiness, goodness and satisfaction with various aspects of their lives and environment[9-11]. What is apparent is that QoL is a multi-dimensional concept 'just as is life itself'[12]. A wide range of domains is suggested for inclusion as QoL indicators, including physical and mental health, intellectual and emotional function, social and role function, activities of daily living, economic aspects, and job and life satisfaction[13-15]. The expression QoL may also overlap with the terms 'health status' and 'functional status', and have been considered interchangeable[16]. Perceptions of well-being may, however, be influenced by psychological factors unrelated to health or function[17].

DEFINITIONS AND CONCEPTUALIZATIONS OF QoL

There are several meanings of the term QoL, which remains a vague, elusive concept for which there is no single widely accepted definition. The definitions provided are broad and varied; indeed, there may be as many QoL definitions as there are people[18]. QoL is viewed as 'a concept which incorporates all aspects of an individual's existence'[19] and as 'an abstraction which integrates and summarizes all those features of our lives that we find more or less desirable and satisfying'[20]. The inclusion of the terms life satisfaction, morale and happiness are debated but may be considered to be transient states which should be distinguished from QoL as they differ in their degree of subjectivity[21]. Alternatively, life satisfaction, self-esteem and physical health are argued to be key dimensions of QoL[22]. Lawton[23] defines QoL as 'the multidimensional evaluation, by both intrapersonal and social-normative criteria, of the person–environment system of an individual in time past, current and anticipated' and hypothesizes four dimensions of QoL: behavioural competence, perceived QoL, objective environment, and psychological well-being. Each sector is intrinsic and considered core to the concept of QoL and also interlinked. Fundamentally, QoL is perceived as being continuous and dynamic in nature and may be evaluated negatively or positively depending on the individual's own internal perceptions and response to their environment.

HEALTH-RELATED QoL

Within the context of health, QoL is defined as a reflection of patients' perception and response to their health status and to other non-medical aspects that have an impact on patients' lives, and within health-related quality of life (HRQoL) this includes physical,

Principles and Practice of Geriatric Psychiatry, 3rd edn. Edited by Mohammed T. Abou-Saleh, Cornelius Katona and Anand Kumar
© 2011 John Wiley & Sons, Ltd

psychological and social perspectives[24,25]. This definition is in keeping with that given by the World Health Organization Quality of Life Group (WHOQOL), as 'the individuals' perception of their position in life in the context of the culture and value systems in which they live and in relation to their goals, expectations, standards and concerns'[26]. This broad description encompasses the complex nature of the person's physical, psychological and social well-being in relation to their environment. The recognition of cultural factors is particularly important when considering the QoL of the ageing population and especially those people with dementia. Memory impairment is not regarded as so important in all cultures[27]. Similarly, functional disability may seem less important in cultural contexts where independence and autonomy in activities of daily living are a less central part of the older person's role[28]. Older people are frequently marginalized as society holds a negative view of their QoL, and health and social research tends to focus on decline and disability[29]. There are, however, both positive and negative elements that impact on an older person's QoL, and Hughes[30] identifies the key domains that should be evaluated when measuring older people's QoL. These include physical environment, social environment, socioeconomic, cultural and health status, personality and personal autonomy factors.

MEASURING QoL IN HEALTH

Lerner[31] argues that 'health is more than just a biomedical phenomenon; it involves a social human-being functioning in a social environment with social roles they need to fulfil'. The use of QoL as an outcome measure focuses the impact of the patient's condition and treatment on their emotional and physical functioning and lifestyle[3]. Hence, health-related QoL has become important in measuring the impact of chronic disease[16]. This is of particular significance as patients with the same clinical symptoms often differ in their evaluation of what the illness means to their life. The term 'disability paradox' is used to describe how patients with significant health and functional problems frequently have high QoL scores despite their health status[32]. QoL measures can be used to evaluate human and financial costs-benefits of interventions and care provided through assessing change in physical, functional, mental and social health[33].

Calman[34] suggests that people perceive QoL in relationship to their past experiences, current lifestyle, hopes and ambitions for the future. QoL measures the gap between the individual's present experience and their expectations for the future. QoL can therefore be improved by narrowing this gap, either by improving experience or lowering expectations[34]. Importantly, the model recognizes the highly individual nature of QoL and the influence of culture and past experience[35]. Carr et al.[36] further propose a model of the relation between expectations and experience and identify three areas of difficulty in measuring QoL: people have different expectations; people are at different stages of their illness when QoL is measured; and expectations may change over time. By providing health education, information and increasing awareness of risks, patients are helped to adapt to their disability through changing their health expectations. The impact of the disability on their QoL may thus be reduced[36].

SUBJECTIVE AND OBJECTIVE DIMENSIONS OF QoL

Testa and Simonson[33] recommend that measures of QoL should cover the objective and subjective components important to the relevant patient group that may be affected positively or negatively

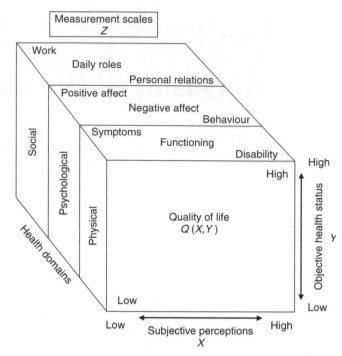

Figure 35.1 Conceptual scheme of the domains and variables involved in a QoL assessment
Source: Reproduced with permission from Testa & Simonson (1996), *New England Journal of Medicine*, 334: 834–840. Copyright ©1996 Massachusetts Medical Society. All rights reserved.

by interventions. Objective factors are primarily needs based and incorporate basic needs that determine people's well-being in society, such as environment and material resources, including levels of income, crime, pollution, transport, housing type, access to amenities and employment[2,37]. Subjective factors include life satisfaction and psychological well-being, morale, individual fulfilment, happiness and self-esteem, and are expressed in terms of satisfaction, values and perceptions of individual life circumstances[1]. While health status is defined through the objective components, QoL is determined through subjective perception and expectations (Figure 35.1)[33]. The subjective perceptions thus translate that objective assessment into the actual QoL experienced.[33] Nevertheless, Bowling[3] cautions that subjective measures are not designed to be used as substitutes for traditional measures of clinical endpoints but to complement existing measures and provide a fuller picture of health state.

Variation among QoL scales is often due to the different emphasis placed on objective and subjective dimensions, which domains are covered and the question format rather than differences in how QoL is defined[33]. The overall satisfaction an individual has with life is argued to be the most important domain of QoL[2,38]. This means the importance of the individual's personal sense of satisfaction with various areas of life is recognized; these include physical comfort, emotional well-being and interpersonal connections[38].

VALIDITY AND RELIABILITY

QoL scales should be able to demonstrate validity but this is complicated as there is no measure of criterion validity: no scale can provide a full picture of people's life quality or be relevant to all individuals[33,39,40]. Content validity includes evaluation in terms of the applicability of the questionnaire and its comprehensiveness, as well as its clarity, simplicity and likelihood of bias[41]. Scales should also have predictive validity, sensitivity and be responsive to change in QoL, particularly for clinically important changes[3,33,42,43]. This ensures the areas relevant to the patient's QoL are measured and that scales are responsive to the different stages of the disease and interventions or treatment given. Orley et al.[44] argue that QoL is influenced by a broad range of facets and is therefore unlikely to alter markedly from day to day. Fallowfield[45] recommends that QoL measures should discriminate between patient groups and identify those patients experiencing good QoL and those who are not. In addition, QoL measures used in clinical practice must be appropriate and acceptable for their intended use and the results meaningful and amenable to clinical interpretation[43].

GENERIC VERSUS DISEASE-SPECIFIC MEASURES OF QoL

Generic as opposed to disease-specific instruments offer broader measures of health status and are useful for making comparisons with other conditions, while disease-specific instruments are used for assessing disease-related attributes when greater sensitivity to specific aspects of the clinical condition is required[3,33]. Generic measures include single indicators, health profiles and utility measures. Health profiles attempt to measure all aspects of health-related QoL potentially affected by a condition or its treatment. Thus generic instruments tend to be lengthy to ensure sensitivity and adequate psychometric properties[3]. They can be applied irrespective of the underlying condition but may be unresponsive to changes in specific conditions. Disease-specific instruments aim to have greater discrimination between severity levels of a particular disease and thus have increased sensitivity to clinical outcomes[44]. They are more concise and should be able to reflect clinically significant change in health status or disease severity. Therefore in order to detect significant clinical changes, generic measures may need to be supplemented with disease-specific measures[16], particularly for evaluating therapeutic interventions within clinical trials[33]. The use of disease-specific measures may, however, be limited as their narrow focus may not assess the impact of disease or interventions upon wider aspects of life, which could disadvantage arguments for additional resources[24,46].

Essentially the use of both generic and disease-specific measures is recommended to ensure assessment of both disease-specific and wider aspects of life and to detect positive or negative impacts of interventions[3,16,24].

METHODS OF QoL MEASUREMENT

Self-Assessment Scales

The use of visual analogue scales is a common method for measuring subjective experiences such as QoL[47]. They are, however, time consuming to complete and may not be relevant to the experience being considered[45]. Self-reports are obtained using standardized measures that have response formats with closed questions in a categorical dichotomous format (e.g. yes/no) or sequences of categorized responses (e.g. strongly agree, agree, disagree, strongly disagree). Standardized measures have fixed questions and a range of answers; Carr and Higginson[32] caution that these may not measure patients' QoL unless scores are weighted for the individual patient.

Individual weightings are important for obtaining a true assessment of QoL and being responsive to change. Scores may be calculated for each domain separately or combined to provide a composite or index score of overall life satisfaction. The disadvantage of scales that are calculated to produce an overall score is that the total may result from several combinations of responses, thus leading to a loss of information about the individual components of the scale[48]. Muldoon et al.[17] and Lawton[49] both argue that the use of a composite score fails to recognize QoL measures as being multidimensional and that it is illogical to aggregate scores that combine appraisals of objective measures of behaviour, function and subjective well-being; and there is a need to evaluate individual domains separately within research and clinical practice[12,30,49]. Alternatively, Gill and Feinstein[25] advocate the use of a global rating through aggregating the scores of individual QoL domains as this explains QoL more comprehensively, and they encourage more explicit criteria or weighting of the different components that construct QoL. Furthermore global ratings have been considered more acceptable for use in clinical trials as change in QoL could be more easily distinguished.

Direct Observation

Where self-ratings of QoL are difficult to elicit, such as in dementia, observational ratings may be of more benefit[50-52]. Observational methods are undertaken either through direct observation of the person with dementia, which records the frequency at which certain behaviours present, or by applying attribute ratings of observed affect states over time. Direct observation is time consuming and costly but, it has been argued, provides the most objective method of rating QoL in dementia as the subjective component is removed[49,53]. Observation requires a degree of interpretation by the rater and training to reduce any influence on the behaviour observed. In addition, multiple observations of the same individual are needed to achieve a consistent result and cannot be limited to the 'working day' of the observer[54]. Observational tools have, however, been devised that can be used to reliably measure health-related QoL and well-being in people with dementia[55,56], with Dementia Care Mapping[56] being increasingly used to assess the well-being of people with dementia in care settings. Well-being scores were found to be closely associated with QoL[57].

Proxy Ratings

Proxy ratings involve a judgement of the person's QoL being made by another person to whom they are known and may be provided by a paid or family caregiver. Proxy reports may be the only source of information available, particularly for those people with the most severe levels of cognitive impairment[58]. Proxy ratings have been shown to be a reliable and valid indicator of patient QoL[59,60]. Nevertheless, proxies impose their own judgement, and in dementia these are thought to be influenced by feelings of caregiver burden and depression as well as by how the person with dementia is feeling[59,61]. Moreover, QoL is consistently rated lower by caregivers than by patients with mild to moderate dementia[62-66]. While proxy ratings may be considered necessary where cognitive impairment exists, the inclusion of the individual's own rating of QoL is the preferred method for assessment, as QoL ultimately reflects the experience of the person with the disease[67,68].

Utility Assessments (Cost-Effectiveness)

Utility measures of QoL originate from economic and decision theory and are devised to reflect the health status and value of that health status to a patient[16], to assess cost-effectiveness in health care. When applying utility measures, values are placed on different health states, and the preference of a particular health outcome is determined through calculating a single summary score[3]. A common utility measure is quality adjusted life years (QALY), which are used as indicators of health gain for health service resource allocation. QALYs integrate two concepts, life expectancy and life quality, that offer a mathematical outcome for rationing the allocation of health service resources[8]. Although offering a utilitarian argument for determining the greatest health gain for the greatest number, QALYs are criticized as being ageist and for focusing on cure rather than care and their use marginalizes the most disabled, elderly and chronically ill[48]. Older people have a shorter life expectancy in comparison to younger people. A further criticism of using QALYs is that the 'disability paradox', where QoL scores do not appear commensurate with the patient's health status, prevents direct comparisons of different patient groups for allocating resources[43]. There are, however, other measures of cost-effectiveness that consider the cost per unit of health gain and do not involve years. Cost-utility ratios are being calculated in some trials in dementia using utility scores computed from the EQ-5D and societal weights. The National Institute for

Health and Clinical Excellence (NICE) now uses cost-effectiveness in consideration of all interventions in the UK[69].

MEASURING QoL IN OLDER AGE

Early studies identify retirement, bereavement, loneliness and isolation as important influences on older people's lives[70], whereas, more recent studies found that older people define good QoL as family, social contacts, health, mobility/ability, material circumstances, activities, happiness, youthfulness and living environment[71]. Hyde et al.[72] argue that the improved health and financial status of older people means the lives of older people have changed over recent decades, with increased healthy life expectancy and access to personal incomes, such as private pensions, share dividends and rent. The QoL of people entering old age who are younger, healthier and wealthier will differ from those much older people who are more likely to experience chronic and degenerative ill health or require palliative care. Not all older people can be assumed to suffer poor QoL and while health status is an essential component of QoL, it cannot be used as a proxy for QoL in older age[72]. Individual perceptions are therefore essential in assessing health-related QoL in people of all age groups. Magaziner[73] reported that a fifth of older adults living in the community and half of those living in institutions are reluctant or unable to be interviewed. In contrast, Livingston et al.[74] administered the Index of Health-Related Quality of Life (IHQL)[75]

Table 35.1 Generic quality of life instruments for use with older people

QoL measure	Target population	Respondent	Item no.	Domains	Single score	Time taken
EQ-5D EuroQol Group[96]	General	Self-report	5	Mobility Self-care Usual activities Pain/discomfort Anxiety/depression	Yes	5 mins
SF-12 Ware et al.[78]	General	Self-report	12–36	Physical functioning Role – physical Bodily pain General health Vitality Social functioning Role – emotional Mental health Health transition	Yes	10 mins
HSQ – 12 item Radosevich and Pruitt[77]	General	Self-report	12–39	Physical functioning Role – physical Bodily pain Health perception Energy/fatigue Social functioning Role – mental Mental health	Yes	10 mins
CASP-19 Hyde et al.[72]	Early old age	Self-report	19	Control Autonomy Self-realization Pleasure	No	Not specified

Table 35.2 Dementia-specific quality of life instruments

QoL measure	Target population	Respondent	Item. no.	Domains	Single score	Time taken
ADRQL Rabins et al.[88]	Mild/moderate and severe dementia	Caregiver – proxy Formal and informal	47	Social interaction Awareness of self Feeling and mood Enjoyment of activities Response to surroundings	Yes	Not specified
DQOL Brod et al.[51]	Mild/moderate dementia MMSE $\geq$ 12	Self-report	29	Self-esteem Positive affect Negative affect Feeling of belonging Sense of aesthetics	No	15–20 mins
QOL-AD Logsdon et al.[61]	Mild/moderate dementia Severe dementia MMSE $\geq$ 3	Self-report+ Caregiver – proxy	13	Physical health Mental health Personal relationships Finances Overall life quality	Yes	10 mins
C-BS Ready et al.[100]	MCI Mild/moderate dementia MMSE $\geq$ 9	Self-report Caregiver – proxy	19	Negative affectivity Positive affectivity Self-esteem Physical complaints Satisfactions	Yes	15 mins
DEMQOL Smith et al.[99]	Mild/moderate dementia MMSE $\geq$ 10	Self-report	28	Health Well-being Cognitive functioning Social relationships Self-concept	Yes	Not specified

to a community sample of 782 older people aged 65 years and older. Their study found that three quarters of the respondents were able to complete the IHQL and the other measures used; interestingly, this included those people with dementia. Those experiencing somatic symptoms or subjective memory impairment were less likely to complete the questionnaires. They found that the scale was not valid in older people. Pettit et al.[76] administered the 12-item Health Status Questionnaire (HSQ-12)[77] or the 12-item Short Form Health Survey (SF-12)[78] to a community sample of 1 085 older people over 65 years of age. They found that both Health-Related QoL measures were acceptable and valid for use within this population. Completion rates were lower in those people with dementia and the SF-12 was found not to distinguish between people with and without dementia. It is clear, therefore, that most older people and those experiencing dementia are able to complete instruments assessing their own QoL.

MEASURING QoL IN MENTAL ILLNESS

Orley et al.[44] discuss the use of QoL measures in psychiatric patients and consider how QoL ratings may be affected by the impact of the disorder through disturbed affect or thinking and through institutionalization. While psychiatric symptoms such as depression may affect a person's QoL, they do not distort it or make their perceptions invalid. In addition, while institutionalization may mean psychiatric patients perceive a good QoL due to lowered expectations, their assessments are still valid. Proxy ratings for patients with cognitive

impairment may be useful for planning and evaluating care, but they should not be taken as a measure of perceived QoL.[44]

MEASURING QoL IN DEMENTIA

The nature of dementia, which affects cognition and communication, means assessing QoL in dementia offers a unique challenge. The progression of dementia is non-linear; dementia has multiple causes and outcomes and is a complex disorder when compared with other health states[46]. Difficulties are routinely assumed in people with dementia providing subjective assessments of their QoL or care, owing to limitations with comprehension and reliability[79]. Providing an answer does not mean that the question is necessarily understood, and QoL may also be perceived differently as the disease progresses[80]. However, it is logical to assume that people with dementia will have likes and dislikes[55]. Even in the most severe dementia it is possible to display preferences and aversions through emotional expression. Lawton[49] reasons that although subjective measures demand a degree of cognitive skill, people with dementia can provide reliable assessments of their mood and QoL. The patient's subjective ratings of QoL are suggested as the gold standard for measuring QoL.

Several studies have now shown that QoL can be reliably measured in people with mild, moderate and severe dementia using self-rating QoL scales[51,61,81,82]. However, there are differences in QoL ratings as given by caregiver proxies and those given by the person with dementia[62,83–86]. Clinicians should be aware that proxy ratings do not necessarily replicate the QoL views of the person with dementia, and should not be substituted for self-ratings.

Few studies have employed QoL as an outcome measure for interventions in dementia and at present the evidence is not consistent, possibly due to the variety of measures used. Studies have indicated both an increase and a decrease in QoL as dementia advances[65,87,88]. Some studies that have identified cognition and dementia severity as a predictor of QoL in dementia[59,89] were based on caregiver proxy ratings of the person, although more recent studies found caregiver proxy ratings of QoL were strongly associated with depression, disability, and neuropsychiatric symptoms of the person with dementia[64,83,84,90,91]. Depressive symptoms have most consistently been identified as a predictor of lower QoL in dementia[59,62-64,66,81-84]. A review of recent studies of QoL in dementia found that depression was most strongly associated with lower QoL in dementia, but found no consistent association between lower QoL and sociodemographic factors or a decline in cognition and functional ability[92].

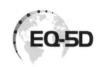

Health Questionnaire

English version for the UK
(validated for Ireland)

By placing a tick in one box in each group below, please indicate which statements best describe your own health state today.

Mobility

I have no problems in walking about ☐
I have some problems in walking about ☐
I am confined to bed ☐

Self-Care

I have no problems with self-care ☐
I have some problems washing or dressing myself ☐
I am unable to wash or dress myself ☐

Usual Activities (*e.g. work, study, housework, family or leisure activities*)

I have no problems with performing my usual activities ☐
I have some problems with performing my usual activities ☐
I am unable to perform my usual activities ☐

Pain/Discomfort

I have no pain or discomfort ☐
I have moderate pain or discomfort ☐
I have extreme pain or discomfort ☐

Anxiety/Depression

I am not anxious or depressed ☐
I am moderately anxious or depressed ☐
I am extremely anxious or depressed ☐

Figure 35.2 EuroQol (EQ-5D) UK English version
Source: Reproduced from the EQ-5D User Guide, Version 1, November 2007 by permission of the EuroQol Foundation

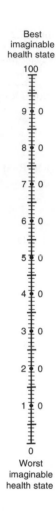

To help people say how good or bad a health state is, we have drawn a scale (rather like a thermometer) on which the best state you can imagine is marked 100 and the worst state you can imagine is marked 0.

We would like you to indicate on this scale how good or bad your own health is today, in your opinion. Please do this by drawing a line from the box below to whichever point on the scale indicates how good or bad your health state is today.

Your own health state today

Figure 35.2 (*continued*)

CHOOSING A QoL MEASURE

There are a broad range of QoL scales that may be used for people with psychiatric disorder[3,93] and for older people[42,94]. The evidence for the validity, reliability and acceptability of generic QoL scales with older people is mixed, although their use is encouraged within research and clinical practice to promote evidence-based health care[1,42,74,94,95]. Table 35.1 gives some examples of generic scales[72,77,78,96] that have been used in studies involving older people with mental health needs[76,97,98]. Haywood *et al.*'s[42,94] review of QoL measures in old age found the SF-36 showed the best reliability and recommended its use where a comprehensive assessment of health is required in older people. Alternatively, the EQ-5D[96] (Figure 35.2) is recommended where a briefer assessment is needed and significant changes in health are anticipated[42,94].

Table 35.2 gives examples of disease-specific QoL scales in dementia[51,61,88,99,100]. Each of the disease-specific QoL scales has been included in previous literature reviews examining the validity and reliability of QoL scales in dementia and their use is supported[68,80,101-105]. The QOL-AD[61] (Figure 35.3) is the preferred measure of choice, as it is brief and has demonstrated sensitivity to psychosocial interventions[101]. However, none of the reviews conclusively identifies a QoL scale for use with people with dementia, and Schölzel-Dorenbos *et al.*[102] state that no QoL scale can be used across all stages of dementia.

ID Number Assessment Number Interview Date

Instructions: Interviewer administer according to standard instructions.
Circle your responses.

1. Physical health	Poor	Fair	Good	Excellent
2. Energy	Poor	Fair	Good	Excellent
3. Mood	Poor	Fair	Good	Excellent
4. Living situation	Poor	Fair	Good	Excellent
5. Memory	Poor	Fair	Good	Excellent
6. Family	Poor	Fair	Good	Excellent
7. Marriage	Poor	Fair	Good	Excellent
8. Friends	Poor	Fair	Good	Excellent
9. Self as a whole	Poor	Fair	Good	Excellent
10. Ability to do chores around the house	Poor	Fair	Good	Excellent
11. Ability to do things for fun	Poor	Fair	Good	Excellent
12. Money	Poor	Fair	Good	Excellent
13. Life as a whole	Poor	Fair	Good	Excellent
Total				

Comments:

Reproduced with permission from © 1996 R.G. Logsdon. Department of Psychosocial and Community Health, Box 357263 University of Washington, Seattle,WA 98195-7263. Logsdon@u.washington.edu

Figure 35.3 Quality of life in Alzheimer's disease (QOL-AD) (participant version)
Source: Reproduced from Logsdon *et al*. (2002), Psychosom. Med. Appendix 1, with permission

Overall, QoL measures should be brief, easy to use, valid and reliable, sensitive to change and useful for both clinical and research settings. In dementia these should where possible include both patient and proxy ratings. It is also possible to generate QALYs from the scores of some QoL scales such as the SF-12, EQ-5D and DEMQOL, to provide an economic evaluation.

CONCLUSION

Within health, HRQoL provides a global measure of well-being in patients and is an appropriate outcome measure for the assessment of disease impact and interventions provided to older people. Moreover, in chronic and disabling disorders where symptomatic and functional recovery is unrealistic, improving quality of life is a particularly worthwhile outcome. QoL is now an established outcome measure for older people and should be routinely included within studies evaluating the effectiveness of care and treatment. Further evidence is needed to show how interventions influence QoL provided to older people with mental health needs. The research undertaken in recent years has established the validity and reliability of a number of QoL measures for use with older people, particularly within dementia. Where possible the individual's perceptions should be sought in preference to the views of others, and this may offer a challenge to health professionals working with older people experiencing increasing physical and mental frailty.

REFERENCES

1. Bowling A. *Ageing Well: Quality of Life in Old Age*. Maidenhead: Open University Press, 2005.
2. Bond J, Corner L. *Quality of Life and Older People*. Maidenhead: Open University Press, 2004.
3. Bowling A. *Measuring Disease: A Review of Disease Specific Quality of Life Measurement Scales*, 2nd edn. Buckingham: Open University Press, 2001.
4. Birren JE, Dieckmann L. Concepts and content of quality of life in the later years: an overview. In Birren JE, Lubben JE, Rowe JC, Deutchman DE (eds), *The Concept and Measurement of Quality of Life in the Frail Elderly*. San Diego, CA: Academic Press, 1991, 344–60.
5. Velarde-Juradon E, Avila-Figuero C. Methods for the quality of life assessment. *Salud Publica Mex* 2002; **44**: 448–63.
6. Fayers PM, de Haes JCJM. Editorial: quality of life assessment in clinical trials. *Lancet* 1995; **346**: 1–2.
7. Bowling A. *Measuring Health: A Review of Quality of Life Measurement Scales*. Milton Keynes: Open University Press, 1991.
8. Oliver J, Huxley P, Bridges K, Mohamad H. *Quality of Life and Mental Health Services*. London: Routledge, 1996.

9. Franklin JL, Simmons J, Solovitz B, Clemons JR, Miller GE. Assessing quality of life of the mentally ill: a three dimensional model. *Eval Health Prof* 1986; **9**(3): 376–88.

10. Lehman AF. The well-being of chronic mental patients: assessing their quality of life. *Arch Gen Psychiatry* 1983; **40**(4): 369–73.

11. Dalkey NC, Rourke DL. Experimental assessment of Delphi procedures with group value judgement. In Dalkey NC, Rourke DL, Lewis R, Snyder D (eds), *Studies in the Quality of Life*. Lexington, MA: Lexington Books, 1972.

12. Lawton M. A multidimensional view of quality of life in frail elders. In Birren JE, Lubben JE, Rowe JC, Deutchman DE (eds), *The Concept and Measurement of Quality of Life in the Frail Elderly*. San Diego, CA: Academic Press, 1991, 3–27.

13. Pearlman RA, Uhlmann RF. Quality of life in chronic diseases: perceptions of elderly patients. *J Gerontol Med Sci* 1988; **43**: 25–30.

14. Ochs J, Mulhern R, Kun L. Quality-of-life assessment in cancer patients. *Am J Clin Oncol* 1988; **11**: 415–21.

15. Spitzer WO, Dobson AJ, Hall J *et al*. Measuring the quality of life in cancer patients: a concise QL index. *J Chron Dis* 1981; **40**: 585–97.

16. Guyatt GH, Feeney DH, Patrick DL. Measuring health-related quality of life. *Ann Intern Med* 1993; **118**(8): 622–9.

17. Muldoon M, Barger SD, Flory JD, Manuck SB. What are quality of life measurements measuring? *Br Med J* 1998; **316**(7130): 542–5.

18. Liu BC. *Quality of Life Indicators in US Metropolitan Areas: A Statistical Analysis*. New York: Praeger, 1976.

19. Torrance GW. Utility approach to measuring health-related quality of life. *J Chron Dis* 1987; **40**: 592–600.

20. Bigelow DM, Brodsky G, Steward LK, Olson MM. The concept and measurement of quality of life as a dependent variable in evaluation of mental health services. In Stahler GJ, Tash WR (eds), *Innovative Approaches to Mental Health Evaluation*. New York: Academic Press, 1982.

21. Gentile KM. A review of the literature on interventions and quality of life in the frail elderly. In Birren JE, Lubben JE, Rowe JC, Deutchman DE (eds), *The Concept and Measurement of Quality of Life in the Frail Elderly*. San Diego, CA: Academic Press, 1991, 74–88.

22. George LK, Bearon LB. *Quality of Life in Older Persons: Meaning and Measurement*. New York: Human Sciences Press, 1980.

23. Lawton MP. Environment and other determinants of well-being in older people. *Gerontologist* 1983; **23**: 349–57.

24. Cheater F. Quality of life measures for the healthcare environment. *Nurs Res* 1998; **5**(3): 17–30.

25. Gill TM, Feinstein AR. A critical appraisal of the quality of quality-of-life measurements. *JAMA* 1994; **272**(8): 619–26.

26. WHOQOL Group. *Measuring Quality of Life: The Development of the World Health Organization Quality of Life Instrument (WHOQOL)*. Geneva: WHO, 1983.

27. Chiu H, Zhang H. Dementia research in China. *Int J Geriatr Psychiatry* 2000; **15**: 947–53.

28. Gureje O, Oguyinni A, Kola L. The profile and impact of probable dementia in a sub-Saharan African community: results from the Ibadan study of aging. *J Psychosom Res* 2006; **61**: 327–33.

29. Gabriel Z, Bowling A. Quality of life in old age from the perspectives of older people. In Walker A, Hennessy C (eds),

Growing Older: Quality of Life in Old Age. Maidenhead: Open University Press, 2004.

30. Hughes B. Quality of life. In Peace SM (ed.), *Researching Social Gerontology: Concepts, Methods and Issues*. London: Sage, 1990, 46–58.

31. Lerner M. Conceptualization of health and social welfare. In Berg RL (ed.), *Health Status Indexes*. Chicago, IL: Hospital Research and Educational Trust, 1973.

32. Carr AJ, Higginson IJ. Measuring quality of life: are quality of life measures patient centred? *Br Med J* 2001; **322**: 1357–60.

33. Testa MA, Simonson DC. Current concepts: assessment of quality-of-life outcomes. *N Engl J Med* 1996; **334**(13): 835–40.

34. Calman KC. Quality of life in cancer patients – an hypothesis. *J Med Ethics* 1984; **10**: 124–7.

35. Higginson IJ. The quality of expectation: healing, palliation or disappointment. *J R Soc Med* 2000; **93**(12): 609–10.

36. Carr AJ, Gibson B, Robinson PG. Measuring quality of life: is quality of life determined by expectations or experience? *Br Med J* 2001; **322**: 1240–43.

37. Delhey J, Bohnke P, Habich R, Zapf W. Quality of life in a European perspective: the EUROMODULE as a new instrument for comparative welfare research. *Soc Indic Res* 2002; **58**: 163–76.

38. Logsdon RG, Albert SM. Assessing quality of life in Alzheimer's disease: conceptual and methodological issues. *J Ment Health Aging* 1999; **5**(1): 3–6.

39. Hickey AM, Bury G, O'Boyle CA *et al*. A new short form individual quality of life measure (SEIQoL-DW): application in a cohort of individuals with HIV/AIDS. *Br Med J* 1996; **313**: 29–33.

40. Hankiss E. *Quality of Life: Problems of Assessment and Measurement*, Socio-economic Studies 5. Paris: UNESCO, 1983.

41. Feinstein AR. *Clinimetrics*. New Haven, CT: Yale University Press, 1987.

42. Haywood KL, Garratt AM, Schmidt LJ, Mackintosh AE, Fitzpatrick R. *Health Status and Quality of Life in Older People: A Structured Review of Patient-reported Health Instruments*, Report from the Patient-reported Health Instruments Group (formerly the Patient-assessed Health Outcomes Programme) to the Department of Health, Oxford, April 2004.

43. Higginson IJ, Carr AJ. Measuring quality of life: using quality of life measures in the clinical setting. *Br Med J* 2001; **322**: 1297–1300.

44. Orley J, Saxena S, Herrman H. Quality of life and mental illness. Reflections from the perspective of the WHOQOL. *Br J Psychiatry* 1998; **172**(4): 291–3.

45. Fallowfield L. *The Quality of Life: The Missing Measurement in Health Care*. London: Souvenir Press, 1990.

46. Mack JL, Whitehouse PJ. Quality of life in dementia: state of the art – Report of the International Working Group for Harmonization of Dementia Drug Guidelines and the Alzheimer's Society satellite meeting. *Alzheimer Dis Assoc Disord* 2001; **15**(2): 69–71.

47. Polit DF, Hungler BP. *Nursing Research: Principles and Methods*, 5th edn. Philadelphia, PA: Lippincott, 1995, 271–300.

48. Bowling A. *Research Methods in Health: Investigating Health and Health Services*. Maidenhead: Open University Press, 1997.

49. Lawton MP. Assessing quality of life in Alzheimer disease research. *Alzheimer Dis Assoc Disord* 1997; **11**(suppl 6): 91–9.

50. Novella JL, Ankri J, Morrone I *et al*. Evaluation of the quality of life in dementia with a generic quality of life questionnaire: the Duke Health Profile. *Dement Geriatr Cogn Disord* 2001; **12**: 158–66.

51. Brod M, Stewart AL, Sands L, Walton P. Conceptualization and measurement of quality of life in dementia: the dementia quality of life instrument (DQOL). *Gerontologist* 1999; **39**: 25–35.

52. Whitehouse P. Measurements of quality of life in dementia. In Wimo A, Jonsson B, Karlsson G, Winblad B (eds), *Health Economics of Dementia*. Chichester: John Wiley & Sons, 1998, 403–17.

53. Whitehouse P. Conclusion: quality of life in Alzheimer's disease: future directions. *J Ment Health Aging* 1999; **5**(1): 107–10.

54. Kane RA. Definition, measurement, and correlates of quality of life in nursing homes: toward a reasonable practice, research, and policy agenda. *Gerontologist* 2003; **43**(special issue II): 28–36.

55. Lawton MP, Van Haitsma K, Perkinson M, Ruckdesschel K. Observed affect and quality of life in dementia: further affirmations and problems. *J Ment Health Aging* 1999; **5**(1): 69–81.

56. Kitwood T, Bredin K. Towards a theory of dementia care: personhood and well being. *Ageing Soc* 1992; **12**: 262–87.

57. Fossey J, Lee L, Ballard C. Dementia Care Mapping as a research tool for measuring quality of life in care settings: psychometric properties. *Int J Geriatr Psychiatry* 2002; **17**: 1064–70.

58. Magaziner J. Use of proxies to measure health and functional outcomes in effectiveness research in persons with Alzheimer disease and related disorders. *Alzheimer Dis Assoc Disord* 1997; **11**(suppl 6): 168–74.

59. Karlawish JHT, Casarett D, Klocinski JL, Clark CM. The relationship between caregivers' global ratings of Alzheimer's disease patients' quality of life, disease severity and the caregiving experience. *J Am Geriatr Soc* 2001; **49**(8): 1066–70.

60. Albert SM, Castillo-Castanada BA, Jacobs DM *et al*. Proxy-reported quality of life in Alzheimer's patients: comparison of clinical and population-based samples. *J Ment Health Aging* 1999; **5**(1): 49–58.

61. Logsdon RG, Gibbons LE, McCurry SM, Teri L. Quality of life in Alzheimer's disease: patient and caregiver reports. *J Ment Health Aging* 1999; **5**: 21–32.

62. Vogel A, Mortensen EL, Hasselbalch SG, Andersen BB, Waldemar G. Patient versus informant reported quality of life in the earliest phases of Alzheimer's disease. *Int J Geriatr Psychiatry* 2006; **21**: 1132–8.

63. Fuh J-L, Wang S-J. Assessing quality of life in Taiwanese patients with Alzheimer's disease. *Int J Geriatr Psychiatry* 2006; **21**: 103–7.

64. Ready RE, Ott BR, Grace J. Patient versus informant perspectives of quality of life in mild cognitive impairment and Alzheimer's disease. *Int J Geriatr Psychiatry* 2004, **19**: 256–65.

65. Logsdon RG, Gibbons LE, McCurry SM, Teri L. Assessing quality of life in older adults with cognitive impairment. *Psychosom Med* 2002; **64**: 510–19.

66. Selai CE, Trimble MR, Rossor MN, Harvey RJ. Assessing quality of life in dementia: preliminary psychometric testing of the quality of life assessment schedule. *Neuropsychol Rehabil* 2001; **11**(3/4): 219–43.

67. Brod M, Stewart AL. Conceptualization of quality of life in dementia. *J Ment Health Aging* 1999; **5**(1): 7–19.

68. Walker MD, Salek SS, Bayer AJ. A review of quality of life in Alzheimer's disease. Part 1: Issues in assessing disease impact. *Pharmacoeconomics* 1998; **14**(5): 499–530.

69. National Institute for Health and Clinical Excellence. *Developing Costing Tools: Methods Guide*. London: NICE, 2008.

70. Tunstall J. *Old and Alone*. London: Routledge & Kegan Paul, 1966.

71. Farquhar M. Definitions of quality of life: a taxonomy. *J Adv Nurs* 1995; **22**(3): 502–8.

72. Hyde M, Wiggins RD, Higgs P, Blane DB. A measure of quality of life in early old age: the theory, development and properties of a needs satisfaction model (CASP-19). *Aging Ment Health* 2003; **73**: 186–94.

73. Magaziner J. The use of proxy respondents in health studies of the aged. In Wallace RB, Woolson RF (eds), *The Epidemiologic Study of the Elderly*. New York: Oxford University Press, 1992, 120–29.

74. Livingston G, Watkin V, Manela M, Rosser R, Katona C. Quality of life in older people. *Aging Ment Health* 1998; **2**(1): 20–23.

75. Rosser RM, Cottee M, Rabin R, Selai C. Index of health related quality of life. In Hopkins A (ed.), *Measures of the Quality of Life and the Uses to which Such Measures May Be Put*. London: Royal College of Physicians, 1992.

76. Pettit T, Livingston G, Manela M *et al*. Validation and normative data of health status measures in older people: the Islington study. *Int J Geriatr Psychiatry* 2001; **16**: 1061–70.

77. Radosevich DM, Pruitt M. Twelve-item health status questionnaire (HSQ-12) cooperative validation project: comparability study. Abstracts from the Academy of Health Services Research Annual Meeting, Atlanta, USA, June 1996, 9–11. *AHSR FHSR Annu Meet Abstr Book* 1996; **13**: 59.

78. Ware JE, Kosinski M, Keller S. A 12 item short form health survey: construction of scales and preliminary tests of reliability and validity. *Med Care* 1996; **34**: 220–33.

79. Stewart A, Sherbourne C, Brod M. Measuring health-related quality of life in older and demented populations. In Spiker B (ed.), *Quality of Life and Pharmacoeconomics in Clinical Trials*, 2nd edn. Philadelphia, PA: Lippincott-Raven, 1996, 819–29.

80. Ettema PT, Dröes R-M, De Lange J, Mellenbergh GJ, Ribbe MW. A review of quality of life instruments used in dementia. *Qual Life Res* 2005; **14**: 675–86.

81. Hoe J, Katona C, Roche B, Livingston G. Use of the QOL-AD for measuring quality of life in people with severe dementia – the LASER-AD study. *Age Ageing* 2005; **34**(2): 130–35.

82. Thorgrimsen L, Selwood A, Spector A *et al*. Whose quality of life is it anyway? The validity and reliability of the quality of life – Alzheimer's disease (QOL-AD) scale. *Alzheimer Dis Assoc Disord* 2003; **17**(4): 201–8.

83. Hoe J, Katona C, Livingston G, Orrell M. Quality of life in dementia: care recipient and caregiver perceptions of quality of life in dementia: the LASER-AD study. *Int J Geriatr Psychiatry* 2007; **22**: 1031–6.

84. Hoe J, Hancock G, Livingston G, Orrell M. Quality of life of people with dementia in residential care homes. *Br J Psychiatry* 2006; **188**: 460–64.

85. Spector A, Orrell M. Quality of life (QoL) in dementia: a comparison of the perceptions of people with dementia and care staff in residential homes. *Alzheimer Dis Assoc Disord* 2006; **20**(3): 160–65.

86. Sands LP, Ferreira MD, Stewart AL, Brod M, Yaffe K. What explains differences between dementia patients' and their caregivers' ratings of patients' quality of life? *Am J Geriatr Psychiatry* 2004; **12**(3): 272–80.

87. Terada S, Ishizu H, Fujisawa Y *et al*. Development and evaluation of a health-related quality of life questionnaire for the elderly with dementia in Japan. *Int J Geriatr Psychiatry* 2002; **17**(9): 851–8.

88. Rabins PV, Kasper JD, Kleinman L, Black BS, Patrick DL. Concepts and methods in the development of the ADRQL: an instrument for assessing health-related quality of life in persons with Alzheimer's disease. *J Ment Health Aging* 1999; **5**(1): 33–48.

89. Albert SM, Jacobs DM, Sano M *et al*. Longitudinal study of quality of life in people with advanced Alzheimer's disease. *Am J Geriatr Psychiatry* 2001; **9**(2): 160–68.

90. Banerjee S, Smith SC, Lamping DL *et al*. Quality of life in dementia: more than just cognition. An analysis of associations with quality of life in dementia. *J Neurol Neurosurg Psychiatry* 2006; **77**: 146–8.

91. Shin I-S, Carter M, Masterman D, Fairbanks L, Cummings JL. Neuropsychiatric symptoms and quality of life in Alzheimer disease. *Am J Geriatr Psychiatry* 2005; **13**(6): 469–74.

92. Banerjee S, Samsi K, Petrie CD *et al*. A review of the emerging evidence on the predictive and explanatory value of disease specific measures of health related quality of life in people with dementia. *Int J Geriatr Psychiatry* 2009; **24**: 15–24.

93. Schmidt LJ, Garratt AM, Fitzpatrick R. *Instruments for Mental Health*, a review report from the Patient-reported Health Instruments Group (formerly the Patient-assessed Health Outcomes Programme) to the Department of Health, September 2000.

94. Haywood KL, Garratt AM, Fitzpatrick R. Quality of life in older people: a structured review of generic self-assessed health instruments. *Qual Life Res* 2005; **14**: 1651–68.

95. Parker SG, Peet SM, Jagger C, Farhan M, Castleden CM. Measuring health status in older patients. The SF-36 in practice. *Age Ageing* 1998; **27**: 13–18.

96. EUROQOL Group. A new facility for the measurement of health related quality of life. *Health Policy* 1990; **16**: 199–208.

97. Wolfs CAG, Dirksen CD, Kessels A *et al*. Performance of the EQ-5D and the EQ-5D+C in elderly patients with cognitive impairments. *Health Qual Life Outcomes* 2007; **5**: 33.

98. Coucill W, Bryan S, Bentham P, Buckley A, Laight A. EQ-5D in patients with dementia: an investigation of inter-rater agreement. *Med Care* 2001; **39**(8): 760–71.

99. Smith SC, Lamping DL, Banerjee S *et al*. Measurement of health-related quality of life for people with dementia: development of a new instrument (DEMQOL) and an evaluation of current methodology. *HTA* 2005; **9**(10): 1–112.

100. Ready RE, Ott BR, Grace J, Fernandez I. The Cornell-Brown scale for quality of life in dementia. *Alzheimer Dis Assoc Disord* 2002; **16**(2): 109–15.

101. Moniz-Cook E, Vernooij-Dassen M, Woods R *et al*., for the Interdem group. European consensus on outcome measures for psychosocial intervention research in dementia care. *Aging Ment Health* 2008; **12**(1): 14–29.

102. Schölzel-Dorenbos CJM, Ettema TP, Bos J *et al*. Evaluating the outcome of interventions on quality of life in dementia: selection of the appropriate scale. *Int J Geriatr Psychiatry* 2007; **22**: 511–19.

103. Ready RE, Ott BR. Quality of life measures for dementia. *Health Qual Life Outcomes* 2003; **1**(11). At www.hqlo.com /content/1/1/11, accessed 23 Jan 2010.

104. Salek SS, Walker MD, Bayer AJ. A review of quality of life in Alzheimer's disease. Part 2: Issues in assessing drug effects. *Pharmacoeconomics* 1998; **14**(6): 613–27.

105. Howard K, Rockwood K. Quality of life in Alzheimer's disease. *Dementia* 1995; **6**: 113–16.

Part D

Degenerative and Related Disorders

36

Delirium

Barbara Kamholz

Department of Psychiatry, Duke University, USA

INTRODUCTION

Delirium is prevalent, dangerous and costly. It is caused by medical or surgical problems and medication burdens that are beyond the physiological tolerance of the patient. Delirium costs between $38 and $152 bn per year[1]. In ICUs, episodes of delirium average 39% higher ICU costs and 31% higher hospital costs[2]. Long considered a reversible epiphenomenon of hospital care, delirium is an independent risk factor for death and dementia[3] and it contributes heavily to lengths of stay, in-hospital complications, and new institutionalization. Deliriums that are more severe or persistent have even more dire outcomes[2]: 22–76% of hospitalized inpatients with delirium die[4]. Delirium occurs in 15–60% of nursing home patients, 14–56% of inpatients and up to 60–80% of ICU patients[5]. Yet delirium can be prevented or mitigated in health care settings that understand it, diagnose it and implement interdisciplinary programmes across the health care spectrum to address it, and there is considerable economic potential in doing so. Progress in the field has been seriously hampered by difficulties with diagnosis; up to 95% of cases are missed[6].

PRESENTATIONS, PHENOMENOLOGY AND IDENTIFICATION OF DELIRIUM

Delirium is misdiagnosed in all settings, including emergency rooms, hospitals, and long term and palliative care settings. The clinical presentation of delirium remains a 'black box'; as of this time we have no explanations for the variations in behavioural, affective, sensory and motor signs of delirium. These signs can change within seconds or hours, and most likely reflect the complex underlying pathophysiologies. The DSM IV-TR diagnostic criteria are shown in Table 36.1[7].

Many rating scales have been developed to assist with the diagnosis, the most widely used including the CAM[8] and CAM-ICU[9]. Inattention and the broad fluctuations of symptoms are characteristics not found in other psychiatric illnesses. At the same time, they are the most difficult to measure and identify. Attention is a complex phenomenon that involves distractibility, vigilance and concentration, and is our most basic interface with the environment. Unless patients are grossly agitated and irrational, the clinical expression of inattention can be very subtle. It is easily mistaken for the withdrawal and lack of environmental engagement found in depression. Fluctuations, unless they are marked, are often written off as fatigue, uncooperativeness, withdrawal, differing responses to different health practitioners, or reactions to procedures. Given changeovers of physicians and nurses in busy hospitals, such indefinite characteristics go largely unrecognized unless staff nursing notes are carefully mined for evidence of these subtle changes. Nurses are the first to recognize early symptoms of delirium, although they do not reliably diagnose it as such, and are a rich source of descriptive information that can greatly assist with diagnosis[10].

Broadly accepted subcategories include 'active', 'mixed', and 'quiet' delirium. These subcategories may have implications for prognosis or pathophysiology. Significant investigation of these subtypes has been done, although these have not provided clear implications for causality, prognosis or intervention. Active delirium is defined as a state marked by agitation, physically aggressive and often violent activity, hyperattentiveness (the inability to suppress responses to the environment or to internal states) and emotional lability. In this condition, deficits in focused attention and fluctuations of presentation are easily identified. Quiet delirium is defined as a state marked by withdrawal, lack of involvement in or communication with the environment, bland or flat affect, and a depressed level of consciousness short of frank stupor. These symptoms reflect an inability to attend appropriately and in sequential fashion to the demands of the environment. Mixed deliriums are considered to be a combination of the two. The prevalence of these subtypes is variably reported but averages 25% for quiet delirium, 45% for mixed delirium, and 30% for active delirium. All subtypes of delirium can present with motor symptoms (dysarthria, difficulty swallowing, gait disturbances), affective symptoms (dysphoria, lability, anxiety), sensory difficulties that are associated with incorrect cerebral processing of sensory data (clinically expressed as difficulties with hearing, appreciation of pain), and illusory phenomena, aphasia (partial or global) and impaired cognitive function (dysexecutive function, disorientation, nonsensical speech). Any of these symptoms may fluctuate, even within seconds. The appreciation and reporting of pain by the delirious patient is particularly problematic, as untreated pain can worsen delirium, yet overtreatment with narcotic agents can have the same result. Psychotic-like symptoms such as disorganized speech and visual hallucinations may also be associated, although the hallucinations in delirium are more illusory than hallucinatory. They commonly involve nonsensical images such as 'clowns on bicycles' or 'tires in the ceiling'. The differentiation of delirium from prominent psychotic illnesses, including schizophrenia, schizoaffective disorder and bipolar disorder, can be problematic. Pre-existing psychiatric diagnoses are a principal cause of poor identification of

Table 36.1 DSM-IV-TR diagnostic criteria for delirium

A. Disturbance of consciousness (i.e. reduced clarity of awareness of the environment) with reduced ability to focus, sustain, or shift attention.

B. A change in cognition (e.g. memory deficit, disorientation, language disturbance) or

C. Development of a perceptual disturbance that is not better accounted for by a pre-existing, established, or evolving dementia.

D. Disturbance develops over a short period of time (usually hours to days) and tends to fluctuate during the course of the day.

E. There is evidence from the history, physical examination, or laboratory findings that the disturbance is caused by the direct physiological consequences of a general medical condition.

delirium, as the patients' symptoms are often attributed to them[11]. In these cases, reliance on clues from the patient's clinical history is critical. Quietly delirious patients are frequently misidentified as depressed. Farrell and Ganzini[12] found that 42% of patients referred to psychiatry consultation services for depression were actually delirious. However, an additional finding was that 60% of patients with delirium have symptoms of dysphoria, and 52% have passive or active thoughts of suicide. Acutely 'suicidal' patients suffering with prolonged hospitalizations and multiple medical problems are prototypically confusing. In such cases, the burden of risk and need for immediate medical intervention rest with delirium rather than depression.

A further consideration is that symptoms of delirium present along a spectrum. Evidence for the existence of subsyndromal delirium has been presented by Levkoff et al., among others[13]. Marcantonio et al. found that patients with subsyndromal delirium had worse outcomes than patients with diagnosable mild delirium[14].

The recognition of delirium remains one of the most prominent problems in the field. The term 'recognition' includes not just diagnosis of the medical condition of delirium, but also the recognition that it is a severe illness that cannot be assumed to resolve on its own with few sequelae. Recent appreciation of this has led to skyrocketing numbers of publications in the field in recent years[15].

THE ETIOLOGY OF DELIRIUM

Population at Risk

A multitude of risk factors have been identified in treatment studies of delirium, often with little overlap. However, most would agree that age, cognitive impairment, medication and medical burden define the characteristics of the population at highest risk[2]. Efforts to advance the field by seeking universal 'causes' of delirium have therefore been very frustrating. It is easiest to conceptualize the aetiology of delirium from the perspective of the syndrome of frailty. Frailty has many definitions, but on a physiological level its most commonly accepted conceptualization is sarcopaenia, or progressive deterioration of skeletal muscle[16]. It is usually found in patients who are older, cognitively impaired and medically ill, and in fact the majority of patients who develop delirium are frail. Some investigators provide a broader view of the components of frailty by including socioeconomic stressors, psychiatric disorders, medication and

home environment as well as medical vulnerabilities, which reference the broad network of resources that frail geriatric patients require to avoid catastrophic illness[17]. The increased vulnerability of frail patients to the catastrophic decline represented by delirium is related to their limited physiological reserve. With ageing, there is diminution of redundant systems such as neurons and neuronal circuits in the brain and excess metabolic capacity in the liver and kidney. Patients with the least reserve are more susceptible to any stressor, however small, than healthier individuals, in a striking resemblance to chemical equations far from equilibrium. The implication is that the patient's underlying vulnerability and disequilibrated status (as opposed to any specific 'last minute' precipitating causes), are the most important predictors of delirium in an individual person. It is then easy to conclude that the prominent precipitating causes of delirium are the most common complications, including iatrogenic ones, found in hospitalized patients. A short list includes hyponatraemia, acute blood loss, pain, acute renal failure, fractures, acute infections (urinary tract or pulmonary), the use of longer term indwelling bladder catheters, dehydration, decubiti, malnutrition and the use of psychotropic medications[2].

Pathophysiology of Delirium

Historically, multiple interacting theories have been proposed to explain the pathophysiology of delirium. Any given delirium may have an unknown number of associated clinical conditions (baseline and precipitating factors), and they do not necessarily occur in the same combinations. It is only when the patient has recovered that there is any clinical certainty that the basic physiological process(es) have been fully addressed. However, many deliriums do not fully resolve. It is also not necessarily the case that two patients who appear to have equal degrees of baseline and precipitating stressors will both become delirious. This lack of reproducibility has wreaked havoc with our investigations of pathophysiology. We are left with broad-based geriatric clinical intervention methods that are helpful but quite non-specific, and this may account for some of our difficulty in making progress in the field.

At a cellular or molecular level, the most compelling evidence indicates that excess dopamine and/or insufficient acetylcholine in the brain could best explain the cascade of metabolic and behavioural complications of delirium. Each has complex and interactive impacts on cellular function within the CNS[18]. Impairments in neuronal membrane function appear to underlie much of the pathophysiology of delirium. Neuroimaging has recently been incorporated to evaluate structural and functional processes in the brain during delirium, although the findings are diverse enough that consistent trends have so far been elusive. Yokota and colleagues, using xenon enhanced CT, found that patients with delirium experienced a 42% reduction in overall cerebral blood flow compared to baseline; after recovery from delirium, the findings normalized[19]. Such findings may explain the multisystem deficits observed, which include cognitive, affective, sensory and motor function. There is not enough evidence at this time to determine whether structural correlates precede or follow delirium.

Major areas of exploration

Inflammation Inflammatory processes such as urinary tract infection, osteomyelitis and pneumonia, are highly associated with delirium. With ageing there is an elevated inflammatory profile[20]. Activated glial cells transmit peripheral inflammatory cytokine responses to the CNS. This is associated with decreased synaptic plasticity, a necessity for the modulation of behaviour, learning and cognition[20]. Inflammatory states as well as hypoxia and hypoglycaemia are associated with impaired mitochondrial function; this might support a hypothesis that disturbed function of endothelial cells could alter the blood–brain barrier. Release of the inflammatory cytokines TNF-alpha and interleukin-1 generates adhesion molecules that disrupt cerebral vasculature, further impacting the integrity of the blood–brain barrier[20].

Extracellular glutamate in normal brain is quickly metabolized. However, in the presence of impaired mitochondrial function, hypoglycaemia hypoxia, and glucose, excess extracellular glutamate results in increases in cellular influx of Ca^{++}. This in turn leads to stimulation of NMDA receptors, which are excitotoxic[2]. Intracellular Ca^{++} appears to be the main trigger of a series of reactions, including mitochondrial injury and activation of catabolic enzymes that lead to cellular dysfunction and potentially death. During states of cerebral ischaemia, further cellular risk is posed by efflux of dopamine. Use of barbiturates, isoflurane and etomidate, common agents associated with anaesthesia, may mitigate these responses[2,21]. Few, if any, studies have linked the risk of delirium to the use of anaesthetic agents.

The acetylcholine hypothesis   Another principal theory involves decreases in the availability to brain cells of adequate amounts of acetylcholine (ACH). ACH is a fundamentally important neurotransmitter in areas serving attention and memory. Among multiple reports, surgical ICU patients with delirium had higher serum anticholinergic levels. A dose-related relationship was identified by Flacker et al.[22], who also identified higher levels of endogenous anticholinergic substances. A number of studies, although not all, have associated anticholinergic medications with delirium.

Impact of excessive dopamine   Another important hypothesis relates to increased extracellular dopamine. The influx of calcium into cells that occurs during hypoxic conditions in brain stimulates the activity of tyrosine hydroxylase. This results in increased production of dopamine, with resulting disruption of ATP production. Decreases in the production of ATP and the increase in toxic metabolites of dopamine then inhibit cathechol O-methyltransferase, the main extracellular deactivator of dopamine. These processes collectively result in increased dopamine levels in brain, up to a factor of $500\times$ during episodes of striatal ischaemia[5]. Further, dopaminergic neurons themselves are known to be highly susceptible to oxidative stress, which may result in massive releases of dopamine into the extracellular space[5]. Agents that increase available dopamine in the brain, such as stimulants, have also been associated with delirium. D2 blockers such as haloperidol are widely known to improve behaviour in patients with delirium, and possibly the syndrome itself.

Other neurotransmitters   The kinetics of neurotransmitters other than acetylcholine and dopamine are also highly sensitive to conditions of hypoxia and hypoglycaemia, as above. Disorders of release, synthesis and degradation of gamma-aminobutyric acid (GABA), serotonin (either in excess or insufficiency), as well as norepinephrine and glutamate, have been linked in various work to delirium[5]. Cerebral oxidative metabolism, as well as cardiovascular and respiratory reserves that support it, decrease with ageing[2].

Glycemic control   Decreased availability of inhibitory neurotransmitters, deposition of neutrophils and mitochondrial damage are associated with poor glycaemic control. Improved glucose control with insulin (specifically) improves the CNS outcomes of critically ill patients[21].

Molecular genetics   Efforts to link the presence of the *APOE4* variant of this gene, which has been well established in association with Alzheimer's disease, have resulted in mixed findings[2]. It has been associated with increased duration of delirium in ICUs. Polymorphisms in DRD3 and the dopamine transporter SLC6A3 are the most commonly polymorphisms associated with delirium tremens[20].

THE IMPACT OF FOCUSED INTERVENTION TRIALS ON RECOGNITION AND MANAGEMENT

A number of intervention programmes have been employed to address the severe long-term outcomes of delirium, which include death, dementia, increased lengths of stay, decreased function, rehospitalization and new institutional placement. These programmes have been studied in hospitalized patients; there are no published trials among outpatients. A number of these trials have found that they are not helpful for the primary outcome of a decrease in incidence[23,24]. Other studies have demonstrated decreases in severity and duration of symptoms of delirium in hospital, both of which have been significantly associated with worsened outcomes. Unfortunately the impact of these interventions on longer term outcomes has been mixed and overall disappointing[25]. In some cases this may be due to the limited time the patient is exposed to the intervention, e.g. when hospitalized as part of a pre-established protocol[14]. In light of this, most studies conclude that prevention of delirium is the primary clinical goal. In a prominent study published in 1999[26], a complex intervention that involved a significant amount of volunteer work as well as a very high level of nursing care was shown to significantly reduce length of stay, number of episodes and, finally, the incidence of delirium. This may have been due to the highly refined identification of risk factors in this population; Inouye distinguished baseline risk factors for delirium from risk factors for triggering of a new episode. Going forward, this two-phased risk assessment method has helped reshape our conceptualization of treatments for delirium by focusing on modifiable, new onset, precipitating risk factors. This innovation has improved our ability to intervene effectively in cases of delirium.

Marcantonio performed a highly organized and comprehensive geriatric medicine programme that also demonstrated a decreased incidence of delirium in post-hip fracture patients[14]. The work of both Inouye and Marcantonio, that has primarily focused on providing basic, but comprehensive care, has demonstrated that the interventions needed in delirium are most often not arcane or difficult to employ, and are largely inexpensive. These interventions highlight an effective level of geriatric care that could be attained in any institution.

DEMENTIA AND DELIRIUM

Delirium is often confused with dementia. A critical part of the diagnosis of delirium involves identifying that the mental status presented by a patient is not the patient's baseline level of cognition and that a relatively rapid change has taken place. Delirium is an acute, catastrophic response to an inciting medical event. The evolution of dementia is significantly more gradual in most cases. Where there is doubt, it is safest to address the clinical situation as a delirium so that any precipitating causes are addressed as soon as possible. The differentiation of these two clinical problems is complex because the precipitating cause(s) of the delirium may not easily be temporally connected with the onset of the syndrome of delirium itself. Patients with delirium superimposed on dementia had more than twice the risk of mortality at 12 months than patients with delirium alone, dementia alone or patients with neither[27]. Assisted living facility residents classically have high rates of dementia and the relative risk of discharge of such patients back to institutional settings after an episode of delirium was 9.1[1]. There may be priming of the immune system as well. Patients with dementia are increasingly understood to have chronic inflammatory processes within the CNS. Acute systemic inflammatory processes that precipitate delirium may have been 'primed' by the underlying inflammatory process[20].

TREATMENT APPROACHES TO DELIRIUM

Priorities of treatment include addressing acute medical contributors to the syndrome as well as stabilizing patient behaviour sufficient to enable the treatment of underlying medical causes. The primary task of clinicians is to identify and address modifiable conditions. In this way the impact of relatively unmodifiable conditions (such as stroke, myocardial infarction end stage renal function etc.) can be minimized. Our effectiveness at treating delirium depends on the extent to which we can provide skilled and sophisticated nursing care that allows time for the multiple interventions required by elderly patients. Avoidance of iatrogenesis that can prolong the delirium is an essential part of this effort. Factors contributing to increased risks of delirium in hospital include the increased pace of health care settings, rapid and increasingly unstable discharges and remarkably limited amounts of time spent with patients. Housestaff may have as little as 3.5 minutes per day per patient[4]. Skilled nursing care alone could provide many of the most effective strategies for minimizing delirium, including mobilization, improvement of cognitive stimulation and minimization of the need for restraints. Up to 50% of cases of delirium can be prevented[4].

Pharmacological Approaches to Behavioural Stabilization

The use of restraints can worsen delirium, as can the overuse of certain medications. Use of benzodiazepines, while standard for obligate alcohol detoxification regimens and for sedation in ICUs, has nonetheless been found in most studies to carry a high risk of inducing or significantly worsening delirium[2]. There are few double-blinded, placebo-controlled, randomized trials of neuroleptics for behavioural management in delirium. Of all these agents, haloperidol remains the most studied. Haloperidol can be effective in low dosages, starting with 0.25 mg po or IM bid, and increasing to the 2–3 mg per day range only in severe cases. Risperidone in doses ranging from 0.5 to 4.0 mg daily and olanzapine in doses of 2.5–11.6 mg daily have been efficacious for the behavioural treatment of delirium with fewer extrapyramidal effects than haloperidol[2]. In addition, case reports or case series regarding quetiapine, aripiprazole and ziprasidone have been published with no

randomized, double-blinded, placebo-controlled studies yet reported. There are very few such medication trials in the field.

Environmental Management for Behavioural Stabilization

Patients with delirium are unable to manage their environment, make appropriate decisions or care for their basic needs, and they cannot problem solve. Therefore, the environment has to adapt to them. Most studies agree that decreasing the complexity of the environment by limiting rotation of personnel caring for the patient, minimizing room changes, providing rest and quiet at night time, feeding the patient, providing a calming 'interpreter' such as a 'sitter' or family member to reorient and guide the patient, limiting distractions (loud conversation, beepers, overhead speakers, televisions, crowded areas), providing hearing aids and glasses, and providing clear-cut and step-by-step instructions are critical. Mobilizing the patient will minimize recovery time, and also may have modulatory impacts on recovering muscle after a critical illness[28]. Patients must be kept safe by limiting dangerous objects in their reach, avoiding falls and using assistive devices to limit the possibility of their pulling at lines or touching wounds. Complex protocols exist for the design of the treating environments that are beyond the scope of this chapter[14].

Treating the Causes

Acute medical conditions

The basic principle of treatment of delirium is to aggressively seek and treat the reversible causes of delirium and to mitigate those that have little room for modulation. Emphasis should be placed on illnesses that result in poor cerebral oxygen availability or that are associated with significant metabolic impairments. Elimination of infectious or inflammatory sources, addressing orthopaedic injuries and removal of offending medications are also essential (see below). Given that most cases of delirium occur in the most vulnerable patients, correcting the most common metabolic and infectious factors, such as serum bun, creatinine, sodium and calcium, and treatment of urinary tract infections and pneumonia are remarkably effective interventions. Identification of metabolic trends by graphing laboratory values can be very helpful to determine original causes as well as indicators of further decline or recovery. Head imaging is not helpful in the absence of focal findings[29].

Removal of offending medications

Removing offending medications, including opiates, anticholinergics, benzodiazepines and dopaminergics, is extremely important. Medications that alter the dopamine/acetylcholine balance within the CNS are a primary focus. A significant number of deliriogenic medications are found in commonly used medications, including digoxin, penicillin, amantadine, quinolone antibiotics, furosemide, nifedipine and warfarin. Further treatment of this topic is beyond the scope of this publication[2].

Pharmacological Approaches

Historically, medications have been used to address behavioural problems, but recent evidence indicates that there may be some gains in disease modification.

Neuroleptics

Recent work (see 'Pathophysiology of Delirium', above) suggests that the use of dopamine blockade is useful for disease modification. Agents that block dopamine have the potential to inhibit many neurotoxic events that occur in the presence of delirium, especially during conditions of hypoxia. Recent studies have focused on the usefulness of prophylactic antipsychotic use to diminish the incidence, severity or persistence of delirium. Kalisvaart was able to demonstrate decreased severity and persistence of delirium, although not incidence, among postoperative hip fracture patients by providing perioperative haloperidol use at 1.5 mg/day preoperatively and 3 days postoperatively. This was the first major study to demonstrate that pharmacological approaches could be used for disease modification[30]. In another randomized, placebo-controlled, double-blinded study of cardiac surgery patients, the incidence of delirium was quite significantly decreased when compared with placebo, even with a single dose of risperidone at 1 mg postoperatively[31]. The use of neuroleptics as preventative or mitigating agents in delirium is not widespread at this time.

Cholinesterase inhibitors

The use of cholinesterase inhibitors has been trialled in delirium. In a randomized, placebo-controlled, double-blinded study by Liptzin et al., the use was not found to have a significant impact on the incidence of delirium among young, relatively healthy patients undergoing elective hip fracture[32]. In a small retrospective study, a population of dementia patients chronically maintained on rivastigmine had significantly less incidence of delirium than a comparable, non-chronically medicated group[33].

Dexemedetomidine

The use of psychopharmacological agents to treat agitation in the ICU has been largely limited to propofol, which is an alcohol that is associated with hypotension and hyperlipidaemia, or to midazolam, which can suppress ventilatory effort and cause hypotension. Both have GABAergic effects that can worsen delirium. Fentanyl, an opiate IV for pain control and sedation, is also frequently utilized, either alone or in combination with propofol or midazolam, with attendant risks of dopaminergic/anticholinergic impacts. Dexemedetomidine, a very selective alpha-2 adrenergic agonist, has analgesic, sympatholytic, sedative and anxiolytic properties. It has increasingly been trialled as an alternative to the older protocols. In a randomized controlled trial of dexemedetomidine versus lorazepam in the ICU setting, while not significant, there was a dramatic difference in post-ICU mortality at 28 days and one year[34].

Delirium is a critical illness that occurs primarily in elderly and frail individuals. Modulation of this very significant problem, however, is increasingly within our reach.

REFERENCES

1. Friedman SM, Mendelson DA, Bingham KW. Hazards of hospitalization: residence prior to admission predicts outcomes. *Gerontologist* 2008; **48**(4): 537–41.
2. Maldonado JR. Delirium in the acute care setting: characteristics, diagnosis and treatment. *Crit Care Clin* 2008; **24**(4): 657–722.
3. Rockwood K, Cosway S, Carver D et al. The risk of dementia and death after delirium. *Age Ageing* 1999; **28**: 551–6.
4. Inouye SK, Schlesinger MJ, Lydon TJ. Delirium: a symptom of how hospital care is failing older persons and a window to improve quality of hospital care. *Am J Med* 1999; **106**: 565–73.
5. Maldonado JR. Pathoetiological model of delirium: a comprehensive understanding of the neurobiology of delirium and an evidence-based approach to prevention and treatment. *Crit Care Clin* 2008; **24**(4): 789–856.
6. Bair BD. Frequently missed diagnosis in geriatric psychiatry. *Psychiatr Clin North Am* 1998; **21**(4): 941–71, viii.
7. American Psychiatric Association. *Diagnostic and Statistical Manual of Mental Disorders*, 4th edn. Washington, DC: American Psychiatric Association, 1994, 129.
8. Inouye SK, Van Dyck CH, Alessi CA et al. Clarifying confusion: the confusion assessment method. A new method for detection of delirium. *Ann Intern Med* 1990; **113**(12): 941–8.
9. Ely EW, Margolin R, Francis J et al. Evaluation of delirium in critically ill patients: validation of the Confusion Assessment Method for the Intensive Care Unit (CAM-ICU). *Crit Care Med* 2001; **29**(7): 1370–79.
10. Steis MR, Fick DM. Are nurses recognizing delirium? A systematic review. *Gerontol Nurs* 2008; **34**(9): 40–48.
11. Kishi Y, Kato M, Okuyama T et al. Delirium: patient characteristics that predict a missed diagnosis at psychiatric consultation. *Gen Hosp Psychiatry* 2007; **29**(5): 442–5.
12. Farrell KR, Ganzini L. Misdiagnosing delirium as depression in medically ill elderly patients. *Arch Intern Med* 1995; **155**(22): 2459–64.
13. Levkoff SE, Liptzin B, Cleary PD et al. Subsyndromal delirium. *Am J Geriatr Psychiatry* 1996; **4**(4): 320–29.
14. Marcantonio ER, Flacker JM, Wright RJ, Resnick NM. Reducing delirium after hip fracture: a randomized trial. *J Am Geriatr Soc* 2001; **49**(5): 516–22.
15. Meagher D. More attention, less confusion: time to lessen the burden of delirium. *Int Rev Psychiatry* 2009; **21**(1): 1–3.
16. Morley JE, Haren MT, Rolland Y, Kim MJ. Frailty. *Med Clin North Am* 2006; **90**: 837–47.
17. Rockwood K, Song X, MacKnight C et al. A global clinical measure of fitness and frailty in elderly people. *CMAJ* 2005; **173**(5): 489–95.
18. Gunther ML, Morandi A, Ely EW. Pathophysiology of delirium in the intensive care unit. *Crit Care Clin* 2008; **24**: 45–65.
19. Yokota H, Ogawa S, Kurokawa A, Yamamoto Y. Regional cerebral blood flow in delirium patients. *Psychiatry Clin Neurosci* 2003; **57**(3): 337–9.
20. Godbout JP, Johnson RW. Age and neuroinflammation: a lifetime of psychoneuroimmune consequences. *Neurol Clin* 2006; **24**: 521–38.
21. Harukuni I, Bhardwaj A. Mechanisms of brain injury after global cerebral ischemia. *Neurol Clin* 2006; **24**: 1–21.
22. Flacker JM, Cummings V, Mach JR et al. The association of serum anticholinergic activity with delirium in elderly medical patients. *Am J Geriatr Psychiatry* 1998; **6**(1): 31–41.
23. Pitkala K, Laurila JV, Strandberg TE, Tilvis RS. Multicomponent geriatric intervention for elderly inpatients with delirium: a randomized, controlled trial. *J Gerontol A Biol Sci Med Sci* 2006; **61**(2): 176–82.
24. Cole MG, Primeau FJ, Laplante J. Systematic detection and multidisciplinary care of delirium in older medical inpatients: a randomized trial. *CMAJ* 2002; **167**(7): 753–9.

25. Milisen K, Lemiengre J, Braes T, Foreman MD. Multicomponent intervention strategies for managing delirium in hospitalized older people: systematic review. *J Adv Nurs* 2005; **52**(1): 79–90.

26. Inouye SK, Bogardus ST, Charpentier PA *et al*. A multicomponent intervention to prevent delirium in hospitalized older patients. *N Engl J Med* 1999; **340**: 669–76.

27. Bellelli G, Frisoni GB, Turco R *et al*. Delirium superimposed on dementia predicts 12-month survival in elderly patients discharged from a postacute rehabilitation facility. *J Gerontol A Biol Sci Med Sci* 2007; **62**(11): 1306–9.

28. Pustavoitau A, Stevens RD. Mechanisms of neurologic failure in critical illness. *Crit Care Clin* 2008; **24**: 1–24.

29. Huschmidt A, Shabarin V. Diagnostic yield of cerebral imaging in patients with acute confusion. *Acta Neurol Scand* 2008; **118**(4): 245–50.

30. Kalisvaart Kees J, deJonghe JFM, Bogaards MJ *et al*. Haloperidol prophylaxis for elderly hip-surgery patients at risk for delirium: a randomized placebo-controlled study. *J Am Geriatr Soc* 2005; **53**: 1658–66.

31. Prakanrattana U, Prapaitrakool S. Efficacy of risperidone for prevention of postoperative delirium in cardiac surgery. *Anaesth Intensive Care* 2007; **35**(5): 714–19.

32. Liptzin B, Laki A, Garb JL, Fingeroth R, Krushell R. Donepezil in the prevention and treatment of post-surgical delirium. *Am J Geriatr Psychiatry* 2005; **13**(12): 1100–106.

33. Dautzenberg PL, Mulder LJ, Olde Rikkert MG, Wouters CJ, Loonen AJ. Delirium in elderly hospitalised patients: protective effects of chronic rivastigmine usage. *Int J Geriatr Psychiatry* 2004; **19**(7): 641–4.

34. Pandharipande PP, Pun BT, Herr DL *et al*. Effect of sedation with dexemedetomidine vs lorazepam on acute brain dysfunction in mechanically ventilated patients: the MENDS randomized controlled trial. *JAMA* 2007; **298**(22): 2644–53.

37

The Nosology of Dementia

Kenneth Rockwood

Division of Geriatric Medicine, Dalhousie University, Halifax, NS, Canada

INTRODUCTION

Nosology is the classification of disease. How the syndrome of dementia has been classified has changed over the years. Recognizing that textbooks are commonly consulted because readers want pragmatic answers to questions, and that understanding nuances first requires understanding the basic facts, this chapter will begin with the current classification of dementia. A second section will provide some historical context. The third section will suggest some areas that remain to be understood or at least, settled on. The focus will be on understanding the basis for the definition of the syndrome of dementia, which historically has been rooted in the diagnosis of Alzheimer's disease. Separate chapters for many of the other dementing disorders will deal with these in separate detail; here we focus on diagnostic criteria for Alzheimer's disease, and how these have influenced the way in which dementia is understood.

CURRENT NOSOLOGY OF DEMENTIA

At present, three references – DSM-IV-TR[1], ICD-10[2] and the NINCDS-ADRDA[3] criteria – provide authoritative approaches to the nosology of dementia. Each is rooted in the formulation codified in an influential textbook by Lishman[4], which proposed that dementia was a global cognitive impairment (memory plus other cognitive features) that was sufficiently severe to interfere with social or occupational function. The newly developed 10/66 criteria, discussed below, have drawn attention to difficulties in the operationalization of the idea that the cognitive impairment must be severe enough to interfere with function, and it may be that their approach will become increasingly influential[5]. Similarly, although largely technically infeasible in the low- and middle-income countries being studied by the 10/66 group, another influential proposal suggests that clinical features beyond demonstrable memory impairment count for little, compared with biomarkers[6]. How these newer trends will play out is not clear.

As a syndrome, dementia must be differentiated from other syndromes in which cognition is (or can be) impaired, including delirium, depression and age-associated cognitive decline. This last is variably conceptualized. Each of the syndromes in which cognition is impaired, but which the cognitive impairment does not meet criteria for dementia, forms part of what has been referred to as 'cognitive impairment, no dementia' (CIND). The prevalence of the heterogeneous group of disorders that is CIND is estimated to be about twice that of the prevalence of dementia[7].

DSM-IV-TR

The Text Revision of the Fourth Edition of the Diagnostic and Statistical Manual of the American Psychiatric Association (DSM-IV-TR) was published in 2000[1]. As with DSM-IV, it gives a general (syndromic) definition of dementia, but the actual dementia diagnostic codes are presented by subtype, based on presumed aetiology. These include Alzheimer's disease, vascular dementia, and separate categories for dementia due to HIV disease, head trauma, Parkinson's disease, Huntington's disease, Pick's disease, Creutzfeldt–Jakob disease, other general medical conditions, substance-induced persisting dementia, dementia of multiple aetiologies, delirium and dementia not otherwise specified.

Within the classification of other general medical conditions are listed a variety of other problems. Some, such as structural brain lesions, including subdural haematomas, and brain tumours, are not infrequently encountered, as are dementia due to multiple sclerosis or to systemic lupus erythematosis. Others are less common, such as dementia due to endocrine disorders (e.g. hypothyroidism or hyperparathyroidism) and CNS infection (neurosyphilis, cryptococcus). Still others are often obscure disorders, such as Kuf's disease and adrenoleukodystrophy.

Note, too, that dementia due to Lewy bodies can be classified in DSM-IV-TR as due to 'other general medical conditions' (or as Parkinson's disease dementia; DSM-IV-TR is in this way up to date in noting controversy over whether Lewy body dementia and Parkinson's disease dementia are aspects of the same disorder, or usefully separable)[8–10]. Frontotemporal dementia, a broader classification than the not unproblematic Pick's disease, can also be recorded under dementia to other general medical conditions.

Although dementia is diagnosed by aetiology, the syndromic aspects said to be 'essential' are repeated for each type. In the criteria for 'Dementia of the Alzheimer's Type' (Table 37.1) these are items A, B, C and E. Item D is adapted to be more disease-specific for each separate dementia classification. Note that DSM-IV-TR maintains the development of DSM-IV in that memory impairment is not further delineated, whereas in DSM-IIIR, impairment had to be demonstrated in both so-called short- and long-term memory.

ICD-10

Chapter V of the 10th revision of the International Classification of Diseases (ICD-10) is the World Health Organization's codification of

Table 37.1   DSM-IV-TR diagnostic criteria for dementia of the Alzheimer's type

A. The development of multiple cognitive deficits manifested by both (1) memory impairment (impaired ability to learn new information or to recall previously learned information) (2) one (or more) of the following cognitive disturbances:
  (a) aphasia (language disturbance)
  (b) apraxia (impaired ability to carry out motor activities despite intact motor function)
  (c) agnosia (failure to recognize or identify objects despite intact sensory function)
  (d) disturbance in executive functioning (i.e., planning, organizing, sequencing, abstracting)
B. The cognitive deficits in Criteria A1 and A2 each cause significant impairment in social or occupational functioning and represent a significant decline from a previous level of functioning.
C. The course is characterized by gradual onset and continuing cognitive decline.
D. The cognitive deficits in Criteria A1 and A2 are not due to any of the following:
  (1) other central nervous system conditions that cause progressive deficits in memory and cognition (e.g., cerebrovascular disease, Parkinson's disease, Huntington's disease, subdural hematoma, normal-pressure hydrocephalus, brain tumor)
  (2) systemic conditions that are known to cause dementia (e.g. hypothyroidism, vitamin B or folic acid deficiency, niacin deficiency, hypercalcemia, neurosyphilis, HIV infection)
  (3) substance-induced conditions
E. The deficits do not occur exclusively during the course of a delirium.
F. The disturbance is not better accounted for by another Axis I disorder (e.g. Major Depressive Episode, Schizophrenia).
Additional coding, based on presence or absence of a clinically significant behavioral disturbance:
294.10 Without Behavioral Disturbance: if the cognitive disturbance is not accompanied by any clinically significant behavioral disturbance.
294.11 With Behavioral Disturbance: if the cognitive disturbance is accompanied by a clinically significant behavioral disturbance. (e.g. wandering, agitation)
Specification of subtype:
With Early Onset: if onset is at age 65 years or below
With Late Onset: if onset is after age 65 years

Source: DSM-IV-TR: Text Revision of the fourth edition of the Diagnostic and Statistical Manual of the American Psychiatric Association.

diagnoses in relation to 'mental and behavioural disorders'. Dementia is included as a so-called 'organic' mental disorder (Table 37.2). The ICD-10 manual states that 'Dementia (F00–F03) is a syndrome due to disease of the brain, usually of a chronic or progressive nature, in which there is disturbance of multiple higher cortical functions, including memory, thinking, orientation, comprehension, calculation, learning capacity, language, and judgment. Consciousness is not clouded. The impairments of cognitive function are commonly accompanied, and occasionally preceded, by deterioration in emotional control, social behaviour, or motivation' (Table 37.2). Its emphasis on impaired behaviour is noteworthy, although in practice this might not be operationalized as distinct from the impaired 'social functioning' seen with DSM. Like DSM-IV-TR, the ICD-10 classifies dementia into an early onset, before age 65 years, and a late onset, after age 65 years. ICD-10 suggests that the early-onset form should have a more rapid onset and progression than the late-onset form. In general, however, in both DSM-IV and ICD-10, the validity of subgroups of dementia has often been found lacking, at least as employed in routine clinical use[11].

The differences in how dementia is operationalized are not inconsequential. Even the minor differences between standard criteria can importantly influence prevalence rates[12,13], especially at very late ages[14]. In general, ICD-10 has been reported to be less sensitive than earlier versions of the DSM criteria, although that is not always the case[15,16].

NINCDS-ADRDA

Even though the diagnostic classification proposed in this 1984 report focuses on Alzheimer's disease, the consensus diagnostic criteria proposed by the National Institute of Neurological and Communicative

Table 37.2   ICD-10 criteria for dementia. Definition of dementia in the ICD-10 (adapted)

G1 There is evidence of each of the following:
  (1) A decline in memory (at least) sufficient to interfere with everyday activities, though not so severe as to be incompatible with independent living
  (2) A decline in other cognitive abilities characterized by deterioration in judgement and thinking, such as planning and organizing, and in the general processing of information (at least) sufficient to cause impaired performance in daily living, but not to a degree that makes the individual dependent on others
G2 Awareness of the environment (i.e. absence of clouding of consciousness)
G3 There is a decline in emotional control or motivation, or a change in social behaviour manifest as at least one of emotional liability, irritability, apathy or coarsening of social behaviour
G4 The symptoms in criterion GI should have been present for at least 6 months

Disorders and Stroke, and the Alzheimer's Disease and Related Disorders Association (NINCDS-ADRDA) has served for many years as the standard for a diagnosis of Alzheimer's disease, and its definition of dementia was also normative[3]. It still heavily influences how research on dementia is conducted, especially as it makes up the usual inclusion criteria for drug trials on Alzheimer's disease (Table 37.3). The original criteria have been adapted somewhat – dementia can be diagnosed with the aid of cognitive screening instruments other than

Table 37.3 NINCDS/ADRDA criteria for Alzheimer's disease

Criteria for clinical diagnosis of Probable AD include:

Dementia established by clinical exam and documented by MMSE or Blessed Dementia scale, confirmed by further neuropsychological tests.

Deficits in two or more areas of cognition.

Progressive worsening of memory and other cognitive functions.

No disturbance of consciousness.

Onset between the ages of 40 and 90.

Absence of systemic diseases or other brain diseases that could explain the cognitive changes.

The diagnosis of Probable AD is supported by:

Progressive deterioration of specific cognitive functions such as language, motor skills, and perception (aphasia, apraxia, agnosia, respectively).

Impaired activities of daily living.

Positive family history, particularly if documented neuropathologically.

Lab results: Normal lumbar puncture, EEG, and evidence of cerebral atrophy on CT or MRI.

Clinical features consistent with diagnosis of Probable AD, after exclusion of other causes of dementia:

Plateaus in clinical course.

Associated symptoms: depression, insomnia, incontinence, delusions, illusions, hallucinations, catastrophic verbal, emotional, or physical outbursts, sexual disorders, and weight loss.

Other neurological abnormalities in some patients, especially with more advanced disease and including motor signs such as increased motor tone, myoclonus, or gait disorder.

Seizures in advanced disease.

CT normal for age.

Features that make the diagnosis of Probable AD unlikely or uncertain:

Sudden apoplectic onset.

Focal neurological findings such as hemiparesis, sensory loss, visual field deficits, and incoordination early in the course of the illness.

Seizures or gait disturbances at the onset or very early in the course of the illness.

Clinical diagnosis of Possible AD.

May be made on the basis of the dementia syndrome, in the absence of other neurologic, psychiatric, or systemic disorders sufficient to cause dementia, and in the presence of variations in the onset, in the presentation, or in the clinical course.

May be made in the presence of a second systematic or brain disorder sufficient to produce dementia, which is not considered to be the cause of the dementia.

Should be used in research studies when a single, gradually progressive severe cognitive deficit is identified in the absence of other identifiable cause.

---

the Mini Mental State Examination (MMSE)[17] or Blessed Dementia Rating Scales[18], and neuropsychological confirmation is not always required. But the key points of a probable cause being the case for a clinical diagnosis, neuropathology providing the definition reference, and the diagnosis being only possible when other disorders are present operate still, even though each is far from an indubitable proposition[19]. Over the years, many proposals have been made for how Alzheimer's disease might be subtyped other than by age at onset. For example, rapidity of progression, focality of onset, presence of additional features such as early extrapyramidal signs each has had adherents, but none has made their way into standard criteria[19].

SOME HISTORICAL CONTEXT FOR THE CURRENT CLASSIFICATION

Dementia as a clinical syndrome has for a long time been distinguished from changes that are often seen as people age – especially problems with memory. Even in the last 30 years, however, there have been major changes in how dementia is conceptualized, and to a large extent these are reflected in ICD-10 and DSM-IV-TR. In the early years of the modern era, much effort was put into making clear that dementia was distinct from normal ageing. Even so, ICD-10 still has a conceptually ancient hold-over in the diagnostic

code (Code R54) of 'senility without mention of psychoses', found in a chapter entitled 'The development of more clinically meaningful outcome measures and laboratory findings, not elsewhere classified'. This code can still appear in certain administrative tabulations, and has the advantage of also being in ICD-9, so that under those circumstances it can allow for the evaluation of trends. Still, the 'senility' diagnosis generally represents an outmoded, obsolete and offensive understanding of dementia – as somehow 'normal' ageing – that has no place in modern care.

Early in the modern era – roughly from the late 1950s, and especially following a series of articles in the mid-to-late 1960s by Martin Roth and colleagues[20-24], a lot of work was put into distinguishing between the neurodegenerative and vascular causes of dementia. They sought to repudiate the view that 'senility' was due to 'hardening of the arteries' and made the case that the changes in cognitive performance in elderly people was a result of plaques and tangles – Alzheimer's disease – or stroke – 'multi-infarct dementia'. While this was true, we have come to understand that the wall between the two is porous – that vascular risk factors are also a risk for Alzheimer's disease, and that the two commonly occur – even in the original series of cases from Newcastle[25] –and can act synergistically (although this last point is disputed)[26-29].

The early descriptions were correct in emphasizing how dementia affected the personality of an individual, through the undoing of what later would be called executive function. For example, a 1971 description of the clinical symptomatology of dementia warned against putting too much emphasis on 'impaired memory and orientation' as an 'undue emphasis on these features may ... obfuscate the richness of the clinical symptomatology. ... an early and frequent complaint is that the patient is "not himself", meaning that the patient and his companions have noted the onset of illness in terms of changes in function that are quite specific to that particular person, whether described in terms of alteration of drive, mood, enthusiasm, capacity to give and receive affection, creativity or other features'[30]. As later – and comparatively recent – calls for an appreciation of the importance of executive function in dementia have made clear[31,32], these descriptions were largely lost soon thereafter. Instead, the view that Alzheimer's disease was predominantly a disorder of memory, that temporal and parietal involvement was early, that frontal lobe involvement was late, and that the standardization offered by psychometric testing would trump the subjectivity of clinical judgement each contributed to the systematic lack of attention to 'what makes a patient him[her]self'.

Another point seen in earlier iterations of dementia criteria that is less commonly emphasized now is that a diagnosis of dementia should only be made in patients in whom consciousness was 'clear'. This was meant to be another way of saying that consciousness should not be clouded, which in DSM-III was seen as a major distinguishing feature of delirium. (In DSM-IV-TR, delirium is again conceptualized as a disorder of consciousness; the only reference that it be clear, however, is the description of 'reduced clarity of awareness of the environment'.) With the recognition of the importance of alterations in levels of consciousness as a hallmark of Lewy body dementia, however[10], this particular requirement has been dropped. Instead, the criteria make reference to the cognitive disorder not being better accounted for by delirium.

FUTURE CHALLENGES IN DEMENTIA NOSOLOGY

The exciting pace of development in the study of dementia means that the field has to look anew at received wisdom. A large number of developments are likely to impact on what will be controversial about the nosology of dementia when the next edition of this textbook appears. Here, a few are sketched out in the barest detail. Even so, they give some hint as to why this most staid of topics is likely to have interest for some time yet.

'Alzheimerization' of Dementia Criteria

Current dementia criteria are, as we have seen, largely modelled on the dementia characteristically seen in Alzheimer's disease. This is a problem for dementias in which memory impairment is not the chief early manifestation. The two most commonly occurring examples are frontotemporal dementia and vascular dementia, especially the so-called 'subcortical' variant[33]. In either, affective and behavioural disturbances can predominate early. The consequences of this problem are many. In the case of vascular dementia, Hachinski has long drawn attention to the opportunities missed in dementia prevention[34] and in understanding the impact of vascular disease on brain function by underestimating its burden in the wait for memory to become impaired. In consequence, he has proposed the concept of vascular cognitive impairment[35]. Over time, this has had great influence[36], but has yet to be reflected in the standard criteria, including in the NINDS-AIREN criteria for vascular dementia[37].

The presentation (and evaluation) of impaired judgement in someone whose memory is reasonably intact can be problematic, especially where social conduct violates legal norms (e.g. theft, sexual impropriety). In some cases, it is clear that a reliable clinical diagnosis of dementia can be made due to other characteristic features in the patient's cognitive profile and how that impacts on function, even if memory is relatively intact. Even so, depending on the literalness of local prosecutors, the understanding that the criteria in real life often are only approximate can be a tricky business. (In such cases, where it is necessary to show that the criteria need not always be applied strictly, I have found it useful to cite Aristotle – who hedged that in biology rules apply 'always or for the most part'[38]. If that seems a bit obscure, it is always possible to resort to the usual disclaimer for hair loss products: 'Your results may vary'.)

Notwithstanding the incompleteness of the criteria, there are other circumstances of late-onset aberrant behaviour, coupled with some evidence of executive dysfunction, in which only the passage of time and progression of the illness to include other dementia features makes the diagnosis clear.

Cognitive Disturbances with Many Causes

Dementia occurs largely in older people who are more likely to have things wrong with them. In consequence, in clinical practice it is common to encounter patients with many things wrong that might contribute to cognitive impairment. For this reason, dementia diagnostic criteria need to give particular attention to how such problems are to be conceptualized and identified. This is relevant in three situations. 'Mixed dementia' refers to co-existing illnesses and especially to the combination of infarction (or, more controversially, ischaemia) with Alzheimer's disease. As noted, given that vascular risk factors are also risks for Alzheimer's disease, not unexpectedly the two often conclude and can be the most common form of dementia encountered[26-29,39,]. In the ICD-10, NINCDS-ADRDA and NINDS-AIREN criteria, the result is a 'possible' diagnosis – e.g. 'possible Alzheimer's disease, with vascular component'. By contrast, DSM-IV-TR allows for 'Dementia due to multiple etiologies'. (From a coding standpoint, multiple codes are allowed – i.e. each of the codes for the given causes is recorded.)

A similar situation occurs when delirium complicates dementia. Again, this is a common situation, as each is a risk for the other[40]. In addition, delirium which does not resolve is a risk for dementia, and results in an indeterminate period (of between 3–6 months) when features of both may be present[41]. The multiple coding approach and the use of codes for delirium-complicating dementia seen in DSM-IV are considered a good way to handle the common co-occurrence of these syndromes, resulting in a proposal that ICD-11 should follow the lead of the DSM[40,42]. The parallel is also seen when depression complicates dementia[43].

Lessons from the 10/66 Experience

The 10/66 Dementia Research group is a collective of dementia researchers worldwide, who are carrying out population-based studies of dementia[44-46]. The title refers to the fact that two-thirds of people with dementia live in low- and middle-income countries and that 10% (or less) of population research is conducted there. An early and important finding of the 10/66 was how poorly standard dementia criteria applied in many parts of the world. In consequence, the 10/66 group developed its own. These criteria differ from the standard criteria chiefly in how they operationalized the impact of cognitive impairment on function (relying less on informant reports of decline) and in the use of detailed procedures for operationalization, which were cross-culturally validated. These criteria yielded results that were both more consistent across sites and strikingly higher than those using DSM-IV dementia criteria (e.g. 10/66 criteria suggested prevalence of 5.6–11.7% by country, compared with 0.4–6.4%)[5]. These last results raised the question of whether the criteria were too sensitive, and thereby not specific enough, or whether 10/66 'pathologizes' mild decline that can be accommodated within many cultures in which less cognitive demand is placed on elders. These questions remain to be resolved.

Alzheimer's Disease without Dementia

At a different spectrum from those who look to diagnose dementia in low- and middle-income countries are groups who are aiming to develop preventive treatment for dementia, or at least ones which could be implemented as early in the disease course as possible[6]. For such groups, the interest is on how to couple the earliest manifestations of dementia with biological markers of the disease. Drawing on a body of work about very early[47] and prodromal Alzheimer's disease, and on the apparent promise of biomarkers, a consortium has proposed that biomarkers, coupled with a memory complaint, should form the basis for a diagnosis of Alzheimer's disease. The clear intent is to provide a test base of people who are at high risk for the development of 'full-blown' Alzheimer's disease, and to see if new interventions might prevent that outcome. How such a proposal will affect more widespread diagnosis of dementia is uncertain. Whether 'prevented Alzheimer's disease' will look like 'no (or mild) cognitive impairment' is also uncertain, but the parallel case might exist now for successfully treated Alzheimer's disease (below).

Executive Dysfunction

As noted, it had been the case that, central to a clinical diagnosis of dementia, was the loss of aspects of an individual's character which made them essentially themselves. This notion largely was lost for a period, before being rediscovered, under the guise of executive function. While the emphasis on executive function is welcome, it is not at all clear that the usual remedy (to employ measures of 'frontal lobe tests') addresses the clinical phenomenon sufficiently well. A cultural bias is at work in rejecting the characterization of an individual's complaints – what makes dementia a problem for them – as too subjective an evaluation process, and instead substituting finger-tapping or clock-drawing tasks as preferable alternatives. Future criteria will need to examine how they view the notion of subjectivity or objectivity. In this, they might be helped by consultation with philosophers who understand the distinctions that are at play here.

Successful Treatment of Dementia

Even though no current treatment cures Alzheimer's disease, many people can be treated successfully, to the extent of having important overall improvement on global clinical measures[48]. Evaluations of the notes from patient interviews in which clinicians rated patients as showing overall improvement have shown that typically in such cases some symptoms improve, most are stabilized and some worsen[49,50]. In short, successful treatment can result not in cure, but in a new state. This state has yet to be operationalized in any terms that could

inform criteria. Even so, it offers a way to retrieve some of the lesson taught by Wells (i.e. the warning that too much emphasis on easily testable cognitive elements might obscure the richness of the clinical symptomology). The approach to this problem that I have used with colleagues is known as goal attainment scaling[51], about which independent reviews suggest it has promise, but needs additional work, chiefly replication and some standardization[52,53]. Whether the results of partially treated (or partially prevented) Alzheimer's disease will be stable enough and common enough to warrant special categorization is a development to be evaluated with some interest.

SUMMARY

The nosology of the dementia syndrome is likely to continue to evolve, reflecting developments in how and where dementia is studied. Important challenges to our understanding of dementia reflect continuing development of our knowledge of these dread illnesses.

REFERENCE

1. American Psychiatric Association. *Diagnostic and Statistical Manual of the American Psychiatric Association Text Revision of the Fourth Edition (DSM-IV-TR)*. Washington, DC. APA Press, 2000.
2. *World Health Organization. The ICD-10 Classification of Mental and Behavioural Disorders. Clinical Descriptions and Diagnostic Guidelines*. Switzerland: World Health Organization, 1992.
3. McKhann G, Drachman D, Folstein M, Katzman R, Price D, Stadlan EM. Clinical diagnosis of Alzheimer's disease: report of the NINCDS-ADRDA work group under the auspices of Department of Health and Human Services Task Force on Alzheimer's Disease. *Neurology* 1984; **34**: 939–44.
4. Lishman WA. *Organic Psychiatry*. Oxford: Blackwell, 1978.
5. Llibre Rodriguez JJ, Ferri CP, Acosta D *et al.* Prevalence of dementia in Latin America, India, and China: a population-based cross-sectional survey. *Lancet* 2008; **372**: 464–74.
6. Dubois B, Feldman HH, Jacova C, *et al.* Research criteria for the diagnosis of Alzheimer's disease: revising the NINCDS-ADRDA criteria. *Lancet Neurol* 2007; **6**: 734–46.
7. Graham JE, Rockwood K, Beattie BL *et al.* Prevalence and severity of cognitive impairment with and without dementia in an elderly population. *Lancet* 1997; **349**: 1793–6.
8. Reveulta GJ, Lippa CF. Dementia with Lewy bodies and Parkinson's disease dementia may best be viewed as two distinct entities. *Int Psychogeriatr* 2009; **21**: 213–16.
9. Aarsland D, Londos E, Ballard C. Parkinson's disease dementia and dementia with Lewy bodies: different aspects of one entity. *Int Psychogeriatr* 2009; **21**: 216–19.
10. McKeith IG, Dickson DW, Lowe J *et al.* Diagnosis and management of dementia with Lewy bodies: third report of the DLB consortium. *Neurology* 2005; **65**: 1863–72.
11. Phung TK, Andersen BB, Hogh P, Kessing LV, Mortensen PB, Waldemar G. Validity of dementia diagnoses in the Danish hospital registers. *Dement Geriatr Cogn Disord* 2007; **24**: 220–8.
12. Erkinjuntti T, Ostbye T, Steenhuis R, Hachinski V. The effect of different diagnostic criteria on the prevalence of dementia. *N Engl J Med* 1997; **337**: 1667–74.
13. Wancata J, Borjesson-Hanson A, Ostling S, Sjogren K, Skoog I. Diagnostic criteria influence dementia prevalence. *Am J Geriatr Psychiatry* 2007; **15**: 1034–45.

14. Pioggiosi P, Forti P, Ravaglia G, Berardi D, Ferrari G, de Ronchi D. Different classification systems yield different dementia occurrence among nonagenarians and centenarians. *Dement Geriatr Cogn Disord* 2004; **17**: 35–41.

15. Riedel-Heller SG, Busse A, Aurich C, Matschinger H, Angermeyer MC. Incidence of dementia according to DSM-III-R and ICD-10: results of the Leipzig longitudinal study of the aged (LEILA75+), part 2. *Br J Psychiatry* 2001; **179**: 255–60.

16. Naik M, Nygaard HA. Diagnosing dementia – ICD-10 not so bad after all: a comparison between dementia criteria according to DSM-IV and ICD-10. *Int J Geriatr Psychiatry* 2008; **23**: 279–82.

17. Folstein MF, Folstein SE, McHugh PR. 'Mini-mental state'. A practical method for grading the cognitive state of patients for the clinician. *J Psychiatr Res* 1975; **12**: 189–98.

18. Blessed G, Tomlinson BE, Roth M. Blessed-roth dementia scale (DS). *Psychopharmacol Bull* 1988; **24**: 705–8.

19. Rockwood K, Camicioli R, Bouchard R, Leger G. Toward a revision of criteria for the dementias. *Alzheimer Dement* 2007; **3**: 428–40.

20. Tomlinson BE, Blessed G, Roth M. Observations on the brains of demented old people. *J Neurol Sci* 1970; **11**: 205–42.

21. Blessed G, Tomlinson BE, Roth M. The association between quantitative measures of dementia and of senile change in the cerebral grey matter of elderly subjects. *Br J Psychiatry* 1968; **114**: 797–811.

22. Tomlinson BE, Blessed G, Roth M. Observations on the brains of non-demented old people. *J Neurol Sci* 1968; **7**: 331–56.

23. Roth M, Tomlinson BE, Blessed G. The relationship between quantitative measures of dementia and of degenerative changes in the cerebral grey matter of elderly subjects. *Proc R Soc Med* 1967; **60**: 254–60.

24. Roth M, Tomlinson BE, Blessed G. Correlation between scores for dementia and counts of 'senile plaques' in cerebral grey matter of elderly subjects. *Nature* 1966; **209**: 109–10.

25. Kalaria RN, Kenny RA, Ballard CG, Perry R, Ince P, Polvikoski T. Towards defining the neuropathological substrates of vascular dementia. *J Neurol Sci* 2004; **226**: 75–80.

26. Snowdon DA, Greiner LH, Mortimer JA, Riley KP, Greiner PA, Markesbery WR. Brain infarction and the clinical expression of Alzheimer's disease. The nun study. *JAMA* 1997; **277**: 813–17.

27. Schneider JA, Arvanitakis Z, Bang W, Bennett DA. Mixed brain pathologies account for most dementia cases in community-dwelling older persons. *Neurology* 2007; **69**: 2197–204.

28. Launer LJ, Petrovitch H, Ross GW, Markesbery W, White LR. AD brain pathology: vascular origins? Results from the HAAS autopsy study. *Neurobiol Aging* 2008; **29**: 1587–90.

29. Schneider JA, Boyle PA, Arvanitakis Z, Bienias JL, Bennett DA. Subcortical infarcts, Alzheimer's disease pathology, and memory function in older persons. *Ann Neurol* 2007; **62**: 59–66.

30. Wells CE. The symptoms and behavioral manifestations of dementia. In Wells CE (ed.), *Dementia*. Philadelphia: FA Davis, 1971, 2.

31. Voss SE, Bullock RA. Executive function: the core feature of dementia? *Dement Geriatr Cogn Disord* 2004; **18**: 207–16.

32. Royall DR, Lauterbach EC, Cummings JL *et al.* Executive control function: a review of its promise and challenges for clinical research. A report from the committee on research of the American Neuropsychiatric Association. *J Neuropsychiatry Clin Neurosci* 2002; **14**: 377–405.

33. Erkinjuntti T, Inzitari D, Pantoni L *et al.* Research criteria for subcortical vascular dementia in clinical trials. *J Neural Transm Suppl* 2000; **59**: 23–30.

34. Hachinski V. Preventable senility: a call for action against the vascular dementias. *Lancet* 1992; **340**: 645–8.

35. Hachinski V. Vascular dementia: a radical redefinition. *Dementia* 1994; **5**: 130–2.

36. Moorhouse P, Rockwood K. Vascular cognitive impairment: current concepts and clinical developments. *Lancet Neurol* 2008; **7**: 246–55.

37. Roman GC, Tatemichi TK, Erkinjuntti T *et al.* Vascular dementia: diagnostic criteria for research studies. report of the NINDS-AIREN International Workshop. *Neurology* 1993; **43**: 250–60.

38. Lennox JG. *Aristotle's Philosophy of Biology*. Cambridge: Cambridge University Press, 2001.

39. Esiri MM, Wilcock GK, Morris JH. Neuropathological assessment of the lesions of significance in vascular dementia. *J Neurol Neurosurg Psychiatry* 1997; **63**: 749–53.

40. Eeles E, Rockwood K. Delirium in the long-term care setting: clinical and research challenges. *J Am Med Dir Assoc* 2008; **9**: 157–61.

41. Cole MG, Ciampi A, Belzile E, Zhong L. Persistent delirium in older hospital patients: a systematic review of frequency and prognosis. *Age Ageing* 2009; **38**: 19–26.

42. Meagher DJ, Maclullich AM, Laurila JV. Defining delirium for the International Classification of Diseases, 11th revision. *J Psychosom Res* 2008; **65**: 207–14.

43. Burns A, Iliffe S. Dementia. *BMJ* 2009; **338**: B75.

44. Ferri CP, Prince M, Brayne C *et al.* Global prevalence of dementia: A Delphi consensus study. *Lancet* 2005; **366**: 2112–17.

45. Jacob KS, Kumar PS, Gayathri K, Abraham S, Prince MJ. The diagnosis of dementia in the community. *Int Psychogeriatr* 2007; **19**: 669–78.

46. Ferri CP, Ames D, Prince M. 10/66 Dementia Research Group. Behavioral and psychological symptoms of dementia in developing countries. *Int Psychogeriatr* 2004; **16**: 441–59.

47. Morris JC. Mild cognitive impairment is early-stage Alzheimer's disease: time to revise diagnostic criteria. *Arch Neurol* 2006; **63**: 15–16.

48. Rockwood K, Wallack M, Tallis R. The treatment of Alzheimer's disease: success short of cure. *Lancet Neurol* 2003; **2**: 630–3.

49. Joffres C, Graham J, Rockwood K. Qualitative analysis of the clinician interview-based impression of change (plus): methodological issues and implications for clinical research. *Int Psychogeriatr* 2000; **12**: 403–13.

50. Joffres C, Bucks RS, Haworth J, Wilcock GK, Rockwood K. Patterns of clinically detectable treatment effects with galantamine: a qualitative analysis. *Dement Geriatr Cogn Disord* 2003; **15**: 26–33.

51. Kiresuk TJ, Sherman R. Goal attainment scaling: a general method for evaluating comprehensive community mental health programs. *Community Ment Health J* 1968; **4**: 443–53.

52. Molnar FJ, Man-Son-Hing M, Fergusson D. Systematic review of measures of clinical significance employed in randomized controlled trials of drugs for dementia. *J Am Geriatr Soc* 2009; **57**: 536–46.

53. Bouwens SF, Van Heugten CM, Verhey FR. Review of goal attainment scaling as a useful outcome measure in psychogeriatric patients with cognitive disorders. *Dement Geriatr Cogn Disord* 2008; **26**: 528–40.

38

Epidemiology of Dementia

Mary Ganguli

University of Pittsburgh School of Medicine and Graduate School of Public Health, WPIC, Pittsburgh, PA, USA

Epidemiology has traditionally been the study of the distribution and determinants of disease in the population. Its principles and approaches are also used to study normal variation, for example changes related to normal ageing in the population at large. Epidemiology helps clinicians by acquainting us with the proportions of given populations that are affected by the conditions we diagnose and treat; the frequency with which different conditions, changes and outcomes occur; and the factors that raise and lower the probability of these conditions occurring. Importantly, epidemiology also completes the clinical picture of disease, demonstrating that patients who seek our services for a given condition are not typical of all individuals in the community with that condition. For example, individuals with dementia who present to a psychiatric clinic may have different characteristics (insight, symptoms, severity, duration, support) than those who are seen in neurological or general practice settings, or who do not seek clinical services at all. As of this writing, efforts are under way to revise the current clinical diagnostic criteria for dementia and its subtypes, including Alzheimer's disease, in the World Health Organization's International Classification of Disease[1] and the American Psychiatric Association's Diagnostic and Statistical Manual of Mental Disorders[2]. More than in previous editions, attention is being paid to epidemiological data that bear on diagnosis: for example, the heterogeneity of dementia and cognitive impairment, and the predictive validity of various diagnostic criteria in population settings.

BASIC DEFINITIONS

Prevalence is a cross-sectional snapshot of the disease burden of the population. It is the proportion of individuals in a defined population who have the disease or condition at a given time (point prevalence) or defined period (period prevalence), regardless of how long these individuals have had the condition.

Incidence is the rate at which new disease occurs in the population. It is the proportion of individuals previously free of disease who develop the disease during a defined period (e.g. one year, or 1 000 person-years), within a defined population.

Overall prevalence and incidence estimates (e.g. for everyone aged 65 years and older) are less useful than age-specific estimates, that is, within defined age groups, such as those aged 65–74, 75–84 and 85+ years.

Prevalence is the product of incidence rate and duration of survival with disease. Thus, high prevalence can be the result of high incidence, long duration, or both. Two groups can have the same dementia incidence, with prevalence being higher in the group in which people with dementia live longer.

GLOBAL AGEING, DEMOGRAPHIC TRANSITION, DEVELOPED VS. DEVELOPING COUNTRIES

The world's population is ageing, as improving living standards have increased life expectancy across the globe. The most affluent countries have the longest average life expectancy, and the greatest proportions of older adults. However, population ageing is occurring faster in the low- and middle-income ('developing') countries than in the wealthier ('developed') countries. It is determined by both birth rates and death rates. Populations with high fertility tend to have low proportions of older people, and vice versa. The 'demographic transition' is the process in which, over time, a high-fertility-high-mortality population becomes a low-fertility-low-mortality population, and its average age increases. As people live longer, the public health concern becomes whether their years of extended life are characterized by relative health and independence or by ill-health, disability and dependence on others. Thus, we measure not only overall life expectancy but healthy life expectancy and disability rates.

In affluent countries, disability rates appear to be decreasing as the population ages. In low- and middle-income countries, it seems likely that disability rates will climb as people live longer with chronic disease. The least affluent countries are the least prepared to deal with the challenges of population ageing, given the rapidity with which the demographic transition is occurring in their societies. However, one factor in their favour is the elderly support ratio, which is the number of elderly people for every 100 younger adults in a given population, with younger individuals assumed to be directly or indirectly supporting older ones. This ratio is increasing rapidly in the affluent countries, with greater numbers of older individuals needing support from a shrinking number of younger persons. In the less affluent countries, this ratio is expected to change quite slowly[3].

Dementia is a major cause of functional disability, dependence and mortality in the elderly. It therefore reduces both overall life expectancy and active (disability-free) life expectancy, although the extent to which it does so might vary across populations. Dementia is also responsible for increasing use and cost of health services,

Principles and Practice of Geriatric Psychiatry, 3rd edn. Edited by Mohammed T. Abou-Saleh, Cornelius Katona and Anand Kumar
© 2011 John Wiley & Sons, Ltd

particularly long-term-institutional care, in countries where such institutions are available and culturally acceptable. The cost to a given society of caring for its members with dementia depends on its age structure, the numbers and proportions of affected individuals, their length of survival and degree of dependency, the availability of appropriate goods and services, and who bears the costs of these items. These direct costs, as well as indirect costs (e.g. loss of income by the patient and family caregiver) will vary according to the affluence and age structure of a given society.

SYNDROMAL DEFINITION OF DEMENTIA: DSM, ICD, EVOLVING CRITERIA; 'CASENESS'

At the time of this writing, the most widely employed diagnostic criteria for dementia at the syndrome level are those of the Tenth Revision of the International Classification of Diseases (ICD-10)[1] and the Fourth Edition of the Diagnostic and Statistical Manual of Mental Disorders (DSM-IV-TR)[2]. Over the years, studies in different countries have used different versions of these criteria. Variations in definitions and criteria can potentially raise and lower estimates of prevalence and incidence across studies and populations. One study demonstrated that the proportion of individuals classified as having dementia varied from 3% using the ICD-10 criteria to 29% using the DSM-III criteria, within the same population[4].

According to current definitions, dementia is a syndrome of acquired, chronic cognitive impairment, occurring in clear consciousness, sufficient to interfere with social and occupational functioning, and characterized by impairment in at least two cognitive domains. For the past few decades, the definition has further required that memory be one of the impaired domains[2], but this requirement may not persist in future revisions of diagnostic criteria. For example, it may be possible that an individual with significant impairments in executive and language functioning can be diagnosed as having dementia, even without memory impairment.

Further, there is currently no standard diagnostic entity reflecting a minor level of cognitive decline that is not accompanied by functional impairment, thus falling short of the threshold for being called dementia. This situation too may change as knowledge evolves and preclinical detection of dementing illnesses becomes a possibility. Besides the functional dimension of the diagnosis, the standard neuropsychological criteria for dementia typically require test performance in two cognitive domains to be at least two standard deviations below the mean for the individual's peer group, as defined by age, education, linguistic/ethnic group and sometimes gender. However, appropriate norms are not always available. Thus, the issue of 'caseness', or what makes an individual a true case, has yet to be universally defined, and will become harder as the demand increases for earlier detection of the dementia syndrome.

DEMENTIA SUBTYPES AND THE ROLE OF CO-MORBIDITY

Alzheimer's disease (AD) is a primary neurodegenerative disease which appears to be the single most common cause of the dementia syndrome in older adults, in most populations which have been studied worldwide. The next single most frequent cause of dementia is cerebrovascular disease; either cortical infarcts or white matter disease, or both, can lead to significant cognitive impairment and decline. Diagnostic criteria for vascular dementia and cognitive impairment have varied as to whether the mere presence of cerebrovascular disease with dementia is sufficient, or whether evidence from neuroimaging is also required, for the diagnosis[2,5]. However, mixed Alzheimer's and vascular pathology is more common than pure vascular disease or pure degenerative disease, as borne out by the few community studies that have been able to conduct autopsies[6]. Although prominent in specialty clinical settings, dementias related to other primary brain disorders such as frontotemporal lobar degeneration, Lewy body disease and Parkinson's disease appear relatively infrequent in the community at large; population-based estimates are scarce. Opinion is moving towards accepting co-morbidity and multiple causes in a given individual with dementia, rather than selecting one subtype over another in the presence of mixed aetiology.

PREVALENCE AND INCIDENCE OF THE DEMENTIAS

The overall prevalence of dementia, based on many studies in affluent countries worldwide, is in the range of 5–10% of individuals aged 65 years and older. One meta-analysis showed a doubling of dementia prevalence with every 5-year increase in age; for AD the doubling occurred with every 4.5 years and for vascular dementia every 5.3 years[7]. Population studies typically do not employ neuroimaging or neuropathology for diagnosis, but rather use operationalized standard clinical diagnostic criteria. In these studies, AD appears to account for two-thirds to three-quarters of observed cases. Previous reports of vascular dementia being more prevalent than degenerative dementia in some Asian populations may have been the result of varying diagnostic criteria. However, prevalence has not been established for the newer, broader entity called vascular cognitive impairment (VCI) which encompasses all levels of cognitive decline from mild deficits to dementia. The prevalence of dementia of Parkinson's disease has been estimated at about 0.5% of the population aged 65 years and older[8].

Although incidence rates vary, one meta-analysis showed rates of AD ranging from 0.33% per year for those aged 65–74 to 8.68% for those aged 95+ years[9]. Evidence is inconclusive as to whether incidence continues to increase after age 90. In a study including MRI scans for the diagnosis, the age-adjusted incidence rate for AD was 19.2, and for vascular dementia 14.6, per 1000 person-years[10]. While many studies have shown higher dementia prevalence among women, many incidence studies have not shown a gender difference. If incidence is indeed the same in men and women, gender difference in prevalence may be due to longer survival in women. There are few population-based data on early-onset dementias.

Based on a handful of studies from Asia, Africa, Central and South America, and Eastern Europe, prevalence in low- and middle-income countries is much lower than in the affluent countries. It is, however, increasing as their populations age, and seems to be divided between Alzheimer's and vascular subtypes as in the rest of the world[11]. The prevalence difference is not solely a function of life expectancy. Opinion is divided as to how much of the discrepancy is due to misclassification, given the difficulties in measurement discussed earlier, and how much reflects true differences in disease occurrence. However, all studies report an exponential increase in both prevalence and incidence with age. With the rapid population ageing of the less affluent countries, among which India and China have very large populations, even a lower proportion affected by dementia will reflect a larger number of individual cases in these countries than in the wealthier countries[12].

NORMAL VS. ABNORMAL COGNITIVE AGEING

To differentiate early dementia from the cognitive changes of normal ageing can be challenging in clinical practice, and is no easier at the population level. The majority of older adults experience some slowing of information processing as part of normal ageing. Memory, visuospatial ability and executive functioning/reasoning also are likely to decline with normal ageing. In contrast, verbal/language abilities tend to remain more stable.

Terms such as age-associated memory impairment and age-related cognitive decline have been used to characterize the cognitive changes of normal ageing. Terms including mild cognitive impairment (MCI)[13] and cognitive impairment, no dementia (CIND)[14] are used to describe states intermediate between normal cognitive ageing and dementia, where individuals experience or exhibit cognitive deficits greater than expected for age, without fulfilling diagnostic criteria for dementia. The prevalence of this variably defined intermediate state in the elderly population is entirely dependent on the definition, and has been shown to vary from 3 to 20% as a function of the criteria employed[15]. The key element is mild cognitive decline with little or no functional change. This state frequently but not inevitably progresses to dementia. The rate of progression to dementia is reported as 12–15% per year in patients actively seeking care for memory problems in specialized settings like memory disorders clinics. The rate is lower in the community at large, when MCI is systematically detected by standardized assessment. In fact, MCI in the community appears to be an unstable and heterogeneous state with many individuals remaining stable or even reverting to normal over time. This discrepancy is inadequately understood, but suggests that it is premature to assume that MCI uniformly represents preclinical dementia. Outside specialty clinical settings, other conditions (e.g. anticholinergic medication effects, depression, heart failure) may contribute substantially to the observed impairments. It is likely that the criteria will undergo further refinement to enhance their predictive validity, possibly by including reliable biomarkers of underlying disease.

It must be firmly recognized that no test of cognitive function is entirely free of the effects of culture and education. Individuals of greater age and lesser education will typically perform worse on most neuropsychological tests than younger and better-educated persons. If not carefully accounted for, these factors can lead to misclassification error in epidemiological studies, potentially inflating prevalence estimates of cognitive impairment and dementia in populations with low literacy and education.

CROSS-CULTURAL ISSUES IN DIAGNOSIS AND EPIDEMIOLOGY

With some caveats, the process and functional consequences of brain ageing are assumed to be fairly similar in all populations, while their personal and social impact may not be the same across societies and cultures. Thus, the clinical thresholds may be different, or the same underlying disease biology may cross the clinical threshold to different extents in different populations. This variation can give rise to varying estimates of prevalence and incidence. Such estimates are also influenced by variation in life expectancy, the presence of co-morbid medical conditions, and local norms and expectations. In many cultures, cognitive impairment is considered an inevitable consequence of ageing, and expectations of the elderly are tailored accordingly. It may be the norm for younger family members to assume most of the older adult's previous responsibilities other than basic self-care. Consider the examples of two older men with AD, one living in a large extended-family setting on a farm, and the other living alone in an urban apartment. Compared to the latter, the former may have to suffer a greater degree of cognitive impairment, and reach a more advanced stage of dementia, before he experiences interference with his own social and occupational functioning or the family reports a problem, resulting in a later diagnosis of dementia. Meanwhile, the second man's environment requires him to independently use household appliances, and manage his own meals, finances and transportation; a lesser degree of cognitive impairment would interfere with his daily functioning and lead to an earlier diagnosis of dementia. Measurements and diagnostic criteria developed in one setting or country may therefore not be entirely appropriate in another; cross-cultural validation is of critical importance as disease concepts and criteria are translated and applied internationally.

RISK AND PROTECTIVE FACTORS AND THE MEANING OF 'RISK'

Going beyond measures of disease distribution (prevalence and incidence), epidemiology also plays a major role in identifying disease determinants (risk and protective factors). As the term 'risk' is most commonly used in epidemiology, it refers to the probability of developing future disease. Thus, ideally, inferences about risk factors should be drawn from prospective studies and not cross-sectional or retrospective studies. Within any population, there are individuals who currently have disease, while the remainder are currently free of disease. A true risk factor is one associated with a significantly higher probability of future disease developing in currently disease-free individuals. The subgroup possessing this risk factor has a higher incidence rate of the disease than the subgroup without that risk factor. Similarly, protective factors are those associated with a lower probability and incidence rate of future disease. It is extremely important to recognize that an identified risk factor may not be the direct cause of the disease. It may be within the causal pathway, or might play a mediating or moderating role between a causal factor and the disease, or may be a surrogate for a causal factor. Further, a risk factor is not necessarily modifiable or preventable. Note that while some studies have singled out risk and protective factors for Alzheimer's disease, many have examined all dementias together, and, other than their genetics, little is known of risk factors for early-onset dementias.

For overall late-onset dementia, which is mostly Alzheimer's or vascular, the strongest known risk factor is greater *age*, as demonstrated by incidence rates increasing with age. Based on similar incidence rates in men and women, at least up until age 90, female *gender* may not be a true risk factor as previously supposed. Several studies have indicated that *lesser education* increases the risk of dementia; the underlying mechanism is not known. Possibilities include education being a reflection of, or a promoter of, greater cognitive 'reserve' capacity that allows the brain to resist or compensate longer for the increasing pathology within it. Alternatively, education could be a surrogate for lifelong socioeconomic status and its consequences, including nutrition and health care; or a confounding variable in the diagnosis of dementia based on cognitive test performance.

A positive *family history of dementia* in a first-degree relative increases the risk of dementia, suggesting a hereditary component. The genetics of AD have been studied the most extensively. While many genes have been reported to play a role in AD, there is, thus far, conclusive evidence for only three deterministic genes and one susceptibility gene. Mutations of the *APP* (amyloid precursor protein) gene on chromosome 21, *PS-1* (presenilin 1) gene on chromosome 14, and the *PS-2* (presenilin 2) gene on chromosome 1 are all associated with early-onset familial AD. Relevant to the *APP* gene, *Down syndrome*, caused by trisomy of chromosome 21, is a well-established risk factor for AD. The one susceptibility gene consistently associated with sporadic cases and late-onset cases is the polymorphic *APOE* (apolipoprotein E) gene, on chromosome 19, also associated with cholesterol elevation. The *E*4* allele of this gene is associated with higher risk and/or earlier onset of Alzheimer's disease in a dose-related fashion, with homozygosity conferring higher risk than heterozygosity. In epidemiological studies, the *APOE*4* genotype is associated with a two- to three-fold elevation of probability of AD. The exceptions are African populations, where the *APOE*4* allele is of high frequency but appears not to increase AD risk, and African American populations, where risk elevation is present but lower. This paradox has been attributed to competing risk of vascular disease. Unlike the mutations, the *APOE*4* genotype only increases susceptibility and does not guarantee that the disease will occur. A comprehensive review of the genetics of AD and other dementias is beyond the scope of this chapter.

There is growing evidence that a host of *cardiovascular risk factors*, including but not limited to *hypertension, hypercholesterolaemia, diabetes mellitus and obesity*, all increase the risk of not only overall dementia and vascular dementia but also of AD. One explanation is that these factors operate primarily by causing cerebrovascular disease, which interacts with degenerative pathology, leading to earlier onset of the dementia syndrome. Another is that they directly influence neurodegeneration, for example by influencing the metabolism or accumulation of amyloid protein in the brain. From the epidemiological perspective, the most striking finding from long-term prospective studies is that dementia risk is elevated by hypertension, elevated serum cholesterol and obesity that are present in middle age, but in not old age. In fact, the onset of dementia in later life is preceded by a period of low blood pressure and cholesterol. These findings suggest, first, that the brain pathology that causes dementia develops over many decades and, second, that it is not only the presence or absence of a given factor but the timing and duration of exposure to the factor that influence the risk of dementia.

Other reported risk factors from the epidemiological literature are based on less consistent evidence. They include, for example, history of *head trauma* with loss of consciousness, possibly acting synergistically with the *APOE*4* genotype, *thyroid* abnormalities, and exposure to certain general *anaesthetic agents*.

Potential protective factors include the rare *APOE*2* genotype, intake of diets rich in *antioxidants*, exposure to the lipid-lowering drugs HMG Co-A reductase inhibitors ('statins'), exposure to nonsteroidal anti-inflammatory drugs (*NSAIDs*), exposure to *oestrogen* supplements, *physical exercise* and *cognitive exercise*. It is difficult to draw firm conclusions about many of these factors because, although they show negative associations in observational studies, intervention studies using them have not revealed benefits in preventing or delaying the onset of dementia. Some observational data suggest that oestrogen supplements taken for several years, starting at menopause, may reduce incidence of Alzheimer's disease at least a decade later. However, clinical trials of oestrogen supplements taken in later life have not shown a protective effect against dementia and in fact suggested an increased risk. As noted earlier, the timing and duration of exposure to risk and protective factors may be critical.

Two examples will be discussed to further illustrate the complexity of putative risk relationships.

Cigarette smoking has been shown in cross-sectional as well as some prospective epidemiological studies of older adults to be associated with a lower probability of Alzheimer's dementia. Short-term trials of transdermal nicotine patches have been inconclusive.

It is certainly plausible that the nicotine use can have cholinergic effects that promote cognitive performance. However, it is also likely that the apparent protective effect is an artefact reflecting survival bias. Smokers who survive into old age without succumbing to heart and lung disease or cancer might be an unusually hardy group with enhanced capacity to resist many diseases including AD; those who died before they could develop dementia cannot participate in these studies.

Depression: in case-control studies, individuals with AD are more likely than healthy controls to have had previous histories of major depression. Older adults with major depression have cognitive deficits which resolve only partially when the depression remits. Major depression in younger adults has been found to be associated with atrophy of the hippocampal cortex, which has been attributed to prolonged hypercortisolaemia caused by depression[16]. The hippocampus and medial temporal lobe are the areas typically affected by AD pathology. An autopsy study of patients with AD showed that those who had suffered major depression earlier in life had greater density of degenerative pathology in their hippocampi than those with no previous history of depression[17]. However, one prospective population study was able to divide elderly participants without dementia into one subgroup which developed dementia over the next several years and another subgroup that remained dementia free. Depressive symptoms at the beginning of the study did not predict rate of cognitive decline in either group; subsequent cognitive decline was primarily explained by the incipient dementia[18]. A potential unifying hypotheses is that depression earlier in life may increase the brain's vulnerability to dementia, while late-onset depression may be merely an early manifestation of the dementing disorder.

BEHAVIOURAL AND PSYCHOLOGICAL SYMPTOMS OF DEMENTIA

Although cognitive impairment is the clinical hallmark of the dementias, Alzheimer's original case report was based on a woman who was brought for care primarily because of her behavioural and psychological disturbances[19]. These are still the symptoms that frequently bring patients with dementia into the mental health care system, but they have not been the focus of much epidemiological work. At least two major population-based studies have shown that the majority of patients with dementia have one or more neuropsychiatric symptoms which add considerably to personal distress and caregiver strain. Irritability and depressed mood are somewhat more common in earlier and milder stages of disease, while wandering, apathy and delusions are more common in more advanced disease[20,21].

STUDY METHODS

For a comprehensive review, readers are directed to any standard epidemiology textbook. A few critical points follow. Different inferences should be drawn from different types of studies: for example, observational vs. experimental; cross-sectional vs. longitudinal; clinical case-control vs. population based. The source of the study sample, its size, and its potential for bias should be taken into account when interpreting the results and generalizing beyond that sample. Statistical significance indicates that the result is unlikely to have occurred by chance, but does not mean that the effect was large in size or that it was clinically significant. Screening tools should be selected after consideration of both sensitivity and specificity, which are usually enhanced at the expense of each other. The same tool, with no change in sensitivity or specificity, can have different predictive value in different populations, depending in part on how prevalent the disease of interest is in a given population.

Brain imaging and other biomarker-based approaches to diagnosis are gaining ground in clinical research as well as clinical practice, especially in the more affluent countries. To a lesser extent, epidemiological studies are incorporating these methods to determine their utility and validity for diagnosis at the population level, and to examine the distribution of these markers in individuals outside the specialty clinical setting. Very few epidemiological studies include *autopsy* data. They have shown the remarkable heterogeneity of neuropathology among individuals with dementia in the community, and also the extent of pathology that exists in relatively old individuals who were cognitively intact until the time of death[6].

FUTURE DIRECTIONS

Future research in the epidemiology of dementia faces both opportunities and challenges. The distribution of dementia and milder forms of cognitive impairment must be understood in a variety of populations, some of which have never been studied. As new tests and biomarkers are developed in specialized research settings, their validity must be ascertained in the community before they are recommended for widespread clinical use. Such research will contribute substantially to improved diagnosis and even preclinical detection of disease. Future studies will also focus on normal ageing, establishing norms for a wide range of populations to help distinguish healthy from pathological ageing. Longer-term population studies must track dementia incidence rates over time, to determine whether or not successive generations are following the same trends as life expectancy increases. They must also examine potential relationships of incidence to the different lifetime exposures in different generations. There is a growing call for 'life-course epidemiology'; that is, studies that start following cohorts of people when they are young or middle aged[22]. These studies will minimize survival bias and allow risk and protective factors to be studied early enough, and for long enough, to shed light on their long-term relationship with the dementias of later life. Such data will provide greatly improved information regarding potentially modifiable risk factors, and provide the basis for strategies to prevent dementia, or at least reduce its incidence, in future generations.

REFERENCES

1. World Health Organization. *The ICD-10 Classification of Mental and Behavioural Disorders: Clinical Descriptions and Diagnostic Guidelines*. Geneva: World Health Organization, 1992.
2. American Psychiatric Association. *Diagnostic and Statistical Manual of Mental Disorders, Fourth Edition, Text Revision: DSM-IV-TR*. Washington DC: American Psychiatric Association, 2000.
3. Kinsella K, Velkoff VA. *An Aging World: 2001*, US Census Bureau International Population Reports P95/01-1. Washington, DC: Government Printing Office, 2001.
4. Erkinjunnti T, Ostbye T, Steenhuis R, Hachinski V. The effect of different diagnostic criteria on the prevalence of dementia. *N Eng J Med* 1997; **337**: 1667–74.
5. Román GC, Tatemichi TK, Erkinjuntti T *et al*. Vascular dementia: diagnostic criteria for research studies. Report of the NINDS-AIREN International Workshop. *Neurology* 1993; **43**: 250–60.
6. Schneider JA, Arvanitakis Z, Bang W, Bennett DA. Mixed brain pathologies account for most dementia cases in community-dwelling older persons. *Neurology* 2007; **69**: 2197–204.
7. Jorm AF, Korten AE, Henderson AS. The prevalence of dementia: a quantitative integration of the literature. *Acta Psychiatr Scand* 1987; **76**: 465–79.
8. Aarsland D, Zaccai J, Brayne C. A systematic review of prevalence studies of dementia in Parkinson's disease. *Move Disord* 2005; **20**: 1255–63.
9. Gao S, Hendrie HC, Hall KS, Hui S. The relationships between age, sex, and the incidence of dementia and Alzheimer disease: a meta-analysis. *Arch Gen Psychiatry* 1998; **55**: 809–15.
10. Fitzpatrick AL, Kuller LH, Ives DG *et al*. Incidence and prevalence of dementia in the Cardiovascular Health Study. *J Am Geriatr Soc* 2004; **52**: 195–204.
11. Kalaria RN, Maetre GE, Arizaga R *et al*. Alzheimer's disease and vascular dementia in developing countries: prevalence, management, and risk factors. *Lancet Neurol* 2008; **7**: 812–26.
12. Ferri CP, Prince M, Brayne C *et al*. Global prevalence of dementia: a Delphi consensus study. *Lancet* 2005; **366**(9503): 2112–17.
13. Winblad B, Palmer K, Kivipelto M *et al*. Mild cognitive impairment – beyond controversies, towards a consensus: report of the International Working Group on Mild Cognitive Impairment. *J Intern Med* 2004; **256**: 240–6.
14. Graham JE, Rockwood K, Beattie BL *et al*. Prevalence and severity of cognitive impairment with and without dementia in an elderly population. *Lancet* 1997; **349**(9068): 1793–6.
15. Busse A, Bischkopf J, Riedel-Heller SG, Angermeyer MC. Mild cognitive impairment: prevalence and incidence according to different diagnostic criteria. Results of the Leipzig Longitudinal Study of the Aged (LEILA75). *Br J Psychiatry* 2003; **182**: 449–54.
16. Sheline YI, Gado MH, Kraemer HC. Untreated depression and hippocampal volume loss. *Am J Psychiatry* 2003; **160**: 1516–8.
17. Rapp MA, Schnaider-Beeri M, Grossman HT *et al*. Increased hippocampal plaques and tangles in patients with Alzheimer disease with a lifetime history of major depression. *Arch Gen Psychiatry* 2006; **63**: 161–7.

18. Ganguli M, Du Y, Dodge HH, Ratcliff GG, Chang CC. Depressive symptoms and cognitive decline in late life: a prospective epidemiologic study. *Arch Gen Psychiatry* 2006; **14**: 419–27.
19. Alzheimer A. Uber eine eigenartige Erkrankung der Hirnrinde. *Allg Z Psychiatr* 1907; **64**: 146–8.
20. Savva GM, Zaccai J, Matthews FE *et al*. Prevalence, correlates, and course of behavioural and psychological symptoms of dementia in the population. *Br J Psychiatry* 2009; **194**: 212–19.
21. Lyketsos CG, Sheppard J-E, Steinberg M *et al*. Neuropsychiatric disturbance in Alzheimer's disease clusters into three groups: the Cache County study. *Int J Geriatr Psychiatry* 2001; **16**: 1043–53.
22. Ben-Shlomo Y, Kuh D. A life course approach to chronic disease epidemiology: Conceptual models, empirical challenges, and interdisciplinary perspectives. *Int. J. Epidemiol* 2002; **31**: 285–93.

39

An Introduction to the Medical Research Council Cognitive Function and Ageing Studies (CFAS) I and II

Fiona E. Matthews[1] and Carol Brayne[2]

[1]MRC Biostatistics Unit, Institute of Public Health, Cambridge, UK
[2]University of Cambridge, Department Public Health and Primary Care, Cambridge, UK

INTRODUCTION

The rise in numbers of older people and the changing proportion of old to young people has been predicted for some time. It has become clear that the potential impact of this ageing phenomenon would have a major impact on population health profiles. Its potential impact on social and economic aspects of the more affluent countries highlights ageing as a sufficiently important issue in resource allocation. Discussion between the UK Department of Health, UK Medical Research Council (MRC), and experts from the scientific and medical communities late last century resulted in the decision that brain changes, most particularly cognitive decline, dementia and their relation to disability were key topics requiring investigation at the population level. This prompted a decision to invest in research into this area and a working group was convened, which included those with epidemiological and biostatistical expertise relevant to such investigation. Out of this working group a successful bid for the study now known as the MRC Cognitive Function and Ageing Study (CFAS) emerged[1].

STUDY DESIGN

The study is a six-centre multidisciplinary multiphased longitudinal design. There are five identical sites and one with a different sampling and interview structure. This centre (Liverpool, also known as the ALPHA study, see Figure 39.1) was already funded at the time of the discussions noted above and thus started earlier than the other five centres[2]. The other five centres (Cambridgeshire, Gwynedd, Newcastle, Nottingham and Oxford) were able to follow a standardized design and are referred to as the five identical sites. Their basic structure was a two-phase design with a screening interview followed by an assessment interview shortly afterwards, with a repeat at two years. The fieldwork began in 1991 to 1993 (centre dependent)[3] (see Figure 39.2 for flow diagram). Additional features are more fully described on the website (www.cfas.ac.uk).

In 2008 additional funding from the MRC enabled the introduction of a new cohort in three of the original CFAS centres (Cambridgeshire, Newcastle and Nottingham). Further funding from the Economic & Social Research Council (ESRC) in 2009 will enable a new cohort to be recruited to the Gwynedd centre (plus a new centre in Neath, Port Talbot) which focuses more on the social aspects of ageing.

THE AIMS OF THE STUDY

The aims of the study (see Box 39.1) have evolved over its existence and cover a wide range including descriptive epidemiology, neuropathology, policy, molecular epidemiology and ethics. The principal neuropathological aim was to determine the contribution of different underlying pathologies to the rates of dementia and the geographical variation in these rates, and to the burden of disability.

Box 39.1 CFAS core aims

CFAS I core aims:
The main descriptive epidemiological aims include:

- the estimation of the prevalence and incidence of cognitive decline and dementia, and geographical variation in those rates;
- the determination of the natural history of dementia, in particular the rate of progression of cognitive decline including the distribution of the interval between the identification of cognitive impairment and death;
- the identification of factors associated with differing rates of cognitive decline and with the risk of dementia.

Principles and Practice of Geriatric Psychiatry, 3rd edn. Edited by Mohammed T. Abou-Saleh, Cornelius Katona and Anand Kumar
© 2011 John Wiley & Sons, Ltd

Additional aims included:

- to determine the prevalence and severity of pathological lesions in the brain of an unselected cohort of older people with and without cognitive impairment;
- to determine the frequency of specific pathological diagnoses in people with cognitive impairment;
- to correlate severity of specific pathologies with patterns of cognition, function and behaviour in life independently of clinical and pathological diagnostic categories. CFAS II core aims include:
- to update profiles of cognitive and physical function, physical and mental health and disability of people aged 65 or over in four of the original CFAS centres: Cambridgeshire, Gwynedd, Newcastle and Nottingham;
- to estimate the cohort change in prevalence and incidence of cognitive impairment and dementia;
- to investigate whether the measures that characterize the intermediate stage (mild cognitive impairment) best within the original CFAS are stable across generations;
- to quantify medication, health, social service use, social support, residential characteristics and care states, including formal and informal care, of people with dementia, frailty or physical disability across the three sites;
- to assess the contribution of different diseases, particularly dementia, to any change in the burden of disability over time, specifically whether diseases have become more or less disabling and estimate the effect of prevention vs. treatment;

- to compare the size of relationship of known genetic factors with frailty, including cognitive impairment, with those found in the earlier cohort;
- to provide a foundation for other collaborative studies that investigates biomarkers and further investigation of early markers, including imaging, for risk of cognitive decline.

The DNA resource was incorporated in a later phase of CFAS I. In CFAS II saliva is collected at baseline. The main molecular epidemiological aim has been to support genetics studies that have sought genes associated with dementia, Alzheimer's disease, mixed and vascular dementia, cognitive impairment and decline. A later aim of the study was to explore the ethical and legal aspects of brain donation within a population-based sample given changing perception surrounding organ donation. The study also aimed to act as a core resource and provide a framework to support specific sub-studies in lone or joint centres. The Resource Implication Study [4-10] used this framework to achieve the core policy aim (see above).

METHODOLOGY

Because the main study is focused on cognition and dementia it has collected the necessary dimensions of physical and mental health to arrive at a study diagnosis of dementia. It now has four major themes: (i) dementia (covering all aspects including cognition); (ii) depression; (iii) disability and healthy life expectancy; and (iv) health policy and health. In addition it has particular strengths in that it is one of

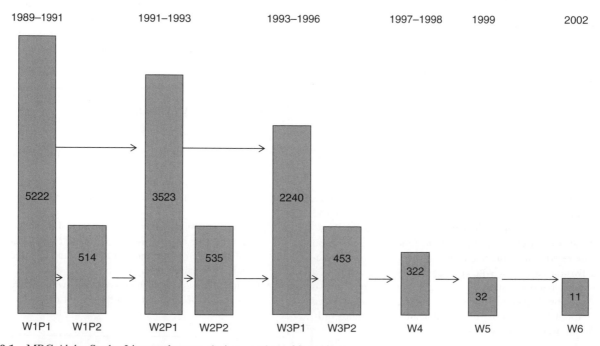

Figure 39.1 MRC Alpha Study: Liverpool centre design number of interviews
Source: Morris, J.C. (1993) The Clinical Dementia Rating (CDR): current version and scoring rules. *Neurology*, **43**, 2412–4

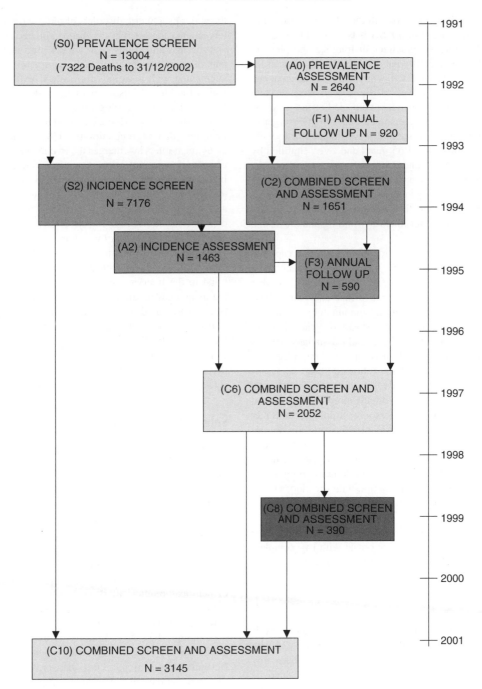

Figure 39.2 CFAS I identical centres study design

the very few truly population-based programmes with a brain donation programme – individuals in the study have indicated whether
they wish to contribute to brain research through the donation of
their brain after death (declaration of intention to donate).

Study Population

The first aim of the study was to estimate age-specific rates of prevalence of cognitive impairment and dementia among those aged 65

and over. The population is thus all those aged 65 years and over
on the index date for centre (1990, 1991), living within a specified
geographical location. Background information on the demographics
of the populations sampled was collected from the Office of Population Censuses and Surveys (OPCS) 1990–91 census, now Office
for National Statistics (ONS), to relate to regional and national data.
Family Health Services Authority (FHSA) lists were used as the sampling frame. The frame would be incomplete if eligible members of
the population were not registered with a GP. However, individuals

in long-stay hospitals remain registered with their GP two years after institutionalization so sampling from FHSA lists ensured their inclusion. Each centre looked into the practices of long-stay hospitals in their area to confirm this. The FHSA list of individuals was used for sampling on a geographical basis. Each centre defined this area, and the study population was drawn from all those who were resident within it. Problems of inaccuracy, patients who died or moved away but were still on the FHSA list, were resolved by asking GP surgeries to check the lists. On this basis, a sample of sufficient size to yield 2500 interviews of individuals aged 65 years and over, stratified by age (equal numbers aged 65–74 and 75 plus) was chosen from the FHSA lists for each selected area (in Liverpool this was 5000 interviews stratified by sex and five-year age band). The population is flagged at ONS for mortality and the database is updated continuously. The follow-up has been determined by funding and the design of associated bolt-on studies.

The main follow-up waves for the identical sites are captured in the audit trail shown in Figure 39.2, which shows the numbers for the main screen, assessment, one-year follow-up and two-year rescreen, new selection for assessment and further one-year follow-up, six-year follow-up of the assessed (with venepuncture), eight-year follow-up of those with intentions to donate, and 10-year follow-up of the total sample. In addition to this the main associated studies are the Resource Implications Study (four centres – Cambridgeshire, Newcastle, Nottingham, Oxford), which followed those who provided care to the physically and cognitively frail at baseline[4–10], the ESRC-funded Healthy Ageing Project, which interviewed in detail those who were not selected into the Resource Implications Study in Nottingham and Cambridgeshire[11–16], the Network Study conducted in Gwynedd and Liverpool to examine individuals' social networks, an embedded case-control study at two-year incidence stage (Cambridgeshire), and the ongoing brain donation programme in all centres. This programme, in combination with the bloods taken at year 6, form the major components of the biological resource of the study.

CFAS II will also have the same sampling frame and study size (at each centre). CFAS II is longitudinal at outset with two complete sweeps of the data planned. Each phase is two years apart.

Interview Method

All interviews were conducted in the respondent's place of residence, using portable computers with customized software. If the interviewer felt that the respondent was frail and tiring, or becoming agitated, the short 'priority mode' set of questions could be invoked manually. Permission was also sought to access GP and hospital notes.

Content

CFAS I screening interview contains questions on residence, marital status, education and occupation, living circumstances, contact with friends and family, health and social care contact, self-reported physical health, instrumental activities of daily living and activities of daily living, cognitive measures (Mini Mental State Examination (MMSE) with augmentation) and medication. The assessment interview is mainly the Geriatric Mental State Examination (GMS) adapted for CFAS[17–19]. This is a structured psychiatric interview, which collects sufficient information for algorithmic 'diagnosis' in

the major psychiatric disorders of old age (dementia, depression, anxiety and psychosis). This has been validated against clinical diagnosis and the instrument has been widely used in Europe and now forms part of the 10/66 international instrument. This interview has been augmented with questions from the CAMDEX (Cambridge Examination for Mental Disorders of the Elderly) including CAMCOG[20], the longer neuropsychological assessment. The relative or carer interview is mainly the History and Aetiology Schedule, the informant interview that accompanies the GMS. The combined screen and assessment interview merges the two interviews but compresses some aspects of data collection. Complete versions of all the interviews including the interview questions and responses are available on the website. CFAS II interview contains all the previous screening and assessment interview information plus additional questions on diet, social activity and objective measures of hearing and physical activity. The neuropathological assessment follows the standardized protocol of the Consortium to Establish a Registry for Alzheimer's Disease (CERAD)[21], with the exception that the neuropathologist is blind to the interview data. This covers in a semiquantitative form the main areas required for the assessment of neurodegenerative and cerebrovascular disorders. The forms are available on the website. The main genetic analyses have been on ApoE and ACE. CFAS II has saliva collection at the outset for genetic comparisons. Data collection in Liverpool was broadly similar to the other five sites except that the screening interview consisted of the GMS plus some of the screening interview questions listed above.

Selected Study Findings

The study has reported on prevalence, incidence (see Figure 39.3) and risk factors of dementia (Table 39.1), and lack of variation in these across the five identical sites[22–24].

It has provided profiles of cognition for MMSE, extended MMSE and CAMCOG, weighted back to the population[25,26]. It has reported on risk for incident dementia including ApoE and ACE (Table 39.2)[27–29].

It has examined the relationship of cognition to mortality[30]. In addition, the study has reported on a variety of impairments to healthy life in old age and their population burden[31–42] and on a variety of neuropathological markers related to dementia and old age (see Table 39.3)[43–54].

Recent publications have also included the investigation of behavioural (BSPD) symptoms of dementia and on stability and population applicability of mild cognitive impairment[55–59]. The Resource Implications Study has provided data for examination of carer burden and the costs of care for the physically and cognitively frail[6,10]. The data have been used for projection forward for these vulnerable groups and also for the costs of long-term care[60]. Liverpool has published on the prevalence of dementia, depression and neurosis, together with incidence of dementia and schizophrenia[2,61–66].

CFAS I AND II AS A RESOURCE

The study is multisite and multidisciplinary. The population is truly representative with high response rates at each stage over diverse sites. Where there is no heterogeneity across sites the study is sufficiently large to provide indicative values for national estimates. The broad scope of measures has allowed the study to contribute to ageing research across a wide range of topics. There are repeat

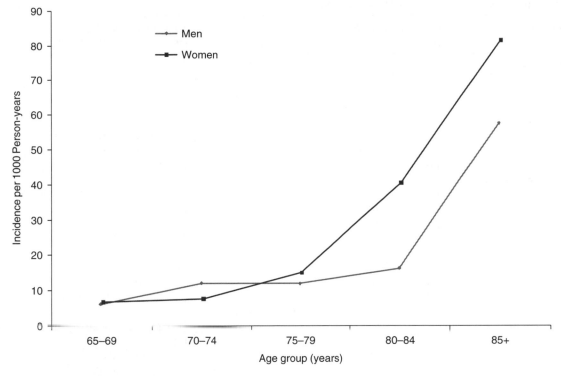

Figure 39.3 Incidence of dementia by sex (five identical centres)
Source: adapted from Matthews[71]

Table 39.1 Risk factors for incident dementia (socio-demographic)

	OR*	(95% CI)
Age (90+ years vs. 65+ years)	25.6	(11.6–56.9)
Sex (women vs. men)	1.6	(1.1–2.4)
Education (<9 vs. 10+)	1.9	(1.3–2.2)
Self-reported health (poor vs. good)	3.9	(2.2–6.4)
Stroke (yes vs. no)	2.1	(1.1–4.2)
Parkinson's disease (Yes vs. No)	3.5	(1.3–9.3)
General anaesthesia (Yes vs. No)	0.6	(0.4–0.9)

*Adjusted for all other factors in the table.
Source: Morris, J.C. (1993) The Clinical Dementia Rating (CDR): current version and scoring rules. *Neurology*, **43**, 2412–4

Table 39.2 Incidence of dementia and ApoE genotype

	Comparison using non-demented controls			
	Adjusted*		Adjusted* and weighted**	
	OR	95% CI	OR	95% CI
Allele				
$\varepsilon2$	0.6	0.3–0.9	0.3	0.1–0.6
$\varepsilon3$	1.0		1.0	
$\varepsilon4$	2.2	1.6–3.0	2.9	1.7–4.9
Genotype				
$\varepsilon2/\varepsilon2$	0.5	0.0–5.7	0.3	0.1–1.7
$\varepsilon2/\varepsilon3$	0.6	0.3–1.1	0.2	0.1–0.7
$\varepsilon2/\varepsilon4$	0.6	0.2–2.3	0.2	0.0–1.3
$\varepsilon3/\varepsilon3$	1.0		1.0	
$\varepsilon3/\varepsilon4$	2.3	1.5–3.6	3.6	1.8–7.3
$\varepsilon4\varepsilon4$	5.0	1.9–13.0	7.9	1.6–39.2

*For age group, sex, education and social class.
**For study design and dropout.
Source: reproduced from Keage[29]

measures on cognition and function, which allows examination of trajectories. There are only two other population-based studies with brain donation in Europe[67]. The study weighted the sample towards the over 75 age group at baseline, which has provided more robust data for the oldest old. As in all epidemiological research in older populations it would be desirable to have higher response and lower dropout between waves, but analysis can adjust for loss between interviews[68–70]. Blood taking and clinical assessment (including imaging) at baseline was not possible because of funding constraints, but venepuncture was included at year 6. The risk measures are self-report, using the available validated measures of the era. The study actively encourages collaboration, and there are established mechanisms for approaching us via the themes mentioned above. Information is available on the website and also through contact with theme leads.

The study website, www.cfas.ac.uk, configures information under themes, documentation, publications and data. There is also a list of study contacts.

CONCLUSION

The methods and results of the Medical Research Council Cognitive Function and Ageing Studies (MRC CFAS) I and II are described

Table 39.3 Neuropathological factors associated with dementia

Neuropathological findings	Age-adjusted analysis			Multivariable analysis			
	OR	(95% CI)	p	OR	(95% CI)	PAR %	(95% CI)
Age at death							
<80 years	1.0			1.0			
80–89 years	3.2	(1.8–5.5)		2.5	(1.1–5.8)	8	(0–16)
≥ 90 years	5.2	(2.9–9.4)	<.001	3.4	(1.4–8.3)	10	(3–16)
Brain weight for sex							
Low	5.7	(3.2–10)		4.1	(1.9–9.2)	12	(5–19)
Average	2.0	(1.2–34)		2.1	(1.0–4.2)	5	(0–11)
High	1.0		<.001	1.0			
Neuritic plaques in neocortex							
None	1.0						
Mild	1.2	(0.7–2.2)		1.0			
Moderate	2.9	(1.7–5.0)					
Severe	18.5	(7.3–47)	<.001	9.7	(2.1–43)	8	(3–14)
NFT in neocortex							
None	1.0			1.0			
Mild	1.3	(0.8–2.1)		1.0	(0.5–1.80)		
Moderate	8.9	(4.0–20)		7.1	(2.3–22)	11	(5–19)
Severe	∞		<.001				
Congophilic angiopathy							
None	1.0			1.0			
Mild	1.9	(1.1–3.3)		1.8	(0.8–3.8)	2	(0–6)
Moderate	4.0	(2.2–7.4)		2.9	(1.2–6.8)	5	(1–10)
Severe	∞		<.001				
Lewy bodies							
No	1.0			1.0			
Yes	3.2	(1.5–6.9)	0.003	3.5	(1.3–9.3)	3	(1–7)
Overall vascular pathology							
None	1.0			1.0			
Infarcts/haemorrhage	1.0	(0.3–3.8)		2.4	(0.4–12)		
SVD/WML/lacunes	2.5	(1.4–4.4)		3.7	(1.5–9.6)	12	(3–19)
Both	2.9	(1.6–5.5)	0.003	4.8	(1.9–12)	9	(3–15)
Hippocampal atrophy							
None	1.0			1.0			
Mild	2.2	(1.3–3.9)		1.8	(0.9–3.7)	2	(0–6)
Moderate	6.9	(3.7–13)		3.4	(1.5–7.5)	8	(2–15)
Severe	11.1	(2.5–50)	<.001				

Source: adapted from MRC CFAS Neuropathology Group[54]

above, as well as the design and aims of these two studies (started in October 2008). CFAS I and CFAS II are population-based studies of individuals aged 65 and above living in England and Wales. CFAS I has produced a range of results and a selection are shown within the chapter. The study data are part of a facilitated managed resource for collaborations, details of which have been described.

ACKNOWLEDGEMENTS

We are grateful to our respondents, their families and their primary care teams. The study has only been possible because of the dedication of a large number of individuals over the years, who are listed on the website. The MRC CFA study has been supported by major awards from the Medical Research Council and the Department of Health. Thanks are also due to the Biological Resource Advisory Group for overseeing this aspect of study.

REFERENCES

1. Brayne C, McCracken C, Matthews FE. Cohort profile: the Medical Research Council Cognitive Function and Ageing Study (CFAS). *Int J Epidemiol* 2006; **35**(5): 1140–5.
2. Saunders PA, Copeland JR, Dewey ME *et al*. Alpha: the Liverpool MRC Study of the incidence of dementia and cognitive decline. *Neuroepidemiology* 1992; **11**(Suppl 1): 44–7.
3. Chadwick C. The MRC Multicentre Study of Cognitive Function and Ageing: a EURODEM incidence study in progress. *Neuroepidemiology* 1992; **11**(Suppl 1): 37–43.
4. Buck D, Gregson BA, Bamford CH *et al*. Psychological distress among informal supporters of frail older people at home and in institutions. The Resource Implications Study Group of the MRC Cognitive Function and Ageing Study. *Int J Geriatr Psychiatry* 1997; **12**(7): 737–44.

5. McNamee P, Gregson BA, Wright K *et al*. Estimation of a multiproduct cost function for physically frail older people. *Health Econ* 1998; **7**(8): 701–10.

6. McNamee P, Gregson BA, Buck D *et al*. Costs of formal care for frail older people in England: the Resource Implications Study of the MRC Cognitive Function and Ageing Study (RIS MRC CFAS). *Soc Sci Med* 1999; **48**(3): 331–41.

7. Bond J, Farrow G, Gregson BA *et al*. Informal caregiving for frail older people at home and in long-term care institutions: who are the key supporters? *Health Soc Care Community* 1999; **7**(6): 434–44.

8. Melzer D, McWilliams B, Brayne C *et al*. Profile of disability in elderly people: estimates from a longitudinal population study. *BMJ* 1999; **318**(7191): 1108–11.

9. Psychological morbidity among informal caregivers of older people: a 2-year follow-up study. The Resource Implications Study Group of the MRC study of Cognitive Function and Ageing (RIS MRC CFAS). *Psychol Med* 2000; **30**(4): 943–55.

10. McNamee P, Bond J, Buck D of the Resource Implications Study of the Medical Research Council Cognitive Function and Ageing Study. Costs of dementia in England and Wales in the 21st century. *Br J Psychiatry* 2001; **179**: 261–6.

11. Huppert FA, Pinto EM, Morgan K, Brayne C. Survival in a population sample is predicted by proportions of lymphocyte subsets. *Mech Ageing Dev* 2003; **124**(4): 449–51.

12. Huppert FA, Pinto EM, Morgan K *et al*. Immune measures which predict 9-year survival in an elderly population sample. *Adv Cell Aging Gerontol* 2003; **13**: 17–28.

13. Pinto EM, Huppert FA, Morgan K *et al*. Neutrophil counts, monocyte counts and cardiovascular disease in the elderly. *Exp Gerontol* 2004; **39**: 615–19.

14. Morgan K, Armstrong GK, Huppert FA *et al*. Healthy ageing in urban and rural Britain: a comparison of exercise and diet. *Age Ageing* 2000; **29**(4): 341–8.

15. Huppert FA, Solomou W, O'Connor *et al*. Aging and lymphocyte subpopulations: whole-blood analysis of immune markers in a large population sample of healthy elderly individuals. *Exp Gerontol* 1998; **33**(6): 593–600.

16. Solomou W, Richards M, Huppert FA *et al*. Divorce, current marital status and well-being in an elderly population. *Int J Law, Policy and the Family* 1998; **12**: 321–42.

17. Copeland JR, Kelleher MJ, Kellett JM *et al*. A semi-structured clinical interview for the assessment of diagnosis and mental state in the elderly: the Geriatric Mental State Schedule. I. Development and reliability. *Psychol Med* 1976; **6**(3): 439–49.

18. Copeland JR, Dewey ME, Griffiths-Jones HM. A computerized psychiatric diagnostic system and case nomenclature for elderly subjects: GMS and AGECAT. *Psychol Med* 1986; **16**(1): 89–99.

19. Copeland JRM. Neuropsychological diagnosis (GMS-HAS-AGECAT package). *Int J Psychogeriatr* 1991; **3**(Suppl 1): 43–9.

20. Huppert FA, Brayne C, Gill C *et al*. CAMCOG – a concise neuropsychological test to assist dementia diagnosis: sociodemographic determinants in an elderly population sample. *Br J Clin Psychol* 1995; **34**(Pt 4): 529–41.

21. Mirra SS, Heyman A, McKeel D *et al*. The Consortium to Establish a Registry for Alzheimer's Disease (CERAD). Part II. Standardization of the neuropathologic assessment of Alzheimer's disease. *Neurology* 1991; **41**(4): 479–86.

22. Yip AG, Brayne C, Matthews FE, Medical Research Council Cognitive Function and Ageing Study (MRC CFAS). Risk factors for incident dementia in England and Wales: The Medical Research Council Cognitive Function and Ageing Study. A population-based nested case-control study. *Age Ageing* 2006; **35**(2): 154–60.

23. Matthews FE, Brayne C, Medical Research Council Cognitive Function and Ageing Study (MRC CFAS). The incidence of dementia in England and Wales: findings from the five identical sites of the MRC CFA Study. *PLoS Med* 2005; **2**(8): 753–63.

24. MRC CFAS. Cognitive function and dementia in six areas of England and Wales: the distribution of MMSE and prevalence of GMS organicity level in the MRC CFA Study. *Psychol Med* 1998; **28**: 319–35.

25. Huppert FA, Cabelli ST, Matthews FE, Medical Research Council Cognitive Function and Ageing Study (MRC CFAS). Brief cognitive assessment in a UK population sample – distributional properties and the relationship between the MMSE and an extended mental state examination. *BMC Geriatr* 2005; **5**(1): 7.

26. Williams JG, Huppert FA, Matthews FE *et al*. Performance and normative values of a concise neuropsychological test (CAMCOG) in an elderly population sample. *Int J Geriatr Psychiatry* 2003; **18**(7): 631–44.

27. Yip AG, Brayne C, Easton D *et al*. Apolipoprotein E4 is only a weak predictor of dementia and cognitive decline in the general population. *J Med Genet* 2002; **39**(9): 639–43.

28. Yip AG, Brayne C, Easton D, Rubinsztein DC. An investigation of ACE as a risk factor for dementia and cognitive decline in the general population. *J Med Genet* 2002; **39**(6): 403–6.

29. Keage HAD, Matthews FE, Yip A *et al*. APOE and ACE polymorphisms and dementia risk in the older population over prolonged follow-up: ten years of incidence in the MRC CFA Study. *Age Ageing* 2009 (under review).

30. Neale R, Brayne C, Johnson AL. Cognition and survival: an exploration in a large multicentre study of the population aged 65 years and over. *Int J Epidemiol* 2001; **30**(6): 1383–8.

31. McDougall FA, Matthews FE, Kvaal K *et al*. Prevalence and symptomatology of depression in older people living in institutions in England and Wales. *Age Ageing* 2007; **36**(5): 562–8.

32. McDougall FA, Kvaal K, Matthews FE *et al*. Prevalence of depression in older people in England and Wales: the MRC CFA Study. *Psychol Med* 2007; **37**(12): 1787–95.

33. Syed A, Chatfield M, Matthews FE *et al*. Depression in the elderly: pathological study of raphe and locus ceruleus. *Neuropathol Appl Neurobiol* 2005; **31**(4): 405–13.

34. Brayne C, Matthews FE, McGee MA *et al*. Health and ill-health in the older population in England and Wales. The Medical Research Council Cognitive Function and Ageing Study (MRC CFAS). *Age Ageing* 2001; **30**(1): 53–62.

35. Jagger C, Matthews F, Medical Research Council Cognitive Function and Ageing Study (MRC CFAS). Gender differences in life expectancy free of impairment at older ages. *J Women Aging* 2002; **14**(1–2): 85–97.

36. Jagger C, Matthews R, Melzer D *et al*. Educational differences in the dynamics of disability incidence, recovery and mortality: findings from the MRC Cognitive Function and Ageing Study (MRC CFAS). *Int J Epidemiol* 2007; **36**(2): 358–65.

37. Jagger C, Matthews R, Matthews F *et al*. The burden of diseases on disability-free life expectancy in later life. *J Gerontol A Biol Sci Med Sci* 2007; **62**(4): 408–14.

38. Matthews FE, Miller LL, Brayne C, Jagger C. Regional differences in multidimensional aspects of health: findings from the

MRC Cognitive Function and Ageing Study. *BMC Public Health* 2006; **6**: 90.

39. Matthews FE, Jagger C, Miller LL, Brayne C. Education differences in life expectancy with cognitive impairment. *J Gerontol A Biol Sci Med Sci* 2009; **64**(1): 125–31.

40. Peres K, Jagger C, Matthews FE. Impact of late-life self-reported emotional problems on Disability-Free Life Expectancy: results from the MRC Cognitive Function and Ageing Study. *Int J Geriatr Psychiatry*, 2007.

41. Spiers NA, Matthews RJ, Jagger C *et al*. Diseases and impairments as risk factors for onset of disability in the older population in England and Wales: findings from the Medical Research Council Cognitive Function and Ageing Study. *J Gerontol A Biol Sci Med Sci* 2005; **60**(2): 248–54.

42. Kvaal K, McDougall FA, Brayne C *et al*. Co-occurrence of anxiety and depressive disorders in a community sample of older people: results from the MRC CFAS (Medical Research Council Cognitive Function and Ageing Study). *Int J Geriatr Psychiatry* 2008; **23**(3): 229–37.

43. Fernando MS, Ince PG. Vascular pathologies and cognition in a population-based cohort of elderly people. *J Neurol Sci* 2004; **226**(1–2): 13–17.

44. Fernando MS, O'Brien JT, Perry RH *et al*. Comparison of the pathology of cerebral white matter with post-mortem magnetic resonance imaging (MRI) in the elderly brain. *Neuropathol Appl Neurobiol* 2004; **30**(4): 385–95.

45. Fernando MS, Simpson JE, Matthews F *et al*. White matter lesions in an unselected cohort of the elderly: molecular pathology suggests origin from chronic hypoperfusion injury. *Stroke* 2006; **37**(6): 1391–8.

46. Ince PG, Fernando MS. Neuropathology of vascular cognitive impairment and vascular dementia. *Int Psychogeriatr* 2003; **15**(Suppl 1): 71–5.

47. MRC CFAS Neuropathology Group. Writing Committee, Esiri M, Matthews F, Brayne C, Ince P. Pathological correlates of late-onset dementia in a multicentre, community-based population in England and Wales. *Lancet* 2001; **357**: 169–75.

48. Simpson JE, Ince PG, Higham CE *et al*. Microglial activation in white matter lesions and nonlesional white matter of ageing brains. *Neuropathol Appl Neurobiol* 2007; **33**(6): 670–83.

49. Simpson JE, Fernando MS, Clark L *et al*. White matter lesions in an unselected cohort of the elderly: astrocytic, microglial and oligodendrocyte precursor cell responses. *Neuropathol Appl Neurobiol* 2007.

50. Simpson JE, Ince PG, Lace G *et al*. Astrocyte phenotype in relation to Alzheimer-type pathology in the ageing brain. *Neurobiol Aging* 2008.

51. Simpson JE, Hosny O, Wharton SB *et al*. Microarray RNA expression analysis of cerebral white matter lesions reveals changes in multiple functional pathways. *Stroke* 2009; **40**(2): 369–75.

52. Wharton SB, Williams GH, Stoeber K *et al*. Expression of Ki67, PCNA and the chromosome replication licensing protein Mcm2 in glial cells of the ageing human hippocampus increases with the burden of Alzheimer-type pathology. *Neurosci Lett* 2005; **383**(1–2): 33–8.

53. Zaccai J, Brayne C, McKeith I *et al*. Patterns and stages of alpha-synucleinopathy: relevance in a population-based cohort. *Neurology* 2008; **70**(13): 1042–8.

54. MRC CFAS Neuropathology Group, Matthews FE, Brayne C, Lowe J, McKeith I, Wharton SB, Ince P. Epidemiological Pathology of Dementia: Attributable-Risks at Death in the Medical Research Council Cognitive Function and Ageing Study. *PLoS Med* 2009; **6**(11): e1000180.

55. Savva GM, Zaccai J, Matthews FE *et al*. Prevalence, correlates and course of behavioural and psychological symptoms of dementia in the population. *Br J Psychiatry* 2009; **194**(3): 212–19.

56. Matthews FE, Stephan BC, McKeith IG *et al*. Two-year progression from mild cognitive impairment to dementia: to what extent do different definitions agree? *J Am Geriatr Soc* 2008; **56**(8): 1424–33.

57. Stephan BC, Brayne C, McKeith IG *et al*. Mild cognitive impairment in the older population: Who is missed and does it matter? *Int J Geriatr Psychiatry* 2008; **23**(8): 863–71.

58. Matthews FE, Stephan BC, Bond J *et al*. Operationalization of mild cognitive impairment: a graphical approach. *PLoS Med* 2007; **4**(10): 1615–19.

59. Stephan BC, Matthews FE, McKeith IG *et al*. Early cognitive change in the general population: how do different definitions work? *J Am Geriatr Soc* 2007; **55**(10): 1534–40.

60. Jagger C, Matthews R, Lindesay J *et al*. The effect of dementia trends and treatments on longevity and disability: a simulation model based on the MRC Cognitive Function and Ageing Study (MRC CFAS). *Age Ageing* 2009; **38**: 319–25.

61. Chen R, Hu Z, Wei L *et al*. Is the relationship between syndromes of depression and dementia temporal? The MRC-ALPHA and Hefei-China studies. *Psychol Med* 2009; **39**(3): 425–30.

62. Copeland JR, Dewey ME, Saunders P. The epidemiology of dementia: GMS-AGECAT studies of prevalence and incidence, including studies in progress. *Eur Arch Psychiatry Clin Neurosci* 1991; **240**(4–5): 212–17.

63. Copeland JR, McCracken CF, Dewey ME *et al*. Undifferentiated dementia, Alzheimer's disease and vascular dementia: age- and gender-related incidence in Liverpool. The MRC-ALPHA Study. *Br J Psychiatry* 1999; **175**: 433–8.

64. Copeland JR, Chen R, Dewey ME *et al*. Community-based case-control study of depression in older people. Cases and sub-cases from the MRC-ALPHA Study. *Br J Psychiatry* 1999; **175**: 340–7.

65. Saunders PA, Copeland JR, Dewey ME *et al*. The prevalence of dementia, depression and neurosis in later life: the Liverpool MRC-ALPHA Study. *Int J Epidemiol* 1993; **22**(5): 838–47.

66. Wilson KC, Chen R, Taylor S *et al*. Socio-economic deprivation and the prevalence and prediction of depression in older community residents. The MRC-ALPHA Study. *Br J Psychiatry* 1999; **175**: 549–53.

67. Zaccai J, Ince P, Brayne C, MRC CFAS. Population-based neuropathological studies of dementia: design, methods and areas of investigation – a systematic review. *BMC Neurol* 2006; **6**: 2.

68. Chatfield MD, Brayne CE, Matthews FE. A systematic literature review of attrition between waves in longitudinal studies in the elderly shows a consistent pattern of dropout between differing studies. *J Clin Epidemiol* 2005; **58**(1): 13–19.

69. Matthews FE, Chatfield M, Freeman C *et al*. Attrition and bias in the MRC Cognitive Function and Ageing Study: an epidemiological investigation. *BMC Public Health* 2004; **4**: 12.

70. Matthews FE, Chatfield M, Brayne C. An investigation of whether factors associated with short-term attrition change or persist over ten years: data from the Medical Research Council Cognitive Function and Ageing Study (MRC CFAS). *BMC Public Health* 2006; **6**: 185.

71. Matthews FE. Incidence estimation in studies of complex design: an example using the Medical Research Council Cognitive Function and Ageing Study (PhD dissertation). University of Cambridge, 2005.

40

The Lundby Study

Mats Bogren, Cecilia Mattisson and Per Nettelbladt

Department of Clinical Sciences, Psychiatry, Lund University Hospital, Sweden

From the Lundby Study, reports on dementias in the elderly for the period 1947–72 have been published. In the EURODERM comparative prevalence studies[1,2], the Lundby prevalence rates of senile dementia of the Alzheimer type (SDAT) in the age intervals 60–69, 70–79 and 80–89 were 0.3%, 2.5% and 10.9%, respectively, and for vascular dementia 0.8%, 3.5% and 6.3%.

In another study[3,4], the cumulative lifetime probability of contracting SDAT was reported to be 25.5% in men and 31.9% in women. For severely impaired cases, the figures were 15.5% and 22.2%, respectively. For vascular dementia the figures were 29.8% in men and 25.1% in women, for severe cases 16.6% and 15.2%, respectively. Background factors to SDAT and vascular dementia have also been studied[5,6]. The last follow-up in 1997 covering the period 1972–97 has now enabled us to compare the population's first incidence of dementia and other organic brain disorders over the two time periods 1947–72 and 1972–97[7].

The Lundby study is a longitudinal investigation of mental disorders in a total population. It originally included all people living in a rural area in 1947 or 1957[8,9]. This population has been investigated in 1947, 1957, 1972 and 1997[8-11] and at each point information has been obtained about the development of the mental and physical health for all individuals alive at the previous investigation providing an opportunity to observe changes of mental disorders in the population over 50 years.

At the inception, the study population lived in two parishes outside the university town Lund in the southern part of Sweden. In 1947 the Lundby area was rural with 2550 inhabitants, aged 0–92 years. In 1957 1013 newcomers were included (one-third born since 1947; and two-thirds immigrated). In all follow-ups, those subjects who had moved out of the area were also investigated. Information was also collected about those who were deceased since the previous follow-up. The present findings apply to the total cohort ($n = 3563$, male 1823, female 1740).

By 1972 gradual urbanization had changed the Lundby area from a farming district into a suburban area[4], which was even more obvious in 1997. Moreover, in 1972, many subjects had moved away from the Lundby area; of the 2827 still alive in 1972, 1424 remained, while 1403 had moved; in 1997, 602 of the 1797 survivors remained, while 1195 had moved.

At the follow-ups the aim has been to obtain as much information as possible about all episodes of mental and somatic disorders in all individuals in the population. Data was gathered from several sources: interviews, case registers, case notes, autopsy reports and key informants[11-14].

Thanks to the many data sources the diagnostic attrition 1947–72 was only 1%; although it was 6% between 1972–97. However, in those over 50 years old in 1972 the attrition 1972–97 was 2% in males and 3% in females.

Psychiatrists have conducted all interviews and evaluations of data. The diagnostic principles have been kept similar and were based on consensus[9-11]. The diagnoses were aimed at getting 'a rough picture of the relative distribution of the main types of mental illness in the population'[9].

Neurotic and psychotic disorders were disorders without evidence of organic aetiopathology. Neurotic, as opposed to psychotic, indicated preserved insight. Organic brain disorders included states with global cognitive dysfunction or gross personality or behavioural disturbance, with obvious organic causation.

Only one diagnosis per episode of disorder was recorded with organic brain disorders ranking higher than psychotic disorders, which in turn takes precedence over neurotic disorders. Furthermore, every episode of disorder was rated along with the degree of dysfunction caused by it (minimal, mild, medium, severe or very severe) according to the criteria defined by Leighton *et al.*[15]. A mild degree of impairment corresponds to a Global Assessment of Functioning (GAF) score of 70–61; medium corresponds to 60–51, and severe to 50–31. Episodes with medium, severe or very severe impairment[16] were chosen to indicate caseness. For all episodes, onset and termination were assessed as closely as possible using all sources of information.

Incidence rates for organic brain disorders in the periods 1947–72 and 1972–97 were obtained as the number of first occurrences of the outcome divided by the total number of person-years under risk for the outcome in individuals who had previously been free from the outcome. Individuals contributed with risk-years until contracting the outcome, dying, dropping out of the study or the end of the study period.

When age- and sex-specific incidences of organic brain disorders in 1947–72 and 1972–97 were compared, the rates had decreased consistently from the first to the last period in all age intervals but 40–49 (Table 40.1). Both male and female age-standardized first-incidence rates decreased significantly from the first to the last period.

Principles and Practice of Geriatric Psychiatry, 3rd edn. Edited by Mohammed T. Abou-Saleh, Cornelius Katona and Anand Kumar
© 2011 John Wiley & Sons, Ltd

In both periods the age-standardized incidence rate of organic brain disorders was higher in males than females. The difference was significant in 1947–72, but not in 1972–97.

When the impairment threshold to indicate caseness was changed from medium to severe, the age-standardized first incidence per 1000 years at risk of organic brain disorders declined from 3.4 to 2.0 in males and from 2.9 to 2.0 in females from 1947–72 to 1972–97. There were no cases of organic brain disorder with impairment level under medium.

In the period 1947–72 dementia constituted 80% and milder organic brain disorders 20% of the category organic brain disorders. In the period 1972–97 the corresponding figures were fairly similar at 83% and 17%, respectively.

When organic brain disorder was divided into dementia and other organic brain disorders not reaching the dementia threshold, one could still, for both groups, see a decrease of the age-standardized first incidences from the first to the second 25-year investigation period. In males the age-standardized first incidence of dementia fell from 5.1 to 2.1 per 1000 years at risk and in females from 4.0 to 2.1. The age-standardized first incidence of organic brain disorders not reaching the dementia threshold fell from 1.2 to 0.6 in males. Among females there was only a marginal decrease from 0.5 to 0.3.

The age interval responsible for the reduction of the age-standardized first incidence of dementia was above all the 70–99 interval, while the age intervals concerned regarding the reduction of milder organic brain disorders were those under 70. In males aged 70–99 the first incidence of dementia decreased from 28.4 to 10.9 per 1000 years at risk. In females the first incidence decreased from 23.4 to 12.6.

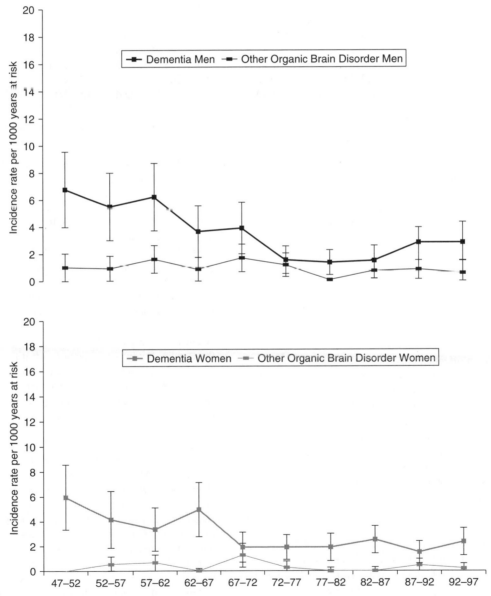

Figure 40.1 Age-standardized first-incidence of dementia and other organic brain disorders of medium + (GAF 60-1) impairment by five-year periods 1947–97
Source: Reproduced with permission from Australian & New Zealand Journal of Psychiatry, 2007; 41(2):178–186

Table 40.1 Organic brain disorders of medium + (GAF 60-1) impairment. First incidence per 1000 years at risk (μ) with 95% confidence intervals (CI)

Age	1947–72				1972–97			
	C	L	μ	95% CI	C	L	μ	95% CI
Men								
15–29	3	8354	0.4	−0.0–0.8	0	1869	0	
30–39	4	5669	0.7	0.0–1.4	2	3862	0.5	−0.2–1.2
40–49	1	5683	0.2	−0.2–0.5	3	5399	0.6	−0.1–1.2
50–59	12	4997	2.4	1.0–3.8	3	5516	0.5	−0.1–1.2
60–69	24	3495	6.9	4.1–9.6	15	4984	3.0	1.5–4.5
70–99	84	2676	31.4	24.7–38.1	60	4445	13.5	10.1–16.9
Total	128	30874	4.2	3.4–4.9	83	26076	3.2	2.5–3.9
			6.4*	**5.3–7.5**			**2.8***	**2.2–3.4**
Women								
15–29	1	8125	0.1	−0.1–0.4	0	1755	0	
30–39	4	5147	0.8	0.0–1.5	0	3872	0	
40–49	0	4974	0		1	5410	0.2	−0.2–0.6
50–59	5	4699	1.1	0.1–2.0	1	5145	0.2	−0.2–0.6
60–69	11	3671	3.0	1.2–4.8	7	4729	1.5	0.4–2.6
70–99	73	2938	24.8	19.2–30.5	80	5593	14.3	11.2–17.4
Total	94	29554	3.2	2.5–3.8	89	26505	3.4	2.7–4.1
			4.5*	**3.6–5.4**			**2.4***	**1.9–3.0**

C = First-incident cases. L = Years at risk. * = Age standardized.
Source: Reproduced with permission from Australian & New Zealand Journal of Psychiatry, 2007; 41(2):178–186

Male and female age-standardized first-incidence rates of dementia and other organic brain disorders every fifth year from 1947–97 are seen in Figure 40.1. In both males and females a trend of decreasing incidences of dementia can be observed from 1947–97, while five-year incidences of other organic brain disorders remained fairly constant through the whole period.

There are a limited number of studies that have tried to ascertain secular trends of dementia incidence. However, in a study from Rochester, Minnesota, no significant change of the incidence of dementia was seen from 1960 to 1984[17,18]. One difference from the Lundby study was the shorter length of the observation period. A long period of study might be needed to be able to see a slow change over many years[18].

The Lundby population offers an opportunity to study the rates of dementia and other organic brain disorders during a period of great transition in society and development of public health. This transition includes changes of lifestyle (e.g. food, smoking) and increased availability of medical care (e.g. antihypertensive and antidiabetic treatment) as well as changes in the physical environment. Thus, the decrease of organic brain disorders in both male and female subjects may be the result of a healthier lifestyle and availability of treatments protecting against the development of organic brain lesions.

REFERENCES

1. Rocca WA, Hofman A, Brayne C *et al*. Frequency and distribution of Alzheimer's disease in Europe. A collaborative study of 1980–1990 prevalence findings. *Ann Neurol* 1991; **30**(3): 381–90.
2. Rocca WA, Hofman A, Brayne C *et al*. The prevalence of vascular dementia in Europe. Facts and fragments from 1980–1990 studies. *Ann Neurol* 1991; **30**(6): 817–24.
3. Hagnell O, Lanke J, Rorsman B *et al*. Current trends in the incidence of senile and multi-infarct dementia. A prospective study of a total population followed over 25 years; the Lundby Study. *Arch Psychiat Nervenkr* 1983; **233**: 423–38.
4. Hagnell O, Lanke J, Rorsman B, Öhman R. The diminishing incidence of chronic organic brain syndromes among the elderly. In *Book of Proceedings from the Third European Symposium on Social Psychiatry in Hanasaari, Finland*, 1983, 253–61.
5. Hagnell O, Franck A, Gräsbeck A *et al*. Senile dementia of the Alzheimer type in the Lundby Study. An attempt to identify possible risk factors. *Eur Arch Psychiat Clin Neurosci* 1992; **241**: 231–5.
6. Hagnell O, Franck A, Gräsbeck A *et al*. Vascular dementia in the Lundby Study. An attempt to identify possible risk factors. *Neuropsychobiology* 1993; **27**: 210–16.
7. Bogren M, Mattisson C, Horstmann V, Bhugra D, Munk-Jørgensen P, Nettelbladt P. Lundby revisited: first incidence of mental disorders 1947–1997. *Aust NZ J Psychiatry* 2007; **41**: 178–86.
8. Essen-Möller E, Larsson H, Uddenberg C-E, White G. *Individual Traits and Morbidity in a Swedish Rural Population*. Copenhagen: Ejnar Munksgaard, 1956.
9. Hagnell O. *A Prospective Study of the Incidence of Mental Disorder*. Lund: Svenska Bokförlaget, 1966.
10. Hagnell O, Essen-Möller E, Lanke J, Öjesjö L, Rorsman B. *The Incidence of Mental Illness over a Quarter of a Century*. Stockholm: Almqvist & Wiksell, 1990.
11. Nettelbladt P, Bogren M, Mattisson C, Öjesjö L, Hagnell O, Hofvendahl E *et al*. Does it make sense to do repeated surveys? – the Lundby Study, 1947–1997. *Acta Psychiatr Scand* 2005; **111**: 444–52.
12. National Board of Health and Welfare (2004). *Patient Register*. Stockholm, 2004.

13. National Board of Health and Welfare. *The Cause of Death Register*. Stockholm, 2004.

14. Community Medicine Institution, Lund University. *The Dalby-Tierp Register*. Lund, 2004.

15. Leighton DC, Harding DC, Macklin DB, Macmillan AM, Leighton AH. *The Character of Danger. The Stirling County Study, Vol III*. New York: Basic Books, 1963.

16. American Psychiatric Association. *Diagnostic and Statistical Manual of Mental Disorders*, 4th edn (DSM-IV). Washington, DC: American Psychiatric Association, 1994.

17. Kokmen E, Chandra V, Schoenberg BS. Trends in incidence of dementing illness in Rochester, Minnesota, in three quinquennial periods, 1960–1974. *Neurology* 1988; **38**: 975–80.

18. Rocca WA, Cha RH, Waring SC, Kokmen E. A Reanalysis of Data from Rochester, Minnesota, 1975–1984. *Am J Epidemiol* 1998; **148**: 51–62.

41

Clinical Features of Alzheimer's Disease: Cognitive and Non-cognitive

Oludamilola Salami and Constantine G. Lyketsos

Johns Hopkins School of Medicine and Johns Hopkins Bayview, Baltimore, USA

Alzheimer's disease is best described as a neurodegenerative brain disease that causes a clinical dementia syndrome. It is the most common neurodegenerative disorder, accounting for over 60% of dementia cases in late life. Alzheimer's dementia is estimated to affect over 4 million Americans and 21 million persons worldwide[1].

The dementia associated with Alzheimer's disease is heterogeneous and diverse. Symptoms and signs vary with the progression and severity of the illness. Progressive cognitive decline with impaired ability to function in the person's usual environment is regarded as the hallmark of the clinical syndrome. Memory is invariably affected. There is also dysfunction in other domains of cognition including language, visuo-spatial, perception, recognition, praxis and executive function. Non-cognitive neuropsychiatric symptoms (NPS) are universal over the course of illness and are themselves diverse. These include affective, perceptual, behavioural, motivational and personality changes. Alzheimer's disease is usually indolent in its early course. Progression of the disease is associated with loss of independent function. The impact on sufferers, caregivers and other loved ones is often profound. Estimates of life expectancy in Alzheimer's disease range from 3 to 9 years[2]. The mortality rate associated with Alzheimer's dementia is on the order of 10.6 deaths per 100 000 person-years in the population[3].

Alzheimer's disease and delirium are clinical syndromes with similarities in clinical features and may be co-morbid. In the early stages of Alzheimer's disease, the key differences are the acute onset, fluctuating symptoms and the prominent sleep–wake cycle fragmentation which are seen in delirium and not in Alzheimer's disease. However, advanced Alzheimer's disease is difficult to differentiate from delirium, except by the clinical history[4]. This section focuses on the clinical presentation of Alzheimer's disease, and the occurrence of its clinical features along a spectrum from early disease to the advanced stages.

COGNITIVE SYMPTOMS

Impairment in cognitive function is the core feature of Alzheimer's disease. Several areas of cognition may be affected and the degree of impairment varies with illness severity (Table 41.1).

Memory

Disturbance of memory is regarded as the hallmark of Alzheimer's disease. Memory impairment is, however, not always the initial symptom. Affective symptoms may often precede memory disturbance[5]. It is important to note that the spouse or close relatives of most patients with Alzheimer's disease are usually the ones who bring the memory deficits to clinical attention, not the patients themselves. Early memory symptoms heralding the onset of dementia include difficulty with the registration and retention of new information, leading to repeating questions or comments. There may also be difficulty manipulating stored information associated with working memory. Delayed spontaneous recall of recently acquired information is impaired in early stages[6]. Immediate recall, recognition and registration of information become increasingly affected with progression of illness. As these symptoms worsen, memory dysfunction affects daily function, which is important in differentiating dementia from memory decline associated with normal ageing. Individuals with early Alzheimer's disease may develop difficulty recalling recent tasks, events, directions and appointments.

Those with advanced education or high intellectual reserve may be able to adapt for some time with minimal impact on their daily function. Some resort to memory cues, such as taking notes or keeping journals, to compensate for decline in memory. In moderate to severe stages, long-term memory becomes impaired. There may be inability to accurately recall details of familiar historic events and personal information, including names of family members, birthdays, special occasions or other aspects of declarative memory.

Language

Both oral and written impairments of language are found in Alzheimer's disease. In the early stages, fluent dysphasia may predominate, often in a pattern similar to transcortical sensory aphasia. Characteristic deficits at this stage include diminished vocabulary and word finding difficulty. Individuals with early dementia often have difficulty selecting words and may lose track during conversations[6]. Word repertoire shrinks and use of language

Principles and Practice of Geriatric Psychiatry, 3rd edn. Edited by Mohammed T. Abou-Saleh, Cornelius Katona and Anand Kumar
© 2011 John Wiley & Sons, Ltd

Table 41.1 Cognitive symptoms associated with Alzheimer's dementia

Memory (working, declarative and procedural impairment)
Language (aphasia, alexia, agraphia, aprosodia, acalculia)
Visuo-spatial dysfunction, recognition impairment or agnosis
Execution of previously learned movements or praxis
Executive dysfunction (planning, sequencing, abstraction,
   set shifting, organizing)

becomes more simplistic, often described as circumlocutory. There may be paraphasic errors with incorrect word substitutions.

In advanced disease, impaired comprehension and word finding difficulties are more pronounced. The ability to communicate effectively becomes impaired. The patient's speech may become non-fluent with mainly short simple phrases or words. Echolalia and palilalia may also occur as affected individuals develop complete loss of verbal expression. These deficits may extend to reading and writing ability. Some affected individuals may retain their ability to understand and respond to non-verbal and emotional cues.

Visuo-spatial Function

Visuo-spatial cognitive impairment and non-verbal visuo-spatial information processing are the characteristic visuo-spatial disturbances observed in Alzheimer's disease. Visual discrimination, visual recognition and visuo-spatial attention deficits may also occur, but less frequently. Although subtle impairments may be seen with early Alzheimer's disease, deficits occur more commonly in moderate to severe stages of dementia and often become progressive. There may be impairment in ability to synthesize, integrate and organize visual sensory stimuli or other environmental information. There may also be difficulty developing strategies for complex construction. Some persons with Alzheimer's disease have impaired right–left orientation and defective re-visualization, which involves internally re-visualizing and imagining a named object and then describing it accurately when prompted. Some may have difficulty with the synthesis of parts of an object into a whole and then properly identifying the whole (classic agnosia). Patients may also have difficulty copying or drawing objects and, with further progression of the illness, lose the ability to construct complex figures or diagrams. Rarely patients present with reduplicative paramnesia, involving the belief that they are in two or more locations simultaneously. Reduplicative paramnesia, more often seen following head injury, can also be regarded as a misidentification syndrome.

Praxis

Impairments with planned motor movements are closely related to executive dysfunction. These deficits are usually seen in advanced stages of Alzheimer's disease dementia. Ideomotor and ideational apraxias may occur earlier. Ideomotor apraxia is characterized by inability to execute learned movements when prompted despite intact comprehension, sensation, motor strength and coordination. There may be difficulty in organizing and sequencing of movements involved in executing an action, e.g. pantomiming combing one's hair or brushing teeth. Individuals with Alzheimer's disease may

exhibit motor perseveration and poor limb positioning. Ideational apraxia is the inability to perform an action comprised of several steps. An example is pantomiming the act of getting dressed or changing the batteries in a remote control. Given the profound limitations to daily function from apraxia, these symptoms can be very distressing to both patients and care providers. There may also be difficulty recalling the ability to perform previously learned tasks such as driving, using utensils, toileting and self-care.

Executive Dysfunction

Impairment of executive function may result in cognitive, mood, behavioural and personality changes. The latter are discussed later as part of NPS. The cognitive symptoms of executive dysfunction are closely related to higher intellectual capacity and involve several aspects of higher intellectual function, including planning, sequencing, abstraction, set shifting and organizing. Features of executive dysfunction arise commonly early in the course of Alzheimer's disease, and may be the primary reason why functioning becomes impaired and care is sought. There is often loss of generative thought, and inability to plan or organize several mental tasks simultaneously without the use of aids. Individuals who previously did not require daily to-do lists to successfully perform tasks may have progressive difficulty completing activities.

It is important to note that there are age-associated declines in executive function; however, the mental flexibility that allows for the adaptive skills in the absence of dementia is often absent with Alzheimer's disease. Ability to solve problems mentally is affected early. In addition, there may be impairment in symbolic and abstract thinking. Thoughts become more concrete and patients may have difficulty accurately interpreting proverbs. Poor response inhibition (e.g. impaired Stroop colour-word interference test), reduced ability to sustain and divide attention, and perseveration of sequential motor tasks can also be seen in Alzheimer's disease at any stage of dementia or in the clinical prodrome to dementia.

NON-COGNITIVE NEUROPSYCHIATRIC SYMPTOMS ASSOCIATED WITH ALZHEIMER'S DISEASE

Neuropsychiatric symptoms such as depression, apathy, agitation and delusions are nearly universal in dementia associated with Alzheimer's disease. Over time, over 98% of individuals with Alzheimer's disease experience at least one NPS disturbance during the course of their illness[7]. In Alzheimer's disease, the presentation, severity and frequency of these symptoms may fluctuate with progression of the illness. NPS can be classified based on individual symptoms or clusters of frequently co-occurring symptoms[8]. The Neuropsychiatric Inventory (NPI) helps distinguish neuropsychiatric symptoms and signs into 12 domains: delusions, hallucinations, agitation, dysphoria, anxiety, apathy, irritability, euphoria, disinhibition, aberrant motor behaviour, night-time behaviour disturbances, and appetite and eating abnormalities[9] (Table 41.2).

NPS may be further differentiated based on a hierarchical approach into clusters of affective disturbance, psychotic disturbance, sleep disturbance, apathetic syndrome and executive dysfunction syndrome[8].

NPS with Prominent Affective Disturbance

Symptoms of disturbed mood are the most common non-cognitive symptoms seen in Alzheimer's disease. These include depression,

Table 41.2 Other neuropsychiatric symptoms associated with Alzheimer's dementia

---

Behavioural disturbance and personality changes (apathy, aggression, agitation, disinhibition and aberrant motor behaviour)
Mood disturbance (depression, anxiety, irritability)
Psychomotor abnormalities (sleep disturbance, appetite dysregulation)
Perceptual disturbance (delusions, hallucinations, illusions)

---

anxiety, irritability, agitation and elation. Depression is the most common mood symptom with an estimated five-year cumulative prevalence of 77%, and an average point prevalence of 31%[10] (Figures 41.1 and 41.2). Depressive symptoms which may also present in the context of a typical major depressive episode are often part of an atypical affective syndrome occurring in Alzheimer's disease referred to as 'depression of Alzheimer's disease' (dAD)[11] or 'affective disorder associated with Alzheimer's disease'[12]. Depression is often co-morbid with apathy. More than 40% of apathetic Alzheimer's disease patients present with depression and 56.4% of those with depression also present with apathy[13]. Other symptoms associated with depression in Alzheimer's disease include impaired sleep, anhedonia, poor concentration, diminished energy and appetite disturbances.

Depressive symptoms may herald the onset of Alzheimer's disease. Mood symptoms are more common in mild to moderate than in advanced dementia[13], although this apparent difference may be a result of difficulties evaluating the mental state of patients with advanced disease. Differentiating Alzheimer's disease with depression from other forms of late life depression (e.g. major depressive disorder) may be challenging as the symptoms overlap. Apathy, anxiety, diminished motivation, sleep disturbance and appetite dysregulation are examples of overlapping symptoms. However, the sustained subjective dysphoria seen with major depressive disorder is not characteristic of depression in Alzheimer's disease. Furthermore, unlike individuals with major depressive disorder, depressed patients with Alzheimer's disease may not report hopelessness, worthlessness and suicidal thinking but rather endorse symptoms of irritability, anxiety, and diminished interest and motivation[14]. Less commonly, elation and mood lability may present in Alzheimer's disease. These mood changes are rarely sustained and are often attenuated by redirection. Delusions may occur in the context of either an affective disturbance or a psychotic disturbance. Delusions are rare in late-life depression but occur in over 30% of patients with dAD.

Individuals with Alzheimer's disease have diminished insight as the disease progresses; however, in the early stages they may become demoralized. Feelings of demoralization often resolve as they adjust to the disease or lose insight with illness progression. Appetite dysregulation affects an estimated 37.8% of patients with Alzheimer's disease[15]. These symptoms are more prominent with

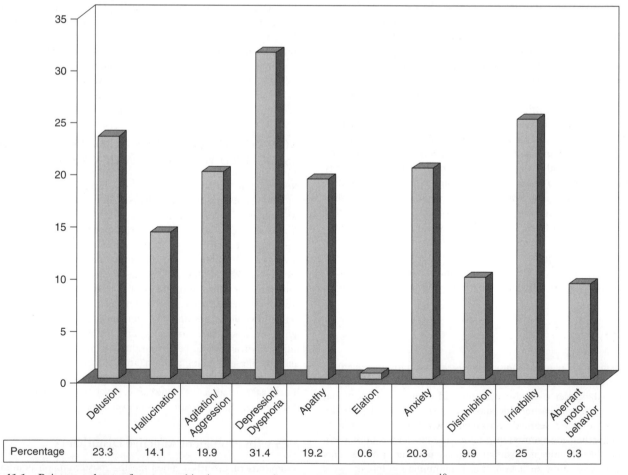

	Delusion	Hallucination	Agitation/ Aggression	Depression/ Dysphoria	Apathy	Elation	Anxiety	Disinhibition	Irriatbility	Aberrant motor behavior
Percentage	23.3	14.1	19.9	31.4	19.2	0.6	20.3	9.9	25	9.3

Figure 41.1 Point prevalence of neuropsychiatric symptoms in a community-based US sample[10]

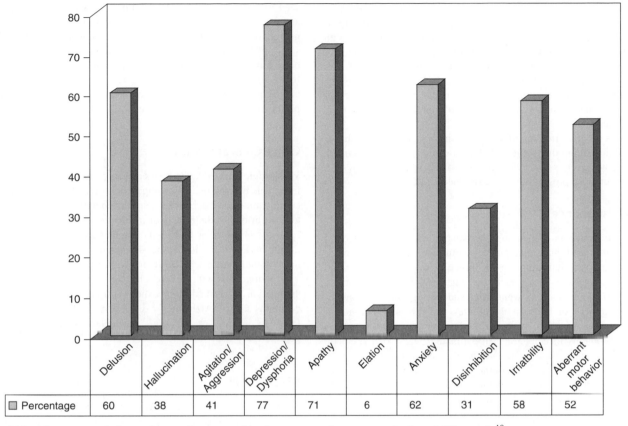

Percentage	Delusion	Hallucination	Agitation/ Aggression	Depression/ Dysphoria	Apathy	Elation	Anxiety	Disinhibition	Irriatbility	Aberrant motor behavior
	60	38	41	77	71	6	62	31	58	52

Figure 41.2 Five-year period prevalence of neuropsychiatric symptoms in a community-based US sample[10]

severe Alzheimer's disease. With progressive decline in independent function, individuals with Alzheimer's disease often exhibit irregular nutritional intake. Behavioural disturbances including irritability, agitation and disinhibition may have a greater impact on eating patterns and the quality of nutritional intake than the level of cognitive impairment[16]. Furthermore, there may be loss of appetite secondary to degeneration of hypothalamic regions associated with feeding and satiety. Nevertheless, without adequate supervision, those with advanced dementia have difficulty maintaining adequate daily nutritional support.

Agitation and aggression in Alzheimer's disease often manifest as emotional excitability, irritability, resistive behaviours, shouting or physical aggression. The estimated prevalence of agitation in Alzheimer's disease is 20–25%[10]. Agitated behaviours are not unique to Alzheimer's disease and may also be a part of other late-life conditions, including primary psychotic, depressive or substance use disorders and unrecognized pain. Agitation may also be provoked by environmental stimuli. Agitation and aggressive behaviours occur more commonly with advanced Alzheimer's disease. These behaviours are often seen in institutionalized Alzheimer's disease patients and frequently precipitate institutionalization in those living in the community.

NPS with Prominent Psychotic Disturbance

Delusions are a common neuropsychiatric symptom of Alzheimer's disease with an estimated point prevalence of 23%[10] and a prevalence range of 15–70%[17]. The wide range in rates may be due to different definitions of psychotic disturbance in Alzheimer's disease[18]. Delusions are unshakable false beliefs that are out of context with the individual's social and cultural background, while hallucinations are false sensory perceptions that are not simply distortions or misinterpretations of actual stimuli. Delusions in Alzheimer's disease have been associated with older age, male gender and a lower level of education[19]. Delusions occur more frequently than hallucinations. The most common types are poorly developed paranoid delusions and misidentification syndromes. The features of paranoid delusions are often related to theft, believing personal objects have been misplaced or stolen, and infidelity. Some characteristic misidentification syndromes may include the belief that family members have been replaced by imposters (Capgras syndrome) or that a stranger (often a misidentified close family member) inhabits their homes (phantom boarder). They may also express the belief that they have been removed from their homes and placed in a foreign environment. There may be differences in cognitive deficits among patients with delusions or delusional misidentification. Patients with delusions often have significantly greater impairment of recent memory, while those with delusional misidentification may have greater impairment of receptive language function. Patients with delusions or delusional misidentification are more likely to have some insight into their psychotic symptoms, unlike those who experience visual hallucinations.[20] Delusions in Alzheimer's disease may be associated with depression, aggression, agitation and anosognosia[21].

Hallucinations are less common in Alzheimer's disease than delusions, occurring in 13–16%[17] of patients with Alzheimer's disease at any point and may occur in up to 38% of these individuals over a cumulative five-year period[10]. Visual misperceptions are the predominant type of hallucinations in Alzheimer's disease. However, if visual hallucinations occur early in the illness, dementia with Lewy bodies should be considered. There is an increase in cognitive impairment, functional decline, placement in institutionalized care and death associated with delusions and hallucinations[22]. Delusions and hallucinations are seen more often in the moderate stages of Alzheimer's disease and may persist and often recur over the course of the illness[17].

Illusions are not often reported in Alzheimer's disease and clinical evidence describing the features of illusions in this disease is limited. There is, however, some evidence that visual illusions, if present, may worsen with progression of Alzheimer's disease[23].

Sleep Disturbance

Sleep disturbance in dementia is associated with significant caregiver distress and may precipitate institutionalization of community dwelling individuals due to its burden on caregivers. Nocturnal insomnia presents a background for unsupervised and potentially unsafe behaviours such as wandering and pacing and may precipitate serious risk of harm to themselves and others. Environmental stimulation may also play a role in aetiology or propagation of sleep problems in dementia. An estimated 59.2% of those with advanced dementia have some evidence of sleep disturbance, with insomnia, excessive daytime somnolence and napping being most prevalent[24]. Other symptoms include increased nocturnal awakenings and fragmented sleep. Insomnia is more common in patients with mild and moderate dementia while daytime sleepiness is more frequently associated with severe dementia[24]. Objective assessments of sleep using wrist actigraphy and polysomnography indicate that individuals with Alzheimer's disease in long-term care facilities may have increased total sleep time, increased sleep latency, increased REM sleep latency, less sleep efficiency, increased N1 non-REM sleep and decreased REM sleep[25].

Apathetic Syndrome

Degeneration of the anterior cingulate gyrus and adjacent medial frontal lobe structures with disruption of the frontal and subcortical circuits is associated with apathy. Apathy is one of the most prevalent psychiatric phenomena in Alzheimer's disease, affecting an estimated 75% of patients over the course of illness[10]. Features of apathy commonly seen include both emotional and motor phenomena. There is decreased emotional range, reduced motivation, diminished volition to initiate new tasks and a decrease in goal-directed behaviour. Comparisons may be drawn with depressed individuals; however, unlike depression, persons with Alzheimer's disease are not distressed or concerned with these symptoms. In rare cases, with severe dementia, there may be severe apathy in which individuals are awake but do not interact with the environment. They do not eat spontaneously unless fed, and do not attend to personal hygiene or maintain voluntary control over bowel and bladder functions.

Executive Dysfunction Syndrome

Changes in behaviour, mood and personality are often associated with the late stages of Alzheimer's disease. It is, however, not uncommon for these symptoms to present early in the clinical course. Other possible underlying causes, particularly the frontotemporal dementias, should be considered if behavioural and personality changes are seen early in the disease. Disinhibition, environmental dependency and verbal or motor perseveration are less prevalent than most other neuropsychiatric symptoms and present more frequently in the late stages of the illness[26]. Behavioural disinhibition and aberrant motor behaviours frequently precipitate placement into a nursing or assisted living home. Pacing and wandering are behaviours seen with increasing frequency with worsening dementia and may also precipitate placement into institutionalized care.

Other Clinical Features

With progression of Alzheimer's disease, there is an increasing risk of falls. This may be related to impairment in balance and gait, or poor coordination caused by the neurodegenerative process. Falls may also occur due to the effects of medications, orthostatic hypotension from cerebrovascular and cardiovascular dysfunction, and environmental hazards[27]. Falls may be associated with scalp injury, subdural haematoma, traumatic brain injury and rarely skull fractures.

In individuals with severe physical debility who have limited ambulation or are bed-bound, there is a significant elevated risk of decubitus ulcers. Alzheimer's disease may also be a predisposing factor in delirium or infections, particularly of the respiratory and genitourinary tract.

REFERENCES

1. Hebert LE, Scherr PA, Bienias JL, Bennett DA, Evans DA. Alzheimer disease in the US population: prevalence estimates using the 2000 census. *Arch Neurol* 2003; **60**(8): 1119–22.
2. Helzner EP, Scarmeas N, Cosentino S *et al*. Survival in Alzheimer disease: a multiethnic, population-based study of incident cases. *Neurology* 2008; **71**(19): 1489–95.
3. Kuller LH, Ives DG. Vital records and dementia. *Neuroepidemiology* 2008; **32**(1): 70–71.
4. Trzepacz PT, Mulsant BH, Dew MA *et al*. Is delirium different when it occurs in dementia? A study using the delirium rating scale. *J Neuropsychiatry Clin Neurosci* 1998; **10**(2): 199–204.
5. Patterson MB, Schnell AH, Martin RJ *et al*. Assessment of behavioral and affective symptoms in Alzheimer's disease. *J Geriatr Psychiatry Neurol* 1990; **3**(1): 21–30.
6. Adelman AM, Daly MP. Initial evaluation of the patient with suspected dementia. *Am Fam Physician* 2005; **71**(9): 1745–50.
7. Treiber KA, Lyketsos CG, Corcoran C *et al*. Vascular factors and risk for neuropsychiatric symptoms in Alzheimer's disease: the Cache County Study. *Int Psychogeriatr* 2008; **20**(3): 538–53.
8. Lyketsos CG. Neuropsychiatric symptoms (behavioral and psychological symptoms of dementia) and the development of dementia treatments. *Int Psychogeriatr* 2007; **19**(3): 409–20.
9. Cummings JL. The Neuropsychiatric Inventory: assessing psychopathology in dementia patients. *Neurology* 1997; **48**(5 suppl 6): S10–16.
10. Steinberg M, Shao H, Zandi P *et al*. Point and 5-year period prevalence of neuropsychiatric symptoms in dementia: the Cache County Study. *Int J Geriatr Psychiatry* 2008; **23**(2): 170–77.
11. Olin JT, Schneider LS, Katz IR *et al*. Provisional diagnostic criteria for depression of Alzheimer disease. *Am J Geriatr Psychiatry* 2002; **10**(2): 125–8.
12. Lyketsos CG, Sheppard JM, Steinberg M *et al*. Neuropsychiatric disturbance in Alzheimer's disease clusters into three groups:

the Cache County study. *Int J Geriatr Psychiatry* 2001; **16**(11): 1043–53.

13. Lyketsos CG, Steinberg M, Tschanz JT *et al*. Mental and behavioral disturbances in dementia: findings from the Cache County Study on memory in aging. *Am J Psychiatry* 2000; **157**(5): 708–14.

14. Rosenberg PB, Onyike CU, Katz IR *et al*. Clinical application of operationalized criteria for 'Depression of Alzheimer's Disease'. *Int J Geriatr Psychiatry* 2005; **20**(2): 119–27.

15. Fernandez-Martinez M, Castro J, Molano A *et al*. Prevalence of neuropsychiatric symptoms in Alzheimer's disease and vascular dementia. *Curr Alzheimer Res* 2008; **5**(1): 61–9.

16. Greenwood CE, Tam C, Chan M *et al*. Behavioral disturbances, not cognitive deterioration, are associated with altered food selection in seniors with Alzheimer's disease. *J Gerontol A Biol Sci Med Sci* 2005; **60**(4): 499–505.

17. Bassiony MM, Lyketsos CG. Delusions and hallucinations in Alzheimer's disease: review of the brain decade. *Psychosomatics* 2003; **44**(5): 388–401.

18. Leroi I, Voulgari A, Breitner JC, Lyketsos CG. The epidemiology of psychosis in dementia. *Am J Geriatr Psychiatry* 2003; **11**(1): 83–91.

19. Bassiony MM, Warren A, Rosenblatt A *et al*. The relationship between delusions and depression in Alzheimer's disease. *Int J Geriatr Psychiatry* 2002; **17**(6): 549–56.

20. Ballard CG, Bannister CL, Patel A *et al*. Classification of psychotic symptoms in dementia sufferers. *Acta Psychiatr Scand* 1995; **92**(1): 63–8.

21. Mizrahi R, Starkstein SE, Jorge R, Robinson RG. Phenomenology and clinical correlates of delusions in Alzheimer disease. *Am J Geriatr Psychiatry* 2006; **14**(7): 573–81.

22. Scarmeas N, Brandt J, Albert M *et al*. Delusions and hallucinations are associated with worse outcome in Alzheimer disease. *Arch Neurol* 2005; **62**(10): 1601–8.

23. Stavitsky K, Brickman AM, Scarmeas N *et al*. The progression of cognition, psychiatric symptoms, and functional abilities in dementia with Lewy bodies and Alzheimer disease. *Arch Neurol* 2006; **63**(10): 1450–56.

24. Rao V, Spiro J, Samus QM *et al*. Insomnia and daytime sleepiness in people with dementia residing in assisted living: findings from the Maryland Assisted Living Study. *Int J Geriatr Psychiatry* 2008; **23**(2): 199–206.

25. Martin JL, Ancoli-Israel S. Sleep disturbances in long-term care. *Clin Geriatr Med* 2008; **24**(1): 39–50, vi.

26. Lyketsos CG, Rosenblatt A, Rabins P. Forgotten frontal lobe syndrome or 'executive dysfunction syndrome'. *Psychosomatics* 2004; **45**(3): 247–55.

27. Shaw FE. Falls in cognitive impairment and dementia. *Clin Geriatr Med* 2002; **18**(2): 159–73.

42

Neuropsychological Assessment of Dementia and Alzheimer's Disease

David Aaron Maroof and Cynthia A. Munro

Department of Psychiatry and Behavioral Sciences, The Johns Hopkins University School of Medicine, Baltimore, USA

INTRODUCTION

Clinical neuropsychology can be conceptualized as both the *study* of affective, behavioural and cognitive manifestations of brain function and the *application* of assessment procedures in quantifying these interrelated processes to inform decisions regarding the causes for dysfunction. The term *neuropsychology* has also been described as a 'merger between experimental psychology and neurological sciences for studying relationships between the brain and behavior'[1] (p. 139). Assessment procedures used by neuropsychologists are tasks that tap various domains of cognition, including, but not limited to, aspects of attention, processing speed, language, visuospatial skills, memory and executive functioning, as well as those assessing mood and aspects of personality. Responses to these tasks provide scores that are used to quantify an individual's functioning in these domains. While we cannot physically observe cognition, we can infer its integrity with the use of standardized psychometric tests. Quantification of an individual's optimal cognitive ability, considering his or her emotional status and personality characteristics and then determining whether one's optimal cognitive ability represents disease, is the cornerstone of the neuropsychological assessment of dementia. In so doing, we improve diagnostic accuracy of dementia above routine clinical evaluation[2]. How we accomplish this is the focus of this chapter.

We have divided this chapter into five sections. First, we will provide a brief introduction to the field of neuropsychology. Second, we will discuss the role of the clinical neuropsychologist in the assessment of dementia. Third, we provide an overview of the basic patterns of cognitive test performance in dementia. Fourth, we discuss some common misconceptions about the practice of neuropsychology. Finally, we present some of the current trends in the neuropsychological assessment of dementia.

INTRODUCTION TO NEUROPSYCHOLOGY

Neuropsychology is an amalgam of many disciplines, influenced by neuroanatomy, neurophysiology, neurochemistry, neuropharmacology, psychology and neurology[3], as well as philosophy, physiology and anatomy[4]. Psychometric theory and application, as they relate to appropriate use of data analyses in test construction and the development of normative data, are the very linchpins of neuropsychological

assessment and substantiate the theoretical and conceptual networks of the discipline.

The nexus between current neuropsychological theory and practice harks back to ancient philosophical thought[3]. Ideas such as aestheticism (e.g., is a theory appealing?), rationalism and empiricism still fuel the practice of clinical neuropsychology[5]. Glozman[6] discusses the influence of Russian contributions dating back to the late 18th century from psychiatrists and neurologists and attributed many changes in neuropsychological practice – including combining both quantitative and qualitative approaches, expansion to include social and personality variables and increasing nosological patient groups – to this influence. A main theme that Glozman[6] noted was '...not so much diagnostic but prognostic...neuropsychological assessment should rather emphasize the subject's strengths which are important...and predict his/her ultimate integration into society' (p. 177). The need for a systematic, valid and reliable method of measuring the manifestations of brain function emerged. Test construction thus came on the heels of conceptual and theoretical models of brain function and organization.

Delineating the inception and progression of various neuropsychological tasks is beyond the scope of this chapter. However, we have selected to discuss one very commonly used method for assessing executive functioning to exemplify the manner in which some of our tests have been developed. Executive functioning is a cognitive process involving one's ability to adapt and respond effectively to environmental demands, novel situations and ultimately deduce efficient and effective ways for completing them. Several 'tributaries' of executive functioning have been promulgated, including sequencing behaviours, abstraction, organization and planning. Eling and colleagues[7] report on the influence of Narziss Ach who designed a paradigm for observing concept formation in the early 20th century. Nonsense words (on cards) were attached on various geometric figures of different shapes and sizes and once these cards were removed, the individual was required to deduce how the words related to the features of the objects. The quintessential element of this task is that one must discover the sorting principle. Goldstein and Scheerer[1] underscored the abstract elements of this task, in which one must be able to abstract from a concrete object, while maintaining insight into other potential 'choices'. The Wisconsin Card Sorting Test (WCST)[8] was developed on the basis of these principles. Brenda Milner[9] ultimately demonstrated that lesions in the

Principles and Practice of Geriatric Psychiatry, 3rd edn. Edited by Mohammed T. Abou-Saleh, Cornelius Katona and Anand Kumar

dorsolateral prefrontal cortex resulted in shifting problems (i.e., perseverating) and subsequent research has repeatedly confirmed that damage to the frontal cortex is associated with poor performance on this task[10].

Integrity of the perforant pathway (the principal source of input to the hippocampal formation) is essential for normal hippocampal function. In Alzheimer's disease, it is the pathological changes in this pathway that preclude its normal operation of acquisition of contextual knowledge, presumably due to a disconnection among the hippocampal formation and input from sensory-specific and multi-modal association cortices[11]. However, as the neuropathology spreads beyond the medial temporal lobe structures to the association cortices of the frontal, temporal and parietal lobes, higher order cognitive deficits result[12]. Regarding cognitive assessment in Alzheimer's disease, it is the juxtaposition of the neuropathological changes along the disease trajectory with administration of specific tests chosen to assess the associated cognitive deficits that is the cornerstone of clinical neuropsychology. The application of statistical methodology provides the intellectual spadework for clinical practice, as the interpretation of test performance requires the understanding of statistical principles underlying test construction and interpretation.

THE ROLE OF THE CLINICAL NEUROPSYCHOLOGIST

The advent of neuroimaging in the 1970s changed the clinical neuropsychologist's role from that of lesion detection to one of description of the cognitive sequelae of disease[13] and/or diagnosis of disease for which imaging is uninformative. In general, there is a chasm between knowledge gleaned from neuroimaging and information gathered through neuropsychological examination. Imaging tells us *what* (e.g. cerebrovascular accident), *where* (e.g. anterior cerebral artery) and *how* (e.g. ruptured aneurysm), whereas neuropsychological examination tells us the consequences, including *how much* (degree of deficit) and *in what way* (memory, language, etc.) functioning has been affected.

Neuropsychological assessment in dementia depends on the context of the referral question. In some cases, the neuropsychologist's role is to determine whether cognitive impairment exists and if so, to assist with the differential diagnosis of its cause. In other cases, diagnosis of the disease causing the dementia has been established and the neuropsychologist is asked to determine areas of cognitive strength and weakness, to assist with the development of compensatory strategies. Neuropsychological assessment is also used to track disease progression through repeated examinations, at times determining whether changes in medication are associated with changes in cognition. In still other cases, neuropsychological assessment provides objective data to assist in determining whether a patient is competent to make independent decisions regarding medical, financial or other matters. Recommendations regarding whether a patient should cease driving or working are also informed by neuropsychological assessment. Thus, the context of the referral, even within the narrow scope of dementia assessment, is important to the information that is provided by the neuropsychologist.

RECOGNIZING PATTERNS OF NEUROCOGNITIVE FUNCTIONING IN THE DEMENTIAS

It is quite often the case that clinical neuropsychologists must disentangle ambiguous complaints of declines in cognitive function. Memory complaints, for example, often dissemble the extent and typology of cognitive deficits. What can present as a memory deficit may be related to the bigger picture of a breakdown in semantic knowledge (e.g. naming), or difficulties with executive function that can affect one's ability to carry out a series of everyday tasks. The pattern of performance exhibited on a neuropsychological examination provides information with regard to these core and peripheral deficits and in conjunction with a comprehensive anamnesis, offers etiological significance.

The cortical–subcortical distinction proffers a heuristically useful model for describing the pattern of neuropsychological performance in various patient groups, despite observations that this is an oversimplified dichotomy[14,15]. This distinction was engendered by the observation of different clinical presentations in patients with cortical compared to subcortical disease[16]. Although the prototypical cortical dementia is that caused by Alzheimer's disease, other diseases, such as frontotemporal lobar degeneration and Creutzfeldt–Jakob disease, are also associated with cortical pathology. Far greater in number, diseases causing subcortical dementia comprise, among others, progressive supranuclear palsy, Parkinson's disease and Huntington's disease and are associated with pathological changes involving the thalamus, basal ganglia and related brain-stem nuclei. Cortical diseases typically develop similar cognitive footprints, including deficits in language, learning and praxis, whereas patients with subcortical dementia typically demonstrate impaired attention/concentration, processing speed and executive function, as well as apathy and depression. Although the cortical/subcortical dichotomy is simplistic and does not account for disorders with both cortical and subcortical features (e.g. cortical-basal degeneration[17]), this distinction remains useful in the differential diagnosis of dementia.

In clinical practice, the neuropsychologist must make several determinations when the question of dementia is being considered. After the tests are administered and the scores are obtained, these scores are compared against a normative sample; that is, a sample of individuals, typically of the same age, but sometimes of the same race, sex and education as the patient. This comparison yields standardized scores (percentiles, z-scores or t-scores) for each raw score. Upon examination of these standardized scores, the neuropsychologist must consider several questions. First, is the examination normal or abnormal? Second, if it is abnormal, does the examination indicate the presence of a cognitive disorder or dementia? Third, is the pattern of cognitive test performance suggestive of cortical or subcortical involvement? Fourth, what disease is underlying the cognitive disorder?

Abnormal scores on individual tests can be defined by several means. In some cases, a score that is obtained by fewer than a particular proportion (often 2%) of the normal population is considered to be abnormal. However, in a large battery of neuropsychological tests, obtaining several scores that are in this 'impaired' range is quite normal[18]. In other instances, an abnormal score is one that is unexpected given a particular patient's premorbid ability. That is, if a patient has limited education or sensory deficits that preclude his or her ability to perform some aspects of a task, then an abnormal score might not represent a decline from premorbid ability. Likewise, if a patient has superior premorbid intellectual functioning, a score in the borderline range on a memory test might be considered an abnormal score for that individual.

A second determination is then made regarding whether the presence of one or more abnormal scores constitutes an abnormal exam. This inference requires one to incorporate other information, such as the patient's or informant's complaints and the overall pattern of test scores. As already mentioned, the presence of one or more abnormal scores often occurs across a battery of neuropsychological tests in normal healthy adults. Thus, the neuropsychologist must determine whether the pattern of abnormal scores is clinically meaningful. This determination is informed by the clinician's knowledge of patterns of test scores that occur in conditions causing dementia. Incorporating measures of emotional functioning are also useful in informing the clinician's determination of whether an abnormal examination is the product of disease or is psychogenic in nature. The practice of interpreting neuropsychological test results is therefore an integrative process, incorporating the patient's history, complaints and test data. Results from neuroimaging and neurological examination, if available, are also considered.

MISCONCEPTIONS ABOUT THE NEUROPSYCHOLOGICAL ASSESSMENT OF DEMENTIA

The assessment of patients with dementia is often multidisciplinary, involving neurologists, psychiatrists, neuroradiologists, geriatric practitioners and/or family practice physicians. Among non-neuropsychologists, several misconceptions regarding the practice of our discipline appear pervasive. We describe several of these misconceptions, as they can hinder one's understanding of the information provided by the neuropsychologist.

Cutoff Scores

Perhaps a result of epidemiological studies that use various scores – such as a Mini Mental State Examination Score of 24 or below – to exclude individuals who are likely to have cognitive difficulties, the notion that a particular score on a given test can be used to indicate dementia is a common misconception. Such scores, when used for research purposes, are often chosen because they are uncommon in healthy individuals. A score that is equal to or below the 2nd or 10th percentiles, that is, a score that represents poorer performance than what 98% or 90%, respectively, of individuals score, are common 'cutoff' scores for research. However, many factors render these cutoff scores inappropriate for use in clinical practice: premorbid ability, effort and number of tests administered all determine whether a particular score is abnormal. Thus, it is inappropriate to apply a cutoff score to an individual, or to use phrases such as 'he scored below the cutoff for dementia', as such scores differ, depending on the individual. For this reason, the use of norms is a cornerstone of the practice of neuropsychology. Such norms are crucial to answering the basic question, 'is this test score normal or abnormal?' Which demographic factors should be considered in the development of normative tables is a topic with particular currency in the field.

Singularity of Domains Assessed by Particular Tests

Another misconception about the practice of neuropsychological assessment is that each test taps a singular ability that is subserved by a discrete brain structure. In practice, two patients might perform poorly on the same task, but for different reasons. For example, if a patient is unable to copy a complex figure, it might be due to poor visual perception, difficulty with constructional praxis or problems

with executive functioning. By administering a battery of tests that assesses these domains in various ways and examining the pattern of test performance, we can then determine which domains are impaired in each patient. It is important to recognize, therefore, that a particular test may require intact functioning in several cognitive domains. It follows that failure to perform a test does not necessarily imply impairment in a single domain.

In addition to the fact that various cognitive processes can subserve performance on the same task, it is also the case that functional networks account for the existence of similar cognitive impairments among individuals with different sites of lesions[19]. A common misconception is that executive functioning is determined by integrity of the frontal lobe. Whereas several executive tasks have been associated with frontal lobe activity[20] and have been shown to be impaired in patients with frontal lobe lesions[21], executive dysfunction can occur in the context of abnormal functioning in other areas as well[22].

Association between Premorbid Ability and Cognitive Test Performance

A third misconception is that individuals with superior premorbid ability should perform in the superior range on all cognitive measures. This logic often leads to the false conclusion that average test performance represents impairment in high-functioning individuals. However, when this notion is tested empirically, it is simply not the case. On the contrary, individuals of above-average intellectual functioning perform better than those with average intelligence on approximately one-third of measures in a test battery. Individuals with lower IQ scores do perform significantly worse, however, than individuals with average intelligence on most measures[23]. Thus, whereas low scores would be expected for individuals with lower intelligence, higher scores on all measures should not be expected among individuals with higher levels of intellectual functioning. While it is possible that average performance across all tests in a domain may represent a decline from premorbid ability in an individual with complaints in that domain, we cannot know this. In such cases, it is important to consider other factors and perhaps even then, the only way we can know whether disease exists is to repeat the examination after some time (usually one year or so) to determine if there is decline in test performance that would suggest the presence of disease.

Time Course of Recovery from Cognitive Deficits in Depression

Depressed individuals can demonstrate cognitive dysfunction in the absence of demonstrable neuropathology[24] and these deficits appear to be more pronounced in depressed elderly compared to younger individuals with depression[25,26]. The most consistently documented deficits among elderly patients with depression involve psychomotor speed, executive functioning and memory for newly learned information[27,28]. Thus, the prototypical cognitive deficits resulting from depression resemble those seen in 'subcortical' dementia[29].

A common misconception concerning the cognitive deficits associated with depression is that they resolve coincident with remission of low mood. Longitudinal studies have shown, however, that cognitive deficits remain during episodes of symptom reduction and even during remission[30]. The more effort a task requires for success, the less well individuals with depression tend to perform on it[31]. Indeed, some evidence suggests that the relationship between depressive symptoms and performance on many cognitive tests is largely mediated by impairments of effortful processing[28,32]. In a study by Hammar and colleagues[33], depressed patients were impaired on cognitively demanding tasks (those requiring effortful processing) when symptomatic and their impairments persisted even after six months, despite significant improvement in symptoms of depression. Similarly, Nebes and colleagues[24] found that depressed elderly patients whose mood symptoms responded to treatment with an antidepressant medication (paroxetine or nortriptyline) showed no greater improvement over baseline performance in any cognitive domain than untreated healthy control subjects on five follow-up examinations taking place over 12 weeks. These studies and others suggest that the cognitive impairment observed among depressed elderly patients may be an enduring feature[34]. Nevertheless, longitudinal assessment of depressed patients can assist in the differential diagnosis between depression and dementia, based on whether there is progressive cognitive decline over time.

RECENT TRENDS IN THE NEUROPSYCHOLOGICAL ASSESSMENT OF DEMENTIA

The evolving field of neuropsychology is witness to numerous developments in the field of dementia and its treatment. These developments have led to changes in the questions we are asked to address and the approaches we use to conduct our evaluations of patients with dementia.

Early Detection of Neurodegenerative Disorder

It is the deliberate use of neuropsychological testing that parallels the course of neuropathology that informs our choice of tests. In so doing, the neuropsychologist makes inferences regarding whether a pattern of test results relates to a pathological process suggestive of a particular disease. However, very early in the course of disease, our tests are not as sensitive in detecting abnormality as they become later in the course of disease. The goal of detecting and distinguishing from among the potential incipient dementias has implications both for prognosis and in determining whether to start relevant disease-specific treatments[12]. This goal has increasing currency in light of recent studies suggesting that some factors, such as diet and exercise, may act as modifiers to the risk of developing dementia and progression of mild cognitive impairment to dementia[35]. Thus, being able to detect the very subtle cognitive changes that are the earliest manifestation of disease has gained more interest in recent years and includes as an objective the detection of a transitional state between normal ageing and dementia. This transitional state has been given several appellations, the most common in the United States being mild cognitive impairment (MCI)[36]. Attempts at identifying this state have included the refinement of diagnostic nomenclature and increased sensitivity of neurocognitive tests to detect abnormality.

Because many of our tests do not have 'ceiling' effects – that is, even normal healthy individuals do not earn perfect scores on them – the tests themselves are sufficiently difficult for even those with subtle cognitive problems. The interest, therefore, is in improving the diagnostic sensitivity of these tests. One way to do this is by improving the similarity between the normative sample and the patient we are assessing. The use of demographically adjusted scores (discussed in the following sections) is one method of achieving this.

Clinical neuropsychologists sometimes reach an impasse when faced with attempting to detect cognitive changes in the behavioural

variant of frontotemporal dementia (FTD). Specifically, the initial symptoms generally include changes in personality and social interaction, as well as disinhibition[37]. Torralva and colleagues[38] demonstrated that while cognitive measures of memory, attention, visuospatial analysis, executive function and language did not significantly differ in patients diagnosed with the behavioural variant of FTD compared to normal healthy individuals, the authors' executive and social cognition battery did distinguish the groups. It is commonly thought that traditional testing environments may fail to induce executive deficits because of the inherent structure provided by the examination process. As such, the development of assessment tools that elicit abnormal behaviour is a challenge for the field.

The Use of Demographically Adjusted Test Scores

Over the past century, neuropsychologists have interpreted individual test scores by comparing an individual's test scores to a normative sample. The field has seen recent controversy regarding the composition of the norms we use. Specifically, which demographic variables should be considered is a matter of debate. The reason we use a normative sample is to determine the degree of deviation from the average, healthy individual, presumably because the patient was pre-morbidly similar to the average, healthy individual. Typically we choose to compare our patient with a sample of comparable age, due to the influence of age on many of our tests. It is sometimes desirable, however, to compare our patient with an individual who is comparable also in education level, due to the effects of education on test performance. Other normative samples include race and sex as well. Brickman and colleagues[39] point out that the value of neuropsychological assessment is contingent on the psychometric properties of the individual tests. If African Americans, for example, have been shown to perform on average lower than Caucasians, a test based on data from the latter group will cause an increase in false positives (i.e. diagnosing someone as impaired, when in fact he or she is performing within normal limits). Such comparisons allow us to determine how similar our patient is to healthy individuals of the same demographic. A similar approach involves the calculation of a predicted score based on a patient's demographic information[40,41]. Both methods take into account demographic variables in informing the decision about whether a particular score is normal or abnormal and improve the sensitivity of our measures in identifying cognitive impairment. Silverberg and Millis[42] have shown that adjusting scores can actually *decrease* the usefulness of test performance for predicting functional outcomes, such as the ability to work. If, for example, a 90-year-old individual is normal compared to other nonagenarians with regard to psychomotor speed, we may interpret his score as normal. However, given that the typical 90-year-old individual is much slower than the typical middle-aged individual, we may interpret the elder's score as rendering him unable to perform tasks that require fast processing speed (e.g. being an air-traffic controller). Thus, whether to use demographic adjustments depends upon the question we seek to answer.

CONCLUDING COMMENTS

The field of neuropsychology, influenced by such disparate areas of study as philosophy, neuroanatomy and psychology, is heavily reliant on statistical methods to substantiate its theoretical and conceptual frameworks. Psychometric theory and application, as they relate to appropriate use of data analyses in test construction and the development of normative data, are the very linchpins of clinical practice. Neuropsychological assessment in patients with suspected dementia provides an important source of diagnostic information, resulting from the empirically based choice of test batteries and the use of statistical methods to interpret these batteries.

Although the role of the clinical neuropsychologist has evolved and depends upon the context of the evaluation, the information provided through neuropsychological assessment remains valuable in the differential diagnosis of dementia and improves diagnostic accuracy above routine clinical examination. The cortical/subcortical distinction, despite its being an oversimplification, remains a useful reference in the decision tree for individual cases. Faulty assumptions about our field relating to how we define abnormality, what our tests measure and the nature of cognitive dysfunction in the presence of low mood, can lead to misunderstandings about what our clinical evaluations can offer.

Current trends in the neuropsychological assessment of dementia include, as in other fields, detection of the very earliest manifestation of disease. Increasing the sensitivity of our tests with the use of increasingly sophisticated statistical methods has resulted from the goal of improving our ability to detect subtle cognitive problems. It is not only the application of knowledge of neuropathological changes and clinical presentation of the various diseases causing dementia that distinguishes neuropsychology as a discipline. It is also the dovetailing of sound clinical judgement with appropriate statistical methodology that is required for good clinical practice.

REFERENCES

1. Goldstein G. Neuropsychology in New York City (1930–1960). *Arch Clin Neuropsychol* 2009; **24**: 137–43.
2. Geroldi C, Canu E, Bruni AC, Dal Forno G, Ferri R, Gabelli C *et al*. The added value of neuropsychologic tests and structural imaging for the etiologic diagnosis of dementia in Italian expert centers. *Alz Dis Assoc Dis* 2008; **22**: 309–20.
3. Adams K. Neuropsychology: past, present and future. In Benton A (ed.), *Exploring the History of Neuropsychology; Selected Papers*. Oxford: Oxford University Press, 2000, 3–40.
4. Kolb B, Whishaw IQ. *Fundamentals of Human Neuropsychology*, 5th edn. New York: Worth, 2003.
5. Viney W, King DB. *A History of Psychology: Ideas and Context*, 3rd edn. London: Allyn & Bacon, 2002.
6. Glozman, JM. A.R. Luria and the history of Russian neuropsychology. *J Hist Neurosci* 2007; **1**: 168–80.
7. Eling P, Derckx K Maes R. On the historical and conceptual background of the Wisconsin Card Sorting Test. *Brain Cognition* 2008; **67**: 247–53.
8. Berg EA. A simple objective for measuring flexibility in thinking. *J Gen Psychol* 1946; **39**: 15–22.
9. Milner B. Effects of different brain lesions on card sorting: the role of the frontal lobes. *Arch Neuro* 1963; **9**: 100–10.
10. Arnett PA, Rao SM, Bernardin L, Grafman J, Yetkin FZ, Lobeck L. Relationship between frontal lobe lesions and Wisconsin Card Sorting Test performance in patients with multiple sclerosis. In Strauss E, Sherman EMS, Spreen, O. (eds), *A Compendium of Neuropsychological Tests: Administration, Norms and Commentary*, 3rd edn. Oxford: Oxford University Press, 2006.
11. Hyman BT, Van Hoesen GW, Kromer LJ, Damasio AR. Perforant pathway changes and the memory impairment of Alzheimer's disease. *Ann Neurol* 1986; **20**: 472–81.
12. Salmon DP, Bondi MW. Neuropsychological assessment of dementia. *Annu Rev Psychol* 2009; **60**: 257–82.
13. Wood RI. The scientist-practitioner model: How do advances in clinical and cognitive neuroscience affect neuropsychology in the courtroom. *J Head Trauma Rehab* 2009; **24**: 88–99.
14. Salmon DP, Filoteo JV. Neuropsychology of cortical versus subcortical dementia syndromes. *Sem Neurology* 2007; **27**: 7–21.
15. Brandt J, Munro, CA. Memory disorders in subcortical dementia. In Baddeley AD, Kopelman MD, Wilson BA. *The Essential Handbook of Memory Disorders for Clinicians*. Hoboken: Wiley, 2004, 591–614.
16. Hodges, JR, Salmon DP, Butters, N. Differential impairment in semantic and episodic in Alzheimer's and Huntington's diseases. *Brain* 1990; **114**: 1547–58.
17. Pillon B, Blin J, Vidailhet M, Deweer B, Sirigu A, Dubois B, Agid Y. The neuropsychological pattern of corticobasal degeneration: comparison with progressive supranuclear palsy and Alzheimer's disease. *Neurology* 1995; **45**; 1477–83.
18. Schretlen DJ, Munro CA, Anthony JC, Pearlson GD. Examining the range of normal intraindividual variability in neuropsychological test performance. *J Int Neuropsych Soc* 2003; **9**: 864–70.
19. Arango-Lasprilla JC, Rogers H, Lengenfelder J, Deluca J, Moreno S, Lopear F. Cortical and subcortical diseases: do true neuropsychological differences exist? *Arch Clin Neuropsychol* 2006; **21**: 29–40.
20. Cummings JL. Frontal-subcortical circuits and human behavior. *Arch Neurol* 1993; **50**: 873–80.
21. Banich M. Executive function: the search for an integrated account. *Curr Dir Psychol Sci* 2009; **18**: 89–94.
22. Huey ED, Goveia EN, Paviol S, Pardini M, Krueger F, Zamboni G *et al*. Executive dysfunction in frontotemporal dementia and corticobasal syndrome. *Neurology* 2009; **72**: 453–9.
23. Diaz-Asper CM, Schretlen DJ, Pearlson GD. How well does IQ predict neuropsychological test performance in normal adults? *J Int Neuropsych Soc* 2004; **10**: 81–90.
24. Nebes RD, Pollock BG, Houck PR, Butters MA, Mulsant BH, Zmuda MD, Reynolds III CF. Persistence of cognitive impairment in geriatric patients following antidepressant treatment: a randomized, double-blind clinical trial with nortriptyline and paroxetine. *J Psychiat Res* 2003; **37**: 99–108.
25. Dotson VM, Resnick SM, Zonderman AB. Differential association of concurrent, baseline and average depressive symptoms with cognitive decline in older adults. *Am J Geriat Psychiatry* 2008; **16**: 3–18.
26. Gualtieri CT & Johnson LG. Age-related cognitive decline in patients with mood disorders. *Prog Neuro Psychoph* 2008; **32**: 962–7.
27. Butters MA, Bhalla RK, Mulsant BH, Mazumdar S, Houck PR, Begley A *et al*. Executive functioning, illness course and relapse/recurrence in continuation and maintenance treatment in late-life depression: is there a relationship? *Am J Geriat Psychiatry* 2004; **12**: 387–94.
28. Nebes RD, Butters MA, Mulsant BH, Pollock BG, Zmuda MD, Houck PR *et al*. Decreased working memory and processing speed mediate cognitive impairment in geriatric depression. *Psychol Med* 2000; **30**: 679–91.
29. Crowe SF, Hoogenraad K. Differentiation of dementia of the Alzheimer's type from depression with cognitive impairment on

the basis of a cortical versus a subcortical pattern of cognitive deficit. *Arch Clin Neuropsych* 2000; **15**: 9–19.

30. Nakano Y, Baba H, Maeshima H, Kitajima A, Sakai Y, Baba K *et al.* Executive dysfunction in medicated, remitted state of major depression. *J Affect Disord* 2008; **111**: 46–51.

31. Roy-Byrne PP, Weingartner H, Bierer LM, Thompson, K, Post R. Effortful and automatic cognitive processes in depression. *Arch Gen Psychiatry* 1986; **43**: 265–7.

32. Butters MA, Whyte EM, Nebes RD, Begley AE, Dew MA, Mulsant BH. The nature and determinants of neuropsychological functioning in late-life depression. *Arch Gen Psychiatry* 2004; **61**: 587–95.

33. Hammar A, Lund A, Hugdal K. Long-lasting cognitive impairment in unipolar major depression: a 6-month follow-up study. *Psychiat Res* 2003; **118**: 189–96.

34. Reischies FM, Neu P. Comorbidity of mild cognitive disorder and depression: a neuropsychological analysis. *Eur Arch Psy Clin N* 2000; **250**: 186–93.

35. Scarmeas N, Luchsinger J A, Schupf N, Brickman AM, Cosentino S, Tang, MX *et al.* Physical activity, diet and risk of Alzheimer' disease. *J Am Med Assoc* 2009; **302**: 627–37.

36. Petersen RC, Doody R, Kurz A, Mohs RC, Morris JC, Rabins PV *et al.* Current concepts in mild cognitive impairment. *Arch Neurol* 2001; **58**: 1985–92.

37. Hodges JR, Miller B. The neuropsychology of frontal variant frontotemporal dementia and semantic dementia. Introduction to the special topic papers: Part II. *Neurocase* 2001; **7**: 113–21.

38. Torralva T, Roca M, Gleichgerrcht E, Bekinschtein T, Manes F. A neuropsychological battery to detect specific executive and social cognitive impairments in early frontotemporal dementia. *Brain* 2009; **132**: 1299–309.

39. Brickman AM, Cabo R, Manly JJ. Ethical issues in cross-cultural neuropsychology. *Appl Neuropsychol* 2006; **13**: 91–100.

40. Crawford JR, Howell DC. Comparing an individual's test score against norms derived from small samples. *Clin Neuropsychol* 1998; **12**: 482–6.

41. Zachary RA, Gorsuch RL. Continuous norming: implications of the WAIS-R. *J Clin Psychol* 1985; **4**: 86–94.

42. Silverberg ND, Millis SR. Impairment versus deficiency in neuropsychological assessment: implications for ecological validity. *J Int Neuropsych Soc* 2009; **15**: 94–102.

43

Genetics of Alzheimer's Disease

Lynn M. Bekris[1], Chang-En Yu[1,2], Thomas D. Bird[1,2] and Debby Tsuang[1,2]

[1]*Departments of Medicine, Neurology and Psychiatry and Behavioral Sciences,*
University of Washington School of Medicine, Seattle, WA, USA
[2]*Geriatric Research, Education and Clinical Center and Mental Illness Research, Education and Clinical Center,*
University of Washington School of Medicine, Seattle, WA, USA

INTRODUCTION

Prevalence and Incidence

Alzheimer's disease (AD) is the most common irreversible, progressive brain disease. It is characterized by a gradual loss of memory and cognitive skills. AD accounts for over 50% of all dementia cases and it presently affects more than 24 million people worldwide. Moreover, over 5 million new cases of AD are reported each year and the incidence is likely to increase as a greater proportion of the population ages[1].

AD prevalence and incidence strongly suggest that age is the most influential known risk factor. Indeed, AD prevalence increases significantly with age and AD incidence increases from 2.8 per 1000 person years for people between 65 and 69 years to 56.1 per 1000 person years for people who are older than 90 years[2]. Approximately 10% of persons older than 70 years have significant memory loss and more than half of these individuals have probable AD. An estimated 25% to 45% of persons older than 85 years have dementia[3]. The duration of disease is typically 8 to 10 years, with a range from 2 to 25 years after diagnosis.

The disease is divided into two subtypes based on the age of onset: early-onset AD (EOAD) and late-onset AD (LOAD). EOAD accounts for approximately 1% to 6% of all cases and ranges roughly from 30 years to 60 or 65 years. On the other hand, LOAD, which is the most common form of AD, is defined as AD with an age at onset later than 60 or 65 years. Both EOAD and LOAD may occur in people with a positive family history of AD. Approximately 60% of EOAD cases have multiple cases of AD within their families and of these familial EOAD cases, 13% are inherited in an autosomal dominant manner with at least three generations affected[4,5]. Early-onset cases can also occur in families with late-onset disease[3]. With the exception of a few autosomal dominant families that are single-gene disorders (see below), most AD cases appear to be a complex disorder that is likely to involve multiple susceptibility genes and environmental factors[3,6-9].

Clinical Symptoms

Both EOAD and LOAD present clinically as dementia that begins with a gradual decline of memory and then slowly increases in severity until the symptoms eventually become incapacitating. Other common symptoms are confusion, poor judgement, language disturbance, agitation, withdrawal and hallucinations. Rare symptoms include seizures, parkinsonism, increased muscle tone, myoclonus, incontinence and mutism. Death commonly occurs from general inanition, malnutrition and pneumonia[3]. Treatment of AD with cholinesterase inhibitors and memantine may result in slowing of cognitive decline in mild to moderate dementia cases, but overall, most patients experience only clinically marginal improvement in measures of cognition and in global assessments of dementia[10,11].

Clinical Diagnosis

Currently, the diagnosis of AD is based on clinical history and neuropsychological tests. The *Diagnostic and Statistical Manual of Mental Disorders, 4th Edition* (DSM-IV), criteria for diagnosing dementia requires the loss of two or more of the following: memory, language, calculation, orientation or judgement[12]. The Mini-Mental State Examination (MMSE) helps to evaluate changes in a patient's cognitive abilities. In addition, a diagnosis of probable AD necessitates the exclusion of other degenerative disorders associated with dementia, such as frontotemporal dementia (including frontotemporal dementia with parkinsonism-17 and Pick's disease), Parkinson's disease, diffuse Lewy body disease, Creutzfeldt–Jakob disease and cerebral autosomal dominant arteriopathy with subcortical infarcts and leukoencephalopathy (CADASIL)[13]. Discriminating AD from other forms of dementia is usually done through clinical history and neuroimaging[3]. In addition, other possible causes of dementia need to be excluded, especially the treatable forms of cognitive impairment, such as impairment due to depression, chronic drug intoxication, chronic central nervous system infection, thyroid disease, vitamin deficiencies (e.g., B12 and thiamine), central nervous system angitis and normal-pressure hydrocephalus[3]. Individuals who do not meet these criteria but have short-term memory loss, have only minimal impairment in other cognitive abilities and are not functionally impaired at work or at home are considered to have 'mild cognitive impairment'[14].

Neuropathological Diagnosis

A definitive diagnosis of AD requires a clinical assessment of probable AD, as well as postmortem confirmation, with the presence of two histopathological features: neurofibrillary tangles and amyloid plaques[15–17]. Before autopsy confirmation, expert clinicians correctly diagnose AD between 80% to 90% of the time[18]. Even though plaques and tangles are often found in cognitively normal age-matched controls, the density and the distribution of these attributes are more severe in patients with AD, according to standardized histological assessments[15]. Amyloid plaques are extracellular with a cross-beta structure that is characteristic of dye-binding (neuritic amyloid plaques contain thioflavin S and Congo red-positive

fibrillar deposits with both $A\beta40$ and $A\beta42$ present)[19,20]. The major component of amyloid plaques is amyloid beta ($A\beta$), which can be stained and detected using $A\beta$ antibodies[21,22]. The most common form of $A\beta$ in humans is 40–amino-acids long and is called $A\beta40$. A 42–amino-acid-long fragment, $A\beta42$, is less abundant than $A\beta40$ and differs only in that it has two additional amino-acid residues at the C-terminus. $A\beta42$ is associated with AD[23].

$A\beta$ is derived from the amyloid precursor protein (APP) by the action of two aspartyl proteases. First, α-secretase (non-neurotoxic 'normal' cleavage) or β-secretase (potential neurotoxic 'abnormal' cleavage) cleave APP (Figure 43.1) and second, γ-secretases cleave APP[24–26]. Upon cleavage by α-secretase, APP releases a large soluble APP alpha fragment (sAPPα) and a membrane-bound C-terminal 83–amino-acid fragment (C83); whereas upon cleavage by β-secretase, APP releases a large soluble APP beta fragment (sAPPβ) and a membrane-bound C-terminal 99–amino-acid fragment (C99)[27,28]. The C99 fragment is subsequently cleaved by γ-secretase to release $A\beta$ and an APP intracellular domain (AICD)[29,30] (Figure 43.1). Thus, depending on the point of cleavage

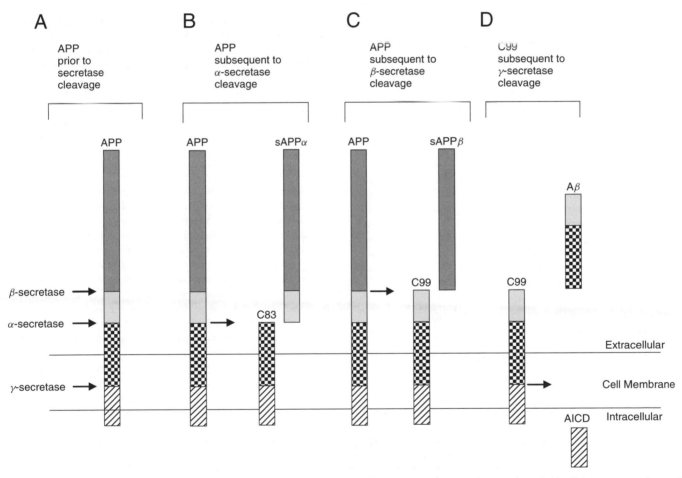

Figure 43.1 APP cleavage. The APP protein can be cleaved by three different secretases; α, β or γ (panel A). Subsequent to 'normal' α-secretase cleavage, sAPPα is produced and released into the extracellular space and the C83 peptide remains in the cell membrane (panel B). Subsequent to β-secretase cleavage, sAPPβ is produced and released into the extracellular space and the C99 peptide remains in the cell membrane (panel C). Subsequent to β-secretase cleavage, the C99 peptide is 'abnormally' cleaved by γ-secretase to yield an $A\beta$ peptide and the AICD peptide (panel D). Scale is approximate

Source: Reproduced from Bekris, Yu, Bird & Tsuang (2010). The Genetics of Alzheimer's and Parkinson's Disease. In: A. Lajtha (Ed.), Handbook of Neurochemistry and Molecular Neurobiology, 3rd edn. Neurochemical Mechanisms in Disease, Vol. 36. New York: Springer-Verlag. With kind permission of Springer Science+Business Media

by γ-secretase, two main forms of Aβ are produced, consisting of either 40 or 42–amino-acid residues (Aβ40 or Aβ42). The proportion of Aβ40 to Aβ42 that is formed is particularly important in AD because Aβ42 is far more prone to oligomerize and form fibrils than the more abundantly produced Aβ40 peptide. Indeed, although it appears that the production of Aβ isoforms is a normal process of unknown function, in a small number of individuals, an increased proportion of Aβ42 appears sufficient to cause EOAD[16,31].

Neurons bearing neurofibrillary tangles are another frequent finding in AD brains[32,33] and the temporal and spatial appearance of these tangles, which contain hyperphosphorylated tau, more closely reflects disease severity than does the presence of amyloid plaques[34,35]. Tangles are formed by hyperphosphorylation of a microtubule-associated protein known as tau, causing it to aggregate in an insoluble form. However, neurofibrillary tangles are also found in other disorders, such as frontotemporal dementia and progressive supranuclear palsy. Moreover, these tangles are not necessarily associated with the cognitive dysfunction and memory impairment that is typical of AD and mutations in the gene that encodes the tau protein (*MAPT*), a main component of neurofibrillary tangles, has not been genetically linked to AD[22].

GENETICS OF ALZHEIMER'S DISEASE

Introduction

Overall, more than 90% of AD cases appear to be sporadic and to have a later age at onset of 60 to 65 years (LOAD)[36]. Although twin studies support the existence of a genetic component in LOAD, no causative gene has been yet identified. Indeed, the only gene that has been consistently found to be associated with sporadic LOAD, across multiple genetic studies, is the apolipoprotein E (*APOE*) gene[37–41] (Table 43.1). However, many carriers of the *APOE* risk allele (ε4) live into their 90s, which suggests the existence of other LOAD genetic and/or environmental risk factors that have yet to be identified. To this end, several unreplicated genetic variants have been reported and these findings suggest that there may be five to seven major LOAD susceptibility genes[3,42,43]. For a catalogue of candidate gene association studies, please refer to the AlzGene online database (www.alzforum.org/res/com/gen/alzgene/default.asp).

Genes Associated with Autosomal Dominant Alzheimer's Disease

AD1: Amyloid precursor protein (APP)

Inheritance and clinical features   In the 1980s, Kang and colleagues purified both plaque and vascular amyloid deposits and isolated their 40-residue constituent peptide (Aβ), which subsequently led to the cloning of the *APP* type I integral membrane glycoprotein from which Aβ is proteolytically derived[44]. The *APP* gene was then mapped to chromosome 21q, which accounted for the observation that Down syndrome patients (trisomy 21) develop amyloid deposits and the neuropathological features of AD when in their 40s[22,45–47].

Since then, over 32 different *APP* missense mutations have been identified in 85 families. Interestingly, most of these mutations are located at the secretase cleavage sites or the *APP* transmembrane domain on exons 16 and 17 (Figure 43.2). Information regarding *APP* mutations are available in the NCBI database and the Alzheimer Disease Mutation Database (www.molgen.ua.ac.be/ADMutations)[48]. Mutations within *APP* account for 10% to 15% of early-onset familial AD (EOFAD)[3,49–51], appear to be family specific and do not occur within the majority of sporadic AD cases. The majority of these EOFAD mutations are in or adjacent to the Aβ peptide sequence (Figure 43.2), the major component of amyloid plaques[52,53]. Most cases containing *APP* mutations have an age of onset in the mid-40s and 50s[54].

Gene location and structure   Sequences encoding APP were first cloned by screening cDNA libraries[44]. The initial full-length cDNA clone encoded a 695–amino-acid protein (APP695)[40] and consisted of 18 exons. The *APP* gene, located on chromosome 21q21, is alternatively spliced into several products, named according to their length in amino-acids (i.e., APP695, APP714, APP751, APP770 and APP563) and expressed differentially by tissue type whereby the three isoforms that are most relevant to AD are restricted to the central nervous system (APP695) or expressed in both the peripheral and CNS tissues (APP751 and APP770)[44,55–61].

Gene function and expression   APP is a type-I integral-membrane protein[44] that resembles a signal-transduction receptor. It is expressed in many tissues and concentrated in the synapses of neurons. Its primary function is not known, though it has been implicated in neural plasticity[62] and as a regulator of synapse formation[63]. APP is synthesized in the endoplasmic reticulum, post-transcriptionally modified in the golgi (N- and O-linked glycosylation, sulfation and phosphorylation) and transported to the cell surface via the secretory pathway. APP is also endocytosed from the cell surface and processed in the endosomal-lysosomal pathway[64,65]. APP and its byproduct Aβ have been found to be translocated inside mitochondria and implicated in mitochondrial dysfunction[66–68].

Proteolysis of APP by α-secretase or β-secretase leads to the secretion of sAPPα or sAPPβ. This proteolysis generates C-terminal fragments of 10 kDa and 12 kDa, respectively, which are inserted into the membrane. These fragments can be cut by γ-secretase to

Table 43.1 Alzheimer's disease (AD) genes. AD genes are located on four different chromosomes and are associated with autosomal dominant or sporadic inheritance

AD loci	Gene symbol	Gene name	Chromosome	Inheritance
AD1	APP	Amyloid Precursor Protein	21q21	Autosomal Dominant
AD2	APOE	Apolipoprotein E	19q13.32	Sporadic
AD3	PSEN1	Presenilin 1	14q24.2	Autosomal Dominant
AD4	PSEN2	Presenilin 2	1q42.13	Autosomal Dominant

Source: Reproduced from Bekris, Yu, Bird & Tsuang (2010). The Genetics of Alzheimer's and Parkinson's Disease. In: A. Lajtha (Ed.), Handbook of Neurochemistry and Molecular Neurobiology, 3rd edn. Neurochemical Mechanisms in Disease, Vol. 36. New York: Springer-Verlag, Table 1. With kind permission of Springer Science+Business Media

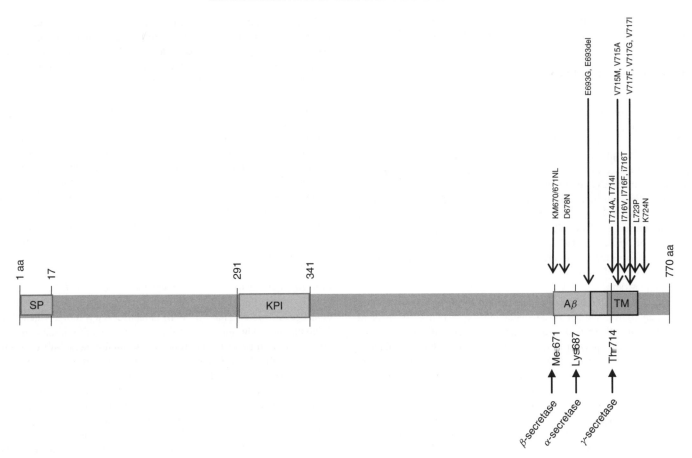

Figure 43.2 AD1: *APP* structure and mutations. SP: Signal peptide. KPI: Kunitz protease inhibitor domain. Aβ: Amyloid beta. TM: Transmembrane domain. Scale is approximate

Source: Reproduced from Bekris, Yu, Bird & Tsuang (2010). The Genetics of Alzheimer's and Parkinson's Disease. In: A. Lajtha (Ed.), Handbook of Neurochemistry and Molecular Neurobiology, 3rd edn. Neurochemical Mechanisms in Disease, Vol. 36. New York: Springer-Verlag. With kind permission of Springer Science+Business Media

extracellularly release the Aβ peptide[69] and intracellularly release a cytoplasmic fragment identified as AICD[70] (Figure 43.1). The majority of EOFAD mutations alter this processing of *APP* in such a way that Aβ42 levels are changed relative to other Aβ isoform levels[71,72]. The function of these *APP* proteolytic fragments is still unclear.

The missense *APP* 'Swedish' mutations (*APP*SW, *APP*K670N, M671L) and the 'London' mutations (*APP*LON, *APP*V717I) are examples of *APP* mutations that lead to increased Aβ production and development of AD[73,74]. Transgenic mouse models of such *APP* mutations (PDAPP, Tg2576, APP23, TgCRND8 and J20) have been developed[75]. Each of these mouse models have different APP expression levels and different neurological abnormalities[75,76]. For example, the Tg2576 mouse model that carries the 'Swedish' mutation has high *APP* levels, high Aβ levels and cognitive disturbances[77] that are progressive and start as early as six months of age[78].

Genetic variation   *APP* transcripts have been identified in which exons 7, 8 and 15 are alternatively spliced. *APP695*, the predominant isoform in neurons[79], contains exon 15 but excludes exons 7 and 8. The *APP751* isoform and the *APP770* isoform both encode Kunitz-type protease inhibitor (KPI)-containing forms of *APP*[58–60,80,], are present in both peripheral tissue and neurons and contain exon 16 and 17 but exclude exons 7, 8 and 15. The gene region that encodes the portion of *APP* that is cleaved to produce the Aβ peptide is located

within exons 16 and 17 of the *APP770* splice variant[81] (Figure 43.2). Other splice variants have been observed that are missing exon 15 in various combinations with exons 7 and 8; these splice variants are referred to as L-*APP*s[80,82]. A number of studies have indicated that alternative splicing of exons 7 and 8 is modulated in brain during ageing and possibly during AD[82–87]. Even though the function of *APP* and its various splice variants is unknown, differential expression of these splice variants between tissues may imply functional differences. It is important to note that while most of the described splice variants contain Aβ-encoding sequences, two additional rare transcripts, APP365 and APP563 do not, implicating additional functionally important variability in *APP* isoform function[55,88].

The first described and best characterized *APP* mutation (V717I) is located within the transmembrane domain near the γ-secretase cleavage site[73] (Figure 43.2). Other substitutions have since been identified at this site and several groups have reported the V717I mutation in families who are unrelated to the initial London family. Many other *APP* mutations have since been identified, especially near the γ-secretase cleavage site, and the bulk of these mutations have been associated with modulation of Aβ levels. For example, a C-terminal L723P mutation was identified in an Australian family; this mutation is reported to generate an increase of Aβ42 peptide levels in CHO cells[89]. The majority of EOFAD mutations alter processing of APP in such a way that the relative level of Aβ42 is increased by increasing Aβ42, decreasing Aβ40 peptide levels or increasing Aβ42 while decreasing Aβ40 peptide levels[71,72].

AD3: Presenilin 1 (PSEN1)

Inheritance and clinical features   Linkage studies established the presence of an AD3 locus on chromosome 14[90], and positional cloning led to the identification of mutations in the presenilin-1 (*PSEN1*) gene, which encodes a polytopic membrane protein[91]. Presenilins are major components of the atypical aspartyl protease complexes that are responsible for the γ-secretase cleavage of *APP*[92,93]. Mutations in *PSEN1* are the most common cause of EOFAD. Indeed, *PSEN1* missense mutations account for 18% to 50% of autosomal dominant EOFAD cases[94]. Over 176 different *PSEN1* mutations have been identified in 390 families. *PSEN1* mutations appear to increase the ratio of Aβ42 to Aβ40 and thereby result in a change in function that leads to reduced γ-secretase activity[95]. It has been suggested that deposition of Aβ42 may be an early preclinical event in *PSEN1* mutation carriers[96].

Defects in *PSEN1* cause the most severe forms of AD, with complete penetrance and an onset occurring as early as 30 years of age. However, there is a wide variability in age of onset as other *PSEN1*-associated AD cases have a mean age of onset greater than 58 years. *PSEN1*-associated AD is an autosomal dominant neurodegenerative disorder characterized by progressive dementia and parkinsonism, notch signalling modulation and Aβ intracellular domain generation[16,97]. There is also considerable phenotypic variability in *PSEN1*-associated AD cases, including some patients who develop spastic paraparesis and other atypical AD symptoms. Some of these variable clinical phenotypes have been associated with specific mutations. Neuropathological studies often confirm the clinical diagnosis of AD with measurement of amyloid plaque and Braak stage (as described above) as well as other neurodegenerative changes in other brain areas according to the presence of specific *PSEN1* mutations[98,99]. For example, researchers found that the clinical and neuropathological features of a Greek family with a *PSEN1* mutation (N135S) included memory loss when the family members were in their 30s, as well as variable limb spasticity and seizures. Upon neuropathological examination of these family members, the diagnosis of AD was confirmed and there was also histological evidence of corticospinal tract degeneration[99]. Moreover, a *PSEN1* mutation (I143M) that lies in a cluster in the second transmembrane domain of the protein has been described in an African family with an age at onset in the early 50s and a short duration of illness of six to seven years. These family members were diagnosed upon autopsy with severe AD pathology characterized by neuronal loss, abundant Aβ neuritic plaques and neurofibrillary tangles and degeneration extending into the brain stem[100].

Gene location and structure   *PSEN1* is located on chromosome 14q24.2. It consists of 12 exons that encode a 467–amino-acid protein that is predicted to traverse the membrane 6 to 10 times; the amino and carboxyl termini are both oriented toward the cytoplasm[101].

Gene function and expression   *PSEN1* is a polytopic membrane protein that forms the catalytic core of the γ-secretase complex[92,102]. Gamma-secretase is an integral membrane protein typically found at the cell surface, but it may also be found in the golgi, endoplasmic reticulum and mitochondria[92,103].

PSEN1, nicastrin (Nct), anterior pharynx defective 1 (Aph-1) and presenilin enhancer 2 (PSENEN) are required for the stability and activity of the γ-secretase complex[104–108]. This complex cleaves many type-I transmembrane proteins, including APP and Notch[92,109], two proteins in the hydrophobic environment of the phospholipid bilayer of the membrane[107].

PSEN1 knockout (KO) mice are not viable[110] but a conditional *PSEN1* KO mouse model, where the loss of the gene is limited to the postnatal forebrain, found that KO mice exhibited mild cognitive impairments in long-term spatial reference memory and retention[111]. These findings suggest that presenilins play a role in cognitive memory. Moreover, knockin mice with missense mutations of the endogenous murine *PSEN1* have high Aβ42 levels and perform poorly on the object recognition test[112,113]. Double *PSEN1/APP* transgenics have been developed and these transgenic suggest that *PSEN1*, *APP* and mutations within these genes play a role in the production of Aβ[76,114].

Genetic variation   To date, there have been 176 *PSEN1* mutations reported (Figure 43.3). A comprehensive list of *PSEN1* mutations is available through the NCBI database (www.molgen.ua.ac.be/ADmutations). The majority of these mutations are missense mutations. These missense mutations cause amino-acid substitutions throughout the *PSEN1* protein and appear to result in a relative increase in the ratio of Aβ42 to Aβ40 peptides; this increase seems to occur through increased Aβ42 production, decreased Aβ40 production, or alternatively, a combination of increased Aβ42 production and decreased Aβ40 production[71]. For example, individuals that carry the *PSEN1* L166P mutation can have an age at onset in adolescence, and *in vitro* studies indicate that this mutation induces exceptionally high levels of Aβ42 production as well as impaired notch intracellular domain production and notch signalling[98].

AD4: Presenilin 2 (PSEN2)

Inheritance and clinical features   A candidate gene for the chromosome 1 AD4 locus was identified in 1995 in a Volga German AD kindred with a high homology to the AD3 locus (*PSEN1*); this gene was later named presenilin 2 (*PSEN2*)[51,115,116]. In contrast to the mutations in the *PSEN1* gene, missense mutations in the *PSEN2* gene are a rare cause of EOFAD, at least in Caucasian populations. The clinical features of *PSEN2*-affected families appear to differ from the clinical features of *PSEN1*-affected families in that the age of onset in these family members is generally older (45–88 years) than for some family members with *PSEN1* mutations (25–65 years). Furthermore, the age of onset is highly variable among *PSEN2*-affected members of the same family, whereas in families with *PSEN1* mutations, the age of onset is generally quite similar among affected family members, and it is even similar among people from different families with the same mutation[5,51,91,116]. Missense mutations in the *PSEN2* gene may be of lower penetrance than in the *PSEN1* gene and therefore may be subject to the modifying action of other genes or environmental influences[51,117].

Gene location and structure   The *PSEN2* gene is located on chromosome 1 (1q42.13) and was identified by sequence homology and then cloned[115,116]. *PSEN2* has 12 exons and is organized into 10 translated exons that encode a 448–amino-acid peptide. The PSEN2 protein is predicted to consist of nine transmembrane domains

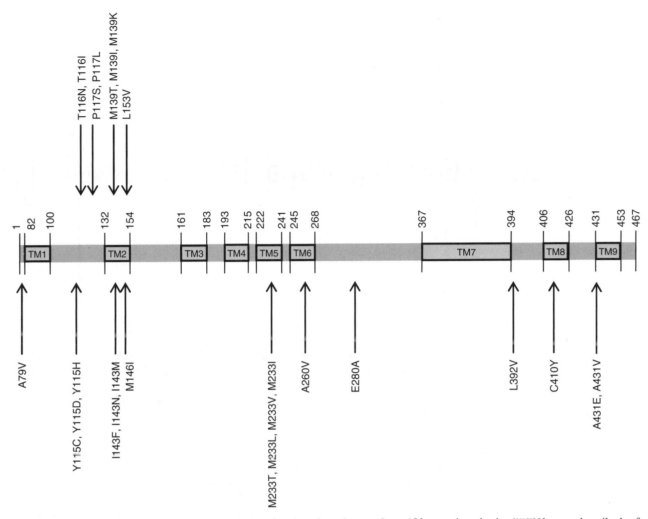

Figure 43.3 AD3: *PSEN1* structure and mutations. Thus far, there have been at least 123 mutations in the *PSEN1* gene described, of which a few are shown. For a more complete list of *PSEN1* mutations see www.molgen.ua.ac.be/ADMutations. TM: Transmembrane domains. Scale is approximate

Source: Reproduced from Bekris, Yu, Bird & Tsuang (2010). The Genetics of Alzheimer's and Parkinson's Disease. In: A. Lajtha (Ed.), Handbook of Neurochemistry and Molecular Neurobiology, 3rd edn. Neurochemical Mechanisms in Disease, Vol. 36. New York: Springer-Verlag. With kind permission of Springer Science+Business Media

and a large loop structure between the sixth and seventh domains (Figure 43.4). *PSEN2* also displays tissue-specific alternative splicing[115,116,118–120].

Gene function and expression

Like PSEN1, PSEN2 has been described as a component of the atypical aspartyl protease called γ-secretase, which is responsible for the cleavage of $A\beta$[92,93]. *PSEN2* is expressed in a variety of tissues, including the brain, where it is expressed primarily in neurons[121]. *PSEN2*-associated mutations have been reported to increase the ratio of $A\beta42$ to $A\beta40$ ($A\beta42/A\beta40$) in mice and humans[71,95], indicating that presenilins might modify the way in which γ-secretase cuts APP.

APP processing at the γ-secretase site has been reported to be differentially affected by specific presenilin mutations. For example, *PSEN1*-L166P mutations cause a reduction in $A\beta$ production whereas *PSEN1*-G384A mutations significantly increase $A\beta42$. In contrast, *PSEN2* appears to be a less efficient producer of $A\beta$ than *PSEN1*[23]. The functions and biological importance of presenilin

splice variants are poorly understood, but it appears that differential expression of presenilin isoforms may lead to differential regulation of the proteolytic processing of the APP protein. For example, aberrant *PSEN2* transcripts lacking exon 5 appear to increase the rate of production of $A\beta$ peptide[122], whereas naturally occurring isoforms without exons 3 and 4 and/or without exon 8 do not affect production of $A\beta$[123].

Genetic variation

Mutations in *PSEN2* are a much rarer cause of familial AD than are *PSEN1* mutations; *PSEN2* mutations have been described in six families, including the Volga-German kindred where a founder effect has been demonstrated[48,51,115,116], whereas *PSEN1* mutations have been found in 390 families. To date as many as 14 *PSEN2* mutations have been identified. One of the first mutations to be identified was a point mutation located within the second transmembrane domain that resulted in the substitution of an isoleucine for an asparagine at residues 141 (N141I)[115]. Most recently, a V393M mutation

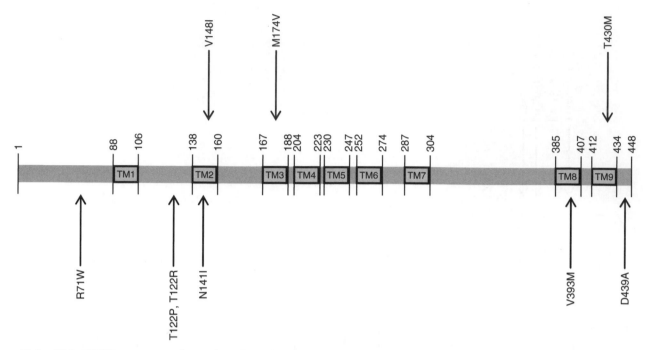

Figure 43.4 AD4: *PSEN2* structure and mutations. Thus far, there have been at least 16 mutations in the *PSEN2* gene described, of which a few are shown. For a more complete list of *PSEN2* mutations see www.molgen.ua.ac.be/ADMutations. TM: Transmembrane domains. The V393M novel mutation was most recently found in one case[124]. Scale is approximate

Source: Reproduced from Bekris, Yu, Bird & Tsuang (2010). The Genetics of Alzheimer's and Parkinson's Disease. In: A. Lajtha (Ed.), Handbook of Neurochemistry and Molecular Neurobiology, 3rd edn. Neurochemical Mechanisms in Disease, Vol. 36. New York: Springer-Verlag. With kind permission of Springer Science+Business Media

located within the seventh transmembrane domain has been described[124] (Figure 43.4). A comprehensive list of *PSEN2* mutations is available through the NCBI database (www.molgen.ua.ac.be/ADmutations).

Genes Associated with Risk in Sporadic Alzheimer's Disease

AD2: APOE

Inheritance and clinical features   The *APOE* gene has been associated with both familial late-onset and sporadic late-onset AD in numerous studies of multiple ethnic groups. The *APOE* ε4 genotype is associated with higher risk of AD[125], earlier age of onset of both AD[126] and Down syndrome (where there is an additional copy of chromosome 21 carrying the *APP* gene)[127] and a worse outcome after head trauma[128] and stroke, both in humans[129] and in transgenic mice expressing human apoE4[130]. The frequency of the *APOE* ε4 allele varies between ethnic groups, but regardless of ethnic group, *APOE* ε4-carriers are more frequently found in controls, and *APOE* ε4+ carriers are more frequently found in AD patients[39–41,131–140].

Gene location and structure   The *APOE* gene is located on chromosome 19q13.2 and consists of four exons that encode a 299–amino-acid protein. The *APOE* gene is in a cluster with other apolipoprotein genes: *APOC1*, *APOC2* and *APOC4*. The *APOE* ε4 loci are located within exon 4 of the gene. The three *APOE* ε4 alleles (ε2, ε3 and ε4) are defined by two single nucleotide polymorphisms, rs429358 and rs7412, which encode three protein

isoforms (E2, E3 and E4). The most frequent apoE isoform is apoE3, which contains cysteine and arginine at amino-acid positions 112 and 158. In contrast, these positions contain only cysteine residues in apoE2 and only arginine residues in apoE4 (Figure 43.5). The cysteine-arginine substitution affects the three-dimensional structure and the lipid-binding properties between isoforms. In apoE4, the amino-acid substitution results in the formation of a salt bridge between an arginine in position 61 and a glutamic acid in 255; whereas apoE3 and apoE2 bind preferentially to high-density lipoproteins (HDLs), this changed structure causes the apoE4 isoform to bind preferentially to very low-density lipoproteins (VLDLs)[141].

Gene function and expression   The mechanisms that govern apoE toxicity in brain tissue are not fully understood. Some proposed mechanisms include isoform-specific toxicity, *APOE* ε4-mediated amyloid aggregation and *APOE* ε4-mediated tau hyperphosphorylation[142].

The *APOE* polymorphism is unique to humans and has been proposed to have evolved as a result of adaptive changes to diet[143,144]. It is known that apoE plays an important role in the distribution and metabolism of cholesterol and triglycerides within many organs and cell types in the human body[141]. Individuals carrying *APOE* ε4 have higher total and LDL cholesterol[145]. Moreover, *in vitro* neurons have a cholesterol uptake that is lower when lipid are bound to apoE4 compared to apoE2 and apoE3[146], and apoE4 appears to be less efficient than the other isoforms in promoting cholesterol efflux from both neurons and astrocytes[147].

As the major apolipoprotein of the chylomicron in the brain, apoE binds to a specific receptor and works through receptor-mediated

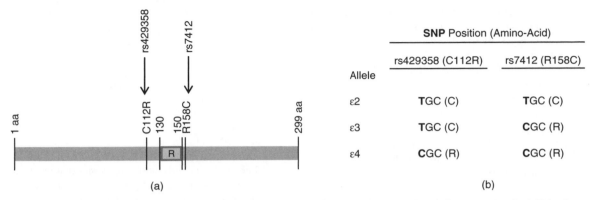

	SNP Position (Amino-Acid)	
Allele	rs429358 (C112R)	rs7412 (R158C)
ε2	**T**GC (C)	**T**GC (C)
ε3	**T**GC (C)	**C**GC (R)
ε4	**C**GC (R)	**C**GC (R)

Figure 43.5 AD2: *APOE* structure and single nucleotide polymorphisms (SNPs). The general protein structure of apoE is shown . The two SNPs and corresponding protein locations are shown (rs429358 and rs7412; C112R and R158C) (panel A). R: Receptor binding domain. Scale is approximate. The *APOE* ε2, ε3, ε4 haplotype is shown in panel B

Source: Reproduced from Bekris, Yu, Bird & Tsuang (2010). The Genetics of Alzheimer's and Parkinson's Disease. In: A. Lajtha (Ed.), Handbook of Neurochemistry and Molecular Neurobiology, 3rd edn. Neurochemical Mechanisms in Disease, Vol. 36. New York: Springer-Verlag. With kind permission of Springer Science+Business Media

endocytosis to rapidly remove chylomicron and VLDL remnants from circulation; this process is essential for the normal catabolism of triglyceride-rich lipoprotein constituents[148]. In the brain, lipidated apoE binds aggregated Aβ in an apoE isoform-specific manner, with apoE4 being much more effective than the apoE3 isoform. Researchers have also proposed that the more efficient binding process of apoE4 enhances the deposition of the Aβ peptide[149].

Brain cells from *APOE* knockout (*APOE*-/-) mice are more sensitive to excitotoxic and age-related synaptic loss[150], and Aβ-induced synaptosomal dysfunction in these mice is also enhanced compared to control animals[151]. When human apoE isoforms (apoE3 and apoE4) are expressed in *APOE*-/- mice, the expression of apoE3, but not apoE4, is protective against age-related neurodegeneration[150] and Aβ toxicity[151]. In addition, astrocytes from *APOE*-/- mice that express human apoE3 release more cholesterol than those expressing apoE4; this suggests that apoE isoforms may modulate the amount of lipid available for neurons. Other studies report apoE-specific effects on Aβ removal from the extracellular space whereby the apoE3 isoform has a higher Aβ-binding capacity than apoE4[152,153]. Animal and *in vitro* models show that, in the brain, astrocytes and microglia are the main producers of secreted apoE[154,155]. ApoE secretion in human primary astrocytes can be reduced by a combination of cytokines[156]; whereas under stress conditions, neurons appear to be the main producers of apoE[157,158]. In a rodent model, moderate injury has been shown to induce enhancement of apoE levels in clusters of CA1 and CA3 pyramidal neurons[159] and in another rodent model, apoE levels have been shown to increase in response to peripheral nerve injury[161].

In addition, individuals carrying *APOE* ε4 have higher amyloid and tangle pathology[160] and an increase in mitochondrial damage[162] compared to those carrying other *APOE* polymorphisms.

Genetic variation   The gene dose of *APOE* ε4 is a major risk factor for AD, with many studies reporting an association between gene dose, age at onset[163] and cognitive decline[164]. After age 65, the risk of AD among individuals with a family member with AD increases depending on the number of ε4 alleles present in the affected individual. Risks to family members with the *APOE* 2/2 and 2/3 genotypes are nearly identical at all ages to risks for family

members with the *APOE* 3/3 genotype. Among family members with *APOE* 3/3, the lifetime risk for AD by age 90 can be as much as three times greater than the expected risk found in *APOE* ε4 carriers, suggesting that factors other than *APOE* contribute to AD risk. In addition, a 44% risk of AD by age 93 among family members of *APOE* 4/4 carriers indicates that as many as 50% of people having at least one ε4 allele do not develop AD. There also appears to be a gender modification effect because the risk to male family members with *APOE* 3/4 is similar to that for the *APOE* 3/3 carriers but is significantly less than the risk for the *APOE* 4/4 carriers, whereas among female family members, the risk for the *APOE* 3/4 carriers is nearly twice that for the *APOE* 3/3 carriers[131,133–140].

SUMMARY

AD is characterized by an irreversible, progressive loss of memory and cognitive skills that can occur in rare familial cases as early as the third decade. Currently, there is no cure for AD, and treatments only manage to slow down the progression of AD progression in some patients[10,11]. The early-onset familial forms of AD have an autosomal dominant inheritance linked to three genes: *APP, PSEN1* and *PSEN2*, whereas the most common sporadic form of AD, which occurs after the age of 60, has thus far been consistently, across numerous studies, associated with only one gene, the *APOE* gene. The mechanistic contribution of these genes in AD pathogenesis has been studied extensively, but the specific biology involved in the progression of AD remains unclear, suggesting that AD is a genetic and environmentally complex disease.

GENETIC TESTING AND COUNSELLING

APOE ε4 is most highly associated with AD for individuals with a family history of dementia and this association is highest for individuals that carry two *APOE* ε4 alleles (ε4/ε4 genotypes). The ε4/ε4 genotype is uncommon and although the ethnicity of the population may alter the expected prevalence, the genotype occurs in about 1% of normal Caucasian controls. In contrast, the ε4/ε4 genotype occurs in nearly 19% of familial LOAD populations. *APOE* ε4-associated risk is also found in African Americans and Caribbean Hispanics[165,166]. Women with an *APOE* ε4/ε4 genotype have a 45% probability of developing AD by age 73 years[167], whereas men have a 25% risk of developing AD by that age[168]. AD risk is also lower for individuals with only one *APOE* ε4 allele (by age 87) or no *APOE* ε4 allele (by age 95)[168]. Approximately 42% of persons with LOAD do not have an *APOE* ε4 allele[169]. Thus, the absence of the *APOE* ε4 allele does not rule out a LOAD diagnosis. First-degree relatives of a person with LOAD have a cumulative lifetime risk of approximately 20% to 25%, whereas the risk in the general population is 10.4%[134,170]. It is still not known whether the age of onset of a LOAD patient changes the risk to first-degree relatives of LOAD patients. But the number of additional affected family members most likely increases the risk to close relatives[171]. Given the low predictive value of the *APOE* ε4 allele, the general consensus is that *APOE* genetic testing has limited value in asymptomatic persons for predicting AD risk[172,173]. Family history may therefore be a better predictor of LOAD risk[171].

In contrast, EOFAD, with an age at onset before 60 to 65 years old, has an autosomal dominant mode of inheritance in which 20% to 70% of cases are estimated to have a *PSEN1* mutation, 10% to 15% of cases are estimated to have an *APP* mutation and *PSEN2* mutations are rare[172,174]. Indeed, approximately 60% of patients with EOAD have another known affected family member. The remaining 40% of EOAD patients may lack a family history because of an early death of a parent, failure to recognize the disorder in family members, or, very rarely, a *de novo* mutation[5]. If an EOAD patient's parent has a mutant allele, then the risk to the patient's sibling of inheriting the mutant allele is 50%. The child of an EOAD patient who carries a mutation (*APP, PSEN1*, or *PSEN2*) has a 50% chance of transmitting the mutant allele to each of their children.

Testing of asymptomatic adults who are at risk for EOAD caused by mutations in the *PSEN1, PSEN2*, or *APP* genes is available clinically. However, genetic testing results for at-risk asymptomatic adults can only be interpreted after the disease-causing mutation has first been identified in the affected family member. It should be emphasized that testing of asymptomatic at-risk individuals with non specific or equivocal symptoms is predictive not diagnostic. In addition, obtaining results from genetic testing can affect an individual's personal relationships as well as their emotional well-being and it may even cause depression. The principal arguments against testing asymptomatic individuals during childhood are that the testing then removes their choice to know or not know this information, it raises the possibility of stigmatization within the family and in other social settings and it could have serious educational and career implications. Thus, the general consensus is that individuals who are at risk for adult-onset disorders should not be tested during childhood. Prenatal genetic testing for mutations in the *PSEN1* gene is possible if the *PSEN1* allele has been identified in an affected family member first. Preimplantation genetic diagnosis is also available for families that have a disease-causing mutation. However, parental requests for prenatal or preimplantation genetic testing of adult-onset diseases is rare[3].

REFERENCES

1. Ferri CP, Prince M, Brayne C, Brodaty H, Fratiglioni L, Ganguli M *et al*. Global prevalence of dementia: a Delphi consensus study. *Lancet* 2005; **366**: 2112–17.

2. Kukull WA, Higdon R, Bowen JD, McCormick WC, Teri L, Schellenberg GD *et al*. Dementia and Alzheimer disease incidence: a prospective cohort study. *Arch Neurol* 2002; **59**: 1737–46.

3. Bird TD. Genetic aspects of Alzheimer disease. *Genet Med* 2008; **10**: 231–9.

4. Brickell KL, Steinbart EJ, Rumbaugh M, Payami H, Schellenberg GD, Van Deerlin V *et al*. Early-onset Alzheimer disease in families with late-onset Alzheimer disease: a potential important subtype of familial Alzheimer disease. *Arch Neurol* 2006; **63**: 1307–11.

5. Campion D, Dumanchin C, Hannequin D, Dubois B, Belliard S, Puel M *et al*. Early-onset autosomal dominant Alzheimer disease: prevalence, genetic heterogeneity and mutation spectrum. *Am J Hum Genet* 1999; **65**: 664–70.

6. Bertram L, Tanzi RE. The current status of Alzheimer's disease genetics: what do we tell the patients? *Pharmacol Res* 2004; **50**: 385–96.

7. Kamboh MI. Molecular genetics of late-onset Alzheimer's disease. *Ann Hum Genet* 2004; **68**: 381–404.

8. Roses AD. On the discovery of the genetic association of Apolipoprotein E genotypes and common late-onset Alzheimer disease. *J Alzheimers Dis* 2006; **9**: 361–6.

9. Serretti A, Artioli P, Quartesan R, De Ronchi D. Genes involved in Alzheimer's disease, a survey of possible candidates. *J Alzheimers Dis* 2005; **7**: 331–53.

10. Raina P, Santaguida P, Ismaila A, Patterson C, Cowan D, Levine M *et al*. Effectiveness of cholinesterase inhibitors and memantine for treating dementia: evidence review for a clinical practice guideline. *Ann Intern Med* 2008; **148**: 379–97.

11. Raschetti R, Albanese E, Vanacore N, Maggini M. Cholinesterase inhibitors in mild cognitive impairment: a systematic review of randomised trials. *PLoS Med* 2007; **4**: e338.

12. Kawas CH. Clinical practice. Early Alzheimer's disease. *N Engl J Med* 2003; **349**: 1056–63.

13. Rogan S, Lippa CF. Alzheimer's disease and other dementias: a review. *Am J Alzheimers Dis Other Demen* 2002; **17**: 11–17.

14. Petersen RC, Doody R, Kurz A, Mohs RC, Morris JC, Rabins PV *et al*. Current concepts in mild cognitive impairment. *Arch Neurol* 2001; **58**: 1985–92.

15. Braak H, Braak E. Frequency of stages of Alzheimer-related lesions in different age categories. *Neurobiol Aging* 1997; **18**: 351–7.

16. Goedert M, Spillantini MG. A century of Alzheimer's disease. *Science* 2006; **314**: 777–81.

17. Nussbaum RL, Ellis CE. Alzheimer's disease and Parkinson's disease. *N Engl J Med* 2003; **348**: 1356–64.

18. Kaye JA. Diagnostic challenges in dementia. *Neurology* 1998; **51**: S45–52; discussion S65–47.

19. Kidd M. Paired helical filaments in electron microscopy of Alzheimer's disease. *Nature* 1963; **197**: 192–3.

20. Terry RD, Gonatas NK, Weiss M. Ultrastructural studies in Alzheimer's presenile dementia. *Am J Pathol* 1964; **44**: 269–97.

21. Glenner GG, Wong CW, Quaranta V, Eanes ED. The amyloid deposits in Alzheimer's disease: their nature and pathogenesis. *Appl Pathol* 1984; **2**: 357–69.

22. Iwatsubo T, Odaka A, Suzuki N, Mizusawa H, Nukina N, Ihara Y. Visualization of A beta 42(43) and A beta 40 in senile plaques with end-specific A beta monoclonals: evidence that

an initially deposited species is A beta 42(43). *Neuron* 1994; **13**: 45–53.

23. Bentahir M, Nyabi O, Verhamme J, Tolia A, Horre K, Wiltfang J *et al*. Presenilin clinical mutations can affect gamma-secretase activity by different mechanisms. *J Neurochem* 2006; **96**: 732–42.

24. Haass C, Koo EH, Mellon A, Hung AY, Selkoe DJ. Targeting of cell-surface beta-amyloid precursor protein to lysosomes: alternative processing into amyloid-bearing fragments. *Nature* 1992; **357**: 500–3.

25. Seubert P, Vigo-Pelfrey C, Esch F, Lee M, Dovey H, Davis D *et al*. Isolation and quantification of soluble Alzheimer's beta-peptide from biological fluids. *Nature* 1992; **359**: 325–7.

26. Shoji M, Golde TE, Ghiso J, Cheung TT, Estus S, Shaffer LM *et al*. Production of the Alzheimer amyloid beta protein by normal proteolytic processing. *Science* 1992; **258**: 126–9.

27. Cai H, Wang Y, McCarthy D, Wen H, Borchelt DR, Price DL, Wong PC. BACE1 is the major beta-secretase for generation of Abeta peptides by neurons. *Nat Neurosci* 2001; **4**: 233–4.

28. Vassar R, Bennett BD, Babu-Khan S, Kahn S, Mendiaz EA, Denis P *et al*. Beta-secretase cleavage of Alzheimer's amyloid precursor protein by the transmembrane aspartic protease BACE. *Science* 1999; **286**: 735–41.

29. De Strooper B. Alzheimer's disease. Closing in on gamma-secretase. *Nature* 2000; **405**: 627, 629.

30. Schroeter EH, Ilagan MX, Brunkan AL, Hecimovic S, Li YM, Xu M *et al*. A presenilin dimer at the core of the gamma-secretase enzyme: insights from parallel analysis of Notch 1 and APP proteolysis. *Proc Natl Acad Sci USA* 2003; **100**: 13075–80.

31. Irvine GB, El-Agnaf OM, Shankar GM, Walsh DM. Protein aggregation in the brain: the molecular basis for Alzheimer's and Parkinson's diseases. *Mol Med* 2008; **14**: 451–64.

32. Kosik KS, Bakalis SF, Selkoe DJ, Pierce MW, Duffy LK. High molecular weight microtubule-associated proteins: purification by electro-elution and amino-acid compositions. *J Neurosci Res* 1986; **15**: 543–51.

33. Wood JG, Mirra SS, Pollock NJ, Binder LI. Neurofibrillary tangles of Alzheimer disease share antigenic determinants with the axonal microtubule-associated protein tau (tau). *Proc Natl Acad Sci USA* 1986; **83**: 4040–3.

34. Braak H, Braak E. Demonstration of amyloid deposits and neurofibrillary changes in whole brain sections. *Brain Pathol* 1991; **1**: 213–16.

35. Thal DR, Capetillo-Zarate E, Del Tredici K, Braak H. The development of amyloid beta protein deposits in the aged brain. *Sci Aging Knowledge Environ* 2006; **6**: re1, Review.

36. Bertram L, Tanzi RE. Alzheimer's disease: one disorder, too many genes? *Hum Mol Genet* 2004; **13**: R135–41.

37. Coon KD, Myers AJ, Craig DW, Webster JA, Pearson JV, Lince DH *et al*. A high-density whole-genome association study reveals that APOE is the major susceptibility gene for sporadic late-onset Alzheimer's disease. *J Clin Psychiatry* 2007; **68**: 613–18.

38. Couzin J. Genetics. Once shunned, test for Alzheimer's risk headed to market. *Science* 2008; **319**: 1022–3.

39. Roses AD, Saunders AM, Alberts MA, Strittmatter WJ, Schmechel D, Gorder E *et al*. Apolipoprotein E E4 allele and risk of dementia. *JAMA* 1995; **273**: 374–5; author reply 375–6.

40. Schellenberg GD. Genetic dissection of Alzheimer disease, a heterogeneous disorder. *Proc Natl Acad Sci USA* 1995; **92**: 8552–9.

41. Selkoe D. Alzheimer's disease: genes, proteins, and therapy. *Physiol Rev* 2001; **81**: 741–66.

42. Chai CK. The genetics of Alzheimer's disease. *Am J Alzheimers Dis Other Demen* 2007; **22**: 37–41.

43. Daw EW, Payami H, Nemens EJ, Nochlin D, Bird TD, Schellenberg GD *et al*. The number of trait loci in late-onset Alzheimer disease. *Am J Hum Genet* 2000; **66**: 196–204.

44. Kang J, Lemaire HG, Unterbeck A, Salbaum JM, Masters CL, Grzeschik KH *et al*. The precursor of Alzheimer's disease amyloid A4 protein resembles a cell-surface receptor. *Nature* 1987; 325: 733–6.

45. Giaccone G, Tagliavini F, Linoli G, Bouras C, Frigerio L, Frangione B *et al*. Down patients: extracellular preamyloid deposits precede neuritic degeneration and senile plaques. *Neurosci Lett* 1989; **97**: 232–8.

46. Lemere CA, Blusztajn JK, Yamaguchi H, Wisniewski T, Saido TC, Selkoe DJ. Sequence of deposition of heterogeneous amyloid beta-peptides and APO E in Down syndrome: implications for initial events in amyloid plaque formation. *Neurobiol Dis* 1996; **3**: 16–32.

47. Mann DM, Prinja D, Davies CA, Ihara Y, Delacourte A, Defossez A *et al*. Immunocytochemical profile of neurofibrillary tangles in Down's syndrome patients of different ages. *J Neurol Sci* 1989; **92**: 247–60.

48. Cruts M, Van Broeckhoven C. Molecular genetics of Alzheimer's disease. *Ann Med* 1998; **30**: 560–5.

49. Janssen JC, Beck JA, Campbell TA, Dickinson A, Fox NC, Harvey RJ *et al*. Early onset familial Alzheimer's disease: Mutation frequency in 31 families. *Neurology* 2003; **60**: 235–9.

50. Raux G, Guyant-Marechal L, Martin C, Bou J, Penet C, Brice A *et al*. Molecular diagnosis of autosomal dominant early onset Alzheimer's disease: an update. *J Med Genet* 2005; **42**: 793–5.

51. Sherrington R, Froelich S, Sorbi S, Campion D, Chi H, Rogaeva EA *et al*. Alzheimer's disease associated with mutations in presenilin 2 is rare and variably penetrant. *Hum Mol Genet* 1996; **5**: 985–8.

52. Esler WP, Wolfe MS. A portrait of Alzheimer secretases–new features and familiar faces. *Science* 2001; **293**: 1449–54.

53. Suzuki N, Cheung TT, Cai XD, Odaka A, Otvos L, Jr., Eckman C *et al*. An increased percentage of long amyloid beta protein secreted by familial amyloid beta protein precursor (beta APP717) mutants. *Science* 1994; **264**: 1336–40.

54. Hardy J. The genetic causes of neurodegenerative diseases. *J Alzheimers Dis* 2001; **3**: 109–16.

55. de Sauvage F, Octave JN. A novel mRNA of the A4 amyloid precursor gene coding for a possibly secreted protein. *Science* 1989; **245**: 651–3.

56. Golde TE, Estus S, Usiak M, Younkin LH, Younkin SG. Expression of beta amyloid protein precursor mRNAs: recognition of a novel alternatively spliced form and quantitation in Alzheimer's disease using PCR. *Neuron* 1990; **4**: 253–67.

57. Goldgaber D, Lerman MI, McBride OW, Saffiotti U, Gajdusek DC. Characterization and chromosomal localization of a cDNA encoding brain amyloid of Alzheimer's disease. *Science* 1987; **235**: 877–80.

58. Kitaguchi N, Takahashi Y, Tokushima Y, Shiojiri S, Ito H. Novel precursor of Alzheimer's disease amyloid protein shows protease inhibitory activity. *Nature* 1988; **331**: 530–2.

59. Ponte P, Gonzalez-DeWhitt P, Schilling J, Miller J, Hsu D, Greenberg B *et al.* A new A4 amyloid mRNA contains a domain homologous to serine proteinase inhibitors. *Nature* 1988; **331**: 525–7.

60. Tanzi RE, McClatchey AI, Lamperti ED, Villa-Komaroff L, Gusella JF, Neve RL. Protease inhibitor domain encoded by an amyloid protein precursor mRNA associated with Alzheimer's disease. *Nature* 1988; **331**: 528–30.

61. Yoshikai S, Sasaki H, Doh-ura K, Furuya H, Sakaki Y. Genomic organization of the human amyloid beta-protein precursor gene. *Gene* 1990; **87**: 257–63.

62. Turner PR, O'Connor K, Tate WP, Abraham WC. Roles of amyloid precursor protein and its fragments in regulating neural activity, plasticity and memory. *Prog Neurobiol* 2003; **70**: 1–32.

63. Priller C, Bauer T, Mitteregger G, Krebs B, Kretzschmar HA, Herms J. Synapse formation and function is modulated by the amyloid precursor protein. *J Neurosci* 2006; **26**: 7212–21.

64. Bossy-Wetzel E, Schwarzenbacher R, Lipton SA. Molecular pathways to neurodegeneration. *Nat Med* 2004; **10**: S2–9.

65. Koo EH, Squazzo SL. Evidence that production and release of amyloid beta-protein involves the endocytic pathway. *J Biol Chem* 1994; **269**: 17386–9.

66. Anandatheerthavarada HK, Biswas G, Robin MA, Avadhani NG. Mitochondrial targeting and a novel transmembrane arrest of Alzheimer's amyloid precursor protein impairs mitochondrial function in neuronal cells. *J Cell Biol* 2003; **161**: 41–54.

67. Devi L, Prabhu BM, Galati DF, Avadhani NG, Anandatheerthavarada HK. Accumulation of amyloid precursor protein in the mitochondrial import channels of human Alzheimer's disease brain is associated with mitochondrial dysfunction. *J Neurosci* 2006; **26**: 9057–68.

68. Lin MT, Beal MF. Alzheimer's APP mangles mitochondria. *Nat Med* 2006; **12**: 1241–3.

69. Walter J, Kaether C, Steiner H, Haass C. The cell biology of Alzheimer's disease: uncovering the secrets of secretases. *Curr Opin Neurobiol* 2001; **11**: 585–90.

70. Sastre M, Steiner H, Fuchs K, Capell A, Multhaup G, Condron MM *et al.* Presenilin-dependent gamma-secretase processing of beta-amyloid precursor protein at a site corresponding to the S3 cleavage of Notch. EMBO 2001; Rep 2: 835–41.

71. Scheuner D, Eckman C, Jensen M, Song X, Citron M, Suzuki N *et al.* Secreted amyloid beta-protein similar to that in the senile plaques of Alzheimer's disease is increased in vivo by the presenilin 1 and 2 and APP mutations linked to familial Alzheimer's disease. *Nat Med* 1996; **2**: 864–70.

72. Walker LC, Ibegbu CC, Todd CW, Robinson HL, Jucker M, LeVine H *et al.* Emerging prospects for the disease-modifying treatment of Alzheimer's disease. *Biochem Pharmacol* 2005; **69**: 1001–8.

73. Goate A, Chartier-Harlin MC, Mullan M, Brown J, Crawford F, Fidani L *et al.* Segregation of a missense mutation in the amyloid precursor protein gene with familial Alzheimer's disease. *Nature* 1991; **349**: 704–6.

74. Mullan M. Familial Alzheimer's disease: second gene locus located. *BMJ* 1992; **305**: 1108–9.

75. Higgins GA, Jacobsen H. Transgenic mouse models of Alzheimer's disease: phenotype and application. *Behav Pharmacol* 2003; **14**: 419–38.

76. Mineur YS, McLoughlin D, Crusio WE, Sluyter F. Genetic mouse models of Alzheimer's disease. *Neural Plast* 2005; **12**: 299–310.

77. Irizarry MC, McNamara M, Fedorchak K, Hsiao K, Hyman BT. APPSw transgenic mice develop age-related A beta deposits and neuropil abnormalities, but no neuronal loss in CA1. *J Neuropathol Exp Neurol* 1997; **56**: 965–73.

78. Westerman MA, Cooper-Blacketer D, Mariash A, Kotilinek L, Kawarabayashi T, Younkin LH *et al.* The relationship between Abeta and memory in the Tg2576 mouse model of Alzheimer's disease. *J Neurosci* 2002; **22**: 1858–67.

79. Weidemann A, Konig G, Bunke D, Fischer P, Salbaum JM, Masters CL *et al.* Identification, biogenesis and localization of precursors of Alzheimer's disease A4 amyloid protein. *Cell* 1989; **57**: 115–26.

80. Sandbrink R, Masters CL, Beyreuther K. Similar alternative splicing of a non-homologous domain in beta A4-amyloid protein precursor-like proteins. *J Biol Chem* 1994; **269**: 14227–34.

81. Lemaire HG, Salbaum JM, Multhaup G, Kang J, Bayney RM, Unterbeck A *et al.* The PreA4(695) precursor protein of Alzheimer's disease A4 amyloid is encoded by 16 exons. *Nucleic Acids Res* 1989; **7**: 517–22.

82. Konig G, Salbaum JM, Wiestler O, Lang W, Schmitt HP, Masters CL *et al.* Alternative splicing of the beta A4 amyloid gene of Alzheimer's disease in cortex of control and Alzheimer's disease patients. *Brain Res Mol Brain Res* 1991; 9: 259–62.

83. Johnson SA, Rogers J, Finch CE. APP-695 transcript prevalence is selectively reduced during Alzheimer's disease in cortex and hippocampus but not in cerebellum. *Neurobiol Aging* 1989; **10**: 755–60.

84. Neve RL, Finch EA, Dawes LR. Expression of the Alzheimer amyloid precursor gene transcripts in the human brain. *Neuron* 1988; **1**: 669–77.

85. Palmert MR, Golde TE, Cohen ML, Kovacs DM, Tanzi RE, Gusella JF *et al.* Amyloid protein precursor messenger RNAs: differential expression in Alzheimer's disease. *Science* 1988; **241**: 1080–4.

86. Sisodia SS, Koo EH, Beyreuther K, Unterbeck A, Price DL. Evidence that beta-amyloid protein in Alzheimer's disease is not derived by normal processing. *Science* 1990; **248**: 492–5.

87. Tanaka S, Nakamura S, Ueda K, Kameyama M, Shiojiri S, Takahashi Y *et al.* Three types of amyloid protein precursor mRNA in human brain: their differential expression in Alzheimer's disease. *Biochem Biophys Res Commun* 1988; **157**: 472–9.

88. Jacobsen JS, Muenkel HA, Blume AJ, Vitek MP. A novel species-specific RNA related to alternatively spliced amyloid precursor protein mRNAs. *Neurobiol Aging* 1991; **12**: 575–83.

89. Kwok JB, Li QX, Hallupp M, Whyte S, Ames D, Beyreuther K *et al.* Novel Leu723Pro amyloid precursor protein mutation increases amyloid beta42(43) peptide levels and induces apoptosis. *Ann Neurol* 2000; **47**: 249–53.

90. Schellenberg GD, Bird TD, Wijsman EM, Orr HT, Anderson L, Nemens E *et al.* Genetic linkage evidence for a familial Alzheimer's disease locus on chromosome 14. *Science* 1992; **258**: 668–71.

91. Sherrington R, Rogaev EI, Liang Y, Rogaeva EA, Levesque G, Ikeda M *et al.* Cloning of a gene bearing missense mutations in early-onset familial Alzheimer's disease. *Nature* 1995; **375**: 754–60.

92. De Strooper B, Saftig P, Craessaerts K, Vanderstichele H, Guhde G, Annaert W *et al.* Deficiency of presenilin-1 inhibits the normal cleavage of amyloid precursor protein. *Nature* 1998; **391**: 387–90.

93. Wolfe MS, Xia W, Ostaszewski BL, Diehl TS, Kimberly WT, Selkoe DJ. Two transmembrane aspartates in presenilin-1 required for presenilin endoproteolysis and gamma-secretase activity. *Nature* 1999; **398**: 513–17.

94. Theuns J, Del-Favero J, Dermaut B, Van Duijn CM, Backhovens H, Van den Broeck MV *et al.* Genetic variability in the regulatory region of presenilin 1 associated with risk for Alzheimer's disease and variable expression. *Hum Mol Genet* 2000; **9**: 325–31.

95. Citron M, Westaway D, Xia W, Carlson G, Diehl T, Levesque G *et al.* Mutant presenilins of Alzheimer's disease increase production of 42-residue amyloid beta-protein in both transfected cells and transgenic mice. *Nat Med* 1997; **3**: 67–72.

96. Lippa CF, Nee LE, Mori H, St George-Hyslop P. Abeta-42 deposition precedes other changes in PS-1 Alzheimer's disease. *Lancet* 1998; **352**: 1117–18.

97. Wolfe MS. When loss is gain: reduced presenilin proteolytic function leads to increased Abeta42/Abeta40. Talking Point on the role of presenilin mutations in Alzheimer disease. *EMBO* 2007; Rep 8: 136–40.

98. Moehlmann T, Winkler E, Xia X, Edbauer D, Murrell J, Capell A *et al.* Presenilin-1 mutations of leucine 166 equally affect the generation of the Notch and APP intracellular domains independent of their effect on Abeta 42 production. *Proc Natl Acad Sci USA* 2002; 99: 8025–30.

99. Rudzinski LA, Fletcher RM, Dickson DW, Crook R, Hutton ML, Adamson J *et al.* Early onset familial Alzheimer Disease with spastic paraparesis, dysarthria and seizures and N135S mutation in PSEN1. *Alzheimer Dis Assoc Disord* 2008; **22**: 299–307.

100. Heckmann JM, Low WC, de Villiers C, Rutherfoord S, Vorster A, Rao H *et al.* Novel presenilin 1 mutation with profound neurofibrillary pathology in an indigenous Southern African family with early-onset Alzheimer's disease. *Brain* 2004; **127**: 133–42.

101. Hutton M, Hardy J. The presenilins and Alzheimer's disease. *Hum Mol Genet* 1997; **6**: 1639–46.

102. Wolfe MS, De Los Angeles J, Miller DD, Xia W, Selkoe DJ. Are presenilins intramembrane-cleaving proteases? Implications for the molecular mechanism of Alzheimer's disease. *Biochemistry* 1999; **38**: 11223–30.

103. Baulac S, LaVoie MJ, Kimberly WT, Strahle J, Wolfe MS, Selkoe DJ *et al.* Functional gamma-secretase complex assembly in Golgi/trans-Golgi network: interactions among presenilin, nicastrin, Aph1, Pen-2 and gamma-secretase substrates. *Neurobiol Dis* 2003; **14**: 194–204.

104. Edbauer D, Winkler E, Regula JT, Pesold B, Steiner H, Haass C. Reconstitution of gamma-secretase activity. *Nat Cell Biol* 2003; **5**: 486–8.

105. Francis R, McGrath G, Zhang J, Ruddy DA, Sym M, Apfeld J *et al.* aph-1 and pen-2 are required for Notch pathway signaling, gamma-secretase cleavage of betaAPP and presenilin protein accumulation. *Dev Cell* 2002; **3**: 85–97.

106. Goutte C, Tsunozaki M, Hale VA, Priess JR. APH-1 is a multipass membrane protein essential for the Notch signaling pathway in Caenorhabditis elegans embryos. *Proc Natl Acad Sci USA* 2002; **99**: 775–9.

107. Kimberly WT, LaVoie MJ, Ostaszewski BL, Ye W, Wolfe MS, Selkoe DJ. Gamma-secretase is a membrane protein complex comprised of presenilin, nicastrin, Aph-1 and Pen-2. *Proc Natl Acad Sci USA* 2003; **100**: 6382–7.

108. Takasugi N, Tomita T, Hayashi I, Tsuruoka M, Niimura M, Takahashi Y *et al.* The role of presenilin cofactors in the gamma-secretase complex. *Nature* 2003; **422**: 438–41.

109. De Strooper B, Annaert W, Cupers P, Saftig P, Craessaerts K, Mumm JS *et al.* A presenilin-1-dependent gamma-secretase-like protease mediates release of Notch intracellular domain. *Nature* 1999; **398**: 518–22.

110. Shen J, Bronson RT, Chen DF, Xia W, Selkoe DJ, Tonegawa S. Skeletal and CNS defects in Presenilin-1-deficient mice. *Cell* 1997; **89**: 629–39.

111. Yu H, Saura CA, Choi SY, Sun LD, Yang X, Handler M *et al.* APP processing and synaptic plasticity in presenilin-1 conditional knockout mice. *Neuron* 2001; **31**: 713–26.

112. Huang XG, Yee BK, Nag S, Chan ST, Tang F. Behavioral and neurochemical characterization of transgenic mice carrying the human presenilin-1 gene with or without the leucine-to-proline mutation at codon 235. *Exp Neurol* 2003; **183**: 673–81.

113. Janus C, D'Amelio S, Amitay O, Chishti MA, Strome R, Fraser P *et al.* Spatial learning in transgenic mice expressing human presenilin 1 (PS1) transgenes. *Neurobiol Aging* 2000, **21**: 541–9.

114. Holcomb L, Gordon MN, McGowan E, Yu X, Benkovic S, Jantzen P *et al.* Accelerated Alzheimer-type phenotype in transgenic mice carrying both mutant amyloid precursor protein and presenilin 1 transgenes. *Nat Med* 1998; **4**: 97–100.

115. Levy-Lahad E, Wijsman EM, Nemens E, Anderson L, Goddard KA, Weber JL *et al.* A familial Alzheimer's disease locus on chromosome 1. *Science* 1995, **269**: 970–3.

116. Rogaev EI, Sherrington R, Rogaeva EA, Levesque G, Ikeda M, Liang Y *et al.* Familial Alzheimer's disease in kindreds with missense mutations in a gene on chromosome 1 related to the Alzheimer's disease type 3 gene. *Nature* 1995; **376**: 775–8.

117. Tandon A, Fraser P. The presenilins. *Genome Biol* 2002; **3**(11): reviews 3014.

118. Anwar R, Moynihan TP, Ardley H, Brindle N, Coletta PL, Cairns N *et al.* Molecular analysis of the presenilin 1 (S182) gene in 'sporadic' cases of Alzheimer's disease: identification and characterisation of unusual splice variants. *J Neurochem* 1996; **66**: 1774–7.

119. Hutton M, Busfield F, Wragg M, Crook R, Perez-Tur J, Clark RF *et al.* Complete analysis of the presenilin 1 gene in early onset Alzheimer's disease. *Neuroreport* 1996; **7**: 801–5.

120. Prihar G, Fuldner RA, Perez-Tur J, Lincoln S, Duff K, Crook R *et al.* Structure and alternative splicing of the presenilin-2 gene. *Neuroreport* 1996; **7**: 1680–4.

121. Kovacs DM, Fausett HJ, Page KJ, Kim TW, Moir RD, Merriam DE *et al.* Alzheimer-associated presenilins 1 and 2: neuronal expression in brain and localization to intracellular membranes in mammalian cells. *Nat Med* 1996; **2**: 224–9.

122. Sato N, Imaizumi K, Manabe T, Taniguchi M, Hitomi J, Katayama T *et al.* Increased production of beta-amyloid and vulnerability to endoplasmic reticulum stress by an aberrant spliced form of presenilin 2. *J Biol Chem* 2001; **276**: 2108–14.

123. Grunberg J, Walter J, Eckman C, Capell A, Schindzielorz A, Younkin S *et al.* Truncated presenilin 2 derived from differentially spliced mRNA does not affect the ratio of amyloid beta-peptide 1-42/1-40. *Neuroreport* 1998; **9**: 3293–9.

124. Lindquist SG, Hasholt L, Bahl JM, Heegaard NH, Andersen BB, Norremolle A *et al.* A novel presenilin 2 mutation (V393M) in early-onset dementia with profound language impairment. *Eur J Neurol* 2008; 15: 1135–9.

125. Corder EH, Saunders AM, Strittmatter WJ, Schmechel DE, Gaskell PC, Small GW *et al.* Gene dose of apolipoprotein E type 4 allele and the risk of Alzheimer's disease in late onset families. *Science* 1993; **261**: 921–3.

126. Tang MX, Maestre G, Tsai WY, Liu XH, Feng L, Chung WY *et al.* Relative risk of Alzheimer disease and age-at-onset distributions, based on APOE genotypes among elderly African Americans, Caucasians and Hispanics in New York City. *Am J Hum Genet* 1996; **58**: 574–84.

127. Schupf N, Sergievsky GH. Genetic and host factors for dementia in Down's syndrome. *Br J Psychiatry* 2002; **180**: 405–10.

128. Nicoll JA, Roberts GW, Graham DI. Apolipoprotein E epsilon 4 allele is associated with deposition of amyloid beta-protein following head injury. *Nat Med* 1995; **1**: 135–7.

129. Liu Y, Laakso MP, Karonen JO, Vanninen RL, Nuutinen J, Soimakallio S *et al.* Apolipoprotein E polymorphism and acute ischemic stroke: a diffusion- and perfusion-weighted magnetic resonance imaging study. *J Cereb Blood Flow Metab* 2002; **22**: 1336–42.

130. Horsburgh K, McCulloch J, Nilsen M, Roses AD, Nicoll JA. Increased neuronal damage and apoE immunoreactivity in human apolipoprotein E, E4 isoform-specific, transgenic mice after global cerebral ischaemia. *Eur J Neurosci* 2000; **12**: 4309–17.

131. Brousseau T, Legrain S, Berr C, Gourlet V, Vidal O, Amouyel P. Confirmation of the epsilon 4 allele of the apolipoprotein E gene as a risk factor for late-onset Alzheimer's disease. *Neurology* 1994; **44**: 342–4.

132. Chauhan NB. Membrane dynamics, cholesterol homeostasis and Alzheimer's disease. *J Lipid Res* 2003; **44**: 2019–29.

133. Farrer LA, Cupples LA, Haines JL, Hyman B, Kukull WA, Mayeux R *et al.* Effects of age, sex and ethnicity on the association between apolipoprotein E genotype and Alzheimer disease. A meta-analysis. APOE and Alzheimer Disease Meta Analysis Consortium. *JAMA* 1997; **278**: 1349–56.

134. Farrer LA, Cupples LA, Van Duijn CM, Kurz A, Zimmer R, Muller U *et al.* Apolipoprotein E genotype in patients with Alzheimer's disease: implications for the risk of dementia among relatives. *Ann Neurol* 1995; **38**: 797–808.

135. Hendrie HC, Hall KS, Hui S, Unverzagt FW, Yu CE, Lahiri DK *et al.* Apolipoprotein E genotypes and Alzheimer's disease in a community study of elderly African Americans. *Ann Neurol* 1995; **37**: 118–20.

136. Liddell M, Williams J, Bayer A, Kaiser F, Owen M. Confirmation of association between the e4 allele of apolipoprotein E and Alzheimer's disease. *J Med Genet* 1994; **31**: 197–200.

137. Lucotte G, Turpin JC, Landais P. Apolipoprotein E-epsilon 4 allele doses in late-onset Alzheimer's disease. *Ann Neurol* 1994; **36**: 681–2.

138. Mayeux R, Stern Y, Ottman R, Tatemichi TK, Tang MX, Maestre G *et al.* The apolipoprotein epsilon 4 allele in patients with Alzheimer's disease. *Ann Neurol* 1993; **34**: 752–4.

139. Poirier J, Davignon J, Bouthillier D, Kogan S, Bertrand P, Gauthier S. Apolipoprotein E polymorphism and Alzheimer's disease. *Lancet* 1993; **342**: 697–9.

140. Tsai MS, Tangalos EG, Petersen RC, Smith GE, Schaid DJ, Kokmen E *et al.* Apolipoprotein E: risk factor for Alzheimer disease. *Am J Hum Genet* 1994; **54**: 643–9.

141. Mahley RW, Weisgraber KH, Huang Y. Apolipoprotein E4: a causative factor and therapeutic target in neuropathology, including Alzheimer's disease. *Proc Natl Acad Sci USA* 2006; **103**: 5644–51.

142. Huang Y. Molecular and cellular mechanisms of apolipoprotein E4 neurotoxicity and potential therapeutic strategies. *Curr Opin Drug Discov Devel* 2006; **9**: 627–41.

143. Finch CE, Stanford CB. Meat-adaptive genes and the evolution of slower aging in humans. *Q Rev Biol* 2004; **79**: 3–50.

144. Mahley RW, Rall SC, Jr. Is epsilon4 the ancestral human apoE allele? *Neurobiol Aging* 1999; **20**: 429–30.

145. Sing CF, Davignon J. Role of the apolipoprotein E polymorphism in determining normal plasma lipid and lipoprotein variation. *Am J Hum Genet* 1985; **37**: 268–85.

146. Rapp A, Gmeiner B, Hüttinger M. Implication of apoE isoforms in cholesterol metabolism by primary rat hippocampal neurons and astrocytes. *Biochimie* 2006; **88**: 473–83.

147. Michikawa M, Fan QW, Isobe I, Yanagisawa K. Apolipoprotein E exhibits isoform-specific promotion of lipid efflux from astrocytes and neurons in culture. *J Neurochem* 2000; **74**: 1008–16.

148. Mahley RW, Huang Y, Rall SC, Jr. Pathogenesis of type III hyperlipoproteinemia (dysbetalipoproteinemia). Questions, quandaries and paradoxes. *J Lipid Res* 1999; **40**: 1933–49.

149. Stratman NC, Castle CK, Taylor BM, Epps DE, Melchior GW, Carter DB. Isoform-specific interactions of human apolipoprotein E to an intermediate conformation of human Alzheimer amyloid-beta peptide. *Chem Phys Lipids* 2005; **137**: 52–61.

150. Buttini M, Orth M, Bellosta S, Akeefe H, Pitas RE, Wyss-Coray T *et al.* Expression of human apolipoprotein E3 or E4 in the brains of Apoe-/- mice: isoform-specific effects on neurodegeneration. *J Neurosci* 1999; **19**: 4867–80.

151. Keller JN, Lauderback CM, Butterfield DA, Kindy MS, Yu J, Markesbery WR. Amyloid beta-peptide effects on synaptosomes from apolipoprotein E-deficient mice. *J Neurochem* 2000; **74**: 1579–86.

152. Canevari L, Clark JB. Alzheimer's disease and cholesterol: the fat connection. *Neurochem Res* 2007; **32**: 739–50.

153. LaDu MJ, Pederson TM, Frail DE, Reardon CA, Getz GS, Falduto MT. Purification of apolipoprotein E attenuates isoform-specific binding to beta-amyloid. *J Biol Chem* 1995; **270**: 9039–42.

154. Pitas RE, Boyles JK, Lee SH, Foss D, Mahley RW. Astrocytes synthesize apolipoprotein E and metabolize apolipoprotein E-containing lipoproteins. *Biochim Biophys Acta* 1987; **917**: 148–61.

155. Uchihara T, Duyckaerts C, He Y, Kobayashi K, Seilhean D, Amouyel P *et al.* ApoE immunoreactivity and microglial cells in Alzheimer's disease brain. *Neurosci Lett* 1995; **195**: 5–8.

156. Baskin F, Smith GM, Fosmire JA, Rosenberg RN. Altered apolipoprotein E secretion in cytokine treated human astrocyte cultures. *J Neurol Sci* 1997; **148**: 15–18.

157. Aoki K, Uchihara T, Nakamura A, Komori T, Arai N, Mizutani T. Expression of apolipoprotein E in ballooned neurons-comparative immunohistochemical study on neurodegenerative disorders and infarction. *Acta Neuropathol* 2003; **106**: 436–40.

158. Xu PT, Gilbert JR, Qiu HL, Ervin J, Rothrock-Christian TR, Hulette C et al. Specific regional transcription of apolipoprotein E in human brain neurons. *Am J Pathol* 1999; **154**: 601–11.

159. Boschert U, Merlo-Pich E, Higgins G, Roses AD, Catsicas S. Apolipoprotein E expression by neurons surviving excitotoxic stress. *Neurobiol Dis* 1999; **6**: 508–14.

160. Gibson GE, Haroutunian V, Zhang H, Park LC, Shi Q, Lesser M et al. Mitochondrial damage in Alzheimer's disease varies with apolipoprotein E genotype. *Ann Neurol* 2000; **48**: 297–303.

161. Ignatius MJ, Gebicke-Harter PJ, Skene JH, Schilling JW, Weisgraber KH, Mahley RW et al. Expression of apolipoprotein E during nerve degeneration and regeneration. *Proc Natl Acad Sci USA* 1986; **83**: 1125–9

162. Nagy Z, Esiri MM, Jobst KA, Johnston C, Litchfield S, Sim E, Smith AD. Influence of the apolipoprotein E genotype on amyloid deposition and neurofibrillary tangle formation in Alzheimer's disease. *Neuroscience* 1995; **69**: 757–61.

163. Blacker D, Haines JL, Rodes L, Terwedow H, Go RC, Harrell LE et al. ApoE-4 and age at onset of Alzheimer's disease: the NIMH genetics initiative. *Neurology* 1997; **48**: 139–47.

164. Martins CA, Oulhaj A, de Jager CA, Williams JH. APOE alleles predict the rate of cognitive decline in Alzheimer disease: a nonlinear model. *Neurology* 2005; **65**: 1888–93.

165. Green RC, Cupples LA, Go R, Benke KS, Edeki T, Griffith PA et al. Risk of dementia among white and African American relatives of patients with Alzheimer disease. *JAMA* 2002; **287**: 329–36.

166. Romas SN, Santana V, Williamson J, Ciappa A, Lee JH, Rondon HZ et al. Familial Alzheimer disease among Caribbean Hispanics: a reexamination of its association with APOE. *Arch Neurol* 2002; **59**: 87–91.

167. Payami H, Zareparsi S, Montee KR, Sexton GJ, Kaye JA, Bird TD et al. Gender difference in apolipoprotein E-associated risk for familial Alzheimer disease: a possible clue to the higher incidence of Alzheimer disease in women. *Am J Hum Genet* 1996; **58**: 803–11.

168. Breitner JC, Wyse BW, Anthony JC, Welsh-Bohmer KA, Steffens DC, Norton MC et al. APOE-epsilon4 count predicts age when prevalence of AD increases, then declines: the Cache County Study. *Neurology* 1999; **53**: 321–31.

169. Mayeux R, Saunders AM, Shea S, Mirra S, Evans D, Roses AD et al. Utility of the apolipoprotein E genotype in the diagnosis of Alzheimer's disease. Alzheimer's Disease Centers Consortium on Apolipoprotein E and Alzheimer's Disease. *N Engl J Med* 1998; **338**: 506–11.

170. Silverman JM, Li G, Zaccario ML, Smith CJ, Schmeidler J, Mohs RC et al. Patterns of risk in first-degree relatives of patients with Alzheimer's disease. *Arch Gen Psychiatry* 1994; **51**: 577–86.

171. Jayadev S, Steinbart EJ, Chi YY, Kukull WA, Schellenberg GD, Bird TD. Conjugal Alzheimer disease: risk in children when both parents have Alzheimer disease. *Arch Neurol* 2008; **65**: 373–8.

172. Tsuang D, Larson EB, Bowen J, McCormick W, Teri L, Nochlin D et al. The utility of apolipoprotein E genotyping in the diagnosis of Alzheimer disease in a community-based case series. *Arch Neurol* 1999; **56**: 1489–95.

173. van der Cammen TJ, Croes EA, Dermaut B, de Jager MC, Cruts M, Van Broeckhoven C et al. Genetic testing has no place as a routine diagnostic test in sporadic and familial cases of Alzheimer's disease. *J Am Geriatr Soc* 2004; **52**: 2110–13.

174. Levy-Lahad E, Tsuang D, Bird TD. Recent advances in the genetics of Alzheimer's disease. *J Geriatr Psychiatry Neurol* 1998; **11**: 42–54.

44

Mouse Models of Alzheimer's Disease

Esther Oh, Constantine Lyketsos and Philip Wong

Johns Hopkins School of Medicine and Johns Hopkins Bayview, Baltimore, USA

Advances in the development of animal models of neurodegenerative diseases have accelerated translation of basic science research into application in humans. While many different animal models are currently being studied in research settings, this chapter will focus on transgenic (tg) mouse models of Alzheimer's disease (AD). There are two main types of tg mouse models of AD: models of amyloidosis and/or of tauopathy. These two types represent the two major pathological changes seen in AD, amyloid plaques and neurofibrillary tangles (NFTs). More recently, a model combining both features has been developed, allowing researchers to study their interaction. Important variations are conditional tg mouse models of AD in which the expression of transgenes can be manipulated – induced or inhibited – by external controls, and models in which normal (or endogenous) genes of interest have been deleted from a selected locus ('knock-outs'). The following sections describe representative models in each category, and discuss advantages and disadvantages of each model. Finally, clinical implications of findings from animal studies are discussed.

TRANSGENIC MOUSE MODELS OF AMYLOID-BETA AMYLOIDOSIS

Although human familial AD (FAD) comprises a small portion of AD cases, the identification of genetic mutations associated with FAD in genes coding for the amyloid precursor protein (APP) or presenilin 1 and 2 (PS1, PS2) led to development of the earliest tg mouse models. APP is cleaved by proteolytic enzymes, β- and γ-secretases, to form amyloid-beta (Aβ) 40 and 42, the main components of the amyloid plaques[1]. Mutations in the APP gene create excess Aβ deposition by enhancing β-secretase cleavage of APP or by altering the pattern of γ-secretase cleavage of APP. This results in a higher Aβ42 to Aβ40 ratio, which in turn enhances Aβ fibrillogenesis.

One of the first strategies to create AD-like pathology in mice was to develop tg mouse models that over-express human APP with FAD mutations. While over-expression of APP is not a general feature of AD, this approach led to tg mice with significant Aβ production and deposition over their lifetime. One such tg mouse model, known as PDAPP, uses a platelet-derived growth factor β (*PDGF β*) promoter to enhance in mice the expression of human APP with V717F mutation[2]. Another early tg mouse model, Tg2576, uses the hamster prion protein promoter (*PrP*) to enhance the expression of human APP with a double Swedish mutation (K670N/M671L)[3]. Both models have been extensively studied as models of Aβ amyloidosis (Table 44.1).

Another approach to developing tg AD mouse models involved the insertion of human presenilin genes with mutations known to cause AD into the mouse genome. Presenilins are part of the γ-secretase complex, which is involved in the cleavage of APP along with β-secretase. However, mouse models with PS1 mutations alone do not develop amyloid pathology[4,5]. When both APP and PS1 mutations are expressed together in tg mice, such as in APPswe/PS1dE9 (Table 44.1)[6], the PS1 mutation increases the ratio of Aβ42 to Aβ40, resulting in more Aβ deposition due to the higher fibrillogenic nature of Aβ42[7].

Many of the tg mouse models of amyloidosis also develop other pathologies seen in the human disease such as neuritic plaques, gliosis or synaptic loss, allowing for observation of the effect of amyloid on neuronal pathologies. Significantly, monoaminergic neurodegeneration, a feature of the human disease, occurs in at least one mouse model[8]. These models have been very useful to the identification of mechanism-based therapeutics, specifically, anti-amyloid therapies. However, a major limitation is that the amyloidosis models do not develop NFTs, one of the hallmark neuropathological changes seen in AD.

TRANSGENIC MOUSE MODELS OF TAUOPATHY

The amyloid cascade hypothesis[1] proposes that Aβ is an early upstream agent that is followed by excess phosphorylation of tau, an intracellular, microtubule-associated protein. Hyperphosphorylation of tau is thought to lead to the formation of paired helical filaments (PHF), which progress to become NFTs in the neuronal cell body. However, as mentioned above, tg mouse models of amyloidosis do not form NFTs. One reason may be differences in tau isoforms across humans and mice. Six human isoforms of tau exist, each derived from alternative splicing in the brain of the same gene. There are only three isoforms in mice, which may result in a lower propensity for hyperphosphorylation[9].

There is currently no known tau mutation in AD. However, independent of amyloid plaques, tau inclusions are found in other neurogenerative diseases such as progressive supranuclear palsy (PSP), corticobasal degeneration (CBD), Pick's disease (PiD) and frontotemporal dementia (FTD). Therefore, tg mouse models of tauopathy have been created using human mutations in the tau

Principles and Practice of Geriatric Psychiatry, 3rd edn. Edited by Mohammed T. Abou-Saleh, Cornelius Katona and Anand Kumar
© 2011 John Wiley & Sons, Ltd

Table 44.1 Examples of mouse models of Alzheimer's disease

Model	Pros	Cons	Best use of model
PDAPP mice (line 109)[2]	Diffuse and neuritic plaques, synaptic loss, astrocytosis and microgliosis; significant impairment on a variety of different learning and memory tests	Some early age-independent memory and behavioural deficits; noncongenic strain background; no NFT or tau aggregates	Studies of passive and active anti-Aβ immunization; interactions between Aβ and apolipoproteins
APPswe (Tg2576)[3]	Numerous Aβ plaques, oxidative lipid and glycoxidative damages; memory deficits seen in 9–10-month-old Tg mice	No NTF or tau aggregates; early deficits in Morris water maze with visible platform; noncongenic strain background	Studies of immunotherapeutic approaches; breeding with other AD models; use of NSAIDs and other treatments
Double transgenic mice: Mo/Hu APPswe/PS1dE9[6]	Exhibit accelerated Aβ deposition despite relatively low level of APPswe over-expression; both transgenes are co-segregated; a similar model, line C3-3/S9, shows age-related deficits in behaviour[31]	Noncongenic strain background; no NFT or tau aggregates	Studies of efficacy of different experimental treatments; breeding of these mice to other transgenic mice is efficient owing to co-segregation of the transgenes
Conditional transgenic mice: rTg4510[14]	These mice express repressible human FTDP-17 mutation P301L (4R0N tau$_{p301L}$); progressive age-related NFT, neuronal loss and functional deficits are present; after the suppression of transgenic tau, memory function recovered and neuron numbers stabilized, but NFTs continued to accumulate	No Aβ accumulation; gross forebrain atrophy, with preservation of hindbrain structures	Studies of reversibility of cognitive and pathological alterations
Conditional transgenic mice: CaMKIIα-tTA × tet-APPswe/ind[13]	These mice express repressible APP transgene with Swedish and Indiana mutations; they develop progressive amyloid plaques	No NFT or tau aggregates; high expression lines are hyperactive	Studies of reversibility of pathological alterations
Triple transgenic mice: 3xTg-AD PS1, APPswe,tau[11]	Amyloid plaque develops before tau pathology, and the regional distribution of amyloid and tau closely mimics human AD pathology; age-dependent decline in both spatial and contextual learning and memory	May be difficult to differentiate the effect of amyloid from tau	Studies of anti-Aβ immunization; understanding the relationship between amyloid and tau pathology; testing the amyloid cascade hypothesis

Source: Adapted from Savonenko *et al*., 2005

gene linked to familial frontotemporal dementia with Parkinsonism on chromosome 17 (FTDP-17). One such model, expressing the FTDP-17 mutation P301L, forms NFTs in diencephalon, brainstem, cerebellum and spinal cord. However, this model also has motor deficits due to spinal cord lesions such as fibrillary gliosis and axonal degeneration[10].

More recently, models which reproduce both amyloid plaques and NFTs have been developed, the triple transgenic mice 3xTg-AD, which carry PS1 (M146V), APP (K670N/M671L) and tau (P301L) transgenes (Table 44.1)[11]. Interestingly, even though both APP and tau transgenes are expressed to similar levels in these mice, Aβ deposits emerge prior to tau pathology, consistent with the amyloid cascade hypothesis. Immunotherapy experiments involving direct injection of anti-Aβ antibodies into the hippocampus showed clearance of Aβ deposits followed by clearance of earlier (non-hyperphosphorylated) forms of tau. Aβ deposits re-emerged by 30 days post-injection, with tau pathology re-emerging at a later time point. Injection of anti-tau antibody had no observable effect on either Aβ or tau deposits. The data from these experiments further support the view that Aβ precedes tau pathology per the amyloid cascade hypothesis[12]. These triple transgenic models are therefore quite useful for studying the role of tau protein in neurodegenerative diseases, and especially its interaction with amyloid pathology.

CONDITIONAL TRANSGENIC MOUSE MODELS

Researchers have also developed variations of the above models in which the expression of APP, tau or both transgenes are temporally controlled. The approach used, commonly known as the 'tet-off system,' creates a tg model in which administration of a tetracycline analogue, such as doxycycline, turns off transcription of the transgene. Conditional tg models allow study of the effects of temporal variation (early vs. late, short vs. long) in the expression of the transgene. Such systems also model pharmaceutical interventions in which the expression of a transgene is suppressed, allowing assessment of potential treatment effect[13]. They can also test the hypothesis of whether certain structural and biochemical changes are related to the expression of the transgene[14].

A well-known conditional APP tg mouse model is CaMKIIα-tTA × tet-APPswe/ind (Table 44.1). This model expresses amyloid plaques starting eight weeks of age, and amyloid deposition is severe by six months of age. APP expression is reduced by greater than 95% two weeks after initiation of doxycycline treatment. When doxycycline was given to examine the effects of Aβ suppression after the onset of deposition, further progression of Aβ deposition was halted, but there was limited to no clearance of previously deposited amyloid plaques even after six months of treatment. These results suggested that inhibition of Aβ production may halt further progression of the pathology, but may not clear the pre-existing amyloid plaques[13].

A tg mouse model with conditional tau expression is rTg4510, in which mutant tau (P301L) expression is suppressed by administration of doxycycline (Table 44.1). This model has age-dependent formation of NFTs, loss of neurons, generalized forebrain atrophy and deficits in spatial memory. While formation of NFTs has been linked to subsequent neuronal loss and cognitive deficits, suppression of mutant tau gene starting at four months of age in these mice did not halt the accumulation of NFTs, even though there was a cessation in the loss of neurons and brain weight[14]. In addition, there was improvement in memory function in these mice, despite progressive NFT accumulation. These findings imply that early memory deficits may be due to reversible neuronal dysfunction rather than irreversible development of NFTs or that there may be neuronal remodelling after the mutant tau gene suppression that allows recovery. Another implication from this study is that NFTs may not entirely account for the neuronal loss[14].

Recently, the conditional triple tg mouse rTg3696AB that harbours two human Swedish APP mutations (K670N and M671L) at the β-secretase site, the London mutation (V717I) at the γ-secretase site (APP$_{NLI}$) and a tau mutation (P301L) has been created. This model shows Aβ deposits from 4 months of age, and NFTs from 11 months of age. Neuronal loss occurs at 13 months of age. Studies of the effects of transgene suppression, mimicking potential human therapeutic strategies, on pathologic and cognitive behavioural outcomes are in progress[15]. This discussion illustrates the advantages of conditional tg mouse models, where temporal variations in the expression of transgenes as well as inhibition of select transgenes can demonstrate the potential role they play in the pathogenesis of neurodegeneration and cognitive behavioural symptoms.

KNOCK-OUT MOUSE MODELS

Knock-out models are mice in which genes of interest have been selectively silenced. They are useful for determining the function of a specific protein or an enzyme, and for studying biological models of the enzyme inhibition.

The APP gene is located on chromosome 21, and has many putative roles. Along with its homologues, the amyloid precursor-like proteins 1 and 2 (APLP1 and APLP 2), APP is thought to have roles in cell adhesion, motility, neuronal survival and neurite outgrowth. Interestingly, one of the APP knock-out mouse models (APP-/-) produces mice that are relatively healthy and fertile, with slightly lower body weight, decreased locomotion and increased reactive gliosis. The ability to maintain a relatively normal litter size was attributed to possible compensation for the loss of APP by its homologues[16]. However, subsequent studies revealed behavioural deficit, defective long-term potentiation and GABA-mediated postsynaptic response in these mice[17].

The microtubule-associated protein tau (MAPT) gene is located on chromosome 17q21. In normal human brain, tau is thought to be involved in stabilizing microtubules, which are located predominantly in axons. MAPT knock-out mice (Mapt -/-) do not have overt histological abnormalities. However, they exhibit muscle weakness on a rod walking (balance coordination) or a wire hanging (traction) test. They also demonstrate impaired contextual fear conditioning in foot shock experiments, which are thought to test amygdala and hippocampal functions. However, these impairments in Mapt -/- mice are thought to be due to hyperactivity of the mice rather than due to memory impairment since they exhibit hyperactivity in open fields but have intact spatial learning tasks[18,19]. As with the APP knock-out models, the lack of significant pathologic deficits in tau knock-out models such as Mapt -/- may be due to compensation by other microtubule-associated proteins that may have overlapping function with MAPT protein[19].

One example of a knock-out mouse model that demonstrates the function of an enzyme while serving as a biological model of enzyme inhibition is the BACE1 knock-out model (BACE1 -/-). This model demonstrates the role of the β-site amyloid precursor cleaving enzyme 1 (BACE1) in APP cleavage. Primary cortical cultures from the BACE1 -/- mouse embryos have undetectable levels of most Aβ40 and 42 species, demonstrating that amyloid is not produced, thus establishing BACE1 as the principal β-secretase in cortical neurons. More importantly, because the BACE1 -/- mouse model was viable, this model suggested that it may be possible to develop therapeutic β-secretase inhibitors to reduce Aβ deposition without mechanism-based adverse effects[20].

While abnormal processing of APP and tau may result in neurotoxic substances, such as Aβ and NFTs, respectively, these knock-out mouse models demonstrate that APP and tau both play important roles in normal neuronal function. In addition, knock-out mouse models of enzymes such as BACE1 demonstrate the biological role of enzymes and the effects of targeting them as part of AD therapy.

DISCUSSION

While Tg mouse models of amyloidosis do not fully reproduce the pathological changes seen in human AD, they have contributed significantly to our understanding of the pathophysiology of AD. Amyloid plaques, along with neurites, neurofibrillary tangles, loss of synapses and death of neurons, are the pathological hallmarks of AD[21,22]. Most tg mouse models express either amyloid or tau pathology, although more recent models express both[12,15]. Many models do not show loss of neurons[23,24], a critical feature of human AD. Several explanations have been proposed, including species variability in neuronal vulnerability, lack of key human-type inflammatory factors[1], species variability in amyloid burden, and differences in types of plaques that accumulate in different tg mouse models[25]. Some tg mouse models also show *age-independent* behavioural deficits *prior* to Aβ deposition in the brain[26], which is different from human AD, in which amyloid deposition begins years before the clinical manifestations are evident.

Model to model variability can also be attributed to the use of different promoters, resulting in different phenotypic expressions. Some tg mouse models have tissue-specific (e.g. brain)[13] or more broadly expressed[3] transgenes, depending on the promoter type. Differences in promoters can also result in differences in transgene expression levels, expression in irrelevant brain areas as well as expression at different times. Differences in background strains can also result in different phenotypic expressions even within the same tg mouse model[19].

Despite limitations, tg mouse models are essential tools for investigating biological mechanisms and assessing potential treatments for AD. AD is characterized by gradual onset and progression of the brain disease over many years. One of the more difficult aspects of human AD research is the long duration of clinical trials, which can become prohibitive due to high patient attrition and costs. In addition, more researchers are focusing their efforts on the period preceding the AD diagnosis, preclinical and mild cognitive impairment (MCI) stages, extending the duration of the study. Tg mouse models have rapid breeding time and lower maintenance costs compared to primate models, allowing accelerated investigation of the mutated gene of interest. This results in shorter lead-time before the development of pathology (e.g. amyloid deposition in the brain) and the resultant behavioural changes. It also enables a researcher to design an intervention and observe pathological and behavioural changes within a short time frame. Many of these models have been used for evaluation of a treatment tool such as immunotherapy[27]. They are also useful for environmental modifications such as enrichment[28] and caloric restriction[29], and direct observation of their effects on behaviour as well as on neuropathology.

Many of the tg mouse models develop impairments in learning and memory as assessed by well-established methods including the Morris water maze task[9,30]. The difficulty of interpreting mouse behaviour partly arises from age-independent behaviours. These behaviours may be due to factors that are unrelated to Aβ toxicity such as transgene insertion and expression levels, strain background and promoter types[9]. Differences in the timing of behavioural onset in relation to the Aβ deposition may also be due to the use of different tasks for behavioural testing as well as assessment of behaviour at different stages of learning[9]. Recently, there have been efforts to elucidate potential soluble Aβ species that may contribute to the behavioural deficits, and that may, in part, explain the age-independent behaviors[26].

Some of the difficulties in human AD research arise from heterogeneity within the study population, which introduces confounders. Tg mouse models allow researchers to minimize the biological heterogeneity that may influence the outcome of interest by repeated backcrosses to an inbred breeding strain of mouse model up to at least tenth generation, creating a 'congenic' strain of the model. In conclusion, tg mouse models are useful for studying molecular mechanisms of a disease as well as for assessing therapeutic effect of drugs or environmental modifications, and continue to make significant contributions towards further understanding of AD.

REFERENCES

1. Hardy J, Selkoe DJ. The amyloid hypothesis of Alzheimer's disease: progress and problems on the road to therapeutics. *Science* 2002; **297**(5580): 353–6.
2. Games D, Adams D, Alessandrini R *et al.* Alzheimer-type neuropathology in transgenic mice overexpressing V717F beta-amyloid precursor protein. *Nature* 1995; **373**(6514): 523–7.
3. Hsiao K, Chapman P, Nilsen S *et al.* Correlative memory deficits, Abeta elevation, and amyloid plaques in transgenic mice. *Science* 1996; **274**(5284): 99–102.
4. Duff K, Eckman C, Zehr C *et al.* Increased amyloid-beta42(43) in brains of mice expressing mutant presenilin 1. *Nature* 1996; **383**(6602): 710–13.
5. Borchelt DR, Ratovitski T, van Lare J *et al.* Accelerated amyloid deposition in the brains of transgenic mice coexpressing mutant presenilin 1 and amyloid precursor proteins. *Neuron* 1997; **19**(4): 939–45.
6. Jankowsky JL, Slunt HH, Ratovitski T *et al.* Co-expression of multiple transgenes in mouse CNS: a comparison of strategies. *Biomol Eng* 2001; **17**(6): 157–65.
7. Jarrett JT, Berger EP, Lansbury PT, Jr. The carboxy terminus of the beta amyloid protein is critical for the seeding of amyloid formation: implications for the pathogenesis of Alzheimer's disease. *Biochemistry* 1993; **32**(18): 4693–7.
8. Liu Y, Yoo MJ, Savonenko A *et al.* Amyloid pathology is associated with progressive monoaminergic neurodegeneration in a transgenic mouse model of Alzheimer's disease. *J Neurosci* 2008; **28**(51): 13805–14.
9. Savonenko AV, Laird FM, Troncoso JC *et al.* Role of Alzheimer's disease models in designing and testing experimental therapeutics. *Drug Discov Today Dis Mod* 2005; **2**(4): 305–12.
10. Lewis J, McGowan E, Rockwood J *et al.* Neurofibrillary tangles, amyotrophy and progressive motor disturbance in mice expressing mutant (P301L) tau protein. *Nat Genet* 2000; **25**(4): 402–5.
11. Oddo S, Caccamo A, Shepherd JD *et al.* Triple-transgenic model of Alzheimer's disease with plaques and tangles: intracellular Abeta and synaptic dysfunction. *Neuron* 2003; **39**(3): 409–21.
12. Oddo S, Billings L, Kesslak JP *et al.* Abeta immunotherapy leads to clearance of early, but not late, hyperphosphorylated tau aggregates via the proteasome. *Neuron* 2004; **43**(3): 321–32.
13. Jankowsky JL, Slunt HH, Gonzales V *et al.* Persistent amyloidosis following suppression of Abeta production in a transgenic model of Alzheimer disease. *PLoS Med* 2005; **2**(12): e355.
14. Santacruz K, Lewis J, Spires T *et al.* Tau suppression in a neurodegenerative mouse model improves memory function. *Science* 2005; **309**(5733): 476–81.
15. Paulson JB, Ramsden M, Forster C *et al.* Amyloid plaque and neurofibrillary tangle pathology in a regulatable mouse model of Alzheimer's disease. *Am J Pathol* 2008; **173**(3): 762–72.
16. Zheng H, Jiang M, Trumbauer ME *et al.* Beta-amyloid precursor protein-deficient mice show reactive gliosis and decreased locomotor activity. *Cell* 1995; **81**(4): 525–31.

17. Zheng H, Koo EH. The amyloid precursor protein: beyond amyloid. *Mol Neurodegener* 2006; **1**: 5.
18. Ikegami S, Harada A, Hirokawa N. Muscle weakness, hyperactivity, and impairment in fear conditioning in tau-deficient mice. *Neurosci Lett* 2000; **279**(3): 129–32.
19. Denk F, Wade-Martins R. Knock-out and transgenic mouse models of tauopathies. *Neurobiol Aging* 2009; **30**(1): 1–13.
20. Cai H, Wang Y, McCarthy D *et al.* BACE1 is the major beta-secretase for generation of Abeta peptides by neurons. *Nat Neurosci* 2001; **4**(3): 233–4.
21. Selkoe DJ. Alzheimer's disease: genotypes, phenotypes, and treatments. *Science* 1997; **275**(5300): 630–31.
22. Price DL, Sisodia SS. Mutant genes in familial Alzheimer's disease and transgenic models. *Annu Rev Neurosci* 1998; **21**: 479–505.
23. Irizarry MC, Soriano F, McNamara M *et al.* Abeta deposition is associated with neuropil changes, but not with overt neuronal loss in the human amyloid precursor protein V717F (PDAPP) transgenic mouse. *J Neurosci* 1997; **17**(18): 7053–9.
24. Irizarry MC, McNamara M, Fedorchak K *et al.* APPSw transgenic mice develop age-related A beta deposits and neuropil abnormalities, but no neuronal loss in CA1. *J Neuropathol Exp Neurol* 1997; **56**(9): 965–73.
25. Bondolfi L, Calhoun M, Ermini F *et al.* Amyloid-associated neuron loss and gliogenesis in the neocortex of amyloid precursor protein transgenic mice. *J Neurosci* 2002; **22**(2): 515–22.
26. Lesne S, Koh MT, Kotilinek L *et al.* A specific amyloid-beta protein assembly in the brain impairs memory. *Nature* 2006; **440**(7082): 352–7.
27. Schenk D, Barbour R, Dunn W *et al.* Immunization with amyloid-beta attenuates Alzheimer-disease-like pathology in the PDAPP mouse. *Nature* 1999; **400**(6740): 173–7.
28. Jankowsky JL, Melnikova T, Fadale DJ *et al.* Environmental enrichment mitigates cognitive deficits in a mouse model of Alzheimer's disease. *J Neurosci* 2005; **25**(21): 5217–24.
29. Halagappa VK, Guo Z, Pearson M *et al.* Intermittent fasting and caloric restriction ameliorate age-related behavioral deficits in the triple-transgenic mouse model of Alzheimer's disease. *Neurobiol Dis* 2007; **26**(1): 212–20.
30. Ashe KH. Learning and memory in transgenic mice modeling Alzheimer's disease. *Learn Mem* 2001; **8**(6): 301–8.
31. Savonenko A, Xu GM, Melnikova T *et al.* Episodic-like memory deficits in the APPswe/PS1dE9 mouse model of Alzheimer's disease: relationships to beta-amyloid deposition and neurotransmitter abnormalities. *Neurobiol Dis* 2005; **18**(3): 602–17.

45

Physiological Neuroimaging in Ageing and Dementia: Metabolic and Molecular Scanning

Markus Donix, Susan Y. Bookheimer and Gary W. Small

David Geffen School of Medicine at UCLA, Los Angeles, USA

INTRODUCTION

It is well recognized that in a process of cognitive decline leading to mild cognitive impairment (MCI) and dementia, detection of the underlying changes in brain structure and function will contribute to establishing an accurate diagnosis, with direct implications for pharmacological and non-pharmacological therapy planning. Since the first positron imaging device in 1950 or the first tomographs from single photon emission data in the 1960s, scientific advances in radionuclide development and detection research have led us to look beyond the brain's regional blood flow (SPECT) or glucose metabolism (FDG-PET) into the patterns of amyloid plaque (PIB-PET) and tau tangle brain deposits (FDDNP-PET) or neuronal disintegrity (MPPF-PET). With new methods entering clinical settings, we will need to balance our expectations for these new tools against availability and costs. Here we review the current state of metabolic and molecular imaging tools used in ageing and dementia, their utility, promise, as well as potential difficulties in bringing them into common practice. We will first review the basic techniques and then discuss their applications, including practical guidelines and results from the most recent studies reporting sensitivity, specificity and optimal uses.

SPECT

Image Acquisition

Single photon emission computed tomography (SPECT) measures the distribution of radioligands in the brain reflecting regional cerebral blood flow (rCBF), which itself is linked to brain metabolism. The tracer accumulates in proportion to the rate of delivery of blood to a distinct volume of brain tissue. Decades ago to patients this would have meant injection of ^{133}Xe or ^{85}Kr into the carotid artery. Today, within the commercial and experimental available radioligands technetium-99m labelled hexamethylpropyleneamine (^{99m}Tc-HMPAO) and ethylcysteinate dimer (^{99m}Tc-ECD) tracers are commonly used in brain SPECT imaging. After intravenous injection, these lipophilic compounds quickly cross the blood–brain barrier by diffusion and, due to slow brain clearance, the distribution of the radioligands then remains stable for hours. The underlying multicompartment clearance ('microsphere') model assumes that the tracer is freely diffusible, completely extracted to the brain and 'fixed' without redistribution. The emitted single photons can be detected by a rotating gamma camera or ring-type imaging system. Spatial resolution is about 10 mm and could reach 5–6 mm using special-purpose detection systems that usually are not available for routine clinical scans.

Spatial resolution in SPECT is only limited by technology (whereas PET resolution also depends on other factors[1]; see below) but today SPECT cannot compete with PET on image resolution and begins to lose its uniqueness within other factors. Cost-effectiveness still remains a controversy from a perspective that would take diagnostic accuracy and secondary costs into account; further, PET has become much more available, which also will make it less expensive. Resulting from physics-based differences, the possibility of simultaneous imaging of more than one radioagent is SPECT territory and a growing field of interest. Since all PET tracers share the same energy level, it would be much more difficult to perform simultaneous multiple tracer studies in PET. Signals would have to be separated based upon half-life or kinetics, which seems feasible in the future[1,2].

Advanced SPECT technology is heavily reliant on detector improvements, use of hybrid imaging (e.g. SPECT/CT) and incorporation of attenuation or collimator-detector response modelling into image reconstruction algorithms (for review see[1]).

The clinical protocol requires the application of 20 mCi (740 MBq) of ^{99m}Tc-HMPAO or ^{99m}Tc-ECD 10 to 20 minutes before imaging with HMPAO and 30 to 60 minutes before image acquisition with ECD. Image acquisition itself will take 30 minutes or less. Total radiation exposure is small (about 9 mSv) and in the range from one to three times of the annual natural background.

Memory Impairment and SPECT Imaging

In the field of dementia and related disorders, SPECT has been used widely for both basic science and clinical applications. Alzheimer's disease patients display a characteristic pattern of posterior temporal and parietal perfusion deficits. Sometimes additional reduced frontal rCBF has been detected, associated with behavioural disturbances, such as depressed mood or apathy[3]. Correlations between neuropsychological performance and rCBF have been reported consistently, especially with focus on language and global functioning[4]. Pharmacological activation studies demonstrated the relationship of, e.g. cholinergic stimulation and rCBF[5].

In addition to clinical assessment, SPECT studies have been shown to improve diagnostic precision. Jagust and colleagues reported that

Principles and Practice of Geriatric Psychiatry, 3rd edn. Edited by Mohammed T. Abou-Saleh, Cornelius Katona and Anand Kumar
© 2011 John Wiley & Sons, Ltd

a positive SPECT result would increase the likelihood of a diagnosis of Alzheimer's disease by a factor of five[6]. In a meta-analysis, 99mTc-HMPAO-SPECT could discriminate between Alzheimer's disease, vascular dementia (VaD), frontotemporal dementia (FTD) and normal controls with sensitivities between 66% and 72% and specificities between 76% and 79%. Diagnostic accuracy is improved especially in patients who present with additional signs of cerebrovascular disease or who do not exactly match clinical criteria[7]. Furthermore, SPECT has been shown to be useful predicting the conversion to Alzheimer's disease in patients with MCI[8].

Measuring cerebral metabolism indirectly using rCBF enhances vulnerability to vascular-related confounders, such as hypertension and other specific cerebrovascular diseases. It has been shown that rCBF differences can be found with respect to gender and advanced age itself[9]. Changes in rCBF are not unique to memory disorders and have been observed in depression[10] and obsessive–compulsive disorder[11] as well.

Currently, most clinical SPECT scans are performed in cardiology. 99mTc-labelled tracers can be used to perform dynamic imaging (e.g. myocardial perfusion SPECT) but in the future, dynamic PET (e.g. 82Rb-based cardiac PET) imaging might have an intrinsic advantage over SPECT since temporal resolution is very closely related to the imaging system's specificity[1].

In addition to regional cerebral perfusion, various neurotransmitter systems have been a target of interest in SPECT tracer development. Dopamine transporter imaging with 123I-2β-carbomethoxy-3β-(4-iodophenyl)-N-(3-fluoropropyl) nortropane (123I-FPCIT), which can be used in the differential diagnosis of Parkinson's disease, could help to distinguish between dementia with Lewy bodies (DLB) and Alzheimer's disease, if the clinical diagnosis remains ambiguous. Since the cholinergic system is of particular interest in dementia, radiolabelled muscarinic and nicotinic acetylcholine SPECT ligands are currently under investigation in preliminary studies.

PET

Image Acquisition

Positron emission tomography (PET) has more diverse applications in imaging in ageing and dementia, as it can be used to generate images of regional cerebral blood flow (e.g. [15O]H2O-PET), metabolic activity (e.g. [18F]FDG-PET), microstructures (e.g. [18F]FDDNP-PET) or neurotransmitter receptor distribution (e.g. [18F]MPPF-PET) in the brain. After being injected intravenously, the isotope emits a positron, which after travelling a few millimetres annihilates with an electron. As a result, two 511 keV gamma photons, moving in almost opposite directions, are produced and then detected using a scintillator material (luminescent when excited by ionizing radiation) in the ring-type scanner. Only coincident arrivals of photons are recognized (within a few nanoseconds' error margin). Because of the peculiar dataset ('coincidence events', each representing a line connecting the two points of detection along which the annihilation occurred) compared to other neuroimaging techniques data, preprocessing and mathematical image reconstruction are challenging. Spatial resolution of PET images is about 3 mm and higher and limited by technological factors (detector-related effects) but also physics-related limitations (positron range and photon non-collinearity)[1]. Improvements in PET technology will be seen in both cases. New scintillators for reduction of random coincidences and silicon-based photodetectors will improve detection. PET/MRI

hybrid imaging systems could be used for monitoring patient motion via MRI to incorporate the data in PET image reconstruction, maybe replacing PET/CT in the future[1,12]. Even ultimate limitations (positron range/photon non-collinearity) have been a target since new statistical reconstruction algorithms could incorporate their probability distributions into image processing or a strong magnetic field (preferably 5 T or higher) of a future PET/MRI system should be able to reduce positron range and therefore enhance scanner resolution[1]. Time-of-flight-PET, as one of the most promising technological advances, uses the nanosecond difference of photon arrival times to restrict the position of the positron emission to a subsection of the photons' connection line, which reduces the statistical noise variance in PET reconstruction[1].

PET isotopes usually have shorter half-lives compared to SPECT ligands. The most common PET isotopes are 11C (half-life: 20 min), 13N (10 min), 15O (2 min) and 18F (110 min). Only a few hospitals have costly on-site cyclotrons, needed to produce them. Third-party suppliers are able to provide 18F because of its relatively long half-life and therefore clinical use is often restricted to 18F-labelled ligands. On the other hand, short half-lives allow the safe injection of higher activities, increasing detectable radiation.

The most common clinical application of PET is in resting measures of glucose metabolism, with [18F]FDG. In the standard clinical procedures, the tracer is injected (usually 5–6 MBq/kg for FDG) after a resting period (15–20 min). [18F]FDG-PET additionally requires at least four hours of fasting before the scan to minimize competitive inhibition of FDG uptake by blood glucose. About 40 min later (uptake phase) scans are performed (at least 20 min for conventional and 4 min for rapid scan procedures[13]).

The number of PET tracers is rapidly growing and we will focus on today's most promising ligands in the field of memory disorders. Thus, we will not further discuss others that may be relevant in the future, such as [18F]-BAY94-9172 (amyloid-β plaque labelling ligand, which has been shown to discriminate Alzheimer's disease from FTD patients and healthy controls), [11C]-nicotine (visualization of nicotine binding sites in patients under cholinesterase inhibitor treatment) or [11C](R)-PK11195 (visualization of microglial activation and immune response) (for review see[14]). Second, certain techniques, such as PET activation measurements, primarily performed in healthy subjects to identify regional brain activation underlying specific cognitive activities, or regional blood flow measurements with [15O]H2O-PET, will not be discussed either because of their decreasing relevance in current diagnostic procedures of memory impairment.

Finally, it must be mentioned that correction for possible confounding parameters is as important as in other neuroimaging techniques. Motion correction must be computed, and limitation in spatial resolution and brain atrophy in the particular patient group discussed here enhances the likelihood of partial volume effects. For adequate correction MRI scans of the subjects should be available.

[18F]FDG-PET

In PET brain imaging the radiolabelled glucose analogue [18F]fluorodeoxyglucose ([18F]FDG) is the most common PET ligand. FDG is transported into cells like glucose but not metabolized after the first step in the glycolytic pathway. Thus, the distribution of [18F]FDG reflects cerebral glucose metabolism, providing information on the distribution of neuronal loss and synapse dysfunction. Glucose provides energy for neurotransmitter synthesis, and synaptic dysfunction and neuronal degeneration cause a decline of glucose metabolism in the affected parts of the brain[15].

In patients with Alzheimer's disease most affected brain regions with reduced FDG uptake are temporoparietal association cortex, posterior cingulate cortex, precuneus and variably also frontolateral association cortex[15]. These highly reproducible findings provide excellent separation of Alzheimer's disease patients from normal controls. Different FDG uptake patterns can also be observed in Alzheimer's disease patients with early (<65 years) versus late onset of the disease or high versus low education profile[16]. Because it is crucially important to identify predictors of future cognitive decline, a growing number of studies is being performed in people carrying risk factors (e.g. genetic) for developing Alzheimer's disease. It has been demonstrated that presymptomatic *APOE4* genotype carriers show abnormal uptake reductions using [^{18}F]FDG-PET in an Alzheimer's disease-like pattern in the absence of cortical atrophy[17]. Although an Alzheimer's disease-like pattern has been found to be predictive for future cognitive decline in normal ageing[18], it remains a controversy if hypometabolism in *APOE4* carriers can be considered a sign of pathology or just a genetic consequence[16].

In patients with MCI, AD-like [^{18}F]FDG-PET patterns are predictive for conversion to Alzheimer's disease[19]. In general, glucose hypometabolism has been reliably observed in MCI subjects, especially in posterior cingulate cortex of amnestic type patients. Metabolic changes in parietotemporal areas seem to be the best predictor for a patient's decline from MCI to Alzheimer's disease[16].

To differentiate Alzheimer's disease from other types of dementia, [^{18}F]FDG-PET can be helpful in addition to a clinical examination, given the typical metabolic deficit patterns (frontal and anterior temporal and/or mesiotemporal in FTD; similar to Alzheimer's disease but less sparing of occipital and cerebellar cortices in DLB; diffuse cortical and subcortical in VaD); however, accuracy of discrimination has rarely been reported[16].

Today, [^{18}F]FDG-PET is the best established and growingly available diagnostic tool to observe the metabolic consequences of structural brain alterations in cognitive decline and it is increasingly accepted for reimbursement in countries' medical systems. In today's comparison to SPECT the superiority of PET is evident. Better spatial resolution allows the investigation of smaller brain regions, like the hippocampus, which is of particular interest in the field of memory disorders. In SPECT the occasional loss of the coupling of cortical metabolism and perfusion due to vascular disorders could bias the findings. The effect of hypometabolism shown with [^{18}F]FDG-PET is generally greater than hypoperfusion effects in SPECT[20] and, most importantly, the achievable diagnostic accuracy with PET (sensitivity/specificity: 93%/93% for moderate and 84%/93% for mild [MMSE 24 or higher] Alzheimer's disease versus controls[21]) is higher than with SPECT (66%/79% for Alzheimer's disease versus controls[6]).

Again, an ultimate limitation of studying metabolic patterns is that different diseases could produce the same pattern of metabolic change. As an example, frontal cortical hypometabolism has been reported in both Alzheimer's disease and depression[22], and the diverse clinical manifestations of Alzheimer's disease, often including behavioural changes or mood abnormalities, underline the importance of a detailed clinical evaluation preceding brain imaging.

[^{11}C]PIB-PET and [^{18}F]FDDNP-PET

Direct detection of Alzheimer's disease's histopathological hallmarks, such as amyloid-β plaques and tau tangles *in vivo* using PET, can be seen as a milestone in PET tracer development. Among more than 10 ligands that have been developed in this respect within the past decade, [^{11}C]N-methyl-2-(4-methylaminophenyl)-6-hydroxybenzothiazole ([^{11}C]PIB) has been most extensively studied. [^{11}C]PIB binds to amyloid-β plaques only, and in several Alzheimer's disease patients who have been followed to autopsy after a [^{11}C]PIB-PET scan, areas of high *in vivo* [^{11}C]PIB retention correspond to postmortem regions showing amyloid-β plaque deposition. Today, the ligand is being used in more than 40 centres worldwide. A disadvantage in terms of commercialization of a [^{11}C]PIB is the short half-life of ^{11}C (20 minutes), which requires on-site cyclotron capabilities, limiting more widespread use. However, in contrast to ^{18}F-labelled tracers (110 minute half-life), different imaging studies (e.g. [^{11}C]PIB followed by [^{18}F]FDG) can be performed on the same day.

In Alzheimer's disease patients, [^{11}C]PIB retention is significantly increased in cortical areas compared to controls, particularly in the frontal cortex. [^{11}C]PIB retention has been shown equivalent in patients and controls in areas known to be relatively unaffected by amyloid-β plaques (e.g. white matter, pons, cerebellum)[23]. To determine sensitivity and specificity, larger studies will be necessary.

[^{11}C]PIB has also been studied in patients with amnestic MCI. About half of those subjects showed higher [^{11}C]PIB retention compared to controls[24]. Recent investigations suggest this MCI subgroup might be at a higher risk of Alzheimer's disease conversion and therefore measuring [^{11}C]PIB retention would improve the identification of possible converters. In addition, a good correlation between [^{11}C]PIB and other biomarkers (e.g. CSF Aβ_{1-42}) has been reported[25].

There could also be a possible role for [^{11}C]PIB in the differential diagnosis of dementia. [^{11}C]PIB retention was lower and more variable in DLB and absent in FTD compared to Alzheimer's disease patients[26].

In a two-year follow-up analysis, Alzheimer's disease patients showed a pronounced decrease in glucose metabolism, measured with [^{18}F]FDG-PET, and cognitive decline but surprisingly stable [^{11}C]PIB retention. It has been argued that only a part of amyloid-β plaques might be accessible to exogenous tracer binding or retention could reach an equilibrium state and that additional processes, such as microglial activation and inflammation, should be taken into account in future PET multitracer binding studies[27]. However, such longitudinal findings of relatively stable levels of [^{11}C]PIB retention[27] despite declines in glucose metabolism and cognitive function may limit its utility as a short-term predictor of future cognitive decline.

[^{11}C]PIB-PET has been shown to detect cerebrovascular amyloid in patients with cerebral amyloid angiopathy, a major cause of haemorrhagic stroke. This raises the possibility of extending the future use of [^{11}C]PIB-PET[28].

2-(1-[{6-[(2-[^{18}F]fluoroethyl)(methyl)amino]-2-naphthyl}ethylidene)malononitrile ([^{18}F]FDDNP) is the only molecular imaging probe known to bind to *both* amyloid-β plaques and tau neurofibrillary tangles. Irrespective of its not yet widespread use compared to [^{11}C]PIB, it might be the more promising candidate from a clinical perspective. Moreover, the longer half-life of ^{18}F could make it more accessible to clinical settings without a cyclotron on site. [^{18}F]FDDNP has been shown to provide good visualization of plaques and tangles in autopsy-obtained human brain tissue specimens, and it clearly distinguishes between Alzheimer's disease and MCI patients and control subjects. Global [^{18}F]FDDNP values were more accurate for diagnostic classification than [^{18}F]FDG-PET or volumetric MRI measurements[29]. [^{18}F]FDDNP-PET signal is highly correlated with cognitive performance, and the agreement between *in vivo* and histopathological postmortem tau and tangle burden maps is remarkable[30].

It has become obvious that tau tangle load and not amyloid-β plaque load is associated with age-related cognitive decline[31]. Direct comparison of [11C]PIB and [18F]FDDNP in the same subjects showed highest [18F]FDDNP but lowest [11C]PIB binding in the medial temporal cortex of Alzheimer's disease patients, again suggesting that tau tangles are the driving pathological factor in this region[32] and maybe in Alzheimer's disease itself.

[18F]MPPF-PET

Changes in neuronal integrity and neuronal loss are a consequence of the molecular processes in AD pathology and are highly correlated with the decline of cognitive abilities. Therefore, any new possibility to (preferably presymptomatically) detect these changes in brain regions known to be the first affected in the development of the disease (e.g. entorhinal cortex and hippocampus CA1 and subicular fields) would be of interest to contribute to diagnostic precision and our understanding of pathology.

The correlation between neuronal death of large pyramidal cells in hippocampus CA1 field and serotonin 1A receptor density (although glutamatergic, these neurons receive high inhibitory serotonergic input via serotonin 1A receptors) has been studied in rodents using autoradiography[33]. With the development of 4-[18F]fluoro-N-{2-[1-(2-methoxyphenyl)-piperazinyl]ethyl}-N-(2-pyridinyl)benzamide ([18F]MPPF) as a serotonin 1A receptor binding PET ligand, *in vivo* measurements of receptor density could be performed in humans. Results indicate that [18F]MPPF-PET clearly distinguishes Alzheimer's disease, MCI and control subjects. Whereas Alzheimer's disease subjects showed the most widespread decrease in [18F]MPPF binding, with primarily hippocampus but also raphe nuclei being affected, the maybe most remarkable finding was that receptor densities were clearly decreased in MCI patients with only mild cognitive decline[34]. Despite the fact that the relationship between serotonin 1A receptor density, possible related compensatory and adaptive processes, and disease progression needs to be further examined, [18F]MPPF-PET, especially in addition to other techniques, such as [18F]FDDNP-PET, could be a next step to an early and exclusive *in vivo* diagnosis of Alzheimer's disease.

CONCLUDING REMARKS

In the years to come, nuclear medicine techniques will face new competitors. Namely, molecular magnetic resonance imaging, using iron oxide based contrast agents, designed with affinity to receptors or cell surface components may provide molecular pathway or receptor distribution mapping with superior spatial resolution[35]. Only a few years ago SPECT brain imaging was believed to undoubtedly persist in brain research and diagnostic procedures but today it struggles to survive in a PET environment. But to draw conclusions about whether one imaging technique would overcome another maybe also means to underestimate the next both hardware- and software-based technological advances.

REFERENCES

1. Rahmim A, Zaidi H. PET versus SPECT: strengths, limitations and challenges. *Nucl Med Commun* 2008; **29**(3): 193–207.

2. Rust TC, Kadrmas DJ. Rapid dual-tracer PTSM+ATSM PET imaging of tumour blood flow and hypoxia: a simulation study. *Phys Med Biol* 2006; **51**(1): 61–75.

3. Sultzer DL. Behavioral syndrome in dementia: neuroimaging insights. *Semin Clin Neuropsychiatry* 1996; **1**(4): 261–71.

4. Montaldi D, Brooks DN, McColl JH *et al.* Measurements of regional cerebral blood flow and cognitive performance in Alzheimer's disease. *J Neurol Neurosurg Psychiatry* 1990; **53**(1): 33–8.

5. Geaney DP, Soper N, Shepstone BJ, Cowen PJ. Effect of central cholinergic stimulation on regional cerebral blood flow in Alzheimer disease. *Lancet* 1990; **335**(8704): 1484–7.

6. Jagust W, Thisted R, Devous MD, Sr *et al.* SPECT perfusion imaging in the diagnosis of Alzheimer's disease: a clinical–pathologic study. *Neurology* 2001; **56**(7): 950–56.

7. Dougall NJ, Bruggink S, Ebmeier KP. Systematic review of the diagnostic accuracy of 99mTc-HMPAO-SPECT in dementia. *Am J Geriatr Psychiatry* 2004; **12**(6): 554–70.

8. Matsuda H. Role of neuroimaging in Alzheimer's disease, with emphasis on brain perfusion SPECT. *J Nucl Med* 2007; **48**(8): 1289–300.

9. Van Laere K, Versijpt J, Audenaert K *et al.* 99mTc-ECD brain perfusion SPET: variability, asymmetry and effects of age and gender in healthy adults. *Eur J Nucl Med* 2001; **28**(7): 873–87.

10. Bench CJ, Friston KJ, Brown RG, Frackowiak RS, Dolan RJ. Regional cerebral blood flow in depression measured by positron emission tomography: the relationship with clinical dimensions. *Psychol Med* 1993; **23**(3): 579–90.

11. Lucey JV, Costa DC, Blanes T *et al.* Regional cerebral blood flow in obsessive–compulsive disordered patients at rest. Differential correlates with obsessive–compulsive and anxious–avoidant dimensions. *Br J Psychiatry* 1995; **167**(5): 629–34.

12. Zaidi H, Mawlawi O, Orton CG. Point/counterpoint. Simultaneous PET/MR will replace PET/CT as the molecular multimodality imaging platform of choice. *Med Phys* 2007; **34**(5): 1525–8.

13. Chen WP, Matsunari I, Noda A *et al.* Rapid scanning protocol for brain (18)F-FDG PET: a validation study. *J Nucl Med* 2005; **46**(10): 1633–41.

14. Small GW, Bookheimer SY, Thompson PM *et al.* Current and future uses of neuroimaging for cognitively impaired patients. *Lancet Neurol* 2008; **7**(2): 161–72.

15. Herholz K. PET studies in dementia. *Ann Nucl Med* 2003; **17**(2): 79–89.

16. Mosconi L. Brain glucose metabolism in the early and specific diagnosis of Alzheimer's disease. FDG-PET studies in MCI and AD. *Eur J Nucl Med Mol Imaging* 2005; **32**(4): 486–510.

17. Small GW, Ercoli LM, Silverman DH *et al.* Cerebral metabolic and cognitive decline in persons at genetic risk for Alzheimer's disease. *Proc Natl Acad Sci U S A* 2000; **97**(11): 6037–42.

18. Small GW, La Rue A, Komo S, Kaplan A, Mandelkern MA. Predictors of cognitive change in middle-aged and older adults with memory loss. *Am J Psychiatry* 1995; **152**(12): 1757–64.

19. Silverman DH, Small GW, Chang CY *et al.* Positron emission tomography in evaluation of dementia: regional brain metabolism and long-term outcome. *JAMA* 2001; **286**(17): 2120–27.

20. Silverman DH. Brain 18F-FDG PET in the diagnosis of neurodegenerative dementias: comparison with perfusion SPECT and

with clinical evaluations lacking nuclear imaging. *J Nucl Med* 2004; **45**(4): 594–607.

21. Herholz K, Salmon E, Perani D *et al*. Discrimination between Alzheimer dementia and controls by automated analysis of multicenter FDG PET. *Neuroimage* 2002; **17**(1): 302–16.

22. Baxter LR, Jr, Schwartz JM, Phelps ME *et al*. Reduction of prefrontal cortex glucose metabolism common to three types of depression. *Arch Gen Psychiatry* 1989; **46**(3): 243–50.

23. Klunk WE, Engler H, Nordberg A *et al*. Imaging brain amyloid in Alzheimer's disease with Pittsburgh Compound-B. *Ann Neurol* 2004; **55**(3): 306–19.

24. Kemppainen NM, Aalto S, Wilson IA *et al*. PET amyloid ligand [11C]PIB uptake is increased in mild cognitive impairment. *Neurology* 2007; **68**(19): 1603–6.

25. Forsberg A, Engler H, Almkvist O *et al*. PET imaging of amyloid deposition in patients with mild cognitive impairment. *Neurobiol Aging* 2008; **29**(10): 1456–65.

26. Rowe CC, Ng S, Ackermann U *et al*. Imaging beta-amyloid burden in aging and dementia. *Neurology* 2007; **68**(20): 1718–25.

27. Engler H, Forsberg A, Almkvist O *et al*. Two-year follow-up of amyloid deposition in patients with Alzheimer's disease. *Brain* 2006; **129**(11): 2856–66.

28. Johnson KA, Gregas M, Becker JA *et al*. Imaging of amyloid burden and distribution in cerebral amyloid angiopathy. *Ann Neurol* 2007; **62**(3): 229–34.

29. Small GW, Kepe V, Ercoli LM *et al*. PET of brain amyloid and tau in mild cognitive impairment. *N Engl J Med* 2006; **355**(25): 2652–63.

30. Braskie MN, Klunder AD, Hayashi KM *et al*. Plaque and tangle imaging and cognition in normal aging and Alzheimer's disease. doi:10.1016/j.neurobiolaging.2008.09.012.

31. Petersen RC, Parisi JE, Dickson DW *et al*. Neuropathologic features of amnestic mild cognitive impairment. *Arch Neurol* 2006; **63**(5): 665–72.

32. Shin J, Lee SY, Kim SH, Kim YB, Cho SJ. Multitracer PET imaging of amyloid plaques and neurofibrillary tangles in Alzheimer's disease. *Neuroimage* 2008; **43**(2): 236–44.

33. Van Bogaert P, de Tiege X, Vanderwinden JM *et al*. Comparative study of hippocampal neuronal loss and in vivo binding of 5-HT1a receptors in the KA model of limbic epilepsy in the rat. *Epilepsy Res* 2001; **47**(1–2): 127–39.

34. Kepe V, Barrio JR, Huang SC *et al*. Serotonin 1A receptors in the living brain of Alzheimer's disease patients. *Proc Natl Acad Sci U S A* 2006; **103**(3): 702–7.

35. Blamire AM. The technology of MRI – the next 10 years? *Br J Radiol* 2008; **81**(968): 601–17.

46

Computational Anatomy in Alzheimer's Disease

Alex D. Leow[1], Liana G. Apostolova[2] and Paul M. Thompson[2]

[1]*Department of Psychiatry, University of Illinois at Chicago, Chicago, IL, USA*
Community Psychiatry Associates, Sacramento, CA, USA
[2]*Department of Neurology, UCLA David Geffen School of Medicine, Los Angeles, CA, USA*

INTRODUCTION

Alzheimer's disease (AD) is the most common form of dementia, afflicting over 24 million people worldwide. In early AD, short-term memory function is typically among the first to be impaired, followed by a progressive decline in other cognitive functions along with emotional/behavioural disturbances. At present, there is no cure for AD, whose natural course is insidious yet gradually debilitating, and is typically fatal at its most advanced stage, usually due to medical complications. In recent years, scientific interest has also focused on mild cognitive impairment (MCI), a pre-dementia stage that carries a four- to six-fold increased risk of future diagnosis of dementia, relative to the general population[1–3].

Many investigators have used MRI and PET imaging to measure longitudinal progression of brain changes in normal aging, MCI and AD, with varying results. As drug candidates that might slow the progression of Alzheimer's pathology began to be developed, the need for robust and sensitive imaging methods to quantify progression of Alzheimer's disease has become increasingly important. As a result, we are starting to see large collaborative multicentre imaging studies on Alzheimer's disease. For example, the National Institute of Aging and pharmaceutical industry funded the Alzheimer's Disease Neuroimaging Initiative[4,5] (ADNI), with the goal of developing improved methods based on imaging and other biomarkers, for AD treatment trials.

Major advances are occurring in scanning techniques and in image analysis, making it easier to track disease progression with greater power. In studies of hundreds of subjects scanned over time, databases of images can now be combined to visualize the disease trajectory, showing the spread of cortical atrophy, impaired metabolism, and even plaque and tangle accumulation. Ultra-high-field MRI reveals early changes in specific hippocampal subfields[4,5], and new PET ligands are emerging to visualize plaque and tangle pathology[6–9].

In this chapter, we review several strategies of computational anatomy in mapping brain deficits in AD and early dementia. These strategies include cortical thickness mapping, tensor-based morphometry (TBM) and hippocampal surface modelling. Mathematical concepts from surface modelling, non-linear three-dimensional volume registration, fluid mechanics and multivariate statistics are used across subjects for group and interval comparisons. They can be exploited to distinguish diseases from normal variations in brain structure, and help yield insights into the dynamics of AD and MCI.

COMPUTATIONAL ANATOMY

Computational anatomy is a general term covering a broad class of mathematical methods that model anatomical structures in images as three-dimensional curves, surfaces and volumes, and combine them across subjects to create statistical maps of brain structural differences.

Cortical Thickness Mapping

In this approach, in order to precisely quantify the amount of tissue loss, overall grey and white matter volumes can be computed from brain MRI scans. Tissue classification methods can assign each image voxel to a specific tissue class. If grey matter maps from many subjects are aligned to a standard three-dimensional digital brain atlas, on which lobar subdivisions have been labelled, regional statistics for subdivisions can be derived. These region-of-interest measures, in conjunction with manual tracings of the hippocampus and other subcortical structures, have been the mainstay of morphometric analysis for nearly two decades.

One approach for cortical thickness mapping is presented in Figure 46.1, which shows a computational pipeline for processing MRI scans as described by Thompson *et al.*[10]. For each scan, a three-dimensional map is first computed quantifying the distance of cortical grey matter voxels to the grey/white matter interface. Thickness values are calculated from the inner cortical surface to the outer cortical surface, and are plotted at each point on a cortical surface model extracted from the scan. To combine thickness data across subjects (Figure 46.1, second row), a spherical coordinate system is imposed onto each subject's cortical surface. This serves as a reference grid so that thickness data can be compared at a given surface-based coordinate across subjects. If sulcal/gyral landmarks are traced onto the cortical models, data from corresponding cortical regions can be averaged across subjects using a technique known as cortical pattern matching[10] (CPM), where the sulcal pattern is digitized and matched across subjects using a flow field in spherical coordinates. By doing so, an average cortical model can be created

Principles and Practice of Geriatric Psychiatry, 3rd edn. Edited by Mohammed T. Abou-Saleh, Cornelius Katona and Anand Kumar

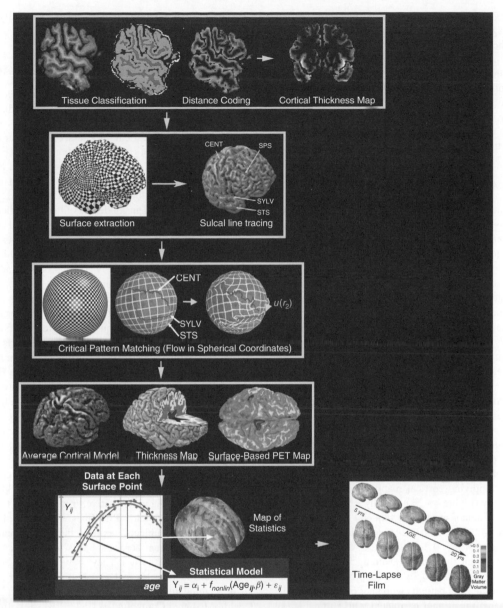

Figure 46.1 Flowchart showing an image analysis pipeline (adapted from[10]) that can map changes of various neuroanatomical measures in the cortex, such as grey matter atrophy. Cortical thickness profiles, for example, can be averaged across subjects or compared across time. Tissue classification techniques can be used to identify grey and white matter and to produce cortical thickness maps (row 1). The CPM approach can be applied by tracing sulcal landmarks on extracted brain surface models (row 2) that serve as anchors to guide a flow field matching gyral regions across subjects (row 3). Then maps of cortical thickness, or other cortical signals (such as co-registered PET images, shown here), can be fluidly aligned to an average cortical model (row 4). Statistical models are fitted to data from all the subjects at each cortical point. This can assess whether imaging signals are associated with age (bottom row), or other parameters of interest. Effects of ageing on cortical measures – or changes relative to baseline – may be animated as a time-lapse film to reveal the disease trajectory. *A full colour version of this figure appears in the colour plate section*

for a group of subjects (such as an AD or MCI population), with well-defined sulcal features in their mean spatial locations (Figure 46.1, fourth row). Moreover, maps of cortical thickness in each individual can be transferred onto this average model while adjusting for the individual gyral pattern differences across subjects. This method allows pixel-by-pixel averaging of values within each delineated region across all subjects, allowing comparisons of patients with controls. Lastly, a statistical model can be fitted to the thickness measures from all subjects at each surface point

(Figure 46.1, bottom row). In brain mapping studies, it is common to fit statistical models to data at each location in an image, to assess effects of age, diagnosis or experimental parameters (an approach known as statistical parametric mapping; SPM[11]). The results are displayed in the form of a three-dimensional map of statistics, and the overall significance of the map can be colour-coded to show the distribution of atrophy[10].

Cortical thickness mapping is related to several simpler but widely used methods. For example, the 'boundary shift integral' technique quantifies differences between two successive co-registered 3D MRIs by examining the magnitude of the shifting of grey–white junction[12]. Before algorithms became widely available for computing cortical thickness accurately from MRI scans, it was more common to compute a local measure of grey matter volume called 'grey matter density' (GMD). This is defined, at each point in an image, as the proportion of tissue segmented as grey matter in a small spherical region (typically of 10–12 mm radius) centred at that point[13,14]. GMD and thickness are highly correlated[15], except at the temporal lobe tips, where cortical curvature is high.

Cortical Maps in AD and MCI

Cortical mapping methods have distinguished patterns of atrophy typical of late- versus early-onset AD[16], and different dementia subtypes[17]. Sowell et al.[18] applied cortical pattern matching to 176 scans of subjects aged 7 to 87, and compiled trajectories of grey matter thinning, for each cortical point, over the life span. Encouragingly, there was close regional correspondence between the cortical thickness maps created from in vivo MRI and the 1929 postmortem data of von Economo. The cortex does not age in a homogeneous way; each cortical region has a somewhat distinctive trajectory[18,19]. A related study by Gogtay et al.[20] created a time-lapse map of cortical development from ages 4 to 22, and showed the earliest maturing cortex is least vulnerable to aging and AD.

Apostolova et al.[21] compared grey matter profiles in 26 amnestic MCI and 31 mild AD subjects, showing strikingly greater atrophy in mild AD (Figure 46.2A), conforming to the pattern of spread of AD pathology observed postmortem through the brain. A related VBM study found significantly greater parietal, anterior and posterior cingulate atrophy in mild to severe AD relative to MCI[23].

In Apostolova et al.[22], we also examined the structural correlates of apathy in AD, by applying cortical mapping to 35 AD patients with and without apathy (Figure 46.2B). Apathy severity was associated with cortical grey matter atrophy in bilateral anterior cingulate (Brodmann area BA 24; $r = 0.39$–0.42, $p = 0.01$) and left medial frontal cortex (BA 8 and 9; $r = 0.4$, $p < 0.02$). A subsequent study found associations between the Boston Naming Test and the animal fluency tests and cortical atrophy in 19 probable AD and 5 multiple-domain amnestic MCI patients who later converted to AD[24]. The degree of language impairment correlated with cortical atrophy in the left temporal and parietal lobes, especially in the perisylvian language cortices.

Time-Lapse Maps and the Trajectory of AD

The cortical pattern matching approach may be extended to time-varying or functional imaging data. If longitudinal scans are available, a time-lapse movie of disease progression can be created by fitting a trajectory to cortical thickness, or any other imaging parameter, at each cortical point (Figure 46.1, bottom right)[25]. A movie 'frame' can then be written out for each time-point and the series of frames can be animated. An example of this type of dynamic map may be viewed at www.loni.ucla.edu/~thompson/AD_4D/dynamic.html. Here, a time-dependent model was fitted to cortical grey matter density in 14 AD patients and 12 controls scanned longitudinally for 4 years. Maps of the degree of deficits – either as a percentage or as a significance map – show that the cortex is thinner in medial and lateral temporal lobes in early AD and deficits advance anteriorly to engulf the cingulate and frontal cortex.

Figure 46.3 shows two time-points from this animation, showing that cortical atrophy on MRI proceeds in approximately the same anatomical sequence as plaque and tangle burden in histopathological studies of AD. Plaque and tangle deposition starts in medial temporal regions[26] and affects the posterior limbic system first due to its close connections to the posterior cingulate gyrus[27]. Hypometabolism of the posterior cingulate is observed early in AD, even when no atrophy is detected in this region[28]. On the other hand, in frontotemporal lobar degeneration, neuronal loss is first observed in the frontal regions closely connected to the anterior cingulate cortex[29].

Cortical pattern matching can also be used to understand how amyloid load spreads in the living brain. Braskie et al.[8,30] applied cortical pattern matching to 23 subjects (10 controls, 6 amnestic MCI, 7 AD) scanned with both MRI and [18F]FDDNP, a recently developed PET ligand sensitive to plaque and tangle pathology[7,31]. They aligned parametric PET images of amyloid load to MRI scans from the same subjects, textured the PET signals onto the cortex, and combined them across subjects using cortical pattern matching (Figure 46.1, fourth row). They showed that the advancing pathology also follows the classical Braak trajectory for neurofibrillary tangle accumulation. Related work by Mintun et al.[9] and Rowe et al.[32] with Pittsburgh Compound-B ([11C]PIB) show frontal lobe labelling

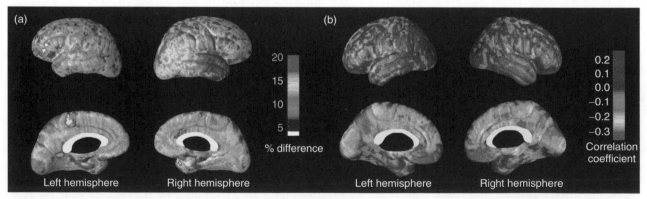

Figure 46.2 (A) Cortical thinning of up to 20% occurs between MCI and AD, in widely distributed cortical areas (greatest tissue loss is coded in red). (B). Grey matter atrophy in the anterior cingulate and supplementary motor cortices is correlated with the presence or absence of apathy in AD. Regions where structural variation correlates with clinical or behavioural differences can be identified using correlation maps such as these (strong associations are shown here in red colours). Data adapted from[21,22]. *A full colour version of this figure appears in the colour plate section*

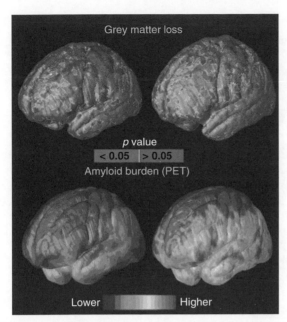

Figure 46.3 Progression of AD based on MRI and [^{18}F]FDDNP PET. On MRI (top row), the areas with grey matter deficits in mild AD (left panel) include primarily the temporal lobe, but in moderate AD (right panel) these deficits have spread to involve the frontal cortex (adapted from a longitudinal study by Thompson *et al.*[25]). Finally, cerebral amyloid estimated *in vivo* from the PET ligand FDDNP is low in controls, but higher in those with impaired cognition (bottom row; adapted from Braskie *et al.*[8]). The anatomical agreement is striking between these *in vivo* maps and the well-established post-mortem maps for the staging of AD. In all maps, the sensorimotor cortex shows least disease-related degeneration. *A full colour version of this figure appears in the colour plate section*

early in the degenerative sequence. The PIB progression pattern is consistent with the Braak trajectory for amyloid deposition, which, unlike tangle deposition, shows early increases in the basal neocortex, particularly in frontal and temporal lobes and primarily in poorly myelinated regions such as the perirhinal cortex.

Tensor-Based Morphometry

While the methods described so far provide detailed maps of changes in cortical measures, tensor-based morphometry (TBM) can identify regional volumetric differences in the structure of the brain, both cross-sectionally and longitudinally, from the gradients of the deformation fields that align, or 'warp', images. In a longitudinal design, TBM can track structural changes between serial 3D MRI images, by producing rates of atrophy over time (in percentage points per year). In a cross-sectional design, TBM can compare structural scans of two different groups, such as AD versus controls or MCI versus controls.

Figure 46.4 shows the premise of TBM. If a pair of scans is collected from the same subject over time, they can be aligned with each other, using a fluid transformation that applies compressions and expansions at a local level throughout the anatomy. One class of registration methods models the baseline image as a deformable elastic medium or as a viscous fluid, and applies distributed internal forces to reconfigure the earlier scan to match the later one. The spatial gradient of this transformation (deformed grid in Figure 46.4) provides information on how much tissue is lost over the time interval between the scans, and can be plotted and colour-coded. Applied to a sequence of scans acquired over time from the same patient, these voxel expansion/compression maps[12], also known as Jacobian maps, can reveal the extent and spread of atrophy. They are also amenable to voxel-by-voxel averaging, to make a map of the average voxel-wise atrophy rate.

As part of the ADNI project, Thompson and Leow have applied the TBM approach and analysed the ADNI dataset using both cross-sectional and longitudinal designs. Leow *et al.*[33] studied the serial high-resolution MRI scans (12 months apart) from 40 normal controls, 40 MCI, and 20 AD patients from ADNI. These individual Jacobian maps, representing annual atrophy rates, are then nonlinearly registered to a common template, followed by voxel-wise statistical testing to detect group differences. These maps can also be correlated, on a voxel level, with biomarkers and neuropsychological measures. Moreover, these Jacobian maps can also be summarized on an ROI level to give overall atrophy rates in regions of interest (Figure 46.5; right panel). In the MCI group, temporal lobe atrophy rates were correlated with changes in mini-mental state exam

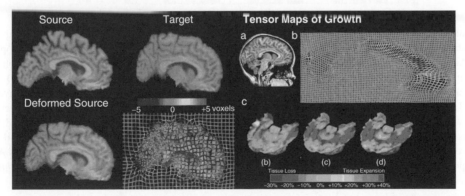

Figure 46.4 Tensor-based morphometry. In TBM, a fluid transformation (*deformed grid*) is applied to a baseline scan (*source*) to reconfigure it (*deformed source*) into the shape of a follow-up scan (*target*). The local expansions (*red colours*) or atrophies (*blue colours*) can be plotted in brain regions such as the corpus callosum (shown in the green box in [a]). Voxel expansions (*red colours*) or contractions (*blue colours*) can be plotted onto a sequence of scans collected from the same subject (shown here in axial view illustrating progressive temporal lobe atrophy in a subject with frontotemporal lobe atrophy) during a degenerative brain disease, emphasizing regions with progressive atrophy. These maps may be averaged across subjects or compared across populations to assess factors that influence degenerative rates in each region of the brain. *A full colour version of this figure appears in the colour plate section*

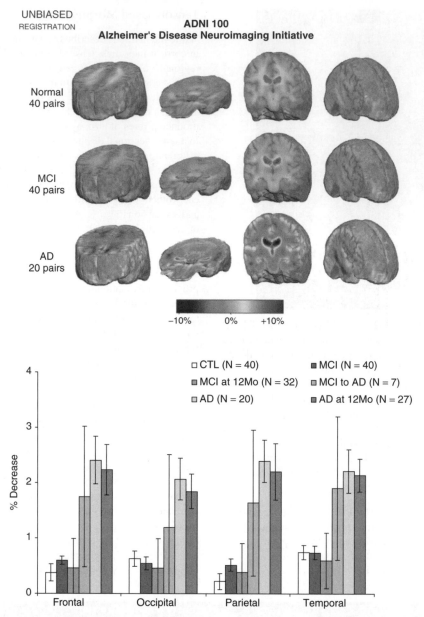

Figure 46.5 (Top panel) average longitudinal tissue atrophy/expansion rate for 40 normal, 40 MCI and 20 AD subjects, using serial MRI scans from the ADNI dataset scanned at 12 months apart. Ventricular expansion (third column) and temporal lobe atrophy (fourth column) are most prominent in the AD group. (Bottom panel) Percentage brain tissue loss from baseline to follow-up within each lobe can be computed by averaging the maps in the left panel for each region of interest (with CSF excluded). The diagnoses for the AD, MCI and CTL groups were determined at baseline. Here, MCI at 12Mo denotes subjects diagnosed as MCI at baseline who did not convert to AD at 12-month follow-up, whereas MCI to AD signifies those who had converted to AD at 12-month follow-up. One MCI subject's diagnosis converted back to control at follow-up, and thus was excluded from the MCI subgroups. The first bar in each group (coloured *white*) shows mild but significant progressive atrophy in controls. The second bar (*turquoise*) denotes MCI subjects at baseline, and is followed by bars denoting converters and non-converters. Mean rates are typically higher in the converters, comparable to subjects diagnosed as AD at both time-points, or AD at the last time-point (*last two bars*). This figure is adapted from the results in[33]. *A full colour version of this figure appears in the colour plate section*

(MMSE) scores, clinical dementia rating (CDR) and logical/verbal learning memory scores. In the AD group, temporal atrophy rates were correlated with several biomarker indices, including a higher CSF level of p-tau protein, and a greater CSF tau/beta amyloid 1–42 (ABeta42) ratio. Temporal lobe atrophy rate was significantly higher in MCI subjects who converted to AD than in non-converters. Serial MRI scans can therefore be analysed with TBM to relate ongoing neurodegeneration to a variety of pathological biomarkers, cognitive changes and conversion from MCI to AD, tracking disease progression in three-dimensional detail.

Using a cross-sectional design, Hua *et al.*[34] computed the statistical maps of group differences using 40 normal controls, 40 MCI subjects

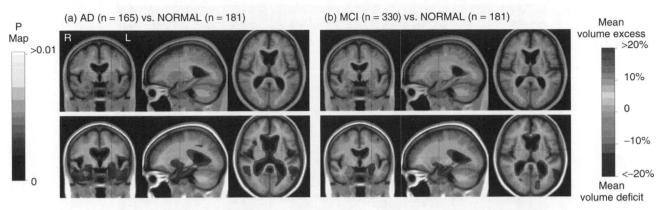

Figure 46.6 3D maps of brain atrophy comparing group differences between MCI ($n = 330$) versus normal ($n = 181$), and AD subjects ($n = 165$) versus normal. The top rows of panels (a) and (b) show the mean level of atrophy as a percentage reduction in volume. The bottom rows show the significance of these reductions, revealing highly significant atrophy in AD but a more anatomically restricted atrophic pattern in MCI. In MCI (b), atrophy is most prominent in the left hippocampus; ventricular expansion is also substantial. When AD is compared with MCI (not shown here), additional temporal lobe degeneration is evident. The overall level of ventricular expansion is about 10–15% for MCI and greater than 20% for the AD group. This figure is adapted from the results in[35]. *A full colour version of this figure appears in the colour plate section*

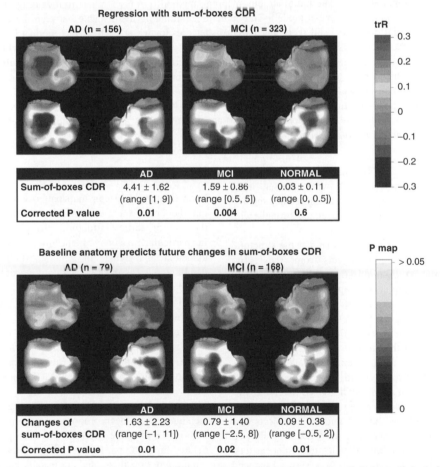

Figure 46.7 Temporal lobe atrophy correlates with sum-of-boxes clinical dementia rating and future clinical decline. Top row negative correlations are detected between temporal lobe atrophy and higher CDR scores at the time of the initial scan (i.e. a higher CDR score correlates with a faster rate of atrophy). The corrected *P* values in the table (inset) provide an overall estimate of significance, corrected for multiple comparisons. Bottom row atrophy of the temporal lobe also predicts future cognitive decline, as reflected by an increase in CDR scores, which indicates deteriorating cognitive function over the following year. trR denotes partial correlation coefficient. This figure is adapted from the results in[35]. *A full colour version of this figure appears in the colour plate section*

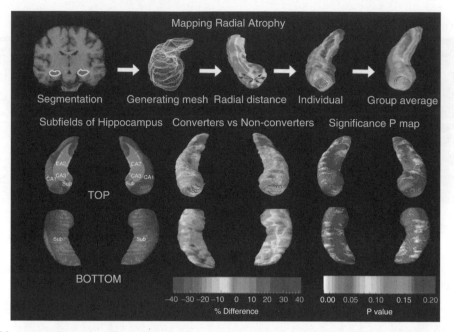

Figure 46.8 Mapping hippocampal atrophy. The radial atrophy mapping method (*top row*) relies on manually or automatically segmenting the hippocampus, computing a 3D parametric mesh model of the structure, estimating the distance between the central core of the structure to each surface point (i.e. the radial distance), and recording radial distance estimates at each surface point to create individual and group average colour-coded maps of the radial distance. These are then statistically compared between groups or conditions. One longitudinal 3D MRI study[50] compared baseline hippocampal atrophy in MCI subjects who converted to AD versus MCI subjects who remained stable or improved cognitively during three years of clinical follow-up. Greater atrophy at baseline was seen in the CA1 and subicular areas in subjects who subsequently convert to clinically probable AD (*bottom right panels*). The bottom panels show a schematic representation of the hippocampal subfields (*left*), the proportional difference in atrophy levels between converters and non-converters (in percentage points; *middle panels*), and the significance of these differences taking into account normal structural variation (*bottom right panel*). *A full colour version of this figure appears in the colour plate section*

and 40 AD subjects enrolled in ADNI, and reported widespread medial temporal and limbic atrophy in AD, with a lesser, more restricted distribution in MCI. Moreover, correlation studies showed that atrophy and CSF space expansion both correlated strongly with MMSE scores and CDR.

Hua *et al.*[35] increased the sample size and mapped the structural differences between groups using 676 subjects from ADNI (165 AD, 330 MCI and 181 controls). Figure 46.6 visualizes these group differences, revealing highly significant atrophy in AD but a more anatomically restricted atrophic pattern in MCI. These maps can also be correlated with neuropsychological test results or biomarkers. In Figure 46.7, these correlations (between atrophy rates and sum-of-box CDR scores) are plotted on the surface of the temporal lobes. Using this 676-subject sample, baseline temporal lobe atrophy is shown to be correlated with current cognitive performance, future cognitive decline and conversion from MCI to AD over the following year; it predicted future decline even in healthy subjects. In this particular sample, over half of the AD and MCI subjects carried the *APOE4* gene, which increases risk for AD; they showed greater hippocampal and temporal lobe deficits than non-carriers. *APOE2* gene carriers – 1/6 of the normal group – showed reduced ventricular expansion, suggesting a protective effect.

Compared to manual tracing employed in cortical pattern matching, TBM is attractive for clinical trials, as large samples can be studied with no manual interaction. Power is also slightly increased if all brains are aligned to a common brain template that is representative of the mean anatomy of all subjects in the population.

Hippocampal Radial Mapping

Even though TBM can map patterns of atrophic changes throughout the brain, the fact remains that the medial temporal lobe is the site of earliest structural change in AD. The hippocampus, in particular, is one of the most researched brain regions in dementia and aging. In general, studies have shown that AD pathology is associated with hippocampal shrinkage[36], and is linked to memory decline. In normal aging, hippocampal volume loss is on average 1.6–1.7% per year[37,38] while that of the entorhinal cortex is ~1.4% per year[39]. Much higher hippocampal rates are observed in MCI and AD, with faster atrophy rates in MCI subjects who progress to AD relative to those who remain stable (annual hippocampal atrophy rate for MCI patients who remain stable = 2.8%, for MCI converters = 3.7% and for AD = 3.5–4%[36]).

In addition to manual tracing on high resolution MRI, several techniques have been proposed for segmenting the hippocampus. A deformable template approach has been proposed that utilizes a predefined hippocampal template[40–43]. Fully automatic methods do not require any user input, and are usually based on extracting and combining some set of image features. For example, Powell *et al.*[44] used artificial neural networks and Golland *et al.*[45] proposed to use a large feature pool, and principal component analysis (PCA) to reduce the size of the feature pool. Another fully automated approach for subcortical segmentation is FreeSurfer by Fischl *et al.*[46,47]. FreeSurfer uses a Markov random field to approximate the posterior distribution for anatomical labellings. Morra *et al.* recently developed a new and powerful hippocampal segmentation approach based on adaptive boosting or AdaBoost. AdaBoost is highly underutilized in medical imaging, although it has generated great interest in pattern recognition and other related fields[48].

Once the hippocampus is segmented, it can serve as a basis for other advanced surface- or volume-based computational anatomy techniques. In an effort to localize these changes to specific hippocampal sectors, Thompson *et al.*[49] proposed a radial atrophy mapping (RAM) approach, which creates surface models to represent the hippocampus, imposes a regular grid structure on anatomical models from different individuals, and uses this structure to compute average shape models for different groups. As a local index of atrophy, the distance of each surface point to a centreline threading down the centre of the structure is plotted on the surface (Figure 46.8). Surface-based statistics on this measure can then be used to identify regions where atrophy is associated with diagnosis, cognition, genotype or medication.

CONCLUSION

Here we surveyed a range of computational anatomy methods to monitor dementia progression, each focusing on specific features of the degenerative process. Cortical thickness maps, for example, localize changes relative to gyral and sulcal landmarks, and can be used to create time-lapse movies, but require some time investment in extracting cortical surface models. If data collection is time-consuming and power requirements are high, this approach is still useful even in a clinical trial, as it may detect disease-related changes over short time intervals. Higher-throughput methods, such as TBM and automated hippocampal mapping, are well suited to very large-scale studies. These may be the first mapping methods to routinely analyse databases of images from thousands of subjects. As such, they are natural approaches to use in epidemiological studies of potential risk factors or protective factors that may influence disease onset, conversion or the normal aging process.

REFERENCES

1. Petersen RC, Smith GE, Waring SC *et al.* Mild cognitive impairment: clinical characterization and outcome. *Arch Neurol* 1999; **56**(3): 303–8.
2. Petersen RC. Aging, mild cognitive impairment, and Alzheimer's disease. *Neurol Clin* 2000; **18**(4): 789–806.
3. Petersen RC, Doody R, Kurz A *et al.* Current concepts in mild cognitive impairment. *Arch Neurol* 2001; **58**(12): 1985–92.
4. Augustinack JC, van der Kouwe AJ, Blackwell ML *et al.* Detection of entorhinal layer II using 7Tesla [corrected] magnetic resonance imaging. *Ann Neurol* 2005; **57**(4): 489–94.
5. Mueller SG, Stables L, Du AT *et al.* Measurement of hippocampal subfields and age-related changes with high resolution MRI at 4T. *Neurobiol Aging* 2007; **28**(5): 719–26.
6. Klunk WE, Engler H, Nordberg A *et al.* Imaging brain amyloid in Alzheimer's disease with Pittsburgh Compound-B. *Ann Neurol* 2004; **55**(3): 306–19.
7. Small GW, Kepe V, Ercoli LM *et al.* PET of brain amyloid and tau in mild cognitive impairment. *N Engl J Med* 2006; **355**(25): 2652–63.
8. Braskie MN, Klunder AD, Hayashi KM *et al.* Dynamic trajectory of cortical plaque and tangle load correlates with

9. Mintun MA, Larossa GN, Sheline YI *et al.* [11C]PIB in a non-demented population: potential antecedent marker of Alzheimer disease. *Neurology* 2006; **67**(3): 446–52.
10. Thompson PM, Hayashi KM, Sowell ER *et al.* Mapping cortical change in Alzheimer's disease, brain development, and schizophrenia. *Neuroimage* 2004; **23**(suppl 1): S2–18.
11. Friston KJ, Holmes A, Poline JB, Price CJ, Frith CD. Detecting activations in PET and fMRI: levels of inference and power. *Neuroimage* 1996; **4**(3pt 1): 223–35.
12. Fox NC, Cousens S, Scahill R, Harvey RJ, Rossor MN. Using serial registered brain magnetic resonance imaging to measure disease progression in Alzheimer disease: power calculations and estimates of sample size to detect treatment effects. *Arch Neurol* 2000; **57**(3): 339–44.
13. Thompson PM, Mega MS, Woods RP *et al.* Cortical change in Alzheimer's disease detected with a disease-specific population-based brain atlas. *Cereb Cortex* 2001; **11**(1): 1–16.
14. Wright IC, McGuire PK, Poline JB *et al.* A voxel-based method for the statistical analysis of grey and white matter density applied to schizophrenia. *Neuroimage* 1995; **2**(4): 244–52.
15. Narr KL, Bilder RM, Toga AW *et al.* Mapping cortical thickness and gray matter concentration in first episode schizophrenia. *Cereb Cortex* 2005; **15**(6): 708–19.
16. Frisoni GB, Pievani M, Testa C *et al.* The topography of grey matter involvement in early and late onset Alzheimer's disease. *Brain* 2007; **130**(3): 720–30.
17. Ballmaier M, O'Brien JT, Burton EJ *et al.* Comparing gray matter loss profiles between dementia with Lewy bodies and Alzheimer's disease using cortical pattern matching: diagnosis and gender effects. *Neuroimage* 2004; **23**(1): 325–35.
18. Sowell ER, Peterson BS, Thompson PM *et al.* Mapping cortical change across the human life span. *Nat Neurosci* 2003; **6**(3): 309–15.
19. Salat DH, Buckner RL, Snyder AZ *et al.* Thinning of the cerebral cortex in aging. *Cereb Cortex* 2004; **14**(7): 721–30.
20. Gogtay N, Giedd JN, Lusk L *et al.* Dynamic mapping of human cortical development during childhood through early adulthood. *Proc Natl Acad Sci U S A* 2004; **101**(21): 8174–9.
21. Apostolova LG, Steiner CA, Akopyan GG, 3D gray matter atrophy mapping in mild cognitive impairment and mild Alzheimer's disease. *Arch Neurol* 2007; **64**(10): 1489–95.
22. Apostolova LG, Akopyan GG, Partiali N, Steiner CA, Dutton RA, Hayashi KM, *et al.* Structural correlates of apathy in Alzheimer's disease. *Dement Geriatr Cogn Disord.* 2007; 24(2): 91–7.
23. Karas GB, Scheltens P, Rombouts SA *et al.* Global and local gray matter loss in mild cognitive impairment and Alzheimer's disease. *Neuroimage* 2004; **23**(2): 708–16.
24. Apostolova LG, Lu PH, Rogers S *et al.* 3D mapping of language networks in clinical and pre-clinical Alzheimer's disease. *Brain Lang* 2008; **104**(1): 33–41.
25. Thompson PM, Hayashi KM, de Zubicaray G *et al.* Dynamics of gray matter loss in Alzheimer's disease. *J Neurosci* 2003; **23**(3): 994–1005.
26. Braak H, Braak E. Neuropathological staging of Alzheimer-related changes. *Acta Neuropathol* 1991; **82**(4): 239–59.
27. Vogt BA, Crino PB, Vogt LJ. Reorganization of cingulate cortex in Alzheimer's disease: neuron loss, neuritic plaques, and muscarinic receptor binding. *Cereb Cortex* 1992; **2**(6): 526–35.

cognitive impairment in normal aging and Alzheimer's disease. doi:10.1016/j.neurobiolaging.2008.09.012.

28. Mosconi L, Pupi A, De Cristofaro MT. Functional interactions of the entorhinal cortex: an 18F-FDG PET study on normal aging and Alzheimer's disease. *J Nucl Med* 2004; **45**(3): 382–92.

29. Kril JJ, Halliday GM. Clinicopathological staging of frontotemporal dementia severity: correlation with regional atrophy. *Dement Geriatr Cogn Disord* 2004; **17**(4): 311–15.

30. Braskie MN, Klunder AD, Hayashi KM *et al*. Plaque and tangle imaging and cognition in normal aging and Alzheimer's disease. doi:10.1016/j.neurobiolaging.2008.09.012.

31. Small GW, Protas HD, Huang SC *et al*. (eds). FDDNP-PET binding values from cortical hemispheric surface maps correlate with MMSE scores. *Alzheimers Dement* 2007; **3**(3 suppl 1): S186.

32. Rowe CC, Ng S, Ackermann U *et al*. Imaging beta-amyloid burden in aging and dementia. *Neurology* 2007; **68**(20): 1718–25.

33. Leow AD, Yanovsky I, Parikshak N *et al*. Alzheimer's disease neuroimaging initiative: a one-year follow up study using tensor-based morphometry correlating degenerative rates, biomarkers and cognition. *Neuroimage* 2009; **45**(3): 645–55.

34. Hua X, Leow A, Lee SE *et al*. 3D characterization of brain atrophy in Alzheimer's disease and mild cognitive impairment using tensor-based morphometry. *Neuroimage* 2008; **41**(1): 19–34.

35. Hua X, Leow AD, Parikshak N *et al*. Tensor-based morphometry as a neuroimaging biomarker for Alzheimer's disease: an MRI study of 676 AD, MCI, and normal subjects. *Neuroimage* 2008; **43**(3): 458–69.

36. Jack CR, Jr, Shiung MM, Gunter JL *et al*. Comparison of different MRI brain atrophy rate measures with clinical disease progression in AD. *Neurology* 2004; **62**(4): 591–600.

37. Jack CR, Jr, Petersen RC, Xu Y *et al*. Rates of hippocampal atrophy correlate with change in clinical status in aging and AD. *Neurology* 2000; **55**(4): 484–9.

38. Jack CR, Jr, Petersen RC, Xu Y *et al*. Rate of medial temporal lobe atrophy in typical aging and Alzheimer's disease. *Neurology* 1998; **51**(4): 993–9.

39. Du AT, Schuff N, Kramer JH *et al*. Higher atrophy rate of entorhinal cortex than hippocampus in AD. *Neurology* 2004; **62**(3): 422–7.

40. Hogan RE, Mark KE, Choudhuri I *et al*. Magnetic resonance imaging deformation-based segmentation of the hippocampus in patients with mesial temporal sclerosis and temporal lobe epilepsy. *J Digit Imaging* 2000; **13**(2 suppl 1): 217–18.

41. Carmichael OT, Aizenstein HA, Davis SW *et al*. Atlas-based hippocampus segmentation in Alzheimer's disease and mild cognitive impairment. *Neuroimage* 2005; **27**(4): 979–90.

42. Chupin M, Hammers A, Bardinet E *et al*. Fully automatic segmentation of the hippocampus and the amygdala from MRI using hybrid prior knowledge. *Med Image Comput Comput Assist Interv* 2007; **10**(pt 1): 875–82.

43. Shen D, Moffat S, Resnick SM, Davatzikos C. Measuring size and shape of the hippocampus in MR images using a deformable shape model. *Neuroimage* 2002; **15**(2): 422–34.

44. Powell S, Magnotta VA, Johnson H *et al*. Registration and machine learning-based automated segmentation of subcortical and cerebellar brain structures. *Neuroimage* 2008; **39**(1): 238–47.

45. Golland P, Grimson WE, Shenton ME, Kikinis R. Detection and analysis of statistical differences in anatomical shape. *Med Image Anal* 2005; **9**(1): 69–86.

46. Fischl B, Salat DH, Busa E *et al*. Whole brain segmentation: automated labeling of neuroanatomical structures in the human brain. *Neuron* 2002; **33**(3): 341–55.

47. Fischl B, Salat DH, van der Kouwe AJ *et al*. Sequence-independent segmentation of magnetic resonance images. *Neuroimage* 2004; **23**(suppl 1): S69–84.

48. Morra JH, Tu Z, Apostolova LG *et al*. Validation of a fully automated 3D hippocampal segmentation method using subjects with Alzheimer's disease mild cognitive impairment, and elderly controls. *Neuroimage* 2008; **43**(1): 59–68.

49. Thompson PM, Hayashi KM, de Zubicaray GI *et al*. Mapping hippocampal and ventricular change in Alzheimer disease. *Neuroimage* 2004; **22**(4): 1754–66.

50. Apostolova LG, Dutton RA, Dinov ID *et al*. Conversion of mild cognitive impairment to Alzheimer disease predicted by hippocampal atrophy maps. *Arch Neurol* 2006; **63**(5): 693–9.

47

Alzheimer's Disease: Risk Factors and Preventive Strategies

JoAnn T. Tschanz[1] and John C. S. Breitner[2]

[1]Department of Psychology and Center for Epidemiologic Studies, Utah State University, Logan, UT, USA
[2]GRECC, VA Puget Sound Health Care System, University of Washington School of Medicine, Seattle, WA, USA

INTRODUCTION

Dementia is a significant cause of disability and mortality among the elderly[1], accounting for nearly 30% of the population-attributable risk of death after age 85[2]. With the continued growth of the world's oldest population segments, the numbers affected by dementia are expected to rise exponentially, reaching 81.1 million by the year 2040[3]. The most common form of late-life dementia, Alzheimer's disease (AD) accounts for about 50% of dementia among people in their 60s, but may represent as much as 80% in those over age 80[4,5]. The annual cost of caring for one person with AD is estimated to range from $9000 early in the disease course to nearly $20 000 in mid-course[6]. Given the rapid growth in the proportion of those who survive into the latest stages of AD, in the United States alone, the total annual economic burden of the disorder is estimated at $100 billion[7], making it the country's third most costly health condition after cancer and heart disease[8].

With the exception of familial, early-onset forms of AD, there is no single identified cause of the disorder. Current treatments are largely symptomatic, providing only temporary improvement in cognition and neuropsychiatric symptoms. The past several decades have witnessed an explosion of research into risk and protective factors for AD, which someday may yield effective strategies for prevention. This chapter will review the current evidence for risk and protective factors associated with AD and end with a discussion of preventive strategies.

IMMUTABLE RISK FACTORS

Age and Sex

In discussion of prevention, it is useful to dichotomize those risk or protective factors for AD that are potentially subject to intervention versus others. The latter, immutable risk factors are age, female sex and family history. Family history and genetic risk are reviewed by Tsuang (Chapter 43) and are not addressed here. Age is the single strongest risk factor for AD. After age 65, the prevalence and incidence of the condition appear to double with every five years of additional age until 90[9], when the rates either plateau or decline. In the Cache County, Utah, population, for example, prevalence estimates ranged between 0.61% at ages 65–69 to nearly 19% at ages 85–89[10]. Incidence rates exhibited a similar trend[11]. Although data are scarce for persons older than age 90, some studies have suggested a plateau or even a decline in incidence rates in extreme old age.

Second only to age in importance is genotype at the polymorphic locus *APOE* that encodes the cholesterol transport protein apoE. The onset of AD is strongly accelerated among individuals homozygous for allele $\varepsilon 4$ (about 2% of most populations), but also tends to be earlier in people with a single $\varepsilon 4$ allele (typically 25–30%). These allele-specific modifications in onset result in increased AD incidence at younger ages, which appear as an overall increase in risk estimates that are typically adjusted for age[12].

Sex differences in the prevalence and incidence for AD have also been reported, with higher percentages observed in females in some (e.g. see[10,11,13,14]) but not all populations (e.g. see[15,16]). Whether this trend is found in any one study may depend on its relative proportions of very old subjects, among whom rates in women may be disproportionately elevated[11,14].

The mechanisms underlying the sex-specific difference in AD risk are of interest, but are presently unknown. Some authors have attributed the difference in risk to the greater longevity of women or the higher prevalence of vascular dementia in men (possibly deterring a diagnosis of AD even in the presence of its characteristic pathology), possible hormonal effects, or even the notion that current cohorts of elderly women have less neural or cognitive reserve than men, owing to fewer years of formal education[17]. The last explanation seems to us not only contentious but unlikely.

The increasing risk of AD with age (and in women) may instead reflect a host of background physiological changes that accompany ageing including programmed 'intrinsic' factors such as apoptosis, dysfunction of repair processes by progenitor cells in the dentate gyrus of the hippocampus or vascular endothelium, chromosome telomere shortening which signals apoptosis and damage to mitochondrial DNA (reviewed by Drachman[18]). 'Extrinsic' factors that occur as the result of normal wear and tear or exposures that accumulate over the lifetime may also contribute. These processes include oxidative stress and the glycation of proteins which interact with reactive oxygen species to form advanced glycation endproducts (AGE). AGE may trigger inflammatory cytokines that damage the

Principles and Practice of Geriatric Psychiatry, 3rd edn. Edited by Mohammed T. Abou-Saleh, Cornelius Katona and Anand Kumar

vascular endothelium. Chaperone proteins that normally repair or eliminate misfolded proteins may fail[18], leading to myelin breakdown. Cortico-cortical association fibres are especially vulnerable, and correspond to brain regions most affected in AD (reviewed by Bartzokis[19]). The degree to which individuals experience these age-related changes likely varies according to their genes, environmental exposures and lifestyle factors, at least some of which may be related to biological sex or gender roles.

MODIFIABLE RISK FACTORS

Neural and Cognitive Reserve

The notion of neural and cognitive reserve reflects an underlying idea that the brain can withstand some degree of compromise while still maintaining normal cognitive and behavioural functions through the recruitment of alternative neural networks[20,21]. Cognitive reserve (first proposed by Robert Katzman) is a concept whereby various cognitive strategies may be used to compensate for deficits. Both forms of reserve are malleable and may be built up through the accumulation of life experiences. Years of occupational and educational attainment are thus seen as predictors of reserve. Theoretically, higher levels of reserve could provide some degree of protection against the expression of clinical AD symptoms in the face of a specified burden of pathological change. Indeed, many epidemiological studies have reported an inverse relation between educational or occupational attainment and risk of AD, but studies have also failed to find this association (reviewed by Stern)[21]. The discrepant results may reflect inadequate assessment, particularly of activities in late life that continue to build neural and cognitive reserve. There is some evidence that stimulating activities in late life may reduce the risk of AD or dementia (see lifestyle factors under preventive strategies). Other explanations are possible, however, particularly when the studies employ two-stage screening and examination for dementia[22].

Traumatic Brain Injury (TBI)

Several epidemiological studies have reported an increased risk of AD among persons with a history of head trauma. A meta-analysis of case-control studies reports a 1.8-fold increase in risk among those with TBI with loss of consciousness. Adjusting for other factors, the higher AD risk was found only among men (relative risk of 2.7[23]), a result confirmed by a subsequent meta-analysis[24]. Interactions of TBI with APOE genotype have been reported by some[25] but not others[26]. The mechanism underlying the association between TBI and AD is unclear. Studies have reported an increase in beta-amyloid deposition and AD pathology following TBI[27], and higher frequency of APOE ε4 carriers among those with cortical plaques[28]. In animal studies, results have varied according to species and genetic variation. Increased beta-amyloid deposition was found later in the course of recovery in rodents, but earlier in pigs. In Alzheimer's PDAPP transgenic mice, beta-amyloid levels increased acutely, but without an increase in deposition, whereas in Tg2576 APP transgenic mice, repeated trauma resulted in greater beta-amyloid deposition[29]. Compounds that reduce beta-amyloid deposition after brain trauma are under active investigation to reduce the neurocognitive sequelae post injury and the risk of AD (e.g. see[30,31]).

VASCULAR RISK FACTORS

A number of risk factors for cardiovascular disease have been associated with AD. Hypertension, high cholesterol, diabetes, smoking and atherosclerosis have all been associated with increased risk. For hypertension, studies report a 1.2- to 4.5-fold increase in risk for AD, depending upon the age at measurement and whether systolic or diastolic measures are taken[32-35]. The relation between blood pressure and AD may be non-linear, as *low* diastolic blood pressure in mid-life has also been associated with an elevated risk[33]. Elevated cholesterol is associated with a 1.4- to 2-fold increase in AD risk[32], diabetes, nearly a 2- to 3.4-fold increase[34,36,37], smoking, a 1.6- to 2-fold increase[34,38] and severe atherosclerosis, a 3-fold increase in risk[39]. With each additional vascular risk factor, there is a corresponding increase in risk[34,35].

Interestingly, some studies report that the relation between cardiovascular risk factors and later dementia risk varies according to the timing of measurement relative to the onset of dementia as well as genotype at APOE. Although elevated blood pressure or cholesterol levels predict later AD onset, measurements of each decline prior to the onset of dementia[37,40]. This phenomenon may explain the negative findings reported by some studies (reviewed by Launer[41]). APOE genotype may also modify the association between vascular factors and AD. In a large Dutch population study of dementia and cognitive decline, the risk of AD with significant atherosclerosis (two or more indicators of plaques in the carotid artery, thickening of the intima media wall of the carotid artery, or evidence of peripheral artery disease) varied according to APOE genotype: among those with at least one APOE ε4 allele, the risk of AD was 3.9, and for others, 1.4[39]. For smoking, increased risk of AD was found only among those without ε4[38]. Further study of the interaction between vascular risk factors and APOE genotype is needed.

The mechanism underlying the relation between vascular risk factors and AD risk is unclear. Cerebrovascular pathology is common in AD brains, and includes such changes as amyloid angiopathy, cerebrovascular atherosclerosis, endothelial damage and periventricular white matter lesions[42]. Co-existing vascular lesions occur in approximately 24–28% of individuals with AD[43,44] and also contribute to the dementia syndrome[45]. However, vascular risk factors may also promote the formation of AD lesions or otherwise contribute to toxic physiological processes. In autopsies of participants of the Honolulu Asia Aging Study, mid-life elevations in systolic and diastolic blood pressure were associated with number of senile plaques and neurofibrillary tangles, respectively[46,47]. In the absence of dementia, increased plaques and tangles have also been reported in middle-aged hypertensive individuals[48]. Cholesterol has also been found to promote the accumulation of beta-amyloid[49,50].

Hypertension damages blood vessel walls and contributes to atherosclerosis[47]. When combined with the diminished elasticity of arterial walls, atherosclerosis reduces the brain's capacity to eliminate beta-amyloid. Normally, beta-amyloid is cleared from brain parenchyma by drainage through the cerebral arteries. A reduction in the elasticity of the arterial walls diminishes the force needed to drain the substance[51]. Furthermore, damage to arterial walls may also result in a variety of negative consequences including accumulation of amyloid precursor protein (APP), oxidative stress and dysfunction of the blood–brain barrier[47].

In addition to increasing the risk for adverse vascular outcomes, diabetes may affect AD risk through other mechanisms. The location of insulin receptors in the hippocampus and temporal cortex implicates insulin's involvement in long-term potentiation and other memory-related functions[52]. Normally, insulin crosses the blood–brain barrier and is thought to promote beta-amyloid clearance. In diabetics, however, insulin resistance and hyperinsulinemia in the periphery can result in reduced brain insulin levels, therefore affecting the rate of beta-amyloid clearance[53]. However, at autopsy, several studies report no association between diabetes and AD neuropathological markers[54,55], but an association with microvascular infarcts instead[55]. Furthermore, diabetes is associated with the production of advanced glycation endproducts, oxidative stress and inflammation[52].

Obesity

Obesity is typically measured by body mass index (BMI), which is a ratio of weight to height or kg to metres squared, waist circumference (a measure of central obesity), or a hip-to-waist ratio[53]. A number of studies have examined the relation between BMI and risk for dementia (reviewed by Gufstafson[56]). A majority of the studies indicates an elevated risk for dementia, and specifically for AD, in those with high BMI. Similar to the effects of blood pressure, the relation between BMI and AD appears to vary according to the timing of measurement in relation to dementia onset. The majority of studies examining BMI 10 or more years prior to dementia diagnosis report an increase in risk. For individuals meeting a definition of obese (BMI $\geq$ 30) the risk of dementia is approximately two-to-five times that of normal weight individuals. A few studies have reported no association or an increase in AD risk with *lower* BMI. However, most of those studies have used a relatively short follow-up period (e.g. within five years of dementia onset), and this raises the possibility that weight loss in this context is an indicator of incipient dementia rather than a risk factor[56].

The relationship between obesity and AD risk may operate through several pathways. First, obesity is a risk factor for a number of other adverse health outcomes including insulin resistance, diabetes and cardiovascular risk factors and conditions, and these in turn are risk factors for AD and vascular dementia[53]. Second, in the USA, obesity is associated with demographic characteristics that are also associated with AD. These include lower education and socioeconomic status and Hispanic or black race. Third, obesity is associated with higher consumption of dietary fat and calories and lower physical activity levels, which also have been associated with AD[53].

Psychosocial Stress

Several studies have reported an association between psychosocial stress and dementia. A prospective, Swedish population-based cohort study of 70 year olds examined the effects of 18 stressful life events experienced in childhood, early adulthood and late adulthood in predicting incident dementia. Death of a parent in childhood and physical illness in a spouse or serious illness in a child in late life were each associated with a 6- to 7-fold increase in dementia risk. Experience of manual labour was associated with a 26-fold increase. The number of risk factors experienced was associated with increasing risk[57]. Similarly, the Cache County (UT) population study reported a 3-fold increase in dementia risk with early-life death of a father[58]. This effect was not observed with mother's death, and it was hypothesized that the association reflected the effects of socioeconomic adversity, limited access to health care and other lost opportunities. Although the outcome examined was all-cause dementia, the predominant form of dementia in this population is AD[10,11].

In a case-control study from a large health maintenance organization (HMO) in Washington state, number of siblings was associated with increased risk of AD. The risk increased with each additional child so that having five or more siblings was associated with a 39%

increase in risk, seven to nine siblings with a 72% increase, and 10 or more siblings with more than a 2-fold increase in risk[59]. Residence in the suburbs was associated with a reduction in risk. Drawing from the same HMO database and linking to US Census records and birth certificates, Moceri and colleagues examined the subsequent risk of AD associated with a number of psychosocial factors. Father's work in unskilled manual labour and number of persons in household were each associated with greater risk. Furthermore, these early life experiences interacted with *APOE* genotype. Among those with one or more $\varepsilon 4$ alleles, those whose fathers worked in manual labour had an odds ratio for AD of 2.35 (95% CI = 1.07–5.16), but those without $\varepsilon 4$ had an odds ratio of 1.40 (95% CI = 0.78–2.52). Compared to individuals with neither the early-life risk factors nor the $\varepsilon 4$ allele, having father's work in manual labour, a household size exceeding six members and having an $\varepsilon 4$ allele was associated with an odds ratio of 14.80 (95% CI = 4.90–46) for AD[60]. A similar interaction between *APOE* genotype and early-life risk factors was reported in a large sample of Japanese Americans living in King County, Washington. Here, more than four children in household and smaller head circumference were associated with increased risk of AD among bearers of an *APOE* $\varepsilon 4$ allele[61].

Other studies have examined the influence of experiences later in life such as loneliness or lack of social support, the latter of which can potentially mitigate the effects of stressful events. Individuals scoring at the 90th percentile of a loneliness questionnaire exhibited a 2-fold increase in risk for AD as compared to those reporting few feelings of loneliness. The elevated risk for loneliness was also associated with more rapid cognitive decline and persisted when controlling for the effects of social network and activity. Interestingly, these effects were independent of the degree of AD neuropathology[62].

Additional work has examined personality traits, particularly distress proneness or neuroticism. In a sample of elderly Catholic clergy, distress proneness was associated with increased risk for AD. Because personality traits are considered to be relatively stable, the measure of distress proneness was thought to reflect cumulative, psychological distress experienced over the life span. Relative to those with a low level on this trait, individuals at the 90th percentile exhibited a 2-fold increase in AD risk. The effects remained after statistical control for depressive symptoms and engagement in cognitive activities. Distress proneness was also associated with more rapid cognitive decline, particularly in episodic memory. Again, baseline scores on distress proneness were not associated with degree of AD neuropathology at death[63], suggesting that the relationship with dementia works through other mechanisms[64].

Activation of the hypothalamic-pituitary-adrenal (HPA) axis has been suggested to underlie the association between psychosocial stress and AD. Broadly speaking, this process mobilizes resources in response to a 'stressor' by releasing glucocorticoids that promote energy metabolism and modulate immune functions[65]. However, with chronic and excessive activation of the HPA axis, high levels of glucocorticoids may lead to cell death in regions of the hippocampus, and this phenomenon in turn can diminish the normal inhibitory feedback loop, leading to further activation and release of glucocorticoids. This 'glucocorticoid cascade' (see Sapolsky[66]) has been invoked to underlie the hippocampal damage and corresponding cognitive impairment observed with chronic stress in aged organisms[66]. In relation to AD risk, hippocampal damage from chronic glucocorticoid release may functionally reduce the brain's capacity (reserve) to compensate for the neuronal degeneration that accompanies AD. Alternatively, animal studies suggest that glucocorticoids can directly promote the development of AD-type pathology. In transgenic mouse models of AD, the administration of an experiental stressor or direct glucocorticoid challenge increased beta-amyloid deposition[67,68] and tau pathology. Clearly, more research examining the role of stress and physiological changes in the brain is warranted.

Early-life stressors may also have their effects through the limitation of financial resources. Early parental death, lower parental socioeconomic occupations and higher sibling density may limit the financial resources available during critical periods of brain development. Nutritional or environmental deprivation associated with low socioeconomic resources may limit brain growth and maturation, and therefore, neural reserve. Access to health care and educational and vocational opportunities may also be curtailed. In addition, the accessibility of emotional resources may be limited, particularly in the case of early parental death. Such non-normative loss may plausibly result in psychological growth and maturation under less than ideal circumstances, potentially leading to maladaptive coping strategies and stress reactivity, that affect brain development[69]. Later, in the face of AD pathology, less neural reserve and poor coping strategies may result in a lower threshold for the clinical expression of dementia.

STRATEGIES FOR THE PREVENTION OF AD

Any of the modifiable risk factors discussed above may present a potential target for intervention. The following sections will briefly summarize the literature regarding potential strategies to reduce the risk of AD. Some of these strategies involve pharmacological compounds that theoretically reduce AD-related neuropathology, whereas others are intended to build neural reserve or promote cardiovascular health. None of these potential prevention strategies has been proven efficacious, but a number are of sufficient promise to warrant discussion here. These include anti-inflammatory drugs, lipid-lowering agents, hormone replacement therapy, antioxidants and lifestyle factors including diet, social support and engagement in physical, cognitive and social activities.

Pharmacological Interventions

Non-steroidal anti-inflammatory drugs

Interest in the use of anti-inflammatory agents in the prevention of AD began with the observation of a lower-than-expected frequency of AD in patients with rheumatoid arthritis[70]. It was speculated that this association reflected the widespread use of non-steroidal anti-inflammatory drugs (NSAIDs) by patients with this condition. The inverse association of AD and NSAID use has subsequently been examined in numerous observational studies, many of which report a reduction in AD risk among NSAID users. Animal studies provide further support for the possibility that NSAIDs may protect against AD pathogenesis (reviewed by Cole et al.[71]). Despite early signs of promise, the results of randomized controlled treatment trials have been disappointing. Except for encouraging results of a pilot AD treatment trial[72], trials with NSAIDS[73–77], low dose corticosteroids[78] and hydroxychloroquine[79] have shown no benefit. A secondary prevention trial to prevent progression from mild cognitive impairment to AD was not beneficial, and suggested harm in the treatment group[80]. Notably, however, all of these trials tested the effect of the drugs on individuals who already exhibited symptoms of dementia or cognitive deterioration – a topic not addressed by the observational literature on NSAIDs and AD *incidence*. In fact, recent studies had

suggested that any protection was limited to NSAID use initiated more than two years before AD onset[81–83]. To date, the only large-scale NSAID primary prevention trial is the Alzheimer's Disease Anti-inflammatory Prevention Trial (ADAPT) in which celecoxib or naproxen was tested against placebo in subjects with a family history of AD. Owing to unexpected cardiovascular safety concerns, the treatments were stopped after an average of two years of treatment. Analyses at that time showed no reduction in incidence of AD in participants assigned to either celecoxib or naproxen, but instead a suggestion of increased risk[84–86]. Compounding the disappointment from these results, a recent community-based study that utilized pharmacy records to assess NSAID exposure showed an *increase* in AD incidence with NSAID use, regardless of the recency of such use. The authors of this study speculated that, because the participants in this study were considerably older than those examined previously, the beneficial effects of NSAIDs might be limited to younger individuals, before the onset of AD neuropathology. Alternatively, they conjectured that NSAID use effected a *delay in the onset* of dementia, thereby increasing the numbers of AD cases in older age groups[87].

Lipid-lowering agents

Based on observations suggesting an increased risk of AD among those with high cholesterol, the use of lipid-lowering agents such as 3-hydroxy-methyl-glutaryl-CoA reductase inhibitors (statins) have been studied as potential protective agents. As previously mentioned, cholesterol promotes beta-amyloid production[49,50] and reduction in cholesterol levels might inhibit it[88]. Statins have other effects as well, such as prevention of atherothrombosis or reduction of inflammation.

Several case-control studies have reported a reduction in AD risk among users of lipid-lowering agents, typically with statins[89–93]. However, most of these studies have been cross-sectional in nature. Prospective studies examining statin use and subsequent dementia onset have been disappointing, with negative findings reported from the Cardiovascular Health Study Cognition Study, the Cache County Study and the Adult Changes in Thought Study[94–96]. Three published randomized controlled trials have found no evidence of a protective effect against cognitive decline as an outcome[97–99]. Further research is needed to determine whether the effectiveness of statins may differ by *APOE* genotype[94].

Hormone replacement therapies

Several observational studies have reported a reduction of AD incidence among women treated with postmenopausal oestrogen replacement therapy (e.g. see[100–103]), but negative findings have been reported as well (e.g. see[104,105]). Oestrogen has noted beneficial neurotrophic and neuroprotective effects (see review by Morrison et al.[106]). Thus a strong rationale exists for potential protection against AD. However, the results of randomized controlled trials have been disappointing. No benefit was reported in treatment trials with women with AD[107–109], with the exception of one study using 17-beta estradiol administered by a transdermal patch[110]. The well-known Women's Health Initiative randomized controlled trials examined hormone users for the prevention of AD, finding no benefit and a suggestion of harm in both treatment groups[111–113]. Although these results are disappointing, there is limited evidence to suggest that oestrogen may yield positive effects, but only if administered well *prior to* the onset of AD symptoms, and perhaps when there is little or no accumulated AD neuropathology. Thus, observational studies in which exposure and case detection were constrained to a 10-year window report no effect for oestrogen replacement therapy[104,105], but protective effects have been reported for use exceeding 10 years[103,114]. Consistent with this notion are studies of cell cultures in which oestrogen protects against apoptotic cell death, but promotes cell death in the presence of beta-amyloid$_{42}$[115,116].

Lifestyle Factors

Diet and nutritional supplements

A number of observational studies have reported certain beneficial effects of nutrients from food sources or dietary supplements. Consumption of fish[117,118], intake of omega 3 fatty acids[117], a Mediterranean style diet[119], light-to-moderate alcohol consumption[120,121] and the antioxidant vitamins, E and C (e.g. see[122,123]) have been associated with a reduction in AD risk in observational studies. Inconsistent findings have also been reported, for example, with antioxidant vitamins (e.g. see[124]). The underlying mechanisms are unclear but may involve improvements in cardiovascular health, reduced insulin insensitivity, antioxidant and anti-inflammatory effects, and improvement in neuronal lipid membrane function (e.g. see[120,125–127]). Furthermore, the associations between nutrients and risk of AD may vary by APOE genotype. For example, in some studies, higher total calorie and fat intake was associated with increased risk of AD, but only among those with an APOE ε4 allele[125,128]. This finding is consistent with the observation that moderate intake of saturated fat in mid-life increased the risk of AD among APOE ε4 carriers[129].

Few randomized controlled prevention trials have been conducted with dietary supplements, but two have examined n-3 polyunsaturated fatty acids, docosahexaenoic acid (DHA) and eicosapentaenoic acid (EPA). As reviewed in Cunnane et al.[127], a four-month trial was conducted with DHA with and without lutein (an antioxidant) vs. placebo. Verbal fluency scores improved in both treatment arms, whereas memory functions improved only in the DHA + lutein arm. A 26-week trial of combined EPA and DHA supplements (1800 mg/day or 400 mg/day) provided no benefit on cognitive outcomes, except that among APOE ε4-positive individuals there was suggestion of improved attention[130].

A few treatment trials have also been conducted with antioxidant supplements. In a large intervention trial of antioxidants and heart disease, the vitamin E arm of the United Kingdom Heart Protection Study showed no differences after five years, in percent of individuals who developed dementia or who were classified as cognitively impaired on a telephone cognitive screening test[131]. Additionally, high dose treatment with vitamin E had no benefit in delaying the onset of AD among those with mild cognitive impairment[132]. These findings appear to contradict those of observational studies. It is commonly conjectured that the latter have been vulnerable to error from a variety of confounding factors, but another possible explanation is that neuroprotective effects are observed only with a combination of lipid-soluble and water-soluble agents such as vitamins E and C in combination[123]. Additional intervention trials are needed to examine the effectiveness of dietary and supplement interventions for the primary prevention of AD.

Physical activity

Many studies report significant benefits of physical activity with respect to maintenance of cognitive ability (e.g. see[133,134]) and

a reduction in risk of AD and other dementias (e.g. see[135–137]). The reduction in risk varies by degree of activity. For example a 50% reduction in cognitive decline was seen in those with high levels of exercise (more than three times per week of moderate to high intensity activity[135], or more than four activities per week[136]). Interactions between activity and APOE status are inconsistent: one study reports reduction in risk among non-carriers of the APOE ε4 allele[136] while another reports greater effects among carriers[137]. Mechanisms purported to underlie the beneficial effects of physical activity on cognitive outcomes include improved cardiovascular health, increased cerebral blood flow and increased attention[138,139]. A recent randomized controlled trial of individuals aged 50 or older reported significant differences between an exercise intervention as compared with education controls on a global measure of cognitive ability (Alzheimer's Disease Assessment Scale-Cognitive (ADAS-Cog) subscale) and a measure of delayed recall[140]. The intervention was conducted over a 24-week period among individuals with subjective memory complaint, and follow-ups were obtained at 6, 12 and 18 months. Improved performance was also observed on a measure of delayed recall and functional ability. Post-hoc comparisons indicated greater effects among those without an APOE ε4 allele[140].

Leisure activity

Active engagement in leisure activities in late life may continue to build neurocognitive reserve and thereby reduce the risk of dementia. Several observational studies report beneficial effects of high engagement in leisure-time activities such as social interaction, physical conditioning, volunteer work and cognitive activities such as reading or playing games. In a large community based study with up to seven years follow-up, greater engagement in total activities was associated with reduced dementia risk (RR = 0.88, 95% CI = 0.83–0.93)[141]. When activities were combined with accrued reserve (as reflected in educational or occupational attainment), the risk of dementia among those with low accrued reserve and low engagement in late-life activities was approximately 1.9–2.3 times that of high reserve and high engagement in late-life activities[141]. Similar effects have been reported for those with limited social networks[142,143].

The mechanisms underlying such positive effects of leisure-time activities include building of neurocognitive reserve, increased synaptogenesis promoted by stimulating activities and stress reduction associated with greater activity and social support (see review by Fratiglioni et al.[144]). Although there are no randomized controlled trials of leisure interventions, one large trial examined the effects of a cognitive intervention on cognitive and functional outcomes in elderly individuals. Over 2000 individuals between the ages of 65–94 were randomly assigned to one of four training groups: memory, reasoning, speed of information processing and a no-contact control. The interventions (and booster session) resulted in significant improvements in each of the targeted cognitive domains immediately after training and after two years follow-up[145]. No effect was observed on the functional outcome measure, although this was thought to reflect limited change in that domain.

CONCLUSION

The scientific literature identifies numerous risk factors that are putatively associated with AD. These processes are not necessarily specific to the disease, but may be changes associated with ageing that effectively reduce the neurocognitive reserve and resources built over the life span. Other risk factors may affect vascular factors and neuroendocrine response to stress which are purported to promote AD neuropathology or negatively impact vulnerable brain regions important for learning and memory. The large number of risk factors and biological processes that increase the risk of AD suggests the disorder results from multiple causes. As a result, the search for prevention strategies may similarly need to consider multiple factors.

ACKNOWLEDGEMENTS

Supported by funding from the National Institute on Aging (R01AG11380 and R01AG21136) and the U.S. Department of Veterans Affairs.

REFERENCES

1. Aguero-Torres H, Fratiglioni L, Winblad B. Natural history of Alzheimer's disease and other dementias: review of the literature in the light of the findings from the Kungsholmen Project. *Int J Geriatr Psychiatry* 1998; **13**(11): 755–66.

2. Tschanz JT, Corcoran C, Skoog I, Khachaturian AS, Herrick J, Hayden KM *et al*. Dementia: the leading predictor of death in a defined elderly population: the Cache County Study. *Neurology* 2004; **62**(7): 1156–62.

3. Ferri CP, Prince M, Brayne C, Brodaty H, Fratiglioni L, Ganguli M *et al*. Global prevalence of dementia: a Delphi consensus study. *Lancet* 2005; **366**(9503): 2112–7.

4. Breteler MM, Claus JJ, Van Duijn CM, Launer LJ, Hofman A. Epidemiology of Alzheimer's disease. *Epidemiol Rev* 1992; **14**: 59–82.

5. Hofman A, Rocca WA, Brayne C, Breteler MM, Clarke M, Cooper B *et al*. The prevalence of dementia in Europe: a collaborative study of 1980–1990 findings. Eurodem Prevalence Research Group. *Int J Epidemiol* 1991; **20**(3): 736–48.

6. Zhu CW, Scarmeas N, Torgan R, Albert M, Brandt J, Blacker D *et al*. Longitudinal study of effects of patient characteristics on direct costs in Alzheimer disease. *Neurology* 2006; **67**(6): 998–1005.

7. Ernst RL, Hay JW. The US economic and social costs of Alzheimer's disease revisited. *Am J Public Health* 1994; **84**(8): 1261–4.

8. Winblad B, Jonsson L, Wimo A. The worldwide costs of dementia. Presented at the Alzheimer's Association International Conference on Prevention of Dementia, Washington, DC, June 2005.

9. Jorm AF, Jolley D. The incidence of dementia: a meta-analysis. *Neurology* 1998; **51**(3): 728–33.

10. Breitner JC, Wyse BW, Anthony JC, Welsh-Bohmer KA, Steffens DC, Norton MC *et al*. APOE-epsilon4 count predicts age when prevalence of AD increases, then declines: the Cache County Study. *Neurology* 1999; **53**(2): 321–31.

11. Miech RA, Breitner JC, Zandi PP, Khachaturian AS, Anthony JC, Mayer L. Incidence of AD may decline in the early 90s for men, later for women: the Cache County Study. *Neurology* 2002; **58**(2): 209–18.

12. Khachaturian AS, Corcoran CD, Mayer LS, Zandi PP, Breitner JC. Apolipoprotein E epsilon4 count affects age at onset of Alzheimer disease, but not lifetime susceptibility: the Cache County Study. *Arch Gen Psychiatry* 2004; **61**(5): 518–24.

13. Gao S, Hendrie HC, Hall KS, Hui S. The relationships between age, sex, and the incidence of dementia and Alzheimer disease: a meta-analysis. *Arch Gen Psychiatry* 1998; **55**(9): 809–15.

14. Ruitenberg A, Ott A, Van Swieten JC, Hofman A, Breteler MM. Incidence of dementia: does gender make a difference? *Neurobiol Aging* 2001; **22**(4): 575–80.

15. Hebert LE, Scherr PA, McCann JJ, Beckett LA, Evans DA. Is the risk of developing Alzheimer's disease greater for women than for men? *Am J Epidemiol* 2001; **153**(2): 132–6.

16. Ganguli M, Dodge HH, Chen P, Belle S, DeKosky ST. Ten-year incidence of dementia in a rural elderly US community population: the MoVIES Project. *Neurology* 2000; **54**(5): 1109–16.

17. Baum LW. Sex, hormones, and Alzheimer's disease. *J Gerontol A Biol Sci Med Sci* 2005; **60**(6): 736–43.

18. Drachman DA. Aging of the brain, entropy, and Alzheimer disease. *Neurology* 2006; **67**(8): 1340–52.

19. Bartzokis G. Age-related myelin breakdown: a developmental model of cognitive decline and Alzheimer's disease. *Neurobiol Aging* 2004; **25**(1): 5–18; author reply 49–62.

20. Katzman R. Education and the prevalence of dementia and Alzheimer's disease. *Neurology* 1993; **43**(1): 13–20.

21. Stern Y. Cognitive reserve and Alzheimer disease. *Alzheimer Dis Assoc Disord* 2006; **20**(2): 112–17.

22. Crane PK, Gibbons LE, Jolley L, Van Belle G, Selleri R, Dalmonte E *et al*. Differential item functioning related to education and age in the Italian version of the Mini-mental State Examination. *Int Psychogeriatr* 2006; **18**(3): 505–15.

23. Mortimer JA, Van Duijn CM, Chandra V, Fratiglioni L, Graves AB, Heyman A *et al*. Head trauma as a risk factor for Alzheimer's disease: a collaborative re-analysis of case-control studies. EURODEM Risk Factors Research Group. *Int J Epidemiol* 1991; **20** Suppl 2: S28–35.

24. Fleminger S, Oliver DL, Lovestone S, Rabe-Hesketh S, Giora A. Head injury as a risk factor for Alzheimer's disease: the evidence 10 years on; a partial replication. *J Neurol Neurosurg Psychiatry* 2003; **74**(7): 857–62.

25. Mayeux R, Ottman R, Maestre G, Ngai C, Tang MX, Ginsberg H *et al*. Synergistic effects of traumatic head injury and apolipoprotein-epsilon 4 in patients with Alzheimer's disease. *Neurology* 1995; **45**(3Pt 1): 555–7.

26. O'Meara ES, Kukull WA, Sheppard L, Bowen JD, McCormick WC, Teri L *et al*. Head injury and risk of Alzheimer's disease by apolipoprotein E genotype. *Am J Epidemiol* 1997; **146**(5): 373–84.

27. Jellinger KA. Traumatic brain injury as a risk factor for Alzheimer's disease. *J Neurol Neurosurg Psychiatry* 2004; **75**(3): 511–12.

28. DeKosky ST, Abrahamson EE, Ciallella JR, Paljug WR, Wisniewski SR, Clark RS *et al*. Association of increased cortical soluble abeta42 levels with diffuse plaques after severe brain injury in humans. *Arch Neurol* 2007; **64**(4): 541–4.

29. Szczygielski J, Mautes A, Steudel WI, Falkai P, Bayer TA, Wirths O. Traumatic brain injury: cause or risk of Alzheimer's disease? A review of experimental studies. *J Neural Transm* 2005; **112**(11): 1547–64.

30. Loane DJ, Pocivavsek A, Moussa CE, Thompson R, Matsuoka Y, Faden AI *et al*. Amyloid precursor protein secretases as therapeutic targets for traumatic brain injury. *Nat Med* 2009; **15**(4): 377–9.

31. Abrahamson EE, Ikonomovic MD, Dixon CE, DeKosky ST. Simvastatin therapy prevents brain trauma-induced increases in beta-amyloid peptide levels. *Ann Neurol* 2009; **66**(3): 407–14.

32. Kivipelto M, Helkala EL, Laakso MP, Hanninen T, Hallikainen M, Alhainen K *et al.* Midlife vascular risk factors and Alzheimer's disease in later life: longitudinal, population based study. *BMJ* 2001; **322**(7300): 1447–51.

33. Launer LJ, Ross GW, Petrovitch H, Masaki K, Foley D, White LR *et al.* Midlife blood pressure and dementia: the Honolulu-Asia aging study. *Neurobiol Aging* 2000; **21**(1): 49–55.

34. Luchsinger JA, Reitz C, Honig LS, Tang MX, Shea S, Mayeux R. Aggregation of vascular risk factors and risk of incident Alzheimer disease. *Neurology* 2005; **65**(4): 545–51.

35. Whitmer RA, Sidney S, Selby J, Johnston SC, Yaffe K. Midlife cardiovascular risk factors and risk of dementia in late life. *Neurology* 2005; **64**(2): 277–81.

36. Ott A, Stolk RP, Van Harskamp F, Pols HA, Hofman A, Breteler MM. Diabetes mellitus and the risk of dementia: The Rotterdam Study. *Neurology* 1999; **53**(9): 1937–42.

37. Notkola IL, Sulkava R, Pekkanen J, Erkinjuntti T, Ehnholm C, Kivinen P *et al.* Serum total cholesterol, apolipoprotein E epsilon 4 allele, and Alzheimer's disease. *Neuroepidemiology* 1998; **17**(1): 14–20.

38. Reitz C, den Heijer T, Van Duijn C, Hofman A, Breteler MM. Relation between smoking and risk of dementia and Alzheimer disease: the Rotterdam Study. *Neurology* 2007; **69**(10): 998–1005.

39. Hofman A, Ott A, Breteler MM, Bots ML, Slooter AJ, Van Harskamp F *et al.* Atherosclerosis, apolipoprotein E, and prevalence of dementia and Alzheimer's disease in the Rotterdam Study. *Lancet* 1997; **349**(9046): 151–4.

40. Skoog I, Lernfelt B, Landahl S, Palmertz B, Andreasson LA, Nilsson L *et al.* 15-year longitudinal study of blood pressure and dementia. *Lancet* 1996; **347**(9009): 1141–5.

41. Launer LJ. Demonstrating the case that AD is a vascular disease: epidemiologic evidence. *Ageing Res Rev* 2002; **1**(1): 61–77.

42. Kalaria RN, Ballard C. Overlap between pathology of Alzheimer disease and vascular dementia. *Alzheimer Dis Assoc Disord* 1999; **13** (Suppl 3): S115–23.

43. Massoud F, Devi G, Stern Y, Lawton A, Goldman JE, Liu Y *et al.* A clinicopathological comparison of community-based and clinic-based cohorts of patients with dementia. *Arch Neurol* 1999; **56**(11): 1368–73.

44. Gearing M, Mirra SS, Hedreen JC, Sumi SM, Hansen LA, Heyman A. The Consortium to Establish a Registry for Alzheimer's Disease (CERAD). Part X. Neuropathology confirmation of the clinical diagnosis of Alzheimer's disease. *Neurology* 1995; **45**(3Pt 1): 461–6.

45. Snowdon DA, Greiner LH, Mortimer JA, Riley KP, Greiner PA, Markesbery WR. Brain infarction and the clinical expression of Alzheimer disease. The Nun Study. *JAMA* 1997; 277(10): 813–7.

46. Petrovitch H, White LR, Izmirilian G, Ross GW, Havlik RJ, Markesbery W *et al.* Midlife blood pressure and neuritic plaques, neurofibrillary tangles, and brain weight at death: the HAAS. Honolulu-Asia Aging Study. *Neurobiol Aging* 2000; **21**(1): 57–62.

47. Skoog I, Gustafson D. Hypertension and related factors in the etiology of Alzheimer's disease. *Ann N Y Acad Sci* 2002; **977**: 29–36.

48. Sparks DL, Scheff SW, Liu H, Landers TM, Coyne CM, Hunsaker JC, 3rd. Increased incidence of neurofibrillary tangles (NFT) in non-demented individuals with hypertension. *J Neurol Sci* 1995; **131**(2): 162–9.

49. Frears ER, Stephens DJ, Walters CE, Davies H, Austen BM. The role of cholesterol in the biosynthesis of beta-amyloid. *Neuroreport* 1999; **10**(8): 1699–705.

50. Refolo LM, Malester B, LaFrancois J, Bryant-Thomas T, Wang R, Tint GS *et al.* Hypercholesterolemia accelerates the Alzheimer's amyloid pathology in a transgenic mouse model. *Neurobiol Dis* 2000; **7**(4): 321–31.

51. Weller RO, Yow HY, Preston SD, Mazanti I, Nicoll JA. Cerebrovascular disease is a major factor in the failure of elimination of Abeta from the aging human brain: implications for therapy of Alzheimer's disease. *Ann N Y Acad Sci* 2002; **977**: 162–8.

52. Craft S. The role of metabolic disorders in Alzheimer disease and vascular dementia: two roads converged. *Arch Neurol* 2009; **66**(3): 300–5.

53. Luchsinger JA. Adiposity, hyperinsulinemia, diabetes and Alzheimer's disease: an epidemiological perspective. *Eur J Pharmacol* 2008; **585**(1): 119–29.

54. Beeri MS, Silverman JM, Davis KL, Marin D, Grossman HZ, Schmeidler J *et al.* Type 2 diabetes is negatively associated with Alzheimer's disease neuropathology. *J Gerontol A Biol Sci Med Sci* 2005; **60**(4): 471–5.

55. Sonnen JA, Larson EB, Brickell K, Crane PK, Woltjer R, Montine TJ *et al.* Different patterns of cerebral injury in dementia with or without diabetes. *Arch Neurol* 2009; **66**(3): 315–22.

56. Gustafson D. A life course of adiposity and dementia. *Eur J Pharmacol* 2008; **585**(1): 163–75.

57. Persson G, Skoog I. A prospective population study of psychosocial risk factors for late onset dementia. *Int J Geriatr Psychiatry* 1996; **11**: 15–22.

58. Norton MC, Ostbye T, Smith KR, Munger RG, Tschanz JT. Early parental death and late-life dementia risk: findings from the Cache County Study. *Age Aging* 2009; **38**(3): 340–3.

59. Moceri VM, Kukull WA, Emanuel I, Van Belle G, Larson EB. Early-life risk factors and the development of Alzheimer's disease. *Neurology* 2000; **54**(2): 415–20.

60. Moceri VM, Kukull WA, Emanual I, van Belle G, Starr JR, Schellenberg GD *et al.* Using census data and birth certificates to reconstruct the early-life socioeconomic environment and the relation to the development of Alzheimer's disease. *Epidemiology* 2001; **12**(4): 383–9.

61. Borenstein AR, Wu Y, Mortimer JA, Schellenberg GD, McCormick WC, Bowen JD *et al.* Developmental and vascular risk factors for Alzheimer's disease. *Neurobiol Aging* 2005; **26**(3): 325–34.

62. Wilson RS, Krueger KR, Arnold SE, Schneider JA, Kelly JF, Barnes LL *et al.* Loneliness and risk of Alzheimer disease. *Arch Gen Psychiatry* 2007; **64**(2): 234–40.

63. Wilson RS, Evans DA, Bienias JL, Mendes de Leon CF, Schneider JA, Bennett DA. Proneness to psychological distress is associated with risk of Alzheimer's disease. *Neurology* 2003; **61**(11): 1479–85.

64. Breitner JC, Costa PT. 'At my wits' end': neuroticism and dementia. *Neurology* 2003; **61**(11): 1468–9.

65. Pedersen WA, Wan R, Mattson MP. Impact of aging on stress-responsive neuroendocrine systems. *Mech Ageing Dev* 2001; **122**(9): 963–83.

66. Sapolsky RM, Krey LC, McEwen BS. The neuroendocrinology of stress and aging: the glucocorticoid cascade hypothesis. *Endocr Rev* 1986; **7**(3): 284–301.

67. Green KN, Billings LM, Roozendaal B, McGaugh JL, LaFerla FM. Glucocorticoids increase amyloid-beta and tau pathology in a mouse model of Alzheimer's disease. *J Neurosci* 2006; **26**(35): 9047–56.

68. Jeong YH, Park CH, Yoo J, Shin KY, Ahn SM, Kim HS *et al.* Chronic stress accelerates learning and memory impairments and increases amyloid deposition in APPV717I-CT100 transgenic mice, an Alzheimer's disease model. *FASEB J* 2006; **20**(6): 729–31.

69. Tarullo AR, Quevedo K, Gunnar MR. The LHPA System and Neurobehavioral Development. In Nelson CA, Luciana M (eds), *Handbook of Developmental Cognitive Neuroscience*, 2nd edn. Cambridge: Massachusetts Institute of Technology, 2008, 63–82.

70. McGeer PL, Akiyama H, Itagaki S, McGeer EG. Activation of the classical complement pathway in brain tissue of Alzheimer patients. *Neurosci Lett* 1989; **107**(1–3): 341–6.

71. Cole GM, Morihara T, Lim GP, Yang F, Begum A, Frautschy SA. NSAID and antioxidant prevention of Alzheimer's disease: lessons from in vitro and animal models. *Ann N Y Acad Sci* 2004; **1035**: 68–84.

72. Rogers J, Kirby LC, Hempelman SR, Berry DL, McGeer PL, Kaszniak AW *et al.* Clinical trial of indomethacin in Alzheimer's disease. *Neurology* 1993; **43**(8): 1609–11.

73. Aisen PS, Schmeidler J, Pasinetti GM. Randomized pilot study of nimesulide treatment in Alzheimer's disease. *Neurology* 2002; **58**(7): 1050–4.

74. Aisen PS, Schafer KA, Grundman M, Pfeiffer E, Sano M, Davis KL *et al.* Effects of rofecoxib or naproxen vs. placebo on Alzheimer disease progression: a randomized controlled trial. *JAMA* 2003; **289**(21): 2819–26.

75. Reines SA, Block GA, Morris JC, Liu G, Nessly ML, Lines CR *et al.* Rofecoxib: no effect on Alzheimer's disease in a 1-year, randomized, blinded, controlled study. *Neurology* 2004; **62**(1): 66–71.

76. Scharf S, Mander A, Ugoni A, Vajda F, Christophidis N. A double-blind, placebo-controlled trial of diclofenac/misoprostol in Alzheimer's disease. *Neurology* 1999; **53**(1): 197–201.

77. Soininen H, West C, Robbins J, Niculescu L. Long-term efficacy and safety of celecoxib in Alzheimer's disease. *Dement Geriatr Cogn Disord* 2007; **23**(1): 8–21.

78. Aisen PS, Davis KL, Berg JD, Schafer K, Campbell K, Thomas RG *et al.* A randomized controlled trial of prednisone in Alzheimer's disease. Alzheimer's Disease Cooperative Study. *Neurology* 2000; 54(3): 588–93.

79. Van Gool WA, Weinstein HC, Scheltens P, Walstra GJ. Effect of hydroxychloroquine on progression of dementia in early Alzheimer's disease: an 18-month randomised, double-blind, placebo-controlled study. *Lancet* 2001; **358**(9280): 455–60.

80. Thal LJ, Ferris SH, Kirby L, Block GA, Lines CR, Yuen E *et al.* A randomized, double-blind, study of rofecoxib in patients with mild cognitive impairment. *Neuropsychopharmacology* 2005; **30**(6): 1204–15.

81. Etminan M, Gill S, Samii A. Effect of non-steroidal anti-inflammatory drugs on risk of Alzheimer's disease: systematic review and meta-analysis of observational studies. *BMJ* 2003; **327**(7407): 128.

82. in't Veld BA, Launer LJ, Hoes AW, Ott A, Hofman A, Breteler MM *et al.* NSAIDs and incident Alzheimer's disease. The Rotterdam Study. *Neurobiol Aging* 1998; **19**(6): 607–11.

83. Zandi PP, Anthony JC, Hayden KM, Mehta K, Mayer L, Breitner JC. Reduced incidence of AD with NSAID but not H2 receptor antagonists: the Cache County Study. *Neurology* 2002; **59**(6): 880–6.

84. Group AR. Cardiovascular and cerebrovascular events in the randomized, controlled Alzheimer's Disease Anti-Inflammatory Prevention Trial (ADAPT). *PLoS Clin Trials* 2006; **1**(7): e33.

85. Group AR, Lyketsos CG, Breitner JC, Green RC, Martin BK, Meinert C *et al.* Naproxen and celecoxib do not prevent AD in early results from a randomized controlled trial. *Neurology* 2007; **68**(21): 1800–8.

86. Martin BK, Szekely C, Brandt J, Piantadosi S, Breitner JC, Craft S *et al.* Cognitive function over time in the Alzheimer's Disease Anti-inflammatory Prevention Trial (ADAPT): results of a randomized, controlled trial of naproxen and celecoxib. *Arch Neurol* 2008; **65**(7): 896–905.

87. Breitner JC, Haneuse SJ, Walker R, Dublin S, Crane PK, Gray SL *et al.* Risk of dementia and AD with prior exposure to NSAIDs in an elderly community-based cohort. *Neurology* 2009; 22 Apr.

88. Simons M, Keller P, de Strooper B, Beyreuther K, Dotti CG, Simons K. Cholesterol depletion inhibits the generation of beta-amyloid in hippocampal neurons. *Proc Natl Acad Sci U S A* 1998; **95**(11): 6460–4.

89. Jick H, Zornberg GL, Jick SS, Seshadri S, Drachman DA. Statins and the risk of dementia. *Lancet* 2000; **356**(9242): 1627–31.

90. Wolozin B, Kellman W, Ruosseau P, Celesia GG, Siegel G. Decreased prevalence of Alzheimer disease associated with 3-hydroxy-3-methyglutaryl coenzyme A reductase inhibitors. *Arch Neurol* 2000; **57**(10): 1439–43.

91. Rockwood K, Kirkland S, Hogan DB, MacKnight C, Merry H, Verreault R *et al.* Use of lipid-lowering agents, indication bias, and the risk of dementia in community-dwelling elderly people. *Arch Neurol* 2002; **59**(2): 223–7.

92. Hajjar I, Schumpert J, Hirth V, Wieland D, Eleazer GP. The impact of the use of statins on the prevalence of dementia and the progression of cognitive impairment. *J Gerontol A Biol Sci Med Sci* 2002; **57**(7): M414–8.

93. Rodriguez EG, Dodge HH, Birzescu MA, Stoehr GP, Ganguli M. Use of lipid-lowering drugs in older adults with and without dementia: a community-based epidemiological study. *J Am Geriatr Soc* 2002; **50**(11): 1852–6.

94. Li G, Higdon R, Kukull WA, Peskind E, Van Valen Moore K, Tsuang D *et al.* Statin therapy and risk of dementia in the elderly: a community-based prospective cohort study. *Neurology* 2004; **63**(9): 1624–8.

95. Rea TD, Breitner JC, Psaty BM, Fitzpatrick AL, Lopez OL, Newman AB *et al.* Statin use and the risk of incident dementia: the Cardiovascular Health Study. *Arch Neurol* 2005; **62**(7): 1047–51.

96. Zandi PP, Sparks DL, Khachaturian AS, Tschanz J, Norton M, Steinberg M *et al.* Do statins reduce risk of incident dementia and Alzheimer disease? The Cache County Study. *Arch Gen Psychiatry* 2005; **62**(2): 217–24.

97. Santanello NC, Barber BL, Applegate WB, Elam J, Curtis C, Hunninghake DB *et al.* Effect of pharmacologic lipid lowering on health-related quality of life in older persons: results from

the Cholesterol Reduction in Seniors Program (CRISP) Pilot Study. *J Am Geriatr Soc* 1997; **45**(1): 8–14.

98. Group HPSC. MRC/BHF Heart Protection Study of cholesterol lowering with simvastatin in 20,536 high-risk individuals: a randomised placebo-controlled trial. *Lancet* 2002; **360**(9326): 7–22.

99. Shepherd J, Blauw GJ, Murphy MB, Bollen EL, Buckley BM, Cobbe SM *et al.* Pravastatin in elderly individuals at risk of vascular disease (PROSPER): a randomised controlled trial. *Lancet* 2002; **360**(9346): 1623–30.

100. Waring SC, Rocca WA, Petersen RC, O'Brien PC, Tangalos EG, Kokmen E. Postmenopausal estrogen replacement therapy and risk of AD: a population-based study. *Neurology* 1999; **52**(5): 965–70.

101. Kawas C, Resnick S, Morrison A, Brookmeyer R, Corrada M, Zonderman A *et al.* A prospective study of estrogen replacement therapy and the risk of developing Alzheimer's disease: the Baltimore Longitudinal Study of Aging. *Neurology* 1997; **48**(6): 1517–21.

102. Tang MX, Jacobs D, Stern Y, Marder K, Schofield P, Gurland B *et al.* Effect of oestrogen during menopause on risk and age at onset of Alzheimer's disease. *Lancet* 1996; **348**(9025): 429–32.

103. Zandi PP, Carlson MC, Plassman BL, Welsh-Bohmer KA, Mayer LS, Steffens DC *et al.* Hormone replacement therapy and incidence of Alzheimer disease in older women: the Cache County Study. *JAMA* 2002; **288**(17): 2123–9.

104. Brenner DE, Kukull WA, Stergachis A, Van Belle G, Bowen JD, McCormick WC *et al.* Postmenopausal estrogen replacement therapy and the risk of Alzheimer's disease: a population-based case-control study. *Am J Epidemiol* 1994; **140**(3): 262–7.

105. Seshadri S, Zornberg GL, Derby LE, Myers MW, Jick H, Drachman DA. Postmenopausal estrogen replacement therapy and the risk of Alzheimer disease. *Arch Neurol* 2001; **58**(3): 435–40.

106. Morrison JH, Brinton RD, Schmidt PJ, Gore AC. Estrogen, menopause, and the aging brain: how basic neuroscience can inform hormone therapy in women. *J Neurosci* 2006; **26**(41): 10332–48.

107. Henderson VW, Paganini-Hill A, Miller BL, Elble RJ, Reyes PF, Shoupe D *et al.* Estrogen for Alzheimer's disease in women: randomized, double-blind, placebo-controlled trial. *Neurology* 2000; **54**(2): 295–301.

108. Mulnard RA, Cotman CW, Kawas C, Van Dyck CH, Sano M, Doody R *et al.* Estrogen replacement therapy for treatment of mild to moderate Alzheimer disease: a randomized controlled trial. Alzheimer's Disease Cooperative Study. *JAMA* 2000; **283**(8): 1007–15.

109. Resnick SM, Henderson VW. Hormone therapy and risk of Alzheimer disease: a critical time. *JAMA* 2002; **288**(17): 2170–2.

110. Asthana S, Baker LD, Craft S, Stanczyk FZ, Veith RC, Raskind MA *et al.* High-dose estradiol improves cognition for women with AD: results of a randomized study. *Neurology* 2001; **57**(4): 605–12.

111. Rapp SR, Espeland MA, Shumaker SA, Henderson VW, Brunner RL, Manson JE *et al.* Effect of estrogen plus progestin on global cognitive function in postmenopausal women: the Women's Health Initiative Memory Study: a randomized controlled trial. *JAMA* 2003; **289**(20): 2663–72.

112. Shumaker SA, Legault C, Rapp SR, Thal L, Wallace RB, Ockene JK *et al.* Estrogen plus progestin and the incidence of dementia and mild cognitive impairment in postmenopausal women: the Women's Health Initiative Memory Study: a randomized controlled trial. *JAMA* 2003; **289**(20): 2651–62.

113. Shumaker SA, Legault C, Kuller L, Rapp SR, Thal L, Lane DS *et al.* Conjugated equine estrogens and incidence of probable dementia and mild cognitive impairment in postmenopausal women: Women's Health Initiative Memory Study. *JAMA* 2004; **291**(24): 2947–58.

114. Breitner JC, Zandi PP. Effects of estrogen plus progestin on risk of dementia. *JAMA* 2003; **290**(13): 1706–7; author reply 7–8.

115. Chen S, Nilsen J, Brinton RD. Dose and temporal pattern of estrogen exposure determines neuroprotective outcome in hippocampal neurons: therapeutic implications. *Endocrinology* 2006; **147**(11): 5303–13.

116. Nilsen J, Chen S, Irwin RW, Iwamoto S, Brinton RD. Estrogen protects neuronal cells from amyloid beta-induced apoptosis via regulation of mitochondrial proteins and function. *BMC Neurosci* 2006; **7**: 74.

117. Morris MC, Evans DA, Bienias JL, Tangney CC, Bennett DA, Wilson RS *et al.* Consumption of fish and n-3 fatty acids and risk of incident Alzheimer disease. *Arch Neurol* 2003; **60**(7): 940–6.

118. Morris MC, Evans DA, Tangney CC, Bienias JL, Wilson RS. Fish consumption and cognitive decline with age in a large community study. *Arch Neurol* 2005; **62**(12): 1849–53.

119. Scarmeas N, Stern Y, Tang MX, Mayeux R, Luchsinger JA. Mediterranean diet and risk for Alzheimer's disease. *Ann Neurol* 2006; **59**(6): 912–21.

120. Letenneur L. Risk of dementia and alcohol and wine consumption: a review of recent results. *Biol Res* 2004; **37**(2): 189–93.

121. Peters R, Peters J, Warner J, Beckett N, Bulpitt C. Alcohol, dementia and cognitive decline in the elderly: a systematic review. *Age Ageing* 2008; **37**(5): 505–12.

122. Morris MC, Beckett LA, Scherr PA, Hebert LE, Bennett DA, Field TS *et al.* Vitamin E and vitamin C supplement use and risk of incident Alzheimer disease. *Alzheimer Dis Assoc Disord* 1998; **12**(3): 121–6.

123. Zandi PP, Anthony JC, Khachaturian AS, Stone SV, Gustafson D, Tschanz JT *et al.* Reduced risk of Alzheimer disease in users of antioxidant vitamin supplements: the Cache County Study. *Arch Neurol* 2004; **61**(1): 82–8.

124. Luchsinger JA, Tang MX, Shea S, Mayeux R. Antioxidant vitamin intake and risk of Alzheimer disease. *Arch Neurol* 2003; **60**(2): 203–8.

125. Hooijmans CR, Kiliaan AJ. Fatty acids, lipid metabolism and Alzheimer pathology. *Eur J Pharmacol* 2008; **585**(1): 176–96.

126. van der Beek EM, Kamphuis PJ. The potential role of nutritional components in the management of Alzheimer's Disease. *Eur J Pharmacol* 2008; **585**(1): 197–207.

127. Cunnane SC, Plourde M, Pifferi F, Begin M, Feart C, Barberger-Gateau P. Fish, docosahexaenoic acid and Alzheimer's disease. *Progress in Lipid Research* 2009.

128. Luchsinger JA, Tang MX, Shea S, Mayeux R. Caloric intake and the risk of Alzheimer disease. *Arch Neurol* 2002; **59**(8): 1258–63.

129. Laitinen MH, Ngandu T, Rovio S, Helkala EL, Uusitalo U, Viitanen M *et al.* Fat intake at midlife and risk of dementia and

Alzheimer's disease: a population-based study. *Dement Geriatr Cogn Disord* 2006; **22**(1): 99–107.

130. Van de Rest O, Geleijnse JM, Kok FJ, Van Staveren WA, Dulle-meijer C, Olderikkert MG *et al*. Effect of fish oil on cognitive performance in older subjects: a randomized, controlled trial. *Neurology* 2008; **71**(6): 430–8.

131. Study MBHP. MRC/BHF Heart Protection Study of antioxidant vitamin supplementation in 20,536 high-risk individuals: a randomised placebo-controlled trial. *Lancet* 2002; **360**: 23–33.

132. Petersen RC, Thomas RG, Grundman M, Bennett D, Doody R, Ferris S *et al*. Vitamin E and donepezil for the treatment of mild cognitive impairment. *N Engl J Med* 2005; **352**(23): 2379–88.

133. Albert MS, Jones K, Savage CR, Berkman L, Seeman T, Blazer D *et al*. Predictors of cognitive change in older persons: MacArthur studies of successful aging. *Psychol Aging* 1995; **10**(4): 578–89.

134. Weuve J, Kang JH, Manson JE, Breteler MM, Ware JH, Grodstein F. Physical activity, including walking, and cognitive function in older women. *JAMA* 2004; **292**(12): 1454–61.

135. Laurin D, Verreault R, Lindsay J, MacPherson K, Rockwood K. Physical activity and risk of cognitive impairment and dementia in elderly persons. *Arch Neurol* 2001; **58**(3): 498–504.

136. Podewils LJ, Guallar E, Kuller LH, Fried LP, Lopez OL, Carlson M *et al*. Physical activity, APOE genotype, and dementia risk: findings from the Cardiovascular Health Cognition Study. *Am J Epidemiol* 2005; **161**(7): 639–51.

137. Rovio S, Kareholt I, Helkala EL, Viitanen M, Winblad B, Tuomilehto J *et al*. Leisure-time physical activity at midlife and the risk of dementia and Alzheimer's disease. *Lancet Neurol* 2005; **4**(11): 705–11.

138. Swain RA, Harris AB, Wiener EC, Dutka MV, Morris HD, Theien BE *et al*. Prolonged exercise induces angiogenesis and increases cerebral blood volume in primary motor cortex of the rat. *Neuroscience* 2003; **117**(4): 1037–46.

139. Colcombe SJ, Kramer AF, Erickson KI, Scalf P, McAuley E, Cohen NJ *et al*. Cardiovascular fitness, cortical plasticity, and aging. *Proc Natl Acad Sci U S A* 2004; **101**(9): 3316–21.

140. Lautenschlager NT, Cox KL, Flicker L, Foster JK, Van Bockxmeer FM, Xiao J *et al*. Effect of physical activity on cognitive function in older adults at risk for Alzheimer disease: a randomized trial. *JAMA* 2008; **300**(9): 1027–37.

141. Scarmeas N, Levy G, Tang MX, Manly J, Stern Y. Influence of leisure activity on the incidence of Alzheimer's disease. *Neurology* 2001; **57**(12): 2236–42.

142. Fratiglioni L, Wang HX, Ericsson K, Maytan M, Winblad B. Influence of social network on occurrence of dementia: a community-based longitudinal study. *Lancet* 2000; **355**(9212): 1315–9.

143. Bassuk SS, Glass TA, Berkman LF. Social disengagement and incident cognitive decline in community-dwelling elderly persons. *Ann Intern Med* 1999; **131**(3): 165–73.

144. Fratiglioni L, Paillard-Borg S, Winblad B. An active and socially integrated lifestyle in late life might protect against dementia. *Lancet Neurol* 2004; **3**(6): 343–53.

145. Ball K, Berch DB, Helmers KF, Jobe JB, Leveck MD, Marsiske M *et al*. Effects of cognitive training interventions with older adults: a randomized controlled trial. *JAMA* 2002; **288**(18): 2271–81.

48

Down Syndrome: Genetic and Clinical Overlap with Dementia

Giles M.Y. Tan and Declan G.M. Murphy

Department of Forensic and Neurodevelopmental Sciences, Institute of Psychiatry at the Maudsley, King's College London, UK

Down syndrome (DS) or trisomy 21 is the most common chromosomal abnormality associated with learning disability and affects approximately 1 per 650–1 000 live births. People with DS are more likely to develop Alzheimer's disease (AD) when compared to the general population. There is a well-established link between the neuropathology of AD and DS[1,2].

EPIDEMIOLOGY

Age of onset for dementia is typically between 50 and 55 years with a median age of onset of dementia of 55.5 years and an age range of 45 to 74 years[3]. Prevalence rates of clinical AD in DS vary substantially depending on the population studied, which ranges from 4% in a community sample[4] to 88% in an institution-based sample[5]. Many of the studies suffered from small sample sizes especially in the numbers of elderly DS persons included. A population-based study found that prevalence rates of AD increased with age – 8.9% (age 45–49), 17.7% (age 50–54), 32.1% (age 55–59) – up to age 60 years then decreased again – 25.6% (age above 60) – with an overall prevalence of 16.8%. The decrease was possibly accounted for by the increased mortality among the elderly demented DS persons[6].

While congenital malformations and especially congenital heart defects are the commonest cause of mortality in early life, survival rates for people with DS have improved significantly over the years with advances in medical care and more are now living longer and into old age. Life expectancy was 9 years in 1929 and 12 in 1949 but more recent data indicate that the median age at death has increased from 25 years in 1983 to 49 years in 1997, an average increase of 1.7 years per year studied[7]. Survival beyond 60 years of age has also improved, with 44.4% and 13.6% of live born DS individuals now surviving to 60 and 68 years, respectively[8]. Recent evidence suggests that age, presence of dementia and mobility restrictions predict mortality in DS. When compared with the general population, it was found that impaired mobility, severity of learning disability, the presence of epilepsy and visual impairment, but not cardiovascular risk factors or sex, predicted survival[9]. There is mounting evidence that the presence of the APOEε2 allele increases longevity[10] while non-demented DS individuals with at least one APOEε4 allele have increased mortality and up to five times the risks of dying within a 5- to 7-year follow-up period than those without an APOEε4 allele[11].

NEUROPATHOLOGY AND GENETICS

The neuropathological manifestation of AD in DS has been attributed to the triplication and over-expression of the APP gene located on chromosome 21[12]. This neuropathology is invariably found in the brains of individuals with DS over the age of 40 years[13]. The characteristic neuropathological changes in AD include the deposition of beta-amyloid (Aβ) as both extracellular diffuse and neuritic plaques as well as in meningeal and cerebral blood vessels and the intracellular accumulation of neurofibrillary tangles (NFTs) consisting of hyperphosphorylated tau in the form of paired helical filaments[1]. The accumulation of the diffuse plaques, which contain non-fibrillar amyloid, are commonly seen in DS before age 50 years and are not associated with AD whereas the neuritic plaques, which contain fibrillized amyloid and accumulate most commonly after age 50 years in DS, are associated with neuronal degeneration and loss of function[10]. NFTs occur at a later age in DS brains than amyloid plaques[14] and have been associated with dementia status in DS[3].

Aβ, which consists of the two major species Aβ1-40 and Aβ1-42, is produced from β-amyloid precursor protein (APP) by sequential proteolytic cleavage by β- and γ- secretases[15]. Starting from a young age, Aβ1-42 precedes Aβ1-40 in the course of amyloid deposition in the brains of people with DS[16]. Plasma Aβ levels are also elevated in DS persons from childhood[17]. Plasma levels of Aβ1-40 and Aβ1-42 may be correlated with age in older DS adults[18] and plasma Aβ1-42 levels were found to be higher in DS persons with dementia compared to those without in some studies[19] but not others, which found no association between plasma Aβ1-40 and Aβ1-42 levels and the presence of dementia, APOE genotype or duration of dementia[20] or age of onset[21].

Genetic Factors

Studies in the general population with AD have identified mutations in APP, presenilin 1 (PS-1) and presenilin 2 (PS-2) to be associated with early-onset familial forms of AD and the *APOE* gene polymorphisms with the more common late-onset AD. However, in DS persons, PS-1 polymorphisms do not appear to have the same detrimental effects and are not associated with the development of dementia[22].

Apolipoprotein E, which is involved in cholesterol transport and lipid metabolism and occurs in three allelic forms as ε2, ε3 and ε4

Principles and Practice of Geriatric Psychiatry, 3rd edn. Edited by Mohammed T. Abou-Saleh, Cornelius Katona and Anand Kumar
© 2011 John Wiley & Sons, Ltd

on chromosome 19, has been shown to modulate the risk of AD in the general population[23] with the APOEε4 allele associated with both late-onset familial and sporadic AD and the APOEε2 allele conferring a protective effect on the risk of developing AD[24]. In persons with DS, the relationship between APOEε4 and risk of AD remains controversial. Some studies have shown APOEε4 allele to be associated with increased risk of AD in persons with DS[25,26] while others have not[27,28]. A recent meta-analysis showed APOEε4 to be significantly associated with the prevalence of AD in DS[29].

The extended tau haplotype occurs in two forms, as H1 and H2, and has been associated with earlier onset of AD in the presence of the APOEε4 allele in the general population. Individuals with DS are at increased risk of developing dementia before age 45 years if they are heterozygous for the extended tau haplotype. Its lack of association with the APOE genotype suggests that it may be an independent risk factor for early onset dementia in DS[30].

The genes for proteins that regulate tau phosphorylation, *DYRK1A* (dual-specificity tyrosine-regulated kinase 1A) and calcipressin, are located on chromosome 21 and their increased expression in DS may promote NFT formation. Furthermore, increased expression of both occur in response to increased Aβ load and helps explain why NFTs occur at a later stage in the dementia process[31].

Tetranucleotide repeat in intron 7 of APP (attt5-8) has been associated with earlier age of onset of dementia by up to 13 years in DS[21].

GENDER AND THE ROLE OF OESTROGENS

Women in the general population are at increased risk of developing AD compared with men and oestrogen deficiency has been implicated in the cascade of pathological processes leading to AD. This has been reviewed recently[32].

The evidence for the effect of gender on risk of AD in DS is contradictory, with some studies finding no differences in age of onset[33], earlier onset[34] or later onset[35]. Postmenopausal DS women with low levels of bioavailable oestradiol have been found to have an increased risk of developing AD[36]. The average age of menopause in DS women was younger than in the general population and the age of onset of AD correlated with the age of menopause, hence it has been suggested that oestrogen deficiency may be a possible independent risk factor for AD in DS[37].

BRAIN METABOLITES: THE POTENTIAL ROLE OF MYO-INOSITOL

The Na+/*myo*-inositol co-transporter gene (SCL5A3) is located on chromosome 21 and *myo*-inositol significantly affects neuronal development and survival, neuronal osmolarity, membrane metabolism, signal transduction, protein kinase C activation and amyloid deposition[38].

Proton magnetic resonance spectroscopy studies in healthy DS persons have reported significant increases in brain choline and *myo*-inositol, but no differences in brain NAA or creatine, and it has been suggested that the abnormal membrane turnover/degradation and increase in *myo*-inositol reflect a 'predementia' phase in which the neuropathology of AD is accumulating and precedes the loss of neurons[39,40]. The increased brain *myo*-inositol concentrations in healthy DS persons have been shown to be negatively correlated with overall cognitive and memory abilities[41].

In a study comparing brain metabolites in demented, mild cognitively impaired (MCI) and healthy controls in the general population

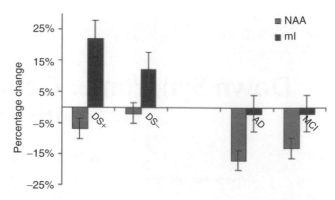

Figure 48.1   The percentage change in unadjusted averages of hippocampal concentrations of NAA and mI by group comparisons (i.e. DS+ to DS−, AD to HC, DS− to HC and MCI to HC)

with demented (DS+) and non-demented (DS−) DS individuals, NAA concentrations were found to be reduced in persons with AD and MCI in the general population but not in either the demented or non-demented DS persons, suggesting that dementia in DS is associated with comparatively small reductions in viable neuronal function (as measured by NAA). In contrast, it was found that brain *myo*-inositol (mI) concentration was only increased in the demented DS group (see Figure 48.1), suggesting that elevated brain *myo*-inositol modifies the risk of dementia in people with DS possibly by interacting synergistically with other risk factors for dementia in this vulnerable population[42]. Research is currently under way to determine if manipulation of brain *myo*-inositol in DS by the use of lithium could offer a novel target for intervention in the dementia process in DS.

OXIDATIVE STRESS

Free radicals produced by metabolic processes are kept in check by antioxidant defences and if this balance is disturbed, results in the highly reactive free radicals reacting with lipids in cell membranes to cause cellular damage, which contributes to neurodegeneration. The genetic locus for Cu,Zn-superoxide dismutase (SOD1), a key enzyme in free radical metabolism, is located on chromosome 21[43] and has been suggested to have particular relevance to neurodegeneration in DS[44].

NEUROINFLAMMATION

There is increasing evidence to suggest that cytokines have an important role to play in the development and/or progression of AD in the general population. The inflammatory component of AD is dominated by the presence of activated microglial cells[45]. Studies have shown some support for the hypothesis that cytokines may act as a risk factor for the development of dementia in DS[46,47]. A small study found positive correlations between serum IL-6 levels with age and severity of AD in people with DS[48], and there is preliminary evidence to indicate that serum TNF-α levels are elevated in DS persons with AD[49], suggesting a disease-stage-dependent general activation of the immune system.

NEUROIMAGING

Using magnetic resonance imaging (MRI) based measurements of grey matter atrophy as a surrogate marker of neuronal density, various neuroimaging studies have described the macroscopic neuroanatomy of DS. More recent studies using sensitive quantitative measures of region-specific atrophy based on high-resolution MRI have suggested that age-specific atrophy in DS resembles the pattern of brain atrophy in the early stages of AD[50].

In DS persons, overall brain volume including the cerebellum and cerebral grey and white matter, ventral pons, mammillary bodies and hippocampus is reduced whereas the parahippocampal gyrus are enlarged[51]. Reductions in cerebral volume are prominent in the frontal and occipital lobes and there is relative preservation of parietal lobe grey and temporal lobe white matter[52].

As they age, non-demented DS individuals show volumetric reductions in most cortical brain regions[53], hippocampus, parahippocampal gyrus and corpus callosum. Demented DS individuals show volumetric reductions in total brain, total grey matter, frontal, temporal and parietal cortices, hippocampus and parahippocampal gyrus and enlarged ventricles when compared to non-demented DS individuals[50]. A recent study showed volumetric reductions of the hippocampus and caudate bilaterally, right amygdala and putamen in demented DS individuals. Hippocampal and caudate volumes both correctly categorized 92% of DS persons without AD as well as 75% and 80%, respectively, of DS persons with AD, suggesting that they may act as markers of clinical AD[34].

COGNITIVE AND BEHAVIOURAL FEATURES

Pre-Existing Cognitive Ability

Low education and low lifetime occupational attainment have been associated with increased risk of AD in the general population possibly by the lack of cognitive reserve, which hastens the onset of clinical manifestations[55]. In DS persons, higher cognitive functioning has been associated with fewer cases of dementia[56] and the rate of cognitive deterioration increased with age and degree of pre-existing cognitive impairment[57].

Executive Dysfunction

The presentation of the early stages of AD in persons with DS differs from that in the general population and is characterized by prominent personality and behaviour changes associated with executive dysfunction rather than declines in episodic memory, which may suggest impairments in frontal lobe functions[58].

Selective Attention

Progressive impairment in selective attention, as measured by cancellation tasks, has been detected in DS adults in the preclinical stage of AD and the performance in this group could be differentiated from their healthy DS peers who do not go on to develop AD[59].

CO-MORBIDITY

Physical Health

As in the general population, people with DS experience more health problems as they age. With the onset of AD, there is an increase in the frequency and severity of the co-morbidities. Visual and hearing impairments, gastric concerns, depression, epilepsy, lung disease and mobility problems have all been reported to be increased in DS with AD compared to those without AD and additionally have also been reported to be associated with the stage of AD, with the co-morbidities being more severe at the later stages of the dementia process[60]. Some of these co-morbidities are significantly more severe in the DS population with AD than those with AD in the general population who do not have DS, e.g. epilepsy[5].

Maladaptive Behaviours and Mental Ill Health

AD is characterized by progressive decline in cognitive and functional skills and is often accompanied by maladaptive behaviours and psychiatric symptoms. A recent longitudinal cohort study showed point prevalence of mental ill health in non-demented DS adults to be between 10.8% and 23.7% while the 2-year incidence varied from 3.7% to 14.9% depending on the diagnostic criteria used. The highest incidence was for depressive episode and dementia/delirium. Mental ill health was found to be lower in DS when compared with other adults with learning disability[61]. An earlier study found that most depressed DS persons were still symptomatic at one year and those with early onset depression were associated with better treatment outcomes[62].

Non-demented elderly DS persons show less initiative and more apathy compared to individuals with other causes of learning disability, and when compared to younger DS persons, showed more irritation, fear, restlessness at night, sadness, suspiciousness and loss of appetite[63]. In DS persons with AD, there was a higher prevalence of low mood, restlessness/excessive overactivity, disturbed sleep, being excessively uncooperative and auditory hallucinations, but they were less aggressive when compared to demented learning disabled individuals without DS[61]. In a more recent study, differences in maladaptive behaviours at various stages of dementia were found, with the non-demented DS individuals displaying fewer and less severe maladaptive behaviours than individuals in the early and mid-stages of dementia. Furthermore, those non-demented DS individuals who were transitioning into the early stages of dementia displayed increased aggression, fearfulness, sadness, sleep problems, social inadequacy, stealing and general regressive behaviours[65].

In a study on referral characteristics, it was found that DS individuals who were referred for specialist dementia assessment showed more behavioural excess, but not deficits, and lower socialization and coping skills when compared to those who were not referred. Their carers also reported the behaviours as having a greater impact on them than on the individual with DS[66].

DIAGNOSTIC ISSUES

There are significant difficulties associated with diagnosing AD in people with DS. The large intra-individual variability in cognitive functioning, lack of standard diagnostic and methodological procedures and difficulties with obtaining baseline cognitive function with which to assess cognitive and behavioural change in DS persons make early diagnosis of AD especially difficult in this population[67]. Further difficulties arise from the fact that many individuals with DS suffer from underdevelopment of social and cognitive skills and high rates of co-morbidity (e.g. depression and hypothyroidism).

The pre-existing learning disability often results in floor effects on many of the standard assessment tests used, and available screening instruments vary in their reliability[68]. Among the informant-rated instruments, the Dementia Questionnaire for Persons with Mental

Retardation (DMR)[69], later revised as the Dementia Questionnaire for people with Learning Disabilities (DLD), is widely used in people with learning disability but had variable sensitivity in single assessments and poor specificity in people with DS, while the Dementia Scale for Down Syndrome (DSDS) had good specificity but mediocre sensitivity. Of the direct assessment instruments, the Test for Severe Impairment (TSI) and Severe Impairment Battery (SIB) have been used but require further evaluation in people with DS. More recently, the CAMDEX-DS, a modified version of the Cambridge Examination for Mental Disorders of the Elderly (CAMDEX) informant interview, has been developed for assessing people with DS suspected of having dementia[70]. As to the different diagnostic criteria in use, the DSM-IV dementia criteria has been shown to be more inclusive than that of the ICD-10, which excluded DS persons with even moderate dementia[71].

TREATMENT

Established antidementia drug treatments for AD in the general population include the cholinesterase inhibitors donepezil, rivastigmine and galantamine as well as the NMDA antagonist memantine. There is limited evidence available on drug therapies for dementia in DS[72]. Recent Cochrane reviews on the subject found only one randomized controlled trial of suitable quality for donepezil, and none for galantamine, rivastigmine and memantine[73-76]. That study on donepezil suggested some limited benefit of donepezil treatment at 24 weeks[77], and an open label extension of that study showed that those continued on donepezil showed less deterioration at two years, which may suggest benefits of longer-term use[78]. Drug therapy should form part of the broader multidisciplinary management of persons with DS and AD, incorporating carer support, psychological and behavioural therapies and ongoing assessment of and management of physical and mental health.

CONCLUSIONS

There is considerable neuropathological, genetic and clinical overlap between the AD in DS and in the general population but also some subtle differences. The occurrence of dementia in people with DS is expected to rise proportionately with the increase in their life expectancy. This has implications for health and social care provisions both for them and their carers, and further research into better understanding the neurobiology of the disease in DS and potential treatments for them are warranted.

REFERENCES

1. Wisniewski KE, Wisniewski HM, Wen GY. Occurrence of neuropathological changes and dementia of Alzheimer's disease in Down's syndrome. *Ann Neurol* 1985; **17**(3): 278–82.
2. Mann DM. The pathological association between Down syndrome and Alzheimer disease. *Mech Ageing Dev* 1988; **43**(2): 99–136.
3. Margallo-Lana ML, Moore PB, Kay DWK *et al*. Fifteen-year follow-up of 92 hospitalized adults with Down's syndrome: incidence of cognitive decline, its relationship to age and neuropathology. *J Intellect Disabil Res* 2007; **51**(6): 463–77.
4. Devenny DA, Silverman WP, Hill AL *et al*. Normal ageing in adults with Down's syndrome: a longitudinal study. *J Intellect Disabil Res* 1996; **40**(3): 208–21.
5. Evenhuis HM. The natural history of dementia in Down's syndrome. *Arch Neurol* 1990; **47**(3): 263–7.
6. Coppus A, Evenhuis H, Verberne, G-J *et al*. Dementia and mortality in persons with Down's syndrome. *J Intellect Disabil Res* 2006; **50**(10): 768–77.
7. Yang Q, Rasmussen SA, Friedman JM. Mortality associated with Down's syndrome in the USA from 1983 to 1997: a population-based study. *Lancet* 2002; **359**(9311): 1019–25.
8. Baird PA, Sadovnick AD. Life expectancy in Down syndrome adults. *Lancet* 1988; **2**(8624): 1354–6.
9. Coppus AM, Evenhuis HM, Verberne GJ. Survival in elderly persons with Down syndrome. *J Am Geriatr Soc* 2008; **56**(12): 2311–16.
10. Schupf N, Sergievsky GH. Genetic and host factors for dementia in Down's syndrome. *Br J Psychiatry* 2002; **180**: 405–10.
11. Zigman WB, Jenkins EC, Tycko B, Schupf N, Silverman W. Mortality is associated with apolipoprotein E epsilon4 in nondemented adults with Down syndrome. *Neurosci Lett* 2005; **390**(2): 93–7.
12. Rumble B, Retallack R, Hilbich C *et al*. Amyloid A4 protein and its precursor in Down's syndrome and Alzheimer's disease. *N Engl J Med* 1989; **320**(22): 1446–52.
13. Wisniewski KE, Dalton AJ, McLachlan C, Wen GY, Wisniewski HM. Alzheimer's disease in Down's syndrome: clinicopathologic studies. *Neurology* 1985; **35**(7): 957–61.
14. Murphy GM, Jr, Eng LF, Ellis WG *et al*. Antigenic profile of plaques and neurofibrillary tangles in the amygdala in Down's syndrome: a comparison with Alzheimer's disease. *Brain Res* 1990; **537**(1–2): 102–8.
15. Selkoe DJ. Normal and abnormal biology of the beta-amyloid precursor protein. *Annu Rev Neurosci* 1994; **17**: 489–517.
16. Teller JK, Russo C, DeBusk LM *et al*. Presence of soluble amyloid beta-peptide precedes amyloid plaque formation in Down's syndrome. *Nature Med* 1996; **2**(1): 93–5.
17. Mehta PD, Capone G, Jewell A, Freedland RL. Increased amyloid beta protein levels in children and adolescents with Down syndrome. *J Neurol Sci* 2007; **254**(1–2): 22–7.
18. Mehta PD, Mehta SP, Fedor B *et al*. Plasma amyloid beta protein 1-42 levels are increased in old Down Syndrome but not in young Down Syndrome. *Neurosci Lett* 2003; **342**(3): 155–8.
19. Schupf N, Patel B, Silverman W *et al*. Elevated plasma amyloid beta-peptide 1-42 and onset of dementia in adults with Down syndrome. *Neurosci Lett* 2001; **301**(3): 199–203.
20. Jones EL, Hanney M, Francis PT, Ballard CG. Amyloid beta concentrations in older people with Down syndrome and dementia. *Neurosci Lett* 2009; **451**(2): 162–4.
21. Margallo-Lana M, Morris CM, Gibson AM *et al*. Influence of the amyloid precursor protein locus on dementia in Down syndrome. *Neurology* 2004; **62**(11): 1996–8.
22. Tyrrell J, Cosgrave M, McPherson J *et al*. Presenilin 1 and alpha-1-antichymotrypsin polymorphisms in Down syndrome: no effect on the presence of dementia. *Am J Med Genet* 1999; **88**(6): 616–20.
23. Saunders AM, Strittmatter WJ, Schmechel D *et al*. Association of apolipoprotein E allele epsilon 4 with late-onset familial and sporadic Alzheimer's disease. *Neurology* 1993; **43**(8): 1467–72.
24. Corder EH, Saunders AM, Risch NJ *et al*. Protective effect of apolipoprotein E type 2 allele for late onset Alzheimer disease. *Nat Genet* 1994; **7**(2): 180–84.

25. Deb S, Braganza J, Norton N et al. APOE epsilon 4 influences the manifestation of Alzheimer's disease in adults with Down's syndrome. Br J Psychiatry 2000; 176: 468–72.

26. Prasher VP, Sajith SG, Rees SD et al. Significant effect of APOE epsilon 4 genotype on the risk of dementia in Alzheimer's disease and mortality in persons with Down syndrome. Int J Geriatr Psychiatry 2008; 23(11): 1134–40.

27. Lai F, Kammann E, Rebeck GW et al. APOE genotype and gender effects on Alzheimer disease in 100 adults with Down syndrome. Neurology 1999; 53(2): 331–6.

28. Prasher VP, Chowdhury TA, Rowe BR et al. ApoE genotype and Alzheimer's disease in adults with Down syndrome: meta-analysis. Am J Ment Retard 1997; 102(2): 103–10.

29. Coppus AM, Evenhuis HM, Verberne GJ et al. The impact of apolipoprotein E on dementia in persons with Down's syndrome. Neurobiol Aging 2008; 29(6): 828–35.

30. Jones EL, Margallo-Lana M, Prasher VP, Ballard CG. The extended tau haplotype and the age of onset of dementia in Down syndrome. Dement Geriatr Cogn Disord 2008; 26(3): 199–202.

31. Kimura R, Kamino K, Yamamoto M et al. The DYRK1A gene, encoded in chromosome 21 Down syndrome critical region, bridges between beta-amyloid production and tau phosphorylation in Alzheimer disease. Hum Molec Genet 2007; 16(1): 15–23.

32. Craig MC, Maki PM, Murphy DG. The Women's Health Initiative Memory Study: findings and implications for treatment. Lancet Neurol 2005; 4(3): 190–94.

33. Visser FE, Aldenkamp AP, Van Huffelen AC et al. Prospective study of the prevalence of Alzheimer-type dementia in institutionalized individuals with Down syndrome. Am J Ment Retard 1997; 101(4): 400–12.

34. Schupf N, Pang D, Patel BN et al. Onset of dementia is associated with age at menopause in women with Down's syndrome. Ann Neurol 2003; 54(4): 433–8.

35. Schupf N, Kapell D, Nightingale B et al. Earlier onset of Alzheimer's disease in men with Down syndrome. Neurology 1998; 50(4): 991–5.

36. Schup N, Winsten S, Patel B et al. Bioavailable estradiol and age at onset of Alzheimer's disease in postmenopausal women with Down syndrome. Neurosci Lett 2006; 406(3): 298–302.

37. Cosgrave MP, Tyrrell J, McCarron M, Gill M, Lawlor BA. Age at onset of dementia and age of menopause in women with Down's syndrome. J Intellect Disabil Res 1999; 43(5): 461–5.

38. McLaurin J, Franklin T, Chakrabartty A, Fraser PE. Phosphatidylinositol and inositol involvement in Alzheimer amyloid-beta fibril growth and arrest. J Mol Biol 1998; 278(1): 183–94.

39. Shonk T, Ross BD. Role of increased cerebral myo-inositol in the dementia of Down syndrome. Magn Reson Med 1995; 33(6): 858–61.

40. Huang W, Alexander GE, Daly EM et al. High brain myo-inositol levels in the predementia phase of Alzheimer's disease in adults with Down's syndrome: a[1] H MRS study. Am J Psychiatry 1999; 156(12): 1879–86.

41. Beacher F, Simmons A, Daly E et al. Hippocampal myo-inositol and cognitive ability in adults with Down syndrome: an in vivo proton magnetic resonance spectroscopy study. Arch Gen Psychiatry 2005; 62(12): 1360–65.

42. Lamar M, Foy CML, Beacher F et al. Dementia in Down's syndrome: a ^{1}H-MRS comparison with Alzheimer's disease and mild cognitive impairment (under review).

43. Brugge KL, Nichols S, Delis D, Saitoh T, Truaner D. The role of alterations in free radical metabolism in mediating cognitive impairments in Down's syndrome. EXS 1992; 62: 190–98.

44. Bush A, Beail N. Risk factors for dementia in people with Down syndrome: issues in assessment and diagnosis. Am J Ment Retard 2004; 109(2): 83–97.

45. McGeer EG, McGeer PL. Brain inflammation in Alzheimer disease and the therapeutic implications. Curr Pharm Des 1999; 5(10): 821–36.

46. Carta MG, Serra P, Ghiani A et al. Chemokines and pro-inflammatory cytokines in Down's syndrome: an early marker for Alzheimer-type dementia? Psychother Psychosom 2002; 71(4): 233–6.

47. Licastro F, Chiappelli M, Ruscica M, Carnelli V, Corsi MM. Altered cytokine and acute phase response protein levels in the blood of children with Downs syndrome: relationship with dementia of Alzheimer's type. Int J Immunopathol Pharmacol 2005; 18(1): 165–72.

48. Kálmán J, Juhász A, Laird G et al. Serum interleukin-6 levels correlate with the severity of dementia in Down syndrome and in Alzheimer's disease. Acta Neurol Scand 1997; 96(4): 236–40.

49. Tan GMY, Nicholls S, Holmes C. Cytokine production and cognitive decline in people with Down's syndrome – a pilot study (under review).

50. Teipel SJ, Hampel H, Neuroanatomy of Down syndrome in vivo: a model of preclinical Alzheimer's disease. Behav Genet 2006; 36(3): 405–15.

51. Raz N, Torres IJ, Briggs SD et al. Selective neuroanatomic abnormalities in Down's syndrome and their cognitive correlates: evidence from MRI morphometry. Neurology 1995; 45(2): 356–66.

52. Pinter JD, Eliez S, Schmitt JE, Capone GT, Reiss AL. Neuroanatomy of Down's syndrome: a high-resolution MRI study. Am J Psychiatry 2001; 158(10): 1659–65.

53. Beacher F, Daly E, Simmons A et al. Brain anatomy and ageing in non-demented adults with Down's syndrome: an in vivo MRI study. Psychol Med 2010; 40(4): 611–19.

54. Beacher F, Daly E, Simmons A et al. Alzheimer's disease and Down's syndrome: an in vivo MRI study. Psychol Med 2009; 39(4): 675–84.

55. Stern Y, Gurland B, Tatemichi TK et al. Influence of education and occupation on the incidence of Alzheimer's disease. JAMA 1994; 271(13): 1004–10.

56. Temple V, Jozsvai E, Konstantareas MM, Hewitt TA. Alzheimer dementia in Down's syndrome: the relevance of cognitive ability. J Intellect Disabil Res 2001; 45(1): 47–55.

57. Oliver C, Crayton L, Holland A, Hall S, Bradbury J. A four year prospective study of age-related cognitive change in adults with Down's syndrome. Psychol Med 1998; 28(6): 1365–77.

58. Ball SL, Holland AJ, Hon J et al. Personality and behaviour changes mark the early stages of Alzheimer's disease in adults with Down's syndrome: findings from a prospective population-based study. Int J Geriatr Psychiatry 2006; 21(7): 661–73.

59. Krinsky-McHale SJ, Devenny DA, Kittler P, Silverman W. Selective attention deficits associated with mild cognitive impairment and early stage Alzheimer's disease in adults with Down syndrome. Am J Ment Retard 2008; 113(5): 369–86.

60. McCarron M, Gill M, McCallion P, Begley C. Health co-morbidities in ageing persons with Down syndrome and Alzheimer's dementia. *J Intellect Disabil Res* 2005; **49**(7): 560–66.

61. Mantry D, Cooper S-A, Smiley E *et al.* The prevalence and incidence of mental ill-health in adults with Down syndrome. *J Intellect Disabil Res* 2008; **52**(2): 141–55.

62. Prasher V, Hall W. Short-term prognosis of depression in adults with Down's syndrome: association with thyroid status and effects on adaptive behaviour. *J Intellect Disabil Res* 1996; **40**(1): 32–8.

63. Haveman MJ, Maaskant MA, van Schrojenstein Lantman HM, Urlings HF, Kessels AG. Mental health problems in elderly people with and without Down's syndrome. *J Intellect Disabil Res* 1994; **38** (3): 341–55.

64. Cooper SA, Prasher V. Maladaptive behaviours and symptoms of dementia in adults with Down's syndrome compared with adults with intellectual disability of other aetiologies. *J Intellect Disabil Res* 1998; **42** (4): 293–300.

65. Urv TK, Zigman WB, Silverman W. Maladaptive behaviors related to dementia status in adults with Down syndrome. *Am J Ment Retard* 2008; **113**(2): 73–86.

66. Adams D, Oliver C, Kalsy S *et al.* Behavioural characteristics associated with dementia assessment referrals in adults with Down syndrome. *J Intellect Disabil Res* 2008; **52**(4): 358–68.

67. Nieuwenhuis-Mark RE. Diagnosing Alzheimer's dementia in Down syndrome: problems and possible solutions. *Res Dev Disabil* 2009; **30**(5): 827–38.

68. Strydom A, Hassiotis A. Diagnostic instruments for dementia in older people with intellectual disability in clinical practice. *Aging Ment Health* 2003; **7**(6): 431–7.

69. Evenhuis HM. Further evaluation of the Dementia Questionnaire for Persons with Mental Retardation (DMR). *J Intellect Disabil Res* 1996; **40**(4): 369–73.

70. Ball SL, Holland AJ, Huppert FA *et al.* The modified CAMDEX informant interview is a valid and reliable tool for use in the diagnosis of dementia in adults with Down's syndrome. *J Intellect Disabil Res* 2004; **48**(6): 611–20.

71. Strydom A, Livingston G, King M, Hassiotis A. Prevalence of dementia in intellectual disability using different diagnostic criteria. *Br J Psychiatry* 2007; **191**: 150–57.

72. Prasher VP. Review of donepezil, rivastigmine, galantamine and memantine for the treatment of dementia in Alzheimer's disease in adults with Down syndrome: implications for the intellectual disability population. *Int J Geriatr Psychiatry* 2004; **19**(6): 509–15.

73. Mohan M, Carpenter PK, Bennett C. Donepezil for dementia in people with Down syndrome. *Cochrane Database Syst Rev* 2009 Jan 21; (1): CD007178.

74. Mohan M, Bennett C, Carpenter PK. Galantamine for dementia in people with Down syndrome. *Cochrane Database Syst Rev* 2009 Jan 21; (1): CD007656.

75. Mohan M, Bennett C, Carpenter PK. Rivastigmine for dementia in people with Down syndrome. *Cochrane Database Syst Rev* 2009 Jan 21; (1): CD007658.

76. Mohan M, Bennett C, Carpenter PK. Memantine for dementia in people with Down syndrome. *Cochrane Database Syst Rev* 2009 Jan 21; (1): CD007657.

77. Prasher VP, Huxley A, Haque MS. A 24-week, double-blind, placebo-controlled trial of donepezil in patients with Down syndrome and Alzheimer's disease – pilot study. *Int J Geriatr Psychiatry* 2002; **17**(3): 270–78.

78. Prasher VP, Adams C, Holder R. Long term safety and efficacy of donepezil in the treatment of dementia in Alzheimer's disease in adults with Down syndrome: open label study. *Int J Geriatr Psychiatry* 2003; **18**(6): 549–51.

49

The Molecular Neuropathology of Alzheimer's Disease

Orly Lazarov

Department of Anatomy and Cell Biology, The University of Illinois at Chicago, IL, USA

INTRODUCTION

It is yet to be discovered what induces the high vulnerability exhibited by specific groups of neurons in Alzheimer's disease (AD), leading to their progressive degeneration. Vulnerable neurons are located in brain areas that are functionally linked to various forms and aspects of learning and memory, including the hippocampal formation, olfactory system and neocortex (for review see[1]). The parahippocampal regions are the earliest to be affected (Braak stages I and II). In particular, the entorhino-hippocampal circuit exhibits an early and significant neuropathology. Neuropathology in this region correlates significantly with degree of dementia. The hallmark lesions of the disease, most pronounced in the affected brain areas, are neurofibrillary tangles and amyloid deposits. Neurofibrillary tangles are intracellular aggregates of bundled paired helical filaments. The principal component of neurofibrillary tangles is hyperphosphorylated tau. The microtubule-associated group of tau proteins consists of alternatively spliced cytoplasmic proteins that bear either three or four microtubule-binding domains and co-assemble with tubulin onto microtubules, where they stabilize these organelles. As such, tau is implicated in numerous critical cellular processes, such as cell proliferation, neuronal maturation, process elongation and axonal transport. Thus, preceding neurofibrillary tangle formation, hyperphosphorylation of tau may interfere with crucial cellular and neuronal functions. The mechanism underlying hyperphosphorylation of tau in AD is not fully understood, as discussed below. Amyloid deposits are aggregates of β-amyloid (Aβ) peptides released from a large precursor termed amyloid precursor protein (APP) upon enzymatic cleavage. Upon increase production or fibrillogenic properties, Aβ undergoes conformational changes to form β-sheet structures that tend to form oligomers and subsequently insoluble aggregates. One form of amyloid aggregates is neuritic plaque, an extracellular core of amyloid fibrils surrounded by dystrophic dendrites, degenerating axons and reactive gliosis. Neuritic plaques are abundant in the molecular layer of the dentate gyrus of the hippocampus, the amygdala, the association cortices of the frontal, temporal and parietal lobes, and within certain deep brain nuclei that project to these regions. In addition to neuritic plaques, several other forms of Aβ aggregates exist, including abundant 'diffuse plaques' in the limbic and association cortices and even in non-conventionally affected regions, such as cerebellum. Increased fibrillogenesis and/or levels of Aβ is caused by either mutagenesis or ageing-linked unknown pathogenesis. In rare, familial, early onset form of AD (FAD), increased fibrillogenesis and/or levels of Aβ are caused by mutations in APP, presenilin-1 (PS1) and presenilin-2 (PS2). These mutations cause misprocessing and trafficking of APP by β-secretase or γ-secretase, the aspartyl protease of which PS is the catalytic core, yielding an increased amount and/or ratio of the fibrillogenic forms of Aβ (e.g. Aβ$_{42}$), that consequently aggregate in the form of amyloid deposits. Both hallmark lesions are the result of misfolding and polymerization of otherwise soluble proteins. The progressive emergence of altered conformations of originally soluble proteins and subsequently insoluble aggregates, intra- and extracellularly, is associated with profound neuronal dysfunction and death.

FAMILIAL ALZHEIMER'S DISEASE-LINKED CENTRAL PLAYERS

Amyloid Precursor Proteins

Amyloid precursor proteins encompass a family of membrane-anchored type I glycoproteins that are ubiquitously expressed and particularly abundant in the brain (for review see[2]). APP full length are 110–130 kDa proteins that are synthesized in the endoplasmic reticulum. *APP* maps to chromosome 21 in humans and is transcribed to three isoforms, APP$_{695}$, APP$_{750}$ and APP$_{771}$ with the former being predominantly expressed in neurons and the latter two in glia. APP$_{770}$ is encoded by 18 exons, where exon 17 resembles the membrane-spanning domain. APP$_{695}$ is lacking both exon 7 and exon 8, and is the most abundant APP transcript in the brain. APP$_{751}$ (lacking exon 8), APP$_{714}$ (lacking exon 7) and APP$_{770}$ are expressed in the peripheral and central nervous system. Exon 7 encodes an amino acid fragment that exhibits substantial homology to the Kunitz-type serine protease inhibitor (KPI) while exon 8 shares some homology with the MRC OX-2 antigen. Two additional members of the APP family are amyloid precursor-like protein 1 and 2 (APLP1 and APLP2). They are truncated at the carboxyl terminus and lack the Aβ region. The APLPs map to chromosome 19 in humans. The APLP2 but not APLP1 contains a KPI domain. Nevertheless, neither mutations in APLP1 nor in APLP2 are causative of FAD, supporting the notion that Aβ plays a major role in the disease. Indeed, FAD-linked mutations introduce amino acid substitutions within or flanking the Aβ region of APP, around the cleavage sites of α-, β- and γ-secretase. APP undergoes a complex set of tightly linked trafficking and processing. From the endoplasmic reticulum, APP is transported to the plasma membrane through Golgi apparatus. However, only a small fraction of APP molecules reaches the plasma membrane. During this journey APP undergoes multi post-translation modifications of N- and O-glycosylation, ectodomain and cytoplasmic phosphorylation, and tyrosine sulphation. The presence of the YENPTY internalization motif near the C terminus of APP enables APP endocytosis shortly after it reaches the plasma membrane. Then APP is delivered to endosomes, and a fraction of endocytosed molecules is recycled to the cell surface. Some of internalized APP undergoes lysosomal degradation. During its journey, APP is subject to a complex processing by multiple enzymatic activities (Figure 49.1), most of which are around the 4 kDa region of the Aβ peptide (for review see[1]). In the nonamyloidogenic pathway, APP is cleaved by α-secretase at amino acid 16–17 of the Aβ region, preventing the formation of Aβ. In the amyloidogenic pathway, APP is cleaved by the β-secretase enzymatic activity at the carboxyl terminus of the Aβ region, followed by a cleavage by γ-secretase enzymatic complex at the amino terminus of the Aβ region, leading to the release of Aβ.

Following shedding of APP by α- and β-secretase, the soluble product (sAPPα and sAPPβ) is released to the extracellular space, while a membrane-anchored fragment is subject to an intramembranous cleavage by γ-secretase, releasing APP carboxyl terminus fragments (AICD) into the cytoplasm. AICD can form a transcriptionally active complex with Fe65 and Tip60. While the role of AICD in regulation of gene transcription is yet to be confirmed, several genes are thought to be regulated by AICD: *KAI1*, the Aβ-degrading enzyme *neprilysin*, *LRP1*, and epidermal growth factor (EGF) receptor. Many adaptor proteins with phosphotyrosine-binding domains, including Fe65, Fe65L1, Fe65L2, Mint1 (i.e. X11), Mint2, Mint3, Dab1, and c-Jun N-terminal kinase (JNK)-interacting protein family members bind this motif and the flanking region. Overexpression of these adaptors reduces Aβ production and deposition in the brains of transgenic mice, suggesting that these adaptors play a role in regulation of APP processing (for review see[3]). Interestingly, Fe65 serves as a functional linker between APP and LRP in modulating endocytic APP trafficking and Aβ production. Mutations within the YENPTY endocytosis motif inhibit APP internalization and decrease Aβ production, suggesting that APP is processed to yield Aβ following internalization.

The phenotype of mice with homozygous ablation of APP appeared rather mild compared to presenilin-1 knockout phenotype. Some

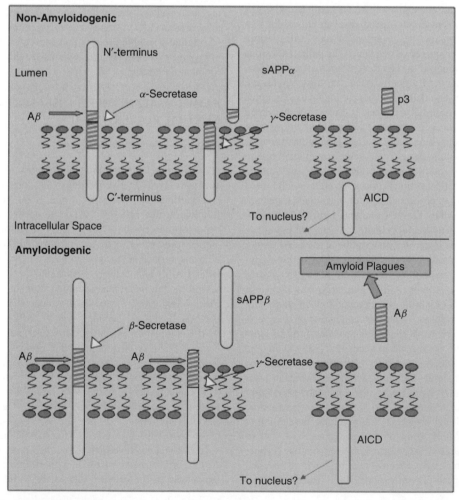

Figure 49.1 Schematic presentation of APP processing in its amyloidogenic and nonamyloidogenic pathways. AICD = APP carboxyl terminus fragments
Image generation by courtesy of Michael Demars

synaptic markers are thought to be reduced in APP-deficient mice, and this reduction correlates with deficits in learning and memory and in synaptic plasticity. APLP2 knockout mice appear normal, while APLP1 knockout exhibit some growth impairments. This mild phenotype might be due to partial functional redundancy among the family members. In support of this notion, *APLP2/APLP1* and *APP/APLP2* double knockouts die right after birth, suggesting that APLP2 functionally overlaps with APP and APLP1. Examination of the central and peripheral nervous system of the double knockout mice confirmed significant deficits in synapse formation, deformed pre- and post-synaptic element distribution, reduced number of synaptic vesicles and aberrant localization of the choline transporter at neuromuscular junctions. Deficiency of all three *App* genes led to death shortly after birth, exhibiting cortical dysplasia suggestive of migration abnormalities of the neuroblasts and partial loss of cortical Cajal–Retzius cells. Taken together, these findings suggest that the *APP* gene family plays important roles in the development of the nervous system, such as synapse formation and regulation of neural progenitor cells.

Presenilins and γ-Secretase

Presenilins (PS1 and PS2) are multipass membrane proteins that are predominantly localized to the endoplasmic reticulum. PS undergo endoproteolysis by an unknown enzymatic activity termed Presenilase, and the resulting amino-terminal and carboxy-terminal fragments that remain closely associated, are thought to be the active form of the protein. PS are thought to play numerous roles in the cell, but are best known for their central role as the catalytic core of the intramembranous, γ-secretase aspartyl protease that cleaves numerous membrane proteins, including APP. γ-secretase is a unique membrane protease complex. Presenilin 1,2 are thought to be the catalytic subunit of γ-secretase. PS contain two essential aspartate residues in putatively adjacent transmembrane domains (for review see[4]). Substitution of either of the two aspartate residues buried within the sixth and seventh transmembrane domains of PS abolishes γ-secretase activity. The proteolytic cleavage, which takes place in the middle of the transmembrane region of the substrate, occurs after ectodomain shedding of the target protein and is amino acid sequence independent. Experiments using transition state analogue inhibitors suggest that γ-secretase has separate sites for substrate binding and catalysis. Another unusual characteristic of the γ-secretase cleavage is the multiplicity of the cleavage sites: one in the middle of the transmembrane domain that creates the carboxy-terminus of Aβ, and another one that liberates intracellular domain of the substrate into the cytoplasm, for example NICD (notch site-3 cleavage) or APP ICD (AICD ε-cleavage of APP). While the composition of the γ-secretase complex is still under intense investigation, three additional proteins, nicastrin, aph-1 and pen-2, have been identified so far as cofactors in the γ-secretase multicomponent complex[5]. Co-expression of these components with presenilin appears to be critical for γ-secretase activity. The first cofactor of the γ-secretase complex to be identified was nicastrin (NCT), a type I membrane glycoprotein comprising 709 amino acid residues in humans. Ablation of NCT in *Drosophila* resulted in embryonic lethality, and knockdown of NCT homolog aph-2 in *C. elegans* resulted in hypoplasia of the anterior pharynx. A point mutation in aph-1 gene identified in *C. elegans* caused an abnormality in anterior pharynx development, similar to that seen in aph-2 mutants. Disruption of the GXXXG motif within the fourth transmembrane domain of APH-1 caused by the mutation

leads to failure in assembly and activation of the γ-secretase complex. Two homologues of aph-1 genes were identified in human aph-1a and aph-1b, both encoding membrane proteins predicted to span the membrane seven times. The identification of presenilin enhancer genes pen-1 and pen-2 revealed that pen-1 is identical to aph-1, while pen-2 encodes a membrane protein that spans the membrane twice. Experiments using RNAi established that suppression of the *Drosophila* homologues of nicastrin, APH-1 or PEN-2 result in the loss of Psn fragments and of γ-secretase activity, as indicated by lack of Aβ production. Based on systematic examination of downregulation of the different components of the γ-secretase using combinations of RNAi, it is thought that APH-1 and NCT team up to stabilize PS holoprotein, while PEN-2 induces PS endoproteolysis, eliciting maturation of the active form of the γ-secretase complex. Reconstitution of γ-secretase activity in yeast by over-coexpression of human PS1, NCT, APH-1a and PEN-2 in yeast, components which otherwise are not endogenously expressed in yeast, strongly suggests that these four cofactors are sufficient to the generation of γ-secretase activity. In contrast to other known proteases, γ-secretase is composed of a high molecular weight multicomponent complex. However, the stoichiometry of the γ-secretase is still under an intensive investigation. It is yet to be determined what other components are associated with the γ-secretase. γ-secretase regulates the second step in a two-step proteolytic cleavage event of membrane proteins known as regulated intramembrane proteolysis (RIP). This process starts with an ectodomain shedding resulting in the proteolytic processing of membrane proteins to their soluble counterparts. Ectodomain shedding is carried out by members of the ADAM family and matrix metalloproteases, and to a lesser extent by BACE1 and BACE2 (see below). Following shedding, the resulting membrane-bound CTF undergoes a second cleavage event within its transmembrane domain, called intramembrane proteolysis that is catalyzed by the γ-secretase complex.

β-Secretase

A decade ago, the enzymatic activity termed β-secretase that cleaves APP at the N' of the Aβ region was identified as the aspartyl protease β-site APP cleaving enzyme I (BACE1; also known as memapsin and Asp2) (for review see[6]). A 501 amino acid type I membrane protein, BACE1 resides on the cell surface and in intracellular compartments of the secretory pathway, with its active site within the lumen of these compartments. BACE1 is predominantly expressed in neural tissues with the highest activity level exhibited in neurons. Genetic ablation of BACE1 provided an explicit evidence that BACE1 is the principal neuronal protease required for cleavage of APP at the +1 and +11 site of Aβ and the main β-secretase in the brain. BACE1 cleaves APP in its extracellular domain at a site close to the membrane surface, the Asp+1 residue, generating a secreted APP ectodomain, soluble APPβ (sAPPβ), and a membrane-bound APP C-terminal fragment of 99 amino acid residues (C99). This highly sequence-specific cleavage is a prerequisite for Aβ formation and is followed by endoproteolysis within the transmembrane domain of C99 by γ-secretase, yielding Aβ. BACE1 also cleaves the APP homologues, amyloid precursor-like proteins, APLP1 and APLP2. BACE1 exhibits classical characteristics of an aspartyl protease with two active site motifs. Mutating either aspartic acid inactivates the protease. A signal sequence (residues 1–21) and a pro-peptide domain (residues 22–45) are in its N-terminus, and are removed post-translationally. Near its C-terminus (residues 455–480) there is a single transmembrane domain and a palmitoylated cytoplasmic tail. Possible regulators of BACE1 may include several stress-induced transcription factors that bind to its promoter, such as Sp1, GATA-1, AP1, AP2, CREB, oestrogen and glucocorticoid receptors, NFκB, STAT1, HIF-1 and HSF-1. Other potential regulators are several cytokines, such as IL-1, and Aβ itself (for review see[6]). BACE1 cleavage of APP is the first critical step for Aβ production. Therefore, alterations in BACE1 activity manifests in changes in levels of Aβ production. Indeed, FAD-linked Swedish mutation in APP causes enhanced BACE1 activity, leading to increased Aβ production and amyloid deposition. In that regard, age-dependent increase in BACE1 activity occurs in the brains of mammals, and correlates with levels of Aβ. Likewise, an increase in BACE1 activity is detected in AD and correlates with amyloid deposition and Aβ_{1-x} and Aβ_{1-42} production. Apparently a mild increase in BACE1 expression results in a significant elevation in Aβ levels until a plateau is reached. In turn, increased levels or ratio of Aβ_{1-42} may trigger an upregulation in BACE1 activity. As BACE1 is primarily enriched in neurons, it is expected that amyloid plaque-induced elevated BACE1 level is manifested primarily in neurons. An additional contribution of increased BACE1 activity is expected from activated glia, especially at the stage of disease in which inflammation in the brain is upregulated. Intriguingly, reduced BACE1 activity ameliorates amyloidosis and memory impairments in FAD mice. Thus, cross-breeding BACE1 KO mice with FAD-linked mice exhibiting high levels of Aβ and amyloid deposition abolished any traces of Aβ formation or aggregation and learning and memory impairments. Nevertheless, it should be noted that BACE1 knockout mice exhibit some abnormalities in cognitive and emotional functions, such as spatial and reference memories and impairments in temporal associative memory, suggesting that BACE1 is required for some aspects of hippocampal memory, and that a complete inhibition of the enzyme may have unfavourable cognitive side effects. Recent studies show that APP is modulated by the interaction of BACE1 with the neurite growth inhibitor NOGO, a member of the reticulon protein family and a component of myelin, which may imply that BACE1 plays a role in myelination. In support of that, high BACE1 expression levels are observed in early postnatal stages when myelination takes place. Like APP, BACE1 cycles between compartments of the secretory pathway and BACE1 activity resides in both the endosomes and secretory pathway. The immature precursor of BACE1 is synthesized in the endoplasmic reticulum (proBACE1). Through the addition of complex carbohydrates and the removal of the propeptide domain, ProBACE1 rapidly matures into a 70 kDa form, which undergoes extensive post-translational modifications. The majority of BACE1 is produced as an integral membrane protein, while a minor portion of BACE1 undergoes ectodomain shedding. Inhibition of shedding does not influence processing of APP at the β-site. However, co-expression of APP and the soluble ectodomain of BACE1 in cells increase the generation of Aβ, suggesting the enhanced BACE1 ectodomain shedding may enhance amyloidogenic processing of APP. Mature BACE1 localizes largely within cholesterol-rich lipid rafts. BACE1 is capable of forming stable homodimers that exhibit enhanced catalytic activity.

α-Secretase

In its non-amyloidogenic cleavage pathway, APP is cleaved by α-secretase. This cleavage takes place within the Aβ domain at Leu+17, thus preventing Aβ formation. Evidence suggests that BACE2 cleaves APP at a novel θ-site Phe+19 and Phe+20 sites of APP, downstream of the α-secretase cleavage site[7].

α-secretase cleavage produces sAPPα ectodomain, and an APP-CTF, C83, which in turn is cleaved by γ-secretase to form a 3 kDa fragment, p3. While an increase in non-amyloidogenic APP metabolism was shown in some studies to be coupled to a reciprocal decrease in the amyloidogenic processing pathway, as α- and β-secretase compete for the same APP substrate, other studies show that these activities may not necessarily be coupled. The identity of α-secretase is unknown. Four putative enzymes were shown to have α-secretase activity: TACE (TNF-α converting enzyme), ADAM (a disintegrin and metalloprotease domain protein)-9 and ADAM-10, and BACE 2[8,9]. BACE2 is an aspartyl protease and a homologue of BACE1. The amino acid sequences of BACE1 and BACE2 are ~45% identical and 75% homologous. BACE2 is expressed at low levels in most human peripheral tissues, but very low or undetectable levels in the brain. *In vitro*, BACE2 can cleave APP at the β-secretase cleavage site[9]. However, it seems that BACE2 functions mainly as an alternative α-secretase and as an antagonist of BACE1. In support of that, BACE2 is not upregulated as a compensatory mechanism following downregulation of BACE1 and its overexpression reduces Aβ production in neuronal cultures.

Aβ MISFOLDING AND OLIGOMERIZATION, SYNAPTIC FAILURE AND MEMORY LOSS

γ-secretase can cleave APP in multiple sites, leading to the formation of numerous size forms of Aβ. The main form is Aβ_{40}, however, Aβ_{38-43} have been identified as well. While its physiological role is yet to be determined, it is important to note that under normal conditions, Aβ is secreted from neurons throughout life. The most abundant 40 amino acid species (Aβ_{40}) is not thought to be harmful, whereas the less abundant Aβ_{42} variant aggregates faster and is thus linked to disease neuropathology (for a review see[10]). It is not clear how the addition of the two amino acids at the C-terminus of Aβ changes the properties of the peptide in a way that makes it more aggregation-prone. However, it is thought that an increase in the Aβ_{42}/Aβ_{40}, an upregulation of Aβ levels and/or reduced Aβ degradation or clearance lead to neuropathology. Aβ_{42} tends to generate soluble oligomers that can range in size between dimers to dodecamers. These oligomers were found in human brains lacking amyloid deposits or fibrillary tangles, suggesting that accumulation of oligmeric species of Aβ occur early in the disease. Many studies have shown that FAD-linked transgenic mice with amyloid pathology have impairments in learning and memory paradigms including acquisition of long-term spatial memory, spatial reversal learning, utilization of spatial working memory, acquisition of social recognition memory, object recognition memory and contextual fear conditioning (for review see[11]). In some cases, the severity of the impairment has been correlated to Aβ levels in the brains of individual mice and treatments that reduce Aβ levels (e.g. immunization with Aβ or Aβ antibodies) can reverse learning deficits. Most of these tasks are dependent on the hippocampus and deficits in hippocampal synaptic plasticity, i.e. long-term potentiation (LTP) in the transgenic mice are possible causes for the learning impairments (for review see[11]). However, the cues used in these learning paradigms are complex and require processing in multiple brain networks before reaching the hippocampus. This makes it difficult to establish where and how in the brain learning breaks down in the affected animals. Several studies have reported impairments in hippocampal LTP in FAD-linked transgenic mice. However, the role of Aβ deposition and the presence or absence of amyloid plaques remains unclear. Some studies have reported impaired synaptic function or LTP deficits prior to amyloid deposition, some deficits only after amyloid deposition, and some preserved LTP in the face of extensive amyloid deposition. These disparate results no doubt reflect strain-specific differences in transgene expression and other factors. Most studies agree that functional synaptic density, measured electrophysiologically, is reduced in hippocampus of mice with extensive Aβ deposits. This accords with other indicators of synaptic degeneration and the toxic effects of Aβ monomers, oligomers, protofibrils and fibrils on synapses. Compelling evidence for the role of soluble Aβ oligomers in memory loss was provided by studies showing that a single intraperitoneal injection of anti-Aβ antibodies can reverse memory impairments in APP transgenic mice without affecting amyloid deposition, suggesting that the antibodies target soluble Aβ. In support of that, recent evidence suggests that these are the oligomeric forms of Aβ that are cytotoxic, interfering with numerous cellular functions as well as interfering with aspects of learning and memory and synaptic function. Synaptic dysfunction takes place before synaptic loss, which precedes neuronal loss.

MEMORY LOSS, ALTERATIONS AND IMPAIRMENTS IN NEUROGENESIS

Neurogenesis and Alzheimer's Disease: Cross-Talk and Effects

The contribution of impaired neurogenesis to memory disorders and to AD in particular is increasingly acknowledged. In the adult brain there are two discrete areas where neural stem cells are maintained and differentiate into new neurons and glia throughout life: the subventricular zone (SVZ), adjacent to the walls of the lateral ventricle, and the subgranule layer (SGL) of the dentate gyrus. Both neurogenic areas are part of the olfactory-hippocampal and entorhino-hippocampal circuits that are most affected in AD. Neurogenesis in the adult brain plays a role in numerous aspects of learning and memory (for review see[12]). Numerous studies have suggested that the rate of neurogenesis in both SVZ and SGL declines with age, raising the possibility that reduced neurogenesis may account for, at least in part, impaired learning and memory and cognitive deterioration in the elderly (for example see[13]). Examination of neurogenesis in brain tissue of AD patients revealed increased expression of immature neuronal marker proteins. However, these observations have been challenged recently. Other reports suggest that in the aged and AD brain, there is a dramatic decline in both proliferative capacity of progenitor cells and in the pool of NSCs in the SGL, and that this decline may be attributed to loss in growth factors (for review see[14]). Information obtained using animal models of the disease reveals that the vast majority of studies using transgenic mice harbouring FAD-linked mutant PS1 report that neurogenesis is impaired on a steady-state level and upon enriched environment stimulation (for review see[15]). Nevertheless, the interpretation of observations obtained in transgenic mice harbouring FAD-linked APP variants is challenging. This may result in the fact that APP is processed to numerous metabolites, that convey different effects on neurogenesis as described below. It is important to keep in mind that the organization composition and dynamics in the neurogenic niches may change as AD progresses, according to the dynamics of neuropathological cues, such as oligomeric Aβ and amyloid deposition. Another fascinating aspect of the cross-talk between AD and neurogenesis, adding

another level of complexity, is that players that cause FAD regulate neurogenesis, as discussed in the next paragraph.

PS1 Regulates Embryonic and Postnatal Neurogenesis

γ-secretase cleaves other membrane proteins in addition to APP, such as the receptor tyrosine kinases ErbB4, IGF-1R and insulin receptor, as well as of the neurogenic signals Notch1, L1 and E-cadherin (for review see[15]). A large number of these substrates are neurogenic signalling that regulate embryonic and postnatal neurogenesis, suggesting that alterations in PS1/γ-secretase expression, activity or function may directly affect neurogenesis. In support of that PS1 is a homologue of the *C. elegans* sel-12 – a protein that plays a major role in cell-fate decisions. Recent evidence suggests that PS1/γ-secretase acts as a tumour suppressor in epithelia and that epidermal growth factor receptor (EGFR) levels inversely correlate with PS1/γ-secretase activity. Intriguingly, EGFR signalling plays a major role in regulation of neural stem proliferation, migration and survival (for review see[16]). PS1 is further implicated in the Wnt/β-catenin signalling pathway that regulates adult hippocampal neurogenesis. The first indication that PS1 may play a role in neurogenesis has been provided by experiments in mice with genomic deletions of *PSEN1* exhibiting severely abnormal somitogenic and neurogenic processes in the brain. These mice die in late embryogenesis. This has hampered further studies of the role of PS1 in a natural brain setting in postnatal life. Some studies in transgenic mice harbouring FAD-linked PS1 variants reveal that expression of FAD-linked mutant PS1P117L, PS1M146V or conditional ablation of PS1 in the forebrain induce impaired hippocampal neurogenesis. In addition, experience of mice in an enriched environment does not upregulate neurogenesis in transgenic mice harbouring PS1 mutant variants. In contrast, other studies suggest that expression of FAD-linked PS1A246E enhances proliferation of progenitor cells in the adult DG. However, these animals express mutant PS1 ubiquitously, including in fully mature neurons. Further studies using mice expressing mutant PS1 in the neurogenic areas solely will be needed to determine the role of PS1 in postnatal neurogenesis.

TAU HYPERPHOSPHORYLATION, AXONAL TRANSPORT, KINASE AND PHOSPHATASE ACTIVITY

Another inevitable cause of synaptic degeneration is impaired communication synapse-cell body, which may result in dysfunctional axonal transport. APP is axonally transported by anterograde fast axonal transport (FAT) in both peripheral and central nerves (for review see[17]). Interference with the tightly regulated and complex trafficking of APP might have detrimental effects on its processing and consequently on neuronal homeostasis. A large body of evidence supports the notion that axonal transport is impaired in neurons harbouring FAD-linked mutant PS1 (for review see[18]). Thus, for example, budding of endoplasmic reticulum- and *trans*-Golgi network (TGN)-derived APP-containing vesicles is increased in PS1-deficient cells, or cells expressing a dominant negative PS1 D385A variant. In addition, increased steady-state levels of APP were observed on the surface of cells lacking PS1 or expressing PS1 D385A, while vesicle biogenesis and the extent of cell-surface APP is reduced in membrane preparations from cells expressing FAD-linked PS1 variants. Other recent studies show that the PS1-interacting protein phospholipase D1 plays a role in PS1-regulated APP trafficking in neuronal cultures. Significantly, FAT of both

APP and Trk receptors is markedly impaired in the sciatic nerves of transgenic mice expressing FAD-linked PS1 mutants, accompanied by a reduction in both steady-state levels and accumulation of kinesin-1 in nerves of mice expressing mutant PS1 relative to nerves of mice expressing human wild-type PS1[19]. These findings are consistent with and extend previous observations that expression of FAD-linked PS1 mutants in embryonic cultured neurons leads to increased glycogen synthase kinase 3 (GSK-3) activity and reductions in kinesin-1-based transport of selected membrane proteins[18]. Taken together, the evidence suggests that expression of FAD-linked PS1 variants leads to deficient supply of both neurotrophin receptors and presynaptic membrane components at nerve terminals, resulting in compromised neuronal function. This evidence further implies that misregulation of phosphatase and kinase activity might underlie impaired axonal transport. In that regard, misregulation of phosphatase and kinase activity may underlie hyperphosphorylation of tau. Tau is a multifunctional microtubule-associated protein that plays major roles in the assembly of microtubules, the stabilization of microtubules against dynamic instability, axonal transport and in polymer interaction with other cytoskeletal filaments. The equilibrium between phosphorylations and dephosphorylations of tau modulates the stability of the cytoskeleton and consequently axonal morphology and transport. Recent studies provide interesting information concerning the course of tau pathology in relation to amyloid pathology in the 3XTg-AD mice and shed new light on the pathological effects of tau hyperphosphorylation and aggregation (for review see[20]). Function-associated phosphorylation sites of tau are reportedly on serine and threonine, suggesting the role of serine and threonine kinases and phosphatases in AD. For example, the epitope at Ser-396/Ser-404 of tau, thought to be preferentially phosphorylated by GSK3, is hyperphosphorylated in AD. There are more than 10 serine/threonine protein kinases that have been shown to phosphorylate tau *in vitro*. According to the motif-specificity, these kinases can be divided into two major groups, i.e. the proline-directed protein kinases (PDPKs) and nonproline- directed protein kinases (NPDPKs). Among these kinases, GSK-3β is among the most implicated in the abnormal hyperphosphorylation of tau in AD brains. Glycogen synthase kinase 3 (GSK3) is a component of the WNT signalling pathway, which plays a major role in adult neurogenesis, microtubule dynamics and fast axonal transport[21]. GSK3 is inactivated by phosphorylation at serine 9 (Ser9) in its N'-terminus. Among GSK3's numerous substrates are PS1, β-catenin, tau and kinesin-I light chains (KLC) (for review see[22]). Previous studies suggest that FAD-linked PS1 mutations affect GSK3 kinase activity in transfected cell lines. Significantly, phosphorylation of KLC by GSK3 promotes the release of kinesin-I from membrane-bound organelles, leading to a reduction in fast anterograde axonal transport[21]. A separate study showed an interplay between cyclin-dependent kinase 5 (Cdk5), previously shown to be central for tau phosphorylation and GSK3β in mice overexpressing p25. While Cdk5 activity increases APP processing, GSK3β activity induces tau phosphorylation. Interestingly, inhibition of Cdk5 activates GSK3β activity. Cdk5 is activated by factors like p35 and p39, and is involved in tau phosphorylations in neurogenesis. Cdk5 activation is concomitant with degeneration of hippocampal neurons and tau hyperphosphorylation, while its inhibition is neuroprotective, suggesting that misregulation of Cdk5 activity plays a role in the formation of neurofibrillary tangles. Recent intriguing studies shed light on a possible role for casein kinase 2 (CK2) activation in the pathogenesis of the disease. Future studies will determine the sequence of events in these signalling pathways in the course of the disease.

PERTURBED CALCIUM HOMEOSTASIS AND INTRACELLULAR CALCIUM SIGNALING

As a primary resident of the ER, it may not be surprising that dysfunctional PS affect ER calcium dynamics on multiple levels, imposing mostly 'gain of function' effects on these processes (for review, see[23,24]). This effect on intracellular calcium homeostasis may also be associated with altered glutamate uptake, leading to neurotoxicity. Expression of FAD-linked mutant PS results in increased ER calcium release in fully mature neurons (for review see[23]). Mutant PS enhance IP$_3$-mediated calcium release from the ER stores, as well as perturb calcium entry through store-operated channels. In addition, it appears that ryanodine receptor (RyR) function is predominantly upregulated. IP$_3$R alterations or direct effects of mutant PS on endoplasmic reticulum store levels may play a role in the observed calcium dysregulation as well. Nevertheless, it should be noted that mutant PS have also shown a reduction in ER calcium load and ER release with SERCA inhibition. Thus it is not clear whether all mutations have the same effect on ER calcium regulation. Overexpression of mutant PS increases IP$_3$ channel activity in suboptimal and saturated IP$_3$ levels by prolonging the channel open time, while wild-type PS mildly affect IP$_3$ channel activity. PS physically interact with IP$_3$ receptors and thus modulate them directly. IP$_3$ receptors modulate gating activity and affect overall calcium dynamics. Indeed, fibroblasts derived from mutant PSKI1 mice exhibit increased sensitivity to IP$_3$ receptor agonists. A recent report suggests that mutant PS reduces endogenous calcium leak from the ER, which may result in an increased ER calcium load and overfilled ER stores. Presenilin knockout cells exhibit perturbed ER calcium stores. Overexpression of PS accelerates the sequestration of cytosolic calcium, an effect that can be blocked by pharmacological inhibition of SERCA, suggesting that PS modulate SERCA function. In support of that, PS1KO/PS2KO cells exhibit a phenotype similar to SERCA KO, suggesting that PS may interact and modulate calcium influx into the endoplasmic reticulum via SERCA, and calcium extrusion from the endoplasmic reticulum via interactions with the ryanodine and IP3 receptors as well as through endogenous leak channels. While a link to Aβ regulation is provided by studies suggesting that knocking out IP$_3$ receptor or SERCA results in a dramatic reduction in Aβ production further studies will be required in order to determine the intracellular sequence of events that lead to calcium imbalance and subsequently neuronal death.

OXIDATIVE STRESS

Oxidative stress refers to circumstances in which oxidant production surpasses the endogenous antioxidant capabilities of the cell, leading to damage of the tissue. Such conditions occur either following increased production of cellular oxidants and/or decreased concentrations of cell antioxidants including glutathione, vitamin E, ascorbate, the glutathione peroxidase system, superoxide dismutase (SOD) and catalase. Overproduction of reactive oxygen and nitrogen species such as superoxide, hydrogen peroxide, nitric oxide and peroxynitrite occurs in AD and is considered to mediate cell damage and subsequently death (for review see[25]). Studies suggest that Aβ induces the formation of high concentrations of oxygen and nitrogen-reactive species and a depletion of endogenous antioxidants. In brain tissue from AD patients, there are increased levels of markers of oxidative stress including oxidized proteins, membrane lipids, DNA and nitrotyrosine immunoreactivity. Additionally, antioxidants including vitamin E, idebenone, uric acid and glutathione are effective in preventing Aβ neurotoxicity *in vitro*. Aβ induces the generation of reactive oxygen species, including the generation of hydrogen peroxide, peroxyl radical and superoxide that in turn may initiate a series of secondary reactions. As oxidative stress might have an accumulative effect that is environment and ageing linked, it may contribute to the initiation and development of neuropathology in sporadic AD.

GENETIC LINKS AND RISK FACTORS UNDERLYING LATE-ONSET SPORADIC AD

Ageing is the greatest risk factor for sporadic Alzheimer's disease, and the vast majority of AD cases are the sporadic late-onset form. The cause of late-onset AD is unknown. Several genetic loci have been identified that predispose individuals to late-onset AD (for review see[26]) and it has been suggested that some of the encoded polypeptides might play roles in modulating the clearance and/or degradation of Aβ peptides. For example, studies that have implicated the low-density lipoprotein receptor-related protein (LRP) in regulating the efflux of Aβ from the brain to plasma have received support from the identification of DNA variants in LRP, apolipoprotein E (ApoE) and α-2-macroglobulin (α2M) in late-onset AD. LRP was recently identified as a substrate of BACE1. Polymorphisms in the apolipoprotein E (apoE) gene show the most significant effects on relative genetic risk of sporadic AD. The ε4 isoform (Cyc112-Arg) of apoE is associated with increased risk of developing AD, while ε2 (Arg158-Cys) is associated with protection from the disease compared to the normal ε3 allele (for review see[27]). ApoE binds to members of the low-density lipoprotein receptor family (LDLR) (for review see[28]). These receptors are known to function in cholesterol and lipid transport and as signal transducers. Numerous reports established that LDLR linked cellular signalling pathways modulate AD pathology. Reelin and its homologue F-spondin are recognized by the very-low density lipoprotein receptor (VLDLR) and apolipoprotein E receptor-2 (apoE-R2), two members of the LDLR family. Interestingly, mice lacking reelin, double-knockouts lacking VLDLR and ApoER2 and mice lacking disabled-1 (Dab1) exhibit tau hyperphosphorylation. Based on that it was suggested that the reelin-ApoE receptor complex initiates a signalling cascade that regulates phosphorylation of tau by GSK3. F-spondin and reelin are thought to regulate APP processing through their interaction with APP and ApoER-2. ApoER-2 has also been shown to be neuroprotective during ageing, and F-spondin was reported to protect against Aβ toxicity. Other LDLR family members including LRP1, LRP1B and LR11/sorLA have also been shown to modulate APP processing. Furthermore, DNA variants have been identified in a gene on chromosome 10, encoding insulin degrading enzyme (IDE), a $\sim$110 kDa thiol zinc-metalloendopeptidase shown earlier to degrade several peptides, including insulin, glucagon, atrial naturetic peptide and TGFα. Interestingly, IDE-deficient mice exhibit increased levels of Aβ in the brain, and transgenic overexpression of IDE results in reduced Aβ burdens in brains of transgenic mice that develop Aβ deposits. Finally, numerous studies during the last 10 years have reported the beneficial effect of the experimental model 'enriched environment' on AD neuropathology, including reductions in Aβ levels and deposition and learning and memory (for review see[11]), suggesting that genetic environmental factors play in concert to induce or prevent sporadic AD.

REFERENCES

1. Selkoe DJ. Alzheimer's disease: genes, proteins, and therapy. *Physiol Rev* 2001; **81**(2): 741–66.
2. Thinakaran G, Koo EH. Amyloid precursor protein trafficking, processing, and function. *J Biol Chem* 2008; **283**(44): 29615–19.
3. Miller CC, McLoughlin DM, Lau KF, Tennant ME, Rogelj B. The X11 proteins, Abeta production and Alzheimer's disease. *Trends Neurosci* 2006; **29**(5): 280–5.
4. Selkoe DJ, Wolfe MS. Presenilin: running with scissors in the membrane. *Cell* 2007; **131**(2): 215–21.
5. De Strooper B. Aph-1, Pen-2, and nicastrin with presenilin generate an active gamma-secretase complex. *Neuron* 2003; **38**(1): 9–12.
6. Cole SL, Vassar R. BACE1 structure and function in health and Alzheimer's disease. *Curr Alzheimer Res* 2008; **5**(2): 100–20.
7. Sun X, He G, Song W. BACE2, as a novel APP theta-secretase, is not responsible for the pathogenesis of Alzheimer's disease in Down syndrome. *Faseb J* 2006; **20**(9): 1369–76.
8. Reiss K, Saftig P. The 'A Disintegrin And Metalloprotease' (ADAM) family of sheddases: physiological and cellular functions. *Sem Cell Development Biol* 2009; **20**(2): 126–37.
9. Farzan M, Schnitzler CE, Vasilieva N, Leung D, Choe H. BACE2, a beta-secretase homolog, cleaves at the beta site and within the amyloid-beta region of the amyloid-beta precursor protein. *Proc Natl Acad Sci USA* 2000; **97**(17): 9712–17.
10. Haass C, Selkoe DJ. Soluble protein oligomers in neurodegeneration: lessons from the Alzheimer's amyloid beta-peptide. *Nat Rev Mol Cell Biol* 2007; **8**(2): 101–12.
11. Lazarov O, Larson J. Environmental enrichment: from mouse AD model to AD therapy. In Sun M (ed.), *Research Progress in Alzheimer's Disease and Dementia*, Vol. 3. Nova Science, 2007, 303–28.
12. Zhao C, Deng W, Gage FH. Mechanisms and functional implications of adult neurogenesis. *Cell* 2008; **132**(4): 645–60.
13. Kempermann G, Gast D, Gage FH. Neuroplasticity in old age: sustained fivefold induction of hippocampal neurogenesis by long-term environmental enrichment. *Ann Neurol* 2002; **52**(2): 135–43.
14. Brinton RD, Wang JM. Therapeutic potential of neurogenesis for prevention and recovery from Alzheimer's disease: allopregnanolone as a proof of concept neurogenic agent. *Curr Alzheimer Res* 2006; **3**(3): 185–90.
15. Lazarov O, Marr RA. Neurogenesis and Alzheimer's disease: at the crossroads. *Exp Neurol* 2009; ahead of print.
16. Ayuso-Sacido A, Graham C, Greenfield JP, Boockvar JA. The duality of epidermal growth factor receptor (EGFR) signaling and neural stem cell phenotype: cell enhancer or cell transformer? *Curr Stem Cell Res Ther* 2006; **1**(3): 387–94.
17. Sheetz MP, Pfister KK, Bulinski JC, Cotman CW. Mechanisms of trafficking in axons and dendrites: implications for development and neurodegeneration. *Prog Neurobiol* 1998; **55**(6): 577–94.
18. Morfini G, Pigino G, Beffert U, Busciglio J, Brady ST. Fast axonal transport misregulation and Alzheimer's disease. *Neuromolecular Med* 2002; **2**(2): 89–99.
19. Lazarov O, Morfini GA, Pigino G, Gadadhar A, Chen X, Robinson J *et al.* Impairments in fast axonal transport and motor neuron deficits in transgenic mice expressing familial Alzheimer's

disease-linked mutant presenilin 1. *J Neurosci* 2007; **27**(26): 7011–20.

20. Binder LI, Guillozet-Bongaarts AL, Garcia-Sierra F, Berry RW. Tau, tangles, and Alzheimer's disease. *Biochim Biophys Acta* 2005; **1739**(2–3): 216–23.

21. Morfini G, Szebenyi G, Elluru R, Ratner N, Brady ST. Glycogen synthase kinase 3 phosphorylates kinesin light chains and negatively regulates kinesin-based motility. *Embo J* 2002; **21**(3): 281–93.

22. Frame S, Cohen P. GSK3 takes centre stage more than 20 years after its discovery. *Biochem J* 2001; **359**(Pt 1): 1–16.

23. Green KN, LaFerla FM. Linking calcium to Abeta and Alzheimer's disease. *Neuron* 2008; **59**(2): 190–4.

24. Mattson MP. Calcium and neurodegeneration. *Aging Cell* 2007; **6**(3): 337–50.

25. Mattson MP. Oxidative stress, perturbed calcium homeostasis, and immune dysfunction in Alzheimer's disease. *J Neurovirol* 2002; **8**(6): 539–50.

26. Tanzi RE, Bertram L. Twenty years of the Alzheimer's disease amyloid hypothesis: a genetic perspective. *Cell* 2005; **120**(4): 545–55.

27. Bu G. Apolipoprotein E and its receptors in Alzheimer's disease: pathways, pathogenesis and therapy. *Nat Rev Mol Cell Biol* 2009; **10**(5): 333–44.

28. Herz J. The LDL receptor gene family: (un)expected signal transducers in the brain. *Neuron* 2001; **29**(3): 571–81.

50

Neurochemistry of Alzheimer's Disease

Paul T. Francis

King's College London, Wolfson Centre for Age-Related Diseases, UK

INTRODUCTION

Alzheimer's disease (AD) is characterized by gross and progressive impairments of cognitive function, which are often accompanied by behavioural disturbances such as aggression, depression, psychosis, apathy and wandering. Cell and synapse loss together with neuronal dysfunction affecting a number of neuronal systems are considered to result in the development of these typical symptoms of the disorder. In particular, non-cognitive behavioural symptoms are also considered to relate to structural and functional alterations in neurotransmission. Carers find behavioural disturbances difficult to cope with and the presence of such behaviours in AD patients often leads to the need for institutionalization[1]. The challenge has been to identify changes in specific neurotransmitter systems that underlie cognitive impairment and particular behavioural problems and to develop rational therapeutic strategies.

NEUROCHEMICAL CHANGES IN ALZHEIMER'S DISEASE

The majority of biochemical studies of AD have relied on information derived from postmortem brain, which typically represents the late stage of the disease (8–10 years after onset of symptoms). In these studies there is considerable evidence of gross brain atrophy, histopathological features and multiple neurotransmitter abnormalities affecting many brain regions. However, investigations of biopsy tissue taken from AD patients 3–5 years (on average) after the onset of symptoms indicate that a selective neurotransmitter pathology occurs early in the course of the disease[2].

Acetylcholine

Changes affecting many aspects of the cholinergic system in patients with AD have been reported since the initial discovery of deficits in choline acetyltransferase activity in postmortem brains[3–5]. In biopsy samples from AD patients, presynaptic markers of the cholinergic system were also uniformly reduced[2]. Thus, choline acetyltransferase activity, choline uptake and acetylcholine synthesis are all reduced to 30–60% of control values. The clinical correlate of this cholinergic deficit in AD was, until recently, considered to be cognitive dysfunction. Such a conclusion was supported by clinicopathological studies in AD and parallel experiments in non-human primates or rodents, which demonstrated disruptive effects of basal forebrain cholinergic lesions on cognitive functions. Furthermore, cholinergic deficits in AD occur to the greatest extent in cortical areas primarily concerned with memory and cognition – the hippocampus, adjacent temporal lobe regions and select frontal areas. Such studies led to the 'cholinergic hypothesis of geriatric memory dysfunction'[6].

Neuropathologically, loss of neurons from the nucleus of Meynert (nbM; Ch4 cholinergic nucleus) is well documented in AD, although the extent of the loss reported varies from moderate to severe, and it has been suggested that in AD cholinergic dysfunction exceeds degeneration[7]. Detailed analysis of subpopulations of cholinergic perikarya in the nbM have been reported by Mesulam and Geula[8], who identified selective cell loss in Ch4p (the posterior section projecting to temporal cortex). In the intermediate sector, Ch4id, which includes projections to the frontal cortex, neuron loss is not as extensive, consistent with the moderate loss of cholinergic enzyme activity.

On the basis of the above evidence, neocortical cholinergic innervation appears to be lost at an early stage of the disease and this is supported by a study in which the cholinergic deficit (reduced ChAT activity) has been related to Braak staging[9]. Braak stages I and II are considered to represent the earliest presentation of AD, with neurofibrillary tangles in the entorhinal cortex, and a 20–30% loss of ChAT activity was reported in brains from patients at these stages of AD[10]. However, another study using the Clinical Dementia Rating Scale (CDR) suggests that the greatest reduction in markers of the cholinergic system occurs between moderate (CDR 2.0) and severe (CDR 5.0) disease, with little change between non-demented and the mild stage (CDR 0–2)[11]. Finally, tau and tangle pathology occurs in cholinergic neurons of the nbM during normal ageing and to a greater extent in patients with mild cognitive impairment (MCI), indicating functional changes in cholinergic neurotransmission[12].

There has been a recent shift of emphasis regarding the clinical significance of cholinergic deficits. Non-cognitive or neuropsychiatric, in addition to cognitive, symptoms also appear to have a cholinergic component[13]. For example, visual hallucinations relate to neocortical cholinergic deficits[14], such deficits (e.g. loss of ChAT) being greater in dementia of Lewy bodies (DLB), where hallucinations are common, than in AD, where they are less common[15]. Reductions in cortical ChAT activity in patients with dementia, in addition to correlating with cognitive decline, are also related to overactivity and aggressive behaviour[16].

Principles and Practice of Geriatric Psychiatry, 3rd edn. Edited by Mohammed T. Abou-Saleh, Cornelius Katona and Anand Kumar
© 2011 John Wiley & Sons, Ltd

Glutamate

Approximately 70% of cortical neurons use glutamate as a neurotransmitter and hence the glutamatergic system plays an important role in all regions of the cortex and hippocampus. Evidence for a pivotal role of glutamate in learning and memory is long-established[2]; indeed, it is likely that any function of a particular cortical region will depend on glutamate neurotransmission at some level. Loss of synapses and pyramidal cell perikarya (both considered to be markers of glutamatergic neurons) from the neocortex of AD patients correlate with measures of cognitive decline[2]. From a biochemical perspective studying the glutamatergic system is more difficult since the amino acid is present at high concentrations in all cells. However, certain proteins related to glutamatergic neurotransmission provide vital clues to the status of this system in AD. For example, reduced glial glutamate uptake is reported in AD[17], probably reflecting oxidative damage to the transporters[18,19]. Additionally, there is loss of the vesicular glutamate transporter (VGluT) in several cortical regions[20,21]. Such changes are likely to generate an elevated baseline level of glutamate at the synapse, triggering inappropriate Ca^{2+} influx. These raised background levels of glutamate impair the usual detection of physiological signals (low signal-to-noise ratio), disrupting normal cognitive processes[22]. Furthermore, the disruption of vesicular glutamate transport results in less glutamate being stored in presynaptic vesicles, reducing the level of signal upon neurotransmitter release[20].

In addition, soluble oligomers of beta amyloid ($A\beta$) can reduce glutamatergic transmission by inducing the internalization of NMDA receptors[23]. This pathological effect has been shown to disrupt NMDA-induced receptor currents, inhibiting long-term potentiation (LTP – synaptic plasticity) and signalling to downstream targets such as Akt (also known as protein kinase B)[23–25].

Other Neurotransmitters

Using biopsy samples from AD patients, serotonergic and some noradrenergic markers are affected, whereas markers for dopamine, γ-aminobutyric acid (GABA) or somatostatin are not altered. When postmortem studies of AD brain are considered, many neurotransmitter systems, including GABA and somatostatin, are involved or are affected to a greater extent[2]. Based on postmortem studies, however, changes in serotonergic neurotransmission may be linked to the behavioural disturbances of AD, such as depression, rather than cognitive dysfunction. For example, patients with AD who were also depressed had lower numbers of serotonin re-uptake sites in the neocortex than did patients without this symptom[26]. Furthermore, both reduced serotonergic[27,28] and increased noradrenergic activities and sensitivity[29,30] have been linked to aggressive behaviour.

Neurotransmitter Receptors

Many neurotransmitter receptors appear to be unaltered in AD; however, studies have demonstrated a reduction in the number of nicotinic and muscarinic (M2) ACh receptors, most of which are considered to be located on presynaptic cholinergic terminals. Despite continuing, often unconfirmed, reports of changes in one or more of the muscarinic receptor subtypes (M–M5), it is generally agreed, on the basis of autopsy studies, that the M1 subtype is unchanged until later in the disease, when it may decline, probably in relation to cholinoceptive (postsynaptic) neurodegeneration. The status of the

other subtypes is not clearly established, primarily due to the lack of specific pharmacological labels. Results using antibodies against the different receptor subtypes, while specific, are complicated by discrepancies between the distribution and density of immunoreactive proteins and localized functional receptors. With respect to muscarinic receptor coupling to G-proteins, most studies using a variety of investigative procedures have identified some degree of uncoupling, especially to the M1 receptor[31,32] that correlated with cognitive decline.

A highly consistent receptor abnormality in AD is the loss of the nicotinic receptor[33,34], which appears to primarily reflect loss of the α4-containing subtype (generally associated with β2) as opposed to α3 or α7 subtypes[35]. Immunohistochemically, loss of α4 and β2 reactive fibres has been observed in temporal cortex, associated with reactive neuropil threads, tangles and plaques[36].

The density of 5-HT$_{2A}$ receptors was reduced in AD patients compared to age-matched controls and this reduction also correlated with the rate of decline of Mini-Mental State Examination (MMSE) scores, suggesting that loss of neocortical 5-HT$_{2A}$ receptors may predict for faster cognitive decline[37]. By contrast, density of 5HT$_{1A}$ receptors in frontal cortex was negatively correlated with cognitive decline[38], consistent with an inhibitory action of these receptors on cortical pyramidal function[2]. It is interesting to note that in temporal cortex loss of 5-HT$_{1A}$ receptors was associated with aggressive behaviour[39].

NEUROCHEMICAL BASIS FOR APPROACHES TO TREATMENT

Biochemical studies of postmortem brains from AD patients showing evidence of a substantial presynaptic cholinergic deficit, which correlated with cognitive impairment[40], together with the emerging role of ACh in learning and memory[6], clearly suggested a rational approach to treatment. However, more recent studies have identified a role for the cholinergic system in attentional processing rather than simply memory.

A prediction of the cholinergic hypothesis is that drugs that potentiate central cholinergic function should improve cognition in AD patients. There are a number of approaches to the treatment of the cholinergic deficit; however, the use of acetylcholinesterase inhibitors is the most well developed approach to the treatment of AD to date[41].

During the late 1980s and early 1990s, the first cholinomimetic compound, tacrine, underwent large-scale clinical studies and established clearly the benefits of cholinesterase inhibition treatment in patients with a diagnosis of probable AD. Tacrine was subsequently approved for use in some, but not all, countries. Statistically significant, dose-related improvements on objective performance-based tests of cognition, clinician- and caregiver-rated global evaluations of patient well-being and also quality of life measures have been reported[42]. Unfortunately, potentially serious adverse side effects have limited the use of this compound.

A so-called second generation of cholinesterase inhibitors has been developed, including donepezil, rivastigmine and galantamine[41]. Such compounds demonstrate a clinical effect and magnitude of benefit of at least that reported for tacrine, but with a more favourable clinical profile[43]. Furthermore, evidence is emerging from clinical trials of cholinomimetics that such drugs may improve the abnormal non-cognitive, behavioural symptoms of AD[44]. The cholinesterase inhibitors physostigmine, tacrine, rivastigmine and metrifonate have variously been reported in placebo-controlled trials to decrease psychoses (hallucinations and delusions), agitation, apathy, anxiety, disinhibition, pacing and aberrant motor behaviour, and lack of cooperation in AD. The most recent studies indicate that cholinesterases inhibitors have the greatest effect on apathy and mood in AD, rather than agitation and aggressive behaviour[45,46].

Targeting the acknowledged glutamatergic deficit in AD has been more problematical since direct agonists would be expected to be toxic and there is no analogous enzyme (cf. cholinesterase) to inhibit. Indirect approaches such as AMPAKines, positive modulators of the AMPA glutamate receptor, have undergone clinical trials with mixed results[47,48]. The only licensed treatment targeting this system is the NMDA glutamate receptor antagonist memantine. In clinical trials this drug has been shown to improve cognition and activities of daily living[49,50] and some troublesome behaviours, in particular agitation and aggressive behaviour[51]. It is proposed that the cognitive benefits of this drug flow from improving 'signal-to-noise ratio' at NMDA receptors[52] while the improvement in behaviour may be because of inhibition of the hyperphosphorylation of tau[53].

CONCLUSIONS

In AD many different pathological manifestations, such as cortical and subcortical β amyloidosis (plaques), abnormal tau (tangles and dystrophic neurites), neuronal and synapse loss and various transmitter deficits, provide an increasingly complex framework for clinical–neuropathological correlations. Based upon detailed knowledge of the neurochemical changes that occur in AD, two main symptomatic treatments have emerged, cholinesterase inhibitors and memantine. These drugs provide some benefit to patients and in particular the improvements in behaviour are important to carers. Such therapy is all that is available at present and may well still be required as new therapies designed to slow disease progression come into the clinic.

REFERENCES

1. Esiri MM. The basis for behavioural disturbances in dementia. *J Neurol Neurosurg Psychiatry* 1996; **61**: 127–30.
2. Francis PT, Sims NR, Procter AW, Bowen DM. Cortical pyramidal neurone loss may cause glutamatergic hypoactivity and cognitive impairment in Alzheimer's disease: investigative and therapeutic perspectives. *J Neurochem* 1993; **60**: 1589–604.
3. Bowen DM, Smith CB, White P, Davison AN. Neurotransmitter-related enzymes and indices of hypoxia in senile dementia and other abiotrophies. *Brain* 1976; **99**: 459–96.
4. Davies P, Maloney AJF. Selective loss of central cholinergic neurones in Alzheimer's disease. *Lancet* 1976; **ii**: 1403.
5. Perry EK, Gibson PH, Blessed G, Perry RH, Tomlinson BE. Neurotransmitter abnormalities in senile dementia. *J Neurol Sci* 1977; **34**: 247–65.
6. Bartus RT, Dean RL, Beer B, Lippa AS. The cholinergic hypothesis of geriatric memory dysfunction. *Science* 1982; **217**: 408–17.
7. Perry RH, Candy JM, Perry EK *et al.* Extensive loss of choline acetyltransferase activity is not reflected by neuronal loss in the nucleus of Meynert in Alzheimer's disease. *Neurosci Lett* 1982; **33**: 311–15.
8. Mesulam MM, Geula G. Nucleus basalis (Ch4) and cortical cholinergic innervation in the human-brain – observations based on the distribution of acetylcholinesterase and choline-acetyltransferase. *J Comp Neurol* 1988; **275**: 216–40.

9. Braak H, Braak E. Neuropathological stageing of Alzheimer-related changes. *Acta Neuropatholol* 1991; **82**: 239–59.
10. Beach TG, Kuo YM, Spiegel K *et al.* The cholinergic deficit coincides with A beta deposition at the earliest histopathologic stages of Alzheimer disease. *J Neuropathol Exp Neurol* 2000; **59**: 308–13.
11. Davis KL, Mohs RC, Marin D *et al.* Cholinergic markers in elderly patients with early signs of Alzheimer disease. *J Am Med Assoc* 1999; **281**: 1401–6.
12. Mesulam M, Shaw P, Mash D, Weintraub S. Cholinergic nucleus basalis tauopathy emerges early in the aging–MCI–AD continuum. *Ann Neurol* 2004; **55**(6): 815–28.
13. Cummings JL, Kaufer DI. Neuropsychiatric aspects of Alzheimer's disease: the cholinergic hypothesis revisited. *Neurology* 1996; **47**: 876–83.
14. Perry EK, Marshall E, Thompson P *et al.* Monoaminergic activities in Lewy-body-dementia – relation to hallucinosis and extrapyramidal features. *J Neural Transm* 1993; **6**: 167–77.
15. Perry EK, Haroutunian V, Davis KL *et al.* Neocortical cholinergic activities differentiate Lewy body dementia from classical Alzheimer's disease. *Neuroreport* 1994; **5**: 747–9.
16. Minger SL, Esiri MM, McDonald B *et al.* Cholinergic deficits contribute to behavioural disturbance in patients with dementia. *Neurology* 2000; **55**: 1460–7.
17. Procter AW, Francis PT, Holmes C *et al.* APP isoforms show correlations with neurones but not with glia in brains of demented subjects. *Acta Neuropathol* 1994; **88**: 545–52.
18. Lovell MA, Ehmann WD, Mattson MP, Markesbery WR. Elevated 4-hydroxynonenal in ventricular fluid in Alzheimer's disease. *Neurobiol Aging* 1997; **18**: 457–61.
19. Ferrarese C, Begni B, Canevari C *et al.* Glutamate uptake is decreased in platelets from Alzheimer's disease patients. *Ann Neurol* 2000; **47**(5): 641–3.
20. Kirvell SL, Esiri MM, Francis PT. Down regulation of vesicular glutamate transporters precede cell loss and pathology in Alzheimer's disease. *J Neurochem* 2006; **98**: 939–50.
21. Kashani A, Lepicard E, Poirel O *et al.* Loss of VGLUT1 and VGLUT2 in the prefrontal cortex is correlated with cognitive decline in Alzheimer disease. *Neurobiol Aging* 2008; **29**(11): 1619–30.
22. Parsons CG, Danysz W, Quack G. Memantine is a clinically well tolerated N-methyl-D-aspartate (NMDA) receptor antagonist – a review of preclinical data. *Neuropharmacology* 1999; **38**(6): 735–67.
23. Snyder EM, Nong Y, Almeida CG *et al.* Regulation of NMDA receptor trafficking by amyloid-beta. *Nat Neurosci* 2005; **8**(8): 1051–8.
24. Klyubin I, Walsh DM, Cullen WK *et al.* Soluble Arctic amyloid beta protein inhibits hippocampal long-term potentiation in vivo. *Eur J Neurosci* 2004; **19**(10): 2839–46.
25. Abbott JJ, Howlett DR, Francis PT, Williams RJ. Aβ1-42 modulation of Akt phosphorylation via a7 nAChR and NMDA receptors. *Neurobiol Aging* 2008; **29**: 992–1001.
26. Chen CPL-H, Alder JT, Bowen DM *et al.* Presynaptic serotonergic markers in community-acquired cases of Alzheimer's disease: correlation with depression and neuroleptic medication. *J Neurochem* 1996; **66**: 1592–8.
27. Coccaro EF. Central serotonin and impulsive aggression. *Br J Psychiatry* 1989; **155**(suppl 8): 52–62.

28. Procter AW, Francis PT, Stratmann GC, Bowen DM. Serotonergic pathology is not widespread in Alzheimer patients without prominent aggressive symptoms. *Neurochem Res* 1992; **17**: 917–22.

29. Peskind ER, Wingerson D, Murray S *et al.* Effects of Alzheimer's disease and normal aging on cerebrospinal-fluid norepinephrine responses to yohimbine and clonidine. *Arch Gen Psychiatry* 1995; **52**: 774–82.

30. Raskind MA. Evaluation and management of aggressive behavior in the elderly demented patient. *J Clin Psychiatry* 1999; **60**: 45–9.

31. Jope RS, Song L, Li X, Powers R. Impaired phosphoinositide hydrolysis in Alzheimer's disease brain. *Neurobiol Aging* 1994; **15**: 221–6.

32. Tsang SW, Lai MK, Kirvell S *et al.* Impaired coupling of muscarinic M(1) receptors to G-proteins in the neocortex is associated with severity of dementia in Alzheimer's disease. *Neurobiol Aging* 2006; **27**: 1216–23.

33. Aubert I, Araujo DM, Cecyre D *et al.* Comparative alterations of nicotinic and muscarinic binding-sites in Alzheimer's and Parkinson's diseases. *J Neurochem* 1992; **58**: 529–41.

34. Perry EK, Morris CM, Court JA *et al.* Alteration in nicotine binding sites in Parkinson's disease, Lewy body dementia and Alzheimer's: possible index of early neuropathology. *Neuroscience* 1995; **64**: 385–95.

35. Martin-Ruiz CM, Court JA, Molnar E *et al.* Alpha 4 but not alpha 3 and alpha 7 nicotinic acetylcholine receptor subunits are lost from the temporal cortex in Alzheimer's disease. *J Neurochem* 1999; **73**: 1635–40.

36. Sparks DL, Beach TG, Lukas RJ. Immunohistochemical localization of nicotinic β2 and α4 receptor subunits in normal human brain and individuals with Lewy body and Alzheimer's disease: preliminary observations. *Neurosci Lett* 1998; **256**: 151–4.

37. Lai MK, Tsang SW, Alder JT *et al.* Loss of serotonin 5-HT2A receptors in the postmortem temporal cortex correlates with rate of cognitive decline in Alzheimer's disease. *Psychopharmacology* 2005; **179**: 673–7.

38. Lai MK, Tsang SW, Francis PT *et al.* Postmortem serotoninergic correlates of cognitive decline in Alzheimer's disease. *Neuroreport* 2002; **13**(9): 1175–8.

39. Lai MK, Tsang SW, Francis PT *et al.* Reduced serotonin 5-HT1A receptor binding in the temporal cortex correlates with aggressive behavior in Alzheimer disease. *Brain Res* 2003; **974**(1–2): 82–7.

40. Francis PT, Palmer AM, Sims NR *et al.* Neurochemical studies of early-onset Alzheimer's disease. Possible influence on treatment. *N Engl J Med* 1985; **313**: 7–11.

41. Francis PT, Palmer AM, Snape M, Wilcock GK. The cholinergic hypothesis of Alzheimer's disease: a review of progress. *J Neurol Neurosurg Psychiatry* 1999; **66**: 137–47.

42. Davis KL, Thal LJ, Gamzu ER *et al.* A doule-blind, placebo-controlled multicenter study of tacrine for Alzheimer's disease. *N Engl J Med* 1992; **327**: 1253–9.

43. Evans JG, Wilcock G, Birks J. Evidence-based pharmacotherapy of Alzheimer's disease. *Int J Neuropsychopharmacol* 2004; **7**(3): 351–69.

44. Wynn ZJ, Cummings JL. Cholinesterase inhibitor therapies and neuropsychiatric manifestations of Alzheimer's disease. *Dement Geriatr Cogn Disord* 2004; **17**(1–2): 100–108.

45. Gauthier S, Feldman H, Hecker J *et al.* Efficacy of donepezil on behavioral symptoms in patients with moderate to severe Alzheimer's disease. *Int Psychogeriatr* 2002; **14**(4): 389–404.

46. Howard RJ, Juszczak E, Ballard CG *et al.* Donepezil for the treatment of agitation in Alzheimer's disease. *N Engl J Med* 2007; **357**(14): 1382–92.

47. Chappell AS, Gonzales C, Williams J *et al.* AMPA potentiator treatment of cognitive deficits in Alzheimer disease. *Neurology* 2007; **68**(13): 1008–12.

48. Black MD. Therapeutic potential of positive AMPA modulators and their relationship to AMPA receptor subunits. A review of preclinical data. *Psychopharmacology (Berl)* 2005; **179**(1): 154–63.

49. Reisberg B, Doody R, Stoffler A. Memantine in moderate-to-severe Alzheimer's disease. *N Engl J Med* 2003; **348**(14): 1333–41.

50. McShane R, Areosa SA, Minakaran N. Memantine for dementia. *Cochrane Database Syst Rev* 2006; (2): CD003154.

51. Gauthier S, Wirth Y, Mobius HJ. Effects of memantine on behavioural symptoms in Alzheimer's disease patients: an analysis of the Neuropsychiatric Inventory (NPI) data of two randomised, controlled studies. *Int J Geriatr Psychiatry* 2005; **20**(5): 459–64.

52. Parsons CG, Stoffler A, Danysz W. Memantine: a NMDA receptor antagonist that improves memory by restoration of homeostasis in the glutamatergic system – too little activation is bad, too much is even worse. *Neuropharmacology* 2007; **53**(6): 699–723.

53. Francis PT. Altered glutamate neurotransmission and behaviour in dementia: evidence from studies of memantine. *Curr Mol Pharmacol* 2009; **2**: 77–82.

51

Antemortem Markers

Susan J. van Rensburg[1], Felix C.V. Potocnik[2], Maritha J. Kotze[2] and Dan J. Stein[3]

[1]Division of Chemical Pathology, National Health Laboratory Service, Cape Town, South Africa
[2]Faculty of Health Sciences, Stellenbosch University, Cape Town, South Africa
[3]Department of Psychiatry and Mental Health, University of Cape Town, South Africa

INTRODUCTION

It has become increasingly clear that the disease process of Alzheimer's disease (AD) is multifaceted. Because AD appears to be a complex disorder involving several genes interacting with environmental influences, it is difficult to single out any one factor as the root cause of the disease. Apart from the familial forms of the disease, in which the gene mutations have been elucidated, many post-translational factors are involved in the process of neurodegeneration, in the formation of plaques and tangles and in the development of an inflammatory state of the brain. Although some of these have been found to be altered in AD patients compared with controls, very few markers suitable for antemortem diagnostic purposes have emerged, since many of the alterations are not specific for AD, while others pertain only to subsets of AD[1].

While it has been argued that the most powerful antemortem marker in AD is a clinical diagnosis based on an adequate range of observations[2], such diagnosis is at present largely one of exclusion. An ideal biological marker would allow for greater specificity and sensitivity than a clinical diagnosis on its own, and be readily obtainable. While neuropathological biopsy diagnosis of AD allows high specificity and sensitivity, it is typically only available postmortem.

The neurobiological alterations present in AD may be reflected in changes in cerebrospinal fluid (CSF) neurotransmitters or neurochemicals, or changes in systemic tissues including blood constituents. It should be borne in mind, however, that CSF measurements are influenced by a variety of factors, including CSF gradients, age, gender, diurnal and seasonal variations, state of the blood–brain barrier, blood contamination, contributions from the spinal cord, phase of illness, psychomotor activity, stress and diet. Measurement of blood constituents may also reflect concentration differences due to diurnal rhythms and other factors.

In this chapter on antemortem markers, we will briefly review neurotransmitters, neurochemistry and systemic pathology. We will also briefly address findings in brain imaging, and genomic and proteomic methods.

NEUROTRANSMITTERS AND NEUROCHEMISTRY

The Cholinergic System

Cholinesterase inhibitors (ChEIs) were introduced for the treatment of AD following the discovery that cholinergic neurons were depleted, and that cholinergic function was significantly decreased in the basal forebrain of AD patients[3]. Interestingly, the latter research group recently reported that ChEIs increased the phosphorylation of tau protein[4], resulting in a possible decrease in long-term clinical responsiveness to ChEIs. The depletion of membrane choline may also play a role[5]. CSF markers of cholinergic function, as well as erythrocyte and plasma choline, have been studied as biomarkers for AD, but have not yielded consistent results[6]. Studies, however, indicate differences in the dynamics of RBC choline uptake, consistent with a vulnerability of cholinergic neurons in patients with AD[7].

The Noradrenergic System

Autopsy studies of AD brains demonstrate that loss of cells in the locus coeruleus (LC), the major nucleus of origin of noradrenergic fibres, may undergo even greater degeneration than the nucleus basalis of Meynert[8]. This raises the question whether the degeneration of the noradrenergic system would provide markers for AD. Reduced noradrenaline (norepinephrine; NE) in autopsy samples of AD brains has been a fairly consistent finding, although it may be hypothesized that increased activity and turnover of the noradrenergic system may compensate for cell loss and that a limited number of NE cells remain highly active in AD patients. Loss of NE innervation would in addition lead to peripheral effects, such as decreased control of vasoconstriction[8]. Some patients with advanced AD have biochemical and physiological indices of noradrenergic hyperactivity, including higher heart rate and blood pressure. Severe neuronal loss in advanced AD may lead to a compensatory increase in LC firing rate, contributing to symptoms such as pacing, agitation, insomnia and weight loss. Haglund et al.[8] developed a scale for the evaluation of LC degeneration in patients with AD, vascular dementia and non-focal ischaemic deep white matter disease (WMD), as part of the ongoing Lund Longitudinal Dementia study. They found that LC degeneration was significantly higher in AD than in vascular dementia cases, and that there was a significant correlation with white matter pathology severity. However, there was no correlation between the degree of LC degeneration and duration of dementia or AD pathology[8].

The Serotonergic System

Numerous autopsy studies of AD brains have suggested a serotonergic deficit. Although there have been reports that the major serotonin metabolite, 5-hydroxyindoleacetic acid (5-HIAA), is unchanged in the CSF of AD patients, most studies indicate a reduction in CSF 5-HIAA. In a study by Stuerenburg et al., CSF 5-HIAA correlated with CSF Aβ42, but not with CSF tau. There was also a significant positive correlation between CSF 5-HIAA and homovanillic acid (HVA) in AD, but neither 5-HIAA nor HVA could differentiate between mild cognitive impairment (MCI), depression and AD[9].

Although CSF measures of monoamines have not proven sufficiently specific and sensitive for clinical diagnosis, the degree of pineal calcification (DOC) can be used as an intra-individual melatonin deficit marker[10]. Melatonin, the pineal hormone biosynthesized from serotonin, declines with age and more so in AD patients due to calcification of the pineal gland. Mahlberg et al.[10] measured the DOC, as well as the size of uncalcified tissue, with computed tomography (CT) in 279 consecutive memory clinic outpatients. The DOC was significantly higher in AD than in patients with other types of dementia, depression or controls, while the size of uncalcified pineal tissue in AD patients was significantly smaller than in patients of the other three groups[10].

Wu and Swaab found that pineal melatonin secretion and pineal clock gene oscillation were disrupted in AD patients, as well as in non-demented controls with early signs of AD neuropathology (neuropathological Braak stages I–II), in contrast to non-demented controls without AD neuropathology[11]. Furthermore, a functional disruption of the suprachiasmatic nucleus (SCN) was observed from the earliest AD stages onwards, as shown by decreased vasopressin mRNA, a clock-controlled major output of the SCN.

Taken together, measures of neurotransmitter systems have not provided sufficient sensitivity and specificity to be used for diagnostic purposes in the clinic. Nevertheless, such work has been useful in investigating the pathophysiology of AD.

SYSTEMIC PATHOLOGY

It is possible to view AD as a systemic illness. Thus, if AD were a genetic disorder, then disturbances at the molecular level may be expressed in non-neural tissue, with systemic effects. Using blood cells for biomarkers has the added advantage of being relatively non-invasive, and techniques such as flow cytometry provide a convenient platform for such analyses. Uberti et al. found that the expression of a conformational mutant of p53 in mononuclear cells was significantly higher in AD patients compared to non-AD subjects. The expression of mutant p53 did not, however, correlate with the duration of illness or disease severity[12].

Zainaghi et al. found that an alteration of amyloid precursor protein (APP) fragments in platelets, as measured by Western blot analysis, correlated with cognitive decline in patients with AD[13]. Platelets contain more than 95% of circulating APP and enzymatically produce both soluble APP and amyloid-beta peptides. It was found that the ratio of 130- to 110-kDa APP fragments in platelets from patients with AD was significantly lower compared to patients with mild cognitive impairment and elderly controls. There was no difference between the latter two groups. The alteration in APP also correlated with membrane fluidity of the platelets[13].

Membrane fluidity of platelets as a biomarker for AD has been extensively studied. Increased fluidity was demonstrated in patients with AD compared to patients with vascular dementia and elderly controls. Only about 50% of AD patients, however, demonstrate this abnormality. Increased platelet membrane fluidity (PMF) appears to be a familial trait, and the subgroup of AD patients in whom it manifests suffers from an earlier onset and a more rapidly progressive decline. In a prospective longitudinal study evaluating PMF as a putative risk factor for AD, 9 of 330 people with increased PMF (initially asymptomatic first-degree relatives of probands with AD) developed AD after 7.5 years[14]. On a biochemical level, it was found that free radical induced lipid peroxidation increased the fluidity of platelet membranes, providing a possible mechanism underlying increased PMF[15]. This putative marker of AD would hence also be subject to modulation by environmental factors such as a diet rich in antioxidants.

In fibroblasts, abnormalities in enzymatic activity, glucose metabolism, abnormal calcium metabolism, impaired DNA repair as well as potassium channel dysfunction[16] have been observed. While studies on blood cells and fibroblasts have advanced our understanding of the mechanisms relevant to AD, they are not sufficiently sensitive or specific for clinical use, once more raising the question of environmental influences.

Protein Abnormalities

The hallmark lesions of Alzheimer's disease are neurofibrillary tangles, which contain tau protein, and the plaques with deposition of β-amyloid (Aβ). Given that the clinical phase of AD may be preceded by a 15–30 year period of deposition of amyloid and tau protein, markers to predict the development of AD should ultimately be obtainable. Several studies have found increased levels of tau protein (total tau as well as phosphorylated tau) and decreased levels of Aβ(1–42) in CSF[17], while the ratio of these two measures has been found to be a highly sensitive discriminator of AD from normal ageing. Maddalena et al. found that the ratio of CSF phospho-tau to Aβ42 was significantly increased in patients with AD and provided high diagnostic accuracy in distinguishing patients with AD from healthy control subjects (sensitivity, 86%; specificity, 97%), subjects with non-AD dementias (sensitivity, 80%; specificity, 73%), and subjects with other neurological disorders (sensitivity, 80%; specificity, 89%)[18].

Inflammation

Neuropathological findings in AD brains demonstrate an inflammatory response, including activated microglia. Several studies have measured concentrations of inflammatory markers such as C-reactive protein (CRP) and cytokines in the blood and CSF of AD patients. In the Framingham study, peripheral blood mononuclear cell (PBMC) cytokine production was related to the risk of incident AD. It was concluded that higher spontaneous production of IL-1 or TNF-alpha by PBMCs may be a marker for the future risk of AD in older individuals. These data strengthen the evidence for a pathophysiological role of inflammation in the development of clinical AD[19]. Although these markers are too non-specific for AD diagnosis, drugs aimed at diminishing inflammation and the activity of microglia are currently still being investigated.

A range of other research areas in AD can conveniently be mentioned in this section. These include studies of visual system dysfunctions, olfactory deficits, extrapyramidal dysfunction, atypical dermatoglyphic patterns, altered sweat response, abnormal glucose tolerance and vitamin B12 deficiency. Such work, although interesting, has not yet led to a sensitive and specific antemortem marker.

Environmental Factors in Alzheimer's Disease

Although AD has been linked to a genetic aetiology, studies with monozygotic twins revealed variability in age at onset of as much as 9, 15 or 20 years[20]. This led to the suspicion that some environmental factor(s) ingested from food and water, or a deficiency of some protective element, or increased oxidation status resulting from stress[21] may accelerate disease expression in susceptible individuals. Several metals have been investigated in AD in the hope of finding a marker for the disease. Iron metabolism is altered and levels of the iron transport protein transferrin are decreased in the serum of AD patients. Previous reports of elevated levels of the iron binding protein p97 (melanotransferrin) in AD patients were not confirmed in a later study[22]. Blood mercury levels are significantly raised in AD patients[23] and zinc and copper are decreased in AD compared to controls. Decreased activity of the copper-containing protein ceruloplasmin may be linked to iron deposition in the brains of patients with AD[24]. Although CSF diagnostic markers $A\beta42$, tau and phospho-tau correlate with lower plasma copper and ceruloplasmin levels in AD patients, supplementation with copper has not improved cognition in AD[25], whereas in our experience supplementing AD patients with zinc improves cognition, especially if augmented by vitamins A and D[26].

Wu *et al.* investigated the effect of infantile exposure to lead on markers of AD-like pathology in monkeys, and found that epigenetic imprinting in early life influenced the expression of AD-related genes with the effect that a causative environmental marker could be undetectable by the time of disease expression[27]. Indeed, to date environmental markers have insufficient sensitivity and specificity to serve as useful in the diagnosis of AD.

BRAIN IMAGING

There has been considerable interest in the use of brain imaging in the diagnosis of AD and follow-up during drug trials. Initial promising neuroimaging candidate markers obtained from CT scans and MRI have been confirmed and extended with new techniques, such as measuring hippocampal and entorhinal cortex volumes, basal forebrain nuclei, cortical thickness, deformation-based and voxel-based morphometry, as well as the use of diffusion tensor imaging tractography and functional MRI[28].

There are ongoing attempts to validate MR and PET imaging and other biomarkers for use in clinical trials to distinguish between elderly controls, subjects with mild cognitive impairment, and subjects with AD[29]. C-11 Pittsburgh compound B (PIB) PET (amyloid imaging) represents a particularly promising avenue of exploration, potentially providing a direct window on the pathological processes that underlie AD. A combination of PET, MRI and mutation analysis

of APOEε4 has been found to be effective in determining grey matter volume and quantification of $A\beta$ plaque load for patient inclusion and follow-up in anti-amyloid therapy trials[30]. High-resolution PET also allows *in vivo* visualization of changes in amyloid after administration of Pittsburg Compound-B, and microglial activation after administration of [18F]fluoroethyl-DAA1106[31].

GENOMICS AND PROTEOMICS

Advances in genomic and proteomic methods raise the question of whether these may provide clinically useful antemortem markers. The greatest potential impact arguably lies in the detection of early stages of the disease, monitoring of AD progression, and assessment of response to existing and future active and preventative treatments.

Genomics has to date not been helpful in providing accurate diagnostic markers for AD. Structural genomic studies indicated that more than 200 genes may be involved in the pathogenesis of AD. Mutations in the *APP, PSEN1* and *PSEN2* genes directly associated with the amyloid cascade account for AD in much less than 5% of affected patients. The most consistent susceptibility factor for late-onset AD[32], the ε4 allele of the *APOE* gene, underlies dementia in 40% of Caucasian patients with late onset disease; however, the APOEε4 allele does not (yet) influence dementia progression in sub-Saharan Africans[33]. Could this indicate that effects of the environment on individuals may change their susceptibility to AD and the expression of genes involved with AD predisposition, causing divergent results when putative markers are compared in different populations? Notably, alcohol consumption increases the risk of dementia specifically in those individuals carrying the APOEε4 allele[34].

Another genetic marker, a genetic variant of transferrin, TfC2, has an increased allele frequency in AD in some populations[35,36], but not in others, such as a French population of the Bordeaux region[37]. TfC2 is associated with diseases attributed to free radical damage, therefore it could be hypothesized that increased dietary intake of antioxidants in certain populations would be protective against the effects of the oxidative allele. The predominantly Mediterranean diet and red wine, which is consumed in the Bordeaux region of France, is known to be antioxidative. Robson *et al.* found that carriers of TfC2 and the C282Y allele of the haemochromatosis gene were at a five times greater risk of AD, while co-inheritance of APOEε4 conferred an even higher risk of AD in cases from the OPTIMA cohort in the UK[38]. In the Bordeaux study, in contrast, such an effect was not observed.

While genomics may not at present provide a reliable diagnostic marker for AD, it is estimated that genetic variation accounts for between 20% and 95% of the variability in therapeutic response in AD patients. The pharmacogenetic response in AD depends on the interaction of genes involved in disease pathogenesis (such as APOEε4) and genes involved in drug metabolism (such as the cytochrome P450 [CYP] system). The CYP2D6 enzyme isoforms affect the metabolism of more than 20% of drugs used to treat CNS disorders, and gene variation may cause drug side effects. Of the four genotype-related metabolizer types defined by CYP2D6, the extensive and intermediate metabolizers are the best responders, while the ultra-rapid and poor metabolizers are the worst responders to pharmacologic treatments in AD.

Genetic markers not suitable for diagnostic purposes may therefore still be useful in providing knowledge of the disease process, for disease prognosis and to guide treatment, e.g. to detect responders to treatment with ChEIs by testing for the *APOE* genotype. The incorporation of pharmacogenetic protocols into AD research and clinical practice potentially helps to optimize therapeutics by developing cost-effective pharmaceuticals and improving drug efficacy and safety.

Gene expression profiling with microarrays has also yielded some useful evaluations of pathomechanisms and systemic manifestations in AD, using blood mononuclear cell (BMC) transcriptomes of sporadic AD subjects and aged-matched controls. The AD BMCs exhibited a significant decline in the expression of genes concerned with cytoskeletal maintenance, cellular trafficking, cellular stress response, redox homeostasis, transcription and DNA repair, as well as those genes which may impact on Aβ production and the processing of tau. The microarray results also revealed gender differences in the levels of altered gene expression[39].

Proteomic research has not fared better than genomics when it comes to providing markers for the diagnosis of AD. Several markers that were initially promising (such as complement factor H precursor and alpha-2-macroglobulin) did not provide the specificity and sensitivity required for biomarkers[40]. In a European task force consensus document, it was also stated that no marker had been validated to reliably measure a change in response to therapy, not even the rate of change in hippocampal volume[41]. It was recommended that future trials should include assessment of biomarkers in order to advance our knowledge about their usefulness. Proteomics is an attractive technique for prospecting protein biomarkers, since it involves plasma proteins and peptides that are readily obtained.

Ravid has commented that although plasma could be a useful source of markers, it is also one of the most complex media to work with[17]. Dealing with sample-to-sample variations, variations among individuals, and separating 'noise' from a true signal require the processing of thousands of samples. Moreover, only 13% of peptides reproducibly change significantly with the changes in the patient's disease state. Some new technologies that are being used to deal with the complexities of the plasma proteome include a combination of mass spectrometry, affinity chromatography and liquid chromatography to produce unbiased identification and quantification of signature peptides. This author has confirmed that the gap between discovery and diagnostics is still wide. Some of the outstanding issues include finding ways to reduce the costs associated with the validation of biomarkers or proteomic platforms, demonstration of biomarkers' clinical significance, minimizing technical complexity, gaining regulatory approvals, and reaching pharmaceutical levels of reproducibility and sensitivity. He also emphasized the need for collaboration between different disciplines.

Zellner *et al.*, on a more optimistic note, have predicted that the constraints on proteomics will be overcome by developing more advanced technologies, including the design of AD-related protein panels, on which established markers such as tau and Aβ42 will be used in combination with novel markers. Laser capture microdissection and fluorescence saturation labelling will overcome the limitations of homogeneous sample collection[42].

CONCLUSION

It is clear that a number of difficulties face the researcher interested in finding an antemortem marker for AD. Many of the techniques used in this search have important limitations: for example, CSF measurements are influenced by a variety of factors; brain imaging findings often show group differences only; and genetic and proteomic studies reveal multiple small effects. Diagnosis of AD, even at autopsy, may not always be definitive, leading to heterogeneity of patient samples. In addition, AD may be a heterogeneous disorder, certainly with different manifestations in the older age group. A marker may be present in a control with the AD trait who has not yet developed AD; and if a marker is related to the severity of AD, it may not distinguish between mild cases and controls. Other dementias may overlap with AD not only in phenomenology but also in pathogenesis, and therefore display similar markers. There are also mixed cases, where patients, for example, have both AD and vascular dementia. In addition, biomarkers are currently only of value when they form part of the clinical diagnostic work-up of the patient, emphasizing the expertise of the clinician and collaboration between disciplines.

Nevertheless, the work discussed here does suggest that some combination of measures may ultimately correlate strongly with biopsy diagnosis. Measures from molecular and genetic biology and brain imaging seem particularly promising and are consistent with our growing knowledge of neurochemistry and neuropathology. Genomic and proteomic advances have the potential to ultimately translate into clinically meaningful biomarkers and to result in advances in patient care.

ACKNOWLEDGEMENTS

The authors are supported by the National Health Laboratory Service, the Universities of Stellenbosch and Cape Town and the Medical Research Council of South Africa.

REFERENCES

1. Zubenko GS. Biological correlates of clinical heterogeneity in primary dementia. *Neuropsychopharmacology* 1992; **6**: 77–93.
2. Roth M. Antemortem markers of Alzheimer's disease: a commentary. *Neurobiol Aging* 1986; **7**: 402–5.
3. Perry EK, Tomlinson BE, Blessed G *et al.* Correlation of cholinergic abnormalities with senile plaques and mental test scores in senile dementia. *Br Med J* 1978; **2**: 1457–9.
4. Chalmers KA, Wilcock GK, Vinters HV *et al.* Cholinesterase inhibitors may increase phosphorylated tau in Alzheimer's disease. *J Neurol* 2009; **256**(5): 717–20.
5. Wurtman RJ. Choline metabolism as a basis for the selective vulnerability of cholinergic neurons. *Trends Neurosci* 1992; **15**(4): 117–22.
6. Marksteiner J, Pirchl M, Ullrich C *et al.* Analysis of cerebrospinal fluid of Alzheimer patients. Biomarkers and toxic properties. *Pharmacology* 2008; **82**(3): 214–20.
7. Kanof PD, Breenwald BS, Mohs RC, Davis KL. Red cell choline II: Kinetics in Alzheimer's disease. *Biol Psychiatry* 1985; **20**(4): 375–83.
8. Haglund M, Sjöbeck M, Englund E. Locus ceruleus degeneration is ubiquitous in Alzheimer's disease: possible implications for diagnosis and treatment. *Neuropathology* 2006; **26**(6): 528–32.
9. Stuerenburg HJ, Ganzer S, Müller-Thomsen T. 5-Hydroxyindoleacetic acid and homovanillic acid concentrations in cerebrospinal fluid in patients with Alzheimer's disease, depression and mild cognitive impairment. *Neuro Endocrinol Lett* 2004; **25**(6): 435–7.
10. Mahlberg R, Walther S, Kalus P *et al.* Pineal calcification in Alzheimer's disease: an in vivo study using computed tomography. *Neurobiol Aging* 2008; **29**(2): 203–9.

11. Wu YH, Swaab DF. Disturbance and strategies for reactivation of the circadian rhythm system in aging and Alzheimer's disease. *Sleep Med* 2007; **8**(6): 623–36.

12. Uberti D, Lanni C, Racchi M, Govoni S, Memo M. Conformationally altered p53: a putative peripheral marker for Alzheimer's disease. *Neurodegener Dis* 2008; **5**(3–4): 209–11.

13. Zainaghi IA, Forlenza OV, Gattaz WF. Abnormal APP processing in platelets of patients with Alzheimer's disease: correlations with membrane fluidity and cognitive decline. *Psychopharmacology (Berl)* 2007; **192**(4): 547–53.

14. Zubenko GS, Winwood E, Jacobs B *et al*. Prospective study of risk factors for Alzheimer's disease: results at 7.5 years. *Am J Psychiatry* 1999; **156**(1): 50–7.

15. Van Rensburg SJ, Daniels WMU, Van Zyl J *et al*. Lipid peroxidation and platelet membrane fluidity – implications for Alzheimer's disease? *Neuroreport* 1994; **5**(17): 2221–4.

16. Etcheberrigaray R, Ito E, Oka K *et al*. Potassium channel dysfunction in fibroblasts identifies patients with Alzheimer's disease. *Proc Natl Acad Sci U S A* 1993; **90**(17): 8209–13.

17. Ravid R. Biobanks for biomarkers in neurological disorders: the Da Vinci bridge for optimal clinico-pathological connection. *J Neurol Sci* 2009; **283**(1): 119–26.

18. Maddalena A, Papassotiropoulos A, Müller-Tillmanns B *et al*. Biochemical diagnosis of Alzheimer disease by measuring the cerebrospinal fluid ratio of phosphorylated tau protein to beta-amyloid peptide42. *Arch Neurol* 2003; **60**(9): 1202–6.

19. Tan ZS, Beiser AS, Vasan RS *et al*. Inflammatory markers and the risk of Alzheimer disease: the Framingham Study. *Neurology* 2007; **68**(22): 1902–8.

20. Breitner JCS, Murphy EA, Folstein MF, Magruder-Habib K. Twin studies of Alzheimer's disease: an approach to etiology and prevention. *Neurobiol Aging* 1990; **11**(6): 641–8.

21. Van Rensburg SJ, Van Zyl JM, Potocnik FCV *et al*. The effect of stress on the antioxidative potential of serum: implications for Alzheimer's disease. *Metab Brain Dis* 2006; **21**(2–3): 171–9.

22. Desrosiers RR, Bertrand Y, Nguyen QT *et al*. Expression of melanotransferrin isoforms in human serum: relevance to Alzheimer's disease. *Biochem J* 2003; **374**(2): 463–71.

23. Hock C, Drasch G, Golombowski S *et al*. Increased blood mercury levels in patients with Alzheimer's disease. *J Neural Transm* 1998, **105**(1). 59–60.

24. Castellani RJ, Smith MA, Nunomura A, Harris PL, Perry G. Is increased redox-active iron in Alzheimer disease a failure of the copper-binding protein ceruloplasmin? *Free Radic Biol Med* 1999; **26**(11–12): 1508–12.

25. Kessler H, Bayer TA, Bach D *et al*. Intake of copper has no effect on cognition in patients with mild Alzheimer's disease: a pilot phase 2 clinical trial. *J Neural Transm* 2008; **115**(8): 1181–7.

26. Potocnik FC, Van Rensburg SJ, Hon D *et al*. Oral zinc augmentation with vitamins A and D increases plasma zinc concentration: implications for burden of disease. *Metab Brain Dis* 2006; **21**(2–3): 139–47.

27. Wu J, Basha MR, Brock B *et al*. Alzheimer's disease (AD)-like pathology in aged monkeys after infantile exposure to environmental metal lead (Pb): evidence for a developmental origin and environmental link for AD. *J Neurosci* 2008; **28**(1): 3–9.

28. Hampel H, Bürger K, Teipel SJ *et al*. Core candidate neurochemical and imaging biomarkers of Alzheimer's disease. *Alzheimers Dement* 2008; **4**(1): 38–48.

29. Weiner MW, Aisen PS, Jack CR Jr *et al*. The Alzheimer's disease neuroimaging initiative: progress report and future plans. *Alzheimers Dement* 2010; **6**(3): 202–11.e7.

30. Drzezga A, Grimmer T, Henriksen G *et al*. Effect of *APOE* genotype on amyloid plaque load and gray matter volume in Alzheimer disease. *Neurology*. 2009; **72**(17): 1487–94.

31. Higuchi M. Visualization of brain amyloid and microglial activation in mouse models of Alzheimer's disease. *Curr Alzheimer Res* 2009; **6**(2): 137–43.

32. Li H, Wetten S, Li L *et al*. Candidate single-nucleotide polymorphisms from a genomewide association study of Alzheimer disease. *Arch Neurol* 2008; **65**: 45–53.

33. Kalaria RN, Maestre GE, Arizaga R *et al*. World Federation of Neurology Dementia Research Group. Alzheimer's disease and vascular dementia in developing countries: prevalence, management, and risk factors. *Lancet Neurol* 2008; **7**(9): 812–26.

34. Anttila T, Helkala EL, Viitanen M. Alcohol drinking in middle age and subsequent risk of mild cognitive impairment and dementia in old age: a prospective population based study. *Br Med J* 2004; **329**(7465): 539.

35. Van Rensburg SJ, Carstens ME, Potocnik FCV, Aucamp AK, Taljaard JJF. Increased frequency of the transferrin C2 subtype in Alzheimer's disease. *Neuroreport* 1993; **4**(11): 1269–71.

36. Zambenedetti P, de Bellis G, Biunno I, Musicco M, Zatta P. Transferrin C2 variant does confer a risk for Alzheimer's disease in Caucasians. *J Alzheimers Dis* 2003; **5**(6): 423–7.

37. Rondeau V, Iron A, Letenneur L *et al*. Analysis of the effect of aluminum in drinking water and transferrin C2 allele on Alzheimer's disease. *Eur J Neurol* 2006; **13**(9): 1022–5.

38. Robson KJ, Lehmann DJ, Wimhurst VL *et al*. Synergy between the C2 allele of transferrin and the C282Y allele of the haemochromatosis gene (*HFE*) as risk factors for developing Alzheimer's disease. *J Med Genet* 2004; **41**(4): 261–5.

39. Maes OC, Xu S, Yu B *et al*. Transcriptional profiling of Alzheimer blood mononuclear cells by microarray. *Neurobiol Aging* 2007; **28**(12): 1795–809.

40. Hye A, Lynham S, Thambisetty M *et al*. Proteome-based plasma biomarkers for Alzheimer's disease. *Brain* 2006; **129**(11): 3042–50.

41. Vellas B, Andrieu S, Sampaio C, Coley N, Wilcock G; European Task Force Group. Endpoints for trials in Alzheimer's disease: a European task force consensus. *Lancet Neurol* 2008; **7**(5): 436–50.

42. Zellner M, Veitinger M, Umlauf E. The role of proteomics in dementia and Alzheimer's disease. *Acta Neuropathol* 2009; **118**(1): 181–95.

52

Pharmacological Therapies in Alzheimer's Disease

Martin Steinberg and Constantine G. Lyketsos

Johns Hopkins Bayview Medical Center, Baltimore, MD, USA

INTRODUCTION

Alzheimer's disease (AD) is a progressive neurodegenerative disorder that causes deterioration in cognition and functioning and is associated with a high frequency of neuropsychiatric co-morbidity. The emotional and financial costs of AD for patients and their caregivers are enormous. To date, no treatment is available to cure the disease or halt its progression, nor is any disease-modifying. Available symptomatic therapies, which include cholinesterase inhibitors and memantine, attenuate cognitive and functional decline and may also improve neuropsychiatric symptoms. This chapter will review the rationales for these therapies, summarize research pertaining to their cognitive, functional and neurobehavioural efficacy, and discuss current prescription and monitoring guidelines. Available evidence concerning the use of unapproved therapies such as vitamin supplementation and *Ginkgo biloba* will also be discussed.

RATIONALE FOR CHOLINERGIC THERAPIES

The deteriorations in cognition and function that occur in AD have been linked to the degeneration of numerous neuronal systems. Evidence is especially strong, however, for an association between these symptoms and the loss of cholinergic neurons. Therefore, increasing available levels of brain acetylcholine may be expected to attenuate decline in AD. Three approaches to increasing cholinergic transmission have been subject to research: increasing availability of the chemical precursors of acetylcholine (e.g. lecithin), enhancing cholinergic transmission by direct receptor stimulation, and inhibiting the breakdown of acetylcholine at its receptor site[1,2]. Early studies involving the use of acetylcholine precursors were not encouraging. Lecithin, phosphatidylcholine and acetyl-L-carnitine were ineffective, with the former also causing significant body odour[1,2]. While modest cognitive and behavioural benefits were demonstrated in trials of two cholinomimetic agents, milameline and xanomeline, the frequent occurrence of sweating, gastrointestinal symptoms and syncope limited their usefulness[2]. While the first two strategies have to date been unsuccessful, both efficacy and safety have been established for cholinesterase inhibitors, which increase the availability of acetylcholine for neurotransmission by inhibiting the enzyme acetylcholinesterase. Four cholinesterase inhibitors are currently approved by the FDA for the treatment of AD. Three of these are discussed in detail below. The fourth, tacrine, is now rarely used due to both its complex titration schedule and risks of hepatotoxicity.

DONEPEZIL

Cognitive Benefits

A reversible acetylcholinesterase inhibitor, donepezil has been FDA-approved since 1997 for the treatment of mild to moderate Alzheimer's disease. In one double-blind, placebo-controlled study of 468 participants with mild to moderately severe Alzheimer's disease[3], those in the donepezil group improved significantly compared to placebo on a 70-point cognitive battery. The improvement, however, was modest: 2.5 points in the 5 mg/d group and 3.1 in the 10 mg/d group. On the 30-point Mini-Mental State Examination (MMSE), this improvement was 1.0 and 1.3 points respectively. On a scale of global impression of function, 32% and 38% respectively in the donepezil group improved, compared to only 18% with placebo. Correlation was found between clinical improvement and the degree of red blood cell acetylcholinesterase inhibition. Comparable benefits were found in additional trials up to 24 weeks[4]. In an open-label extension trial of two 15–30 week studies[5], benefits were observed to possibly persist for up to 2.8 years. Donepezil's benefits have been demonstrated in the nursing home setting[6], and in one study[7], treatment delayed nursing home placement by 18 months. A one-year, double-blind study[8] found donepezil to be both cost effective and to reduce the time caregivers spent providing care by 400 hours annually. The sustained benefits of long-term treatment remain controversial, however. One study suggested no significant benefits compared to placebo persisting after three years[9], while another study[10] did demonstrate sustained benefits over three years, particularly in participants who began treatment immediately, as opposed to receiving placebo for the first year.

Donepezil's benefits have been found to extend to the severe stages of AD as well. In one six-month, placebo-controlled, double-blind study of participants with MMSE scores less than or equal to 10[11], those receiving donepezil performed better on measures of cognitive function and activities of daily living. In 2006, donepezil received FDA approval for the treatment of severe AD and is currently the only acetylcholinesterase inhibitor approved for treatment during all disease stages.

Side Effects

Donepezil's side-effects profile and those of the other marketed cholinesterase inhibitors are similar. Gastrointestinal symptoms

Table 52.1 Common and less common side effects of cholinesterase inhibitors and memantine

Medication class	Common side effects	Less common side effects
Cholinesterase inhibitors	Nausea Vomiting Diarrhoea	Anorexia Muscle cramps Insomnia Nightmares Bradycardia Syncope
Memantine	None	Dizziness Constipation Headaches

(e.g. nausea, loose stool) are most common and usually mild and transient, though in some cases these symptoms can be severe. Patients sometimes experience vivid nightmares; discussion of this with patients and caregivers is important as they may not automatically associate these unpleasant experiences with a medication side effect. Muscle cramps and diaphoresis may also occur. Due to its cholinergic properties, caution should be used in patients with pre-existing bradycardia. These cholinergic effects are the likely cause of the most serious side effect, syncope, which may occur in 1% of patients. Table 52.1 displays common and less common side effects for donepezil and other approved AD therapies.

Dosing

The starting dose of donepezil is 5 mg/d. The dose is usually increased to 10 mg/d after four weeks. Side effects are dose dependent and should be monitored. Some clinicians have found doses of 15 mg and 20 mg/d to be tolerated and to confer additional benefit; however, these doses have not been systematically studied and are unapproved. Table 52.2 displays typical dosing guidelines for donepezil and other approved AD therapies.

GALANTAMINE

Cognitive Benefits

Galantamine was FDA approved in 2001 for the treatment of mild to moderately severe AD. A reversible, competitive inhibitor of

Table 52.2 Starting and optimal treatment doses for cholinesterase inhibitors and memantine

Medication	Starting dose	Optimal dose
Donepezil	5 mg daily	10 mg daily
Galantamine	4 mg bid immediate release	12 mg bid immediate release
	8 mg daily extended release	24 mg daily extended release
Rivastigmine	1.5 mg bid immediate release	6 mg bid immediate release
	4.6 mg/24 hours for patch	9.5 mg/24 hours for patch
Memantine	5 mg daily	10 mg bid

acetylcholinesterase derived from the snowdrop variety of daffodils, galantamine is also an allosteric modulator of nicotinic acetylcholine receptors. Although nicotinic receptors may increase cholinergic transmission, any additional cognitive benefits specifically conferred by this mechanism remain theoretical. In one six-month, double-blind, placebo-controlled study[12] of 636 participants with mild to moderate AD, those treated with galantamine at doses of 24 mg/d and 32 mg/d scored 3.9 and 3.8 points higher on the 70-point ADAS-Cog scale than those in the placebo group. At the end of a 6-month, open-label extension with all participants receiving 24 mg/d, ADAS-Cog scores for those treated for the entire 12 months with 24 mg/d remained stable, with less benefit seen in those who started on 32 mg/d and then decreased to 24 mg/d, possibly due to a rebound effect. Although the six-month, double-blind phase showed no benefit on the Disability Assessment for Dementia (DAD) measurement of activities of daily living (ADLs), at the end of the open-label extension, ADL scores for participants receiving galantamine remained at pre-treatment baseline. A later double-blind, placebo-controlled study of 653 participants demonstrated the benefit of galantamine on DAD scores[13]. In a 36-month, open-label trial of galantamine[14], the 194 participants with mild to moderate AD were assessed as experiencing 50% less cognitive decline than would be expected without treatment. An extended-release form of galantamine was FDA approved in late 2004, and has been shown to have similar bioavailability to the immediate-release galantamine. The benefits of galantamine in severe AD are less certain than is the case for donepezil. In a recent placebo-controlled, double-blind study of 407 participants with severe AD, those treated with galantamine demonstrated improvement in cognitive function, but not in activities of daily living. Galantamine remains approved for treatment of mild to moderate AD only. Galantamine is also currently the only acetylcholinesterase inhibitor available in generic form.

Dosing

The starting dose for immediate-release galantamine is 4 mg twice daily. This is increased after one month to 8 mg twice daily. Depending on response, patients can remain at this dose, or increase to 12 mg twice daily after one month. Extended-release galantamine is begun at 8 mg/d and is increased to 16 mg/d after one month, with the option after at least one month to increase to 24 mg/d. Galantamine should be taken with food to reduce gastrointestinal side effects.

Side Effects

The side effects of galantamine are essentially identical to those of donepezil (see above). Gastrointestinal side effects may be slightly more frequent with galantamine than donepezil. For many patients, however, the cost savings due to its availability in generic form may offset this minor disadvantage.

RIVASTIGMINE

Rivastigmine was approved in 2000 and, unlike donepezil and galantamine, is a reversible inhibitor of both acetylcholinesterase and butyrylcholinesterase. Although research suggests that butyrylcholinesterase plays a role in acetylcholine breakdown in AD, as is the case for the allosteric nicotinic properties of galantamine, the clinical significance of this additional mechanism of action remains unclear. Like galantamine, rivastigmine is currently approved for the treatment of mild to moderate AD. In a placebo-controlled, double-blind study of 725 participants with mild to moderate AD[15], the treatment group was randomized to either 1–4 mg/d or 6–12 mg/d, and more participants in the 6–12 mg/d group improved by ≥ 4 points on the ADAS-Cog; improvement compared to the other groups was also seen in a scale of progressive deterioration. Nearly a quarter of participants discontinued the higher dose treatment due to side effects, however, mostly gastrointestinal. In a study demonstrating similar clinical outcomes[16], only 55% tolerated the 12 mg/d dose. In a 26-week, open-label extension of a 26-week, double-blind study of rivastigmine at 6–12 mg/d[17], participants treated with rivastigmine for the entire 52-week study duration had improved cognition compared to those initially receiving placebo. Open-label data suggest benefit for rivastigmine over even longer durations. Using a baseline-dependent mathematical model, Small et al.[18] demonstrated that patients treated with rivastigmine for up to five years experienced less decline on the MMSE than would be expected in a modelled untreated group.

Since 2007, a rivastigmine 24-hour transdermal patch has also been approved by the FDA for the treatment of mild to moderate AD. The efficacy of the transdermal patch appears to be similar to that of 12 mg/d oral rivastigmine, with three-fold *fewer* gastrointestinal side effects[19].

Side Effects

While oral rivastigmine has been associated with a high occurrence of gastrointestinal side effects, with the 24-hour transdermal patch, these side effects now appear comparable to those of donepezil and galantamine. Side effects otherwise are similar to donepezil (see above) and galantamine. Rare cases of oesophageal rupture have been reported, and restarting rivastigmine at higher than the minimum dose after several weeks or more off from the medication may place patients at increased risk for this. Oral rivastigmine should be taken with food.

Dosing

Oral rivastigmine is usually begun at 1.5 mg twice daily. At minimum two-week intervals, the dose is gradually increased in 1.5 mg twice-daily increments up to a maximum dose of 6 mg twice daily. Increasing the dose titration intervals from two weeks to four weeks may decrease side effects, and rivastigmine should be taken with food[2]. The rivastigmine 24-hour transdermal patch is started at 4.6 mg/24 hours, and after one month can be increased to 9.5 mg/24 hours. Switching from oral rivastigmine to transdermal patch typically does not require delay, and most patients taking 9–12 mg of oral rivastigmine daily can immediately switch to the 9.5 mg/24 hours patch[2].

COMPARATIVE EFFICACY AND TOLERABILITY

Several studies have compared the efficacy and tolerability of cholinesterase inhibitors in the treatment of AD. In one 12-week, open-label study of donepezil and oral rivastigmine in the treatment of mild to moderate AD[20], similar improvements were noted in both groups on the ADAS-Cog. Tolerability favoured donepezil. Only 47% of the rivastigmine group remained on the maximum dose (6 mg twice daily), compared to 88% for donepezil (at 10 mg/d). The rivastigmine group was also twice as likely to discontinue treatment due to side effects (22% vs. 11%). Another study compared donepezil to oral rivastigmine in 994 participants with moderate to moderately severe AD over a two-year period[21] and found that while cognitive benefits were similar, the rivastigmine group performed better in activities of living and daily functioning, though only in the intention-to-treat population. Although adverse events, especially gastrointestinal, were more frequent with rivastigmine during the titration phase, no difference was evident in the maintenance phase, and serious adverse events were nearly identical at 32%.

In a 52-week comparison of donepezil and galantamine in 182 AD participants[22], galantamine treatment trended to fewer declines in MMSE score and, in the subgroup of participants with MMSE scores between 12 and 18, fewer declines on the ADAS-Cog. Although no difference was found in performance of activities of daily living, caregivers from the galantamine group reported larger reductions in burden. In contrast, a recent meta-analysis of comparison trials among acetylcholinesterase inhibitors found that, while cognitive profiles among the three were similar, the relative risk of global response favoured donepezil and rivastigmine over galantamine (relative risks 1.63 and 1.42 respectively). Adverse events were lowest for donepezil and highest for rivastigmine, although with the introduction of the rivastigmine transdermal patch, which has improved tolerability, this difference may be less relevant. In interpreting the above inconsistent research, clinicians would be wise to consider Farlow and Boustani's[2] observation that the companies sponsoring comparison trials often have conflicts of interest, and the results 'must be judged with caution'.

SWITCHING ACETYLCHOLINESTERASE INHIBITORS

Given the similar mechanisms of action among acetylcholinesterase inhibitors, it might be anticipated that patients failing to benefit from one of these agents would be unlikely to benefit from switching to another. Research, however, has suggested that non-responders may benefit from such a medication change. Most studies have focused on a switch from donepezil or galantamine to rivastigmine and have been open label, which limits interpretation of results. In one recent study[23], 270 participants with mild to moderate AD who had not adequately responded to donepezil were immediately switched to rivastigmine and followed for 26 weeks. Seventy percent of these donepezil non-responders either improved or showed no deterioration in global functioning, although only 69% completed the trial and 54% experienced at least one adverse event, mostly gastrointestinal. One hundred and forty six of these participants entered a 26-week, open-label extension[16] in which rivastigmine was generally well tolerated, and 80% completed the trial. Similar results have been found in other studies of non-responders who switch from donepezil or galantamine to rivastigmine[24]. Unfortunately, no published research has evaluated switching from another acetylcholinesterase inhibitor to donepezil or galantamine; nor has any study evaluated the benefits of a medication change for rivastigmine non-responders.

PRESCRIBING AND MONITORING ACETYLCHOLINESTERASE INHIBITORS

When to Begin

All acetylcholinesterase inhibitors are approved for the treatment of mild AD. Some research points to the benefits of starting treatment as early as possible after the diagnosis is made; in several clinical trials, participants who began on placebo and switched to a cholinesterase inhibitor were never able to 'catch up' to study peers who received treatment all along[25]. In patients who do not yet meet criteria for dementia but are diagnosed with mild cognitive impairment (MCI), evidence does not support the use of cholinesterase inhibitors. Potential benefits have been described as 'minor, short-lived and associated with significant side effects'[26]. If a clinician chooses to begin a cholinesterase inhibitor in an MCI patient (e.g. at the patient's request), disclosure to the patient about the limited known benefits as well as side-effect risks is essential.

Which Cholinesterase Inhibitor to Choose

As reviewed above, limited comparison data are available and research suggests that the three medications are roughly equivalent in efficacy. Most clinicians decide which drug to use based on side-effect profile and patient convenience. For a patient vulnerable to gastrointestinal upset, for example, donepezil may be preferable as gastrointestinal symptoms are likely mildest. If cost is a concern, galantamine is currently the only cholinesterase inhibitor available as a generic. The rivastigmine 24-hour transdermal patch might be an appropriate choice for patients who do not wish to or have difficulty taking oral medication. Because oral rivastigmine is associated with frequent gastrointestinal symptoms and confers no benefit over the patch, it is now uncommonly prescribed.

How Long to Continue Treatment

Guidance in this regard is limited. Most studies demonstrating benefit after six months of treatment have been open label; instead of placebo-controlled, participant outcomes are compared against the expected outcomes of a theoretical untreated cohort. Many clinicians, including the authors, recommend a trial of at least six months, with use of at least one and preferably several outcome measures (e.g. MMSE, opinion of caregivers)[1]. If no clear improvement or stabilization is evident after six months, a trial off the medication should be strongly considered, with close observation for decline and a plan to reinitiate treatment if such occurs. Reinitiation should occur promptly, as some research suggests that after a washout of more than several weeks, patients may not regain full treatment benefits after restarting the drug[27]. If no difference is seen off the medication, consideration should be given to switching to another cholinesterase inhibitor. As reviewed above, most available evidence supports the benefit of switching to rivastigmine from another cholinesterase that has not provided benefit.

MEMANTINE

Rationale

Glutamate excitotoxicity may play an important role in the death of neurons in AD. It is hypothesized that injured glutamate-producing neurons release excessive amounts of glutamate, resulting in injury and death to downstream neurons. This likely occurs via glutamate's activation of calcium channels, leading to influx of calcium into downstream neurons. Memantine, a non-competitive antagonist of the *N*-methyl-D-aspartate (NMDA) receptor of glutamate, is believed to protect these neurons by preventing the glutamate-mediated cascade of neuronal damage.

Cognitive Benefits

Memantine has been FDA approved since 2003 for the treatment of moderate to severe Alzheimer's disease. In one 28-week, placebo-controlled, double-blind trial of memantine at 20 mg/d in 252 participants with moderate to severe AD[28], participants treated with memantine had improved outcomes compared to placebo on measurements of global assessment of change, activities of daily living and cognitive functioning. Another placebo-controlled, 12-week study in participants with moderately severe dementia (either AD or vascular dementia) found memantine use to be associated with a significant decrease in care dependence[29]. A 24-week, open-label extension of the above-mentioned 28-week study[30] demonstrated benefits both in participants who remained on memantine for the entire study duration and those who switched from memantine to placebo. One study suggests that the addition of memantine to donepezil may confer additional advantages in cognition, activities of daily living, global outcome and behaviour[31]. A more recent study suggests that addition of memantine to a cholinesterase inhibitor delays time to nursing home admission[32]. A third study of memantine addition to a cholinesterase inhibitor, however, found no benefit over placebo[33]. Although some evidence suggests benefits in mild AD, memantine is not FDA approved for this purpose.

Side Effects

Memantine is well tolerated by most patients and side effects are uncommon. These can include dizziness, constipation and headaches. The presence of severe renal impairment is a contraindication, and the dose should be reduced in the presence of moderate renal insufficiency.

Dosing

Memantine is started at 5 mg/d and the dose is increased by 5 mg/d weekly until a total dose of 20 mg/d is reached, typically using a commercially available 'titration starter pack'. After initial titration, memantine is administered in a divided dose of 10 mg twice daily.

Prescribing and Monitoring Memantine

A memantine trial should be considered in patients with moderate to severe AD who are able to tolerate such. Memantine can be prescribed in combination with a cholinesterase inhibitor which, as indicated above, may confer additional advantages. Negligible guidance exists as to how long to continue a memantine trial. Most clinicians, including the authors, recommend re-evaluating use every six months, as with the cholinesterase inhibitors. Because cognitive measures (i.e. MMSE) are less useful in advanced dementia, increased emphasis should be placed on the report of caregivers, including professional providers in the assisted living and nursing home setting.

NEUROPSYCHIATRIC EFFECTS OF CHOLINESTERASE INHIBITORS AND MEMANTINE

Neuropsychiatric symptoms (e.g. apathy, agitation, delusions) are nearly universal in patients with Alzheimer's disease, with over 90% experiencing at least one such symptom over the illness course. While these symptoms are often distressing to patients and caregivers, conventional treatments such as antipsychotics, antidepressants and mood stabilizers are often inadequately effective or cause significant side effects. Studies reporting positive neurobehavioural effects of cholinesterase inhibitors and memantine are therefore of particular interest. In a study by Holmes et al.[34], 134 participants with mild to moderate AD and significant neuropsychiatric co-morbidity (defined as a neuropsychiatric inventory (NPI) score >11) were randomized to donepezil or placebo for 12 weeks (following a 12-week, open-label donepezil trial). At the end of 12 weeks, NPI scores were 6.2 points lower in the donepezil group compared to placebo. Similar improvement has been demonstrated in trials of galantamine[35] and rivastigmine[36]. Another 12-week study of 272 AD patients with significant agitation[37], however, showed no benefit with donepezil treatment compared to placebo. In studies showing positive benefits of donepezil, apathy and mood symptoms appear most likely to respond. The addition of memantine to a cholinesterase inhibitor may confer additional benefit. In a 24-week, placebo-controlled, double-blind study of 404 participants with moderate to severe AD[38], those treated with memantine and donepezil demonstrated improvement on the NPI compared to those treated with donepezil alone. Memantine's benefits were most pronounced on agitation, eating behaviour and irritability.

Despite the above encouraging findings, cholinesterase inhibitors and memantine currently have at best a limited role in the treatment of neuropsychiatric symptoms in AD. Although most clinical trials report positive treatment effects, these effects are typically modest. Heterogeneity among studies also exists regarding which symptoms are most likely to respond[38], making decisions to target a specific neuropsychiatric symptom with an antidementia drug difficult. Another factor limiting the applicability of these findings to clinical care is that, in most published studies, improvement of neuropsychiatric symptoms was a secondary outcome. A review by Cummings et al.[39] notes that of 13 placebo-controlled, double-blind trials, only 4 included behavioural change as a primary outcome. For these reasons, the authors do not recommend cholinesterase inhibitors as first-line treatment for any neuropsychiatric symptom causing severe distress. However, in situations where symptoms are mild to moderate in severity and an immediate intervention is not required, a trial of a cholinesterase inhibitor or memantine is a reasonable first step before resorting to pharmacotherapy (e.g. antipsychotics, mood stabilizers) that carries higher side-effect risks. An antidementia drug trial may be particularly appropriate for apathy and irritability both because studies suggest that these symptoms may be most responsive and because alternative effective pharmacotherapy options are especially limited.

ALTERNATIVE THERAPIES FOR ALZHEIMER'S DISEASE

The cholinesterase inhibitors and memantine are currently the only FDA-approved treatments for AD. Various unapproved alternative treatments which have been proposed include vitamin B12, folic acid, vitamin E, Ginkgo biloba and serotonergic augmentation with serotonin-specific re-uptake blockers (SSRIs). None of these treatments are supported by sufficient evidence to be recommended by clinicians. Patients and caregivers often inquire about these, however, and they are reviewed below.

Vitamin B12 and Folate

Elevated homocysteine levels have been linked to Alzheimer's disease, and studies have demonstrated an association between high levels of homocysteine and cognitive dysfunction even in the non-demented elderly. Because vitamin B12 and folate are linked to reduction in homocysteine levels, they have been proposed as treatments for AD. Unfortunately, trials to date do not support clinical benefit. A recent double-blind trial of 409 participants with mild to moderate AD randomized to placebo or high-dose vitamin supplementation (folate, B6 and B12)[40] demonstrated that, although vitamin supplementation was associated with decreased homocysteine levels, no clinical improvements were evident. This is consistent with prior studies showing no cognitive benefit from folic acid supplementation with or without vitamin B12[41]. Vitamin supplementation in the above study was also associated with an increase in depression reaching marginal significance. Thus, vitamin B12 or folate cannot be recommended as treatments for AD.

Ginkgo Biloba

Oxidative stress has been linked to the neuropathological changes in AD, and Ginkgo biloba has been proposed as a putative therapy due to its antioxidant properties; recent evidence suggests some anti-amyloid aggregation effects as well. Despite these theoretical rationales, clinical benefits are unclear. One placebo-controlled, double-blind study of 513 participants with mild to moderate AD[42] found no difference between placebo and treatment groups. However, the authors note that this study may have been compromised by the negligible decline observed in the placebo group. Also, participants with neuropsychiatric symptoms did appear to benefit cognitively compared to placebo. A recent Cochrane review[43] of 36 trials describes the evidence for ginkgo as 'inconsistent and unreliable'. Ginkgo is generally well tolerated, but carries a small risk of intracranial bleeding. The authors do not recommend use of ginkgo to treat AD, but would not strongly discourage patients who wish to take it[1].

Vitamin E

Similar to Ginkgo biloba, vitamin E has antioxidant properties hypothesized to be of benefit in treating AD. One placebo-controlled, double-blind trial suggested that high-dose vitamin E (2000 international units daily) may slow functional decline in moderate AD[44]. These findings have been considered controversial because clinical significance was found only after adjustment for higher MMSE score in the placebo group. More recent findings have suggested that high-dose vitamin E may be associated with a small increased mortality risk in the elderly. The authors therefore do not recommend vitamin E supplementation in AD, but would not discourage patients wishing to start vitamin E in doses of 1000 international units daily or less.

SSRI Augmentation

Although acetylcholine is the neurotransmitter most highly linked to the cognitive deficits of AD, other neurotransmitters are presumed to play important roles as well. Despite uncertainty about the relationship between serotonin and cognition in AD, some clinicians have observed a modest increase in functional performance in patients treated with SSRIs[2]. In a study by Mowla of 122 participants with mild to moderate AD[45], cognition improved equally whether subjects were treated with rivastigmine or rivastigmine plus fluoxetine. However, those treated with the combination therapy performed better in activities of daily living and global functioning.

Some of the functional improvement clinicians report with SSRI treatment may actually reflect improvement in underlying depression; Lyketsos et al.[46], for example, found functional decline to be attenuated in depressed AD participants who responded to antidepressant therapy.

FUTURE THERAPIES FOR AD

To date, only symptomatic pharmacotherapies are available for the treatment of AD. Despite the consistently demonstrated efficacy of these medications, their benefit remains frustratingly modest in degree. Current research focuses on the development of novel therapeutic strategies which are disease modifying. Although the pathological mechanisms leading to neuronal loss in AD remain only partially understood, abnormal amyloid processing appears to be a crucial early step. When amyloid precursor protein (APP), which is normally cleaved by alpha secretase, is instead cleaved by beta and then gamma secretase, insoluble extracellular amyloid plaques occur. These plaques have been implicated in neuronal death. Some treatments under development therefore aim to either inhibit beta or gamma secretase, or to enhance alpha secretase activity. Other proposed treatments target the aggregation of amyloid into plaques. Neprolysin, an amyloid-degrading enzyme, is one such target under study. Immunotherapies have also been designed with the intent to clear abnormally processed amyloid from the brain. Although an early clinical trial of an active amyloid-beta vaccine was discontinued after several participants developed meningoencephalitis, modified versions of this vaccine believed less likely to have this adverse effect have since been developed and are being tested.

Neurofibrillary tangles of phosphorylated tau protein are another hallmark AD pathology. These tangles are hypothesized to cause neuronal death by interfering with microtubule function. Proposed therapies to promote microtubule stability include tau kinase inhibitors and the anticancer compound paclitaxel. Although still in early development, viral vectors to deliver genes to modify AD neuropathology are another hopeful area of research.

The results of recent clinical trials for novel AD therapies have unfortunately been discouraging. The failure to demonstrate benefit may at least in part reflect that some AD therapies will work best in certain 'subtypes' of the disease, in certain stages of severity, or in individuals with specific characteristics (e.g. gender, apolipoprotein E status). Increasing attention has therefore focused on biomarkers, which may differentiate which patients are most likely to benefit from different therapies. Such biomarkers may also assist in determining drug response in pre-symptomatic patients, serve as outcome measures in clinical trials of symptomatic patients, and aid in determining whether further development of a treatment is warranted[47].

CONCLUSION

Although a cure for AD remains elusive, available symptomatic therapies may slow cognitive and functional decline, delay the need for a higher level of care and decrease caregiver burden. Donepezil is currently approved for the treatment of all AD stages, galantamine and rivastigmine for mild to moderate AD, and memantine for moderate to severe. These medications are typically well tolerated. Severe side effects are more common with cholinesterase inhibitors and are mostly gastrointestinal in nature. Although none of the available pharmacological treatments can presently be recommended as

a first-line therapy for any neuropsychiatric symptom, some patients may experience behavioural benefits, especially in regards to mood and apathy. Negligible evidence exists for vitamin supplementation, Ginkgo biloba or SSRI augmentation as treatments for AD. When a patient or caregiver inquires about beginning an unapproved therapy, a careful discussion of the available evidence and potential risks is warranted. Current research focuses on the development of treatments which are disease-modifying. The investigation of valid biomarkers for AD may be pivotal in determining which treatments are most promising, and in which subgroups of AD patients they are most likely to be effective.

REFERENCES

1. Rabins PV, Lyketsos CG, Steele CD. *Practical Dementia Care*. Oxford: Oxford University Press, 2006.
2. Farlow MR, Boustani M. Pharmacologic treatment of Alzheimer disease and mild cognitive impairment. In Weiner MF, Lipton AM (eds), *The American Psychiatric Publishing Textbook of Alzheimer Disease and Other Dementias*. Arlington, VA: American Psychiatric Publishing, 2009, 317–31.
3. Rogers SL, Doody RS, Mohs RC, Friedhoff LT. Donepezil improves cognition and global function in Alzheimer disease: a 15-week, double-blind, placebo-controlled study. Donepezil Study Group. *Arch Intern Med* 1998; **158**: 1021–31.
4. Burns A, Rossor M, Hecker J et al. The effects of donepezil in Alzheimer's disease – results from a multinational trial. *Dement Geriatr Cogn Disord* 1999; **10**: 237–44.
5. Doody RS, Geldmacher DS, Gordon B et al. Open-label, multicenter, phase 3 extension study of the safety and efficacy of donepezil in patients with Alzheimer disease. *Arch Neurol* 2001; **58**: 427–33.
6. Tariot P, Cummings JL Katz IR et al. A randomized, double-blind, placebo-controlled study of the efficacy and safety of donepezil in patients with Alzheimer's disease in the nursing home setting. *J Am Geriatr Soc* 2001; **49**: 1590–9.
7. Geldmacher DS, Provenzano G, McRae T, Mastey V, Ieni JR. Donepezil is associated with delayed nursing home placement in patients with Alzheimer's disease. *J Am Geriatr Soc* 2003; **51**: 937–44.
8. Wimo A, Winblad B, Shah SN et al. Impact of donepezil treatment for Alzheimer's disease on caregiver time. *Curr Med Res Opin* 2004; **20**: 1221–5.
9. Courtney C, Farrell D, Gray R et al. Long-term donepezil treatment in 565 patients with Alzheimer's disease (AD2000): randomised double-blind trial. *Lancet* 2004; **363**: 2105–15.
10. Winblad B, Wimo A, Engedal K et al. 3-year study of donepezil therapy in Alzheimer's disease: effects of early and continuous therapy. *Dement Geriatr Cogn Disord* 2006; **21**: 353–63.
11. Winblad B, Kilander L, Eriksson S et al. Donepezil in patients with severe Alzheimer's disease: double-blind, parallel-group, placebo-controlled study. *Lancet* 2006; **367**: 1057–65.
12. Raskind MA, Peskind ER, Wessel T, Yuan W. Galantamine in AD: a 6-month randomized, placebo-controlled trial with a 6-month extension. The Galantamine USA-1 Study Group. *Neurology* 2000; **54**: 2261–8.
13. Wilcock GK, Lilienfeld S, Gaens E. Efficacy and safety of galantamine in patients with mild to moderate Alzheimer's disease: multicentre randomised controlled trial. *BMJ* 2000; **321**: 1–7.

14. Raskind MA, Peskind ER, Truyen L, Kershaw P, Damaraju CV. The cognitive benefits of galantamine are sustained for at least 36 months: a long-term extension trial. *Arch Neurol* 2004; **61**: 252–6.

15. Rösler M, Anand R, Cicin-Sain A *et al*. Efficacy and safety of rivastigmine in patients with Alzheimer's disease: international randomised controlled trial. *BMJ* 1999; **318**: 633–8.

16. Corey-Bloom J, Anand R, Veach J. A randomized trial evaluating the efficacy and safety of ENA 713 (rivastigmine tartrate), a new acetylcholinesterase inhibitor, in patients with mild to moderately severe Alzheimer's disease. *In J Psychopharmacol* 1998; **2**: 55–65.

17. Figiel GS, Koumaras B, Meng X, Strigas J, Gunay I. Long-term safety and tolerability of rivastigmine in patients with Alzheimer's disease switched from donepezil: an open-label extension study. *Prim Care Companion J Clin Psychiatry* 2008; **10**: 363–7.

18. Small GW, Kaufer D, Mendiondo MS, Quarg P, Spiegel R. Cognitive performance in Alzheimer's disease patients receiving rivastigmine for up to 5 years. *Int J Clin Pract* 2005; **59**: 473–7.

19. Cummings J, Winblad B. A rivastigmine patch for the treatment of Alzheimer's disease and Parkinson's disease dementia. *Expert Rev Neurother* 2007; **11**: 1457–63.

20. Wilkinson DG, Passmore AP, Bullock R *et al*. A multinational, randomised, 12-week, comparative study of donepezil and rivastigmine in patients with mild to moderate Alzheimer's disease. *Int J Clin Pract* 2002; **56**: 441–6.

21. Bullock R, Touchon J, Bergman H *et al*. Rivastigmine and donepezil treatment in moderate to moderately-severe Alzheimer's disease over a 2-year period. *Curr Med Res Opin* 2005; **21**: 1317–27.

22. Wilcock G, Howe I, Coles H *et al*. A long-term comparison of galantamine and donepezil in the treatment of Alzheimer's disease. *Drugs Aging* 2003; **20**: 777–89.

23. Figiel GS, Sadowsky CH, Strigas J *et al*. Safety and efficacy of rivastigmine in patients with Alzheimer's disease not responding adequately to donepezil: an open-label study. *Prim Care Companion J Clin Psychiatry* 2008; **10**: 291–8.

24. Bartorelli L, Giraldi C, Saccardo M *et al*. Effects of switching from an AChE inhibitor to a dual AChE-BuChE inhibitor in patients with Alzheimer's disease. *Curr Med Res Opin* 2005; **21**: 1809–18.

25. Singh B, O'Brien JT. When should drug treatment be started for people with dementia? *Maturitas* 2009; **62**: 230–4.

26. Birks J, Flicker L. Donepezil for mild cognitive impairment. *Cochrane Database Syst Rev* 2006; **3**: CD006104.

27. Homma A, Imai Y, Tago H *et al*. Long-term safety and efficacy of donepezil in patients with severe Alzheimer's disease: results from a 52-week, open-label, multicenter, extension study in Japan. *Dement Geriatr Cogn Disord* 2009; **27**: 232–9.

28. Reisberg B, Doody R, Stoffler A *et al*. Memantine in moderate-to-severe Alzheimer's disease. *N Engl J Med* 2003; **348**: 1333–41.

29. Bullock R. Efficacy and safety of memantine in moderate-to-severe Alzheimer disease: the evidence to date. *Alzheimer Dis Assoc Disord* 2006; **20**: 23–9.

30. Reisberg B, Doody R, Stoffler A, Schmitt F, Ferris S. A 24-week open-label extension study of memantine in moderate to severe Alzheimer disease. *Arch Neurol* 2006; **63**: 49–54.

31. Tariot PN, Farlow MR, Grossberg GT *et al*. Memantine treatment in patients with moderate to severe Alzheimer disease already receiving donepezil: a randomized controlled trial. *JAMA* 2004; **291**: 317–24.

32. Lopez OL, Becker JT, Wahed AS *et al*. Long-term effects of the concomitant use of memantine with cholinesterase inhibition in Alzheimer disease. *J Neurol Neurosurg Psychiatry* 2009; **80**: 600–7.

33. Porsteinsson AP, Grossberg GT, Mintzer J, Olin JT; Memantine MEM-MD-12 Study Group. Memantine treatment in patients with mild to moderate Alzheimer's disease already receiving a cholinesterase inhibitor: a randomized, double-blind, placebo-controlled trial. *Curr Alzheimer Res* 2008; **5**: 83–9.

34. Holmes C, Wilkinson D, Dean C *et al*. The efficacy of donepezil in the treatment of neuropsychiatric symptoms in Alzheimer disease. *Neurology* 2004; **63**. 214–9.

35. Cummings JL, Schneider L, Tariot PN, Kershaw PR, Yuan W. Reduction of behavioral disturbances and caregiver distress by galantamine in patients with Alzheimer's disease. *Am J Psychiatry* 2004; **161**: 532–8.

36. Cummings JL, Koumaras B, Chen M, Mirski D; Rivastigmine Nursing Home Study Team. Effects of rivastigmine treatment on the neuropsychiatric and behavioral disturbances of nursing home residents with moderate to severe probable Alzheimer's disease: a 26-week, multicenter, open-label study. *Am J Geriatr Pharmacother* 2005; **3**: 137–48.

37. Howard RJ, Juszczak E, Ballard CG *et al*. Donepezil for the treatment of agitation in Alzheimer's disease. *N Engl J Med* 2007; **357**: 1382–92.

38. Cummings JL, Schneider E, Tariot PN, Graham SM; Memantine MEM-MD-02 Study Group. Behavioral effects of memantine in Alzheimer disease patients receiving donepezil treatment. *Neurology* 2006; **67**: 57–63.

39. Cummings JL, Mackell J, Kaufer D. Behavioral effects of current Alzheimer's disease treatments: a descriptive review. *Alzheimers Demen* 2008; **4**: 49–60.

40. Aisen PS, Schneider LS, Sano M *et al*. High-dose B vitamin supplementation and cognitive decline in Alzheimer disease: a randomized controlled trial. *JAMA* 2008; **300**: 1774–83.

41. Malouf R, Grimley Evans J. Folic acid with or without vitamin B12 for the prevention and treatment of healthy elderly and demented people. *Cochrane Database Syst Rev* 2008; **8**: CD004514.

42. Scheider LS, DeKosky ST, Farlow MR *et al*. A randomized, double-blind, placebo-controlled trial of two doses of *Ginkgo biloba* extract in dementia of the Alzheimer's type. *Curr Alzheimer Res* 2005; **2**: 541–51.

43. Birks J, Grimley Evans J. *Ginkgo biloba* for cognitive impairment and dementia. *Cochrane Database Syst Rev* 2009; **1**: CD003120.

44. Sano M, Ernesto C, Thomas RG *et al*. A controlled trial of selegiline, alpha-tocopherol, or both as treatment for Alzheimer's disease. The Alzheimer's Disease Cooperative Study. *N Engl J Med* 1997; **33**: 1216–22.

45. Mowla A, Mosavinasab M, Haghshenas H, Haghighi AB. Does serotonin augmentation have any effect on cognition and activities of daily living in Alzheimer's dementia? A double-blind, placebo-controlled clinical trial. *J Clin Psychopharmacol* 2007; **5**: 484–7.

46. Lyketsos CG, DelCampo L, Steinberg M *et al*. Treating depression in Alzheimer disease: efficacy and safety of sertraline therapy, and the benefits of depression reduction: the DIADS. *Arch Gen Psychiatry* 2003; **60**: 737–46.

47. Lyketsos CG, Szekely CA, Mielke MM, Rosenberg PB, Zandi PP. Developing new treatments for Alzheimer's disease: the who, what, when, and how of biomarker-guided therapies. *Int Psychogeriatr* 2008; **5**: 871–89.

53

Behavioural Management in Alzheimer's Disease – Pharmacology

David A. Merrill and David L. Sultzer

Department of Psychiatry and Biobehavioral Sciences, David Geffen School of Medicine at UCLA and VA Greater Los Angeles Healthcare System,
Supported by the Department of Veterans Affairs (Merit Review) and the NIMH (Contract N01 MH9001)

INTRODUCTION

Behavioural symptoms are common in patients with Alzheimer's disease (AD) and contribute substantially to morbidity[1-3]. As many as 80% of Alzheimer's patients develop behavioural changes, typically with increasing frequency as the disease progresses[4]. Estimates range from between 30–50% for delusions or hallucinations and up to 70% for agitated or aggressive behaviors[5]. Behavioural symptoms have long been known to contribute to caregiver distress[5,6]. More recent work has found that 46% of caregivers cite dementia-related behaviours as a primary reason for institutionalization[7]. Behavioural symptoms in patients with AD significantly increase direct costs of care, a cost which may be lessened by appropriate psychopharmacological management[8,9]. In this chapter, descriptions of the most common behavioural disturbances observed in AD and other dementias are provided, followed by examples of common measurement tools used in research to study these symptoms. The currently available pharmacological options for treating the behavioural symptoms of dementia are then reviewed, highlighting areas in which data can help guide targeted treatment of specific symptoms. This chapter concludes with a discussion of general treatment principles, intended to aid clinicians in an era when there are not clearly benign and beneficial treatment options available to address the ongoing severe and complex behavioural symptoms of dementia[10].

The psychosis of AD typically consists of delusions, misidentification syndromes and, less frequently, visual or auditory hallucinations[3,11]. Delusions of dementia tend to be simple, non-bizarre and often reflective of misinterpretation of the environment. The delusion of stealing is most prevalent, followed by persecutory delusions, delusions of reference, infidelity, grandiosity and somatic delusions[12]. Delusions are more common in moderate stages of the illness and are associated with greater cognitive impairment. Likewise, hallucinations are rare in the early stages of AD and become more common in the later stages[13]. The most common misidentification syndromes include failure to recognize one's home ('this is not my home' phenomenon), the belief that strangers are living in the home (phantom boarder syndrome) and imposter loved ones (Capgras phenomenon)[14]. Psychosis in AD clearly represents a syndrome distinct from schizophrenia in elderly patients, with only rare presence of first-rank Schneiderian symptoms and a higher rate of eventual remission of psychosis. In contrast to treatment of older adults with schizophrenia, antipsychotic treatment of psychosis in AD, described in detail below, is characterized by lower doses of medication, shorter duration of treatment and greater vulnerability to extrapyramidal symptoms (EPS).

Agitation in dementia has been defined as inappropriate verbal, vocal or motor behaviours not judged by an outside observer to result directly from the needs or confusion of the agitated individual. Increasing agitation is associated with advanced dementia, pre-morbid aggression and rapid decline. AD patients often also develop depression and anxiety, which in general are managed with antidepressant medications. While these topics will not be addressed in depth during this chapter, it is important to note that, similar to the contrast between schizophrenia and the psychosis of AD, substantial differences exist between primary mood and anxiety disorders versus dementia-related psychological symptoms in terms of aetiology, manifestations and treatment response.

Several standard neuropsychiatric symptom rating scales are used, primarily in research settings, to categorize the common behavioural and psychological symptoms in dementia (BPSD) (Table 53.1). Four of the most widely used general rating instruments include the Neuropsychiatric Inventory (NPI), the Brief Psychiatric Rating Scale (BPRS), the Neurobehavioral Rating Scale (NBRS) and the Cohen–Mansfield Agitation Inventory (CMAI). The NPI measures the frequency and severity of 12 psychiatric symptoms on the basis of caregiver report[15]. The items are delusions, hallucinations, agitation/aggression, depression/dysphoria, anxiety, elation, apathy/indifference, disinhibition, irritability/lability, aberrant motor behaviour, sleep disturbance, and appetite and eating disorder. The BPRS measures the severity of 18 psychiatric and behavioural symptoms, typically scored by a trained clinician after a semi-structured patient interview and collection of additional information from caregivers[16]. The NBRS has 28 items, covering areas including agitation (aggression, agitation, hostility) and psychosis (suspiciousness, hallucinations, delusions) and is completed by an observer on a 7-point scale[17]. The CMAI rates the frequency of 29 agitated behaviours in four factors on 7-point scales[18].

Principles and Practice of Geriatric Psychiatry, 3rd edn. Edited by Mohammed T. Abou-Saleh, Cornelius Katona and Anand Kumar
© 2011 John Wiley & Sons, Ltd

Table 53.1 Neuropsychiatric symptom rating scales

Agitated Behavior Inventory for Dementia (ABID)
Agitation-Calmness Evaluation Scale (ACES)
Alzheimer Disease Assessment Scale, non-cognitive portion
  (ADAS–noncog)
Bech–Rafaelsen Mania Scale (BRMS)
Behavior Observation Scale for Intramural Psychogeriatric
  Patients (GIP)
Behavior Rating Scale for Dementia (BRSD)
Behavioral Pathology in Alzheimer Disease Rating Scale
  (BEHAVE–AD)
Brief Psychiatric Rating Scale (BPRS)
Caregiver Burden Questionnaire (CBQ)
Clinical Global Impression of Change (CGIC)
Clinical Global Impression Scale (CGIS)
Clinicians Interview Based Impression of Change plus caregiver
  input (CIBIC–plus)
Cohen–Mansfield Agitation Inventory (CMAI)
Hamilton Rating Scale for Depression (HAM–D)
Iowa Caregiver Stress Inventory (CSI)
Neurobehvaioral Rating Scale (NBRS)
Neuropsychiatric Inventory (NPI)
Neuropsychiatric Inventory–Nursing Home version (NPI–NH)
Neuropsychiatric Inventory minus 5 'mood' items (NPI–NM)
Overt Aggression Scale (OAS)
Positive and Negative Syndrome Scale–Excited Component
  (PANSS–EC)
Revised Memory and Behavior Problem Checklist (RMBPC)
Screen for Caregiver Burden (SCB)
Social Dysfunction and Aggression Scale (SDAS-9)

When approaching behavioural disturbances in dementia, the overall preferred approach to management includes: (i) assessing to characterize the specific psychiatric or behavioural symptoms; (ii) developing an appropriate set of nonpharmacological behavioural interventions; and (iii) considering medication treatment if there are immediate safety concerns or insufficient response to behavioural interventions. To date, there are no FDA approved medications for behavioural management of AD. The largest amount of available evidence studying psychosis and/or agitation associated with dementia suggests a modest efficacy of antipsychotic medications in symptom reduction, in the context of these medications now carrying a 'black box' warning regarding use in elderly patients with dementia. What follows is a review of the options available for pharmacological management of behavioural symptoms of dementia. See Tables 53.2 and 53.3 for dosing and side-effect information for agents discussed below.

ANTIPSYCHOTIC MEDICATIONS

Efficacy Trials

The majority of data examining the psychopharmacological management of behavioural symptoms in dementia exist for the use of antipsychotic medications. Historically, short-term (6–12 week), double-blind, placebo-controlled, randomized controlled trials (RCTs) were completed using standardized neuropsychiatric symptom rating scales. These trials have been reviewed in depth in prior publications; here, the reader is referred to Table 53.4 for a summary of published trial results.

In total, efficacy trials of antipsychotic medications have demonstrated a modest benefit for treatment of agitated behaviour and psychosis in AD and other dementias. However, there is heterogeneity of these findings, with multiple studies also showing no benefit of antipsychotic treatment on primary or secondary outcome measures. Efficacy trials in this arena have typically had high placebo response rates, underscoring the likely importance of several general effects, including the passage of time, increased attention and the expectation of therapeutic intervention. Medication benefit has further been counteracted by adverse events.

As discussed in more detail at the end of this chapter, the decision to use medication and antipsychotic medications in particular should be made in parallel to the process of ongoing optimization of the social and environmental setting of each patient. Concerning results from meta-analyses and a recent large effectiveness trial underscore the importance of completing a thorough individualized risk–benefit analysis prior to initiating psychopharmacological management of behavioural disturbances in dementia with antipsychotic or other medications. However, despite the potential risks involved, antipsychotic medications continue to be used to manage particularly severe and persistent symptoms in patients with dementia, due in large part to a lack of available alternative with substantial supporting evidence.

Meta-Analyses

Schneider et al. reported a meta-analysis of RCT data on the efficacy and adverse effects of atypical antipsychotic medications for dementia[19]. Using a combination of published and drug company data, they reported on 15 RCTs (three on aripiprazole, five on olanzapine, three on quetiapine and five on risperidone) with a total of 3353 patients assigned to active treatment versus 1757 patients treated with placebo. The majority of patients had AD (87%), were female (70%) and averaged 81 years of age. Mean MMSE score was 11. Eleven trials were conducted in nursing homes and four were completed on outpatients. While approximately half of included trials were designed to recruit subjects with psychosis and the other half agitation, the authors found that most studies had a mixture of

Table 53.2 Dosage and adverse effects of atypical antipsychotics in dementia

Medication	Initial dose (mg/day)	Usual dosage range (mg/day)	Sedation	Hypo-tension	Anti-cholinergic	EPS	Weight gain
Risperidone	0.5	0.5–2	++	++	+/–	+	++
Olanzapine	2.5–5	5–10	+++	++	+	+	+++
Quetiapine	25	25–250	++	++	+/–	–	++
Aripiprazole	5	5–15	+	+	+/–	–	+/–

Table 53.3 Dosage and adverse effects of other agents in dementia

Medication	Initial dose (mg/day)	Usual dosage range (mg/day)	Common adverse effects	Precautions
Cognitive enhancers				
Donepezil	5	5–10	Nausea, diarrhoea	Bradycardia
Galantamine	8	16–24	Nausea, diarrhoea	Bradycardia
Rivastigmine	3	6–12	Nausea, diarrhoea	Bradycardia
Memantine	5	10–20	Sedation	Dose reduction with kidney impairment
Antidepressants				
Citalopram	10	10–40	Nausea, diarrhoea	Hyponatremia, EPS
Sertraline	25	50–200	Nausea, diarrhoea, insomnia	Hyponatremia, EPS
Trazodone	25	50–200	Sedation, orthostasis	Priapism (rare)
Mood stabilizers				
Divalproex sodium	125–250	250–1000	Nausea, sedation	Liver function abnormalities, thrombocytopenia, pancreatitis
Carbamazepine	50–100	200–1000	Nausea, sedation, ataxia	Hyponatremia, pancytopenia, drug interactions

patients with psychosis and agitation, a subject pool likely to reflect typical clinical populations.

After combining the trials, symptomatic efficacy was observed for aripiprazole and risperidone while olanzapine was not associated with efficacy overall. The available quetiapine trials used different selection criteria and outcomes and thus could not be statistically combined. In general, there was heterogeneity of findings across trials. Larger effect sizes were seen in patients without psychosis (vs. with psychosis), for those in nursing homes (vs. outpatients) and in patients with more severe cognitive impairment (MMSE less than 10). Approximately one-third of subjects dropped out of the trials, without significant difference between drug and placebo groups. The most common adverse events were somnolence and urinary tract infections or incontinence; increased incidence of extra-pyramidal symptoms and gait abnormalities were seen with risperidone and olanzapine. The authors noted a significant risk for cerebrovascular events, especially with risperidone. In addition, an increased risk for overall death was observed, which will be discussed in more detail below.

Two meta-analyses of typical antipsychotic medications found that neuroleptics are significantly more effective than placebo for behavioural disturbances in dementia, albeit with a small effect size and without differential efficacy between particular agents. For example, results from a meta-analysis of six studies comparing thioridazine with another neuroleptic and five studies comparing haloperidol with another neuroleptic, did not show that these two medications differed significantly from comparison medications[20]. In another meta-analysis, Lonergan et al. examined five RCTs comparing haloperidol to placebo and found that aggression decreased among patients with agitated dementia treated with haloperidol; other aspects of agitation were not affected significantly in treated patients, compared with controls[21].

A recent meta-analysis of patients with psychosis of AD from four large placebo-controlled clinical trials of risperidone in dementia demonstrated that risperidone significantly improved scores on the BEHAVE-AD Psychosis subscale and CGI scale compared with placebo[22]. Secondary analyses demonstrated that patients with more severe symptoms showed a more pronounced response to treatment with risperidone compared with placebo than those patients with less severe symptoms. Extra-pyramidal symptoms and somnolence were

more frequent with risperidone than placebo ($p = 0.04$). Cerebrovascular adverse events and all-cause mortality were observed more frequently, although not statistically significantly, with risperidone versus placebo.

Effectiveness Data: NIMH CATIE-AD Trial

The National Institute of Mental Health (NIMH) Clinical Antipsychotic Trials of Intervention Effectiveness–Alzheimer's Disease (CATIE–AD) project compared the effectiveness of antipsychotic medications versus placebo in treating AD-associated psychosis or agitated/aggressive behaviour[23]. CATIE–AD included outpatients in usual care settings and assessed treatment outcome on several clinical measures over nine months. Initial CATIE–AD treatment (olanzapine, quetiapine, risperidone or placebo) was randomized and masked, yet the protocol allowed medication dose adjustments or a switch to a different treatment at any time on the basis of the clinician's judgement. The primary CATIE–AD phase 1 outcome was time to discontinuation of the initially assigned medication for any reason, which was intended as an overall measure of effectiveness that incorporated the judgements of patients, caregivers and clinicians about therapeutic benefits in relation to undesirable effects.

The two primary hypotheses were that (i) there would be pair-wise differences between the three antipsychotic treatment groups and the placebo group in the time to discontinuation for any reason and (ii) among antipsychotic medications that were different from placebo, none would be inferior to the others. The results revealed no pair-wise treatment differences in all-cause discontinuation. The benefits of olanzapine and risperidone, i.e. longer times to discontinuation for lack of efficacy in comparison to placebo (Kaplan–Meier estimate of median time: olanzapine, 22.1 weeks; quetiapine, 9.1 weeks; risperidone, 26.7 weeks; placebo, 9.0 weeks), were offset by shorter times to discontinuation due to adverse effects in the antipsychotic groups (discontinuations due to intolerability: olanzapine, 24%; quetiapine, 16%; risperidone, 18%; placebo, 5%)[24]. The mean last prescribed medication dose was 5.5 mg/day olanzapine, 56.5 mg/day quetiapine and 1.0 mg/day risperidone.

A secondary data analysis of phase 1 in CATIE–AD found that some clinical symptoms improved with atypical antipsychotic

Table 53.4 Published randomized double-blind, placebo-controlled trials of atypical antipsychotics for dementia related psychosis or agitation

Study	Medication(s)	Sample size	Length (weeks)	Primary outcome(s)	Secondary outcomes	Primary outcome significance	Results/Comments	Adverse events (AEs)
Katz et al.[65]	Risperidone (0.5–2 mg/d)	625	12	BEHAVE-AD (50% reduction)	BEHAVE-AD psychosis subscale, CMAI, CGIS	Yes	Significant primary outcome (50% or more reduction of BEHAVE-AD in 45% of risperidone 1 mg group and 50% of 2 mg group compared to 33% of placebo group)	More EPS with risperidone 2 mg; dose-dependent increase in somnolence
De Deyn et al.[66]	Risperidone (mean dose: 1.1 mg/d), haloperidol (mean dose: 1.2 mg/d)	344	13	BEHAVE-AD (30% reduction)	BEHAVE-AD, CMAI	No	Negative primary outcome – no difference between groups; several positive results for secondary outcomes of risperidone vs. haloperidol and placebo	More somnolence with risperidone than placebo; more EPS with haloperidol than risperidone or placebo
Street et al.[67]	Olanzapine (5, 10 or 15 mg/d)	206	6	Sum of NPI-NH agitation/ aggression, hallucinations, delusion scores	NPI-NH, BPRS	Yes	5 mg and 10 mg but not 15 mg had a significant effect on the primary outcome; only 5 mg yielded improved NPI-NH total score	Somnolence and gait disturbance were increased significantly; not EPS
Meehan et al.[59]	Olanzapine (2.5 or 5 mg IM), lorazepam (1 mg IM)	204	24 h	PANSS-EC	CMAI, ACES	Yes	Significant mean change in primary outcome at 2 and 24 h for both olanzapine doses; lorazepam with significant effect at 2 h but not 24 h	Not significantly different across groups
Brodaty et al.[68]	Risperidone (mean dose: 1.0 mg/d)	345	12	CMAI total aggression score	CMAI, BEHAVE-AD, CGIS, CGIC	Yes	Risperidone improved CMAI-aggression subscale more than placebo (4.4 point difference, $P < .001$); similar results for other outcomes	Sedation, urinary tract infections with risperidone

Table 53.4 (continued)

Study	Medication(s)	Sample size	Length (weeks)	Primary outcome(s)	Secondary outcomes	Primary outcome significance	Results/Comments	Adverse events (AEs)
De Deyn et al.[69]	Olanzapine (1–7.5 mg/d)	652	10	NPI-NH psychosis subscale, CGIC	NPIH-NH total and item scores	No	No significant difference on primary outcome between any olanzapine dose and placebo	Weight gain, anorexia and urinary incontinence
Ballard et al.[70]	Quetiapine (50–100 mg/d), rivastigmine (6–12 mg/d)	93	26	CMAI	SIB (Severe Impairment Battery)	No	Rivastigmine, quetiapine and placebo equivalent	Statistically significant negative effect on cognition with quetiapine
Deberdt et al.[71]	Risperidone (mean dose: 1.0 mg/d), olanzapine (mean dose: 5.2 mg/d)	494	10	NPI, CGIS		No	Improvement regardless of treatment group	EPS with risperidone, weight gain and higher rate of discontinuation due to AEs with olanzapine
De Deyn et al.[72]	Aripiprazole (5, 10 or 15 mg/d)	208	10	NPI psychosis subscale, BPRS	BPRS	No	No difference in NPI psychosis subscale decline between aripiprazole (−6.5) and placebo (−5.5). BPRS psychosis and core subscale scores improved significantly with aripiprazole vs. placebo	Mild somnolence, not associated with falls or injury; no increase in EPS
Mintzer et al.[73]	Risperidone (mean dose 1.0 mg/d)	473	8	BEHAVE-AD psychosis subscale, CGIC		No	Both placebo and risperidone improved without significant difference	Somnolence occurred significantly more with risperidone
Tariot et al.[74]	Quetiapine (mean dose 97 mg/d), haloperidol (mean dose 1.9 mg/d)	284	10	BPRS total, CGIS	BPRS factors, NPI	No	All groups improved without significant differences on primary outcomes	Somnolence with quetiapine and haloperidol; EPS with haloperidol

Table 53.4 (*continued*)

Study	Drug (dose)	N		Primary outcome	Secondary outcomes	Significant?	Results	Comments
Zhong et al.[75]	Quetiapine (100 mg/d or 200 mg/d)	333	10	PANSS-EC	NPI-NH, CMAI	Yes	No significant effect on primary outcome with 100 mg group alone or when combined with 200 mg group, but a significant effect with the 200 mg/day group alone; no effect of quetiapine on CMAI	
Kurlan et al.[76]	Quetiapine (mean dose 120 mg/d)	40	10	BPRS score		No	No significant difference in primary or secondary outcomes	Quetiapine did not worsen Parkinsonism; trend towards decline on a measure of daily functioning
Mintzer et al.[77]	Aripiprazole (2, 5 or 10 mg/d)	487	10	NPI-NH psychosis subscale	NPI-NH total; CGIS, BPRS, CMAI	Yes	Aripiprazole 10 mg/d but not 2 or 5 mg/d significantly improved the primary outcome	CVAEs were present with aripiprazole ($N = 7$) but not placebo ($N = 0$)
Paleacu et al.[78]	Quetiapine (mean dose 200 mg/d)	40	6	NPI, CGIC		No	Reductions in NPI did not differ between placebo and quetiapine; CGIC did decrease significantly in the quetiapine ($P = 0.009$) but not placebo ($P = 0.48$) group	No differences between groups
Streim et al.[79]	Aripiprazole (mean dose 9 mg/d)	256	10	NPI-NH psychosis subscale, CGIS	NPI-NH total, BPRS total, CGIC, CMAI	No	No significant difference in co-primary outcomes; improvements in several secondary outcomes	Somnolence increased (14% vs. 4% placebo), no increase in EPS

medications[25]. Data from the last phase 1 observation indicated greater improvement with olanzapine or risperidone on NPI total scores and the BPRS hostile suspiciousness factor, as well as for risperidone alone on the BPRS psychosis factor and the CGIC. There was worsening with olanzapine on the BPRS withdrawn depression factor. Among patients continuing phase 1 treatment at 12 weeks, there were no significant differences between antipsychotic medications and placebo on functioning, care needs or quality of life, except for worsened functioning on an activities of daily living (ADL) scale with olanzapine compared to placebo. These results suggest that specific symptoms, rather than global changes, may be more realistic treatment targets for antipsychotic medications when used in dementia and that anger, aggression and paranoia may improve preferentially with treatment. These and other treatment guidelines will be discussed in more detail at the conclusion of the chapter.

Analysis of the entire 36-week trial revealed that, metabolically, atypical antipsychotic use was associated with a significant weight gain (0.08 lb/week) and increase in BMI (0.02 kg/m^2 per week), with the likelihood of weight gain increasing with longer use of antipsychotic medication[26]. In sub-group analysis, change in weight reached significance for olanzapine (0.12 lb/week) and quetiapine (0.14 lb/week), but not risperidone (0.10 lb/week); similar findings were present for BMI. When examined by gender, these changes in weight and BMI were significant in women (0.14 lb/week and 0.02 kg/m^2 per week, respectively), but not in men (−0.02 lb/week and −0.003 kg/m^2, respectively). Further analysis revealed unfavourable overall changes in HDL cholesterol (−0.19 mg/dl/wk) and waist circumference (0.07 inches/wk) with olanzapine.

Cognitively, patients declined significantly over the course of the trial (e.g. mean total decline in MMSE 2.4 points); a decline apparently increased by antipsychotic treatment[27]. Patients on antipsychotic medications declined more than patients on placebo on all 11 cognitive measures completed in the study, though the majority of differences between active treatment groups and placebo were non-significant. Statistically significant differences included greater decline on the MMSE in the olanzapine group, greater decline on the BPRS cognitive subscale in the quetiapine group and greater decline on a cognitive summary score in the risperidone and olanzapine groups.

Safety Issues with Antipsychotic Medications

Usual side effects of antipsychotic medications include sedation, hypotension, anti-cholinergic effects, extrapyramidal symptoms and weight gain. The general frequency of these side effects varies based on the dose and agent used, as listed in Table 53.2.

Two major safety issues concerning antipsychotic use in dementia, namely cerebrovascular adverse events (CVAEs) and risk of death, have come into focus over the last several years. In 2003, the FDA issued a warning about CVAEs (e.g. stroke, transient ischaemic attack), including fatalities, in patients (mean age 85 years; range 73–97) in trials of risperidone in elderly patients with dementia-related psychosis. In placebo-controlled trials, there was a significantly higher incidence of CVAEs in patients treated with risperidone compared to patients treated with placebo: in combining data from three controlled trials of risperidone, 12 of 744 (1.6%) risperidone-treated patients compared to 4 of 562 (0.7%) placebo-treated patients developed serious cerebrovascular events. Risperidone prescribing information was adjusted to include this risk. A similar warning was issued for olanzapine and aripiprazole by the manufacturers based on similar data. For example, in a pooled analysis of five controlled trials of olanzapine in patients with dementia, 15 patients of the 1178 randomly assigned in the trials to receive olanzapine suffered CVAEs (1.3%), compared with 2 out of the 478 randomly assigned to placebo (0.4%). For the subgroup of patients who had vascular dementia, there was a five-fold higher likelihood of experiencing a CVA. Overall, a meta-analysis found that pooled rates of CVAEs were 1.9% in atypical antipsychotic treated patients versus 0.9% in placebo-treated patients, yielding an odds ratio of 2.1 (95% CI, 1.2–3.8)[19]. Typical antipsychotics appear to be similar to atypical antipsychotics in stroke risk[28,29].

Regarding risk of death, in 2005 the FDA reported that atypical antipsychotic medications were associated with a significantly (1.6–1.7 times) greater mortality risk compared with placebo, based on several analyses of 17 RCTs of 5106 elderly patients with dementia[30]. Most deaths were due to either cardiac or infectious causes, the two most common immediate causes of death in dementia in general. A meta-analysis of 15 RCTs found a risk of death with atypical antipsychotics of 3.5%, compared to 2.3% for placebo, resulting in an odds ratio of 1.5 (95% CI, 1.1–2.2)[31]. Data on typical antipsychotic medications demonstrated a similar elevated risk of death[31,32]. In 2008, the FDA required manufacturers of typical antipsychotic drugs to make safety-related changes to prescribing information to warn about an increased risk of death associated with the off-label use of these drugs to treat behavioural problems in older people with dementia[33].

These safety concerns are highlighted in warnings now on all antipsychotic medications stating that these drugs are not approved for treatment of dementia-related psychosis. This has resulted in efforts to re-evaluate the prescription of antipsychotic medications to patients with dementia. In addition, there is a renewed level of interest in the discovery and development of alternatives to the use of antipsychotic medications in treating the behavioural disturbances found in dementia, as discussed below.

Antipsychotic Withdrawal Trials

In AD patients initially prescribed antipsychotic medications for treatment of behavioural disturbance for at least three months, the DART–AD trial found no significant difference between those randomized to receive continued treatment and those receiving placebo (antipsychotic medication discontinued) in the change of global cognitive function on the Severe Impairment Battery (SIB) or behavioural symptoms (as measured by the NPI) after six months follow-up[34]. A later analysis of this same population found a significantly increased risk of mortality in the patients who continued to receive antipsychotic medications compared to those who received placebo[35]. A similar lack of negative impact on NPI scores with stopping antipsychotic drug therapy in demented nursing home patients was observed in the briefer four-week BEDNURS trial[36].

COGNITIVE ENHANCERS

Cholinesterase Inhibitors

Given the high proportion of patients with advancing dementia placed on cholinesterase inhibitors, several recent studies have examined the possible clinical utility of cognitive enhancers in ameliorating emergent behavioural symptoms. A meta-analysis of

26 trials to quantify the efficacy of cholinesterase inhibitors for neuropsychiatric and functional outcomes in patients with mild to moderate AD found at best a very modest beneficial impact of these drugs[37]. For neuropsychiatric outcomes, six used the NPI and 10 of the trials used the ADAS-noncog. Compared with placebo, patients randomized to cholinesterase inhibitors improved 1.72 points on the NPI (95% CI, 0.87–2.57) and 0.03 points on the ADAS-noncog (95% CI, 0.00–0.05). For functional outcomes, 14 trials used activities of daily living (ADL) and 13 trials used independent-ADL (IADL) scales. Compared with placebo, patients randomized to cholinesterase inhibitors improved 0.1 SDs on ADL scales (95% CI, 0.00–0.19) and 0.09 SDs on IADL scales (95% CI, 0.01–0.17)[37]. There was no difference in efficacy among the various currently available cholinesterase inhibitors. Importantly, these trials did not specifically seek to include patients with behavioural disturbance and the findings may best apply to patients with very mild symptoms.

In contrast, a notable recent negative study was the 2007 CALM-AD trial examining donepezil treatment of agitation in AD[38]. Howard *et al.* examined the potential benefits of cholinesterase inhibitors for behavioural disturbances in 272 patients with AD who had clinically significant agitation and no response to a brief psychosocial treatment programme. There was no significant difference between the effects of 12 weeks of donepezil (128 patients) versus placebo (131 patients) on scores of the Cohen–Mansfield Agitation Inventory (CMAI). Twenty-two of 108 patients (20.4%) in the placebo group and 22 of 113 patients (19.5%) in the donepezil group had a reduction of 30% or greater in the CMAI. Likewise, there were also no significant differences between the placebo and donepezil groups in scores for the NPI, the Neuropsychiatric Inventory Caregiver Distress Scale or the CGIC. An earlier nursing-home study of 208 patients with advanced AD also failed to show a significant benefit of donepezil on total NPI scores, although there was benefit of donepezil on the agitation measure specifically[39].

Memantine

Data investigating the behavioural effects of memantine on behavioural disturbances in dementia are limited. A recent exploratory analysis of a 24-week, double-blind, placebo-controlled trial comparing memantine (20 mg/day) with placebo in subjects with moderate to severe AD on stable donepezil treatment was completed[40]. Authors used NPI measurements at baseline, week 12 and week 24, to assess the effects of memantine on behaviour. Treatment with memantine reduced agitation/aggression, irritability and appetite/eating disturbances. While the studies did not seek to include patients with behavioural symptoms and mean rating scores suggested mild symptoms, memantine reduced agitation/aggression in patients who were agitated at baseline and delayed its emergence in those who were free of agitation at baseline.

ANTIDEPRESSANTS

Available data on antidepressants and behavioural disturbance in dementia are limited, but do show some possible benefit. The findings discussed below need to be replicated in expanded study populations before antidepressants can be confidently recommended as alternatives to antipsychotic medications for the treatment of agitation or psychotic symptoms associated with dementia. Adverse effects may be more benign than with antipsychotic treatment, although there is very little comparison data and more complete understanding of the antidepressant side-effect profile in this population will require larger trial samples.

Citalopram

In a moderately sized study, citalopram was found to be more efficacious than placebo in the short-term hospital treatment of psychotic symptoms and behavioural disturbances in non-depressed, demented patients[41]. This study also included a treatment arm with perphenazine, which did not differ from citalopram or placebo groups. In a later study, when citalopram was compared to risperidone, agitation symptoms (aggression, agitation or hostility) and psychotic symptoms (suspiciousness, hallucinations or delusions) decreased in both treatment groups, but the improvement did not differ significantly between the two groups[42]. There was, however, a significant increase in side-effect burden with risperidone but not with citalopram.

Sertraline

An initial small trial of sertraline showed a 38% overall response rate, which was equivalent to placebo and a trend for decreased aggression ($P = 0.08$)[43]. A later trial of sertraline, in this case added to donepezil treatment, in outpatient AD patients with behavioural problems found no primary effect, but post hoc analyses demonstrated a modest but statistically significant advantage of sertraline over placebo augmentation in mixed-model analyses and in a subgroup of patients with moderate-to-severe symptoms as measured on CGI and NPI scales[44].

Fluvoxamine

The initial published trial on fluvoxamine use in dementia did not show significant benefit on cognitive functioning or behavioural changes in elderly dementia patients[45]. However, given that fluvoxamine can increase antipsychotic blood levels, another small trial examined fluvoxamine augmentation of perphenazine in AD patients and found that perphenazine plus fluvoxamine was better than perphenazine plus placebo on lowering total BPRS scores[46].

Trazodone

Sultzer *et al.* 1997 found that trazodone was equally efficacious as haloperidol in reducing agitation and aggression in a small mixed population of inpatient dementia subjects over a 9-week trial period[47]. Further analysis found that the presence of delusions did not predict a greater behavioural improvement with haloperidol treatment than in subjects without signs of psychosis, while mild depressive symptoms were associated a with greater improvement in trazodone-treated patients[48]. However, a larger ($n = 149$) randomized, placebo-controlled, multicentre trial comparing the efficacy of trazodone, haloperidol, behavioural management and placebo found modest but non-significantly different improvement in all four groups of the study[49]. Post hoc analysis of placebo responders demonstrated that the reduction observed was of the same magnitude as predicted by regression to the mean; patients exhibiting greater improvement had more severe baseline behavioural disturbances[50]. A small ($n = 26$) study of frontotemporal dementia patients found trazodone to be effective in reducing behavioural disturbances; 10 of the trazodone treated patients had a greater than 50% reduction of NPI scores[51].

MOOD STABILIZERS

Valproate/Divalproex Sodium

Despite preliminary promise, results from controlled trials published to date essentially show very limited effect of valproate/divalproex sodium over placebo in the treatment of behavioyral disturbances in dementia. The first RCT published using divalproex sodium in nursing-home patients with agitation and dementia ($n = 56$) found the drug/placebo difference in BPRS agitation scores at the threshold of significance ($P = 0.05$), while differences in CGI did not reach significance ($P = 0.06$)[52]. In a second trial, in aggressive demented inpatients ($n = 42$), there was no primary effect of valproate[53]. Secondary improvement was shown on restless, melancholic and anxious behaviours – with the caveat that no correction was made for multiple comparisons. A third study of divalproex in nursing-home patients with AD associated agitation ($n = 153$), found no difference from placebo over six weeks of treatment[54]. More recently, Herrmann et al. found that valproate was poorly tolerated and significantly worsened agitation and aggression on NPI and CMAI measures in a small population ($n = 14$) of institutionalized AD patients, when compared with placebo treatment for six weeks[55].

Given the negative results in trials targeting existent behavioural symptoms in dementia, the Alzheimer's Disease Cooperative Study (ADCS) has been conducting a clinical trial to address whether chronic valproate treatment can delay emergence of behavioural symptoms in outpatients with AD. Divalproex sodium has been shown to be better tolerated in these AD patients in doses less than 1000 mg/day, with doses of 1500 mg/day causing worse cognitive performance[56].

Carbamazepine

Two small positive efficacy trials have been published using carbamazepine to treat behavioural symptoms of dementia. The first involved nursing-home patients with dementia with agitation who showed improvement on BPRS and CGI measures over six weeks when compared to a parallel placebo group[57]. The second examined outpatient AD patients who had failed treatment with antipsychotic medications and again found relatively greater improvement in carbamazepine-treated patients compared to placebo but also a trend for worsened hallucinations[58].

Other Medications

A few small studies have examined other pharmacological approaches for treatment of behavioural disturbances in dementia, including oral or intramuscular benzodiazepines[59,60], diphenhydramine[61], propranolol[62], buspirone[63] and transdermal oestrogen[64].

GENERAL PRINCIPLES FOR PHARMACOLOGY OF BEHAVIOURAL DISTURBANCES

At the current time, no uniform treatment algorithm can be applied to elderly patients with behavioural disturbance in dementia. However, some general treatment guidelines for medication use can be discussed. Medications should be prescribed only for specifically defined target signs and symptoms. Prior to initiating psychopharmacological management, one must identify underlying contributing factors. Modifiable causes, such as environmental issues or co-morbid medical conditions, should be addressed and corrected prior to medication treatment. A review of the patient's medication regimen should be undertaken to discontinue unnecessary drugs and those that may dull cognition, such as sedative-hypnotic, opiate and anti-cholinergic medications. Superimposed delirium due to acute change in medical condition or medications is common in patients with dementia and often promotes behavioural disturbances.

Behavioural interventions (see related chapter in this book) should be initiated prior to medication use and monitored for effectiveness and modification throughout the treatment process. Given the known risks of medication use in patients with dementia, only behavioural symptoms that are recurrent and severe should be considered for pharmacological treatment. Examples of such behaviours would include those which put patient or caregiver safety at risk, such as psychosis contributing prominently to behavioural disturbance. Medication management may also be considered for psychotic symptoms that are prominently distressing to the patient or for behaviours that interfere with basic care needs.

The treatment plan should be guided by an individualized assessment of specific symptoms and the possible benefits and potential risks to the individual of a particular intervention. Clinicians should recognize the value of evidence from controlled clinical trials that is derived from studies of specific patient groups and settings, yet must also consider the individual patient's particular circumstances, needs and goals in developing a personalized treatment plan. When initiating psychotropic drug trials, micro-doses may be a good starting point but this needs to be monitored, as some patients respond well to low doses but may need increases over time. In general, the minimally effective dose should be used over the shortest duration of time possible to address the target symptom being treated. Medication effects need to be monitored over time and the treatment adjusted to match ongoing goals. This should include regular attempts at dose reduction and medication discontinuation trials. Lack of improvement or presence of significant adverse effects may require medication discontinuation or switching to another agent within or between classes of psychotropic agents.

Psychopharmacological management works best when coordinated with caregivers and treatment team members in an active collaboration. The consultant model of treatment has been found to be least effective when compared to alternative models such as interdisciplinary treatment teams which include active input not only from treating specialists, but internists, nurses, social workers, therapists and other care partners.

Following the above guidelines, one can typically look for improvement within 2–4 weeks of treatment initiation and if not observed, this requires re-evaluation of target symptoms and treatment goals. Such goals should typically be shared decisions, based on the patient and family values expressed regarding quality of life and other relevant matters. Documented sharing of information regarding known risks and benefits of proposed drug treatments should be completed with patients and caregivers. Information should be delivered in a manner appropriate to each familiy's education level and knowledge base.

REFERENCES

1. Lopez OL, Becker JT, Sweet RA, Klunk W, Kaufer DI, Saxton J et al. Psychiatric symptoms vary with the severity of dementia in probable Alzheimer's disease. J Neuropsychiatry Clin Neurosci 2003; 15(3): 346–53.

2. Lyketsos CG, Steinberg M, Tschanz JT, Norton MC, Steffens DC, Breitner JC. Mental and behavioral disturbances in dementia: findings from the Cache County Study on Memory in Aging. *Am J Psychiatry* 2000; **157**(5): 708–14.

3. Ropacki SA, Jeste DV. Epidemiology of and risk factors for psychosis of Alzheimer's disease: a review of 55 studies published from 1990 to 2003. *Am J Psychiatry* 2005; **162**(11): 2022–30.

4. Jost BC, Grossberg GT. The evolution of psychiatric symptoms in Alzheimer's disease: a natural history study. *J Am Geriatr Soc* 1996; **44**(9): 1078–81.

5. Craig D, Mirakhur A, Hart DJ, McIlroy SP, Passmore AP. A cross-sectional study of neuropsychiatric symptoms in 435 patients with Alzheimer's disease. *Am J Geriatr Psychiatry* 2005; **13**(6): 460–8.

6. Schulz R, O'Brien AT, Bookwala J, Fleissner K. Psychiatric and physical morbidity effects of dementia caregiving: prevalence, correlates and causes. *Gerontologist* 1995; **35**(6): 771–91.

7. Buhr GT, Kuchibhatla M, Clipp EC. Caregivers' reasons for nursing home placement: clues for improving discussions with families prior to the transition. *Gerontologist* 2006; **46**(1): 52–61.

8. Murman DL, Chen Q, Powell MC, Kuo SB, Bradley CJ, Colenda CC. The incremental direct costs associated with behavioral symptoms in AD. *Neurology* 2002; **59**(11): 1721–9.

9. Murman DL, Colenda CC. The economic impact of neuropsychiatric symptoms in Alzheimer's disease: can drugs ease the burden? *Pharmacoeconomics* 2005; **23**(3): 227–42.

10. Jeste DV, Blazer D, Casey D, Meeks T, Salzman C, Schneider L et al. ACNP White Paper: update on use of antipsychotic drugs in elderly persons with dementia. *Neuropsychopharmacology* 2008; **33**(5): 957–70.

11. Jeste DV, Finkel SI. Psychosis of Alzheimer's disease and related dementias. Diagnostic criteria for a distinct syndrome. *Am J Geriatr Psychiatry* 2000; **8**(1): 29–34.

12. Bassiony MM, Lyketsos CG. Delusions and hallucinations in Alzheimer's disease: review of the brain decade. *Psychosomatics* 2003; **44**(5): 388–401.

13. Devanand DP, Brockington CD, Moody BJ, Brown RP, Mayeux R, Endicott J et al. Behavioral syndromes in Alzheimer's disease. *Int Psychogeriatr* 1992; **4**(suppl 2): 161–84.

14. Rubin EH, Drevets WC, Burke WJ. The nature of psychotic symptoms in senile dementia of the Alzheimer type. *J Geriatr Psychiatry Neurol* 1988; **1**(1): 16–20.

15. Cummings JL, Mega M, Gray K, Rosenberg-Thompson S, Carusi DA, Gornbein J. The Neuropsychiatric Inventory: comprehensive assessment of psychopathology in dementia. *Neurology* 1994; **44**(12): 2308–14.

16. Overall JE, Rhoades HM. Clinician-rated scales for multidimensional assessment of psychopathology in the elderly. *Psychopharmacol Bull* 1988; **24**(4): 587–94.

17. Sultzer DL, Berisford MA, Gunay I. The Neurobehavioral Rating Scale: reliability in patients with dementia. *J Pyschiatr Res* 1995; **29**: 185–91.

18. Cohen-Mansfield J, Marx MS, Rosenthal AS. A description of agitation in a nursing home. *J Gerontol* 1989; **44**(3): M77–84.

19. Schneider LS, Dagerman K, Insel PS. Efficacy and adverse effects of atypical antipsychotics for dementia: meta-analysis of randomized, placebo-controlled trials. *Am J Geriatr Psychiatry* 2006; **14**(3): 191–210.

20. Schneider LS, Pollock VE, Lyness SA. A meta-analysis of controlled trials of neuroleptic treatment in dementia. *J Am Geriatr Soc* 1990; **38**(5): 553–63.

21. Lonergan E, Luxenberg J, Colford J. Haloperidol for agitation in dementia. *Cochrane Database Syst Rev* 2002(2): CD002852.

22. Katz I, de Deyn PP, Mintzer J, Greenspan A, Zhu Y, Brodaty H. The efficacy and safety of risperidone in the treatment of psychosis of Alzheimer's disease and mixed dementia: a meta-analysis of 4 placebo-controlled clinical trials. *Int J Geriatr Psychiatry* 2007; **22**(5): 475–84.

23. Schneider LS, Ismail MS, Dagerman K, Davis S, Olin J, McManus D et al. Clinical Antipsychotic Trials of Intervention Effectiveness (CATIE): Alzheimer's disease trial. *Schizophr Bull* 2003; **29**(1): 57–72.

24. Schneider LS, Tariot PN, Dagerman KS, Davis SM, Hsiao JK, Ismail MS et al. Effectiveness of atypical antipsychotic drugs in patients with Alzheimer's disease. *N Engl J Med* 2006; **355**(15): 1525–38.

25. Sultzer DL, Davis SM, Tariot PN, Dagerman KS, Lebowitz BD, Lyketsos CG et al. Clinical symptom responses to atypical antipsychotic medications in Alzheimer's disease: phase 1 outcomes from the CATIE–AD effectiveness trial. *Am J Psychiatry* 2008; **165**(7): 844–54.

26. Zheng L, Mack WJ, Dagerman KS, Hsiao JK, Lebowitz BD, Lyketsos CG et al. Metabolic changes associated with second–generation antipsychotic use in Alzheimer's disease patients: The CATIE–AD Study. *Am J Psychiatry* 2009; **166**(5): 583–90.

27. Schneider LS, Vigen CL, Mack WJ, Dagerman KS, Keefe R, Sano M et al. Cognitive effects of atypical antipsychotics in patients with Alzheimer's disease: outcomes from CATIE–AD. *Am J Geriatr Psychiatry* 2009; **17**(3, suppl 1): A76.

28. Herrmann N, Mamdani M, Lanctot KL. Atypical antipsychotics and risk of cerebrovascular accidents. *Am J Psychiatry* 2004; **161**: 1113–15.

29. Gill SS, Rochon PA, Herrmann N, Lee PE, Sykora K, Gunraj N. Atypical antipsychotic drugs and risk of ischaemic stroke: population based retrospective cohort study. *BMJ* 2005; **330**: 445.

30. US FDA. FDA Public Health Advisory: Deaths with antipsychotics in elderly patients with behavioral disturbances. US FDA, 2005.

31. Schneider LS, Dagerman KS, Insel P. Risk of death with atypical antipsychotic drug treatment for dementia. *JAMA* 2005; **294**: 1934–43.

32. Wang PS, Schneeweiss S et al. Risk of death in elderly users of conventional vs. atypical antipsychotic medications. *N Engl J Med* 2005; **353**: 2335–41.

33. US FDA. FDA News: FDA requests boxed warnings on older class of antipsychotic drugs. US FDA, 2008.

34. Ballard C, Hanney ML, Theodoulou M, Douglas S, McShane R, Kossakowski K et al. The dementia antipsychotic withdrawal trial (DART–AD): long-term follow-up of a randomised placebo-controlled trial. *Lancet Neurol* 2009; **8**(2): 151–7.

35. Ballard C, Lana MM, Theodoulou M, Douglas S, McShane R, Jacoby R et al. A randomised, blinded, placebo-controlled trial in dementia patients continuing or stopping neuroleptics (the DART–AD trial). *PLoS Med* 2008; **5**(4): e76.

36. Ruths S, Straand J, Nygaard HA, Aarsland D. Stopping antipsychotic drug therapy in demented nursing home patients: a randomized, placebo-controlled study – the Bergen District Nursing

Home Study (BEDNURS). *Int J Geriatr Psychiatry* 2008; **23**(9): 889–95.

37. Trinh NH, Hoblyn J, Mohanty S, Yaffe K. Efficacy of cholinesterase inhibitors in the treatment of neuropsychiatric symptoms and functional impairment in Alzheimer disease: a meta–analysis. *JAMA* 2003; **289**(2): 210–16.

38. Howard RJ, Juszczak E, Ballard CG, Bentham P, Brown RG, Bullock R *et al*. Donepezil for the treatment of agitation in Alzheimer's disease. *N Engl J Med* 2007; **357**(14): 1382–92.

39. Tariot PN, Cummings JL, Katz IR, Mintzer J, Perdomo CA, Schwam EM *et al*. A randomized, double-blind, placebo-controlled study of the efficacy and safety of donepezil in patients with Alzheimer's disease in the nursing home setting. *J Am Geriatr Soc* 2001; **49**(12): 1590–9.

40. Cummings JL, Schneider E, Tariot PN, Graham SM. Behavioral effects of memantine in Alzheimer disease patients receiving donepezil treatment. *Neurology* 2006; **67**(1): 57–63.

41. Pollock BG, Mulsant BH, Rosen J, Sweet RA, Mazumdar S, Bharucha A *et al*. Comparison of citalopram, perphenazine and placebo for the acute treatment of psychosis and behavioral disturbances in hospitalized, demented patients. *Am J Psychiatry* 2002; **159**(3): 460–5.

42. Pollock BG, Mulsant BH, Rosen J, Mazumdar S, Blakesley RE, Houck PR *et al*. A double-blind comparison of citalopram and risperidone for the treatment of behavioral and psychotic symptoms associated with dementia. *Am J Geriatr Psychiatry* 2007; **15**(11): 942–52.

43. Lanctot KL, Herrmann N, Van Reekum R, Eryavec G, Naranjo CA. Gender, aggression and serotonergic function are associated with response to sertraline for behavioral disturbances in Alzheimer's disease. *Int J Geriatr Psychiatry* 2002; **17**(6): 531–41.

44. Finkel SI, Mintzer JE, Dysken M, Krishnan KR, Burt T, McRae T. A randomized, placebo-controlled study of the efficacy and safety of sertraline in the treatment of the behavioral manifestations of Alzheimer's disease in outpatients treated with donepezil. *Int J Geriatr Psychiatry* 2004; **19**(1): 9–18.

45. Olafsson K, Jorgensen S, Jensen HV, Bille A, Arup P andersen J. Fluvoxamine in the treatment of demented elderly patients: a double-blind, placebo-controlled study. *Acta Psychiatr Scand* 1992; **85**(6): 453–6.

46. Levkovitz Y, Bloch Y, Kaplan D, Diskin A, Abramovitchi I. Fluvoxamine for psychosis in Alzheimer's disease. *J Nerv Ment Dis* 2001; **189**(2): 126–9.

47. Sultzer DL, Gray KF, Gunay I, Berisford MA, Mahler ME. A double-blind comparison of trazodone and haloperidol for treatment of agitation in patients with dementia. *Am J Geriatr Psychiatry* 1997; **5**(1): 60–9.

48. Sultzer DL, Gray KF, Gunay I, Wheatley MV, Mahler ME. Does behavioral improvement with haloperidol or trazodone treatment depend on psychosis or mood symptoms in patients with dementia? *J Am Geriatr Soc* 2001; **49**(10): 1294–300.

49. Teri L, Logsdon RG, Peskind E, Raskind M, Weiner MF, Tractenberg RE *et al*. Treatment of agitation in AD: a randomized, placebo-controlled clinical trial. *Neurology* 2000; **55**(9): 1271–8.

50. Cummings JL, Tractenberg RE, Gamst A, Teri L, Masterman D, Thal LJ. Regression to the mean: implications for clinical trials of psychotropic agents in dementia. *Curr Alzheimer Res* 2004; **1**(4): 323–8.

51. Lebert F, Stekke W, Hasenbroekx C, Pasquier F. Frontotemporal dementia: a randomised, controlled trial with trazodone. *Dement Geriatr Cogn Disord* 2004; **17**(4): 355–9.

52. Porsteinsson AP, Tariot PN, Erb R, Cox C, Smith E, Jakimovich L *et al*. Placebo-controlled study of divalproex sodium for agitation in dementia. *Am J Geriatr Psychiatry* 2001; **9**(1): 58–66.

53. Sival RC, Haffmans PM, Jansen PA, Duursma SA, Eikelenboom P. Sodium valproate in the treatment of aggressive behavior in patients with dementia – a randomized placebo controlled clinical trial. *Int J Geriatr Psychiatry* 2002; **17**(6): 579–85.

54. Tariot PN, Raman R, Jakimovich L, Schneider L, Porsteinsson A, Thomas R *et al*. Divalproex sodium in nursing home residents with possible or probable Alzheimer's disease complicated by agitation: a randomized, controlled trial. *Am J Geriatr Psychiatry* 2005; **13**(11): 942–9.

55. Herrmann N, Lanctot KL, Rothenburg LS, Eryavec G. A placebo-controlled trial of valproate for agitation and aggression in Alzheimer's disease. *Dement Geriatr Cogn Disord* 2007; **23**(2): 116–19.

56. Profenno LA, Jakimovich L, Holt CJ, Porsteinsson A, Tariot PN. A randomized, double-blind, placebo-controlled pilot trial of safety and tolerability of two doses of divalproex sodium in outpatients with probable Alzheimer's disease. *Curr Alzheimer Res* 2005; **2**(5): 553–8.

57. Tariot PN, Erb R, Podgorski CA, Cox C, Patel S, Jakimovich L *et al*. Efficacy and tolerability of carbamazepine for agitation and aggression in dementia. *Am J Psychiatry* 1998; **155**(1): 54–61.

58. Olin JT, Fox LS, Pawluczyk S, Taggart NA, Schneider LS. A pilot randomized trial of carbamazepine for behavioral symptoms in treatment-resistant outpatients with Alzheimer disease. *Am J Geriatr Psychiatry* 2001; **9**(4): 400–5.

59. Meehan KM, Wang H, David SR, Nisivoccia JR, Jones B, Beasley CM, Jr. *et al*. Comparison of rapidly acting intramuscular olanzapine, lorazepam and placebo: a double-blind, randomized study in acutely agitated patients with dementia. *Neuropsychopharmacology* 2002; **26**(4): 494–504.

60. Christensen DB, Benfield WR. Alprazolam as an alternative to low-dose haloperidol in older, cognitively impaired nursing facility patients. *J Am Geriatr Soc* 1998; **46**(5): 620–5.

61. Coccaro EF, Kramer E, Zemishlany Z, Thorne A, Rice CM, 3rd, Giordani B *et al*. Pharmacologic treatment of noncognitive behavioral disturbances in elderly demented patients. *Am J Psychiatry* 1990; **147**(12): 1640–5.

62. Peskind ER, Tsuang DW, Bonner LT, Pascualy M, Riekse RG, Snowden MB *et al*. Propranolol for disruptive behaviors in nursing home residents with probable or possible Alzheimer disease: a placebo-controlled study. *Alzheimer Dis Assoc Disord* 2005; **19**(1): 23–8.

63. Cantillon M, Brunswick R, Molina D, Bahro M. Buspirone vs. haloperidol: A double-blind trial for agitation in a nursing home population with Alzheimer's disease. *Am J Geriatr Psychiatry* 1996; **4**: 263–7.

64. Hall KA, Keks NA, O'Connor DW. Transdermal estrogen patches for aggressive behavior in male patients with dementia: a randomized, controlled trial. *Int Psychogeriatr* 2005; **17**(2): 165–78.

65. Katz IR, Jeste DV, Mintzer JE, Clyde C, Napolitano J, Brecher M. Comparison of risperidone and placebo for psychosis and behavioral disturbances associated with dementia: a randomized, double-blind trial. Risperidone Study Group. *J Clin Psychiatry* 1999; **60**(2): 107–15.

66. de Deyn PP, Rabheru K, Rasmussen A, Bocksberger JP, Dautzenberg PL, Eriksson S *et al.* A randomized trial of risperidone, placebo and haloperidol for behavioral symptoms of dementia. *Neurology* 1999; **53**(5): 946–55.

67. Street JS CW, Gannon KS *et al.* Olanzapine treatment of psychotic and behavioral symptoms in patients with Alzheimer disease in nursing care facilities: a double-blind, randomized, placebo-controlled trial. *Arch Gen Psychiatry* 2000; **57**: 968–76.

68. Brodaty H, Ames D, Snowdon J, Woodward M, Kirwan J, Clarnette R *et al.* A randomized placebo-controlled trial of risperidone for the treatment of aggression, agitation and psychosis of dementia. *J Clin Psychiatry* 2003; **64**(2): 134–43.

69. de Deyn PP, Carrasco MM, Deberdt W, Jeandel C, Hay DP, Feldman PD *et al.* Olanzapine versus placebo in the treatment of psychosis with or without associated behavioral disturbances in patients with Alzheimer's disease. *Int J Geriatr Psychiatry* 2004; **19**(2): 115–26.

70. Ballard C, Margallo-Lana M, Juszczak E, Douglas S, Swann A, Thomas A *et al.* Quetiapine and rivastigmine and cognitive decline in Alzheimer's disease: randomised double blind placebo controlled trial. *BMJ* 2005; **330**(7496): 874.

71. Deberdt WG, Dysken MW, Rappaport SA, Feldman PD, Young CA, Hay DP *et al.* Comparison of olanzapine and risperidone in the treatment of psychosis and associated behavioral disturbances in patients with dementia. *Am J Geriatr Psychiatry* 2005; **13**(8): 722–30.

72. De Deyn P, Jeste DV, Swanink R, Kostic D, Breder C, Carson WH *et al.* Aripiprazole for the treatment of psychosis in patients with Alzheimer's disease: a randomized, placebo-controlled study. *J Clin Psychopharmacol* 2005; **25**(5): 463–7.

73. Mintzer J, Greenspan A, Caers I, Van Hove I, Kushner S, Weiner M *et al.* Risperidone in the treatment of psychosis of Alzheimer disease: results from a prospective clinical trial. *Am J Geriatr Psychiatry* 2006; **14**(3): 280–91.

74. Tariot PN, Schneider L, Katz IR, Mintzer JE, Street J, Copenhaver M *et al.* Quetiapine treatment of psychosis associated with dementia: a double-blind, randomized, placebo-controlled clinical trial. *Am J Geriatr Psychiatry* 2006; **14**(9): 767–76.

75. Zhong KX, Tariot PN, Mintzer J, Minkwitz MC, Devine NA. Quetiapine to treat agitation in dementia: a randomized, double-blind, placebo-controlled study. *Curr Alzheimer Res* 2007; **4**(1): 81–93.

76. Kurlan R, Cummings J, Raman R, Thal L. Quetiapine for agitation or psychosis in patients with dementia and parkinsonism. *Neurology* 2007; **68**(17): 1356–63.

77. Mintzer JE, Tune LE, Breder CD, Swanink R, Marcus RN, McQuade RD *et al.* Aripiprazole for the treatment of psychoses in institutionalized patients with Alzheimer dementia: a multicenter, randomized, double-blind, placebo-controlled assessment of three fixed doses. *Am J Geriatr Psychiatry* 2007; **15**(11): 918–31.

78. Paleacu D, Barak Y, Mirecky I, Mazeh D. Quetiapine treatment for behavioural and psychological symptoms of dementia in Alzheimer's disease patients: a 6-week, double-blind, placebo-controlled study. *Int J Geriatr Psychiatry* 2008; **23**(4): 393–400.

79. Streim JE, Porsteinsson AP, Breder CD, Swanink R, Marcus R, McQuade R *et al.* A randomized, double-blind, placebo-controlled study of aripiprazole for the treatment of psychosis in nursing home patients with Alzheimer disease. *Am J Geriatr Psychiatry* 2008; **16**(7): 537–50.

54

Behavioural Management: Non-Pharmacological

Jiska Cohen-Mansfield

George Washington University Medical Center and School of Public Health, Washington DC, USA
Tel Aviv University Herczeg Institute on Aging and Sackler Faculty of Medicine, Tel-Aviv, Israel

The discussion of non-pharmacological interventions to treat dementia has increased in recent years. Such interventions can be used to reduce agitation and problem behaviours, enhance affect, cognition and activities of daily living (ADL), and reduce delusions and hallucinations. These interventions most often change the physical and social environment of the person with dementia by improving the level and quality of stimulation in the environment, providing social contact, or adapting the environment to increase comfort and ease in daily activities. In this way, non-pharmacological interventions can address unmet needs of persons with dementia and enhance their quality of life.

THEORETICAL FRAMEWORKS

Several theoretical frameworks describe the manifestations of the behavioural, affective, cognitive and psychotic impairments associated with dementia from an environmental and psychosocial perspective. Three such theories that explain behaviour problems are the behavioural model, the environmental vulnerability model and the unmet needs model. Some of the theories that explain affect include the learned helplessness model and the reduced reinforcement model. There are also various theories relating pain and loneliness to affect. Each theoretical framework has different implications for intervention.

Behaviour

The behavioural model states that a problem behaviour is controlled by its antecedents and consequences. Antecedents include triggers that initiate the behaviour, such as the view of the exit door eliciting an attempt to exit the institution; consequences refer to the reaction to the behaviour, such as when screaming is followed by attention from staff members, a response that reinforces the screaming behaviour. Alternatively, the environmental vulnerability model asserts that dementia results in an increased vulnerability to the environment, which leads to a lower threshold at which stimuli affect behaviour. A stimulus that may elicit an appropriate response in a person without cognitive impairment, such as a movie or magazine, may overwhelm a person with cognitive impairment and therefore generate an inappropriate behaviour. This model is based on the concepts of person–environment congruence[1] and the environment-behavioural model, which suggest that, for optimal functioning, a

match is needed between the person's needs and abilities and the demands of the environment as they relate to those needs and abilities. A related concept is that dementia results in a progressively lowered stress threshold[2]. Accordingly, persons with dementia progressively lose their coping abilities, and therefore perceive their environment as increasingly stressful. Since their threshold for tolerating this stress is also decreasing, anxiety and inappropriate behaviour can result as environmental stimuli exceed the person's stress threshold.

According to the unmet needs model, a person with dementia has difficulty meeting his/her needs because of a decreased ability to communicate needs and provide for oneself. The loss in the ability to communicate and perform tasks. The combination of the loss of ability to communicate and perform tasks, inability to effectively utilize the environment, and deficiencies in individualizing care results in unmet needs[3,4]. Problem behaviours emerge as an attempt to meet or to communicate those needs.

The different models are not mutually exclusive and may be complementary. An environmental vulnerability may make the person who suffers from dementia more susceptible to environmental antecedents and consequences. The environmental vulnerability may also produce an unmet need when normal levels of stimulation are perceived as over-stimulation. Furthermore, different models may account for different behaviours in different people.

Affect

Depressed affect has been conceptualized as resulting from lack of control and a sense of helplessness, from insufficient level of control over one's environment[5], or from an insufficient level of reinforcing activities, i.e. pleasurable experiences[6]. Depressed affect has also been linked to loneliness[7] and to physical pain.

Delusions/Hallucinations

Delusions can represent a misinterpretation of reality, which may stem from actual environmental changes for which the person is not adequately prepared. This may be the case when an older person becomes frightened by a caregiver who comes to get her dressed, and whom the older person may perceive as a total stranger. Hallucinations have been associated with visual impairments, and may therefore represent a natural reaction to sensory deprivation[8].

Principles and Practice of Geriatric Psychiatry, 3rd edn. Edited by Mohammed T. Abou-Saleh, Cornelius Katona and Anand Kumar
© 2011 John Wiley & Sons, Ltd

INTERVENTIONS

The following describes non-pharmacological interventions used for alleviating behavioural, affective, cognitive and psychotic symptoms of dementia.

Behavioural

Interventions for behavioural problems that are based on the unmet needs model most often focus on three types of unmet needs: need for social support and contact, need for stimulation and activities, and need for relief from discomfort. At the most basic level, providing social support and contact involves talking to persons with dementia, even if the caregiver conducts the majority of the conversation. One-on-one interaction is a potent intervention that can be performed by relatives, paid caregivers or volunteers. Alternatively, simulated social interventions can be useful when live social contact is not available; such interventions include videotapes of family members[9], simulated presence therapy[10], in which an audiotape of a family member's side of a telephone conversation is played repeatedly to the person with dementia, or commercially produced interaction videos for persons with dementia, in which viewers are invited to sing along to familiar music or to remember past events. Training staff members to view all interactions with those in their care (such as during ADL) as opportunities for social contact is also an opportunity to provide social support.

Pet therapy is another option[11], which may include visits with dogs, cats or fish, or simulated pet therapy using plush stuffed animals or robotic pets[12]. In addition to interaction with the animal, pet therapy provides a topic for interaction with other people. Dolls have also been used to simulate companions/babies, and massage may be an effective mechanism for social contact with non-verbal persons with advanced dementia.

In order to address the need for activity or stimulation, many different types of activities or stimuli have been used. Stimulation includes music, aromatherapy, touch therapy, 'Snoezelen' programmes, massages and white noise. Structured activities, such as manipulation of objects, sorting, cooking, sewing and sensory interventions, may be helpful. Montessori-based activities are a set of activities based on Maria Montessori's principles[13], such as task breakdown, immediate feedback, and use of everyday, real-world materials. Other options for activities include exercise, art therapy, including drawing and painting, where participants can express themselves by choosing colours and themes, and adaptations of ADL, like setting the table or cooking.

Activities can include cognitive tasks that can be done individually or within a group. Group examples include 'Question Asking Readings', in which a group reads a script accompanied by questions typed on cards that encourage participants to discuss related topics. Another group memory task is memory bingo, a game in which participants match beginnings and endings of popular sayings, which can also stimulate group discussion[14]. Individual cognitive tasks involve sorting cards or objects by category.

An alternative to addressing the need for stimulation by providing stimuli is to accommodate the behaviour that provides activity and stimulation. For example, interventions for accommodating pacing or wandering behaviour include outdoor walks[15] and the use of wandering areas[16]. Inappropriate handling or the constant manipulation of objects can be accommodated by providing appropriate materials, such as books and pamphlets for handling, or activity aprons (aprons that have buttons, zippers and other articles sewn on) as appropriate and safe items for persons to handle. Similarly, rocking chairs and gliding swings have been used to accommodate restless behaviour and provide more acceptable stimulation.

Regarding relief of discomfort, interventions such as pain management, light therapy to improve sleep, and reduction of discomfort by improved seating or positioning and removal of physical restraints have all been related to improvement in behaviour. Changes in the methods and environment of providing ADL have also been associated with reduction in inappropriate behaviours. For example, tape recordings and pictures of birds, flowing water and small animals in baths as well as offering food during bathing have been associated with a decrease of agitated behaviours during bathing. Person-centred showering and towel baths resulted in decreased agitation in comparison with usual bathing routines[17].

In order to provide for the unmet needs of the person with dementia, caregivers need to understand the needs and how to address them. Staff training is a category of non-pharmacological interventions, which includes training in skills such as communication and providing assistance in ADL, or in techniques to handle inappropriate behaviours. Many such programmes focus on improved understanding of the older person and the impact of dementia. Person-centred care and the use of dementia care mapping are care principles that have been associated with decreased levels of behaviour problems[18]. Changing caregiver behaviour through training is, however, a complex and difficult challenge, and often requires ongoing instruction, modeling, monitoring, feedback and support of the caregiver. Therefore, in institutional settings, staff training is closely tied to management.

The most common intervention based on the behavioural theoretical framework is differential reinforcement, which changes the contingencies that are supposed to maintain or reinforce the behaviour. This consists of positive reinforcement contingent on non-agitated behaviour, such as moving the person to a quiet area when agitated for time out, or restriction, where the person is denied goods (e.g. cigarettes), activities or access to a location or another person when agitated. In contrast, reinforcement is provided when not agitated.

The interventions based on the environmental vulnerability theoretical framework include reduced stimulation units, which aim to eliminate the stimuli that, according to the theory, activate the low stress threshold and result in the problem behaviours. These units have been modified to appear less obstructive to those with dementia. They typically have small group sizes at tables for eating and small groups for activities, neutral colours on pictures and walls, no televisions, radios or telephones (except for emergencies), an educational programme for staff and visitors concerning the use of touch, eye contact and slow, soft speech, use of quiet voices by staff at all times, and a consistent daily routine[19].

Affect

Based on the theoretical model of learned helplessness, interventions to decrease depressed affect focus on increasing the older person's sense of control, such as allowing the person to make his/her own decisions about meals or clothes or to care for a plant. The intervention approach based on the alternative theoretical framework of reduced reinforcing events is that of providing older persons with pleasant activities, individualized to the preferences of each person[20]. Loneliness is highly correlated with depressed affect, and social interventions described above, including both live and simulated social activities, are also appropriate for improving affect. Group activities can also be used as vehicles to promote social contacts. Additionally, combined interventions that merge outdoor experience with social contact, such as combining a wheelchair bicycle with small-group activity therapy and one-to-one bike rides with a staff member, have been applied to reduce depression in nursing home residents[21].

Self-affirming interventions also target improving affect. These include reminiscence therapy, which encourages persons with dementia to talk about their pasts, and may utilize audiovisual aids, such as old family photos and objects. Reminiscence can enhance individuals' sense of identity, sense of worth or general well-being[22], and may also stimulate memory processes. Validation therapy, in which a therapist accepts the disorientation of a person with dementia and validates his or her feelings, can improve affect by acceptance rather than rejection of the experiences of the person with dementia[23].

Cognition

Several cognitive principles underlie cognitive interventions for persons with dementia. These include: (i) long-term memory is usually maintained better than short-term memory; (ii) procedural memory remains more intact than declarative memory; and (iii) new learning is possible in dementia and is achieved through the same principles as other memory, but often requires more aids or repetition. Cognitive interventions have been used to improve general cognitive function or the performance of specific tasks. Interventions for improving general cognitive function include memory training[24], maintaining lifelong habits that have been over-learned through long-term practice, general problem solving, use of mnemonic devices, word games and puzzles, computer programs with cognitive exercises, and/or the use of external memory aids such as notebooks, lists, calendars or alarms. Computer-based memory training has the advantage of adapting to the level of the older person and to the type of cognitive stimulation most needed[25]. Physical exercise has also been shown to have a positive effect on cognitive performance in older adults with dementia[26]. For persons with more advanced cognitive impairment, reality orientation has been used, where staff members present orienting information such as information about time, place and person, usually in a group setting[27].

The use of cognitive interventions for more specific procedures often includes procedural memory training, using spaced-retrieval (a procedure where a task, such as placing the walker in a specific location, is learned through repetition over increasingly longer retention intervals[28]), cueing and similar techniques. In the later stages of dementia, memory books, which contain autobiographical, daily schedule and problem resolution information, can assist with communication[29]. Technological aids, such as the use of electronic memory devices or environmental sensors[30], are expected to play an increasing role in the future as prostheses for cognitive losses.

FUNCTION

Non-pharmacological interventions to improve function often include environmental interventions and task simplification. These are used to optimize the performance of activities of daily living by adjusting the surroundings (including physical access, temperature, colour, furniture, wall design and cues) to facilitate the activity for both patient and caregiver. The extent of environmental adaptation varies, from decreasing clutter to providing grab bars or handrails. As a means to decrease the risk of falling, lowering bed height, placing mattresses on the floor, using hip protectors, improving light on the way to the bathroom, and improving call systems have been used. Enhanced visibility of toilets increased their utilization[31], and eating behaviour improved with better light and increased contrast between plates and the table[32].

An alternative intervention is task simplification or cognitive prosthesis, which utilizes task breakdown, enhanced instruction, modeling, rehearsal, cueing and gradual approximations of a task. The notion of simplifying tasks can also be applied across daily activities, such as by providing consistency in caregiver assignment, which helps orient older persons across different tasks. A combination of these interventions and others has been included in occupational therapy interventions to enhance function in dementia[33].

Delusions/Hallucinations

Non-pharmacological interventions for psychotic symptoms are based on the understanding of the aetiology of the symptom.

- *Misinterpretation of stimuli or reality*. At times, the diagnosed 'delusion' or 'hallucination' is triggered by an environmental stimulus. For example, a loudspeaker system may sound like voices from outside or an image seen through a mirror may be interpreted as someone being in the room. This is facilitated by the combination of sensory deficits and cognitive limitations that occur with dementia giving rise to an incorrect interpretation of an initially vague or unclear stimulus. Interventions to minimize this confusion would most often remove or change the stimulus so as not to elicit the mistaken interpretation. Delusion can also be a representation of reality. Examples are delusions of theft, as theft is common in many nursing homes, or the delusions of abandonment that may occur when a person enters a nursing home. Whether this feeling reflects reality from the point of view of the caregiver is irrelevant, as the move into a strange environment represents abandonment from the point of view of the person with dementia. The goal of interventions to alleviate this feeling is to re-establish trust in the relationship. Older persons may eventually change their perceptions when they become comfortable with their care and when they sense consistent caring by the family, such as with social contact (real or simulated, described above), which may provide a sense of love and familiarity, thus countering the feelings of abandonment and betrayal.
- *Delusion as confabulation in the face of memory loss*. Many delusions are misinterpretations of actual events in the environment. When a person with dementia complains that an object has been stolen, she may be forgetting where she has placed her personal belongings and interpreting her inability to find them as theft. A number of potential solutions can be offered to older persons, including marking personal belongings in clear ways so that they are easily identifiable, attaching a finder such as a KeyRinger™ to a personal belonging, or purchasing multiple inexpensive copies of personal articles so they may be easily replaced when necessary. Similarly, the delusion that a caregiver is an impostor is often the result of an individual's inability to recognize the caregiver. In that case, an intervention should work toward improving the individual's relationship with the caregiver.
- *Other reasons*. Delusions have at times been reported to result from delirium associated with acute medical conditions that should be treated, or from bright light therapy, which, in those cases, should be removed. Delusions have also been linked to depressed

affect in many studies[34,35]. It is unclear whether the delusions lead to depression or the depression leads to delusions (e.g., through inactivity and isolation), or if both are caused by other factors. Depression may be controlled by treating the depression non-pharmacologically, as described above.

- *Pleasant 'psychotic symptoms'*. At times hallucinations are pleasurable. Some people talk with deceased relatives and derive happiness from these encounters. If a person seems to enjoy such hallucinations and does not suffer any ill effects, an optimal intervention may be to explain this situation to caregivers in a manner that will make the practice acceptable to them.
- *Visual and auditory problems/sensory deprivation*. Hallucinations are more likely to occur in persons with visual problems[8,35,36], and may be linked to sensory deprivation[37]. Additionally, there is evidence that in the absence of the stimulation of sensory areas by external objects, people may experience hallucinations[38]. Correction of visual problems through medical intervention or through aids such as eyeglasses, enhanced contrast, larger type/object or improved lighting is a first step in addressing hallucinations among persons with visual impairments. To the extent that sensory deprivation may be a contributing cause of hallucinations, sensory stimulation, such as music, massage and aromatherapy, may be beneficial.
- *Cultural differences between caregivers and persons with dementia*. Some behaviours perceived by caregivers as psychotic symptoms may actually be culturally based, such as 'talking' to the dead or singing, or praying in a loud voice.

INDIVIDUALIZATION OF INTERVENTIONS

A crucial principle in applying non-pharmacological interventions to persons with dementia is that of individualizing these interventions to fit the person's needs and abilities. Some of the dimensions to consider in tailoring interventions are listed below:

1. Current and past sense of identity, which usually include some retained aspects of previously held identities, such as work role, family relationship or preference for a certain type of leisure activity.
2. Current sensory abilities, which include visual, auditory, smell and touch modalities. Mechanisms for augmentation of sensory abilities should be explored, including simple ones, such as better fitting eyeglasses, an auditory amplifier, better fitting hearing aids etc.
3. An enhanced understanding of current needs, including social contact of any kind, longing for family, for daytime activity, for stimulation, for physical exercise or for a specific meaningful activity, such as helping or working.
4. Cognitive and communication abilities.

EFFICACY OF INTERVENTIONS

Many reviews have tried to clarify the evidence regarding the efficacy of non-pharmacological interventions, despite many methodological and other difficulties in the research in this area[39-43]. Many non-pharmacological approaches resulted in a statistically and clinically meaningful improvement in the manifestation of behaviour problems, function and affect. With few exceptions, most studies are small and have methodological problems, often due to insufficient funding. There are, however, some larger studies

that used valid comparison groups and showed the efficacy of non-pharmacological approaches[44]. For some areas, however, such as delusions and hallucinations, no studies were found regarding the efficacy of non-pharmacological approaches. While results vary, non-pharmacological approaches to intervention are a promising option when treating specific symptoms and when aiming to improve quality of life in dementia.

PREREQUISITES AND BARRIERS TO THE PRACTICE OF INTERVENTIONS

The actual utilization of non-pharmacological interventions in dementia falls far short of its potential. A number of systemic issues are responsible for this gap. Funding is lacking both for the practice of non-pharmacological interventions and for the acquisition of knowledge about these through systematic research. The commonly used alternative intervention of psychoactive medication is reimbursed, and the underlying structure for its delivery, including physicians, medicine aids, pharmacies, and monitoring and quality control systems, is largely in place. In contrast, the provision of non-pharmacological interventions is generally not reimbursed, and a system for providing them is often absent. Similarly, funding for non-pharmacological research is limited, because, unlike pharmacological interventions, there is no financial entity that is likely to benefit financially from this knowledge. Such limited funding results in many of the studies on these interventions having small samples and other methodological limitations, further limiting the faith in this approach and the willingness to fund it.

Yet, the most obvious barrier to the implementation of the non-pharmacological approaches described is that the current structure of care does not promote such non-pharmacological assessment and intervention. In most cases, the physician prescribes antipsychotic or antidepressant medication based on informant reports. No one in the care system is currently responsible for assessing, observing and analysing inappropriate behaviour or psychotic symptoms in order to determine their aetiology and their impact on individuals' lives. Thus, clinicians most often do not witness the event and do not have the ability to verify or question the interpretation of the diagnosis. The ability of caregivers to provide non-pharmacological interventions is further limited by lack of staff member knowledge, insufficient staffing levels and insufficient support within and outside the care situation. In order to provide non-pharmacological interventions for dementia, the system of care needs to promote an atmosphere and practice of caring that goes beyond what is currently available in most care settings. Attentive listening and observation are needed to differentiate between the various needs expressed by behavioural and psychotic symptoms. Knowledge of the disease, as well as of specific symptoms and their aetiology, meaning and management, will allow caregivers to better understand the individual's behaviours rather than attributing them to resistance, difficult personality, malicious intent, craziness or indifference. Compassion and empathy by caregivers allow them to better understand the needs of the person with dementia and to clarify appropriate avenues for interventions. In order to allow alternative interventions, the system of care needs to promote autonomy and respect for the person with dementia and to maximize flexibility in procedures for caregiver and care-receiver alike. A transformation in the system of care is therefore needed in order to allow an optimal use of non-pharmacological interventions to promote quality of life for persons with dementia.

REFERENCES

1. Kahana E. A congruence model of person–environment interaction. In Lawton MP, Windley PG, Byerts TO (eds), *Aging and the Environment: Theoretical Approaches*. New York: Springer, 1982, 97–121.
2. Hall GR. Caring for people with Alzheimer's disease using the conceptual model of progressively lowered stress threshold in the clinical setting. *Nurs Clin North Am* 1994; **29**(1): 129–41.
3. Cohen-Mansfield J, Werner P. Environmental influences on agitation: an integrative summary of an observational study. *Am J Alzheimers Care Relat Disord Res* 1995; **10**(1): 32–7.
4. Cohen-Mansfield J, Deutsch L. Agitation: subtypes and their mechanisms. *Semin Clin Neuropsychiatry* 1996; **1**(4): 325–39.
5. Seligman MEP. *Helplessness: On Depression, Development, and Death*. San Francisco, CA: WH Freeman, 1975.
6. Lewinsohn PM, Youngren MA. The symptoms of depression. *Compr Ther* 1976; **2**(8): 62–9.
7. Cohen-Mansfield J, Parpura-Gill A. Loneliness in elderly persons: a theoretical model and empirical findings. *Int Psychogeriatr* 2007; **19**(2): 279–94.
8. Cohen-Mansfield J. Nonpharmacologic interventions for psychotic symptoms in dementia. *J Geriatr Psychiatry Neurol* 2003; **16**(4): 219–24.
9. Cohen-Mansfield J, Werner P. Management of verbally disruptive behaviors in nursing home residents. *J Gerontol A Biol Sci Med Sci* 1997; **52A**(6): M369–77.
10. Camberg L, Woods P, Ooi WL *et al.* Evaluation of simulated presence: a personalized approach to enhance well-being in persons with Alzheimer's disease. *J Am Geriatr Soc* 1999; **47**(4): 446–52.
11. Churchill M, Safaoui J, McCabe B, Baun M. Using a therapy dog to alleviate the agitation and desocialization of people with Alzheimer's disease. *J Psychosoc Nurs Ment Health Serv* 1999; **37**(4): 16–24.
12. Libin A, Cohen-Mansfield J. Therapeutic robocat for nursing home residents with dementia: preliminary inquiry. *Am J Alzheimers Dis Other Demen* 2004; **19**(2): 111–16.
13. Camp C, Cohen-Mansfield J, Capezuti E. Nonpharmacological interventions for dementia: enhancing and maintaining mental health in long-term care residents. *Psychiatr Serv* 2002; **53**(11): 1397–1404.
14. Camp CJ, Foss JW, O'Hanlon AM, Stevens AB. Memory interventions for persons with dementia. *Appl Cogn Psychol* 1996; **10**(3): 193–210.
15. Cohen-Mansfield J, Werner P. Visits to an outdoor garden: impact on behavior and mood of nursing home residents who pace. In Vellas B, Fitten J, Frisoni G (eds), *Research and Practice in Alzheimer's Disease*. Paris: Serdi, 1998, 419–36.
16. Cohen-Mansfield J. Outdoor wandering parks for persons with dementia. *J Housing Elderly* 2007; **21**(1/2): 35–53.
17. Sloane PD, Hoeffer B, Mitchell CM *et al.* Effect of person-centered showering and the towel bath on bathing-associated aggression, agitation, and discomfort in nursing home residents with dementia: a randomized, controlled trial. *J Am Geriatr Soc* 2004; **52**(11): 1795–804.
18. Chenoweth L, King MT, Jeon YH *et al.* Caring for aged dementia care resident study (CADRES) of person-centered care, dementia-care mapping, and usual care in dementia: cluster-randomised trial. *Lancet Neurol* 2009; **8**(4): 317–25.
19. Cleary TA, Clamon C, Price M, Shullaw G. A reduced stimulation unit: effects on patients with Alzheimer's disease and related disorders. *Gerontologist* 1988; **28**(4): 511–14.
20. Teri L, Logsdon RG, Uomoto J, McCurry SM. Behavioral treatment of depression in dementia patients: a controlled clinical trial. *J Gerontol B Psychol Sci Soc Sci* 1997; **52B**(4): 159–66.
21. Buettner LL, Fitzsimmons S. AD-venture program: therapeutic biking for the treatment of depression in long-term care residents with dementia. *Am J Alzheimers Dis Other Demen* 2002; **17**(2): 121–7.
22. Brooker D, Duce L. Wellbeing and activity in dementia: a comparison of group reminiscence therapy, structured goal-directed group activity and unstructured time. *Aging Ment Health* 2000; **4**(4): 354–8.
23. Feil N. *Validation: The Feil Method*. Cleveland, OH: Feil Productions, 1982.
24. Spector A, Thorgrimsen L, Woods B *et al.* Efficacy of an evidence-based cognitive stimulation therapy programme for people with dementia: randomised controlled trial. *Br J Psychiatry* 2003; **183**: 248–54.
25. Galante E, Venturini G, Fiaccadori C. Computer-based cognitive intervention for dementia: preliminary results of a randomized clinical trial. *G Ital Med Lav Ergon* 2007; **29**(3 suppl B): B26–32.
26. Heyn P, Abreu BC, Ottenbacher KJ. The effects of exercise training on elderly persons with cognitive impairment and dementia: a meta-analysis. *Arch Phys Med Rehabil* 2004; **85**: 1694–704.
27. Zanetti O, Oriani M, Geroldi C *et al.* Predictors of cognitive improvement after reality orientation in Alzheimer's disease. *Age Ageing* 2002; **31**(3): 193–6.
28. Cherry KE, Hawley KS, Jackson EM, Boudreaux EO. Booster sessions enhance the long-term effectiveness of spaced retrieval in older adults with probable Alzheimer's disease. *Behav Modif* 2009; **33**(3): 295–313.
29. Bourgeois M, Dijkstra K, Burgio L, Allen-Burge R. Memory aids as an augmentative and alternative communication strategy for nursing home residents with dementia. *Augment Altern Commun* 2001; **17**(3): 196–210.
30. Cohen-Mansfield J, Creedon MA, Malone TB *et al.* Electronic memory aids for community dwelling elderly persons: attitudes, preferences, and potential utilization. *J Appl Gerontol* 2005; **24**(1): 3–20.
31. Namazi KH, Johnson BD. Environmental effects on incontinence problems in Alzheimer's disease patients. *Am J Alzheimer's Care Rel Dis Res* 1991; **6**(6): 16–21.
32. Koss E, Gilmore GC. Environmental interventions and functional ability of AD patients. Vellas B, Fritten J, Frisoni G, eds, *Research and Practice in Alzheimer's Disease*. Paris, France: Serdi, 1998.
33. Graff MJ, Vernooij-Dassen MJ, Thijssen M *et al.* Community based occupational therapy for patients with dementia and their care givers: randomised controlled trial. *Br Med J* 2007; **62**: 1002–9.
34. Bassiony MM, Warren A, Rosenblatt A *et al.* The relationship between delusions and depression in Alzheimer's disease. *Int J Geriatr Psychiatry* 2002; **17**(6): 549–56.
35. Cohen-Mansfield J, Taylor L, Werner P. Delusions and hallucinations in an adult day care population: a longitudinal study. *Am J Geriatr Psychiatry* 1998; **6**(2): 104–21.

36. Forsell Y. Predictors for depression, anxiety and psychotic symptoms in a very elderly population: data from a 3-year follow-up study. *Soc Psychiatry Psychiatr Epidemiol* 2000; **35**(6): 259–63.

37. Holroyd S, Sheldon-Keller A. A study of visual hallucinations in Alzheimer's disease. *Am J Geriatr Psychiatry* 1996; **3**(3): 198–205.

38. Zubek JP, Pushkar DSW, Gowing J. Perceptual changes after prolonged sensory isolation (darkness and silence). *Can J Psychol* 1961; **15**(2): 83–100.

39. Cohen-Mansfield J. Nonpharmacologic interventions for inappropriate behaviors in dementia: a review, summary, and critique. *Am J Geriatr Psychiatry* 2001; **9**(4): 361–81.

40. Zec RF, Burkett NR. Non-pharmacological and pharmacological treatment of the cognitive and behavioral symptoms of Alzheimer's disease. *NeuroRehabilitation* 2008; **23**(5): 425–38.

41. Overshott R, Byrne J, Burns A. Nonpharmacological and pharmacological interventions for symptoms in Alzheimer's disease. *Expert Rev Neurother* 2004; **4**(5): 809–21.

42. Acevedo A, Loewenstein DA. Nonpharmacological cognitive interventions in aging and dementia. *J Geriatr Psychiatry Neurol* 2007; **20**(4): 239–49.

43. O'Connor DW, Ames D, Gardner B, King M. Psychosocial treatments of psychological symptoms in dementia: a systematic review of reports meeting quality standards. *Int Psychogeriatr* 2009; **21**(2): 242–51.

44. Cohen-Mansfield J, Libin A, Marx MS. Non-pharmacological treatment of agitation: a controlled trial of systematic individualized intervention. *J Gerontol A Biol Sci Med Sci* 2007; **62A**(8): 908–16.

55

Emerging Applications of Gene and Somatic Cell Therapy in Geriatric Neuropsychiatry

Eric Wexler

David Geffen School of Medicine at UCLA, Los Angeles, USA

'Men do not quit playing because they grow old; they grow old because they quit playing.'

Oliver Wendell Holmes

INTRODUCTION

Startling advances in medicine have extended our lives and given us healthier bodies, but not healthier minds. The mere fact that we are living longer consigns more of us to enduring our final years ravaged by diseases like Alzheimer's or stroke, and suffering all the psychiatric manifestations that are part and parcel of these diseases. Currently available treatments do little. Therapies that replace the damaged brain tissue, either by regeneration or by transplantation, are needed. Unfortunately, both a poor theoretical understanding of neuronal generation/regeneration, and a lack of practical tools to effectively deliver these genes to the right cells, in the right amounts, continue to hamper the field of regenerative medicine. Similarly, harnessing the therapeutic potential of stem cell transplants remains a promise unfulfilled because neural stem cells (NSCs) simply do not function properly when transplanted into regions other than those that normally support adult neurogenesis. Worse yet, even those few privileged environments that normally support neurogenesis are rendered inhospitable to newly implanted NSCs by many of the same conditions that make someone a candidate for neural transplantation in the first place.

The idea of transplanting neurons to repair damaged brain is not new; the first trials, using foetal tissue, in Parkinson's patients were performed more than two decades ago. Initial optimism gave way to the harsh reality that this was not the cure many had hoped for. Many hypothesized that more mature cells simply had lost the ability to learn how to adapt to their new host environment. Naturally, waves of enthusiasm have heralded discoveries from foetal NSCs to human embryonic stem cells (hESCs), with their uncanny pluripotency. Still, somatic cell therapy remains an elusive prospect because transplanted cells do not properly engraft, either failing to properly differentiate, dying or not integrating into the local circuitry. Developing therapies that provide real clinical improvement requires leveraging our new-found appreciation of the microenvironment within which neurons normally develop.

Since the field of neural repair remains in its infancy, any review of this field (including this one) must contain a fair degree of educated

guessing about the future, some of which will turn out to be wrong. To minimize the impact this might have, we will focus on communicating the essentials of current thinking in the field, rather than trying to divine what approach(es) will ultimately be successful. To this end we have broken this chapter down into three sections. The first section aims to supply the reader with a historical understanding of early clinical repair trials, highlighting some of their limitations and questions raised. The second section provides a primer on the regenerative capacity of the adult brain. In this section we introduce the concept of an adult stem cell niche. To the clinician, some of these sections may seem technically dense; we have made every attempt to minimize the use of unnecessary jargon. However, the reader should recognize that an under-appreciation of the importance of the niche goes a long way towards explaining the shortcomings of previous trials. Conversely, understanding how disease or ageing alters the functioning of these microenvironments will be absolutely critical for understanding the rational of any future neuroregenerative therapy trials. The third section introduces the clinical reader to some of the current and emerging tools at the gene therapist's disposal. Finally, we will provide some plausible scenarios where the discussed concepts and tools can be integrated to produce workable future clinical trials. In sum, this chapter should empower the reader with the necessary framework for understanding ongoing developments, rather than trying to divine which approaches will ultimately be successful.

BIRTH OF REGENERATIVE MEDICINE

Molecular strategies for functionally repairing the damaged brain fall into one of three categories: (i) replace/repair circuitry; (ii) potentiate function of remaining cells; and (iii) halt disease progression[1]. The cell replacement strategy has the longest track record with the first foetal neuron transplants being reported in 1989[2]. The lion's share of transplantation trials was performed on patients suffering from either Huntington's or Parkinson's disease. However, the technique has also been applied to patients with macular degeneration, stroke and, most recently approved, children with Batten's disease. More recently, there has been some forays into gene-therapy-based approaches. Below we will review the finding from these previous transplantation trials, with an emphasis on calling out those features that are amenable to improvement in future studies.

Principles and Practice of Geriatric Psychiatry, 3rd edn. Edited by Mohammed T. Abou-Saleh, Cornelius Katona and Anand Kumar
© 2011 John Wiley & Sons, Ltd

Parkinson's Disease

Parkinson's disease (PD) is characterized by relatively selective loss of the dopaminergic neurons in the nigrostriatal tract, though all brain regions are ultimately affected in later stages. Nigrostriatal degeneration results in a well-characterized syndrome of progressive rigidity, bradykinesia, tremors, poor gait/balance, and later dementia in many patients. The first human neural transplants involved unilateral stereotactic injection of mesencephalic dopamine neurons, obtained from 7 to 9 weeks gestational age human foetuses, into the putamen of long-term Parkinson's patients[2–11]. These trials delivered initially encouraging results. Imaging studies (PET or MRI) revealed graft viability and recipients exhibited motor improvement, with reduced medication doses.

Because initial trials were all unblended, concerns over the placebo effect prompted more sophisticated trials. These included sham surgery and blinded rating of imaging results. In a larger trial reported by Freed and colleagues[12] 40 PD patients, ranging in age from 34 to 75 years old, received either embryonic mesencephalic neuroblasts/neurons or sham surgeries and were followed, double-blind, for the succeeding 12 months. They found that although the transplanted cells survived transplantations, the procedure only seemed to clinically benefit younger (younger than 60 years of age) PD patients. Unfortunately, the more carefully this promising therapy was evaluated, the less 'promising' it appeared[13]. Some patients developed uncontrollable dyskinesia, presumably due to aberrant axon regrowth; many showed limited improvement. However, this approach has fallen out of favour because it neither slows disease progression, not is it more effective than aggressive medication, and probably less effective than deep brain stimulation. With a guide to designing future therapies, it is interesting to note that on analysis some transplanted neurons developed Lewy bodies[14,15]. This finding suggests that merely placing new tissue into an inhospitable (deteriorating) brain is not a viable solution. The most recent regenerative trials for PD have focused on changing this environment by providing additional trophic support. Specifically, there have been attempts to augment glial-cell-derived growth factor (GDNF) levels in the striatum, as this protein has shown a significant ability to protect dopaminergic neurons from a variety of experimental insults. The farthest along trial involved direct infusion of GDNF into the putamen[16]. The preliminary results of these studies are again promising, but only time will tell[16–18]. The current trend in PD trials is towards use of adeno-associated virus (AAV) to deliver and induce production of the therapeutic factor (neurturin, a GDNF-like ligand[19]) or enzyme (glutamic acid decarboxylase[20]; aromatic l-amino acid decarboxylase[21]).

Alzheimer's Disease

In constrast to PD, only one group has made any progress towards applying regenerative medicine to Alzheimer's patients. The two trials differed in their technical approach, but shared the goal of delivering nerve growth factor (NGF), a survival factor for cholinergic neurons, to the brain regions suffering cholinergic neuron loss. Using an *ex vivo* gene therapy approach, they implanted fibroblasts that were engineered to secrete NGF[22]. The other study used *in vivo* gene therapy, utilizing AAV to induce local NGF production[23]. The initial results seem promising, but the long-term benefit and safety is an open question.

Huntington's Disease

Huntington's disease (HD) serves as a model neuropsychiatric disorder, despite being a relatively rare disease (7 per 100 000 persons). A toxic gain-of-function mutation (polyglutamine trinucleotide repeat expansion) in the huntingtin protein causes this dominantly inherited movement disorder. Huntingtin is widely expressed throughout the brain, resulting in personality changes or other psychiatric manifestations that may precede overt motor symptoms by almost a decade. However, it is the striking degeneration of the striatum that burdens patients with its characteristic choreoathetoid movements. Eventually, all patients will suffer major psychiatric symptoms, and if they live long enough, dementia will ensue (DSM-IV; 294.1 Dementia Due to Huntington's Disease).

Transplantation trials in HD were contemplated soon after the purported 'success' of foetal neural transplant in PD patients. These open label trials (i.e. no sham surgery) entailed transplantation of committed neuroblasts from foetal human striatum into the brains of moderately affected HD patients[24,25] (and later[26,27]). The results of these trials appeared mixed. Bachoud-Lévi and colleagues reported that on two-year follow-up, three out of five transplant recipients exhibited improvement of both motor and cognitive symptoms[28,29]. These improvements correlated recovery of metabolic activity in the specific striatal location of the transplants, as well as connected regions of the cortex. In contrast, another group following seven patients used PET to examine graft survival. They found evidence of poor graft survival/function. Moreover, they could not demonstrate a significant relationship between changes in PET and clinical function, forcing them to conclude that there was no benefit from transplantation[30].

On longer-term follow-up, Bachoud-Lévi and colleagues found mixed results with regard to improvements in motor symptoms. Among those patients who displayed an improvement at two years, chorea remained stable at an improved level for the following four years[31]. While chorea was improved, dyssomnia became steadily more prominent, paralleling the results in PD transplant trials. More encouraging were their observations of limited cognitive decline among initial responders. They showed no worsening on the Mattis dementia rating scale and only slight worsening on the Trails A. Although the relatively small numbers of these follow-up studies makes it difficult to draw any major conclusions, they suggest that transplants in HD may be more beneficial than in PD. Unlike PD, there are very few pharmacological interventions for HD, making an invasive procedure like cell transplant more appealing. Still, it seems apparent that transplantation is not going to become more pervasive until concomitant neuroprotective treatment becomes available. On a more general cautionary note, there are at least two documented cases of tumour formation among patients who have received cell transplants[32,33], raising the spectre of additional safety concerns.

REGENERATIVE CAPACITY OF ADULT BRAIN

A Brief History of Adult Neurogenesis

For nearly the entire twentieth century the regenerative capacity of the adult brain was considered to be almost nil. It was dogma that the number of neurons in the adult mammalian brain was fixed near birth. This sentiment was reflected by the great neuroanatomist Santiago Ramón y Cajal, who wrote, 'Once development was ended, the fonts of growth and regeneration of the axons and dendrites dried up irrevocably. In adult centers, the nerve paths are something fixed, and immutable: everything may die, nothing may be regenerated'[34]. As early as 1897 there was evidence for undifferentiated cells in the adult brain that had the potential to become either neurons or glia; however, this view was not accepted for almost another century. (Charles Gross provides a fascinating historical accounting of this cautionary tale of scientific sophistry and denial[35].)

In the early 1990s, Reynolds and Weiss demonstrated that one could easily isolate multipotent progenitors from the adult mouse striatum. These precursors expanded in culture by application of epidermal growth factor (EGF) and then directed towards differentiating into neurons or glia[36,37]. More than anything, the ease with which other laboratories could replicate their findings ushered in the acceptance of adult neurogenesis. Subsequently, Eriksson and colleagues examined the postmortem brains of cancer patients who received BrdU as part of their chemotherapy regimen. They found that this thymidine analogue, which is incorporated into replicating DNA, was present in adult borne hippocampal neurons[38]. This elegant study was later extended and replicated, demonstrating a similar neurogenic zone in the subventricular zone (SVZ), neatly paralleling previous animal studies[39–41].

The lingering question of why all mammals retain this form of plasticity has yet to be answered satisfactorily. That the hippocampus plays a critical role in short-term memory formation and is implicated in emotional regulation suggests that adult neurogenesis plays an evolutionarily conserved role in these processes. The most straightforward evidence suggests that adult neurogenesis plays a role in memory formation. For example, the two most potent stimulators of adult neurogenesis, exercise and environmental enrichment, increase hippocampal neurogenesis and improve performance on cognitive tasks like the Morris water maze, even among aged animals. These improvements are only seen with tasks that are hippocampus-dependent (e.g. the water maze), but not with hippocampus-independent learning (e.g. active shock avoidance or delayed eye blink) (reviewed by [42–45]).

Neural Stem Cells and Their Environment

What is a neural stem cell?

Throughout our lifetime new neurons are generated from nascent precursors termed neural stem cells. 'Stem cells' have garnered tremendous popular and scientific attention over the past several years, but this raises the question of what is a neural stem cell? Since the discovery and acceptance of adult neurogenesis over 10 years ago, the field has been mired by confusing language and inconsistent definitions of what it means to be a neural stem cell[46]. In order to avoid such confusion, the following definitions will apply throughout this chapter: a neural stem cell is one that self-renews and has the potential to give rise to multiple cell lineages. Precursors (e.g. adult hippocampal precursor; AHP) are proliferating multipotent cells that do not self-renew. It is often difficult to experimentally distinguish NSCs from multipotential precursors. Therefore, in the absence of data showing that a cell truly self-renews, it is more conservative to refer to multipotent cells as precursors, and not stem cells. In contrast, lineage committed progenitors (e.g. neural progenitors) are rapidly proliferating cells whose differentiation potential is limited to one cell type.

Emergence of adult NSCs

The earliest NSCs begin their life as a thin layer of symmetrically dividing neuroepithelium lining the neural tube. In later embryonic development, these neuroepithelia become radial glia, which support the migration of migrating neuroblasts. These radial glia persist in the neonatal brain and ultimately transform into an astrocytic subtype with the properties of an NSC[47]. These NSC appear to constitute two preserved germinal centres in the adult mammalian brain, one in the SVZ and the other in the subgranular zone (SGZ) of the hippocampal dentate gyrus. The former migrate through the rostral migratory stream (RMS) to take up residence in the olfactory bulb, while the latter migrate a short distance to form the dentate granule cells[47].

Neurogenic stem cell niche

The anatomy of these two neurogenic region shares many similarities. Both constitute thin strips containing small clusters of proliferating cells (types A/G, B, C/D) in close opposition to vascular endothelium[48,49]. The type B cells are slowly proliferating, self-renewing astrocytes that are the real NSCs in these regions. The C (SVZ) and D (SGZ) cells are more rapidly dividing neural progenitors (transit amplifying), while the A (SVZ) and G (SGZ) cells are the immature neurons. The intricacies of the anatomy and the developmental process are far too complex for this discussion and are reviewed extensively elsewhere[47,49]. What is important is to recognize that the NSCs, their progeny and their blood supply reside in close opposition, creating a somewhat self-contained microenvironment. This specialized milieu is termed the stem cell niche[50].

Three compartments comprise this niche: ultrastructure, cells and milieu. (i) Ultrastructure: extracellular matrix and other cellular scaffolding maintain the gross cytoarchitecture of specific brain regions. Since guidance molecules are immobilized on these scaffolds, their loss can cause aberrant dendritic arborization and impaired axonal pathfinding of transplanted/regenerating neurons. (ii) Cellular components include NSCs, astrocytes (supportive and immunological), neurons, oligodendrocytes, microglia, and vascular endothelium and smooth muscle. (iii) The milieu is a metastructure composed of the many dynamically regulated, diffusible factors released by the constituent cells. Gradients of these factors are responsible for coordinating: (i) homing of immune cells; (ii) migration of neuroblast during foetal development (or transplanted neural stem cells); and (iii) neuritogenesis and synaptogenesis.

Niche Function

The niche, like a womb, creates a uniquely nurturing environment to support the birth and development of NSCs into full-fledged neurons. In addition to this supportive function, it serves to insulate the NSCs from the greater milieu. The constituent cells create this environment and generate the milieu, and in turn, each is impacted by it. Therefore, no cell is an island (with apologies to John Donne), the fate of each intimately affected by its neighbours. *In toto*, the niche preserves the delicate balance between NSC maintenance and differentiation and directs lineage decisions.

How is the niche regulated?

The SVZ/SGZ niche contains cells in various stages of development, from stem cells to committed progenitors to maturing neurons, as well as vasculature and ependyma (SVZ). As such, the developing NSCs are subjects to a host of intrinsic (e.g. neighbouring

Table 55.1 Niche targets for future gene therapy trials

Secreted proteins	Niche effects
Bone morphogenic protein4 [BMP4]	Astroglial differentiation
Brain derived neurotrophic factor [BDNF][a]	NPC/neuron survival
Ciliary neurotrophic factor [CNTF][a]	Astroglial differentiation
CCL5 (Rantes)	NSC quiescence
CXCL12 (SDF1α)	NPC chemoattractant, NSC
CX3CL1 (Fractaline)	NPC differentiation
Epidermal growth factor [EGF]	NSC/NPC survival and proliferation
Erythropoietin[b]	NPC differentiation
Fibroblast growth factors [FGF-2/FGF-20][a]	NPC proliferation
Glial-derived neurotrophic factor [GDNF][a]	Neuron survival
Granulocyte macrophage colony stimulating factor [GM-CSF][b]	Neuronal differentiation
Hepatocyte growth factor (HGF)[a]	NPC/neuron survival
Insulin-like growth factor 1 [IGF-1][b]	NPC proliferation, neuron survival
Leukaemia inhibitory factor [LIF]	NSC proliferation and survival
Neurotrophin 3,4/5 [NT3, NT4/5]	Neuron survival
Nerve growth factor [NGF[a]][a]	Neuron survival
Platelet-derived growth factor [PDGF][b]	OPC proliferation and survival
Progranulin [PGRN]	Neuronal survival (?), anti-inflammatory(?)
R-spondin [RSPO[a]]	NPC proliferation (?)
Transforming growth factor beta [TGFβ]	Neuronal differentiation, anti-inflammatory
Vascular endothelial growth factor [VEGF][a]	Angiogenesis, NPC/neuron survival
Wnt3,Wnt7a, Wnt8b	NSC/NPC proliferation and survival
Wnt5a, Wnt7b	Neuronal differentiation

NSC, neural stem cell; NPC, neural progenitor; OPC, oligodendrocyte progenitor.
[a] Used in clinical trials.
[b] FDA approved (alternate indication).

cells) and extrinsic (e.g. from blood or CSF) cues. These 'niche players' represent the prime targets of proposed gene therapy protocols. Formally, there are three forms of signalling at play: (i) externally derived signals conveyed via the blood (endocrine) or CSF (exocrine); these include diffusible factors like muscle-derived IGF-1 or VEGF, or inflammatory cytokines (e.g. interleukin-6, IL-1β or tumour necrosis factor alpha; TNFα); (ii) paracrine factors produced by local astrocytes or neurons (e.g. BDNF, FGF-2, Wnt, neurotransmitters); and (C) cell-autonomous signalling, which includes autocrine factors like Wnt or PDGF as well as genetically preprogrammed differentiation[51–53].

Table 55.1 summarizes some of the most prominent modulators of the adult NSC niche; however, the full panoply of secreted factors influencing the niche is far too extensive for the confines of this chapter (for review see[54–62]).

'Normally' aging niche

Neurogenesis reduces by more than 50% with advancing age. Some of the non-mutually exclusive hypotheses put forth to explain this observation include (i) functional, active downregulation[63]; (ii) inflammation[64]; (iii) burnout/depletion of stem cells (e.g. secondary to reduced Wnt[61]); (iv) niche changes that directly suppress trophic support[65]; (v) reduced circuit activity, which in turn could decrease BDNF/trophic support[66]; (vi) elevated cortisol, which accompanies normal ageing[63]; (vii) reduced physical activity, which reduces IGF-1, again, limiting trophic support[67–71]; and (viii) less intellectual stimulation might functionally reduce need for neurogenesis or might limit circuit activity indirectly (intellectual

reserve hypothesis[72]). Intriguingly, exercise, environmental enrichment, cortisol reduction and inflammatory blockade all improve neurogenesis in older animals to near youthful levels and improve cognition[73–76]. Therefore, even though the aged brain exhibits lower baseline plasticity, it retains the capacity for regeneration, if properly stimulated. These provide additional scientific unpinning for ongoing trials of their efficacy in patients with cognitive impairment. (The reader should consult[77] for a systematic review of neurogenesis and ageing. However, for a more general review of age-related plasticity changes, consider[78,79].)

Neurogenesis and psychiatric illness

There is conflicting evidence about whether aberrant hippocampal neurogenesis underlies the aetiology of major depression or anxiety disorder. However, there is mounting evidence that neurogenesis is required for the beneficial effects of antidepressants. Without exception, all effective treatments for depression, including all classes of antidepressants, lithium and electroconvulsive therapy, stimulate neurogenesis, while chronic stress, which predisposes depression suppresses neurogenesis in animal models. Similarly, infusion of neurogenic stimulators like BDNF, IGF-1, FGF-2 and VGF produces antidepressant/anxiolytic effects, with the expected delay in onset. More recently, it was shown that ablation of neurogenesis blocks the beneficial effects of antidepressants on mood and cognition[80–85].

Niche and neurodegenerative disease

A host of pathologies, many associated with older age, can comprise niche function. Broadly, they do so in three ways: (i) generation of an actively toxic environment by inflammation, increased expression of trophic antagonists or neurotoxins (e.g. soluble Aβ); (ii) development of a passively non-permissive environment through loss of trophic support (e.g. reduced BDNF, WNT, IGF-1, VEGF etc.) or vascular insufficiency; and (iii) structural damage from trauma or stroke. Because each neuropsychiatric disease differs in its underlying pathology, lesions to the neurogenic niche will differ as well. Since any cellular replacement/repair strategy requires recreating the niche (see below), an understanding of how the niche is compromised is an absolute prerequisite for the development of effective treatments.

Alzheimer's is the most common progressive neurodegenerative disease. It is characterized by early loss of short-term memory. Hippocampal involvement occurs early in the disease course, unlike PD or HD. As recently reviewed[86], there are conflicting reports in the literature as to whether hippocampal neurogenesis is increased or decreased early in the disease course[87-89]. The emerging picture suggests that early on modest cell loss triggers a compensatory increase in neurogenesis, probably via increases in FGF-2. However, the underlying pathology prevents survival of sufficient neurons to have a clinical impact. Later on, neurogenesis is uniformly impaired, paralleling the clinical picture. From the perspective of future therapies, it is interesting to note that exercise and environmental enrichment improve neurogenesis and cognitive performance, despite equal β-amyloid plaque loads[90,91].

A common feature of patients with AD, PD, HD and even non-specific mild cognitive impairment (MCI) is that they exhibit significantly impaired olfaction before the onset of more defining features (e.g. abnormal movements in PD)[92-96]. It is tempting to speculate that the cause is alterations in the SVZ niche, since the primary role of adult SVG neurogenesis is to supply new neurons to the olfactory bulb. Interestingly, when one examines the SVZ in patients with these three diseases, each displays a unique cytoarchitectural pathology. In AD, there is diffuse cell loss in regions with Aβ accumulation. In contrast, in PD, there is an SVZ thinning and 30% reduction in NSC proliferation, primarily reflecting a loss of type C (transit amplifying) progenitors and type A (immature) neurons. Examination of the SVZ in HD provides us with the most illuminating observation. The SVZ in HD is more than twice as thick as in age-matched healthy brains, even though AD, PD and HD are all characterized by profound neuronal loss. This increase is due almost exclusively to a doubling in the number of type B cells (radial glia/NSCs). Unlike in stroke patients, it appears that these cells never mature enough to leave the niche, hence never migrating to the lesioned area (i.e. striatum)[97].

Neurogenesis and stroke

Stroke represents a physiologically unique aetiology of cognitive impairment and mood dysregulation in the elderly. Up until the time of the ischaemic event, baseline regenerative mechanisms are unimpaired, unlike progressive neurodegenerative diseases like AD or PD. For this reason, the post-insult neurogenesis is far more robust than in AD, PD or HD. Initially, neural progenitors from the striatal SVZ migrate towards the area of inflammation created by the infarct. Neurogenesis in the region of the infarct can persist for upwards of four months in both humans and animal models[98-101], while the damage in younger patients can be mitigated by administration of erythropoietin[102] or GM-CSF[103] (as reviewed in[104]).

ADVANCED THERAPEUTIC TECHNOLOGIES

The terminology used for describing new technique or technologies can often be confusing; regenerative medicine is no exception. For simplicity's sake, let us define a few of these terms. *In vivo* gene therapy is the introduction of a novel gene into the patient. Most often, the goal is to raise above baseline the endogenous levels of some beneficial protein (e.g. infecting the striatum with a virus that over-expresses GDNF: see above). Somatic cell therapy is where primitive cells are engrafted into a region with the hope that they will integrate and subserve some function. The early foetal tissue transplants were an example of this type of therapy. *Ex vivo* gene therapy is a hybrid of the gene and cell therapy. In this model, cells (e.g. stem cells, fibroblasts) are engineered to express and release the protein of interest. In other words, they serve as living, implantable minipumps. Finally, there are advanced pharmaceuticals, which includes just about everything else. These can be engineered proteins (e.g. recombinant IGF-1 which is FDA approved for use in children with growth defects), small molecules (classic drugs), therapeutic antibodies, vaccines, interfering RNAs etc. In this section we will introduce cutting edge reagents and vectors that are being deployed in the coming generation of neural-repair trials

Cell-based Therapy

Cell-based therapy has received tremendous attention in recent years, as judged by both the volume of published review articles extolling its virtues and the volume of political debate regarding its use. People conceive of these cells as a ready source of spare parts that could be used to replace the damaged tissue. This conceptual simplicity belies quite significant technical challenges.

Newer transplantation trials propose using one of the following types of stem cells: (i) neural stem cells (NSC): possess the ability to differentiate into neurons, astrocytes or oligodendrocytes, but no other tissues; (ii) embryonic stem cells (hESC): blastocyst-derived pluripotent cells can give rise to any cell type in the body (in theory); and (iii) induced pluripotent stem cells (iPSC): pluripotent cells derived from a more mature cell type by genetic reprogramming with a panel of transcription factors. Since iPSCs can be derived from living patients, they hold great prospective value for modelling disease, as well as holding therapeutic potential. However, they are a less than two-year-old technology and many clinicians may be unfamiliar with them. Smith and colleagues provide a fuller discussion comparing and contrasting iPSCs and hESCs[105].

Even though no successful stem cell trial has been completed, the reader should already have a sense that no type of stem cell is the 'magic bullet' many had hoped for[106]. Each has significant limitations, as well as advantages, some of which are summarized in Table 55.2. Any pronouncement on which prove to be therapeutically useful would be mere speculation. Instead, the clinician and translational researcher should focus on what it would take to make any therapeutically useful.

First, we need to understand what we expect of these transplanted cells. (i) The transplanted stem cells must differentiate into the proper cell type and subtype (e.g. dopaminergic neurons, rather than glia); (ii) they must migrate into the correct position to integrate with the intact circuitry; (iii) they must survive in an environment already compromised by the underlying disease (i.e. survive immune attack, inflammation, apoptosis secondary to inadequate trophic support etc); and (iv) they need to remain differentiated and not

Table 55.2 Resources for cell-based therapy

	Source	Application	Advantages	Disadvantages
Foetal neural stem cells	Abortus	Replacement	Large expansion capacity	Heterologous donor
			Steady supply of tissue	Difficult to sort tissue
			Low transformation potential	
			High differentiation potential	
Adult NSC	Postmortem brain, biopsy (?)	Replacement	Autologous (potentially)	Limited expansion capacity
			Limited tissue supply	
Embryonic stem cell	Derived from discarded blastocycts	Replacement	Pluripotent	High teratoma risk
				Heterologous donor
				Chromosomal instability
				Religious/political complications
				Few available lines
Induced pleuripotent stem cells	Skin biopsy or hair samples (fibroblast-keratinocyte)	Replacement	Autologous	Potential transformation
Hematopoetic stem cell	Blood sample	Create vascular niche, anti-inflammatory	Easily purified	May be useless
			Easily acquired	
			Autologous grafing	
Engineered fibroblast-keratinocyte	Skin biopsy or hair samples	Ex-vivo gene therapy (minipumps)	Autologous	May not migrate sufficiently
Immortalized cell-lines	Mixed	Replacement	Easy to grow	Poor function
				High tumour risk
				Archaic technology

NSC, neural stem cell.

malignantly transform as occurred in several early gene therapy and foetal cell trials[32,107].

Second, getting transplanted stem cells to differentiate and integrate in non-neurogenic regions represents the greatest technical hurdle that must be overcome (points i and ii above). When foetal NSCs, and later hESCs, were first derived, there was a fanciful belief that being fully plastic (i.e. pluripotent) meant that they could be engrafted into a brain region. Once there they would grow into the region, as the native cells had done during foetal development. Since this was another case of wishful thinking, a limitation common to all three stem cell types is that they will require cellular programming prior to engraftment. As a field, we have made the greatest strides towards converting stem cells into dopaminergic neurons[1,108,109]. However, even here the programming efficiencies are low, and the developmental programme traversed is poorly understood. (The reader wishing a better understanding of these complexities should consult the following recent reviews[110,111].) Unfortunately, even less is known about coaxing these cells to properly integrate into the existing neuronal network. In short, the first few steps in making stem cells therapeutically useful are, truly, big steps indeed.

Third, safety concerns by the FDA and individual IRBs have been the primary holding up to initiation of many stem cell trials. Because hESCs universally form teratomas when injected into animals, it is unlikely that they, in their unadulterated form, will ever be used in human trials. Even the very first clinical trial of an hESC-derived progenitor was on an extended hold by the FDA until early 2009[112,113]. How real these safety concerns are is a matter of debate, but one that is sure to continue for several years.

Gene Therapy Vectors

W. French Anderson reported in the autumn of 1990 the first gene therapy trial on a patient suffering from a form of severe combined immunodeficiency (SCID). Almost three decades later, the only broadly successful application of gene therapy has been in the treatment of SCID[114]. It is hard to overstate the disappointment that, with over 1 500 approved clinical trials worldwide (many prematurely aborted), successes are so few and setbacks all too prominent[115,116]. The darker side of its major 'success' is that in the European trial, four patients who had received retroviral-based gene therapy for X-linked SCID went on to develop leukaemia. These malignancies were

Table 55.3 Most common gene therapy vectors

Vectors	Advantages	Limitations
Virus		
Retrovirus	Integrating	Dividing cells ONLY
Integrating	Broad tropism	Preferential insertion in active genes, particularly those regulating cell proliferation
	Moderate transgene size	High oncogenic potential
	Long-term expression	
Lentivirus	Integrating	Oncogenic potential
Integrating	Infects quiescent cells	Modest diffusion
	Broad tropism	
	Moderate transgene size	
	Long-term expression	
Herpes virus	Large transgene size	High inflammatory potential
Episomal		Transient expression in non-neuronal cells
AAV	High-titres	Smallest transgene capacity
Episomal (90%)	Highly-specific tropsim	Highly-specific tropsim
Integrating (10%)	Low inflammatory potential	
	Serotype-9 crosses blood–brain barrier	
Adenovirus	Large payload	High inflammatory potential
Episomal	Efficient transduction	Poor diffusion
		Short-term expression
Naked plasmid DNA-liposome[139]	Large payload	Poor transduction
	Easy to purify	
Blood-brain barrier translocators		
Carrier-mediated peptide transport	IGF-1, EGF	No carrier for most proteins
Receptor-mediated transcytosis	Highly adaptable to different proteins	Unproven in clinical trials
	RMT-BDNF entering clinical trials	
Cell-penetrating peptides	Highly adaptable to different proteins	Unproven in clinical trials
Intranasal delivery	Positive clinical improvement in clinical trials of stroke and Alzheimer's	Highly variable dosing and penetration

the result of the retrovirus preferentially inserting into the promoter of the *LMO2* gene (in two cases), a known T-cell oncogene.

Most gene therapy trials were designed to treat cancer (65%), where the goal is to arrest proliferation and foster death in the target cells. As neuropsychiatrists, our goals for gene therapy are diametrically opposite; preservation of neurons forces us to develop our own 'personalize toolbox'. To illustrate the shortcoming of applying previous trials' technique to problems of neurodegeneration, consider the following. The earliest (and only successful) trials used Moloney murine leukaemia virus (MMLV) based retroviral vectors. Like all oncoretroviruses, they only infect dividing cells, making them almost useless for treating the CNS (i.e. mature neurons do not divide). The alternative for initial trials, adenoviral vectors, can infect CNS, but have demonstrated extremely limited CNS penetration and the potential for severe inflammation. (Such inflammatory induced multi-organ failure led to the high-profile death of a relatively healthy clinical trial volunteer in 1999[117].) Together these help to explain why just 1.8% ($n = 27$) of clinical gene therapy trials have been approved for neurological disease, and only half of those for treatment of the brain (see the Gene Therapy Clinical Trials Worldwise database[118]).

These recognized shortcomings help define the requirements for the next generation of neuro-gene therapy tools. CNS gene therapy vectors must (i) possess the ability to infect non-dividing cells; (ii) carry the gene of interest to the intended target; (iii) be able to express the gene and resist the cell's natural defences, thereby preventing it from being turned off; and (iv) be safe (i.e. not induce malignancy transformation or severe inflammation, two primary causes of morbidity and mortality in previous gene therapy patients[107,117]).

Engineered viruses carrying a therapeutic gene remain the mainstay of proposed trials. Lentivirus (HIV-based) and adeno-associated virus (AAV) vectors are the two most popular viral vectors for current trials. They possess the desirable traits of low inflammatory response, good gene transduction and long-term gene expression. Table 55.3 summarizes the strengths and weaknesses of these and other gene therapy vectors (reviewed by[115,119–123]).

Interfering RNA

Until recently it was thought that most RNA transcribed from our genomes was either translated into protein or incorporated into ribosome function (i.e. rRNA, tRNA). Now, it is believed that much, if not most, RNA is actually regulatory in nature. These short RNA species (RNAi) are able to complex with coding RNAs, thereby regulating protein production. The therapeutic potential of RNAi for treating cancer or HIV has garnered a great deal of press (and the 2006 Nobel Prize). In brief, the utility of RNAi is to reduce expression of some undesired mutant gene (a.k.a. toxic or gain-of-function mutation) like the bcr-abl fusion mutant found in chronic myeloid leukaemia. In psychiatric disease, some examples include AAV-delivered RNAi targeting the tau, and APP mutations found in

AD and frontotemporal dementia (FTD) or mutant huntingtin[124–126]. At the time of this writing no RNAi-based therapy for a CNS disorder has reached the stage of approved clinical trial; however, this is likely to change in the coming years. This subject has been reviewed extensively elsewhere[127–129].

Rethinking Clinical Trials

This section title begs the question, why do we need to change how we conduct clinical trials? Even though the mathematics behind selecting trial sample sizes is well understood[130], the psychiatry literature suffers from an unfortunately large number of studies being 'underpowered' for their purpose (power being the probability of concluding a benefit when there actually is one.) The primary culprit is not academic laziness, but arises from the fact that the statistical design of most trials requires that end-points and sample sizes must be fixed ahead of time. The more complex a trial, the more likely that these *pre hoc* assumptions will be wrong. While space limitations prevent a lengthy discussion of clinical trial design, it is important for the reader to understand that there is an alternative to designing exploratory trials around proving or disproving a null hypothesis. These Bayesian designs provide several advantages, including (i) allowing adaptive sizing of arms, midway in trial; (ii) measuring probabilities for non-directly observable events; (iii) incorporating prior knowledge; (iv) allowing smaller trials with the same statistical power; and (v) cross-arm information sharing, allowing more treatment variables. All of these will be invaluable for future gene therapy trials where such trials will require multifactor treatments and small sample sizes. For a more complete discussion of Bayesian statistics and their application to clinical trial design, the reader is referred to one of the following[131–136].

Neural Repair Finds Its Niche: Where Do We Begin Putting All the Pieces Together?

Many would begin by asking the question: what do we want to treat? However, we should ask: what are we willing to treat? It was proposed several years ago to apply gene therapy towards the treatment of anxiety/stress disorder[137]. The great philosopher (and baseball player) Yogi Berra reportedly quipped, 'In theory there is no difference between theory and practice. In practice there is.' Many illnesses we confront in geriatric psychiatry could, in theory, be treated with gene therapy or stem cells, but would we? All proposed gene- or cell-based therapy trials are invasive and present a high risk of morbidity. As with our anxiety example, when would we recommend brain surgery with gene therapy over a larger dose of diazepam? The risk versus benefit calculation has always been such that we will only consider these treatments for the worst afflicted patients (i.e. the ones with little to lose). Since these are the hardest patients to treat, we have made the already daunting task of perfecting regenerative therapy even harder.

To resolve our conundrum and bring these therapies into clinical practice, we need to complete many, many more clinical trials. Therefore, we need to make the trials less invasive, and thus less risky, thereby allowing us to treat less sick individuals. An example might be a regenerative trial in patients with early stage HD. Preclinical studies demonstrate that viral cotransduction of BDNF to promote survival and Noggin to block astrocytosis regenerates medium spiney neurons in the striatum[138]. Directly translating these animal studies into a clinical trial would be the 'sexy' approach. The theoretical grounds for such a trial are sound, but in practice it would be *extremely* difficult to obtain IRB approval for a two-gene therapy trial. A pragmatic, though less flashy, alternative is to determine whether some combination of available drugs might induce the same regeneration (see Table 55.4). For illustration purposes, we are

Table 55.4 FDA approved drugs with neuroregenerative potential

	Target	NSC	NPC	OPC	Mature neurons/oligos
Drug					
Antidepressants (↑ 5HT/NE/DA)	Increased circuit activity Increased BDNF		S	S	D, S
Indomethicin	Anti inflammatory			S	S
Lithium	GSK-3β	P	P	P	
Lovastatin (?)	GSK-3β (?)		P (?)	P (?)	
Milrinone, rolipram	PDE3/4				D, S
Rosiglitazone	PPARγ				D
Valproic acid	HDAC GSK-3β (?)	I	I	I	D, S
Peptide					
IGF-1		P (?)	P, S	P, S	D, S
Erythropoietin					D Angiogenesis (?)
GM-CSF					D
PDGF				D, S	
Other					
ECT	Increased circuit activity Increased BDNF		P	?	D,S
DBS/rTMS	Increased circuit activity		P (?)	?	?

NSC, neural stem cell; NPC, neural progenitor; OPC, oligodendrocyte progenitor.
I, inhibits proliferation; D, promotes differentiation; S, promotes survival; P, increases proliferation.

finalizing the Bayesian framework for such a trial comparing IGF-1 treatment paired with combinations of VPA, lithium, rosaglitazone and indomethicin.

The list of approved drugs with regenerative potential is growing, but is still quite limited. Therefore, most approaches to neuro-repair will ultimately require either gene therapy and/or cell-based therapy. The process needs to be a rational one, not relying on serendipity. In its most basic form it should entail

1. *Careful target selection*: identifying the biological target in need of correction (e.g. loss of dopaminergic nigral neurons);
2. *Payload*: design the actual treatment. A good basis for selecting these comes from our previous discussion of the neural stem cell niche, in health and disease;
3. *Vector/delivery*: engineer a means of getting it to the right place;
4. *Surveillance*: devise a way of monitoring the treatment (i.e. is it working?).

In summary, the best guide for future trials may be simply not to repeat the naïve mistakes of the past, most notable ignoring the essential role of the neurovascular niche in supporting and guiding neural regeneration. If we take such care then future editions of this text will likely contain more discussion of treatments at hand, and less hand-waving about the treatments of the future.

REFERENCES

1. Ormerod BK, Palmer TD, Caldwell MA. Neurodegeneration and cell replacement. *Philos Trans R Soc Lond B Biol Sci* 2008; **363**(1489): 153–170.
2. Lindvall O, Bjorklund A. Transplantation strategies in the treatment of Parkinson's disease: experimental basis and clinical trials. *Acta Neurol Scand Suppl* 1989; **126**: 197–210.
3. Freed CR, Breeze RE, Rosenberg NL *et al*. Transplantation of human fetal dopamine cells for Parkinson's disease. Results at 1 year. *Arch Neurol* 1990; **47**(5): 505–12.
4. Lindvall O, Brundin P, Widner H *et al*. Grafts of fetal dopamine neurons survive and improve motor function in Parkinson's disease. *Science* 1990; **247**(4942): 574–7.
5. Freed CR, Breeze RE, Rosenberg NL *et al*. Survival of implanted fetal dopamine cells and neurologic improvement 12 to 46 months after transplantation for Parkinson's disease. *N Engl J Med* 1992; **327**(22): 1549–55.
6. Widner H. Immature neural tissue grafts in Parkinson's disease. *Acta Neurol Scand Suppl* 1993; **146**: 43–5.
7. Widner H, Tetrud J, Rehncrona S *et al*. Bilateral fetal mesencephalic grafting in two patients with parkinsonism induced by 1-methyl-4-phenyl-1,2,3,6-tetrahydropyridine (MPTP). *N Engl J Med* 1992; **327**(22): 1556–63.
8. Spencer DD, Robbins RJ, Naftolin F *et al*. Unilateral transplantation of human fetal mesencephalic tissue into the caudate nucleus of patients with Parkinson's disease. *N Engl J Med* 1992; **327**(22): 1541–8.
9. Breeze RE, Wells TH, Jr, Freed CR. Implantation of fetal tissue for the management of Parkinson's disease: a technical note. *Neurosurgery* 1995; **36**(5): 1044–7; discussion 7–8.
10. Freed CR, Breeze RE, Schneck SA. Transplantation of fetal mesencephalic tissue in Parkinson's disease. *N Engl J Med* 1995; **333**(11): 730–1.
11. Bluml S, Kopyov O, Jacques S, Ross BD. Activation of neurotransplants in humans. *Exp Neurol* 1999; **158**(1): 121–5.
12. Freed CR, Greene PE, Breeze RE *et al*. Transplantation of embryonic dopamine neurons for severe Parkinson's disease. *N Engl J Med* 2001; **344**(10): 710–9.
13. Clarkson ED. Fetal tissue transplantation for patients with Parkinson's disease: a database of published clinical results. *Drugs Aging* 2001; **18**(10): 773–85.
14. Kordower JH, Chu Y, Hauser RA, Freeman TB, Olanow CW. Lewy body-like pathology in long-term embryonic nigral transplants in Parkinson's disease. *Nat Med* 2008; **14**(5): 504–6.
15. Kordower JH, Brundin P. Lewy body pathology in long-term fetal nigral transplants: is Parkinson's disease transmitted from one neural system to another? *Neuropsychopharmacology* 2009; **34**(1): 254.
16. Gill SS, Patel NK, Hotton GR *et al*. Direct brain infusion of glial cell line-derived neurotrophic factor in Parkinson disease. *Nat Med* 2003; **9**(5): 589–95.
17. Patel NK, Bunnage M, Plaha P *et al*. Intraputamenal infusion of glial cell line-derived neurotrophic factor in PD: a two-year outcome study. *Ann Neurol* 2005; **57**(2): 298–302.
18. Love S, Plaha P, Patel NK *et al*. Glial cell line-derived neurotrophic factor induces neuronal sprouting in human brain. *Nat Med* 2005; **11**(7): 703–4.
19. NCT00400634. Multicenter, Randomized, Double-Blind, Sham Surgery-Controlled Study of CERE-120 (Adeno-Associated Virus Serotype 2 [AAV2]-Neurturin [NTN]) to Assess the Efficacy and Safety of Bilateral Intraputaminal (IPu) Delivery in Subjects with Idiopathic Parkinson's Disease.
20. Kaplitt MG, Feigin A, Tang C *et al*. Safety and tolerability of gene therapy with an adeno-associated virus (AAV) borne GAD gene for Parkinson's disease: an open label, phase I trial. *Lancet* 2007; **369**(9579): 2097–105.
21. Eberling JL, Jagust WJ, Christine CW *et al*. Results from a phase I safety trial of hAADC gene therapy for Parkinson disease. *Neurology* 2008; **70**(21): 1980–3.
22. Tuszynski MH, Thal L, Pay M *et al*. A phase 1 clinical trial of nerve growth factor gene therapy for Alzheimer disease. *Nat Med* 2005; **11**(5): 551–5.
23. NCT00087789. A Phase I, Dose-Escalating Study to Assess the Safety and Tolerability of CERE-110 [Adeno-Associated Virus (AAV)-Based Vector-Mediated Delivery of Beta-Nerve Growth Factor (NGF)] in Subjects With Mild to Moderate Alzheimer's Disease.
24. Kopyov OV, Jacques S, Lieberman A, Duma CM, Eagle KS. Safety of intrastriatal neurotransplantation for Huntington's disease patients. *Exp Neurol* 1998; **149**(1): 97–108.
25. Ross BD, Hoang TQ, Bluml S *et al*. *In vivo* magnetic resonance spectroscopy of human fetal neural transplants. *NMR Biomed* 1999; **12**(4): 221–36.
26. Hauser RA, Furtado S, Cimino CR *et al*. Bilateral human fetal striatal transplantation in Huntington's disease. *Neurology* 2002; **58**(5): 687–95.
27. Rosser AE, Barker RA, Harrower T *et al*. Unilateral transplantation of human primary fetal tissue in four patients with Huntington's disease: NEST-UK safety report ISRCTN no 36485475. *J Neurol Neurosurg Psychiatry* 2002; **73**(6): 678–85.
28. Bachoud-Lévi AC, Remy P, Nguyen JP *et al*. Motor and cognitive improvements in patients with Huntington's disease after neural transplantation. *Lancet* 2000; **356**(9246): 1975–9.
29. Bachoud-Lévi A, Bourdet C, Brugières P *et al*. Safety and tolerability assessment of intrastriatal neural allografts in five

patients with Huntington's disease. *Exp Neurol* 2000; **161**(1): 194–202.

30. Furtado S, Sossi V, Hauser RA *et al*. Positron emission tomography after fetal transplantation in Huntington's disease. *Ann Neurol* 2005; **58**(2): 331–7.

31. Bachoud-Lévi AC, Gaura V, Brugières P *et al*. Effect of fetal neural transplants in patients with Huntington's disease 6 years after surgery: a long-term follow-up study. *Lancet Neurol* 2006; **5**(4): 303–9.

32. Amariglio N, Hirshberg A, Scheithauer BW *et al*. Donor-derived brain tumor following neural stem cell transplantation in an ataxia telangiectasia patient. *PLoS Med* 2009; **6**(2): e1000029.

33. Keene CD, Chang RC, Leverenz JB *et al*. A patient with Huntington's disease and long-surviving fetal neural transplants that developed mass lesions. *Acta Neuropathol* 2009; **117**(3): 329–38.

34. Ramón y Cajal S. *Degeneration and Regeneration of the Nerve Centres*, trans May RM. Oxford: Oxford University Press, 1991. Originally published 1959.

35. Gross CG. Neurogenesis in the adult brain: death of a dogma. *Nat Rev Neurosci* 2000; **1**(1): 67–73.

36. Reynolds BA, Tetzlaff W, Weiss S. A multipotent EGF-responsive striatal embryonic progenitor cell produces neurons and astrocytes. *J Neurosci* 1992; **12**(11): 4565–74.

37. Reynolds BA, Weiss S. Generation of neurons and astrocytes from isolated cells of the adult mammalian central nervous system. *Science* 1992; **255**(5052): 1707–10.

38. Eriksson PS, Perfilieva E, Bjork-Eriksson T *et al*. Neurogenesis in the adult human hippocampus [see comments]. *Nat Med* 1998; **4**(11): 1313–17.

39. Kam M, Curtis MA, McGlashan SR *et al*. The cellular composition and morphological organization of the rostral migratory stream in the adult human brain. *J Chem Neuroanat* 2009; **37**(3): 196–205.

40. Qui nones-Hinojosa A, Sanai N, Soriano-Navarro M *et al*. Cellular composition and cytoarchitecture of the adult human subventricular zone: a niche of neural stem cells. *J Comp Neurol* 2006; **494**(3): 415–34.

41. Curtis MA, Kam M, Nannmark U *et al*. Human neuroblasts migrate to the olfactory bulb via a lateral ventricular extension. *Science* 2007; **315**(5816): 1243–9.

42. Leuner B, Gould E, Shors TJ. Is there a link between adult neurogenesis and learning? *Hippocampus* 2006; **16**(3): 216–24.

43. Kempermann G, Wiskott L, Gage FH. Functional significance of adult neurogenesis. *Curr Opin Neurobiol* 2004; **14**(2): 186–91.

44. Aimone JB, Wiles J, Gage FH. Potential role for adult neurogenesis in the encoding of time in new memories. *Nat Neurosci* 2006; **9**(6): 723–7.

45. Zhao C, Deng W, Gage FH. Mechanisms and functional implications of adult neurogenesis. *Cell* 2008; **132**(4): 645–60.

46. Seaberg RM, van der KD. Stem and progenitor cells: the premature desertion of rigorous definitions. *Trends Neurosci* 2003; **26**(3): 125–31.

47. Merkle FT, Alvarez-Buylla A. Neural stem cells in mammalian development. *Curr Opin Cell Biol* 2006; **18**(6): 704–9.

48. Palmer TD, Willhoite AR, Gage FH. Vascular niche for adult hippocampal neurogenesis. *J Comp Neurol* 2000; **425**(4): 479–94.

49. Doetsch F. A niche for adult neural stem cells. *Curr Opin Genet Dev* 2003; **13**(5): 543–50.

50. Wurmser AE, Palmer TD, Gage FH. Neuroscience. Cellular interactions in the stem cell niche. *Science* 2004; **304**(5675): 1253–5.

51. Ming GL, Song H. Adult neurogenesis in the mammalian central nervous system. *Annu Rev Neurosci* 2005; **28**: 223–50.

52. Riquelme PA, Drapeau E, Doetsch F. Brain micro-ecologies: neural stem cell niches in the adult mammalian brain. *Philos Trans R Soc Lond B Biol Sci* 2008; **363**(1489): 123–37.

53. Binder DK. Neurotrophins in the dentate gyrus. *Prog Brain Res* 2007; **163**: 371–97.

54. Grote HE, Hannan AJ. Regulators of adult neurogenesis in the healthy and diseased brain. *Clin Exp Pharmacol Physiol* 2007; **34**(5–6): 533–45.

55. Toledo EM, Colombres M, Inestrosa NC. Wnt signaling in neuroprotection and stem cell differentiation. *Prog Neurobiol* 2008; **86**(3): 281–96.

56. Bauer S. Cytokine control of adult neural stem cells. *Ann N Y Acad Sci* 2009; **1153**: 48–56.

57. Martino G, Pluchino S. The therapeutic potential of neural stem cells. *Nat Rev Neurosci* 2006; **7**(5): 395–406.

58. Zacchigna S, Lambrechts D, Carmeliet P. Neurovascular signalling defects in neurodegeneration. *Nat Rev Neurosci* 2008; **9**(3): 169–81.

59. Krathwohl MD, Kaiser JL. Chemokines promote quiescence and survival of human neural progenitor cells. *Stem Cells* 2004; **22**(1): 109–18.

60. Kruger C, Laage R, Pitzer C, Schabitz WR, Schneider A. The hematopoietic factor GM-CSF (granulocyte-macrophage colony-stimulating factor) promotes neuronal differentiation of adult neural stem cells in vitro. *BMC Neurosci* 2007; **8**: 88.

61. Wexler EM, Paucer A, Kornblum HI, Palmer TD, Geschwind DH. Endogenous Wnt signaling maintains neural progenitor cell potency. *Stem Cells* 2009; **27**(5): 1130–41.

62. Battista D, Ferrari CC, Gage FH, Pitossi FJ. Neurogenic niche modulation by activated microglia: transforming growth factor beta increases neurogenesis in the adult dentate gyrus. *Eur J Neurosci* 2006; **23**(1): 83–93.

63. Jessberger S, Gage FH. Stem-cell-associated structural and functional plasticity in the aging hippocampus. *Psychol Aging* 2008; **23**(4): 684–91.

64. Monje ML, Toda H, Palmer TD. Inflammatory blockade restores adult hippocampal neurogenesis. *Science* 2003; **302**(5651): 1760–65.

65. Shetty AK, Hattiangady B, Shetty GA. Stem/progenitor cell proliferation factors FGF-2, IGF-1, and VEGF exhibit early decline during the course of aging in the hippocampus: role of astrocytes. *Glia* 2005; **51**(3): 173–86.

66. Deisseroth K, Singla S, Toda H. Excitation-neurogenesis coupling in adult neural stem/progenitor cells. *Neuron* 2004; **42**(4): 535–52.

67. Duman CH, Schlesinger L, Terwilliger R *et al*. Peripheral insulin-like growth factor-I produces antidepressant-like behavior and contributes to the effect of exercise. *Behav Brain Res* 2009; **198**(2): 366–71.

68. van Praag H, Shubert T, Zhao C, Gage FH. Exercise enhances learning and hippocampal neurogenesis in aged mice. *J Neurosci* 2005; **25**(38): 8680–5.

69. van Praag H, Kempermann G, Gage FH. Running increases cell proliferation and neurogenesis in the adult mouse dentate gyrus. *Nat Neurosci* 1999; **2**(3): 266–70.

70. Anderson MF, Aberg MA, Nilsson M, Eriksson PS. Insulin-like growth factor-I and neurogenesis in the adult mammalian brain. *Brain Res Dev Brain Res* 2002; **134**(1–2): 115–22.

71. Mattson MP, Maudsley S, Martin B. A neural signaling triumvirate that influences ageing and age-related disease: insulin/IGF-1, BDNF and serotonin. *Ageing Res Rev* 2004; **3**(4): 445–64.

72. Lautenschlager NT, Cox KL, Flicker L *et al.* Effect of physical activity on cognitive function in older adults at risk for Alzheimer disease: a randomized trial. *JAMA* 2008; **300**(9): 1027–37.

73. Cameron HA, McKay RD. Restoring production of hippocampal neurons in old age. *Nat Neurosci* 1999; **2**(10): 894–7.

74. Kempermann G, Kuhn HG, Gage FH. Experience-induced neurogenesis in the senescent dentate gyrus. *J Neurosci* 1998; **18**(9): 3206–12.

75. Trejo JL, Llorens-Martin MV, Torres-Aleman I. The effects of exercise on spatial learning and anxiety-like behavior are mediated by an IGF-I-dependent mechanism related to hippocampal neurogenesis. *Mol Cell Neurosci* 2008; **37**(2): 402–11.

76. Pereira AC, Huddleston DE, Brickman AM *et al.* An *in vivo* correlate of exercise-induced neurogenesis in the adult dentate gyrus. *Proc Natl Acad Sci U S A* 2007; **104**(13): 5638–43.

77. Drapeau E, Nora Abrous D. Stem cell review series: role of neurogenesis in age-related memory disorders. *Aging Cell* 2008; **7**(4): 569–89.

78. Burke SN, Barnes CA. Neural plasticity in the ageing brain. *Nat Rev Neurosci* 2006; **7**(1): 30–40.

79. Mattson MP, Magnus T. Ageing and neuronal vulnerability. *Nat Rev Neurosci* 2006; **7**(4): 278–94.

80. Santarelli L, Saxe M, Gross C *et al.* Requirement of hippocampal neurogenesis for the behavioral effects of antidepressants. *Science* 2003; **301**(5634): 805–9.

81. Surget A, Saxe M, Leman S *et al.* Drug-dependent requirement of hippocampal neurogenesis in a model of depression and of antidepressant reversal. *Biol Psychiatry* 2008; **64**(4): 293–301.

82. Sahay A, Hen R. Adult hippocampal neurogenesis in depression. *Nat Neurosci* 2007; **10**(9): 1110–15.

83. Sen S, Duman R, Sanacora G. Serum brain-derived neurotrophic factor, depression, and antidepressant medications: meta-analyses and implications. *Biol Psychiatry* 2008; **64**(6): 527–32.

84. Levi A, Eldridge JD, Paterson BM. Molecular cloning of a gene sequence regulated by nerve growth factor. *Science* 1985; **229**(4711): 393–5.

85. Krishnan V, Nestler EJ. The molecular neurobiology of depression. *Nature* 2008; **455**(7215): 894–902.

86. Kuhn HG, Cooper-Kuhn CM, Boekhoorn K, Lucassen PJ. Changes in neurogenesis in dementia and Alzheimer mouse models: are they functionally relevant? *Eur Arch Psychiatry Clin Neurosci* 2007; **257**(5): 281–9.

87. Rodriguez JJ, Jones VC, Tabuchi M *et al.* Impaired adult neurogenesis in the dentate gyrus of a triple transgenic mouse model of Alzheimer's disease. *PLoS ONE* 2008; **3**(8): e2935.

88. Jin K, Galvan V, Xie L *et al.* Enhanced neurogenesis in Alzheimer's disease transgenic (PDGF-APPSw,Ind) mice. *Proc Natl Acad Sci U S A* 2004; **101**(36): 13363–7.

89. Jin K, Peel AL, Mao XO *et al.* Increased hippocampal neurogenesis in Alzheimer's disease. *Proc Natl Acad Sci U S A* 2004; **101**(1): 343–7.

90. Catlow BJ, Rowe AR, Clearwater CR. Effects of environmental enrichment and physical activity on neurogenesis in transgenic PS1/APP mice. *Brain Res* 2009; **1256**: 173–9.

91. Mirochnic S, Wolf S, Staufenbiel M, Kempermann G. Age effects on the regulation of adult hippocampal neurogenesis by physical activity and environmental enrichment in the APP23 mouse model of Alzheimer disease. *Hippocampus* 2009; **19**(10): 1008–18.

92. Moberg PJ, Pearlson GD, Speedie LJ *et al.* Olfactory recognition: differential impairments in early and late Huntington's and Alzheimer's diseases. *J Clin Exp Neuropsychol* 1987; **9**(6): 650–64.

93. Devanand DP, Michaels-Marston KS, Liu X *et al.* Olfactory deficits in patients with mild cognitive impairment predict Alzheimer's disease at follow-up. *Am J Psychiatry* 2000; **157**(9): 1399–405.

94. Williams SS, Williams J, Combrinck M *et al.* Olfactory impairment is more marked in patients with mild dementia with Lewy bodies than those with mild Alzheimer disease. *J Neurol Neurosurg Psychiatry* 2009; **80**(6): 667–70.

95. Schubert CR, Carmichael LL, Murphy C *et al.* Olfaction and the 5-year incidence of cognitive impairment in an epidemiological study of older adults. *J Am Geriatr Soc* 2008; **56**(8): 1517–21.

96. Djordjevic J, Jones-Gotman M, de Sousa K, Chertkow H. Olfaction in patients with mild cognitive impairment and Alzheimer's disease. *Neurobiol Aging* 2008; **29**(5): 693–706.

97. Curtis MA, Faull RL, Eriksson PS. The effect of neurodegenerative diseases on the subventricular zone. *Nat Rev Neurosci* 2007; **8**(9): 712–23.

98. Arvidsson A, Collin T, Kirik D, Kokaia Z, Lindvall O. Neuronal replacement from endogenous precursors in the adult brain after stroke. *Nat Med* 2002; **8**(9): 963–70.

99. Parent JM, Vexler ZS, Gong C, Derugin N, Ferriero DM. Rat forebrain neurogenesis and striatal neuron replacement after focal stroke. *Ann Neurol* 2002; **52**(6): 802–13.

100. Jin K, Wang X, Xie L *et al.* Evidence for stroke-induced neurogenesis in the human brain. *Proc Natl Acad Sci U S A* 2006; **103**(35): 13198–202.

101. Thored P, Arvidsson A, Cacci E *et al.* Persistent production of neurons from adult brain stem cells during recovery after stroke. *Stem Cells* 2006; **24**(3): 739–47.

102. Chang YS, Mu D, Wendland M *et al.* Erythropoietin improves functional and histological outcome in neonatal stroke. *Pediatr Res* 2005; **58**(1): 106–11.

103. Schabitz WR, Schneider A. New targets for established proteins: exploring G-CSF for the treatment of stroke. *Trends Pharmacol Sci* 2007; **28**(4): 157–61.

104. Zhang RL, Zhang ZG, Chopp M. Ischemic stroke and neurogenesis in the subventricular zone. *Neuropharmacology* 2008; **55**(3): 345–52.

105. Smith KP, Luong MX, Stein GS. Pluripotency: toward a gold standard for human ES and iPS cells. *J Cell Physiol* 2009; **220**(1): 21–9.

106. NCT00337636. A Phase I Study of the Safety and Preliminary Effectiveness of Human CNS Stem Cells (HuCNS-SC) in

Patients with Neuronal Ceroid Lipofuscinosis Caused by Palmitoyl Protein Thioesterase 1 (PPT1) or Tripeptidyl Peptidase 1 (TPP-I) Deficiency.

107. Hacein-Bey-Abina S, von Kalle C, Schmidt M *et al*. A serious adverse event after successful gene therapy for X-linked severe combined immunodeficiency. *N Engl J Med* 2003; **348**(3): 255–6.

108. Lindvall O, Kokaia Z. Stem cell therapy for human brain disorders. *Kidney Int* 2005; **68**(5): 1937–9.

109. Parish CL, Castelo-Branco G, Rawal N *et al*. Wnt5a-treated midbrain neural stem cells improve dopamine cell replacement therapy in parkinsonian mice. *J Clin Invest* 2008; **118**(1): 149–60.

110. Smidt MP, Burbach JP. How to make a mesodiencephalic dopaminergic neuron. *Nat Rev Neurosci* 2007; **8**(1): 21–32.

111. Wexler EM, Geschwind DH. Out FOXing Parkinson disease: where development meets neurodegeneration. *PLoS Biol* 2007; **5**(12): e334.

112. Alper J. Geron gets green light for human trial of ES cell-derived product. *Nat Biotechnol* 2009; **27**(3): 213–14.

113. NCT01005004. Phase I Study of the Safety and Preliminary Efficacy of Intracerebral Transplantation of HuCNS-SC® Cells for Connatal Pelizaeus-Merzbacher Disease (PMD).

114. Cavazzana-Calvo M, Hacein-Bey S, de Saint Basile G *et al*. Gene therapy of human severe combined immunodeficiency (SCID)-X1 disease. *Science* 2000; **288**(5466): 669–72.

115. Thomas CE, Ehrhardt A, Kay MA. Progress and problems with the use of viral vectors for gene therapy. *Nat Rev Genet* 2003; **4**(5): 346–58.

116. Scollay R. Gene therapy: a brief overview of the past, present, and future. *Ann N Y Acad Sci* 2001; **953**. 26–30.

117. Committee RDA. Assessment of adenoviral vector safety and toxicity: report of the National Institutes of Health Recombinant DNA Advisory Committee. *Hum Gene Ther* 2002; **13**(1): 3–13.

118. Gene Therapy Clinical Trials Worldwide [database]. At www.wiley.co.uk/genmed/clinical, accessed 30 Jan 2010.

119. Brasnjevic I, Steinbusch HW, Schmitz C, Martinez-Martinez P. Delivery of peptide and protein drugs over the blood–brain barrier. *Prog Neurobiol* 2009; **87**(4): 212–51.

120. Ma M, Ma Y, Yi X *et al*. Intranasal delivery of transforming growth factor-beta1 in mice after stroke reduces infarct volume and increases neurogenesis in the subventricular zone. *BMC Neurosci* 2008; **9**: 117.

121. Benedict C, Hallschmid M, Schmitz K *et al*. Intranasal insulin improves memory in humans: superiority of insulin aspart. *Neuropsychopharmacology* 2007; **32**(1): 239–43.

122. Mathias NR, Hussain MA. Non-invasive systemic drug delivery: developability considerations for alternate routes of administration. *J Pharm Sci*. 2010; **99**(1): 1–20.

123. Waehler R, Russell SJ, Curiel DT. Engineering targeted viral vectors for gene therapy. *Nat Rev Genet* 2007; **8**(8): 573–87.

124. Miller VM, Gouvion CM, Davidson BL, Paulson HL. Targeting Alzheimer's disease genes with RNA interference: an efficient strategy for silencing mutant alleles. *Nucleic Acids Res* 2004; **32**(2): 661–8.

125. Boudreau RL, McBride JL, Martins I *et al*. Nonallele-specific silencing of mutant and wild-type huntingtin demonstrates therapeutic efficacy in Huntington's disease mice. *Mol Ther* 2009; **17**(6): 1053–63.

126. Franich NR, Fitzsimons HL, Fong DM *et al*. AAV vector-mediated RNAi of mutant huntingtin expression is neuroprotective in a novel genetic rat model of Huntington's disease. *Mol Ther* 2008; **16**(5): 947–56.

127. Whitehead KA, Langer R, Anderson DG. Knocking down barriers: advances in siRNA delivery. *Nat Rev Drug Discov* 2009; **8**(2): 129–38.

128. Mittal V. Improving the efficiency of RNA interference in mammals. *Nat Rev Genet* 2004; **5**(5): 355–65.

129. Kim DH, Rossi JJ. Strategies for silencing human disease using RNA interference. *Nat Rev Genet* 2007; **8**(3): 173–84.

130. Kraemer HC, Thiemann S. *How Many Subjects? Statistical Power Analysis in Research.* Newbury Park, CA; Sage, 1987.

131. Eddy SR. What is Bayesian statistics? *Nat Biotechnol* 2004; **22**(9): 1177–8.

132. Howard G, Coffey CS, Cutter GR. Is Bayesian analysis ready for use in phase III randomized clinical trials? Beware the sound of the sirens. *Stroke* 2005; **36**(7): 1622–3.

133. Howard G. Nonconventional clinical trial designs: approaches to provide more precise estimates of treatment effects with a smaller sample size, but at a cost. *Stroke* 2007; **38**(2 suppl): 804–8.

134. Spiegelhalter DJ, Abrams KR, Myles JP. *Bayesian Approaches to Clinical Trials and Health Care Evaluation*. Chichester: John Wiley & Sons, 2004.

135. Berry DA. Bayesian clinical trials. *Nat Rev Drug Discov* 2006; **5**(1): 27–36.

136. Needham CJ, Bradford JR, Bulpitt AJ, Westhead DR. Inference in Bayesian networks. *Nat Biotechnol* 2006; **24**(1): 51–3.

137. Sapolsky RM. Is impaired neurogenesis relevant to the affective symptoms of depression? *Biol Psychiatry* 2004; **56**(3): 137–9.

138. Cho SR, Benraiss A, Chmielnicki E *et al*. Induction of neostriatal neurogenesis slows disease progression in a transgenic murine model of Huntington disease. *J Clin Invest* 2007; **117**(10): 2889–902.

139. Hedman M, Muona K, Hedman A *et al*. Eight-year safety follow-up of coronary artery disease patients after local intracoronary VEGF gene transfer. *Gene Ther* 2009; **16**(5): 629–34.

56

Vascular Dementia

Ingmar Skoog

*Institute of Neuroscience and Physiology, Unit of Neuropsychiatric Epidemiology,
Sahlgrenska Academy at the University of Gothenburg, Gothenburg, Sweden*

BACKGROUND

Cerebrovascular disorders are generally believed to be the second most common cause of dementia, after Alzheimer's disease (AD). Dementia caused by cerebrovascular disease is often labelled vascular dementia (VaD). AD and cerebrovascular disease often co-exist in the same patient. This condition is termed mixed dementia[1]. Cerebrovascular disorders are also associated with cognitive decline which does not reach diagnostic thresholds for dementia[2-6]. The term vascular cognitive impairment was introduced by Bowler and Hachinski in 1995[7] to capture the whole range of cognitive dysfunction associated with vascular disease. This term thus includes VaD, mixed dementia and other forms of cognitive decline caused by cerebrovascular and cardiovascular diseases. It is important to recognize that cognitive impairment associated with cerebrovascular or cardiovascular disorders is potentially preventable or treatable.

DIAGNOSTIC CRITERIA AND DEFINITIONS

The most often used criteria for VaD were developed almost two decades ago. ICD-10 was published in 1993[8], DSM-IV in 1994[9], and the National Institute of Neurological Disorders and Stroke and the Association Internationale pour la Recherché et l'Enseignement en Neurosciences (NINDS-AIREN) criteria were published 1993[10]. These criteria show inconsistencies, and give rise to very different rates of VaD[11,12].

Definition of Dementia and Cognitive Decline

Cognitive function declines with increasing age. The decline may be accelerated by a range of insults to the brain, such as AD, cerebrovascular disease, other brain disorders, and various peripheral disorders such as cardiovascular diseases (CVDs). When the cognitive function reaches a certain threshold, and gives rise to difficulties in everyday life, the term dementia is used.

In criteria such as those of the ICD-10[8] and DSM-IV[9], dementia is a global decline in intellectual function involving memory, orientation, visuospatial abilities, executive function, language, thinking and often changes in personality and emotions. One problem with these criteria is that they state that memory impairment is mandatory for a diagnosis of dementia. This concept is based on the symptoms of AD, and misses a large proportion of individuals with severe cognitive dysfunction associated with impairments in activities of daily living (ADLs) and personal function, as cerebrovascular disease may cause significant cognitive dysfunction with relatively preserved memory function[7].

Definition of Cerebrovascular Disease

Many different cerebrovascular diseases may cause cognitive decline and dementia, including stroke, silent infarcts, ischaemic white matter lesions (WMLs), hereditary cerebral haemorrhage with amyloidosis, granular cortical atrophy, hypertensive encephalopathy, cerebral amyloid angiopathy and cerebral vasculitis (Table 56.1). Most cases of VaD have a mixture of cerebrovascular changes, which could be expected, as different cerebrovascular diseases share similar risk factors. The two most common causes of VaD are stroke and WMLs. However, most criteria highlight clinical strokes in their definitions of cerebrovascular disease. Thus, the definition of cerebrovascular disease is based on the presence or history of focal neurological motor symptom/signs, or brain imaging findings of cerebrovascular disease. DSM-IV lists examples of signs, while the ICD-10 specifies that at least one should be unilateral spastic weakness of the limbs, unilateral increased tendon reflexes, extensor plantar response or pseudobulbar palsy.

The DSM-IV requires that there should be signs *and* symptoms *or* laboratory evidence of cerebrovascular disease (i.e. that brain imaging reveals 'multiple infarctions in the cortex and subcortical white matter'), while ICD-10 requires evidence from history, examination *or* tests of significant cerebrovascular disease (i.e. history of stroke or evidence of cerebral infarction on brain imaging). In the NINDS-AIREN criteria[10], a diagnosis of probably VaD requires that focal signs consistent with stroke *and* relevant cerebrovascular disease by brain imaging should be present. One of the authors of the NINDS-AIREN criteria published a modified version a year later[13], in which this criterion was changed to focal signs consistent with stroke *or* relevant cerebrovascular disease by brain imaging. The first version is far too strict and underestimates the occurrence of VaD[11], since it will exclude individuals without stroke symptoms (including those with silent infarcts or white matter lesions). In a study on 85-year-olds[14], 13% of the demented had VaD based on the first version (i.e. 'focal signs consistent with stroke *and* relevant cerebrovascular disease by

Principles and Practice of Geriatric Psychiatry, 3rd edn. Edited by Mohammed T. Abou-Saleh, Cornelius Katona and Anand Kumar
© 2011 John Wiley & Sons, Ltd

Table 56.1 Causes of vascular dementia

Stroke
Silent infarcts
Ischaemic white matter lesions (WMLs)
CADASIL
Hereditary cerebral haemorrhage with amyloidosis
Granular cortical atrophy
Hypertensive encephalopathy
Cerebral amyloid angiopathy
Cerebral vasculitis

CADASIL, cerebral autosomal dominant arteriopathy with subcortical infarcts and leukoencephalopathy.

brain imaging'), while 47% had VaD with the second version (i.e. 'focal signs consistent with stroke *or* relevant cerebrovascular disease by brain imaging'). In a study conducted on 100 demented patients, the prevalence of VaD was 14% using the first NINDS-AIREN criteria and 76% using DSM-III-R (which uses 'focal signs consistent with stroke *or* relevant cerebrovascular disease by brain imaging')[12]. The NINDS-AIREN criteria allow for a diagnosis of 'possible' VaD in patients with dementia and focal neurological signs in whom brain imaging is missing, and in patients with subtle onset and variable course.

Definition of an Association between Cerebrovascular Disease and Dementia

The influence of a stroke or an infarct on the cognitive symptoms is not easy to decide in the individual case, even if epidemiological studies suggest a strong statistical relationship[6,15–19]. The temporal relationship between symptoms of stroke and onset of dementia is often regarded as strengthening the possibility that the two disorders are related. The recent reports that non-symptomatic infarcts are common in the elderly and related to an increased risk for dementia and stroke[20,21] may question this statement. The NINDS-AIREN criteria suggest an arbitrary limit of three months for onset of dementia after stroke. However, a stroke which occurred years ago indicates the presence of cerebrovascular disease, including silent infarcts. The NINDS-AIREN criteria allow for a diagnosis of 'possible' VaD in the absence of a clear temporal relationship between dementia and clinical symptoms of stroke.

Both DSM-IV and ICD-10 criteria leave the clinician to decide on whether cerebrovascular disease and dementia are related, as both state that 'CVD should be (reasonably) judged to be etiologically related to the disturbance'. There are no specifications as to what this judgement should be based on.

EPIDEMIOLOGY

Almost all epidemiological studies reporting on the frequency of VaD are concerned with the subtype related to clinically manifest stroke or transitory ischaemic attacks (TIA). The proportion of vascular dementia varies widely between studies: between 15 and 45%. The variation may reflect disparities in diagnostic criteria, or differences in the rate of cerebrovascular disorders in different geographical areas[22]. It may also reflect differences in the efforts made to detect and diagnose cerebrovascular disease, and if brain imaging has been used. Although the prevalence of dementia is similar in most parts

of the world, there are differences regarding the type of dementia. Stroke-related dementia is traditionally reported to be more common in Finland, the former Soviet Union and Asian countries, including Japan and China, than in Western Europe and the USA, where AD is generally reported to be the most common type of dementia. However, more recent studies report proportions of VaD in China and Japan similar to western countries[23]. Whether this is due to changes in diagnostic procedures or in risk factors for stroke is not clear.

Stroke

As mentioned, all criteria for VaD encompass history of stroke. Stroke patients typically have history of stroke or TIA including acute focal neurological symptoms and signs, such as hemiparesis or acute aphasia. Other cardiovascular manifestations, including myocardial infarction and hypertension, are common in the patients. Stroke is most often caused by cortical infarcts due to thromboembolism from extracranial arteries and the heart, and is often related to large vessel disease.

The typical clinical course of stroke-related dementia includes sudden onset, stepwise deterioration and a fluctuating course. In the early stages, the expression of cognitive impairment is variable and depends on the site of the lesions. A large proportion of patients with cerebrovascular disease have a gradual onset of dementia with a slowly progressive course[24], with or without focal signs or infarcts on brain imaging, which makes it difficult to differentiate from AD or other types of dementia. It has even been suggested that individuals with cortical strokes show less decline in cognitive function than those with subcortical cerebrovascular disease[25].

Stroke is an essential part of most criteria for VaD or vascular cognitive impairment. In line with this, most epidemiological studies report an increased frequency of dementia in individuals with stroke (Table 56.2). In the studies by Tatemichi *et al.*[15–17], relatively young individuals with ischaemic stroke had at least nine-times greater risk for dementia than stroke-free controls, and those with dementia had a higher mortality rate and worse prognosis which was independent of stroke severity. Also Pohjasvaara *et al.*[18] reported an increased prevalence of dementia in stroke victims, as well as a decrease in independent living for those with dementia. Lindén *et al.*[6] reported that stroke victims aged above 70 had an odds ratio (OR) of 4.7 for dementia. The odds for dementia were higher in those aged 70–80 (OR 6.7) than in those aged above 80 (OR 4.8), but the frequency of dementia after stroke was higher after age 80 (34% versus 18%). In addition, 60% of non-demented stroke victims had some cognitive dysfunction, showing that very few elderly stroke victims are free from cognitive disturbances. In a population study on 85-year-olds, Liebetrau *et al.*[19] reported that the odds ratio for dementia in stroke was 4.3, but the prevalence of dementia in those with stroke was

Table 56.2 Prevalence of dementia in stroke patients and in the general population

Age group	Stroke (%)	Population (%)
60–64	10	1
65–69	20	1
70–74	25	2
75–79	30	5
80+	50	20–30

57%. It may be that the increased risk for dementia with stroke decreases with age although the prevalence increases.

The most important risk factors for stroke are hypertension, diabetes mellitus, atherosclerosis, atrial fibrillation, smoking, being overweight, and hypercholesterolaemia, especially high levels of low-density lipoprotein (LDL) cholesterol[26]. All these risk factors are potentially preventable or treatable. Changing risk factor patterns (e.g. decrease in smoking, more treatment of hypertension) have decreased the incidence of stroke, and may thus decrease the frequency of VaD. On the other hand, more individuals survive after stroke, which may act in the opposite direction. It is not yet known if the prevalence or incidence of VaD is increasing or decreasing.

The pathogenesis of stroke-related dementia has not been established. The main hypothesis is that dementia is related to the location or the volume of the infarcts, but there are also other possibilities. The risk factors for VaD can be divided into stroke-related and non-stroke-related[27]. The stroke-related are similar to those in stroke, for example male sex, hypertension, diabetes mellitus, smoking and cardiac diseases. Non-stroke-related risk factors are similar to those found in sporadic AD and include higher age, lower level of formal education, family history of dementia and the presence of cerebral atrophy. This combination of risk factors supports the view that stroke-related dementia often is a consequence of both stroke and pre-existing AD pathology. According to neuropathological studies, pure VaD, without any AD brain changes, is rare[28].

Silent Cerebrovascular Disease

Most cerebrovascular disease is not related to focal symptoms, aphasia or other distinct clinical manifestation, but may be detected on brain imaging. The relevance of this silent cerebrovascular disease has been debated, but recent research has shown that it is related both to dementia and later manifestations of clinical stroke. The most common 'silent' disorders are silent infarcts and ischaemic white matter lesions.

Silent infarcts

Cerebral infarcts often occur without focal symptoms. The frequency of these so-called silent infarcts increases with age[29]. These lesions were until recently believed to be benign incidental findings on brain imaging, when researchers from the Rotterdam Study reported that individuals with silent infarcts were at increased risk of developing clinical stroke[29] and dementia[20]. Among 85-year-olds, 10% have silent infarcts on CT, and these lesions double the prevalence of dementia[21]. It is important to detect these lesions, as treatment of vascular risk factors, such as hypertension, may decrease the risk of new strokes and thus potentially delay dementia in these high-risk patients.

Subcortical white matter lesions

Another important cerebrovascular disease causing dementia and cognitive decline is subcortical white matter lesions (WMLs)[30]. These have been suggested to be the most common cause of VaD. Subcortical areas of both hemispheres are affected by marked or diffuse ischaemic demyelination and moderate loss of axons with astrogliosis and incomplete infarction. In addition, arteriosclerotic changes with hyalinization or fibrosis and thickening of the vessel walls and narrowing of the lumina of the small penetrating arteries and arterioles are also present[31,32]. The cortex, the subcortical U fibres and corpus callosum are generally well preserved, probably due to the construction of the blood supply.

The pathogenesis behind WMLs is probably that long-standing hypertension causes lipohyalinosis and thickening of the vessel walls with narrowing of the lumen of the small perforating arteries and arterioles which nourish the deep white matter[31]. Episodes of hypotension may lead to further hypoperfusion and hypoxia-ischaemia, leading to more loss of myelin in subcortical areas. The deep white matter has few collaterals, which makes it more vulnerable to ischaemia than the cortex. Furthermore, myelin is probably more vulnerable than axons to ischaemia[33].

WMLs may be detected on brain imaging. On computerised tomography (CT) scans they appear as low-density areas, and on magnetic resonance imaging (MRI) as hyperdense areas. MRI and CT may not always capture the same changes. WMLs on MRI correspond to several different histological findings, most often état criblé, and often show no correlation with cognitive decline and dementia. On the other hand, in 55 cases of WMLs on CT, the histopathological picture described in the previous paragraph was reported at autopsy in 53 of the cases[34]. Thus, MRI is more sensitive than CT for detecting changes in the white matter, but has a lower specificity.

MRI studies generally report much higher rates of WMLs than CT studies. The Rotterdam population study[3] reported that 11% in the age strata 65–69 years, 21% in those aged 70–74 years, 27% in 70–79-year-olds and 54% in those aged 80–84 years had WMLs, and the Helsinki Aging Brain Study[35] reported periventricular hyperintensities in 21% of those aged 55–75 years, and 65% in those above that age. A recent population-based neuropathological study reported that 94% of demented subjects had WMLs[30].

The cognitive decline related to WMLs is suggested to be due to disconnection of subcortical–cortical pathways, producing a decline in abilities related to subcortical or frontal lobe structures. Subcortical symptoms in individuals with WMLs include psychomotor slowness and retardation[4,5] and extrapyramidal signs. Frontal lobe symptoms[36] include executive dysfunction, apathy, loss of drive and emotional blunting. Other symptoms are bilateral or unilateral pyramidal tract signs, and hemi- or motor anaesthesia, pseudobulbar palsy, depression, early urinary incontinence and early gait dysfunction. Memory dysfunction is often mild.

The dementia often has an insidious onset and a slowly progressive course[25,31], which makes it difficult to distinguish from AD. Initially, there may be transient and fleeting attacks of focal neurological symptoms, with a subacute accumulation of deficits. WMLs seldom occur as the sole cause of dementia, and the clinical picture may vary depending on what other causes contribute to the dementia. Punctate WMLs on MRI do not progress, while confluent white matter abnormalities are progressive, and thus more malignant in the long term[37].

The main risk factors for WMLs are high age, hypertension, and hypertension clustering factors. It has been suggested that the arterial changes are due to exposure of vessel walls to increased pressure over time. The greater the pressure and/or life span, the more likely are these changes to be present. This may be one reason for the observed increase with age reported in most studies.

It was recently shown that diastolic blood pressure and mean arterial pressure in midlife was related to the presence of white matter lesions in late life, supporting both the theory that long-standing high blood pressure is important and that resistance of the smaller arteries and microvascular network is important[38].

Mixed Dementias

The common co-occurrence of AD and VaD is becoming increasingly recognized[1,30]. This may even be the most common cause of dementia, especially in the oldest ages. As already mentioned, cerebrovascular disease increases the risk of developing dementia[6,15–19,34], but to evaluate the relative contribution of cerebrovascular disease towards the dementia symptoms in the individual patient is almost impossible. Cerebrovascular disease may be the sole cause of dementia in an individual; it may be the event that finally overcomes the brain's compensatory capacity in a subject whose brain is already affected by not-yet clinically manifest Alzheimer pathology, and in many instances minor manifestations of both disorders which individually would not be enough to produce dementia may produce it together[39,40]. On a clinical basis, it is often almost impossible to differentiate mixed dementia from pure VaD. Cerebrovascular disease as a contributing cause of dementia may be overlooked as onset is sometimes insidious, the course gradual, and the infarctions clinically silent or not detectable by brain imaging. Pure VAD may also be overdiagnosed, as the presence of stroke, WMLs or other cardiovascular disease does not mean that they caused the dementia.

Even the histopathological diagnoses of AD and VaD are uncertain. Extensive AD encephalopathy[41–43] and cerebrovascular disease[41,44] are reported in individuals with no signs of dementia during life. The MRC-FAS study[43], and the Nun Study[45] both found that only about half of those fulfilling neuropathological criteria for AD were demented during life. Similar results are reported in PET (positron emission tomography) studies using the PiB (Pittsburgh compound B) to detect amyloid deposition[46]. This shows that presence of extensive AD in the brain does not always result in dementia. A substantial proportion of individuals fulfilling the NINCDS-ADRDA (National Institute of Neurological and Communicative Disorders and Stroke, and the Alzheimer's Disease and Related Disorders Association) criteria for probable AD or NINDS-AIREN criteria for probable VaD have mixed pathologies[28,47,48]. Also, WMLs have been described on both brain imaging and at autopsy in about two-thirds of cases of Alzheimer's disease[32,34,49]. The Nun study[45] showed that presence of cerebrovascular disease increased the risk that individuals with AD lesions in their brains would express a dementia syndrome, from 57% in those without cerebrovascular disease to 93% in those with 1–2 lacunar infarcts and 75% in those with large infarcts[45]. In addition, patients with VaD may have cholinergic deficits similar to those seen in AD, caused by ischaemia of basal forebrain nuclei and of cholinergic pathways[50,51]. Also other markers of AD, such as high tau[52] and low beta-amyloid[53] in cerebrospinal fluid may appear in VaD. Finally, similar vascular risk factors have been reported both for AD and VaD[54], which also may explain the common co-occurrence of these disorders.

DIAGNOSIS

The first step in the diagnostic work-up is to determine the extent of cognitive dysfunction, the nature of this dysfunction, and its consequences. This should be done in all elderly patients with a recent stroke, or other cerebrovascular disease. A simple screening instrument may be used, for example the Mini-Mental State Examination. Other tests include examinations of executive function, the Clock Test, word fluency, naming ability and five-item memory test. It needs to be emphasized that patients with dementia related to CVD are often difficult to test due to language dysfunction.

The second step aims to identify cerebrovascular and other causes of the dementia. In the elderly, there are often multiple causes of dementia, and every contributing treatable cause that can be diagnosed may be important in the treatment of the patient. Besides cerebrovascular disease, other conditions that might contribute to cognitive decline include, for example, cardiovascular diseases, deficiency states, infections and depression. Brain imaging is necessary in this step, not only to identify cerebrovascular disease (white matter lesions and cerebral infarcts), but also to diagnose low pressure hydrocephalus, subdural haematoma, and brain tumours. The examinations should also include careful history-taking, interview of a close informant, neurological, psychiatric and physical examinations, chest X-ray, ECG and biochemical screening. This last includes cholesterol (total cholesterol, s-high-density lipoprotein cholesterol, s-low-density lipoprotein, triglycerides), screening for diabetes mellitus (fasting P-glucose, B-HbA1c), P-homocystein, vitamin B12, a thyroid function test and thrombocytes, leukocytes and haemoglobin. Cerebrospinal fluid (CSF) examinations should be performed for analyses of beta-amyloid, tau protein, inflammation and CSF/blood ratio (for blood–brain barrier function).

An ECG should be performed to detect arrhythmias and other cardiac diseases. A carotis Doppler should be done to detect atherosclerosis in this vessel.

Traditionally AD has been a diagnosis of exclusion and VaD has often been assigned if the patient has a history of stroke thought to be etiologically related to dementia. From a clinical standpoint, it is neither important nor possible to differentiate between AD and VaD in most cases with cerebrovascular disease. Most cases of VaD are probably of a mixed aetiology, and older patients with AD may often have concomitant cerebrovascular disease, which needs treatment. Therefore the diagnostic procedure should detect evidence for AD and cerebrovascular disease and direct the treatment to both disorders.

TREATMENT POSSIBILITIES

The general strategy in the treatment of VaD is to prevent new strokes or infarcts. Detection and treatment of risk factors is essential. Some risk factors are listed in Table 56.3. Treatment of cardiac arrhythmias, diabetes mellitus, hypertension and hypercholesterolaemia is also essential. Regarding white matter dementia, antihypertensive treatment may potentially prevent the changes in the small vessels. Recently it was shown that treatment of hypertension prevented stroke also in individuals above the age of 80[55]. Although no formal studies have been performed, the use of anticoagulant agents, for

Table 56.3 Risk factors for vascular dementia

Hypertension
Atherosclerosis
Arteriolosclerosis
Heart disease (infarction, arrhythmias)
Hypotension
Diabetes mellitus
Hyperlipidaemia
Smoking
Overweight
Hyperviscosity

example low-dose treatment with salicylates, is often used. Patients with VaD often have concomitant AD. In these cases, one should initiate treatment with an acetylcholinesterase inhibitor[50,56].

REFERENCES

1. Langa KM, Foster NL, Larson EB. Mixed dementia. Emerging concepts and therapeutic implications. *JAMA* 2004; **292**: 2901–8.
2. Breteler MMB, Claus JJ, Grobbee DE, Hofman A. Cardiovascular disease and distribution of cognitive function in elderly people: the Rotterdam study. *BMJ* 1994; **308**: 1604–8.
3. Breteler MMB, Van Swieten JC, Bots ML *et al.* Cerebral white matter lesions, vascular risk factors, and cognitive function in a population-based study: the Rotterdam study. *Neurology* 1994; **44**: 1246–52.
4. Breteler MMB, Van Amerongen NM, Van Swieten JC *et al.* Cognitive correlates of ventricular enlargement and cerebral white matter lesions on magnetic resonance imaging. The Rotterdam study. *Stroke* 1994; **25**: 1109–15.
5. Skoog I, Berg S, Johansson B, Palmertz B, Andreasson L-A. The influence of white matter lesions on neuropsychological functioning in demented and non-demented 85-year-olds. *Acta Neurol Scand* 1996; **93**: 142–8.
6. Lindén T, Skoog I, Fagerberg B, Steen B, Blomstrand C. Cognitive impairment and dementia 20 months after stroke. *Neuroepidemiology* 2004; **23**: 45–52.
7. Bowler JV, Hachinski V. Vascular cognitive impairment: a new approach to vascular dementia. *Baillieres Clin Neurol* 1995; **4**: 357–76.
8. World Health Organization. *The ICD-10 Classification of Mental and Behavioural Disorders. Diagnostic Criteria for Research.* Geneva: WHO, 1993.
9. American Psychiatric Association. *Diagnostic and Statistical Manual of Mental Disorders, Fourth Edition.* Washington, DC: American Psychiatric Association, 1994.
10. Román GC, Tatemichi TK, Erkinjuntti T *et al.* Vascular dementia: diagnostic criteria for research studies. Report of the NINDS-AIREN international workshop. *Neurology* 1993; **43**: 250–60.
11. Skoog I, Copeland JRM. Nosology of dementia. In Copeland JRM, Abou-Saleh MT, Blazer DG (eds), *Principles and Practice of Geriatric Psychiatry*, 2nd edn. Chichester: John Wiley & Sons, Ltd, 2002, 185–9.
12. Wetterling T, Kanitz R-D, Borgis K-J. Comparison of different diagnostic criteria for vascular dementia (ADDTC, DSM-IV, ICD-10, NINDS-AIREN). *Stroke* 1996; **27**: 30–6.
13. Tatemichi TK, Sacktor N, Mayeux R. Dementia associated with cerebrovascular disease, other degenerative diseases, and metabolic disorders. In Terry RD, Katzman R, Bick KL (eds), *Alzheimer Disease*. New York: Raven Press Ltd, 1994.
14. Skoog I, Nilsson L, Palmertz B, Andreasson L-A, Svanborg A. A population-based study of dementia in 85-year-olds. *N Engl J Med* 1993; **328**: 153–8.
15. Tatemichi TK, Desmond DW, Mayeux R *et al.* Dementia after stroke: baseline frequency, risks, and clinical features in a hospitalized cohort. *Neurology* 1992; **42**: 1185–93.
16. Tatemichi TK, Desmond DW, Paik M *et al.* Clinical determinants of dementia related to stroke. *Ann Neurol* 1993; **33**: 568–75.

17. Tatemichi TK, Paik M, Bagiella E *et al.* Dementia after stroke is a predictor of long-time survival. *Stroke* 1994; **25**: 1915–19.
18. Pohjasvaara T, Erkinjuntti T, Vataja R, Kaste M. Dementia three months after stroke. Baseline frequency and effect of different definitions of dementia in the Helsinki Stroke Aging Memory (SAM) cohort. *Stroke* 1997; **28**: 785–92.
19. Liebetrau M, Steen B, Skoog I. Stroke in 85-year-olds. Prevalence, incidence, risk factors and relation to mortality and dementia. *Stroke* 2003; **34**: 2617–22.
20. Vermeer SE, Prins ND, Den Heijer T *et al.* Silent brain infarcts and the risk of dementia and cognitive decline. *N Engl J Med* 2003; **348**: 1215–22.
21. Liebetrau M, Steen B, Hamann GF, Skoog I. Silent and symptomatic infarcts on cranial computerized tomography in relation to dementia and mortality. A population-based study in 85-year-olds. *Stroke* 2004; **35**: 1816–20.
22. Skoog I, Aevarsson O. Epidemiology of vascular dementia in Europe. In O'Brien J, Ames D, Gustafson L, Folstein M, Chiu E (eds), *Cerebrovascular Disease, Cognition and Dementia*, 2nd edn. London: Martin Dunitz Ltd, 2004, 35–48.
23. Zhang ZX, Zahner GE, Roman GC *et al.* Dementia subtypes in China: prevalence in Beijing, Xian, Shanghai, and Chengdu. *Arch Neurol* 2005; **62**: 447–53.
24. Fischer P, Gatterer G, Marterer A, Simanyi M, Danielczyk W. Course characteristics in the differentiation of dementia of the Alzheimer type and multi-infarct dementia. *Acta Psychiatr Scand* 1990; **81**: 551–3.
25. Gunstad J, Brickman AM, Paul RH *et al.* Progressive morphometric and cognitive changes in vascular dementia. *Arch Clin Neuropsychology* 2005; **20**: 229–41.
26. Qiu C, Skoog I, Fratiglioni L. Occurrence and determinants of vascular cognitive impairment. In Erkinjuntti T, Gauthier S (eds), *Vascular Cognitive Impairment*. London: Martin Dunitz Ltd, 2002, 61–83.
27. Skoog I. Guest editorial. Status of risk factors for vascular dementia. *Neuroepidemiology* 1998; **17**: 2–9.
28. Barker WW, Luis CA, Kashuba A *et al.* Relative frequencies of Alzheimer disease, Lewy body, vascular and frontotemporal dementia, and hippocampal sclerosis in the State of Florida Brain Bank. *Alzheimer Dis Assoc Disord* 2002; **16**: 203–12.
29. Vermeer SE, Koudstaal PJ, Oudkerk M, Hofman A, Breteler MM. Prevalence and risk factors of silent brain infarcts in the population-based Rotterdam Scan Study. *Stroke* 2002; **33**: 21–5.
30. Fernando MS, Ince PG, on behalf of the MRC Cognitive function and Ageing Neuropathology Study Group. Vascular pathologies and cognition in a population-based cohort of elderly people. *J Neurol Sciences* 2004; **226**: 13–17.
31. Román GC. Senile dementia of the Binswanger type. A vascular form of dementia in the elderly. *JAMA* 1987; **258**: 1782–88.
32. Brun A, Englund E. A white matter disorder in dementia of the Alzheimer type: a pathoanatomical study. *Ann Neurol* 1986; **19**: 253–62.
33. Englund E, Brun A. White matter changes in dementia of Alzheimer's type. The difference in vulnerability between cell compartments. *Histopathology* 1990; **16**: 433–9.
34. Skoog I, Palmertz B, Andreasson L-A. The prevalence of white matter lesions on computed tomography of the brain in demented and non-demented 85-year-olds. *J Geriatr Psychiatry Neurol* 1994; **7**: 169–75.
35. Ylikoski A, Erkinjuntti T, Raininko R *et al.* White matter hyperintensities on MRI in the neurologically non-diseased elderly.

Analysis of cohorts of consecutive subjects aged 55 to 85 years living at home. *Stroke* 1995; **26**: 1171–7.

36. Boone KB, Miller BL, Lesser BL *et al.* Neuropsychological correlates of white-matter lesions in healthy elderly subjects. A threshold effect. *Arch Neurol* 1992; **49**: 549–54.

37. Schmidt R, Enzinger C, Ropele S, Schmidt H, Fazekas F. Austrian Stroke Prevention Study. Progression of cerebral white matter lesions: 6-year results of the Austrian Stroke Prevention Study. *Lancet* 2003; **361**: 2046–8.

38. Guo X, Pantoni L, Simoni M *et al.* Midlife blood pressure and late-life white matter lesions: the prospective population study of women in Gothenburg, Sweden. *Hypertension* 2009; **54**: 57–62.

39. Erkinjuntti T, Hachinski V. Dementia post stroke. In Teasell RW (ed.), *Physical Medicine and Rehabilitation: State of the Art Reviews*, vol. 7. Philadelphia, PA: Hanley & Belfus Inc, 1993, 195–212.

40. Erkinjuntti T, Hachinski V. Rethinking vascular dementia. *Cerebrovasc Dis* 1993; **3**: 3–23.

41. Tomlinson BE, Blessed G, Roth M. Observations on the brains of demented old people. *J Neurol Sci* 1970; **11**: 205–42.

42. Arriagada P, Marzloff K, Hyman B. Distribution of Alzheimer-type pathologic changes in nondemented elderly individuals matches the pattern in Alzheimer's disease. *Neurology* 1992; **42**: 1681–8.

43. Neuropathology Group. Medical Research Council Cognitive Function and Aging Study. Pathological correlates of late-onset dementia in a multicentre, community-based population in England and Wales. Lancet 2001; 357: 169–75.

44. Del Ser T, Bermejo F, Portera A *et al.* Vascular dementia. A clinicopathological study. *J Neurol Sci* 1990; **96**: 1–17.

45. Snowdon DA, Greiner LH, Mortimer JA *et al.* Brain infarction and the clinical expression of Alzheimer disease. The Nun Study. *JAMA* 1997; **277**: 813–17.

46. Aizenstein HJ, Nebes RD, Saxton JA *et al.* Frequent amyloid deposition without significant cognitive impairment among the elderly. *Arch Neurol* 2008; **65**: 1509–17.

47. Holmes C, Cairns N, Lantos P, Mann A. Validity of current clinical criteria for Alzheimer's disease, vascular dementia and dementia with Lewy bodies. *Br J Psychiatry* 1999; **174**: 45–50.

48. Lim A, Tsuang D, Kukull W *et al.* Clinico-neuropathological correlation of Alzheimer's disease in a community-based case series. *J Am Geriatr Soc* 1999; **47**: 564–9.

49. De la Monte SM. Quantitation of cerebral atrophy in preclinical and end-stage Alzheimer's disease. *Ann Neurol* 1989; **25**: 450–9.

50. Erkinjuntti T, Roman G, Gauthier S. Treatment of vascular dementia – evidence from clinical trials with cholinesterase inhibitors. *J Neurol Sci* 2004; **226**: 63–6.

51. Roman GC. Cholinergic dysfunction in vascular dementia. *Curr Psychiatry Rep* 2005; **7**: 18–26.

52. Skoog I, Vanmechelen E, Andreasson L-A *et al.* A population-based study of tau protein and ubiquitin in cerebrospinal fluid in 85-year-olds: relation to severity of dementia and cerebral atrophy, but not to the apolipoprotein E4 allele. *Neurodegeneration* 1995; **4**: 433–42.

53. Skoog I, Davidsson P, Aevarsson O *et al.* Cerebrospinal fluid beta-amyloid 42 is reduced before the onset of sporadic dementia: a population-based study in 85-year-olds. *Dement Geriatr Cogn Disord* 2003; **15**: 169–76.

54. Kalaria R, Skoog I. Overlap with Alzheimer's disease. In Erkinjuntti T, Gauthier S (eds), *Vascular Cognitive Impairment*. London: Martin Dunitz Ltd, 2002, 145–66.

55. Skoog I. Antihypertensive treatment and dementia prevention. *Lancet Neurology* 2008; **7**: 664–5.

56. Erkinjuntti T, Kurz A, Gauthier S *et al.* Efficacy of galantamine in probable vascular dementia and Alzheimer's disease combined with cerebrovascular disease: a randomised trial. *Lancet* 2002; **359**: 1283–90.

57

The Frontotemporal Dementia Syndromes

Mario F. Mendez

VA Greater Los Angeles Healthcare System and David Geffen School of Medicine at UCLA, Los Angeles, USA

INTRODUCTION

The frontotemporal dementia (FTD) syndromes are related disorders resulting from neurodegeneration of the frontal and anterior temporal lobes. In 1892, Arnold Pick, a Prague neuropsychiatrist, described the first known patient and subsequently published a series of three patients with left anterior temporal atrophy[1,2]. In 1911, Alois Alzheimer, a German neuropathologist, described the characteristic inclusion bodies of what came to be known as 'Pick's disease.' The field was nearly quiescent until the late 1980s when investigators in Lund, Sweden reported on an autopsy series of 158 patients with dementia[3,4], 20 (13%) of whom proved to have frontal lobe degeneration. In the past two to three decades, progress has been rapid. In the 1990s, there were several clinicopathological studies of FTD[5,6] and the eventual demonstration of a linkage of some cases to the tau gene region on chromosome 17[7]. Finally, in the past few years, researchers discovered an association of FTD with mutations in the progranulin gene (*PGRN*) and identified one of the major ubiquitinated proteins in FTD as the TAR DNA-binding protein 43 (TDP-43)[8-11].

The three principal FTD syndromes are the behavioural variant (bvFTD), which comprises over half of these patients, and the language-predominant syndromes of progressive non-fluent aphasia (PNFA) and semantic dementia (SD). Although often underdiagnosed[12,13], these three FTD syndromes comprise the third most common neurodegenerative dementia after Alzheimer's disease (AD) and dementia with Lewy bodies (DLB). Clinical reports describe frequencies of FTD of 5–13% among dementia outpatients[14,15]. In possibly the best population-based series, there was a calculated annual (1990–1994) incidence of FTD in Rochester, MN, of 2.2 per 100 000 in the age group 40–49 years, 3.3 for 50–59, and 8.9 for 60–69[15].

On average, the FTD syndromes have a presenile age of onset, are equally common among men and women, and lack a proven ethnic predisposition. The age of onset of bvFTD averages around 57 years with a usual range of 51–63 years, but patients have presented from the 20s to the 80s[16-18]. The age of onset of SD is similar to that of bvFTD, but PNFA patients are often slightly older[17]. FTD syndromes are common among dementia patients with an age of onset of less than 65 years, accounting for approximately 15–20% of young-onset dementias[18-20], with prevalences in the 45–64 year age group of 15 per 100 000 in the UK and 6.7 per 100 000 in the Netherlands[20-22].

CLINICAL PRESENTATIONS

Behavioural Variant FTD

The clinical syndrome of FTD presents with several 'core' and 'supportive' behavioural changes in mid-life (Table 57.1)[23-26]. The most common behavioural changes are apathy or decreased spontaneity and interest, and disinhibition or impulsivity[25,27,28]. Second, bvFTD patients violate social and moral norms, conventions or rules[25,26]. They may inappropriately touch others or violate their personal space, talk to strangers or children that they do not know, make sexual comments, forgo tact or table manners, and even manifest sociopathic behaviour such as theft. Third, they have 'emotional blunting' with a loss of empathy and awareness of the needs of others. Basic emotional appreciation is decreased, particularly for negative facial or vocal emotions[29,30]. Fourth, patients lose insight into their behavioural changes and lack self-referential behaviours such as embarrassability or shame. Fifth, they frequently have changes in dietary or eating behaviour, most commonly a carbohydrate craving[25]. Sixth, bvFTD patients have a range of repetitive behaviours from simple motor stereotypies to complex compulsive-like acts[25]. Finally, a supportive criterion is neglect or loss of interest in personal hygiene with failure to wash, bathe, groom or dress appropriately. In comparison, psychotic symptoms such as delusions and hallucinations are much less common among bvFTD patients compared to other dementia syndromes[25,31].

Cognitive functions

Patients with bvFTD develop frontal-executive deficits. This is reflected in their lack of insight and loss of awareness or distress at their disability or the consequences of their behaviour. Their judgement is abnormal, and they are often concrete on idiom and proverb interpretation. Occasionally, patients have stimulus-bound behaviour such as echolalia and utilization behaviour (grasping and repeatedly using objects that they see or tending to read aloud anything they see). On language examination, bvFTD patients often have progressively decreased verbal output and mutism in advanced stages. They also manifest reiterative speech or verbal stereotypies. In contrast, early bvFTD patients have relatively spared memory with better free recall, cued recall and recognition than

Table 57.1 Behavioural variant frontotemporal dementia

I. Core diagnostic features
- A. Progressive deterioration of behaviour, cognition or both
- B. Early apathy or inertia
- C. Early behavioural disinhibition with abnormal sociomoral behaviour
- D. Early 'emotional blunting' or loss of sympathy or empathy
- E. Loss insight or and self-referential behaviours

II. Supportive diagnostic features
- A. Dietary or eating behaviour, most commonly a carbohydrate craving
- B. Repetitive (stereotypic or compulsive) behaviour
- C. Executive deficits with relative sparing of memory and visuo-spatial functions
- D. Decline in personal hygiene and grooming
- E. Brain imaging: predominant frontal and/or anterior temporal abnormality

Source: Modified from Neary *et al.*[61]

Table 57.2 Progressive non-fluent aphasia

I. Core diagnostic features
- A. Insidious onset and gradual progression
- B. Agrammatism
  1. Grammatical morpheme and functor word omission
  2. Reduced mean length of utterance
  3. Phonemic paraphasias
- C. Motor speech abnormalities
  1. Articulatory struggle and stuttering
  2. Dyarthria and/or dysprosody
  3. Apraxia of speech

II. Supportive diagnostic features
- A. Impaired syntactical comprehension
- B. Impaired repetition
- C. Alexia and agraphia
- D. Brain imaging: asymmetric abnormality predominantly affecting left hemisphere

Source: Modified from Neary *et al.*[61]

do AD patients[18,32,33]. Furthermore, they have preserved visuospatial skills such as spatial localization and orientation in familiar surroundings[34,35]. Rare bvFTD patients even have a facilitation of artistic and musical ability[36].

On neurological examination, bvFTD patients are usually normal early in their course but can develop primitive reflexes and motor changes as the disease progresses. A major subgroup of bvFTD patients develops parkinsonism, dystonia and ideomotor apraxia, or fasciculations and muscle wasting. Many of those who develop parkinsonism eventually evolve to the related syndromes of progressive supranuclear palsy (PSP) and corticobasal syndrome (CBS)[37–43]. A second major subgroup of about 10–15% of bvFTD patients develop motor neuron disease (MND), primarily with bulbar and proximal upper extremity impairment[44–47].

On neuropsychological testing, bvFTD patients perform particularly poorly on tests of executive functions[48–52]. They are often impaired on digit span backwards, verbal fluency, Trail Making Test B, and the Tower Test. They do poorly on the Iowa Gambling Task, where they fail to improve when offered monetary rewards[53]. Patients with bvFTD cannot do tasks of abstraction and have poor verb comprehension relative to nouns[54–56]. They may be impaired on paradigms where they must infer other people's mental states, thoughts and feelings, referred to as 'theory of mind'[57], and the ability to process social rule violations is impaired along with their sense of 'personal' morality[30,58]. In comparison, as previously noted, there is relative preservation of amnesia or visuo-spatial impairments on neuropsychological measures.

Progressive Nonfluent Aphasia

PNFA is characterized by an initial two or more year period of relatively isolated difficulty in verbal expression with agrammatism, difficulty with sentence syntax, shortened phrase length, and motor speech difficulties in the presence of relatively preserved comprehension (Table 57.2)[59–62]. Patients have difficulty with verbs and with sentence processing[63]. They also have apraxia of speech, with hesitant, broken and effortful output and phonologic (phonemic paraphasic) errors, particularly in repetition of polysyllabic words. Speech changes include progressive dysarthria with stuttering and

oral apraxia[64]. Reading and writing is correspondingly impaired, and patients with PNFA are aware of their language and speech deficits.

In PNFA, there is asymmetric atrophy of the left frontotemporal lobes[61]. Magnetic resonance imaging (MRI) with voxel-based morphometry (VBM) and functional imaging reveal marked atrophic changes or hypometabolism and decreased blood flow in the left perisylvian, inferior frontal and anterior insular areas[59,65]. Most patients with PNFA have frontotemporal neuropathology, but some patients have a language variant of AD at postmortem[62,66].

Semantic Dementia

This FTD syndrome produces a multimodal loss of conceptual knowledge, particularly in word comprehension and facial recognition (Table 57.3). In contrast to PNFA, patients with SD have fluent speech and normal grammar but cannot understand words[67]. They have relative preservation of repetition, phonology, syntax, the ability to read aloud and the ability to write orthographically regular words. Their speech output becomes progressively empty, however, as they lose substantive words and their meanings. On testing, they have problems with single word comprehension on pointing commands, word definitions and matching of objects or pictures with words. On reading, there is a characteristic disorder termed 'surface dyslexia' with inability to read irregularly spelled words but preserved ability to sound them out[68]. The rest of their cognitive profile reflects semantic loss in other domains. There may be an impairment in the recognition of familiar faces (prosopagnosia) and impairment of object meaning or identity (object agnosia) that cannot be attributed to naming difficulties. Despite these deficits, SD patients can continue to learn (episodic memory) and have intact visuo-spatial skills[69].

In SD there is circumscribed atrophy of the anterior inferior temporal gyri[70]. The cortical atrophy involves the left inferolateral temporal lobe and fusiform gyrus, right temporal pole, bilateral ventromedial frontal cortex, and the amygdaloid complex with sparing of the hippocampus[70]. Most SD patients have greater atrophy in the left anterior temporal region compared to the right. The asymmetric involvement is often evident on MRI imaging and correlates

Table 57.3 Semantic dementia: consensus criteria

I. Core diagnostic features
  A. Insidious onset and gradual progression
  B. Poor confrontational naming, particularly for unfamiliar items
  C. Loss of word comprehension, particularly for unfamiliar items
  D. Intact word repetition
  E. Intact motor speech
AND/OR
  A. Perceptual disorder characterized by
    1. Prosopagnosia: impaired recognition of identity of familiar faces
    2. Object agnosia: impaired recognition of object identity
  B. Preserved perceptual matching and drawing reproduction
Supportive diagnostic feature
  Brain imaging: predominant anterior temporal abnormality-bilaterally or asymmetric

Source: Modified from Neary *et al.*[61]

with relative impairments for word meaning (left temporal lobe) versus prosopagnosia or object recognition (right temporal lobe)[71]. The function of the anterior inferior temporal region appears to be to bind information together.

CLINICAL EVALUATION AND DIAGNOSIS

With the exception of the identifiable mutations, there are as yet no definitive tests for the FTD syndromes. In bvFTD, the behavioural changes outlined above usually precede or overshadow any cognitive deficits[6,18,19,72]. Suspicion for bvFTD arises when there is a change in personality, usually in mid-life[19,73,74]. Suspicion for PNFA or SD arises when there is new speech or word-finding difficulty in mid-life. Clinical criteria for diagnosing the three main FTD syndromes are the FTD Consensus Criteria (see Tables 57.1–57.3)[61]. These criteria have proven imperfect, with about 33–56% of bvFTD patients failing to meet Core Consensus Criteria on presentation (see Table 57.1)[12,13,75]. They are particularly deficient when it comes to a subgroup of bvFTD patients who lack changes on neuroimaging and who fail to progress after years of follow-up[50,51,76]. Currently, the FTD Consensus Criteria are undergoing revision by an international team of experts in the field.

Brain MRI can help confirm the presence of an FTD syndrome (Figure 57.1)[77]. Although often normal in early stages[78,79], MRI scans eventually show frontal and anterior temporal atrophy, enlargement of the Sylvian fissures, and anterior callosal atrophy[80–86]. There is temporal polar, amygdalar and lateral temporal and fusiform gyral involvement but relative sparing of the hippocampi[83,87–90]. FTD patients may have additional MRI evidence of bilateral caudate atrophy, and others have changes in the substantia nigra and putamen or high signal changes in white matter[91]. VBM studies in autopsy-confirmed patients have confirmed the mesial frontal, anterior insular and anterior temporal regional atrophy[92–96]. Finally, recent studies suggest that the neuropathological variants of FTD may have different patterns of frontotemporal atrophy on neuroimaging[95,97].

Functional imaging may be more sensitive than MRI for the diagnosis of FTD. Positron emission tomography (PET) and single-photon emission tomography scans show decreased regional

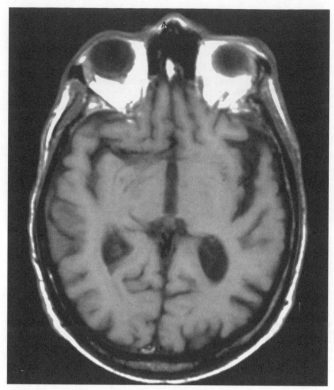

Figure 57.1 MRI (T2-weighted) image of progressive non-fluent aphasia (PNFA). Asymmetric atrophy of the left Sylvian fissure with reciprocal enlargement of the left frontal horn

metabolism and cerebral blood flow in the frontal cortex and anterior temporal lobes (Figure 57.2)[72,82,98,99]. On fluorodeoxyglucose (FDG) PET, glucose uptake is reduced primarily in dorsolateral and ventrolateral prefrontal cortices and in frontopolar and anterior cingulate regions[100]. Although PET scan changes are not specific for FTD syndromes[101], worsening functional changes over time favour the diagnosis of a neurodegenerative dementia such as FTD[102,103]. Furthermore, new functional imaging technologies, such as Pittsburgh Compound-B (PIB), hold great promise for distinguishing FTD syndromes from AD and other neurodegenerative disorders with amyloid-related pathology[104,105].

There are important brain–behaviour relationships between symptoms and specific regions of involvement in FTD. Patients with bvFTD have greater right than left-sided atrophy[106,107]. The initial pathology in bvFTD involves the ventromedial frontal cortex, orbitofrontal region and anterior insula[108,109]. Abnormalities in social and moral conduct correlate with changes in these regions on functional neuroimaging[26]. Apathy correlates with mesial frontal atrophy on both MRI VBM and on FDG-PET[28,110]. Disinhibition correlates with atrophy of the subcallosal part of the frontal lobe, orbitofrontal region and adjacent temporal areas[28,106,110]. PFNA and apraxia of speech correlate with left peri-Sylvian and anterior insular involvement[92]. SD correlates with anterior temporal atrophy[88,111]. Moreover, in SD, impaired word comprehension corresponds to left anterior temporal atrophy, and right temporal atrophy corresponds to impaired recognition of faces (Figure 57.3).

Most other biomarkers, such as plasma TDP-43 or tau levels, have not yet proven to be clinically useful for the diagnosis of FTD syndromes. Cerebrospinal (CSF) biomarkers hold the most promise for

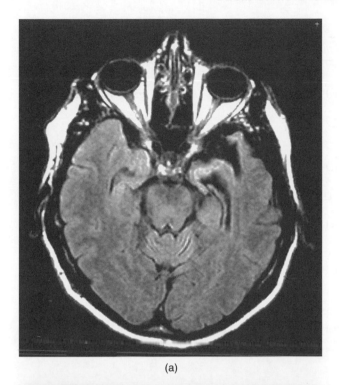

(a)

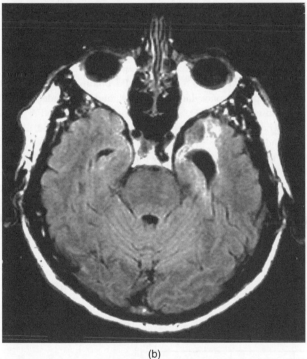

(b)

Figure 57.2 FDG-PET imaging of FTD patient. (a) Horizontal and (b) saggital views demonstrate frontal and anterior temporal hypometabolism

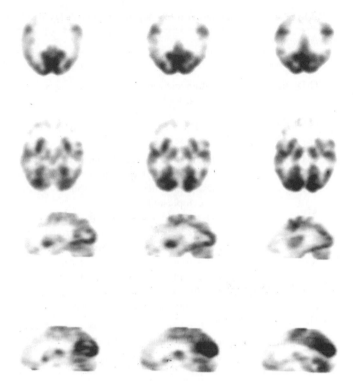

Figure 57.3 MRI (T2-weighted) images from patient with semantic dementia (SD). There is bilateral anterior temporal atrophy disproportionately affecting the left temporal lobe and associated with impaired word comprehension

PRGN protein in FTD patients with these mutations may be useful in screening for this specific genetic form of FTD (see below)[121].

PATHOLOGY AND NEUROGENETICS

There is frontotemporal lobar degeneration on gross pathology. The ventromedial frontal region and the anterior temporal areas have the most severe atrophic changes. Initially, the cortical degeneration is usually asymmetric and involves the mesial frontal regions including the anterior cingulate gyrus and the anterior insula. The frontotemporal cortex has neuronal and synaptic loss and astrogliosis with spongiosis (minute cavities or microvacuolation) of the outer, supra-granular (II–III) layers, with variable involvement of subcortical and limbic structures[122–124]. Specific loss of von Economo neurons occurs in the anterior cingulate and anterior insulae[124]. Finally, the serotoninergic and dopaminergic systems are decreased with relative sparing of cholinergic systems[125,126].

The FTD syndromes include pathological variants that have intraneuronal inclusions that are either tau-positive or tau-negative, ubiquitin-positive (Table 57.4)[127]. FTD is most commonly due to tau protein, with tau-positive inclusions, or to the neuronal accumulation of TAR DNA-binding protein-43 (TDP-43) protein, with tau-negative, ubiquitin-positive inclusions. Among a cohort of 26 bvFTD patients, there were equal numbers with tau-positive and tau-negative pathology[128], and among another 74 bvFTD patients, 55% were associated with a TDP-43 proteinopathy[60,129]. Tau is a microtubule-associated protein (MAPT) that stabilizes microtubules and promotes microtubule assembly by binding to tubulin[130].

eventually helping distinguish FTD from AD[112]. Among patients with bvFTD, some have found a significant decrease of CSF tau protein[113], but most report normal or only slightly increased CSF total tau and phospho-tau levels[114–120]. Overall, the literature indicates significantly lower total tau and tau/Aβ42 amyloid ratios in FTD compared to AD. In addition, decreased plasma levels of the

Table 57.4 Frontotemporal lobar degeneration (FTLD) neuropathology[127,141]

Histopathology		Clinical syndromes	Genetic association
Tau-positive			
FTLD-tau	Intranuclear tau-positive inclusions, e.g. Pick bodies	bvFTD, PNFA, PSP, CBS	*MAPT* gene abnormities
Tau-negative, ubiquitin-positive			
FTLD-TDP			
U1	Dystrophic neurites (elongated, long); neuronal cytoplasmic inclusions (few)	SD	None known
U2	Dystrophic neurites (few, short); neuronal cytoplasmic inclusions	FTD-MND, MND	Intraflagellar transport 74
U3	Dystrophic neurites (short); neuronal cytoplasmic inclusions; neuronal intranuclear inclusions	bvFTD, PNFA	*PRGN*
U4	Dystrophic neurites; few neuronal cytoplasmic inclusions; neuronal intranuclear inclusions	bvFTD	*VCP*
FTDP-UPS	Ubiquitin proteosome system	bvFTD	*CHMP2B*
FTDP-U 'atypical'		Very young onset bvFTD	
Tau-negative, ubiquitin-negative			
FTDP-IF	Neuronal intermediate filament inclusion disease		
FTDP-ni	No inclusions	bvFTD	
BIBD	Basophilic inclusion body disease	bvFTD	

It is abnormal if hyperphosphorylated, resulting in a breakdown of microtubules and an impairment of axonal transport. TDP-43 is a nuclear protein whose function is not entirely clear, but appears to have a role in the regulation of transcription and mRNA splicing[131]. It is normal for TDP-43 to be ubiquinated, but it is abnormal when phosphorylated[131].

Many patients with FTD syndromes have the intraneuronal accumulation of MAPT with tau-positive inclusions[132-134]. Six different isoforms of this tau protein result from alternative splicing, particularly of exon 10, which affects the number of carboxyl-terminal repeats[135,136]. An FTD 'tauopathy' may result from tau-positive inclusions due to either an imbalance in the ratio of tau isoforms with 3 or 4 microtubular binding repeats or to the abnormal hyperphosphorylation of tau. A tauopathy underlies nearly half of those with bvFTD, most of those with the PNFA variant, and all who develop parkinsonism, including the related disorders of PSP and CBS[60,92,128,129,137].

More than half of patients with FTD syndromes have tau-negative, ubiquitin-positive inclusions which contain TDP-43 (Figure 57.4)[127,138-140]. TDP-43 is expressed when there is neuronal injury, resulting in caspase-dependent cleavage of TDP-43 and its deposition in insoluble neuronal inclusions. These ubiquitin-positive inclusions include different ubiquitin subtypes (U1–U4) depending on the distribution of ubiquitin positivity (Table 57.4)[141-144]. About

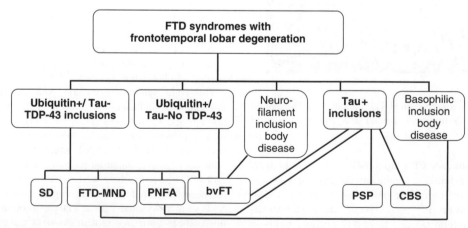

Figure 57.4 The relationships among the different pathologic and clinical variants of FTD syndromes with frontotemporal lobar degeneration

a quarter of FTLD-TDP cases are U1, half are U2, a quarter are U3, and a very small number are U4. A ubiquitin-positive, TDP-43 proteinopathy underlies over half of those with bvFTD, most of those with the SD variant, and FTD patients who develop MND[60,128,129,145]. In addition, abnormal TDP-43 immunoreactivity also occurs in other neurodegenerative disorders including AD[94,146].

A small proportion of FTD cases are associated with pathologies other than a tauopathy or a TDP-43 proteinopathy (Table 57.4). Some patients have ubiquitin-positive inclusions without TDP-43. A subset of these shows immunostaining against proteins of the ubiquitin proteosome system (FTDP-UPS). Another subset is ubiquitin-positive, TDP-43-negative without any positive immunostaining to an identified target protein. These 'atypical' FTLD-U patients have a very early age of onset and lack a clear family history for the disorder[127]. Other patients are both tau-negative and ubiquitin-negative. One, known as neuronal intermediate filament inclusion body disease, results from an accumulation of intraneuronal inclusions that are immunoreactive to neurofilament and α-internexin (FTDP-IF)[127,147,148]. Another has no inclusions whatsoever evident on immunohistochemistry (FTDP-ni). This term replaces the formerly described FTD cases of 'dementia lacking distinctive histology'[139,140,149,150]. A further subset associated with FTD-MND is basophilic inclusion body disease, which results in the identification of basophilic round neuronal inclusions that show variable immunoreactivity to ubiquitin but are unreactive to other stains (BIBD)[151,152].

Some estimates state that 38–50% of patients with FTD may have a positive family history[153,154], but direct autosomal dominant inheritance is present in only about 15%[155]. These autosomal dominant cases are due to MAPT mutations in 7–21% and PGRN mutations in 5–26%, both linked to chromosome 17[10,156–158].

MAPT mutations may result in neurodegeneration from tau aggregation in neurons and glia resulting in interference with axonal transport[159,160]. This aggregation often follows from missplicing of exon 10 and the surrounding intronic 'stem-loop'. There are over 40 known potential pathogenic MAPT mutations including 27 missense mutations, 4 silent mutations, 2 in-frame single codon deletions and 8 intronic mutations[161].

In 2006, researchers reported mutations in the PGRN gene in association with FTD and ubiquitin-positive (FTLD-TDP U3) inclusions[9,10,140,162]. Since then, researchers have found 40 to 50 different PGRN mutations that lead to degradation of mutant RNA[9,156,161]. Progranulin is a 593-amino acid, secreted glycosolated protein. It has many roles, including in brain development, as a growth factor and as an anti-inflammatory agent with functions in wound healing. The relationship between PRGN and TDP-43 remains to be elucidated. Paradoxically, investigators have identified mutations in the gene encoding for TDP-43 in familial amyotrophic lateral sclerosis, but not in FTD or FTD-MND families[163,164].

In addition to MAPT and PGRN, there are rare genetic mutations associated with FTD syndromes. Mutations in the valosin-containing protein linked to chromosome 9 result in bvFTD with inclusion body myopathy or Paget's disease (VCP)[165]. VCP is an ATPase associated with multiple cellular activity, and, at autopsy, there are widespread ubiquitin- and TDP-43-positive intranuclear inclusions (FTLD-TDP U4)[141,166]. Mutations in the charged multivesicular body protein 2B (CHMP2B) linked to chromosome 3 result in early onset bvFTD with severe cognitive deficits[167]. CHMP2B plays a role in efficient autophagy, and, at autopsy, there are ubiquitin-positive inclusions that are not immunoreactive to TDP-43 but that appear to stain for other ubiquitin proteosome system proteins (FTLD-UPS)[168].

Finally, the clinical bvFTD-like syndrome may result from an alternative transcription of the presenilin 1 mutation associated with familial AD[169].

COURSE AND MANAGEMENT

The duration of FTD syndromes can be quite variable, depending on subtype and the presence or absence of complications, such as parkinsonism or MND. The usual duration of the three uncomplicated syndromes, bvFTD, PNFA and SD, is about 8–11 years with death resulting from terminal pulmonary, urinary tract or decubitus infections or complications[6,170]. Those with FTD-MND have a much shorter, more malignant course of about 1–3 years[18]. There may be a decreased survival if there is an underlying tauopathy, as opposed to a TDP43 proteinopathy[171]. As FTD syndromes progress, syndromes may transform and evolve. For example, bvFTD or PNFA patients with an underlying tauopathy may evolve to parkinsonism and PSP or CBS. Regardless of phenotypic evolution, all, except for a subgroup of non-progressors ('phenocopies'), eventually accumulate cognitive deficits, develop profound dementia, and have a tendency to late mutism. The non-progressive phenocopies are an enigmatic group of patients who fulfil criteria for bvFTD but show little change in their symptoms over time[50,51,172].

The treatment of bvFTD primarily involves managing the behavioural symptoms with psychoactive medications. Selective serontonin-receptor inhibitors, such as sertraline, paroxetine or fluoxetine, can decrease disinhibition–impulsivity, repetitive behaviours and eating disorders[173]. Trazodone or an atypical antipsychotic such as aripriprazole can also help manage significantly disturbed or agitated behaviour, disinhibition or verbal outbursts. Antipsychotics, however, carry some risk in dementia and in bvFTD, and the US Food and Drug Administration has required warning labels because these medications may increase mortality in elderly patients. Moreover, similar to patients with dementia with Lewy bodies, some patients with bvFTD can have an unusual neuroleptic hypersensitivity[12,174]. The acetylcholinesterase inhibitors, such as donepezil, galantamine or rivastigmine, have not had significant efficacy for patients with bvFTD and can worsen disinhibition or compulsions[169]. Memantine, another dementia medication, is under investigation for the treatment of this disorder, but has not yet shown clinically significant efficacy[175,176]. Most recently, investigators have developed measures for monitoring of clinical drug trials and rational drug treatment for FTD syndromes[177]. This approach holds great promise for an eventual treatment that targets the underlying pathophysiology of FTD, particularly the abnormalities in tau protein and TDP-43[176].

The non-pharmacological management of patients with FTD syndromes focuses on behavioural interventions and care of the caregivers. Behavioural disturbances are particularly distressing to caregivers, who are prone to significant depression[27,178,179]. Family support and education is critical, including the availability of psychosocial counselling and community resources. Some behavioural disturbances may respond to retraining or to rehabilitation techniques[180,181], and speech therapy may benefit PNFA and SD patients. Special attention is needed for safety issues among FTD patients[182], and, when hyperorality is present, restrictions are necessary to prevent lethal ingestion behaviours[183]. As immobility occurs, FTD patients, like all advanced dementia patients, become susceptible to pulmonary emboli, aspiration pneumonia, urinary tract infections and decubitus ulcers.

CONCLUSIONS

The FTD syndromes are neurodegenerative disorders that are rapidly being elucidated. Research has now shown that they are clinical, pathological and genetically heterogeneous conditions. The three classic syndromes are bvFTD, with apathy, disinhibition and other behavioural changes, and PNFA and SD, with early predominant language or word comprehension difficulty. These FTD syndromes can be associated or evolve into the parkinsonian syndromes of PSP and CBS or into FTD with MND. In recent years, basic science research has also made great strides in uncovering the underlying neuropathology and neurogenetics of these syndromes. We now know that they are primarily due to abnormalities in tau or in TDP-43 protein and that these may result from mutations of the *MAPT, PRGN* or other genes. The future looks extremely promising for the discovery of pathophysiological mechanisms and disease-modifying therapies for the FTD syndromes.

REFERENCES

1. Baldwin B, Forstl H. 'Pick's disease' – 101 years on still there, but in need of reform. *Br J Psychiatry* 1993; **163**: 100–104.
2. Pick A. Über die Beziehungen der senilen Hirnatrophie zur Aphasie. *Prager Med Wochenschr* 1892; **17**: 165–7.
3. Brun A, Passant U. Frontal lobe degeneration of non-Alzheimer type. Structural characteristics, diagnostic criteria and relation to other frontotemporal dementias. *Acta Neurol Scand Suppl* 1996; **168**: 28–30.
4. Gustafson L. Clinical picture of frontal lobe degeneration of non-Alzheimer type. *Dementia* 1993; **4**(3–4): 143–8.
5. Knopman DS, Mastri AR, Frey WH, 2nd, Sung JH, Rustan T. Dementia lacking distinctive histologic features: a common non-Alzheimer degenerative dementia. *Neurology* 1990; **40**(2): 251–6.
6. Mendez MF, Selwood A, Mastri AR, Frey WH, 2nd. Pick's disease versus Alzheimer's disease: a comparison of clinical characteristics. *Neurology* 1993; **43**(2): 289–92.
7. Wilhelmsen KC, Lynch T, Pavlou E, Higgins M, Nygaard TG. Localization of disinhibition–dementia–parkinsonism–amyotrophy complex to 17q21–22. *Am J Hum Genet* 1994; **55**(6): 1159–65.
8. Arai T, Hasegawa M, Akiyama H *et al*. TDP-43 is a component of ubiquitin-positive tau-negative inclusions in frontotemporal lobar degeneration and amyotrophic lateral sclerosis. *Biochem Biophys Res Commun* 2006; **351**(3): 602–11.
9. Baker M, Mackenzie IR, Pickering-Brown SM *et al*. Mutations in progranulin cause tau-negative frontotemporal dementia linked to chromosome 17. *Nature* 2006; **442**(7105): 916–19.
10. Cruts M, Gijselinck I, van der Zee J *et al*. Null mutations in progranulin cause ubiquitin-positive frontotemporal dementia linked to chromosome 17q21. *Nature* 2006; **442**(7105): 920–24.
11. Neumann M, Sampathu DM, Kwong LK *et al*. Ubiquitinated TDP-43 in frontotemporal lobar degeneration and amyotrophic lateral sclerosis. *Science* 2006; **314**(5796): 130–33.
12. Mendez MF, Perryman KM. Neuropsychiatric features of frontotemporal dementia: evaluation of consensus criteria and review. *J Neuropsychiatry Clin Neurosci* 2002; **14**(4): 424–9.
13. Piguet O, Hornberger M, Shelley BP, Kipps CM, Hodges JR. Sensitivity of current criteria for the diagnosis of behavioral variant frontotemporal dementia. *Neurology* 2009; **72**(8): 732–7.
14. Ikeda M, Ishikawa T, Tanabe H. Epidemiology of frontotemporal lobar degeneration. *Dement Geriatr Cogn Disord* 2004; **17**(4): 265–8.
15. Knopman DS, Petersen RC, Edland SD, Cha RH, Rocca WA. The incidence of frontotemporal lobar degeneration in Rochester, Minnesota, 1990 through 1994. *Neurology* 2004; **62**(3): 506–8.
16. Coleman LW, Digre KB, Stephenson GM, Townsend JJ. Autopsy-proven, sporadic Pick disease with onset at age 25 years. *Arch Neurol* 2002; **59**(5): 856–9.
17. Johnson JK, Diehl J, Mendez MF *et al*. Frontotemporal lobar degeneration: demographic characteristics of 353 patients. *Arch Neurol* 2005; **62**(6): 925–30.
18. Pasquier F, Delacourte A. Non-Alzheimer degenerative dementias. *Curr Opin Neurol* 1998; **11**(5): 417–27.
19. Clinical and neuropathological criteria for frontotemporal dementia. The Lund and Manchester Groups. *J Neurol Neurosurg Psychiatry* 1994; **57**(4): 416–18.
20. Ratnavalli E, Brayne C, Dawson K, Hodges JR. The prevalence of frontotemporal dementia. *Neurology* 2002; **58**(11): 1615–21.
21. Harvey RJ, Skelton-Robinson M, Rossor MN. The prevalence and causes of dementia in people under the age of 65 years. *J Neurol Neurosurg Psychiatry* 2003; **74**(9): 1206–9.
22. Rosso SM, Landweer EJ, Houterman M. Medical and environmental risk factors for sporadic frontotemporal dementia: a retrospective case-control study. *J Neurol Neurosurg Psychiatry* 2003; **74**(11): 1574–6.
23. Bathgate D, Snowden JS, Varma A, Blackshaw A, Neary D. Behaviour in frontotemporal dementia, Alzheimer's disease and vascular dementia. *Acta Neurol Scand* 2001; **103**(6): 367–78.
24. Bozeat S, Gregory CA, Ralph MA, Hodges JR. Which neuropsychiatric and behavioural features distinguish frontal and temporal variants of frontotemporal dementia from Alzheimer's disease? *J Neurol Neurosurg Psychiatry* 2000; **69**(2): 178–86.
25. Mendez MF, Lauterbach EC, Sampson SM. An evidence-based review of the psychopathology of frontotemporal dementia: a report of the ANPA Committee on Research. *J Neuropsychiatry Clin Neurosci* 2008; **20**(2): 130–49.
26. Kipps CM, Nestor PJ, Acosta-Cabronero J, Arnold R, Hodges JR. Understanding social dysfunction in the behavioural variant of frontotemporal dementia: the role of emotion and sarcasm processing. *Brain* 2009; **132**(3): 592–603.
27. Mioshi E, Kipps CM, Hodges JR. Activities of daily living in behavioral variant frontotemporal dementia: differences in caregiver and performance-based assessments. *Alzheimer Dis Assoc Disord* 2009; **23**(1): 70–76.
28. Massimo L, Powers C, Moore P *et al*. Neuroanatomy of apathy and disinhibition in frontotemporal lobar degeneration. *Dement Geriatr Cogn Disord* 2009; **27**(1): 96–104.
29. Keane J, Calder AJ, Hodges JR, Young AW. Face and emotion processing in frontal variant frontotemporal dementia. *Neuropsychologia* 2002; **40**(6): 655–65.
30. Lough S, Kipps CM, Treise C *et al*. Social reasoning, emotion and empathy in frontotemporal dementia. *Neuropsychologia* 2006; **44**(6): 950–58.
31. Omar R, Sampson EL, Loy CT *et al*. Delusions in frontotemporal lobar degeneration. *J Neurol* 2009; **256**(4): 600–607.

32. Glosser G, Gallo JL, Clark CM, Grossman M. Memory encoding and retrieval in frontotemporal dementia and Alzheimer's disease. *Neuropsychology* 2002; **16**(2): 190–96.

33. Nestor PJ, Graham KS, Bozeat S, Simons JS, Hodges JR. Memory consolidation and the hippocampus: further evidence from studies of autobiographical memory in semantic dementia and frontal variant frontotemporal dementia. *Neuropsychologia* 2002; **40**(6): 633–54.

34. Hodges JR, Gurd JM. Remote memory and lexical retrieval in a case of frontal Pick's disease. *Arch Neurol* 1994; **51**(8): 821–7.

35. Neary D. Neuropsychological aspects of frontotemporal degeneration. *Ann N Y Acad Sci* 1995; **769**: 15–22.

36. Miller BL, Boone K, Cummings JL, Read SL, Mishkin F. Functional correlates of musical and visual ability in frontotemporal dementia. *Br J Psychiatry* 2000; **176**: 458–63.

37. Boeve BF, Maraganore DM, Parisi JE *et al.* Corticobasal degeneration and frontotemporal dementia presentations in a kindred with nonspecific histopathology. *Dement Geriatr Cogn Disord* 2002; **13**(2): 80–90.

38. Henderson JM, Gai WP, Hely MA. Parkinson's disease with late Pick's dementia. *Mov Disord* 2001; **16**(2): 311–19.

39. Jendroska K, Rossor MN, Mathias CJ, Daniel SE. Morphological overlap between corticobasal degeneration and Pick's disease: a clinicopathological report. *Mov Disord* 1995; **10**(1): 111–14.

40. Kertesz A, Hudson L, Mackenzie IR, Munoz DG. The pathology and nosology of primary progressive aphasia. *Neurology* 1994; **44**(11): 2065–72.

41. Kertesz A, Martinez-Lage P, Davidson W, Munoz DG. The corticobasal degeneration syndrome overlaps progressive aphasia and frontotemporal dementia. *Neurology* 2000; **55**(9): 1368–75.

42. Mathuranath PS, Xuereb JH, Bak T, Hodges JR. Corticobasal ganglionic degeneration and/or frontotemporal dementia? A report of two overlap cases and review of literature. *J Neurol Neurosurg Psychiatry* 2000; **68**(3): 304–12.

43. Miyamoto K, Ikemoto A, Akiguchi I *et al.* A case of frontotemporal dementia and parkinsonism of early onset with progressive supranuclear palsy-like features. *Clin Neuropathol* 2001; **20**(1): 8–12.

44. Caselli RJ, Windebank AJ, Petersen RC *et al.* Rapidly progressive aphasic dementia and motor neuron disease. *Ann Neurol* 1993; **33**(2): 200–207.

45. Ferrer I, Roig C, Espino A, Peiro G, Matias Guiu X. Dementia of frontal lobe type and motor neuron disease. A Golgi study of the frontal cortex. *J Neurol Neurosurg Psychiatry* 1991; **54**(10): 932–4.

46. Neary D, Snowden JS, Mann DM *et al.* Frontal lobe dementia and motor neuron disease. *J Neurol Neurosurg Psychiatry* 1990; **53**(1): 23–32.

47. Sam M, Gutmann L, Schochet SS, Jr, Doshi H. Pick's disease: a case clinically resembling amyotrophic lateral sclerosis. *Neurology* 1991; **41**(11): 1831–3.

48. Hodges JR. Frontotemporal dementia (Pick's disease): clinical features and assessment. *Neurology* 2001; **56**(11 suppl 4): S6–10.

49. Hodges JR, Miller B. The neuropsychology of frontal variant frontotemporal dementia and semantic dementia. Introduction to the special topic papers: Part II. *Neurocase* 2001; **7**(2): 113–21.

50. Hornberger M, Piguet O, Kipps C, Hodges JR. Executive function in progressive and nonprogressive behavioral variant frontotemporal dementia. *Neurology* 2008; **71**(19): 1481–8.

51. Hornberger M, Shelley BP, Kipps CM, Piguet O, Hodges JR. Can progressive and non-progressive behavioural variant frontotemporal dementia be distinguished at presentation? *J Neurol Neurosurg Psychiatry* 2009; **80**(6): 591–3.

52. Huey ED, Garcia C, Wassermann EM, Tierney MAM, Grafman J. Stimulant treatment of frontotemporal dementia in 8 patients. *J Clin Psychiatry* 2008; **69**(12): 1981–2.

53. Torralva T, Kipps CM, Hodges JR *et al.* The relationship between affective decision-making and theory of mind in the frontal variant of fronto-temporal dementia. *Neuropsychologia* 2007; **45**(2): 342–9.

54. Cappa SF, Binetti G, Pezzini A *et al.* Object and action naming in Alzheimer's disease and frontotemporal dementia [see comment]. *Neurology* 1998; **50**(2): 351–5.

55. Rhee J, Antiquena P, Grossman M. Verb comprehension in frontotemporal degeneration: the role of grammatical, semantic and executive components. *Neurocase* 2001; **7**(2): 173–84.

56. Snowden JS, Neary D. Progressive anomia with preserved oral spelling and automatic speech. *Neurocase* 2003; **9**(1): 27–43.

57. Gregory C, Lough S, Stone V *et al.* Theory of mind in patients with frontal variant frontotemporal dementia and Alzheimer's disease: theoretical and practical implications. *Brain* 2002; **125**(4): 752–64.

58. Mendez MF, Anderson E, Shapira JS. An investigation of moral judgement in frontotemporal dementia. *Cogn Behav Neurol* 2005; **18**(4): 193–7.

59. Gorno-Tempini ML, Dronkers NF, Rankin KP *et al.* Cognition and anatomy in three variants of primary progressive aphasia. *Ann Neurol* 2004; **55**(3): 335–46.

60. Kertesz A, McMonagle P, Blair M, Davidson W, Munoz DG. The evolution and pathology of frontotemporal dementia. *Brain* 2005; **128**(9): 1996–2005.

61. Neary D, Snowden JS, Gustafson L *et al.* Frontotemporal lobar degeneration: a consensus on clinical diagnostic criteria. *Neurology* 1998; **51**(6): 1546–54.

62. Rogalski E, Mesulam M. An update on primary progressive aphasia. *Curr Neurol Neurosci Rep* 2007; **7**(5): 388–92.

63. Grossman M. Progressive aphasic syndromes: clinical and theoretical advances. *Curr Opin Neurol* 2002; **15**(4): 409–13.

64. Santens P, Van Borsel J, Foncke E *et al.* Progressive dysarthria. Case reports and a review of the literature. *Dement Geriatr Cogn Disord* 1999; **10**(3): 231–6.

65. San Pedro EC, Deutsch G, Liu HG, Mountz JM. Frontotemporal decreases in rCBF correlate with degree of dysnomia in primary progressive aphasia. *J Nucl Med* 2000; **41**(2): 228–33.

66. Green J, Morris JC, Sandson J, McKeel DW, Jr, Miller JW. Progressive aphasia: a precursor of global dementia? *Neurology* 1990; **40**(3pt 1): 423–9.

67. Adlam AL, Patterson K, Rogers TT *et al.* Semantic dementia and fluent primary progressive aphasia: two sides of the same coin? *Brain* 2006; **129**(11): 3066–80.

68. Noble K, Glosser G, Grossman M. Oral reading in dementia. *Brain Lang* 2000; **74**(1): 48–69.

69. Nestor PJ, Fryer TD, Hodges JR. Declarative memory impairments in Alzheimer's disease and semantic dementia. *Neuroimage* 2006; **30**(3): 1010–20.

70. Mummery CJ, Patterson K, Price CJ. A voxel-based morphometry study of semantic dementia: relationship between temporal

lobe atrophy and semantic memory. *Ann Neurol* 2000; **47**(1): 36–45.

71. Hodges JR, Patterson K, Ward R *et al*. The differentiation of semantic dementia and frontal lobe dementia (temporal and frontal variants of frontotemporal dementia) from early Alzheimer's disease: a comparative neuropsychological study. *Neuropsychology* 1999; **13**(1): 31–40.

72. Miller BL, Cummings JL, Villanueva-Meyer J *et al*. Frontal lobe degeneration: clinical, neuropsychological, and SPECT characteristics. *Neurology* 1991; **41**(9): 1374–82.

73. Knopman DS, Christensen KJ, Schut LJ *et al*. The spectrum of imaging and neuropsychological findings in Pick's disease. *Neurology* 1989; **39**(3): 362–8.

74. Neary D, Snowden JS, Mann DM. Familial progressive aphasia: its relationship to other forms of lobar atrophy. *J Neurol Neurosurg Psychiatry* 1993; **56**(10): 1122–5.

75. McKhann GM, Albert MS, Grossman M *et al*. Clinical and pathological diagnosis of frontotemporal dementia: report of the Work Group on Frontotemporal Dementia and Pick's Disease. *Arch Neurol* 2001; **58**(11): 1803–9.

76. Huey ED, Goveia EN, Paviol S *et al*. Executive dysfunction in frontotemporal dementia and corticobasal syndrome. *Neurology* 2009; **72**(5): 453–9.

77. Knopman DS. The initial recognition and diagnosis of dementia. *Am J Med* 1998; **104**(4A): 2S–12S; discussion 39S–42S.

78. Kirshner HS. Frontotemporal dementia. *Neurology* 1999; **52**(7): 1516.

79. Rossor MN. Differential diagnosis of frontotemporal dementia: Pick's disease. *Dement Geriatr Cogn Disord* 1999; **10**(suppl 1): 43–5.

80. Rosen HJ, Gorno-Tempini ML, Goldman WP *et al*. Patterns of brain atrophy in frontotemporal dementia and semantic dementia. *Neurology* 2002; **58**(2): 198–208.

81. Duara R, Barker W, Luis CA. Frontotemporal dementia and Alzheimer's disease: differential diagnosis. *Dement Geriatr Cogn Disord* 1999; **10**(suppl 1): 37–42.

82. Friedland RP, Koss E, Lerner A *et al*. Functional imaging, the frontal lobes, and dementia. *Dementia* 1993; **4**(3–4): 192–203.

83. Frisoni GB, Laakso MP, Beltramello A *et al*. Hippocampal and entorhinal cortex atrophy in frontotemporal dementia and Alzheimer's disease. *Neurology* 1999; **52**(1): 91–100.

84. Kaufer DI, Miller BL, Itti L *et al*. Midline cerebral morphometry distinguishes frontotemporal dementia and Alzheimer's disease. *Neurology* 1997; **48**(4): 978–85.

85. Kitagaki H, Mori E, Yamaji S *et al*. Frontotemporal dementia and Alzheimer disease: evaluation of cortical atrophy with automated hemispheric surface display generated with MR images. *Radiology* 1998; **208**(2): 431–9.

86. Yamauchi H, Fukuyama H, Nagahama Y *et al*. Comparison of the pattern of atrophy of the corpus callosum in frontotemporal dementia, progressive supranuclear palsy, and Alzheimer's disease. *J Neurol Neurosurg Psychiatry* 2000; **69**(5): 623–9.

87. Galton CJ, Gomez-Anson B, Antoun N *et al*. Temporal lobe rating scale: application to Alzheimer's disease and frontotemporal dementia. *J Neurol Neurosurg Psychiatry* 2001; **70**(2): 165–73.

88. Galton CJ, Patterson K, Graham K *et al*. Differing patterns of temporal atrophy in Alzheimer's disease and semantic dementia. *Neurology* 2001; **57**(2): 216–25.

89. Jack CR, Jr, Dickson DW, Parisi JE *et al*. Antemortem MRI findings correlate with hippocampal neuropathology in typical aging and dementia. *Neurology* 2002; **58**(5): 750–57.

90. Laakso MP, Frisoni GB, Kononen M *et al*. Hippocampus and entorhinal cortex in frontotemporal dementia and Alzheimer's disease: a morphometric MRI study. *Biol Psychiatry* 2000; **47**(12): 1056–63.

91. Varma AR, Laitt R, Lloyd JJ *et al*. Diagnostic value of high signal abnormalities on T2 weighted MRI in the differentiation of Alzheimer's, frontotemporal and vascular dementias. *Acta Neurol Scand* 2002; **105**(5): 355–64.

92. Josephs KA, Duffy JR, Strand EA *et al*. Clinicopathological and imaging correlates of progressive aphasia and apraxia of speech. *Brain* 2006; **129**(6): 1385–98.

93. Josephs KA, Whitwell JL, Dickson DW *et al*. Voxel-based morphometry in autopsy proven PSP and CBD. *Neurobiol Aging* 2008; **29**(2): 280–9.

94. Josephs KA, Whitwell JL, Duffy JR *et al*. Progressive aphasia secondary to Alzheimer disease vs FTLD pathology. *Neurology* 2008; **70**(1): 25–34.

95. Whitwell JL, Josephs KA, Rossor MN *et al*. Magnetic resonance imaging signatures of tissue pathology in frontotemporal dementia. *Arch Neurol* 2005; **62**(9): 1402–8.

96. Whitwell JL, Jack CR, Jr, Baker M *et al*. Voxel-based morphometry in frontotemporal lobar degeneration with ubiquitin-positive inclusions with and without progranulin mutations. *Arch Neurol* 2007; **64**(3): 371–6.

97. Whitwell JL, Jack CR, Jr, Boeve BF *et al*. Voxel-based morphometry patterns of atrophy in FTLD with mutations in MAPT or PGRN. *Neurology* 2009; **72**(9): 813–20.

98. Alexander GE, Prohovnik I, Sackeim HA, Stern Y, Mayeux R. Cortical perfusion and gray matter weight in frontal lobe dementia. *J Neuropsychiatry Clin Neurosci* 1995; **7**(2): 188–96.

99. Charpentier P, Lavenu I, Defebvre L *et al*. Alzheimer's disease and frontotemporal dementia are differentiated by discriminant analysis applied to (99m)Tc HmPAO SPECT data. *J Neurol Neurosurg Psychiatry* 2000; **69**(5): 661–3.

100. Garraux G, Salmon E, Degueldre C *et al*. Comparison of impaired subcortico-frontal metabolic networks in normal aging, subcortico-frontal dementia, and cortical frontal dementia. *Neuroimage* 1999; **10**(2): 149–62.

101. Pasquier F, Lavenu I, Lebert F *et al*. The use of SPECT in a multidisciplinary memory clinic. *Dement Geriatr Cogn Disord* 1997; **8**(2): 85–91.

102. Sjogren M, Gustafson L, Wikkelso C, Wallin A. Frontotemporal dementia can be distinguished from Alzheimer's disease and subcortical white matter dementia by an anterior-to-posterior rCBF-SPET ratio. *Dement Geriatr Cogn Disord* 2000; **11**(5): 275–85.

103. Golan H, Kremer J, Freedman M, Ichise M. Usefulness of follow-up regional cerebral blood flow measurements by single-photon emission computed tomography in the differential diagnosis of dementia. *J Neuroimaging* 1996; **6**(1): 23–8.

104. Cummings J. Primary progressive aphasia and the growing role of biomarkers in neurological diagnosis. *Ann Neurol* 2008; **64**(4): 361–4.

105. Engler H, Santillo AF, Wang SX *et al*. In vivo amyloid imaging with PET in frontotemporal dementia. *Eur J Nucl Med Mol Imaging* 2008; **35**(1): 100–106.

106. Rosen HJ, Allison SC, Schauer GF *et al.* Neuroanatomical correlates of behavioural disorders in dementia. *Brain* 2005; **128**(11): 2612–25.

107. Williams GB, Nestor PJ, Hodges JR. Neural correlates of semantic and behavioural deficits in frontotemporal dementia. *Neuroimage* 2005; **24**(4): 1042–51.

108. Broe M, Hodges JR, Schofield E *et al.* Staging disease severity in pathologically confirmed cases of frontotemporal dementia. *Neurology* 2003; **60**(6): 1005–11.

109. Seeley WW. Selective functional, regional, and neuronal vulnerability in frontotemporal dementia. *Curr Opin Neurol* 2008; **21**(6): 701–7.

110. Zamboni G, Huey ED, Krueger F, Nichelli PF, Grafman J. Apathy and disinhibition in frontotemporal dementia: Insights into their neural correlates. *Neurology* 2008; **71**(10): 736–42.

111. Snowden JS, Thompson JC, Neary D. Knowledge of famous faces and names in semantic dementia. *Brain* 2004; **127**(4): 860–72.

112. Ingelson M, Blomberg M, Benedikz E *et al.* Tau immunoreactivity detected in human plasma, but no obvious increase in dementia. *Dement Geriatr Cogn Disord* 1999; **10**(6): 442–5.

113. Roks G, Dermaut B, Heutink P *et al.* Mutation screening of the tau gene in patients with early-onset Alzheimer's disease. *Neurosci Lett* 1999; **277**(2): 137–9.

114. Fabre SF, Forsell C, Viitanen M *et al.* Clinic-based cases with frontotemporal dementia show increased cerebrospinal fluid tau and high apolipoprotein E epsilon4 frequency, but no tau gene mutations. *Exp Neurol* 2001; **168**(2): 413–18.

115. Green AJ, Harvey RJ, Thompson EJ, Rossor MN. Increased tau in the cerebrospinal fluid of patients with frontotemporal dementia and Alzheimer's disease. *Neurosci Lett* 1999; **259**(2): 133–5.

116. Riemenschneider M, Wagenpfeil S, Diehl J *et al.* Tau and Abeta42 protein in CSF of patients with frontotemporal degeneration. *Neurology* 2002; **58**(11): 1622–8.

117. Rosengren LE, Karlsson JE, Sjogren M, Blennow K, Wallin A. Neurofilament protein levels in CSF are increased in dementia. *Neurology* 1999; **52**(5): 1090–93.

118. Sjogren M, Minthon L, Davidsson P *et al.* CSF levels of tau, beta-amyloid(1-42) and GAP-43 in frontotemporal dementia, other types of dementia and normal aging. *J Neural Transm* 2000; **107**(5): 563–79.

119. Sjogren M, Rosengren L, Minthon L *et al.* Cytoskeleton proteins in CSF distinguish frontotemporal dementia from AD. *Neurology* 2000; **54**(10): 1960–64.

120. Sjogren M, Wallin A. Pathophysiological aspects of frontotemporal dementia – emphasis on cytoskeleton proteins and autoimmunity. *Mech Ageing Dev* 2001; **122**(16): 1923–35.

121. Bird TD. Progranulin plasma levels in the diagnosis of frontotemporal dementia. *Brain* 2009; **132**(3): 568–9.

122. Hooten WM, Lyketsos CG. Frontotemporal dementia: a clinicopathological review of four postmortem studies. *J Neuropsychiatry Clin Neurosci* 1996; **8**(1): 10–19.

123. Schmitt HP, Yang Y, Forstl H. Frontal lobe degeneration of non-Alzheimer type and Pick's atrophy: lumping or splitting? *Eur Arch Psychiatry Clin Neurosci* 1995; **245**(6): 299–305.

124. Seeley WW. Frontotemporal dementia neuroimaging: a guide for clinicians. *Front Neurol Neurosci* 2009; **24**: 160–7.

125. Rinne JO, Laine M, Kaasinen V *et al.* Striatal dopamine transporter and extrapyramidal symptoms in frontotemporal dementia. *Neurology* 2002; **58**(10): 1489–93.

126. Sparks DL, Danner FW, Davis DG *et al.* Neurochemical and histopathologic alterations characteristic of Pick's disease in a non-demented individual. *J Neuropathol Exp Neurol* 1994; **53**(1): 37–42.

127. Mackenzie IR, Foti D, Woulfe J, Hurwitz TA. Atypical frontotemporal lobar degeneration with ubiquitin-positive, TDP-43-negative neuronal inclusions. *Brain* 2008; **131**(5): 1282–93.

128. Hodges JR, Davies RR, Xuereb JH *et al.* Clinicopathological correlates in frontotemporal dementia. *Ann Neurol* 2004; **56**(3): 399–406.

129. Josephs KA, Petersen RC, Knopman DS *et al.* Clinicopathologic analysis of frontotemporal and corticobasal degenerations and PSP. *Neurology* 2006; **66**(1): 41–8.

130. Hirokawa N. Microtubule organization and dynamics dependent on microtubule-associated proteins. *Curr Opin Cell Biol* 1994; **6**(1): 74–81.

131. Buratti E, Baralle FE. Multiple roles of TDP-43 in gene expression, splicing regulation, and human disease. *Front Biosci* 2008; **13**: 867–78.

132. Adamec E, Chang HT, Stopa EG, Hedreen JC, Vonsattel JP. Tau protein expression in frontotemporal dementias. *Neurosci Lett* 2001; **315**(1–2): 21–4.

133. Neary D, Snowden JS, Mann DM. Classification and description of frontotemporal dementias. *Ann N Y Acad Sci* 2000; **920**: 46–51.

134. Poorkaj P, Grossman M, Steinbart E *et al.* Frequency of tau gene mutations in familial and sporadic cases of non-Alzheimer dementia. *Arch Neurol* 2001; **58**(3): 383–7.

135. Andreadis A, Brown WM, Kosik KS. Structure and novel exons of the human tau gene. *Biochemistry* 1992; **31**(43): 10626–33.

136. Goedert M, Spillantini MG, Potier MC, Ulrich J, Crowther RA. Cloning and sequencing of the cDNA encoding an isoform of microtubule-associated protein tau containing four tandem repeats: differential expression of tau protein mRNAs in human brain. *EMBO J* 1989; **8**(2): 393–9.

137. Boeve BF, Lang AE, Litvan I. Corticobasal degeneration and its relationship to progressive supranuclear palsy and frontotemporal dementia. *Ann Neurol* 2003; **54**(suppl 5): S15–19.

138. Freeman SH, Spires-Jones T, Hyman BT, Growdon JH, Frosch MP. TAR-DNA binding protein 43 in Pick disease. *J Neuropathol Exp Neurol* 2008; **67**(1): 62–7.

139. Lipton AM, White CL, 3rd, Bigio EH. Frontotemporal lobar degeneration with motor neuron disease-type inclusions predominates in 76 cases of frontotemporal degeneration. *Acta Neuropathol* 2004; **108**(5): 379–85.

140. Mackenzie IR, Bigio EH, Ince PG *et al.* Pathological TDP-43 distinguishes sporadic amyotrophic lateral sclerosis from amyotrophic lateral sclerosis with SOD1 mutations. *Ann Neurol* 2007; **61**(5): 427–34.

141. Cairns NJ, Bigio EH, Mackenzie IR *et al.* Neuropathologic diagnostic and nosologic criteria for frontotemporal lobar degeneration: consensus of the Consortium for Frontotemporal Lobar Degeneration. *Acta Neuropathol* 2007; **114**(1): 5–22.

142. Grossman M, Wood EM, Moore P *et al.* TDP-43 pathologic lesions and clinical phenotype in frontotemporal lobar degeneration with ubiquitin-positive inclusions. *Arch Neurol* 2007; **64**(10): 1449–54.

143. Mackenzie IR, Baborie A, Pickering-Brown S *et al.* Heterogeneity of ubiquitin pathology in frontotemporal lobar degeneration: classification and relation to clinical phenotype. *Acta Neuropathol* 2006; **112**(5): 539–49.

144. Snowden J, Neary D, Mann D. Frontotemporal lobar degeneration: clinical and pathological relationships. *Acta Neuropathol* 2007; **114**(1): 31–8.
145. Knibb JA, Xuereb JH, Patterson K, Hodges JR. Clinical and pathological characterization of progressive aphasia. *Ann Neurol* 2006; **59**(1): 156–65.
146. Amador-Ortiz C, Lin WL, Ahmed Z *et al.* TDP-43 immunoreactivity in hippocampal sclerosis and Alzheimer's disease. *Ann Neurol* 2007; **61**(5): 435–45.
147. Cairns NJ, Grossman M, Arnold SE *et al.* Clinical and neuropathologic variation in neuronal intermediate filament inclusion disease. *Neurology* 2004; **63**(8): 1376–84.
148. Josephs KA, Holton JL, Rossor MN *et al.* Neurofilament inclusion body disease: a new proteinopathy? *Brain* 2003; **126**(10): 2291–303.
149. Josephs KA, Holton JL, Rossor MN *et al.* Frontotemporal lobar degeneration and ubiquitin immunohistochemistry. *Neuropathol Appl Neurobiol* 2004; **30**(4): 369–73.
150. Josephs KA, Jones AG, Dickson DW. Hippocampal sclerosis and ubiquitin-positive inclusions in dementia lacking distinctive histopathology. *Dement Geriatr Cogn Disord* 2004; **17**(4): 342–5.
151. Aizawa H, Kimura T, Hashimoto K. Basophilic cytoplasmic inclusions in a case of sporadic juvenile amyotrophic lateral sclerosis. *J Neurol Sci* 2000; **176**(2): 109–13.
152. Matsumoto S, Kusaka H, Murakami N. Basophilic inclusions in sporadic juvenile amyotrophic lateral sclerosis: an immunocytochemical and ultrastructural study. *Acta Neuropathol* 1992; **83**(6): 579–83.
153. Chow TW, Miller BL, Hayashi VN, Geschwind DH. Inheritance of frontotemporal dementia. *Arch Neurol* 1999; **56**(7): 817–22.
154. Stevens M, Van Duijn CM, Kamphorst W *et al.* Familial aggregation in frontotemporal dementia. *Neurology* 1998; **50**(6): 1541–5.
155. Josephs KA. Frontotemporal dementia and related disorders: deciphering the enigma. *Ann Neurol* 2008; **64**(1): 4–14.
156. Gass J, Cannon A, Mackenzie IR *et al.* Mutations in progranulin are a major cause of ubiquitin-positive frontotemporal lobar degeneration. *Hum Mol Genet* 2006; **15**(20): 2988–3001.
157. Le Ber I, van der Zee J, Hannequin D *et al.* Progranulin null mutations in both sporadic and familial frontotemporal dementia. *Hum Mutat* 2007; **28**(9): 846–55.
158. Pickering-Brown SM, Rollinson S, Du Plessis D *et al.* Frequency and clinical characteristics of progranulin mutation carriers in the Manchester frontotemporal lobar degeneration cohort: comparison with patients with MAPT and no known mutations. *Brain* 2008; **131**(3): 721–31.
159. Foster NL, Wilhelmsen K, Sima AA *et al.* Frontotemporal dementia and parkinsonism linked to chromosome 17: a consensus conference. Conference Participants. *Ann Neurol* 1997; **41**(6): 706–15.
160. Hutton M, Lendon CL, Rizzu P *et al.* Association of missense and 5'-splice-site mutations in tau with the inherited dementia FTDP-17. *Nature* 1998; **393**(6686): 702–5.
161. Rademakers R, Hutton M. The genetics of frontotemporal lobar degeneration. *Curr Neurol Neurosci Rep* 2007; **7**(5): 434–42.
162. Josephs KA, Ahmed Z, Katsuse O *et al.* Neuropathologic features of frontotemporal lobar degeneration with ubiquitin-positive inclusions with progranulin gene (PGRN) mutations. *J Neuropathol Exp Neurol* 2007; **66**(2): 142–51.
163. Gitcho MA, Baloh RH, Chakraverty S *et al.* TDP-43 A315T mutation in familial motor neuron disease. *Ann Neurol* 2008; **63**(4): 535–8.
164. Sreedharan J, Blair IP, Tripathi VB *et al.* TDP-43 mutations in familial and sporadic amyotrophic lateral sclerosis. *Science* 2008; **319**(5870): 1668–72.
165. Watts GD, Wymer J, Kovach MJ *et al.* Inclusion body myopathy associated with Paget disease of bone and frontotemporal dementia is caused by mutant valosin-containing protein. *Nat Genet* 2004; **36**(4): 377–81.
166. Neumann M, Mackenzie IR, Cairns NJ *et al.* TDP-43 in the ubiquitin pathology of frontotemporal dementia with VCP gene mutations. *J Neuropathol Exp Neurol* 2007; **66**(2): 152–7.
167. Skibinski G, Parkinson NJ, Brown JM *et al.* Mutations in the endosomal ESCRTIII-complex subunit CHMP2B in frontotemporal dementia. *Nat Genet* 2005; **37**(8): 806–8.
168. Holm IE, Englund E, Mackenzie IR, Johannsen P, Isaacs AM. A reassessment of the neuropathology of frontotemporal dementia linked to chromosome 3. *J Neuropathol Exp Neurol* 2007; **66**(10): 884–91.
169. Mendez MF, McMurtray A. Frontotemporal dementia-like phenotypes associated with presenilin-1 mutations. *Am J Alzheimers Dis Other Demen* 2006; **21**(4): 281–6.
170. Snowden JS, Gibbons ZC, Blackshaw A *et al.* Social cognition in frontotemporal dementia and Huntington's disease. *Neuropsychologia* 2003; **41**(6): 688–701.
171. Xie SX, Forman MS, Farmer J *et al.* Factors associated with survival probability in autopsy-proven frontotemporal lobar degeneration. *J Neurol Neurosurg Psychiatry* 2008; **79**(2): 126–9.
172. Davies RR, Kipps CM, Mitchell J *et al.* Progression in frontotemporal dementia: identifying a benign behavioral variant by magnetic resonance imaging. *Arch Neurol* 2006; **63**(11): 1627–31.
173. Swartz JR, Miller BL, Lesser IM, Darby AL. Frontotemporal dementia: treatment response to serotonin selective reuptake inhibitors. *J Clin Psychiatry* 1997; **58**(5): 212–16.
174. Janssen JC, Warrington EK, Morris HR *et al.* Clinical features of frontotemporal dementia due to the intronic tau 10(+16) mutation. *Neurology* 2002; **58**(8): 1161–8.
175. Diehl-Schmid J, Forstl H, Perneczky R, Pohl C, Kurz A. A 6-month, open-label study of memantine in patients with frontotemporal dementia. *Int J Geriatr Psychiatry* 2008; **23**(7): 754–9.
176. Vossel KA, Miller BL. New approaches to the treatment of frontotemporal lobar degeneration. *Curr Opin Neurol* 2008; **21**(6): 708–16.
177. Knopman DS, Kramer JH, Boeve BF *et al.* Development of methodology for conducting clinical trials in frontotemporal lobar degeneration. *Brain* 2008; **131**(11): 2957–68.
178. Mioshi E, Bristow M, Cook R, Hodges JR. Factors underlying caregiver stress in frontotemporal dementia and Alzheimer's disease. *Dement Geriatr Cogn Disord* 2009; **27**(1): 76–81.

179. Rosness TA, Haugen PK, Engedal K. Support to family carers of patients with frontotemporal dementia. *Aging Ment Health* 2008; **12**(4): 462–6.

180. Ikeda M, Tanabe H, Horino T *et al.* [Care for patients with Pick's disease – by using their preserved procedural memory]. *Seishin Shinkeigaku Zasshi* 1995; **97**(3): 179–92.

181. Robinson KM. Rehabilitation applications in caring for patients with Pick's disease and frontotemporal dementias. *Neurology* 2001; **56**(11 suppl 4): S56–8.

182. Talerico KA, Evans LK. Responding to safety issues in frontotemporal dementias. *Neurology* 2001; **56**(11 suppl 4): S52–5.

183. Mendez MF, Foti DJ. Lethal hyperoral behaviour from the Klüver–Bucy syndrome. *J Neurol Neurosurg Psychiatry* 1997; **62**(3): 293–4.

58

The Lewy Body Dementia Spectrum (Alpha Synucleinopathies)

J.-P. Taylor and I. G. McKeith

Wolfson Research Centre, Newcastle General Hospital, Newcastle upon Tyne, UK

INTRODUCTION

The alpha synucleinopathies encompass a diverse range of neurodegenerative entities with the common neuropathological hallmark of abnormal accumulation in the brain of aggregates of insoluble alpha-synuclein. Major members of this club include Parkinson's disease (PD), the associated Parkinson's disease dementia (PDD), dementia with Lewy bodies (DLB), multisystem atrophy (MSA), pure autonomic failure and rapid eye movement (REM) sleep behaviour disorder. The clinico-pathological manifestation of each of these conditions appears to depend upon the pattern of insoluble alpha-synuclein deposition in specific neuronal and glial populations[1].

Of particular relevance to geriatric practitioners, and the focus of the present chapter, are the Lewy body dementias (LBDs) PDD and DLB, given that, combined, these diseases represent the second commonest cause of dementia in the elderly[2].

NEUROPATHOLOGY OF LEWY BODY DEMENTIAS

As intimated by their appellation, the common histopathological feature of LBDs is Lewy bodies (LBs). These spherical neural inclusions were first described by Friederich Lewy in 1912 in the substantia nigra, locus coerulus and dorsal nucleus of vagus as well as in the hypothalamus, nucleus basalis of Meynert and sympathetic ganglia of PD patients[3,4]. However, interest in the role of LB formation in dementia did not arise until the latter half of the twentieth century when Japanese neuropathologists described a number of cases of dementia with severe extrapyramidal signs, who on autopsy had significant cortical LB deposition[5-8]. These cortical LBs can now be relatively easily visualized by the use of advanced neuropathological techniques including antiubiquitin and, more recently, specific alpha-synuclein immunohistochemical staining.

Histopathologically, LBs are eosinophilic neuronal inclusion bodies whose major constituent is aggregated alpha-synuclein bound together with ubiquitin and neurofilament. Cortical LBs tend to be smaller and less eosinophilic than LBs seen in the brainstem. It has been proposed by Braak and colleagues[9] that in PD, LBs appear initially in the brainstem and then ascend progressively along the neuroaxis, with this pattern corresponding to the clinical development of parkinsonism. Later cognitive and neuropsychiatric symptoms emerge then as a consequence of LB cortical involvement.

The temporal order of progression appears to be less clear in DLB although neuropathologically three categories, based on LB deposition, have been proposed[3]: a brainstem-predominant DLB, a limbic (or transitional) DLB, and a predominantly cortical DLB. Correlation of these categories or the distribution of alpha-synuclein with dementia development, extrapyramidal signs or neuropsychiatric symptoms, however, is lacking[10]. In addition, current pathological criteria probably do not explain the full range of potential pathological distributions that can occur, as up to 20% of older patients with LBs at autopsy have a cortical predominant pattern of distribution that does not conform to either the Braak or DLB Consortium schemas[11].

Neuropathological assessments of DLB are further complicated by the presence of co-existent Alzheimer's disease (AD) pathology as high senile plaque counts are found in 80–90% of DLB cases; this is a comparable level to that found in pure AD. Conversely, LB pathology has been found in the amygdalae of individuals who have widespread AD pathology[12] although these cases seldom display any clinical characteristics of DLB and thus should be regarded separately from LBDs[3]. These observations have, however, contributed to the sustained belief that AD and LBDs are caused by the same underlying disease as reflected in the use of terms such as 'the Lewy body variant of AD' for these mixed pathology cases[13]. This is inappropriate, since 80–90% of DLB cases neuropathologically do not have the typical AD-associated neocortical neurofibrillary tangles which are now known to be integral to the pathophysiology of AD[14]. More recently clinico-pathological data have suggested that the expression of a DLB clinical phenotype is related to the severity of LB pathology and inversely related to the severity of Alzheimer type pathology[3,15].

CLASSIFICATION OF LEWY BODY DEMENTIAS

Existing nosological systems such as DSM-IVR have been poorly operationalized with regard to PDD and DLB. PDD in DSM-IV-R is only briefly referenced and its syndromal definition is imprecise requiring the presence of PD with associated cognitive and motoric deficits, executive dysfunction and impairment in memory retrieval, which may be exacerbated by depression. DLB as a disease entity is not even listed in DSM-IV-R and this probably reflects the presumed association with AD as well as the various and confusing diagnostic labels which have been attached to this condition over the years, including Lewy body dementia, Lewy body variant of AD, senile dementia of Lewy body type and diffuse cortical Lewy body disease.

Principles and Practice of Geriatric Psychiatry, 3rd edn. Edited by Mohammed T. Abou-Saleh, Cornelius Katona and Anand Kumar
© 2011 John Wiley & Sons, Ltd

An important step forward to address these issues has been the formulation of operationalized criteria for both PDD[16] and DLB[5,6] (see Tables 58.1, 58.2 and 58.3), with the latter undergoing a revision in 2005[3]. These have allowed clinicians to make more precise diagnoses and develop clearer management strategies. From the perspective of research, operational criteria have begun to facilitate in a systemized manner a better understanding of the natural history of these conditions and improved clinico-pathological correlations, as well as allowing clinical trials to be conducted to standards accepted by drug regulatory authorities. Overall, however, it is important to recognize that the criteria for DLB and PDD are still under development and will require further refinement (e.g. neuropathological criteria), as well as being complemented by effective disease biomarkers to improve early detection (see later discussion).

As presented in Tables 58.1 and 58.2, the diagnosis of probable or possible PDD depends primarily upon the presence of core symptoms of (i) diagnosis of parkinsonism, (ii) a dementia with an insidious onset and slow progression in the context of established PD and (iii) the absence of features which could suggest other conditions as the cause of mental impairment[16]. The diagnosis of probable PDD depends upon the presence of the core symptoms as well as a cognitive profile typical for PDD (e.g. attention, visuo-spatial) and at least one behavioural symptom (e.g. visual hallucinations). The diagnosis of possible PDD is less rigorous; while still requiring the core features, the associated cognitive impairment may be, for example, atypical; behavioural symptoms may or may not be present and there may be features which make the diagnosis less robust, e.g. evidence for vascular disease on imaging. For a diagnosis of probable or

Table 58.1 Features of dementia associated with Parkinson's disease

I. **Core features**
   1. Diagnosis of Parkinson's disease according to Queen Square Brain Bank criteria
   2. A dementia syndrome with insidious onset and slow progression, developing within the context of established Parkinson's disease and diagnosed by history, clinical, and mental examination, defined as:
      * Impairment in more than one cognitive domain
      * Representing a decline from premorbid level
      * Deficits severe enough to impair daily life (social, occupational, or personal care), independent of the impairment ascribable to motor or autonomic symptoms

II. **Associated clinical features**
   1. Cognitive features:
      * Attention: Impaired. Impairment in spontaneous and focused attention, poor performance in attentional tasks; performance may fluctuate during the day and from day to day
      * Executive functions: Impaired. Impairment in tasks requiring initiation, planning, concept formation, rule finding, set shifting or set maintenance; impaired mental speed (bradyphrenia)
      * Visuo-spatial functions: Impaired. Impairment in tasks requiring visual-spatial orientation, perception, or construction
      * Memory: Impaired. Impairment in free recall of recent events or in tasks requiring learning new material, memory usually improves with cueing, recognition is usually better than free recall
      * Language: Core functions largely preserved. Word finding difficulties and impaired comprehension of complex sentences may be present
   2. Behavioral features:
      * Apathy: decreased spontaneity; loss of motivation, interest, and effortful behaviour
      * Changes in personality and mood including depressive features and anxiety
      * Hallucinations: mostly visual, usually complex, formed visions of people, animals or objects
      * Delusions: usually paranoid, such as infidelity, or phantom boarder (unwelcome guests living in the home) delusions
      * Excessive daytime sleepiness

III. **Features which do not exclude PD-D, but make the diagnosis uncertain**
   * Co-existence of any other abnormality which may by itself cause cognitive impairment, but judged not to be the cause of dementia, e.g. presence of relevant vascular disease in imaging
   * Time interval between the development of motor and cognitive symptoms not known

IV. **Features suggesting other conditions or diseases as cause of mental impairment, which, when present make it impossible to reliably diagnose PD-D**
   * Cognitive and behavioral symptoms appearing solely in the context of other conditions such as:
     Acute confusion due to
       a. Systemic diseases or abnormalities
       b. Drug intoxication
     Major Depression according to DSM IV
   * Features compatible with "Probable Vascular dementia" criteria according to NINDS-AIREN (dementia in the context of cerebrovascular disease as indicated by focal signs in neurological exam such as hemiparesis, sensory deficits, and evidence of relevant cerebrovascular disease by brain imaging AND a relationship between the two as indicated by the presence of one or more of the following: onset of dementia within 3 months after a recognized stroke, abrupt deterioration in cognitive functions, and fluctuating, stepwise progression of cognitive deficits)

Source: From Emre *et al*. (2007); Clinical diagnostic criteria for dementia associated with Parkinson's disease. Movement Disorders **22**(12):1689–1707. Reprinted with permission of John Wiley & Sons, Inc.

Table 58.2   Criteria for the diagnosis of probable and possible PD-D

Probable PD-D
  A. Core features: Both must be present
  B. Associated clinical features:
   • Typical profile of cognitive deficits including impairment in at least two of the four core cognitive domains (impaired attention which may fluctuate, impaired executive functions, impairment in visuo-spatial functions, and impaired free recall memory which usually improves with cueing)
   • The presence of at least one behavioral symptom (apathy, depressed or anxious mood, hallucinations, delusions, excessive daytime sleepiness) supports the diagnosis of Probable PD-D, lack of behavioral symptoms, however, does not exclude the diagnosis
  C. None of the group III features present
  D. None of the group IV features present

Possible PD-D
  A. Core features: Both must be present
  B. Associated clinical features:
   • Atypical profile of cognitive impairment in one or more domains, such as prominent or receptive-type (fluent) aphasia, or pure storage-failure type amnesia (memory does not improve with cueing or in recognition tasks) with preserved attention
   • Behavioral symptoms may or may not be present
  OR
  C. One or more of the group III features present
  D. None of the group IV features present

Source: From Emre *et al*. Clinical diagnostic criteria for dementia associated with Parkinson's disease. *Movement Disorders* **22**(12): 1689–1707. Reprinted with permission of John Wiley & Sons, Inc.

Table 58.3   Consensus criteria for the clinical diagnosis of probable and possible DLB

1. Central feature (essential for a diagnosis of possible or probable DLB): Dementia defined as a progressive cognitive decline of sufficient magnitude to interfere with normal social or occupational function. Prominent or persistent memory impairment may not necessarily occur in the early stages but is usually evident with progression. Deficits on tests of attention, executive function and visuo-spatial ability may be especially prominent.
2. Core features (two core features are sufficient for a diagnosis of probable DLB, one for possible DLB):
   • Fluctuating cognition with pronounced variations in attention and alertness
   • Recurrent visual hallucinations that are typically well formed and detailed
   • Spontaneous features of parkinsonism.
3. Suggestive features (if one or more of these is present in the presence of one or more core features, a diagnosis of probable DLB can be made. In the absence of any core features, one or more suggestive features is sufficient for the diagnosis of possible DLB. Probable DLB should not be diagnosed on the basis of suggestive features alone):
   • REM sleep behaviour disorder
   • Severe neuroleptic sensitivity
   • Low dopamine transporter uptake in basal ganglia demonstrated by SPECT or PET imaging.
4. Supportive features (commonly present but not proven to have diagnostic specificity):
   • Repeated falls and syncope
   • Transient, unexplained loss of consciousness
   • Severe autonomic dysfunction, e.g. orthostatic hypotension, urinary incontinence
   • Hallucinations in other modalities
   • Systematized delusions
   • Depression
   • Relative preservation of medial temporal lobe structures on structural imaging
   • Generalized low uptake on SPECT/PET perfusion scan with reduced occipital activity
   • Abnormal (low uptake) MIBG myocardial scintigraphy
   • Prominent slow wave activity on EEG with temporal lobe sharp waves.
5. A diagnosis of DLB is less likely:
   • In the presence of cerebrovascular disease evident as focal neurological signs or on brain imaging
   • In the presence of any other physical illness or brain disorder sufficient to account in part or in total for the clinical picture
   • If parkinsonism only appears for the first time at a stage of severe dementia.
6. Temporal sequence of symptoms:
   DLB should be diagnosed when dementia occurs before or concurrently with parkinsonism (if present). In research studies, when a distinction needs to be made between DLB and PDD, the one-year rule between the onset of dementia and parkinsonism should be applied.

Source: Adapted from McKeith *et al*. Diagnosis and management of dementia with Lewy bodies. Third report of the DLB consortium, *Neurology* 2005; **65**: 1863–72. Reprinted with permission from Wolters Kluwer Health.

possible DLB (Table 58.3), consensus criteria demand that the core features of fluctuating cognitive impairment, recurrent visual hallucinations and parkinsonism should be present (two or more core features for a diagnosis of probable DLB and one core feature for a diagnosis of possible DLB). DLB criteria also provide supportive and suggestive features that may make the diagnosis more likely. Clinical assessment of these features is discussed in more detail later.

The development of these criteria has, however, not been without difficulties:

Deciding if it is DLB or PDD

The diagnostic separation of DLB from PDD, on the basis of when the motor features occur relative to the dementia has caused controversy[17-20]. Currently both the consensus criteria for DLB and PDD recommend that for a diagnosis of PDD, the extrapyramidal motor features need to be present for at least 12 months or more before the onset of the dementia, but if the dementia precedes the motor symptoms or occurred within 12 months of the motor features then the diagnosis should be DLB. This boundary delineation has been considered useful in research for determining the epidemiology and natural history of these conditions as well as providing clinicians with clear categorical labels for diagnosis. However, separation of PDD and DLB on a temporal arbitrariness has no strong clinical or pathological basis. Indeed, as will be discussed below, while minor differences do exist between DLB and PDD, they demonstrate remarkably similar cognitive profiles as well as similar neuropsychiatric features, neuroleptic sensitivities, sleep symptoms, autonomic dysfunction and responsiveness to cholinesterase inhibitors[21]. Overall unitary approaches have proven useful for study of common neurobiological and genetic processes in these conditions, and, indeed, the term Lewy body disease, which encompasses PD, PDD and DLB, and the term Lewy body dementias, which includes PDD and DLB, have been particularly helpful in this regard (see Figure 58.1). Therefore, while separating the dementias, PDD from DLB, avoids confusion clinically and helps stream patients depending upon the clinical setting in which they are first diagnosed (e.g. movement disorder clinics for PDD and dementia clinics for DLB), in certain cases, particularly when the temporal ordering of motor to cognitive symptoms is not clear, the umbrella term LBDs is likely to be more useful (Table 58.4).

Problems with Validation of DLB Consensus Criteria

Neuropathological validation studies using the 1996 DLB consensus criteria[6] suggested that while the specificity of the clinical diagnosis

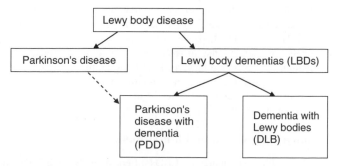

Figure 58.1 Classification of Lewy body diseases

Table 58.4 Key points in classification

- Parkinson's disease with dementia (PDD) should be used to describe dementia that occurs in well-defined Parkinson's
- Dementia with Lewy bodies (DLB) should be diagnosed when the dementia occurs before or concurrently with parkinsonism
- In research, the parkinsonism needs to be present for at least one year before the onset of dementia to make a diagnosis of PDD, but if the dementia occurs within 12 months of the motor symptoms, or indeed precedes it, then the diagnosis should be DLB
- Lewy body disease includes PD, PDD and DLB
- Lewy body dementias (LBDs) are part of the Lewy body disease spectrum and include PDD and DLB

When it is difficult to diagnostically separate PDD from DLB, the generic term LBDs might be more helpful clinically.

of probable DLB, i.e. LB pathology found at autopsy, is high at >80%, the sensitivity ≈60%, which suggests that many LB pathology cases do not present with the typical features of fluctuations, visual hallucinations or parkinsonism. Difficulties in clinically discerning core symptoms in certain individuals, particularly when the dementia is severe, the fact that significant LB pathology may occur later in the disease course such that its clinical effects are limited, or the co-occurrence of Alzheimer pathology, which modifies the clinical presentation, are all possible explanations for this reduced sensitivity in DLB detection. Importantly, it means that a significant proportion of potential DLB cases are missed; however, biomarkers and, in particular imaging techniques (see below), which enhance sensitivity in atypical/uncertain cases, may help overcome this problem.

AETIOLOGY

The aetiology of LBDs remains unclear. However, a number of biological candidates have been proffered, including LB formation, alpha-synuclein pathology and neurochemical deficits.

LB and Alpha-Synuclein Pathology

Initially LBs were hypothesized as the core neurotoxic lesion involved in the aetiology of LBDs given their association in PD with nigro-striatal dopaminergic cell loss. However LBs are only sparsely distributed in the cortex in LBDs and their density does not appear to correlate strongly with disease duration or symptom[22]. More recent thinking has been to view LBs as a neuroprotective response by vulnerable neurons attempting to sequester toxic alpha-synuclein species. An earlier stage in the neurodegenerative process appears to be the accumulation of small aggregates of alpha-synuclein. These aggregates, which are enormous in number, appear to be more widely distributed in the brains of patients with PDD and DLB than LBs and their presence in presynaptic terminals is thought to severely impair synaptic function[23]. The presence of amyloid beta in the neocortex has also been associated with more extensive alpha-synuclein lesions and thus it has been speculated that amyloid beta may have a role in the genesis of alpha-synuclein deposition in LBDs. This is an intriguing finding as it may provide evidence of a link between LBDs and AD pathology but further work is required to clarify this interaction[24].

Recently, a great deal of interest has been focused on the role of the enzyme glucocebebrosidase (GBA) in LBDs. GBA deficiency as a result of an autosomal recessive mutation has long been known to be associated with Gaucher's disease, where there is marked cellular accumulation of the GBA lipid substrate, glucocerebroside. However, it has become evident that while the severe manifestations of Gaucher's occur when there is less than 20% GBD activity, milder heterozygous mutant variants can have little deleterious effect in early life but can cause the later development of PD or DLB (see below for further discussion)[25]. Currently it is unclear in what way GBA mutations are related to PD and LBDs although it has been speculated that impaired ceramide metabolism (in which GBA is involved) and lysosomal recycling interact with the process of alpha-synuclein formation.

Neurochemical Changes

In addition to the neuropathological changes, there are severe deficits in monoaminergic and cholinergic systems in LBDs (see O'Brien et al. for further elaboration[2]). While the link between nigro-striatal dopaminergic neuronal degeneration and parkinsonism is established, it is also speculated that abnormal dopamine transmission, particularly in the striatum and frontal areas, contributes to the executive dysfunction[26]. Cell loss in raphe nuclei (serotonin) and locus coerulus (norepinephrine) may explain the mood symptoms, apathy and attentional dysfunction evident in LBDs. Cholinergic deficits in LBDs have been suggested to contribute to the global cognitive impairment and attentional dysfunction as well as hallucinosis; amelioration of these symptoms by cholinesterase inhibitors (ChEis) strongly supports the involvement of cholinergic dysfunction in LBDs pathology.

EPIDEMIOLOGY

Parkinson's Disease Dementia

The prevalence of dementia in PD has been estimated at between 24% and 31%, and the incidence rate is at least four to six times that of the rate of dementia in age-matched controls[27,28]. It is becoming increasingly recognized that cognitive impairment is present even in the earliest stages of PD; in two recent studies it was estimated that between 19% and 24% of newly diagnosed PD patients appear to have some degree of cognitive impairment[29,30]. The nature of these deficits varies, but subtle deficits in executive function, including attention shifting and working memory, as well as deficits in visuo-spatial function and episodic memory, have been noted. With time there appears to be a broadening and exacerbation of these deficits and it has been suggested that the mean duration from onset of PD to the development of PDD is around ten years; indeed one longitudinal study suggested that the cumulative prevalence was up to 78% after eight years of follow-up[31]. Risk factors for the development of PDD include older age, mild cognitive and attentional impairments at the initial diagnosis of PD, the severity of motor manifestations, and, in particular, the presence of rigidity, postural instability and gait disturbance[32-35]. While PD incidence is twice as common in men as women it is not clear if male gender predisposes PD patients to the development of PDD. Smoking may also be a risk factor but the presence of apolipoprotein E4 (APOE4) genotype, unlike AD, does not appear to be a risk factor for PDD[36-39]. Recent large-scale autopsy studies have demonstrated that between 4% and 10% of PD patients have evidence for GBA mutations. These individuals tend to display early-onset parkinsonism and at least half had hallucinations and cognitive decline; it has recently been suggested that GBA mutations represent the most common genetic risk factor for the development of PD or LBDs[40].

Dementia with Lewy Bodies

Community prevalence figures for DLB have ranged from 0% to 30.5% of dementia cases depending on the sample cohort[41]. This wide range can be explained by a small number of studies with low patient numbers, differences in case criteria used and the presence of significant sampling biases. However, studies have suggested approximately 15–30% of all dementia cases meet neuropathological criteria for DLB at autopsy, emphasizing that a significant proportion of DLB cases are probably being missed clinically[42]. There are very few studies examining the incidence of DLB; two longitudinal studies, one US-based and the other Japanese-based, estimated the incidence as 0.57 per 1 000 person years and 1.4 per 1 000 person years, respectively[43,44]. Risk factors for DLB are unclear as prevalence studies have been too small. It has, however, been suggested that APOE4 status reduces survival rate in DLB (as with AD) although its presence has little effect on disease onset or duration[45]. With regard to GBA, an autopsy study that included 95 patients with pathological confirmed DLB noted that 28% of subjects had GBA mutations. Those patients with AD co-pathology had substantially less at 10%, suggesting that GBA mutations tend to lead to more pathologically pure forms of LBDs[46]. There may be an increased prevalence of DLB with older age and some case series have suggested a male preponderance although more recent studies have refuted this. Of note, however, is a recent neuropathological study suggesting that while the prevalence of LBs is almost the same between the sexes, the severity of LB pathology may differ, with males having a more brainstem/limbic pattern compared to a more diffuse neocortical pattern seen in women[15].

CLINICAL FEATURES

LBDs have a distinctive constellation of symptoms and signs, including progressive cognitive impairment, neuropsychiatric alterations, parkinsonism, sleep behaviour disturbances and autonomic dysfunction. In PDD, parkinsonism is the initial complaint with the subsequent development over many years of an insidiously progressive cognitive impairment. Neuropsychiatric symptoms such as visual hallucinations are often initially viewed as a side effect of dopamine replacement therapy, but later, particularly as the cognitive impairment advances, they often arise independent of any anti-parkinson treatment. DLB patients, on the other hand, often have less prominent parkinsonism at initial presentation; instead, they tend to present with an evolving dementia that is often associated with attentional/cognitive fluctuations as well as visual hallucinations. These differences in the clinical presentation of the PDD versus DLB, particularly earlier in the disease course, are likely to relate to the differences in pathological spread and distribution of LBs and alpha-synuclein between the two conditions, as previously discussed. However, symptom and feature convergence occur between PDD and DLB later in the disease course, reflecting the commonality at this point in terms of neuropathology.

Cognitive and Attentional Impairment

Clinicians with experience in LBDs often state that they get an inherent 'feel' of how the cognitive profile of patients with LBDs differs from that of patients with AD. Patients with LBDs have been suggested to display 'subcortical' features such as bradyphrenia and attentional deficits as well as visuo-perceptual problems (disproportionate to the global cognitive impairment), and this contrasts with the more 'cortical' feel of AD, where language and memory deficits predominant. Thus on the Mini-Mental State Examination, a patient with DLB or PDD might be well orientated to time and place, score two out of three points on the delayed recall, but be unable to perform the serial sevens or copy the double pentagons.

This clinical impression of a difference is certainly supported by detailed neuropsychological testing. Patients with LBDs tend to perform better on verbal memory tests; indeed, in the early stages of the disease, episodic recall tends to be preserved, in contrast to AD, where short-term memory deficits are the presenting complaint. However, psychomotor speed is much slower in patients with LBDs compared to AD patients. In addition, patients with LBDs tend to have much more marked executive and attentional dysfunction[47,48] and this appears to be associated with fluctuations in cognitive function. These fluctuations, which may vary in duration in terms of minutes, hours or days, occur in up to 85% of patients with LBDs[49]. Fluctuations in cognition can occur in other dementias, such as AD and vascular dementia, but they appear qualitatively distinct in LBDs, where there appears to be an interruption of awareness that is often associated with transient episodes of confusion and communicative difficulties. Remission of near-normal cognitive function can then occur spontaneously in the absence of clear environmental triggers, suggesting that the fluctuations in LBDs are internally driven. A major problem, however, which has affected the accurate diagnosis of LBDs, is how to clinically define what cognitive fluctuations actually are. In DLB, various caregiver/observer inventories have been created to answer this issue. Importantly, Forman et al.[49] found that four characteristics of the fluctuations appear to be particularly useful in reliably distinguishing DLB from AD:

- daytime drowsiness and lethargy
- daytime sleep of two or more hours
- staring into space for long periods
- episodes of disorganized speech.

Patients with LBDs also display more marked visuo-perceptual impairments on testing than AD patients, and this may tie in with the finding that there is marked parietal and occipital hypoperfusion in LBDs on functional neuroimaging. Within LBDs, the profile of cognitive deficits is broadly similar in PDD and DLB although it has been suggested that DLB patients suffer more severe executive and attentional dysfunction than PDD patients[50].

Neuropsychiatric Symptoms

Visual hallucinations are a common symptom in LBDs: 45–65% of PDD patients have visual hallucinations; their occurrence is higher in DLB with 60–80% displaying visual hallucinations[16]. These rates contrast with the low rates of visual hallucinations reported in AD (less than 10%) and hence the importance which is attached to the presence of visual hallucinations in the diagnostic criteria for both PDD and DLB. Visual hallucinations also tend to be persistent in LBDs, which helps differentiate them from those which occur in AD or delirium. In terms of phenomenology, the majority of hallucinations tend to be complex and formed, and are typically of people (often children), animals and body parts that are either animate or static. The hallucinations can provoke emotional responses ranging from amusement through to indifference and outright fear. Insight is often variable and dependent upon the severity of the concurrent dementia although patients often have better insight into the unreality of the episode when it is over. Auditory hallucinations can also occur, but less frequently than visual hallucinations, in about 20% of patients with LBDs. Delusions are very common in DLB patients (rates of up to 78% have been reported) although their prevalence in PDD patients is lower at about 20–25%[16]. They are often based around experienced hallucinations and visuo-perceptual disturbances. They are typically complex and bizarre and their content often includes persecutory, spouse infidelity and 'phantom boarder' themes. Misidentification syndromes such as Capgras appear to occur almost exclusively in DLB compared to PDD[16].

Depressive symptoms also appear to be common in PDD and DLB patients although prevalence estimates vary considerably from 7% up to 76% depending upon the population studied and the definition used[42]. It can be difficult to make the diagnosis of depression as the clinical picture is often complicated by associated apathy, bradykinesia and attentional dysfunction.

Sleep disorders, in particular REM sleep behaviour disorder, are frequently associated with LBDs. This parasomnia is characterized by a loss of skeletal muscle atonia during REM sleep and its onset often precedes the onset of LBDs by many years. With associated daytime somnolence and noctural restlessness, it has been suggested that REM sleep behaviour disorder may contribute to the cognitive fluctuations and hallucinations seen in LBDs[49].

Parkinsonism

PD is a prerequisite for the diagnosis of PDD; in contrast, in DLB, parkinsonism is only present in about 25–50% of patients at time of diagnosis, although the majority (75–80%) will go on to develop motor features sometime during their disease course. Postural gait instability with less tremor dominance appears to be the typical presenting motor phenotype in both PDD and DLB[51]. Symmetric extrapyramidal symptoms, greater axial rigidity and suboptimal levodopa responsivity (especially evident in DLB) in comparison to PD are also features[52].

Autonomic Dysfunction

Autonomic dysfunction that affects both sympathetic and parasympathetic systems is a significant and common feature of PD through to PDD and DLB. The dysfunction leads to a variety of clinical manifestation including orthostatic hypotension, carotid sinus hypersensitivity, reduced secretions (lacrimal, mouth, sweat), urinary retention, erectile dysfunction and bowel problems (both constipation and diarrhoea). Orthostatic hypotension and carotid sinus sensitivity occur more commonly in LBDs than AD or age-matched controls[53,54] and are likely to contribute to the high rates of syncope and falls that occur in this population.

Alpha-synuclein and LB deposition appear to be widespread within the autonomic system. This and the associated acetylcholine deficiency, which impairs effective preganglionic and parasympathetic synaptic neurotransmission, have been speculated as possible causes of the autonomic dysfunction[53].

Neuroleptic Sensitivity

Neuroleptics can provoke a severe adverse reaction in 30–50% of patients with LBDs[55] even when low doses are used. These reactions can either be acute or subacute and they generally manifest as an abrupt worsening of parkinsonism with associated increased sedation and confusion. The severity of these reactions is such that they can prove fatal within days or weeks. Acute D2 blockade is thought to mediate these effects and they can occur with the use of both typical and atypical antipsychotics[56].

Gait Instability, Falls and Loss of Consciousness

Gait dysfunction and falls are extremely common in the LBDs; the causes are probably multifactorial and related to motor symptoms, attentional impairments and autonomic dysfunction. Transient losses of consciousness occur in patients with LBDs where they are found mute and unresponsive for several minutes but do not obviously display any focal neurological signs. These may relate to autonomic mechanisms such as orthostatic hypotension or carotid sinus sensitivity although they may be an extreme expression of fluctuating attention and arousal.

CLINICAL DIAGNOSIS

The availability of clear, internationally recognized consensus criteria for both PDD[16] and DLB[3,5,6] provides a rigorous scaffold on which clinicians can formulate their diagnosis; however, this places an onus on the clinician to:

- Take a detailed history from both the patient and a reliable informant, which is inclusive of the severity of impairment in daily living activities;
- Compile a problem list which will aid management decisions;
- Perform a mental state examination as well as cognitive testing which encompasses multiple domains;
- Carry out a full neurological examination;
- Arrange for appropriate investigations such as brain imaging or assessment of dopaminergic function.

DIFFERENTIAL DIAGNOSIS

Aside from the difficulties of diagnostically separating PDD from DLB there are a number of other differentials that should be considered. Often the question for PD versus PDD is: when does the dementia become clinically evident? To address this, the movement task force[57] provided a five-point guideline that recommends there should be:

1. a clear diagnosis of PD according to Queen's Square Brain Bank criteria;
2. the PD develops before the onset of dementia;
3. there is a global decline in cognitive efficiency (Mini-Mental State score <26);
4. cognitive deficiency is sufficient to impair daily life;
5. impairment occurs in more than one cognitive domain (e.g. attention, executive, visuo-constructive or memory).

For both PDD and DLB, other atypical Parkinson syndromes such as MSA, progressive supranuclear palsy, and corticobasal degeneration should be considered in the differential. However, for DLB the main differential diagnosis is other dementias, in particular AD; up to 65% of autopsy-confirmed DLB cases also meet the clinical NINCDS-ADRDA criteria for probable or possible AD[58]. Vascular dementias

frequently present with fluctuations in cognition, which can cause diagnostic confusion with DLB. Although rare, Creutzfeldt–Jakob disease should be considered, particularly if myoclonus is evident.

DLB has often been re-elaborated as 'delirium with Lewy bodies'; therefore, intermittent delirium is another important differential; the diagnosis of DLB should therefore only be considered after appropriate clinical investigation to exclude infective, metabolic, medication or other related causes has been carried out. Occasionally DLB may present atypically, initially, as a late-onset delusional disorder or a depressive psychosis. Development of cognitive decline or parkinsonism should raise suspicions of DLB as the underlying cause.

INVESTIGATIONS AND POTENTIAL BIOMARKERS

Electroencephalography

Although not specific, the EEG in LBDs can show generalized slowing with transient temporal sharp waves; indeed, this EEG pattern is incorporated into the supportive features described in the DLB consensus criteria.

Imaging

Generalized atrophy as well as white matter changes occurs in LBDs. However, their presence does not help clinically in making the differential diagnosis. Nevertheless, in DLB there appears to be a relative preservation of hippocampal and medial temporal lobe volume on MRI, which can help differentiate it from AD[59]. Functionally, occipital hypoperfusion has been noted in LBDs in single photon emission computerized tomography (SPECT)/positron emission tomography (PET). However, while specificity in SPECT/PET is often greater than 80% for distinguishing DLB from Alzheimer's, sensitivities tend to be lower. For example, Lobotesis et al.[60] noted a sensitivity of only 68%. An important recent development for the diagnosis of DLB is the visualization of presynaptic dopaminergic deficits in the striatum using ^{123}I-radiolabelled 2β-carbomethoxy-3β-(4-iodophenyl)-N-(3-fluoropropyl)nortropane (FP-CIT, trade name DaTSCAN). This technique demonstrates high sensitivity (78%) and specificity (90%) in identifying probable DLB versus non-DLB dementia[61]. However, although the current regulatory approval for FP-CIT imaging is in distinguishing probable DLB from AD, this discrimination can often be adequately made on clinical grounds alone. Rather, a longitudinal study has suggested that FP-CIT appears to be much more useful in determining clinically uncertain, i.e. 'possible', cases[62]. In this study of 19 people with an initial diagnosis of possible DLB who subsequently were diagnosed with probable DLB 1 year later, 12 had had abnormal FP-CIT scans at baseline (63% sensitivity).

Another potentially useful imaging modality is that of cardiac scintigraphy with ^{123}iodine metaiodobenzyl guanidine (^{123}I-MIBG); this provides a measure of the degree of postganglionic sympathetic cardiac innervation and it has been used to discriminate PD from other motor disorders such as MSA[63]. Additionally, ^{123}I-MIBG uptake is markedly reduced in DLB in contrast to non-demented PD patients[64] and AD patients, and it has been advocated as a means of improving sensitivity in discriminating DLB from AD, particularly if SPECT perfusion imaging is equivocal[65].

Cerebrospinal Fluid and Plasma Markers

There is increasing interest in the use of cerebrospinal fluid (CSF) and serum markers in the diagnosis of dementias. CSF levels of alpha-synuclein species and p-tau, as well as a large number of other neurochemicals, have all been mooted as potential markers of LBDs (see Mollenhauer and Trenkwalder for further elaboration[66]), in particular the differentiation of DLB from AD. However, study results have been mixed, with poor replication between studies, variable sensitivities and specificities with frequent overlap in concentration levels between disease groups (e.g. DLB versus AD), and a lack of neuropathological confirmed diagnoses. Recently, serum proteomic array methods, which identify multiple potential diagnostic protein markers, have been used to diagnostically separate DLB from AD[67], and RNA expression patterns in blood have been suggested to be helpful in the diagnosis of early PD[68].

Genetics

A large number of genes have been associated with rare forms of familial PD; for example, *LRRK2*, *PINK1*, *SNCA* and *PARK2*, to name a few. As noted previously, GBA mutations appear to be strongly associated with the development of PD and LBDs. However, aside from this, specific gene linkages to PDD and DLB are less clear although a gene–dose effect with triplication of the associated alpha-synuclein gene (*SNCA*) has been suggested to give rise to familial variants of DLB and PDD whereas duplication is associated only with motor PD[69]. However, sporadic LBDs have not been found to be associated with over-expression of alpha-synuclein genes. Butylcholinesterase allelic variants in conjunction with the presence of APOE ε4 alleles have been suggested, in individuals who will go on to develop LBDs, to increase the likelihood than they will express the DLB clinical phenotype rather than PDD phenotype, i.e. dementia before the onset of parkinsonism[70].

Conclusion

Biomarkers are useful in early diagnosis, separation of the disease from other differentials, understanding the natural history of the disease and providing objective biological correlates of treatment response. However, while a number of modalities, including fluid markers and genetics, are potentially promising, they will require significant further research before they are clinically useful. Currently, best evidence probably exists for imaging markers, in particular, FP-CIT SPECT.

COURSE, PROGNOSIS AND PSYCHOSOCIAL EFFECTS

The annual decline in cognitive and motor function scores in DLB and PDD patients is about 10%[35]. The survival duration from symptom onset (either parkinsonism or dementia) to death is between five and eight years in DLB and PDD patients depending upon the population studied[71,72]. However, some patients display a much more rapid disease course and adverse predictors may include older age at onset, greater neuropsychiatric symptom severity (hallucinations and depressive symptoms), cognitive fluctuations and the presence of co-morbid Alzheimer pathology. Conversely, a long latency between parkinsonism onset and dementia onset in PDD patients has been suggested to predict longer survival after dementia onset.

The psychosocial impact of LBDs is high: cognitive, neuropsychiatric and motor impairments cause significant difficulties for patients and their caregivers. Nursing home placement is often a frequent outcome and is particularly common when psychotic symptoms are present. One study which examined quality of life indices in DLB patients suggested that DLB patients had lower quality of life scores and used more resources than AD patients; indeed, almost 25% of DLB patients included had negative scores on the EQ-5D utility index, a level which has been defined as a state worse than death[73]. Determinants of poor quality of life in DLB patients included the presence of apathy, delusions, poor activities of daily living and absence of a caregiver; cognitive scores had no impact.

MANAGEMENT

Initial diagnosis of AD is often straightforward; in contrast, awareness of LBDs among clinicians and the general public is often very limited and this has previously led to patients being misdiagnosed, given incorrect information and treated inappropriately. Fortunately, the establishment of the consensus criteria, diagnostic neuroimaging and an increasing evidence base for the symptomatic treatment of LBDs has improved this situation. Furthermore, dissemination of knowledge is also now being supported by organizations such as the Lewy Body Dementia Association (www.lewybodydementia.org) and Lewy Body Society (www.lewybody.org).

Overall, LBDs are complex conditions in which there are multiple management issues including those of early diagnosis, treatment of cognitive impairments, assessment and management of neuropsychiatric and behavioural symptoms as well as treatment of parkinsonism, autonomic dysfunction and sleep disorders[3]. Treatments include pharmacological therapy, but non-pharmacological approaches, psychoeducation to patients and family about the various neuropsychiatric symptoms and a multidisciplinary approach to management which encompasses occupational therapy, good nursing care, and social and carer groups are also very important. Table 58.5 provides a summary of the management approach. However, currently there is insufficient data for evidence-based guidelines for PDD and DLB management although it should be noted that the Third Consortium report by McKeith and colleagues does provide the first authoritative recommendations based on expert consensus for the latter condition[3].

NON-PHARMACOLOGICAL TREATMENTS

Systematic evaluation of non-pharmacological interventions in LBDs is lacking. In the case of visual hallucinations, clear explanations as to their origin to patients who still have insight and the caregivers can be helpful. Hallucinations also appear to be exacerbated by visuo-perceptual disturbances, which can be secondary to eye disease or environmental issues; cataract removal, improved illumination and removal of patterned furnishings (e.g. carpets, curtains) that can provoke illusionary experiences all may be helpful. In addition, low levels of arousal and cognitive fluctuations appear to respond to enhanced environmental novelty and improved social interaction.

PHARMACOLOGICAL TREATMENTS

Management of Cognitive Impairments

The profound cholinergic deficits which occur in the central nervous system of patients with LBDs have provided the scientific rationale that restoration of acetylcholine may help ameliorate some of the cognitive and neuropsychiatric dysfunction that occurs in LBDs. Three ChEis – donepezil (Aricept), rivastigmine (Exelon) and galantamine (Reminyl) – which block the breakdown of acetylcholine within the synapse and thus prolong its effect postsynaptically have been used

Table 58.5 Symptom management in LBDs

General management

Provide psychoeducation to patient and relatives, including explanation of the intrinsic features of LBDs including cognitive effects (attention and cognitive fluctuations), neuropsychiatric symptoms such as hallucinations, and any associated motor symptoms

Establish from the patient and carer which symptoms are most problematic, impair quality of life and need active treatment

Consider firstly what non-pharmacological and social care interventions can be implemented e.g. environmental stimulation for fluctuations; care package and occupational therapy assessment for cognitive and motor impairments

Specific treatment

Cognitive impairment

Perform baseline assessment of cognitive function; this may need to be done on several occasions given the tendency to fluctuate in LBDs

Review medication chart; stop any unnecessary drugs with a propensity to anticholinergic or sedative effects

Consider, provided there are no contraindications, a gradual introduction of a ChEi; response should be evident within several weeks. This may include specific improvements in test scores, but also be alert to more global improvements in activities of daily living and attention

Memantine, in addition, or as an alternative, should also be considered

Neuropsychiatric symptoms

Treat symptoms only if they are causing distress and/or are functionally impairing; for example, many patients are able to tolerate their visual hallucinations without the need for active treatment

Review any antiparkinson medication; gradually reduce and, if possible, stop the medications in the following order: anticholinergics, amantadine, direct dopamine agonists, COMT inhibitors and L-dopa

ChEi, in addition to their cognitive benefit, may help ameliorate neuropsychiatric symptoms such as visual hallucinations, delusions, and apathy

If psychotic symptoms persist, consider a cautious trial of an antipsychotic:

Warn both patient and carers about the potential for severe adverse reactions

Start low and go slow

Review antipsychotic use regularly, looking for side effects; be alert that most neuroleptic reactions occur in the first two weeks and it may be appropriate to admit patients during this period for monitoring

If parkinsonism is worsened or occurs for the first time (in the case of some DLB patients) stop the antipsychotic

Do not prescribe the antipsychotic for prolonged periods. Regularly re-assess the need for the drug; can alternative interventions be applied now the situation is containable?

Depression may respond to SSRIs or SNRI. Avoid antidepressants with major anticholinergic effects (e.g. tricyclics) as this can adversely affect cognition and cause confusion

Clonazapam may help noctural hallucinations and RBD

Motor symptoms

Balance the need for treatment of motor dysfunction versus the potential for exacerbation of neuropsychiatric symptoms; use the minimal antiparkinson medication required for benefit

Autonomic dysfunction/orthostatic hypotension

Discontinue any unnecessary antihypertensives. Orthostatic hypotension may respond to the addition of midodrine or fludrocortisone

---

in LBDs treatment. There is some evidence for all three medications with regard to improvement in global cognitive function, attentional function and activities of daily living, although to date, only the efficacy of rivastigmine has been examined in large, robust placebo control trials in DLB and PDD patients[74,75] and as such it is the only ChEi which is currently licensed for treatment in PDD. Nevertheless, there is no evidence to suggest that any one ChEi is better than another[76]. Generally the treatment effect size for cognitive impairment appears to be larger in LBDs than AD and this probably reflects the greater cholinergic deficit seen in the former[77].

Overall, ChEis are reasonably tolerated in patients with LBDs; notable side effects include gastrointestinal disturbance, urinary frequency, insomnia, leg cramps, hypersalivation and lacrimation. Given the reciprocal interplay between dopamine and acetylcholine in the striatum, one might expect an exacerbation of motor symptoms with ChEi treatment; surprisingly a dose-dependent worsening only occurs in a minority of patients[78].

There is limited data for the long-term effect of ChEi treatment in LBDs although benefits appear to be sustained for up to two years[79,80]. However, there is no data with regard to any potential disease modifying effects.

Memantine, which has a low side effect profile, may also be useful treatment in LBDs; a recent study in PDD and DLB patients by Aarsland *et al.* noted some improvement in a clinical global impression of change scale and improved speed on attentional tasks in patients receiving memantine for 24 weeks in comparison to placebo, and within the memantine receiving group there was a 1.4 point improvement in MMSE scores[81].

Management of Neuropsychiatric Symptoms

Visual hallucinations are the most frequently occurring symptom in LBDs and they are often accompanied by delusions, agitation and behavioural disturbance. As noted above for cognition, ChEis have also been shown to be effective in open-labelled studies for treating visual hallucinations although placebo-controlled data is available only for rivastigmine[74,75]. Symptom reduction in frequency and intensity seems to be, in part, mediated by improvements in attentional function. Conversely, the presence of visual hallucinations predicts a better cognitive response to ChEi, perhaps as a result of greater cholinergic deficits in those individuals who experience them[82].

ChEi should be considered first line; however, if they are ineffective it is sometimes necessary to consider the use of an atypical antipsychotic. Clozapine or quetiapine have been advocated in the literature as preferred agents. However, clozapine has notable side effects (e.g. agranulocytosis) and needs regular blood monitoring. Clinical trial data for quetiapine is equivocal; one study noted that while quetiapine did not worsen parkinsonism, it did not have any demonstrable benefits with regard to agitation or psychosis in DLB or PDD patients[83].

However, there are substantial risks associated with antipsychotic use. Aside from the high risk of severe neuroleptic reaction, the Food and Drugs Administration in 2008 issued an alert that both typical and atypical antipsychotics are associated with increased mortality in older patients with dementia related psychosis[84]. Additionally both risperidone and olanzapine have warnings about increased risk of cerebrovascular disease[85]. Overall, therefore, a high level of caution needs to be applied to the use of antipsychotics in LBDs.

Treatment of depression and apathy in LBDs is empirical as there is no clear evidence base. Preferred agents include SSRIs and SNRIs with the avoidance of tricyclics given their anticholinergic propensity. Apathy and drowsiness may respond to ChEis, and some have advocated the use of modafinil or methylphenidate although there is no evidence to support the effectiveness of these agents.

Low dose clonazepam before bed may be helpful in the management of associated REM behaviour disorder (RBD) in LBDs[86].

Management of Parkinsonism

It is well established that antiparkinsonian medications can exacerbate psychotic symptoms in LBDs and often there needs to be a clinical compromise between a relatively mobile and active patient with psychosis and one who is non-psychotic but immobile. In PDD, it is often necessary to have some level of anti-parkinsonian medication given the greater motor impairments that occur in this condition relative to DLB. Medications should be used at the lowest dose possible, and anticholinergic, antiglutaminergic and direct dopamine agonists should be avoided if possible. In DLB, only a third of patients show significant motor response to L-dopa; therefore treatment of parkinsonism should only be instituted if motor symptoms interfere with function.

REFERENCES

1. Galvin JE, Lee VMY, Trojanowski JQ. Synucleinopathies: clinical and pathological implications. *Arch Neurol* 2001; **58**, 186–90.
2. O'Brien JT, McKeith IG, Ames D *et al. Dementia with Lewy Bodies and Parkinson's Disease Dementia*. Oxford: Taylor and Francis, 2006.
3. McKeith IG, Dickson DW, Lowe J *et al*. Diagnosis and management of dementia with Lewy bodies. Third report of the DLB consortium. *Neurology* 2005; **65**: 1863–72.
4. Lewy FH. Paralyis Agitans: I. Pathologische Anatomie. In Lewandowsky M (ed.) *Handbuch der Neurologie*. Julius Springer, Berlin, 1912, 920–33.
5. McKeith IG, Perry RH, Fairbairn AF *et al*. Operational criteria for senile dementia of Lewy body type (SDLT). *Psychol Med* 1992; **22**: 911–22.
6. McKeith IG, Galasko D, Kosaka K *et al*. Consensus guidelines for the clinical and pathologic diagnosis of dementia with Lewy bodies (DLB): report of the consortium on DLB international workshop. *Neurology* 1996; **47**: 1113–24.
7. Okazaki H, Lipton LS, Aronson SM. Diffuse intracytoplasmatic ganglionic inclusions (Lewy type) associated with progressive dementia and quadriparesis in flexion. *J Neuropathol Exp Neurol* 1961; **20**: 237–44.
8. Kosaka K, Oyanagi S, Matsushita M, Hori A. Presenile dementia with Alzheimer-, Pick- and Lewy-body changes. *Acta Neuropathol* 1976; **36**: 221–33.
9. Braak H, Del Tredici K, Rub U *et al*. Staging of brain pathology related to sporadic Parkinson's disease. *Neurobiol Aging* 2003; **24**: 197–211.
10. Parkkinen L, Kauppinen T, Pirttilä T *et al*. (2005) Alpha-synuclein pathology does not predict extrapyramidal symptoms or dementia. *Ann Neurol* 2005; **57**: 82–91.
11. Zaccai J, Brayne C, McKeith I *et al*. Patterns and stages of alpha-synucleinopathy: relevance in a population-based cohort. *Neurology* 2008; **70**: 1042–8.
12. Uchikado H, Lin WL, DeLucia MW *et al*. Alzheimer disease with amygdala Lewy bodies: a distinct form of alpha-synucleinopathy. *J Neuropathol Exp Neurol* 2006; **65**: 685–97.
13. Hansen L, Salmon D, Galasko D *et al*. The Lewy body variant of Alzheimer's disease: a clinical and pathologic entity. *Neurology* 1990; **40**: 1–8.
14. Lippa CF, McKeith I. Dementia with Lewy bodies: improving diagnostic criteria. *Neurology* 2003; **60**: 1571–3.
15. Fujimi K, Sasaki K, Noda K *et al*. Clinicopathological outline of dementia with Lewy bodies applying the revised criteria: the Hisayama study. *Brain Pathol* 2008; **18**: 317–25.
16. Emre M, Aarsland D, Brown R *et al*. Clinical diagnostic criteria for dementia associated with Parkinson's disease. *Mov Disord* 2007; **22**: 1689–1707.
17. McKeith I. Dementia with Lewy bodies and Parkinson's disease with dementia: where two worlds collide. *Pract Neurol* 2007; **7**: 374–82.
18. Revuelta GJ, Lippa CF. Dementia with Lewy bodies and Parkinson's disease dementia may best be viewed as two distinct entities. *Int Psychogeriatr* 2009; **21**: 213–16.
19. Aarsland D, Londos E, Ballard C. Parkinson's disease dementia and dementia with Lewy bodies: different aspects of one entity. *Int Psychogeriatr* 2009; **21**: 216–19.
20. McKeith I. Commentary: DLB and PDD: the same or different? Is there a debate? *Int Psychogeriatr* 2009; **21**: 220–24.
21. McKeith I, Mintzer J, Aarsland D *et al*. Dementia with Lewy bodies. *Lancet Neurol* 2004; **3**: 19–28.
22. Gomez-Tortosa E, Newell K, Irizarry MC *et al*. Clinical and quantitative pathologic correlates of dementia with Lewy bodies. *Neurology* 1999; **53**: 1284–91.
23. Kramer ML, Schulz-Schaeffer WJ. Presynaptic {alpha}-synuclein aggregates, not Lewy bodies, cause neurodegeneration in dementia with Lewy bodies. *J Neurosci* 2007; **27**: 1405–10.

24. Pletnikova O, West N, Lee MK *et al*. Aβ deposition is associated with enhanced cortical α-synuclein lesions in Lewy body diseases. *Neurobiol Aging* 2005; **26**: 1183–92.

25. Hardy J, Lewis P, Revesz T *et al*. The genetics of Parkinson's syndromes: a critical review. *Curr Opin Genet Dev* 2009; **19**: 254–65.

26. Goldmann Gross R, Siderowf A, Hurtig HI. Cognitive impairment in Parkinson's disease and dementia with Lewy bodies: a spectrum of disease. *Neurosignals* 2008; **16**: 24–34.

27. Aarsland D, Zaccai J, Brayne C. A systematic review of prevalence studies of dementia in Parkinson's disease. *Mov Disord* 2005; **20**: 1255–63.

28. Aarsland D, Andersen K, Larsen JP *et al*. Risk of dementia in Parkinson's disease: a community-based, prospective study. *Neurology* 2001; **56**: 730–36.

29. Muslimovic D, Post B, Speelman JD *et al*. Cognitive profile of patients with newly diagnosed Parkinson disease. *Neurology* 2005; **65**: 1239–45.

30. Aarsland D, Bronnick K, Larsen JP *et al*. Cognitive impairment in incident, untreated Parkinson disease: the Norwegian Park-West Study. *Neurology* 2009; **72**: 1121–6.

31. Aarsland D, Andersen K, Larsen JP *et al*. Prevalence and characteristics of dementia in Parkinson disease: an 8-year prospective study. *Arch Neurol* 2003; **60**: 387–92.

32. Zgaljardic DJ, Foldi NS, Borod JC. Cognitive and behavioral dysfunction in Parkinson's disease: neurochemical and clinicopathological contributions. *J Neural Transm* 2004; **111**: 1287–1301.

33. Taylor JP, Rowan EN, Lett D *et al*. Poor attentional function predicts cognitive decline in patients with non-demented Parkinson's disease independent of motor phenotype. *J Neurol Neurosurg Psychiatry* 2008; **79**: 1318–23.

34. Hughes TA, Ross HF, Musa S *et al*. A 10-year study of the incidence of and factors predicting dementia in Parkinson's disease. *Neurology* 2000; **54**: 1596–1602.

35. Burn DJ, Rowan EN, Allan LM *et al*. Motor subtype and cognitive decline in Parkinson's disease, Parkinson's disease with dementia, and dementia with Lewy bodies. *J Neurol Neurosurg Psychiatry* 2006; **77**: 585–9.

36. Marc G, Weisskopf FGAA. Smoking and cognitive function in Parkinson's disease. *Mov Disord* 2007; **22**: 660–65.

37. Jasinska-Myga B, Opala G, Goetz CG *et al*. Apolipoprotein E gene polymorphism, total plasma cholesterol level, and Parkinson disease dementia. *Arch Neurol* 2007; **64**: 261–5.

38. Levy G, Schupf N, Tang MX *et al*. Combined effect of age and severity on the risk of dementia in Parkinson's disease. *Ann Neurol* 2002; **51**: 722–9.

39. Inzelberg R, Chapman J, Treves TA *et al*. Apolipoprotein E4 in Parkinson disease and dementia: new data and meta-analysis of published studies. *Alzheimer Dis Assoc Disord* 1998; **12**: 45–8.

40. Neumann J, Bras J, Deas E *et al*. Glucocerebrosidase mutations in clinical and pathologically proven Parkinson's disease. *Brain* 2009; **132**: 1783–94.

41. Zaccai J, McCracken C, Brayne C. A systematic review of prevalence and incidence studies of dementia with Lewy bodies. *Age Ageing* 2005; **34**: 561–6.

42. Dodel R, Csoti I, Ebersbach G *et al*. Lewy body dementia and Parkinson's disease with dementia. *J Neurol* 2008; **255**: 39–47.

43. Miech RA, Breitner JCS, Zandi PP *et al*. Incidence of AD may decline in the early 90s for men, later for women: the Cache County study. *Neurology* 2002; **58**: 209–18.

44. Matsui Y, Tanizaki Y, Arima H *et al*. Incidence and survival of dementia in a general population of Japanese elderly: the Hisayama study. *J Neurol Neurosurg Psychiatry* 2009; **80**: 366–70.

45. Singleton AB, Wharton A, O'Brien KK *et al*. Clinical and neuropathological correlates of apolipoprotein E genotype in dementia with Lewy bodies. *Dement Geriatr Cogn Disord* 2002; **14**: 167–75.

46. Clark LN, Kartsaklis LA, Wolf Gilbert R *et al*. Association of glucocerebrosidase mutations with dementia with Lewy bodies. *Arch Neurol* 2009; **66**: 578–83.

47. Ballard CG, Aarsland D, McKeith I *et al*. Fluctuations in attention: PD dementia vs DLB with parkinsonism. *Neurology* 2002; **59**: 1714–20.

48. Beatty WW, Ryder KA, Gontkovsky ST *et al*. Analyzing the subcortical dementia syndrome of Parkinson's disease using the RBANS. *Arch Clin Neuropsychol* 2003; **18**: 509–20.

49. Ferman TJ, Smith GE, Boeve BF *et al*. DLB fluctuations: specific features that reliably differentiate DLB from AD and normal aging. *Neurology* 2004; **62**: 181–7.

50. Aarsland D, Ballard CG, Halliday G. Are Parkinson's disease with dementia and dementia with Lewy bodies the same entity? *J Geriatr Psychiatry Neurol* 2004; **17**: 137–45.

51. Burn DJ, Rowan EN, Minett T *et al*. Extrapyramidal features in Parkinson's disease with and without dementia and dementia with Lewy bodies: a cross-sectional comparative study. *Mov Disord* 2003; **18**: 884–9.

52. Molloy S, McKeith IG, O'Brien JT *et al*. The role of levodopa in the management of dementia with Lewy bodies. *J Neurol Neurosurg Psychiatry* 2005; **76**: 1200–203.

53. Allan LM, Ballard CG, Allen J *et al*. Autonomic dysfunction in dementia. *J Neurol Neurosurg Psychiatry* 2007; **78**: 671–7.

54. Kenny RA, Shaw FE, O'Brien JT *et al*. Carotid sinus syndrome is common in dementia with Lewy bodies and correlates with deep white matter lesions. *J Neurol Neurosurg Psychiatry* 2004; **75**: 966–71.

55. Aarsland D, Perry R, Larsen JP *et al*. Neuroleptic sensitivity in Parkinson's disease and parkinsonian dementias. *J Clin Psychiatry* 2005; **66**: 633–7.

56. Piggott MA, Perry EK, McKeith IG *et al*. Dopamine D2 receptors in demented patients with severe neuroleptic sensitivity. *Lancet* 1994; **343**: 1044–5.

57. Bruno D, David B, Christopher G *et al*. Diagnostic procedures for Parkinson's disease dementia: recommendations from the Movement Disorder Society task force. *Mov Disord* 2007; **22**: 2314–24.

58. McKeith IG, Fairbairn AF, Perry RH *et al*. The clinical diagnosis and misdiagnosis of senile dementia of Lewy body type (SDLT). *Br J Psychiatry* 1994; **165**: 324–32.

59. Burton EJ, Barber R, Mukaetova-Ladinska EB *et al*. Medial temporal lobe atrophy on MRI differentiates Alzheimer's disease from dementia with Lewy bodies and vascular cognitive impairment: a prospective study with pathological verification of diagnosis. *Brain* 2009; **132**: 195–203.

60. Lobotesis K, Fenwick JD, Phipps A *et al*. Occipital hypoperfusion on SPECT in dementia with Lewy bodies but not AD. *Neurology* 2001; **56**: 643–9.

61. McKeith I, O'Brien J, Walker Z *et al*. Sensitivity and specificity of dopamine transporter imaging with 123I-FP-CIT SPECT in dementia with Lewy bodies: a phase III, multicentre study. *Lancet Neurol* 2007; **6**: 305–13.

62. O'Brien JT, McKeith IG, Walker Z et al. Diagnostic accuracy of ^{123}I-FP-CIT SPECT in possible dementia with Lewy bodies. Br J Psychiatry 2009; 194: 34–9.

63. Braune S, Reinhardt M, Schnitzer R et al. Cardiac uptake of [^{123}I]MIBG separates Parkinson's disease from multiple system atrophy. Neurology 1999; 53: 1020–25.

64. Suzuki M, Kurita A, Hashimoto M et al. Impaired myocardial ^{123}I-metaiodobenzylguanidine uptake in Lewy body disease: comparison between dementia with Lewy bodies and Parkinson's disease. J Neurol Sci 2006; 240: 15–19.

65. Hanyu H, Shimizu S, Hirao K et al. Comparative value of brain perfusion SPECT and [123I]MIBG myocardial scintigraphy in distinguishing between dementia with Lewy bodies and Alzheimer's disease. Eur J Nucl Med Mol Imaging 2006; 33: 248–53.

66. Mollenhauer B, Trenkwalder C. Neurochemical biomarkers in the differential diagnosis of movement disorders. Mov Disord 2009; 24: 1411–26.

67. Wada-Isoe K, Michio K, Imamura K et al. Serum proteomic profiling of dementia with Lewy bodies: diagnostic potential of SELDI-TOF MS analysis. J Neural Transm 2007; 114: 1579–83.

68. Scherzer CR, Eklund AC, Morse LJ et al. Molecular markers of early Parkinson's disease based on gene expression in blood. Proc Natl Acad Sci 2007; 104: 955–60.

69. Singleton A, Gwinn-Hardy K. Parkinson's disease and dementia with Lewy bodies: a difference in dose? Lancet 2004; 364: 1105–7.

70. Lane R, He Y, Morris C et al. BuChE-K and APOE ε4 allele frequencies in Lewy body dementias, and influence of genotype and hyperhomocysteinemia on cognitive decline. Mov Disord 2009; 24: 392–400.

71. Jellinger KA, Wenning GK, Seppi K. Predictors of survival in dementia with Lewy bodies and Parkinson dementia. Neurodegener Dis 2007; 4: 428–30.

72. Walker Z. Progression of cognitive impairment and duration of illness. In O'Brien JT, McKeith IG, Ames D, Chiu E (eds), Dementia with Lewy Bodies and Parkinson's Disease Dementia. Oxford: Taylor and Francis, 2006, 141–7.

73. Bostrom F, Jonsson L, Minthon L et al. Patients with dementia with Lewy bodies have more impaired quality of life than patients with Alzheimer disease. Alzheimer Dis Assoc Disord 2007; 21: 150–54.

74. McKeith I, Del Ser T, Spano P et al. Efficacy of rivastigmine in dementia with Lewy bodies: a randomised, double-blind, placebo-controlled international study. Lancet 2000; 356: 2031–6.

75. Emre M, Aarsland D, Albanese A et al. Rivastigmine for dementia associated with Parkinson's disease. N Engl J Med 2004; 351: 2509–18.

76. Bhasin M, Rowan E, Edwards E et al. Cholinesterase inhibitors in dementia with Lewy bodies – a comparative analysis. Int J Geriatr Psychiatry 2007; 22: 890–95.

77. Samuel W, Caligiuri M, Galasko D et al. Better cognitive and psychopathologic response to donepezil in patients prospectively diagnosed as dementia with Lewy bodies: a preliminary study. Int J Geriatr Psychiatry 2000; 15: 794–802.

78. Thomas AJ, Burn DJ, Rowan EN et al. A comparison of the efficacy of donepezil in Parkinson's disease with dementia and dementia with Lewy bodies. Int J Geriatr Psychiatry 2005; 20: 938–44.

79. Grace J, Daniel S, Stevens T et al. Long-term use of rivastigmine in patients with dementia with Lewy bodies: an open-label trial. Int Psychogeriatr 2001; 13: 199–205.

80. Werner P, Erik W, Murat E et al. Long-term benefits of rivastigmine in dementia associated with Parkinson's disease: an active treatment extension study. Mov Disord 2006; 21: 456–61.

81. Aarsland D, Ballard C, Walker Z et al. Memantine in patients with Parkinson's disease dementia or dementia with Lewy bodies: a double-blind, placebo-controlled, multicentre trial. Lancet Neurol 2009; 8: 613–18.

82. McKeith IG, Wesnes KA, Perry E et al. Hallucinations predict attentional improvements with rivastigmine in dementia with Lewy bodies. Dement Geriatr Cogn Disord 2004; 18: 94–100.

83. Kurlan R, Cummings J, Raman R et al. Quetiapine for agitation or psychosis in patients with dementia and parkinsonism. Neurology 2007; 68: 1356–63.

84. Anon. FDA Alert. Information for Healthcare Professionals – Antipsychotics, 2009. At www.fda.gov/Drugs/DrugSafety/PostmarketDrugSafetyInformationforPatientsandProviders/ucm124830.htm, accessed 31 Jan 2010.

85. Anon. Medicines CftSo. Atypical Antipsychotic Drugs and Stroke, 2008. At www.mhra.gov.uk/Safetyinformation/Safetywarningsalertsandrecalls/Safetywarningsandmessagesformedicines/CON1004298, accessed 31 Jan 2010.

86. Boeve BF, Silber MH, Ferman TJ. REM sleep behavior disorder in Parkinson's disease and dementia with Lewy bodies. J Geriatr Psychiatry Neurol 2004; 17: 146–57.

59

Prion Diseases

Brian S. Appleby

Division of Geriatric Psychiatry and Neuropsychiatry, The Johns Hopkins Hospital, Baltimore, USA

PRION THEORY AND BIOLOGY

Cellular Prion Protein

The native cellular prion protein (PrP^c) is located throughout the human body, predominantly in the brain and gut. PrP^c is a glycosyl phosphatidyl inositol-linked glycoprotein that is anchored on lipid rafts. The tertiary structure of PrP^c is primarily composed of α-helixes with few β-sheets. The prion protein gene (*PRNP*) was identified in 1986 and its identification has led to the development of *PRNP* knock-out mice, which do not appear to behave differently from wild-type mice. However, PrP^c null mice exhibit impaired synaptic inhibition and it has been proposed that PrP^c has stress-protective functions. Divalent cations including copper, zinc and manganese have also been shown to bind to PrP^c, though the significance of this is unclear. There has been emerging evidence that PrP^c may be associated with Alzheimer's disease and psychiatric illnesses as part of the stress diathesis.

Pathological Prion Protein

In contrast to the native prion protein, the pathological prion protein's (PrP^{res}) structure is primarily composed of β-sheets that aggregate and form amyloid plaques. The high β-sheet content of PrP^{res} leads to its partial resistance to proteinase K, resulting in proteinase-resistant protein fragments (i.e. PrP$^{'res'}$) called prions, which stands for '*pr*oteinaceous *in*fectious particle.'

There are three aetiologies of PrP^{res}: (i) sporadic, (ii) genetic and (iii) acquired. Although the exact mechanism for the formation of sporadic PrP^{res} is unknown, it is widely believed to be the result of a posttranslational mutation. This has recently been demonstrated using *in vitro* protein misfolding cyclic amplification (PMCA) techniques[1]. PrP^{res} can also be generated *de novo* by mutations within the prion protein gene (*PRNP*). Lastly, PrP^{res} can be acquired from an outside source and introduced into the body, precipitating the formation of additional PrP^{res}.

Prion Theory (The Protein-Only Hypothesis)

Prions are transmissible agents that lack the nucleic acids that bacteria and viruses use to infect other organisms. In lieu of nucleic acids, the transmissibility of prions is accomplished via an autocatalytic mechanism, a theory coined the 'protein-only hypothesis' (Figure 59.1). This process was first postulated by the mathematician J. S. Griffith

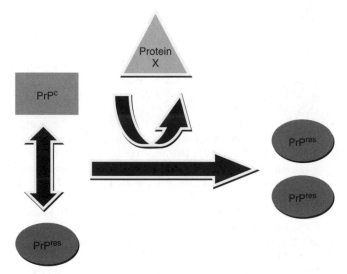

Figure 59.1 The prion conversion process. PrP^{res} replicates via an autocatalytic mechanism. PrP^{res} uses PrP^c as a substrate for the production of further PrP^{res} proteins. An uncharacterized protein (protein X) is postulated to facilitate the transformation process

in 1967[2] and was later described by Stanley Prusiner, who was subsequently granted a Nobel Prize for his work[3]. PrP^{res} interacts with PrP^c, using itself as a template to change the conformation of PrP^c into another PrP^{res} protein. Mouse studies have found that the presence of PrP^c is a requirement for the conversion process to occur. As evidence of this fact, PrP^c-null mice do not develop prion disease when they are inoculated with PrP^{res}, as the conversion process does not occur without the PrP^c substrate.

HUMAN PRION DISEASES

Kuru

Human prion diseases, or transmissible spongiform encephalopathies (TSEs), were initially described in detail by Nobel Prize laureate Carlton Gajdusek through his research on kuru[4]. Believed to be a 'slow virus', kuru was an endemic illness in the Fore tribe of Papua New Guinea. Kuru was characterized by rapidly progressive ataxia, oculomotor impairment, myoclonus and dementia with death typically occurring within two years of the illness onset. Gajdusek later found that kuru was transmitted among the tribe via its cannibalistic rituals of consuming their deceased, particularly their brains. Tribal members who consumed brain matter of relatives with kuru were exposed to the illness and incubated it for several years, sometimes decades, until they eventually developed the illness. It is generally accepted that the kuru epidemic has since subsided and no longer exists.

Creutzfeldt–Jakob Disease

The most common human prion disease is Creutzfeldt–Jakob disease (CJD), which was first described by two neuropsychiatrists, Hans Gerhard Creutzfeldt[5] and Alfons Maria Jakob[6]. Both Creutzfeldt and Jakob described patients with a rapid neurodegenerative illness who

had a spongiform appearance of their brain at postmortem analysis. CJD is recognized at autopsy by the neuropathological triad of astrogliosis, spongiform changes and neuronal death (Figure 59.2a). Immunostaining with monoclonal 3F4 antibodies also shows prion deposition within the brain (Figure 59.2b). Abnormal prion proteins can also be detected by pre-treating brain homogenate with proteinase K and performing Western blot analyses that typically detect proteinase-resistant protein fragments (PrP$^{27-30}$).

CJD is a rare cause of dementia. The worldwide incidence of CJD is one per million people per year and is slightly higher in females than in males, although the age-adjusted incidence is slightly higher in males. CJD is rare in blacks for unclear reasons, but ascertainment problems may be one reason for the low incidence. Researchers have discovered a genetic propensity towards the development of CJD in relation to the codon 129 polymorphism of the *PRNP* gene. Individuals who are homozygous (Met-Met or Val-Val) at codon 129, especially Met-Met, are more likely to develop CJD. The *PRNP* codon 129 polymorphism is also associated with differences in clinical presentations and survival times.

CJD can be divided by aetiological subtypes. There are three main aetiologies of CJD: (i) sporadic CJD (sCJD), (ii) genetic CJD (gCJD), and (iii) acquired forms of CJD. The latter group includes the iatrogenic transmission of CJD (iCJD) and human transmission of bovine spongiform encephalopathy (BSE) called variant CJD (vCJD). In addition to different aetiologies, these subclasses of CJD also demonstrate different demographic, clinical, diagnostic, neuropathological

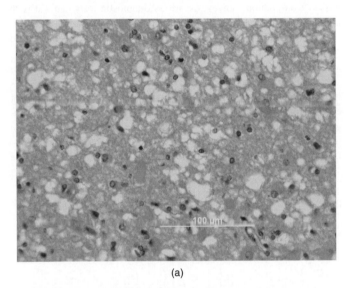

(a)

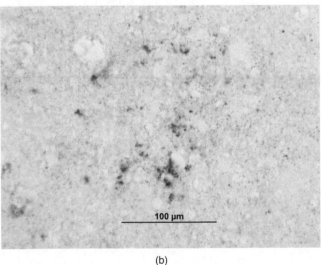

(b)

Figure 59.2 (a) Haematoxylin and eosin (H&E) stain of the temporal cortex and (b) monoclonal 3F4 antibody immunostaining of the hippocampus in a patient with Creutzfeldt–Jakob disease. The neuropathology is characterized by a spongiform appearance, astrogliosis and neuronal cell death. Immunostaining (b) reveals abnormal prion protein deposits (dark brown). *A full colour version of this figure appears in the colour plate section*

Table 59.1 Characteristics of Creutzfeldt–Jakob disease by aetiological subtypes

CJD subtype	Cases (%)	Mean age of onset (years)	Mean illness duration (months)
Sporadic	85	61	4
Genetic	15	56	14
Iatrogenic	<1	43	11
Variant	<1	32	13

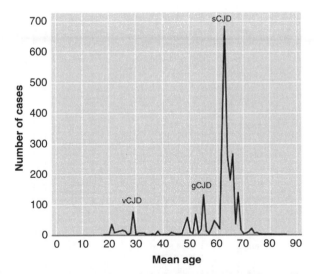

Figure 59.3 Age of onset of Creutzfeldt–Jakob disease. The age of onset follows a bell-shaped curve with a mean age of onset in sporadic CJD (sCJD) of 61 years, 56 years in genetic CJD (gCJD), and 32 years in variant CJD (vCJD). Adapted from Appleby *et al.*[8]

Table 59.2 Presenting symptoms of sporadic Creutzfeldt–Jakob disease

Presenting symptom	Cases (%)
Cognitive impairment	72
Ataxia	44
Visual/oculomotor impairment	35
Mood disorder	28
Vertigo	26
Behaviour/personality change	23
Psychosis/agitation	20
Sleep disorder	18

Source: Adapted from Appleby *et al*.[8]

Table 59.3 Diagnostic test results in sporadic CJD

Diagnostic test	Characteristics
EEG	Periodic sharp wave complexes
CSF analyses	+14-3-3 protein
Brain MRI (DWI/FLAIR)	Hyperintensity in the basal ganglia and/or cortical ribbon

and molecular characteristics. Table 59.1 lists the characteristics of the CJD subtypes[7,8].

Sporadic Creutzfeldt–Jakob disease

The exact aetiology of sCJD is unknown, but is largely believed to be a consequence of a posttranslational mutation of PrP^c. Comprising 85% of all human prion diseases, sCJD is the most common human prion disease. The age of onset follows a bell-shaped curve with a mean age of onset of 61 years (Figure 59.3). The average survival time is four months and a very small percentage of individuals survive for more than two years. Although the cardinal symptoms of sCJD are dementia, ataxia, myoclonus, akinetic mutism and visual disturbances, the clinical presentation is widely variable and can include many different neuropsychiatric symptoms (Table 59.2)[9].

A definitive diagnosis of CJD is only possible via neuropathological examination; however, various diagnostic tests can aid with an antemortem diagnosis (Table 59.3). CJD is a diagnosis of exclusion; hence, all other possible aetiologies should be considered and ruled out first. An electroencephalogram (EEG) may help to arrive at a diagnosis should it show the classic periodic sharp wave complexes (PSWCs) that are characteristic of CJD (Figure 59.4). A lumbar puncture must always be performed to exclude other causes of encephalopathy but the cerebrospinal fluid (CSF) can also be examined for the presence of the 14-3-3 protein, a native neuronal protein that is a marker of neuronal cell death. Although a sensitive diagnostic test, the 14-3-3 protein is non-specific and can be detected in the

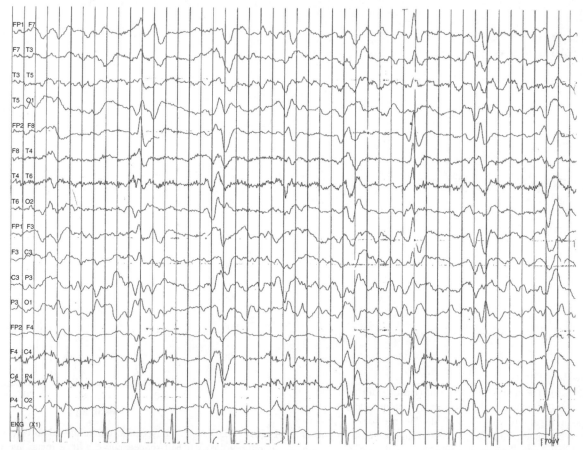

Figure 59.4 Electroencephalogram (EEG) of a sporadic Creutzfeldt–Jakob disease patient. The diffuse and synchronous periodic sharp wave complexes (PSWCs) seen in this EEG are characteristic of CJD

CSF of patients with multiple sclerosis, transverse myelitis and brain tumours. The presence of 14-3-3 in combination with tau is highly specific for a diagnosis of sCJD. Brain magnetic resonance imaging (MRI) can also be helpful in establishing a diagnosis of CJD. Hyperintensity in the cortical ribbon and/or basal ganglia are frequently observed on diffusion weighted and FLAIR image sequences, as shown in Figure 59.5.

Genetic Creutzfeldt–Jakob disease

Genetic CJD accounts for approximately 15% of human prion diseases and it is caused by a pathological mutation in the prion protein gene (*PRNP*) that results in the production of PrP^{res}. To date, over 30 different mutations in the *PRNP* gene are known to result

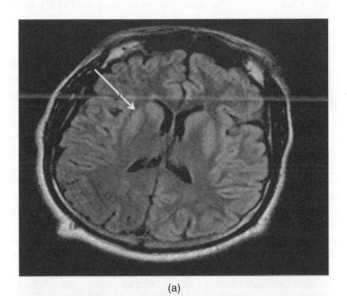

(a)

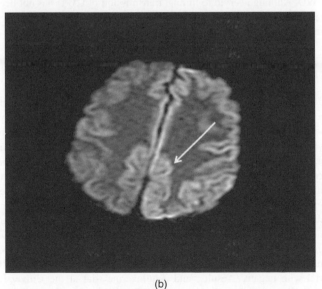

(b)

Figure 59.5 Brain magnetic resonance imaging of a patient with Creutzfeldt–Jakob disease. (a) Basal ganglia hyperintensity is seen on FLAIR sequences and (b) hyperintensity in the cortical ribbon is seen on diffusion-weighted imaging

in prion diseases. The majority of mutations are autosomal dominant point mutations, but insertion and deletion mutations have also been described. All mutations demonstrate near complete penetrance by the ninth decade of life. The age of onset is usually mid-life (Figure 59.3) and disease duration is typically longer than other prion diseases and can be several years in duration. Clinical and neuropathological phenotypes vary and are determined by the mutation site, codon 129 polymorphism, and PrP^{res} type[10]. Diagnostic test results also differ between mutation types. The most common gCJD haplotype is E200K-129M. Other common mutations and their characteristics are listed in Table 59.5.

Iatrogenic Creutzfeldt–Jakob disease

Iatrogenic CJD is pre-empted by the transmission of prions through several possible medical interventions[11]. Table 59.4 lists the known risk factors for iCJD, including cadaveric dura grafts, gonadotrophins, corneal transplants, neurosurgical depth electrodes and neurosurgical instrument contamination. Direct contact with the central nervous system is necessary for transmission to occur in the majority of cases. Very low levels of prion proteins have been detected in the blood and urine of CJD patients, though the amounts are not significant enough to cause transmission with the exception of vCJD. There have been four recognized cases of vCJD transmission via blood transfusions; three died of CJD and one was pre-symptomatic at the time of death. There has been no known blood-borne transmission of the other prion diseases. Because of iCJD, cadaveric dura mater grafts and corneas are no longer used and neurosurgical instruments undergo extensive autoclaving procedures to prevent the transmission of prions. The ages of onset and survival times are variable given the groups' varied demographic features.

Variant Creutzfeldt–Jakob disease

Although it is the most publicized form of CJD, vCJD is quite rare. Fewer than 300 total cases have been described to date, nearly exclusively in European countries (e.g. UK, France, Spain, Italy and the Netherlands). Variant CJD is caused by ingesting foodstuffs tainted with a form of prion disease found in cows, termed bovine spongiform encephalopathy (BSE). During the 1990s, Bob Will and colleagues at the UK National Creutzfeldt–Jakob Disease Surveillance Centre noted an increased incidence of CJD in younger people, who also exhibited atypical neuropathological features at autopsy. Individuals with vCJD tended to be in their 20s or 30s (Figure 59.3) and had amyloid plaques in their brains, termed 'kuru plaques'[12]. Individuals with vCJD primarily presented with psychiatric (e.g. mood and anxiety disorders) and sensory symptoms and their illness duration was typically longer than sCJD. Until December 2008, all cases of vCJD

Table 59.4 Risk factors for iatrogenic Creutzfeldt–Jakob disease

Risk factors
Dural mater grafts
Cadaveric gonadotrophins (e.g. hGH, hCG)
Corneal transplants
Neurosurgical depth electrodes
Neurosurgical instrument contamination

Table 59.5 Clinical characteristics and EEG findings of familial prion diseases by mutation

PRNP genotype	Clinical characteristics	EEG findings
E200K	Rapidly progressive dementia, ataxia and myoclonus	PSWCs
V210I	Memory impairment, behavioural changes, and ataxia	PSWCs
D178N-129V	Cognitive impairment, depression and irritability	Lack of PSWCs
D178N-129M (fatal familial insomnia)	Insomnia, dysautonomia, pyrexia and dementia late in illness	Loss of sleep architecture
P102L (Gerstmann–Sträussler–Scheinker disease)	Gait and limb ataxia, nystagmus and dysarthria	Slowing

have been homozygous for methionine at codon 129 (129Met-Met), which led many to believe that the *PRNP* codon 129Met-Met genotype was necessary for the development of vCJD. Many researchers cautioned that, similar to iCJD, the codon 129 polymorphism may affect incubation period and that other polymorphisms may also be at risk, though they may display a prolonged incubation period. With the discovery of the first codon 129 Met-Val vCJD case in December 2008[13], many are concerned that there may be another cluster of vCJD cases from the 1990s BSE exposure.

Fatal Familial Insomnia

Fatal familial insomnia (FFI) is a hereditary prion disease first described by Pierluigi Gambetti and colleagues[14]. FFI is caused by the D178N-129M mutation of the *PRNP* gene in contrast to one of the more common gCJD mutations, D178N-129V (Table 59.5). The different haplotypes differ in their codon 129 polymorphism of the mutant allele, resulting in different clinical and neuropathological phenotypes. FFI typically occurs in mid-life with the onset of progressive insomnia, fatigue, dysautonomia (e.g. labile blood pressure and pulse, pyrexia) and hypervigilance. Dementia typically does not manifest until late in the disease. EEGs and sleep studies show a characteristic loss of sleep architecture, including the absence of sleep spindles and K complexes. The neuropathology of FFI also differs from conventional CJD in that spongiform changes are found predominantly in the thalamus. There have also been several cases of sporadic fatal insomnia (sFI) described in the literature.

Gerstmann–Sträussler–Scheinker Disease

Gerstmann–Sträussler–Scheinker disease (GSS) is the least common heritable prion disease and it is caused by several different mutations in the *PRNP* gene, the P102L mutation being the most common[15] (Table 59.5). The initial symptoms of GSS include global cerebellar impairment (e.g. limb and gait ataxia, dysmetria, scanning speech). The survival time of individuals with GSS can be several years in duration. The unique pathological prion protein, Pr^{7-8}, is also a characteristic feature of GSS.

SAFEGUARDS

Despite the name 'transmissible spongiform encephalopathies,' prion diseases are not infectious in the usual clinical environment. Only universal precautions are necessary when providing routine care to individuals with prion diseases. Prion precautions, which consist of special autoclaving and sterilization procedures, are necessary when

there is exposure to the central nervous system. Scenarios in which prion precautions would be necessary include neurosurgery, postmortem examinations, and general surgery in individuals who have a family history of familial prion disease and suspected vCJD. In the United States, individuals who have a relative who has been diagnosed with a prion disease or those who spent time in the UK during the 1990s cannot give blood.

In relation to the zoonotic forms of acquired prion disease, care must be taken when handling central nervous system tissue of any mammal. Consuming brain matter, which is considered a delicacy in some cultures, is a high-risk activity for acquiring prion diseases. Not all animal prion diseases are transmissible to humans. Scrapie, a prion disease in sheep, has not been demonstrated to cross the animal–human species barrier. Some prion diseases in other species, such as cows, have shown the potential for human transmission. Because of vCJD, national governments and agricultural regulatory agencies should prohibit the return of 'downer cows' into the feed. Genetic forms of BSE have recently been discovered, strongly discouraging any re-feeding of animals as they have the potential to be presymptomatic carriers of prion disease. Chronic wasting disease (CWD), a prion disease that is rampant in cervids (e.g. deer and elk), has recently become a concern in the US. Researchers have estimated that up to 30% of deer in certain locales are incubating CWD. Although cervid to human transmission of CWD has not been demonstrated in the laboratory, hunters are encouraged to have their game tested for CWD prior to its consumption.

TREATMENTS

Unfortunately, human prion diseases are invariably fatal with no current treatment or cure. Several investigational treatments have been and are currently being explored. Carsten Korth, a psychiatrist who trained in Stanley Prusiner's laboratory, discovered the antiprion effects of chlorpromazine and other phenothiazine antipsychotics that led to the two largest clinical trials in prion diseases to date[16]. Korth uncovered that many compounds with antiprion activity were based on tricyclic structures with an aliphatic side chain at the middle ring moiety. Chlorpromazine, imipramine and quinacrine were among these compounds, quinacrine having approximately 10-fold greater antiprion activity compared to the others. This discovery led to two major trials of quinacrine for the treatment of CJD: PRION-1, a UK trial with negative results, and a quinacrine trial at the University of California at San Francisco (UCSF), the results of which have not been published. Besides quinacrine, several other compounds are being investigated as potential treatments for prion diseases, including intraventricular pentosan polysulphate (PPA) and doxycycline. Both compounds exhibit antiprion activity *in vitro*, although human studies have demonstrated that neither drug will likely be a cure. Future studies are planned to examine the use of antiprion protein antibodies, gene therapy and iRNA.

Until better treatments are available for individuals with prion disease, the clinician is left with the all-important symptomatic treatment of the disease. Certain symptoms can be particularly upsetting to the patient and the family. Myoclonus, especially startle myoclonus, can greatly decrease quality of life, yet can be easily managed with behavioural interventions (e.g. decreased touching, turning and decreased sensory input in general) and benzodiazepines or anticonvulsants. Both drugs can also address seizures, which are sometimes present in the end stages of the illness. Insomnia can also be treated with benzodiazepines. Visual hallucinations and paranoid delusions are common due to visual impairments and disorientation in the setting of a relatively normal level of alertness. These symptoms can be treated with antipsychotics, with a preference towards quetiapine and clozapine due to the high prevalence of extrapyramidal symptoms in this patient population. Pyrexia, another end-stage symptom, can be managed with cold compresses and acetaminophen. Finally, hospice care is usually recommended, which includes palliative care as well as treating pain and agonal breathing with morphine or other opiates.

PRION DISEASES AND OTHER PROTEIN-MISFOLDING DISORDERS

Prion diseases posit a unique situation for studying protein-misfolding disorders, also known as proteinopathies. Proteinopathies are diseases caused by the formation of an abnormal isomer of a native protein. Through toxicity and/or loss of function mechanisms, proteinopathies cause neurodegenerative diseases including Alzheimer's disease (amyloid beta), frontotemporal dementia (tau), Parkinson's disease (alpha-synuclein) and Huntington's disease (huntingtin). Most of the above illnesses have familial forms caused by gene mutations (e.g. PS-1 and -2, APP, MAPT, TDP-43 and PGRN), but the majority of cases are of sporadic aetiology. Basic science research typically focuses on transgenic animal models, which may ignore the disease mechanisms that are responsible for the majority of these populations. Prion diseases are unique in that they are sporadic, familial and transmissible. Whereas transgenic mice can also be used to study prion diseases, PrP^res can be used to inoculate normal animals, causing them to become ill without any genetic modification. Hence, prion diseases are a unique proteinopathy because PrP^res is both necessary and sufficient to cause disease in a normal population. Prions also aggregate and form amyloid plaques, a process called nucleation. Other proteinopathies follow this pattern: amyloid-beta forms amyloid plaques in Alzheimer's disease, tau proteins aggregate into neurofibrillary tangles in frontotemporal dementia, and alpha-synuclein forms Lewy bodies in Parkinson's disease and dementia with Lewy bodies. Protein misfolding cyclic amplification (PMCA), as used in prion diseases, can also be used to study other protein misfolding disorders, which may share similar features such as abnormal chaperone activity. Although one of the rarest protein misfolding disorders, much more is known about prion diseases than most of the other proteinopathies. Prion diseases thus serve as an opportunity to study these diseases from a much different, and perhaps easier, perspective. Additionally, the prion protein gene (PRNP) is routinely listed in the top 20 genes implicated in Alzheimer's disease and the native prion protein has recently been shown to inhibit beta site APP-cleaving enzyme (BACE-1), an enzyme associated with Alzheimer's disease.

REFERENCES

1. Supattapone S. Prion protein conversion *in vitro*. *J Mol Med* 2004; **82**(6): 348–56.
2. Griffith JS. Self-replication and scrapie. *Nature* 1967; **215**(5105): 1043–4.
3. Prusiner SB. Novel proteinaceous infectious particles cause scrapie. *Science* 1982; **216**(4542): 136–44.
4. Gajdusek C, Gibbs CJ, Alpers M. Slow-acting virus implicated in kuru. *JAMA* 1967; **199**(7): 34.
5. Creutzfeldt H. Uber eine eigenartige herdformige Erkrankung des Zentralnervensystems. Vorlaufige Mitteilung. *Z Gesamte Neurol Psychiatr* 1920; **57**: 1–18.
6. Jakob A. Uber eigenartige Erkrankungen des Zentralnervensystems mit bemerkenswerten anatomischen Befunden (spastische Pseudosklerose-Encephalomyelopathie mit disseminierten Degenerationsherden). *Z Gesamte Neurol Psychiatr* 1921, **64**. 147–228.
7. Will R, Alpers M, Dormont D, Schonberger L. Infectious and sporadic prion diseases. In Prusiner SB (ed.), *Prion Biology and Diseases*, 2nd edn. New York: Cold Spring Harbor Laboratory Press, 2004, 629–72.
8. Appleby BS, Appleby KK, Rabins PV. Does the presentation of Creutzfeldt–Jakob disease vary by age or presumed etiology? A meta analysis of the past 10 years. *J Neuropsychiatry Clin Neurosci* 2007; **19**(4): 428–35.
9. Appleby BS, Appleby KK, Crain BJ *et al.* Characteristics of established and proposed sporadic Creutzfeldt–Jakob disease variants. *Arch Neurol* 2009; **66**(2): 208–15.
10. Gambetti P, Parchi P, Chen SG. Hereditary Creutzfeldt–Jakob disease and fatal familial insomnia. *Clin Lab Med* 2003; **23**(1): 43–64.
11. Will RG. Acquired prion disease: iatrogenic CJD, variant CJD, kuru. *Br Med Bull* 2003; **66**(1): 255–65.
12. Will R, Ironside J. A new variant of Creutzfeldt–Jakob disease in the UK. *Lancet* 1996; **347**(9006): 921–5.
13. Devlin K. Hundreds could die as scientists identify first case of 'second wave' vCJD, *Daily Telegraph* 18 Dec 2008. At www.telegraph.co.uk/health/healthnews/3815384/Hundreds-could-die-as-scientists-identify-first-case-of-second-wave-vCJD.html, accessed 3 Feb 2010.
14. Gambetti P, Petersen R, Monari L *et al.* Fatal familial insomnia and the widening spectrum of prion diseases. *Br Med Bull* 1993; **49**(4): 980–94.
15. Hsiao K, Prusiner SB. Inherited human prion diseases. *Neurology* 1990; **40**(12): 1820–27.
16. Korth C, May BC, Cohen FE, Prusiner SB. Acridine and phenothiazine derivatives as pharmacotherapeutics for prion disease. *Proc Natl Acad Sci U S A* 2001; **98**(17): 9836–41.

60

Alcoholic and Other Toxic Dementias

Eileen M. Joyce

Professor of Neuropsychiatry, UCL Institute of Neurology, Queen Square, London, UK

ALCOHOLIC DEMENTIA

The concept of a dementia consequent upon the neurotoxic effects of long-term alcohol abuse developed from clinical observations of a gradual deterioration in personality and intellect in many alcoholics. Subsequent research suggested that this is age related, is milder in degree than other forms of dementia and constitutes 11–24% of all demented patients[1,2]. To put this in further perspective, of the estimated 18 million alcoholics in the USA, approximately 40% will have mild cognitive impairment which is potentially reversible with abstinence, but a further 10% will have persisting severe cognitive impairment requiring institutional care, comprising patients mainly with dementia and amnesia[3,4].

Amnesia in alcoholics is known as the Wernicke-Korsakoff syndrome. This is the result of thiamine malnutrition which causes subcortical periventricular vascular lesions in diencephalic structures, the mamillary body and thalamus, known to be critically involved in new memory formation[5]. Alcoholic dementia was originally thought to be distinct from the Wernicke-Korsakoff syndrome and due to the direct neurotoxic effect of alcohol on the cerebral cortex. Horvath[6] prospectively examined 100 chronic alcoholics presenting clinically with a dementia syndrome and concluded that alcoholic dementia was different from the Wernicke-Korsakoff syndrome and that other non-amnesic organic syndromes exist in alcoholics characteristic of frontal, parietal or global cortical damage. Cutting[7] performed a retrospective case-note analysis of alcoholic patients with cognitive impairment and found two forms of clinical presentation. One consisted of a rapidly developing illness in younger patients with preserved intellect, akin to the traditional Wernicke-Korsakoff syndrome, whereas the other was more characteristic of dementia, being a gradual and global cognitive deterioration in older patients.

Although these studies support the concept of alcoholic dementia as a distinct entity, other evidence suggests a more complex picture with there being several different neuropathological 'routes' to the development of brain damage sufficient to cause the diffuse cognitive impairment recognized clinically as dementia. Torvik and colleagues[8] examined the clinical records of patients who at autopsy had diencephalic lesions characteristic of thiamine malnutrition; that is, Wernicke-type lesions. Seventy five percent of these were considered to be demented in life rather than amnesic and the majority had no additional neuropathological hallmarks of a neurodegenerative dementia. They concluded that the diencephalic lesions of thiamine deficiency can result in the clinical picture of both 'alcoholic dementia' and the Wernicke-Korsakoff syndrome. Victor and Adams[9]

then pointed out that 10% of their pathologically proven cases of the Wernicke-Korsakoff syndrome developed cognitive abnormalities insidiously rather than acutely[5] and that cognitive impairment other than amnesia and behavioural abnormalities such as inertia and apathy can be demonstrated in these patients[10]. Thus they argued that, depending on the severity of the non-mnemonic deficits or the mode of presentation, cases of the Wernicke-Korsakoff syndrome may be misattributed as cases of alcoholic dementia. The neuropathological studies of Harper and colleagues[11-13] are in agreement with this view. They found that two thirds of the alcoholics coming to postmortem in their unit had lesions of thiamine deficiency; of these, only a third had received a clinical diagnosis of the Wernicke-Korsakoff syndrome in life and, in the remainder, the most common diagnosis was dementia.

This evidence points to the conclusion that subcortical lesions caused by thiamine malnutrition can be sufficient to explain both amnesia and dementia witnessed in alcoholics. However, Victor and Adams[9] and Torvik and colleagues[8] did not suggest that *all* cases of alcoholic dementia are unrecognized cases of the Wernicke-Korsakoff syndrome. Both considered that superadded cerebral lesions may explain the dementia-like presentation of a proportion of patients with the Wernicke-Korsakoff syndrome. Because these additional lesions can be attributed to a variety of pathological processes, including chronic hepatocerebral degeneration, communicating hydrocephalus, Alzheimer's disease and ischaemic infarction, they argued that there is no need to invoke a special process of alcohol neurotoxicity. Some studies have supported this hypothesis. For example, Kasahara and colleagues[14] compared young and old alcoholics and found evidence of dementia only in the older group; most of these patients had additional medical diagnoses including hypertension, liver disease and cardiomyopathy and no case of dementia could be accounted for by the direct effect of alcohol alone.

Although these clinical studies suggest that dementia in alcoholics can be caused by factors other than the direct effect of alcohol on brain function, the neuropathological evidence is that alcohol is neurotoxic. The question therefore still remains as to whether this is sufficient to cause cortical damage and frank dementia. Carefully controlled neuropathological studies have frequently found whole brain atrophy involving grey and white matter in chronic alcoholics with and without evidence of thiamine depletion as indicated by the presence or absence of subcortical Wernicke-type lesions[15-18]. This atrophy appears to reflect reductions of white matter volume, neuronal loss in the dorsal frontal association cortex and neuronal shrinkage in other cortical areas such as the cingulate gyrus and the precentral motor cortex[19-23]. The contribution of liver failure to this neuropathology has been assessed in several studies and the bulk of evidence suggests that cirrhosis alone does not account for the brain atrophy witnessed in alcoholics[16,17,24]. Other findings suggest that thiamine depletion in the context of alcohol ingestion may contribute to this neuropathological picture even when this is insufficient to cause the subcortical lesions of the Wernicke-Korsakoff syndrome.

Thiamine is an essential co-enzyme for three enzyme complexes (pyruvate dehydrogenase, alpha-ketoglutarate dehydrogenase and transketolase) involved in mitochondrial oxidative phosphorylation and a number of cellular synthetic processes. Animal models have shown that lack of thiamine leads to mitochondrial dysfunction and cell death consequent upon oxidative stress, glutamatergic excitotoxicity and inflammatory responses; as these mechanisms are also active in other forms of neurodegenerative dementia, it is possible that thiamine depletion, as well as causing diencephalic vascular lesions, also directly causes cortical cell damage secondary to these actions[25]. Animal models have also shown that alcohol alone can lead to cell damage via oxidative stress[26-28] and that cortical cell death is greater in the presence of both alcohol and thiamine depletion than either factor alone[29].

Thiamine deficiency is common in alcoholics due to a combination of inadequate diet, poor absorption secondary to the effect of alcohol on the gastrointestinal tract and poor cellular utilization due to the direct action of alcohol on intracellular mechanisms[30,31]. Thus it is likely that, even in alcoholics who have not developed Wernicke-Korsakoff syndrome, reduced thiamine availability will be present in a significant proportion and that this contributes to the development of dementia along with alcohol via a joint action on cortical neurones. Evidence that alcohol and thiamine deficiency are synergistic in man also comes from findings that the cortical pathological changes witnessed in alcoholics without evidence of thiamine depletion are similar to but less severe than those with co-existent subcortical Wernicke lesions[16,18,21,24,32-34].

In summary, it can be concluded from these studies that: (i) alcohol itself can cause neuronal damage including cell death; (ii) liver disease *per se* is not a major factor in the aetiology of the neuropathological cerebral changes seen in alcoholics; and (iii) thiamine malnutrition potentiates the neurotoxic effect of alcohol on the brain and it is likely that frank dementia in alcoholics is due to this combined action rather than the effect of alcohol alone.

What is the relationship between alcohol ingestion and the more common, milder cognitive impairment seen in alcoholics? The advent of *in vivo* neuroimaging has enabled clinicopathological correlational studies to clarify the consequences of alcohol consumption on brain function and cognition in alcoholics uncomplicated by liver disease or thiamine depletion. Well-controlled, prospective studies using both CT and MRI have reliably confirmed the presence of cerebral shrinkage in such alcoholics in life involving both cortical grey and subcortical white matter[35-42], which is more pronounced in older patients[43] and more apparent in the frontal lobe[44,45]. One early imaging study highlighted the possibility that women are more vulnerable to the effects of alcohol in that brain atrophy was equivalent in age-matched men and women despite the women having shorter or less severe drinking histories[46]. This remains controversial, however, as some later studies[47,48] but not all[49,50] have replicated this finding.

The development of the MRI modality of diffusion tensor imaging (DTI) has allowed a more detailed assessment of the white matter volume reductions found in postmortem and conventional MRI studies.

DTI depends on water diffusion being constrained by cell membranes or myelin sheaths and, when abnormal, may reflect pathology of myelin microstructure. Studies of alcoholics without complications of liver disease or a history of Wernicke's encephalopathy have found that white matter abnormalities are widespread in life, being present in areas not previously detected by conventional MRI[51-53]. DTI data can also be used to examine specific fibre pathways using the technique of tractography. When applied to alcoholics, abnormalities in the frontal forceps, internal and external capsules, fornix, and superior cingulate and longitudinal fasciculi have been detected, and the severity of these abnormalities was found to correlate with lifetime alcohol consumption[54]. In the same study, when matched for alcohol exposure, alcoholic women showed more DTI signs of white matter degradation than alcoholic men in several fibre bundles, suggesting that any sex differences in the vulnerability to alcohol may be neural tissue specific[54].

An important observation is that the percentage of alcoholics with evidence of cerebral damage on brain scans is far in excess of that noted in neuropathological studies[15]. This discrepancy is probably explained by the finding that brain changes are reversible with continuing abstinence[37,41,42,46,55-63], thus indicating that neuroimaging findings may not accurately reflect the permanent neuropathological changes previously described in postmortem studies. However, because some studies have found that neuroimaging changes worsen in patients who continue to drink, and may not be entirely reversible with abstinence in heavier drinkers[56,64,65], and others have found that greater total alcohol consumption is associated with greater decrease in cortical grey matter, particularly in the frontal[62,66] and temporal lobes[62], these neuroimaging abnormalities may represent neurotoxic processes which may ultimately lead to more permanent neuropathology if abstinence is not achieved.

Like dementia, the characteristic cognitive impairment witnessed in uncomplicated alcoholics is diffuse in nature but much milder. Parsons[67], following decades of his own research, concluded that both male and female sober adult alcoholics have deficits on tests of learning, memory, executive functions and speed of information processing which are equivalent to those found in other patients with known brain dysfunction of a mild to moderate nature. Similar findings have repeatedly been demonstrated by others (see[68]). Like neuroimaging studies, controlled neuropsychological studies have shown that cognitive deficits are largely reversible following abstinence[69] although, again, these may not be reversible in those with severe and long-term alcohol abuse[67]. Early studies attempting to relate cognitive and structural changes in alcoholics found weak and inconsistent correlations, the majority of which were explained mainly by age and premorbid IQ[35,36,38,70-72]. However, the use of novel MRI techniques has produced stronger evidence for a link between cognitive impairment on the one hand and brain structural and functional abnormalities on the other. For example, studies have combined structural MRI and MR spectroscopy to demonstrate concomitant brain atrophy and metabolic abnormalities in the context of cognitive deficits, all of which improve together with abstinence[60,61,73]. Precise volumetric analyses have also confirmed the neuropathological finding that the dorsal frontal association cortex is the area most vulnerable to alcohol, in that this undergoes the greatest reduction in volume, but that other areas such as the temporal cortex, insula and cerebellum are also affected, as well as widespread areas of white matter[74]. In the same study, neuropsychological impairments correlated with the grey and white matter volume reductions even in detoxified patients with well-preserved social function[74].

These studies of uncomplicated alcoholics suggest that chronic alcohol ingestion can cause damage to widespread areas of the cerebral cortex and subcortical white matter sufficient to cause cognitive impairment even in people who otherwise appear to be functioning well. Such findings, although reversible with sustained abstinence if caught early enough, seem to herald more permanent brain damage and possibly dementia in those who continue to drink heavily, especially if there is co-existent thiamine depletion. Together with the recent findings of the combined action of alcohol and thiamine deficiency on cortical viability in animal studies[25,29], this underscores the need to suspect and treat thiamine malnutrition even in apparently healthy alcoholics.

OTHER TOXIC DEMENTIAS IN THE ELDERLY

The long-term neuropsychiatric effects of ingestion of drugs of abuse are unclear and probably differ depending on the compound; however, there is little evidence to suggest that these generally cause significant brain damage enough to produce dementia. For example, benzodiazepines, perhaps the most relevant substance in elderly populations, do not produce diffuse cognitive impairment or brain damage[75]. As ageing populations will now include people with other forms of long-term drug abuse or dependence, it is also important to consider other substances. Although there is some evidence that opiate addiction can result in grey matter volume reductions, these studies have been contaminated by including subjects with co-morbid alcohol abuse, and at least one of these suggests that alcohol rather than opiates *per se* was responsible for their findings[76]. There is one notable exception to the lack of strong evidence that substances of abuse cause dementia and that is the phenomenon of toxic leukencephalopathy seen in heroin, cocaine and amphetamine abuse. This usually occurs in the context of an overdose via the intravenous route or by inhalation, and is thought to be due to a direct toxic effect causing impaired intracellular energy metabolism[77-79].

The neuropsychiatric effects of long-term occupational solvent exposure are also relevant to the elderly. Although there is controversy concerning whether solvents *per se* produce long-lasting effects, most studies find evidence for lasting neuropsychological abnormalities[80-82]. Of particular interest is that these studies also found that a combination of long-term solvent exposure and alcohol abuse is a particular risk factor for the development of dementia. Of final relevance to this age group is the identification of bismuth encephalopathy which results from the over-ingestion of bismuth-containing compounds commonly taken for gastric irritation and sold without prescription. Following an acute organic reaction characterized by delirium, seizures and neurological abnormalities, persistent sequelae of diffuse cognitive impairment and cerebral atrophy has been documented[83,84].

REFERENCES

1. Carlen PL, McAndrews MP, Weiss RT *et al*. Alcohol-related dementia in the institutionalized elderly. *Alcohol Clin Exp Res* 1994; **18**(6): 1330–4.
2. Woodburn K, Johnstone E. Measuring the decline of a population of people with early-onset dementia in Lothian, Scotland. *Int J Geriatr Psychiatry* 1999; **14**(5): 355–61.
3. Oscar-Berman M, Marinkovic K. Alcoholism and the brain: an overview. *Alcohol Res Health* 2003; **27**(2): 125–33.
4. Rourke S, Loberg T. The neurobehavioral correlates of alcoholism. In Grant I, Adams K (eds), *Neuropsychological Assessment of Neuropsychiatric Disorders*, 2nd edn. New York: Oxford University Press, 1996, 423–85.
5. Victor M, Adams R, Collins G. *The Wernicke-Korsakoff Syndrome and Related Neurological Disorders Due to Alcoholism and Malnutrition*, 2nd edn. Philadelphia: FA Davis and Company, 1989.
6. Horvath TB. Clinical spectrum and epidemiological features of alcoholic dementia. In Rankin J (ed.), *Alcohol, Drugs and Brain Damage*. Toronto: Addiction Research Foundation of Ontario, 1975.
7. Cutting J. The relationship between Korsakov's syndrome and 'alcoholic dementia'. *Br J Psychiatry* 1978; **132**: 240–51.
8. Torvik A, Lindboe CF, Rogde S. Brain lesions in alcoholics. A neuropathological study with clinical correlations. *J Neurol Sci* 1982; **56**(2-3): 233–48
9. Victor M, Adams R. The alcoholic dementias. In Vinken P, Bruyn H, Klawans H (eds), *Handbook of Clinical Neurology*. Amsterdam: Elsevier, 1985, 335–52.
10. Talland G. *Deranged Memory*. New York: Academic Press, 1965.
11. Harper C, Kril J. Pathological changes in alcoholic brain shrinkage. *Med J Aust* 1986; **144**(1): 3–4.
12. Harper C. Wernicke's encephalopathy: a more common disease than realised. A neuropathological study of 51 cases. *J Neurol Neurosurg Psychiatry* 1979; **42**(3): 226–31.
13. Harper C. The incidence of Wernicke's encephalopathy in Australia – a neuropathological study of 131 cases. *J Neurol Neurosurg Psychiatry* 1983; **46**(7): 593–8.
14. Kasahara H, Karasawa A, Ariyasu T *et al*. Alcohol dementia and alcohol delirium in aged alcoholics. *Psychiatry Clin Neurosci* 1996; **50**(3): 115–23.
15. Harper C, Kril J. Brain atrophy in chronic alcoholic patients: a quantitative pathological study. *J Neurol Neurosurg Psychiatry* 1985; **48**(3): 211–7.
16. Harper C, Kril J. If you drink your brain will shrink. Neuropathological considerations. *Alcohol Alcohol Suppl* 1991; **1**: 375–80.
17. de la Monte SM. Disproportionate atrophy of cerebral white matter in chronic alcoholics. *Arch Neurol* 1988; **45**(9): 990–2.
18. Jensen GB, Pakkenberg B. Do alcoholics drink their neurons away? *Lancet* 1993; **342**(8881): 1201–4.
19. Harper C, Kril J, Daly J. Are we drinking our neurones away? *Br Med J (Clin Res Ed)* 1987; **294**(6571): 534–6.
20. Harper C, Kril J. Patterns of neuronal loss in the cerebral cortex in chronic alcoholic patients. *J Neurol Sci* 1989; **92**(1): 81–9.
21. Kril JJ, Halliday GM, Svoboda MD, Cartwright H. The cerebral cortex is damaged in chronic alcoholics. *Neuroscience* 1997; **79**(4): 983–98.
22. Ferrer I, Fabregues I, Rairiz J, Galofre E. Decreased numbers of dendritic spines on cortical pyramidal neurons in human chronic alcoholism. *Neurosci Lett* 1986; **69**(1): 115–9.
23. Harper C, Corbett D. Changes in the basal dendrites of cortical pyramidal cells from alcoholic patients – a quantitative Golgi study. *J Neurol Neurosurg Psychiatry* 1990; **53**(10): 856–61.
24. Kril JJ. The contribution of alcohol, thiamine deficiency and cirrhosis of the liver to cerebral cortical damage in alcoholics. *Metab Brain Dis* 1995; **10**(1): 9–16.
25. Hazell AS, Butterworth RF. Update of cell damage mechanisms in thiamine deficiency: focus on oxidative stress, excitotoxicity and inflammation. *Alcohol Alcohol* 2009; **44**(2): 141–7.

26. Chen G, Ma C, Bower KA *et al*. Ethanol promotes endoplasmic reticulum stress-induced neuronal death: involvement of oxidative stress. *J Neurosci Res* 2008; **86**(4): 937–46.

27. Gibson GE, Blass JP, Beal MF, Bunik V. The alpha-ketoglutarate-dehydrogenase complex: a mediator between mitochondria and oxidative stress in neurodegeneration. *Mol Neurobiol* 2005; **31**(1-3): 43–63

28. Park LC, Calingasan NY, Uchida K, Zhang H, Gibson GE. Metabolic impairment elicits brain cell type-selective changes in oxidative stress and cell death in culture. *J Neurochem* 2000; **74**(1): 114–24.

29. Ke ZJ, Wang X, Fan Z, Luo J. Ethanol promotes thiamine deficiency-induced neuronal death: involvement of double-stranded RNA-activated protein kinase. *Alcohol Clin Exp Res* 2009; **33**(6): 1097–103.

30. Martin PR, Singleton CK, Hiller-Sturmhofel S. The role of thiamine deficiency in alcoholic brain disease. *Alcohol Res Health* 2003; **27**(2): 134–42.

31. Matsumoto I. Proteomics approach in the study of the pathophysiology of alcohol-related brain damage. *Alcohol Alcohol* 2009; **44**(2): 171–6.

32. Alvarez I, Gonzalo LM, Llor J. Effects of chronic alcoholism on the amygdaloid complex. A study in human and rats. *Histol Histopathol* 1989; **4**(2): 183–92.

33. Harding AJ, Wong A, Svoboda M, Kril JJ, Halliday GM. Chronic alcohol consumption does not cause hippocampal neuron loss in humans. *Hippocampus* 1997; **7**(1): 78–87.

34. Korbo L. Glial cell loss in the hippocampus of alcoholics. *Alcohol Clin Exp Res* 1999; **23**(1): 164–8.

35. Bergman H, Borg S, Hindmarsh T, Idestrom CM, Mutzell S. Computed tomography of the brain, clinical examination and neuropsychological assessment of a random sample of men from the general population. *Acta Psychiatr Scand Suppl* 1980; **286**: 47–56.

36. Cala LA, Jones B, Wiley B, Mastaglia FL. A computerized axial tomography (C.A.T.) study of alcohol induced cerebral atrophy – in conjunction with other correlates. *Acta Psychiatr Scand Suppl* 1980; **286**: 31–40.

37. Carlen PL, Wilkinson DA. Alcoholic brain damage and reversible deficits. *Acta Psychiatr Scand Suppl* 1980; **286**: 103–18.

38. Ron MA. The alcoholic brain: CT scan and psychological findings. *Psychol Med Monogr Suppl* 1983; **3**: 1–33.

39. Hayakawa K, Kumagai H, Suzuki Y *et al*. MR imaging of chronic alcoholism. *Acta Radiol* 1992; **33**(3): 201–6.

40. Moore JW, Dunk AA, Crawford JR *et al*. Neuropsychological deficits and morphological MRI brain scan abnormalities in apparently healthy non-encephalopathic patients with cirrhosis. A controlled study. *J Hepatol* 1989; **9**(3): 319–25.

41. Schroth G, Naegele T, Klose U, Mann K, Petersen D. Reversible brain shrinkage in abstinent alcoholics, measured by MRI. *Neuroradiology* 1988; **30**(5): 385–9.

42. Zipursky RB, Lim KC, Pfefferbaum A. MRI study of brain changes with short-term abstinence from alcohol. *Alcohol Clin Exp Res* 1989; **13**(5): 664–6.

43. Pfefferbaum A, Sullivan EV, Rosenbloom MJ *et al*. Increase in brain cerebrospinal fluid volume is greater in older than in younger alcoholic patients: a replication study and CT/MRI comparison. *Psychiatry Res* 1993; **50**(4): 257–74.

44. Jernigan TL, Butters N, DiTraglia G *et al*. Reduced cerebral grey matter observed in alcoholics using magnetic resonance imaging. *Alcohol Clin Exp Res* 1991; **15**(3): 418–27.

45. Pfefferbaum A, Sullivan EV, Mathalon DH, Lim KO. Frontal lobe volume loss observed with magnetic resonance imaging in older chronic alcoholics. *Alcohol Clin Exp Res* 1997; **21**(3): 521–9.

46. Jacobson R. The contributions of sex and drinking history to the CT brain scan changes in alcoholics. *Psychol Med* 1986; **16**(3): 547–59.

47. Hommer D, Momenan R, Kaiser E, Rawlings R. Evidence for a gender-related effect of alcoholism on brain volumes. *Am J Psychiatry* 2001; **158**(2): 198–204.

48. Mann K, Ackermann K, Croissant B *et al*. Neuroimaging of gender differences in alcohol dependence: are women more vulnerable? *Alcohol Clin Exp Res* 2005; **29**(5): 896–901.

49. Pfefferbaum A, Rosenbloom M, Deshmukh A, Sullivan E. Sex differences in the effects of alcohol on brain structure. *Am J Psychiatry* 2001; **158**(2): 188–97.

50. Pfefferbaum A, Rosenbloom M, Serventi KL, Sullivan EV. Corpus callosum, pons, and cortical white matter in alcoholic women. *Alcohol Clin Exp Res* 2002; **26**(3): 400–6.

51. Rosenbloom M, Sullivan EV, Pfefferbaum A. Using magnetic resonance imaging and diffusion tensor imaging to assess brain damage in alcoholics. *Alcohol Res Health* 2003; **27**(2): 146–52.

52. Pfefferbaum A, Adalsteinsson E, Sullivan EV. Supratentorial profile of white matter microstructural integrity in recovering alcoholic men and women. *Biol Psychiatry* 2006; **59**(4): 364–72.

53. Harris GJ, Jaffin SK, Hodge SM *et al*. Frontal white matter and cingulum diffusion tensor imaging deficits in alcoholism. *Alcohol Clin Exp Res* 2008; **32**(6): 1001–13.

54. Pfefferbaum A, Rosenbloom M, Rohlfing T, Sullivan EV. Degradation of association and projection white matter systems in alcoholism detected with quantitative fiber tracking. *Biol Psychiatry* 2009; **65**(8): 680–90.

55. Carlen PL, Wortzman G, Holgate RC, Wilkinson DA, Rankin JC. Reversible cerebral atrophy in recently abstinent chronic alcoholics measured by computed tomography scans. *Science* 1978; **200**(4345): 1076–8.

56. Muuronen A, Bergman H, Hindmarsh T, Telakivi T. Influence of improved drinking habits on brain atrophy and cognitive performance in alcoholic patients: a 5-year follow-up study. *Alcohol Clin Exp Res* 1989; **13**(1): 137–41.

57. Ron MA, Acker W, Shaw GK, Lishman WA. Computerized tomography of the brain in chronic alcoholism: a Survey and follow-up study. *Brain* 1982; **105** (Pt 3): 497–514.

58. Mann K, Mundle G, Strayle M, Wakat P. Neuroimaging in alcoholism: CT and MRI results and clinical correlates. *J Neural Transm Gen Sect* 1995; **99**(1-3): 145–55

59. Sullivan EV, Rosenbloom MJ, Lim KO, Pfefferbaum A. Longitudinal changes in cognition, gait, and balance in abstinent and relapsed alcoholic men: relationships to changes in brain structure. *Neuropsychology* 2000; **14**(2): 178–88.

60. Ende G, Welzel H, Walter S *et al*. Monitoring the effects of chronic alcohol consumption and abstinence on brain metabolism: a longitudinal proton magnetic resonance spectroscopy study. *Biol Psychiatry* 2005; **58**(12): 974–80.

61. Bartsch AJ, Homola G, Biller A *et al*. Manifestations of early brain recovery associated with abstinence from alcoholism. *Brain* 2007; **130**(Pt 1): 36–47.

62. Cardenas VA, Chao LL, Studholme C et al. Brain atrophy associated with baseline and longitudinal measures of cognition. *Neurobiol Aging* 2010, in press.

63. Wobrock T, Falkai P, Schneider-Axmann T et al. Effects of abstinence on brain morphology in alcoholism: a MRI study. *Eur Arch Psychiatry Clin Neurosci* 2009; **259**(3): 143–50.

64. Pfefferbaum A, Sullivan EV, Mathalon DH et al. Longitudinal changes in magnetic resonance imaging brain volumes in abstinent and relapsed alcoholics. *Alcohol Clin Exp Res* 1995; **19**(5): 1177–91.

65. Shear PK, Jernigan TL, Butters N. Volumetric magnetic resonance imaging quantification of longitudinal brain changes in abstinent alcoholics. *Alcohol Clin Exp Res* 1994; **18**(1): 172–6.

66. Pfefferbaum A, Sullivan EV, Rosenbloom MJ, Mathalon DH, Lim KO. A controlled study of cortical gray matter and ventricular changes in alcoholic men over a 5-year interval. *Arch Gen Psychiatry* 1998; **55**(10): 905–12.

67. Parsons OA. Neurocognitive deficits in alcoholics and social drinkers: a continuum? *Alcohol Clin Exp Res* 1998; **22**(4): 954–61.

68. Oscar-Berman M, Marinkovic K. Alcohol: effects on neurobehavioral functions and the brain. *Neuropsychol Rev* 2007; **17**(3): 239–57.

69. Mann K, Gunther A, Stetter F, Ackermann K. Rapid recovery from cognitive deficits in abstinent alcoholics: a controlled test-retest study. *Alcohol Alcohol* 1999; **34**(4): 567–74.

70. Lee K, Moller L, Hardt F, Haubek A, Jensen E. Alcohol-induced brain damage and liver damage in young males. *Lancet* 1979; **2**(8146): 759–61.

71. Wilkinson DA, Carlen PL. Relation of neuropsychological test performance in alcoholics to brain morphology measured by computed tomography. *Adv Exp Med Biol* 1980; **126**: 683–99.

72. Carlen PL, Wilkinson DA, Wortzman G et al. Cerebral atrophy and functional deficits in alcoholics without clinically apparent liver disease. *Neurology* 1981; **31**(4): 377–85.

73. Bendszus M, Weijers HG, Wiesbeck G et al. Sequential MR imaging and proton MR spectroscopy in patients who underwent recent detoxification for chronic alcoholism: correlation with clinical and neuropsychological data. *AJNR Am J Neuroradiol* 2001; **22**(10): 1926–32.

74. Chanraud S, Martelli C, Delain F et al. Brain morphometry and cognitive performance in detoxified alcohol-dependents with preserved psychosocial functioning. *Neuropsychopharmacology* 2007; **32**(2): 429–38.

75. Lishman WA. *Organic Psychiatry*, 3rd edn. Oxford: Blackwell, 1998.

76. Reid AG, Daglish MR, Kempton MJ et al. Reduced thalamic grey matter volume in opioid dependence is influenced by degree of alcohol use: a voxel-based morphometry study. *J Psychopharmacol* 2008; **22**(1): 7–10.

77. Bartlett E, Mikulis DJ. Chasing "Chasing the dragon" with MRI: leukoencephalopathy in drug abuse. *Br J Radiol* 2005; **78**: 997–1004.

78. Kondziella D, Danielsen ER, Arlien-Soeberg P. Fatal encephalopathy after an isolated overdose of cocaine. *J Neurol Neurosurg Psychiatry* 2007; **78**: 437–8.

79. Gottfried JA, Mayer SA, Shungu DC et al. Delayed posthypoxic demyelination. Association with arylsulfatase A deficiency and lactic acidosis on protein MR spectroscopy. *Neurology* 1997; **49**: 1400–4.

80. Tsai SY, Chen JD, Chao WY, Wang JD. Neurobehavioral effects of occupational exposure to low-level organic solvents among Taiwanese workers in paint factories. *Environ Res* 1997; **73**(1-2): 146–55

81. Daniell WE, Claypoole KH, Checkoway H et al. Neuropsychological function in retired workers with previous long-term occupational exposure to solvents. *Occup Environ Med* 1999; **56**(2): 93–105.

82. Albers JW, Wald JJ, Garabrant DH, Trask CL, Berent S. Neurologic evaluation of workers previously diagnosed with solvent-induced toxic encephalopathy. *J Occup Environ Med* 2000; **42**(4): 410–23.

83. Collignon R, Bruyer R, Rectem D, Indekeu P, Laterre EC. [Semiology of bismuth encephalopathy. Comparison with seven personal cases (author's transl.)]. *Acta Neurol Belg* 1979; **79**(2): 73–91.

84. Buge A, Supino-Viterbo V, Rancurel G, Pontes C. Epileptic phenomena in bismuth toxic encephalopathy. *J Neurol Neurosurg Psychiatry* 1981; **44**(1): 62–7.

61

Reversible Dementias

Michael Philpot

Mental Health of Older Adults, South London and Maudsley NHS Foundation Trust, Maudsley Hospital, London, UK

INTRODUCTION

The aim of this chapter is to review the causes of 'reversible' dementias, their prevalence, methods of investigation and response to treatment. Given the right circumstances, almost any illness can affect cognition, so the objective is to identify those treatable conditions that most commonly present in this way. The early literature on this subject included numerous case studies or series of 'dementia' that appeared to resolve completely following treatment of the associated physical or psychiatric condition. Undoubtedly many of the patients described were actually suffering from delirium or other organic brain syndromes[1]. Also, the concept of 'reversible' dementia appears at odds with the term 'dementia', denoting an insidiously progressive disorder[2]. This confusion extends to psychiatric disorders such as depression and schizophrenia that may present as 'pseudo-dementia'[3]. Lastly, many patients, indeed probably the majority, with 'real' dementias will have concomitant conditions that, while not being aetiologically related to the dementia, may reduce cognitive function.

AETIOLOGY

The timely investigation of patients presenting with symptoms of dementia is a keystone of many clinical protocols[4-6]. Diagnosis of 'probable' Alzheimer's disease is largely by exclusion of other causes of dementia – including those reckoned to be reversible. A list of what are considered the classic potentially reversible causes of dementia (PRD) is given in Table 61.1. Table 61.2 lists PRD that have been described in the past 10 years – usually in either single cases or small case series. The identification of the latter can depend crucially on how intensively a case is investigated. They include conditions sometimes grouped together as the 'rapidly progressive' dementias[7].

PREVALENCE

Despite the extensive lists in Tables 61.1 and 61.2, the frequency with which PRD occur in everyday clinical practice is an important factor in determining the rigour with which contributory physical disorders or other causes are pursued. The overall prevalence identified in case series or clinic surveys can vary depending on the setting (inpatient, outpatient or community), the medical specialty involved (geriatric psychiatry, geriatrics, neurology or neuropsychi-

atry) and the disease pattern of the country in which the study is carried out (e.g. neurological infections are more prevalent in developing countries). Early studies generally failed to provide follow-up data to confirm whether the identified PRD were actually reversible or not. Previous reviews[24,25] concluded that approximately 11–12% of patients presenting to a variety of specialist services with symptoms of dementia during the 1970s and 1980s had PRD. Philpot and Burns[24] found that the rate was 18% in patients under the age of 65 years but only 5% in those over 65, an observation that has been supported[26,27]. However, few of the early studies provided follow-up data to confirm recovery. Clarfield[28] has reviewed the literature for studies published between 1987 and 2000 and identified 39 that fulfilled meta-analysis criteria. He found that recent studies were more often community or outpatient based, but that only 9% of cases had PRD. These figures represented a fall in prevalence from a previous review examining studies published in the 1970s and early 1980s when 13% of dementias were potentially reversible[25].

Table 61.3 lists more recent studies of PRD since 2001. The frequency of each underlying cause is compared to Clarfield[28]. Mental disorders (chiefly depression) comprise the most prevalent category, with alcohol-related disorders also being more prominent than in previous reviews. Space-occupying lesions, endocrine/metabolic disease and drug toxicity appear less frequently.

INVESTIGATION PROTOCOLS

A number of organizations have published guidelines for routine investigations used in the assessment of dementia, and the recommendations of three such are listed in Table 61.4[4-6]. Chui and Zhang[39] examined the added value of using investigations routinely. After a thorough clinical assessment, blood tests and neuroimaging results changed management in only 13% and 15%, of cases respectively. Van Crevel et al.[40] found that the number of patients requiring investigation to find one case of PRD was approximately 100, and the financial saving on care costs was insignificant. Foster et al.[41], in a detailed examination of the cost-effectiveness of brain computed tomography, concluded that scans should only be performed routinely if symptom duration was less than one year, symptoms were rapidly progressive, presentation was atypical or the patient was under 65 years. However, the hard facts of health economics need to be balanced against the imperative to do one's best for the patient, so consensus protocols tend not to specify limiting investigations to particular age groups.

Principles and Practice of Geriatric Psychiatry, 3rd edn. Edited by Mohammed T. Abou-Saleh, Cornelius Katona and Anand Kumar

Table 61.1 Classification of potentially reversible dementias (after Lishman[2])

Reversible dementias	Common clinical examples
Degenerative	Normal pressure hydrocephalus, Wilson's disease
Space-occupying lesions	Cerebral tumour, subdural haematoma
Infection	Neurosyphilis, chronic meningitis and encephalitis, HIV-associated dementia
Collagen-vascular	Cerebral vasculitis systemic lupus erythematosus, sarcoidosis
Metabolic/endocrine	Liver disease, uraemia, remote effects of carcinoma, hypo- and hyperthyroidism, hypopituitarism, hypo- and hyperparathyroidism, hypoglycaemia, Cushing's disease, Addison's disease
Toxic	Primary alcoholic dementia, Wernicke-Korsakoff syndrome, chronic intoxication with sedative drugs, heavy metals
Anoxic	Chronic obstructive airways disease, sleep apnoea syndrome, chronic carbon monoxide poisoning, post-cardiac arrest, congestive cardiac failure
Nutritional	Anaemia, deficiencies of vitamin B12, folate, thiamine
Psychiatric	Depression, late-onset schizophrenia

Table 61.2 Recently reported reversible dementias

Reversible dementias	Common clinical examples
Autoimmune encephalopathies	Anti-NMDA receptor[8], anti-neuronal antibodies (limbic and extralimbic paraneoplastic syndromes)[7], potassium channel antibody-associated[9], non-vasculitic meningoencephalitis[10], Hashimoto's disease[11,12]
Space-occupying lesions	Dural arteriovenous fistulae[13]
Infection	Neurocysticercosis[14], cryptococcal meningitis[15], enteroviral meningo-encephalitis[16], Whipple's disease[17]
Collagen-vascular	Cerebral amyloid inflammatory vasculopathy[18], antiphospholipid syndrome[19], other CNS vasculitides (multiple causes)[7]
Metabolic/endocrine	Paget's disease[20], Cushing's syndrome[21]
Toxic	Steroids[22]
Anoxic	Spontaneous intracranial hypotension[23]

RESPONSE TO TREATMENT IN ORGANIC DISORDERS

A minority of studies identifying the prevalence of PRD actually include follow-up data reporting the response to treatment. Individual retrospective studies from the 1980s (e.g. Byrne[1]) found some improvement in two thirds of patients and complete recovery in 40%. However, Clarfield[25,28] suggested a much less optimistic outcome: 15% of PRD showed some response to treatment, 8% with full recovery, the remainder only partial recovery. Overall, some degree of recovery was shown in only 0.6% of patients with dementia[28]. In more recent studies listed in Table 61.3, treatment outcome was only reported in two studies. Takada et al.[33] found that 55% showed some degree of reversibility. Of the 10 patients with neurosyphilis, only one fully recovered: full recovery was also seen in a patient with normal pressure hydrocephalus (NPH) and partial recovery in a patient with a subdural haematoma (SDH). All the potentially reversible cases identified in Sheng et al.[38] showed some degree of recovery. However, 63% had functional psychiatric disorders, mainly depression. Clearly, the lack of reversibility revealed by these studies suggests that most of the potentially reversible disorders are actually *concomitant* with real dementia[42]. Treatment of concomitant disorders may have some clinical benefits, improving overall function while not eliminating the underlying cause. Some problems may also be secondary to the dementia itself, e.g. anaemia as a result of malnutrition. The response rates of a selection of disorders are now discussed in more detail.

Vitamin B12 Deficiency

Strachan and Henderson[43] first described dementia in association with B12 deficiency. Treatment with cobalamin brought about complete remission of cognitive impairment. However, there have been mixed results in prospective studies of replacement in patients with dementia and B12 deficiency, some showing improvement[44,45] and others showing little benefit[46–48]. Patients with mild cognitive impairment and B12 deficiency fare better[44,47,48].

Thyroid Dysfunction

The propensity for thyroid deficiency to lead to memory impairment and psychomotor slowing has been known since the nineteenth century[49] and hypo- and hyperthyroidism are among the traditionally accepted causes of PRD[2]. However, a clear reversibility of cognitive impairment sufficient to be considered dementia is rare[28]. Hypo- and hyperthyroidism are found in approximately 0.4% and 0.3% of older people, but subclinical thyroid dysfunction is found five or six times more often[50,51]. There is a complex relationship between this condition and incident dementia. An increased risk of dementia has been associated with subclinical hyperthyroidism[52,53] and hypothyroidism[54], while a U-shaped relationship with thyroid function has also been demonstrated[55]. However, the association found between high free T4, T3 levels and atrophy in the hippocampus and amygdala in otherwise healthy elderly people might suggest a preclinical phase of cognitive impairment[56].

Table 61.3 Outcome of investigation in patients presenting with clinical symptoms of dementia: studies published since 2001

Source	Total with dementia	Cases of potentially reversible dementia, N (%)									
		Total	NPH	Brain tumour	SDH	CNS infection	Endocrine/ metabolic	Alcohol	Mental disorder	Drugs	Misc
Van Hout et al.[29]	96	5	2	1				2		1	2
Luce et al.[30]	132	38[a]					2	5	28		
Hejl et al.[31]	432	18	15	3							
Vale and Miranda[32]	186	32	10			4	2	16	2		0
Takada et al.[33]	275	22	5		1	9		6			1
Stratford et al.[34]	369	51	NR	NR	NR	NR	NR	18	19	1	18
Knopman et al.[35]	560	32		7		1		7	11		6
Shelley and Al Khabouri[36]	100	10	2			1		1			6
Van der Flier et al.[37]	358	94	1	NR	NR	NR	NR		58		35
Sheng et al.[38]	385	24					2		15		7
Total	**2893 (100)**	**326 (11.2)**	**35 (1.2)**	**11 (0.4)**	**1 (0.04)**	**15 (0.5)**	**4 (0.1)**	**55 (1.9)**	**133 (4.6)**	**2 (0.07)**	**75 (2.6)**
Data from Clarfield[28]: 39 studies published between 1987 and 2000	3940 (100)	355 (9)	57 (1.4)	53 (1.3)	17 (0.4)	15 (0.4)	64 (1.6)	36 (0.9)	52 (1.3)	4 (0.1)	57 (1.4)

Source: Adapted from Clarfield[28].
NPH, normal pressure hydrocephalus; SDH, subdural haematoma; Misc, assorted conditions or studies not listing systemic physical disorders; NR, not reported.
[a]Includes patients with mild cognitive impairment.

Table 61.4   Physical investigations for the assessment of patients presenting with cognitive impairment

Routine investigations (all cases)	Special investigations (atypical cases or clinically indicated)
Full blood count[a,b,c]	Electroencephalogram[b]
Electrolytes[a,b,c]	Chest X-ray[b]
Renal function[a,b,c]	Electrocardiogram[b]
Liver function[b,c]	Lumber puncture[a,b]
Thyroid function[a,b,c]	Brain biopsy[b]
Calcium[b,c]	SPECT or PET[b]
Vitamin B12[a,b,c]	Syphilis serology[a,b]
Folate[a,b,c,d]	
Glucose[a,b,c]	
Brain computed tomography or magnetic resonance imaging[a,b,c]	
Urine for culture[a,b]	

[a] American Academy of Neurology[4].
[b] NICE (UK) guidance for dementia[5].
[c] Third Canadian Consensus Conference[6].
[d] Test is optional in Canada.

Brain Lesions

NPH is the single most common organic cause of PRD[28]. Hakim and Adams[57] described two patients who presented with dementia, gait disturbance and incontinence in association with ventricular enlargement and normal cerebrospinal fluid (CSF) pressure. Most cases are idiopathic but NPH can follow meningitis, bleed or head injury. The treatment is shunt insertion diverting CSF from the lateral ventricles to the peritoneum. Good outcome in terms of an improvement in cognition can vary from 20% to 80%[58-61]. Features associated with a good prognosis include younger age, shorter duration of symptoms, and whether temporary improvement occurs as a result of pre-operative CSF drainage[59-61].

SDH occur usually as a result of head injuries or anticoagulant drugs but can occur spontaneously. A chronic SDH may present solely with progressive cognitive impairment but this is usually accompanied by fluctuating confusion, drowsiness and headache. Bleeding occurs from the veins between the dura and arachnoid mater and the resulting fluid collection may exert localizing neurological signs[62]. Clots are removed via burr holes and a good prognosis is found in more than half the cases thought to have dementia preoperatively[63,64]. Again, good prognosis is associated with younger age (under 74), milder cognitive impairment and less handicap[64].

The increasing prevalence and incidence of malignant brain tumours with age is well documented in surveillance studies[65-67] and may relate to increasing population in the older age groups[65,67]. Late-onset epilepsy, focal neurological signs or evidence of raised intracranial pressure raise the suspicion of a space-occupying lesion. Elderly patients may be less likely than younger ones to present with headache or seizures, but more likely to present with confusion, aphasia or memory impairment[66]. Dementia is usually associated with slowly growing lesions that can develop without localizing signs, but may be accompanied by mood disorder, personality change, apathy or fatigue[2]. In older patients, slowly growing meningiomas may indeed be largely asymptomatic and 'watchful waiting' with repeat neuroimaging annually may be the best approach[68].

With regard to malignant tumours, although the outcome of surgical and/or radiotherapy treatment can be less favourable than in young patients[66,69], aggressive approach to treatment is still advocated[69].

DEPRESSION AND DEMENTIA

The syndromes of depression and dementia interact in a complex way. Depression may be a risk factor for Alzheimer's disease[70], and is commonly found in association with established dementia[71]. Depression can be a reaction to the early symptoms of dementia[72]. Depression in late life is associated with impaired cognition[73,74]. Impairment is in multiple areas – attention, working memory, visual and verbal memory, and executive function[73] – but slowed information processing might underline all difficulties[74]. For the most part, cognitive dysfunction is relatively mild but in some patients it can be extreme. Although, in practice, it can be difficult distinguishing between these disorders, depressive 'pseudo-dementia' has traditionally been viewed as a treatable condition with a distinct clinical history and symptoms that distinguish it from 'true' dementia[3]. Patients have a relatively short clinical course and a clearly defined onset. They complain of a poor memory, poor concentration or difficulty thinking, emphasize their disability, and communicate distress and low mood. They may frequently answer 'don't know' to direct questions and be slow to respond. There is often a past or family history of depression. For the individual patient, physical investigations including brain imaging[75] and neurophysiological studies[76] are of little use in differentiating between pseudo-dementia and 'real' dementia.

Traditional teaching holds that treatment of the underlying depression with antidepressant therapy results in complete recovery in depressive pseudo-dementia[1-3]. However, some degree of cognitive impairment may persist after treatment[73,77], and longitudinal studies tend to support the view that severe cognitive impairment in depression is a harbinger of true dementia in between 25% and 50% of patients[78-80]. Indeed, elderly patients who develop cognitive impairment during depression are at four to five times increased risk of developing dementia within five years[79,80].

CONCLUSION

Reversible dementias are relatively uncommon but their identification is important from the individual patient's perspective. As investigative techniques improve and new treatments are developed, the range of potentially reversible conditions grows. However, the literature encompasses a polarization of views. Depression aside, the evidence-based view would suggest that given the rarity and poor response to treatment, extensive investigation is unnecessary. The more traditional, patient-centred view, perhaps coloured by the early literature and the fear of litigation, would demand the continued use of routine investigations in the hope of excluding treatable aetiologies, however rare. The introduction of care protocols reached by consensus should guide clinicians and ensure patients have equity of access to appropriate assessment.

REFERENCES

1. Byrne EJ. Reversible dementias. *Int J Geriatr Psychiatry* 1987; **2**: 72–81.
2. Lishman WA. *Organic Psychiatry*, 3rd edn. Oxford: Blackwell, 1998.

3. Wells CE. Pseudodementia. *Am J Psychiatry* 1979; **37**: 336–51.

4. Knopman DS, DeKosky ST, Cummings JL *et al*. Practice parameter: diagnosis of dementia (an evidence-based review). *Neurology* 2001; **56**: 1143–53.

5. National Institute for Health and Clinical Excellence, and Social Care Institute for Excellence. *Dementia: Supporting People with Dementia and Their Carers in Health and Social Care*, NICE clinical guideline 42. London: NICE/SCIE, 2006.

6. Feldman HH, Jacova C, Robillard A *et al*. Diagnosis and treatment of dementia: 2. Diagnosis. *CMAJ* 2008; **178**: 825–36.

7. Geschwind MD, Shu H, Haman A, Sejvar JJ, Miller BL. Rapidly progressive dementia. *Ann Neurol* 2008; **64**: 97–108.

8. Dalmau J, Gleichman AJ, Hughes EG *et al*. Anti-NMDA receptor encephalitis: case series and analysis of the effects of antibodies. *Lancet Neurol* 2008; **7**: 1091–8.

9. McKeon A, Marnane M, O'Connell M *et al*. Potassium channel antibody associated encephalopathy presenting with a frontotemporal dementia like syndrome. *Arch Neurol* 2007; **64**: 1528–30.

10. Lyons MK, Caselli RJ, Parisi JE. Nonvasculitic autoimmune inflammatory meningo-encephalitis as a cause of potentially reversible dementia: report of 4 cases. *J Neurosurg* 2008; **108**: 1024–7.

11. Nieuwenhuis L, Santens P, Vanwalleghem P, Boon P. Subacute Hashimoto's encephalopathy, treated with plasmapheresis. *Acta Neurol Belg* 2004; **104**: 80–83.

12. Spiegel J, Hellwig D, Becker G, Muller M. Progressive dementia caused by Hashimoto's encephalopathy – report of two cases. *Eur J Neurol* 2004; **11**: 711–13.

13. Waragai M, Takeuchi H, Fukushima T, Haisa T, Yonemitsu T. MRI and SPECT studies of dural arteriovenous fistulas presenting as pure progressive dementia with leukoencephalopathy: a cause of treatable dementia. *Eur J Neurol* 2006; **13**: 754–9.

14. Ramirez-Bermudez J, Higuera J, Sosa AL *et al*. Is dementia reversible in patients with neurocysticercosis? *J Neurol Neurosurg Psychiatry* 2005; **76**: 1164–6.

15. Ala TA, Doss RC, Sullivan CJ. Reversible dementia: a case of crytococcal meningitis masquerading as Alzheimer's disease. *J Alzheimer's Dis* 2004; **6**: 503–8.

16. Valcour V, Haman A, Cornes S *et al*. A case of enteroviral meningo-encephalitis presenting as rapidly progressive dementia. *Nat Clin Pract Neurol* 2008; **4**: 399–403.

17. Benito-Leon J, Sedano LF, Louis ED. Isolated central nervous system Whipple's disease causing reversible frontotemporal-like dementia. *Clin Neurol Neurosurg* 2008; **110**: 747–9.

18. Harkness KA, Coles A, Pohl U *et al*. Rapidly reversible dementia in cerebral amyloid inflammatory vasculopathy. *Eur J Neurol* 2004; **11**: 59–62.

19. Gomez-Puerta JA, Cervera R, Calvoi LM *et al*. Dementia associated with the antiphospholipid syndrome: clinical and radiological characteristics of 30 patients. *Rheumatology (Oxford)* 2005; **44**: 95–9.

20. Chan YP, Shui KK, Lewis RR, Kinirons MT. Reversible dementia in Paget's disease. *J R Soc Med* 2000; **93**: 595–6.

21. Guldiken S, Guldiken B. Subclinical Cushing's syndrome is a potential cause of metabolic dementia and rapidly progressive Alzheimer-type dementia. *Med Hypotheses* 2009; **71**: 703–5.

22. Sacks O, Shulman M. Steroid dementia: an overlooked diagnosis? *Neurology* 2005; **64**: 707–9.

23. Hong M, Shah GV, Adams KM, Turner RS, Foster NL. Spontaneous intracranial hypotension causing reversible frontotemporal dementia. *Neurology* 2002; **58**: 1285–7.

24. Philpot MP, Burns A. Reversible dementias. In Katona CLE (ed.), *Dementia Disorders: Advances and Prospects*. Chapman and Hall, London, 1989, 142–59.

25. Clarfield AM. The reversible dementias: do they reverse? *Ann Intern Med* 1988; **109**: 476–86.

26. Farina E, Pornati S, Mariani C. Observations on dementia with possibly reversible symptoms. *Aging (Milano)* 1999; **11**: 323–8.

27. Hejl A, Hogh P, Waldemar G. Potentially reversible conditions in 1000 consecutive memory clinic patients. *J Neurol Neurosurg Psychiatry* 2002; **73**: 390–94.

28. Clarfield AM. The decreasing prevalence of reversible dementias: an updated meta-analysis. *Arch Intern Med* 2003; **163**: 2219–29.

29. Van Hout H, Teunisse S, Derix M *et al*. CAMDEX, can it be more efficient? Observational study on the contribution of four screening measures to the diagnosis of dementia by a memory clinic team. *Int J Geriatr Psychiatry* 2001; **16**: 64–9.

30. Luce A, McKeith I, Swann A, Daniel S, O'Brien J. How do memory clinics compare with traditional old age psychiatry services? *Int J Geriatr Psychiatry* 2001; **16**: 837–45.

31. Hejl A, Hogh P, Waldemar P. Potentially reversible conditions in 1000 consecutive memory clinic patients. *J Neurol Neurosurg Psychiatry* 2002; **73**: 390–94.

32. Vale FA, Miranda SJ. Clinical and demographic features of patients with dementia attended in a tertiary outpatient clinic. *Arq Neuropsiquiatr* 2002; **60**: 548–52.

33. Takada LT, Caramelli P, Radanovic M *et al*. Prevalence of potentially reversible dementias in a dementia outpatient clinic of a tertiary university-affiliated hospital in Brazil. *Arq Neuropsiquiatr* 2003; **61**: 925–9.

34. Stratford JA, Logiudice D, Flicker L *et al*. A memory clinic at a geriatric hospital: a report on 577 patients assessed with CAMDEX over 9 years. *Aus N Z J Psychiatry* 2003; **37**: 319–26.

35. Knopman DS, Petersen RC, Cha RH, Edland SD, Rocca WA. Incidence and causes of nondegenerative nonvascular dementia: a population-based study. *Arch Neurol* 2006; **63**: 218–21.

36. Shelley BP, Al Khabouri J. The spectrum of dementia: frequency, causes and clinical profile. A national referral hospital-based study in Oman. *Dement Geriatr Cogn Disord* 2007; **24**: 280–87.

37. Van der Flier WM, Pijenburg YAL, Schoonenboom SNM *et al*. Distribution of APOE genotypes in a memory clinic cohort. *Dement Geriatr Cogn Disord* 2008; **25**: 433–8.

38. Sheng B, Law CB, Yeung KM. Characteristics and diagnostic profile of patients seeking dementia care in a memory clinic in Hong Kong. *Int Psychogeriatr* 2009; **21**: 392–400.

39. Chui H, Zhang Q. Evaluation of dementia: a systematic study of the usefulness of the American Academy of Neurology's Practice Parameters. *Neurology* 1997; **49**: 925–35.

40. van Crevel H, van Gool WA, Walstra GJM. Early diagnosis of dementia: which tests are indicated? What are their costs? *J Neurol* 1999; **246**: 73–8.

41. Foster GR, Scott DA, Payne S. The use of CT scanning in dementia. *Int J Technol Assess Health Care* 1999; **15**: 406–23.

42. Hogh P, Waldemar G, Knudsen GM *et al*. A multidisciplinary memory clinic in a neurological setting: diagnostic evaluation of 400 consecutive patients. *Eur J Neurol* 1999; **6**: 279–88.

43. Strachan RW, Henderson JG. Psychiatry syndromes due to avitaminosis B12 with normal blood and marrow. *Q J Med* 1965; **34**: 303–17.

44. Teunisse S, Bollen AE, van Gool WA, Walstra GJ. Dementia and subnormal levels of vitamin B12: effects of replacement therapy on dementia. *J Neurol* 1996; **243**: 522–9.

45. Eastley R, Wilcock GK, Bucks RS. Vitamin B12 deficiency in dementia and cognitive impairment: the effects of treatment on neuropsychological function. *Int J Geriatr Psychiatry* 2000; **15**: 226–33.

46. Hin H, Clarke R, Sherliker P *et al*. Clinical relevance of low serum vitamin B12 concentrations in older people: the Banbury B12 study. *Age Ageing* 2006; **35**: 416–22.

47. Aaron S, Kumar S, Vijayan J *et al*. Clinical and laboratory features and responses to treatment in patients presenting with vitamin B12 deficiency-related neurological syndromes. *Neurol India* 2005; **53**: 55–8.

48. Osimini A, Berger A, Friedman J, Porat-Katz BS, Abaranel JM. Neuropsychology of vitamin B12 deficiency in elderly dementia patients and control subjects. *J Geriatr Psychiatry Neurol* 2005; **18**: 33–8.

49. Olivaris BF, Roder E. Reversible psychosis and dementia in myxoedema. *Acta Psychiatr Scand* 1970; **46**: 1–13.

50. Wilson S, Parle JV, Roberts LM *et al*. Prevalence of subclinical thyroid dysfunction and its relation to socioeconomic deprivation in the elderly: a community-based cross-sectional survey. *J Clin Endocrinol Metab* 2006; **91**: 4809–16.

51. Hollowell JG, Staeling NW, Flanders WD *et al*. Serum TSH, T(4), and thyroid antibodies in the United States population (1988 to 1994): National Health and Nutrition Examination Survey (NHANES III). *J Clin Endocrinol Metab* 2002; **87**: 489–99.

52. Kalmijn S, Mehta KM, Pols HA *et al*. Subclinical hyperthyroidism and the risk of dementia. The Rotterdam study. *Clin Endocrinol (Oxf)* 2000; **53**: 733–7.

53. Hogervorst E, Huppert F, Matthews FE, Brayne C. Thyroid function and cognitive decline in the MRC Cognitive Function and Ageing Study. *Psychoneuroendocrinology* 2008; **33**: 1013–22.

54. Volpato S, Guralnik JM, Fried LP *et al*. Serum thyroxine level and cognitive decline in euthyroid older women. *Neurology* 2002; **58**: 1055–61.

55. Tan ZS, Beiser A, Vasan RS *et al*. Thyroid function and the risk of Alzheimer's disease: the Framingham Study. *Arch Intern Med* 2008; **168**: 1514–20.

56. De Jong FJ, den Heijer T, Visser TJ *et al*. Thyroid hormones, dementia, and atrophy of the medial temporal lobe. *J Clin Endocrinol Metab* 2006; **91**: 2569–73.

57. Hakim S, Adams RD. The special clinical problems of symptomatic hydrocephalus with normal cerebral spinal fluid pressure. *J Neurol Neurosurg Psychiatry* 1965; **2**: 307–27.

58. Aygok G, Marmarou A, Young HF. Three-year outcome of shunted idiopathic NPH patients. *Acta Neurochir Suppl* 2005; **95**: 241–5.

59. Chang S, Agarwal S, Williams MA, Rigamonti D, Hillis AE. Demographic factors influence cognitive recovery after shunt for normal-pressure hydrocephalus. *Neurologist* 2006; **12**: 39–42.

60. Chaudhry P, Kharkar S, Heidler-Gary J *et al*. Characteristics and reversibility of dementia in normal pressure hydrocephalus. *Behav Neurol* 2007; **18**: 149–58.

61. Kahlon B, Sjunnesson J, Rehncrona S. Long-term outcome in patients with suspected normal pressure hydrocephalus. *Neurosurgery* 2007; **60**: 327–32.

62. Schebesch KM, Woertgen C, Rothoerl RD, Ulrich OW, Brawanski AT. Cognitive decline as an important sign for an operable cause of dementia: chronic subdural haematoma. *Zentralbl Neurochir* 2008; **69**: 61–4.

63. Patrick D, Gates PC. Chronic subdural haematoma in the elderly. *Age Ageing* 1984; **13**: 367–9.

64. Ishikawa E, Yanaka, K, Sugimoto K, Ayuzawa S, Nose T. Reversible dementia in patients with chronic subdural haematomas. *J Neurosurg* 2002; **96**: 680–83.

65. Riggs JE. Rising primary malignant brain tumor mortality in the elderly. A manifestation of differential survival. *Arch Neurol* 1995; **52**: 571–6.

66. Lowry JK, Snyder JJ, Lowry PW. Brain tumors in the elderly: recent trends in a Minnesota cohort study. *Arch Neurol* 1998; **55**: 922–8.

67. Flowers A. Brain tumors in the older person. *Cancer Control* 2000; **7**: 523–38.

68. Olivero WC, Lister JR, Elwood PW. The natural history and growth rate of asymptomatic meningiomas: a review of 60 patients. *J Neurosurg* 1995; **83**: 222–4.

69. Myint PK, May HM, Baillie-Johnson H, Vowler SL. CT diagnosis and outcome of primary brain tumours in the elderly: a cohort study. *Gerontology* 2004; **50**: 235–41.

70. Devanand DP, Sano M, Tang MX *et al*. Depressed mood and the incidence of Alzheimer's disease in the elderly living in the community. *Arch Gen Psychiatry* 1996; **53**: 175–82.

71. Zubenko GS, Zubenko WN, McPherson S *et al*. A collaborative study of the emergence and clinical features of the major depressive syndrome of Alzheimer's disease. *Am J Psychiatry* 2003; **160**: 857–66.

72. Amieva H, Le Goff M, Millet X *et al*. Prodromal Alzheimer's disease: successive emergence of the clinical symptoms. *Ann Neurol* 2008; **64**: 492–8.

73. O'Brien JT, Lloyd A, McKeith I, Gholkar A, Ferrier N. A longitudinal study of hippocampal volume, cortisol levels, and cognition in older depressed subjects. *Am J Psychiatry* 2004; **161**: 2081–90.

74. Butters MA, Whyte EM, Nebes RD *et al*. The nature and determinants of neuropsychological functioning in late-life depression. *Arch Gen Psychiatry* 2004; **61**: 587–95.

75. Schweitzer I, Tuckwell V, Ames D, O'Brien J. Structural neuroimaging studies in late-life depression: a review. *World J Biol Psychiatry* 2001; **2**: 83–8.

76. Philpot M. The neurophysiology of dementia. In O'Brien J, Ames D, Burns A (eds), *Dementia*, 3rd edn. Arnold, London, 2005, 179–92.

77. Bhalla RK, Butters MA, Becker JT *et al*. Patterns of mild cognitive impairment after treatment of depression in the elderly. *Am J Geriatr Psychiatry* 2009; **17**: 308–16.

78. Copeland JRM, Davidson IA, Dewey ME *et al*. Alzheimer's disease, other dementias, depression and pseudodementia: prevalence, incidence and three-year outcome in Liverpool. *Brit J Psychiatry* 1992; **161**: 230–39.

79. Alexopoulos GS, Meyers BS, Young RC, Mattis S, Kakuma T. The course of geriatric depression with 'reversible dementia': a controlled study. *Am J Psychiatry* 1993; **150**: 1693–9.

80. Saez-Fonseca JA, Lee L, Walker Z. Long-term outcome of depressive pseudodementia in the elderly. *J Affect Disord* 2007; **101**: 123–9.

62

Cognitive Domains Affected by Conditions of Ageing and the Role of Neuropsychological Testing

Heather R. Romero, Scott M. Hayes and Kathleen A. Welsh-Bohmer

Joseph and Kathleen Bryan Alzheimer's Disease Research Center, Department of Psychiatry (Div Medical Psychiatry), Department of Medicine (Div Neurology), Center of Cognitive Neurosciences, Department of Psychology, Duke University, Durham, NC, USA

INTRODUCTION

Memory loss and dementia are nearly universal concerns in the ageing sector of our population[1]. In practice, differentiating the normal age changes from those of early Alzheimer's disease can be daunting. Advances in clinical diagnostics and laboratory imaging methodologies facilitate this process[2]; however, there remains no definitive diagnostic biological test for Alzheimer's disease or for other related neurodegenerative conditions. Ultimately, the diagnosis of a cognitive disorder rests on an informed clinical examination. A thorough neurobehavioural examination and more detailed neuropsychological assessment, when indicated, allow the clinician to determine the integrity of various mental processes. Using this information, diagnostic inferences can be made regarding the presence or absence of brain disease and the potential confounding influences of depression, anxiety and other medical factors. The purpose of this chapter is to provide an overview of the cognitive domains assessed by a standard neuropsychological evaluation with focused consideration of the domains specifically affected by normal brain ageing, mild cognitive impairment, Alzheimer's disease and geriatric depression.

PRINCIPAL COGNITIVE DOMAINS IN THE GERIATRIC EVALUATION

When patients present with memory or other cognitive complaints, objective verification of the nature and extent of these problems and the determination of their functional impact are goals of the neuropsychological evaluation. To ascertain this, the evaluation will assess eight major areas of cognitive function along with aspects of mood and personality. The basic areas assessed or 'cognitive domains' include: (i) general orientation and alertness, (ii) attention/concentration, (iii) intellect, (iv) memory, (v) language, (vi) executive functions, (vii) visuoperception/spatial judgement, and (viii) sensorimotor control. A brief discussion of each of these domains and the tests commonly used to measure each are described in the sections that follow. More detailed discussion of the range of instruments available to clinicians can be found in other sources[3].

General Orientation

Orientation is a particularly important function that can be disrupted by a number of medical (e.g. delirium), psychiatric (e.g. depression) and neurological disorders[4]. In assessing general personal awareness, the neuropsychologist will establish the patient's ability to orient to time (e.g. year, date, time of day), place (e.g. current location), personal information (e.g. name, age) and situation (e.g. why they are having a doctor's appointment). Commonly, the examining clinician may use mental status tests in which orientation screening is included, such as the Mini-Mental State Examination (MMSE)[5] or more detailed batteries, such as the Mattis Dementia Rating Scale[6] and the comprehensive memory battery of the Wechsler Memory Scale[7]. Targeted, well-validated measures of orientation, such as the Temporal Orientation Test (TOT)[8], are often selected and preferred by neuropsychologists over mental status screening tests, in order to streamline the evaluation and allow comprehensive evaluation of domains only cursorily measured in a screening metric.

Attentional Functions

The components of attention tapped within the neuropsychological examination include visual and auditory: (i) simple attention span, (ii) selective attention, (iii) vigilance or sustained attention, (iv) divided attention and (v) alternating attention[9]. There are a number of well-validated tests from which to choose when assessing attention and concentration, some of which are now computerized.

Simple attention span, the number of units held in immediate memory, is commonly assessed by tests such as the Digit Span subtest from the Wechsler Adult Intelligence Scale III (WAIS-III)[10] or the Spatial Span test of the Wechsler Memory Scale III[7]. *Selective attention* requires the ability to respond to relevant stimuli while simultaneously inhibiting response to irrelevant, distracting stimuli, such as in speeded target identification tasks (e.g. Symbol Search of the WAIS-III) or the Ruff 2 and 7 Selective Attention Test[10,11]). *Vigilance* requires that stimuli be attended to over a period of time, commonly assessed by computerized continuous performance tests (CPTs), such

Principles and Practice of Geriatric Psychiatry, 3rd edn. Edited by Mohammed T. Abou-Saleh, Cornelius Katona and Anand Kumar

as the Test of Variables of Attention (T.O.V.A.)[12]. *Divided attention* requires response to multiple competing tasks that occur simultaneously, such as tasks involving the simultaneous performance of both verbal repetition and visual search tasks. *Alternating attention* requires an individual to shift between tasks, such as the Trails B task, which requires switching between number and letters. It should be noted that tests of attention are easily influenced by a number of factors.

Failure on any single attentional test, or any neuropsychological test for that matter, can occur for a myriad of reasons. Consequently, it is important to consider confounds (e.g. sensory or motor limitations) and factors that may modify performance (e.g. educational experience) before drawing conclusions regarding impairments. Typically a neuropsychologist will look for consistency of performance across at least two tests measuring the same cognitive function before drawing an inference of compromised function.

Intelligence

Intelligence is a multifaceted construct that examines capacities of reasoning, problem solving, creative thought and abstraction, measured both verbally and non-verbally. Significant impairments in this domain result in compromised function, a defining feature of dementia. The tests most commonly used for the purpose of assessing intelligence are those of the Wechsler Adult Intelligence Scale IV (WAIS-IV)[13] (and its predecessors, WAIS-III and the WAIS-R), due to the well-established psychometric properties (reliability, validity and clinical utility) and extensive normative information for a broad age range (age 16–89). The WAIS tests also afford a comprehensive survey of a number of complex cognitive processes, including calculation, verbal and non-verbal abstraction, fund of knowledge, comprehension, reasoning and problem solving, spatial judgement, and sensorimotor integration. In situations where administration of an entire intelligence battery may be impractical, shorter versions are available (e.g. Wechsler Abbreviated Scale of Intelligence, WASI[14]). Alternatively, the neuropsychologist may sample specific areas of concern. Subtests of the WAIS, such as Block Design and Similarities, are sensitive indicators of brain

disease and are often selected to quickly assess non-verbal and verbal abstraction, respectively.

Learning and Memory

A considerable portion of the neuropsychological evaluation is generally devoted to the in-depth characterization of the different components involved in the learning and retention of new information as depicted in Figure 62.1. The pattern of deficit across these varying learning and memory processes can suggest one medical condition over another. In a standard neuropsychological evaluation of dementia there will be measures of *semantic memory*, the recall of well-learned facts and world knowledge, and *episodic memory*, the rich person-specific memory that records all new occurring daily events. Tests of semantic memory include category or semantic fluency tests, which require the patient to generate items to a category or group items that are related to one another along specific dimensions (living vs. non-living; instruments vs. tools). Other tests tap recall of world knowledge and are built into larger memory batteries[7].

Episodic memory and its component processes of encoding, storing and retrieving new information are determined using tests aimed at verbal and visual learning and memory functions. Acquisition of new information over multiple trials examines the efficacy of encoding whereas assessment of memory retention over short intervals (less than 3 minutes) and extended delay periods (30+ minutes) allow inferences regarding consolidation. Recognition memory allows determinations of the integrity of retrieval when cueing is provided.

Tests commonly used to assess memory are summarized in Table 62.1 and include comprehensive batteries such as the Wechsler Memory Scale (WMS-III)[7]. Targeted verbal learning and memory measures include the California Verbal Learning Test II[15], the Hopkins Verbal Learning Test-Revised[16] and the Rey Auditory Verbal Learning Test (Rey AVLT)[17]. Complementary visual memory tests include the Brief Visuospatial Memory Test-Revised[18] and the Benton Visual Retention Test[19]. An entire listing of all available memory tests is beyond the scope of this review. However, a summary of commonly used metrics in current practice is presented in Table 62.1, and the reader is referred to other comprehensive sources[3].

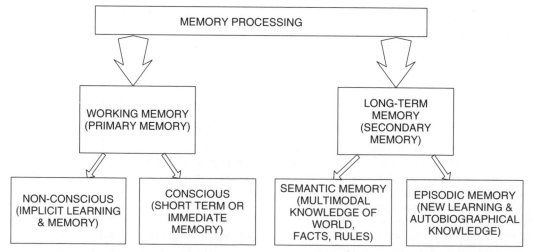

Figure 62.1 Neuropsychological conceptualization of learning and memory organization. Conscious aspects of working memory that require immediate, short-term processing of information and processes of semantic and episodic memory are typically assessed in the geriatric evaluation. Non-conscious learning and memory (e.g. motor memory, habits) are not typically assessed directly in the clinical neuropsychological examination

Table 62.1 Domains and common tests used to measure memory

Domain	Common tests
Orientation	Temporal Orientation Test[8]
	Mini-Mental State Examination[5]
	Mattis Dementia Rating Scale II[6]
	Wechsler Memory Scale III[7]
Attention	Wechsler Adult Intelligence Scale III[10]
	Cancellation Tests (Ruff 2&7 test)[11]
	Test of Variables of Attention (TOVA)[12]
Intellect and premorbid function	Wechsler Adult Intelligence Scale (WAIS)
	WAIS-R, WAIS-III, WAIS-IV[10,13,31]
	Wechsler Abbreviated Scale of Intelligence (WASI)[14]
	Wechsler Test of Adult Reading (WTAR)
Memory	Wechsler Memory Scale (WMS): WMS-R, WMS III, WMS-IV[7,13,69]
	Rey Auditory Verbal Learning Test[17]
	California Verbal Learning Test-II[15]
	Hopkins Verbal Learning Test – Revised[16]
	Rey Osterrith Complex Figure Test[30]
	Brief Visuospatial Memory Test[18]
	Benton Visual Retention Test – 5th Edition[70]
Language	Multilingual Aphasia Examination (MAE)[21]
	Boston Naming Test 2 (BNT2)[20]
	Boston Diagnostic Aphasia Examination – Third Ed (BDAE-3)[20]
Executive function	Wisconsin Card Sort Test (WCST)[71]
	Halstead Category Test[72]
	Stroop Color-Word Test[23]
	Trail Making Test A and B
	Tests of Verbal and Design Fluency[21,73]
	Delis-Kaplan Executive Function System (D-KEFS)[22]
Visuospatial/perceptual	Judgment of Line Orientation Test[28]
	Benton Facial Recogniton Test[28]
	Hooper Visual Organization Test[32]
	Clock Drawing Test[20]
Sensorimotor	Finger Tapping Test/Finger Oscillation
	Reitan Battery – Grip Strength
	Grooved Pegboard
	Purdue Pegboard
	Reitan Battery – Tactile Performance Test

Language

Verbal communication in day-to-day life relies on the individual's ability to express and comprehend oral and written speech. Formal neuropsychological evaluation focuses on spoken and written expressive language and on comprehension or 'receptive' language abilities. The Boston Diagnostic Aphasia Exam[20] and the Multilingual Aphasia Exam[21] are two comprehensive batteries of language function commonly used. Administered in their entirety, each aphasia battery takes approximately 30–60 minutes to administer. Unless language disorder is the referral issue, more focused brief testing of specific functions is frequently a preferred approach. Expressive language will be assessed with fluency measures, such as the Controlled Oral Word Association Task (generating words beginning with a specified letter, e.g. 'R'), and with tests of 'semantic fluency' in which participants provide examples to a given category (e.g. sports). The Boston Naming Test, a visual naming procedure, is used to formally assess word-finding difficulty. Impairments in aural and written comprehension, if not detected during the interview, are often assessed with subtests of the Wechsler Adult Intelligence Scale, including Comprehension, Vocabulary, Similarities or Information (see section on Intelligence).

Executive Functions

Executive functions, commonly referred to as higher order cognitive functions, comprise a number of supervisory processes that provide some control over many fundamental cognitive abilities and in the organization of general behaviour. The basic components of executive function include planning and organization abilities, monitoring and inhibition of responses, set shifting and cognitive flexibility, and verbal or non-verbal abstract reasoning. Attention and concentration processes, discussed previously, are also subsumed under the broad category of executive control; however, typically, these very specific functions are assessed separately.

There are a number of neuropsychological measures used to tap executive disorders. Comprehensive, all-in-one batteries of executive abilities include the Delis-Kaplan battery, which examines flexible behaviour, problem solving, judgement, personality and abstraction[22]. Targeted measures of decision making and flexible behaviour include sorting tasks, such as the Wisconsin Card Sorting Test (WCST), or alternating letter–number sequencing procedures, such as the Trail Making Test. Measures commonly used to examine behavioural control and response inhibition include tests such as the Stroop Color Word test[23]. Finally, assessment of abstract reasoning is commonly accomplished using subtests from the WAIS-III, such as the Similarities and Matrix Reasoning, or tests requiring the development of visual or verbal analogies, such as the Halstead Category Test.

Detection of executive deficits can be extraordinarily difficult, particularly in situations of subtle impairment and within the structured clinical setting, which is unlike the real world, where the patient must determine rules, contingencies and adjust behaviour accordingly. Consequently, in cases of suspected frontal lobe dementia, where executive disorders are prominent, and in neurodegenerative conditions (such as Alzheimer's disease and Parkinson's disease), where executive dysfunction emerges over the course of disease, the combined use of neuropsychological performance-based measures of executive function and informant-based measures of daily function, can be enormously helpful in determining the presence of problems in this domain and can help guide management approaches. Computerized tests of decision making and planning, such as the Cambridge Neuropsychological Tests Automated Battery (CANTAB), can augment the diagnostic process[24]. Self-report and informant-report measures such as the Frontal System Behavioral Examination (FrSBe)[25] or the Behavioral Rating Inventory of Executive Function – Adult version (BRIEF-A)[26] are also useful for assessing personality change and patient insight.

Visuospatial Function

Neuropsychological assessment of visual–spatial function focuses on object perception, spatial appreciation, constructional praxis and complex visual integrative capacities[27]. Object perception is often determined through tests such as the Facial Recogniton Task[28], in which the patient is required to discriminate between faces presented from different views or under different lighting conditions. Spatial perception ability is determined via tests assessing judgement of angular relationships, locations of objects in space and detection of movement. Praxis will be assessed either through the copy of simple (e.g. CERAD battery[29]) and visually complicated geometric figures (e.g. Rey-Ostereith Complex Figure Test[30]) or via three-dimensional constructional tasks (e.g. block design[31]). Integrating visual information into a meaningful whole is often determined with tests such as the Hooper Visual Organization test, which require visual processing and conceptualization[32].

In clinical practice, visuo-spatial problems are often less obvious on screening evaluation than either memory or language disorders. Consequently, incorporation of simple visuo-spatial measures, such as the Clock Drawing test[20], to the neurobehaviour examination can augment the detection and tracking of these disorders and can improve the sensitivity of the Alzheimer's disease diagnosis[33]. The information from a detailed neuropsychological evaluation of visuo-spatial function may be very useful for arriving at recommendations concerning daily activities, such as driving[34].

Sensorimotor Function

The neuropsychological examination of motor function will begin with the enumeration of any obvious motor signs, such as evident hemiplegia, tremor, dyskinesia or chorea. Tests for subtle problems in fine motor control are then typically administered and can be highly instructive in pointing to potential lateralized central nervous system deficits[35]. A number of standardized tests of manual strength and speed are available for quantifying and interpreting sensorimotor functions (Table 62.1). Typically, function with both the dominant and non-dominant hands is assessed using any of a number of metrics, permitting an evaluation of hand grip strength, rapid finger movement or fine motor dexterity (e.g. manipulation of small objects). Easy to administer, the measures are a sensitive indicator of general cognitive integrity and lateralized deficits in the nervous system, and can be useful in tracking disease progression and medication effects, particularly those treatments directly effecting extrapyramidal motor function[36].

Mood and Personality

The assessment of mood and personality begins with a psychological interview, allowing the neuropsychologist to assess the range of symptoms, level of functional impairment and relationship of the problems to the onset of cognitive dysfunction. This interview will then be augmented by objective metrics to determine changes from a pre-existing level and longstanding traits. Patient self-report measures of mood state include the Beck Depression Inventory II (BDI-II) or the Geriatric Depression Scale[37,38]. More detailed measures, such as the Minnesota Multiphasic Personality Inventory 2 (MMPI-2), survey broad psychiatric symptoms and are used in situations where psychiatric or personality issues are considered primary to the complaint[39].

Informant report questionnaires are particularly helpful in dementia as patient insight into their own behavioural change may be impaired. The Neuropsychiatric Inventory (NPI) assesses eight different domains of behaviour affected in brain disease (depression, apathy, anxiety, disinhibition, hallucinations, paranoia, delusions, agitation) from an informed observer perspective[40]. Changes in personality can also be assessed by questionnaires such as the FrSBe, discussed previously, which is an inventory that has both self and informant report forms and focuses on areas such of apathy, disinhibition and executive dysfunction[25].

COGNITIVE PROFILES ASSOCIATED WITH COMMON CONDITIONS OF AGEING

With performance across various cognitive domains established, consideration of the impairment profile and its relationship to underlying neural systems and brain disease is required for diagnosis. In the next section we review the typical neuropsychological profiles of normal ageing, Alzheimer's disease, mild cognitive impairment and geriatric depression.

Normal Cognitive Ageing

The profile of cognitive change due to normal brain ageing can be fairly easily distinguished from impairments due to neurodegenerative conditions, such as Alzheimer's disease, particularly in individuals who are 85 years of age or younger[41]. The neuropsychological findings of ageing reveal a spectrum of modest decline within a number of cognitive domains (Figure 62.2)[42]. Selective losses occur on tests of psychomotor speed and sensorimotor functions. Other functions affected include memory retrieval, attentional capacity, executive function and working memory[43]. Semantic knowledge

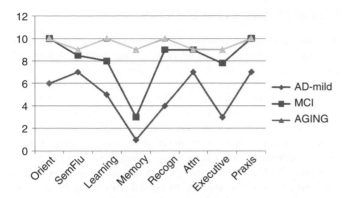

Figure 62.2 Neuropsychological performance in Alzheimer's disease, mild cognitive impairment and normal ageing. Presented are prototypical cognitive profiles of mild-staged Alzheimer's disease (AD), mild cognitive impairment (MCI) and normal ageing when considered relative to the performance of young adults on domains of Orientation, Expressive language (Semantic fluency), Learning, Delayed memory, Recognition memory, Praxis, and Executive function. Compared to young adults, normal older aged adults will demonstrate modest declines on tests of delayed free recall (Memory), word fluency (SemFlu), and higher order executive functions involving flexible behaviour (Executive). These rather modest changes in performance are exacerbated in MCI and AD. Delayed memory is particularly poor and there are also deficits in new learning and recognition memory. Verbal semantic fluency (SemFlu), simple attention, and praxis are also affected by the AD process, but become particularly problematic later in the course of the disease

and crystallized intelligence, which are acquired over the life span, are typically spared from age-related decline. Large cross-sectional comparisons across diverse cohorts aged 18–90 demonstrate monotonic declines across the broad domains noted, beginning as early as age 30; improved function is seen on tests of general knowledge and verbal comprehension[44]. These findings are robust and are confirmed in longitudinal, within-person studies[45]. In fact, within these within-subject comparisons there is evident test–retest improvement in test performance over time (i.e. practice effect)[46]. It has been suggested that the absence of the practice effect on re-evaluation may be an important indicator of an early neurocognitive condition[47], an observation important to consider on repeated evaluation with mental status screens, such as the MMSE.

Alzheimer's disease

In contrast to normal ageing, the cognitive disorder of Alzheimer's disease is characterized, early and throughout the disorder, by a profound impairment in memory consolidation (i.e. effectively storing new information for recall later), making it exceptionally difficult to learn and retain new information. On neuropsychological evaluation this problem is manifest by rapid forgetting of new information, measured with delayed recall procedures administered 10–30 minutes after the individual has already effectively demonstrated ability to successful encode new information on tests of immediate recall[48]. Characteristically, the memory deficit is facilitated very little by structural support, such as recognition cuing. Recall becomes vague, and patients will commit errors on recognition tests, showing a tendency to over-endorse items as recognized targets (i.e. false positive errors[49]). The failure to

benefit from cueing in Alzheimer's disease contrasts the memory disorders of normal brain ageing, depression, Lewy body dementia and vascular cognitive impairment. In each of the latter situations, retrieval cueing is beneficial and assists recall[50–52].

Although memory impairment is the prominent clinical sign of Alzheimer's disease, it is not the only deficit characterizing this neurodegenerative dementia. There are also highly characteristic problems in expressive language evident early in the illness. Later, problems in complex problem solving, executive control and abstraction are more clearly evident as well as disorders in visuo-spatial analysis and motor praxis (organization of skilled motor movements – such as writing, drawing, dressing, etc.). As each of these cognitive domains become more impaired, deficits in activities of daily function unfold[29].

On formal neuropsychological evaluation, the early language disorder of Alzheimer's disease is characterized by difficulties on tests of visual confrontation naming and on measures of semantic fluency, assessed by asking the patient to generate exemplars to a category (e.g. household tools, cars). Qualitatively, there may be a vacuous nature to speech output. With an absence of content words in their discourse, patients may resort to 'circumlocution' (i.e. description phrases) rather than easily accessing the precise word needed. Word substitutions and paraphasia errors also become common. Despite these difficulties in expression, comprehension of speech and repetition tend to be spared until later in the illness.

Praxis difficulties, impaired geographical orientation, and visuo-spatial errors may manifest as problems in spatial navigation, judgement of distances and difficulties locating and correctly identifying objects in the environment. On formal neuropsychological testing, these deficits are revealed using tests requiring visual integrative functions, judgement of spatial relationships between objects and form perception[53,54]. Atypical presentations of pronounced and relatively isolated visuo-spatial deficits are noted on occasion in Alzheimer's disease and are common in the Lewy body variant of Alzheimer's disease[53,55]. Similar presentations can also be seen in other progressive dementias, such as posterior cortical atrophy or 'Benson's Syndrome', multisystem atrophy, corticobasal dementia, forms of Creutzfeldt–Jakob disease[56]. In making distinctions between aetiologies, consideration must be given to other salient clinical features including presence or absence of motor signs, history of symptom expression and disease course[52].

Mild Cognitive Impairment

The concept of mild cognitive impairment (MCI) has emerged as a construct describing a transitional stage between normal ageing and the dementia syndrome common in Alzheimer's disease. The original MCI criteria specified: (i) a pronounced and rather isolated deficit in recent memory function, and (ii) preserved activities of daily living capabilities[57]. MCI appears to be a risk factor for later dementia, with a 12% rate of conversion per year compared with 1–2% in normal ageing. The operationalization of this construct has greatly facilitated early Alzheimer's disease identification; however, it has been criticized as too restrictive and not capturing the broad range of sub-syndromal symptoms leading ultimately to Alzheimer's disease and to other closely aligned dementias. In addition, the construct has been found in many settings to be diagnostically unstable. Many individuals characterized as MCI in community settings and epidemiological surveys have been reported to revert back to normal function at later observation points, therefore, calling into question the validity of the diagnosis as a prodrome to neurodegenerative dementia[58].

Revised criteria now in use recognize that mild cognitive impairments may be a prelude to a number of different types of dementias, not only Alzheimer's disease[59]. The new criteria have been broadened to include four subcategories of subsyndromal states, each of which share the core criteria of: (i) cognitive complaint, (ii) objective evidence of cognitive deficit beyond expectation for age (variably defined as either -1.0 SD or -1.5 SD below age, education mean), and (iii) activities of daily living are preserved and instrumental functions are either intact or are minimally impaired. With the new criteria, MCI can be dichotomized into an 'amnesic' and 'non-amnesic form', which is further dichotomized into 'single domain' affected vs. 'multiple cognitive domains' impaired. The four resulting subcategories are: 'amnesic MCI', corresponding to the original criteria; 'amnesic- multiple domain MCI', a situation where memory involvement is prominent but another domain (such as executive function or language) is also impaired; 'non-amnesic single-domain MCI', which captures conditions such as an early pronounced visuo-spatial, executive or language-based disorders; and 'non-amnesic multiple domain MCI', which captures multiple deficit disorders in which memory is by and large spared.

The predictive utility of the new subcategories of MCI for Alzheimer's disease and other dementias has yet to be fully demonstrated[60]; however, initial information suggests that the amnesic forms of MCI are predictive of later Alzheimer's disease development[61]. Other non-amnesic forms may be more predictive of other forms of chronic, degenerative disorders, such as vascular dementia[62]. However, there is no universal information on the latter point, and some studies suggest that all categories are equally predictive of later dementia[63,64]. This topic is an evolving area of clinical research, which will be facilitated as the pathobiology of the various chronic diseases and their interactions with one another are better understood.

Geriatric Depression

The neuropsychological profile in geriatric depression reveals highly specific cognitive disturbances in general cognitive efficiency. The entire profile of performance may be suppressed or there can be deficits confined to tests of executive processes of attention, working memory and processing speed[65,66]. On detailed characterization, specific impairments are commonly detected in selective attention, sustained attention, organization, set shifting, initiation and response inhibition. Visuo-spatial deficits and deficient memory performance are also possible; however, unlike the disorder of Alzheimer's disease these impairments tend to result from executive and processing speed deficits, rather than being a problem in spatial ability or memory consolidation. Very poor acquisition of new information in the context of shifting attention leads to memory complaints and subsequent impairment on tests of delayed free recall. However, when memory tasks are more structured and less reliant on executive abilities, delayed recall improves in the depressed patient, sometimes to the normal level, underscoring the role of the initial processing deficits.

Treatment of depression can lead to some reversibility of cognitive deficits and improved function[67]. Persisting cognitive impairment following adequate treatment may be due to underlying neuropathology, which is contributing to both depression symptoms and cognitive deficits, such as cerebrovascular disease or neurodegenerative conditions[68]. Careful evaluation of mood is therefore essential both for differential diagnosis of memory disorder and also for optimizing patient outcomes.

SUMMARY AND CONCLUSIONS

By understanding the common profiles of neurocognitive dysfunction typical of the major disorders of ageing, such as Alzheimer's disease and geriatric depression, the examining physician is given valuable information that complements the more abbreviated mental status assessment. In enhancing the detection of dementia cases in everyday clinical practice, the application of targeted measures of episodic memory (recall after a delay) and executive function (flexible thought) can be quite useful while also providing adequate profile information for tracking the clinical progress of patients over time. To facilitate the recognition of subtle disorders such as MCI, the addition of a screen of functional ability may be necessary in order to establish the impact of a cognitive complaint on the patient's ability to carry out normal, routine activities of daily living. Although the current pharmacological treatments for Alzheimer's disease offer little hope in terms of disease reversal, early diagnosis allows the clinician to treat contributing conditions in an effort to optimize function and prevent excess disability. It also permits the anticipation of problems before they occur and allows inclusion of patients in care decisions, enhancing their sense of autonomy and self-determination in their illness.

REFERENCES

1. Harris Interactive. *Alzheimer's: What America Thinks*. Survey conducted by Harris Interactive, 2006. At www.metlife.org.
2. Dubois B, Feldman HH, Jacova C *et al*. Research criteria for the diagnosis of Alzheimer's disease: revising the NINCDS-ADRDA criteria. *Lancet Neurol* 2007; **6**: 734–46.
3. Strauss E, Sherman EMS, Spreen O. *A Compendium of Neuropsychological Tests: Administration, Norms, and Commentary*, 3rd edn. Oxford: Oxford University Press, 2006.
4. Levin HS, Benton AL. Temporal orientation in patients with brain disease. *Appl Neurophysiol* 1975; **38**: 56–60.
5. Folstein MF, Folstein SE, Mchugh PR. Mini-Mental State – practical method for grading cognitive state of patients for clinician. *J Psychiatr Res* 1975; **12**: 189–98.
6. Mattis S, Jurica PJ, Leitten CL. *Dementia Rating Scale-2 (DRS-2) Professional Manual*. Odessa, FL: Psychological Resources, 2002.
7. Weshler D. *Wechsler Memory Scale III Manual*. San Antonio, TX: Psychological Corporation, 1997.
8. Benton AL, Vanallen MW, Fogel ML. Temporal orientation in cerebral disease. *J Nerv Ment Dis* 1964; **139**: 110–19.
9. Lezak MD. *Neuropsychological Assessment*, 4th edn. Oxford: Oxford University Press, 2004.
10. Weshler D. *Wechsler Intelligence Scale III Manual*. San Antonio, TX: Psychological Corporation, 1997.
11. Ruff RM, Niemann H, Allen CC, Farrow CE, Wylie T. The Ruff 2 and 7 Selective Attention Test – a neuropsychological application. *Percept Motor Skill* 1992; **75**: 1311–19.
12. Greenberg LM, Kindschi CL, Dupuy TR, Hughes SJ. *T.O.V.A. Clinical Manual. Test of Variables of Attention Continuous Performance Test*. Los Alamitos, CA: TOVA Company; 2007.
13. Weshler D. *Wechsler Adult Intelligence Scale IV*. San Antonio, TX: Psychological Corporation, 2008.
14. Psychological Corporation. *Wechsler Abbreviated Scale of Intelligence (WASI) Manual*. San Antonio, TX: Psychological Corporation, 1999.

15. Delis DC, Kramer JH, Kaplan E, Ober BA. *California Learning Tests*, 2nd edn, Adult Version. San Antonio, TX: Psychological Corporation, 2000.

16. Brandt J, Benedict RHB. *Hopkins Verbal Learning Test-Revised*. Odessa, FL: Psychological Assessment Resources, 2001.

17. Schmidt M. *Rey Auditory and Verbal Learning Test. A Handbook*. Los Angeles: Western Psychological Services, 1996.

18. Benedict RHB. *Brief Visuospatial Memory Test – Revised*. Odessa, FL: Psychological Assessment Resources, 1997.

19. Benton AL. *Revised Visual Retention Test*. New York: Psychological Corporation, 1974.

20. Goodglass H, Kaplan E, Barresi B. *Boston Diagnostic Aphasia Examination*, 3rd edn (BDAE). Lutz, FL: Psychological Assessment Resources, 2000.

21. Benton AL, Hamsher K, Sivan AB. *Multilingual Aphasia Examination*, 3rd edn. Lutz, FL: Psychological Assessment Resources, 2000.

22. Delis DC, Kaplan E, Kramer JH. *Delis-Kaplan Executive Function System*. San Antonio, TX: Psychological Corporation, 2001.

23. Golden CJ. *Stroop Color and Word Test: A manual for clinical and experimental uses*. Chicago: Stoelting Co, 1978.

24. De Luca CR, Wood SJ, Anderson V *et al*. Normative data from the CANTAB. I: development of executive function over the lifespan. *J Clin Exp Neuropsychol* 2003; **25**: 242–54.

25. Grace J, Malloy P. *Frontal Systems Behavior Scale Professional Manual*. Lutz, FL: Psychological Assessment Resources, 2001.

26. Roth RM, Isquith PK, Gioia GA. *Behavioral Rating Inventory of Executive Function*. Lutz, FL: Psychological Assessment Resources, 2005.

27. Tranel D, Vianna E, Manzel K, Damasio H, Grabowski T. Neuroanatomical correlates of the Benton Facial Recognition Test and Judgment of Line Orientation Test. *J Clin Exp Neuropsychol* 2009; **31**: 219–33.

28. Benton AL, Sivan AB, Hamsher K, Varney NR, Spreen O. *Contributions to Neuropsychlogical Assessment: A clinical manual*, 2nd edb. New York: Oxford University Press, 1994.

29. Welsh KA, Butters N, Hughes JP, Mohs RC, Heyman A. Detection and staging of dementia in Alzheimer's disease. Use of the neuropsychological measures developed for the Consortium to Establish a Registry for Alzheimer's Disease. *Arch Neurol* 1992; **49**: 448–52.

30. Osterrieth PA. Le test de copie d'une figure complexe. *Arch Psychol* 1944; **30**: 206–356.

31. Weshler D. *Wechsler Adult Intelligence Scale – Revised*. San Antonio, TX: Psychological Corporation, 1987.

32. Hooper HE. *The Hooper Visual Organization Test: Manual*. Los Angeles: Western Psychological Services, 1983.

33. Solomon PR, Hirschoff A, Kelly B *et al*. A 7 minute neurocognitive screening battery highly sensitive to Alzheimer's disease. *Arch Neurol-Chicago* 1998; **55**: 349–55.

34. Dubinsky RM, Stein AC, Lyons K. Practice parameter: risk of driving and Alzheimer's disease (an evidence-based review): report of the quality standards subcommittee of the American Academy of Neurology. *Neurology* 2000; **54**: 2205–11.

35. Demakis GJ, Mercury MG, Sweet JJ, Rezak M, Eller T, Vergenz S. Motor and cognitive sequelae of unilateral pallidotomy in intractable Parkinson's disease: electronic measurement of motor steadiness is a useful outcome measure. *J Clin Exp Neuropsychol* 2002; **24**: 655–63.

36. Yang YK, Chiu NT, Chen CC, Chen M, Yeh TL, Lee IH. Correlation between fine motor activity and striatal dopamine D-2 receptor density in patients with schizophrenia and healthy controls. *Psychiatr Res Neuroimaging* 2003; **123**: 191–97.

37. Beck AT, Steer RA, Brown GK. *BDI-II, Beck Depression Inventory: Manual*, 2nd edn. San Antonio, TX: Psychological Corporation, 1996.

38. Yesavage JA, Brink TL, Rose TL *et al*. Development and validation of a geriatric depression screening scale: a preliminary report. *J Psychiatr Res* 1982; **17**: 37–49.

39. Butcher JN, Dahlstrom W, Graham JR, Tellegen A, Kaemmer B. *Manual for the Restardized Minnesota Multiphasic Personality Inventory: MMPI-2*. Minneapolis, MN: University of Minnesota Press, 1989.

40. Cummings JL, Mega M, Gray K, Rosenberg-Thompson S, Carusi DA, Gornbein J. The Neuropsychiatric Inventory: comprehensive assessment of psychopathology in dementia. *Neurology* 1994; **44**: 2308–14.

41. Bondi MW, Houston WS, Salmon DP *et al*. Neuropsychological deficits associated with Alzheimer's disease in the very-old: Discrepancies in raw vs. standardized scores. *J Int Neuropsychol Soc* 2003; **9**: 783–95.

42. Welsh-Bohmer KA, Ostbye T, Sanders L *et al*. Neuropsychological performance in advanced age: influences of demographic factors and apolipoprotein E: Findings from the Cache County Memory Study. *Clin Neuropsychol* 2009; **23**: 77–99.

43. Hedden T, Gabrieli JDE. Insights from the ageing mind: a view from cognitive neuroscience. *Nature Rev* 2004; **5**: 87–97.

44. Park DC, Reuter-Lorenz P. The adaptive brain: ageing and neurocognitive scaffolding. *Annu Rev Psychol* 2009; **60**: 173–96.

45. Salthouse TA. When does age-related cognitive decline begin? *Neurobiol Aging* 2009; **30**: 507–14.

46. Ivnik RJ, Smith GE, Lucas JA *et al*. Testing normal older people three or four times at 1- to 2-year intervals: defining normal variance. *Neuropsychology* 1999; **13**: 121–27.

47. Zehnder AE, Blasi S, Berres M, Spiegel R, Monsch AU. Lack of practice effects on neuropsychological tests as early cognitive markers of Alzheimer disease? *Am J Alzheimers Dis Other Demen* 2007; **22**: 416–26.

48. Welsh K, Butters N, Hughes J, Mohs R, Heyman A. Detection of abnormal memory decline in mild cases of Alzheimers-disease using Cerad neuropsychological measures. *Arch Neurol* 1991; **48**: 278–81.

49. Brandt J, Corwin J, Krafft L. Is verbal recognition memory really different in Huntingtons and Alzheimers-disease. *J Clin Exp Neuropsychol* 1992; **14**: 773–84.

50. Spaan PE, Raaijmakers JG, Jonker C. Alzheimer's disease versus normal ageing: a review of the efficiency of clinical and experimental memory measures. *J Clin Exp Neuropsychol* 2003; **25**: 216–33.

51. Gaffett KD, Browndyke JN, Whelihan W *et al*. The neuropsychological profile of vascular cognitive impairment – no dementia: comparisons to patients at risk for cerebrovascular disease and vascular dementia. *Arch Clin Neuropsychol* 2004; **19**: 745–57.

52. Tiraboschi P, Salmon DP, Hansen LA, Hofstetter RC, Thal LJ, Corey-Bloom J. What best differentiates Lewy body from Alzheimer's disease in early-stage dementia? *Brain* 2006; **129**: 729–35.

53. Metzler-Baddeley C. A review of cognitive impairments in dementia with Lewy bodies relative to Alzheimer's disease and Parkinson's disease with dementia. *Cortex* 2007; **43**: 583–600.

54. Cronin-Golomb A, Amick M. Spatial abilities in ageing, Alzheimer's disease and Parkinson's disease. In: Boller F, Cappa S (eds), *Handbook of Neuropsychology*. Amsterdam: Elsevier, 2001, 119–43.

55. Ferman TJ, Smith GE, Boeve BF *et al*. Neuropsychological differentiation of dementia with Lewy bodies from normal ageing and Alzheimer's disease. *Clin Neuropsychol* 2006; **20**: 623–36.

56. Renner JA, Burns JM, Hou CE, McKeel DW, Jr., Storandt M, Morris JC. Progressive posterior cortical dysfunction: a clinicopathologic series. *Neurology* 2004; **63**: 1175–80.

57. Petersen RC, Smith GE, Waring SC, Ivnik RJ, Tangalos EG, Kokmen E. Mild cognitive impairment: clinical characterization and outcome. *Arch Neurol* 1999; **56**: 303–308.

58. Ritchie K, Artero S, Touchon J. Classification criteria for mild cognitive impairment: a population-based validation study. *Neurology* 2001; **56**: 37–42.

59. Petersen RC, Morris JC. Mild cognitive impairment as a clinical entity and treatment target. *Arch Neurol* 2005; **62**: 1160–63.

60. Jak AJ, Bangen KJ, Wierenga CE, Delano-Wood L, Corey-Bloom J, Bondi MW. Contributions of neuropsychology and neuroimaging to understanding clinical subtypes of mild cognitive impairment. *Int Rev Neurobiol* 2009; **84**: 81–103.

61. Yaffe K, Petersen RC, Lindquist K, Kramer J, Miller B. Subtype of mild cognitive impairment and progression to dementia and death. *Dement Geriatr Cogn Disord* 2006; **22**: 312–19.

62. Busse A, Hensel A, Guhne U, Angermeyer MC, Riedel-Heller SG. Mild cognitive impairment: long-term course of four clinical subtypes. *Neurology* 2006; **67**: 2176–85.

63. Rountree SD, Waring SC, Chan WC, Lupo PJ, Darby EJ, Doody RS. Importance of subtle amnestic and nonamnestic deficits in mild cognitive impairment: prognosis and conversion to dementia. *Dement Geriatr Cogn Disord* 2007; **24**: 476–82.

64. Fischer P, Jungwirth S, Zehetmayer S *et al*. Conversion from subtypes of mild cognitive impairment to Alzheimer dementia. *Neurology* 2007; **68**: 288–91.

65. Butters MA, Whyte EM, Nebes RD *et al*. The nature and determinants of neuropsychological functioning in late-life depression. *Arch Gen Psychiatry* 2004; **61**: 587–95.

66. Lockwood KA, Alexopoulos GS, van Gorp WG. Executive dysfunction in geriatric depression. *Am J Psychiatry* 2002; **159**: 1119–26.

67. Saito H, Ichikawa K, Nomiyama T *et al*. Changes in activities of daily living during treatment of late-life depression. *Psychogeriatrics* 2008; **8**: 12–18.

68. Taylor WD, Steffens DC, Krishnan KR. Psychiatric disease in the twenty-first century: The case for subcortical ischemic depression. *Biol Psychiatry* 2006; **60**: 1299–303.

69. Weshler D. *Wechsler Memory Scale – Revised*. San Antonio, TX: Psychological Corporation; 1987.

70. Sivan AB. *Benton Visual Retention Test*, 5th edn. San Antonio, TX: Psychological Corporation, 1992.

71. Grant DA, Berg EA. A behavioural analysis of degree of impairment and ease of shifting to new responses in Weigl type cart sorting problem. *J Exp Psychol* 1948; **29**: 404–11.

72. DeFillippis NA, McCampbell E. *Manual for the Booklet Category Test*. Odessa, FL: Psychological Assessment Resources, 1997.

73. Ruff R. *Ruff Figural Fluency Test*. Odessa, FL: Psychological Assessment Resources, 1998.

63

Memory Training for Older Adults

Karen Miller, Linda Ercoli, Jeanne Kim and Gary W. Small

Semel Institute for Neuroscience and Human Behavior,
David Geffen School of Medicine at UCLA, Los Angeles, CA, USA

Normal ageing is typically associated with a decline in select domains of cognitive functioning, including processing speed, memory and executive functioning[1,2]. In addition, non-pharmacological interventions such as cognitive training and rehabilitation are being developed to enhance existing cognitive capacities, prolong independence in functional activities and promote healthy ageing. However, there is controversy as to whether cognitive stimulation enhances mental function[3] or decreases risk for Alzheimer's disease[4].

This chapter will present an overview of cognitive interventions that have been used with older adults, including healthy individuals with age-related memory changes, those with mild cognitive impairment (MCI), and persons with dementia, such as Alzheimer's disease (AD), and will include discussion of memory systems, metamemory, self-perceptions of memory, and interventions.

MEMORY SYSTEMS

Accumulated knowledge from studies in humans and animals has led to a widely accepted model of memory as being composed of multiple separate but parallel systems[5]. These multiple memory systems can be conceptualized as being either *declarative* or *non-declarative*[5]. Non-declarative memory is a general term for memory systems that do not involve conscious recollections but actions and performance-based tasks. Non-declarative memory is often targeted in rehabilitation interventions for skill maintenance, teaching skills, or functional abilities[6]. Declarative memory is the conscious recollection of information such as facts (*semantic memory*) and experienced single events linked to time and place (*episodic memory*)[7]. Individuals with progressive memory disorders, such as amnesic MCI and mild AD, present with deficits in declarative memory[8], which is the target of most memory enhancement strategies for non-demented persons and persons with milder forms of cognitive impairment.

Another conceptualization of memory relevant to cognitive enhancement interventions is the *levels of processing* approach, which comes from learning theory[9]. Levels of processing is the concept that memory is a function of the degree to which a stimulus is analysed. The deeper and more meaningful the analysis, the better the stimulus is remembered. In memory training, forming associations, images or stories can be considered deep processing strategies. It renders the information more distinctive, and helps integrate new information with a framework of pre-existing knowledge that provides cues for later retrieval[10].

METAMEMORY AND SELF-PERCEPTION OF MEMORY

A person's subjective understanding of their memory functioning is called *metamemory*. Most individuals have some understanding of their memory strengths, which might guide subsequent behaviours[11]. In non-depressed individuals, memory self-perceptions have been found to be accurate indicators of memory difficulties on objective tests[12], and may be indicators of underlying brain processes[13]. Several studies indicate that memory training interventions improve self-perceptions of memory ability and reduce memory complaints[14–16]. In healthy older adults, memory training may result in self-reported improvements in stability of memory functioning, and reduced anxiety and stress about memory functioning[15]. Effects of memory training on self-perceived memory are typically small, but nevertheless significant[14,17]. However, self-perceived memory ability is not always accurate. Persons with developing dementia may lose awareness of memory dysfunction as memory impairment advances[18,19].

TYPES OF COGNITIVE INTERVENTIONS

There are three primary approaches to cognitive training intervention: *cognitive stimulation*, *cognitive rehabilitation* and *cognitive training*[20]. The choice of approach depends on the degree and nature of deficits.

- **Cognitive stimulation** typically involves participation in group activities and/or discussions aimed at general enhancement of cognitive and social functioning[21]. These types of interventions are non-specific to a cognitive domain, and include such activities as discussions of current events, supervised recreational activities, and group reminiscence therapies. Cognitive stimulation is typically used for demented patients and often as a control condition in studies investigating the effects of cognitive training.
- **Cognitive rehabilitation** is an individualized intervention designed for patients with a specific brain injury or neurological disorder. Health-care providers work collaboratively with patients and their families or caregivers in order to identify personally relevant goals in day-to-day living and to develop strategies[20] that enhance functional tasks and activities of daily living, rather than increasing performance on a specific cognitive task[22].

The focus of this chapter is *cognitive training*, which involves learning and practising strategies to improve specific cognitive

Principles and Practice of Geriatric Psychiatry, 3rd edn. Edited by Mohammed T. Abou-Saleh, Cornelius Katona and Anand Kumar

functions, such as memory, attention, or problem-solving. Cognitive training is often administered to people with mild forms of difficulties associated with normal ageing, and to clinical populations, including persons with MCI, dementia or schizophrenia. The goals of cognitive training are to maintain or improve cognitive function, and to learn to compensate for deficits. Cognitive training is based on the assumption that, with intensive training, people will apply the strategies they learn to real-life situations beyond the training session. Cognitive training typically involves teaching skills and strategies in a standardized and structured fashion to individuals or to small groups[12]. Strategies vary in difficulty level and can be traditional paper–pencil tasks, classroom instruction or computerized activities[20].

MEMORY TRAINING APPROACHES

Many training techniques have been developed to specifically improve learning and recall. The techniques vary with respect to complexity, structure and application. One example is *errorless learning*, which is based on the premise that remembering new information will be more efficient if errors during learning are minimized and/or immediately corrected[23–25]. *Spaced retrieval*[26], which is also known as expanded rehearsal[27], is another common technique and involves learning and retaining new information by recalling the information over increasingly longer periods of time[28,29].

Mnemonic strategies have been one of the primary memory interventions used within clinical settings. Generally, mnemonic strategies facilitate encoding and aid retrieval by enhancing the meaningfulness or personal relevance of information. Mnemonic strategies involve organizing information in meaningful ways, forming associations, or forming visual images. Examples include: (i) verbal organization (i.e. forming acronyms), (ii) semantic clustering and elaboration (i.e. categorizing lists of words into subgroups or clusters of items that share something in common; or creating a story linking all target words on a list), and (iii) visual imagery strategies (i.e. method of loci, face-name association, creating a mental picture of a target)[11].

One of the most popular and oldest mnemonic strategies is the *method of loci* technique, which was used by ancient orators to remember long speeches. The method of loci involves imagining a familiar path and identifying unique landmarks along the path. Visual imagery is used to associate items on a list with each landmark along the imagined path. To remember the list, simply take a mental 'walk' along the path, recalling each image at each landmark.

Another popular mnemonic strategy is *face-name association*[30]. Individuals can use the face-name method for remembering someone they just met. The face-name strategy involves three steps: (i) looking at a person's face and identifying a prominent facial feature, (ii) transforming the person's name into something imaginative or that sounds concrete or meaningful, and (iii) developing a visual image integrating the prominent facial feature with the transformed name.

The efficacy of mnemonic or memory training strategies has been examined in a number of studies. Factors associated with memory improvement in one meta-analysis included younger age, higher cognitive functioning, group setting (versus individual training), shorter duration of sessions, education and 'pretraining'[17]. Pretraining allows the participant to get comfortable with visualization and move beyond their comfort zone of thinking about ordinary or logical images. In addition, the number of sessions did not appear to limit the efficacy of memory training[17]. In fact, interventions as short as 4 weeks

can be just as effective as programmes that are 8 weeks, or even 6–12 months long[31,32]. Most research demonstrating effectiveness of mnemonic techniques has focused on healthy adults, both young and old, but persons over 75 years of age show less improvement[33]. The few studies of efficacy in MCI populations have yielded mixed results[34,35]. A subset of subjects from the ACTIVE study (Advanced Cognitive Training for Independent and Vital Elderly) who were identified as 'memory impaired'(comparable to MCI) showed no significant benefit from memory training when compared to a no-contact control group, but had gains in speed of processing and inductive reasoning[36].

COMPUTER-ASSISTED COGNITIVE INTERVENTIONS

With the advancement of technology, researchers and clinicians are interested in computer-assisted training interventions for both healthy older adults and people with memory impairments. Initial studies have demonstrated that computer-based cognitive training has improved learning efficiency in healthy older adults[37], and supported cognitive and functional improvements in patients with AD[38]. Computer-based software technology has also recently been introduced in rehabilitative and training settings for patients with AD and MCI. Results seemed to suggest that the individualized rehabilitative intervention could have different effects according to a patient's diagnosis[39]. Cognitively intact older adults who received computer-based training demonstrated improvements in information processing, working memory and verbal learning/memory, and these gains were maintained over a five-month follow-up[40]. In mildly demented patients, computer-based training improved immediate recall of visual information and delayed retention of topographical information[38]. Combining a cognitive seminar and computer-assisted training in demented patients resulted in short-term improvement on measures of global cognitive functioning and short-term memory, as well as behavioural and social improvements[41].

Posit Science has developed a cognitive training program that contains increasingly difficult tasks of stimulus recognition, discrimination, sequencing and memory. Participants with mild cognitive changes associated with age demonstrated a significant increase on all computer tasks, with maintenance of improvements in attention over three months, when compared to active and no-contact controls[42]. In a subsequent larger trial, the Improvement in Memory with Plasticity-based Adaptive Cognitive Training (IMPACT) study[43], subjects demonstrated improvement in auditory memory and attention as compared to a general cognitive stimulation program that functioned as the active control condition.

Additionally, pilot studies have evaluated a computerized program, Brain Fitness by Dakim, which provides cognitive training and stimulation in language, visual processing, and memory domains. Results indicated improvement in memory functioning for those who could participate in the higher levels of the program, in addition to improved encoding and delayed recall for verbal pairs after just 10 sessions[44,45]. Presently, a clinical trial is underway to investigate the short- and long-term impact of this computer program on memory functioning in a larger sample of older adults with mild memory complaints as compared to wait-list controls.

As people become more technologically aware, computer programs are likely to become an important conduit for simulating real-life environments and integrating goal-directed behaviours in order to increase ecological validity[38]. These newer computer-based cognitive training interventions, however, have both advantages and limitations. Many of the tasks included in these interventions are laboratory based and likely lack ecological validity for functional activities. Moreover, many older adults have not had regular exposure to modern technology and thus may be hesitant or cautious in using them. Some of the advantages to using computer-assisted cognitive training programs are their flexibility and ability to tailor interventions to specific aspects of cognitive impairments, as well as the ability of the computer to provide immediate and specific feedback regarding performance[40].

The effects of computer-based training on brain function have not been widely studied. To date, one study has shown that computer use (via internet searching) may involve more than a two-fold increase in brain activation (as measured by functional magnetic resonance imaging) for the areas of the brain that are associated with vision, complex reasoning and decision making[46].

COMPREHENSIVE PROGRAMMES

Comprehensive or 'multifactorial' memory training programmes address non-cognitive factors in addition to teaching cognitive enhancement strategies. Non-cognitive factors include: (i) self-efficacy, expectations, and beliefs about one's ability to improve cognition; (ii) anxiety; and (iii) general education about memory[10,14,17,47,48]. Comprehensive training programmes may include interventions for stress or anxiety reduction, and cognitive restructuring to counter negative and self-deprecating thoughts about memory ability. Most programmes include pre-training because this facilitates learning more complex cognitive techniques. Overall, these integrative approaches take into account the multiple factors that impact an individual's receptiveness, or response to cognitive enhancement interventions.

There is recent evidence that the role of lifestyle and environmental factors can be neuroprotective and possibly lower the risk for developing AD[49]; therefore, some researchers have developed comprehensive healthy lifestyle programmes that incorporate aspects of diet, physical exercise, relaxation strategies and mental exercise[50]. Small and colleagues[51] developed a 14-day lifestyle programme consisting of memory mnemonics, mental puzzles, cardiovascular exercises, diet and recipe suggestions and relaxation strategies. Subjects in the healthy lifestyle intervention group demonstrated significant improvement on objective measures of verbal fluency, and FDG-PET imaging revealed a 5% decrease in activity in the left dorsolateral pre-frontal cortex, an area associated with working memory, semantic organization skills, anxiety and verbal fluency. This decrease in activity was interpreted as greater cognitive efficiency. This 14-day programme was then expanded into a classroom-based Memory Fitness curriculum, which has recently been implemented and studied in retirement homes[52,53]. Participants in the memory fitness programme had fewer memory concerns and better performance on immediate and delayed recall measures as compared to controls.

Researchers have developed similar programmes for individuals with amnesic MCI[34,35]. These programmes are typically comprised of multifaceted group-training sessions that include relaxation techniques, education regarding memory and ageing, memory skills training, cognitive restructuring of memory-related beliefs, information regarding appropriate diet and recreational activities, and availability of community resources[35]. Intervention programmes for those with MCI typically focus on improving memory for daily tasks and maintaining a level of functional independence[54]. A four-week multi-component rehabilitation programme resulted in improvement in activities of daily living, memory functioning and mood compared to a wait-list control group[55]. An additional programme utilized occupational therapy and behavioural training with computerized cognitive training; results showed improvement in cognitive and affective status of patients with MCI and mild dementia[56].

Another area of research to consider is the combination of medication with a computer-based cognitive training programme, suggesting that a combination of pharmacological and non-pharmacological treatment in MCI might maximize the effects of acetylcholinesterase inhibitors and delay memory deterioration and conversion to AD[32,57,58]. Gains may be maintained for approximately six months to one year, but individuals tend to experience a gradual deterioration by year two[57]. Although the effects are time limited, these findings suggest a complementary relationship between cognitive interventions and drug therapy for both cognitive and psychosocial disturbances.

LONG-TERM OUTCOMES

Few studies have evaluated the long-term effects of cognitive interventions in healthy older adults. Overall, the effects of memory training interventions have been found to last from six months to five years[59-62], although the benefits tend to attenuate over time. The largest clinical trial to date is the ACTIVE study ($n = 2832$), which evaluated the effectiveness and durability of cognitive interventions on objective cognitive tests and on subjective and objective instrumental activities of daily living (e.g. financial management, driving)[62,63]. This longitudinal study incorporated 3 cognitive training groups receiving a 10-session training programme for memory, reasoning, or speed of processing, and a wait list control group. Subjects also received periodic refresher courses, called 'booster sessions', on the skills initially trained. Follow-up results from two[63] and five years[62] revealed that the cognitive interventions in each group helped increase performance on objective measures of cognitive ability for which they were trained. According to self-report measures, this effect was significant only for the reasoning group, although the effect sizes for memory and processing speed were similar in magnitude to the reasoning effect sizes. Performance-based results demonstrated significant speed of processing benefits after additional booster sessions[62]. It is important to note that the lasting impact of cognitive interventions is still dependent on the individual's effort and motivation to maintain the use of the strategies. Future research in this area may consider factors such as motivation and maintenance in order to preserve treatment gains.

FUTURE DIRECTIONS

Overall, cognitive interventions are effective in improving cognition in subjects with mild age-related cognitive declines. However, there are important aspects of cognitive training that deserve more scrutiny. For instance, there is a need for more studies of persons with mild cognitive impairment and additional longitudinal studies in healthy older adults, in order to address whether cognitive training can delay dementia onset. Future studies should include functional outcome measures, to better address whether training can generalize beyond laboratory tests and improve practical, day-to-day functions[34,35]. In addition, there are still unaddressed questions, such as how engaging in stimulating everyday activities (also called an engaged lifestyle) is as effective as specific cognitive training[64,65].

Another important area for study is non-compliance, which may partially account for the lack of generalization and maintenance of cognitive strategy use. The key to long-term benefit appears to be continued use of cognitive strategies after initial training ends[60]. One solution to improve compliance is the implementation of periodic 'booster sessions', which may further help individuals use techniques with greater consistency and in more generalized situations (e.g. daily 'to-do' lists)[62,63].

Another limitation is the knowledge-base for the impact of 'brain games' and programmes targeted at stimulating cognition (e.g. crossword puzzles, sudoku problems, hand-held computerized games) on facilitating memory improvement. Although epidemiological studies suggest an association between engaging in cognitively stimulating activities and lower dementia risk[4,66], these studies do not prove a cause and effect relationship.

Finally, the effect of cognitive training on brain function has received minimal attention. In the few studies available, cognitive training does affect brain activation or resting state brain activity, including areas associated with encoding and retrieval[50,67,68], and training may also result in changes in neurochemistry[69]. Including brain function outcome measures will be important in addressing the more direct effects of cognitive training on neural circuitry and the mechanisms of action in cognitive enhancement interventions.

CONCLUSIONS

In sum, the research to date suggests that cognitive training is beneficial to individuals with memory complaints associated with normal ageing. The effectiveness in demented individuals is less consistent compared to persons with normal ageing. Even less is known about the effects of training on persons with MCI. There are a number of factors to consider before implementing a treatment trial, including the design of the training, the duration of the training, long-term compliance and the possible necessity of concurrent medication for those with cognitive impairment. Many options and designs are available to tailor programmes to the needs of individuals, or to develop programmes for small groups. Additional studies on the effectiveness of cognitive training in persons with MCI will help clarify the outcomes for this growing patient group.

REFERENCES

1. Park DC, Lautenschlager G, Hedden T et al. Models of visuospatial and verbal memory across the adult lifespan. Psychol Aging 2002; 17(2): 299–320.
2. Salthouse TA. When does age-related cognitive decline begin? Neurobiol Aging 2009; 30(4): 507–14.
3. Salthouse TA, Berish DE, Miles JD. The role of cognitive stimulation on the relations between age and cognitive functioning. Psychol Aging 2002; 17(4): 548–57.
4. Wilson RS, Scherr PA, Schneider JA, Tang Y, Bennett DA. Relation of cognitive activity to risk of developing Alzheimer disease. Neurology 2007; 69: 1911–20.
5. Squire LR. Memory systems of the brain: a brief history and current perspective. Neurobiol Learn Mem 2004; 82: 171–7.
6. Cohen NJ, Squire LR. Preserved learning and retention of pattern analyzing skill in amnesia: dissociation of knowing how and knowing that. Science 1980; 210: 207–9.
7. Tulving E. Elements of Episodic Memory. Oxford: Oxford University Press, 1983.
8. Cummings JL. The Neuropsychiatry of Alzheimer's Disease and Related Dementias. Independence, KY: Martin Dunitz Taylor and Francis Group, 2003.
9. Craik F, Lockhart RS. Levels of processing: a framework for memory research. J Verb Learn Verb Behav 1972; 11L: 71–84.
10. Yesavage J, Rose TL. Semantic elaboration and the method of loci: a new trip for older learners. Exp Aging Res 1984; 10: 155–9.
11. Sohlberg MM, Mateer CA. Cognitive Rehabilitation: An Integrative Neuropsychological Approach. New York: Guilford Press, 2001.
12. Belleville S, Chertkow H, Gauthier S. Working memory and control of attention in persons with Alzheimer's disease and mild cognitive impairment. Neuropsychology 2007; 21: 458–69.
13. Ercoli LM, Siddarth P, Huang S-C et al. Perceived loss of memory ability and cerebral metabolic decline in persons with the apolipoprotein E-4 genetic risk for Alzheimer's disease. Arch Gen Psychiatry 2006; 63: 442–8.
14. Floyd M, Scogin F. Effects of memory training on the subjective memory functioning and mental health of older adults: a meta-analysis. Psychol Aging 1997; 12: 150–61.
15. Valentijn SA, van Hooren SA, Bosma H et al. The effect of two types of memory training on subjective and objective memory performance in healthy individuals aged 55 years and older: a randomized controlled trial. Patient Educ Couns 2005; 57(1): 106–14.
16. Lachman ME, Weaver SL, Bandura M, Elliott E, Lewkowicz CJ. Improving memory and control beliefs through cognitive restructuring and self-generated strategies. J Gerontol 1992; 47(5): P293–9.
17. Verhaeghen P, Marcoen A, Goossens L. Improving memory performance in the aged through mnemonic training: a meta-analytic study. Psychol Aging 1992; 7: 242–51.
18. Correa DD, Graves RE, Costa L. Awareness of memory deficit in Alzheimer's disease patients and memory-impaired older adults. Neuropsychol Dev Cogn B Aging Neuropsychol Cogn 1996; 3: 215–28.
19. Vogel A, Stokholm J, Gade A et al. Awareness of deficits in mild cognitive impairment and Alzheimer's disease: do MCI patients have impaired insight? Dement Geriatr Cogn Disord 2004; 17: 181–7.
20. Clare L, Woods B. Cognitive rehabilitation and cognitive training for early-stage Alzheimer's disease and vascular dementia. Cochrane Database Syst Rev 2003; 4: CD003260.
21. Boylin W, Gordon S, Nehrke M. Reminiscence and ego integrity in institutionalized elderly. Gerontologist 1976; 16: 118–24.
22. Wilson BA. Towards a comprehensive model of cognitive rehabilitation. Neuropsychol Rehabil 2002; 12(2): 97–110.
23. De Vreese LP, Mirco N, Fioravanti M, Belloi L, Zanetti O. Memory rehabilitation in Alzheimer's disease: a review of progress. Int J Geriatr Psychiatry 2001; 16: 794–809.
24. Evans J, Levine B, Bateman A. Errorless learning. Neuropsychol Rehabil 2004; 4(4): 467–76.
25. Baddeley AD, Wilson BA. When implicit learning fails: amnesia and the problem of error elimination. Neuropsychologia 1994; 32: 53–68.
26. Landauer TK, Bjork RA. Optimal rehearsal patterns and name learning. In Gruneberg MM, Harris PE, Sykes RN (eds), Practical Aspects of Memory. New York: Academic Press, 1978, 625–32.

27. Moffat NJ. Home-based cognitive rehabilitation with the elderly. In Poon LW, Rubin DC, Wilson BC (eds), *Everyday Cognition in Adulthood and Late Life*. New York: Cambridge University Press, 1989, 659–80.

28. Bjork RA. Retrieval practice and the maintenance of knowledge. In Gruneberg MM, Morris PE, Sykes RN (eds), *Practical Aspects of Memory: Current Research and Issues*, vol. 1. New York: John Wiley & Sons, Inc., 1988, 396–401.

29. Logan JM, Balota DA. Expanded vs. equal interval spaced retrieval practice: exploring different schedules of spacing and retention interval in younger and older adults. *Neuropsychol Dev Cogn B Aging Neuropsychol Cogn* 2008; **15**: 257–80.

30. McCarty DL. Investigation of a visual imagery mnemonic device for acquiring face-name associations. *J Exp Psychol Hum Learn* 1980; **6**: 145–55.

31. Becker H, McDougall Jr GJ, Douglas NE, Arheart KL. Comparing the efficiency of eight-session versus four-session memory intervention for older adults. *Arch Psychiatr Nurs* 2008; **22**(2): 87–94.

32. Rozzini L, Costardi D, Chilovi BV *et al.* Efficacy of cognitive rehabilitation in patients with mild cognitive impairment treated with cholinesterase inhibitors. *Int J Geriatr Psychiatry* 2007; **22**: 356–60.

33. Singer T, Lindenberger U, Baltes PB. Plasticity of memory for new learning in very old age: a story of major loss? *Psychol Aging* 2003; **18**(2): 306–17.

34. Rapp S, Brenes G, Marsh AP. Memory enhancement training for older adults with mild cognitive impairment: a preliminary study. *Aging Ment Health* 2002; **6**(1): 5–11.

35. Troyer AK, Murphy KJ, Anderson ND, Moscovitch M, Craik FI. Changing everyday memory behaviour in amnesic mild cognitive impairment: a randomized controlled trial. *Neuropsychol Rehabil* 2008; **18**(1): 65–88.

36. Unverzagt FW, Kasten L, Johnson KE *et al.* Effect of memory impairment on training outcomes in ACTIVE. *J Int Neuropsychol Soc* 2007; **13**: 953–60.

37. Hickman JM, Rogers W, Fisk A. Training older adults to use new technology. *J Gerontol B Psychol Sci Soc Sci* 2007; **62B**: 77–84.

38. Schreiber M, Schweizer A, Lutz K, Kalveram KT, Jancke L. Potential of an interactive computer based training in the rehabilitation of dementia: an initial study. *Neuropsychol Rehabil* 1999; **9**(2): 155–67.

39. Cipriani G, Bianchetti A, Trabucchi M. Outcomes of a computer-based cognitive rehabilitation program on Alzheimer's disease patients compared with those on patients affected by mild cognitive impairment. *Arch Gerontol Geriatr* 2006; **43**: 327–35.

40. Gunther VK, Schafer P, Holzner BJ, Kemmler GW. Long-term improvements in cognitive performance through computer-assisted cognitive training: a pilot study in a residential home for older people. *Aging Ment Health* 2003; **7**(3): 200–6.

41. Mate-Kole CC, Fellows RP, Said PC *et al.* Use of computer assisted and interactive cognitive training programmes with moderate to severely demented individuals: a preliminary study. *Aging Ment Health* 2007; **11**(5): 485–95.

42. Mahncke HE, Connor BB, Appelman J *et al.* Memory enhancement in healthy older adults using a brain plasticity-based training program: a randomized, controlled study. *Proc Natl Acad Sci U S A* 2006; **103**(33): 12523–8.

43. Smith GE, Housen P, Yaffe K *et al.* A cognitive training program based on principles of brain plasticity: results from the Improvement in Memory with Plasticity-based Adaptive Cognitive Training (IMPACT) study. *J Am Geriatr Soc* 2009; **57**(4): 594–603.

44. Miller KJ, Siddarth P, O'Toole E *et al.* [M]Power® by Dakim: evaluating the effects of a computer fitness system for older adults. Poster session presented at 13th Annual UCLA Research Conference on Aging, 2008, Los Angeles.

45. Miller KJ, Siddarth P, O'Toole E *et al.* A computer fitness system for older adults: evaluating the effects of [M]Power® by Dakim. Poster session presented at 37th Annual Meeting of the International Neuropsychological Society, 2009, Altanta, GA.

46. Small, GW, Moody TD, Siddarth P, Bookheimer SY. Your brain on Google: patterns of cerebral activation during Internet searching. *Am J Geriatr Psychiatry* 2009; **17**(2): 116–26.

47. Stigsdotter-Neely A. Multifactorial memory training in normal aging: in search of memory improvement beyond the ordinary. In Hill RD, Backman L, Stigsdotter-Neely A (eds), *Cognitive Rehabilitation in Old Age*. New York: Oxford University Press, 2000, 63–80.

48. West RL, Bagwell DK, Dark-Freudeman A. Self-efficacy and memory aging; the impact of a memory intervention based on self efficacy. *Neuropsychol Dev Cogn B Aging Neuropsychol Cogn* 2008; **15**(3): 302–29.

49. Kramer AF, Bherer L, Colcombe SJ, Dong W, Greenough WT. Environmental influences on cognitive and brain plasticity during aging. *J Gerontol A Biol Sci Med Sci* 2004; **59**: 940–57.

50. Small GW, Silverman DHS, Siddarth P *et al.* Effects of a 14-day healthy longevity lifestyle program on cognitive and brain function. *Am J Geriatr Psychiatry* 2006; **14**(6): 538–45.

51. Small GW, Vorgan G. *The Memory Prescription*. New York: Hyperion, 2004.

52. Miller KJ, Gaines JM, Parrish JM *et al.* The memory fitness study: effects of a healthy aging intervention program on older adults. Poster session presented at 12th Annual UCLA Research Conference on Aging, 2007, Los Angeles.

53. Miller KJ, Siddarth P, Gaines J *et al.* The memory fitness study: healthy lifestyle choices improve memory. Poster session presented at 36th Annual Meeting of the International Neuropsychological Society, 2008, Big Island, HI.

54. Petersen RC. Mild cognitive impairment as a diagnostic entity. *J Intern Med* 2004; **256**: 183–94.

55. Kurz A, Pohl C, Ramsenthaler M, Sorg C. Cognitive rehabilitation in patients with mild cognitive impairment. *Int J Geriatr Psychiatry* 2009; **24**: 163–8.

56. Talassi E, Guerreschi M, Feriani M *et al.* Effectiveness of a cognitive rehabilitation program in mild dementia (MD) and mild cognitive impairment (MCI): a case control study. *Arch Gerontol Geriatr* 2007; **44**(Suppl 1): 391–9.

57. Requena C, Maestu F, Campo P, Fernandez A, Ortiz T. Effects of cholinergic drugs and cognitive training on dementia: 2-year follow-up. *Dement Geriatr Cogn Disord* 2006; **22**: 339–45.

58. Olazaran J, Muniz R, Reisberg B *et al.* Benefits of cognitive-motor intervention in MCI and mild to moderate Alzheimer disease. *Neurology* 2004; **63**: 2348–53.

59. Brooks JO, Friedman L, Pearman AM, Gray C, Yesavage JA. Mnemonic training in older adults: effects of age, length of training, and type of cognitive pretraining. *Int Psychogeriatr* 1999; **11**(1): 75–84.

60. O'Hara R, Brooks JO 3rd, Friedman L *et al.* Long-term effects of mnemonic training in community-dwelling older adults. *J Psychiatr Res* 2007; **41**(7): 585–90.

61. Bottiroli S, Cavallini E, Vecchi T. Long-term effects of memory training in the elderly: a longitudinal study. *Arch Gerontol Geriatr* 2008; **47**: 277–89.

62. Willis SL, Tennstedt SL, Marsiske M *et al.* Long-term effects of cognitive training on everyday functional outcomes in older adults. *JAMA* 2006; **296**: 2805–14.

63. Ball K, Berch DB, Helmers KF *et al.* Effects of cognitive training interventions with older adults: a randomized controlled trial. *JAMA* 2002; **288**: 2271–81.

64. Carlson MC, Saczynski JS, Rebok GW *et al.* Exploring the effects of an "everyday" activity program on executive function and memory in older adults: Experience Corps. *Gerontologist* 2008; **48**(6): 793–801.

65. Stine-Morrow EAL, Parisi JM, Morrow DG, Park DC. The effects of an engaged lifestyle on cognitive vitality: a field experiment. *Psychol Aging* 2008; **23**(4): 778–86.

66. Wilson RS, Medes de Leon CF, Barnes LL *et al.* Participation in cognitively stimulating activities and risk of incident Alzheimer disease. *JAMA* 2002; **287**(6): 742–8.

67. Nyberg L, Sandblom J, Jones S *et al.* Neural correlates of training-related memory improvement in adulthood and aging. *Proc Natl Acad Sci U S A* 2003; **100**(23): 13728–33.

68. Kondo Y, Suzuki M, Mugikura S *et al.* Changes in brain activation associated with use of a memory strategy: a functional MRI study. *Neuroimage* 2005; **24**(4): 1154–63.

69. Valenzuela MJ, Jones M, Wen W *et al.* Memory training alters hippocampal neurochemistry in healthy elderly. *Neuroreport* 2003; **14**(10): 1333–7.

Complementary and Alternative Medicine Approaches to Memory Improvement in the Elderly

Helen Lavretsky

Department of Psychiatry and Biobehavioral Sciences, and Semel Institute for Neuroscience and Human Behavior, David Geffen School of Medicine at UCLA, Los Angeles, USA

THE TRENDS IN USE OF COMPLEMENTARY AND ALTERNATIVE MEDICINE IN THE US

The use of complementary and alternative medicine (CAM) in the US is increasing rapidly, exceeding a prevalence of 60% in a nationally representative survey conducted by the National Center for Health Statistics in 2002. CAM therapies are defined by the National Center for Complementary and Alternative Medicine as a group of diverse medical and health systems, practices and products that are not currently considered to be part of conventional medicine. An alternative approach to mental health care is one that emphasizes the interrelationship between mind, body and spirit. A national US survey noted a 47% increase in total visits to CAM practitioners, from 427 million in 1990 to 629 million in 1997. These figures surpass total visits to primary care physicians[1]. Estimated expenditures for CAM professional services were conservatively estimated at $21.2 billion in 1997, with at least $12.2 billion of out-of-pocket expenditures, exceeding out-of-pocket expenditures for all US hospitalizations. In a more recent nationwide survey, 36% of US adults aged 18 years and over were found to use some form of CAM[1], and ageing baby boomers are expected to accelerate the use of CAM in the coming years[2]. Barnes and colleagues noted that nearly 33% of older adults used CAM in the preceding year (2004)[2]. In a survey, 42% of the patients in a managed care organization reported using at least one CAM therapy, most commonly relaxation techniques (18%), massage (12%), herbal medicine (10%) or megavitamin therapy (9%). Perceived efficacy of CAM was very high, ranging from 98% (energy healing) to 76% (hypnosis)[1].

With the increasing public use of complementary and alternative medicine for preventive and therapeutic purposes, including a very active 'anti-ageing' movement, a significant effort is now devoted to the integration of alternative methods of treatment into mainstream health care practice and research[3]. The principal uses in older adults include anti-ageing effects of CAM for memory enhancement, and treatment of various neuropsychiatric symptoms, such as depression, anxiety, insomnia and pain. This chapter is devoted to the description of the existing CAM interventions applied to the care of older adults with late-life cognitive disorders.

DIET AND THE USE OF NUTRITIONAL AND HERBAL SUPPLEMENTS

Adjusting both diet and nutrition may help some people with mental illnesses manage their symptoms and promote recovery. For example, research suggests that eliminating milk and wheat products can reduce the severity of symptoms for some people who have schizophrenia and some children with autism. Similarly, some holistic/natural physicians use herbal treatments, B-complex vitamins, riboflavin, magnesium and thiamine to treat anxiety, depression, drug-induced psychoses and memory loss. A number of herbs and dietary supplements have demonstrable effects on memory, mood, and insomnia[4]. There is a significant amount of evidence supporting the use of *Gingko biloba* and omega-3 fatty acids for dementia, as reviewed below. Many users of CAM may take a variety of herbal products[5].

Gingko Biloba

Ginkgo biloba leaf extract is among the most widely sold herbal dietary supplements in the United States. Its purported biological effects include scavenging free radicals, lowering oxidative stress, reducing neural damage, reducing platelet aggregation, and anti-inflammatory, anti-tumour and anti-ageing activities. Clinically, it has been prescribed to treat CNS disorders such as Alzheimer's disease and cognitive deficits. It elicits allergy and changes in bleeding time. Its components, quercetin, kaempferol and rutin, have been shown to be genotoxic[6] but the mutagenicity or carcinogenicity of *Gingko biloba* itself has not been reported. There are no standards or guidelines regulating the constituent components of *Gingko biloba* leaf extract, nor are exposure limits imposed. Safety evaluation of *Gingko biloba* leaf extract is being conducted by the US National Toxicology Program.

Ginkgo biloba has been widely used for many years by people with symptoms attributed to 'cerebrovascular insufficiency,' despite the lack of evidence of a causal role. Many placebo-controlled trials of *Ginkgo biloba* in patients with various types of dementia have yielded contradictory results. Of the studies that revealed any

Principles and Practice of Geriatric Psychiatry, 3rd edn. Edited by Mohammed T. Abou-Saleh, Cornelius Katona and Anand Kumar
© 2011 John Wiley & Sons, Ltd

cognitive improvement, the effect was minor and did not last more than six months. Some studies reported haemorrhaging, indicating that it is necessary to use caution when prescribing *Ginkgo biloba* for cognitive deficits, especially in patients with increased risk of haemorrhage[7]. The recommended doses range widely, but in a trial of Alzheimer's disease prevention, 120 mg of *Gingko biloba* twice a day was not effective in reducing the overall incidence rate of dementia or Alzheimer's disease in elderly individuals with normal cognition or those with mild cognitive impairment[8]. Its short-term use is acceptable under some conditions, but the potential risk of bleeding must be seriously considered. *Gingko biloba* has been reported to reduce depression in dementia patients and counteract sexual side effects of antidepressants[9].

The Use of Nutritional Supplements

In addition to herbal remedies, consumers use a variety of nutritional supplements (including vitamins, amino acids and fish oil) that may affect mood and functioning.

Elevated plasma homocysteine concentrations have been implicated with risk of cognitive impairment and dementia, but it is unclear whether low vitamin B12 or folate status is responsible for cognitive decline or can protect against it[10,11]. Most studies reporting associations between cognitive function and homocysteine or B vitamins have used a cross-sectional or case-control design and have been unable to determine whether such associations are causal or merely a result of the disease. The homocysteine hypothesis of dementia has attracted considerable interest, as homocysteine can be easily lowered by folic acid and vitamin B12, raising the prospect that B-vitamin supplementation could lower the risk of dementia[10]. Incident dementia is more strongly associated with changes in folate, vitamin B12 and homocysteine, than with previous concentrations. These changes may be linked to other somatic manifestations of early dementia, such as weight loss[12]. However, in a trial of high dose vitamin B in patients with Alzheimer's disease, the supplement did not slow cognitive decline in individuals with mild to moderate Alzheimer's disease[13]. Two other placebo-controlled trials of treatment with B12, folic acid and B6 showed no advantage of vitamins over placebo at reducing the severity of depressive symptoms or the incidence of clinically significant depression over a period of two years in older men[14]. Similarly, a recent Cochrane review found no evidence for short-term benefit from vitamin B6 in improving mood (depression, fatigue and tension symptoms) or cognitive functions. For the older people included in one of the two trials mentioned in the review, oral vitamin B6 supplements improved biochemical indices of vitamin B6 status, but potential effects on blood homocysteine levels were not assessed in either study. This review found evidence that there is scope for increasing some biochemical indices of vitamin B6 status among older people[15]. The limited available evidence suggests folate may have a potential role as a supplement to other treatments for depression. It is currently unclear if this is the case both for people with normal folate levels and for those with folate deficiency. More randomized controlled trials are needed to explore possible benefits from vitamin B6 supplementation for healthy older people and those with cognitive impairment or dementia.

Omega-3 Fatty Acids

Fish oil and omega-3 fatty acids are also commonly used supplements. Reductions in cardiovascular risk, depression and rheumatoid arthritis symptoms have been correlated with omega-3 fatty acid

intake, and there is increased interest in the use of omega-3 fatty acid supplementation for other psychiatric illnesses and prevention of Alzheimer's disease. Reported health benefits include improvements in cognition and mood in unipolar and bipolar mood disorders. Omega-3 fatty acids are found principally in fish and seafood although some can be derived from green vegetables. By contrast, omega-6 fatty acids are found in soft margarine, most vegetable oils and animal fat. Omega-6 is plentiful in most modern Western diets while omega-3 is often relatively lacking. A high dietary ratio of omega-6 to omega-3 has been linked to vulnerability to many physical and mental disorders[1]. Most studies recommend omega-3 essential fatty acids with a ratio of eicosapentaenoic acid (EPA) to docosahexaenoic acid (DHA) of 7:1. PUFA DHA 22:6(n - 3), a dietary essential, is important for maintaining normal nervous system function and cellular structure. A lack of DHA is associated with cognitive decline during ageing and neurodegenerative disease[16]. DHA-derived neuroprotectin D1 (NPD1) has recently been shown to provide homeostatic regulation of brain cell survival and repair involving neurotrophic, antiapoptotic and anti-inflammatory signalling[16]. Research suggests that growth factors and neurotrophins activate the synthesis of NPD1, which interacts with the molecular-genetic mechanisms affecting beta-amyloid precursor protein (betaAPP) and amyloid beta (Abeta) peptide neurobiology. Deficits in DHA or its peroxidation may play a role in inflammatory signalling, apoptosis and neuronal dysfunction in Alzheimer's disease[17,18].

In a well-designed trial of the effect of EPA and DHA on mental well-being using a double-blind, placebo-controlled design in the general older population, the study failed to find drug–placebo difference in improving cognition or well-being[18]. In a meta-analysis, the authors concluded that available data are insufficient to draw strong conclusions about the effects of omega-3 fatty acids on cognitive function in normal ageing or on the incidence or treatment of dementia[19]. However, limited evidence suggests a possible association between omega-3 fatty acids and reduced risk of dementia.

In summary, omega-3 fatty acids may have a role in the treatment of late-life dementia, cognitive impairment and neuropsychiatric disorders. Future studies should clarify the function and the optimal dose of omega-3 fatty acids or EPA in the treatment of cognitive decline and address lingering questions regarding the purity of marketed supplements.

S-ADENOSYL-L-METHIONINE (SAME)

S-adenosyl-L-methionine (SAMe) is one of the CAM products that has been studied under rigorous controlled conditions. SAMe is a methyl donor involved in the synthesis of monoaminergic neurotransmitters derived from the amino acid L-methionine through the one-carbon cycle. SAMe has been investigated for its antidepressant properties in both open[1] and randomized controlled[20] trials. SAMe dosages of 200–1600 mg/day (orally or parenterally) have been shown to be superior to placebo and as effective as tricyclic antidepressants in alleviating depression, although some individuals may require higher doses[20]. At this time, the recommended doses range from SAMe 200 mg bid up to 800 mg bid. Oral dosages of SAMe up to 1600 mg/day appear to be significantly bioavailable and safe. SAMe has been associated with minor adverse effects, e.g. gastrointestinal symptoms and headaches[1], and an occasional induced mania[21].

SAMe plays an essential role in maintaining neuronal health, and may prove to be an effective neuroprotective dietary supplement in Alzheimer's disease. This disease is accompanied by reduced glutathione S-transferase (GST) activity, diminished SAMe, and increased S-adenosyl homocysteine (SAH), the downstream metabolic product resulting from SAMe-mediated transmethylation reactions. Panza *et al.* confirmed that SAMe can exert a direct effect on GST activity, thereby making SAMe an ideal neuroprotective candidate to slow the progression of Alzheimer's disease[22]. It remains unclear if such supplements can reduce the risk for cognitive decline in very mild Alzheimer's disease and mild cognitive impairment.

CULTURALLY BASED HEALING ARTS

Culturally based healing includes traditional Oriental medicine (such as acupuncture, shiatsu and reiki), Indian systems of health care (such as Ayurveda and yoga) and Native American healing practices (such as the sweat lodge and talking circles). All incorporate the beliefs that (i) wellness is a state of balance between the spiritual, physical and mental/emotional 'selves'; (ii) an imbalance of forces within the body is the cause of illness; and (iii) herbal/natural remedies, combined with sound nutrition, exercise and meditation/prayer will correct this imbalance.

Acupuncture

Acupuncture is the Chinese practice of inserting needles into the body at specific points to manipulate the body's flow of energy in order to balance the endocrine system. This manipulation regulates functions such as heart rate, body temperature and respiration, as well as sleep patterns and emotional changes. Acupuncture has been used in clinics to assist people with substance abuse disorders through detoxification; to relieve stress and anxiety; to treat attention deficit and hyperactivity disorder in children; to reduce symptoms of depression; and to help people with physical ailments. There have been only a few studies of acupuncture for dementia compared to studies of depression or stress. There is accumulating evidence from animal models of dementia that acupuncture can be useful for memory improvement. In a Chinese study, Zhou and Jin performed acupuncture on the scalp in areas corresponding to brain regions involved in Alzheimer's disease[23]. Twenty-six patients with clinically diagnosed Alzheimer's disease underwent functional magnetic resonance imaging (fMRI) while undergoing acupuncture at four acupoints. Activation occurred in both the right main hemisphere and the left hemisphere in locations consistent with brain regions frequently impaired in Alzheimer's disease. These areas are closely correlated with cognitive function (memory, reason, language, executive etc.), providing evidence that acupuncture has a potential effect on Alzheimer's disease[23].

Despite promising results, there is insufficient evidence to determine the efficacy of acupuncture compared to medication, wait list control or sham acupuncture in the management of depression. Scientific study design is generally poor and the number of people studied is relatively small. One of the barriers to conducting appropriate studies of acupuncture is the difference between diagnostic systems in Western and Chinese medicine, precluding fair comparison.

In a vascular dementia model using rats, the effect of electro-acupuncture was tested on the formation system of free radicals in brain tissues. The researchers used the Morris's water labyrinth for testing learning ability and memory in rats receiving electro-acupuncture and rats assigned to the control group. The mean escape latency in the electro-acupuncture group was much shorter in several cognitive tests compared with the control group. This research suggests that electro-acupuncture can improve learning and memory ability in vascular dementia rat models[24].

Ayurveda

Ayurveda is a natural health care approach that originated in India more than 5000 years ago. It is still widely used in India as a system of primary health care, and is growing in popularity worldwide. Ayur means 'life' or 'longevity' and Veda means 'knowledge or science.' Combined, Ayurveda means 'the science of life' and the practice of Ayurvedic medicine is described as 'knowledge of how to live'[25]. As a form of complementary and alternative medicine, Ayurveda is commonly used as a method to enhance memory, combat ageing and as nerve tonic. It is also used as an anxiolytic, anti-inflammatory and immunopotentive remedy. Ayurveda incorporates an individualized treatment regimen, such as diet, yoga, meditation, herbal preparations or other techniques to facilitate lifestyle changes and to teach people how to release stress and tension. It is often used as a treatment for depression. There are some preliminary encouraging results for its effectiveness in treating various ailments, including chronic disorders associated with the ageing process. Pilot studies of depression, anxiety, sleep disorders, hypertension, diabetes mellitus, Parkinson's disease and Alzheimer's disease yielded positive results[26]. However, no extensive controlled studies of Ayurveda in older adults are available to date.

There is an increasing number of publications on antioxidant, neuroprotective and memory enhancing properties of various herbal Ayurvedic preparations in rat and mice models of Alzheimer's disease[27]. The part of the Ayurvedic system that provides an approach to prevention and treatment of degenerative diseases is known as Rasayana, and plants used for this purpose are classed as rejuvenators. Traditional medicinal plants in various countries, particularly in India, have been used for centuries for various ailments; however, there has been little scientific effort to validate these anecdotal uses mentioned in the literature.

A number of these traditionally used plant extracts and various 'Ayurvedic medicines' have been screened using the National Institute of Mental Health Synthetic Screening Program for scientific validation and the development of new leads of psychotherapeutic compounds[28]. In young and ageing mice models, Anwala churna produced a dose-dependent improvement in memory scores. Furthermore, it reversed the amnesia induced by scopolamine and diazepam. Anwala churna may prove to be a useful remedy for the management of Alzheimer's disease because of its diverse beneficial effects, including its memory improving property, cholesterol lowering property and anticholinesterase activity[26]. *Ocimum sanctum*, a plant widely used in Ayurveda, has been shown to possess anti-inflammatory, antioxidant and cognition-enhancing properties[29]. In rats, the effect of methanolic extract from *Ocimum sanctum* leaves was studied in cerebral reperfusion injury as well as long-term hypoperfusion. Treatment significantly prevented long-term hypoperfusion-induced functional and structural disturbances. The results suggest that *Ocimum sanctum* may be useful in treatment of cerebral reperfusion injury and cerebrovascular insufficiency states[29].

Trasina is a herbal formulation of some Indian medicinal plants classified in Ayurveda as Medhyarasayanas, or drugs reputed to improve memory and intellect[21]. In a rodent model of Alzheimer's disease, subchronic administration of Trasina reversed deficits in acetylcholine after 14 and 21 days of treatment. Thus the herbal formulation exerts a significant nontropic effect after subchronic treatment that may be due to reversal of perturbed cholinergic function[30].

Research that compares Ayurveda's comprehensive treatment approach, Western allopathic treatment and an integrated approach combining both the Ayurvedic and allopathic treatments would shed light on which treatment system is the most effective for the benefit of the patient.

YOGA AND MEDITATION

Practitioners of yoga, the ancient Indian system of health care, use breathing exercises, posture, stretch and meditation to balance the body's energy centres. Mindful physical exercise is a special kind of physical exercise with an additional element that focuses on one's state of mind. It has recently emerged as a therapeutic intervention for improving the psychosocial well-being of individuals. According to the IDEA Mind–body Fitness Committee (1997–2001), a mindful physical exercise is characterized by 'physical exercise executed with a profound inwardly directed contemplative focus.' A physical exercise is considered mindful if it: (i) has a meditative/contemplative component that is non-competitive and non-judgmental; (ii) has proprioceptive awareness that involves low to moderate level of muscular activity with mental focus on muscular movement; (iii) is breath centering; (iv) focuses on anatomic alignment, such as spine, trunk and pelvis, or proper physical form; and (v) concerns energy centric awareness of individuals' flow of intrinsic energy, vital life force, qi etc. With the above framework, yoga and qigong are two major streams of mindful physical exercise based on the literature. Yoga is used in combination with other treatments for depression, anxiety and stress-related disorders.

The principle of yoga is to achieve integration of mind, body and spirit. There are twenty-two types of yoga and many more modifications. The most popular in the US is Hatha yoga, a branch of yoga that requires a vast repertoire of physical postures during sitting, standing or lying on the floor, along with specific breathing patterns. Other than physical movement, participants are required to maintain a 'homeostasis' of mind and body, which refers to the relaxation of body tension with quieting of thoughts. The qigong exercise is a system of self-practising physical exercise, which includes healing posture, movement, self-massage, breath work and meditation. All forms of qigong are featured on balance, relaxation, breathing and good posture. The movements of qigong are executed at very low energy expenditure levels. A specific breathing pattern also applies to qigong. Similar to yoga, the breathing style of qigong is slow and deep in order to achieve body relaxation, clearing of mind and maintenance of health. Combining all of the above components, mindful physical exercise has been shown to provide an immediate source of relaxation and mental quiescence. Scientific evidence shows that medical conditions such as hypertension, cardiovascular disease, insulin resistance, depression and anxiety disorders respond favorably to mindful physical exercises[31]. Despite a growing body of evidence to show the effects of mindful physical exercises such as qigong, tai chi and yoga on depression, there is a dearth of review that examined mindful physical exercise as to its effects on memory enhancement. A review on complementary and alternative treatments on older adults shows that mind–body interventions were effective in treating depression, anxiety and insomnia in 10 out of 12 studies reviewed[32]. Some studies demonstrated improvement in functioning

on a spatial cognitive task while breathing through the left nostril. Performance improved in the cerebral hemisphere contralateral to the patent nostril[33]. An integrated approach of yoga therapy in menopausal women improved cognitive functions such as remote memory, mental balance, attention and concentration, delayed and immediate recall, verbal retention and recognition tests[34].

RELAXATION AND STRESS REDUCTION TECHNIQUES, BIOFEEDBACK

Learning to control muscle tension and 'involuntary' body functioning, such as heart rate and skin temperature, can be a path to mastering one's fears. It is used in combination with, or as an alternative to, medication to treat disorders such as anxiety, panic and phobias. For example, a person can learn to 'retrain' his or her breathing habits in stressful situations to induce relaxation and decrease hyperventilation. Some preliminary research indicates it may offer an additional tool for treating depression.

Although there are no data in geriatric depression, an increasing number of publications describe the use of biofeedback for memory training and cognitive enhancement using neurofeedback. This is an electroencephalographic (EEG) technique for training individuals to alter their brain activity using operant conditioning. Research has shown that neurofeedback helps reduce symptoms of several neurological and psychiatric disorders. Ongoing research is currently investigating its application in the treatment of other disorders and for enhancing non-disordered cognition[35].

Angelakis et al. used EEG peak alpha frequency for neurofeedback because it has been shown to correlate positively with cognitive performance and to correlate negatively with age[35]. In a pilot double-blind study of neurofeedback training in older individuals, they observed that peak alpha frequency neurofeedback improved cognitive processing speed and executive function, but had no clear effect on memory. Kotchoubey et al. reported the results of two groups of subjects, aged 20–28 and 50–64 years, matched for health status and verbal abilities[36]. They described how subjects learned to control their slow cortical potentials in a feedback paradigm by producing, on command, shifts in these potentials in either the positive or negative direction. Both groups were able to differentiate significantly between the positivity task and the negativity task. Older subjects had only explicit, but not implicit, learning deficits. Elderly subjects showed consistently more negative slow cortical potential shifts, which may indicate their impaired cortical inhibition. This pattern is likely due to brain ageing. The question remains if biofeedback could be helpful in reducing cognitive deficits associated with ageing or dementia[36].

EXERCISE

Human and other animal studies demonstrate that exercise targets many aspects of brain function, providing broad effects on overall brain health. The benefits of exercise have been best defined for learning and memory, protection from neurodegeneration and alleviation of depression, particularly in elderly populations. Exercise increases synaptic plasticity by directly affecting synaptic structure and potentiating synaptic strength, and by strengthening the underlying systems that support plasticity including neurogenesis, metabolism and vascular function. In addition, exercise reduces peripheral risk factors such as diabetes, hypertension and cardiovascular disease, which converge to cause brain dysfunction and neurodegeneration. Such exercise-induced structural and functional change has been documented in various brain regions but has been best studied in the hippocampus[37].

Randomized and crossover clinical trials demonstrate the efficacy of aerobic or resistance training exercise (2–4 months) as a treatment for depression in both young and older individuals that may have an effect on cognitive function[38]. The benefits are similar to those achieved with anti-depressants[38]. They are also dose dependent, and greater improvements are seen with higher levels of exercise[38,39].

In a study of exercise in early Alzheimer's disease, cardiorespiratory fitness was modestly reduced in subjects with Alzheimer's disease compared to subjects without dementia[40]. The results were associated with whole brain volume and white matter volume reductions after controlling for age. In participants without dementia, there was no relationship between fitness and brain atrophy[40]. Therefore, cardiovascular fitness may moderate brain atrophy related to Alzheimer's disease; however, further studies are needed to resolve inconsistent findings.

A key mechanism involved in the benefits of exercise on the brain is induction of central and peripheral growth factors and growth factor cascades. These growth factors instruct downstream structural and functional change. Inflammation, which can impair growth factor signalling both systemically and in the brain, is a common mechanism relating to the central and peripheral effects of exercise. Thus, through regulation of growth factors and reduction of peripheral and central risk factors, exercise ensures successful brain function[37].

In summary, cognitive ageing is one of the most common reasons for using complementary and alternative therapies in older adults. The amount of rigorous scientific data to support the efficacy of complementary therapies in the treatment of cognitive impairment is extremely limited. The areas with the most evidence for beneficial effects are exercise, herbal therapy (*Gingko biloba*), the use of fish oil, and, to a lesser extent, acupuncture and relaxation therapies (see Table 64.1). There is a need for further research involving randomized controlled trials to investigate the efficacy of complementary and alternative therapies in the treatment of dementia and cognitive impairment in late life. This research may lead to the development

Table 64.1 Complementary and alternative medicine interventions for the treatment of cognitive impairment and dementia[41]

Mode of intervention	Postulated mechanism of action	Dementia, cognition	Main adverse effects and drug interactions
Omega-3 fatty acids (fish oil)	Mood stabilization, memory enhancement, neuroprotection, reduction in amyloid production	Several RCTs are mixed or negative in the effect on cognition	Fishy aftertaste; gastrointestinal distress; increased effect of warfarin and NSAIDs
SAMe	Cofactor in neurotransmitter synthesis, methylation homocysteine to methionine	Animal studies are suggestive of potential use; no human studies available	Mania; gastrointestinal distress; headache interaction with SSRIs
Folate and B12	Cofactor in neurotransmitter synthesis, methylation homocysteine to methionine, precursor to SAMe	RCTs are suggestive of usefulness in prevention of cognitive decline and improved memory performance	Mania induction, interaction with SSRIs
Gingko biloba	Scavenging free radical; lowering oxidative stress; reducing neural damages; increased blood flow to the brain	Mixed and negative results in RCTs of dementia and other cognitive disorders	Increased bleeding time, allergic reactions
Ayurveda	Indian treatment system with the use of herbs, diet and lifestyle to achieve balance in cognition and well-being	Few RCTs; suggestive of positive effect; positive antiamyloid animal studies	Consistent with above side effect of herbals
Acupuncture	Balancing energy flow through the meridians in the body	In a few trials improved memory and other cognitive tests in Alzheimer's disease and vascular dementia	Needle phobia, bleeding
Yoga	Postures, breath, meditation; rebalancing the mind–body connections	A few uncontrolled studies showed improved attention and memory in nondemented adults	None
Biofeedback	Retraining of the autonomic nervous system or alpha brain waves	Alpha peak in brain waves is associated with enhanced cognitive performance	None
Spirituality	Lowers stress and enhances cognition via church attendance and prayer	Enhances cognitive performance in those who attend church	None
Exercise	Improved cardiovascular function, release of endorphins, increased energy, mental stimulation	Modest improvement in cognition in dementia and in ageing	None

SAMe, S-adenosyl-L-methionine; RCT, randomized controlled trial.

of effective treatment and preventive approaches for these serious conditions.

ACKNOWLEDGEMENT

This work was supported by the NIH grants R01 MH077650 and R-21 AT003480 to Dr Lavretsky.

Adapted from Aging Health (2009) **5**(1), 61–78 with permission of Future Medicine Ltd.

REFERENCES

1. Andreescu C, Mulsant BH, Emanuel JE. Complementary and alternative medicine in the treatment of bipolar disorder – a review of the evidence. *J Affect Disord* 2008; **110**(1–2): 16–26.
2. Barnes PM, Powell-Griner E, McFann K, Nahin RL. Complementary and alternative medicine use among adults: United States, 2002. *Adv Data* 2004; **343**: 1–19.
3. Astin JA. Why patients use alternative medicine: results of a national study. *JAMA* 1998; **279**(19): 1548–53.
4. Fugh-Berman A, Cott JM. Dietary supplements and natural products as psychotherapeutic agents. *Psychosom Med* 1999; **61**(5): 712–28.
5. Werneke U, Turner T, Priebe S. Complementary medicines in psychiatry: review of effectiveness and safety. *Br J Psychiatry* 2006; **188**: 109–21.
6. Chan PC, Xia Q, Fu PP. Ginkgo biloba leave extract: biological, medicinal, and toxicological effects. *J Environ Sci Health C Environ Carcinog Ecotoxicol Rev* 2007; **25**(3): 211–44.
7. Ginkgo and Alzheimer's disease: little or no different from placebo. *Prescrire Int* 2007; **16**(91): 205–7.
8. DeKosky ST, Williamson JD, Fitzpatrick AL *et al.* Ginkgo biloba for prevention of dementia: a randomized controlled trial. *JAMA* 2008; **300**(19): 2253–62.
9. Scripnikov A, Khomenko A, Napryeyenko O. Effects of Ginkgo biloba extract EGb 761 on neuropsychiatric symptoms of dementia: findings from a randomised controlled trial. *Wien Med Wochenschr* 2007; **157**(13–14): 295–300.
10. Clarke R. B-vitamins and prevention of dementia. *Proc Nutr Soc* 2008; **67**(1): 75–81.
11. Smith AD. The worldwide challenge of the dementias: a role for B vitamins and homocysteine ? *Food Nutr Bull* 2008; **29** (2 suppl): S143–72.
12. Kim JM, Stewart R, Kim SW *et al.* Changes in folate, vitamin B12 and homocysteine associated with incident dementia. *J Neurol Neurosurg Psychiatry* 2008; **79**(8): 864–8.
13. Aisen PS, Schneider LS, Sano M *et al.* High-dose B vitamin supplementation and cognitive decline in Alzheimer disease: a randomized controlled trial. *JAMA* 2008; **300**(15): 1774–83.
14. Ford AH, Flicker L, Thomas J *et al.* Vitamins B12, B6, and folic acid for onset of depressive symptoms in older men: results from a 2-year placebo-controlled randomized trial. *J Clin Psychiatry* 2008; **69**(8): 1203–9.
15. Malouf R, Grimley Evans J. The effect of vitamin B6 on cognition. *Cochrane Database Syst Rev* 2003(4): CD004393.
16. Lukiw W, Bazan N. Docosahexaenoic acid and the aging brain. *J Nutr* 2008; **138**(12): 2510–14.
17. Smith DG, Cappai R, Barnham KJ. The redox chemistry of the Alzheimer's disease amyloid beta peptide. *Biochim Biophys Acta* 2007; **1768**: 1976–90.
18. van de Rest O, Geleijnse JM, Kok FJ *et al.* Effect of fish-oil supplementation on mental well-being in older subjects: a randomized, double-blind, placebo-controlled trial. *Am J Clin Nutr* 2008; **88**(3): 706–13.
19. Issa AM, Mojica WA, Morton SC *et al.* The efficacy of omega-3 fatty acids on cognitive function in aging and dementia: a systematic review. *Dement Geriatr Cogn Disord* 2006; **21**(2): 88–96.
20. Mischoulon D, Fava M. Role of S-adenosyl-L-methionine in the treatment of depression: a review of the evidence. *Am J Clin Nutr* 2002; **76**(5): 1158S–61S.
21. Gören JL, Stoll AL, Damico KE, Sarmiento IA, Cohen BM. Bioavailability and lack of toxicity of S-adenosyl-L-methionine (SAMe) in humans. *Pharmacotherapy* 2004; **24**(11): 1501–7.
22. Panza F, Frisardi V, Capurso C *et al.* Possible role of S-adenosylmethionine, S-adenosylhomocysteine, and polyunsaturated fatty acids in predementia syndromes and Alzheimer's disease. *J Alzheimers Dis* 2009; **16**(3): 467–70.
23. Zhou Y, Jin J. Effect of acupuncture given at the HT 7, ST 36, ST 40 and KI 3 acupoints on various parts of the brains of Alzheimer's disease patients. *Acupunct Electrother Res* 2008; **33**(1–2): 9–17.
24. Wang L, Tang C, Lai X. Effects of electroacupuncture on learning, memory and formation system of free radicals in brain tissues of vascular dementia model rats. *J Tradit Chin Med* 2004; **24**(2): 140–43.
25. Vasudevan M, Parle M. Memory enhancing activity of Anwala churna (Emblica officinalis Gaertn.): an Ayurvedic preparation. *Physiol Behav* 2007; **91**(1): 46–54.
26. Sharma H, Chandola HM, Singh G, Basisht G. Utilization of Ayurveda in health care: an approach for prevention, health promotion, and treatment of disease. Part 2: Ayurveda in primary health care. *J Altern Complement Med* 2007; **13**(10): 1135–50.
27. Auddy B, Ferreira M, Blasina F *et al.* Screening of antioxidant activity of three Indian medicinal plants, traditionally used for the management of neurodegenerative diseases. *J Ethnopharmacol* 2003; **84**(2–3): 131–8.
28. Misra, R. Modern drug development from traditional medicinal plants using radioligand receptor-binding assays. *Med Res Rev* 1998; **18**(6): 383–402.
29. Yanpallewar SU, Rai S, Kumar M, Acharya SB. Evaluation of antioxidant and neuroprotective effect of Ocimum sanctum on transient cerebral ischemia and long-term cerebral hypoperfusion. *Pharmacol Biochem Behav* 2004; **79**(1): 155–64.
30. Bhattacharya SK, Kumar A. Effect of Trasina, an ayurvedic herbal formulation, on experimental models of Alzheimer's disease and central cholinergic markers in rats. *J Altern Complement Med* 1997; **3**(4): 327–36.
31. Khalsa SB. Yoga as a therapeutic intervention: a bibliometric analysis of published research studies. *Ind J Physiol Pharmacol* 2004; **48**: 269–85.
32. Meeks TW, Wetherell JL, Irwin MR, Redwine LS, Jeste DV. Complementary and alternative treatments for late-life depression, anxiety, and sleep disturbance: a review of randomized controlled trials. *J Clin Psychiatry* 2007; **68**(10): 1461–71.
33. Joshi M, Telles S. Immediate effects of right and left nostril breathing on verbal and spatial scores. *Indian J Physiol Pharmacol* 2008; **52**(2): 197–200.
34. Chattha R, Nagarathna R, Padmalatha V, Nagendra HR. Effect of yoga on cognitive functions in climacteric syndrome: a randomised control study. *BJOG* 2008; **115**(8): 991–1000.

35. Angelakis E, Stathopoulou S, Frymiare JL *et al*. EEG neurofeedback: a brief overview and an example of peak alpha frequency training for cognitive enhancement in the elderly. *Clin Neuropsychol* 2007; **21**(1): 110–29.

36. Kotchoubey B, Haisst S, Daum I, Schugens M, Birbaumer N. Learning and self-regulation of slow cortical potentials in older adults. *Exp Aging Res* 2000; **26**: 15–35.

37. Cotman CW, Berchtold NC, Christie L. Exercise builds brain health: key roles of growth factor cascades and inflammation. *Trends Neurosci* 2007; **30**(9): 464–72. Erratum in *Trends Neurosci* 2007; **30**(10): 489.

38. Blumenthal JA, Babyak MA, Moore KA *et al*. Effects of exercise training on older patients with major depression. *Arch Intern Med* 1999; **159**(19): 2349–56.

39. Duman RS. Neurotrophic factors and regulation of mood: role of exercise, diet and metabolism. *Neurobiol Aging* 2005; **26**(suppl 1): 88–93.

40. Burns JM, Cronk BB, Anderson HS *et al*. Cardiorespiratory fitness and brain atrophy in early Alzheimer disease. *Neurology* 2008; **71**(3): 210–16.

41. Lavretsky H. The use of complementary and alternative medicine for treatment of late-life neuropsychiatric disorders. *Aging Health* 2009; **5**(1): 61–78.

65

Ethics of Dementia Care

Eran Klein[1] and Jason Karlawish[2]

[1] *The Johns Hopkins Berman Institute of Bioethics, Baltimore, USA*
[2] *University of Pennsylvania Institute on Aging, Philadelphia, USA*

The stages of dementia, from presymptomatic concerns to diagnosis to death, present clinicians, patients and families with numerous ethical challenges. These challenges may stand out as acute problems or crises, while others simply form the background of living with chronic and progressive loss of cognition. Clinicians who aspire to provide the best care possible for their patients and patients' families need to recognize and respond appropriately to the ethical dimension of dementia. This chapter will present the major ethical challenges typical of each stage of dementia care – presymptomatic, symptomatic and end of life – and suggest ways to approach them.

AN OVERALL FRAMEWORK

The approach to the patient with dementia starts with identifying the goals of care. These vary with the stage of the disease. Early in the disease, the goal is to maximize autonomous decision making. The patient's own vision of what constitutes a life well lived should guide decisions. The clinician should help sustain this vision to the extent possible through pharmacotherapy, provision of patient and family education and support, treatment of co-morbid conditions, and an honest assessment of disease progression and what to expect in the future. As the patient's ability for autonomous decision making diminishes, the goals of care shift to those focused on what will maximize the patient's dignity and quality of life. Accurate assessment of quality of life relies on a complex interplay of expressed patient preferences as well as clinician and family observations and interpretations of patient moods and behaviours. To facilitate a commonsense discussion of quality of life, a clinician can ask both the patient and the family *what is a typical day?* The answers to this question will not only indicate the patient's abilities and disabilities but also the nature and character of the patient's social and emotional engagement in the world. The shift in goals of care tracks a shift in the role of the patient within the patient–caregiver–clinician relationship from being a co-participant in the decision making to a non-participant[1].

The patient, family and medical team all bring different perspectives and commitments that need to be taken into account. Sometimes these fit seamlessly together, such as when patients and families express a mutual preference for care that prioritizes comfort over longevity. At other times, disagreements may be evidence of deep differences in values, such as when a patient directs that care at a future stage of dementia be minimal out of a concern for preserving dignity but the family is committed to sustaining life when at all possible. Various methodological tools are available for working through some of these deep disagreements[2-5]. For instance, the appeal to – and balancing or specification of – the principles of respect for autonomy and beneficence is a common starting point for working through such cases[6].

MANAGING UNCERTAINTY

As researchers uncover more about the genetic and biological markers of the common causes of dementia, such as Alzheimer's disease[7], clinicians will have to address the ethical challenges of the presymptomatic stage of dementia. Can genes, biomarkers or imaging[8] – or some combination of these – reliably predict a person's risk of developing dementia? Communicating such prediction models to patients presents clinicians with real challenges. For example, the use of the apolipoprotein E4 allele in predictive testing – which initially indicated a threefold increased chance of developing Alzheimer's disease if heterozygous for the allele but with quite poor specificity[9] – already suggests that significant challenges face both the clinician in interpreting the meaning of predictive tests for patients and patients in applying probabilistic knowledge to future decisions. Similar questions and challenges apply to so-called biomarkers of common causes of neurodegenerative dementia such as tau protein in spinal fluid.

An approach to presympotomatic testing that addresses these issues is as follows. Patients are entitled to good quality predictive testing, if available, given the value that this information may have for some. In accordance with the Genetic Nondiscrimination Act of 2008 (GINA), this information has at least the same legal protections as other medical information[10]. The clinician (and the medical system) are only obligated to provide tests, however, that significantly improve upon current predictive information (e.g. family history, neuropsychiatric testing) and which the patient can understand and reasonably make use of (e.g. not make dramatic changes to future plans based on small differences in probability). The decision to provide a predictive test is an important clinical decision and, like the provision of other tests or treatments, requires clinical judgement. An essential clinical skill in exercise of this judgement is how to assess a patient's understanding and appreciation of such information. Below, we discuss techniques to do this.

DISCLOSING THE DIAGNOSIS

The first ethical issue that many clinicians face with regard to the detection of dementia is when, how and if to deliver a diagnosis of dementia[11]. The question of 'if' is largely settled as a matter of policy. Patients are morally and legally entitled to their diagnosis. Although this approach has been widely endorsed by the Alzheimer's Association[12], the AMA[13] and a consensus statement[14], studies suggest that this policy has not fully filtered down to practice. Surveys of caregivers suggest that some physicians often do not disclose the diagnosis to the patient[15]. Instead, they disclose the diagnosis to the family[16]. And many generalists[17] and dementia specialists[18-20] choose not to disclose a diagnosis of dementia, particularly at a more advanced stage when comprehension is seriously compromised. This practice persists despite evidence that most cognitively intact adults say they would want to know if they were diagnosed with dementia[21] (though the strength of this desire seems to wane with the increasing age at which this diagnosis would be made[22]). This obviously paternalistic practice reflects the complexity of a disease with progressive cognitive decline that impairs a person's ability to adequately understand relevant information. The most compelling reason to disclose even at later stages of disease is that the patient with dementia is owed the chance, however small in some cases, of understanding (or gaining a glimpse of) why the things that are happening are happening and what this portends for the future. To deny the patient this, whether to make things easier for a caregiver or to prevent purported psychological harm to the patient ('therapeutic privilege'), is to deny an opportunity, perhaps the most important and last opportunity, for self-knowledge left to the patient with dementia.

A reasonable approach to guide whether to disclose a diagnosis to a patient is to converse with the patient about his or her awareness of cognitive problems, and, if the patient is aware of these problems, about the patient's desire to know what is their cause[23]. Useful questions to elicit these symptoms include *Are you having problems with your memory?* and *Do your memory problems bother you?* If a patient endorses these symptoms, a follow-up question is *Would you like to know what is the cause of these problems?* In the case of a patient who has awareness of problems with memory and a desire to know the cause of these problems, a clinician has a clear warrant to disclose the diagnosis. Two useful techniques include asking the patient what he or she knows about Alzheimer's disease and clarifying any misunderstandings about the disease (*One of the most common causes of memory problems is Alzheimer's disease. Have you ever heard of that? Tell me what you know about it?*). This needs to be done in a way that balances truth with kindness. For example, after disclosing a diagnosis to a patient, it is sensible to ask how the patient feels about this diagnosis and whether any questions or concerns remain.

ASSESSING DECISIONAL CAPACITY AND MANAGING INCAPACITY

The central issue that is at the heart of many of the ethical concerns during the symptomatic stage of dementia care is the loss of decision-making capacity. Dementia progressively undermines the abilities necessary for competent medical decision making (e.g. understanding, appreciation, reasoning and expression of choice[24]) and consequently undermines the capacity for giving informed consent or refusal for treatment or research. While the development of some clinical instruments has shown some promise for aiding the assessment of capacity[25-27], the determination of whether someone has sufficient capacity is still ultimately a clinical judgement.

When a clinician does judge that a patient has lost the capacity to make a decision, the appointment of a surrogate provides a way to protect and promote the patient's interests. In clinical practice, a surrogate tends to appear naturally as part of that person's other roles as knowledgeable informant and caregiver. Often this person is a spouse, partner, adult child or sibling. A surrogate can be designated preemptively by the patient (via an advance directive) or appointed through established (often state) standards for next of kin. The *raison d'être* of the surrogate is to make decisions on the patient's behalf.

Acceptable standards for how the surrogate makes decisions vary[28]. Traditionally, ethics has posited a hierarchy of standards. The surrogate can try to decide *as the patient would have decided* given what is known of her previous beliefs, values, character and so on (called the *substituted judgement standard*). Absent the ability to fulfil this standard, the surrogate should decide based on what the surrogate believes is in the best interest of the patient (*best interest standard*). Studies suggest that most older adults do not want a surrogate to practice this hierarchy of standards, but instead to exercise a leeway that balances the two standards. In a study of 150 dialysis patients, two thirds preferred that their surrogate exercise at least 'a little leeway' in interpreting their advance directives to withdraw dialysis were they to develop advanced Alzheimer's disease[29]. This has substantial implications for clinicians when they talk with surrogates. Specifically, it suggests a useful approach to guiding surrogates in decision making; consideration should be given both to what preferences, if any, their relative told them, and what they think will maximize their relative's dignity and quality of life. A surrogate decision should be challenged, in court if necessary, if clear evidence suggests that the surrogate is not acting with the patient's interests in mind. In the absence of such, the presumption lies in favour of the surrogate knowing how best to act on the patient's behalf.

Patients with dementia can formulate *instructional* advance directives. These advance directives spell out how a person wishes to be treated when, at some future time, a decision needs to be made but capacity for making that decision is no longer present. These have great intuitive appeal but variable practical usefulness. Where next of kin knows little of the patient or of the patient's end of life wishes, however, these can be helpful. And they can be useful when instruction is categorical (e.g. under no circumstances perform CPR). Where one would want instructional advance directives to be their most useful, however, they often cannot be. To anticipate and fully articulate the myriad variables that a particular decision will involve one year, five years or ten years into the future is unrealistic. If a decision is truly difficult and contested, it will be *because* there is disagreement about whether the particularities of a situation – some variable or variables – make it different than what is spelled out in the advance directive. This does not entail that instructional advance directives are useless, just that they need to be approached in a particular way. In designing them, one should help patients communicate how in general they want the end of life to go. Is more or less aggressive treatment preferable? Should pain relief or longevity be afforded priority? Where they can be categorical (e.g. do not attempt resuscitation; DNAR), they should be, but where they cannot be they should provide examples as guideposts for decision makers (e.g. 'no feeding tube unless likely to need for fewer than two weeks'). The ideal should not be to spell out decision rules in so detailed a manner that exercising judgement is unnecessary; this is impossible. The goal should be to provide decision makers a tool for knowing the spirit in which judgements should be made.

LIVING WITH DEMENTIA: THE CASE OF PARTICIPATING IN RESEARCH

Those with dementia constitute a vulnerable research population, like other vulnerable populations (e.g. children[30], pregnant women[31], the mentally ill[32], the incarcerated[33]). The status of people with dementia as a vulnerable population has afforded needed protection from exploitation, but at some cost. It has exposed persons with dementia to the risks of medications for non-dementia ailments – risks that are largely unknown given the group's exclusion from most drug approval trials. And it has deprived a segment of the population that might be uniquely motivated to participate in research of the opportunity to do so and, in turn, closed off a way of giving expression to deeply held values. Though vigilance continues to be needed in protecting this vulnerable population in research, there is also a growing appreciation of the costs of excluding persons with dementia from research as well[34].

Surrogates face the decision of whether to enrol demented individuals in research. In the case of research procedures that involve the potential for therapeutic benefit to patients, the decision is made analogously to a surrogate treatment decision with a weighing of harms and benefits. In contrast, research procedures that do not involve direct therapeutic benefit present a challenge as exposure to these risks cannot be justified on the basis of benefits to the patient but rather on the value of the knowledge the research may realistically produce. In such a circumstance, a common set of proposals permit surrogate consent only if (i) the research presents minimal risk or some minor increment over minimal risk, (ii) the subject gives assent or lack of dissent, (iii) institutional review board (IRB) approval is obtained, and (iv) the surrogate gives consent on the subject's behalf consistent with the patient's previous preferences[35]. Difficult issues remain as to how to define 'minimal risk', whether assent is necessary or even meaningful, and whether surrogates accurately reflect subjects' views on acceptable risk[36], but the current protections allow those with dementia to participate in limited forms of research while still acknowledging their status as a vulnerable population.

LIVING WITH DEMENTIA: THE CASE OF DRIVING

For many patients, the restriction of driving privileges marks a turning point in the disease process and often in the patient–clinician relationship as well. For many patients, driving is essential for their involvement in the larger social world. It allows freedom of movement and independence, and is central to a sense of self. When clinicians seek to restrict driving, confrontation can arise. Patients with dementia can lack the insight necessary to recognize their deficits and fail to appreciate that restrictions align their safety with the public's safety. And even when they do recognize some deficits, the value of driving may outweigh for them the added risks to self and others.

In the case of driving, clinicians are not only advocates for their patients, but stewards of the public health. They are obligated to step in and restrict driving even when this threatens individual patient–clinician relationships. Strategies can help minimize this threat. Frank, early discussion of driving and dementia can prepare patients for future restrictions, and timely neuropsychiatric and driving performance testing can help convince patients of unappreciated and evolving deficits. While the Mini-Mental State Examination (MMSE) only roughly predicts driving performance[37], substantial evidence correlates Clinical Disease Rating (CDR) scores

with driving performance. A CDR of 0.5 correlates with mildly impaired driving (akin to a 16- to 21-year-old) and a CDR of 1 with significant traffic safety risk[38]. At a CDR of 0.5, patients should be encouraged not to drive or to restrict driving (e.g. shorter distance, time of day), and patients at a CDR of 1 should be advised not to drive. Where required by state law, a report should be made to the appropriate driving authority (with full disclosure to the patient), and where not required by law, one should clearly and without equivocation advise against driving, with mention, if appropriate, of possible financial or legal ramifications from driving against medical advice. Although not always acknowledged as such, driving is a privilege and responsibility, not a civil right.

A useful strategy to address driver safety issues is to ask the patient's family if they would be comfortable with the patient driving the grandchildren or someone else's grandchildren. If the answer is short of a resounding 'yes', then a driver's assessment is warranted.

LIVING WITH DEMENTIA: THE CASE OF VOTING

Voting *is* a civil right that is threatened both by dementia and by how those with dementia are treated. The elderly form a significant and growing proportion of the eligible (and active) voting population in many industrialized countries. Given the incidence of dementia in this population, the disease poses a significant challenge to those interested in protecting and promoting the right to vote. States determine voter qualifications and already restrict voting (e.g. based on criminal convictions)[39] and mandate certain kinds of assistance with voting (e.g. for the blind). Many states have been slow to provide voting assistance for those with dementia. This needs to change as methods of voting shift from traditional in-person polling stations to more private venues (e.g. absentee ballots mailed from private homes or nursing homes, home electronic voting). Studies suggest wide and worrisome variation in the access that people with dementia have to the vote and in systemic opportunities for voter fraud[40]. At minimum, we owe to those with dementia an aggressive effort to extend the ease of voting (e.g. using mobile polling in nursing homes) and to all citizens simple safeguards against voter fraud (e.g. monitoring of absentee voting at large nursing homes).

DECIDING ON THERAPY

The decision to either pursue or to forgo therapy in dementia raises ethical concerns. Where potential therapies for dementia carry mild side effects and promise moderate benefits, such concerns may seem uncomplicated weighing of costs and benefits. However, as therapies are developed that promise significant improvement but at a cost of substantial inconvenience (e.g., intravenous medication infusion) or potentially seriously side effects (e.g. meningoencephalitis in an early beta amyloid vaccine trial[41]), the ethical importance of such decisions becomes more substantial. It is all the more important to clarify issues of capacity and surrogacy, and at an early stage, when potentially large risks and pay-offs are in the balance.

The need to clarify these issues arises as well for decisions about life-prolonging therapy (e.g. surgery, chemotherapy) for co-morbid conditions (e.g. oesophageal cancer). When capacity to make these decisions is lacking, a surrogate has to weigh the costs of potential side effects, including the cost of enduring side effects that the patient does not understand. In the case of incapacity, potentially life-prolonging therapy should be pursued if (i) the patient has previously clearly expressed a prioritization for longevity over comfort and (ii) the therapy involves only mild to moderate time-limited discomfort in return for a substantially improved quality and quantity of life. Where these conditions are met, a complicated, expensive treatment should be regarded the same as a cheap, routine one (e.g. antibiotics). The aim of treatment in dementia should not be to prolong life for the sake of prolonging life; it should be to prolong life when the quality of that life falls within the range of that which someone could value.

The choice of whether to pursue enteral nutritional support in patients who have lost (or are soon to lose) the ability to swallow oral nutrition and hydration is one of the most difficult therapy decisions that surrogates face. Eating has deep symbolic and cultural meaning. The presumption has been that enteral nutritional support extends life, reduces respiratory infections by reducing aspiration, wards off other infections (e.g. skin ulcers) by improving nutritional status and provides a comfortable satiety. However, such presumptions, held by both physicians[42] and surrogates[43], are not borne out by evidence[44]. The emerging consensus is that since enteral nutritional support for the severely demented entails harms and provides little or no medical benefit, it can (and often should) be refused if requested by family or surrogates. Instead, the conversation should focus on what is good palliative care and how best to provide it for the patient.

PROMOTING SAFETY AND PRESERVING QUALITY OF LIFE

Personal safety can be an issue both for patients and for caregivers. Patients with impaired memory, insight, judgement and inhibition can wander out of beds, rooms and homes and exhibit other behaviour (e.g. aggression) that endangers themselves or others[45]. Traditionally, the options for ensuring safety have been restraints such as bed rails, medications and locked wards. However, these interventions carry harms[46,47] and may also mask the need to identify the underlying and potentially reversible causes of these behaviours (e.g. boredom, pain or thirst in the case of wandering and agitation). Recently, techniques of surveillance (such as video, electronic) have become increasingly popular. As valuable as these may be to limit concerns of safety, they must be balanced against other important harms (e.g. violations of privacy, infringements of liberty, indignity) that may result from their use.

Securing the physical safety of persons with dementia and those around them is a balance of freedom and control. Just as medical interventions (e.g. chemotherapy) have a cost in terms of suffering, so too do many safety measures. They should be judged in basically the same way. If these measures so distress the patient that it significantly diminishes whatever quality of life they are able to maintain, then one should seriously question their value. The goal in dementia care is not to prolong life by providing safety at all costs. It is to provide whatever safety is possible – balanced in terms of its costs – so that patients can enjoy the maximal quality of life of which they are able.

An appreciation of the ethical challenges in dementia care is important. It allows the clinician the opportunity for a more thoughtful and systematic approach to questions that are often the most vexing and meaningful for patients and families. There may be few easy answers in these areas but there are ways to approach problems that yield better results than others. Clinicians have an obligation to provide dementia patients with the best care possible and this includes attention to the ethical dimension of the care being provided.

REFERENCES

1. Karlawish JH, Casarett D, Propert KJ, James BD, Clark CM. Relationship between Alzheimer's disease severity and patient participation in decisions about their medical care. *J Geriatr Psychiatry Neurol* 2002; **15**(2): 68–72.
2. Beauchamp TL, Childress JF. *Principles of Biomedical Ethics*, 6th edn. New York: Oxford University Press, 2009.
3. Gert B, Culver CM, Clouser KD. *Bioethics: A Systematic Approach*, 2nd edn. Oxford: Oxford University Press, 2006.
4. Jonsen AR, Toulmin SE. *The Abuse of Casuistry: A History of Moral Reasoning*. Berkeley, CA: University of California Press, 1988.
5. Tong R. *Feminist Approaches to Bioethics: Theoretical Reflections and Practical Applications*. Boulder, CO: Westview, 1997.
6. Degrazia D. Moving forward in bioethical theory: theories, cases, and specified principlism. *J Med Philos* 1992; **17**(5): 511–39.
7. Shaw LM, Vanderstichele H, Knapik-Czajka M *et al.* Cerebrospinal fluid biomarker signature in Alzheimer's disease neuroimaging initiative subjects. *Ann Neurol* 2009; **65**(4): 403–13.
8. Mosconi L, Tsui WH, Herholz K *et al.* Multicenter standardized 18F-FDG PET diagnosis of mild cognitive impairment, Alzheimer's disease, and other dementias. *J Nucl Med* 2008; **49**(3): 390–8.
9. Seshadri S, Drachman DA, Lippa CF. Apolipoprotein E ε4 allele and the lifetime risk of Alzheimer's disease: what physicians know, and what they should know. *Arch Neurol* 1995; **52**(11): 1074–9.
10. Public Law no. 110-233, 122 Stat. 881 (May 21, 2008).
11. Drickamer MA, Lachs MS. Should patients with Alzheimer's disease be told their diagnosis? *N Engl J Med* 1992; **326**(14): 947–51.
12. Alzheimer's Association. Diagnostic disclosure, 2007. At www.alz.org/professionals_and_researchers_diagnostic_disclosure.asp, accessed 1 Mar 2009.
13. Guttman R, Seleski M (eds). *Diagnosis, Management and Treatment of Dementia*. Chicago, IL: American Medical Association, 1999.
14. Post SG, Whitehouse PJ. Fairhill guidelines on ethics of the care of people with Alzheimer's disease: a clinical summary. Center for Biomedical Ethics, Case Western Reserve University and the Alzheimer's Association. *J Am Geriatr Soc* 1995; **43**(12): 1423–9.
15. Brodaty H, Griffin D, Hadzi-Pavlovic D. A survey of dementia carers: doctors' communications, problem behaviours and institutional care. *Aust N Z J Psychiatry* 1990; **24**(3): 362–70.
16. Holroyd S, Turnbull Q, Wolf AM. What are patients and their families told about the diagnosis of dementia? Results of a family survey. *Int J Geriatr Psychiatry* 2002; **17**(3): 218–21.
17. Vassilas CA, Donaldson J. Telling the truth: what do general practitioners say to patients with dementia or terminal cancer? *Br J Gen Pract* 1998; **48**(428): 1081–2.
18. Clafferty RA, Brown KW, McCabe E. Under half of psychiatrists tell patients their diagnosis of Alzheimer's disease. *Br Med J* 1998; **317**(7158): 603.
19. Rice K, Warner N. Breaking the bad news: what do psychiatrists tell patients with dementia about their illness? *Int J Geriatr Psychiatry* 1994; **9**(6): 467–71.

20. Rice K, Warner N, Tye T, Bayer A. Telling the diagnosis to patients with Alzheimer's disease. Geriatricians' and psychiatrists' practice differs. *Br Med J* 1997; **314**(7077): 376.

21. Holroyd S, Snustad DG, Chalifoux ZL. Attitudes of older adults on being told the diagnosis of Alzheimer's disease. *J Am Geriatr Soc* 1996; **44**(4): 400–3.

22. Erde EL, Nadal EC, Scholl TO. On truth telling and the diagnosis of Alzheimer's disease. *J Fam Pract* 1988; **26**(4): 401–6.

23. Karlawish J. On telling someone she has Alzheimer's disease, 2006. At www.uphs.upenn.edu/ADC/info-disclosure.shtml, accessed 27 Mar 2009.

24. Appelbaum PS. Clinical practice. Assessment of patients' competence to consent to treatment. *N Engl J Med* 2007; **357**(18): 1834–40.

25. Grisso T, Appelbaum P. *MacArthur Competency Assessment Tool for Treatment (MacCAT-T)*. Sarasota, FL: Professional Resource Press, 1998.

26. Marson DC, Ingram KK, Cody HA, Harrell LE. Assessing the competency of patients with Alzheimer's disease under different legal standards. A prototype instrument. *Arch Neurol* 1995; **52**(10): 949–54.

27. Edelstein B. *Hopemont Capacity Assessment Interview Manual and Scoring Guide*. Morgantown, WV: West Virginia University, 1999.

28. Buchanan AE, Brock DW. *Deciding for Others: The Ethics of Surrogate Decision Making*. Cambridge: Cambridge University Press, 1989.

29. Sehgal A, Galbraith A, Chesney M et al. How strictly do dialysis patients want their advance directives followed? *JAMA* 1992; **267**(1): 59–63.

30. Kopelman LM. Children as research subjects: a dilemma. *J Med Philos* 2000; **25**(6): 745–64.

31. Lyerly AD, Little MO, Faden RR. Pregnancy and clinical research. *Hastings Cent Rep* 2008 (Nov–Dec); **38**(6): inside back cover.

32. Dresser R. Mentally disabled research subjects. The enduring policy issues. *JAMA* 1996; **276**(1): 67–72.

33. Hoffman S. Beneficial and unusual punishment: an argument in support of prisoner participation in clinical trials. *Indiana Law Rev* 2000; **33**(2): 475–515.

34. National Bioethics Advisory Commission. Research involving persons with mental disorders that may affect decision-making capacity, vol. 1: Report and Recommendations of the National Bioethics Advisory Commission, Dec 1998. At http://bioethics.georgetown.edu/nbac/capacity/TOC.htm, accessed 5 Feb 2010.

35. Wendler D, Prasad K. Core safeguards for clinical research with adults who are unable to consent. *Ann Intern Med* 2001; **135**(7): 514–23.

36. Stocking CB, Hougham GW, Danner DD et al. Speaking of research advance directives: planning for future research participation. *Neurology* 2006; **66**(9): 1361–6.

37. Fox GK, Bowden SC, Bashford GM, Smith DS. Alzheimer's disease and driving: prediction and assessment of driving performance. *J Am Geriatr Soc* 1997; **45**(8): 949–53.

38. Dubinsky RM, Stein AC, Lyons K. Practice parameter: risk of driving and Alzheimer's disease (an evidence-based review): report of the quality standards subcommittee of the American Academy of Neurology. *Neurology* 2000; **54**(12): 2205–11.

39. *The National Voter Registration Act of 1993* ('The Motor Voter Act'). Pub L No. 103-31, 107 Stat 77 (codified as amended at 42 USC 1973gg).

40. Karlawish JH, Casarett DA, James BD, Propert KJ, Asch DA. Do persons with dementia vote? *Neurology* 2002; **58**(7): 1100–2.

41. Orgogozo JM, Gilman S, Dartigues JF et al. Subacute meningoencephalitis in a subset of patients with AD after Abeta42 immunization. *Neurology* 2003; **61**(1): 46–54.

42. Shega JW, Hougham GW, Stocking CB, Cox-Hayley D, Sachs GA. Barriers to limiting the practice of feeding tube placement in advanced dementia. *J Palliat Med* 2003; **6**: 885–93.

43. Mitchell SL, Berkowitz RE, Lawson FM. A cross-national survey of tube-feeding decisions in cognitively impaired older persons. *J Am Geriatr Soc* 2000; **48**: 391–7.

44. Finucane TE, Christmas C, Travis K. Tube feeding in patients with advanced dementia: a review of the evidence. *JAMA* 1999; **282**: 1365–70.

45. Marks W. Physical restraints in the practice of medicine. Current concepts. *Arch Intern Med* 1992; **152**(11): 2203–6.

46. Miles S. A case of death by physical restraint: new lessons from a photograph. *J Am Geriatr Soc* 1996; **44**(3): 291–2.

47. Tinetti ME, Liu WL, Marottoli RA, Ginter SF. Mechanical restraint use among residents of skilled nursing facilities. Prevalence, patterns, and predictors. *JAMA* 1991; **265**(4): 468–71.

66

Successful Interventions for Family Caregivers

L. McKenzie Zeiss[1], Yookyung Kwon[2], Renee Marquett[2] and Dolores Gallagher-Thompson[2]

[1]*University of California, Irvine, CA, USA*
[2]*Stanford Geriatric Education Center, Palo Alto, CA, USA*

INTRODUCTION

In the United States, an estimated 5.3 million people have Alzheimer's disease today[1]; that number is projected to grow to 13.2 million by 2050[2]. In the UK, approximately 700 000 people have some form of dementia, and that number is expected to top 1 million by 2025[3]. Most dementia patients will eventually need some form of care, and informal caregivers (usually family members) provide most of that care. It is estimated that there are about 9 million informal caregivers in the United States[1] and 4 million in England[3]. Family caregiving, although it allows dementia patients to stay in their homes with their loved ones longer and is less financially costly than nursing home care, places an immense strain on the caregivers.

Caregiving is difficult work, and dementia caregiving is particularly stressful[4]. Dementia family caregivers have higher rates of nearly every form of psychiatric and psychological distress, especially depression – several studies that used psychiatric interviews to evaluate caregivers found that rates of major depressive disorder were around 30% – considerably higher than anticipated in the general adult population[5]. Caregivers also report more physical health problems than non-caregivers, and numerous studies have found that compromised immune system function, changes in blood pressure and disrupted HPA axis function are common[6]. Although these indicators of stress are well documented, the development and careful evaluation of theoretically grounded interventions to address these problems and symptoms have been slow. Recent studies have begun to use better methodology and to show significant decreases in caregiver stress and depression. This chapter will describe assessment of caregiver distress, then review evidence-based treatments (EBTs) and other promising approaches emerging in the field today.

CAREGIVER STRESS

Dementia caregiving is stressful for many reasons. Caregivers are watching the inevitable decline of a loved one, often their significant other. They are often elderly themselves and face their own declining health. Family caregivers shoulder the intense burden of daily care activities, ranging from taking over the care recipient's finances to feeding and toileting. The constantly increasing level of care required over the course of a progressive illness like Alzheimer's disease deprives caregivers of time for their own activities and opportunities

for social support, and can even compromise their jobs and their ability to meet obligations to other family members. Yet many caregivers also feel there are positive aspects of caregiving that tremendously benefit their lives[7].

The 'stress process' model has guided our understanding of caregiving for almost 20 years[9]. This model describes how caregivers use resources (both internal and external) to respond to the demands of their caregiving situation and other life circumstances (e.g. job, spouse, children). This process takes place within a sociocultural context. Perceived stress is a function of the extent to which demands exceed resources and the requisite coping skills to manage these demands are no longer adequate to the tasks at hand.

One must also take into account such 'individual difference' variables as age, gender, ethnicity, relationship and socioeconomic status, which interact with objective stressors and resources and play important roles in determining which caregivers develop physical and/or emotional problems in response to their situations. For example, spousal caregivers are particularly susceptible to depression and stress[10]. Being female and being married to the care recipient tend to be related to lower levels of both physical health and psychological well-being[11]. A caregiver's age is also significant: younger caregivers and non-spouses are more likely to experience role strain, which is usually magnified by lack of resources and perceived intensity of caregiving-related stressors[11].

Cultural diversity is another important dimension that adds heuristic value to the stress process model. Many studies find that cultural differences affect multiple aspects of caregiving. Racial/ethnic groups vary greatly in how they perceive objective and subjective stressors, the knowledge they have and the use they make of resources, and the kinds of coping skills they prefer to employ to help them manage their situations[11–14].[i] For example, Caucasian/white caregivers are

---

[i]There is great divergence in empirical findings on cultural differences, and to date there have been only a small number of studies on Asian-American and Hispanic caregivers. In order to give equal balance to each ethnic group and resolve heterogeneous or conflicting results, we rely here on available meta-analyses and reviews rather than individual studies. Note also that the terms 'Asian-American' and 'Hispanic' refer to very heterogeneous groups in terms of language, cultural heritage and socioeconomic status. These terms are used in this chapter because they are current designations used in the US Census; however, for clinical purposes, information about specific sub-groups is needed to work effectively – rather than relying on broad generalizations that may or may not be accurate or apply to the individual caregiver in your office.

Principles and Practice of Geriatric Psychiatry, 3rd edn. Edited by Mohammed T. Abou-Saleh, Cornelius Katona and Anand Kumar
© 2011 John Wiley & Sons, Ltd

more likely to be married to the care recipient and report higher levels of caregiver stress, burden and depression than African-American caregivers[14]. They tend to use more formal support, such as attending support groups and receiving help from professionals, than non-white caregivers. However, Caucasian/white caregivers also tend to report lower levels of confidence and mastery and less positive appraisal of caregiving compared to ethnic minority caregivers[11,13,14].

African-American caregivers often report more role strain, such as more cognitive and physical impairment of the care recipient and a higher number of caregiving tasks, than white caregivers[11]. Their use of religious coping and their sharing of caregiving responsibilities with extended family and non-family members seem to buffer the impact of objective stressors. They express lower subjective burden, higher levels of mastery and greater satisfaction, and fewer depressive symptoms than white or Asian caregivers[12,13].

Asian-American and Hispanic/Latino caregivers may have language limitations, strong beliefs in filial obligation and low levels of both acculturation and health literacy. Combined, these factors make caregiving more stressful. Such caregivers are often reluctant to admit their distress openly, relying instead on more indirect means of expression. For example, Chinese-American caregivers tend to present with a high level of somatic complaints; Mexican-American caregivers often present with depression and guilt[13]. Those who have limited knowledge of English for both reading and writing also have less accurate information about dementia and less access to the health-care system in general and use fewer formal support services than do their Caucasian/white counterparts[11].

While cultural beliefs and practices, such as strong family ties and religiosity, can buffer and protect caregivers from negative health outcomes of caregiving, other cultural premises such as filial obligation, the priority of family needs over individual needs, and face saving carry special hazards. Many ethnic minority caregivers regard it as shameful or a 'loss of face' to admit caregiving-related distress. They are likely to under-report care recipients' behavioural and other problems, and to be reluctant to use formal services for elderly family members. Asian-Americans and Hispanics, in particular, may have low levels of acculturation, language barriers, and inadequate health literacy, which may lead to cultural isolation and inability to access services that are currently available in the US health-care system.

ASSESSMENT OF FAMILY CAREGIVERS

Current psychiatric practice emphasizes assessment and treatment of the patient with dementia[15]. We recommend a dyadic focus in which caregivers are also assessed and treated. Dementia family caregivers (across all racial and ethnic groups studied to date) are at risk of poor physical health and increased mortality, depression, anxiety, anger, frustration and feelings of grief and loss. A clinician should first assess a caregiver for serious difficulty in one or more areas; any diagnosable psychiatric disorders should be treated promptly with either pharmacotherapy or psychotherapy.

Existing guidelines suggest a variety of approaches for assessing the psychosocial and psychiatric status of the dementia family caregiver[15]. We suggest reviewing the Family Caregiver Alliance's recommendations on domains to assess[16,17]. An easily downloaded 'kit' of these resources, including actual measures and the 'Caregivers Count Too!' toolkit for practitioners[18], is available free from its website. These provide materials needed to follow up problem areas with detailed assessment and begin directing caregivers towards treatment.

Key Domains to Assess

First: Assess the caregiver's *knowledge of dementia*. A crucial part of understanding the disease process is knowledge of what to expect as a caregiver. Practitioners should assess medical knowledge of the dementing illness and familiarity with problems caregivers commonly face. It is helpful to have brochures on hand to send home with caregivers, and to have a list of specific websites, such as the Family Caregiver Alliance (www.caregiver.org), Alzheimer's Disease Education and Referral Center (ADEAR, sponsored by the National Institute on Aging in the US) (www.nia.nih.gov/Alzheimers/), National Alliance for Caregiving (www.caregiving.org), and the national website of the Alzheimer's Association in the US (www.alz.org). Several of these groups provide free, downloadable materials about dementia, managing caregiver stress and handling common behaviour problems, in multiple languages besides English. Local chapters of many of these organizations also offer free support groups.

Second: Assess *basic safety needs* of both caregiver and care recipient. Driving, for instance, is a common safety concern, and caregivers are often grateful for physicians' insistence that care recipients give up their car keys permanently. Other environmental issues – can the care recipient be safely left alone and for how long? Does he/she smoke? – are also essential points to cover. Hints of abuse by either the caregiver or care recipient are also important targets that must be followed up with referrals to Adult Protective Services or similar agencies whose role is to investigate such claims and seek remedies for the situation.

Third: Assess caregivers' *emotional and physical well-being*. Several measures are available starting with the brief 'Caregiver Self-Assessment Questionnaire'[19] developed by the American Medical Association as a screening tool for caregiver stress. It is free and downloadable from the AMA website.

The new 16-item Risk Appraisal Measure (RAM) was developed specifically for culturally diverse dementia caregivers and designed to provide a clear view of what treatments are indicated for a particular caregiver[20]. Short enough to be administered to the caregiver in the waiting room, it addresses depression, burden, self-care and health, social support and patient problem behaviours. It also assesses safety, focusing on risks associated with both caregiver behaviours (those suggesting an abuse risk) and care recipient behaviours (e.g. continued driving). Caregivers' answers indicate areas for further assessment or treatment. The RAM is available free of charge and can be obtained in English or Spanish from the study authors.

Other common areas to assess are depressive symptoms and extent of perceived burden. Depressive symptoms can be evaluated quickly and reliably using the CES-D scale[21] or the Geriatric Depression Scale[22]. The CES-D measures the frequency of occurrence of common symptoms of depression in the past week. The CES-D is not copyrighted and is available free of charge from numerous online sources.

The Geriatric Depression Scale is widely used in the US and other countries as a screen for depression. It was designed to tap psychological aspects of depression. Its simple 'yes/no' response format makes it easy to use with low-literacy caregivers. It is available free of charge and can be downloaded in many languages from the website: www.stanford.edu/~yesavage/GDS.html.

Perceived burden can be assessed using the Zarit Burden Inventory[23]. Many other scales exist to assess this and other relevant domains, but due to space constraints we cannot describe them all; see citations 15 and 16 for details.

Fourth: Assess the care recipient's *cognitive status* and ability to perform activities of daily living. As dementia progresses and cognitive impairment increases, the care recipient's functional abilities will decline, resulting in increased hours of care and increasingly demanding tasks. Often caregivers of patients in the middle stage of dementia are the most stressed since behavioural problems are most common then. They need to learn flexibility and creative problem solving. They must be willing to accept the level of care the patient requires, and must have the personal, social and socioeconomic resources to provide that care. While advanced skills for dealing with problem behaviours are a common target of effective intervention programmes even for highly skilled caregivers, a caregiver who does not recognize that a patient can no longer be safely left alone, or who is not able to help with the patient's basic needs, is not able to provide adequate care.

Fifth: Assess the caregiver's perception of instrumental and emotional *social support*. Such support can substantially decrease stress and also improve the quality of care the care recipient receives. Often, caregivers are unaware of available community- or hospital-based support services or feel too overwhelmed to research them; however, day and respite care are invaluable adjuncts to treatment for distressed caregivers[24]. Resources to assess include help from family and friends, transportation, legal and other professional services and financial assistance. The Administration on Aging's Eldercare Locator (www.eldercare.gov/eldercare.net/public/home.aspx) directs caregivers to the resources available to them locally. The Alzheimer's Association CareFinder service (www.alz.org/carefinder) is also an excellent guide.

Assessing Diverse Caregivers

Clinicians' cultural competence leads to more or less effective interactions with ethnically diverse patients and caregivers. 'Cultural competence' encompasses both clinicians' attitudes and knowledge about ethnic groups and their specific skills for interacting with them. The Stanford Geriatric Education Center (http://sgec.stanford.edu) provides online training in improving communication with ethnically diverse elderly; the *Diversity Toolbox* (Alzheimer's Association, www.alz.org) is likewise a useful resource. The book *Ethnicity and the Dementias*[25] is also a good source of information about working with ethnically diverse dementia patients and caregivers. A few points apply broadly to many minority groups: (i) health-care providers need to include the family unit. Ethnic elders generally prefer to be cared for by family, who often see caring for elderly parents and relatives as a family responsibility[26]; (ii) assess ethnic minority caregivers' health literacy and cultural and linguistic competency. Low education levels, language barriers and low levels of acculturation are related to lower health literacy, which in turn affects ability to comply with treatment plans and access appropriate services. There are explicit assessment tools to measure health literacy[27] and implicit screening strategies such as asking caregivers to bring all medications and explain them, or handing caregivers a written document upside down to see if they turn it over to read; (iii) practitioners need to enhance the comprehensibility of health messages, use culturally appropriate examples and materials, and use a team approach involving practitioners, family, culturally and linguistically competent counsellors and translators.

BEST PRACTICES FOR HELPING CAREGIVERS WITH STRESS

What are the Evidence-Based Treatments?

The most recent reviews[28,29] of evidence-based psychological treatments (EBTs) note that three modalities show consistent effectiveness: psychoeducational small group programmes focused on teaching caregivers skills for coping with depression, frustration and common behavioural problems; cognitive behavioural psychotherapy (for those in need of more extensive treatment); and multi-component interventions combining several approaches. Other approaches, particularly respite care, show some promising results but have not yet met criteria for EBT. Support groups are important pieces to consider in multimodal approaches but are not empirically supported standalone treatments for caregiver distress. Gallagher-Thompson and Coon[28] found that evidence-based psychoeducational and psychotherapeutic treatments had the most empirical support, and in general produced large effect sizes. They further concluded that interventions combining support with skills building and targeting specific quality-of-life components were the most effective overall.

From our review of this literature, we propose that five key factors delineate the most effective treatments. They are:

1. **Treatment should be drawn from evidence-based practice.** Treating dementia caregivers is particularly difficult because of the intense stress they face in daily life. The most successful interventions for caregivers' distress are drawn from the same pool as those most successful with other patients. Well-supported modalities rooted in cognitive behavioural therapy and stress-management theory work well with caregivers. For example, individual cognitive behaviour therapy is an effective treatment for caregivers with a diagnosable disorder such as major depressive disorder. Psychoeducational programmes work well to teach behavioural management[30], depression management[31], effective communication and relaxation and stress management[32].

2. **Treatment should require active participation.** Some educational interventions consist of giving caregivers printed materials to complement a lecture delivered to the group. Others take a more 'Socratic' pedagogical approach, actively soliciting input from group members and encouraging them to discuss and question the materials. While both approaches might increase knowledge, neither does much to guide caregivers in the implementation of that knowledge – a feature that some researchers[33] suggest is far more important than what precise materials are covered or what pedagogical style a leader takes. 'Active participation' consists of participation in discussion of new skills and actively putting those skills into practice, with regular check-ins to ensure caregivers are using what they have learned. Using role-playing exercises and 'homework' assignments are ways to support this learning.

3. **Treatment should be tailored to meet individual needs.** Effective treatment begins with assessing a caregiver's areas of strength and weakness, setting specific goals and determining which avenues to pursue most vigorously. Imagine a caregiver who complains of depressed mood and low social support, and

has trouble getting her care recipient's physician to address her concerns, but who has no other pressing complaints. Skills training tailored to managing depression, increasing social support and communicating assertively (especially with medical professionals) is recommended. She would benefit less from a one-size-fits-all programme stressing relaxation exercises, for example, or from a programme that covers quality of life as a general domain without any specific targets. Some other specific guidelines suggested by the reviews and analyses include referring depressed caregivers for treatment. For those with sub-clinical distress, refer to a psychoeducational group; for those whose stress is very high, refer to a stress-management programme[28]. Likewise, caregivers with more severe distress tend to require longer periods of treatment[8]. Finally, as Alzheimer's and other dementias are progressive illnesses, caregivers' specific profiles are likely to change over time as their caregiving situations change. Support groups are useful for learning about this process.

4. **Treatment should be tailored to caregivers' individual differences.** These include gender, age, family relationship, education, socioeconomic resources, ethnicity and language issues.

   – Gender: Although female caregivers are generally more distressed and show greater levels of distress initially, male caregivers remain more distressed after treatment[34] and so may require more intensive treatment to achieve the same improvement. More research is needed with male caregivers since intervention studies are few.

   – Age and family relationship: Spousal caregivers are usually older than adult child caregivers. Even when controlling for age, spousal caregivers show higher levels of depression[35] and are less responsive to treatment[28,34]. There are, as yet, no studies showing a solid basis for preferring specific treatments for spousal caregivers as opposed to other caregivers, though preliminary research[8] suggests that couples and family therapies may be of more help for them.

   – Education and socioeconomic status: Numerous studies have found that caregivers who begin treatment with low education and resources improve more quickly and dramatically than their more-educated peers[34,35]. Caregivers who have more knowledge about dementia and more access to support resources, but are still distressed, may not be helped much by extra information. They are therefore more likely to require psychotherapy or extended psychoeducational/skills-building programmes. At the same time, caregivers of lower socioeconomic status are less likely to avail themselves of services in the first place, so for these populations outreach is especially important.

   – Ethnicity and cultural issues: Intervention with dementia caregivers is an active process that consists of conceptualizing individual caregiving contexts, identifying specific demands and vulnerabilities, and designing and implementing interventions for individuals of different cultural backgrounds. For example, REACH II, the largest randomized control trial on caregiver interventions to date and the only one meeting CONSORT standards, suggested different intervention targets for each race/ethnic group[11]. Overall, the interventions produced statistically significant improvement on all short-term outcomes. Among African-American caregivers, however, only spousal caregivers benefited from the treatment. Furthermore, while all intervention groups except African-American non-spousal caregivers had lower depression scores, only white caregivers showed lower rates of clinical depression at

six months. Based on these outcomes, REACH researchers have suggested refining treatments further. White caregivers were more likely to experience intrapsychic strain, and to benefit most from interventions that target this (e.g., learning to regulate negative emotions). In contrast, Hispanic caregivers might benefit from psychoeducational interventions that increase knowledge of dementia processes, resources and services, and that train them to respond effectively to memory and behaviour problems. African-Americans tend to experience financial strain, and might benefit from interventions that provide financial support, e.g. respite-type services.

Finally, because minorities often place particular emphasis on familism and filial duty, family-based interventions may be particularly useful. They have been found to improve family communication and sharing of the caregiving role[8,11,36,37]. Further research is needed to support the usefulness of this approach with ethnically diverse caregivers.

5. **Consider multi-component treatments.** Although there is not a great deal of empirical data on multi-component treatments, it seems reasonable to expect a greater 'yield' from combining two or more approaches when possible. For examples, findings from Mittelman[38] and REACH I[37] suggest that multi-component treatments may be particularly effective at delaying nursing home placement and at reaching otherwise inaccessible groups.

One of the difficulties with this is that, precisely because they do combine multiple approaches, these interventions are a heterogeneous group and it can be challenging to figure out which component is really having the main effect. For example, a novel delivery system (such as the telephone-computer technology used in Miami during REACH I) counts as a 'component', even though a telephone or computer is not a means of treatment in and of itself. Yet because some caregivers face difficulties in attending appointments, telephone-based treatments may make interventions more accessible to them. New programmes along these lines that need more study include the Savvy Caregiver Program[39], which includes take-home information for use at home, and Powerful Tools for Caregivers, a web-based psychoeducational programme[40]. New web-based programmes are currently in development and may be very useful at replacing at least some individual or small group meetings. Whether they should be viewed as 'supplements' or 'standalone' interventions requires additional research.

OTHER SUPPORT SERVICES FOR CAREGIVERS

Support groups are immensely popular, are usually free, have a long history and are readily available in most communities. However, support groups are not EBTs, as they simply do not have an empirical basis consistently demonstrating effectiveness.

Gallagher-Thompson and Coon[28] noted in their review that no methodologically sound study has shown support groups to be effective unless combined with another active therapy. Some studies have even shown worse outcomes for support-group participants[41]. Pinquart and Sorensön found in their meta-analyses[34,35,42] that support group interventions generally underperformed on all measures of caregiver distress, concluding that they had fewer positive effects for dementia caregivers than they did for other types of caregivers studied. At the same time, support groups are recognized as a valuable adjunct to EBTs. When possible, clinicians should direct caregivers to other treatment options as well as support groups, and should clarify caregivers' expectations about what they may get out of a support group. Many caregivers subjectively report that support groups are extremely valuable to them for the social support and 'normalization' they provide. Used in combination with EBTs, support groups can be very helpful as dementia progresses.

Many other services are available to caregivers, including pharmacotherapy, case management, respite care, environmental management/modification and technology-based programmes. At least two studies support case management for improving caregivers' quality of life[43,44]. Respite care has been shown to be effective in reducing caregiver burden when used at least twice a week for at least three months. Its cost-effectiveness improves with increased use, suggesting that higher levels of funding for respite care to allow regular, long-term use might be a cost-effective public health policy[45-47]. Respite care can delay nursing home placement[45], especially among minorities. Even in low doses, many find respite care extremely welcome as an occasional relief.

Programmes focused on modifying the home environment and teaching caregivers skills for engaging the care recipient in everyday pleasurable activities have also shown promise[48]. This approach improves safety in the home and encourages positive interaction between caregiver and care recipient. It was especially helpful for elderly, poor, inner-city African-American families who would not otherwise have funds to make environmental modifications (e.g. installing grab bars in the bathroom, removing slippery rugs that could contribute to falls).

New technology-based programmes may be helpful for rural caregivers who are unable to travel to city centres for programmes. Although there are limitations to what these programmes can provide, they may meet the needs of some caregivers who otherwise would not have assistance[49,50]. These and other programmes show promise, and it is likely that additional research will support their efficacy, at least to some extent.

WHERE IS THIS FIELD GOING IN THE NEXT DECADE?

While we are gaining in our knowledge of 'what works' to reduce depression, improve adaptive coping skills and reduce caregiving-related burden, there is still considerable room for improvement. For example, the patchwork of services that can be found in one state or region of the US may not be available in other states, there is little coordination of care, and there are still very few culturally appropriate services and programmes for caregivers (and care recipients) who are mono-lingual or whose primary language is not English. Given the fact that ethnic minority older adults are a rapidly increasing segment of the US population, their needs will only continue to grow. Programmes that meet their needs *and* are evidence-based are sorely lacking at this time.

A particular challenge facing this field is the lack of research to develop 'practice guidelines' for working with caregivers similar to those that now exist in other areas of medicine. There is also a lack of substantial data on how to match effectively the client/patient in your office with existing programmes and providers. The study of what level of care and what kinds of services are needed to adequately treat a given caregiver is just beginning – but it is being pushed forward at a rapid pace because of the expected onslaught of the baby boomers. From a public policy perspective, progress in this area is essential.

A final area for study is how long-term caregiving affects caregivers' physical health. Although we have some information, it is not extensive, due in part to the difficulty securing funding to conduct long-term follow-up studies with caregivers at high risk for development of, say, type II diabetes or coronary artery disease. Since these conditions typically develop over a period of years, long-term follow-up is needed. New programmes that focus on modification of caregiver health habits are underway; it may be the combination of interventions focused on improving both physical *and* mental health that will have the greatest success with this population in the long run.

REFERENCES

1. Alzheimer's Association. 2009 Alzheimer's disease facts and figures. *Alzheimers Dement* 2009; **5**(3): 234–70.
2. Herbert LE, Sherr PA, Bienias JL *et al*. Alzheimer disease in the US population: prevalence estimates using the 2000 census. *Arch Neurol* 2003; **60**(8): 1119–22.
3. Alzheimer's Society. *Dementia UK: The Full Report*. London: Alzheimer's Society, 2007.
4. Ory MG, Hoffman RR, Yee JL *et al*. (1999) Prevalence and impact of caregiving: a detailed comparison between dementia and nondementia caregivers. *Gerontologist*; **39**: 177–85.
5. Pinquart M, Sorensön S. Differences between caregivers and noncaregivers in psychological health and physical health: a meta-analysis. *Psychol Aging* 2003; **18**: 250–67.
6. Vitaliano PP, Zhang J, Scanlan JM. Is caregiving hazardous to one's physical health? A meta-analysis. *Psychol Bull* 2003; **20**: 946–72.
7. Tarlow BJ, Wisniewski SR, Belle SH, Rubert M, Ory MG, Gallagher-Thompson, D. Positive aspects of caregiving: Contributions of the REACH project to the development of new measures for Alzheimer's caregiving. *Res Aging* 2004; **26**(4): 429–53.
8. Sorensön S, King D, Pinquart M. Care of the caregiver: Individual and family interventions. In Sheila ML (ed.), *Supporting the Caregiver in Dementia: A Guide for Health Care Professionals*. Baltimore: Johns Hopkins Press, 2006, 168–91.
9. Pearlin LI, Mullan JT, Semple SJ *et al*. Caregiving and the stress process: an overview of concepts and their measures. *Gerontologist* 1990; **30**: 583–94.
10. George LK, Gwyther LP. Caregiver well-being: a multidimensional examination of family caregivers of demented adults. *Gerontologist* 1986; **26**: 253–9.
11. Hilgeman MM, Durkin DW, Sun F, DeCoster J, Allen RS, Gallagher-Thompson D, Burgio LD. Testing a theoretical model of the stress process in Alzheimer's caregivers with race as a moderator. *Gerontologist* 2009; **49**: 248–61.
12. Knight BG, Silverstein M, McCullum TJ, Fox LS. A sociocultural stress and coping model for mental health outcomes among African-American caregivers in Southern California. *J Gerontol Psychol Sci* 2000; **55**: 142–50.
13. Pinquart M, Sorensön S. Ethnic differences in stressors, resources, and psychological outcomes of family caregiving: a meta-analysis. *Gerontologist* 2005; **45**: 90–106.
14. Connell CM, Gibson GD. Racial, ethnic, cultural differences in dementia caregiving: review and analysis. *Gerontologist* 1997; **37**: 355–64.
15. Thompson LW, Spira AP, Depp CA, McGee JS, Gallagher-Thompson D. The geriatric caregiver. In Agronin ME, Maletta GJ (eds.), *Principles and Practice of Geriatric Psychiatry*. Philadelphia: Lippincott Williams & Wilkins, 2006, 37–48.

16. Family Caregiver Alliance. *Caregiver Assessment, Principles, Guidelines and Strategies for Change: Volume 1*. San Francisco, CA: Family Caregiver Alliance, April 2006.

17. Family Caregiver Alliance. *Caregiver Assessment: Voices and Views from the Field: Volume II*. San Francisco, CA: Family Caregiver Alliance, April 2008.

18. Family Caregiver Alliance. *Caregivers Count Too!* At www.caregiver.org/caregiver/jsp/content_node.jsp?nodeid=1695, accessed 25 June 2009.

19. American Medical Association. Caregiver Self-Assesment. At www.ama-assn.org/ama/pub/physician-resources/public-health/promoting-healthy-lifestyles/geriatric-health/caregiver-health/caregiver-self-assessment.shtml, accessed 25 June 2009.

20. Czaja SJ, Gitlin LN, Schulz R, Zhang S, Burgio LD, Stevens AB *et al.* Development of the risk appraisal measure: a brief screen to identify risk areas and guide interventions for dementia caregivers. *J Am Geriatr Soc* 2009; **57**: 1064–72.

21. Radloff L. The CES-D scale: a self-report scale for research in the general population. *Appl Psychol Meas* 1977; 1: 385–401.

22. Yesavage JA, Brink TL, Rose TL, Lum O, Huang V, Adey M Leirer VO. Development and validation of a geriatric depression screening scale: a preliminary report. *J Psychiatr Res* 1982; **17**: 37–49.

23. Zarit SH, Todd PA, Zarit JM. Subjective burden of husbands and wives as caregivers: a longitudinal study. *Gerontologist* 1986; **26**: 260–70.

24. Zarit SH, Gaugler JE, Jarrott SE. Useful services for families: research findings and directions. *Int J Geriatr Psychiatry* 1999; **14**: 165–81.

25. Yeo G, Gallagher-Thompson D (eds), *Ethnicity and the Dementias*, 2nd edn. New York: Routledge, 2006.

26. Gallagher-Thompson D. The family as the unit of assessment and treatment in work with ethnically diverse older adults with dementia. In Yeo G, Gallagher-Thompson D (eds), *Ethnicity and the Dementias*, 2nd edn. New York: Routledge, 2006.

27. Davis TC, Long SW, Jackson RH, Mayeaux EJ, George RB, Murphy PW. Rapid estimate of adult literacy in medicine: a shortened screening instrument (REALM). *Fam Med* 1993; **25**: 391–5.

28. Gallagher-Thompson D, Coon DW. Evidence-based psychological treatments for distress in family caregivers of older adults. *Psychol Aging* 2007; **22**(1): 37–51.

29. United States Administration on Aging. Alzheimer's disease supportive services program (ADSSP) resource compendium, 2009. At http://www.aoa.gov/AoARoot/AoA_Programs/HCLTC/Alz_Grants/compendium.aspx#toolkits, accessed 25 June 2009.

30. Bourgeois MS, Schulz R, Burgio L, Beach S. Skills training for spouses of patients with Alzheimer's disease: outcomes of an intervention study. *J Clin Geropsychol* 2002; **8**: 53–73.

31. Coon D, Thompson LW, Steffen S, Sorocco K, Gallagher-Thompson D. Anger and depression management: psychoeducational skill training interventions for women caregivers of a relative with dementia. *Gerontologist* 2003; **43**: 678–89.

32. Steffen AM. Anger management for dementia caregivers: a preliminary study using video and telephone interviews. *Behav Ther* 2000; **31**: 281–99.

33. Belle SH, Czaja SJ, Schulz R, Zhang S, Burgio L, Gitlin LN *et al.*) Using a new taxonomy to combine the uncombinable: integrating results across diverse interventions. *Psychol Aging* 200; **318**: 396–405.

34. Pinquart M, Sorensön S. Helping caregivers of persons with dementia: which interventions work and how large are their effects? *International Psychogeriatrics* 2006; **18**(4): 577–95.

35. Pinquart M, Sorensön S. Caregiving distress and psychological health of caregivers. In Oxington KV (ed.), *Psychology of Stress*. New York: Nova Science, 2005, 165–206.

36. Gitlin LN, Belle SH, Burgio LD *et al.* Effect of multi-component interventions on caregiver burden and depression: the REACH multisite initiative at 6-month follow-up. *Psychol Aging* 2003; **18**: 361–74.

37. Qualls SH. Caregiver family therapy. In Laidlaw K, Knight B (eds), *Handbook of Emotional Disorders in Later Life*. Oxford: Oxford University Press, 2008, 183–209.

38. Mittelman MS, Haley WE, Clay OJ, Roth DL. Improving caregiver well-being delays nursing home placement of patients with Alzheimer disease. *Neurology* 2006; **67**: 1592–9.

39. Hepburn KW, Lewis M, Sherman CW, Tornatore J. The Savvy Caregiver Program: developing a transportable dementia family caregiver training program. *Gerontologist* 2003; **43**: 908–15.

40. Mather LifeWays Institute. *Proven Benefits for Family Caregivers*, 2006. At www.matherlifeways.com/re_ptcbenefits.asp, accessed 25 June 2009.

41. Gonyea JG. Alzheimer's disease support group participation and caregiver well-being. *Clin Gerontol* 1990; **10**: 17–34.

42. Sorensön S, Pinquart M, Duberstein P. How effective are interventions with caregivers? An updated meta-analysis. *Gerontologist* 2002; **42**(3): 356–72.

43. Callahan CM, Boustani MA, Unverzagt FW, Austrom MC, Damush TM, Perkins AJ *et al.* Effectiveness of collaborative care for older adults with Alzheimer disease in primary care: a randomized controlled trial. JAMA 2006; 295: 2148–57.

44. Bass DM, Clark PA, Looman WJ, McCarthy CA, Eckert S. The Cleveland Alzheimer's Managed Care Demonstration: outcomes after 12 months of implementation. *Gerontologist* 2003; **43**: 73–85.

45. Wilson RS, McCann JJ, Li Y, Aggarwal NT, Gilley DW, Evans DA. Nursing home placement, day care use, and cognitive decline in Alzheimer's disease. *Am J Psychiatry* 2007; **164**: 910–15.

46. Gaugler JE, Zarit SH, Townsend A, Stephens MAP, Greene R. Evaluating community-based programs for dementia caregivers: the cost implications of adult day services. *J Appl Gerontol* 2003; **22**: 118–33.

47. Zarit SH, Stephens MAP, Townsend A, Greene R, Femia EE. Give day care a chance to be effective: A commentary. *Journal of Gerontology: Psychol Sci* 2003; **58B**: P195–9.

48. Gitlin LN, Winter L, Earland TV, Herge EA, Chernett NL, Piersol CV *et al.* The Tailored Activity Program to reduce behavioral symptoms in individuals with dementia: feasibility, acceptability, and replication potential. *Gerontologist* 2009; **49**: 428–39.

49. Glueckauf RL, Ketterson TU. Telehealth interventions for individuals with chronic illness: research review and implications for practice. *Prof Psychol Res Pract* 2004; **35**: 615–27.

50. Glueckauf RL, Young ME, Stine C, Bourgeois M, Pomidor A, Massey A *et al.* Alzheimer's Rural Care Healthline: Linking rural dementia caregivers to cognitive-behavioural interventions for depression. *Rehab Psychol* 2005; **50**: 346–54.

67

The Role of Alzheimer Societies in the United States

Ruth O'Hara[1,2] and Bevin Powers[1,2]

[1]*Department of Psychiatry and Behavioral Sciences, Stanford University School of Medicine, USA*
[2]*VA Sierra-Pacific Mental Illness Research Education and Clinical Center, Palo Alto, USA*

Alzheimer's disease (AD) is listed by the Center for Disease Control and Prevention (CDC) as the sixth leading cause of death in the United States. Currently there are 5.3 million people diagnosed with AD[1], and it is estimated that one in eight people aged 65 or older will develop AD[2]. As the baby-boomer generation approaches older age, the need for medical care and caregivers will be immense. Incidence rates are projected to double every 20 years with the aging of the baby boomers, therefore, it is predicted that 7.7 million people will be diagnosed with AD by 2030, and by 2050, AD is estimated to reach between 11 million and 16 million people[1]. The psychological, social and financial costs of this illness are substantial, with approximately $148 billion per year in medical expenses[1].

Alzheimer's disease societies can be traced back to the 1950s with the forming of the National Counsel of Aging whose aim was to improve the lives of aging Americans[3]. From that point forward additional AD societies in the United States were created for multiple reasons, however largely humanitarian. Table 67.1 lists AD societies in the United States. As the prevalence of AD increases, the need for caregivers and services will be astronomical.

Approximately 54% of the US population has been touched in some way by AD, either having a family member diagnsed with AD, or knowing someone who has been diagnosed with AD[1]. In 2009 alone, AD contributed to the death of 660 000 Americans which continues to climb each year. AD produces more deaths compared to AIDS (16 316), prostate cancer (27 350), Parkinson's disease (17 898) and hepatitis C (12 000)[4]. Yet, the disparity of funds allotted to AD research compared to other diseases is striking. In 2007, the National Institute of Health (NIH) awarded AIDS research $2.9 billion, while AD research received $644 million[4]. As the frequency of AD diagnosis continues to climb with the growing aging population, the lack of caregivers, health-care professionals and burden on family and services will generate a national crisis.

Over the decades, AD societies have been developed in many ways to address these issues and gaps in service. These societies are dedicated to implementing and disseminating more effective treatments, assessment and supportive interdisciplinary services. The majority of AD societies particularly focus on the community need for resources, family needs and early detection and diagnosis. Some are more clinical and research oriented exploring prevention, the pathophysiological mechanisms and disease process, and ultimately, a cure. However, all provide levels of hope and support for victims of AD, their families and caregivers.

Alzheimer's disease societies have been shown to result in stress reduction in those diagnosed with AD or a caregiver for an individual with AD[5]. The burden of the disease and the quality of life are of great relevance to those who suffer from an illness or disease, and warrant careful consideration and comprehensive care. A number of AD societies aim to target care planning and other support needs required by the patient and their caregivers. However, it is estimated that those diagnosed with AD and caregivers do not seek support from AD societies for three years after diagnosis, and the support is often sought out only in a time of crisis[1]. Frequently, by the time support is obtained, patients with AD may be at a disadvantage; missing an opportunity to explore research options or other available treatments, advanced care planning, taking advantage of caregiver and family education and training, and establishing support before stress and burden have taxed the family and caregiver.

FEDERAL AGENCIES

As a federal agency of the United States Department of Health and Human Services agency, the Administration on Aging (AoA) has supported the Older Americans Act (OAA) of 1965 mandated programmes[6]. Also, the AoA awards research grants that support the needs of an aging population. Centers for Medicare and Medicaid Services also receive support from the AoA.

The AoA's primary interest is the aging population and caregiving, and it aims to invest in research, aging programmes and policy, including improvement of health care, aging in place, optimal aging and protecting the rights of older people. Some programmes are focused to provide home and community-based services such as home-delivered meals or nutrition services in congregate settings, or transportation, adult day care, legal assistance, health promotion programmes and local ombudsman[6]. In addition, AoA provides funding for a range of support services for family caregivers.

The US National Institutes of Health National Institute on Aging (NIA) is the aging and health scientific based agency of the NIH. By an act of Congress in 1974, the NIA was authorized to lead aged-focused research, training and health information distribution[7]. The NIA is the leading federal agency supporting research on Alzheimer's disease and other neurodegenerative disorders.

Through research, the NIA supports the well-being of older Americans with a primary focus on the aging processes, age-related diseases and distinct needs of the aged. The NIA train, develop and

Principles and Practice of Geriatric Psychiatry, 3rd edn. Edited by Mohammed T. Abou-Saleh, Cornelius Katona and Anand Kumar
© 2011 John Wiley & Sons, Ltd

Table 67.1 Alzheimer's disease societies in the US

Agency	Funding source	Description
Administration on Aging (AoA)	Federal	Awards research grants, provides home and community-based services including nutrition services, transportation, adult day care, legal assistance, health promotion programmes, ombudsman and support services for family caregivers
National Institute on Aging (NIA)	Federal	Health- and science-based agency focused on research, training and health information distribution
Alzheimer's Disease Cooperative Study (ADCS)	Federal	Primary aim is to conduct clinical trials on cognitive and behavioural treatments and interventions for AD
Alzheimer's Disease Neuroimaging Initiative (ADNI)	Federal	Primary aim is a worldwide clinical trial on MCI and AD, and to establish a database to improve future treatment trials
Alzheimer's Disease Centers (ADC)	Federal	Research focused on the mechanisms of AD, prevention, management and improvement of patient care. Also provides clinical and community programmes and services
National Alzheimer's Coordinating Center (NACC)	Federal	Provides collaborative research data collection, database, analysis, methodological and technical support.
The National Cell Repository for Alzheimer's disease (NCRAD)	Federal	National resource for clinical and genetic research, specifically housing a genetic databank
Alzheimer's Disease Education and Referral Center (ADEAR)	Federal	National archive centre for publications, audiovisual material. Responsible for dissemination for AD treatment and diagnostic information
The Geriatric Research, Education, Clinical Center (GRECC)	Federal	Primarily focused on research, education and clinical advancements for the care programmes and advancements in the quality of life of the aging veteran.
The Stanford Geriatric Education Center (SGEC)	Federal	Through academic and community educational dissemination the SGEC offers ethnogeriatric multidisciplinary education and didactics including health literacy, caregiving for dementia patients and other chronic disease, hospice and spirituality, ethics in geriatric care and emergency preparedness.
The National Association of Area Agencies on Aging (n4a)	Federal	Supports Agencies on Aging (AAA) to address support initiatives to assist older Americans through community-based and home services.
Stanford/VA/NIA Aging Clinical Research Center (ACRC)	Federal	Investigates normal cognitive aging and AD through medical and neuroscience disciplines to improve the lives of patients with memory loss
Memory and Aging Center	Federal/Private	Coordinating site for ADRC, conducts research, provides clinical services, education and outreach
Alzheimer's Disease Research Center (ADRC)	Federal	Focuses on laboratory and clinical studies in dementia and aging, improvements in diagnosis and treatments, and community education
Alzheimer's Caregiver Support Online (Alzonline)	Federal/Private	Provides online support for caregivers through education, information and support networks
Alzheimer's Association (AA)	Non-profit	Funds advance research, provides community support for AD or other dementias
Alzheimer's Foundation of America (AFA)	Non-profit	Several collaborating agencies dedicated to providing AD patients and families educational, social and emotional support
Association for Frontotemporal Dementias (AFTD)	Non-profit	Promotes and funds research and education for frontotemporal dementias
Alzheimer's Research & Prevention Foundation (ARPF)	Non-profit	Through the 4 Pillars of Alzheimer's Prevention programme, the agency provides training and educational opportunities for professionals and communities
Family Caregiver Alliance (FCA)	Non-profit	Supports caregivers with caring for those with AD or other chronic illnesses with local services tailored to each individual
The National Family Caregivers Association (NFCA)	Non-profit	Provides caregiver education, support and empowerment
The Lewy Body Dementia Association (LBDA)	Non-profit	Community support for family and caregivers, and research focused on scientific advances

Table 67.1 (*continued*)

Agency	Funding source	Description
National Council on Aging (NCOA)	Non-profit	Implements and disseminates programmes into communities to improve lives of older adults. Dedicates effort to raising awareness and lobbying for funding and programmes for the aging population
International Longevity Center	Non-profit	Research, education and policy driven to advance healthy aging, promotes productive engagement and to eliminate ageism
Institute on Aging (IOA)	Non-profit	Improves the quality of live for aging Americans in diverse community settings. Promotes independent living for older and disabled adults
National Alliance for Caregiving	Non-profit	Conducts research, analyses policy and produces programmes devoted to improving the quality of live for care recipients
Dementia Advocacy and Support Network (DASN)	Non-profit	Internet-based support group for individuals with dementia
American Federation for Aging Research (AFAR)	Non-profit	Research aimed at exploring the aging process and age-related diseases

support researchers in the field of aging, and place a funding priority on those research endeavours that will likely help illuminate the mechanisms underlying the pathological features of AD.

In 1991, the Alzheimer's Disease Cooperative Study (ADCS) was established by the National Institute on Aging's (NIA) Neuroscience and Neuropsychology of Aging Program, and the University of California San Diego[8]. Funded by the Federal Alzheimer's Disease Prevention Initiative, the ADCS clinical trials focus on cognitive and behavioural treatments for AD in response to an increased need to development of drugs that might be useful for treating patients with AD. The ADCS employs a multi-site approach to conduct pharmaceuticals clinical trials to test new treatments that may improve cognition, decrease decline and delay the onset or progression of AD. The ADCS offers over 30 research studies nationally which are disseminated though the media and journal publications. A strength of this approach is that the investigators across the different sites comply a core set of identical assessment tools in order to achieve the maximum leverage for ongoing research projects.

The Alzheimer's Disease Neuroimaging Initiative (ADNI) was built upon the resources of the ADCS. ADNI is funded through NIH, National Institute of Bioimaging and Bioengineering, the pharmaceutical industry and several foundations. The ADNI's aim was to produce, conduct and report the results of a worldwide study designed to 'define the rate of progress of mild cognitive impairment (MCI) and Alzheimer's disease, to develop improved methods for clinical trials in this area, and to provide a database which will improve design of treatment trials'[9]. Using a national network of centers engaged in AD research, ADNI employs a common protocol to assess cognition, function, biomarkers and brain structure in the elderly with mild cognitive impairment, and AD across the multiple sites. This allows investigators to have sufficient numbers of subjects enrolled to be able to get a better scientific picture of the pathology, course and symptoms of this disorder.

The NIA funds the Alzheimer's Disease Centers (ADCs) at major medical institutions across the United States[10,11]. Research at ADCs focus on the basic mechanisms of AD, prevention, management of symptoms and improvement in patient care[10,11]. Each ADC has a unique focus within a common goal shared by all centres, to enhance research on AD. ADC programmes offer collaborative clinical, research and community programmes, such as, diagnosis and medical management, information about the disease, services

and resources, opportunities to participate in drug trials and clinical research projects. Additionally ADCs offer diagnostic and treatment services and research opportunities in underserved, rural and minority communities.

Created by NIA, the National Alzheimer's Coordinating Center (NACC) was founded in 1999 to promote collaborative research and offer technical support throughout the 29 nationwide NIA-funded ADCs[12]. The NACC encourages ADC collaborative research and data collection, and maintains a primary database of clinical and neuropathological research data collected from each ADC. From the NACC-maintained database, data analysis is conducted to generate descriptive and hypothesis within specific areas, and develop methodological areas of study.

The National Cell Repository for Alzheimer's Disease (NCRAD) was also founded and funded by the NIA in 1989[13]. The Repository serves as a national resource for clinical and genetic research. The Repository's mission is to help identify the genes that lead to the development AD which can lead to more effective treatment and eventually prevention[13]. Programmes offered by the Repository are primarily research based and focused on families with a history of AD. This databank is instrumental in storing genetic data from Alzheimer's patients and their families for future use and current scientific exploration.

The Alzheimer's Disease Education and Referral Center (ADEAR) is the information centre and library on AD and is also operated under the NIA umbrella. It provides access to publications and audiovisual materials that can be retrieved online or through mail. ADEAR was created in 1990 to 'compile, archive, and disseminate information concerning Alzheimer's disease' for health professionals and the community[10,11]. This federally funded agency has the most updated, comprehensive information about the cause, treatment and diagnostic advancements of AD. As a community resource for information, the ADEAR services include free publications, referrals for services and AD specialized centres, literature and educational materials.

Within the Veteran Health Administration (VHA) system are 20 Geriatric Research, Education, and Clinical Centers (GRECC)[14]. In the mid-1970s, the VHA focused awareness on the aging veterans and their care[14]. The GRECCs were designed to advance and integrate research, education and clinical achievement in geriatrics and gerontology into the VHA health-care system. GRECCs have developed and expanded clinical models such as Geriatric Evaluation and Management (GEM) programmes, Palliative Care Programs for Late-Stage Dementia patients, education and training products[14].

The National Association of Area Agencies on Aging (n4a) supports the 629 Area Agencies on Aging (AAA) and 244 Title VI programmes. AAA was created in 1973 by the Older Americans Act (OAA) to address the needs of aging Americans[15]. The n4a oversees programmes to support initiatives that help older adults age in place through community-based and home services. The n4a advocates in large for services and resources for older adults and persons living with disabilities.

Beyond federal-supported enterprises, there are several state-supported centres dedicated to AD. For example, in 2000, Alzheimer's Caregiver Support Online (Alzonline) was established to support the caregiver community through daily challenges and provide expanded caregiver education, information and support[16]. Alzonline continues to receive funding through the State of Florida Department of Elder Affairs and the University of Florida (UF) Center for Telehealth[16]. Alzonline provides caregivers of Alzheimer's patients support, education and up-to-date information on caregiving.

NON-PROFIT AGENCIES

The Alzheimer's Association (AA) was started in 1980 by Jerome Stone in Chicago, IL, as it merged with the Alzheimer's Disease and Related Disorders Association[1]. Beginning with only seven chapters, the Alzheimer's Association has developed into one of the most prominent non-profit health associations focused on Alzheimer's care, support and research. Appropriately, Alzheimer's Association's vision is a 'world without Alzheimer's disease'[1]. Its purpose is to promote prevention and elimination of AD through advances in research, and to provide and improve care and support for all those affected by AD, or other dementias[1]. The programmes offer vast community outreach, support and education through local chapters, including telephone hotlines, support groups for caregivers and those in the early stages of the disease, personal consultations, referrals to local health-care services and facilities, online services and caregiver workshops.

The Alzheimer's Foundation of America (AFA) is a non-profit organization consisting of a number of agencies across the nation. These collaborating agencies are committed to providing AD patients and their families, educational, social and emotional support. The AFA promotes community awareness about the disease and contributes expertise and grants to health-care professionals and other organizations to enhance services[17]. The AFA was established in 1999 to oversee quality of care and services nationally that are provided to individuals with AD, their caregivers and families. They strive to improve the quality of life and public awareness of AD for those affected by the debilitating disease[17].

The AFA offers educational, social, emotional and practical needs of individuals with AD and related illnesses, and their caregivers and families with 950 member organizations untied under the AFA's umbrella[17]. Some of the AFA's member organizations include Dementia Care Professionals of America, Teens for Alzheimer's Awareness, AFA Quilt to Remember and National Memory Screening Day for early diagnosis[17]. The National Memory Screening Day for early diagnosis and detection of AD and other dementia began in 2003, and is dedicated to early recognition of AD to provide patients and families the opportunity to explore treatment and care-planning options. Frequently early symptoms of AD

are mistaken for cognitive decline associated with normal aging. Failure to recognize early symptoms of dementia may lead to possible harmful and unsafe behaviours displayed by the patient as the disease progresses. Moreover, early detection can help lessen the burden on the family and/or caregiver(s) and can provide opportunities for research and other medical interventions to help slow the progression of the disease.

The community services accessible are social work case managers, resource and referral centres, educational conferences and workshops, Early-stage and middle-stage programmes, adult day services, family services, respite and telephone support, and memory assessments.

The Association for Frontotemporal Dementias (AFTD) was created in 2002 by a caregiver who lost her husband to Pick's disease and saw the need to address the requirements of all those with frontotemporal dementias with treatment and cure promotion and education[18]. The AFTD is a national non-profit organization that promotes and funds research and education for the cure of frontotemporal dementias[18]. AFTD provides information, education and support to those afflicted with frontotemporal dementias (FTD), their families and caregivers.

The academic research based Alzheimer's Research & Prevention Foundation (ARPF) was founded as a first of its kind in implementing a prevention programme for memory loss and AD through the 4 Pillars of Alzheimer's Prevention[19]. The 4 Pillars of Alzheimer's Prevention combines training conferences on preventing memory loss and AD for medical professionals, educational opportunities for communities and medical professionals, and conducts research for the possible prevention of AD[19].

PATIENT AND CAREGIVER SUPPORT ORGANIZATIONS

Although all of the organizations previously mentioned provide excellent support and education, several organizations were founded to specifically provide ongoing services and resources for AD patients and their caregivers. Founded in 2000, Dementia Advocacy and Support Network (DASN) has formed an internet-based support network for people with dementia. DASN establishes a forum for autonomy, respect and support for persons with dementia[20]. Through educational services, counselling, advocacy and local service connection, DASNI promotes quality of life for those diagnosed with dementia.

In 1977, the Family Caregiver Alliance (FCA), a non-profit organization, was founded to assist and support caregivers of those with AD and other chronic conditions[21]. The FCA is a national community-based programme funded through corporate and foundation grants, the State of California, Area Agencies on Aging, and program participants and donations, which promotes services for caregivers and families providing care for those with chronic illnesses[21].

The FCA established the National Center on Caregiving (NCC) to develop national programmes and policies for caregivers[21]. The FCA acts as a concierge for services and programmes, helping caregivers locate support services in their communities. It offers a broad array of services from caregiver service and programmes, publications, education and training programmes, direct services, online information and support programmes, research and policy development. The National Family Caregivers Association (NFCA) was founded in 2003 to educate, support and empower caregivers of those who are living with a chronic illness or disability[22]. The community-based NFCA raises awareness about the caregiver's role and helps empower caregivers with education and support to lead full, productive and healthy lives.

The National Alliance for Caregiving was established in 1996 as a non-profit association in collaboration with other national organizations dedicated to caregiving[23]. In union with grassroots organizations, professional associations, service organizations, disease-specific organizations, a government agency and corporations, the National Alliance for Caregiving conducts research, analyses policy, pioneers national programmes and continues public awareness of family caregiving challenges[23]. Moreover, the Alliance remains devoted to improving the quality of life for families and care recipients. The Alliance has implemented the National Caregiver Survey, the Family Care Resource Connection, a National Caregiving Agenda and international conferences on family caregiving.

OTHER ORGANIZATIONS PROVIDING SUPPORT FOR AD

There are several other programmes and centres, that do not specifically focus on AD, but who still consider it under the boarder umbrella of their mandates. In 1950, the National Council on Aging (NCOA), a non-profit organization, was formed to develop, implement and disseminate innovative programmes to improve the lives of older adults[3]. NCOA collaborates with organizations nationally to provide older adults affordable and independent living, employments and activities. Although the NCOA does not have a primary focus on AD, it does consider the impact of AD. This is important as this organization has been instrumental in shaping public policy. The NCOA has had a congressional hand in Medicare, the Age Discrimination in Employment Act (ADEA), and the Older Americans Act (OAA)[3]. Furthermore, the NCOA is dedicated to raising awareness of the challenges older Americans with limited income and resources face.

Other such organizations include the International Longevity Center, a research and educational organization, devoted to the development of science-based policies[24], the Institute on Aging (IOA) a community-based, non-profit organization, which embraces diverse aging communities' need for health, social service, creative arts, spiritual support and education programmes, as well as continuous research. Today the IOA is one of the largest providers for community-based services for the aging population[25].

The American Federation for Aging Research (AFAR), established in the 1980s, has been a leader in a 'revolutionary approach to the science of healthier aging'[26]. AFAR explores aging and the aging processes in understanding age-related diseases. By studying the components of disease that are related to aging and the underlying mechanisms of aging and how they regulate the processes in our bodies, AFAR has contributed to the understanding of aging and mechanisms of age-related disease. AFAR funds 2500 early-career scientists from prominent institutions each year, and together explores the fundamental mechanisms of aging and aging with age-related diseases[26].

REFERENCES

1. Alzheimer's Association. *2009 Alzheimer's Disease Facts and Figures*. At www.alz.org/national/documents/report_alzfacts figures2009.pdf, accessed 24 Oct 2009.

2. Center for Disease Control and Prevention (CDC). At www.cdc.gov, accessed 19 Dec 2009.

3. National Council on Aging. At www.ncoa.org, accessed 24 Oct 2009.

4. Third Age. *Shocking New Alzheimer's Statistics: Why doesn't the NIH Allocate fair funding?*, 2008. At www.thridage.com/today/caregiving/shocking-new-alzheimer-statistics-why-doesnt-the-nih-allocate-fair-funding, accessed 24 Oct 2009.

5. Pillai JA, Verghese J. Social networks and their role in preventing dementia. *Indian J Psychiatry* 2009; **5**: 22–8.

6. Administration on Aging. At www.aoa.gov/AoARoot/Index.aspx, accessed 24 Oct 2009.

7. US National Institutes of Health. National Institute on Aging. At www.nia.nih.gov, accessed 24 Oct 2009.

8. Alzheimer's Disease Cooperative Study (ADCS). At www.adcs.org, accessed 24 Oct 2009.

9. Alzheimer's Disease Neuroimaging Initiative (ADNI). At www.adni-info.org, accessed 24 Oct 2009.

10. National Institute of Aging. AD Research Centers. At www.nia.nih.gov/nia.nih.gov, accessed 24 Oct 2009.

11. National Institute of Aging. The Alzheimer's Disease Education and Referral Center. At www.nia.nih.gov/alzheimers, accessed 24 Oct 2009.

12. National Alzheimer's Coordinating Center (NACC). At www.alz.washington.edu, accessed 24 Oct 2009.

13. The National Cell Repository for Alzheimer's disease. At http://ncrad.iu.edu, accessed 24 Oct 2009.

14. United States Department of Veterans Affairs. Geriatric Research Education and Clinical Centers (GRECCs). At www1.va.gov/GRECC, accessed 24 Oct 2009.

15. National Association of Area Agencies on Aging (n4a). At www.n4a.org, accessed 24 Oct 2009.

16. Alzheimer's Caregiver Support Online. At http://alzonline.phhp.ufl.ed/, accessed 24 Oct 2009.

17. Alzheimer's Foundation of America. At www.alzfdn.org, accessed 24 Oct 2009.

18. Association for Frontotemporal Dementias. At www.ftd-picks.org, accessed 24 Oct 2009.

19. Alzheimer's Research & Prevention Foundation. At www.alzheimersprevention.org, accessed 24 Oct 2009.

20. Dementia Advocacy and Support Network (DASN) International. At www.dasninternational.org, accessed 24 Oct 2009.

21. Family Caregiver Alliance. (2009). At www.caregiver.org/caregiver/jsp/home.jsp, accessed 24 Oct 2009.

22. National Family Caregivers Association. At www.nfcacares.org, accessed 24 Oct 2009.

23. National Alliance for Caregiving. At www.caregiving.org, accessed 24 Oct 2009.

24. International Longevity Center. At www.ilcusa.org, accessed 24 Oct 2009.

25. Institute on Aging. At www.ioaging.org, accessed 24 Oct 2009.

26. American Federation for Aging Research (AFAR). At www.afar.org, accessed 24 Oct 2009.

68

Psychiatric Manifestations of Nervous System Infections

Jeffrey T. Guptill and E. Wayne Massey

Duke University School of Medicine, Duke University Medical Center, Durham, USA

This chapter highlights nervous system infections that may masquerade as psychiatric disease or may be coincident in the geriatric patient with psychiatric disorders. This is not meant to be an exhaustive discussion, but rather emphasizes a few conditions that may enter into the differential diagnosis of patients presenting with psychiatric symptoms.

A thorough history and clinical examination are paramount to recognizing the neurological origin for patients presenting with psychiatric symptoms. Rapidly progressive symptoms, alteration in the patient's level of consciousness, seizures, focal weakness or numbness, slurred speech, tremor, vision change or diplopia, difficulty walking or falls, and headache are symptoms that should raise the suspicion for neurological disease and should be investigated further. The reader is encouraged to refer to the provided references for in-depth reviews of each topic.

Subacute and chronic infections are more likely to have manifestations confused with primary psychiatric disease. We have limited our discussion to the neurological manifestations, diagnosis, and treatment of tuberculosis, Lyme disease, syphilis, cryptococcosis, and herpes virus.

MYCOBACTERIUM TUBERCULOSIS

Although relatively uncommon in the United States, the incidence of tuberculosis has been increasing since the mid-1980s related, in part, to the increased prevalence of HIV infection. Other than patients with HIV, tuberculosis infection in the USA is mostly seen in substance abusers, immigrants from underdeveloped countries (35% of new cases in the USA), and the elderly (25%)[1]. In Europe 80% of infected individuals are over the age of 50 and similar figures have been reported in Asia[2]. The incidence in the USA is estimated at 4.4 per 100 000[3], but it is more common in developing nations, particularly Africa and Asia. Approximately one third of the world population, about 2 billion people, is infected with *Mycobacterium tuberculosis*. One in ten will develop active disease[4].

Three important, and occasionally overlapping, presentations occur with central nervous system (CNS) tuberculosis infection. A myeloradiculitis may result in pathologic hyperreflexia, spasticity, paraplegia, sensory level, and/or radicular weakness and numbness with depressed reflexes. Next, tuberculomas of the brain parenchyma are composed of inflammatory cells and granulation tissue and often behave like tumours due to mass effect. Tuberculomas are often multiple but can be single and large. Symptoms and signs are usually related to location and size. If located in a periventricular location, hydrocephalus may develop. Tuberculomas are more likely to be confused with psychiatric disease, particularly with involvement of the frontal lobes or with the gradual development of hydrocephalus[5]. Finally, tuberculous meningitis may present with slowly progressive headache, confusion, lethargy and meningeal signs or as an acute meningoencephalitis. Multiple cranial neuropathies are not infrequent due to basilar leptomeningeal involvement[6]. Hydrocephalus with increased intracranial pressure, develops later in the course and results in progressive lethargy and confusion. Importantly, meningitis may occur in patients with inactive lung nodules, no other evidence of infection, and a negative purified protein derivative (PPD) test[7]. As expected, the patient with HIV co-infection tends to have a more fulminant presentation. Rapid clinical deterioration may also be associated to HIV/AIDS.

Although 75% of geriatric patients present with pulmonary tuberculosis, extrapulmonary presentations increase with age[1]. Atypical presentations of tuberculosis, including meningitis, are well described in the elderly. However, the prevalence is not well known. Geriatric patients may present with non-specific symptoms such as fatigue, cognitive impairment, encephalopathy, and impaired activities of daily living[2]. As a result of co-morbid conditions, tuberculosis is often not initially considered in the elderly, resulting in delayed diagnosis, more advanced disease and lower cure rates with higher mortality.

When the diagnosis of tuberculous meningitis is suspected a lumbar puncture should be performed following computed tomography (CT) scan of the brain evaluating for impending herniation. The cerebrospinal fluid (CSF) profile typically shows an elevated opening pressure, high protein content, lymphocytic pleocytosis and a mildly low glucose. Rarely, acid-fast bacilli are identified. Early in the disease process polymorphonuclear (PMN) cells may be the predominant immune cell type, but if the lumbar puncture is repeated several days later, the typical lymphocytic pleocytosis will usually be observed[5]. Paradoxically, the lymphocytic pleocytosis may shift towards a PMN predominance following initiation of treatment. This shift is felt by some experts as nearly pathognomonic of tuberculous meningitis and has been utilized in developing countries to direct therapy[6]. Methods of identifying the organism include

Principles and Practice of Geriatric Psychiatry, 3rd edn. Edited by Mohammed T. Abou-Saleh, Cornelius Katona and Anand Kumar
© 2011 John Wiley & Sons, Ltd

standard culture, rapid culture techniques and polymerase chain reaction (PCR) with DNA amplification. The diagnostic yield of culture is highly dependent on the amount of fluid sent for analysis (10 cc recommended). Growth with standard culture techniques would not be expected before about four weeks and rapid culture techniques may yield results in a week or slightly less. Treatment is often begun without isolating the organism when there is a high clinical suspicion and a compatible CSF profile. Brain CT or magnetic resonance imaging (MRI) may show evidence of hydrocephalus or infarct. Imaging obtained with contrast often shows strong enhancement of the basilar meninges and cranial nerves. Tuberculomas have imaging characteristics suggestive of primary brain tumours such as peripheral enhancement and vasogenic oedema.

Therapy of CNS tuberculosis typically consists of a three- or four-drug regimen, usually rifampin (10 mg/kg/d, maximum 600 mg daily), isoniazid (5 mg/kg/d), ethambutol (15 mg/kg/d), ± pyrazinamide (20–35 mg/kg/d) or ethionamide (15–25 mg/kg/d in divided doses). Streptomycin (10 mg/kg, maximum 750 mg daily) may be considered with isoniazid, rifampin and pyrazinamide in multidrug-resistant strains. Antimicrobial therapy typically lasts 12–18 months, but may extend up to two years and should be tailored to the presence/absence of drug-resistant mycobacterium[5]. Pyridoxine (50 mg daily) is typically added to prevent the neuropathy associated with isoniazid. Corticosteroids may be used to reduce inflammation and are recommended in cases of hydrocephalus, spinal block or impending herniation. Rifampin, streptomycin and ethambutol penetrate the CSF better in the presence of meningeal inflammation, whereas isoniazid and pyrazinamide are unaffected. Mortality may be reduced with dexamethasone treatment, but morbidity appears unaffected[6]. Large tuberculomas exerting significant mass effect or spinal osteomyelitis/granulomas resulting in cord compression may require surgical intervention. In the immunocompetent population mortality is about 10% and is greatest in children and the elderly. In the HIV-infected population mortality is higher, at 20%. Residual neurological deficits are seen in a quarter to one third of patients[5].

BORRELIA BURGDORFERI: LYME DISEASE

In the USA, Lyme disease is contracted from Ixodes ticks harbouring the spirochete Borrelia burgdorferi. Borrelia garinii and Borrelia afzelii account for the overwhelming majority of organisms isolated in Europe in cases of neuroborreliosis. Lyme neuroborreliosis is felt to occur in Asia and has been documented in Russia. Currently, there is no evidence of the disease in South America or Africa[8]. The majority of cases in the USA occur in northeastern, mid-Atlantic and north-central states. The number of cases reported to the Centers for Disease Control (CDC) in Atlanta, Georgia has climbed steadily since it became a reportable disease in 1991[9]. In 1992 approximately 10 000 cases were reported, while 2007 produced more than 27 000 cases with an incidence of 9.1/100 000. In the 10 states reporting the most cases, the incidence was significantly higher at 34.7/100 000[10]. Mandatory reporting does not exist in Europe, so obtaining accurate epidemiological data is more difficult. The eastern central region of Europe probably has the highest incidence of neuroborreliosis[8].

Early manifestations of Borrelia burgdorferi infection include an expanding 'bullseye' rash, also known as erythema migrans, as well as headache, fever, myalgia or arthralgia, and fatigue[11]. CDC review of cases from 2003 to 2005 demonstrated that erythema migrans was present historically in about 70% of cases[9], while other sources cite 90% of cases with rash, about 40% of which have central clearing[12]. The rash typically appears within 30 days of Ixodes tick exposure. In the European form, rash is much less common. Other early presentations include facial palsy, radiculopathy, meningitis/encephalitis and heart block. European Lyme neuroborreliosis most commonly presents with a painful radiculitis (86%), which is called Bannwarth's syndrome[8]. Onset of symptoms in the USA is typically during the months of June, July or August, and less than 8% of cases occurred from December to March[9]. Rickettsial infections, including Rocky Mountain spotted fever, can also present with acute encephalitis and patients may have cranial neuropathies, focal neurological signs and seizures.

Patients with untreated Borrelia burgdorferi infections often develop a subacute to chronic disease with musculoskeletal, cardiovascular or neurological symptoms. Arthritis is typically oligoarticular and most commonly involves the knee joint (60%). Cardiovascular involvement occurs in about 8% of patients and is typically a pericarditis or myocarditis producing conduction abnormalities[5]. Chronic skin manifestations are more common in European Lyme neuroborreliosis and take the form of acrodermatitis chronica atrophicans and lymphocytoma. Neurologic symptoms and signs develop in about 15% of patients and include cranial neuropathy, painful radiculopathy, peripheral neuropathy and meningoencephalitis. The most common cranial nerve affected in Lyme neuroborreliosis is the facial nerve, causing a 'Bell's palsy'. Between 25% and 50% of patients developing meningitis will have multiple radiculopathies or peripheral nerve lesions. The peripheral neuropathy is typically axonal and not severe[8]. Myelitis, cerebellar ataxia, seizures and chorea are rare[5].

Manifestations of chronic infection may overlap with its subacute features and include fatigue, dermatitis, arthritis and neuropsychiatric symptoms such as depression and cognitive dysfunction. Patients with chronic Lyme disease may report poor concentration and attention, irritability and memory complaints. Other considerations in the differential diagnosis typically include fibromyalgia and chronic fatigue syndrome. Importantly, symptoms and signs suggestive of early disseminated disease should have been present at an earlier point[13]. Other reported psychiatric symptoms include mania, delirium, dementia, psychosis, panic attacks, personality change, obsessions/compulsions and catatonia[14,15]. There is no clear evidence that Lyme disease causes the majority of these reported symptoms.

Cerebrospinal fluid examination in patients with Lyme disease typically shows a mild lymphocytic pleocytosis with a mildly elevated protein and normal glucose. In patients with a history of tick exposure, erythema migrans and suggestive symptoms and signs, the enzyme linked immunosorbent assay (ELISA) is a helpful screening test. A positive test with a rise in IgM occurs in about 90% of patients who have acute and chronic serum samples tested[5]. The presence of elevated IgG without IgM suggests a chronic exposure. A positive ELISA test must be confirmed with Western blot due to the possibility of false positive screening tests. In Europe where multiple strains cause neuroborreliosis, an antibody index comparing CSF and serum antibody levels is typically used for diagnosis[8]. CSF culture has a yield of about 5% and is not useful, while CSF PCR is positive in about 30–40% of cases, usually early in the disease. CT and MRI are usually most helpful in ruling out other neurological diseases, but may rarely demonstrate multifocal periventricular white matter lesions in advanced cases[5]. These lesions are not specific for Lyme disease and are seen in several other neurological diseases, including demyelinating disease, migraine and cerebrovascular disease.

Treatment of acute disease is typically with oral doxycycline (100–200 mg bid) or amoxicillin (500 mg tid) for 2–4 weeks. Options for neuroborreliosis include intravenous ceftriaxone (2 g daily) for 2–4 weeks, high-dose penicillin (20 million units daily) for 2–4 weeks or tetracycline (500 mg qid) for 30 days[16]. A recent European trial demonstrated similar efficacy when comparing two weeks of therapy with intravenous ceftriaxone 2 g daily versus oral doxycycline 200 mg daily[17]. Following treatment, patients may report continued fatigue, difficulty concentrating and memory difficulty. This is the so-called 'post-Lyme syndrome.' These patients have often been given extended courses of treatment with oral or intravenous antibiotics in an attempt to clear their 'chronic infection'. Typically, there are alternative explanations for their symptoms, and there is a little data to support prolonged antimicrobial treatment in individuals who have received adequate treatment[8,16,18].

TREPONEMA PALLIDUM: NEUROSYPHILIS

Close to 37 000 cases of syphilis were reported in the continental United States in 2006 and the majority occurred in the southeastern region. Late and latent syphilis accounted for over 17 000 of the total cases[19]. During that same year, it was noted that 64% of cases occurred in men who have sex with men. Cases occur predominantly in young adults, and there has been a steady increase in syphilis cases in patients with HIV. Syphilitic chancres increase the risk of acquiring HIV when exposed to the virus between two and five times[20].

Neurosyphilis may occur at any point after exposure to *Treponema pallidum* and is most commonly an asymptomatic meningitis. The meningitis occurs in about 25% of syphilis cases and may remain asymptomatic for years before becoming symptomatic or regressing. Early nervous system involvement with *Treponema pallidum* typically affects the meninges, blood vessels and cranial nerves. Late CNS infection typically involves the parenchyma of the brain and spinal cord[5]. The classical late presentations of 'tabes dorsalis' and 'general paresis of the insane' (dementia paralytica) have become exceptionally rare following the widespread availability and general use of antibiotics[21,22]. General paresis is a progressive dementia with prominent neuropsychiatric features, including psychosis. Tabes dorsalis affects the dorsal columns of the spinal cord and sensory nerve roots and manifests with sensory ataxia, urinary incontinence, lancinating pain and lower extremity hyporeflexia[23]. Recent reviews and case series emphasize the atypical presentations of neurosyphilis and its preponderance in the HIV-positive population. The remainder of this discussion focuses on 'modern neurosyphilis' in the antibiotic era. The reader is encouraged to refer to Ropper and Brown[5] for further information on paretic and tabetic neurosyphilis.

Meningovascular neurosyphilis may present with stroke symptoms such as hemiparesis, aphasia, sensory disturbance or visual loss. The symptoms are commonly referable to medium and small branch arteries of the anterior and middle cerebral arteries. Confusion, psychosis, delirium and dementia have been increasingly reported. About 50% (82 of 161) of neurosyphilis cases in a recent South African retrospective review had neuropsychiatric presentations defined as psychosis, delirium or dementia. 15% presented with stroke, 12% with ocular symptoms, with myelopathy, 9% with seizure, about 9% with seizure and 5% with cranial neuropathy or other brainstem symptoms. Overlapping presentations occurred predominantly with seizure, neuropsychiatric features and stroke[21]. Other series from Europe and the USA have emphasized neuropsychiatric presentations of neurosyphilis, including psychosis, atypical depression and memory loss[24,25].

Ocular and otologic infections are often included in discussions of neurosyphilis. Ocular syphilis may involve any eye structure and can occur at any time during the course of infection. Overall, however, ocular involvement tends to occur early and uveitis is the most common clinical diagnosis. Though otologic syphilis with sensorineural hearing loss has traditionally been associated with chronic *Treponema* infection, more recent studies have reported early otologic involvement with sensorineural hearing loss and occasionally tinnitus and vertigo. Treatment of ocular and otologic syphilis is the same as neurosyphilis, though the addition of steroids is recommended by many experts for ocular syphilis[22].

CSF examination typically shows a lymphocytic pleocytosis and elevated protein with a normal glucose. An elevated IgG index and oligoclonal bands are often present[23]. According to the CDC, the diagnosis of neurosyphilis is confirmed with a reactive CSF Venereal Disease Research Laboratory (VDRL) test and syphilis of any stage. Probable neurosyphilis is defined as syphilis of any stage, a nonreactive VDRL, symptoms and signs consistent with neurosyphilis and no other known cause, and an elevated CSF protein or WBC count without another explanation[26]. The CSF-VDRL test is very specific but not sensitive and, therefore, may be negative in cases of neurosyphilis. The fluorescent treponemal antibody (FTA-ABS) is a direct treponemal test with very high sensitivity and less specificity. Many experts advocate using the FTA-ABS to essentially exclude the diagnosis of neurosyphilis with a negative test due to its high sensitivity. All patients with syphilis should be tested for HIV[22]. Neuroimaging may be normal or show meningeal, nerve root or cranial nerve enhancement, cerebral atrophy or stroke.

Traditionally, treatment is with aqueous penicillin G (3–4 million units every 4 hours or 24 million units daily) for 10–14 days. Procaine penicillin (2.4 million units IM daily) with probenecid (500 mg orally qid) is an alternative[27]. Patients with penicillin allergy may be desensitized, but ceftriaxone (2 g daily) is more convenient and appears effective. Lumbar puncture should be repeated every six months after treatment until a normal CSF profile is demonstrated. The CDC recommends re-treatment if the WBC count has not normalized six months after adequate treatment or other CSF abnormalities persist after two years. Other experts recommend re-treatment with an increase in CSF WBC count or a four-fold rise in the CSF-VDRL titre[22].

CRYPTOCOCCOSIS

Cryptococcal infection was once rare, but it is now one of the most common fungal infections of the nervous system due to the HIV epidemic and more widespread availability of organ transplantation. Although it is most prevalent in immunocompromised patients with solid organ transplant or HIV/AIDs, it may also occur in immunocompetent individuals[28]. In the HIV-positive population, cryptococcal infection typically occurs with a CD4+ count less than 50, and approximately 10% of AIDS patients will develop cryptococcal CNS infection. Worldwide, 80% of patients infected with *Cryptococcus* are HIV positive, and cryptococcal meningitis may be the presenting illness in patients with undiagnosed HIV infection. The highest incidence of cryptococcal meningitis occurs in Africa and Asia where HIV is most common, and 20–30% of

HIV patients in Africa die from cryptococcal meningitis[29]. In the USA, the incidence is about 4.9/100 000.

Cryptococcosis is usually acquired through the respiratory tract or occasionally through mucus membranes or wounds. Two species cause disease in humans, *Cryptococcus neoformans* and *C. gattii*. The nearly ubiquitous *C. neoformans* is present in soil and is associated with bird nesting sites. *C. gattii* is unique in that it is more geographically limited, typically affects immunocompetent patients, presents more insidiously, and is associated with a delayed response to treatment. *Cryptococcus* can infect any organ, though the central nervous and respiratory systems and skin are common sites of clinical involvement[28].

Cryptococcal CNS infection commonly presents as a chronic granulomatous meningitis or meningoencephalitis developing over days to weeks or months. Headache, encephalopathy, dementia, nausea and vomiting, and cranial neuropathy are common[5]. Importantly, headache may be the only symptom and cryptococcal meningitis should be considered in the adult patient without a prior headache history developing a chronic, unremitting headache[28]. Patients may also have gait difficulty, and case reports have described new-onset psychosis and mania[30,31]. Fever is documented on presentation in less than 50% of immunocompetent patients. In a recent French prospective study French of 230 patients with cryptococcosis, neurological abnormalities were present in 46% of patients diagnosed with meningoencephalitis at the time of initial evaluation, independent of HIV status; 77% of the patients were HIV positive. Mental status changes (33%), seizures (10%) and cranial neuropathy (15%) were the most common abnormalities[32]. Another series of 43 adult patients with neoplastic disease (predominantly leukaemia and lymphoma) reported 90% had altered consciousness on presentation, which varied from mild behavioural change to psychosis or coma[33]. More rarely, cryptococcomas, consisting of small cortical gelatinous cystic nodules or large predominantly subcortical granulomas, may occur and cause focal neurological symptoms. Due to meningovascular infiltration, strokes may rarely occur[5].

Lumbar puncture in cryptococcal CNS infection may show an elevated opening pressure, lymphocytic pleocytosis and elevated protein. The CSF glucose level is low in about 75% of cases. However, the glucose and cell count may be normal in AIDS patients. India ink preparation often shows the thickly encapsulated organism and cultures often become positive, but take days to yield results. Microscopy and culture are labour and time intensive and have a sensitivity of 50–80%. Furthermore, large volumes of CSF may need to be analysed and cultured if the burden of the organism is relatively low. A capsular polysaccharide antigen forms the basis of the widely available latex agglutination test. It is a rapid test and has a sensitivity of 93–100% and a specificity of 93–98%, though false positives are well described in the literature[28]. A titre of >1 : 8 should be considered a positive test. Finally, enzyme immunosorbent assays have been compared to the polysaccharide antigen agglutination test with promising results[34]. This test is not widely available, however. Neuroimaging is usually normal but may show parenchymal lesions, hydrocephalus, meningeal enhancement, dilated Virchow–Robin spaces and cystic lesions (see Figure 68.1). Abnormal brain imaging generally confers a poorer prognosis.

Treatment is with amphotericin B (0.5–0.7 mg/kg/d), typically with flucytosine (150 mg/kg/d) for 2 weeks, followed by fluconazole for at least 10 weeks. In the AIDS patient, maintenance fluconazole therapy is generally continued for life unless the CD4+ count rises above 100–200 cells/μl for 3–6 months at which time the asymptomatic

patient with sterile spinal fluid may be discontinued. Historically, a lumbar puncture has been performed after the first two weeks of therapy to confirm therapeutic response, although some authorities now forgo the second lumbar puncture if the patient is clinically responding and has a normal neurological examination. If the initial lumbar puncture showed an elevated opening pressure and the patient has symptoms of increased intracranial pressure, a lumbar puncture should be repeated daily until the patient becomes asymptomatic or the pressure normalizes for a minimum of two days. HIV patients with low CD4+ counts who are started on highly active antiretroviral therapy at the time of diagnosis of a cryptococcal CNS infection are at risk for immune reconstitution inflammatory syndrome (IRIS)[35]. Independent risk factors for treatment failure regardless of HIV status include high serum antigen titres, widespread dissemination at the time of diagnosis, and the absence of flucytosine during the induction phase of treatment. Three-month survival is reduced in patients with an abnormal neurological exam or brain imaging at baseline and haematological malignancy[32,33]. The three-month mortality rate of CNS cryptococcal infection is at least 20%, and 40% of survivors have lasting neurological impairment.

HERPES SIMPLEX ENCEPHALITIS

Herpes simplex virus type 1 (HSV-1) is the most common sporadic viral encephalitis in the USA and accounts for about 10% of all encephalitis cases. Over 2000 cases occur annually in the USA and the worldwide incidence is estimated at 2–4 cases per million per year[36]. HSV-2, associated with genital infection, also causes neurological disease, which is most commonly aseptic meningitis and occasionally acute encephalitis. The remainder of the discussion will focus on HSV-1 CNS infection due to its prevalence (HSV-1 accounts for 90% of herpes encephalitis cases)[37] and significant morbidity and mortality. Herpes simplex encephalitis (HSE) occurs more commonly in individuals with recurrent HSV infection. It has been hypothesized that propagation of the virus from the trigeminal ganglion, where it lies dormant, along the ophthalmic division of the trigeminal nerve results in its tropism for the orbital frontal lobes, insular cortex and medial temporal lobes[38].

HSE usually presents acutely with fever and seizures, behavioural changes, altered mentation, aphasia or other focal neurological deficits. Olfactory hallucinations may occur. Without treatment the patient usually progresses to obtundation and coma[20]. Although HSE typically has a fulminant course, cases progressing over several weeks to months occur, and merit mention due to the potential diagnosis of psychiatric disease. In a series of 24 adult patients with HSE, 4 (17%) reportedly had atypical presentations, consisting of slowly progressive encephalitis often with a non-focal clinical exam[40]. Patients with several months of memory impairment, confusion, lethargy and progressive headache have been reported in the literature[41]; these patients may or may not have focal signs.

Examination of the CSF shows a lymphocytic pleocytosis with normal glucose and elevated protein. The opening pressure may be elevated. Although HSE causes haemorrhagic pathology in the brain, xanthochromia and red blood cells are only occasionally present on CSF examination. HSV PCR, which is sensitive and specific, should be sent. Imaging classically shows temporal lobe hypointensities on CT (see Figure 68.2) and areas of T2 prolongation on MRI. Abnormalities may extend contiguously to the insular cortex and orbitofrontal lobes, as well as into the rostral midbrain. Enhancement usually occurs following administration of contrast (indicating disruption of the blood–brain barrier)[5]. Electroencephalography may

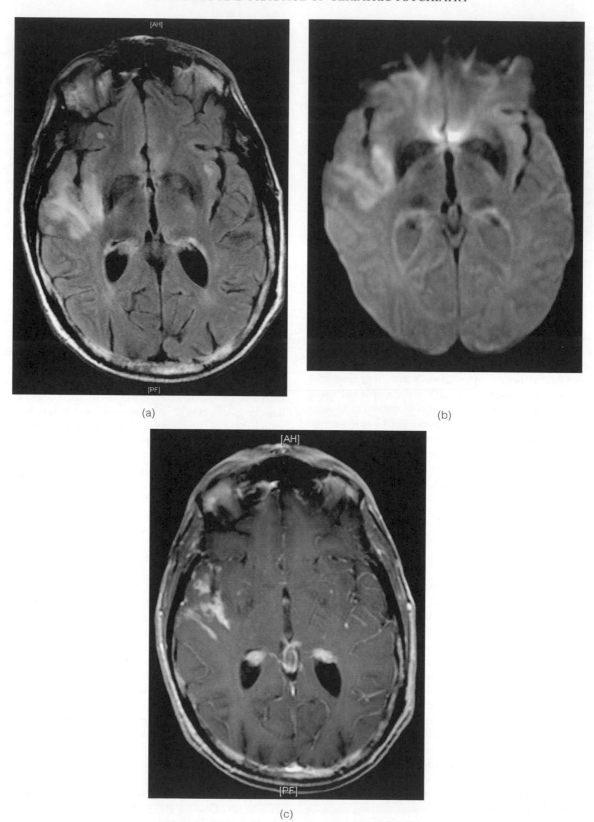

Figure 68.1   A 60-year-old male with hepatic cirrhosis from alcoholism presented with eight months of progressive headache, several months of intermittent left arm numbness and new onset gait difficulty. Neurological exam revealed encephalopathy and gait ataxia. MRI of the brain showed A) prominent T2/FLAIR signal prolongation in the right temporal lobe with B) restricted diffusion. C) Contrast enhancement was present in the right temporal lobe and diffuse leptomeningeal enhancement was also seen. Lumbar puncture showed 83 nucleated cells, glucose <20, 3 red blood cells, protein 584. Opening pressure was normal. Cryptococcal antigen was positive (1:16) in the CSF and serum. HIV testing was negative.

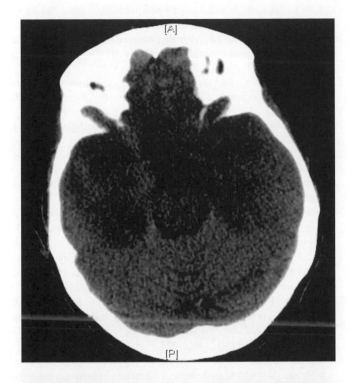

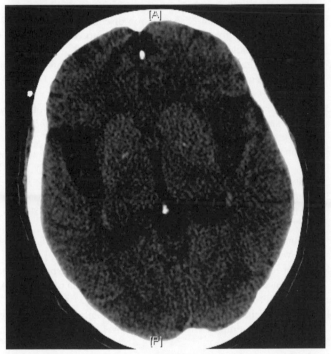

Figure 68.2 A 70-year-old female presented with four days of progressive confusion, lethargy and fatigue. Sodium on presentation was 110, and neurologic exam was non-focal. Non-contrasted head CT on presentation was read as normal. Repeat head CT 10 days after onset of symptoms (shown above) shows bilateral temporal, insular and inferior frontal lobe hypodensities. Lumbar puncture showed 69 nucleated cells (94% lymphocytes), protein 78, and glucose 53. HSV PCR was positive. EEG showed slowing in the theta and delta range with interspersed GPED activity.

show focal temporal slowing or more generalized slowing. These findings often evolve into periodic lateralized epileptiform discharges (PLEDS) at two to three per second intervals or generalized periodic epileptiform discharges (GPEDS)[38].

Treatment with acyclovir (30 mg/kg per day divided three times daily) should be started as soon as possible in suspected cases and should not be delayed for PCR results. Treatment is continued for 10–14 days[5], and some experts emphasize 14 days of treatment to reduce the risk of relapse[39]. Other management includes medical treatment of seizures, supportive ventilation and possibly corticosteroids to control cerebral oedema. There is scant evidence to support worsening of infection with administration of steroids. The mortality from untreated HSE is 60–70%. Treatment reduces mortality to about 20–30% in some series[38]. Practically, the patient's age and level of consciousness at the time of treatment initiation strongly predict outcome[5].

Neuropsychiatric and cognitive sequelae of HSV-1 encephalitis occur in up to 80% of patients[38]. In one series of 34 patients, the most common long-term effects included memory impairment (69%), behavioural and personality change (45%) and epilepsy (24%). Clinical examination following HSE infection revealed short term memory loss (70%), anosmia (65%) and aphasia (41%)[42]. The memory impairment following HSE is typically anterograde, resulting from damage to medial temporal structures. Other reported sequelae include visuo-spatial, executive function and retrograde memory deficits, as well as aggression, disinhibition, catatonia and Klüver–Bucy syndrome (behavioural and cognitive deficit, placidity, apathy, hypersexuality, hyperorality and visual/auditory agnosia)[38]. Although imaging typically reveals evidence of infection in both hemispheres, residual deficits may be relatively lateralized, and right hemispheric infection tends to produce less severe functional impairments. Hokkanen and Launes[36] recently published a comprehensive review of the neuropsychological sequelae of acute viral encephalitis. Typical and atypical antipsychotics, antidepressants, benzodiazepines, stimulants and anticonvulsants have been used to manage the behavioural and cognitive sequelae. Treatment, however, remains empirical due to a paucity of data[38].

REFERENCES

1. Van den Brande P. Revised guidelines for the diagnosis and control of tuberculosis: impact on management in the elderly. *Drugs Aging* 2005; **22**(8): 663–86.
2. Rajagopalan S. Tuberculosis and aging: a global health problem. *Clin Infect Dis* 2001; **33**(7): 1034–9.
3. Centers for Disease Control and Prevention. *Reported Tuberculosis in the United States, 2007*. Atlanta, GA: US Department of Health and Human Services, 2008. At www.cdc.gov/tb/statistics/reports/2007/pdf/fullreport.pdf, accessed 18 Mar 2009.
4. World Health Organization. *Tuberculosis*, Fact Sheet no. 104. Geneva: World Health Organization, 2007. At www.who.int/mediacentre/factsheets/fs104/en, accessed 18 Mar 2009.
5. Ropper AH, Brown RH. *Adams and Victor's Principles of Neurology: Infections of the Nervous System and Sarcoidosis*, 8th edn. New York: McGraw-Hill, 2005.
6. Roos KL. Neuroinfectious diseases. In *Global Health Challenges: Neurology in Developing Countries*, American Academy of Neurology Annual Meeting, 14 Apr 2008, Chicago, IL. Seattle, WA: American Academy of Neurology, 1–5.

7. Rock RB, Olin M, Baker CA, Molitor TW, Peterson PK. Central nervous system tuberculosis: pathogenesis and clinical aspects. *Clin Microbiol Rev* 2008; **21**(2): 243–61.

8. Pachner AR, Steiner I. Lyme neuroborreliosis: infection, immunity, and inflammation. *Lancet Neurol* 2007; **6**: 544–52.

9. Centers for Disease Control and Prevention. Lyme Disease – United States, 2003–2005. *MMWR Morb Mortal Wkly Rep* 2007; **56**(23): 573–6.

10. Centers for Disease Control and Prevention. Reported cases of Lyme disease by year – United States, 1992–2007. Atlanta, GA: US Department of Health and Human Services, 2008. At www.cdc.gov/ncidod/dvbid/lyme/resources/Lyme07Cases.pdf accessed 1 Apr 2009.

11. Nadelman RB, Nowakowski J, Forseter G *et al.* The clinical spectrum of early Lyme borreliosis in patients with culture-confirmed erythema migrans. *Am J Med* 1996; **100**: 502–8.

12. Steere AC, Bartenhagen NH, Craft JE *et al.* The early clinical manifestations of Lyme disease. *Ann Intern Med* 1983; **99**: 76–82.

13. Schneider RK, Robinson MJ, Levenson JL. Psychiatric presentations of non-HIV infectious diseases. *Psychiatr Clin North Am* 2002; **25**(1): 1–16.

14. Fallon BA, Nields JA. Lyme disease: a neuropsychiatric illness. *Am J Psychiatry* 1994; **151**: 1571–83.

15. Fallon BA, Nields JA, Parsons B, Liebowitz MR, Klein DF. Psychiatric manifestations of Lyme borreliosis. *J Clin Psychiatry* 1993; **54**(7): 263–8.

16. Halperin JJ, Shapiro ED, Logigian E *et al.* Practice parameter: treatment of nervous system Lyme disease (an evidence-based review): report of the quality standards subcommittee of the American Academy of Neurology. *Neurology* 2007; **69**(1): 91–102.

17. Ljøstad U, Skogvoll E, Eikeland R. Oral doxycycline versus intravenous ceftriaxone for European Lyme neuroborreliosis: a multicentre, non-inferiority, double-blind, randomized trial. *Lancet Neurol* 2008; **7**(8): 690–5.

18. Klempner MS, Hu LT, Evans J *et al.* Two controlled trials of antibiotic treatment in patients with persistent symptoms and a history of Lyme disease. *N Engl J Med* 2001; **345**(2): 85–92.

19. Centers for Disease Control and Prevention. *Sexually Transmitted Disease Surveillance 2006 Supplement*, Syphilis Surveillance Report. Atlanta, GA: US Department of Health and Human Services, 2007. At www.cdc.gov/std/syphilis2006/Syphilis2006Short.pdf, accessed 15 Mar 2009.

20. Centers for Disease Control and Prevention. Syphilis *and MSM (Men Who Have Sex with Men)*, CDC Fact Sheet. Atlanta, GA: US Department of Health and Human Services, 2007. At www.cdc.gov/std/syphilis/STDFact-MSM&Syphilis.htm, accessed 20 Apr 2009.

21. Timmermans M, Carr J. Neurosyphilis in the modern era. *J Neurol Neurosurg Psychiatry* 2004; **75**: 1727–30.

22. Marra CM. Update on neurosyphilis. *Curr Infect Dis Rep* 2009; **11**: 127–34.

23. Golden MR, Marra CM, Holmes KK. Update on syphilis: resurgence of an old problem. *JAMA* 2003; **290**(11): 1510–14.

24. Kararizou E, Mitsonis C, Dimopoulos E *et al.* Psychosis or simply a new manifestation of neurosyphilis? *J Int Med Res* 2006; **34**: 335–7.

25. Lair L, Naidech AM. Modern neuropsychiatric presentation of neurosyphilis. *Neurology* 2004; **63**: 1331–3.

26. Wharton M, Chorba TL, Vogt RL, Morse DL, Buehler JW. Case definitions for public health surveillance. *MMWR Recomm Rep* 1990; **39**: 1–43.

27. Workowski KA, Berman SM. Sexually transmitted diseases treatment guidelines, 2006. *MMWR Recomm Rep* 2006; **55**: 1–94.

28. Chayakulkeeree M, Perfect JR. Cryptococcosis. *Infect Dis Clin North Am* 2006; **20**(3): 507–44.

29. Park BJ, Wannemuehler KA, Marston BJ, Govender N, Pappas PG, Chiller TM. Estimation of the current global burden of cryptococcal meningitis among persons living with HIV/AIDS. *AIDS* 2009; **23**: 525–30.

30. Johnson FY, Naraqi S. Manic episode secondary to cryptococcal meningitis in a previously healthy adult. *P N G Med J* 1993; **36**(1): 59–62.

31. Sa'adah MA, Araj GF, Diab SM, Nazzal M. Cryptococcal meningitis and confusional psychosis. A case report and literature review. *Trop Geogr Med* 1995; **47**(5): 224–6.

32. Dromer F, Mathoulin-Pélissier S, Launay O, Lortholary O, French Cryptococcus Study Group. Determinants of disease presentation and outcome during cryptococcosis: the cryptoA/D study. *PLoS Med* 2007; **4**(2): e21.

33. Kaplan MH, Rosen PP, Armstrong D. Cryptococcosis in a cancer hospital: clinical and pathological correlates in forty-six patients. *Cancer* 1977; **39**(5): 2265–74.

34. Saha DC, Xess I, Jain N. Evaluation of conventional and serological methods for rapid diagnosis of cryptococcosis. *Indian J Med Res* 2008; **127**(5): 483–8.

35. Saag MS, Graybill RJ, Larsen RA *et al.* Practice guidelines for the management of cryptococcal disease. *Clin Infect Dis* 2000; **30**(4): 710–18.

36. Hokkanen L, Launes J. Neuropsychological sequelae of acute-onset sporadic viral encephalitis. *Neuropsychol Rehabil* 2007; **17**(4): 450–77.

37. Kennedy PG. Viral encephalitis: causes, differential diagnosis, and management. *J Neurol Neurosurg Psychiatry* 2004; **75**(suppl): i10–15.

38. Arcinegas DB, Anderson CA. Viral encephalitis: neuropsychiatric and neurobehavioral aspects. *Curr Psychiatry Rep* 2004; **6**: 372–9.

39. Kennedy PG, Chaudhuri A. Herpes simplex encephalitis. *J Neurol Neurosurg Psychiatry* 2002; **73**: 237–8.

40. Fodor PA, Levin MJ, Weinberg A *et al.* Atypical herpes simplex virus encephalitis diagnosed by PCR amplification of viral DNA from CSF. *Neurology* 1998; **51**: 554–9.

41. Sage JJ, Weinstein MP, Miller DC. Chronic encephalitis possibly due to herpes simplex virus: two cases. *Neurology* 1985; **35**(10): 1470–72.

42. McGrath N, Anderson NE, Croxson MC, Powell KF. Herpes simplex encephalitis treated with acyclovir: diagnosis and long term outcome. *J Neurol Neurosurg Psychiatry* 1997; **63**: 321–6.

69

Magnetic Resonance Imaging and Computed Tomography

Howard Aizenstein and Vijay Venkatraman

University of Pittsburgh School of Medicine, Pittsburgh, USA

COMPUTED TOMOGRAPHY

Computed tomography (CT) is a general term for several radiographic techniques that result in a series of images showing slices of an organ or body region, such as the brain. The CT systems measure the attenuation of X-ray beams passing through target tissue; this is done using a small X-ray device that rotates around the body region of interest in a fixed plane. Various absorption and scattering processes are utilized in CT: coherent scattering, photoelectric absorption and Compton scattering. The X-ray tubes provide incident X-rays yielding a spectrum of X-rays with a transmission of the signals. The signals are sent to a computer that produces the corresponding cross-sectional slice for that plane. The image is composed of a set of individual pixels, which represent the attenuation of the X-ray at the corresponding point. These attenuation values are referred to as the CT number or Hounsfield units. The computer can create sections in axial, coronal and sagittal alignments using an image reconstruction process. The three major paradigms of image reconstruction are (i) simple back-projection, (ii) filtered back-projection, and (iii) iterative reconstruction.

In a single CT scan across one section in a patient, thousands of X-ray transmission measurements are obtained along many different angular projections. From these measurements, utilizing a variety of mathematical paradigms, a matrix of CT numbers can be computed for the cross-sectional plane through the patient and then displayed as a grey-scale image. There are a number of artefacts that affect the performance of CT scanning and the quality of the acquired data. These artefacts lead to streak patterns on the image display or appear in the form of CT number inaccuracies. Some of the artefacts are caused during the X-ray transmission phase (e.g. patient motion, polychromatic effects), X-ray detection and measurement (e.g. detector imbalance, scatter collimation), data acquisition (e.g. slice geometry, profile sampling) and data processing (e.g. algorithm effects). CT scans require the use of a limited amount of radiation, which presents a potential health risk for those undergoing CT scans. The estimated radiation exposure varies by the particular type of CT scan performed. It is estimated that a head CT is associated with 1.5 millisieverts, which is equivalent to the radiation exposure from 75 chest X-rays. This amount of radiation exposure is considered an acceptable risk when the CT is medically indicated. CT studies should follow the radiation recommendation, including the special cases for multiple exposures and overlapping scanning techniques.

With advances in scanning, software and display systems, the quality of CT images improved (i.e. better resolution) and has led to many useful clinical applications, including virtual CT colonoscopy or angiography. Neuroimaging with CT is used for studying various psychiatric populations including schizophrenia and depression, as well as aging and dementia.

CT imaging is used to examine brain structure; it allows for the ready identification of many structures, although it does have limitations. By measuring differences in density, it can distinguish among CSF, blood, bone, grey matter and white matter. CT is particularly useful for demonstrating injuries such as skull fractures (bone abnormalities), subdural haematoma (haemorrhage regions) and different lesions (mass effect). CT is also used to study variation in atrophy or ventricular enlargement. However, CT studies are restricted by location of the structures like the brain stem because of surrounding bone. CT has been used to measure cerebral atrophy and grey matter (secondary loss of neurons) since 1974[1]. CT has been widely used in the identification of dementia[2]. Many studies were performed to study age variation in geriatric populations[3-6], normal ageing[7] and the effect of presence of dementia[8,9].

With improvement in resolution of CT, it was used to distinguish some pathological processes, which primarily affect white matter (i.e. demyelination)[10,11]. A large number of CT studies of white-matter diseases in the geriatric population were published[12-16]. CT measurements of the cerebrospinal fluid (CSF) spaces from patients with geriatric depression, normal control subjects and patients with primary degenerative dementia have been compared and studied also[17].

CT is widely available and well understood, but is nowadays supplemented with magnetic resonance imaging (MRI) to use the advantages of both techniques.

MAGNETIC RESONANCE IMAGING

In 2003, Paul C. Lauterbur and Peter Mansfield were awarded the Nobel Prize in Medicine for their discovery of MRI. MRI revolutionized *in vivo* human brain imaging, allowing for remarkably clear high-resolution images of the brain. MRI is based on the concept of nuclear magnetic resonance (NMR), where the measurement of the signals comes from the nuclei in response to radio waves that have the same frequency as the nuclei themselves[18,19]. For a comprehensive review, please refer to[18,19].

Principles and Practice of Geriatric Psychiatry, 3rd edn. Edited by Mohammed T. Abou-Saleh, Cornelius Katona and Anand Kumar
© 2011 John Wiley & Sons, Ltd

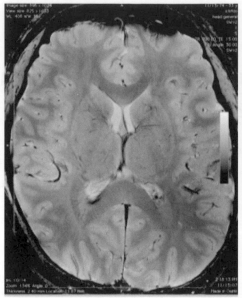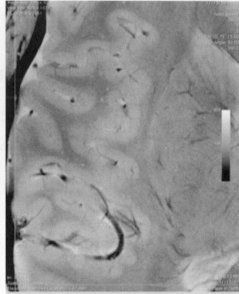

Figure 69.1   SWI image using 7 T Siemens scanner

The relaxation time (T1) is a property of a tissue at a given magnetic field strength. With each excitation pulse, the longitudinal magnetization begins to recover and reduces to steady state after several pulses. The time between repetitions of the excitation pulse is called the repetition time (TR). The repetition time and flip angle are the two major parameters varied to control the T1 weighting of an image. The transverse magnetization decays at the rate of T2 relaxation time. The delay between the creation of the transverse magnetization and the measurement of the resulting echo is called the echo time (TE). The images where signal intensity is largely dependent on T2 differences (or TE values) are called T2-weighted images. The various pulse sequences are designed based on TR, TE and other parameters to obtain the necessary contrast variation in the magnetic resonance image. The magnetic resonance image can have different artefacts, such as motion-induced artefacts, susceptibility, wrap around, edge artefacts (partial volume, chemical shift edge, truncation, relaxation), ghost artefacts, altered signal intensity, stripes and image distortion. The different pulse sequences used in imaging sequences, such as T2*, echo planar imaging used in BOLD fMRI, fluid-attenuated inversion-recovery imaging (FLAIR), diffusion weighted imaging, magnetization transfer imaging and others, are novel variations obtained from optimization of the various parameters.

Difference between 1.5 T, 3 T vs. 7 T Images

Typically the MRI scanner is built around a permanent magnet, which is the most expensive and important component of the scanner[18,19]. The strength of the main magnet and its precision (homogeneity of the field strength) is important. Magnetic field strength is an important factor in determining image quality. Higher magnetic fields increase signal-to-noise ratio, permitting higher resolution or faster scanning. The higher field strengths have drawbacks such as more costly magnets, higher maintenance costs, increased safety concerns and increases in certain artefacts compared to lower field strengths. The 1.0–1.5 T field strengths are a good option for general medical use. Field strengths up to 3.0 T may be desirable for research

(such as brain imaging) and the latest research studies use 7 T field strengths. Figure 69.1 provides the susceptibility-weighted imaging (SWI) using a 7 T Siemens imaging scanner.

Structural MRI

Structural MRI methods can be used to identify and quantify patterns of changes in volumetric neuroimaging studies. The various structural MRI sequences enable the identification of structural alterations such as (i) volume in grey matter, white matter and cerebrospinal fluid from high resolution T1-weighted images[20–22], (ii) white matter hyperintensities (WMH) from FLAIR images[23,24], (iii) white matter integrity from diffusion weighted imaging[25,26], and (iv) myelination from magnetization transfer imaging[27] (Figure 69.2). Advanced neuroimaging sequences such as diffusion spectrum imaging (DSI) and Q-ball imaging are currently been used for studying the white matter tracts[28].

Structural MRI is useful for studying the patterns of neuroanatomical changes in geriatric research. Structural MRI is important for studies in normal ageing, late-life depression, dementia, Alzheimer's disease and other cognitive disorders to examine how age-associated changes in neuroanatomy are associated with specific age-related changes, such as the changes in cognition.

Functional MRI

In the 1960s and 1970s a number of investigators showed that not only could MRI be used to visualize neuroanatomy and structural

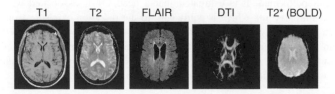

Figure 69.2   T1, T2, FLAIR, DTI and T2* images from 3 T scanner

pathology, but by tuning the MRI contrast appropriately, MRI could be used to visualize the dynamic changes in blood oxygenation across the brain; this was the beginning of functional MRI (fMRI). Over the subsequent years, a number of studies have shown that this blood oxygenation level dependent (BOLD) signal could be used to map brain activity on a variety of cognitive and affective tasks.

Functional MRI has been a major advance for the fields of cognitive and affective neuroscience by allowing investigators to test theories of the underlying neural pathways controlling cognitive and emotional processes. This approach is often referred to as 'human brain mapping'. In addition to studying 'normal' human brain function, fMRI can also be used to characterize the functional activation patterns in patient groups. This area of clinical fMRI research has recently led to a number of new insights into the nature of psychopathology and treatment – including recognition of a dorsal versus ventral processing imbalance in depression[29], overlap in response patterns with placebo as with medication[30], and paradoxical non-linear activation patterns in mild cognitive impairment[31], suggesting a compensatory stage prior to the onset of dementia.

The functional circuit involved in a particular task can be identified by contrasting the MRI images acquired while someone is doing the task versus when they are doing a control task. There are two main ways this can be done: (i) blocked design, where the subject performs several minutes of task and then several minutes of control, and the images during these blocks are compared; and (ii) event-related design, where the subject performs discrete events during the scanning session, and the images during discrete events are compared. The task could also be a mixed design of block and event designs. Several studies have examined the statistical advantages between block design and event-related fMRI, and the general view is that for the same amount of time spent scanning (on the same task), the observed effect size is larger for a block design study as compared to an event-related study[32].

Perfusion MRI: An Alternative to BOLD

A significant limitation in BOLD fMRI is concern that the BOLD haemodynamic response is inherently relative. That is, the raw BOLD signal does not provide a reliable estimate of regional blood flow in a region. Rather, it is contrast of the BOLD signal on alternating experimental versus control tasks that provides the meaningful signal. In contrast to this limitation, PET imaging with an O15 radioligand is capable of providing quantitative blood flow measures. In MRI, a technique analogous to O15 PET is also available, and is referred to as arterial spin label (ASL) imaging, or perfusion imaging[33,34]. In perfusion MRI the MRI excitation signal is inverted to provide a 'tagged' signal, which is alternated with an 'untagged' image. Comparing the tagged and untagged images provides a quantitative measure of the perfusion of the region. Full-brain voxel-wise perfusion images acquired can provide a quantitative image of the perfusion across the brain. Investigators have recently used perfusion imaging to demonstrate similar findings as with PET blood flow studies, e.g. decreased parietal-temporal resting perfusion with Alzheimer's disease[35]. In addition to providing quantitative resting perfusion, ASL has also recently been used for investigating the blood flow changes associated with tasks. For instance, Fernandez-Seara et al.[36] have used ASL to show medial temporal lobe activity on an encoding task. The two primary methods for perfusion imaging are referred to as continuous arterial spin labelling (CASL) and pulsed arterial spin labelling (PASL). CASL is believed to provide

better signal quality, but generally requires special hardware for providing the continuous tagging pulse.

Methodological Challenges of fMRI in Geriatric Psychiatry

In order to appropriately interpret fMRI results in geriatric psychiatry, it is important to consider whether differences in brain structure may impact the resulting fMRI signal, and similarly it is important to consider whether changes in brain physiology may influence assumptions about the BOLD fMRI signal. These concerns about brain morphometric changes in the elderly and age-related changes in the BOLD signal are the two primary methodological challenges of fMRI in geriatric psychiatry.

The change in brain volume with age and with the diseases of ageing presents a particular challenge for fMRI studies in these populations: how should these structural changes be accounted for when comparing the functional signal? In a standard fMRI analysis plan, the functional signals from all the subjects in a study are lined up with each other (referred to as normalization). If the brains have significantly different shapes and sizes then this brain alignment may bias the results by contributing more CSF (due to the larger sulci and ventricles) of the more atrophic brains as compared to more grey matter from the less atrophic brains. The standard alignment algorithms vary in their ability to account for the variability in brain structure[37]. Some investigators have addressed this problem by using a larger smoothing kernel in studies of ageing subjects (e.g. 10 mm instead of standard smoothness of 6 mm or 8 mm full-width half-maximum Gaussian). An alternative approach that other investigators have used involves avoiding the registration problems altogether, by focusing on a region-of-interest (ROI)-based analysis[38].

SUMMARY

There has been tremendous increase in the use of CT and MRI (functional and structural) in studying the brain. The neuroimaging studies have provided insight into normal ageing and the neuropsychiatric diseases of ageing. In this chapter we reviewed the basis of CT and MRI (structural and functional).

REFERENCES

1. Hughes CP, Gado M. Computed tomography and aging of the brain. *Radiology* 1981; **139**: 391–6.
2. Soininen H, Puranen M, Riekkinen PJ. Computed tomography findings in senile dementia and normal aging. *J Neurol Neurosurg Psychiatry* 1982; **45**: 50–54.
3. Gyldensted C, Kosteljanetz M. Measurements of the normal hemispheric sulci with computer tomography: a preliminary study on 44 adults. *Neuroradiology* 1975; **10**: 147–9.
4. Barron SA, Jacobs L, Kinkel WR. Changes in size of normal lateral ventricles during aging determined by computerized tomography. *Neurology* 1976; **26**: 1011–13.
5. Haug G. Age and sex dependence of the size of normal ventricles on computed tomography. *Neuroradiology* 1977; **14**: 201–4.
6. Jacoby RJ, Levy R, Dawson JM. Computed tomography in the elderly: I. The normal population. *Br J Psychiatry* 1980; **136**: 249–55.

7. Laffey PA, Peyster RG, Nathan R, Haskin ME, McGinley JA. Computed tomography and aging: results in a normal elderly population. *Neuroradiology* 1984; **26**: 273–8.

8. Jacoby RJ, Levy R. Computed tomography in the elderly. II. Senile dementia: diagnosis and functional impairment. *Br J Psychiatry* 1980; **136**: 256–69.

9. Kaszniak AW, Fox J, Gandell DL *et al.* Predictors of mortality in presenile and senile dementia. *Ann Neurol* 1978; **3**: 246–52.

10. Huckman MS, Fox JH, Ramsey AG. Computed tomography in the diagnosis of degenerative diseases of the brain. *Semin Roentgenol* 1977; **12**: 63–75.

11. Rao CVGK, Brennan TG, Garcia JH. Computed tomography in the diagnosis of Creutzfeldt–Jacob disease. *J Comput Assist Tomogr* 1977; **1**: 211–15.

12. Eiben RM, Di Chiro G. Computer assisted tomography in adrenoleukodystrophy. *J Comput Assist Tomogr* 1977; **1**: 308–14.

13. Carroll BA, Lane B, Norman D, Enzmann D. Diagnosis of progressive multifocal leukoencephalopathy by computed tomography. *Radiology* 1977; **122**: 137–41.

14. Peylan-Ramu N, Poplack DG, Blei CL *et al.* Computer assisted tomography in methotrexate encephalopathy. *J Comput Assist Tomogr* 1977; **1**: 216–21.

15. Heinz ER, Drayer BP, Haenggeli CA, Painter MJ, Crumnine P. Computed tomography in white-matter disease. *Radiology* 1979; **130**: 371–8.

16. Goto K, Ishli N, Fukasawa H. Diffuse white-matter disease in the geriatric population: a clinical, neuropathobogical, and CT study. *Radiology* 1981; **141**: 687–95.

17. Wurthmann C, Bogerts B, Falkai P. Brain morphology assessed by computed tomography in patients with geriatric depression, patients with degenerative dementia, and normal control subjects. *Psychiatry Res* 1995; **61**: 103–11.

18. Liang ZP, Lauterbur PC. *Principles of Magnetic Resonance Imaging: A Signal Processing Perspective*. Bellingham, WA: SPIE Optical Engineering Press, 2000.

19. Mitchell DG. *MRI principles*. Philadelphia, PA: WB Saunders, 1999.

20. Raz N. The aging brain observed in vivo: differential changes and their modifiers. In Cabeza R, Nyberg L, Park D (eds), *Cognitive Neuroscience of Aging*. New York: Oxford University Press, 2005, 19–57.

21. Raz N. Neuroanatomy of aging brain: evidence from structural MRI. In Bigler ED (ed.), *Neuroimaging II: Clinical Applications*. New York: Academic Press, 1996, 153–82.

22. Rosano C, Becker J, Lopez O *et al.* Morphometric analysis of gray matter volume in demented older adults: exploratory analysis of the cardiovascular health study brain MRI database. *Neuroepidemiology* 2005; **24**(4): 221–9.

23. Gunning-Dixon FM, Raz N. The cognitive correlates of white matter abnormalities in normal aging: a quantitative review. *Neuropsychology* 2000; **14**(2): 224–32.

24. Soderlund H, Nyberg L, Adolfsson R, Nilsson LG, Launer LJ. High prevalence of white matter hyperintensities in normal aging: relation to blood pressure and cognition. *Cortex* 2003; **39**(4–5): 1093–1105.

25. Pfefferbaum A, Adalsteinsson E, Sullivan EV. Frontal circuitry degradation marks healthy adult aging: evidence from diffusion tensor imaging. *Neuroimage* 2005; **26**(3): 891–9.

26. Salat DH, Tuch DS, Greve DN *et al.* Age-related alterations in white matter microstructure measured by diffusion tensor imaging. *Neurobiol Aging* 2005; **26**(8): 1215–27.

27. Van Es AC, van der Flier AW, Admiraal-Behloul F *et al.* Magnetization transfer imaging of gray and white matter in mild cognitive impairment and Alzheimer's disease. *Neurobiol Aging* 2006; **27**(12): 1757–62.

28. Schmahmann JD, Pandya DN, Wang R, Dai G, D'Arceuil HE. Association fibre pathways of the brain: parallel observations from diffusion spectrum imaging and autoradiography. *Brain* 2007; **130**: 630–53.

29. Phillips ML, Drevets WC, Rauch SL, Lane R. Neurobiology of emotion perception II: Implications for major psychiatric disorders. *Biol Psychiatry* 2003; **54**(5): 515–28.

30. Mayberg HS, Silva JA, Brannan SK *et al.* The functional neuroanatomy of the placebo effect. *Am J Psychiatry* 2002; **159**(5): 728–37.

31. Wierenga CE, Bondi MW. Use of functional magnetic resonance imaging in the early identification of Alzheimer's disease. *Neuropsychology Rev* 2007; **17**(2): 127–43.

32. Friston KJ, Holmes AP, Price CJ, Buchel C, Worsley KJ. Multisubject fMRI studies and conjunction analyses. *Neuroimage* 1999; **10**: 385–96.

33. Detre JA, Leigh JS, Williams DS, Koretsky AP. Perfusion imaging. *Magn Reson Med* 1992; **23**(1): 37–45.

34. Aguirre GK, Detre JA, Wang J. Perfusion fMRI for functional neuroimaging. *Int Rev Neurobiol* 2005; **66**: 213–36.

35. Alsop DC, Detre JA, Grossman M. Assessment of cerebral blood flow in Alzheimer's disease by spin-labeled magnetic resonance imaging. *Ann Neurol* 2000; **47**(1): 93–100.

36. Fernandez-Seara MA, Wang J, Wang Z *et al.* Imaging mesial temporal lobe activation during scene encoding: comparison of fMRI using BOLD and arterial spin labeling. *Hum Brain Mapp* 2007; **28**(12): 1391–1400.

37. Reuter-Lorenz PA, Lustig C. Brain aging: reorganizing discoveries about the aging mind. *Curr Opin Neurobiol* 2005; **15**(4): 245–51.

38. Aizenstein HJ, Clark KA, Butters MA. The BOLD hemodynamic response in healthy aging. *J Cogn Neurosci* 2004; **16**(5): 786–93.

70

Functional MRI Studies in Ageing and Early Alzheimer's Disease

Ottavio V. Vitolo[1,2,5,7] **and Reisa A. Sperling**[1,2,3,4,5,6,7]

[1]*Memory Disorders Unit, Harvard Medical School, USA*
[2]*Brigham and Women's Hospital, Harvard Medical School, USA*
[3]*Alzheimer's Disease Research Center, Harvard Medical School, USA*
[4]*Gerontology Research Unit, Harvard Medical School, USA*
[5]*Massachusetts General Hospital, Harvard Medical School, USA*
[6]*Department of Neurology, Harvard Medical School, USA*
[7]*Psychiatry, Harvard Medical School, USA*

INTRODUCTION

The last few years have seen a rapid upsurge in the number of functional magnetic resonance imaging (fMRI) studies of Alzheimer's disease (AD). The increasing popularity of fMRI is likely due to the tremendous need to find early markers for this devastating illness, prior to the point of irreversible neuronal loss. The clinical course of AD is typically insidious, characterized by episodic memory impairment beginning years prior to the time a clinical diagnosis is established. Evidence from postmortem and antemortem molecular imaging studies of subjects at risk for AD suggests that underlying pathology of AD may begin more than a decade prior to onset of dementia[1]. The link between the pathophysiological process of AD and the earliest clinical manifestations remains to be fully elucidated. Animal studies indicate that amyloid-related synaptic dysfunction precedes the onset of neuron loss and may account for early memory deficits[2,3]; however, autopsy studies suggest that tangle pathology and neuronal loss may correlate better with clinical dementia severity at later stages of the disease[4,5].

The lack of reliable diagnostic biomarkers, which can detect AD early in its course, continues to limit our ability to effectively develop and initiate disease-modifying therapies. In this respect, fMRI has the potential to elucidate the pathophysiological process that ultimately leads to AD and could prove to be an invaluable tool for early detection of the disease and to assist in monitoring the effectiveness of new therapies.

This chapter will focus on recent findings from fMRI research on ageing and early AD, focusing on potential applications of fMRI for the diagnosis of AD and development of therapeutic agents.

POTENTIAL APPLICATIONS OF FUNCTIONAL IMAGING

Functional imaging techniques, in particular those that study brain activity during cognitive processes, have the potential to detect the earliest impact of pathophysiological changes on the functional integrity of neural networks. Although volumetric magnetic resonance imaging is presumably quite sensitive to loss of neurons and surrounding neuropil, it may not be able to detect changes until there is significant neuronal loss in specific medial temporal lobe (MTL) structures[6], at a point too late to intervene with disease-modifying therapies. Functional imaging techniques that observe the brain at rest, such as fludeoxyglucose (^{18}F) (18-fluorodeoxyglucose, FDG) positron emission tomography (PET), perfusion MRI[7,8] and resting-state fMRI[9,10], have shown evidence of regional abnormalities in early AD and may prove valuable in predicting subsequent decline in at-risk subjects. In order to detect brain dysfunction in individuals with very subtle cognitive impairment, and even asymptomatic individuals with early pathology of AD, we may need to employ more sensitive measures that probe the brain during exactly the types of cognitive processes that will become clinically impaired as the disease progresses. Task-related functional MRI may be able to detect alterations in the brain's functional capacity prior to neuronal loss, or even evidence of dysfunction at rest.

PHYSIOLOGICAL BASIS OF fMRI

The fMRI technique most widely used to investigate neural activity is based on imaging of the blood-oxygen-level-dependent (BOLD) contrast[11]. This depends on the magnetic properties of haemoglobin, which differ depending on whether or not it is bound to oxygen. The ratio between oxygenated haemoglobin, which is a diamagnetic substance with zero magnetic moment, and deoxyhaemoglobin, which instead is a natural paramagnetic substance, in capillary beds and larger blood vessels subserving neural tissue creates an image contrast detected by the MRI machine. Neuronal activity affects the ratio by increasing oxygen consumption and blood supply. Since the blood supply exceeds the oxygen demand, this results in an increase of the amount of deoxyhaemoglobin and therefore of the MR signal[12]. Thus, BOLD fMRI is an indirect measure of neuronal activity but

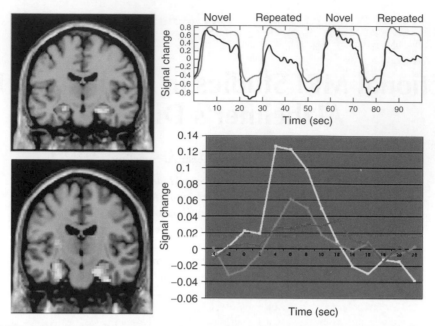

Figure 70.1   Functional MRI data during a face-name encoding paradigm. The top left figure demonstrates a statistical parametric map (SPM) of the hippocampus showing greater MR signal response to novel (N) face-name pairs compared to repeated (R) face-name pairs in a block-design fMRI paradigm. The top right shows a representative time course of the MR signal in the block-design paradigm, with marked increase in signal during novel blocks compared to blocks of visual fixation (+) or repeated blocks. The bottom left demonstrates significant hippocampal activation for an event-related face-name paradigm comparing successful vs. failed encoding. The bottom right graph shows the MR signal change in the right hippocampus for those face-name pairs correctly remembered with high confidence (yellow line), low confidence (pink line) or forgotten (blue line). *A full colour version of this figure appears in the colour plate section*

can provide an important 'window' into the neural underpinnings of complex cognitive processes.

Typically BOLD fMRI is almost always reported as a 'relative measure', comparing the MR signal during one task (e.g. memory encoding) to a control task (e.g. viewing familiar stimulus) or a 'baseline condition' (e.g. visual fixation). Stimuli of each cognitive condition can be either grouped together in blocks lasting 20–40 s, as in a 'block-design' paradigm (see Figure 70.1), or can be interspersed with single stimuli of different conditions as in 'event-related' paradigms. The peak haemodynamic response is typically observed 4–6 s after the stimulus onset. Comparisons between conditions are performed using statistical packages that analyse the raw data of each voxel according to a general linear model (Statistical Parametric Mapping (SPM) and Brain Voyager are some commonly used analysis toolboxes). This type of analysis considers all the variables that can affect signal within each voxel and ultimately translates in either increased BOLD signal, referred to as 'fMRI activation', or decreased BOLD signal, referred to as 'fMRI deactivation' in one condition compared to another. Deactivations or negative BOLD responses have been shown to reflect task-related decreases in neuronal activity below levels detected during spontaneous activity[13], but it remains unclear whether this phenomenon is due to specific inhibitory influences.

At the present there is no way to determine an absolute measure of fMRI signal at 'baseline', and even resting fMRI scans investigate the correlations between regional MR signal over time to measure resting activity. Arterial spin labelling (ASL) perfusion fMRI techniques may provide a more robust baseline measurement of perfusion, but most task-related fMRI studies utilizing ASL techniques still rely on the 'subtraction' of MR signal in one condition versus another.

Intrinsic or resting connectivity studies examine the inter-regional correlations in the MR signal time course[14].

In the future, information from multiple imaging modalities, particularly perfusion MR, FDG-PET, and task-related BOLD fMRI, may be useful in determining whether the observed functional changes in patient populations relate primarily to alterations in 'baseline' function vs. the neural requirements of the cognitive task, or perhaps to a combination of both factors.

A few studies have demonstrated fMRI alterations in sensorimotor areas in both cognitively normal older and AD patients[15–17]. These findings have invited caution in the interpretation of fMRI study results in ageing and AD, and raised concerns that changes in BOLD response could be due to a global decoupling of the haemodynamic response related to ageing and pathological processes of the vascular system.

Multiple studies have now demonstrated that the fMRI alterations in subjects with mild and moderate AD reflect regional changes specific to the memory task and that the BOLD response in unaffected brain regions is quite similar in magnitude and extent to that seen in age-matched normal older control subjects[18,19].

NEUROIMAGING IN NORMAL AGEING

In recent years, fMRI studies have provided important insights into the neural underpinnings of the cognitive changes associated with ageing. Neuroimaging studies of non-demented older subjects compared to normal young adults have demonstrated group differences in the activation of brain regions responsible for the cognitive task in study. These findings have led to the formulation of the functional compensation theory and the dedifferentiation theory to explain the observed changes. The first theory postulates that decreased activation of brain regions in older compared to younger adults may represent less efficient processing. Instead, increased activity reflects compensatory mechanisms recruited to maintain efficient performance. Both PET and fMRI studies of memory performance have found loss of hemispheric asymmetry activation in older adults who have performances similar to those of young adults. Cabeza renamed this phenomenon 'hemispheric asymmetry reduction in older adults' (HAROLD). In one fMRI study of a word recognition task controlled for performance[20], older participants showed increased activation of bilateral regions. In addition to increased bilateral activation to maintain performance, additional evidence points to age-related increased activation of the prefrontal cortex (PFC) associated with successful performance. This mechanism has been called 'posterior–anterior shift in ageing' (PASA)[21] and is thought to compensate for deficient perceptual processing in the sensory areas seen in ageing. According to the dedifferentiation theory, the more widespread engagement of brain areas, not found to be involved in the execution of the same task in younger individuals, represents loss of efficiency of networks activated in younger subjects. To further support this view, some authors propose that various cognitive processes possess a higher degree of interdependence in older individuals[22]. These changes can be thought of as lying on a continuum that moves from lack of differentiation in childhood, to differentiation in adulthood, then to dedifferentiation in older adults.

The adaptive nature of the changes described above is at the core of what Park and Reuter-Lorenz have termed the 'scaffolding theory of ageing and cognition' (STAC). They define scaffolding as 'a process that results in changes of brain function through strengthening of existing connections, formation of new connections, and disuse of connections that have become weak or faulty'. In their view, both HAROLD and PASA can be conceptualized as part of the same compensatory process that reallocates tasks to preserved circuitries unaffected by ageing and possibly pathology to meet the task demands[23].

NEURAL NETWORKS SUPPORTING MEMORY FUNCTION

The use of fMRI can be extended to investigate the brain networks involved in memory formation and how they are affected in AD. In particular, those studies using a 'subsequent memory' paradigm have demonstrated that greater fMRI activity in the MTL, as well as the left inferior prefrontal cortex, during encoding is associated with the likelihood of subsequent successful retrieval of the information[24–28]. This is further supported by the observation that compounds with known amnesic effects, such as benzodiazepines and anticholinergics, induce decreased activation in the hippocampus and prefrontal regions[29,30].

Our own fMRI work has focused primarily on associative memory processes and, in particular, face-name associations. One primary role of the hippocampal formation in episodic encoding is to form new associations between previously unrelated items of information[31,32]. Learning the relationship between a name and a face is a particularly difficult cross-modal, non-contextual, paired associate memory task, and difficulty remembering proper names is the most common memory complaint of older individuals visiting memory clinics[33,34]. Tasks that tap into this cognitive process may be particularly useful in detecting the earliest memory impairment in AD[1,35,36]. Several fMRI

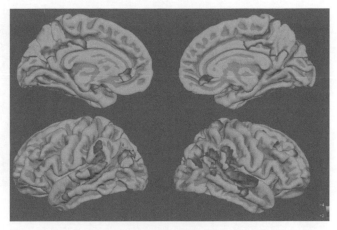

Figure 70.2   The default network, a set of regions that demonstrate higher fMRI activity during rest compared to challenging cognitive tasks. In this group fMRI data map, regions in blue demonstrate greater MR signal during rest (visual fixation) compared to novel face-name encoding. *A full colour version of this figure appears in the colour plate section*

studies, including our own in young subjects using a face-name associative encoding task[27,29,37] show that associative memory paradigms produce robust activation of the anterior hippocampal formation[38–40].

While activation in the anterior hippocampal formation is required for successful memory formation, a similar task-induced decrease in MR signal (i.e. deactivation), particularly in medial and lateral parietal regions, is also associated with successful encoding[41,42]. These lateral and medial parietal regions, including the precuneus and posterior cingulate, are central components of the 'default-mode network' (see Figure 70.2), characterized by Raichle and colleagues in a series of both PET and fMRI studies[43,44]. These regions typically exhibit increased activity at rest and decreased activity during externally focused task performance[44]. These parietal regions also appear to have significant connectivity with the hippocampus in resting-state network analyses[14,45], and overlap with a 'retrospenial memory system' that typically activates during memory retrieval tasks[46,47]. Our own work in cognitively normal young and older adults suggests that the MTL system and the default-network system can be conceptualized as the 'yin–yang' of a distributed memory network. Successful encoding appears to require coordinated activity between these components, such that the lateral and medial parietal regions need to deactivate, while the MTL regions are activated[42,48] (Figure 70.3).

fMRI STUDIES IN PATIENTS WITH CLINICALLY DIAGNOSED ALZHEIMER'S DISEASE

Since episodic memory impairment is an early finding of AD, the majority of fMRI studies to date have focused on episodic memory tasks[18,19,49–57]. These studies have employed a variety of unfamiliar visual stimuli, including faces[17,49], face-name pairs[19,55], scenes[54], line-drawings[50,57], geometric shapes[51] and verbal stimuli[56], and have consistently reported decreased hippocampal and parahippocampal activity in AD patients compared to healthy older controls during the encoding of novel stimuli. In our own studies using the block-design face-name paradigm, we found evidence that AD patients demonstrate significantly less hippocampal activation in the novel vs. repeated comparison than normal older controls[19,53]. Instead,

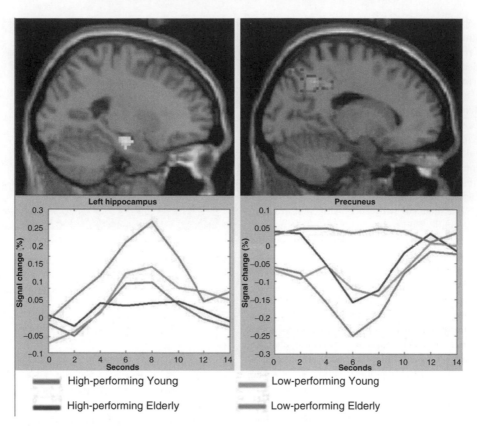

Figure 70.3 Group fMRI data maps (top) with MR signal time courses (bottom) for Young and Elderly controls show hippocampal activation (left) and precuneus deactivation (right) during the successful encoding of face-name pairs. Low-performing Elderly failed to deactivate the precuneus and demonstrated increased hippocampal and prefrontal activation for successful but not failed encoding trials, perhaps as a compensatory response to failure of default network activity. *A full colour version of this figure appears in the colour plate section*

during repeated stimuli exposure, AD patients continue to demonstrate increased MTL activation to stimuli that are highly familiarized to normal older controls[58], and the degree of hyperactivation relates to poor post-scan memory performance. These findings indicate that intact MTL response suppression is an integral part of successful memory encoding and consolidation process and that failure of repetition suppression may be a sensitive marker of hippocampal dysfunction early in the course of AD[59]. Interestingly, in addition to MTL hyperactivation, several fMRI studies have also found evidence of increased activation in frontal and parietal regions in AD patients compared to controls, which, as described before, may represent a compensatory process in the setting of hippocampal failure[19,55,56,60].

Abnormal patterns of fMRI activity have also been found in the default-mode network regions of AD patients[17,47,61,62]. Buckner *et al.*[47] were the first to note that these regions are strikingly similar to those regions that typically demonstrate evidence of fibrillar amyloid deposition binding with Pittsburgh compound B (PiB) in PET studies in AD[63], as well as to the pattern of hypometabolism found on FDG-PET studies of AD patients[64–66] and subjects at-risk for AD[67–69]; and of hypoperfusion on resting MR perfusion studies in AD[7,8]. More recently, we have also noted that the pattern of intrinsic connectivity, or 'hubs' also overlaps the pattern of amyloid deposition[70], supporting the hypothesis that amyloid-beta deposition is dependent on neuronal activity[71].

The alterations in hippocampal activation and parietal deactivation over the course of mild cognitive impairment (MCI) and AD appear to be strongly correlated[72]. Similarly, resting-state fMRI data has

demonstrated alterations in parietal and hippocampal connectivity in MCI and AD[9]. Thus, converging evidence suggests that a distributed memory network is disrupted by the pathophysiological process of AD, which includes both medial temporal lobe systems and medial and lateral parietal regions involved in default-mode activity. Future studies to probe alterations in connectivity between these systems, which combine fMRI with other techniques such as diffusion tensor imaging, may prove particularly valuable in elucidating the early functional alterations in AD[73]. Of particular interest is a recent study by Seeley *et al.*[74], combining functional and structural network mapping in patients with AD and other neurodegenerative disorders. This study evidences how each neurodegenerative disorder affects a specific intrinsic connectivity network. The regions showing the greatest atrophy and functional connectivity disruption in AD corresponded to the 'default-mode network' involved in episodic memory, thus further confirming the previous findings of the fMRI studies described above.

fMRI ALTERATIONS IN MEDIAL TEMPORAL LOBE ACTIVITY IN MILD COGNITIVE IMPAIRMENT

We began this chapter by describing the realm of possibilities available through the use of fMRI as a diagnostic tool for early diagnosis of AD and for establishing the effectiveness of disease-modifying treatments. Unfortunately, the use of fMRI to characterize the cognitive changes of mild cognitive impairment is still in its infancy. This is due to several limitations including: (i) the heterogeneity of MCI as a diagnostic category, and (ii) the lack of standardized criteria until very recently developed and implemented in large-scale clinical trials and imaging studies[75]. Although we conceptualize MCI as a transitional state between normal ageing and mild AD[76], in reality MCI includes a diverse group of subjects, some of whom will never develop clinical AD. Most studies suggest that 15–18% of individuals with MCI convert to clinical AD within one year of follow-up. Interestingly, both autopsy and amyloid imaging studies have not demonstrated evidence of AD pathology in a large proportion of MCI patients, suggesting that the mechanisms for cognitive impairment in those who do not convert to AD may be different[77,78].

It is not surprising, then, that the few fMRI studies in MCI which have been published to date have shown heterogeneous findings, with some studies reporting hyperactivation and others hypoactivation of MTL. In part this apparent discrepancy could be ascribed to the broad definition of MCI, the wide range of cognitive impairment allowed in these studies and the type of cognitive tasks employed. In addition, we hypothesize that the MCI subjects' ability to perform the specific cognitive tasks has contributed to the variability in the published literature.

Studies Showing MTL Hypoactivation

Several studies[18,49,62,79] have reported hypoactivation in the MTL of MCI subjects similar to that seen in AD subjects during novel pictures encoding[18], face-encoding paradigm[49] and forced-choice recognition (retrieval) condition[62]. In addition, the study by Small et al. also found a group of impaired subjects with entorhinal and hippocampal activation similar to controls, and decreased activation in the subiculum. In the study by Petrella et al.[62], hypoactivation disappeared when memory performance was included as a covariate in the analysis. One of our own studies also found evidence of decreased MTL activation during face-name encoding in subjects who were thought to be at late stages of MCI with significant functional impairment as assessed by a high Clinical Dementia Rating Sum of Box score (CDR-SB)[72,80]. Other examples of hypoactivation findings include two studies by Johnson et al.[59,79]. In the first one, using a paradigm involving face repetition, MCI patients failed to show the same slope of decreasing hippocampal activation with stimulus repetition seen in control subjects, suggesting disruption of the habituating response to familiar stimuli in MCI[59]. The second study instead found right hippocampal hypoactivation in MCI patients compared to controls during a recognition paradigm for novel compared to previously learned items[79].

Studies Showing MTL Hyperactivation

In contrast, several studies have reported increased MTL activation in MCI subjects[53,57,81–83]. Using a visual object encoding paradigm, Hämäläinen et al. found greater activation in the caudal hippocampal formation, parahippocampal gyrus and fusiform cortex. Based on MMSE (mini-mental state examination) and neuropsychological data, this group had intermediate impairment between AD and mild MCI. Our own group has showed evidence of increased MTL activation in MCI subjects, using an associative face-name encoding paradigm. One study compared subjects across a range of clinical impairment assessed with CDR-SB and controls, using a scene encoding fMRI paradigm[83]. The results indicated a positive correlation between the degree of clinical impairment and the extent of activation in the posterior hippocampus and parahippocampal regions, such that subjects

with more impairment had a greater extent of MTL activation. A multivariate analysis showed that increasing impairment (CDR-SB) was related to older age, *decreased* volume of the left hippocampus, and *increased* extent of activation in the right parahippocampal gyrus. Greater MTL activation and larger MTL volume correlated with better performance on the post-scan recognition memory test. Importantly, two years later, those subjects with greater MTL activation were more likely to demonstrate clinical decline. We recently published a longer follow-up study, which further suggested that greater hippocampal activation at baseline predicted faster rate of clinical decline up to four years later[84]. The phenomenon of hippocampal hyperactivation in MCI subjects compared to controls was further confirmed by one of our studies which used the face-name encoding paradigm to compare MTL activation in subjects with very mild MCI (vMCI), AD and controls[53]. Compared with controls, the vMCI subjects showed a greater extent of hippocampal activation, and only minimal atrophy of the hippocampus. These very mild MCI subjects also performed in the same range as controls on post-scan memory test. The AD patients had smaller MTL volumes, decreased activation in these regions, and performed below controls on the post-scan memory test. Post-scan memory task performance of each group correlated with extent of activation in the hippocampus. Another one of our studies confirmed evidence of greater activation in the vMCI subjects compared to controls, particularly in the MTL (Figure 70.4) using the same face-name paradigm. A subset of subjects from the first study was analysed, applying independent component analyses to explore the alterations in larger memory networks in older controls, two groups of MCI subjects, one on the milder end and one on the more impaired end, and a group of mild AD patients[72]. In line with the previous findings, the significantly impaired MCI (sMCI) group showed significantly decreased activation down to levels similar to those found in AD. The MTL hypoactivation paralleled changes in medial and lateral parietal regions of the default network so that performance on the post-scan memory task was directly related to activation in the MTL and deactivation in the default network.

Further confirmation of the validity of the finding of MTL hyperactivation in MCI comes from fMRI studies that have applied an event-related design. This type of design allows the division of stimuli on the basis of successful vs. failed memory processes and can better control for the effects of memory performance. In one study, Kircher et al.[82] found that while performing similarly to controls, MCI subjects activated the left hippocampus and surrounding cortical regions to a greater degree than controls. This result was echoed by the evidence from an event-related verbal memory retrieval task, in which Heun et al. also found evidence of increased activation in MCI subjects compared to normal older controls when specifically examining successful retrieval trials[85].

How to Reconcile Hyperactivation and Hypoactivation?

Despite variability related to demographic, clinical and neuropsychological data, there is evidence that less-impaired MCI subjects, who perform better on the fMRI memory tasks, show greater MTL activation, whereas subjects who have more cognitive impairment perform worse and display less MTL activation. Thus, these differences may lie on a continuum, with MTL hyperactivation at one end happening early in the course of MCI, representing a compensatory mechanism to counteract the network dysfunction early in its course and to maintain an efficient memory performance. On the other hand, subjects with more severe MCI, whose pathology

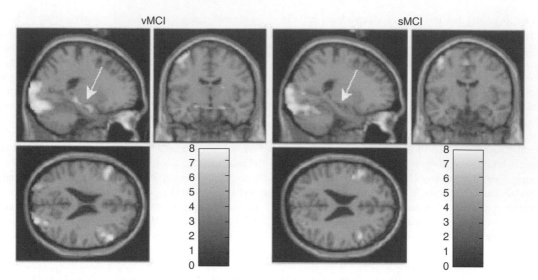

Figure 70.4 Group fMRI data from 15 very mildly impaired MCI (vMCI) and 12 significantly impaired MCI (sMCI) subjects on a face-name encoding task. The vMCI subjects showed evidence of hippocampal 'hyperactivation' compared to controls. The sMCI subjects showed significantly decreased hippocampal activation at levels similar to those seen in mild AD patients. *A full colour version of this figure appears in the colour plate section*

is closer to that found in AD, fail to perform well on the memory task and have MTL hypoactivation. This may represent an inability to compensate for the overwhelming pathological changes that have irreparably damaged the memory network with extensive synaptic and neuronal loss. We can assimilate the course of these changes to an 'inverse U-shaped curve' which goes progressively from normal to hyper to hypoactivation, paralleling changes in behavioural and neuropsychological performance.

PHARMACOLOGICAL fMRI IN MCI AND AD

A relatively new but promising area of application for fMRI is that of clinical trials of pharmacological agents. fMRI may provide a faster and more sensitive approach to assess efficacy of new therapies without the need to await for the completion of large and long trials. As of today, there have been few published studies that use fMRI to assess pharmacological effects of the available cholinesterase inhibitors for the treatment of AD, but their number is expected to grow as soon as other ongoing trials are completed.

One of these studies[86] looked at the effects of donepezil in patients with amnesic MCI compared to matched controls using working memory tasks. The results showed improvement of activation in the frontoparietal regions, which were found to be hypoactive before initiation of treatment. The changes occurred in the presence of preserved hippocampal integrity and were visible after only an average of six weeks of treatment. Another study[87] investigated the effects of acute rivastigmine treatment in patients with mild AD using fMRI with both a face encoding and a working memory task. The results indicated that rivastigmine increased bilateral activation in the fusiform gyrus during the face encoding task and in the prefrontal cortex in the working memory task. When working memory load was further increased, not only was increased activation seen, but in certain areas there was also decreased activation.

In a following study, Goekoop *et al.*[88] compared patients with AD to subjects with MCI using a face recognition task before and after a single dose of, or five-day treatment with, the cholinesterase inhibitor galantamine. Acute exposure to the drug produced strong activation in both groups. In particular, MCI subjects showed increased activation in the posterior cingulate, left inferior parietal and anterior temporal lobe. Prolonged exposure decreased activation in similar posterior cingulate areas and in bilateral prefrontal areas. In AD, acute exposure increased bilateral hippocampal activation, while prolonged treatment led to decreased activation in the same areas. The authors argued that differential response to cholinergic stimulation in MCI and AD could suggest differences in the functional status and integrity of the cholinergic system and provide a useful biomarker to monitor disease progression and treatment response.

More recently, Petrella *et al.*[89] published the first double-blind placebo-controlled fMRI study of the effect of a cholinesterase inhibitor, donepezil, on brain function in subjects with MCI. The subjects were assessed at baseline and following 12 or 24 weeks of therapy with an event-related delayed-response visual memory task for novel faces. The imaging findings were correlated with ADAS-Cog score, a commonly used clinical outcome measure in trials of therapies for dementia and MCI. The results indicated that donepezil increases activation in the ventrolateral prefrontal cortex, compared with baseline, and in both the bilateral dorsal and ventrolateral prefrontal cortices, compared with the placebo group post-treatment. The authors conclude that donepezil, when administered during a three to six month period to subjects with MCI, may potentially induce brain activation in the left inferior frontal gyrus during memory processing, thus improving performance.

CONCLUSIONS

Functional MRI has begun to establish itself as an important tool to probe the neural underpinnings of cognitive functions in the living brain. Although the use of fMRI in the study of MCI and AD is relatively new, it holds great potential for illuminating the black box between the pathophysiological process of AD and the early clinical symptomatology. A lot of questions remain to be answered, particularly regarding the early phases of MCI and how to identify subjects who will ultimately develop dementia. This can be done only with a rigorous methodological approach that reduces intergroup variability[90]. Integrating different imaging modalities including volumetric MRI, FDG-PET and PiB-PET with neuropathological analysis, will expand our knowledge of the temporal and spatial course of the pathophysiological changes involving the affected brain networks. Ultimately, fMRI may prove particularly valuable in early 'proof of concept' studies for novel pharmacological approaches to treating AD, predicting long-term response to potential disease-modifying therapies for this devastating illness.

REFERENCES

1. Morris JC, McKeel DW Jr, Storandt M *et al.* Very mild Alzheimer's disease: informant-based clinical, psychometric, and pathologic distinction from normal aging. *Neurology* 1991; **41**(4): 469–78.

2. Selkoe DJ. Alzheimer's disease is a synaptic failure. *Science* 2002; **298**(5594): 789–91.

3. Walsh DM, Selkoe DJ. Deciphering the molecular basis of memory failure in Alzheimer's disease. *Neuron* 2004; **44**(1): 181–93.

4. Ingelsson M, Fukumoto H, Newell KL *et al.* Early Abeta accumulation and progressive synaptic loss, gliosis, and tangle formation in AD brain. *Neurology* 2004; **62**(6): 925–31.

5. Markesbery WR, Schmitt FA, Kryscio RJ *et al.* Neuropathologic substrate of mild cognitive impairment. *Arch Neurol* 2006; **63**(1): 38–46.

6. Gomez-Isla T, Price JL, McKeel DW Jr *et al.* Profound loss of layer II entorhinal cortex neurons occurs in very mild Alzheimer's disease. *J Neurosci* 1996; **16**(14): 4491–500.

7. Alsop DC, Detre JA, Grossman M. Assessment of cerebral blood flow in Alzheimer's disease by spin-labeled magnetic resonance imaging. *Ann Neurol* 2000; **47**(1): 93–100.

8. Johnson NA, Jahng GH, Weiner MW *et al.* Pattern of cerebral hypoperfusion in Alzheimer disease and mild cognitive impairment measured with arterial spin-labeling MR imaging: initial experience. *Radiology* 2005; **234**(3): 851–9.

9. Greicius MD, Srivastava G, Reiss AL, Menon V. Default-mode network activity distinguishes Alzheimer's disease from healthy aging: evidence from functional MRI. *Proc Natl Acad Sci U S A* 2004; **101**(13): 4637–42.

10. Rombouts SA, Barkhof F, Goekoop R, Stam CJ, Scheltens P. Altered resting state networks in mild cognitive impairment and mild Alzheimer's disease: an fMRI study. *Hum Brain Mapp* 2005; **26**(4): 231–9.

11. Ogawa S, Lee TM, Nayak AS, Glynn P. Oxygenation-sensitive contrast in magnetic resonance image of rodent brain at high magnetic fields. *Magn Reson Med* 1990; **14**(1): 68–78.

12. Logothetis NK, Pauls J, Augath M, Trinath T, Oeltermann A. Neurophysiological investigation of the basis of the fMRI signal. *Nature* 2001; **412**(6843): 150–7.

13. Shmuel A, Augath M, Oeltermann A, Logothetis NK. Negative functional MRI response correlates with decreases in neuronal activity in monkey visual area V1. *Nat Neurosci* 2006; **9**(4): 569–77.

14. Vincent JL, Snyder AZ, Fox MD *et al.* Coherent spontaneous activity identifies a hippocampal-parietal memory network. *J Neurophysiol* 2006; **96**(6): 3517–31.

15. D'Esposito M, Zarahn E, Aguirre GK, Rypma B. The effect of normal aging on the coupling of neural activity to the bold hemodynamic response. *Neuroimage* 1999; **10**(1): 6–14.

16. Buckner RL, Koutstaal W, Schacter DL, Rosen BR. Functional MRI evidence for a role of frontal and inferior temporal cortex in amodal components of priming. *Brain* 2000; **123**(Pt 3): 620–40.

17. Rombouts SA, Goekoop R, Stam CJ, Barkhof F, Scheltens P. Delayed rather than decreased BOLD response as a marker for early Alzheimer's disease. *Neuroimage* 2005; **26**(4): 1078–85.

18. Machulda MM, Ward HA, Borowski B *et al.* Comparison of memory fMRI response among normal, MCI, and Alzheimer's patients. *Neurology* 2003; **61**(4): 500–6.

19. Sperling R, Bates J, Chua E *et al.* fMRI studies of associative encoding in young and elderly controls and mild AD patients. *J Neurol Neurosurg Psychiatry* 2003; **74**: 44–50.

20. Anderson KE, Perera GM, Hilton J *et al.* Functional magnetic resonance imaging study of word recognition in normal elders. *Prog Neuropsychopharmacol Biol Psychiatry* 2002; **26**(4): 647–50.

21. Davis SW, Dennis NA, Daselaar SM, Fleck MS, Cabeza R. Que PASA? The posterior-anterior shift in aging. *Cereb Cortex* 2008; **18**(5): 1201–9.

22. Li SC, Lindenberger U, Sikstrom S. Aging cognition: from neuromodulation to representation. *Trends Cogn Sci* 2001; **5**(11): 479–86.

23. Park DC, Reuter-Lorenz P. The adaptive brain: aging and neurocognitive scaffolding. *Annu Rev Psychol* 2009; **60**: 173–96.

24. Brewer JB, Zhao Z, Desmond JE, Glover GH, Gabrieli JD. Making memories: brain activity that predicts how well visual experience will be remembered. *Science* 1998; **281**(5380): 1185–7

25. Wagner AD, Schacter DL, Rotte M *et al.* Building memories: remembering and forgetting of verbal experiences as predicted by brain activity. *Science* 1998; **281**(5380): 1188–91.

26. Kirchhoff BA, Wagner AD, Maril A, Stern CE. Prefrontal-temporal circuitry for episodic encoding and subsequent memory. *J Neurosci* 2000; **20**(16): 6173–80.

27. Sperling R, Chua E, Cocchiarella A *et al.* Putting names to faces: successful encoding of associative memories activates the anterior hippocampal formation. *Neuroimage* 2003; **20**(2): 1400–10.

28. Chua EF, Schacter DL, Rand-Giovannetti E, Sperling RA. Evidence for a specific role of the anterior hippocampal region in successful associative encoding. *Hippocampus* 2007; **17**(11): 1071–80.

29. Sperling R, Greve D, Dale A *et al.* fMRI detection of pharmacologically induced memory impairment. *Proc Natl Acad Sci U S A* 2002; **99**(1): 455–60.

30. Schon K, Atri A, Hasselmo ME *et al.* Scopolamine reduces persistent activity related to long-term encoding in the parahippocampal gyrus during delayed matching in humans. *J Neurosci* 2005; **25**(40): 9112–23.

31. Squire LR, Zola-Morgan S. The medial temporal lobe memory system. *Science* 1991; **253**(5026): 1380–6.

32. Eichenbaum H, Schoenbaum G, Young B, Bunsey M. Functional organization of the hippocampal memory system. *Proc Natl Acad Sci U S A* 1996; **93**(24): 13500–7.

33. Zelinski EM, Gilewski MJ. Assessment of memory complaints by rating scales and questionnaires. *Psychopharmacol Bull* 1988; **24**(4): 523–9.

34. Leirer VO, Morrow DG, Sheikh JI, Pariante GM. Memory skills elders want to improve. *Exp Aging Res* 1990; **16**(3): 155–8.

35. Fowler KS, Saling MM, Conway EL, Semple JM, Louis WJ. Paired associate performance in the early detection of DAT. *J Int Neuropsychol Soc* 2002; **8**: 58–71.

36. Gallo DA, Sullivan AL, Daffner KR, Schacter DL, Budson AE. Associative recognition in Alzheimer's disease: evidence for impaired recall-to-reject. *Neuropsychology* 2004; **18**(3): 556–63.

37. Sperling RA, Bates J, Cocchiarella A *et al*. Encoding novel face-name associations: a functional MRI study. *Hum Brain Mapp* 2001; **14**: 129–39.

38. Small SA, Nava AS, Perera GM *et al*. Circuit mechanisms underlying memory encoding and retrieval in the long axis of the hippocampal formation. *Nat Neurosci* 2001; **4**(4): 442–9.

39. Zeineh MM, Engel SA, Thompson PM, Bookheimer SY. Dynamics of the hippocampus during encoding and retrieval of face-name pairs. *Science* 2003; **299**(5606): 577–80.

40. Kirwan CB, Stark CE. Medial temporal lobe activation during encoding and retrieval of novel face-name pairs. *Hippocampus* 2004; **14**(7): 919–30.

41. Daselaar SM, Prince SE, Cabeza R. When less means more: deactivations during encoding that predict subsequent memory. *Neuroimage* 2004; **23**(3): 921–7.

42. Miller SL, Celone K, DePeau K *et al*. Age-related memory impairment associated with loss of parietal deactivation but preserved hippocampal activation. *Proc Natl Acad Sci U S A* 2008; **105**(6): 2181–6.

43. Raichle ME, MacLeod AM, Snyder AZ *et al*. A default mode of brain function. *Proc Natl Acad Sci U S A* 2001; **98**(2): 676–82.

44. Fox MD, Snyder AZ, Vincent JL *et al*. The human brain is intrinsically organized into dynamic, anticorrelated functional networks. *Proc Natl Acad Sci U S A* 2005; **102**(27): 9673–8.

45. Greicius MD, Krasnow B, Reiss AL, Menon V. Functional connectivity in the resting brain: a network analysis of the default mode hypothesis. *Proc Natl Acad Sci U S A* 2003; **100**(1): 253–8.

46. Wheeler ME, Buckner RL. Functional-anatomic correlates of remembering and knowing. *Neuroimage* 2004; **21**(4): 1337–49.

47. Buckner RL, Snyder AZ, Shannon BJ *et al*. Molecular, structural, and functional characterization of Alzheimer's disease: evidence for a relationship between default activity, amyloid, and memory. *J Neurosci* 2005; **25**(34): 7709–17.

48. Sperling R. Functional MRI studies of associative encoding in normal aging, mild cognitive impairment, and Alzheimer's disease. *Ann N Y Acad Sci* 2007; **1097**: 146–55.

49. Small SA, Perera GM, DeLaPaz R, Mayeux R, Stern Y. Differential regional dysfunction of the hippocampal formation among elderly with memory decline and Alzheimer's disease. *Ann Neurol* 1999; **45**: 466–72.

50. Rombouts SA, Barkhof F, Veltman DJ *et al*. Functional MR imaging in Alzheimer's disease during memory encoding. *AJNR Am J Neuroradiol* 2000; **21**(10): 1869–75.

51. Kato T, Knopman D, Liu H. Dissociation of regional activation in mild AD during visual encoding: A functional MRI study. *Neurology* 2001; **57**: 812–6.

52. Gron G, Bittner D, Schmitz B, Wunderlich AP, Riepe MW. Subjective memory complaints: objective neural markers in patients with Alzheimer's disease and major depressive disorder. *Ann Neurol* 2002; **51**(4): 491–8.

53. Dickerson BC, Salat D, Greve D *et al*. Increased hippocampal activation in mild cognitive impairment compared to normal aging and AD. *Neurology* 2005; **65**: 404–11.

54. Golby A, Silverberg G, Race E *et al*. Memory encoding in Alzheimer's disease: an fMRI study of explicit and implicit memory. *Brain* 2005; **128**(Pt 4): 773–87.

55. Pariente J, Cole S, Henson R *et al*. Alzheimer's patients engage an alternative network during a memory task. *Ann Neurol* 2005; **58**(6): 870–9.

56. Remy F, Mirrashed F, Campbell B, Richter W. Verbal episodic memory impairment in Alzheimer's disease: a combined structural and functional MRI study. *Neuroimage* 2005; **25**(1): 253–66.

57. Hämäläinen A, Pihlajamaki M, Tanila H *et al*. Increased fMRI responses during encoding in mild cognitive impairment. *Neurobiol Aging* 2007; **28**(12): 1889–903.

58. Pihlajamaki M, Depeau KM, Blacker D, Sperling RA. Impaired medial temporal repetition suppression is related to failure of parietal deactivation in Alzheimer disease. *Am J Geriatr Psychiatry* 2008; **16**(4): 283–92.

59. Johnson SC, Baxter LC, Susskind-Wilder L *et al*. Hippocampal adaptation to face repetition in healthy elderly and mild cognitive impairment. *Neuropsychologia* 2004; **42**(7): 980–9.

60. Grady CL, McIntosh AR, Beig S *et al*. Evidence from functional neuroimaging of a compensatory prefrontal network in Alzheimer's disease. *J Neurosci* 2003; **23**(3): 986–93.

61. Lustig C, Snyder AZ, Bhakta M *et al*. Functional deactivations: change with age and dementia of the Alzheimer type. *Proc Natl Acad Sci U S A* 2003; **100**(24): 14504–9.

62. Petrella J, Krishnan S, Slavin M *et al*. Mild cognitive impairment: evaluation with 4-T functional MR imaging. *Radiology* 2006; **240**: 177–86.

63. Klunk WE, Engler H, Nordberg A *et al*. Imaging brain amyloid in Alzheimer's disease with Pittsburgh Compound-B. *Ann Neurol* 2004; **55**(3): 306–19.

64. Meltzer CC, Zubieta JK, Brandt J *et al*. Regional hypometabolism in Alzheimer's disease as measured by positron emission tomography after correction for effects of partial volume averaging. *Neurology* 1996; **47**(2): 454–61.

65. Silverman DH, Small GW, Chang CY *et al*. Positron emission tomography in evaluation of dementia: regional brain metabolism and long-term outcome. *JAMA* 2001; **286**(17): 2120–7.

66. Alexander GE, Chen K, Pietrini P, Rapoport SI, Reiman EM. Longitudinal PET evaluation of cerebral metabolic decline in dementia: a potential outcome measure in Alzheimer's disease treatment studies. *Am J Psychiatry* 2002; **159**(5): 738–45.

67. Reiman EM, Chen K, Alexander GE *et al*. Functional brain abnormalities in young adults at genetic risk for late-onset Alzheimer's dementia. *Proc Natl Acad Sci U S A* 2004; **101**(1): 284–9.

68. Small GW, Ercoli LM, Silverman DH *et al*. Cerebral metabolic and cognitive decline in persons at genetic risk for Alzheimer's disease. *Proc Natl Acad Sci U S A* 2000; **97**(11): 6037–42.

69. Jagust W, Gitcho A, Sun F *et al*. Brain imaging evidence of preclinical Alzheimer's disease in normal aging. *Ann Neurol* 2006; **59**(4): 673–81.

70. Buckner RL, Sepulcre J, Talukdar T *et al*. Cortical hubs revealed by intrinsic functional connectivity: mapping, assessment of stability, and relation to Alzheimer's disease. *J Neurosci* 2009; **29**(6): 1860–73.

71. Cirrito JR, Yamada KA, Finn MB *et al*. Synaptic activity regulates interstitial fluid amyloid-beta levels in vivo. *Neuron* 2005; **48**(6): 913–22.

72. Celone KA, Calhoun VD, Dickerson BC *et al.* Alterations in memory networks in mild cognitive impairment and Alzheimer's disease: an independent component analysis. *J Neurosci* 2006; **26**(40): 10222–31.

73. Wierenga CE, Bondi MW. Use of functional magnetic resonance imaging in the early identification of Alzheimer's disease. *Neuropsychol Rev* 2007; **17**(2): 127–43.

74. Seeley WW, Crawford RK, Zhou J, Miller BL, Greicius MD. Neurodegenerative diseases target large-scale human brain networks. *Neuron* 2009; **62**(1): 42–52.

75. Grundman M, Petersen RC, Ferris SH *et al.* Mild cognitive impairment can be distinguished from Alzheimer disease and normal aging for clinical trials. *Arch Neurol* 2004; **61**(1): 59–66.

76. Petersen RC, Stevens JC, Ganguli M *et al.* Practice parameter: early detection of dementia: mild cognitive impairment (an evidence-based review). Report of the Quality Standards Subcommittee of the American Academy of Neurology. *Neurology* 2001; **56**(9): 1133–42.

77. Petersen RC, Parisi JE, Dickson DW *et al.* Neuropathologic features of amnestic mild cognitive impairment. *Arch Neurol* 2006; **63**(5): 665–72.

78. Kemppainen NM, Aalto S, Wilson IA *et al.* PET amyloid ligand and [11C]PIB uptake is increased in mild cognitive impairment. *Neurology* 2007; **68**(19): 1603–6.

79. Johnson SC, Schmitz TW, Moritz CH *et al.* Activation of brain regions vulnerable to Alzheimer's disease: the effect of mild cognitive impairment. *Neurobiol Aging* 2006; **27**(11): 1604–12.

80. Morris JC. The Clinical Dementia Rating (CDR): current version and scoring rules. *Neurology* 1993; **43**(11): 2412–4.

81. Trivedi MA, Murphy CM, Goetz C *et al.* fMRI activation changes during successful episodic memory encoding and recognition in amnestic mild cognitive impairment relative to cognitively healthy older adults. *Dement Geriatr Cogn Disord* 2008; **26**(2): 123–37.

82. Kircher TT, Weis S, Freymann K *et al.* Hippocampal activation in patients with mild cognitive impairment is necessary for successful memory encoding. *J Neurol Neurosurg Psychiatry* 2007; **78**(8): 812–8.

83. Dickerson BC, Salat DH, Bates JF *et al.* Medial temporal lobe function and structure in mild cognitive impairment. *Ann Neurol* 2004; **56**(1): 27–35.

84. Miller SL, Fenstermacher E, Bates J *et al.* Hippocampal activation in adults with mild cognitive impairment predicts subsequent cognitive decline. *J Neurol Neurosurg Psychiatry* 2008; **79**(6): 630–5.

85. Heun R, Freymann K, Erb M *et al.* Mild cognitive impairment (MCI) and actual retrieval performance affect cerebral activation in the elderly. *Neurobiol Aging* 2007; **28**(3): 404–13.

86. Saykin AJ, Wishart HA, Rabin LA *et al.* Cholinergic enhancement of frontal lobe activity in mild cognitive impairment. *Brain* 2004; **127**(Pt 7): 1574–83.

87. Rombouts SA, Barkhof F, Van Meel CS, Scheltens P. Alterations in brain activation during cholinergic enhancement with rivastigmine in Alzheimer's disease. *J Neurol Neurosurg Psychiatry* 2002; **73**(6): 665–71.

88. Goekoop R, Scheltens P, Barkhof F, Rombouts SA. Cholinergic challenge in Alzheimer patients and mild cognitive impairment differentially affects hippocampal activation – a pharmacological fMRI study. *Brain* 2006; **129**(Pt 1): 141–57.

89. Petrella JR, Prince SE, Krishnan S *et al.* Effects of donepezil on cortical activation in mild cognitive impairment: a pilot double-blind placebo-controlled trial using functional MR imaging. *AJNR Am J Neuroradiol* 2009; **30**(2): 411–6.

90. Samanez-Larkin GR, D'Esposito M. Group comparisons: imaging the aging brain. *Soc Cogn Affect Neurosci* 2008; **3**(3): 290–7.

71

Magnetic Resonance Spectroscopy

Olusola Ajilore[1], Brent Forester[2], Matthew R. Woodward[2] and Anand Kumar[1]

[1]*Department of Psychiatry, University of Illinois-Chicago, IL, USA*
[2]*Geriatric Psychiatry Research Program, McLean Hospital, Belmont, MA, USA*

BASIC PRINCIPLES OF MAGNETIC RESONANCE SPECTROSCOPY

In vivo magnetic resonance spectroscopy (MRS) is a non-invasive technique that allows for the measurement of brain biochemicals in particular regions of the brain. In magnetic resonance imaging, the image is generated from the signal derived from water hydrogen nuclei. MRS suppresses the water signal to measure metabolites in the tissue fluid. It takes advantage of the chemical shift effect, a property that describes the notion that the same nuclei in different molecules respond differently to a magnetic field. Magnetic field strengths usually range from 1.5 Tesla (T) to 4 T in human studies. The chemical shift is typically measured in parts per million relative to the nuclear frequency and plotted on the horizontal axis of a spectrum with the vertical axis displaying the amplitude or intensity of a peak (Figure 71.1). Each peak represents a metabolite of interest for a given nucleus, with the area under the peak reflecting the concentration of that metabolite in the measured region.

There are several signal detection parameters that determine the shape of a spectrum. One is the voxel size which determines the region of tissue being studied and the concentration of metabolites measured. Another important parameter is relaxation time represented by T1 and T2. T1 is the time necessary for hydrogen nuclei to emit 63% of the energy from the stimulating pulse, while T2 is the time for 63% of the transverse energy pulse to be lost due to dephasing. These parameters affect signal strength since long T1s and short T2s are typically found in intracellular molecules with high molecular weights and thus can lead to weak signals. As a result, MRS is particularly useful for measuring low molecular weight molecules that are highly concentrated. Typical concentrations of metabolites detected by MRS are in the range of 4–10 mM. It is difficult to detect metabolites under 1 mM. These concentrations can be reported in absolute measures or as ratios to creatine concentrations, using creatine as an internal control.

NUCLEAR ISOTOPES USED IN MRS

Phosphorous

^{31}P-MRS (Figure 71.2) can be used to measure the following metabolites: adenosine triphosphate (ATP), phosphomonoesters (phosphoryl choline, phosphoryl ethanolamine and glycerophos-

Table 71.1 Summary of metabolites detected using proton MRS

Metabolite	Measure
N-acetylaspartate	Neuronal density and viability, mitochondrial function
Choline and choline-containing metabolites	Neuronal membrane integrity
Myo-inositol	Glial function
Glutamate/glutamine	Excitatory neurotransmitter
GABA	Inhibitory neurotransmitter

phate), phosphodiesters (glyceryl phosphoryl ethanolamine, glyceryl phosphoryl serine and glyceryl phosphoryl inositol), phosphocreatine and inorganic phosphate. This is a useful isotope to measure the bioenergetics of neuronal processes.

Proton

Hydrogen or proton MRS is used to probe for the following neurochemicals: choline (Cho), creatine (Cr), *N*-acetylaspartate (NAA), myo-inositol (mI), glutamate/glutamine and gamma amino butyrate (GABA) (Table 71.1). NAA is generally viewed as a marker of neuronal viability and may represent a measure of neuronal volume, number and/or function. However, some evidence suggests that it may more specifically reflect mitochondrial function[1,2]. The choline signal represents a composite of choline-containing metabolites such as phosphocholine, glycerophosphocholine and phosphotidylcholine. These metabolites are involved in cell membrane integrity. Myo-inositol is seen as a marker of gliosis and is the storage form of the inositol phosphate second messenger system. Glutamate/glutamine and GABA are the most ubiquitous excitatory and inhibitory neurotransmitters, respectively.

Other less commonly used nuclei include carbon, lithium, fluorine and sodium. Often, studies utilizing these nuclei involve measuring the impact of pharmaceutical agents containing these metabolites.

NORMAL AGEING

Several studies have used MRS to study neurochemical changes associated with normal, healthy ageing. Perhaps due to methodological

Principles and Practice of Geriatric Psychiatry, 3rd edn. Edited by Mohammed T. Abou-Saleh, Cornelius Katona and Anand Kumar

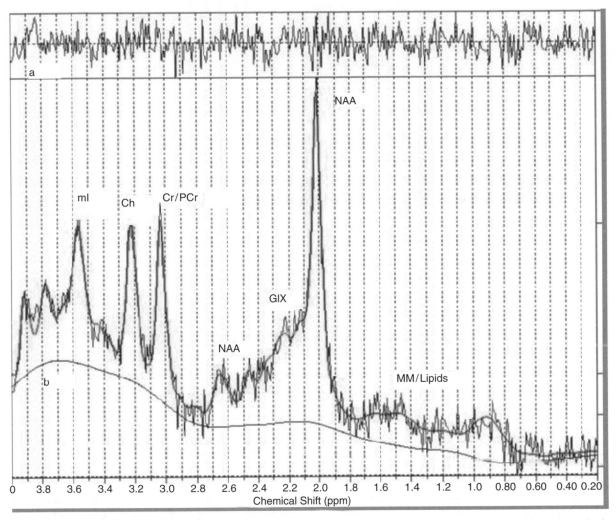

Figure 71.1 Sample proton MRS spectrum. Each peak represents a different metabolite with the area under the peak equivalent to the concentration of the metabolite

limitations, early studies using MRS to examine brain alterations associated with normal ageing failed to find significant changes over time[3,4]. However in a study by Cohen and colleagues comparing brain uptake of choline using proton MRS in younger subjects (mean age 32) and older subjects (mean age 73), it was shown that older subjects had decreased choline uptake[5]. In a 2001 study, Brooks et al. showed a significant decline in frontal lobe NAA comparing subjects from age 20 to 70 with an overall decrease of 12%[6]. This decline was interpreted as a decrease in neuronal volume, number or function as NAA is thought to be a marker of neuronal viability. In addition to decreases in NAA, increases in myo-inositol have also been seen in white matter associated with normal ageing. Kaiser et al. found a significant increase in both absolute levels and myo-inositol ratios in older subjects (mean age 56 years) compared with younger subjects (mean age 26 years)[7].

The impact of these neurochemical changes associated with ageing in frontal white matter have been explored in correlational studies examining the relationship between metabolite levels and cognitive function. For example, in a study by Valenzuela et al., frontal white matter NAA/Cr ratios were significantly correlated with cognitive tasks of executive function[8]. In a study by Elderkin-Thompson et al., choline, myo-inositol and phosphocholine ratios were correlated with performance on learning and recognition tasks[9].

The neurochemical changes described above are not limited to frontal white matter as demonstrated in a study that showed age-related decreases in NAA, NAA/Cho and NAA/Cr ratios across 30 different voxels[10]. In a longitudinal study examining similar measures over a three-year period, Ross et al. demonstrated that there were no significant changes in brain metabolites (with the exception of myo-inositol) or cognitive function over the time period studied[11]. In a comprehensive review and meta-analysis of MRS studies in normal ageing, while the majority of studies showed no significant change in metabolites with age, the authors did note a trend towards an increase in frontal and parietal choline with increasing age and a trend towards increases in parietal and occipital creatine with increasing age[12].

The studies above describe whole brain or cortical measurements of metabolites associated with normal ageing. However, age-related neurochemical changes in subcortical regions have also been demonstrated. For example, significant decreases in NAA/Cr and increases in choline/Cr in the genu of the corpus callosum have been shown when older subjects have been compared with younger subjects[13]. In the pons, decreases in NAA and increases in choline and creatine were noted in subjects over 50 years of age compared with subjects under 50[14]. In a study of the hippocampus, age-related decreases in NAA were measured by Szentkuti et al.[15]. These changes appear

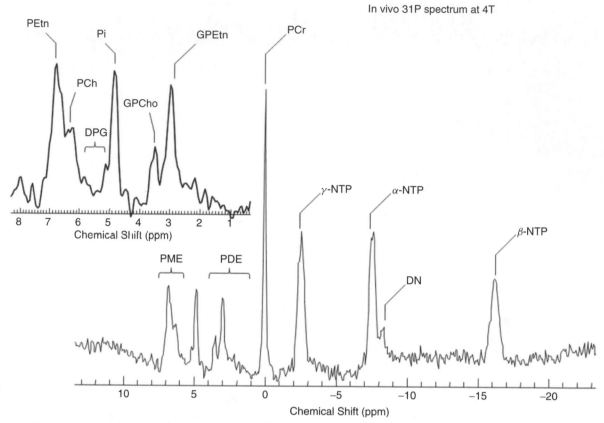

Figure 71.2 ^{31}P sample spectra. PEtn, phosphoryl ethanolamine; PCh, phosphoryl choline; DPG, diphosphatidylglycerol; GPEtn, glyceryl phosphoryl ethanolamine; PME, phosphomonoesters; PDE, phosphodiesters; PCr, phosphocreatine; NTP, nucleoside triphosphate; Pi, inorganic phosphate; DN, dinucleotides. Reprinted courtesy of Dr Eric Jensen

to have a functional impact as well, noted by a correlational study showing that hippocampal NAA/Cr was a significant predictor of performance on a verbal memory task[16].

GERIATRIC DEPRESSION AND BIPOLAR DISORDER

MRS has been used increasingly to study mood disorders in geriatric populations (Table 71.2). Comparing older adults with depression or bipolar disorder with healthy control subjects may offer insight into the pathophysiology of geriatric depression and predictors of treatment response and aid the development of more specific therapeutic interventions.

Most of the studies of geriatric depression utilize proton MRS. Changes in myo-inositol, choline and NAA have been observed in association with major depression. In the prefrontal region, increased myo-inositol and decreased NAA have been observed[17-19]. These findings are hypothesized to be associated with changes in myelination and/or neuronal loss. However, there have been differing findings for choline in which Venkatraman et al.[17] found a significant decrease and Kumar et al.[18] a significant increase. Two proposed reasons for these differences include differing severity of depression and region of interest. The subjects in the Venkatraman study were depressed older adults who were responsive to treatment and had only residual symptoms, whereas Kumar and colleagues studied acutely depressed older adults. Additionally, Venkatraman et al. focused on the anterior cingulate while Kumar's findings were located in the dorsolateral prefrontal cortex. An additional novel finding for Venktraman and

colleagues was increased NAA in the left medial temporal lobe, which may result in increased amygdala activity via diminished frontal lobe inhibition. Furthermore, changes in metabolite concentrations were found in the basal ganglia, where NAA was decreased in the caudate and choline was increased in the putamen[20].

A negative correlation was found between magnetization transfer ratio (MTR) and NAA+NAAG/Cr (N-acetylaspartylglutamate) and between myo-inositol/Cr and MTR[21] in white matter. MTR is associated with structural tissue integrity and it is hypothesized that changes in myo-inositol and NAA pools may result in the observed changes in macromolecular protein pools. Decreases in NAA were also found to be positively correlated with increased severity of white matter hyperintensities[22].

Changes in glutamate and glutamine have also been observed in geriatric depressed subjects. In comparing older adults with major depression, diabetes mellitus and healthy controls, subcortical nuclei glutamate and glutamine levels were significantly decreased in subjects with diabetes mellitus and depression compared with diabetic subjects and healthy controls. It is hypothesized that reduced glutamate and glutamine may be a result of glial dysfunction as well as impaired glucose metabolism. Also of note, myo-inositol was significantly increased in both depressed patients and depressed patients with diabetes mellitus versus controls[23]. In another study examining myo-inositol levels and visuo-spatial functioning, it was found that increased frontal white matter myo-inositol levels, present in both depressed and non-depressed diabetes mellitus subjects, were correlated with visuo-spatial dysfunction[24]. Patients with diabetes are

Table 71.2 Brain MRS findings in geriatric depression and bipolar disorder

Author	MRS type	Findings
Venkatraman[17]	[1]H	NAA decreased in prefrontal cortex
		NAA increased in left medial temporal lobe
		Cho decreased in prefrontal cortex
		Cre decreased in prefrontal cortex
		mI increased in left medial temporal lobe
Binesh[19]	[1]H	mI increased in dorsolateral prefrontal region
		PE increased in dorsolateral prefrontal region
		Glx increased in dorsolateral prefrontal region
Kumar[18]	[1]H	mI/Cr increased in frontal white matter
		Cho/Cr increased in frontal white matter
Vythilingam[20]	[1]H	NAA decreased in caudate
		Cho increased in putamen
Wyckoff[21]	^{1}H, MT and MRS	Inverse relationship between MTR and mI/Cr in left dorsolateral white matter
		Inverse relationship between MTR and (NAA+NAAG)/Cr in left dorsolateral white matter
Murata[22]	[1]H	Correlation b/t increased WMH severity and decreased NAA/Cr in frontal white matter
Ajilore[23]	[1]H	Significantly decreased Glu and Gln for DM+MDD and DM vs. HC in subcortical nuclei
Haroon[24]	[1]H	Increased mI in DM and DM+MDD correlated with visuo-spatial dysfunction in frontal white matter
Moore[29]	[31]P	Beta NTP decreased in basal ganglia
		Total NTP decreased in basal ganglia
Volz[30]	[31]P	Beta NTP decreased in frontal lobes
		Total NTP decreased in frontal lobes
Renshaw[31]	[1]H and [31]P	Average purine levels were not different between depressed and comparison groups in basal ganglia; however, female responders to fluoxetine treatment had 30% lower purine levels than non-responders
		Beta NTP 21% lower in beta NTP of responders to fluoxetine than non-responders, correlated with purine levels
Iosifescu[32]	[31]P	Mg^{2+} decreased at baseline in frontal and parietal slice superior to corpus callosum of depressed subjects
		Total NTP increased in frontal and parietal slice superior to corpus callosum of T3 responders
		PCr decreased in frontal and parietal slice superior to corpus callosum of T3 responders
Pettegrew[33]	[31]P	Prefrontal phosphomonoester levels increased at baseline; decreased with ALCAR treatment, trend between HDRS and phosphomonoester
		ALCAR increased PCr in prefrontal region, PCr levels correlated with HDRS
Forester[34]	[31]P	Whole brain total NTP decreased in geriatric depressed, difference in WM, not GM, total NTP decreased with treatment
		Whole brain beta NTP decreased in MDD
		Whole brain pH increased in GM for pretreatment depressed; pH decreased following treatment
Forester[35]	[7]Li	Increased brain Li in the superior edge of the corpus callosum associated with increased HDRS scores and frontal lobe dysfunction
Forester[36]	[7]Li	Brain Li levels in the anterior cingulate gyrus associated with increased NAA in BP
		Brain Li levels in the anterior cingulate gyrus associated with increased mI in BP

ALCAR, acetyl-L-carnitine; BP, bipolar disorder; Cho, choline; Cre, creatine; DM, diabetes mellitus; Gln, glutamine; Glu, glutamate; Glx, glutamate + glutamine; GM, grey matter; H, hydrogen; HDRS, Hamilton Depression Rating Scale; Li, lithium; MDD, major depressive disorder; Mg^{2+}, magnesium ion; mI, myo-inositol; MT, magnetization transfer; MTR, magnetization transfer ratio; NAA, *N*-acetylaspartate; NAAG, *N*-acetylaspartylglutamic acid; NTP, nucleoside triphosphate; P, phosphorous; PCr, phosphocreatine; T3, triiodothyronine.

at increased risk of suffering from depression and increased medical burden may be a risk factor for poor response to antidepressant treatment[25].

These metabolic changes associated with major depression seem to be clinically relevant as demonstrated by treatment effect studies. For example, an increase in amygdala region NAA was seen in depressed patients who exhibited a positive response to electroconvulsive therapy[26]. In addition, Glx concentrations (a composite of glutamate and glutamine) in left dorsal lateral prefrontal cortex were negatively correlated with severity of depression and increased significantly after electroconvulsive treatment[27]. In a report examining the effect of antidepressant treatment, it was shown that decreased NAA levels in the anterior cingulate cortex in depressed patients were reversed with venlafaxine treatment[28].

In addition to using proton MRS in depression, ^{31}P-MRS allows for examination of membrane phospholipids and high-energy phosphorous-containing molecules, such as ATP and phospho-creatine (PCr). Previous ^{31}P-MRS studies have demonstrated lower levels of beta and total NTP in the basal ganglia[29] and the frontal lobes[30] of depressed adults. Bioenergetic changes have also been demonstrated to correlate with response to pharmacological treatment[31,32]. Earlier studies have been inconclusive regarding whether differences in bioenergetic metabolism reflect a trait condition for those individuals at risk for depression or a state condition related to depression severity[32].

Studies examining changes in high-energy phosphate metabolites with treatment in geriatric depression are limited. In prefrontal tissue, phosphomonoester concentration was increased in two male older depressed subjects compared with six male controls of similar age. In the depressed group, prefrontal phosphomonoester levels decreased with acetyl-L-carnitine (ALCAR) treatment[33]. In addition, following ALCAR treatment there was a significant increase in PCr levels. In this study a trend level correlation was also found between phosphomonoester levels and Hamilton Depression Rating Scale (HDRS) scores[33]. A recent ^{31}P-MRS study of 13 older depressed adults and 10 healthy older controls at 4 T demonstrated that both total NTP (nucleoside triphosphate) and β-NTP (which primarily reflects levels of ATP) were decreased in the geriatric depressed subjects. More specifically, total NTP among depressed subjects was significantly decreased in white matter, but there was no significant difference in grey matter vs. controls. Following sertraline treatment, there was a significant decrease (2%) in total NTP. In addition, intracellular pH in grey matter, which was significantly greater in depressed subjects vs. controls pretreatment, was decreased to levels similar to that of healthy controls following treatment[34]. The authors propose that further study of high-energy phosphate alterations in geriatric depression is warranted and this may lead to bioenergetically based treatment approaches in late life major depression.

MRS studies in late-life bipolar disorder are more limited, though recent findings using ^{7}Li-MRS hold promise for a clinical application of this method to help regulate lithium dosing more accurately in older bipolar adults. Examining the superior edge of the corpus callosum in a 4 T MRS study of older adults with bipolar disorder treated with lithium, increased brain but not serum Li levels were associated with increased depression symptoms (measured by the HDRS) as well as frontal executive dysfunction (measured by the Stroop Interference Tests, Trails B and Wisconsin Card Sort)[35]. In addition, brain Li levels were associated with increased myo-inositol and NAA levels[36]. Increased NAA suggests potential neuroprotective and neurotropic effects of lithium treatment while increased myo-inositol levels were thought to reflect increased inositol monophosphatase activity in the setting of chronic lithium treatment.

Studies utilizing proton (^{1}H) MRS have identified changes in cerebral concentrations of NAA, Glx, choline-containing compounds, myo-inositol and lactate in adult bipolar subjects compared with normal controls[37]. Other studies using ^{31}P-MRS have examined additional alterations in levels of PCr, phosphomonoesters and intracellular pH (pH_i)[37]. Based on these findings, some have hypothesized that the majority of MRS findings in bipolar disorder can be fit into a cohesive bioenergetic and neurochemical model that is focused on central nervous system (CNS) energy metabolism[19]. Treatment studies examining bioenergetic changes in geriatric bipolar depressed individuals utilizing both ^{1}H- and ^{31}P-MRS at 4 T are currently underway and may provide further insight into the pathophysiology of late-life bipolar disorder.

DEMENTIA AND COGNITIVE DISORDERS

Mild Cognitive Impairment/Cognitively Impaired Non-Demented

MRS studies in mild cognitive impairment (MCI) have been used to distinguish MCI from normal ageing, as well as more advanced forms of cognitive dysfunction. An early study by Kantarci et al. examined regional metabolic changes associated with MCI. They found that increases in myo-inositol/Cr ratios in the posterior cingulate were the metabolic change unique to patients with MCI and Alzheimer's disease, while decreases in NAA/Cr and Cho/Cr only seemed present in the patients with more progressive disease[38]. Subsequent studies have shown a similar pattern of changes associated with MCI compared with control subjects[39]. Other regions have been shown to demonstrate metabolic perturbations restricted to MCI. For example in a study by Ackl et al., hippocampal decreases in NAA occurred in MCI and Alzheimer's patients, but NAA changes in the parietal region seemed to only occur in more advanced patients[40]. MRS has been studied as a predictor of developing dementia in a number of studies. For example, cognitively impaired non-demented (CIND) patients have been shown to have reduced NAA in the medial temporal lobe, hippocampus and neocortical grey matter compared with controls. There was also a difference between stable CIND patients and CIND patients who developed dementia over 3.6 years of follow-up[41]. In another study, changes in occipital NAA/Cr ratios predicted conversion to dementia with 100% sensitivity and 75% specificity[42]. Thus, MRS has been a useful tool in determining the early metabolic profiles that distinguish MCI from more advanced dementia and the changes that predict the development of more advanced dementia.

Alzheimer's Disease

The majority of studies using MRS to measure brain metabolites associated with dementia have been in Alzheimer's disease. The most consistent finding is reduced NAA, a marker of neuronal viability, and increased myo-inositol. This has been demonstrated in a number of cross-sectional studies[43–46]. These patterns also occur longitudinally as demonstrated in a brief report from Adalsteinsson et al. They showed that grey matter NAA levels (on average) declined 12.26% over the course of year in Alzheimer's disease patients, whereas controls had no significant change over the same time period[47]. Metabolic alterations associated with AD have associated with cognitive function as well. For example, NAA reductions in the left medial temporal lobe were associated with impairment in verbal memory, while myo-inositol increases in the right parietotemporal cortex were associated with impairment in visuoconstructional performance[48].

There have been several studies looking at the effects of treatment of Alzheimer's disease on brain metabolic profiles. In a study on donepezil, the authors found that patients receiving treatment demonstrated higher NAA concentrations compared to patients receiving placebo over a 24-week period[49]. In a subsequent study, these types of changes were shown to be significantly correlated with cognitive improvement associated with donepezil treatment[50]. Rivastigmine has also been shown to positively affect the metabolic profile associated with Alzheimer's disease. Patients treated with rivastigmine over a four-month period exhibited significant increases in frontal cortex NAA/Cr ratio[51].

The newest pharmaceutical agent in the treatment of Alzheimer's disease, memantine, is thought to exert an anti-excitotoxic effect by the inhibition of the glutamate-receptor agonist, n-methyl D-aspartate

(NMDA). In keeping with this mechanism, a recent proton MRS study has shown that memantine decreases hippocampal glutamate in Alzheimer's disease[52]. Thus, with the evidence from these treatment effect studies, it appears the metabolic alterations seen in Alzheimer's disease appear to be related to the underlying pathophysiology of the disease and in the case of memantine may reflect pharmaceutical mechanisms.

Vascular Dementia

While a number of studies have attempted to use MRS to distinguish Alzheimer's disease from vascular dementia[53,54], there are more similarities in the patterns of change than differences. The main distinguishing feature of vascular dementia is the subcortical predominance of metabolic alterations versus more cortical changes in Alzheimer's disease. However, as with Alzheimer's disease, patients with vascular dementia have been shown to have decreased NAA as well as increased myo-inositol[54].

Frontotemporal Dementia

As to be expected with frontotemporal dementia, metabolic changes in this disorder are associated with more frontal structures, as evidenced by a study showing decreased NAA in frontal areas compared with more posterior regional changes in Alzheimer's disease patients[55]. In a study comparing patients with frontotemporal dementia patients with those with Alzheimer's disease and controls, frontal lobe NAA and Glx concentrations were decreased in conjunction with increases in myo-inositol[56]. The NAA results have been replicated in a later study examining metabolites in the posterior cingulate cortex of frontotemporal dementia patients[57].

Lewy Body Dementia

A few studies have used MRS to examine brain changes associated with Lewy body dementia. One report including 20 patients with Lewy body dementia showed Cho/Cr ratios were significantly elevated compared with healthy controls[58]. In another study, white matter changes were detected with significantly lower mean NAA/Cr, Glx/Cr and Cho/Cr ratios in patients with Lewy body dementia compared with controls[59].

SUMMARY

Overall, the studies outlined above demonstrate a general pattern that applies to most of the neurodegenerative diseases. Dementia subtypes appear to differ only in terms of the neuroanatomical regions affected. In a number of areas, including grey and white matter and cortical and subcortical regions, NAA tends to be decreased compared to controls, while increases in myo-inositol and choline have been detected. This is thought to reflect the loss of neurons (with NAA), membrane breakdown (choline) and reactive gliosis (detected by myo-inositol) associated with these diseases.

STRENGTHS AND LIMITATIONS OF MRS

The major strength of MRS is that it allows for the measurement of specific metabolites in a particular region of the brain. Thus, the selection of crucial brain regions plays a vital role in the understanding of the pathophysiology underlying late-life mental illness. This is also a potential limitation as many studies choose different brain regions to study the same illness, thus generalizability and broad interpretation across studies are difficult to achieve.

Another limitation is poor resolution of specific peaks. Often, GABA, glutamate and glutamine peaks overlap, making it difficult to determine exact concentrations of these metabolites. One technique designed to surmount this limitation is two-dimensional magnetic resonance spectroscopy (2D-MRS).

TWO-DIMENSIONAL MAGNETIC RESONANCE SPECTROSCOPY

Two-dimensional (2D) spectroscopy is a technique that allows for greater resolution. The advantage of 2D spectroscopy is that is allows for the detection of GABA which is typically masked by the spectral peaks of other metabolites such as N-acetylaspartate and glutamate/glutamine. One of the first papers to apply 2D-MRS techniques to brain chemistry was done by Thomas and colleagues showing the feasibility of the 2D J-coupled point-resolved spectroscopy (JPRESS) technique in human subjects[60]. They were able to detect peaks representing NAA, glutamate/glutamine and lactate in occipital cortex.

Two-dimensional J-resolved spectroscopy has been successfully applied to measure previously hard-to-detect levels of GABA[61]. This technique has also been used to measure grey matter/white matter differences. In a study by Jensen et al., it was shown that GABA levels are significantly higher in grey matter than in white matter[62].

Localized two-dimensional chemical shift correlated magnetic resonance spectroscopy (2D-COSY) is a method that presents certain advantages over the JPRESS and J-resolved techniques. This method was successfully used in human brain in a study by Thomas et al, where peaks for N-acetylaspartate (NAA), glutamate/glutamine (Glx), myo-inositol (mI), creatine (Cr), choline, aspartate, GABA, taurine, glutathione, threonine and macromolecules were identified[63]. The authors demonstrated that 2D-COSY generates spectra with better resolution and less overlap of peaks. 2D-COSY has also shown to be highly reliable and reproducible[64].

The advantage of this technique is that it allows for the detection of important metabolites that are difficult to measure by traditional MRS methods. In particular, it allows for better resolution of aspartate and GABA, important neurotransmitters that have been implicated in mood disorders.

CONCLUSION

MRS is an important tool for the localized measurement of brain metabolites that has been successfully applied to the understanding of geriatric mental illness. Despite its limitations, the method continues to evolve more sophisticated techniques for the improved measurement of clinically important neurochemicals to better understand pathophysiology, functional impact and treatment effects.

REFERENCES

1. Clark JB. N-Acetyl aspartate: a marker for neuronal loss or mitochondrial dysfunction. *Dev Neurosci* 1998; **20**: 271–76.
2. De SN, Matthews PM, Arnold DL. Reversible decreases in N-acetylaspartate after acute brain injury. *Magn Reson Med* 1995; **34**: 721–27.

3. Saunders DE, Howe FA, van den BA, Griffiths JR, Brown MM. Aging of the adult human brain: in vivo quantitation of metabolite content with proton magnetic resonance spectroscopy. *J Magn Reson Imaging* 1999; **9**: 711–16.

4. Chang L, Ernst T, Poland RE, Jenden DJ. In Vivo proton magnetic resonance spectroscopy of the normal ageing human brain. *Life Sci* 1996; **58**: 2049–56.

5. Cohen BM, Renshaw PF, Stoll AL, Wurtman RJ, Yurgelun-Todd D, Babb SM. Decreased brain choline uptake in older adults. An in vivo proton magnetic resonance spectroscopy study. *JAMA* 1995; **274**: 902–907.

6. Brooks JC, Roberts N, Kemp GJ, Gosney MA, Lye M, Whitehouse GH. A proton magnetic resonance spectroscopy study of age-related changes in frontal lobe metabolite concentrations. *Cereb Cortex* 2001; **11**: 598–605.

7. Kaiser LG, Schuff N, Cashdollar N, Weiner MW. Scyllo-inositol in normal ageing human brain: 1H magnetic resonance spectroscopy study at 4 Tesla. *NMR Biomed* 2005; **18**: 51–55.

8. Valenzuela MJ, Sachdev PS, Wen W, Shnier R, Brodaty H, Gillies D. Dual voxel proton magnetic resonance spectroscopy in the healthy elderly: subcortical-frontal axonal N-acetylaspartate levels are correlated with fluid cognitive abilities independent of structural brain changes. *Neuroimage* 2000; **12**: 747–56.

9. Elderkin-Thompson V, Thomas MA, Binesh N *et al*. Brain metabolites and cognitive function among older depressed and healthy individuals using 2D MR spectroscopy. *Neuropsychopharmacology* 2004; **29**: 2251–57.

10. Angelie E, Bonmartin A, Boudraa A, Gonnaud PM, Mallet JJ, Sappey-Marinier D. Regional differences and metabolic changes in normal ageing of the human brain: proton MR spectroscopic imaging study. *AJNR Am J Neuroradiol* 2001; **22**: 119–27.

11. Ross AJ, Sachdev PS, Wen W, Brodaty H. Longitudinal changes during ageing using proton magnetic resonance spectroscopy. *J Gerontol A Biol Sci Med Sci* 2006; **61**: 291–98.

12. Haga KK, Khor YP, Farrall A, Wardlaw JM. A systematic review of brain metabolite changes, measured with ^{1}H magnetic resonance spectroscopy, in healthy ageing. *Neurobiol Aging* 2009; **30**: 353–63.

13. Bozgeyik Z, Burakgazi G, Sen Y, Ogur E. Age-related metabolic changes in the corpus callosum: assessment with MR spectroscopy. *Diagn Interv Radiol* 2008; **14**: 173–76.

14. Moreno-Torres A, Pujol J, Soriano-Mas C, Deus J, Iranzo A, Santamaria J. Age-related metabolic changes in the upper brainstem tegmentum by MR spectroscopy. *Neurobiol Aging* 2005; **26**: 1051–59.

15. Szentkuti A, Guderian S, Schiltz K *et al*. Quantitative MR analyses of the hippocampus: unspecific metabolic changes in ageing. *J Neurol* 2004; **251**: 1345–53.

16. Zimmerman ME, Pan JW, Hetherington HP *et al*. Hippocampal neurochemistry, neuromorphometry, and verbal memory in nondemented older adults. *Neurology* 2008; **70**: 1594–600.

17. Venkatraman TN, Krishnan RR, Steffens DC, Song AW, Taylor WD. Biochemical abnormalities of the medial temporal lobe and medial prefrontal cortex in late-life depression. *Psychiatry Res* 2009; **172**: 49–54.

18. Kumar A, Thomas A, Lavretsky H *et al*. Frontal white matter biochemical abnormalities in late-life major depression detected with proton magnetic resonance spectroscopy. *Am J Psychiatry* 2002; **159**: 630–36.

19. Binesh N, Kumar A, Hwang S, Mintz J, Thomas MA. Neurochemistry of late-life major depression: a pilot two-dimensional MR spectroscopic study. *J Magn Reson Imaging* 2004; **20**: 1039–45.

20. Vythilingam M, Charles HC, Tupler LA, Blitchington T, Kelly L, Krishnan KR. Focal and lateralized subcortical abnormalities in unipolar major depressive disorder: an automated multivoxel proton magnetic resonance spectroscopy study. *Biol Psychiatry* 2003; **54**: 744–50.

21. Wyckoff N, Kumar A, Gupta RC, Alger J, Hwang S, Thomas MA. Magnetization transfer imaging and magnetic resonance spectroscopy of normal-appearing white matter in late-life major depression. *J Magn Reson Imaging* 2003; 537–43.

22. Murata T, Kimura H, Omori M *et al*. MRI white matter hyperintensities, ^{1}H-MR spectroscopy and cognitive function in geriatric depression: a comparison of early- and late-onset cases. *Int J Geriatr Psychiatry* 2001; **16**: 1129–35.

23. Ajilore O, Haroon E, Kumaran S *et al*. Measurement of brain metabolites in patients with type 2 diabetes and major depression using proton magnetic resonance spectroscopy. *Neuropsychopharmacology* 2007; **32**: 1224–31.

24. Haroon E, Watari K, Thomas A *et al*. Prefrontal myo-inositol concentration and visuo-spatial functioning among diabetic depressed patients. *Psychiatry Res* 2009; **171**: 10–19.

25. Iosifescu DV, Clementi-Craven N, Fraguas R *et al*. Cardiovascular risk factors may moderate pharmacological treatment effects in major depressive disorder. *Psychosom Med* 2005; **67**: 703–706.

26. Michael N, Erfurth A, Ohrmann P, Arolt V, Heindel W, Pfleiderer B. Neurotrophic effects of electroconvulsive therapy: a proton magnetic resonance study of the left amygdalar region in patients with treatment-resistant depression. *Neuropsychopharmacology* 2003; **28**: 720–25.

27. Michael N, Erfurth A, Ohrmann P, Arolt V, Heindel W, Pfleiderer B. Metabolic changes within the left dorsolateral prefrontal cortex occurring with electroconvulsive therapy in patients with treatment resistant unipolar depression. *Psychol Med* 2003; **33**: 1277–84.

28. Gonul AS, Kitis O, Ozan E *et al*. The effect of antidepressant treatment on N-acetyl aspartate levels of medial frontal cortex in drug-free depressed patients. *Prog Neuropsychopharmacol Biol Psychiatry* 2006; **30**: 120–25.

29. Moore CM, Christensen JD, Lafer B, Fava M, Renshaw PF. Lower levels of nucleoside triphosphate in the basal ganglia of depressed subjects: a phosphorous-31 magnetic resonance spectroscopy study. *Am J Psychiatry* 1997; **154**: 116–18.

30. Volz HP, Rzanny R, Riehemann S *et al*. ^{31}P magnetic resonance spectroscopy in the frontal lobe of major depressed patients. *Eur Arch Psychiatry Clin Neurosci* 1998; **248**: 289–95.

31. Renshaw PF, Parow AM, Hirashima F *et al*. Multinuclear magnetic resonance spectroscopy studies of brain purines in major depression. *Am J Psychiatry* 2001; **158**: 2048–55.

32. Iosifescu DV, Bolo NR, Nierenberg AA, Jensen JE, Fava M, Renshaw PF. Brain bioenergetics and response to triiodothyronine augmentation in major depressive disorder. *Biol Psychiatry* 2008; **63**: 1127–34.

33. Pettegrew JW, Levine J, Gershon S *et al*. ^{31}P-MRS study of acetyl-L-carnitine treatment in geriatric depression: preliminary results. *Bipolar Disord* 2002; **4**: 61–66.

34. Forester BP, Harper DG, Jensen JE *et al*. ^{31}Phosphorus magnetic resonance spectroscopy study of tissue specific changes in high energy phosphates before and after sertraline treatment of geriatric depression. *Int J Geriatr Psychiatry* 2009;. **24**: 788–97.

35. Forester BP, Streeter CC, Berlow YA *et al.* Brain lithium levels and effects on cognition and mood in geriatric bipolar disorder: a lithium-7 magnetic resonance spectroscopy study. *Am J Geriatr Psychiatry* 2009; **17**: 13–23.

36. Forester BP, Finn CT, Berlow YA, Wardrop M, Renshaw PF, Moore CM. Brain lithium, *N*-acetyl aspartate and myo-inositol levels in older adults with bipolar disorder treated with lithium: a lithium-7 and proton magnetic resonance spectroscopy study. *Bipolar Disord* 2008; **10**: 691–700.

37. Stork C, Renshaw PF. Mitochondrial dysfunction in bipolar disorder: evidence from magnetic resonance spectroscopy research. *Mol Psychiatry* 2005; **10**: 900–19.

38. Kantarci K, Jack CR, Jr., Xu YC *et al.* Regional metabolic patterns in mild cognitive impairment and Alzheimer's disease: A 1H MRS study. *Neurology* 2000; **55**: 210–17.

39. Catani M, Cherubini A, Howard R *et al.* ¹H-MR spectroscopy differentiates mild cognitive impairment from normal brain ageing. *Neuroreport* 2001; **12**: 2315–17.

40. Ackl N, Ising M, Schreiber YA, Atiya M, Sonntag A, Auer DP. Hippocampal metabolic abnormalities in mild cognitive impairment and Alzheimer's disease. *Neurosci Lett* 2005; **384**: 23–28.

41. Chao LL, Schuff N, Kramer JH *et al.* Reduced medial temporal lobe N-acetylaspartate in cognitively impaired but nondemented patients. *Neurology* 2005; **64**: 282–89.

42. Modrego PJ, Fayed N, Pina MA. Conversion from mild cognitive impairment to probable Alzheimer's disease predicted by brain magnetic resonance spectroscopy. *Am J Psychiatry* 2005; **162**: 667–75.

43. Shiino A, Matsuda M, Morikawa S, Inubushi T, Akiguchi I, Handa J. Proton magnetic resonance spectroscopy with dementia. *Surg Neurol* 1993; **39**: 143–47.

44. Parnetti L, Tarducci R, Presciutti O *et al.* Proton magnetic resonance spectroscopy can differentiate Alzheimer's disease from normal ageing. *Mech Ageing Dev* 1997; **97**: 9–14.

45. Frederick BB, Satlin A, Yurgelun-Todd DA, Renshaw PF. In Vivo proton magnetic resonance spectroscopy of Alzheimer's disease in the parietal and temporal lobes. *Biol Psychiatry* 1997; **42**: 147–50.

46. Lazeyras F, Charles HC, Tupler LA, Erickson R, Boyko OB, Krishnan KR. Metabolic brain mapping in Alzheimer's disease using proton magnetic resonance spectroscopy. *Psychiatry Res* 1998; **82**: 95–106.

47. Adalsteinsson E, Sullivan EV, Kleinhans N, Spielman DM, Pfefferbaum A. Longitudinal decline of the neuronal marker N-acetyl aspartate in Alzheimer's disease. *Lancet* 2000; **355**: 1696–97.

48. Chantal S, Labelle M, Bouchard RW, Braun CMJ, Boulanger Y. Correlation of regional proton magnetic resonance spectroscopic metabolic changes with cognitive deficits in mild Alzheimer disease. *Arch Neurol* 2002; **59**: 955–62.

49. Krishnan KRR, Charles HC, Doraiswamy PM *et al.* Randomized, placebo-controlled trial of the effects of donepezil on neuronal markers and hippocampal volumes in Alzheimer's disease. *Am J Psychiatry* 2003; **160**: 2003–11.

50. Jessen F, Traeber F, Freymann K, Maier W, Schild HH, Block W. Treatment monitoring and response prediction with proton MR spectroscopy in AD. *Neurology* 2006; **67**: 528–30.

51. Modrego PJ, Pina MA, Fayed N, Diaz M. Changes in metabolite ratios after treatment with rivastigmine in Alzheimer's disease: a nonrandomised controlled trial with magnetic resonance spectroscopy. *CNS Drugs* 2006; **20**: 867–77.

52. Glodzik L, King KG, Gonen O, Liu S, De SS, de Leon MJ. Memantine decreases hippocampal glutamate levels: a magnetic resonance spectroscopy study. *Prog Neuropsychopharmacol Biol Psychiatry* 2008; **32**: 1005–12.

53. Kattapong VJ, Brooks WM, Wesley MH, Kodituwakku PW, Rosenberg GA. Proton magnetic resonance spectroscopy of vascular- and Alzheimer-type dementia. *Arch Neurol* 1996; **53**: 678–80.

54. Herminghaus S, Frolich L, Gorriz C *et al.* Brain metabolism in Alzheimer disease and vascular dementia assessed by in vivo proton magnetic resonance spectroscopy. *Psychiatry Res Neuroimag* 2003; **123**: 183–90.

55. Mihara M, Hattori N, Abe K, Sakoda S, Sawada T. Magnetic resonance spectroscopic study of Alzheimer's disease and frontotemporal dementia/Pick complex. *Neuroreport* 2006; **17**: 413 16.

56. Ernst T, Chang L, Melchor R, Mehringer CM. Frontotemporal dementia and early Alzheimer disease: differentiation with frontal lobe H-1 MR spectroscopy. *Radiology* 1997; **203**: 829–36.

57. Kizu O, Yamada K, Ito H, Nishimura T. Posterior cingulate metabolic changes in frontotemporal lobar degeneration detected by magnetic resonance spectroscopy. *Neuroradiology* 2004; **46**: 277–81.

58. Kantarci K, Petersen RC, Boeve BF *et al.* 1H MR spectroscopy in common dementias. *Neurology* 2004; **63**: 1393–98.

59. Molina JA, Garcia-Segura JM, ito-Leon J *et al.* Proton magnetic resonance spectroscopy in dementia with Lewy bodies. *Eur Neurol* 2002; **48**: 158–63.

60. Ryner LN, Sorenson JA, Thomas MA. Localized 2D J-resolved 1H MR spectroscopy: strong coupling effects in vitro and in vivo. *Magn Reson Imaging* 1995; **13**: 853–69.

61. Jensen JE, Frederick BD, Wang L, Brown J, Renshaw PF. Two-dimensional, J-resolved spectroscopic imaging of GABA at 4 Tesla in the human brain. *Magn Reson Med* 2005; **54**: 783–88.

62. Jensen JE, Frederick BB, Renshaw PF. Grey and white matter GABA level differences in the human brain using two-dimensional, J-resolved spectroscopic imaging. *NMR Biomed* 2005; **18**: 570–76.

63. Thomas MA, Yue K, Binesh N *et al.* Localized two-dimensional shift correlated MR spectroscopy of human brain. *Magn Reson Med* 2001; **46**: 58–67.

64. Binesh N, Yue K, Fairbanks L, Thomas MA. Reproducibility of localized 2D correlated MR spectroscopy. *Magn Reson Med* 2002; **48**: 942–48.

Part E

Affective Disorders

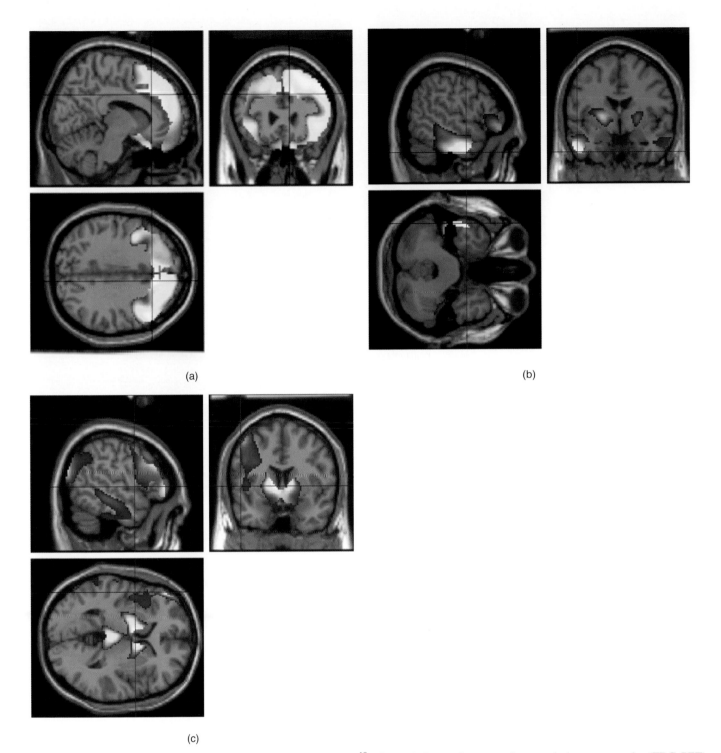

(a)

(b)

(c)

Figure 5.1 Reductions of regional cerebral glucose metabolism in ^{18}F-fluoro-2-deoxy-glucose positron emission tomography (FDG PET) studies of patients with (a) frontotemporal dementia, (b) semantic dementia and (c) progressive non-fluent aphasia compared with healthy control subjects (sagittal, axial, and coronal slices; areas with reduced metabolism are displayed in colour).

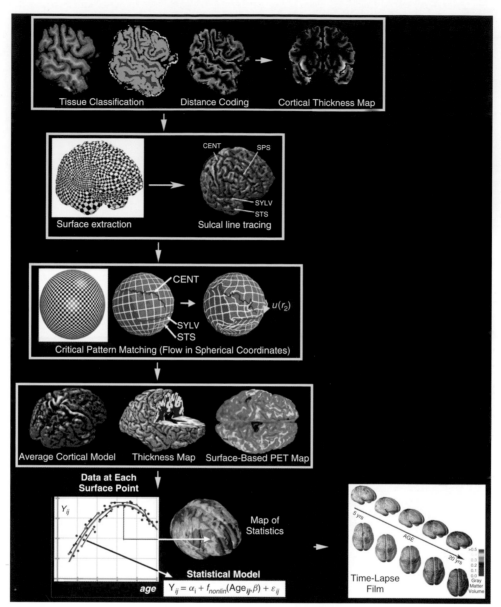

Figure 46.1 Flowchart showing an image analysis pipeline (adapted from[10]) that can map changes of various neuroanatomical measures in the cortex, such as grey matter atrophy. Cortical thickness profiles, for example, can be averaged across subjects or compared across time. Tissue classification techniques can be used to identify grey and white matter and to produce cortical thickness maps (row 1). The CPM approach can be applied by tracing sulcal landmarks on extracted brain surface models (row 2) that serve as anchors to guide a flow field matching gyral regions across subjects (row 3). Then maps of cortical thickness, or other cortical signals (such as co-registered PET images, shown here), can be fluidly aligned to an average cortical model (row 4). Statistical models are fitted to data from all the subjects at each cortical point. This can assess whether imaging signals are associated with age (bottom row), or other parameters of interest. Effects of ageing on cortical measures – or changes relative to baseline – may be animated as a time-lapse film to reveal the disease trajectory.

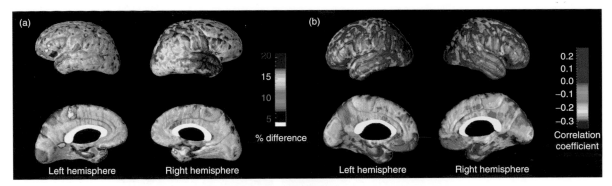

Figure 46.2 (A) Cortical thinning of up to 20% occurs between MCI and AD, in widely distributed cortical areas (greatest tissue loss is coded in red). (B). Grey matter atrophy in the anterior cingulate and supplementary motor cortices is correlated with the presence or absence of apathy in AD. Regions where structural variation correlates with clinical or behavioural differences can be identified using correlation maps such as these (strong associations are shown here in red colours). Data adapted from[21,22].

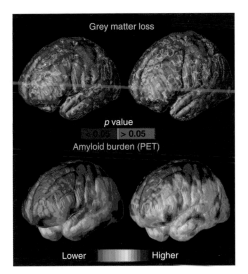

Figure 46.3 Progression of AD based on MRI and [18F]FDDNP PET. On MRI (top row), the areas with grey matter deficits in mild AD (left panel) include primarily the temporal lobe, but in moderate AD (right panel) these deficits have spread to involve the frontal cortex (adapted from a longitudinal study by Thompson et al.[25]). Finally, cerebral amyloid estimated in vivo from the PET ligand FDDNP is low in controls, but higher in those with impaired cognition (bottom row; adapted from Braskie et al.[8]). The anatomical agreement is striking between these in vivo maps and the well-established postmortem maps for the staging of AD. In all maps, the sensorimotor cortex shows least disease-related degeneration.

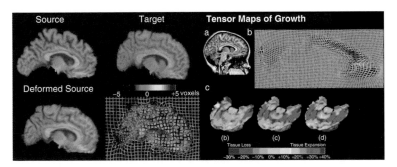

Figure 46.4 Tensor-based morphometry. In TBM, a fluid transformation (deformed grid) is applied to a baseline scan (source) to reconfigure it (deformed source) into the shape of a follow-up scan (target). The local expansions (red colours) or atrophies (blue colours) can be plotted in brain regions such as the corpus callosum (shown in the green box in [a]). Voxel expansions (red colours) or contractions (blue colours) can be plotted onto a sequence of scans collected from the same subject (shown here in axial view illustrating progressive temporal lobe atrophy in a subject with frontotemporal lobe atrophy) during a degenerative brain disease, emphasizing regions with progressive atrophy. These maps may be averaged across subjects or compared across populations to assess factors that influence degenerative rates in each region of the brain.

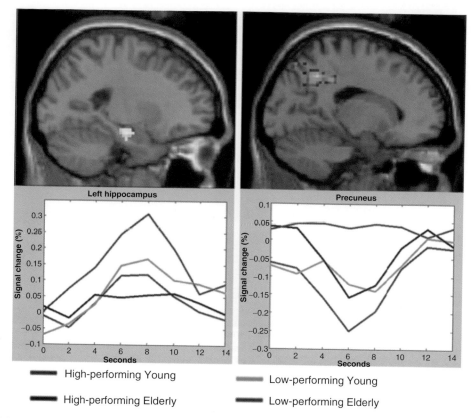

Figure 70.3 Group fMRI data maps (top) with MR signal time courses (bottom) for Young and Elderly controls show hippocampal activation (left) and precuneus deactivation (right) during the successful encoding of face-name pairs. Low-performing Elderly failed to deactivate the precuneus and demonstrated increased hippocampal and pre-frontal activation for successful but not failed encoding trials, perhaps as a compensatory response to failure of default network activity.

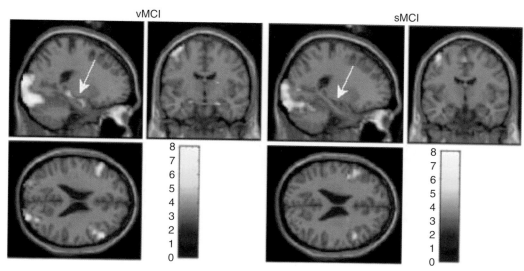

Figure 70.4 Group fMRI data from 15 very mildly impaired MCI (vMCI) and 12 significantly impaired MCI (sMCI) subjects on a face-name encoding task. The vMCI subjects showed evidence of hippocampal 'hyperactivation' compared to controls. The sMCI subjects showed significantly decreased hippocampal activation at levels similar to those seen in mild AD patients.

72

Nosology and Classification of Mood Disorders

Dan Blazer

Duke University School of Medicine, Duke University Medical Center, Durham, USA

The mood or affective disorders are a group of disorders characterized by disturbance of mood and accompanied by a partial or complete change in mood or affect that is either manic (or hypomanic) or depressed (or mildly dysphoric). These disorders are classified in both the ICD[1] and the DSM[2] diagnostic systems in the three-digit rubric (296.xx in DSM-IV and F30.x–F39.x in ICD-10). With some exceptions noted below, the nosology of mood disorders in ICD-10 and DSM-IV is appropriate for the classification of mood disturbances in older adults. The classification of the disorders will therefore be described below, with specific comments related to older adults.

It should be noted at the outset of this chapter that DSM-IV is unchanged since the second edition of this text. A new version, DSM-V, is due for publication in 2012. ICD-10 has been instituted since the second edition, yet many changes in ICD-10 and the desire to bring the classification systems into closer concert were anticipated in the chapter from the second edition. It should also be noted that, despite the many advances in the pathophysiological investigation of late life mood disorders and new studies of therapies (pharmacological, psychological and social), DSM-IV and ICD-10 classifications have been accepted by investigators and clinicians alike. Some suggestions of new syndromes, such as 'depression in Alzheimer's Disease', have emerged and will be discussed briefly though none of these are widely employed.

MANIC EPISODE (F30, 296.4–7)

A manic episode is characterized by an elevated mood that is unrelated to the patient's circumstances. This elevated mood usually varies from an expansive or irritable syndrome to an almost uncontrollable excitement and psychotic agitation. Changes in mood are accompanied by increased energy, a decreased need for sleep, a decline in normal social inhibitions, as well as inflated and grandiose ideas, which frequently become delusional. Older persons can experience a typical episode of mania as well as hypomania (a less severe elevation of mood) but are more likely to suffer a so-called 'irritable' or 'angry' manic episode. Joviality and elation are replaced by irritability and agitation (as described elsewhere in this text). Nevertheless, older persons who suffer manic episodes usually meet both ICD-10 and DSM-IV criteria, even when the predominant symptoms are irritability and anger, as other diagnostic criteria are met.

ICD-10 defines a hypomanic episode as a disorder characterized by a persistent mild elevation of mood, increased energy and activity, and usually marked feelings of well-being and both physical and mental efficiency. Increased sociability, talkativeness, over-familiarity, increased sexual energy and a decreased need for sleep are often present but not to the extent that they lead to severe disruption of work or result in social rejection. Older adults, however, often experience irritability and anger as with a full episode. A parallel diagnosis is bipolar II disorder in DSM-IV.

DEPRESSIVE (F32) OR MAJOR DEPRESSIVE (296.2, 3) EPISODE

A major depressive episode is characterized by a depressed, disinterested or irritable mood, associated with the loss of interest or pleasure in all or almost all activities, accompanied by a number of other symptoms. These additional symptoms include a reduced capacity for enjoyment, reduced interest in surroundings, difficulty concentrating, lethargy, sleep disturbances, appetite disturbances, decreased self-esteem and self-confidence, and frequent ideas of guilt or worthlessness. Although older persons are somewhat less likely to report a specific decrease in their mood, they almost always describe a loss of interest in usual activities (anhedonia) in the midst of a major depressive episode. The categories of severe depressive episode in ICD-10 and major depressive episode in DSM-IV are very similar. DSM-IV and ICD-10 permit the diagnosis of a minor depressive episode (in the appendix of DSM-IV and categorized as mild in ICD-10); that is, a depressive episode which fulfils some of the symptom criteria for a major depressive episode and/or dysthymia and which lasts two weeks or longer. The more severe consequences of a depressive episode, such as a successful suicide or a retardation that progresses to stupor, would be characteristic of a severe but not a mild depressive episode in ICD-10.

Older persons who suffer a complicated, severe depression are easily diagnosed according to both ICD-10 and DSM-IV criteria. Problems do arise, however, when the episode experienced by older persons is accompanied by a severe medical illness or significant cognitive impairment. The frequency of psychobiologic symptoms in more severe depressions renders the distinction between symptoms of depression and symptoms of physical illness/functional impairment difficult in the midst of a depressed mood associated with medical illness. The current nosology is not helpful in disaggregating mood disorders from either the symptoms of physical illness or normal psychological reactions to physical illness. Some have suggested that a unique criterion for older persons with depression and cognitive impairment should be instituted (but this is yet to be included in

Principles and Practice of Geriatric Psychiatry, 3rd edn. Edited by Mohammed T. Abou-Saleh, Cornelius Katona and Anand Kumar
© 2011 John Wiley & Sons, Ltd

any extant diagnostic system). The co-morbidity of depressive symptoms in cognitive disorders such as dementia, Parkinson's disease and small strokes renders such an approach potentially useful in improving the current nosology. Two examples are presented below.

'Vascular depression' has been proposed as the diagnostic entity secondary to vascular lesions in the brain and appears to increase in frequency with age[3]. The clinical presentation may differ from major depression, even if only in subtle ways. Elders with vascular depression exhibit impairment in set shifting, verbal fluency, psychomotor speed, recognition memory and planning (executive cognitive function), a 'depression–executive dysfunction syndrome' characterized by psychomotor retardation, and reduced interest in activities. Vascular depression is associated with an absence of psychotic features, less likelihood of a family history, more anhedonia and greater functional disability when compared with nonvascular depression.

Others have proposed a depression of Alzheimer's disease[4]. The criteria are as follows. In persons who meet criteria for dementia of the Alzheimer's type, three of a series of symptoms that includes depressed mood, anhedonia, social isolation, poor appetite, poor sleep, psychomotor changes, irritability, fatigue or loss of energy, feelings of worthlessness and suicidal thoughts must be present for the diagnosis to be made.

BIPOLAR (F31, 296.4–7) AND UNIPOLAR DISORDER (F32, 296.2, 3)

In both ICD-10 and DSM-IV, individuals who present with a history of recurrent mood disorder (at least two), in which mood and activity were profoundly disturbed and at least one of the episodes was manic, are classified as suffering from bipolar mood disorder. Bipolar disorder usually has an early age of onset, although it can have its onset later in life, and the categorization is useful in older as well as younger persons. Bipolar disorders are classified as manic (the individual is currently in a manic episode), depressed (the individual is currently in a depressed episode and has at least one well-authenticated manic episode in the past) or mixed (the individual's current episode involves a full symptomatic picture of both manic and depressed episode, except for the duration requirement of two weeks of depressed episodes). Symptoms are often intermixed or rapidly alternating within hours or days in the latter category.

Bipolar II disorder (F31.8 and 296.89) is characterized by at least one hypomanic episode and at least one episode of major depression. These disorders are probably more common among older persons than the more classic bipolar disorder described above. Older persons frequently experience depression and occasionally mania secondary to medical illness or medications, categories that are specified in DSM-IV as mood disorder due to a general medical disorder and substance-induced mood disorder. Common examples of causes of these secondary mood disorders in the elderly include hypothyroidism, Parkinson's disease, chronic obstructive pulmonary disease, various forms of cancer, alcohol, β-adrenergic blockers and L-dopa. Mood disorders with a seasonal pattern are less frequent in the elderly[5].

Individuals who never experience an episode of mania or hypomania but nevertheless suffer episodes of major depression are generally classified as 'single-episode' or 'recurrent'. Most depressive disorders are recurrent; that is, distinct episodes of major depression followed by distinct episodes of normal functioning may be the exception rather than the rule. For this reason, additional diagnostic categories have been instituted in the nosology to disaggregate the classification of the natural history of depressive episodes. In ICD-10, a category of 'recurrent severe depressive disorder' (F33.3) is analogous to the DSM-IV category of 'major depression recurrent' (296.3). Recurrent mild depressive disorder (F33.0) is categorized in ICD-10 by repeated episodes of depression, the majority of which fulfil the description given for mild depressive episode above. These recurrent mild episodes may or may not be associated with environmental stress and may be either acute or insidious in onset. Recovery is usual, although not always complete.

Cyclothymia is included in both DSM-IV (301.13) and ICD-10 (F34.0). According to ICD-10, cyclothymia is a persistent instability of mood involving numerous periods of mild depression and mild elation. The instability usually develops early in adult life and pursues a chronic course, although at times mood may be normal and stable for months. Cyclothymia is difficult to establish without a prolonged period of observation or an unusually good account of the subject's past behaviour. In DSM-IV, cyclothymia must persist for at least two years to be diagnosed and involve numerous hypomanic episodes.

Yet another phenomenon has emerged in the study of the natural history of depression – rapid cycling[6,7]. Rapid cycling is the occurrence of four or more episodes of depression or mania per year, with either two weeks of normal mood between episodes, or a shift directly from mania to depression, or vice versa. Others have classified rapid cycling as involving either mixed mood states, or frequent mood fluctuation without discrete intermorbid periods, or involving 24- or 48-hour cycles of mood disturbance. Rapid cycling occurs in persons regardless of age, although there may be some tendency for individuals to decrease their propensity to rapid cycling with increased age. Rapid cycling appears to be more common in individuals with bipolar disorder than unipolar disorder, but it is not limited to individuals with bipolar disorder. Rapid cycling is a specific type of bipolar mood disorder in DSM-IV (296.8) and major depression (311). Research criteria are proposed in the appendix of DSM-IV-TR.

DYSTHYMIA (F34.1, 300.4)

Dysthymia is a category included in both ICD-10 and DSM-IV. Dysthymia is a chronic depression of mood that does not fulfil the description and guidelines of mild recurrent depressive disorders (in ICD-10) and is characterized by periods of days or weeks at a time when patients feel tired and depressed, where everything is an effort and where nothing is enjoyed. They 'brood and complain', sleep badly and feel inadequate, but are usually able to cope with the basic demands of everyday life. This description is similar to the description of dysthymia in DSM-IV, where the essential feature is a chronic disturbance of mood, involving a depressed mood for most of the day and more days than not for at least two years (the two-year minimum duration is not a criterion in ICD-10 but rather is to last at least several years). In addition, individuals suffering dysthymia suffer many of the symptoms of the more severe depression but with less severity, such as poor appetite, insomnia, low energy and low self-esteem. Older persons often meet criteria for a dysthymic disorder (in terms of duration of symptoms) when diagnosed with major depression. It is difficult to determine, however, whether the dysthymic disorder is a separate entity or whether it is part of the same syndrome which 'waxes and wanes' in severity. Recent studies have suggested that dysthymic disorder may exist most often in the elderly as an entity not associated with major depression. Dysthymic disorder has usually been equated with depressive neuroses, as described in earlier versions of both the ICD and DSM diagnostic systems, which assumes that the depressed mood results from psychoneurotic and stress-related difficulties.

Yet another category that has been suggested is minor or mild depression. Criteria for minor depression can be found in the appendix of DSM-IV and variants can be found in the Research Diagnostic Criteria and in ICD-10 (F32.0). There is virtually no data to substantiate a specific entity for minor depressions, except that persons who experience minor depression (that is, symptoms less severe than major depression for at least two weeks, according to DSM-IV) exhibit a similar risk factor profile and are at much greater risk for developing major depression over time. There have been a number of studies of minor depression among the elderly. The renewed interest in minor depression once again brings the categorical vs. continuum controversy to the forefront in the phenomenology of depression.

ADJUSTMENT DISORDER WITH DEPRESSED MOOD (F43.2, 309.0)

In the DSM-IV system of classification, an adjustment disorder is a reaction to an identifiable psychosocial stressor that leads to maladaptive reactions, including impairment in occupational functioning and symptoms that are in excess of normal and expected reaction to this stressor. The maladaptive reaction may take many forms and an exaggerated depressed mood is one of the forms.

Symptoms of adjustment disorder with depressed mood include tearfulness and feelings of hopelessness. By definition, the maladaptive reaction can persist no longer than six months, does not meet criteria for other disorders and does not represent uncomplicated bereavement.

ICD-10 includes the category of adjustment disorder (but depressed type is not specifically coded) and the clinical form may take the characteristic of a 'prolonged depressive reaction'; that is, a mild depressive state occurring in response to prolonged exposure to a stressful situation but of a duration not lasting six months. The categories of adjustment disorder are therefore very similar for both diagnostic systems. In theory, the stressor may include physical illness and therefore this category is most relevant to depressive episodes in later life. A lack of acceptable longitudinal data on the association of depressive symptoms with physical illness renders it difficult to determine whether older persons do recover from the depressive episode, which often accompanies a physical illness, within the six months required by the diagnostic category of adjustment disorder.

CONCLUSION

In general, the current classificatory systems of both DSM-IV and ICD-10 work relatively well for classifying older persons suffering from mood disorders. A number of distinct exceptions must be recognized, however. Categories such as dysthymic disorder, adjustment disorder and minor depression in DSM-IV do not appear to be adequate, and therefore more exploration of the ICD-10 construct of mild depression (but possibly not utilizing the specific diagnostic criteria of ICD-10) would appear in order. A major problem with the current classification systems is the inability to take into account co-morbidity, especially co-morbid depression and physical illness. Co-morbid depression and physical illness is a grossly unstudied area, compared to the clinical relevance of the condition. To what extent do our current classification systems accommodate individuals suffering mild or even severe depressive symptoms in the midst of physical illness? In addition, depression is often co-morbid with other psychiatric symptoms, especially anxiety disorders and somatic complaints. Neither ICD-10 nor DSM-IV adequately accommodates the co-morbid psychiatric syndromes that are frequently seen in older adults.

Finally, when classifying mood disorders many individuals suffer a depressed mood in late life that is not disordered. Uncomplicated bereavement is an expected accompaniment of older persons who experience a significant loss in old age. In addition, other older persons may become demoralized, given the current circumstances in their lives. Such persons should not be classified in a disease-oriented classification system. Nevertheless, these human experiences are not to be ignored by the clinician working with the older adult suffering a mood disorder.

REFERENCES

1. World Health Organization. *International Statistical Classification of Diseases and Related Health Problems*, 10th edn. Geneva: World Health Organization, 2007.
2. American Psychiatric Association. *Diagnostic and Statistical Manual of Mental Disorders*, 4th edn, text revision. Washington, DC: American Psychiatric Association, 2000.
3. Alexopoulos G, Meyers B, Young R *et al.* 'Vascular depression' hypothesis. *Arch Gen Psychiatry* 1997; **54**: 915–22.
4. Olin J, Schneider L, Katz I *et al.* Provisional diagnostic criteria for depression of Alzheimer disease. *Am J Geriatr Psychiatry* 2002; **10**: 125–8.
5. Akiskal HS. The clinical management of affective disorders. In Michels R (ed.), *Psychiatry*, vol. 1. Philadelphia, PA: Lippincott, 1989, ch 61.
6. Dunner DL, Patric V, Fieve RR. Rapid cycling manic depressive patients. *Compr Psychiatry* 1977; **18**: 561–6.
7. Wolpert EA, Goldberg JF, Harrow M. Rapid cycling in unipolar and bipolar affective disorders. *Am J Psychiatry* 1990; **147**: 725–8.

73

Genetics of Affective Disorders

Carolina Aponte Urdaneta and John L. Beyer

Duke University Medical Center, Durham, NC, USA

INTRODUCTION

With the completion of the Human Genome Project, the field of genetics has vastly changed. Even our current definitions of disorders and treatment of diseases are anticipated to evolve pending the interpretation of our new genetic data[1]. However, rather than just narrowly looking at genetic associations in persons with affective disorders, the contributions obtained from the wider body of research examining the genetic basis of psychiatric disorders need to be interpreted in the context of environmental influences and the heterogeneous nature of these disorders[2,3]. This is especially true for late-life disorders, in which simple Mendelian genetics do not apply, and multiple genes each likely play a small role, together with co-morbid illnesses, earlier life insults and environmental factors[4,5].

Genetic studies can be classified into linkage studies, gene–disease association studies (looking at specific single nucleotide polymorphisms (SNPs)), and the more recent genome-wide association studies (GWAs). Other more classic forms of genetic studies include familial aggregation studies, twin studies, adoption studies, and linkage studies of an illness with a genetic marker. Finally, an area of recent intense research that may soon show significance in late-life psychiatric disorders is that of copy-number variations (CNVs). Findings have suggested that CNVs may cause disease due to genomic rearrangements that result in altered number of copies. These disorders have primarily been associated with neurodevelopmental and neurodegenerative disease processes[6,7], a classification in which late-life affective disorders could well be included.

In this chapter, we will review the current understanding of genetic influences in late-life affective disorders. However, before looking at specifics, it is important to highlight the intricacies of examining the associations of genetic variations with complex diseases such as late-life affective disorders; researchers have had difficulty replicating associations[8]. Therefore, many of the findings reviewed here may be considered suggestive, but not fully verified. It will be up to future research to clarify and reveal the developing story of genetic influences in late-life mood disorders.

LATE-LIFE AFFECTIVE DISORDERS

As with affective disorders in the early and mid-life ages, late-life mood disorders are quite heterogeneous. Age of onset appears to be an important clinical variable in the genetic study of affective illness. Therefore, two groups of affectively ill elderly patients are usually differentiated: those who had an early onset of illness with continued symptoms or episodes in their later life, and those who had a late onset of illness (usually defined as a first onset after the age of 60 years)[9]. When differentiated by age of onset, late-onset depressive disorders have qualities suggesting that they may be genetically different from early onset forms, including clinical differences in expression and non-conformity to expected genetic models[10].

For example, basic genetic models propose that diseases with strong genetic influences are most often found in earlier onset and/or more severe forms of an illness. However, late-onset affective syndromes are typically among the most severe and most refractory to treatment[11,12]. Further, many studies have consistently found that patients with late-onset depression and bipolar disorders have less familial aggregation of mood disorders than those with the early onset affective disorders[13–18]. Also, late-onset mood disorders are also less likely to display the gender disparity present in early onset mood disorders[13]. These considerations challenge our models of genetic influence for late-life affective disorders.

Two explanations have been proposed for the age-related variation in genetic influence for affective illnesses: multifactorial inheritance and increased phenocopy expression with age. Multifactorial inheritance (also called polygenic inheritance) suggests that inheritance patterns are a result of a combination between multiple interacting genes and environmental factors. Examples of traits that have multifactorial inheritance include stature, intelligence or blood pressure[10]. According to the multifactorial theory, the onset of an affective disorder results from the additive effects of several genetic and environment factors. One could also assume that early onset illnesses probably result from greater genetic loading, while late-onset illnesses may have less genetic loading but increased occurrence of environmental events with age.

The second explanation, increased phenocopies, may explain the limited specificity of the affective disorders diagnosis. Both bipolar disorder and major depressive disorder are syndrome diagnoses; that is, the diagnosis is based on the presence of a collection of observed symptoms (phenotypes) rather than an etiological cause. In this theory, late-onset affective illness is a collection of phenocopies. Phenocopies are illnesses with a characteristic phenotype but different underlying causes.

It has long been known that depressive syndromes are very common in neurological disorders such as Parkinson's disease, Alzheimer's disease and stroke; more recently added to this list would be the proposed subtype of depression called 'vascular

Principles and Practice of Geriatric Psychiatry, 3rd edn. Edited by Mohammed T. Abou-Saleh, Cornelius Katona and Anand Kumar
© 2011 John Wiley & Sons, Ltd

depression'[19,20]. Taking these into account, the age-related variation in late-life affective disorders may be explained by increasing phenocopies in older adults who have late-onset affective disorders. Patients with early onset affective disorders (which would include elderly patients with previous diagnosis of affective disorders) may be, therefore, more likely to have a genetic cause. As research sharpens our understanding of these diseases, the 'heterogeneous' group of affective disorders will be differentiated into various subtypes, each with a more specifically defined course, prognosis and treatment. Each new subtype will also suggest new ways that genes and the environment may contribute to the expression of the illness.

There is one further consideration in studying genetic contributions to late-life affective disorders. This is the fact that not all subjects with higher or lower genetic susceptibility may reach the developmental age of expression. Competing causes of death must be taken into account (i.e. individuals at high risk of developing a disorder may not express the disease symptoms during their lifetime). This in turn means that the actual risk of developing a disease is decreased when other causes of mortality are in play[21].

GENETICS OF LATE-LIFE DEPRESSION

First-degree relatives (parents, siblings, offspring) of depressed adult patients are twice as likely to develop depression as those in the general population[22-26]. In two twin studies of adult populations, the relative risk for monozygotic twins to develop depression was 1.9, while the risk for dizygotic twins was 1.2[27,28]. Adoption studies have suggested that certain environmental influences, especially parental loss and parental alcoholism, may be predictors of depression[29]. Heritability, therefore, is estimated at around 40% in the adult population[30]; however, it has also been estimated to be lower in the elderly[31,32]. Evidence of only limited heritability (16%) was found in a sample of elderly reared-apart and reared-together Swedish twins studied for characteristics of depression[4]. In contrast, a sample of Danish twins 75 years of age and older revealed that depression symptomatology is moderately heritable in late life (approximately 35%)[5]. Moreover, both studies consistently implicated environmental factors as the major source of variance in depression symptoms among the elderly.

Large-scale family linkage studies of major depression to chromosomal loci have been conducted focusing predominantly on early onset major depression, with some consistency of findings[33]. In the area of candidate genes mainly drawn from monoamine theory of depression, study findings have suggested that 44 base pair deletions or insertions in the serotonin transporter (SLC6A4) may result in dysfunction or reduced expression of the transporter and, possibly, depressive symptoms or major depression[34,35]. In the same area, the gene SLC6A4 has been associated in several studies with increase risk for depression induced by life stresses[35,36]. However, caution is still warranted about these associations because, as in repeated cases of genetic association findings in psychiatric disorders, several studies have failed to replicate the findings on SLC6A4 and stress reactivity[37,38]. Still, SLC6A4 variations may be implicated in functional effects[39]. As with most findings, further research is required.

Other candidate genes that have been proposed and received attention in the field of late-life depression are the genes associated with brain-derived neurotrophic factor (BDNF), tryptophan hydroxylase 2 (TPH2), and APOE (apolipoprotein E). Studies in BDNF and TPH2 genetic associations have reported mixed results[35,40,41]. Since one of the major complications of Alzheimer's disease is the development of a major depressive disorder, researchers have been especially interested in the APOE genes. Research has suggested that the presence of one of the APOE alleles may predispose patients to the development of major depression[42]. Other researchers have not supported this finding[43-45].

GENETICS OF LATE-LIFE BIPOLAR DISORDER

Bipolar disorder has been widely recognized as having a strong genetic component[46]. Heritability has been estimated at over 80%[47]. Depending on which particular study is cited, first-degree relatives of adult bipolar patients may have a 3.7 to 17.5% risk for developing bipolar disorder[22-26]. The risk of bipolar disorder diminishes in second-degree relatives (grandparents, grandchildren, aunts, uncles) of bipolar patients, though still elevated over the general population. The average concordance rate for bipolar disorders in monozygotic twins is 60%, while the concordance rate in dizygotic twins is 12%. This five-fold greater rate of concordance strongly indicates the importance of genetic factors in the familial aggregation[48].

Large samples for genetic analyses have been obtained by combining family data sets. These studies have found consistent evidence of a linkage region on chromosome 6q. Other regions that seem to be implicated include chromosomes 4q and 8q[46,49-51]. Associations with the schizophrenia risk genes D-amino acid oxidase activator (DAOA), disrupted in schizophrenia 1 (DISC1), neuregulin 1 (NRG1) and catechol-O-methyltransferase (COMT) have been reported[46,47,52,53]. Meta-analyses of bipolar disorder genetic association studies have also identified small effect sizes for BDNF, MTHFR, and SLC6A4[54]. However, even these candidate genes appear to explain a small proportion of bipolar disorder's heritability since the odds ratios for individual susceptibility variants typically are less than 1.5. Specific associations for genetics in late-life bipolar disorder are unknown.

CONCLUSIONS

Late-life affective disorders are genetic complex diseases, resulting from the interplay of multiple genes, environmental factors, comorbid illnesses and life stressors. This complexity makes the results obtained from the various studies difficult to interpret and replicate. Furthermore, translating the findings into clinically useful data that results in advancements in treatment is at this point still elusive. This is especially true given that these diagnoses are syndromal, not necessarily clearly and cleanly elucidated, and therefore likely to represent a conglomerate of diseases (each with its own genetic make-up). Moreover, most of the research to date, including that discussed in this chapter, is not specific to late-life affective disorders but also to early onset affective disorders. Despite the biases and difficulties mentioned above, genetic research in late-life affective disorders remains a very exciting field of study, where new advances and breakthroughs are paving the way for future research in this area. With the advent of GWAs, there is increased hope that susceptibility loci will be identified, and that the ultimate identification and characterization of affective disorder susceptibility genes will clarify the biological mechanism of the disorders and lead to new treatment strategies.

REFERENCES

1. Guttmacher AE, Collins FS. Genomic medicine – a primer. N Engl J Med 2002; 347(19): 1512–20.

2. Risch N, Herrell R, Lehner T et al. Interaction between the serotonin transporter gene (5-HTTLPR), stressful life events, and risk of depression: a meta-analysis. *JAMA* 2009; **301**(23): 2462–71.

3. Kendler KS, Kessler RC, Walters EE et al. Stressful life events, genetic liability, and onset of an episode of major depression in women. *Am J Psychiatry* 1995; **152**(6): 833–42.

4. Gatz M, Pedersen NL, Plomin R, Nesselroade JR, McClearn GE. Importance of shared genes and shared environments for symptoms of depression in older adults. *J Abnorm Psychol* 1992; **101**(4): 701–8.

5. McGue M, Christensen K. Genetic and environmental contributions to depression symptomatology: evidence from Danish twins 75 years of age and older. *J Abnorm Psychol* 1997; **106**(3): 439–48.

6. Redon R, Ishikawa S, Fitch KR et al. Global variation in copy number in the human genome. *Nature* 2006; **444**(7118): 444–54.

7. Sebat J, Lakshmi B, Malhotra D et al. Strong association of de novo copy number mutations with autism. *Science* 2007; **316**(5823): 445–9.

8. NCI-NHGRI Working Group on Replication in Association Studies, Chanock SJ, Manolio T et al. Replicating genotype-phenotype associations. *Nature* 2007; **447**(7145): 655–60.

9. Beyer JL, Steffens DC. Genetics of affective disorders. In Copeland JRM, Abou-Saleh MT, Blazer DG (eds), *Principles and Practice of Geriatric Psychiatry*, 2nd edn. Chichester: John Wiley & Sons, Ltd, 2002, 375–8.

10. Mendlewicz J. Juvenile and late onset forms of depressive disorder: genetic and biological characterization of bipolar and unipolar illness – a review. *Maturitas* 1979; **1**(4): 229–34.

11. Post F. The management and nature of depressive illnesses in late life: a follow-through study. *Br J Psychiatry* 1972; **121**(563): 393–404.

12. Murphy E. The prognosis of depression in old age. *Br J Psychiatry* 1983; **142**: 111–9.

13. Krishnan KR, Hays JC, Tupler LA, George LK, Blazer DG. Clinical and phenomenological comparisons of late-onset and early-onset depression. *Am J Psychiatry* 1995; **152**(5): 785–8.

14. Rice J, Reich T, Andreasen NC. The familial transmission of bipolar illness. *Arch Gen Psychiatry* 1987; **44**(5): 441–7.

15. Bland RC, Newman SC, Orn H. Recurrent and nonrecurrent depression. A family study. *Arch Gen Psychiatry* 1986; **43**(11): 1085–9.

16. Baron M, Mendlewicz J, Klotz J. Age-of-onset and genetic transmission in affective disorders. *Acta Psychiatr Scand* 1981; **64**(5): 373–80.

17. Mendlewicz J, Baron M. Morbidity risks in subtypes of unipolar depressive illness: differences between early and late onset forms. *Br J Psychiatry* 1981; **139**: 463–6.

18. Hopkinson G. A genetic study of affective illness in patients over 50. *Br J Psychiatry* 1964; **110**: 244–54.

19. Krishnan KR, Hays JC, Blazer DG. MRI-defined vascular depression. *Am J Psychiatry* 1997; **154**(4): 497–501.

20. Alexopoulos GS, Meyers BS, Young RC. Clinically defined vascular depression. *Am J Psychiatry* 1997; **154**(4): 562–5.

21. Blazer DG, Steffens DC. *Textbook of Geriatric Psychiatry*, 4th edn. Arlington, VA: American Psychiatric Publishing, Inc., 2009.

22. Gershon ES, Hamovit J, Guroff JJ. A family study of schizoaffective, bipolar I, bipolar II, unipolar, and normal control probands. *Arch Gen Psychiatry* 1982; **39**(10): 1157–67.

23. Tsuang MT, Winokur G, Crowe RR. Morbidity risks of schizophrenia and affective disorders among first degree relatives of patients with schizophrenia, mania, depression and surgical conditions. *Br J Psychiatry* 1980; **137**: 497–504.

24. Winokur G, Crowe RR. Bipolar illness. The sex-polarity effect in affectively ill family members. *Arch Gen Psychiatry* 1983; **40**(1): 57–8.

25. Maier W, Lichtermann D, Minges J et al. Continuity and discontinuity of affective disorders and schizophrenia. Results of a controlled family study. *Arch Gen Psychiatry* 1993; **50**(11): 871–83.

26. Weissman MM, Merikangas KR, John K et al. Family-genetic studies of psychiatric disorders. Developing technologies. *Arch Gen Psychiatry* 1986; **43**(11): 1104–16.

27. McGuffin P, Katz R, Rutherford J. Nature, nurture and depression: a twin study. *Psychol Med* 1991; **21**(2): 329–35.

28. Kendler KS, Neale MC, Kessler RC, Heath AC, Eaves LJ. A population-based twin study of major depression in women. The impact of varying definitions of illness. *Arch Gen Psychiatry* 1992; **49**(4): 257–66.

29. Cadoret RJ, Cunningham L, Loftus R, Edwards J. Studies of adoptees from psychiatrically disturbed biological parents. III. Medical symptoms and illnesses in childhood and adolescence. *Am J Psychiatry* 1976; **133**(11): 1316–8.

30. Sullivan PF, Neale MC, Kendler KS. Genetic epidemiology of major depression: review and meta-analysis. *Am J Psychiatry* 2000; **157**(10): 1552–62.

31. Jansson M, Gatz M, Berg S et al. Gender differences in heritability of depressive symptoms in the elderly. Psychol Med, 2004. **34**(3): p. 471–9.

32. Johnson W, McGue M, Gaist D, Vaupel JW, Christensen K. Frequency and heritability of depression symptomatology in the second half of life: evidence from Danish twins over 45. *Psychol Med* 2002; **32**(7): 1175–85.

33. Camp NJ, Cannon-Albright LA. Dissecting the genetic etiology of major depressive disorder using linkage analysis. *Trends Mol Med* 2005; **11**(3): 138–44.

34. Lesch KP, Bengel D, Heils A et al. Association of anxiety-related traits with a polymorphism in the serotonin transporter gene regulatory region. *Science* 1996; **274**(5292): 1527–31.

35. Levinson DF. The genetics of depression: a review. *Biol Psychiatry* 2006; **60**(2): 84–92.

36. Caspi A, Sugden K, Moffitt TE et al. Influence of life stress on depression: moderation by a polymorphism in the 5-HTT gene. *Science* 2003; **301**(5631): 386–9.

37. Gillespie NA, Whitfield JB, Williams B, Heath AC, Martin NG. The relationship between stressful life events, the serotonin transporter (5-HTTLPR) genotype and major depression. *Psychol Med* 2005; **35**(1): 101–11.

38. Surtees PG, Wainwright NW, Willis-Owen SA et al. Social adversity, the serotonin transporter (5-HTTLPR) polymorphism and major depressive disorder. *Biol Psychiatry* 2006; **59**(3): 224–9.

39. Hahn MK, Blakely RD. The functional impact of SLC6 transporter genetic variation. *Annu Rev Pharmacol Toxicol* 2007; **47**: 401–41.

40. Zhang X, Gainetdinov RR, Beaulieu JM *et al.* Loss-of-function mutation in tryptophan hydroxylase-2 identified in unipolar major depression. *Neuron* 2005; **45**(1): 11–6.

41. Zhou Z, Peters EJ, Hamilton SP *et al.* Response to Zhang *et al.* (2005): loss-of-function mutation in tryptophan hydroxylase-2 identified in unipolar major depression. Neuron 45, 11–16. *Neuron* 2005; **48**(5): 702–3; author reply 705–6.

42. Holmes C, Russ C, Kirov G *et al.* Apolipoprotein E: depressive illness, depressive symptoms, and Alzheimer's disease. *Biol Psychiatry* 1998; **43**(3): 159–64.

43. Zubenko GS, Henderson R, Stiffler JS *et al.* Association of the APOE epsilon 4 allele with clinical subtypes of late life depression. *Biol Psychiatry* 1996; **40**(10): 1008–16.

44. Schmand B, Hooijer C, Jonker C, Lindeboom J, Havekes LM. Apolipoprotein E phenotype is not related to late-life depression in a population-based sample. *Soc Psychiatry Psychiatr Epidemiol* 1998; **33**(1): 21–6.

45. Papassotiropoulos A, Bagli M, Jessen F *et al.* Early-onset and late-onset depression are independent of the genetic polymorphism of apolipoprotein E. *Dement Geriatr Cogn Disord* 1999; **10**(4): 258–61.

46. Farmer A, Elkin A, McGuffin P. The genetics of bipolar affective disorder. *Curr Opin Psychiatry* 2007; **20**(1): 8–12.

47. Craddock N, O'Donovan MC, Owen MJ. The genetics of schizophrenia and bipolar disorder: dissecting psychosis. *J Med Genet* 2005; **42**(3): 193–204.

48. Merikangas KR, Kupfer DJ. Mood disorders: genetic aspects. In Kaplan HI, Sadock BJ (eds), *Comprehensive Textbook of Psychiatry*. Baltimore, MD: Williams & Wilkins, 1995, 1102–16.

49. McQueen MB, Devlin B, Faraone SV *et al.* Combined analysis from eleven linkage studies of bipolar disorder provides strong evidence of susceptibility loci on chromosomes 6q and 8q. *Am J Hum Genet* 2005; **77**(4): 582–95.

50. Lambert D, Middle F, Hamshere ML *et al.* Stage 2 of the Wellcome Trust UK-Irish bipolar affective disorder sibling-pair genome screen: evidence for linkage on chromosomes 6q16-q21, 4q12-q21, 9p21, 10p14-p12 and 18q22. *Mol Psychiatry* 2005; **10**(9): 831–41.

51. Schumacher J, Kaneva R, Jamra RA *et al.* Genomewide scan and fine-mapping linkage studies in four European samples with bipolar affective disorder suggest a new susceptibility locus on chromosome 1p35-p36 and provides further evidence of loci on chromosome 4q31 and 6q24. *Am J Hum Genet* 2005; **77**(6): 1102–11.

52. Chen YS, Akula N, Detera-Wadleigh SD *et al.* Findings in an independent sample support an association between bipolar affective disorder and the G72/G30 locus on chromosome 13q33. *Mol Psychiatry* 2004; **9**(1): 87–92; image 5.

53. Hattori E, Liu C, Badner JA *et al.* Polymorphisms at the G72/G30 gene locus, on 13q33, are associated with bipolar disorder in two independent pedigree series. *Am J Hum Genet* 2003; **72**(5): 1131–40.

54. Smoller JW, Gardner-Schuster E. Genetics of bipolar disorder. *Neuroscience* 2009; **164**(1): 331–43.

Environmental Factors, Life Events and Coping Abilities

Toni C. Antonucci and James S. Jackson

Institute for Social Research, University of Michigan, Ann Arbor, USA

Understanding physical and social environmental factors, life events and coping abilities in the lives of older people is best accomplished by applying both a life-span and a life-course perspective. The life-span framework allows one to incorporate information about individual experiences over the life course, the successes and failures that individuals have coping with these experiences, the tangible and human resources that have or have not been helpful, as well as the organizational or societal events that have influenced their development[1]. Thus, understanding how the elderly cope with environmental factors and life events must also be considered within a dynamic family and friendship context that is multigenerational, influenced by ageing, cohort differences and historical events [1,2].

These intersecting contexts are characterized by exchanges which are perceived as either reciprocal or non-reciprocal over time. These transactions have been described as being of three types: those earmarked by the anticipation of linear downward transfers, i.e. from older to younger generations; those characterized by curvilinear exchanges, from the middle to younger and older generations; and resource-based exchange networks, which assume that resources will be exchanged based on availability rather than generational lineage membership. Akiyama et al.[3] have argued that cultural and resource differences affect how generations exchange goods and services. But this argument can also be extended to expectations based on lifetime affective relationships and competencies. These resource exchanges also contribute to the individual's experience of the physical and social environments, life events they encounter and their coping capacities and abilities. Each model predicts a certain expectation or resource availability. The degree to which individuals have positively experienced these exchanges will directly affect their successful adaptation to old age.

It is clear that individuals vary in their ability to cope with the stresses and strains of life. As individuals age, it has been assumed that they are faced with more negative experiences, that the environment in terms of both physical and psychological characteristics becomes more difficult. One therefore seeks to understand the mechanisms individuals use to cope with these events.

Education has been linked to health, a well-documented finding indicating that those with higher levels of education enjoy better health. However, Antonucci et al.[4] showed that this relationship can be attenuated for specific groups and levels of support; less-educated men enjoyed the same good health as men with higher levels of education if they had key social supports. Less-educated men with larger networks, emotional, financial and sick care support from a child have better health than less-educated men without these supports. Interestingly, these findings were not found for women. The findings can be interpreted as illustrating the protective potential of social relations, though the gender differences highlight the complexity of the relationships.

Another important question is whether as people age they become better able to cope with relationships over time. Research thus far, although cross-sectional, suggests this is the case at least for most relationships[5]. Social relations with parents, children and friends do tend to decrease in negativity over time. Spousal negativity, however, remained stable over time, well into old age. It appears that part of the successful coping strategy seemed to be reduced contact with the 'difficult' party. This is less easily accomplished with a spouse living in the same household. Strained spousal relationships can be devastating, since they tend to be one of the most significant long-term relationships of adulthood, understanding what factors allow an individual to cope with stressful spousal relationships is important. Birditt and Antonucci[6] examined relationship profiles of married people. They were able to demonstrate that married individuals with two high-quality relationships had higher well-being, if one of these was a best friend, regardless of whether they reported a positive relationship with their spouse. However, if the married individual did not have a best friend, quality of spousal relationship was singularly and significantly related to well-being. Thus, as previous research has shown, while spousal relationship is an important predictor of well-being, the potentially negative influence of a poor spousal relationship can be offset by other significant and high-quality relationships.

Coyne and Downey[7] argue that people evidencing depressive symptoms generate a negative exchange loop for their support network. The life-span perspective is useful because individuals do not suffer isolated single depressive episodes, but rather a series of depressive episodes over time. Network members may come to recognize the negative aspects of these episodes and as Coyne and Downey argue, subsequently distance themselves from the individual in crisis. It is speculated that knowledgeable network members recognize this crisis as one of many that have negative consequences. In an effort to protect themselves from the unsuccessful and frustrating experience of attempting to be helpful, network members may ignore, isolate or abandon the individual in crisis. This is most likely to happen, unfortunately, when the individual has a history of being maladaptive. Thus, in the case of the individual in need, but with a history of depressive episodes or other series of crises events, it may be difficult to activate a support network. On the other hand, for individuals who have a more successful history of coping with crises, their support networks are likely to respond to a crisis with both affective and instrumental support.

Recent work suggests that it is vital to consider the realistic viability of various coping behaviours[8,9,10]. Socioeconomic status (SES) and the challenging nature of physical and social environments, especially in large urban areas, simultaneously help to afford greater opportunities for engaging in what we have termed 'negative' coping behaviours (e.g. smoking, drinking alcohol and drug use) and fewer opportunities for relying on positive coping alternatives, a traditional focus of the coping literature. Studies report that lower SES individuals have a more limited set of coping resources at their disposal compared to those with more income or education[10]; these findings suggest that some coping choices may not be readily available to poor populations, particularly those living in urban centres. Limited access to exercise and public recreation facilities and perceived poor neighbourhood safety have been linked to reduced physical activity levels and increased obesity in lower income neighbourhoods[11,12]. Lower levels of education, unskilled and semi-skilled versus professional occupations and lower levels of income, have all been associated with lower levels of emotional support, less contact with friends and lower frequency of disclosing problems[13].

At the same time, people of low SES and traditionally disadvantaged ethnic minority populations are more likely to smoke, use alcohol and be obese[14,15]. They are more likely to live in close proximity to liquor stores[16]. They are also more likely to have limited access to healthy foods, putting them at greater risk for obesity and obesity-related diseases[15,17]. This suggests that the physical and social environments characterizing the urban poor may facilitate certain negative coping mechanisms that are effective at relieving psychological symptoms of stress over more positive behaviours that may be less accessible to these populations, especially in middle and older ages[8,9].

Comprehending the effectiveness of potential stress-reducing strategies has important implications for understanding the epidemiology of chronic diseases that are more prevalent among low SES and certain race and ethnic groups. A variety of coping strategies may help reduce the body's response to chronic stressors; some linked to those having negative health consequences and others linked to more neutral or positive health outcomes. It is clear that more research needs to be conducted to understand the role of positive coping behaviours in alleviating the physiological responses to stressful events among different social and economic groups and at different ages and at different points in the life course[2].

Although it is clearly true that some people experience more crises than others, it is not always the case that those who experience a great many crises are the ones overwhelmed by them. The same environmental conditions or life events which might devastate one person may have much fewer negative effects on another. As noted above we have some information about risk factors or vulnerabilities, but we actually know very little about what makes some people capable of coping with stress and others incapable of coping with the same events. Among the explanatory hypotheses which have been offered are personality characteristics, supportive interactive exchanges, self-concept and self-efficacy. We are not at a point where there is clear evidence in support of one explanatory concept over another and it may, of course, be some combination of these influences. Nevertheless, a series of studies by Taylor and his colleagues[18] offers interesting insights about the interactive basis of coping strategies. In their studies of men recovering from uncomplicated myocardial infarction (MI), they found that wives who believed in their husbands' ability to recover were more likely to have husbands who did recover. It is especially interesting that these husbands were no less disabled by their MI than others in the study. The researchers were able to experimentally augment the wife's view of her husband's potential for recovery, which in turn directly affected the husband's actual recovery. This series of studies, replicating the impressions of many clinicians, dramatically demonstrate that individuals can be fundamentally influenced in how they face life conditions and events which confront them. The mechanisms through which these influences occur are not well understood. Bandura[19] has argued that the relevant characteristic is self-efficacy. Whether self-efficacy is the critical variable or not, it is clearly evident that 'objective' facts or events are influenced by very 'subjective' factors.

Social support is not always or solely considered a coping ability or strategy. In fact, it may be best considered as a resource that individuals may call upon if needed to cope with particular environmental stressors. Moreover, successful coping is the ability to activate the kinds of support needed to meet the needs of a specific situation and to help the individual achieve a positive affective disposition. We know that people vary in their ability to develop a supportive entourage or network; in their ability to mobilize or activate this network once established; and in their ability to benefit from this support. We can best understand these differences as indications of how older people differentially experience their environments and life events; and how they cope with these experiences.

Once again it is critical to recognize the life span and life-course contexts because the individual old person confronts a specific event with a history of either positive or negative coping experiences. A related issue is the question of how frequently the individual experiences crises and at what points in their lifetime. The now classic work of Brown and Harris[20] established both the lifetime vulnerability of people who experience the loss of significant intimate others early in their lives and their frequent lack of healthy, positive adult intimate relationships. Others have also established the influence on depression and overall affective well-being of negative relationships with close supportive others.

The life-course and life-span perspectives[1,21] emphasize that people evolve throughout their lifetime and become more heterogeneous with age. As people grow older the separate experiences of their lifetime combine uniquely to shape the individual. There is every reason to believe that this is especially important to the question of how individuals cope with the challenges of old age. Although major theoretical and empirical questions have not been resolved, research concerning social support as a coping strategy does provide insights into how people manage the stresses and strains that they face in late life. It has been suggested that an individual's ability to cope with specific environmental conditions and life events is best understood through a consideration of the resources and experiences available to that person. One simplistic way to consider this is that successfully coping with stresses and strains in early life is the best predictor of the individual's ability to cope with stressful situations in later life. This is likely to be true, even if the exact nature of the stressful event varies. There is also reason to believe that individuals develop coping styles over their lifetime which can be seen to be generally successful and adaptive while others develop coping styles which are generally unsuccessful or maladaptive. These coping strategies, at their best, match the environmental conditions and life events that the individual experiences. It is proabable that, although the specific nature of these experiences will change with age, an individual's ability to cope with these events is likely to show fairly stable life-span continuity. As research clearly demonstrates, however, individual coping and adaptation competency can be improved through informal and professional intervention at all points in the individual life course.

It is also important to consider the influence of non-psychiatric factors on the experience of events in old age and how one copes with stressors and stress. Jackson et al.[22] have noted that different racial, cultural and other socio-demographic factors fundamentally affect how a situation is experienced. If an individual is one of many suffering the same negative experience(s), the aetiology of that experience may not be devastatingly personalized. On the other hand, if everyone else in one's reference group is significantly more successful, the relative comparison can be devastating, even if 'objectively' the situation is quite positive. Similarly empirical evidence indicates that different national groups appear to vary considerably in the degree to which they respond negatively to environmental factors and life events. Recent profile analysis of social relations and relationships among different groups has suggested interesting similarities, but also differences. Using almost identical measures in the US, Germany and Japan, three sets of profile analyses were conducted. Interesting similarities and differences emerged. Cross-cultural work[23] examined social relations and mental health among older men and women in the US, Japan, France and Germany. Findings indicate that women experience more resource deficits, i.e. widowhood, illness, financial strain, than men in all these countries. In addition, the social relations of women in France and Japan were shown to offset the effects of these deficits on depressive symptoms and well-being, but this was not the case for women in the US and Germany or for men in any of the four countries. Apparently not only gender, but also the unique cultural environment, influences how well an individual copes with even the same life events.

One additional approach to understanding environmental factors, life events and coping is through the study of relationship profiles among individuals of different cultures. Studies in the US[24] and Israel[25] indicate that common network types could be conceptualized as diverse (including both family and friends), predominantly family, predominantly friends and restricted (very limited). While all four existed in both cultures there were actually two types of restricted networks in the US, those restricted to only family and those restricted to only friends. Diverse networks were associated with the highest levels of well-being, whereas restricted networks were associated with the lowest levels. Interestingly, in the US, sample individuals who might be seen as vulnerable because of the limited number of family members in their networks were shown to be less so if there were friends in the network. Among those with limited friends in their networks, however, their vulnerability was not mediated by the presence of family members. In keeping with the increased awareness of the importance of the quality of relationships, the US study also demonstrated that quality of relationship, not just the existence of the relationship, influenced mental health and depressive symptoms. Additional profile studies[26,27] in the US, Japan and Germany reinforce these findings. The same four types of clusters were found, although each country also had additional unique clusters. The frequencies of these clusters and their associations with well-being varied by country: in the US the diverse network was the most prevalent, but this was less true in Japan and Germany.

Nevertheless, only in the US and Germany was there an association between clusters and well-being. In the US and Germany, the diverse networks were associated with better mental health and the restricted networks were associated with poorer mental health. The unique, country-specific clusters and associations with well-being are interesting and informative. For example, in Germany people with friend-focused supportive networks had relatively high levels of depressive symptoms, perhaps suggesting that the lack of family support cannot be compensated for among this post World War II cohort of elders. The lack of association between network type and well-being in Japan and the poor well-being among those with high levels of friend support in Germany suggests that there may be deep-seated cultural differences that require explanation.

Further work is needed to better elucidate which aspects of social support are more important as strategies to cope with chronic stressors (e.g. a large social network, or higher quality support received regardless of quantity) in specific environments. In addition, more research is needed to develop a better understanding of the physiological mechanisms through which social support may exert its mental and physical health benefits[8,9].

Finally, several researchers have shown that the size of social networks and the frequency of contact with network members change over the life course. In general, older adults tend to have smaller social networks and have less frequent contact with members than younger adults, though this depends on how social networks are assessed. It is possible that these smaller networks represent a voluntary diminution because of perceived growing time constraints, as well as an increasing awareness of their own pending mortality among elders. Research suggests that this awareness may lead older adults to build deeper relationships with a small group of friends with whom they feel emotionally close rather than maintaining a large network. These changes in the nature of social support in later life may influence its utilization and effectiveness as a coping resource over the life course among different socioeconomic and ethnic groups, but more work among diverse groups at different points in the life course is needed[4,22].

REFERENCES

1. Fuller-Iglesias H, Antonucci TC, Smith J. Theoretical perspectives on life span and life course development. In Antonucci TC, Jackson JS (eds), *Annu Rev Gerontol Geriatr*, 2009; **29**, 3–25.
2. Antonucci TC, Jackson JS (eds). *Life-Course Perspectives on Late-Life Health Inequalities*. New York: Springer, 2010.
3. Akiyama H, Antonucci TC, Campbell R. Exchange and reciprocity among two generations of Japanese and American women. In Sokolovsky J (ed.), *Cultural Context of Aging: Worldwide Perspectives*, 2nd edn. Westfort, CT: Greenwood Press, 1997, 127–38.
4. Antonucci TC, Ajrouch KJ, Janevic MR. The effect of social relations with children on the education-health link in men and women aged 40 and over. *Soc Sci Med* 1997; **56**: 949–60.
5. Akiyama H, Antonucci TC, Takahashi K, Langfahl ES. Negative interactions in close relationships across the lifespan. *J Gerontol B Psychol Sci Soc Sci* 2003; **58**: 70–9.
6. Birditt KS, Antonucci TC. Relationship quality profiles and well-being among married adults. *J Fam Psychol* 2007; **21**: 595–604.
7. Coyne JC, Downey G. Social factors and psychopathology: stress, social support and coping processes. *Ann Rev Psych* 1991; **42**: 401–26.

8. Jackson JS, Knight KM. Race and self-regulatory health behaviors: the role of the stress response and the HPA axis in physical and mental health disparities. In Schaie KW, Cartensen L (eds), *Social Structures, Aging and Self-Regulation in the Elderly*. New York: Springer, 2006, 189–207.

9. Kershaw KN, Rafferty JA, Abdou CM, Colbert SJ, Knight KM, Jackson JS. Chronic stress and the role of coping behaviors in health inequalities. Antonucci TC, Jackson JS (eds). *Life-Course Perspectives on Late-Life Health Inequalities*. New York: Springer, 2010, 161–80.

10. McEwen BS. Protective and damaging effects of stress mediators. *N Engl J Med* 1998; **338**: 171–9.

11. Powell LM, Slater S, Chaloupka FJ, Harper D. Availability of physical activity-related facilities and neighborhood demographic and socioeconomic characteristics: a national study. *Am J Public Health* 2006; **96**(9): 1676–80.

12. Wilson DK, Kirtland KA, Ainsworth BE, Addy CL. Socioeconomic status and perceptions of access and safety for physical activity. *Ann Behav Med* 2004; **28**(1): 20–8.

13. Mickelson KD, Kubzansky LD. Social distribution of social support: the mediating role of life events. *Am J Community Psychol* 2003; **32**(3–4): 265–81.

14. Gilman SE, Abrams DB, Buka SL. Socioeconomic status over the life course and stages of cigarette use: initiation, regular use and cessation. *J Epidemiol Community Health* 2003; **57**: 802–8.

15. Robert SA, Reither EN. A multilevel analysis of race, community disadvantage and body mass index among adults in the US. *Soc Sci Med* 2004; **59**(12): 2421–34.

16. LaVeist TA, Wallace JM Jr. Health risk and inequitable distribution of liquor stores in African American neighborhood. *Soc Sci Med* 2000; **51**(4): 613–17.

17. Moore LV, Diez Roux AV. Associations of neighborhood characteristics with the location and type of food stores. *Am J Public Health* 2006; **96**(2): 325–31.

18. Taylor CB, Bandura A, Ewart CK, Miller NH, DeBusk RF. Raising spouse's and patient's perception of his cardiac capabilities after clinically uncomplicated acute mycoardial infarction. *Am J Cardiol* 1985; **55**: 628–36.

19. Bandura A. *Social Foundations of Thought and Actions*. New York: Prentice Hall, 1986.

20. Brown G, Harris TD. *Social Origins of Depression: a Study of Psychiatric Disorder in Women*. New York: Free Press, 1978.

21. Baltes PB, Reese HW, Lipsitt LP. Life-span developmental psychology. *Annu Rev Psychol* 1980; **31**: 65–110.

22. Jackson JS, Brown E, Antonucci TC. A cultural lens on biopsychosocial models of aging. *Adv Cell Aging Gerontol* 2004; **15**: 221–41.

23. Antonucci TC, Lansford JE, Akiyama H, Smith J, Baltes MM, Takahashi K *et al*. Differences between men and women in social relations, resource deficits and depressive symptomatology during later life in four nations. *J Soc Issues* 2002; **58**: 767–83.

24. Fiori KL, Antonucci TC, Cortina KS. Social network typologies and mental health among older adults: a replication. *J Gerontol B Psychol Sci Soc Sci* 2002; **61B**: P25–32.

25. Litwin H. Social network type and morale in old age. *Gerontologist* 2001; **41**: 516–24.

26. Fiori KL, Antonucci TC, Akiyama H. Profiles of social relations among older adults: a cross-cultural approach. *Ageing Soc* 2008; **28**: 203–31.

27. Fiori KL, Smith J, Antonucci TC. Social network types among older adults: a multidimensional approach. *J Gerontol B Psychol Sci Soc Sci* 2007; **62**: P322–30.

75

Vascular Disease and Late-Life Depressive Disorder

Robert Baldwin

Manchester Mental Health & Social Care Trust, Manchester Royal Infirmary, Manchester, UK

DEPRESSION COMPLICATING VASCULAR DISEASE

Stroke and Mood Disorder

Stroke is associated with a high risk of depression as well as pathological laughing or crying and emotionalism. These are covered in Chapter 82.

Heart Disease

Soon after a coronary event about 15–20% of patients develop depressive symptoms[1]. By two months, out of 804 patients with stable coronary heart disease (CHD), 7.1% met criteria for major depression and 5.3% for generalized anxiety disorder[2]. These rates are at least double that expected in the general population.

Diabetes

The frequency of type 2 diabetes increases with age. In a cohort of patients aged 70–79 years followed for about six years those with diabetes had an increased rate of depression which attenuated after adjustment for diabetes-related co-morbidities, although this still represented a significantly increased risk compared to controls[3]. In this study HbA1c was a predictor of recurrent depression.

Blood Pressure and Depression

Whether the prevalence of depression increases as blood pressure rises is controversial. Rabkin *et al.*[4] found a three-fold higher frequency of major depression in 452 patients treated for hypertension whereas Jones-Webb *et al.*[5] found no association between resting blood pressure and self-rated depression in 4352 young subjects. Scalco *et al.*[6] suggest that a link between depression and hypertension may be mediated by hyperreactivity of the sympathetic nervous system. There is also a potential link between low blood pressure and depression. An inverse relationship between low diastolic blood pressure (below 75 mmHg) and depressive symptoms (such as fatigue, pessimism and sadness) was shown in a study of 846 elderly men without a psychiatric diagnosis[7].

Vascular Depression

Central to the notion of vascular depression is that vascular brain disease may predispose to depression, precipitate it or perpetuate it[8]. Features include reduced depressive ideation, more psychomotor retardation, poor insight, executive dysfunction (see below), greater disability and often an age of onset over 60. Magnetic resonance imaging (MRI) has shown higher rates of hyperintensities in the deep white matter and basal ganglia compared with control subjects, an effect seen most in late-onset cases[9]. Epidemiological studies confirm that the severity and location (especially in the basal ganglia) of white matter lesions (WMLs) seem to be causally related to late-life depression[10,11]. Pathological data show that WMLs in the brains of depressed patients are more likely to be ischaemic compared to those seen in the brains of non-depressed subjects[1].

A clear-cut association between the symptoms of vascular depression and common cerebrovascular risk factors (such as hypertension, smoking, hyperlipidaemia and diabetes) has not been shown and the vascular depression hypothesis has its critics. McDougall and Brayne[12] analysed 13 studies comparing depressive symptoms in subjects with and without co-morbid vascular conditions and concluded there was insufficient evidence to agree an operational definition of vascular depression. However, Sneed *et al.*[13] applied the statistical technique of latent class analysis to two naturalistic clinical trials of treatment in late-life depression. WML burden was the most accurate indicator of vascular vs. non-vascular depression. This internal consistency is important for confirming vascular depression as a distinct entity.

Chronic hypoperfusion (rather than small vessel infarction) may be another cause of vascular depression. Hypoperfusion might be secondary to hypotension (as discussed above), damage to blood pressure regulating mechanisms or arterial stiffness and/or failed compensation by the brain[14]. Brain hypoperfusion is not readily detectable by 'bedside' measures of cerebrovascular function other than perhaps by assessing postural hypotension.

The 'Depression–executive dysfunction syndrome' is an important feature of vascular depression[15]. Deficits involve executive tasks (planning, initiation and task persistence) and speed of information processing[16]. Clinically, these patients present with slow inefficient thinking, patchy memory impairment and are often apathetic.

DEPRESSION AS A RISK FACTOR FOR VASCULAR DISEASE

A number of studies have demonstrated that depression is a risk factor for cardiovascular and cerebrovascular events. However, the quality of evidence has been variable, for example fully accounting for factors which might explain such an association (such as severity of cardiac disease and vascular risk factors) markedly attenuates the association.

Stroke

Whether depression is a risk factor for stroke is controversial. In the Framingham study[17] participants aged 65 or below with raised depression scores on a rating scale were four times more likely to experience a stroke or transient ischemic attack compared with those of the same age without depression, after controlling for smoking status and education. The effect was not seen among those who were 65 or older. A positive association between the presence of depression and the risk of stroke across the entire adult age range was, however, found in another study[18].

Wouts *et al.*[19] reported that patients with baseline cardiac disease and depression were most at risk of later stroke and that there was a dose–response relationship: greater severity and chronicity of depression increased the risk. This may reflect the synergistic effect of depression and vascular disease or it may be that depressive symptomatology merely reflects the severity of underlying vascular disease (reverse causality).

Heart Disease

A meta-analysis concluded that depressed mood moderately increases the risk of myocardial infarction, coronary heart disease and cerebrovascular diseases by about the same amount (odds ratio between 1.43 and 1.63)[20] and adversely affects the prognosis of CHD to about the same degree[21]. The evidence for depression as an *independent* risk factor for vascular events has been sufficiently robust for the American Heart Association to recommend screening for depression in cardiac patients[22]. As a risk factor for cardiovascular disease, depression may rank somewhere between active and passive smoking[23]. However; adjustment for baseline factors, especially left ventricular function, substantially attenuates this association.

A Dutch epidemiological study of older adults showed that cardiac patients with minor (subthreshold) depression had a relative risk of subsequent cardiac mortality of 1.6 rising to 3.0 for those with major depression, after adjustment for confounding factors[24], an effect replicated by Ariyo and colleagues[25]. Negative effects on cardiac outcome are seen whether or not subjects are healthy at baseline and can last for many years[26] but generally manifest themselves within the first year after an acute myocardial infarct[22].

Diabetes

For diabetes, again there is some evidence that depression is a risk factor for diabetes but this may apply mainly to the non-insulin dependant type[27], the commonest form in older adults. The risk though is only modest once other factors (for example lifestyle) are accounted for. The occurrence of diabetic complications and poorer glycaemic control are more likely in depressed subjects because depression undermines motivation (Figure 75.1). Painful neuropathy

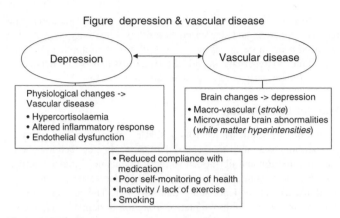

Figure depression & vascular disease

Figure 75.1 Depression and vascular disease

may be another factor in triggering depression. Diabetes can cause small vessel pathology in the brain that leads to subcortical encephalopathy, not unlike that seen in vascular depression. This may lead to both cognitive impairment and depressed mood.

Hypertension

Some evidence suggests that depressed people have higher resting blood pressure than non-depressed people[6]. This may be because depression reduces medication conpliance, but one study of normotensive, non-elderly subjects followed over several years showed that high levels of depressive symptoms doubled the risk of hypertension[28].

Cholesterol

Low cholesterol may reduce serotonin available to the brain, although there is no convincing evidence which links cholesterol and depression via vascular disease. One study of statins did not demonstrate that lowering cholesterol increased depression[29].

POSSIBLE MECHANISMS OF CAUSATION

The relationship between depression and vascular disease is two-way (Figure 75.1) and there are aetiological factors which may be shared, such as genetic risk and lifestyle factors.

Genetic Mechanisms

In a study of older, middle-aged patients with late-onset depression a higher prevalence of the homozygous or heterozygous forms of the C677T mutation of the methylenetetrahydrofolate reductase enzyme (MTHFR) was found compared to those with early-onset depression[30]. This enzyme system is relevant to homocysteine, B_{12} and folate metabolism. A high level of homocysteine has been implicated in depression and in vascular disease[31]. No convincing role has been identified for the apolipoprotein E (*APOE*) gene in late-life depression.

Autonomic Dysfunction

Autonomic imbalance is associated with major depression and leads to sympathetic over-activity and/or parasympathetic under-activity, with decreased heart rate variability, downregulated beta-adrenergic receptor function and decreased baroreflex sensitivity, making the diseased heart more susceptible to arrhythmia. Autonomic imbalance contributes to hypertension and atherosclerosis and is an independent risk factor for early cardiovascular mortality[32].

Platelet Dysfunction

A number of studies have found subtle changes in one or more platelet markers such as increased plasma platelet factor 4, beta-thromboglobulin and fibrinogen suggesting enhanced platelet activation. Platelets seem to be more activated in depressed patients with heart disease than in depressed patients without. The current evidence that antidepressants improve platelet function in depression is inconclusive, but it is known that selective serotonin re-uptake inhibitors (SSRIs) can normalize platelet hyperactivity[33].

Neuroendocrine Abnormality

Dysregulation of the hypothalamic-pituitary-adrenal (HPA) axis and hypercorticolism are two well-known factors seen in major depression and associated with hippocampal damage and insulin resistance. The latter is a feature of the metabolic syndrome (abdominal obesity, hypertension and triglyceride abnormality) which is associated with increased cardio- and cerebrovascular disease as well as hypercoagulation, enhanced inflammatory responses and possibly endothelial damage (see below). The metabolic syndrome may be an intermediary linking depression to vascular disease.

Endothelial Dysfunction and Subclinical Atheroma

The vascular endothelium produces local vasoactive agents including nitric oxide, a vasodilator, and the peptide endothelin, a vasoconstrictor. Endothelial dysfunction is thought to precede and predict atheroma. In non-elderly subjects endothelial function was impaired irrespective of the presence of vascular risk factors[34]. Using carbon dioxide inhalation to assess vasomotor reactivity in the middle cerebral artery, depressive symptoms were associated with lower reactivity, which is a risk factor for cerebrovascular disease[35]. Tiemeier et al.[36] also found that carotid artery distensibility and pulse wave velocity (measures of arterial stiffness) were significantly associated with late-life depression. Lastly, the same group assessed coronary calcification and found that for every standard deviation increase in extracoronary atherosclerosis there was a 30% increase in depression[37].

These studies do not prove that depression causes vascular damage as causality could be in either direction. In a study of 324 adults, mean age 60.6 years[38], measures of carotid intima media thickness (IMT) to detect subclinical atheroma showed that baseline depressive symptoms were associated with a significantly greater three-year worsening in carotid IMT, even after adjusting for potential confounding factors. Similar conclusions were reached in a study of participants aged over 65[39], while another study of women showed that it was those with recurrent depression who were most at risk of subclinical atheroma[40]. Again this is not proof but it is strong evidence that depressive disorder is bad for a person's arteries.

Inflammatory Responses

Inflammatory markers include C-reactive protein (CRP), interlukin-6, tumour necrosis factor (TNF) and fibrinogen. In a two-year study,

Frasure-Smith et al.[41] investigated the relationship between depression and inflammatory markers. Elevated depressive symptoms and raised CRP two months after an acute event were overlapping risk factors for later cardiac events in men. Carney et al.[32] demonstrated that fibrinogen was most associated with altered heart rate variability in depressed CHD patients and proposed that this could be attributable to deficits in parasympathetic modulation of immunity and coagulation. In contrast, another study found that major depression was associated with lower levels of CRP, fibrinogen and interleukin-6[42]. Nevertheless, pro-inflammatory cytokines are known to be expressed in the brains of those with late-life depression[43].

Behavioural and Psychological Factors

Lifestyle factors in depression include a reduced likelihood of taking medication such as antihypertensives and antidepressants, inactivity, lack of exercise, smoking and excessive alcohol intake. Clearly these can act as intermediaries between depression and vascular disease (Figure 75.1). It is also possible that patients with vascular disease subtly recognize that something is wrong before it becomes clinically apparent, thereby triggering depression.

Treatment

The presence of WMLs, especially when numerous, severe in extent or strategically located (as in the basal ganglia) is of relevance to poorer outcomes for depression in later life[44]. One study has shown that in patients with late-life depression nimodipine (a drug with vasoprotective properties) when combined with antidepressant medication led to a reduction in time to remission and a longer time before recurrence compared to placebo augmentation[45]. This needs to be replicated before vasoactive drugs can be recommended. Likewise, statins can improve vascular function[46] but it is not known whether they benefit depression. Omega 3 fatty acid is a promising treatment for vascular disorder but a study of two dosages in patients with late-life depressive symptoms did not show benefit to depression over placebo[47].

There is no evidence that antidepressants have adverse effects on the vasculature; possibly they are protective as SSRIs reduce platelet aggregation[48]. However some SSRIs can interfere with the metabolism of some cardiac drugs. Treatment of vascular depression with electroconvulsive treatment is effective but there is an increased risk of post-treatment confusion; a recent trial showing that repetitive trancranial magnetic stimulation (rTMS) was moderately effective in older patients with clinically defined vascular depression is of interest[49].

Apathy is common in both depression and vascular disease and amphetamines have been used to treat it. There are data showing that augmentation of an SSRI with methylphenidate can improve response rates in late-life depression[50] and that problem-solving treatment for the dysexecutive syndrome associated with depression is effective[51].

Metyrapone reduces adrenal cortisol synthesis. Broadley et al.[52] gave this drug to 30 depressed subjects (mean age 40) and 36 control subjects, showing that cortisol levels reduced in the depressed group and endothelial function improved. More innovative studies like this are needed.

CONCLUSION

The relationship between depression and vascular disease is two-way; that is, depression may lead to vascular disease and vascular disease may trigger depression. The overall burden of vascular disease seems to be the best predictor of subsequent depression[53]. Clinical trials are needed to study whether drugs with vasoprotective properties can improve outcomes in depressive disorder. These will not be easy to conduct but in the meantime the management of depression should encompass the optimum treatment of both affective disorder and vascular disease.

REFERENCES

1. Thomas, AJ, Kalaria, RN, O'Brien, JT. Depression and vascular disease: what is the relationship? *J Affect Disord* 2004; **79**: 81–95.

2. Frasure-Smith N, Lespérance F. Depression and anxiety as predictors of 2-year cardiac events in patients with stable coronary artery disease. *Arch Gen Psychiatry* 2008; **65**: 62–71.

3. Maraldi C, Volpato S, Penninx BW *et al*. Diabetes mellitus, glycemic control, and incident depressive symptoms among 70- to 79-year-old persons: the health, ageing, and body composition study. *Arch Intern Med* 2007; **167**: 1137–44.

4. Rabkin JG, Charles E, Kass F. Hypertension and DSM-III Depression in psychiatric outpatients *Am J Psychiatry* 1983; **140**: 1072–74.

5. Jones-Webb R, Jacobs DR, Flack JM, Liu K. Relationship between depressive symptoms, anxiety, alcohol consumption, and blood pressure: Results from the CARDIA study. *Alcohol Clin Exp Res* 1996; **20**: 420–27.

6. Scalco AZ, Scalco MZ, Azul JBS, Lotufo Neto F. Hypertension and depression. *Clinics* 2005; **60**: 241–50.

7. Barrett-Connor E, Palinkas LA. Low blood pressure and depression in older men: a population based study. *BMJ* 1994; **308**: 446–49.

8. Alexopoulos GS, Meyers BS, Young RC, Campbell S, Silbersweig D, Charlson M. 'Vascular depression' hypothesis. *Arch Gen Psychiatry* 1997; **54**: 915–22.

9. Krishnan KRR, Taylor WD, McQuiod DR *et al*. Clinical characteristics of magnetic resonance imaging-defined subcortical ischemic depression. *Biol Psychiatry* 2004; **55**: 390–97.

10. Steffens DC, Helms MJ, Krishnan KRR, Burke GL. Cerebrovascular disease and depression symptoms in the cardiovascular health study. *Stroke* 1999; **30**: 2159–66.

11. de Groot JC, de Leeuw F-E, Oudkerk M, Hofman A, Jolles J, Breteler MMB. Cerebral white matter lesions and depressive symptoms in elderly adults. *Arch Gen Psychiatry* 2000; **57**: 1071–76.

12. McDougall F, Brayne C. Systematic review of depressive symptoms associated with vascular conditions. *J Affect Disord* 2007; **104**: 25–35.

13. Sneed, JR, Rindskopf, D, Steffens, DC, Krishnan, KRR, Roose, SP. The vascular depression subtype: evidence of internal validity. *Biol Psychiatry* 2008; **64**: 491–97.

14. Naish JH, Baldwin RC, Patankar T *et al*. Abnormalities of CSF flow patterns in the cerebral aqueduct in treatment-resistant late-life depression: a potential biomarker of microvascular angiopathy. *Magn Reson Med*. 2006; **56**: 509–16.

15. Alexopoulos, GS, Kiosses, DN, Klimstra, S, Kalayam, B, Bruce ML. Clinical presentation of the 'depression–executive dysfunction syndrome' of late life. *Am J Geriatr Psychiatry* 2002; **10**: 98–106.

16. Butters MA, Whyte EM, Nebes RD *et al*. The nature and determinants of neuropsychological functioning in late-life depression. *Arch Gen Psychiatry* 2004; **61**: 587–95.

17. Salaycik KJ, Kelly-Hayes M, Beiser A *et al*. Depressive symptoms and risk of stroke. The Framingham study. *Stroke* 2007; **38**: 16–21.

18. Jonas BS, Mussolino ME. Symptoms of depression as a prospective risk factor for stroke. *Psychosom Med*. 2000; **62**: 463–71.

19. Wouts L, Oude Voshaar RC, Bremmer MA *et al*. Cardiac disease, depressive symptoms, and incident stroke in an elderly population. *Arch Gen Psychiatry* 2008; **65**: 596–602.

20. Van der Kooy K, van Hout H, Marwijk H, Marten H, Stehouwer C, Beekman A () Depression and the risk for cardiovascular diseases: systematic review and meta analysis. *Int J Geriatr Psychiatry* 2007; **22**: 613–26.

21. Nicholson A, Kuper H, Hemingway H. Depression as an aetiologic and prognostic factor in coronary heart disease: a meta-analysis of 6362 events among 146538 participants in 54 observational studies. *Eur Heart J* 2006; **27**: 2763–74.

22. Lichtman JH, Bigger JT, Blumenthal JA *et al*. Depression and coronary heart disease: recommendations for screening, referral, and treatment: a science advisory from the American Heart Association Prevention Committee of the Council on Cardiovascular Nursing, Council on Clinical Cardiology, Council on Epidemiology and Prevention, and Interdisciplinary Council on Quality of Care and Outcomes Research. *Circulation* 2008; **118**: 1768–75.

23. Wulsin LR. Is depression a major risk factor for coronary disease? A systematic review of the epidemiologic evidence. *Harv Rev Psychiatry* 2004; **12**: 79–93.

24. Penninx BWJH, Beekman ATF, Honig A, Deeg DJH, Schoevers RA, van Eijk JTM, van Tilburg W. Depression and cardiac mortality results from a community-based longitudinal study. *Arch Gen Psychiatry*. 2001; **58**: 221–27.

25. Ariyo AA, Haan M, Tangen CM *et al*. Depressive symptoms and risks of coronary heart disease and mortality in elderly Americans. Cardiovascular Health Study Collaborative Research Group. *Circulation* 2000; **102**: 1773–79.

26. Janszky I, Ahlbom A, Hallqvist J, Ahnve S. Hospitalization for depression is associated with an increased risk for myocardial infarction not explained by lifestyle, lipids, coagulation, and inflammation: The SHEEP Study. *Biol Psychiatry* 2007; **62**: 25–32.

27. Eaton WW. Epidemiologic evidence on the comorbidity of depression and diabetes. *J Psychosom Res* 2002; **53**: 903–906.

28. Jonas BS, Franks P, Ingram DD. Are symptoms of anxiety and depression risk factors for hypertension? Longitudinal evidence from the National Health and Nutrition Examination Survey I Epidemiologic Follow-up Study. *Arch Fam Med* 1997; **6**: 43–49.

29. Wardle J, Armitage J, Collins R, Wallendszus K, Leech A, Lawson A. Randomised controlled trial of effect on mood of lowering cholesterol concentration. *BMJ* 1996; **313**: 75–78.

30. Hickie I, Scott E, Naismith S *et al*. Late-onset depression: genetic, vascular and clinical contributions. *Psychol Med* 2001; **31**: 1403–12.

31. Folstein M, Liu T, Peter I *et al*. The homocysteine hypothesis of depression. *Am J Psychiatry* 2007; **164**: 861–67.

32. Carney RM, Freedland KE, Stein PK *et al*. Heart rate variability and markers of inflammation and coagulation in depressed patients with coronary heart disease. *J Psychosom Res* 2007; **62**: 463–67.

33. von Känel R. Platelet hyperactivity in clinical depression and the beneficial effect of antidepressant drug treatment: how strong is the evidence? *Acta Psychiatr Scand* 2004; **110**: 163–77.

34. Broadley AJM, Korszun A, Jones CJH, Frenneaux MP. Arterial endothelial function is impaired in treated depression. *Heart* 2002; **88**: 521–24.

35. Tiemeier H, Bakker SLM, Hofman A, Koudstaal PJ, Breteler MMB. Cerebral haemodynamics and depression in the elderly. *J Neurol Neurosurg Psychiatry* 2002; **73**: 34–39.

36. Tiemeier H, Breteler MMB, van Popele NM, Hofman A, Witterman JCM. Late-life depression is associated with arterial stiffness: a population-based study. *J Am Geriatr Soc* 2003; **51**: 1105–10.

37. Tiemeier H, van Dijck W, Hofman A, Witteman JCM, Stijnen T, Breteler MMB. Relationship between atherosclerosis and late-life depression: the Rotterdam Study. *Arch Gen Psychiatry* 2004; **61**: 369–76.

38. Stewart JC, Janicki DL, Muldoon MF, Sutton-Tyrrell K, Kamarck TW. Negative emotions and 3-year progression of subclinical atherosclerosis. *Arch Gen Psychiatry* 2007; **64**: 225–33.

39. Faramawi, MF, Gustat, J, Wildman, RP, Rice, J, Johnson, E, Sherwin, E. Relation between depressive symptoms and common carotid artery atherosclerosis in American persons ⩾ 65 years of age. *Am J Cardiol* 2007; **99**: 1610–13.

40. Jones DJ, Bromberger JT, Sutton-Tyrrell K, Matthews KA. Lifetime history of depression and carotid atherosclerosis in middle-aged women. *Arch Gen Psychiatry* 2003; **60**: 153–60.

41. Frasure-Smith N, Lesperance F, Irwin MR *et al.* Depression, C-reactive protein and two-year major adverse cardiac events in men after acute coronary syndromes. *Biol Psychiatry* 2007; **62**: 302–308.

42. Whooley MA, Caska CM, Hendrickson BE, Rourke MA, Ho J, Ali S. Depression and inflammation in patients with coronary heart disease: findings from the heart and soul study. *Biol Psychiatry* 2007; **62**: 314–20.

43. Thomas AJ, Davis S, Morris C. Increase in interleukin-1beta in late-life depression. *Am J Psychiatry* 2005; **162**: 175–77.

44. Baldwin, RC. Is vascular depression a distinct sub-type of depressive disorder? A review of causal evidence *Int J Geriatr Psychiatry* 2005; **20**: 1–11.

45. Tarangano, FE, Bagnatti, P, Allegri, RF. A double-blind, randomized clinical trial to assess the augmentation with nimodipine of antidepressant therapy in the treatment of vascular depression. *Int Psychogeriatrics* 2005; **17**: 487–98.

46. Landmesser U, Bahlmann F, Mueller M *et al.* Simvastatin versus ezetimibe: pleiotropic and lipid-lowering endothelial function in humans. *Circulation* 2005; **111**: 2356–63.

47. van de Rest O, Geleijnse JM, Kok FJ *et al.* Effect of fish-oil supplementation on mental well-being in older subjects: a randomized, double-blind, placebo-controlled trial. *J Clin Nutr* 2008; **88**: 706–13.

48. Teper E, O'Brien JT. Vascular factors and depression. *Int J Geriatr Psychiatry* 2007; **23**: 993–1000.

49. Jorge RE, Moser DJ, Acion L, Robinson RG. Treatment of vascular depression using repetitive transcranial magnetic stimulation. *Arch Gen Psychiatry* 2008; **65**: 268–76.

50. Lavretsky H, Park S, Siddarth P, Kumar A, Reynolds CF, III. Methylphenidate-enhanced antidepressant response to citalopram in the elderly: a double-blind, placebo-controlled pilot trial. *Am J Geriatr Psychiatry* 2006; **14**: 181–85.

51. Alexopoulos GS, Raue P, Arean P. Problem-solving therapy versus supportive therapy in geriatric major depression with executive dysfunction. *Am J Geriatr Psychiatry* 2003; **11**: 46–52.

52. Broadley AJM, Korszun A, Abdelaal E *et al.* Metyrapone improves endothelial dysfunction in patients with treated depression. *J Am Coll Cardiol* 2006; **48**: 170–75.

53. Mast BT, Miles T, Penninx BW *et al.* Vascular disease and future risk of depressive symptomatology in older adults: findings from the health, aging, and body composition study. *Biol Psychiatry* 2008; **64**: 320–26.

76

Mood Disorders in Parkinson's Disease

John V. Hindle

Senior Clinical Lecturer in Neurodegenerative Diseases, School of Medical Sciences, University of Bangor, North Wales, UK,
Consultant Physician Care of the Elderly, Llandudno Hospital, Llandudno, Conwy, UK

INTRODUCTION

Parkinson's disease is the second commonest cause of chronic neurological disability after stroke. The prevalence of Parkinson's disease increases with increasing age and in the United Kingdom is ~150 per 100 000 population with an incidence of 10.8 cases per 100 000 population. The mean age of onset of Parkinson's disease is in the seventies. The diagnosis is based on the presence of bradykinesia, rest tremor, rigidity and loss of postural reflexes, all of which are likely to be asymmetrical. It is now recognized that Parkinson's disease is much more than a motor disorder, having a spectrum of non-motor symptoms, which may occur prior to the onset of the motor signs. The non-motor symptoms of Parkinson's disease may have more impact on long-term quality of life than the motor symptoms[1]. Non-motor symptoms include autonomic impairment (e.g. constipation, sweating, urinary problems, dribbling and dysphagia), psychiatric problems (e.g. depression, dementia, psychosis), sleep disturbances (e.g. sleep behaviour disorder), sensory disturbances, nutritional problems and problems of balance and falls.

This chapter will focus on depression in Parkinson's disease, which is the most common psychiatric non-motor symptom of Parkinson's disease. Depression in Parkinson's disease is associated with a poor quality of life, excess disability and carer stress, and treatment of depression can reduce functional disability[2].

DIAGNOSIS

Depressive symptoms are common in Parkinson's disease, especially in elderly patients. Recognition of depression in Parkinson's disease can be confounded by the symptoms of Parkinson's disease itself. It is not clear whether the symptoms of depression in Parkinson's disease differ from those of depression in persons without Parkinson's disease. Some have suggested that patients with depression in Parkinson's disease have less guilt and sadness, whereas others have shown no difference when compared with patients with major depression. Anhedonia, or the lack of ability to enjoy, may be a clinical feature of Parkinson's disease and a key symptom of depression in Parkinson's disease. Tearfulness and emotionalism can occur in Parkinson's disease in a similar manner to stroke and must not be confused with depression. Clinicians should be aware of the difficulties in diagnosing mild depression and should have a low threshold for the diagnosis in Parkinson's disease.

Depression in Parkinson's disease probably represents a spectrum of mood disturbances from mood changes before Parkinson's disease motor symptoms through to depression associated with dementia. DSM-IV criteria may not adequately capture the spectrum of mood disorders seen in Parkinson's disease. A broader definition of mood phenotype to include greater levels of psychological distress and particularly anxiety may be more appropriate in Parkinson's disease. DSM-IV criteria for depression have been modified for depression in Parkinson's disease by a consensus group to be more inclusive of symptoms, to include subsyndromal depression, to specify the timing of assessment and to use informants in those who are cognitively impaired[3]. These modified criteria have been validated prospectively[4].

In a prospective cohort study of mood states in Parkinson's disease it has been shown mood disturbance can be divided into depression plus anxiety, depression alone, excessive worry and normal mood[5].

A variety of rating scales have been used to assess depression in Parkinson's disease although they may reflect the presence of depressive symptomatology rather than depressive illness. For screening, the Hamilton Depression Rating Scale (HDRS), Beck Depression Inventory (BDI), Hospital Anxiety and Depression Scale (HADS), Montgomery and Asberg Depression Rating Scale (MADRS) and the Geriatric Depression Scale (GDS) have been shown to be valid. For measurement of severity of depressive symptoms, the HDRS, MADRS, BDI and Zung Self-Rating Depression Scale (SDS) are recommended. The HADS and the GDS include limited motor symptom assessment and may, therefore, be most useful in rating depression severity across a range of Parkinson's disease severity[6]. The HDRS is based on a structured interview whereas the self-rated GDS takes 5 minutes to complete, has been validated against the HDRS and is used commonly in United Kingdom practice in older patients.

EPIDEMIOLOGY

People who are prescribed anti-parkinsonian drugs are more likely than controls or diabetics to be prescribed antidepressant drugs. Recent prescription of antidepressants is associated with an increased risk of developing Parkinson's disease since depression can be a premorbid sign of early Parkinson's disease[7]. A prevalence meta-analysis showed the weighted prevalence of major depressive disorder was 17%, and that of minor depression 22% and dysthymia 13%. Clinically significant depressive symptoms were present in

Principles and Practice of Geriatric Psychiatry, 3rd edn. Edited by Mohammed T. Abou-Saleh, Cornelius Katona and Anand Kumar

35%[8]. In a study of mood disorders in Parkinson's disease in the United Kingdom the prevalence of major depression was 2.8% and minor depression was 7.7% although there was a high prevalence of up to 80% of worry and tension[5]. Depression is often unrecognized. In a survey of 1000 patients, 50% reported depressive symptoms but only 1% identified themselves as depressed[9]. This may be because people do not believe themselves to be depressed unless they feel sad. Similarly doctors can miss depression, in the majority of cases.

Age, psychosis and depression in Parkinson's disease increase mortality, with a relative risk of 2.7 in patients with depression in Parkinson's disease compared with those without depression, with the increased risk not due to suicide. The prevalence of depression is not related to disease duration. The five-year cumulative risk of depression onset is around 10%. Depression in Parkinson's disease has a chronic course, and in one study, 56% of patients with major depression at baseline still had major depression at follow-up, while by combining major and minor forms, depression was chronic in 89% of cases[10]. Minor depression can lead to major depression in 11% of cases over a year and major depression will lead on to minor depression in 33% of cases and will remain chronic in the majority of cases[11].

DEPRESSION IN PARKINSON'S DISEASE AND COGNITION

It is unclear whether cognitive impairment in Parkinson's disease is a risk factor for depression or vice versa, or whether the two sets of symptoms represent a depressive–executive syndrome. Depression in Parkinson's disease may be similar in nature to depression associated with the depression–executive dysfunction syndrome of later life, which is associated with a slow or poor response to antidepressants. Depression and dementia combined may represent a subtype of Parkinson's disease[12]. Studies comparing depression in Parkinson's disease with depression without Parkinson's disease have shown similar cognitive deficits in both conditions, with reduced verbal fluency and attention deficits in depression and problems of abstract reasoning and set shifting in depression in Parkinson's disease. Patients with depressive pseudodementia respond to cueing in a similar manner to Parkinson's disease patients with subcortical dementia, which suggests that similar neural pathways are involved. Defining and diagnosing depression in Parkinson's disease in the presence of dementia are problematic since most rating scales are unsuitable. The Cornell Scale for Depression in Dementia has been used in research but takes 30 minutes to administer and may not be practical for screening in clinical practice[13].

AETIOLOGY

It is still unclear how much the depression in Parkinson's disease is due to the biology of the disease or is the result of psychosocial effects of chronic disease. An organic basis for depression is supported by a number of factors. Depression has been shown to be common in early disease, impairing activities of daily living and increasing the need for symptomatic therapy for Parkinson's disease[14]. One case–control study has shown that initiation of any antidepressant therapy may be associated with a higher risk of Parkinson's disease in the two years after the start of treatment, which suggests that depressive symptoms could be an early manifestation of Parkinson's disease, preceding motor dysfunction[7]. The early pathological stages of Parkinson's disease (Braak stage 1 and 2) with

pathology in the brainstem linking to the limbic system before the onset of motor symptoms may be associated with depression and anxiety. Depressed patients are more likely to develop Parkinson's disease than they are to develop osteoarthritis or diabetes, suggesting some common underlying aetiological factors. At diagnosis, 9.2% of Parkinson's disease patients have a background history of depression compared with 4% of controls, again suggesting a link between depression and Parkinson's disease[15].

There is a possible familial aggregation of unipolar depression and Parkinson's disease. Female gender, young onset, akinesia, postural and gait problems and right hemi-Parkinson's disease have a significantly higher risk of depression in Parkinson's disease. Depression is more pronounced in 'off ' periods, possibly due to the deregulation of the locus caeruleus similar to that found in rapid cycling bipolar affective disorder. Position emission tomography (PET) studies of depression in Parkinson's disease have shown reduced cortical serotonin (5HT) binding and reduced limbic noradrenaline and dopamine but no correlation with basal ganglia dopamine levels[16]. Abnormalities of the mesencephalon on MRI and transcranial ultrasound, frontal cortical under-activity on PET scans, and reduced caudate metabolism all suggest an organic basis for depression in Parkinson's disease.

Cerebrovascular disease is an important determinant in the aetiology of depression, especially in the elderly, and may also be an important contributory factor to the development of depression in the elderly Parkinson's disease patient.

There is no good evidence for a direct correlation between disease severity and depression. There is, however, considerable disadvantage and handicap associated with a chronic neurological disorder. Some workers have gone so far as to suggest a mainly psychosocial model for depression in Parkinson's disease. A particular pattern of negative beliefs and worries described as metacognitive style may increase the risk of depression in Parkinson's disease[17]. It is difficult to attribute functions of the human mind to purely neurochemical and structural changes, and intuitively it seems most likely that depression in Parkinson's disease has a major organic predisposition interacting with psychosocial factors influencing its presentation.

MANAGEMENT

The general principles of management of depression in chronic physical health problems are outlined in the guideline *Depression with a Chronic Physical Health Problem* published by NICE[18].

Psychological Therapies

Provision of support, advice and counselling to both patients and carers may be all that is needed in sub-syndromal and mild cases. A clear explanation that depression is a common intrinsic part of Parkinson's disease is needed in order for patients and carers to accept appropriate help and treatment. Support groups can provide an informal form of group therapy. Counselling and support can be provided for patients and carers by social workers and counsellors with a special interest in Parkinson's disease. In the United Kingdom the Parkinson's disease nurse specialists have a key role in the provision and coordination of these support services in the management of depression. Cognitive behavioural therapy (CBT) can benefit mild or moderate depression in the elderly but there have only been small open studies of CBT in patients with depression in Parkinson's disease[19]. Group-based cognitive therapy or computerized cognitive therapy has not been studied in depression in Parkinson's disease. Bright light therapy has been shown to have a positive effect on mood and motor function in a small study[20]. Exercise interventions may help function in Parkinson's disease but the effects on mood have not been well studied [21].

Drug Treatments

There is insufficient evidence from randomized controlled trials of the safety or efficacy of any antidepressant in depression in Parkinson's disease[22]. In a meta-analysis of the treatment of patients with depression in Parkinson's disease compared with elderly depressed patients without Parkinson's disease, the newer antidepressants were well tolerated in depression in Parkinson's disease. Patients with depression in Parkinson's disease may benefit less from antidepressant treatment, particularly SSRIs, than do elderly patients without Parkinson's disease. The meta-analysis showed a positive effect for depression treatment in patients with depression in Parkinson's disease whether with active drug or placebo[23]. A large placebo effect because of the expectation of reward may be found in Parkinson's disease and this may be caused by placebo-induced dopamine or serotonin release in depression. This placebo effect may be an important consideration in future strategies for the management of depression in Parkinson's disease and emphasizes the need for placebo-controlled trials. In a veterans' study of the impact of a diagnosis of Parkinson's disease on depression treatment the presence of a Parkinson's disease diagnosis had little impact on the frequency and type of antidepressant treatment.

Efforts to improve the care of depressed Parkinson's disease patients should focus on improving recognition, ensuring adequacy of treatment and evaluating the efficacy of existing antidepressants[24].

Dopaminergic Treatment

The first option in the drug treatment of depression in Parkinson's disease is to ensure optimal dopaminergic treatment. Mood elevation and anxiety reduction can be demonstrated using levodopa infusions, and therefore smoothing out fluctuations may be important in the control of depression in Parkinson's disease. Optimization of dopaminergic therapy could include the addition of a non-ergot dopamine agonist. Direct-acting dopamine agonists acting on the D3 receptors (e.g. pramipexole) in the limbic system may have an antidepressant effect, and this may be due partly to an effect on psychomotor retardation. Pramipexole has compared favourably with sertraline[25]. Catechol-O-methyltransferase (COMT) inhibitors may have a similar effect through enhancement of dopaminergic transmission and reduction in motor fluctuation, but this has not been studied in trials. Older reviews suggested that selegeline may be effective; however, later evidence-based reviews have not confirmed this.

Serotonin Re-Uptake Inhibitors

A favourable side effect profile possibly makes selective serotonin re-uptake inhibitor (SSRI) antidepressants the first-line treatment in depression in Parkinson's disease, although trial evidence for efficacy is limited[23]. There is a theoretical risk of increased parkinsonism with SSRI antidepressants, and some case reports exist of akathisia, tardive dyskinesia and dystonia, but there is no clinical evidence that these effects are significant. Possible increased suicide risk need to be considered, especially when treating younger patients. The pattern of liver enzyme induction varies from one SSRI to another, and this may influence the choice of drug. There is no trial evidence that the SSRI antidepressants help symptoms of low mood outside a depressive illness in Parkinson's disease. A generic SSRI such as sertraline may be the best choice for efficacy and tolerability since it has low propensity for interactions[18].

Combined Re-Uptake Inhibitors

The noradrenaline and serotonin combined re-uptake inhibitors may have a role in depression in Parkinson's disease but have yet to show advantages over SSRI drugs. Venlafaxine, a serotonin and noradrenaline re-uptake inhibitor (SNRI) has an anxiolytic effect with a rapid onset of action in the elderly at 1–2 weeks although these effects have not been demonstrated in depression in Parkinson's disease. Mirtazepine, a derivative of mianserin, is a noradrenaline and specific serotonin antidepressant (NaSSA) which may have a rapid onset of action. Theoretically this profile of neurotransmitter action may be useful in depression in Parkinson's disease. Mirtazepine may produce weight gain which can sometimes be used to good effect in depression in Parkinson's disease. There are only a few uncontrolled reports using reboxetine or nafazodone and no studies of duloxetine in patients with depression in Parkinson's disease[18].

Tricyclics

An evidenced-based review suggested that amitriptyline should be considered in the non-demented patient with depression in Parkinson's disease[26]. A trial comparing the short-term efficacy of the predominantly noradrenergic tricyclic desimipramine with citalopram showed a significant improvement in depression at 30 days with a more rapid onset of effect at 14 days with desimipramine. This effect was outweighed by the side effects of desimipramine which can include increased tremor in Parkinson's disease[27]. Other studies show that imipramine is most effective in patients with rigidity and nortriptyline may improve Parkinson's disease. In elderly patients, the anticholinergic side effects of these drugs, including confusion, hallucinosis, urinary retention, blurred vision, faecal impaction and dry mouth, reduce their tolerability. Since anticholinergic drugs are now avoided by most experts in the treatment of Parkinson's disease[22], tricyclic antidepressants are usually reserved for situations where other antidepressants have failed.

Other Drug Treatments

Moclobamide, a reversible monoamine-oxidase A (MAOA) inhibitor is used rarely in depression in Parkinson's disease. Some have combined MAOA inhibition with MAOB inhibition, showing enhanced antidepressant activity with no hypertensive effect. High-dose SSRI regimes have not been studied in depression in Parkinson's disease and are only weakly supported by trial evidence outside Parkinson's disease. From experience the combination of an SSRI in the day and mirtazepine at night may be useful in resistant depression in Parkinson's disease.

Other High-Intensity Therapy of Depression in Parkinson's Disease

Electroconvulsive therapy (ECT) has been shown to be effective in the treatment of depression, motor fluctuations and drug-induced mania. Motor symptoms, especially rigidity, have been shown to respond and relapse more quickly than depression, the response being greater in the elderly. In a randomized controlled trial, repetitive transcranial magnetic stimulation (rTMS) has been shown to improve depression in Parkinson's disease to the same extent as fluoxetine[28]. The effects on depression may last only two weeks, and concurrent antidepressants are needed. In future rTMS may be a useful alternative to ECT since it has a more focal effect, reducing adverse cognitive symptoms and avoiding the need for a general anaesthetic, in addition to improving motor function. Stimulation over the motor cortex can reduce motor slowing and improve cognition in elderly Parkinson's disease patients. rTMS requires further evaluation, but

has a promising future role in the treatment of depression in Parkinson's disease.

Summary of Management of Depression in Parkinson's Disease (Figure 76.1)

Treatment should take into account a patient's needs and preferences. People with depression in Parkinson's disease should have the opportunity to make informed decisions, including advance decisions and advance statements, about their care and treatment, in partnership with their practitioners[18]. It is important to consider both Parkinson's disease-related and non-Parkinson's disease-related

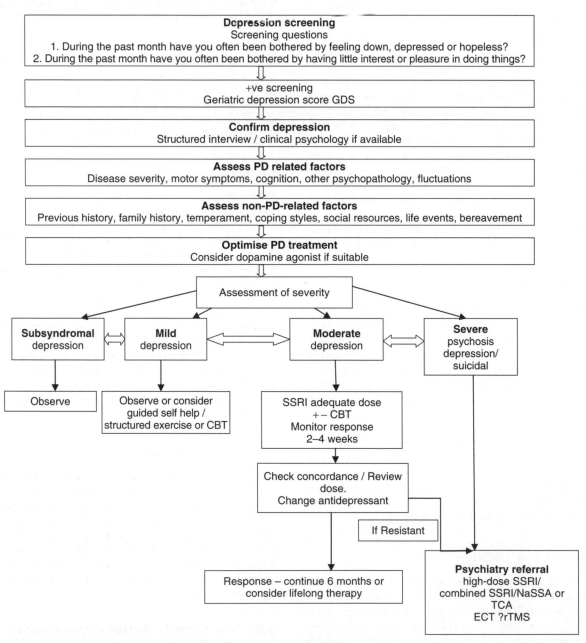

Figure 76.1 Depression screening. PD, Parkinson's disease; CBT, cognitive behavourial therapy; SSRI, selective serotonin re-uptake inhibitor; NaSSA, noradrenaline and specific serotonin antidepressant; TCA, tricyclic antidepressant; ECT, electroconvulsive therapy; rTMS, repetitive transcranial magnetic stimulation

factors. Parkinson's disease-related factors include reviewing and managing disease severity, motor symptoms, cognitive impairments, other disease-related psychopathology, and reviewing psychiatric side effects and fluctuating response to medications[29].

Non-Parkinson's disease-related factors include obtaining insights into previous psychiatric history, family history, temperament, coping styles, social resources and life events which all contribute to the aetiology of depression and may also significantly affect its management[29].

Two screening questions could be used and then if the person responds positively to these a rating such as the GDS completed. Once depression is identified a stepwise collaborative approach to management is based on an assessment of severity and response to interventions[18]. Both the number and severity of symptoms, as well as degree of impairment determine the severity of depression. A clinical assessment of severity of depression, into subsyndromal, mild, moderate and severe based on DSM categories as per the NICE guidelines may help with management decisions[18]. Stepped care encompasses intervention ranging from support, low intensity psychosocial interventions, and medication through to ECT and inpatient management.

In subsyndromal and mild cases a watch and wait approach may be appropriate. Counselling or CBT may be considered in mild cases. In moderate depression, the first step is to optimize dopaminergic therapy and to consider the use of a dopamine agonist if the patient is suitable. If there is no improvement, a trial of an adequate dose of a SSRI antidepressant should be considered with careful monitoring of the patient's mood and motor function. The presence of anxiety may influence the choice of a more sedative antidepressant such as mirtazepine. There is a small risk of producing a serotonin syndrome (hyperpyrexia, agitation, confusion) when selegeline is combined with tricyclics or SSRI antidepressants. The response to an antidepressant is best reviewed after 2–4 weeks of a therapeutic dose[18]. If there is no response after this period, a change of antidepressant can be considered. Patients should be seen on a regular basis at intervals of 2–4 weeks in the first three months and at longer intervals thereafter, if response is good. Antidepressants are usually continued for six months after remission. Two or more episodes of depression have been considered an indication for long-term treatment, but the chronic nature of depression in Parkinson's disease suggests that lifelong therapy may be needed in most cases. Referral to a psychiatrist should be considered if there is a severe depression with psychosis – especially if insight is lost, if there is medication failure in chronic depression or if there are suicidal ideas. The development of suicidal ideas or life-threatening complications, such as refusal to eat, should be taken seriously, and ECT may be considered.

REFERENCES

1. Hely MA, Morris JGL, Reid WGJ *et al*. Sydney multicenter study of Parkinson's disease: Non-L-dopa-responsive problems dominate at 15 years. *Mov Disord* 2005; **20**: 190–99.
2. Schrag A. Quality of life and depression in Parkinson's disease. *J Neurol Sci* 2006; **248**: 151–57.
3. Marsh L, McDonald WM, Cummings J *et al*. Provisional diagnostic criteria for depression in Parkinson's disease: report of a NINDS/NIMH working group. *Mov Disord* 2006; **21**: 148–58.
4. Starkstein S E, Merello M, Jorge R *et al*. A validation study of depressive syndromes in Parkinson's disease. *Mov Disord* 2008; **23**: 538–46.
5. Brown RG, Landau S, Burn DJ *et al*. Defining anxiety and depression-related phenotypes in Parkinson's disease. *Under review JNNP* 2010 (submitted).
6. Schrag A, Barone P, Brown RG *et al*. Depression rating scales in Parkinson's disease: critique and recommendations. *Mov Disord* 2007; **22**: 1077–92.
7. Alonso A, García Rodríguez LA, Logroscino, Hernán MA. Use of antidepressants and the risk of Parkinson's disease: a prospective study. *J Neurol Neurosurg Psychiatry* 2009; **80**: 671–74.
8. Reijnders JS, Ehrt U, Weber WEJ, Aarsland D, Leentjens AFG. Systematic review of prevalence studies of depression in Parkinson's disease. *Mov Disord* 2008; **23**: 183–89.
9. Global Parkinson's Disease Survey Steering Committee. Factors impacting on quality of life in Parkinson's disease: results from an international survey. *Mov Disord* 2002; **17**: 60–67.
10. Sirey JA, Bruce ML, Alexopoulos GS *et al*. Perceived stigma as a predictor of treatment discontinuation in young and older outpatients with depression. *Am J Psych* 2001; **158**: 479–81.
11. Starkstein SE, Mayberg HS, Leiguarada R *et al*. A prospective longitudinal study of depression, cognitive decline, and physical impairments in patients with Parkinson's disease. *J Neurol Neurosurg Psychiatry* 1992; **55**: 377–82.
12. Lewis SJ, Foltynie T, Blackwell AD *et al*. Heterogeneity of Parkinson's disease in the early clinical stages using a data driven approach. *J Neurol Neurosurg Psychiatry* 2005; **76**: 343–48.
13. Alexopoulos GS, Abrams RC, Young RC, Shamoian CA. Cornell scale for depression in dementia. *Biol Psychiatry* 1988; **23**: 271–84.
14. Ravina B, Camicioli R, Como PG *et al*. The impact of depressive symptoms in early Parkinson disease. *Neurology* 2007; **69**: 342–47.
15. Leentjens AF, Van den Akker M, Metsemakers JF *et al*. Higher incidence of depression preceding the onset of Parkinson's disease: a register study. *Mov Disord* 2003; **18**: 414–18.
16. Remy P, Doder M, Lees A *et al*. Depression in Parkinson's disease: loss of dopamine and noradrenaline innervation in the limbic system. *Brain* 2005; **128**: 1314–22.
17. Allott R, Wells A, Morrison AP, Walker R. Distress in Parkinson's disease: contributions of disease factors and metacognitive style. *Br J Psychiatry* 2005; **187**: 182–83.
18. National Institute for Health and Clinical Excellence (NICE). *Depression with a Chronic Physical Health Problem. The treatment and management of depression in adults with chronic physical health problems*. 2009, http://guidance.nice.org.uk/CG91/NICEGuidance/pdf/English accessed June 2010.
19. Dobkin RD, Allen LA, Menza M. Cognitive-behavioral therapy for depression in Parkinson's disease: a pilot study. *Mov Disord* 2007; **22**: 946–95.
20. Paus S, Schmitz-Hubsch T, Wullner U *et al*. Bright light therapy in Parkinson's disease: a pilot study. *Mov Disord* 2007; **22**: 1495–98.
21. Goodwin VA, Richards SH, Taylor RS, Taylor AH, Campbell JL. The effectiveness of exercise interventions for people with Parkinson's disease: a systematic review and meta-analysis. *Mov Disord* 2008; **23**: 631–40.
22. National Institute of Health and Clincal Excellence (NICE). *Clinical Guideline CG035. The Diagnosis and Management of Parkinson's Disease in Primary and Secondary Care*. June 2006. http://guidance.nice.org.uk/CG35/NICEGuidance/pdf/English, accessed June 2010.

23. Weintraub D, Morales KH, Moberg PJ *et al*. Anti-depressant studies in Parkinson's disease: a review and meta-analysis. *Mov Disord* 2005; **20**: 1161–69.

24. Chen P, Kales HC, Weintraub D *et al*. Antidepressant treatment of veterans with Parkinson's disease and depression: analysis of a national sample. *J Geriatr Psychiatry Neurol* 2007; **20**: 161–65.

25. Barone P, Scarzella L, Marconi R *et al*. Pramipexole versus sertaline in the treatment of depression in Parkinson's disease. *J Neurol* 2006; **253**: 555–61.

26. Miyasaki JM, Shannon K, Voon V *et al*. Practice parameter: evaluation and treatment of depression, psychosis and dementia in Parkinson's disease. *Neurology* 2006; **66**: 996–1002.

27. Devos, D, Dujardin K, Poirot I *et al*. Comparison of desipramine and citalopram treatments for depression in Parkinson's disease: a double-blind, randomized, placebo-controlled study. *Mov Disord* 2008; **23**: 850–57.

28. Fregni F, Santos CM, Myczkowski ML *et al*. Repetitive transcranial magnetic stimulation is as effective as fluoxetine in the treatment of depression in patients with Parkinson's disease. *J Neurol Neurosurg Psychiatry* 2004; **75**: 1171–74.

29. Hindle JV. Neuropsychiatry. In Playfer JR, Hindle JV (eds), *Parkinson's Disease in the Older Patient*. Oxford: Radcliffe, 2008.

77

Epidemiology of Depression: Prevalence and Incidence

Ruoling Chen[1] and John Copeland[1,2]

[1]*Centre for Health and Social Care Improvement, School of Health and Wellbeing, University of Wolverhampton, UK*
[2]*Division of Psychiatry, University of Liverpool, UK*

INTRODUCTION

The most common geriatric psychiatric disorder is depression. Depression in older people has become a serious health-care issue worldwide. But it is often ignored, and thus opportunities are lost for prevention and early treatment. Blazer in his introduction to this section in the second edition of this book states, 'Many symptom checklists have been used to estimate the burden of depressive symptoms in community populations. The results of these studies are remarkably consistent, with the range of significant depressive symptoms estimated to be 10–25%'. He quotes from 10 studies. In order to update information on prevalence and incidence of depression, we have now been able to review 38 studies of prevalence and 10 of incidence appearing in the English language during the last 10 years. Blazer continues, 'Lower prevalences of major depression have been found in more rural samples with an estimate of less than 1% in a North Carolina rural sample, whereas urban studies have typically estimated higher prevalence. The prevalence of dysthymic disorder is generally higher than that for major depression, approximately 2–8%, depending on the instrument used in the survey'.

The problem that Blazer highlights including the diverse case-finding methods causing difficulties in drawing comparisons has substantially increased since the second edition. Most of the studies reviewed used at least one of the following instruments to diagnose depression, including those clinically based, replicating a psychiatrist's diagnosis using ICD-10, DSM-III,-R DSM-IV criteria, CSNMD (clinically significant non-major depression) applied to the results of case-finding instruments, others to the results of psychiatrists' clinical examination, CIDI and GMS-AGECAT (Geriatric Mental State-Automated Geriatric Examination for Computer Assisted Taxonomy), and those based on scale cut points such as GDS-30, 15-item GDS (score >5), EURO-D scale, CES-D (Center for Epidemiological Studies Depression Scale). Although there is some correspondence between these methods, precise comparisons are difficult to make. There is also the problem of the type of selection of samples, whether or not they were purely community based, that is to say people living in their own homes or also in residential accommodation, or included hospital admissions, especially in those

countries where hospitals still accommodate large proportions of patients. Are the samples randomly selected and what were the dropout rates? Was a one-stage method of identification used or a two-stage method with loss due to death, illness or refusal between stages (a particular problem in the calculation of incidence rates). Studies report their samples, grouping the data in different ways. Most do not state the kind of case they are trying to identify. The majority are likely to be interested in cases suitable for intervention but use DSM or ICD criteria aimed specifically at improving reliability between psychiatrists, and therefore likely to lead to a narrower more sharply defined concept of a case than would be acceptable to most clinicians who, as a consequence, are tempted to invent their own 'subsyndromal' cases for treatment. Nevertheless, in spite of these difficulties it may be possible to draw broad conclusions.

Blazer warns: 'One of the major tasks facing psychiatric epidemiologists studying depression cross-nationally in the elderly is to explain the residual depressive symptoms in community samples not easily captured by the usual diagnostic categories' and goes on to quote the 34 studies of the prevalence of late-life depression where the prevalence varied from 0.4% to 35%[1]. Arranged according to diagnostic category, major depression was relatively rare (weighted average prevalence of 1.8%), minor depression more common (weighted average prevalence of 9.8%) while all depressive syndromes deemed clinically relevant yield an average prevalence of 13.5%. Depression was more common among women and among older people living under adverse socioeconomic circumstances.

Below, we review 38 studies of the prevalence of depression and 10 of incidence across the world, published over the last 10 years, divided by continent and whether clinically-based diagnosis was used or scale cut scores.

PREVALENCE OF DEPRESSION IN EUROPE (TABLE 77.1)

The EURODEP study[2] (1999) reported the prevalence of depression in nine countries in Europe, which had all used the GMS-AGECAT assessment and computerized differential diagnosis. This instrument was designed to facilitate large epidemiological studies in older people where psychiatrists could not be employed for screening every

Principles and Practice of Geriatric Psychiatry, 3rd edn. Edited by Mohammed T. Abou-Saleh, Cornelius Katona and Anand Kumar
© 2011 John Wiley & Sons, Ltd

case. A case was defined as one requiring some form of intervention. This package was prepared before DSM-III and ICD-10 revisions but AGECAT cases of depression have been shown in a number of studies to equate with major depression, dysthymia and 'depression not otherwise specified'.

In the EURODEP study[2] all subjects were aged 65 or over, randomly selected or total samples in the community except for the Dublin centre which sampled a general practice, to yield a total of 13 803 individuals. Substantial differences in the prevalence of depression were found, with Iceland having the lowest level at 8.8%, followed by Liverpool 10.0%, Zaragoza 10.7%, Dublin 11.9%, Amsterdam 12.0%, Berlin 16.5%, London 17.3%, Verona 18.3% and Munich 23.6%. There was no constant association between prevalence and age. A meta-analysis of the pooled data on the nine European centres yielded an overall prevalence of 12.3% (95% CI, 11.8–12.9%); for women 14.1% (95% CI, 13.5–14.8%) and for men 8.6% (95% CI, 7.9–9.3%).

Using Clinically Based Diagnosis

DSM-IV criteria. Prevalence of major depression in France. Ritchie et al.[3] randomly recruited 1873 non-institutionalized persons aged 65 and over from the Montpellier district electoral rolls to assess current and lifetime depression symptoms using the Mini-International Neuropsychiatric Interview. Cases identified were re-examined by a clinical panel. Major depression was found to be 3% and lifetime prevalence 26.5%. A level consistent with many other studies.

GMS-AGECAT. Como (personal communication) reported the findings of the random community study of participants aged 65 and over in Tirana, Albania, which formed part of the EURODEP study but entered at a later date. Prevalence levels of depression were 19.3%. This is the first EURODEP study from a Muslim state in Europe. de Jonge and colleagues found levels of depression in the second Zaragosa study of persons aged 55 and over of 11.2%[4]. McDougall et al.[5] reported the prevalence of depression in the Medical Research Council Cognitive Function and Ageing Study (MRC-CFAS), and the prevalence of depression and depressive symptoms in those living in institutions[6]. The MRC-CFAS is a population-based cohort comprising 13 004 individuals aged 65 and above from five sites across England and Wales. A stratified random sub-sample of 2640 participants were interviewed by GMS-AGECAT, showing that the prevalence of depression in those living at home was 9.3% (similar to the 9.2% in an earlier Liverpool study (n = 5222)[2] and for those living in institutions was 27.1%. The prevalence increased if subjects with concurrent dementia were included. This is of interest because such cases of dementia are often excluded in surveys of depression but may require treatment for depression. Also, such exclusion may give a spurious impression of a fall in the proportion of people with depression with increasing age as the prevalence of dementia escalates. Depression was more common in women (10.4%) than men (6.5%) and was associated with functional disability, co-morbid medical disorder and social deprivation.

Using Scale Scores

EURO-D based prevalence in 10 European countries. Castro-Costa et al.[7] administered the EURO-D with score ≥ 4 to cross-sectional nationally representative samples of non-institutionalized persons aged 50 years and over (n = 22 777) across 10 European

countries – Denmark, Sweden, the Netherlands, Germany, Austria, Switzerland, France, Spain, Italy and Greece – as part of the SHARE study. The distribution of gender and age did not differ between countries. Educational levels were lowest in the Latin countries (France, Italy and Spain) and in Greece. The highest country-specific depression prevalence rates were found in France (33.7%), Italy (33.7%) and Spain (36.8%), with a 9% difference between the lowest of these (33% in France) and the next lowest (24% in Greece). Prevalence in the remaining countries was 18–19%. Heterogeneity between countries was statistically significant ($p < 0.001$). The pattern and extent of between-country differences were not affected by direct standardization for gender, age, education, verbal fluency or memory. But the SHARE data are limited by the relatively low proportion of households and individuals responding. This may, unfortunately, represent a secular trend in more developed countries. The net effect may be an underestimation of the true prevalence of depression[8,9].

The EURO-D scale was developed in order to include more centres in the EURODEP study. It was shown to have strong conceptual validity and high internal consistency when applied to data from 21 724 subjects. EURO-D scores tended to increase with increasing age, unlike the levels of prevalence of depression[3]. Women had generally higher scores than men, and widowed and separated subjects were higher than those who were currently or never married.

GDS in the Netherlands. Stek et al.[10] assessed the prevalence of depression and correlates from a representative sample of 599 community-based 85-year-old subjects with a MMSE >18. The prevalence of depression, as measured with a GDS-S score of 5 points or more, was 15.4%, not very different from the EURODEP level for Amsterdam of 12.0%.

CES-D in the Netherlands. Van't et al.[11] assessed the prevalence of depressive symptomatology and risk indicators in 2850 participants aged 75 years or more in the PIKO study. The prevalence of depressive symptoms was 31.1% across all participants.

PREVALENCE IN THE AMERICAS (TABLE 77.2)

Using Clinically Based Diagnosis

DSM-IV. One study[15] in the United States examined the current and lifetime prevalence of depressive disorders in 4559 non-demented individuals aged 65 to 100 years. This sample represented 90% of the elderly population of Cache County, Utah. The researchers employed DSM-IV criteria for major depression, dysthymia and sub-clinical depressive disorders using a modified version of the Diagnostic Interview Schedule. The point prevalence of major depression was 4.4% in women and 2.7% in men ($p = 0.003$), similar to the level (3%) found by Ritchie et al.[3] in France using similar criteria. Other depressive syndromes were surprisingly uncommon (combined point prevalence, 1.6%), and the current prevalence of major depression did not change appreciably with age. They also estimated that lifetime prevalence of major depression was 20.4% in women and 9.6% in men ($p < 0.001$) (Ritchie 26.5%), decreasing with age.

In Quebec, Preville et al.[16] used the 'Enquete sur la sante des aines' study, conducted in 2005–6, to obtain a representative sample (n = 2798) of community-dwelling older adults. Of this sample, 12.7% met the criteria for depression, mania, anxiety disorders or benzodiazepine dependency. The 12-month prevalence rate of major depression was 1.1% (again demonstrating the low levels found with these criteria) and the prevalence of minor depression was 5.7%.

Table 77.1 Prevalence of depressive symptoms in community samples of older adults in Europe

Author	Sample	n	Screening method	Findings
Clinically based diagnosis				
Como (personal communication)	Random community sample in Tirana, Albania (65 years and over) part of the EURODEP Consortium	1239	GMS-AGECAT	19.3% depression
de Jonge et al.[4]	Second random community sample in Zaragoza, Spain (55 years and over)	4803 (M2771, F2032)	GMS-AGECAT	11.2% depression, 2.7% men, 9.3% of women
Ritchie et al.[3]	Community sample in France (65 years and over)	1873	Mini-International Neuropsychiatric Interview DSM-IV criteria	3% for major depression (26.5% with major depression lifetime prevalence)
Intorre et al.[12]	Community sample in Rome, Italy (70–85 years)	359 (M167, F192)	Mental health assessment	9% men, 19% women with possible depression
McDougall et al.[5]	Five centre community samples MRC CFAS (England and Wales) (65 years and over)	2640	GMS-AGECAT	9.3% depression (95% CI, 7.8–10.9%) living at home
Score cut point				
Stek et al.[10]	Community sample in the Netherlands (85+) MMSE >18	500	GDS-S (score 5 or more)	15.4% depression (no age, gender or racial difference in prevalence) 25% of participants who were seen by their GP with depressive symptoms
Jansson et al.[13]	Twin pairs in Sweden (50+, mean 72) female monozygotic (MZ), Male MZs, Female DZs, Male DZs, opposite-sex DZs)	959 (123, 90, 207, 109, 430)	CES-D	16% men, 24% women (clinically significant depressive symptoms)
Wilson et al.[14]	Community sample living alone in their own home in UK (80–90)	376	GDS (score 5 or more)	21% depression
Castro-Costa et al.[7]	Community sample in 10 European countries (50+)	22 777	EURO-D (score 4 or more)	The prevalence of symptoms higher in the Latin ethno-lingual group 33.7% France; 33.7% Italy; 36.8% Spain other countries in between these and 24.0% Greece
van't et al.[11]	Community sample in the Netherlands (75+) the PIKO study	2850	CES-D (score 16 or more)	31.1% depression

ICD-10, SCAN. Two studies were conducted in Brazil, and one study in Peru, Mexico and Venezuela. Costa *et al.*[17] investigated the prevalence and correlates of common mental disorders with semi-structured interviews administered by a psychiatrist. During the study, a two-phase population survey of 392 persons aged 75 years and over were screened for depression and mental disorders using the General Health Questionnaire (GHQ-12) and Geriatric Depression Scale (GDS). In the second phase, 20% were evaluated using the SCAN to generate ICD-10 diagnoses. The prevalence of depressive episode was 19.2% with no effect of gender or age. Lay-administered interviews were thought to underestimate the prevalence of mental disorders in older people and they recommended one-month prevalence as more appropriate for the oldest-old given patchy recall of distant experiences.

DSM-IV. Xavier *et al.*[18] described the prevalence of minor depression as 12% of the oldest-old in a random representative sample (*n* = 77 subjects) aged 80 years and over from the Brazilian rural southern region using DSM-IV criteria. A small but interesting study which was found to be consistent with others quoted here concerning younger age groups.

DSM-IV and ICD-10 GMS-AGECAT. Investigating the prevalence in five locations in Latin America, Guerra *et al.*[19] conducted a one-phase cross-sectional survey of 5886 people aged 65 and over from urban and rural locations in Peru and Mexico and an urban site in Venezuela. Depression was identified according to diagnostic criteria, and scale scores with EURO-D cut-off point. DSM-IV major depression prevalence varied between 1.3% and 2.8% by site (consistent with other sites in Europe and North America), ICD-10 depressive episode between 4.5% and 5.1%, GMS-AGECAT all forms of clinical depression between 30.0% and 35.9% (high, because of the low level of education stage one of the algorithm was used, i.e. level of depression in all participants regardless of other diagnoses such as dementia), and for EURO-D depression between 26.1% and 31.2%. The prevalence of EURO-D depression was in a similar range of 24–36.8% in Latin countries in Europe. The prevalence of DSM-IV major depression was lower than that in men in the United States (4.4% in women and 2.7% in men). The authors of this important study (part of 10/66 Dementia Research Group) from low and middle income countries draw several conclusions, 'the population attributable prevalence fractions suggest that 13.6% of the prevalence of severe disability in Peru, 32.4% in Mexico and 31.7% in Venezuela could be independently attributed to depression'; 'a strong and independent association between subsyndromal depression and an established criteria of relative severe disability, 15 or more disability days in the past month, would appear to indicate that DSM-IV and ICD-10 diagnostic criteria might indeed be missing a substantial proportion of clinically significant cases. We have also demonstrated... that the true population burden of depression is significantly under estimated by these very narrow diagnostic definitions'; 'late-life depression in Peru, Mexico and Venezuela is similar to that seen in Europe'.

Using Scale Scores

Alvarado and colleagues[20] in the SABE (Salud Bienestar y Envejecimiento) study interviewed a sample of 10 661 persons aged 60 and over in seven Latin American and Caribbean countries using the GDS. They found the prevalence of depression varied from 0.4–5.2% in men and 0.3–9.5% in women. They concluded that current socioeconomic conditions and health status as well as functional disabilities mainly accounted for gender differences in prevalence.

PREVALENCE IN ASIA – CHINA AND TAIWAN (TABLE 77.3)

Using Clinically Based Diagnosis

GMS-AGECAT studies in mainland China. In urban communities, the prevalence of depression was 2.2% – about five times lower than that of older people in Liverpool including older people of Chinese origin[22] – but in poorer rural communities depression was higher at 6.0%[23]. Could these low levels be due to failure to recognize cultural ways of expressing depression? This would seem unlikely because the GMS-AGECAT diagnosis, as in other studies, was formally validated by local psychiatrists using a translated version and comparing their diagnosis with one provided by computer. Chong *et al.*[24] and Chen *et al.*[25] investigated the one-month prevalence of clinically significant depression in 1500 subjects aged 65 years and older, randomly selected from three communities of urban and rural elderly in southern Taiwan. One-month prevalence of depressive neurosis and major depression were 15.3% and 5.9%, respectively. These results reflect similar differences in prevalence rates from Europe and North America found in surveys of younger adults.

CIDI. In a Beijing study[26] involving urban and rural regions, the overall 12-month prevalence of depression was 4.33% (2.65% in men, 5.83% in women). The overall lifetime prevalence was 7.83% (4.65% in men and 10.66% in women).

Using Scale Scores

CES-D. The prevalence of depression was 9.5% (6.7% men and 11.7% women) in a two-centre study by Pan *et al.*[27]: north China (Beijing) 14.9% rather different from south China (Shanghai) 4.1% (*p* < 0.001). These also appeared to be low rates for a *CES-D* study.

GDS (≥ 8). In Hong Kong, three urban random community samples were undertaken by Li *et al.*[28] examining obesity and depression among 18 750 men and 37 417 women aged 65 or over in health centres using the 15-item Chinese GDS (CGDS; ≥ 8) found 4.9% depression in men and 7.9% for women (*p* < 0.001). Since attendance at the health centre was voluntary severe depressive symptoms may have been under-represented. Chi *et al.*[29] using the same instrument with a random community sample of 917 people aged 60 and over found depression levels of 11.0% men and 14.5% women, a prevalence rate not dissimilar to that in the United States, England and Finland. The same scale was used by Chou *et al.*[30] in a representative community sample of 1903 Chinese aged 60 and above, finding prevalence rates for the oldest-old of 31.1%; for those aged 70–79, 22.4% and for those 60–69, 19.1%. Chiu *et al.*[31] compared depression in urban and rural elders finding that 20.1% of urban elders and 12.8% of rural samples were classified with depressive symptoms. Tsai *et al.*[32] using stratified random sampling of 1200 elderly participants from northern, middle, southern and eastern regions of Taiwan found the prevalence of depression to be 13%, within the range of previous findings 4.9–20.1%[28,31].Overall, the prevalence of depression based on this scale and cut-off point in Taiwan and Hong Kong lay between 4.9–31.1% – an apparently large geographical disparity.

The GMS-AGECAT prevalence of depression was higher in rural than that in urban mainland China, while in Taiwan the urban sample had a relatively higher prevalence of depressive symptoms than that found in rural elders[31].

Table 77.2 Prevalence of depressive symptoms in community samples of older adults in North, South and Central America

Author	Sample	n	Screening method	Findings
North America – Clinically based diagnosis				
Steffens et al.[15]	Community sample in Cache County, Utah (non-demented; 65–100 years)	4559	Diagnostic Interview Schedule	2.7% men, 4.4% women (major depression), prevalence did not change with age. 1.6% with other depressive syndromes 9.6% men, 20.4% women (lifetime depression, decreasing with age)
Heo et al.[21]	Community sample – nationally representative survey data from 2006 BRFSS in US (18+ years)	188 292	Doctor diagnosed	15.7% depression; 11% men, 20.6% women (117% increase from year 2005–50 in older people)
Preville et al.[16]	Community sample in Quebec	2798	DSM-IV	12.7% depression (12-month prevalence: 1.1% major depression, 5.7% minor depression)
South and Central America – Clinically based diagnosis				
Xavier et al.[18]	Community sample of Italian descent in rural Southern Brazil (80+)	77	DSM-IV	12% minor depression (frequency greater in women)
Guerra et al.[19]	Urban and rural community sample in Peru and Mexico and an urban in Venezuela (65+)	5886	DSM-IV GMS- AGECAT EURO-D	1.3–2.8% DSM-IV major depression 4.5–5.1% ICD-10 depressive episode 30.0–35.9% GMS-AGECAT 30.0–35.9% GMS AGECAT depression 26.1–1.2% EURO-D depression
Costa et al.[17]	Community sample in Brazil (75+)	392	SCAN/ICD10 GHQ-12 GDS	19.2% depressive episode No age, gender or racial difference in prevalence
South and Central America – Score cut point				
Alvarado et al.[20]	Urban community sample in Latin America and the Caribbean region		GDS	Overall 0.4–5.2% men depression, 0.3–9.5% women depression Buenos Aires 2.1% men 3.2% women Barbados 0.4% men 0.3% women Havana 1.9% men 6.7% women Mexico City 1.6% men 6.2% women Montevideo 3.4% men 5% women Santiago 5.2% men 9.5% women São Paulo 2.2% men 4.9% women

PREVALENCE IN OTHER ASIAN COUNTRIES (TABLE 77.3)

Using clinically Based Diagnosis

GMS-AGECAT with ICD-10, DSM-IV. Rajkumar et al.[33] investigating 1000 participants aged over 65 years from a rural south Indian community using the Geriatric Mental State, ICD-10 and DSM-IV diagnoses of major depression within the previous one month found 12.7%.

GMS AGECAT with DSM IV. Suh[34] with a community sample of 1241 persons in Korea aged 65 and over found 10.5% depression.

GMS AGECAT. With the community sample of 1156 people aged 65 and over in Nakayama, Japan, Ikeda et al.[35] found a level of depression of of 5.8% (AGECAT) and 4.3% (DSM IV) (personal communication).

GMS AGECAT (Arabic version). Ghubash et al.[36] investigated the prevalence of depression within a random sample of households representing the United Arab Emirates national population. They screened 610 UAE nationals aged 60 years and over, irrespective of the age of other individuals in each household. The researchers found 20.2% with depression at syndrome case level. An important study and the only one so far from Arabic countries. More studies are required from the Islamic world as a whole.

Using Scale Scores

GDS-15 cut-point 5/6. Wada et al.[37] used this scale to assess depression in a 2695 community sample aged 60 and over living in five rural Asian towns. They found 29.0% of depression overall. Indonesia was 33.8%, (sample size 411), Vietnam 17.2% (379) and Japan 30.3% (1905). Malhotra et al.[38] using the same scale and cut-off point with an 1181 community sample of Sri Lankans (aged 60 years and over) found a prevalence of depression of 27.8% overall (24.0%

men, 30.8% women), lower than in Indonesia and Japan and higher than in Vietnam. In Japan, Niu et al.[39] assessed depression in 1058 community-dwelling Japanese individuals aged 70 years and over using the 30-item Geriatric Depression Scale with two cut-off points: 11 (to include most clinical depressions) and 14 (severe depressions) yielding 34.1% and 20.2%, respectively.

GDS (Korean). The majority of studies have rarely examined both urban and rural populations simultaneously. Kim et al.[40]

Table 77.3 Prevalence of depressive symptoms in community samples of older adults in Asia

Author	Sample	n	Screening method	Findings
Clinically based diagnosis				
2. Chong et al.[24]	Community sample in Taiwan (65+)	1500	GMS-AGECA	5.9% major depression (one month) 15.3% depressive neurosis high
Ghubash et al.[36]	Community sample in United Arab Emirates (60+, 68.6 ± 8.3)	610 (M347, F263)	GMS- AGECAT	20.2% depression
Chen et al.[22]	Urban community sample in Hefei City, central-east China (65+)	1736	GMS-AGECAT	2.2% (95% CI, 1.5–2.9%) depression (five times lower than that of older people in Liverpool, UK)
Chen et al.[23]	Rural community sample in China, low income (60+)	M754 F 846	GMS-AGECAT	6.0% (4.8–7.3%) with depression (85.9% living with family members)
Ma et al.[26]	Urban and rural community sample in Beijing, China (60)	1601	CIDI 1.0	4.33% 12-month prevalence 2.65% men, 5.83% women (7.83% lifetime prevalence, 4.65% men, 10.66% women)
Rajkumar et al.[33]	Rural community sample in south Indian (65+)	1000	GMS ICD-10	12.7% One month prevalence (95% CI 10.64–14.76%)
Chen et al.[25]	Community sample in Taiwan (65+)	1500	Assessment by psychiatrists (CSNMD)	8.8% prevalence of 1 month
Suh et al.[34]	Community sample in Korea (65+)	1241	GMS AGECAT/DSM IV	10.5% depression
Ikeda et al.[35]	Community sample in Nakayama, Japan (65+)	1156	GMS-AGECAT	5.8% depression
Score cut point				
Thongtang et al.[41]	Community sample in Thailand	1713	Thai GDS TMSE	12.78% depression 8.23% only depression (5.43% men, 9.63% women) 4.55% both depression and cognitive impairment (male 2.8%, female 5.54%)
Kim et al.[40]	Urban and rural community sample in South Korea (65+)	485(U) 649(R)	Korea form of the GDS (KGDS)	No difference between urban and rural in prevalence
Li et al.[28]	Urban community sample in Hong Kong (65+)	56167 M18750 F37417	GDS	4.9% depression men (4.6–5.2%) 7.9% depression women (7.6–8.1%)
Chou et al.[30]	Community sample in Hong Kong (60+)	1903	GDS-15 (score 8 or more)	(31.1% ± 9.7%) depression for 80+ 22.4% ± 4.2% for 70–79 19.1% ± 2.8% for 60–69

Table 77.3 (continued)

Author	Sample	n	Screening method	Findings
Wada et al.[37]	Rural community sample in three Asian countries (60+)	411 (Ind) 379 (Viet) 1905 (Japan) total 2695	GDS-15 (score 5 or 6)	33.8% Indonesia 17.2% Vietnam 30.3% Japan 29.0% depression overall
Chi et al.[29]	Urban random community sample in Hong Kong (60+)	917	GDS-15 (score 8 or more)	11.0% depression men 14.5% depression women
Chiu et al.[31]	Urban and rural community sample in South Taiwan	678 (urban) 327 (rural)	The Chinese GDS	20.1% depression urban 12.8% depression rural
Tsai et al.[32]	Community sample in northern, middle, southern and eastern regions of Taiwan	1200	GDS-S	27.5% depression
Pan et al.[27]	Community sample in northern and southern China (Beijing and Shanghai) (50–70)	3289	CES-D	14.9% Beijing 4.1% Shanghaih 9.5% depression overall 6.7% men 11.7% women
Niu et al.[39]	Community sample in Japan (70+)	1058	GDS (score ≥11 mild and severe, 14 severe)	34.1% mild and severe depression 20.2% severe
Malhotra et al.[38]	Community sample in Singapore (60+) of elderly Sri Lankans	1181	GDS 15 (score ≥6)	27.8% depression 24.0% men 30.8% women

investigated 485 urban-dwelling and 649 rural-dwelling participants within Kwangju, South Korea for depression. No differences rural/urban were found, findings being consistent with other studies in China.

GDS Thai (TGDS). Thongtang et al.[41] using in addition the Thai Mini Mental State Examination (TMSE), screened 1713 elderly people in 35 communities from four districts finding a prevalence of depression of 12.7% (8.2% depression alone (5.4% men, 9.6% women) and 4.5% depression with cognitive impairment (2.8% men, 5.5% women).

PREVALENCE IN AFRICA (TABLE 77.4)

Using Clinically Based Diagnosis

CIDI DSM IV. Gureje et al.[42] estimated major depressive disorder in a representative sample of 2152 people aged 65 years and older by sampling households in the Yoruba-speaking areas of Nigeria. Twelve- month and lifetime prevalence estimates of major depressive disorder were 7.1% and 26.2%, respectively. The 12-month prevalence estimate of major depressive disorder was higher than the rate of 1.1% in the study in Quebec[16].

Using Scale Scores

GDS. Baiyewu et al.[43] undertook a two-stage study. The community-based samples aged 69 years and over were first screened for

dementia, 2627 individuals in Indianapolis of whom 17.2% underwent clinical assessment including GDS and 2806 in Ibadan with 21.6% having clinical assessment. Prevalence of depression was estimated using weights indicated by the sampling stratification. The prevalence of mild and severe depression was similar for the two sites: 12.3% and 2.2%, respectively in Indianapolis and 19.8% and 1.6% in Ibadan. However, Ibadan men had significantly higher prevalence of mild depression than Indianapolis men. Poor cognitive performance was associated with significantly higher rates of depression in Ibadan.

PREVALENCE IN AUSTRALIA

Using Clinically Based Diagnosis

DSM. Snowdon and Lane[44] re-examined the data from a 1985 survey of 146 elderly people living at home. Depression and cognitive impairment were also assessed in a local hostel (n = 42) and nursing home (n = 74). DSM diagnoses were made by an old-age psychiatrist. In the nursing home, 23 residents could not respond to interview questions and were considered to have severe dementia. Subjects in all three settings were followed up after four years. They found that seven community subjects (4.5%, 95% CI 1.3–8.3%) and three in residential care fulfilled criteria for major depression. The estimated total prevalence of depressive disorders among older people in Botany was between 13.0% and 13.6% (4.6% major depression, 3.6% dementia with depression, 5.4% other depressive disorders).

Table 77.4 Prevalence of depressive symptoms in community samples of older adults in Africa

Author	Sample	n	Screening method	Findings
Clinically based diagnosis				
Gureje et al.[42]	Community sample in Ibadan, Nigeria (65+)	2152	CIDI DSM-IV	7.1% (5.9–8.3) major depressive disorder (12-month prevalence) 26.2% (lifetime prevalence) (95% CI 24.3–28.2%)
Score cut point				
Baiyewu et al.[43]	Community sample in Indianapolis and Ibadan, Nigeria of African Americans and Yoruba (69+)	2627 (451) 2806 (605) total 5433	Screening GDS for sub-sample	19.8% Ibadan (mild depression) and 1.6% (severe depression) 12.3 Indianapolis% (mild depression) and 2.2% (severe depression)

INCIDENCE OF DEPRESSION IN OLDER PEOPLE

In the original chapter for the second edition of this book Blazer wrote, incidence studies of depression in the elderly are extremely rare in the literature. Two studies provide some estimate of incidence, however, Rorsman et al.[45] estimated incident depression from the Lundby cohort in Sweden among 2612 individuals evaluated in 1957 and later in 1972 (i.e. 15-year incidence) until the age of 70. The cumulative probability of suffering a first episode of depression was 27% for men and 45% for women, a very high incidence figure in this cohort (especially compared to lifetime prevalence figures, reported in other studies, of less than 15%). The annual age-standardized first incidence for depression, all degrees of impairment included, was 0.43 for men and 0.76 for women. Incidence appears to decrease in the studies as individuals aged, especially for men. Eaton et al. (1997)[46] estimated the incidence of major depression over 10 years for the ECA cohort from Baltimore. They found an overall estimated annual incidence of 3.0 per 1000 per year, with a peak while subjects were in their 30s, a smaller peak when subjects were in their 50s and a definite lower incidence in the elderly. Prodromal symptoms were present many years before the full criteria for major depression were met, further linking the minor and major depression. Foster et al. (1991) estimated the incidence of depression in long-term care facilities. In a cohort of 104 new admissions followed for a year, they found an incidence of 14%. One-third of these new cases were diagnosed as major depression, two thirds as minor depression.

In the last 10 years, nine important studies on the incidence of depression in older people have been conducted in the Netherlands, UK, London, USA, Austria, Thailand and Republic of Korea. Depression was diagnosed in these studies by using the 15-item GDS?score >4 or 5)? the 10-item CES-D (score >8)? the Geriatric Mental State, SDS (Zung self-rating depression scale) and the Thai Geriatric Depression Scale (TGDS). Participants were generally community-dwelling older people or patients registered with primary care practices participating in community-based cohort studies.

Incidence Rate

After one-year follow-up: Thongtang et al.[47] assessed 1713 elderly people in 35 communities from four districts in Bangkok using the Thai Geriatric Depression Scale (TGDS) and the Thai Mini Mental State Examination (TMSE). The point incidence (one year) of depression was 1.58% in men and 5.68% in women[47].

After two-year follow-up[46,47]: out of 521 people aged 65 years and over from an East Asian population, incident depression was found in 63 (12% or 6% per year). In Austria, 331 non-demented and never-depressed individuals were followed up for 30 months, by which time 31.4% had developed a subsyndromal, minor, or major depressive episode. In a prospective cohort study with index assessment and two-year follow-up of patients initially aged 65 years and over registered with two south London practices (n = 1164), the incidence of depression was 8.4% (4.2% per year)[50].

An eight-year follow-up[51]: A study of a cohort of 5653 community-dwelling elderly free of dementia was conducted in the Netherlands. For depressive syndromes, the incidence rate was 7.0 (95%CI 6.0–8.3) per 1000 person-years which was more than doubled when episodes of depressive symptoms were included. The rate was almost twice as high for women compared with men. The incidence did not appear to change with age.

During a follow-up period of 15 years, depressive symptoms in 464 men aged 64 to 84 years were assessed by the Zung self-rating depression scale (SDS). The cumulative incidence for depressive symptoms was 44%[52].

Among the oldest old, depression is frequent[13,14]. In a population-based prospective study, depressive symptoms were annually assessed in 500 people aged 85 years or above with the 15-item GDS, using a cut-off of 4. During a mean follow-up of 3.9 years, the annual risk for the emergence of depression was 6.8%.

Of 376 participants aged between 80 and 90 years, who lived alone and followed-up for one year, the annual incidence of depression was 12.4%, with the depression identified by GDS of 5 or more.

RISK FACTORS

Risk factors for incidence of depression 'Dispositional optimism' predicted a lower cumulative incidence of depressive symptoms with an odds ratio of 0.23[52]. Poor daily functioning and institutionalization predicted depression[13]. Subsequent development of clinically significant depressive symptoms was associated with baseline increased scores in depression (OR 1.68, 95% CI 1.21–2.34)[14].

Family factors

Risk factors associated with prevalence depression include not living close to family and friends (OR 2.54, 1.44–4.47)[14]. Having severe troubles with relatives and pre-existing cognitive impairments may enhance the probability of developing a late-onset depression[49].

Vascular depression hypothesis

The vascular depression hypothesis suggests that age-related vascular diseases and risk factors contribute to late-life depression. A study of 1796 elders ages 70–79 without depression at baseline were followed-up to assess two-year incidence of elevated depressive symptoms, defined as a score >8 on the 10-item Center for Epidemiologic Studies Depression (CES-D) scale. After adjustment for demographic data and physical and cognitive functioning, increased risk of depressive symptomatology remained associated with several vascular conditions, including metabolic syndrome and its components, coronary heart disease, a positive questionnaire for angina, and high haemoglobin level. Cumulative vascular risk based upon a composite of 10 vascular diseases and risk factors was independently associated with incident elevated depression at two-year follow-up after controlling for demographic data, physical and cognitive functioning, and selected co-morbid medical conditions. These results provide support for the vascular depression hypothesis in demonstrating an association between vascular conditions and risk factors and subsequent risk of depressive symptomatology. The authors suggest older adults with vascular conditions and risk factors require close monitoring of depressive symptoms[53].

CONCLUSIONS

From all this data there emerge certain conclusions. There are major differences between classification schemes. There is a difference between clinically based diagnosis, whether by humans or computers, and those derived from scale scores. The latter tend to be higher if only because they usually include all participants regardless of diagnosis. They give an estimate of morbidity and co-morbidity, and point to a level of suffering in a community. There is a major difference between diagnostic classifications ostensibly aimed at improving reliability between psychiatrists, so necessary in the 1960s and 1970s in the USA and now elsewhere, and diagnostic classifications such as GMS-AGECAT, which aim to identify cases for intervention. Clearly the evidence is now strong that these are quite different types of cases[54]. Those persons concerned with relieving suffering rather than cutting back on health resources need to take up this cause and those responsible for international classification systems may need to reassess their aims. Has the time come to move from improving reliability between doctors to acknowledge that in vast areas of the globe doctors are not particularly active or apparent and that guidance on suitability for intervention must have a higher priority? That after all is what it is about. No longer is it sensible to hide under the shield of 'they may have symptoms, but do they have disability'? Many excluded from the classifications do have serious disability.

The increase in the number of studies in Asia and South America is gratifying but we need more studies in Africa to persuade governments that mental illness, the hidden illness, is behind much human disability and is treatable.

REFERENCES

1. Beekman ATF, Copeland JRM, Prince MJ. Review of community prevalence of depression in later life. *British Journal of Psychiatry* 1999; **174**: 307–11.
2. Copeland JRM, Beekman ATF, Dewey ME, Hooijer C, Jordan A, Lawlor BA et al. Depression in Europe. Geographical distribution among older people. *Br J Psychiatry* 1999; **174**: 312–21.
3. Ritchie K, Artero S, Beluche I et al. Prevalence of DSM-IV psychiatric disorder in the French elderly population. *Br J Psychiatry* 2004; **184**: 147–52.
4. de Jonge P, Roy JF, Saz P et al. Prevalence and incident depression in community-dwelling elderly persons with diabetes: results from the ZARADEMP project. *Diabetologia* 2006; 49: 2627–33.
5. McDougall FA, Kvaal K, Matthews FE et al. Prevalence of depression in older people in England and Wales: the MRC CFA Study. *Psychol Med* 2007; 37: 1787–95.
6. McDougall FA, Matthews FE, Kvaal K. Prevalence and symptomatology of depression in older people living in institutions in England and Wales. *Age Ageing* 2007; **36**: 562–8.
7. Castro-Costa E, Dewey M, Stewart R et al. Prevalence of depressive symptoms and syndromes in later life in ten European countries: the SHARE study. *Br J Psychiatry* 2007; **191**: 393–401.
8. Eaton WW, Anthony JC, Tepper S et al. Psychopathology and attrition in the epidemiologic catchment areas surveys. *Am J Epidemiology* 1992; **135**(9): 1051–9.
9. de Graaf R, Bijil RV, Smit F et al. Psychiatric and sociodemographic predictors of attrition in a longitudinal study: the Netherlands Mental Health Survey and incidence study (NEMESIS). *American Journal of Epidemiology* 2000; **152**(11): 1039–47.
10. Stek ML, Gussekloo J, Beekman AT et al. Prevalence, correlates and recognition of depression in the oldest old: the Leiden 85-plus study. *J Affect Disord* 2004; **78**: 193–200.
11. van't VP, van Marwijk HW, Jansen AP et al. Depression in old age (75+), the PIKO study. *J Affect Disord* 2008; **106**: 295–9.
12. Intorre F, Maiani G, Cuzzolaro M et al. Descriptive data on lifestyle, anthropometric status and mental health in Italian elderly people. *J Nutr Health Aging* 2007; **11**: 165–74.
13. Jansson M, Gatz M, Berg S et al. Gender differences in heritability of depressive symptoms in the elderly. *Psychol Med* 2004; **34**: 471–9.
14. Wilson K, Mottram P, Sixsmith A. Depressive symptoms in the very old living alone: prevalence, incidence and risk factors. *Int J Geriatr Psychiatry* 2007; **22**: 361–6.
15. Steffens DC, Skoog I, Norton MC et al. Prevalence of depression and its treatment in an elderly population: the Cache County study. *Arch Gen Psychiatry* 2000; **57**: 601–7.
16. Preville M, Boyer R, Grenier S et al. The epidemiology of psychiatric disorders in Quebec's older adult population. *Can J Psychiatry* 2008; **53**: 822–32.
17. Costa E, Barreto SM, Uchoa E et al. Prevalence of International Classification of Diseases, 10th Revision common mental disorders in the elderly in a Brazilian community: the Bambui Health Ageing Study. *Am J Geriatr Psychiatry* 2007; **15**: 17–27.
18. Xavier FM, Ferraza MP, Argimon I et al. The DSM-IV 'minor depression' disorder in the oldest-old: prevalence rate, sleep patterns, memory function and quality of life in elderly people of Italian descent in Southern Brazil. *Int J Geriatr Psychiatry* 2002; **17**: 107–16.
19. Guerra M, Ferri CP, Sosa AL et al. Late-life depression in Peru, Mexico and Venezuela: the 10/66 population-based study. *Br J Psychiatry* 2009; **195**: 510–15.
20. Alvarado BE, Zunzunegui MV, Beland F et al. Social and gender inequalities in depressive symptoms among urban older adults

of Latin America and the Caribbean. *J Gerontol B Psychol Sci Soc Sci* 2007; **62**: 226–36.

21. Heo M, Murphy CF, Fontaine KR *et al*. Population projection of US adults with lifetime experience of depressive disorder by age and sex from year 2005 to 2050. *Int J Geriatr Psychiatry* 2008; **23**: 1266–70.

22. Chen R, Hu Z, Qin X *et al*. A community-based study of depression in older people in Hefei, China – the GMS-AGECAT prevalence, case validation and socioeconomic correlates. *Int J Geriatr Psychiatry* 2004; **19**: 407–13.

23. Chen R, Wei L, Hu Z, *et al*. Depression in older people in rural China. *Arch Intern Med* 2005; **165**: 2019–25.

24. Chong M Y, Tsang HY Chen CS *et al*. Community study of depression in old age in Taiwan: prevalence, life events and socio-demographic correlates. *Br J Psychiatry* 2001; **178**: 29–35.

25. Chen CS, Chong MY, Tsang H Y. Clinically significant non-major depression in a community-dwelling elderly population: epidemiological findings. *Int J Geriatr Psychiatry* 2007; **22**: 557–62.

26. Ma X, Xiang YT, Li SR *et al*. Prevalence and sociodemographic correlates of depression in an elderly population living with family members in Beijing, China. *Psychol Med* 2008; **38**: 1723–30.

27. Pan A, Franco OH, Wang YF. Prevalence and geographic disparity of depressive symptoms among middle-aged and elderly in China. *J Affect Disord* 2008; **105**: 167–75.

28. Li ZB, Ho SY, Chan WM *et al*. Obesity and depressive symptoms in Chinese elderly. *Int J Geriatr Psychiatry* 2004; **19**: 68–74.

29. Chi I, Yip PS, Chiu HF *et al*. Prevalence of depression and its correlates in Hong Kong's Chinese older adults. *Am J Geriatr Psychiatry* 2005; **13**: 409–16.

30. Chou KL, Chi I. Prevalence and correlates of depression in Chinese oldest-old. *Int J Geriatr Psychiatry* 2005; **20**: 41–50.

31. Chiu HC, Chen CM, Huang CJ *et al*. Depressive symptoms, chronic medical conditions and functional status: a comparison of urban and rural elders in Taiwan. *Int J Geriatr Psychiatry* 2005; **20**: 635–44.

32. Tsai YF, Yeh SH, Tsai HH. Prevalence and risk factors for depressive symptoms among community-dwelling elders in Taiwan. *Int J Geriatr Psychiatry* 2005; **20**: 1097–102.

33. Rajkumar AP, Thangadurai P, Senthilkumar P *et al*. Nature, prevalence and factors associated with depression among the elderly in a rural south Indian community. *Int J Geriatr Psychiatry* 2009; **21**: 372–8.

34. Suh G-K. A community study of depression in old age. *J Korean Geriatr Soc* 2005; **9**: 291–300.

35. Ikeda *et al*.

36. Ghubash R, El-Rufaie O, Zoubeidi T *et al*. Profile of mental disorders among the elderly United Arab Emirates population: sociodemographic correlates. *Int J Geriatr Psychiatry* 2004; **19**: 344–51.

37. Wada T, Ishine M, Sakagami T *et al*. Depression, activities of daily living, and quality of life of community-dwelling elderly in three Asian countries: Indonesia, Vietnam, and Japan. *Arch Gerontol Geriatr* 2005; **41**: 271–80.

38. Malhotra R, Chan A, Ostbye, T. Prevalence and correlates of clinically significant depressive symptoms among elderly people

in Sri Lanka: findings from a national survey. *Int Psychogeriatr* 2009; 1–10.

39. Niu K, Hozawa A, Kuriyama S. *et al*. Green tea consumption is associated with depressive symptoms in the elderly. *Am J Clin Nutr* 2009; **90**: 1615–22.

40. Kim JM, Shin IS, Yoon JS *et al*. Prevalence and correlates of late-life depression compared between urban and rural populations in Korea. *Int J Geriatr Psychiatry* 2002; **17**: 409–15.

41. Thongtang O, Sukhatunga K, Ngamthipwatthana T *et al*. Prevalence and incidence of depression in the Thai elderly. *J Med Assoc Thai* 2002; **85**: 540–4.

42. Gureje O, Kola L, Afolabi E. Epidemiology of major depressive disorder in elderly Nigerians in the Ibadan Study of Ageing: a community-based survey. *Lancet* 2007; **370**: 957–64.

43. Baiyewu O, Smith-Gamble V, Lane KA *et al*. Prevalence estimates of depression in elderly community-dwelling African Americans in Indianapolis and Yoruba in Ibadan, Nigeria. *Int Psychogeriatr* 2007; **19**: 679–89.

44. Snowdon J, Lane F. The prevalence and outcome of depression and dementia in Botany's elderly population. *Int J Geriatr Psychiatry* 2001; **16**: 293–9.

45. Rorsman B, Gransbeck A, Hagnell O *et al*. Prospective study of first incidence depression: the Lundby study, 1957-1972. *British Journal of psychiatry* 1990; **156**: 336–42.

46. Eaton WW, Anthony JC, Gallo J *et al*. Natural history of Diagnostic Interview Schedule/DSM-IV major depression. The Baltimore Epidemiologic Catchment Area follow-up. *Archives of General Psychiatry* 1997; **54**: 993–9.

47. Thongtang O, Sukhatunga K, Ngamthipwatthana T *et al*.. Prevalence and incidence of depression in the Thai elderly. *J Med Assoc Thai* 2002; **85**: 540–4.

48. Kim JM, Stewart R, Kim SW *et al*. Modification by two genes of associations between general somatic health and incident depressive syndrome in older people. *Psychosom Med* 2009; **71**: 286–91.

49. Mossaheb N, Weissgram S, Zehetmayer S *et al*.. Late-onset depression in elderly subjects from the Vienna Transdanube Aging (VITA) study. *J Clin Psychiatry* 2009; **70**: 500–8.

50. Harris T, Cook DG, Victor C *et al*. onset and persistence of depression in older people – results from a 2-year community follow-up study. *Age Ageing* 2006; **35**: 25–32.

51. Luijendijk HJ, van den Berg JF, Dekker MJ *et al*.. Incidence and recurrence of late-life depression. *Arch Gen Psychiatry* 2008; **65**: 1394–401.

52. Giltay EJ, Zitman FG, Kromhout D. Dispositional optimism and the risk of depressive symptoms during 15 years of follow-up: the Zutphen Elderly Study. *J Affect Disord* 2006; **91**: 45–52.

53. Mast BT, Miles T, Penninx BW *et al*. Vascular disease and future risk of depressive symptomatology in older adults: findings from the Health, Aging, and Body Composition study. *Biol Psychiatry* 2008; **64**: 320–6.

54. Copeland JRM. What is a case, a case for what? In Wing JK, Bebbington P, Robbins LN, McIntyre G. (eds), *What is a Case? The Problems of Definition in Psychiatric Community Surveys*. London, 1981, 7–11.

78

Neuroimaging in Geriatric Depression

Faith M. Gunning

Institute of Geriatric Psychiatry, Department of Psychiatry, Weill Cornell Medical College, USA

OVERVIEW

Geriatric depression is a complex and heterogeneous syndrome that likely has multiple environmental and biological determinants. Among these, structural and functional abnormalities in specific cerebral networks likely confer vulnerability that increases the likelihood of developing geriatric depression. The aetiology of such brain abnormalities may be diverse and likely results from processes commonly occurring in older adults including cerebral ageing, vascular, inflammatory, autoimmune and endocrine processes[1].

Significant effort has been devoted to characterizing alterations that occur in the brains of elderly depressed patients. In this chapter, we discuss work using a number of different neuroimaging modalities to advance our understanding of the neurobiology of late-life depression. In addition, when data exist, we will examine the question of how these neuroimaging correlates of late-life depression relate to specific features of the illness, including the presence of cognitive deficits and the course of the illness.

VOLUMETRIC STUDIES

Volume reductions are often present on T1-weighted magnetic resonance imaging (MRI) in the brains of elderly depressed patients in select frontal, limbic and subcortical regions. These regions include the anterior cingulate cortex, the orbitofrontal cortex, the neostriatum, the hippocampus and the amygdala[2-11]. The anterior cingulate cortex and orbitofrontal regions demonstrate the most consistent alterations. MRI-based parcellation of prefrontal regions in elder depressed patients confirms that relative to elderly control subjects, there are significant attenuations of grey and white matter in the anterior cingulate cortex and the gyrus rectus, as well as reductions of grey matter in the orbitofrontal cortex[12].

In addition to the presence of volumetric differences between elderly depressed patients and non-depressed individuals, there is evidence that specific clinical characteristics of the illness may be related to volumes of select regions[2,7,13-15]. For example, reduced amygdala volumes have been reported in recurrent depression[15]. In addition, one of the early studies to use voxel-based morphometry (VBM), revealed that smaller hippocampal volumes in elderly depressed patients were associated with greater number of years since first depressive episode[13]. Furthermore, apathy has been associated with smaller volume of the right anterior cingulate

cortex in elderly subjects, although this may not be specific to depressed patients[16]. Finally, antidepressant medication itself may impact regional brain volumes. Lavretsky and colleagues[7] observed that orbitofrontal grey-matter volumes were larger in patients with geriatric depression who had been treated with antidepressant medication relative to drug-naive patients, although these volumes were smaller than those of age-matched controls.

Although most of the volumetric studies in late-life depression have focused on specific regions of interest (ROIs), a study by Andreescu and colleagues[2] applied an automatic labelling pathway technique to 24 ROIs to examine the relationship of volumes of grey-matter regions in elderly depressed patients to age of onset and duration of illness. Relative to non-depressed subjects, elderly depressed patients had smaller volumes in 17 of the ROIs examined. Both shorter duration of illness and later age of onset were correlated with smaller volumes of parahippocampal and inferior parietal ROIs. However, a later age of onset was also correlated with smaller volumes of several frontal and temporal ROIs, the cingulum and the putamen. These findings were interpreted to support the hypothesis that small volumes in late-life depression may be more related to neurodegenerative changes than the result of a toxic stress response[2].

In cross-sectional studies of geriatric depression, poor performance on tasks of episodic memory and executive functions have been associated with reduced volume of the hippocampus and select prefrontal regions[8,17]. In one study of late-life depression, volumes from specific ROIs within the prefrontal cortex were calculated and related to performance on a battery of executive measures[17]. Poorer performance on tests of response inhibition was associated with smaller anterior cingulate volumes, whereas poorer performance in nonverbal inductive reasoning tasks were associated with smaller gyrus rectus volumes[17]. Longitudinal studies of the hippocampus, indicate that smaller hippocampal volumes predict MCI and subsequent dementia[8,9].

There is little published data about the relationship of MRI volumes to response of late-life depression to treatment. However, in one study of elderly non-demented depressed patients, the relationship of remission status following treatment with escitalopram and volume of subregions of the anterior cingulate cortex was evaluated. Regional anterior cingulate volumes were manually outlined (dorsal, rostral, anterior subgenual and posterior subgenual) on high-resolution T1-weighted images. Analyses revealed that patients who failed to remit following escitalopram treatment had smaller dorsal

Principles and Practice of Geriatric Psychiatry, 3rd edn. Edited by Mohammed T. Abou-Saleh, Cornelius Katona and Anand Kumar
© 2011 John Wiley & Sons, Ltd

and rostral anterior cingulate grey-matter volumes than patients who remitted, whereas subgenual cortical volumes did not differ between the groups[18].

Volumetric differences in elderly depressed patients tend to be small and the relationship to clinical variables, when significant, tend to be modest in strength. More sophisticated shape analysis and/or 3D surface mapping may be used to better localize structural abnormalities in late-life depression[4]. For example, the caudate nucleus was examined using traditional volumetry and a 3D brain-mapping technique in a group of patients with late-life depression and non-depressed elderly comparison subjects. Relative to comparison subjects, depressed subjects had significantly lower mean caudate volumes bilaterally. Furthermore, the 3D maps localized these reductions in volume to the caudate head and volume reductions were correlated with depression severity[4]. Another study used shape analysis to examine the amygdala in a small group of healthy elderly individuals and elderly depressed individuals. Although no significant volumetric differences were found for either amygdala, regions of specific shape variation were detected. The most notable difference was contraction of the amygdala in depressed patients relative to comparison subjects in a region associated with the basolateral nucleus[19].

A number of methodological issues must be considered when interpreting morphometry studies. The specific neurohistological processes that account for the observed volume reductions in late-life depression cannot be distinguished. In addition, manual ROI morphometry is quite time consuming and a lack of standard guidelines used for delineation of ROIs across laboratories may contribute to differences between studies. VBM can overcome some of these weaknesses because of the relative ease with which it can be carried out, as well as its ability to examine the entire brain at once. However, VBM studies of ageing brains may be particularly problematic because of the requirement that MR images are transformed from native space to standardized stereotaxic space and this space is most often defined by a template that reflects a young, healthy brain. Approaches that apply templated ROI maps to MRI data in native space may increase both reliability and validity of findings from VBM studies.

Even within the context of the limitations of morphometry, the studies to date reveal a pattern of frontostriatal and limbic abnormalities, with some evidence that such abnormalities may be associated with the clinical presentation and perhaps even the course and outcome of the illness. In future studies, advancements in techniques (e.g. shape analysis) may facilitate more precise localization of structural anomalies in late-life depression.

WHITE MATTER INTEGRITY IN LATE-LIFE DEPRESSION

White-Matter Hyperintensities

Traditionally, the most common method to study white-matter abnormalities on MRI has been the examination of white-matter hyperintensities (WMH). These WMH are typically observed in T2-weighted sequences and are taken to indicate white-matter damage. They can be discrete, or punctate, or may appear more confluent with the lateral ventricles.

WMH are more frequent and severe in older depressed individuals than in age-matched controls and occur most often in subcortical grey-matter regions and frontal white-matter projections[10,20–26].

Even in cognitively intact individuals, WMH are often associated with subtle cognitive deficits, particularly executive dysfunction and slowed processing speed[27–30]. Furthermore, in elderly depressed patients, increases in WMH volumes at longitudinal follow-up predict the development of dementia, especially among non-Alzheimer type dementias[31].

Some studies suggest that WMH also may influence the course of affective symptoms in late-life depression. For example, longitudinal CHS data found that large cortical white-matter lesions and severe subcortical lesions were significant risk factors for developing depressive symptoms[9]. Furthermore, WMH burden and subcortical grey-matter hyperintensities have been associated with response to both ECT[32,33] and antidepressant treatment[32,34] although disagreement exists[35,36]. One report indicated that basal ganglia lesions predicted failure to respond to antidepressant monotherapy with a sensitivity of 80% and a specificity of 62%[37].

Neuropathological correlates of WMH in brains of elderly depressed individuals provide rather compelling support for a vascular contribution to the pathophysiology of late-life depression. In a study of neuropathological correlates of WMH in 20 depressed patients and 20 elderly comparison subjects (see[38–40]), all of the deep WMH examined in the depressed subjects showed evidence of ischaemia compared with less than a third of deep WMH in control subjects. Whereas large deep WMH were usually ischaemic in both groups, punctate lesions were typically characterized by ischaemia in depressed patients but not in controls. Periventricular WMH were characterized by ependymal loss, varying degrees of demyelination and cerebral ischaemia with no differences in pathological correlates detected between patients and controls[41]. Furthermore, in the depressed subjects, the ischaemic DWMH showed a striking predilection for the dorsolateral prefrontal white matter[40].

The methods of quantifying WMH are characterized by some of the same limitations as morphometry studies. That is, there are a number of different WMH rating scales and these scales vary widely in reliability and sensitivity. Also, postmortem studies of WMH suggest that such white-matter abnormalities reflect a number of pathological processes; however, MRI scans do not always allow a reliable discrimination among the underlying processes. Although recent advancements in measurement (i.e. volumetric measurements and regional WMH measurements) partially address these limitations, the introduction of newer MRI techniques to examine white-matter integrity may help to achieve not only better differentiation between true white-matter lesions and spurious findings, but will also help to identify the location of white-matter abnormalities and perhaps clarify their underlying causes.

MRI STUDIES OF MICROSTRUCTURAL WHITE-MATTER ABNORMALITIES

Diffusion Tensor Imaging

Diffusion tensor imaging (DTI) offers a promising approach for the examination of cerebral white-matter integrity in geriatric depression. DTI measures the magnitude and direction of self-diffusion of water. When no barriers to such diffusion are present, diffusion occurs equally in all directions (i.e. it is isotropic). However, when barriers to this diffusion are present, the diffusion tends to follow the long axis of those barriers (i.e. diffusion is anisotropic). Barriers to diffusion in the brain include cell membranes, myelin sheaths and white-matter fibre tracts. Diffusion anisotropy can be quantified by a number of different metrics, including fractional anisotropy (FA). FA, which ranges in value from 0 to 1, is a measure of the strength of the directional dependence of diffusion and generally reflects the organization of fibre tracts. In regions with dense, highly organized fibres (e.g. the corpus callosum) FA values are the highest.

Commensurate with the morphometry findings of reduced volumes of select frontostriatal and limbic regions, DTI studies reveal that depressed elderly patients exhibit compromised integrity (i.e. reduced FA) of the white matter of prefrontal regions and the anterior cingulate[42,43], perhaps within the context of more subtle, widespread white-matter abnormalities[44]. A study that explored the relationship of diastolic blood pressure and FA in elderly depressed patients revealed significant associations between FA and diastolic blood pressure throughout the anterior cingulate and in multiple additional frontotemporal and frontostriatal white-matter regions[45]. These findings, albeit preliminary, suggest that reduced microstructural integrity of frontal-subcortical white matter may be one of the mechanisms by which high blood pressure, a known vascular risk factor, confers vulnerability to geriatric depression.

Regarding cognitive correlates of FA in geriatric depression, one study has examined the relationship of FA in depressed elders to performance on an executive task[46]. Response inhibition, one aspect of executive function that has been shown to predict antidepressant response[47], was assessed with the Stroop colour-word task. Voxelwise correlational analysis revealed significant associations between FA and Stroop colour-word interference in multiple frontostriatal-limbic regions, including white matter lateral to the anterior and posterior cingulate cortex and white matter in prefrontal, insular and parahippocampal regions.

In addition to a relationship between FA and response inhibition, there is evidence that lower FA in distributed cerebral networks is associated with poor antidepressant response of geriatric depression[48], although some disagreement exists[49]. Furthermore, a preliminary study of the association of the serotonin transporter gene status to both FA and response to antidepressant treatment indicated that depressed elderly S-allele carriers had lower FA than L homozygotes in frontolimbic brain areas, including the dorsal and rostral anterior cingulate, posterior cingulate, dorsolateral prefrontal and medial prefrontal regions[50]. S-allele carriers also had a lower remission rate than L homozygotes, introducing the possibility that the risk for chronicity of geriatric depression in S-allele carriers may be mediated by frontolimbic white-matter compromise.

Magnetization Transfer Imaging

Magnetization transfer ratio (MTR) is another method that can be used to study white-matter integrity in geriatric depression. MTR imaging provides information about the macromolecular structure of cerebral white matter based on the interaction of the normally observed tissue water signal with protons contained in large macromolecules (including myelin). Macromolecular structures in the brain (e.g. myelinated axons) are ordinarily not detected by MRI because of their extremely short transverse relaxation times. However, protons bound to them can be selectively excited using off-resonance radio-frequency pulses. To achieve MTR contrast, two MR sequences are used. The first is a proton density (PD) weighted sequence, which reflects the total water signal. The second uses an additional pulse prior to the basic proton density sequence and serves to null the signal from water molecules that are associated with macromolecules. The percent contrast difference between the two image

sets is usually expressed as the magnetization transfer ratio: MTR = (M0 − MSAT)/M0. Reduced MTR reflects reduced macromolecular volume fraction. Studies conducted in neurodevelopment and multiple sclerosis suggest that DTI and MTR may provide complementary information about white-matter integrity with DTI mostly reflecting organization of fibre tracts and MTR being particularly sensitive to myelin and axonal integrity[51,52].

Kumar and colleagues[53] were the first to demonstrate the use of MTR in geriatric depression. Their results from a small study of elderly depressed patients suggest that, relative to their elderly counterparts, older depressed patients have lower MTR in the genu and splenium of the corpus callosum, the neostriatum and the occipital white matter. In a larger study of elderly patients with major depression and elderly non-psychiatric comparison subjects, we reported lower MTR in multiple left hemisphere frontostriatal and limbic regions, including dorsolateral, dorsomedial, dorsal anterior cingulate, insula, periamygdalar, subcallosal, posterior cingulate and regions lateral to the lentiform nuclei[54]. However, there have been no studies published to date that have reported the relationship of MTR to features of depressive illnesses in the elderly.

FUNCTIONAL NEUROIMAGING STUDIES

Functional neuroimaging studies in late-life depression reveal a pattern of abnormal activation of frontolimbic regions, generally characterized by hypoactivation of specific dorsal cortical regions and hyperactivation of select limbic regions. One of the first published reports of task-related activation in geriatric depression, reported results of a PET study that compared cerebral blood flow during a word activation task between elderly patients with severe depression and normal elders. During the word activation task, hypoactivation of the dorsal ACC and the hippocampus was detected[55]. This finding of attenuated activation of the dorsal ACC during a verbal fluency task was later replicated by another group in an fMRI study of older depressed individuals in remission who had experienced multiple previous episodes of depression[56]. In depressed elderly patients, relative to age-matched controls, Aizenstein and colleagues[57] reported decreased prefrontal activation in addition to increased caudate activation in response to an explicit sequence learning task.

Emerging evidence from functional neuroimaging studies suggests that select frontolimbic structures are not only abnormally activated in late-life depression, but these abnormalities are related to clinical features of the illness. For example, in a preliminary study of late-life anxious depression, subjects completed an executive control task. Relative to elderly depressed patients, elderly subjects with anxious depression produced a significantly greater and more sustained signal in the dorsal anterior cingulate, posterior cingulate and lateral prefrontal cortex. These preliminary results not only suggest specific activation patterns unique to anxious depression but also demonstrate the utility of using fMRI to examine the neurobiology of clinical subtypes of late-life depression[58].

Regarding the relationship of illness state to frontolimbic activation, an fMRI study of elderly depressed patients using an emotional oddball task reported that relative to healthy comparison subjects, the elderly depressed patients demonstrated attenuated activation in select frontolimbic regions, including the right middle frontal gyrus and the cingulate, as well as the inferior parietal cortex. Activation in the middle frontal gyrus appeared depressive state-related, whereas attenuated activation in the posterior cingulate and inferior parietal regions persisted in the remitted subjects, consistent with a disease-related alteration[59].

In a study examining the relationship of cerebral activation to course of illness, acutely depressed patients exhibited hypoactivation of the ventromedial prefrontal cortex in response to the emotional evaluation of negatively-valenced relative to positively-valenced words. However, this hypoactivation normalized after several months of uncontrolled antidepressant treatment[60]. Furthermore, in a controlled, antidepressant treatment trial, during a cognitive control task elderly depressed patients demonstrated hypoactivation in the dorsolateral prefrontal cortex and diminished functional connectivity between the dorsolateral prefrontal cortex and dorsal ACC prior to treatment[61]. Although this hypoactivity in the right dorsolateral prefrontal cortex subsided after successful antidepressant treatment, the reduced functional connectivity between the dorsal ACC and the DLPFC persisted.

Taken together, the functional neuoroimaging results indicate that abnormal frontolimbic activation is present in elderly depressed patients during the depressed state and these abnormalities may normalize, at least in part, in response to antidepressant treatment.

MAGNETIC RESONANCE SPECTROSCOPY

Magnetic resonance spectroscopy (MRS) provides important information about the neurochemical environment. Different molecules have unique MR spectra that can be quantified by taking the area under the signal curve. In most cases, the values are not absolute, so it is customary to take ratios of the measure of interest to some standard metabolite, for example choline.

Kumar and colleagues[62] used MRS to examine biochemical abnormalities in left frontal WM and bilateral anterior cingulate grey matter of elderly depressed patients. They observed higher choline to creatine as well as myoinositol to creatine ratios in the white, but not grey, matter of patents relative to age-matched comparison subjects. Results from a follow-up MRS study suggested that cognitive performance was associated with levels of metabolites as measured by 2D MRS in healthy controls, but not in patients with geriatric depression[63]. There was a significant difference in the overall pattern of associations between the four measured metabolites and verbal learning and processing speed in elderly depressed patients compared to elderly controls. The weaker relationship between metabolites and specific cognitive domains in patients with late-life major depressive disorder was interpreted by the authors to suggest that cognitive performance in geriatric depression may be associated with biochemical changes in frontostriatal circuitry.

In a recent study of elderly depressed patients and age-matched control subjects, MRS spectra were acquired from voxels that were placed in the left frontal white matter, left periventricular white matter and left basal ganglia. Results indicate that elderly depressed patients had significantly lower NAA/creatine ratio in the left frontal white matter and higher choline/creatine and myoinositol/creatine ratios in the left basal ganglia when compared with the control subjects. Furthermore, the myoinositol correlated with global cognitive function among the patients[64].

Most recently, MRS was used to examine biochemical correlates of response to antidepressant treatment[65]. Using a 3D chemical shift imaging sequence, tissue-specific differences in markers of energy metabolism, including high-energy phosphate compounds (beta and total NTP, PCr) and pH, were examined in 13 older adults with major depression pre and post 12 weeks of treatment with sertraline and 10 age-matched controls. Total NTP was reduced in the white matter, but not in the grey matter, in the depressed group prior to treatment depression group. Intracellular pH was higher in the grey matter of subjects with pre-treatment depression but similar to levels of controls after treatment[65].

Although there are only a handful of published reports that have used MRS to examine the neurochemical environment in geriatric depression, this appears to be a promising technique that, especially if used in combination with other measures of tissue integrity (e.g. DTI), is likely to be a quite powerful tool to advance our understanding of the neurobiology of late-life depression.

CONCLUSIONS AND FUTURE DIRECTIONS

For more than two decades, scientists have taken advantage of the remarkable capacity of neuroimaging to visualize and quantify patterns of cerebral abnormalities in psychiatric illnesses. As with many features of psychiatric illnesses, MRI observations are notable for the variability of findings between studies. However, when considering evidence from multiple MRI modalities across the numerous studies that have been performed, a general pattern of findings has emerged. This pattern is characterized by compromise in the structure of select aspects of frontostriatal and limbic networks coupled with hypoactivation of cortical regions critical for cognitive control and hyperactivation of limbic structures involved in emotional reactivity. Both structural compromise and abnormal activation in frontolimbic systems appear to be associated with poor response to antidepressants. These findings that relate MRI indices to antidepressant response raise the possibility that structural abnormalities may interfere with the normalization of frontolimbic activity in individuals who fail to respond adequately to antidepressants. While each neuroimaging technique alone has limitations, the concurrent application of more than one technique yielding complementary information can increase the information gleaned from future neuroimaging observations and significantly advance our understanding of the pathophysiology of depression in the elderly.

ACKNOWLEDGEMENTS

This work was supported by the National Institute of Mental Health grant K23 MH074818.

REFERENCES

1. Alexopoulos GS. Depression in the elderly. *Lancet* 2005; **365**(9475): 1961–70.
2. Andreescu C, Butters MA, Begley A, Rajji T, Wu M, Meltzer CC et al. Gray matter changes in late life depression – a structural MRI analysis. *Neuropsychopharmacology* 2008; **33**(11): 2566–72.
3. Ballmaier M, Narr KL, Toga AW, Elderkin-Thompson V, Thompson PM, Hamilton L et al. Hippocampal morphology and distinguishing late-onset from early-onset elderly depression. *Am J Psychiatry* 2008; **165**(2): 229–37.
4. Butters MA, Aizenstein HJ, Hayashi KM, Meltzer CC, Seaman J, Reynolds CFr et al. Three-dimensional surface mapping of the caudate nucleus in late-life depression. *Am J Geriatr Psychiatry* 2009; **17**(1): 4–12.
5. Krishnan KR, McDonald WM, Escalona PR, Doraiswamy PM, Na C, Husain MM et al. Magnetic resonance imaging of the caudate nuclei in depression. Preliminary observations. *Arch Gen Psychiatry* 1992; **49**(7): 553–7.

6. Lai T, Payne ME, Byrum CE, Steffens DC, Krishnan KR. Reduction of orbital frontal cortex volume in geriatric depression. *Biol Psychiatry* 2000; **48**(10): 971–5.

7. Lavretsky H, Roybal DJ, Ballmaier M, Toga AW, Kumar A. Antidepressant exposure may protect against decrement in frontal gray matter volumes in geriatric depression. *J Clin Psychiatry* 2005; **66**(8): 694–7.

8. O'Brien JT, Lloyd A, McKeith I, Gholkar A, Ferrier N. A longitudinal study of hippocampal volume, cortisol levels and cognition in older depressed subjects. *Am J Psychiatry* 2004; **161**(11): 2081–90.

9. Steffens DC, Payne ME, Greenberg DL, Byrum CE, Welsh-Bohmer KA, Wagner HR *et al.* Hippocampal volume and incident dementia in geriatric depression. *Am J Geriatr Psychiatry* 2002; **10**(1): 62–71.

10. Taylor WD, Steffens DC, McQuoid DR, Payne ME, Lee SH, Lai TJ *et al.* Smaller orbital frontal cortex volumes associated with functional disability in depressed elders. *Biol Psychiatry* 2003; **53**(2): 144–9.

11. Kumar A, Bilker W, Jin Z, Udupa J. Atrophy and high intensity lesions: complementary neurobiological mechanisms in late-life major depression. *Neuropsychopharmacology* 2000; **22**(3): 264–74.

12. Ballmaier M, Toga AW, Blanton RE, Sowell ER, Lavretsky H, Peterson J *et al.* Anterior cingulate, gyrus rectus and orbitofrontal abnormalities in elderly depressed patients: an MRI-based parcellation of the prefrontal cortex. *Am J Psychiatry* 2004; **161**(1): 99–108.

13. Bell-McGinty S, Butters MA, Meltzer CC, Greer PJ, Reynolds CFr, Becker JT. Brain morphometric abnormalities in geriatric depression: long-term neurobiological effects of illness duration. *Am J Psychiatry* 2002; **159**(8): 1424–7.

14. Egger K, Schocke M, Weiss E, Auffinger S, Esterhammer R, Goebel G *et al.* Pattern of brain atrophy in elderly patients with depression revealed by voxel-based morphometry. *Psychiatry Res* 2008; **164**(3): 237–44.

15. Sheline YI, Gado MH, Price JL. Amygdala core nuclei volumes are decreased in recurrent major depression. *Neuroreport* 1998; **9**(9): 2023–8.

16. Lavretsky H, Ballmaier M, Pham D, Toga A, Kumar A. Neuroanatomical characteristics of geriatric apathy and depression: a magnetic resonance imaging study. *Am J Geriatr Psychiatry* 2007; **15**(5): 386–94.

17. Elderkin-Thompson V, Hellemann G, Pham D, Kumar A. Prefrontal brain morphology and executive function in healthy and depressed elderly. *Int J Geriatr Psychiatry* 2009; **24**(5): 459–68.

18. Gunning FM, Cheng J, Murphy CF, Kanellopoulos D, Acuna J, Hoptman MJ *et al.* Anterior cingulate cortical volumes and treatment remission of geriatric depression. *Int J Geriatr Psychiatry* 2009; **24**(8): 829–36.

19. Tamburo RJ, Siegle GJ, Stetten GD, Cois CA, Butters MA, Reynolds CFr *et al.* Amygdalae morphometry in late-life depression. *Int J Geriatr Psychiatry* 2009; **24**(8): 837–46.

20. Coffey CE, Figiel GS, Djang WT, Weiner RD. Subcortical hyperintensity on magnetic resonance imaging: a comparison of normal and depressed elderly subjects. *Am J Psychiatry* 1990; **147**(2): 187–9.

21. Greenwald BS, Kramer-Ginsberg E, Krishnan RR, Ashtari M, Aupperle PM, Patel M. MRI signal hyperintensities in geriatric depression. *Am J Psychiatry* 1996; **153**(9): 1212–5.

22. Krishnan KR. Neuroanatomic substrates of depression in the elderly. *J Geriatr Psychiatry Neurol* 1993; **6**(1): 39–58.

23. Krishnan KR, Hays JC, Blazer DG. MRI-defined vascular depression. *Am J Psychiatry* 1997; **154**(4): 497–501.

24. O'Brien J, Desmond P, Ames D, Schweitzer I, Harrigan S, Tress B. A magnetic resonance imaging study of white matter lesions in depression and Alzheimer's disease. *Br J Psychiatry* 1996; **168**(4): 477–85.

25. O'Brien JT, Firbank MJ, Krishnan MS, van Straaten EC, van der Flier WM, Petrovic K *et al.* White matter hyperintensities rather than lacunar infarcts are associated with depressive symptoms in older people: the LADIS study. *Am J Geriatr Psychiatry* 2006; **14**(10): 834–41.

26. Tupler LA, Krishnan KR, McDonald WM, Dombeck CB, D'Souza S, Steffens DC. Anatomic location and laterality of MRI signal hyperintensities in late-life depression. *J Psychosom Res* 2002; **53**(2): 665–76.

27. Boone KB, Miller BL, Lesser IM, Mehringer CM, Hill-Gutierrez E, Goldberg MA *et al.* Neuropsychological correlates of white-matter lesions in healthy elderly subjects. A threshold effect. *Arch Neurol* 1992; **49**(5): 549–54.

28. Gunning-Dixon FM, Raz N. The cognitive correlates of white matter abnormalities in normal aging: a quantitative review. *Neuropsychology* 2000; **14**(2): 224–32.

29. Gunning-Dixon FM, Raz N. Neuroanatomical correlates of selected executive functions in middle-aged and older adults: a prospective MRI study. *Neuropsychologia* 2003; **41**(14): 1929–41.

30. Lesser I, Boone K, Mehringer C, Wohl M, Miller B, Berman N. Cognition and white matter hyperintensities in older depressed patients. *Am J Psychiatry* 1996; **153**(10): 1280–7.

31. Steffens DC, Potter GG, McQuoid DR, MacFall JR, Payne ME, Burke JR *et al.* Longitudinal magnetic resonance imaging vascular changes, apolipoprotein E genotype and development of dementia in the neurocognitive outcomes of depression in the elderly study. *Am J Geriatr Psychiatry* 2007; **15**(10): 839–49.

32. Hickie I, Scott E, Mitchell P, Wilhelm K, Austin M, Bennett B. Subcortical hyperintensities on magnetic resonance imaging: clinical correlates and prognostic significance in patients with severe depression. *Biol Psychiatry* 1995; **37**(3): 151–60.

33. Steffens DC, Conway CR, Dombeck CB, Wagner HR, Tupler LA, Weiner RD. Severity of subcortical gray matter hyperintensity predicts ECT response in geriatric depression. *J ECT* 2001; **17**(1): 45–9.

34. Simpson S, Baldwin RC, Jackson A, Burns AS. Is subcortical disease associated with a poor response to antidepressants? Neurological, neuropsychological and neuroradiological findings in late-life depression. *Psychol Med* 1998; **28**(5): 1015–26.

35. Janssen J, Hulshoff Pol HE, Schnack HG, Kok RM, Lampe IK, de Leeuw FE *et al.* Cerebral volume measurements and subcortical white matter lesions and short-term treatment response in late life depression. *Int J Geriatr Psychiatry* 2007; **22**(5): 468–74.

36. Salloway S, Boyle PA, Correia S, Malloy PF, Cahn-Weiner DA, Schneider L *et al.* The relationship of MRI subcortical hyperintensities to treatment response in a trial of sertraline in geriatric depressed outpatients. *Am J Geriatr Psychiatry* 2002; **10**(1): 107–11.

37. Patankar TF, Baldwin R, Mitra D, Jeffries S, Sutcliffe C, Burns A *et al.* Virchow-Robin space dilatation may predict resistance to antidepressant monotherapy in elderly patients with depression. *J Affect Disord* 2007; **97**(1–3): 265–70.

38. Thomas AJ, O'Brien JT, Davis S, Ballard C, Barber R, Kalaria RN et al. Ischemic basis for deep white matter hyperintensities in major depression: a neuropathological study. *Arch Gen Psychiatry* 2002; **59**(9): 785–92.

39. Thomas AJ, Perry R, Barber R, Kalaria RN, O'Brien JT. Pathologies and pathological mechanisms for white matter hyperintensities in depression. *Ann N Y Acad Sci* 2002; **977**: 333–9.

40. Thomas AJ, Perry R, Kalaria RN, Oakley A, McMeekin W, O'Brien JT. Neuropathological evidence for ischemia in the white matter of the dorsolateral prefrontal cortex in late-life depression. *Int J Geriatr Psychiatry* 2003; **18**(1): 7–13.

41. Thomas AJ, O'Brien JT, Barber R, McMeekin W, Perry R. A neuropathological study of periventricular white matter hyperintensities in major depression. *J Affect Disord* 2003; **76**(1–3): 49–54.

42. Bae JN, Macfall JR, Krishnan KR, Payne ME, Steffens DC, Taylor WD. Dorsolateral prefrontal cortex and anterior cingulate cortex white matter alterations in late-life depression. *Biol Psychiatry* 2006; **27**.

43. Taylor WD, MacFall JR, Payne ME, McQuoid DR, Provenzale JM, Steffens DC et al. Late-life depression and microstructural abnormalities in dorsolateral prefrontal cortex white matter. *Am J Psychiatry* 2004; **161**(7): 1293–6.

44. Shimony JS, Sheline YI, D'Angelo G, Epstein AA, Benzinger TL, Mintun MA et al. Diffuse microstructural abnormalities of normal-appearing white matter in late life depression: a diffusion tensor imaging study. *Biol Psychiatry* 2009; **66**(3): 245–52.

45. Hoptman MJ, Gunning-Dixon FM, Murphy CF, Ardekani BA, Hrabe J, Lim KO et al. Blood pressure and white matter integrity in geriatric depression. *J Affect Disord* 2009; **115**(1–2): 171–6.

46. Murphy CF, Gunning-Dixon FM, Hoptman MJ, Lim KO, Ardekani B, Shields JK et al. White-matter integrity predicts stroop performance in patients with geriatric depression. *Biol Psychiatry* 2007; **61**(8): 1007–10.

47. Alexopoulos GS, Kiosses DN, Heo M, Murphy CF, Shanmugham B, Gunning-Dixon F. Executive dysfunction and the course of geriatric depression. *Biol Psychiatry* 2005; **58**(3): 204–10.

48. Alexopoulos GS, Murphy CF, Gunning-Dixon FM, Latoussakis V, Kanellopoulos D, Klimstra S et al. Microstructural white matter abnormalities and remission of geriatric depression. *Am J Psychiatry* 2008; **165**(2): 238–44.

49. Taylor WD, Kuchibhatla M, Payne ME, Macfall JR, Sheline YI, Krishnan KR et al. Frontal white matter anisotropy and antidepressant remission in late-life depression. *PLoS One* 2008; **3**(9): e3267.

50. Alexopoulos GS, Murphy CF, Gunning-Dixon FM, Glatt CE, Latoussakis V, Kelly REJ et al. Serotonin transporter polymorphisms, microstructural white matter abnormalities and remission of geriatric depression. *J Affect Disord* 2009; **119**(1–3): 132–41.

51. Hoptman MJ, Gunning-Dixon FM, Murphy CF, Lim KO, Alexopoulos GS. Structural neuroimaging research methods in geriatric depression. *Am J Geriatr Psychiatry* 2006; **14**(10): 812–22.

52. Wozniak JR, Lim KO. Advances in white matter imaging: a review of in vivo magnetic resonance methodologies and their applicability to the study of development and aging. *Neurosci Biobehav Rev* 2006; **30**(6): 762–74.

53. Kumar A, Gupta RC, Albert Thomas M, Alger J, Wyckoff N, Hwang S. Biophysical changes in normal-appearing white matter and subcortical nuclei in late-life major depression detected using magnetization transfer. *Psychiatry Res* 2004; **130**(2): 131–40.

54. Gunning-Dixon FM, Hoptman MJ, Lim KO, Murphy CF, Klimstra S, Latoussakis V et al. Macromolecular white matter abnormalities in geriatric depression: a magnetization transfer imaging study. *Am J Geriatr Psychiatry* 2008; **16**(4): 255–62.

55. de Asis JM, Stern E, Alexopoulos GS, Pan H, Van Gorp W, Blumberg H et al. Hippocampal and anterior cingulate activation deficits in patients with geriatric depression. *Am J Psychiatry* 2001; **158**(8): 1321–3.

56. Takami H, Okamoto Y, Yamashita H, Okada G, Yamawaki S. Attenuated anterior cingulate activation during a verbal fluency task in elderly patients with a history of multiple-episode depression. *Am J Geriatr Psychiatry* 2007; **15**(7): 594–603.

57. Aizenstein HJ, Butters MA, Figurski JL, Stenger VA, Reynolds CF, 3rd, Carter CS. Prefrontal and striatal activation during sequence learning in geriatric depression. *Biol Psychiatry* 2005; **58**(4): 290–6.

58. Andreescu C, Butters M, Lenze EJ, Venkatraman VK, Nable M, Reynolds CFr et al. fMRI activation in late-life anxious depression: a potential biomarker. *Int J Geriatr Psychiatry* 2009; **24**(8): 820–8.

59. Wang L, Krishnan KR, Steffens DC, Potter GG, Dolcos F, McCarthy G. Depressive state- and disease-related alterations in neural responses to affective and executive challenges in geriatric depression. *Am J Psychiatry* 2008; **165**(7): 863–71.

60. Brassen S, Kalisch R, Weber-Fahr W, Braus DF, Buchel C. Ventromedial prefrontal cortex processing during emotional evaluation in late-life depression: a longitudinal functional magnetic resonance imaging study. *Biol Psychiatry* 2008; **28**.

61. Aizenstein HJ, Butters MA, Wu M, Mazurkewicz LM, Stenger VA, Gianaros PJ et al. Altered functioning of the executive control circuit in late-life depression: episodic and persistent phenomena. *Am J Geriatr Psychiatry* 2009; **17**(1): 30–42.

62. Kumar A, Thomas A, Lavretsky H, Yue K, Huda A, Curran J et al. Frontal white matter biochemical abnormalities in late-life major depression detected with proton magnetic resonance spectroscopy. *Am J Psychiatry* 2002; **159**(4): 630–6.

63. Elderkin-Thompson V, Thomas MA, Binesh N, Mintz J, Haroon E, Dunkin JJ et al. Brain metabolites and cognitive function among older depressed and healthy individuals using 2D MR spectroscopy. *Neuropsychopharmacology* 2004; **29**(12): 2251–7.

64. Chen CS, Chiang IC, Li CW, Lin WC, Lu CY, Hsieh TJ et al. Proton magnetic resonance spectroscopy of late-life major depressive disorder. *Psychiatry Res* 2009; **172**(3): 210–4.

65. Forester BP, Harper DG, Jensen JE, Ravichandran C, Jordan B, Renshaw PF et al. 31Phosphorus magnetic resonance spectroscopy study of tissue specific changes in high energy phosphates before and after sertraline treatment of geriatric depression. *Int J Geriatr Psychiatry* 2009; **24**(8): 788–97.

79

Clinical Features of Depressive Disorders in the Elderly

Davangere P. Devanand and Steven P. Roose

Division of Geriatric Psychiatry, New York State Psychiatric Institute, and the College of Physicians and Surgeons, Columbia University, New York, USA

Late-life depression refers to depressive syndromes in people who are older than 60–65 years. Depression causes considerable personal suffering and adversely affects family members and other caregivers. In elderly subjects, depressive syndromes are often associated with chronic medical illnesses that can precipitate depression. Conversely, the presence of depression can worsen the outcomes of many medical disorders and promote disability. Depression occurs commonly in a variety of other neuropsychiatric syndromes, including mild cognitive impairment, dementia, stroke and Parkinson's disease.

In the elderly, the fear of ageing and its effects are common. Older adults commonly state that since they are getting old it is normal to feel depressed. This view is often shared by family members and even health care providers. However, the vast majority of elderly individuals are not depressed, and therefore depression should not be considered a normal part of the ageing process.

Many elderly patients describe their mood accurately as depressed or anxious, but some tend to deny and suppress it and they come to clinical attention only at the insistence of family members. Somatization is common in older patients, particularly gastrointestinal symptoms like constipation. Some patients are unsure if they are depressed because they have begun to feel less energetic and lose interest in activities in the absence of a clear-cut depressed mood. Some of these patients have dysthymia or minor depression. In the elderly, one important distinction to make is whether the first depressive syndrome began in late life or whether it represents a pattern of recurrent depression throughout adulthood, because the underlying aetiology may differ in these two types of patients. Premorbid personality does carry into old age, but its impact on the presentation of depression varies considerably. Personality itself may change with ageing and life experiences. Psychological changes in the elderly may be environmentally determined, but may also be based on changes in neurobiology; for instance, catecholaminergic neurons in the locus coeruleus decay markedly with ageing and this change may be related to the rarity of late-onset anxiety disorders and lower prevalence of major depression in the elderly population.

PREVALENCE

Depressive syndromes are common in late life[1] and represent the leading cause of poor functioning and disability worldwide that has an overall adverse impact comparable to cardiovascular disease[2]. A low proportion of clinically depressed elderly individuals seek help and typically they present to primary care practitioners. However, primary care physicians correctly diagnose only a minority of depressed patients and consequently few patients receive treatment for this illness. An even smaller proportion is referred for psychiatric care.

Epidemiological studies indicate that among the elderly, milder sub-threshold depressive syndromes may be more common than major depression, which ranges in prevalence from 1 to 3%[3]. However, the rate of major depression changes significantly depending on the setting. Studies of patients in medical clinics report rates of 10% for major depression; in non-psychiatric hospital in-patients the rate increases to 15–25%, and it is even higher in nursing homes[4]. These studies primarily used assessment instruments and diagnostic criteria that were developed for and/or validated in a younger population, and it is not known whether the adoption of age-adjusted diagnostic criteria would produce significantly different results.

DIAGNOSTIC CLASSIFICATION

A depressive disorder may be diagnosed by DSM-IV (or DSM-IV TR) clinical criteria only if the depressive symptoms adversely affect work, family or social functioning, or if the subject seeks or has received treatment for depression. The clinical entities in the current nomenclature identified in young adults that also occur in older adults are major depression (unipolar or bipolar, single episode or recurrent, with or without melancholia, with or without psychotic features); dysthymic disorder; and atypical depression. Disorders that are common in the elderly include mood syndromes secondary to a general medical condition, and subsyndromal depression including minor depression. Depression with cognitive impairment is a common presentation in elderly patients.

MAJOR DEPRESSION IN OLDER PATIENTS

Clinical observations and systematic studies suggest that patients with late-life major depression may well be different in important dimensions from younger adult patients with major depression. Such differences may reflect age-associated physiological changes, the changes associated with depressive illness (the ravages of a depressed life)

Principles and Practice of Geriatric Psychiatry, 3rd edn. Edited by Mohammed T. Abou-Saleh, Cornelius Katona and Anand Kumar
© 2011 John Wiley & Sons, Ltd

and/or the impact of co-morbid medical conditions[5-7]. For example, the differences in young versus old people may manifest in how functional impairment as a symptom of depression is expressed differently through the life cycle. Depression-associated dysfunction in childhood can present as poor performance in school or antisocial behaviour, in young adults as dissatisfaction in work or love, and for older patients as hypochondrias and increased utilization of medical resources[8].

The cumulative impact of depressive illness itself in patients with onset of illness early in life may be a critical factor. By the time a patient with early onset depression reaches age 60, they have already suffered through recurrent episodes. There is increasing evidence that the number of depressive episodes as well as the total amount of time spent 'depressed' in a lifetime is associated with less robust response to treatment and the development of chronic symptoms[6]. Furthermore, some data suggest that the cumulative time spent in a depressed state is correlated with changes in brain structure that may subsequently affect the phenomenology and treatment response in future episodes[5].

Moreover, changes in the brain that occur with age may also affect how the individual interacts with the environment, and can result in increased vulnerability to depression. Regional brain dysfunction, especially in the pre-frontal areas, is associated with instability of temperament, vulnerability to and the intensification of the experience of distress, and a degrading of coping mechanisms. Such alterations in an individual's psychic capacities may result in increased social isolation, loss of independence, and related behaviours that can precipitate, intensify, or prolong a depressive episode. Thus, by the time a patient with recurrent depression reaches late life, the consequences of the disorder itself, and maybe the impact of treatments received, will influence the presentation, psychobiology, treatment response and course of illness during late life.

Alternatively, the differences that exist in younger versus older depressed patients may indicate that late-life depression is a distinct disease entity and, despite some commonality, early onset and late-life depressive illness are significantly different in fundamental aetiological ways. An example of such aetiological heterogeneity is the distinction between the late-life patient with recurrent major depressive illness with onset of the first episode early in life, and the late-life patient with first onset of major depressive illness after the age of 60. The hypothesis that early-onset (before age 50 or 60) and late-onset depression may be, despite similarities, distinct entities is suggested by data from epidemiological, brain imaging, treatment, and long-term outcome studies[9-11]. Patients with late-onset depression have a lower rate of family history of depression, and a greater frequency of MRI abnormalities compatible with ischaemic cerebrovascular disease[10]. These lesions have been associated with symptoms of cognitive impairment, a decreased and slower response to antidepressant medication and a deteriorating course of illness[12,13].

In summary, the label late-life depression may be attached to a group of patients who share some commonalties but who, nonetheless, suffer from a heterogeneous group of disorders that differ in aetiology, pathophysiology and prognosis. Indeed, some of these disorders may be relatively unique to older adults.

Diagnostic Features of Major Depression in Late Life

Whatever the reason, and whether in a medical or psychiatric setting, the age-associated changes in the presentation of depression undoubtedly contribute to the problem of under-diagnosis and inadequate treatment of depression in late-life patients. In general, older patients report fewer emotional symptoms, for example depressed mood, and present with more cognitive/somatic symptoms, for instance sleep disturbance, fatigue, pain and memory or concentration difficulties. In fact, the older-age depressed patient may never complain of, or indeed may deny, being 'depressed'. This presentation of late-life depression has been labelled 'depression without sadness'[14]. Thus, if when making a diagnosis a physician adheres strictly to DSM-IV criteria, than depressive disorder may well be omitted from the differential diagnosis for an older patient presenting with non-specific physical complaints.

Diagnostic Criteria for Major Depression in the Elderly

Despite the compelling evidence that late-life depression and older people are different, the diagnostic criteria for unipolar depression in DSM-IV are not adjusted for age[15]. One of the five required symptoms must be either (i) depressed mood most of the day, nearly every day; or (ii) markedly diminished interest or pleasure in all, or almost all activities. The other symptoms that are counted to the total of five, but not required, are: (iii) significant weight loss, or decrease or increase in appetite nearly every day; (iv) insomnia or hypersomnia; (v) psychomotor agitation or retardation; (vi) fatigue or loss of energy; (vii) feelings of worthlessness or excessive or inappropriate guilt; (viii) diminished ability to think or concentrate, or indecisiveness (older patients with depression often have mild cognitive impairment, including disturbances in attention, speed of mental processing, and executive function); (ix) recurrent thoughts of death, suicidal ideation with or without a plan.

Though there are no separate diagnostic subtypes unique to late life, there are some considerations that are more relevant to late-life depressed patients than younger patients with the same disorder. The DSM-IV precludes the diagnosis of major depression if it can be established that the symptoms counted towards the diagnosis of depression are a direct physiological effect of a different medical disorder. However, this rule is not supported by evidence, and to the contrary, studies have suggested that the inclusive approach (i.e. if a symptom is present it is counted towards the diagnosis of depression) is justified[16].

There is also the belief that unipolar major depression with psychotic features may be a more frequently occurring subtype in older than younger patients. Psychotic depression occurs in 20 to 45% of elderly depressives hospitalized for psychiatric care, and in 3.6% of elderly depressives living in the community[17].

VASCULAR DEPRESSION

Hickie et al.[12] hypothesized that there may exist a vascular depression subtype that is unique to late life; he wrote that 'cerebral vascular insufficiency in elderly people leads to major changes in their subcortical and basal ganglia structure. The resultant late-onset depressive disorders are characterized by deficits in functions that are dependent on intact cortical striatal connections (e.g. psychomotor speed), as well as subcortical hyperintense lesions and reduced basal ganglia volumes.' The hypothesis emanated from studies that reported that patients with late-onset major depressive disorder (MDD) had higher rates of hyperintensities on MRI compared to patients with early onset MDD[10,12,18]. The patients with late-onset depression and hyperintensities also showed deficits on neuropsychological testing including, but not limited to, deficits in executive function[18,19]. Thus, structural brain damage secondary to ischaemia creates a vulnerability to MDD that may be precipitated by negative life events or other stresses. Given that vascular disease of sufficient severity is the cause of the ischaemia, this form of depression will be significantly more prevalent in older adults[20].

Much about the vascular depression hypothesis is compelling. First, the evidence that vascular disease is the cause of the hyperintensities prominent in late-onset depression supports the hypothesis. Second, vascular risk factors, such as smoking, hypertension and high lipid levels, are prevalent in patients with late-onset depression. Actually, early onset depression is itself a very significant risk factor for both ischaemic heart disease and stroke later in life. Increased cortisol, insulin resistance and platelet reactivity, all of which can contribute to vascular damage and ischaemia, may mediate the increased risk of myocardial infarction and stroke associated with depression[7].

Diagnostic Criteria for Vascular Major Depression

Criteria for vascular depression include vascular disease, cognitive impairment, late age of onset, and depression. However, the various research groups who study this syndrome have proposed the variables in many different combinations. For example, one group considers clinical and/or laboratory evidence of vascular disease and depression onset after age 65 as cardinal features and executive dysfunction as secondary[21], whereas another group believes neuroimaging evidence of cerebrovascular disease to be the cardinal feature and age-of-onset over 50 as an additional secondary feature. Krishnan et al.[22] have further refined the notion of vascular depression, requiring only MRI evidence of cerebrovascular pathology to define it, and have referred to this syndrome as subcortical ischaemic depression. Alexopoulos has proposed a depression executive dysfunction disorder of late life that only requires executive dysfunction to meet diagnostic criteria[21,23]. Although the proposed criteria sets are important and have moved the field toward recognizing a potentially important subtype of late-life major depression, this recognition might be premature because there is no agreement on how the construct is defined. Furthermore, most studies only include patients who meet criteria for MDD; however, many patients with vascular disease have dysthymia or subsyndromal symptoms.

SUICIDAL IDEATION

Studies consistently show that elderly males, particularly white males, are the demographic group with the highest risk of committing suicide. Also, the majority of elderly patients who commit suicide have visited their primary care physician a few days to weeks before the act[24]. These findings appear to be present across countries in several continents, although there are cultural differences in the preferred method of committing suicide[25].

ATYPICAL DEPRESSION

Little attention has been paid to the atypical subtype in samples of late-life depressed patients. The term 'atypical' was originally coined to describe a group of depressed patients who characteristically present with 'reverse' vegetative symptoms such as hyperphagia and hypersomnia[26]. The diagnostic criteria and acceptance of this subtype of major depression have evolved over the past 25 years so that they are included in DSM-IV with the atypical features specifier requiring that a patient has (i) mood reactivity and (ii) two or more of the following symptoms: significant weight gain or increase

in appetite, hypersomnia, leaden paralysis, or a long-standing pattern of interpersonal rejection sensitivity[15]. Studies have documented that patients with atypical depression differ from other patients with major depression in a number of parameters besides phenomenology, including biological variables, treatment response, demographic characteristics and age of onset[27,28].

There are two studies of the atypical subtype in late-life patients. The first study has many methodological limitations but is notable because it brought attention to this subtype of depression in late life. In this study, a single practitioner in a private practice reported on 358 consecutive DSM-IV unipolar (major depressive and dysthymic disorder $N = 179$) and bipolar II ($N = 179$) outpatients presenting for treatment of a major depressive episode over the last two years[29]. Depressed patients over the age of 60 had a significantly lower rate of the atypical subtype compared to younger depressed patients, 28 vs. 55% respectively ($p < 0.0001$), and also a significantly lower rate of bipolar II atypical subtype in the late-life patients compared to the younger sample, 35 vs. 67% respectively ($p = 0.01$). Furthermore, in comparison to atypical patients under age 60, atypical patients over age 60 had an older age of onset of illness (44 years vs. 23 years) and a lower rate of rejection sensitivity (55 vs. 83%).

The second study reported on an open trial of venlafaxine in late-life depressed patients with the atypical subtype[30]. The sample was 17 patients, mean age 65.6 ± 7.3 years, 77% female, mean Cumulative Illness Rating Scale-Geriatric score[31] 2.9 ± 2.8, and 43.8% of the subjects had cardiovascular disease. The mean Mini-Mental State Examination (mMMSE) was 28.6 ± 1.4. In this sample, 58% of the patients had recurrent depression and, most strikingly, 53% presented with late onset of depression (defined as first episode after age 50) and only 12% with onset before age 21. Of note, 15/17 patients completed the eight-week venlafaxine trial; intent-to-treat response rate was 65% and the completer response rate was 73%.

CLINICAL RATING SCALES FOR MAJOR DEPRESSION

Patients should be evaluated with a history and clinical evaluation, supplemented by semi-structured interviews, together with additional information from informants and referring physicians and mental health professionals. The Hamilton Depression Rating Scale (17, 21, 24 or 29 item versions) and Montgomery Asberg Depression Rating Scale are commonly used in young adults, and can also be used in elderly patients with depression. Specific instruments that address symptoms likely to occur in the elderly have been developed. The Geriatric Depression Scale[32] has been validated in older depressed patients and can be useful in the overall assessment process. The CES-D (Center for Epidemiological Studies-D) is another short instrument with both 'positive' and 'negative' symptom assessment of depression and is widely used in epidemiological studies. Both these instruments can be completed as self-reports, though interviewer ratings often add to the nature of the information obtained. Some instruments developed for use by primary care practitioners, for instance PRIME-MD, are useful for basic office screening but require follow-up with a more comprehensive evaluation if the initial screen is positive[33]. A weakness of using this type of screening approach in elderly patients is that many depressed patients do not recognize their depression as a symptom of illness or have masked depression with or without somatic symptoms. In such cases, the screen may give a false negative result. There is no objective evidence that any one of these rating instruments is superior to any other instrument in distinguishing diagnostic groups, predicting clinical course or treatment response. Other areas of query to complete the evaluation include assessments of cognitive, nutritional and functional status, social function and general health status. Review of medications, medical work-up and laboratory assessment, if indicated, is necessary to complete the evaluation.

Depression may be reflected in behavioural changes in the elderly, with apathy, anhedonia and occasionally irritability being prominent symptoms. Although several studies show that major depression in the elderly is more likely to become chronic, it remains unclear if the likelihood of chronicity is more common in elderly patients[34]. Some older patients show partial improvement without full remission from an episode of major depression[35], but the STAR-D findings suggest that this may also be the case in many young adults[36]. While the goal is full remission, partial response without full remission remains common. In addition to antidepressant medication treatment, a variety of psychotherapies including interpersonal, cognitive behavioural and problem-solving therapy have been shown to have some efficacy, though well-controlled studies are fairly limited[37]. Other behavioural interventions include exercise and group activity involvement, but systematic controlled studies are lacking.

DYSTHYMIC DISORDER

Dysthymic disorder is a syndrome of depression of mild or moderate severity that lasts at least two years. Dysthymia is a chronic condition that may begin early in life and extend into late life, often interspersed with episodes of major depression. In these patients, the term 'chronic depression' has been used to designate the co-morbid or sequential occurrence of major depression and dysthymic disorder[38]. However, in the elderly, the majority of cases of dysthymic disorder are of late onset by DSM criteria (age of onset > 21 years), and the majority of patients have an age of onset above 50 years[39]. As discussed earlier in this chapter, there is considerable evidence that patients with late-onset (onset after 50–60 years of age) major depression are less likely to have a positive family history of affective disorder and more likely to have evidence of cerebrovascular disease and cerebral atrophy than elderly patients with early onset depressive illness. These features also appear to be present in patients with dysthymic disorder[39,40] who often have a 'pure' dysthymia uncomplicated by a history of major depression[39]. Co-morbid Axis I disorders, particularly anxiety disorders, are far more common in early onset than late-onset patients with dysthymic disorder[39,41]. The gender distribution in late-onset dysthymic disorder does not seem to have the female preponderance that is observed in most types of affective disorder. Personality disorders in elderly dysthymic patients are less common than in young adults with depression, and tend to be of the obsessive-compulsive and avoidant subtypes. Borderline, histrionic, narcissistic and antisocial personality disorders are rare in the elderly[39,42].

Co-morbid general medical conditions, cognitive disorders and frequent adverse life events, for example bereavement, can complicate the diagnosis of dysthymic disorder. Associated features may include the presence of major chronic stressors, increased physical impairment and more symptoms of anxiety. Patients with dysthymia tend to be seen in primary care settings rather than by psychiatric specialists.

DSM-IV describes the symptoms of dysthymic disorder as being similar to those in major depression, with the distinction being the presence of fewer symptoms of lesser severity. However, the DSM-IV field trials revealed a high prevalence of cognitive and social symptoms in patients with dysthymic disorder, and neurovegetative symptoms were less frequent. This led to the alternative symptom criteria for dysthymic disorder that were listed in the DSM-IV appendix. These symptoms include low self-esteem, hopelessness, social withdrawal and lack of interest, fatigue, low productivity, poor concentration and indecisiveness. These symptoms are also more common than classical neurovegetative symptoms in elderly patients with dysthymic disorder[42]. The assessment of dysthymic disorder in the elderly can benefit from the use of the Cornell Dysthymia Rating Scale that emphasizes cognitive and social and motivational difficulties[43].

The optimal treatment of dysthymic disorder in the elderly remains uncertain. Fluoxetine has been shown to have marginal superiority over placebo[44] and there is equivocal evidence on whether psychotherapy or SSRIs should be the first-line treatment[45]. Problem-solving therapy may have limited utility in dysthymic disorder and other types of late-life depression, but there appears to be considerable variability in treatment response when this therapy is not administered by experts[37,45].

OTHER SUBSYNDROMAL DEPRESSIVE DISORDERS

Subsyndromal depression is defined as the presence of depressive symptoms that do not qualify for a formal mood disorder. Subsyndromal depressive disorder tends to be a heterogeneous group of milder forms of depression with symptom patterns qualitatively distinct from more severe forms such as major depression[46]. Subsyndromal depression is often used to describe patients with occasional depressed mood in the absence of other depressive symptoms. Minor depression in elderly people is associated with functional disability, and about 25% of patients develop major depression within two years. These subsyndromal depressive disorders commonly occur in patients with co-morbid medical illness, cognitive impairment, and other Axis I and II psychiatric disorders. There have been few treatment studies in the elderly, partly because the inherent heterogeneity of this set of syndromes makes it difficult to identify consistent treatment effects. Another view is that these patients' symptoms are too mild to require treatment, but the higher than expected likelihood of progression to major depression and the possible detrimental impact of even low levels of depression on medical outcomes suggest that treatment may often be warranted.

GRIEF AND PATHOLOGICAL BEREAVEMENT

Grief, a normal psychological response to the loss of a loved one, possessions or health, or unexpected adverse events, is associated with feelings of sadness, transient somatic symptoms, weight loss and difficulty in sleeping. Symptoms are often intense for several weeks to a few months and then typically begin to improve[47]. Pathological grief refers to the persistence of symptoms of grief at the same intensity more than six months after the event, and may include acquisition of symptoms belonging to the last illness of the deceased, psychosomatic illness, greater interpersonal conflicts and social withdrawal, difficulty in concentration and other cognitive difficulties, low productivity and impaired overall functioning[48,49]. Fear, demoralization and loneliness can occur. Spousal bereavement is common in late life, and is associated with declining mental and physical health and increased risk of mortality[50]. Among elderly widows and widowers, 20% meet the criteria for major depressive syndrome two months after their loss, and one-third of these individuals develop persistent depression for a year or longer[51]. Generally, individuals who are at greatest risk for persistent depression have worse health, more functional and social difficulties and more protracted grief than do bereaved individuals who are not depressed.

There are two schools of thought on whether grief should be treated in its early stages: some believe that it should be treated and others have the view that only persistent and prolonged grief requires intervention. The utility of antidepressant medications or psychotherapy in these contexts is not fully established, but there is some evidence for the efficacy of a specific form of therapy, complicated grief therapy, to treat patients with prolonged and disabling grief symptoms[52].

A relatively new diagnostic concept that is especially relevant to older patients is complicated grief. In this syndrome, the grief that is normally experienced during bereavement does not resolve but instead becomes persistent. The predominant symptoms of complicated grief include recurrent intrusive images of the death, bitter or angry avoidance of situations, activities, or people, intense yearning and/or longing, seeking proximity to items belonging to the deceased, feeling that life has no meaning without the deceased, self-blaming thoughts of not helping the person or not preventing the death. This syndrome is frequently co-morbid with depressive disorder; however, complicated grief itself may be mistaken for major depression. The diagnostic criteria for complicated grief are still in development and treatment studies are ongoing. For obvious reasons this syndrome has special relevance for older patients.

STRESSFUL LIFE EVENTS AND ADJUSTMENT DISORDERS

Older adults face a variety of stresses: medical illnesses, physical disability, sensory impairments in vision and hearing, loss of family and friends, loss of social supports, changes in relationships with children and significant others, alterations in living situation, and loss of income. One or more of these factors may be related to the onset of the clinical syndrome of depression. The death of a spouse is extremely stressful, as is the death of an adult child. Patients with major depression perceive significantly greater negative emotional impact of the same life events than patients with dysthymic disorder and healthy controls, particularly for interpersonal conflicts[53]. The resolution of stressful events probably depends on several factors, including genetic predisposition, prevailing early life experiences, adequacy of previous adaptive and coping mechanisms, patterns and profiles of premorbid personality and, in particular, the presence or absence of a strong support system. A specific scale has been developed to assess a range of stressful life events and their impact on mood and functioning in the elderly[53].

DEPRESSION WITH COGNITIVE IMPAIRMENT

In the elderly, depression is a major cause of suffering and disability, is often co-morbid with medical illnesses, worsens their outcome and increases mortality[2]. Cognitive deficits are common in the elderly, and often precede Alzheimer's disease (AD) and vascular dementia, which are illnesses with enormous costs. Depression and cognitive disorders are the most common neuropsychiatric disorders in the elderly; their co-occurrence may exceed chance.

Apathetic, withdrawn behaviour is common to both depression and dementia. Paucity of speech with long latency is characteristic of major depression, particularly the melancholic subtype. However, there are many symptoms common to both depression and mild cognitive impairment or early dementia: apathy, anhedonia, insomnia, agitation, irritability, memory loss and difficulty concentrating. This overlap in symptoms makes it difficult to make an accurate diagnosis and to estimate prognosis and plan treatment.

In patients with depression plus cognitive decline, the following symptoms commonly occur: difficulties in memory or thinking or concentration, forgetting of recent events, forgetting where things are located, problems in finding the right word to say, getting lost in familiar places, remembering appointments and to take medications, and difficulty in managing finances like balancing the chequebook or paying for items in a shop. These symptoms, especially financial management and remembering appointments or taking medications, may be the first indicators of dementia. The symptom of forgetting names of books and movies and people is common during the normal ageing process and by itself is not indicative of dementia.

The presence of depression of any type appears to be associated with an increased risk of converting to dementia during follow-up[54,55]. Among patients with depression and cognitive impairment, a large proportion of converters to dementia are diagnosed with AD. Autopsy studies show that elderly depressed subjects who have mild cognitive impairment or dementia often have a pathological diagnosis of AD[56].

As already described, 'vascular depression' refers to major depression with higher rates of leukoencephalopathy on MRI and executive function deficits. A number of patients with both depression and cognitive impairment have evidence of cerebrovascular disease, while others have incipient AD. Patients who present clinically with 'pseudodementia', that is, depression masquerading as dementia in its clinical presentation, were thought to be common but in fact are relatively rare[2].

The treatment of patients with depression and cognitive impairment has been poorly studied. In one study, open treatment with sertraline showed improvement in depression with minimal improvement in cognitive deficits[57], and there is preliminary evidence that adding a cholinesterase inhibitor to antidepressant treatment may lead to improvement in cognitive test performance[58]. There are no large-scale studies addressing these issues, and the standard clinical practice remains to first treat with antidepressants and then evaluate if cognition improves along with antidepressant response, even though there is little evidence to support this notion. The literature on the treatment of depression in patients with dementia, primarily AD, suggests a marginal positive effect for antidepressant medication in some studies, while other studies show no advantage of medication over placebo.

MEDICAL CO-MORBIDITY

Depression frequently accompanies other medical illnesses and is associated with considerable dysfunction and disability. Co-morbid medical illness increases the chronicity and refractoriness to treatment and it may slow recovery rates for depressed patients with various conditions, including heart disease, stroke, hip fracture and dementia.

The elderly patient typically suffers from several medical illnesses and takes a large number of medications. Benzodiazepines, steroids and anticholinergics can lead to cognitive impairment and even delirium, L-dopa and dopamine agonists prescribed for Parkinson's disease can lead to psychosis, and the use of some antihypertensives and steroids may be associated with depression.

A variety of medical disorders can first present with disturbances in mood, cognition, or psychotic features, including infections, electrolyte and metabolic imbalances, cardiovascular and cerebrovascular disease. Depression can lead to weight loss, inanition and malnutrition. Dietary history is important in this regard; the older adult living alone may not obtain adequate nutrition and may develop vitamin and other deficiencies.

From a diagnostic classification perspective, the diagnosis of depression due to a general medical condition is given when depressed mood or anhedonia occur in patients already diagnosed with an illness that is associated with depression. A common co-morbidity is depression and cardiovascular disease, and myocardial infarction is frequently associated with depression in the short term to intermediate term.

BIPOLAR DISORDER IN THE ELDERLY

Late-onset mania is not common in the elderly, but can occur as a primary late-onset mania or secondary to dementia or stroke or other neurological insult. Labile affect is believed to be typical of vascular dementia, but it remains unclear if labile affect is more common in vascular compared to other forms of dementia. Elderly patients are prone to the neurological side effects of lithium, and systematic monitoring of lithium and anticonvulsant blood levels when anticonvulsants are used is important, though the optimal treatment strategy for elderly patients with bipolar disorder is not well established. Many younger patients with bipolar disorder are maintained on the same treatment(s) as they age, and dosage reductions and other adjustments depend on the development of side effects.

CONCLUSION

While depression in the elderly shares many clinical features with depression in young adults, there are important differences. Late-onset patients, particularly those with cerebrovascular disease, may have an illness related directly to brain pathology, and those with both depression and cognitive impairment have an increased risk of developing AD. The preponderance of subsyndromal depression, and again the large proportion among them with late age of onset, indicates that the approach to diagnosis and management should not be restricted to the major depression category. Lack of social supports and life stresses do play a role in late-life depression. The high risk of suicide, particularly in elderly males living alone, should be at the forefront of the clinician's mind when evaluating the elderly depressed patient. A comprehensive biopsychosocial approach should take into account the patient's entire history, the social context and medical issues that arise during the ageing process. Medical co-morbidity needs to be addressed, and close communication with the patient's medical providers is important in elderly patients with significant medical illness. Treatment strategies should encompass both medications and psychotherapy, taking into account the reduced tolerability and increased side effects with psychotropic medication use, and the need to emphasize behavioural and problem-solving approaches in therapy when it is utilized.

CONFLICTS OF INTEREST

Dr Devanand – research support: Eli Lilly, Novartis. Consultant: Glaxo Smith Kline, Sanofi-Aventis, Bristol Myers Squibb.
Dr Roose – research support: Forest. Consultant: Eli Lilly.

REFERENCES

1. Blazer D, Williams CD. Epidemiology of dysphoria and depression in an elderly population. *Am J Psychiatry* 1980; **137**(4): 439–44.

2. Alexopoulos GS. Depression in the elderly. *Lancet* 2005; **365**(9475): 1961–70.

3. Blazer D, Hughes DC, George LK. The epidemiology of depression in an elderly community population. *Gerontologist* 1987; **27**: 281–7.

4. Parmelee PA, Katz IR, Lawton MP. Depression among institutionalized aged: assessment and prevalence estimation. *J Gerontol* 1989; **44**: 22–9.

5. Lebowitz BD, Pearson JL, Schneider LS *et al*. Diagnosis and treatment of depression in late life: consensus statement update. *JAMA* 1997; **278**: 1186–90.

6. Sheline YI, Sanghavi M, Mintun MA, Gado MH. Depression duration but not age predicts hippocampal volume loss in medically healthy women with recurrent major depression. *J Neurosci* 1999; **19**: 5034–43.

7. Roose SP, Krishnan, R. Depression comorbid with other illness. In Charney DS, Nestler EJ (eds), *Neurobiology of Mental Illness*, 2nd edn. Oxford: Oxford University Press, 2004.

8. Unutzer J, Katon WJ, Simon G *et al*. Depression, quality of life, and use of health services in primary care patients over 65: a 4-year prospective study. *Psychosomatics* 1996; **37**: 35.

9. Baldwin R, Jeffries S, Jackson A *et al*. Treatment response in late-onset depression: relationship to neuropsychological, neuroradiological and vascular risk factors. *Psychol Med*; 2004 **34**: 125–36.

10. Krishnan KRR, Hays JC, Blazer DG. MRI-defined vascular depression. *Am J Psychiatry* 1997; **154**: 497–500.

11. Krishnan KR, Hays JC, Tupler LA, George LK, Blazer DG. Clinical and phenomenological comparisons of late-onset and early-onset depression. *Am J Psychiatry* 1995; **152**: 785–8.

12. Hickie I, Scott E, Mitchell P *et al*. Subcortical hyperintensities on magnetic resonance imaging: clinical correlates and prognostic significance in patients with severe depression. *Biol Psychiatry* 1995; **37**: 151–60.

13. O'Brien J, Ames D, Chiu E *et al*. Severe deep white matter lesions and outcome in elderly patients with major depressive disorder: follow up study. *BMJ* 1998; **317**(7164): 982–4.

14. Gallo JJ, Rabins PV. Depression without sadness: alternative presentations of depression in late life. *Am Fam Physician* 1999; **60**: 820–6.

15. American Psychiatric Association. *Diagnostic and Statistical Manual of Mental Disorders, Fourth Edition*. Washington, DC: American Psychiatric Association Press, 2000.

16. Foelker GA, Shewchuk RM. Somatic complaints and the CES-D. *J Am Geriatr Soc* 1992; **40**: 259–62.

17. Linjakumpu T, Hartikainen S, Klaukka T *et al*. Psychotropics among the home-dwelling elderly. *Int J Geriatr Psychiatry* 2002; **9**: 874–83.

18. Salloway S, Malloy P, Kohn R *et al*. MRI and neuropsychological differences in early- and late-life-onset geriatric depression. *Neurology* 1996; **46**(6): 1567–74.

19. Alexopoulos GS, Kiosses DN, Klimstra S, Kalayam B, Bruce ML. Clinical presentation of the "depression-executive dysfunction syndrome" of late life. *Am J Geriatr Psychiatry* 2002; **10**: 98–106.

20. Krishnan KR, McDonald WM. Arteriosclerotic depression. *Med Hypotheses* 1995; **44**: 111–15.

21. Alexopoulos GS, Meyers BS, Young RC *et al*. Clinically defined vascular depression. *Am J Psychiatry* 1997; **154**: 562–5.

22. Krishnan KR, Taylor WD, McQuoid DR *et al*. Clinical characteristics of magnetic resonance imaging-defined subcortical ischemic depression. *Biol Psychiatry* 2004; **55**: 390–7.

23. Alexopoulos GS. "The depression-executive dysfunction syndrome of late life": a specific target for D3 agonists? *Am J Geriatr Psychiatry* 2001; **9**: 22–9.

24. Castle K, Duberstein PR, Meldrum S, Conner KR, Conwell Y. Risk factors for suicide in blacks and whites: an analysis of data from the 1993 National Mortality Followback Survey. *Am J Psychiatry* 2004; **161**(3): 452–8.

25. Shah A. A cross-national study of the relationship between elderly suicide rates and urbanization. *Suicide Life Threat Behav* 2008; **38**(6): 714–9.

26. West ED, Dally PJ. Effects of iproniazid in depressive syndromes. *Br Med J* 1959; **1**: 1491–4.

27. Stewart JW, McGrath PJ, Rabkin JG, Quitkin FM. Atypical depression: a valid clinical entity? *Psychiatr Clin North Am* 1993; **16**: 479–95.

28. Nierenberg AA, Alpert JE, Pava J, Rosenbaum JF, Fava M. Course and treatment of atypical depression. *J Clin Psychiatry* 1998; **59** (Suppl 18): 5–9.

29. Benazzi F. Late-life atypical major depressive episode: a 358-case study in outpatients. *Am J Geriatr Psychiatry* 2000; **8**: 117–22.

30. Roose SP, Miyazaki M, Devanand D *et al*. An open trial of venlafaxine for the treatment of late-life atypical depression. *Int J Geriatr Psychiatry* 2004; **19**(10): 989–94.

31. Miller MD, Paradis CF, Houck PR *et al*. Rating chronic medical illness burden in geropsychiatric practice and research: application of the Cumulative Illness Rating Scale. *Psychiatry Res* 1992; **41**(3): 237–48.

32. Yesavage J, Brink T, Rose T. Development and validation of a geriatric depression screening scale; a preliminary report. *J Psychiat Res* **1983**: 17: 37–49.

33. Spitzer RL, Kroenke K, Williams JB. Validation and utility of a self-report version of PRIME-MD: the PHQ primary care study. Primary Care Evaluation of Mental Disorders. Patient Health Questionnaire. *JAMA* 1999; **282**(18): 1737–44.

34. Geerlings SW, Beekman AT, Deeg DJ, Van Tilburg W. Physical health and the onset and persistence of depression in older adults: an eight-wave prospective community-based study. *Psychol Med* 2000; **30**(2): 369–80.

35. Blazer D. Depression in the elderly. *N Engl J Med* 1989; **320**: 164–5.

36. Rush AJ, Trivedi MH, Wisniewski SR *et al*. Acute and longer-term outcomes in depressed outpatients requiring one or several treatment steps: a STAR*D report. *Am J Psychiatry* 2006; **163**(11): 1905–17.

37. Arean P, Hegel M, Vannoy S, Fan MY, Unuzter J. Effectiveness of problem-solving therapy for older, primary care patients with depression: results from the IMPACT project. *Gerontologist* 2008; **48**(3): 311–23.

38. Kocsis JH, Gelenberg AJ, Rothbaum B *et al*. Chronic forms of major depression are still undertreated in the 21st century: systematic assessment of 801 patients presenting for treatment. *J Affect Disord* 2008; **110**(1-2): 55–61.

39. Devanand DP, Nobler MS, Singer T *et al*. Is dysthymia a different disorder in the elderly? *Am J Psychiatry* 1994; **151**: 1592–9.

40. Elderkin-Thompson V, Hellemann G, Pham D, Kumar A. Prefrontal brain morphology and executive function in healthy and depressed elderly. *Int J Geriatr Psychiatry* 2009; **24**(5): 459–68.

41. Devanand DP, Turret N, Moody BJ *et al*. Personality disorders in elderly patients with dysthymic disorder. *Am J Geriatr Psychiatry* 2000; **8**: 188–95.

42. Devanand DP, Adorno E, Cheng J *et al*. Late onset dysthymic disorder and major depression differ from early onset dysthymic disorder and major depression in elderly outpatients. *J Affect Disord* 2004; **78**: 259–67.

43. Mason BJ, Kocsis JH, Leon AC *et al*. Measurement of severity and treatment response in dysthymia may have been limited by the structure and format of existing rating instruments. *Psychiatr Ann* 1993; **23**: 625–31.

44. Devanand DP, Nobler MS, Cheng J *et al*. Randomized, double-blind, placebo-controlled trial of fluoxetine treatment for elderly patients with dysthymic disorder. *Am J Geriatr Psychiatry* 2005; **13**: 59–68.

45. Williams JW Jr, Barrett J, Oxman T *et al*. Treatment of dysthymia and minor depression in primary care: a randomized controlled trial in older adults. *JAMA* 2000; **284**(12): 1519–26.

46. Geiselmann B, Bauer M. Subthreshold depression in the elderly: qualitative or quantitative distinction? *Comp Psychiat* 2000; **41**(2): 32–8.

47. Clayton PJ. Clinical insights into normal grief. *Ri Med J* 1980; **63**: 107–9.

48. Brown JT, Stoudemire A. Normal and pathologic grief. *J Am Med Assoc* 1983; **250**: 378.

49. Bruce ML, Kim K, Leaf PJ, Jacobs S. Depressive episodes and dysphoria resulting from conjugal bereavement in a prospective community sample. *Am J Psychiat* 1990; **147**: 608–11.

50. Kaprio J, Koskenvuo M, Rita H. Mortality after bereavement; prospective study of 95 647 widowed persons. *Am J Publ Health* 1987; **77**: 282–7.

51. Zisook S, Shuchter SR. Major depression associated with widowhood. *Am J Geriatr Psychiat* 1993; **147**: 316–26.

52. Shear K, Frank E, Houck PR, Reynolds CF 3rd. Treatment of complicated grief: a randomized controlled trial. *JAMA* 2005; **293**(21): 2601–8.

53. Devanand DP, Kim MK, Paykina N, Sackeim HA. Adverse life events in elderly patients with major depression or dysthymic disorder and in healthy control subjects. *Am J Geriatr Psychiatry* 2002; **10**(3): 265–74.

54. Devanand DP, Sano M, Tang M-X *et al*. Depressed mood and the incidence of Alzheimer's disease in the elderly living in the community. *Arch Gen Psychiatry* 1996; **53**: 175–82.

55. Bassuk SS, Berkman LF, Wypij D. Depressive symptomatology and incident cognitive decline in an elderly community sample. *Arch Gen Psychiatry* 1998; **55**(12): 1073–81.

56. Sweet RA, Hamilton RL, Butters MA *et al*. Neuropathologic correlates of late-onset major depression. *Neuropsychopharmacology* 2004; **29**(12): 2242–50.

57. Devanand DP, Pelton GH, Marston K *et al*. Sertraline treatment of elderly patients with depression and cognitive impairment. *Int J Geriatr Psychiatry* 2003; **18**: 123–30.

58. Pelton GH, Harper OL, Tabert MH *et al*. Randomized double-blind placebo-controlled donepezil augmentation in antidepressant-treated elderly patients with depression and cognitive impairment: a pilot study. *Int J Geriatr Psychiatry* 2008; **23**: 670–6.

80

The Outcome of Late-life Depressive Disorders

Aartjan T.F. Beekman[1], Harm W.J. van Marwijk[2] and Max L. Stek[1]

[1]*Department of Psychiatry, VUmc Medical Centre, Amsterdam, The Netherlands*
[2]*Department of General Practice, VUmc Medical Centre, Amsterdam, The Netherlands*

THE OUTCOME OF LATE-LIFE DEPRESSION

Around the turn of the nineteenth century Kraepelin changed the face of contemporary psychiatry, primarily by systematically following up his patients after treatment. The outcome or natural history of a disorder is, since that time, decisive for any appreciation of its clinical relevance, treatment or classification, and is a cornerstone of its conceptualization. In some disorders, such as dementia, the rate of progression of the illness may vary, but the eventual outcome is fixed. Other diseases, such as diabetes or osteoarthritis, may have an extremely varied course and prognosis, but are chronic by nature. The eventual outcome of both diabetes and osteoarthritis is by no means fixed. In both disorders the outcome can vary from being a disorder that, although causing considerable discomfort, remains under control, to a debilitating and pernicious disorder. The outcome of depression is even more varied than that. Some patients suffer one episode in life, recover fully, never to run into affective trouble again. For others depression is a severe and chronic disease, omnipresent in all spheres and phases of life and dyscolouring all life's experience. The eventual outcome may vary from the depression having had a minor impact on the patient's life, to suicide. Between these extremes, every type of course and outcome of depression exists. This holds for depression at all ages. Indeed, it may well be that, given the changes that occur in later life, the variability of the outcome of geriatric depression is even more pronounced than in earlier stages of life.

Given the extreme variability of the outcome of depression and the obvious importance this has for our patients, it is surprising how poorly both our theories and our classification of the prognosis of depression have developed. Although a good many studies have been conducted to assess the naturalistic outcome of depression at all ages, this has not led to a well-developed prognostic theory for affective disorders. The primary aim of treatment is to influence the prognosis and outcome of a disorder. Although hundreds of trials have been conducted to test the efficacy of treatments for depression, this also has not led to an integrated theory of the prognosis of affective disorders. The result is that classification has remained where it essentially has been since Kraepelin's time: a purely descriptive system, categorizing what goes on while it goes on.

This chapter contains a reflection of this still rather primitive state of affairs. The first paragraph will discuss essential conceptual issues, relevant to the outcome of late-life depression. Thereafter, we will summarize the available data with regard to the naturalistic outcome of depression in older people. As will become evident, the pioneering studies in this area were conducted from specialized clinical centres, following up patients after discharge from clinical treatment. Later on, larger cohort studies were put together, following patients seen in general practice and in the community. These data will be used to test the hypothesis that the prognosis is generally more favourable in the community as compared with patients referred to specialized treatment centres. A second question is whether the prognosis of depression changes with age. To this end, results of studies conducted among older people will be compared with those in younger adults. Where possible, associations between age and the prognosis will be summarized. One of the myth's surrounding age and ageing is that later life would be an age of melancholy. This myth has been falsified many times. Although some studies do show that the prevalence of depressive symptoms increases with age, this is related to age-related risk factors and not to ageing itself. The same question will be addressed with regard to the prognosis of late-life depression. Is there an effect of age? If so, is this a result of the ageing itself, or a change in age-related prognostic factors?

A related issue is whether the variation in outcomes of depression is increased in later life. If so, the potential benefit of being able to predict the individual prognosis early on in treatment is similarly increased. First episodes of depression may arise at all ages and there are subtypes of depression that generally arise only in later life (such as vascular depression or depression associated with neurodegenerative disease). It is therefore likely that the prognosis becomes more heterogeneous in later life and that there are specific aetiological or prognostic subtypes that are especially relevant to older people. Identifying prognostic factors is therefore a further aim of this chapter.

Co-morbidity is the hallmark of geriatric medicine. Studying disorders in isolation in older people is only rarely helpful or informative. This is especially true for late-life depression. Moreover, for our patients and in terms of public health, more functional and generic outcomes such as well-being, daily functioning and social integration are essential. As these generic outcomes are the product of all the co-morbid disorders the patient has to cope with, the final aim of this chapter is to consider the role the prognosis of depression plays in the overall well-being and functioning of older people.

Principles and Practice of Geriatric Psychiatry, 3rd edn. Edited by Mohammed T. Abou-Saleh, Cornelius Katona and Anand Kumar

OUTCOME BRIEFLY CONSIDERED

There are many ways to define and measure the outcome of depression. As is the case in most areas of medicine, the methods employed have evolved from studies retrospectively and rather loosely classifying each patient in predefined clinical criteria, to prospective studies, rigorously measuring symptom severity at multiple time points. By definition, the more often symptoms are measured, the more likely it is that change will be detected. That would mean that the more recent and sophisticated studies, employing multiple measures over longer periods of time, are less likely to find a patient in sustained recovery and also less likely to conclude that the patient is chronically depressed.

The way the outcome of a disorder is conceptualized has great impact on the way it is studied and treated. Frank et al.[1] described clear criteria for what may be called the episodic model of the outcome of depression. This model, which is summarized briefly in Figure 80.1 has been by far the most influential. Depression is modelled as an episodic disorder, with a clear beginning, symptomatic stage and resolution phase. If, very soon after the symptoms have resolved, the patient suffers a relapse, this is considered part of the illness episode. If the recovery is more sustained and the patient suffers a recurrence, this is then considered to be a new episode. This well-known model has many merits. First, it is an optimistic model. Regardless of age, most patients recover and treatment generally helps to speed up recovery. The episodic model has also been helpful in both organizing our thinking about the prognosis of depression and in designing studies of treatment.

However, longer term follow-up studies employing multiple measurements have shown that patients often do not follow the neat stages of development of the disorder depicted in Figure 80.1[2]. The best known example is the Collaborative Depression Study, in which more than 400 patients were followed up using detailed weekly life charts. Over 12 years of follow-up, it appeared that patients moved in and out of different levels of symptom severity and diagnostic subtypes; the symptoms often waxing and waning[2]. Using an episodic model of outcome it was reported that 70% of the patients had recovered after one year and that the mean duration of episodes was approximately six months[3]. Given the fact that these were patients referred (and motivated) for treatment in a tertiary treatment centre, the outcome was quite optimistic. However, after 12 years of follow-up, using life charts it appeared that these patients spent

almost 60% of the time in a state with clinically relevant levels of depressive symptoms, severe enough to disturb both well-being and functioning[2]. The results have prompted the authors to conclude that the prognosis in depression is pleiomorphic instead of episodic[2]. When accommodating the pleiomorphic model in research, the prognosis of depression appeared less favourable than when adopting an episodic viewpoint. In practice, there are patients in whom depression follows the path of a clearly delineated episode, there are patients in whom the symptoms wax and wane over time and there are patients with a chronic course. This has clinical relevance, as the way treatment and follow-up are organized should be determined by the expected prognosis. Indeed, as was suggested by McCullough, there is good reason to consider more chronic forms of depression as a different disorder from the more benign episodic disorders[4].

When describing the outcome of late-life depression in the next section, both the parameters relevant to an episodic view of outcome (such as the duration of an episode, the percentage of patients remitting within a given time, relapse or recurrence) and those relevant for a pleiomorphic viewpoint (the average symptom severity over time, the percentage of time patients spend in a depressive state) will be discussed.

THE PROGNOSIS OF LATE-LIFE DEPRESSIVE SYMPTOMATOLOGY

Several systematic reviews have recently summarized the prognosis of late-life depression[5–7]. As was mentioned, the earlier studies were conducted as follow-up assessments of patients treated in clinical facilities. Over 20 such studies have been conducted. The outcome was often determined retrospectively in rather loosely defined clinical terms, such as the patient being well, recovery with relapses or being continually ill. Given various methodological shortcomings, Cole et al.[5] concluded that the majority of patients (about 60%) were well or had suffered relapses with recovery, while 14–22% were continually ill. Both Cole et al.[5] and Licht-Strunk et al.[6] in a more recent review have found poorer outcomes when studying depressed patients recruited from the community or primary care. Licht-Strunk et al.[6] summarized the findings of 4 primary care and 17 community-based studies that fulfilled quite rigorous methodological criteria. After a period of one year, 50–75% of patients no longer fulfilled diagnostic criteria for major depression. Taking a longer time-perspective, the available studies would suggest a rule of thirds: about one in three patients has a short-term remission, another one in three develops a chronic course, while the remaining third has a more varied prognosis, with intermittent episodes[6]. Only one study estimated the duration of episodes of major depression among older primary care patients. In a three-year follow-up of 234 older (55+) primary care patients with well-defined major depressive disorder, the average duration of an episode was estimated to be 18 months[7].

Moving from clinically defined outcomes to the more abstract pleiomorphic measures the prognosis looks even worse. In the Longitudinal Aging Study Amsterdam (LASA), which is a community-based study, 277 older depressed people were followed with six-monthly assessments over six years[8]. It appeared that almost half the sample was depressed more than 60% of the time over six years. Only one in three had a true chronic course, but another third of the patients were depressed most of the six years they were followed up, the symptoms waxing and waning over time.

Taking these results together, the prognosis seems rather good for only one in three older patients, while the majority are either

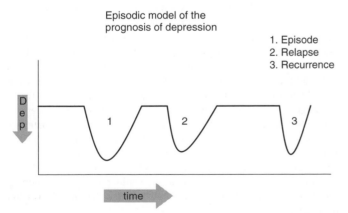

Episodic model of the prognosis of depression

1. Episode
2. Relapse
3. Recurrence

Figure 80.1 Episodic model for the prognosis of depression. From Frank et al.[1]

chronically depressed or have frequent, but intermittent changes in symptoms. It is striking that the data from the community and primary care suggest a less favourable prognosis when compared with data from specialized mental health care facilities. This is not what would be expected, as the more severe, chronic and hard-to-treat patients are referred selectively to specialized mental health. An explanation would be that majority of older depressed patients in the community and in primary care are not treated, while those referred for treatment do receive appropriate care[7].

MAJOR DEPRESSION, MINOR DEPRESSION AND DYSTHYMIA

Most of what is known about the prognosis of depression pertains to major depressive disorder (MDD). However, many older people with depressive symptoms do not fulfil rigorous diagnostic criteria for MDD[9]. What about their prognosis? The term 'dysthymic disorder' was introduced to replace 'neurotic depression'[10]. The underlying idea was that this would be a type of mild, but chronic depression, that was associated with personality disorders and therefore would arise early in life. What about dysthymia in later life? Is this common among older people and is it indeed a chronic, mild type of depression, that is primarily associated with personality problems?

The available data suggest that minor, or other subthreshold types of depressive symptoms, although clinically highly relevant to older people, do tend to have a more favourable prognosis than MDD. The prognosis of dysthymia appears to be worse than the prognosis of MDD. In the LASA study, data concerning the six-year prognoses of minor depression, MDD, dysthymia and double depression (MDD plus dysthymia) were compared[8]. Those with minor depression had the best prognosis (26% remission; 25% chronic course), followed by MDD (22% remission; 35% chronic course), dysthymia (12% remission; 52% chronic course) and finally double depression (only 5% remission and 77% chronic course). Dysthymia is quite common among older people (4.6% in the LASA study), has a symptom profile very similar to that of MDD and an earlier age of onset than MDD (average age at onset of 31 for dysthymia, compared with 53 for MDD)[11].

IS THE PROGNOSIS OF DEPRESSION INFLUENCED BY AGE OR BY AGE-RELATED FACTORS?

To answer this question one would like to be able to compare directly patients of different ages, recruited at similar stages of development of their affective disorder, using identical methods. As no such study is available, conclusions should be drawn cautiously as they are likely to be confounded. Given this caveat, the evidence seems to be overwhelmingly in favour of thinking that outcomes are poorer among older patients.

For instance, in a large community-based study of younger adults, the median duration of an episode of MDD was estimated to be three months, while the average duration among younger adult patients in specialized mental health has been estimated to be six months[13]. This compares very favourably with the 18 months average duration described for older primary care patients[7]. In the LASA study, direct comparisons between young-old (55–65) and older old (75–85) people is possible. It was clear that the oldest age group had a higher average symptom severity over six years of follow-up, a longer duration of symptoms and that they were almost twice as likely to have a chronic course of depression when compared with the youngest group[8].

Cole et al.[5] and Licht-Strunk et al.[6] have synthesized the data on prognostic factors for late-life depression, as described in community- and primary care-based studies. Although methodological differences among studies preclude exact estimates of the prognostic strength of different variables, some conclusions do emerge. The most consistently found prognostic factors are physical illness, impairments (such as pain, loss of hearing and loss of vision), disability and the associated impairment of daily functioning. The effect of cognitive decline and dementia on the prognosis of depression is undecided. Although one would perhaps expect that massive neurodegeneration and the resulting impairments and handicaps would be a powerful factor to prolong depression, moving through different stages of the dementia process may also act as a factor ending a depressive episode.

Another set of prognostic factors that has been studied is the experience of threatening or loss-related life events. Although these are powerful aetiological factors, there is no reason to believe that depression preceded or induced by life events has a different prognosis when compared to other types of depression. A third group of candidate prognostic factors concerns what is often called long-term vulnerability for depression. Examples are genetic factors, severe life events earlier in life, unfavourable personality traits (such as neuroticism), female gender, a lack of education or a lack of adequate social support. The uncovering of genetic subtypes predicting a more chronic course of depression would potentially be of great clinical importance, but has not as yet yielded definitive results. Studies suggest that gender, level of education and social support are not strong prognostic factors[5,6]. Both severe life events earlier in life and maladaptive personality traits have been identified as important unfavourable prognostic factors among younger adults. So far, the limited evidence has confirmed this for older adults, especially with regard to the role of neuroticism[13].

Given the available data on prognostic factors, those that have been uncovered are clearly related to age. This may explain why the prognosis of depression is worse among older people than among younger adults.

IS THE OUTCOME OF DEPRESSION MORE VARIED AMONG OLDER PEOPLE?

As described above, the available data suggest that the outcome of depression is less favourable in older adults than in younger people. This appears from data looking at the average duration of episodes, the rate of recovery, relapse and recurrence and the likelihood of chronic depression. A similar conclusion is drawn when comparing pleiomorphic indices of the outcome, such as the average symptom severity over time or the percentage of time people are depressed. Although many uncertainties remain, it appears that this less favourable outcome is at least partly explained by an increase in exposure to unfavourable prognostic factors. Depression is well known for its aetiological heterogeneity: a myriad of different aetiological factors can play a role in the development of depression. The exposure to such factors increases with age, dramatically changing the palette of risk factors involved. It is likely that the same happens with prognostic factors: the increased variability of the prognosis in part taking responsibility for the overall change in prognosis. This is important, as it would render any sweeping statement with regard to the overall prognosis of late-life depression inadequate.

With more prognostic heterogeneity, being able to reliably predict the prognosis becomes more important. Such data are becoming available slowly. It is clear that, besides the above prognostic, several other markers that may help predict the prognosis in an individual patient are available. The most powerful group of predictors would be the severity, duration and stage of development of the depression (first episode, versus recurrent episode)[6,7,8,12]. Besides this, other clinical factors, such as co-morbid anxiety and substance-related disorders have been shown to predict the prognosis of depression[12].

Overall, the data suggest that old age psychiatry would do well to invest in identifying subgroups of depression by (i) a clinical staging of severity, duration and development of the disorder, (ii) the symptom profile, (iii) biological or other prognostic factors and (iv) treatment response. Examples are the vascular depression hypothesis, which, among other things, would suggest a poorer prognosis and less response to antidepressant therapy, and the recently coined amyloid depression, which would predict cognitive decline and perhaps also a less favourable prognosis[14].

It may be concluded that although much work needs to be done in the area of predicting the prognosis, it is highly likely that variation increases with age and that different prognostic subgroups, highly relevant to clinical work, do exist.

GENERIC OUTCOMES

Excess Morbidity

Co-morbidity between physical health and depression is salient in late life, when both risk for illness and disability rises. Depression in old age can be a consequence of somatic illness and disability but ample research also suggests that depression in the elderly leads to restricted functioning and worsening of co-morbid conditions by a variety of behavioural and biological mediators. The pathways between depression and excess morbidity are complex and bidirectional. Large-scale longitudinal studies have been carried out trying to disentangle this complex interaction. Scott et al.[15] recently found in their review of World Mental Health surveys that although the majority of elderly suffered from chronic physical conditions the large part had no signs of depression and anxiety. By contrast, the majority of those with mental disorders had physical co-morbidity. From another perspective findings suggest that different durations of the presence of depressive symptoms have different impact on physical health. Long-term depression had profound negative effects on illness, a short duration far less[16]. More specifically the association between depression and ischaemic cardiac illness is a frequently studied topic[17]. Depression and cardiac disease often co-occur and this association is likely to be bi-directional[18]. The presence of subclinical atherosclerosis due to exaggerated platelet function, activation of pro-inflammatory pathways and an altered HPA axis state has been suggested as an underlying mechanism[19,20].

A second field that has been studied extensively is co-morbid cognitive impairment, a clinical hallmark in old-age psychiatry because cognitive impairment is one of the immediate consequences of depression. There is a strong association between late-life depression cognitive impairment, cerebrovascular disease and progressive dementia, including Alzheimer's disease. The varied findings suggest that there are probably many pathways to poor cognitive outcomes with multiple aetiological links[14,21]. Research in this field combines data from long-term longitudinal studies with (functional) neuroimaging and biomarkers and should lead to a better understanding of these clinically very important relationships.

Suicide and Other Causes of Excess Mortality

In most countries suicide rates remain highest in old people according to the World Health Organization. In particular, older men act more decisively on their suicidal intent than women, an effect increasing with age, which could be an explanation for the large sex differences in this respect[22]. In a series of psychological autopsy studies from the United States, Scandinavia and the United Kingdom more than 70% of the elderly who died by suicide suffered from a psychiatric condition, mostly depression[23]. Persistent feelings of hopelessness and a long duration of depression and sleep disturbances were the most consistent predictors in the elderly[24]. Notwithstanding the high suicide figures in elderly men the major part of the impressive rates of increased mortality in depressed elderly cannot be explained by suicide, but is related to other causes of death, probably cardiac events in the first place. In a recent study a dose–response relationship was found for late-life depression and early death, suggesting a causal relationship[25]. There are several explanations for this pathway from depression to early death. On a behavioural level depression is generally associated with unhealthy lifestyles like smoking, use of alcohol, physical inactivity and lower compliance with medical treatment. In the elderly cognitive impairment and dieting may add to this negative cascade. Decreased heart rate variability, HPA axis dysregulation and increased pro-inflammatory activity are biological factors which probably play a part in cardiac-related death. At a subclinical level there may be depression-related illness like hypertension and endocrine dysfunctioning leading to early death. In conclusion many pathways in late-life depression lead to early death in complex interacting mechanisms[25,26].

Excess or inadequate use of service

Late-life depression is an important reason for both excess and inadequate utilization of non-mental care resources[27]. Older patients and their care providers frequently persist to attribute depressive symptoms to somatic illness or ageing effects, thus creating diagnostic confusion. In a US national sample of subjects with persistent depressive or anxiety disorder, 87% had a chronic co-morbid medical disorder, most were seeing a primary care practitioner, but only 12% were receiving both appropriate medication and counselling at follow up[28]. In a recent Dutch general practice study, persistent frequent attendance was five times as likely to occur among persons over 65 years of age, and four times as likely when psychological or psychiatric problems were present[29]. Depression plays an especially important role in frequent attendance of the elderly[30]. Up to a quarter of elderly attend frequently, many of whom are depressed[31].

Well-being and Functioning

Older depressed patients have substantial and long-lasting decrements in multiple domains of functioning and well-being that equal or exceed those of patients with chronic medical illnesses such as diabetes mellitus[6,27]. Perhaps this strong relationship is not that surprising as depression is characterized by an absence of well-being and functioning. A prolonged lack of happiness is a key symptom for a diagnosis of major depression. To demonstrate this reciprocal relationship, positive affect, defined as emotional contentment and happiness, was directly correlated over time with social involvement and inversely correlated with negative affect (i.e. depression), instrumental activities of daily living functioning, and somatic co-morbidity[32].

CONCLUSION

All the things that characterize later life also characterize late-life depression. Older people have a lifetime of experience and ageing tends to create more variability among the processes relevant to living. Depressed older people often have a long experience with mood changes and the pathways leading to depression become more complex with age. The available data would suggest that the prognosis of depression, whichever way it is conceptualized, becomes less favourable with ageing. The data also suggest that a large part of this is due to age-related prognostic factors, and much less due to ageing per se. Depressed older people are partly 'graduates': people who have suffered repeated episodes of depression throughout life and who continue to do so when they become old. Their prognosis is a function of the long-term development of their affective disorder and concurrent circumstances or events that happen while ageing. A large minority of our patients have become depressed for the first time in later life. Among them are patients becoming depressed due to life events or circumstances, and patients who become depressed in the context of specific, age-related illnesses. The prognosis of their depression is closely related to the outcome of the underlying cause and treatment more likely to be successful if this is taken into account.

It was argued that geriatric psychiatry would do well to adopt a clinical staging of affective disorders, which should include data on (i) severity, duration and clinical stage (first or recurrent episode), (ii) relevant prognostic factors, including biological markers, (iii) data on specific symptom profiles relevant to treatment or the prognosis and (iv) data on treatment outcome. This would help to build a more definitive database on the outcome of late-life depression, while simultaneously improving treatment.

Depression only rarely occurs in isolation in older people. Although clinicians are prone to focus on the disorders they have specialized in, the more generic outcomes of disorders are likely to be more relevant to our patients than the course of one specific disorder. It was shown that depression has profound impact on most of the generic outcomes that one would consider important for the public health of older people. Although it remains difficult to tease out the unique effect that depression has on these outcomes over and above the effects of co-morbid disorders, the available data suggest that depression often plays a decisive role in tipping the balance towards unfavourable outcomes. The fact that depression remains highly treatable until very late in life should inspire us to work hard to improve both the diagnosis and treatment of depression in older people.

REFERENCES

1. Frank E, Prien RF, Jarret RB. Conceptualisation and rationale for consensus definitions of terms in major depressive disorder. Remission, recovery, relapse and recurrence. *Arch Gen Psychiatry* 1991; **54**: 993–99.
2. Judd LL, Akiskal HS, Maser JD, Zeller PJ, Endicott J, Coryell W. A prospective 12-year study of subsyndromal and syndromal depressive symptoms in unipolar major depressive disorder. *Arch Gen Psychiatry* 1998; **55**: 694–700.
3. Keller MB, Lavori PW, Mueller TI. Time to recovery, chronicity and levels of psychopathology in major depression. *Arch Gen Psychiatry* 1992; **49**: 809–16.
4. McCullough JP. *Treatment for Chronic Depression*. New York: Guilford Press, 2000.
5. Cole MG, Bellavance F, Mansour A. Prognosis of depression in elderly community and primary care populations: a systematic review and meta-analysis. *Am J Psychiatry* 1999; **156**: 1182–89.
6. Licht-Strunk E, van der Windt DA, van Marwijk HW, de Haan M, Beekman AT. The prognosis of depression in older patients in general practice and the community. A systematic review. *Fam Pract* 2007; **24**: 168–80.
7. Licht-Strunk E, van Marwijk HW, Hoekstra T, Twisk JWR, de Haan M, Beekman AT. Outcome of depression in later life in primary care: longitudinal cohort study with three years follow-up. *BMJ* 2009; **338**: a3079.
8. Beekman ATF, Geerlings SW, Deeg DJH et al. () The natural history of late-life depression: a 6-year prospective study in the community. *Arch Gen Psychiatry* 2002; **59**: 605 11.
9. Snowdon J. The prevalence of depression in old age (editorial). *Int J Geriatr Psychiatry* 1990; **5**: 141–44.
10. Akiskal HS. Dysthymic disorder: psychopathology of proposed chronic depressive subtypes. *Am J Psychiatry* 1983; **140**: 11–20.
11. Beekman ATF, Deeg DJH, Smit JH, Comijs HC, de Beurs E, van Tilburg W. Dysthymia in later life: a study in the community. *J Affect Disord* 2004; **81**: 231–40.
12. Spijker J, de Graaf R, Bijl RV, Beekman ATF, Ormel J, Nolen WA. () Duration of major depressive episodes in the general population. Results from the Netherlands Mental Health Survey and Incidence Study (NEMESIS). *Br J Psychiatry* 2002; **181**: 208–13.
13. Steunenberg B, Beekman ATF, Deeg DJH, Bremmer MA, Kerkhof AJFM. Mastery and neuroticism predict recovery of depression in later life. *Am J Geriatr Psychiatry* 2007; **15**: 234–42.
14. Steffens DE, Otey E, Alexopoulos GS. Perspectives on depression, mild cognitive impairment and cognitive decline. *Arch Gen Psychiatry* 2006; **63**: 130–38.
15. Scott KM, Von Korff M, Alonso J. Age patterns in the prevalence of DSM IV depressive/anxiety disorders with and without physical comorbidity. *Psychol Med* 2008; **38**: 1659–69.
16. Meeks S, Murrell SA, Mehl RC. Longitudinal relationships between depressive symptoms and health in normal older and middle-aged adults. *Psychol Aging* 2000; **15**: 100–109.
17. Bremmer MA, Hoogendijk WJG, Deeg DJH, Schoevers RA, Schalk BWM, Beekman AT. Depression in older age is a risk factor for first ischemic cardiac events. *Am J Geriatr Psychiatry* 2006; **14**: 523–30.
18. Schulz R, Drayer RA, Rollman BL. Depression as a risk factor for non-suicide mortality in the elderly. *Biol Psychiatry* 2002; **52**: 205–25.
19. Baldwin RC. Recent understandings in geriatric affective disorder. *Curr Opin Psychiatry* 2007; **20**: 539–43.
20. Bruce EC, Musselman DL. Depression, alterations in platelet functioning and ischaemic heart disease. *Psychosom Med* 2005; **67**: S34–36.
21. Kohler S, Thomas AJ, Barnett NA, O' Brien JT. The pattern and course of cognitive impairment in late-life depression. *Psychol Med* 2009; **6**: 1–12.
22. Dombrovski AY, Szanto K, Duberstein P, Conner KR, Houch PR, Conwell Y. Sex differences in correlates of suicide attempt lethality in late life. *Am J Geriatr Psychiatry* 2008; **16**: 905–13.
23. Waern M, Rubenowitz E, Runeson BS, Skoog I, Wilhelmson K, Allebeck. Burden of illness and suicide in elderly people: a case control study. *BMJ* 2002; **324**: 1355–57.

24. Turvey CL, Conwell Y, Jones MP. Risk factors for late life suicide: a prospective, community based study. *Am J Psychiatry* 2002; **159**: 450–55.

25. Schoevers RA, Geerlings MI, Deeg DJH, Holwerda TJ, Jonker C, Beekman AT. Depression and excess mortality: evidence for a dose response relation in community living elderly. *Int J Geriatr Psychiatry* 2009; **24**: 169–76.

26. Penninx BW, Kritchevsky SB, Yaffe K *et al.* Inflammatory markers and depressed mood in older persons: results from the Health, Aging and Body Composition Study. *Biol Psychiatry* 2003; **54**: 566–72.

27. Beekman AT, Deeg DJH, Braam A, Smit J, van Tilburg W. Consequences of major and minor depression in later life: a study of disability, well-being and service utilization. *Psychol Med* 1997; **6**: 1397–409.

28. Young AS, Klap R, Shoai R, Wells KB. Persistent depression and anxiety in the United States: prevalence and quality of care. *Psychiatry Serv* 2008; **59**: 1391–98.

29. Smits FT, Brouwer HJ, van Weert HC, Schene AH, ter Riet G. Predictability of persistent frequent attendance: a historic 3-year cohort study. *Br J Gen Pract* 2009; **59**: e44–e50.

30. Smits FT, Brouwer HJ, ter Riet G, van Weert HC. Epidemiology of frequent attenders: a 3-year historic cohort study comparing attendance, morbidity and prescriptions of one-year and persistent frequent attenders. *BMC Public Health* 2009; **9**: 36.

31. Menchetti M, Cevenini N, De Ronchi D, Quartesan R, Berardi D. Depression and frequent attendance in elderly primary care patients. *Gen Hosp Psychiatry* 2006; **28**: 119–24.

32. Kurland BF, Gill TM, Patrick DL, Larson EB, Phelan EA. Longitudinal change in positive affect in community-dwelling older persons. *J Am Geriatr Soc* 2006; **54**: 1846–53.

81

Physical Illness and Depression*

Mavis Evans

Elderly Mental Health Directorate, Wirral and West Cheshire Community NHS Trust, Clatter bridge Hospital, Bebington, Wirral, UK

EPIDEMIOLOGY

The prevalence of depression in the general population worldwide is usually found to be 3–8%[1-3]. The prevalence of major depression has been shown to be no higher in the elderly than the young, although these findings do not allow for the co-morbidity of physical illnesses or dementias[4]. The World Health Organization (WHO) World Mental Health surveys[5] of respondents in 10 developed countries ($n = 52\,485$) and 8 developing countries ($n = 37\,265$) showed that 12-month major depressive episodes (MDE) were significantly less prevalent among respondents aged 65+ than in younger respondents in developed but not developing countries. Prevalence of co-morbid mental disorders generally either decreased or remained stable with age, while co-morbidity of MDE with mental disorders generally increased with age. Prevalence of physical conditions, in comparison, generally increased with age, while co-morbidity of MDE with physical conditions generally decreased with age. The surveys concluded that the weakening associations between MDE and physical conditions with increasing age argue against the suggestion that the low estimated prevalence of MDE among the elderly is caused by increased confounding with physical disorders. Future studies are needed to investigate processes that might lead to a decreasing impact of physical illness on depression among the elderly.

Subthreshold or minor depressions have many different names and definitions, which causes widely differing prevalence rates to be quoted. Categorical definitions of depression do not fit well with the range of symptoms and severity seen in normal clinical practice. However, it is generally accepted that the burden of depression among the elderly is high and an accepted measure of diagnosis is necessary to allow communication with patients, relatives and professional colleagues.

'Caseness' can be considered to be the severity of depression at which the majority of professionals would consider some form of intervention appropriate. Prevalence of this degree of depression is reported as 10–15% of the elderly in the community[6,7], 15–30% of those attending primary care facilities[8,9], 15–50% of those in hospital[9-11] and 30–40% of those in institutional care[9,12].

DIAGNOSIS

Depression cannot be diagnosed unless it is first considered a possibility, neither will it be appropriately treated unless it is considered pathological. Depression may be missed when too much emphasis is placed on the presenting complaints of, for example, lethargy, anorexia or pain[13]. Depression and feelings of worthlessness may cause failure to complain of symptoms of physical illness or to ask for help. It may cause non-compliance with medication and other treatments, self-neglect or non-attendance at clinics. Alternatively, the lowering of self-esteem and decreased ability to cope can lead to increased attendance at clinics.

The lack of a concise definition for depression in the elderly makes the establishment of validity a difficult task, which can only be examined by longitudinal follow-up of patients to see what happens to their symptoms[14]. Somatic symptoms, such as lack of energy, poor concentration and weight loss, may be caused by the physical illness or ageing, not depression; even experienced clinicians may have difficulty attributing such symptoms to physical or psychiatric causes. Even feelings of life not being worth living and wishing to die are not always associated with depressed mood; poor subjective health, disability, pain, sensory impairment and living in an institution have been shown to be associated factors in the absence of depressive illness[15].

The elderly tend not to admit to feelings of depression and relatives may be unaware of the condition[16]. Somatization, 'the tendency to experience and communicate somatic distress and somatic symptoms unaccounted for by relevant pathological findings, to attribute them to physical illness and to seek medical help for them'[17], is increasingly recognized. Somatization can still occur in those with genuine physical illness. The somatic symptoms of depression are similar to those of a chronic illness, such as cancer, and it must be remembered that depression and physical illness often co-exist[18].

Hypochondriasis is a recognized symptom of depression in the elderly population[19]. However, in this age group, rigorous steps must be undertaken to exclude physical problems before ascribing symptoms to hypochondriasis or somatization[18,20]. That such patients are depressed is inferred from their good response to standard treatments for depression[21].

The 1991 National Institutes for Health (NIH) Consensus Statement on diagnosis and treatment of depression in late life concluded: 'What makes depression in the elderly so insidious is that neither the victim nor the health provider may recognize its symptoms in the context of the multiple physical problems of many elderly people.' DSM-IV allows somatic symptoms to be counted towards the diagnosis of depression if there is any possibility of psychological aetiology, a more inclusive and accurate means of diagnosis than previously.

*Updated by Mohammed T. Abou-Saleh

Principles and Practice of Geriatric Psychiatry, 3rd edn. Edited by Mohammed T. Abou-Saleh, Cornelius Katona and Anand Kumar
© 2011 John Wiley & Sons, Ltd

MORBIDITY AND MORTALITY

Psychiatric morbidity in hospitals is higher than in the general population. Surveys of wards and clinics do not completely establish an association between psychiatric and physical morbidity because they may be biased for selective referral patterns: psychological symptoms can lead to help-seeking behaviour for physical illness in an individual who had previously been able to tolerate his or her physical problems. Similarly, they may influence a GP on whether or not to refer to hospital. Stress may be as important in triggering help-seeking behaviour as in triggering actual illness. In addition to the degree of distress, many other factors determine whether or not an individual will seek help, including religious and social values, socioeconomic background and personality.

Affective disorder in the elderly is strongly associated with physical ill-health[20]: 'whether or not such an illness has a direct aetiological relationship to the affective disorder, its practical importance must be considered, for it is bound to influence the course and outcome of the psychiatric condition.' Although overall medical burden appears comparable in elderly patients with bipolar and those with major depressive disorder, patients with bipolar disorder have higher body mass index and greater burden of endocrine/metabolic and respiratory disease[22].

Other studies have found that depression leads to increased mortality[23-25] over and above age effects, the prognosis worsening with severity of depression. Chronic illness, physical function and cognitive function all independently predict depressive morbidity in late life. The significance of depressive symptoms was demonstrated by their independent association with all-cause mortality at two-year follow-up[26].

Depression in the elderly may be due partly to a biological ageing process, which would directly increase mortality and morbidity[21,27]. Burvill and Hall[28] showed increased mortality in depressed elderly patients ($n = 103$, aged 60+) followed for five years if they were aged 75+, had impaired mobility or showed poor recovery with residual symptoms or chronicity. There were two peaks of increased mortality, one early in the disease and one late. Cardiovascular or pulmonary disease and malignancies were the predominant causes of death. The results are similar to those of the four-year follow-up by Murphy et al.[29], who also postulate that increased mortality seen in the depressed elderly (especially the men) was not caused by differences in physical health alone. They suggest:

- inadequate treatment of the depression, leading to cardiovascular complications from the antidepressant but no benefit to the patient; the depression itself can also provoke cardiac death, especially in men;
- 'sub-intentional suicide' in those who 'turn their faces to the wall';
- residual depressive invalidism, causing poor nutrition and decreased mobility; with attendant complications of susceptibility to infection, fractures, bedsores, etc., all contributing to the increased mortality.

Mortality in hospital was found to be significantly higher in those depressed but over 30% of those discharged had died within, on average, five months, whether depressed or not[30]. The authors also noted that survivors with depression consumed more health care resources than did the non-depressed survivors. Among the depressed elderly, 40% have chronic poor physical health[31]; they use and need more medical services[32,33] than the non-depressed, but also use fewer social and recreational services[32]. An association has been found between poor mental health and subsequent physical disease, suggesting that positive mental health may significantly retard the decline in physical health with increasing age[34].

Physical illness affects the capacity for independent living, resulting in altered relationships with others, lowered self-esteem and vulnerability to depression. Serious illness may be seen by some as an unpleasant reminder of mortality, bringing apprehension and fear. Continuing physical illness is a poor prognostic factor for depression, although whether this is a result of a biological relationship or the psychological strain of being ill is uncertain.

Mortality in acute medical inpatients is significantly higher in those with associated depression, although the direction of causality is not established. For example, Silverstone[35] followed consecutive admissions for myocardial infarction, subarachnoid haemorrhage, pulmonary embolus or upper gastrointestinal haemorrhage for 28 days post admission; 34% were depressed and 47% of these had life-threatening complications or died, compared with 10% of those not depressed.

PHYSICAL ILLNESS AND DEPRESSION

Mood disturbance can result from structural brain disease, alterations in neurotransmitter concentration or activity caused by drugs or biochemical disturbance. These affective symptoms may present during a physical illness or be the initial symptom of an otherwise occult physical disorder. Depression may be:

- the result of an illness, especially a painful or disabling one;
- iatrogenic (e.g. the result of steroid treatment);
- a symptom of the physical illness (e.g. hypothyroidism);
- an aetiological factor (e.g. alcohol abuse secondary to depression);
- a depressed patient adopting the sick role as a coping mechanism;
- a common aetiological factor, such as bereavement, causing both depression and physical illness; or
- coincidental.

The elderly are particularly susceptible to the side effects of drug treatment[36], especially as they are often subject to polypharmacy[37,38]. Patients with drug-induced depression often have a past or family history of depression and the drug may have precipitated the disease by affecting the levels of available neurotransmitters[37]. Depression can often be alleviated by cessation of the drug, although some patients will also require antidepressant treatment. The combination of a susceptible patient and a depressogenic drug may precipitate a depression sufficiently severe to lead to suicide[37].

Subjective rating of general health has been shown to be independently associated with depression in the elderly, including the very old[39-41]. This can lead to presentation at primary care or emergency facilities, unnecessary investigations and risk of iatrogenic disease, and lower quality of life. Recognition and treatment of the depression may lead to improvement in the patient's subjective perception of his or her health.

Physically ill depressed patients are more likely to be admitted to hospital than those who are not depressed[42]. Depressed patients have higher use of all categories of medical care, including admissions, laboratory tests and emergency department visits[33].

The presence of significant psychiatric disorder has been shown to adversely affect the course of medical admission[43,44], affective disorders in particular prolonging length of stay[45-47] (although the study by Ramsay et al.[48] did not confirm this) and increasing the likelihood of admission to residential care[49]. Psychiatric intervention has been shown to increase recovery rate, reduce duration of stay, reduce the need for residential care after discharge and therefore reduce costs[50,51]. Importantly a diagnosis of major depression in older medical inpatients is independently associated with poor mental health in their informal caregivers six months later[52].

ADJUSTMENT DISORDER

Lipowski[53] has proposed that the subjective significance of an illness and its treatment (e.g. amputation, cancer), combined with the patient's personality and social circumstances, is the key to the psychological response. The variety of physical illnesses found with depression would support this view. Depression may be a reaction to physical problems; it occurs more frequently in those with increasing numbers of medical diagnoses and may be precipitated by developing new physical illnesses[23,54]. All illnesses except the very trivial involve an element of psychological adjustment. Serious medical illness is likely to be a potent psychological stressor, affecting body image, self-esteem, the sense of identity and the capacity to work and to maintain social, family and marital relationships[55]. However, the majority of people adapt their lives to the demands of their illness, maximizing their prospects of recovery and return to previous levels of activity.

In the elderly, physical illness is frequently chronic and may worsen with time. This, combined with the losses suffered by many elderly people, such as loss of status and income on retirement, loss of friends and family by death and the fear of loss of independence and dignity due to the illness itself, can lead to the adjustment disorder merging imperceptibly into a depressive illness. This can be considered secondary depression[56], the depression following or paralleling a life-threatening or incapacitating medical illness. However, the prevalence of this type of depression is unknown, as it is difficult to differentiate from depression related to other stressors and previous history. Patients with this type of depression tend to have fewer suicidal thoughts but have more feelings of helplessness, pessimism and anxiety[57].

SOMATIZED DEPRESSION

This is more common than medical illness presenting as depression, especially in the current generation of elderly, who tend to somatize their psychological symptoms, having been brought up in a society which did not encourage the expression of emotion. Somatic symptoms in the elderly may represent physical illness, depression or emotional responses to physical illness. The somatic symptoms will need investigation, but depression, if suspected, should be treated.

Pseudodementia is a specific type of masked depression. One of the most important differentiating factors is that the severity of cognitive impairment fluctuates in depressed patients, remaining constant or worsening in the evenings in dementia. Depressed patients tend not to try to succeed in tasks, giving up with 'I don't know' or 'I can't'. Demented patients will try, delighting in success but possibly becoming very distressed by failure – the so-called catastrophic reaction. Biological symptoms of appetite and weight loss, sleep disturbance and headache are typical of depression and not dementia. However, depression and dementia can co-exist and the differentiation of the two conditions is not always easy. If in doubt, a trial of antidepressant treatment will help elucidate the diagnosis. The pathognomic symptoms of masked or somatized depression include:

- diurnal variation (symptoms usually worse in the mornings);
- mild impairment of cognitive processes and concentration;
- dysthymic mood changes;
- fatigue, feeling tired, lack of energy;
- sleep disturbance (waking up early and being unable to get back to sleep); and
- an anxious sense of failure or of 'impending disaster'.

LIAISON

Consultation–liaison psychiatry has become well established as an important specialty in general hospitals on both sides of the Atlantic. In an ideal situation, psychiatrists would attend ward rounds in the general hospital, particularly on rehabilitation wards, where prevalence of depression is high and the effect on delayed discharge well documented[45–47]. However, restricted resources prevent this: psychiatric morbidity is too high for a psychiatrist to see all the patients affected – his or her main role should be educational[58], only taking an active part in the management of more difficult cases. In many areas there is increasing development of specialist liaison nurses who are able to advise on diagnosis and treatment, reducing delay before assessments. The liaison nurse is likely to be more permanent than junior doctors on rotation and can often help a patient who refuses to see a psychiatrist or whose physician refuses psychiatric referral[59]. Liaison nurses can educate general nurses in the recognition of psychiatric disorders and can in turn encourage junior medical staff to institute appropriate referral or treatment. Their development and use has been compared with that of community psychiatric nurses[60].

The most common reasons for requesting a psychiatric consultation in a general hospital are[61]:

- diagnostic uncertainty;
- recognition of a gross psychiatric disorder;
- excessive emotional reactions (e.g. fear, anger, depression);
- a patient's deviant behaviour disturbing ward or medical procedures;
- delayed convalescence (i.e. disability incompatible with observed pathology, relapse on mention of discharge);
- crisis in the doctor–patient relationship (e.g. refusing consent!);
- patient's admission of serious psychosocial difficulties;
- selection and/or preparation of patients (e.g. pre-transplant, cosmetic surgery).

It can be seen from the above list that the depressed patient, sitting quiet and withdrawn on the ward or in a home, may not be referred for a psychiatric opinion. In practice, only about 2% of geriatric patients are referred to the liaison services[62–64]. Suggested reasons for the discrepancy between liaison rate and psychiatric morbidity are as follows[62,65]:

- High prevalence of transient self-limiting psychiatric disease.
- Physician's failure to recognize psychiatric disease[66]. Many studies have highlighted the unrecognized psychiatric problems on medical wards[65] and the under-diagnosis of major depression in particular has been well documented[67].
- Medical and nursing staff may actively avoid questioning for psychological problems, due to fear of precipitating emotional distress that they have not been trained to deal with.
- The low priority of psychiatric disease compared to physical, especially in a busy medical ward with acutely ill patients.

- Poor access to, or dissatisfaction with, psychiatric services.
- Physician resistance to psychiatric consultation[50] due to stigma or under-estimating the severity or the potential for treatment.

Use of screening scales is appropriate for assessing depression in the physically ill: it is common, can be a difficult diagnosis and has significant morbidity and mortality if untreated. Care must be taken to differentiate between short-lived adjustment disorders, occurring as a reaction to the admission itself, or the crisis which precipitated it. Diagnosis in acute admissions should therefore include enquiry into symptoms before admission. If none can be elicited, the patient should be reassessed at a later date, either during rehabilitation or after discharge.

Screening scales serve a dual function[68-70] – they identify patients in need of further assessment and also serve as an educational tool if given by general staff during routine admission procedures. They emphasize the associated symptoms and signs of depression in the elderly, who may not show depressed affect and will deny feeling sad. It is important, however, that education about the treatment of depression goes hand in hand with education to recognize it, or the liaison services will be swamped.

TREATMENT

The fact that one can intuitively 'understand' why the physically ill elderly are depressed does not mean that it should be accepted as normal and treatment not attempted. Continuing physical illness is recognized as both a precipitant of depression and a poor prognostic factor, yet despite this, 80% of elderly general hospital patients are not depressed[45,71,72]. Successful coping mechanisms can prevent the emergence of clinical depression. Even in the terminal patient, depression or dysphoria can be relieved by euphoriants, such as oral or parenteral opiates, reducing the distress of patient and relatives[73] without significantly reducing the length of life remaining to the patient.

It is important that the diagnosis is not missed, as this condition usually responds well to treatment, at least initially, thus improving quality of life. Follow-up and early treatment of any relapses will further improve the prognosis. Increased self-esteem and ability to cope will reduce demand on families and possibly on services.

Even when the correct diagnosis is made, the depression may not be treated adequately, if at all: physically ill patients who are also depressed are more likely to be assigned to the 'not to be resuscitated' group, compared with those elderly who are not depressed. The lack of effort and motivation caused by depression may be regarded as 'not trying' or 'giving up' by nurses and rehabilitation staff, who withdraw from this group of patients for more emotionally rewarding non-depressed elderly subjects on the same ward.

The elderly as a group have approximately twice as many adverse drug reactions as younger adults[74]. They are frequently already on polypharmacy, so drug interactions are a real possibility. It is therefore important that physicians are advised and supported by the psychiatric services in the use of safe, well-tolerated antidepressants and other treatments to reduce the impact of this disease on both the individual and society.

Electroconvulsive therapy (ECT) is an effective treatment of depression[75,76]. The response to treatment in older people is better than in the young[77,78]. With the increasing safety of anaesthesia, very few patients, even those with severe physical disease, are unable to tolerate a course of treatment. It is more rapid in effect than medication alone, but the improvement is rarely sustained unless antidepressants are also given to prevent relapse.

A review of psychological treatments in chronic illness[79] found very little empirical evidence of benefit when therapeutic interventions were applied indiscriminately. However, some evidence was found to show benefit in patients with somatization disorders rather than physical illness, and also that brief interventions following the onset of acute physical illness reduced longer term psychological morbidity. A suggested general approach to the treatment of physically ill depressed patients is as follows:

1. Investigate and give appropriate treatment to all physical problems, either curative treatment or to minimize persistent morbidity. Explain the illness, treatment and prognosis to the patient in as much detail as he/she wishes. Make sure the explanation is understood and repeat as often as necessary.
2. Give general social support (e.g. home help services, financial assistance if relevant, or residential or nursing home care).
3. Give psychological support – encouragement, continued interest in the patient (e.g. outpatient follow-up). Support groups are often beneficial for chronic conditions such as rheumatoid arthritis, Parkinson's disease, etc.
4. Consider antidepressant therapy if the symptoms are sufficiently severe that they would be considered to warrant medication if seen in a patient without physical problems. Monitor the response to treatment; this may take 7–8 weeks[80]. If no response is seen to a therapeutic dosage of antidepressant, consider a trial of an alternative antidepressant or adjunctive treatment, or specialist referral.

PROGNOSIS

Little is known of the prognosis of psychiatric disorder identified in the medical setting[81], except that concomitant physical illness is a poor prognostic factor. Psychiatric disturbance often persists[82-84], especially in patients with a previous history of psychiatric disorder. Those with affective disorder on admission have increased mortality and make greater demands on medical, social and psychiatric services[81,85].

In one series of consecutive acute medical admissions[84], fewer than 45% of those patients with concomitant depression had received antidepressants at all, 20% had been given benzodiazepines, and less than 25% had been treated for more than one week. The authors concluded that an effective treatment for depression in elderly patients needed to be found, with widespread education of geriatricians in the diagnosis and treatment of depression.

In psychiatric patients, relapse has been linked with supervening physical illness[86]. The presence or development of cerebral or any other irreversible physical disorder indicates poor future mental health in the great majority of patients, as well as the likelihood of early death[87].

The prognosis of the physical illness, for both morbidity and mortality, is also inextricably linked with that of the depression. Increased mortality from physical illness, especially cardiovascular disease, has been reported[88,89]. This excess of deaths is significantly associated with groups who have been only partially treated (e.g. have not responded to antidepressants[90], especially in older men[91].

Explanations for the apparent association of physical illness with poor treatment outcome might include[92]:

- age as a confounding factor – most of the trials of treatment in the physically ill are in the elderly;

- medically ill patients may be given inadequate doses of antidepressants because of problems with side effects or over-cautious physicians;
- different subtypes of depression exist, some medication responsive, some not. Organic mood disorder (depression induced by physical illness or a specific organic factor) has been shown to have a worse prognosis at four-year follow-up[93].

The prognosis of depression in the physically ill elderly is therefore dependent on accurate diagnosis, intensive treatment, follow-up and early treatment of any relapses[86,88,94]. Increased self-esteem and ability to cope will reduce demand on families and possibly on services. No studies have yet convincingly identified predictors of response in physically ill populations, although pre-existing depression prior to admission with physical problems appears to predict persistent depression, rather than if the depression develops in hospital[82,95].

SUICIDE

Suicide is the most dramatic of poor outcomes, and the elderly are over-represented in suicide statistics. Although the elderly are less likely to attempt suicide, they are more likely to complete it[96,97]. The presence of physical illness, especially if associated with chronic pain and disability, increases the risk; elderly men living alone are at the highest risk. The individual's adjustment to ill-health and his or her associated feelings of hopelessness and demoralization are obviously important[98]. Many elderly suicide victims are suffering from their first episode of major depression, which is typically only moderately severe but the diagnosis is missed[99], and the potential for recovery following intervention therefore lost.

Depression has been linked to decreased compliance and to voluntary refusal of life-saving essential medical treatments[100,101]. This may reflect either conscious or unconscious suicidal motivation.

SERVICE IMPLICATIONS

It is important to note that the ageing population itself is growing older, with large numbers of very old individuals. It is this old-old group who have the highest physical and psychiatric morbidity and who make the greatest demands on services.

Undergraduate teaching programmes must be tightly integrated in order for students to develop a holistic approach to the elderly, together with an understanding of the psychosocial and economic factors that will affect presentation and treatment. Joint postgraduate meetings between the two specialties are becoming more common and should be encouraged, each maintaining their separate identities and training but working closely together in clinical practice.

Interdisciplinary research continues to grow in amount, but is mostly directed at psychiatric problems on medical wards. Little seems to be researched in the other direction, medical illnesses on psychiatric wards. All research is obviously relevant to both specialties and in practice helps to strengthen links between them.

REFERENCES

1. Myers JK, Weissman MM, Tischler GL. Six month prevalence of psychiatric disorders in three communities 1980–1982. *Arch Gen Psychiatry* 1984; **41**: 959–67.
2. Mavreas VG, Beis A, Bouyias A. Psychiatric disorders in Athens: a community study. *Soc Psychiatry* 1986; **21**: 172–81.
3. Bebbington PE, Hurry J, Tennant C. Epidemiology of mental disorders in Camberwell. *Psychol Med* 1981; **11**: 561–79.
4. Blazer D. EURODEP consortium and late life depression. *Br J Psychiatryry* 1999; **174**: 284–85.
5. Kessler RC, Birnbaum HG, Shahly V et al. Age differences in the prevalence and co-morbidity of DSM-IV major depressive episodes: results from the WHO World Mental Health Survey Initiative. *Depress Anxiety* 2009 Dec 27. [Epub ahead of print]
6. Copeland JRM, Dewey ME, Wood N et al. Range of mental illness among the elderly in the community: prevalence in Liverpool using the GMS–AGECAT package. *Br J Psychiatryry* 1987; **150**: 815–23.
7. Blazer D, Williams CD. Epidemiology of dysphoria and depression in an elderly population. *Am J Psychiatry* 1980; **137**: 439–44.
8. Callahan CM, Hendrie HC, Dittus RS et al. Depression in late life: the use of clinical characteristics to focus screening efforts. *J Gerontol* 1994; 9: M9–14.
9. Katona CLE. The epidemiology of depression in old age: the importance of physical illness. *Clin Neuropharmacol* 1992; **15** (suppl): 281–82.
10. Fenton FR, Cole MG, Engelsman N, Mansouri I. Depression in older medical inpatients. *Int J Geriatr Psychiatry* 1994; **9**: 279–84.
11. Hammond MF, Evans ME, Lye M. Depression in medical wards. *Int J Geriatr Psychiatry* 1993; **8**: 957–58.
12. Harrison R, Savla N, Kafetz K. Dementia, depression and physical disability in a London Borough: a survey of elderly people in and out of residential care and implications for future developments. *Age Aging* 1990; **19**: 97–103.
13. Kidd CB. Misplacement of the elderly in hospital. A study of patients admitted to geriatric and mental hospitals. *BMJ* 1962; **253**: 1491–95.
14. Koenig HG, Pappas P, Holsinger T, Bachar JR. Assessing diagnostic approaches to depression in medically ill older adults: how reliably can mental health professionals make judgements about the cause of symptoms? *J Am Geriatr Soc* 1995; **43**: 472–78.
15. Jorm AF, Henderson AS, Scott R et al. Factors associated with the wish to die in elderly people. *Age Ageing* 1995; **24**: 389–92.
16. Hanley I, Baikie E. Understanding and treating depression in the elderly. In Hanley I, Hodge J (eds), *Psychological Approaches to the Care of the Elderly*. New York: Methuen, 1984.
17. Lipowski ZJ. Somatisation: the concept and its clinical application. *Am J Psychiatry* 1988; **145**: 1358–68.
18. Sweer L, Rairin DC, Ladd RA et al. The medical evaluation of elderly patients with major depression. *J Gerontol* 1988; **3**: M53–58.
19. Kramer-Ginsberg E, Greenwald BS, Aisen PS, Brod-Miller C. Hypochondriasis and the elderly depressed. *J Am Geriatr Soc* 1989; **37**: 507–10.
20. Roth M, Kay DWK. Affective disorders arising in the senium II: physical disability as an aetiological factor. *J Ment Sci* 1956; **102**: 141–50.
21. Jacoby RJ. Depression in the elderly. *Br J Hosp Med* 1981; 40–47.
22. Gildengers AG, Whyte EM, Drayer RA et al. Medical burden in late-life bipolar and major depressive disorders. *Am J Geriatr Psychiatry* 2008; **16**: 194–200.

23. Murphy E. The prognosis of depression in old age. *Br J Psychiatry* 1983; **142**: 111–19.

24. Baldwin RC, Jolley DJ. The prognosis of depression in old age. *Br J Psychiatry* 1986; **149**: 574–83.

25. Robinson JR. The natural history of mental disorder in old age: a long term study. *Br J Psychiatry* 1989; **154**: 783–89.

26. Turvey CL, Schultz SK, Beglinger L, Klein DM. A longitudinal community-based study of chronic illness, cognitive and physical function, and depression. *Am J Geriatr Psychiatry* 2009; **17**: 632–41.

27. Post F. The management and nature of depressive illness in late life: a follow-through study. *Br J Psychiatry* 1972; **121**: 393–404.

28. Burvill PW, Hall WD. Predictors of increased mortality in elderly depressed patients. *Int J Geriatr Psychiatry* 1994; **9**: 219–27.

29. Murphy E, Smith R, Lindesay J, Slattery J. Increased mortality rates in late-life depression. *Br J Psychiatry* 1988; **152**: 347–53.

30. Koenig HG, Shelp F, Goli V *et al*. Survival and health care utilization in elderly medical inpatients with major depression. *J Am Geriatr Soc* 1989; **37**: 599–606.

31. Murphy E. Social origins of depression in old age. *Br J Psychiatry* 1982; **141**: 135–42.

32. Badger TA. Depression, physical health impairment and service use among older adults. *Publ Health Nurs* 1998; **15**: 136–45.

33. Unutzer J, Patrick DL, Simon G *et al*. Depressive symptoms and the cost of health services in HMO patients aged 65 years and older. *J Am Geriatr Assoc* 1997; **277**: 1618–23.

34. Vaillant GE. Natural history of male psychologic health. *N Engl J Med* 1979; **301**: 1249–55.

35. Silverstone PH. Depression increases mortality and morbidity in acute life-threatening medical illness. *J Psychosom Res* 1990; **34**: 651–57.

36. Ouslander JG. Physical illness and depression in the elderly. *J Am Geriatr Soc* 1982; **30**: 593–99.

37. Whitlock FA. *Systematic Affective Disorders*. London: Academic Press, 1982.

38. Braithwaite R. The pharmakokinetics of psychotropic drugs in the elderly. In Wheatley D (ed.), *Pharmacology of Old Age*. Oxford. Oxford University Press, 1982.

39. Evans ME, Copeland JRM, Dewey ME. Depression in the elderly in the community: effect of physical illness and selected social factors. *Int J Geriatr Psychiatry* 1991; **6**: 787–95.

40. Meller I, Fichter MM, Schroppel H. Risk factors and psychosocial consequences in depression of octo- and nonagenarians: results of an epidemiological study. *Eur Arch Psychiat Clin Neurosci* 1997; **247**: 278–87.

41. Mulsant BH, Ganguli M, Seaberg EC. The relationship between self rated health and depressive symptoms in an epidemiological sample of community-dwelling older adults. *J Am Geriatr Soc* 1997; **45**: 954–58.

42. Kay DWK, Beamish R, Roth M. Old age mental disorders in Newcastle upon Tyne. Part 1: a study of prevalence. *Br J Psychiatry* 1964; **110**: 146–58.

43. Johnston M, Wakeling A, Graham N, Stokes F. Cognitive impairment, emotional disorder and length of stay of elderly patients in a district general hospital. *Br J Med Psychol* 1987; **60**: 133–39.

44. Coid J, Crome P. Bed blocking in Bromley. *BMJ* 1986; **292**: 1253–56.

45. Bergmann K, Eastham EJ. Psychogeriatric ascertainment and assessment for treatment in an acute medical ward setting. *Age Ageing* 1974; **3**: 174–87.

46. Mossey JM, Mutran E, Knott K, Craik R. Determinants of recovery 12 months after hip fracture: the importance of psychosocial factors. *Am J Publ Health* 1989; **79**: 279–86.

47. Verbosky LA, Franco KN, Zrull JP. The relationship between depression and length of stay in the general hospital patient. *J Clin Psychiatry* 1993; **54**: 177–81.

48. Ramsay R, Wright P, Katz A *et al*. The detection of psychiatric morbidity and its effects on outcome in acute elderly medical admissions. *Int J Geriatr Psychiatry* 1991; **6**: 861–66.

49. Lindesay J, Murphy E. Dementia, depression and subsequent institutionalisation – the effect of home support. *Int J Geriatr Psychiatry* 1989; **4**: 3–9.

50. Steinberg R, Torem M, Saravay SM. An analysis of physician resistance to psychiatric consultations. *Arch Gen Psychiatry* 1980; **37**: 1007–12.

51. Levitan SJ, Kornfeld DS. Clinical and cost benefits of liaison psychiatry. *Am J Psychiatry* 1981; **138**: 790–93.

52. McCusker J, Latimer E, Cole M, Ciampi A, Sewitch M. Major depression among medically ill elders contributes to sustained poor mental health in their informal caregivers. *Age Ageing* 2007; **36**: 400–406.

53. Lipowski ZJ. Review of consultation psychiatry and psychosomatic medicine. I: general principles. *Psychosom Med* 1967; **29**: 153–71.

54. Kukull WA, Koepsall T, Inui T *et al*. Depression and physical illness among elderly general medical clinic patients. *J Affect Disord* 1986; **10**: 153–62.

55. Rodin GM, Voshart K. Depression in the medically ill: an overview. *Am J Psychiatry* 1986; **143**: 696–705.

56. Feighner JP, Robins E, Guze SB *et al*. Diagnostic criteria for use in research. *Arch Gen Psychiatry* 1972; **26**: 57–63.

57. Lloyd GG. Emotional aspects of physical illness. In Granville-Grossman K (ed.), *Recent Advances in Clinical Psychiatry*, vol. 5. London: Churchill Livingstone, 1985.

58. Anderson DN, Philpott RM. The changing pattern of referrals for psychogeriatric consultation in the general hospital: an eight year study. *Int J Geriatr Psychiatry* 1991; **6**: 801–807.

59. Collinson Y, Benbow SM. The role of an old age psychiatry consultation liaison nurse. *Int J Geriatr Psychiatry* 1998; **13**: 159–63.

60. Benbow SM. Liaison services for elderly people. In Benjamin S, House A, Jenkins P (eds), *Liaison Psychiatry: Defining Needs and Planning Services*. London: Gaskell, 1994.

61. Lipowski ZJ. Review of consultation liaison psychiatry and psychosomatic medicine. II: Clinical aspects. *Psychosom Med* 1967; **29**: 201–24.

62. Popkin MK, MacKenzie TB, Callies AL. Psychiatric consultation to geriatric medically ill patients in a university hospital. *Arch Gen Psychiatry* 1984; **41**: 703–707.

63. Ruskin PE. Geropsychiatric consultation in a university hospital: a report on 67 referrals. *Am J Psychiatry* 1985; **142**: 333–36.

64. Poynton AM. Psychiatric liaison referrals of elderly inpatients in a teaching hospital. *Br J Psychiatry* 1988; **152**: 45–47.

65. Maguire GP, Julier DL, Hawton KE, Bancroft JHJ. Psychiatric morbidity and referral on two general medical wards. *BMJ* 1974; **1**: 268–70.

66. Gurland B. The comparative frequency of depression in various adult age groups. *J Gerontol* 1976; **31**: 283–92.

67. Koenig HJ, Meador KG, Cohen HJ, Blazer DG. Self rated depression scales and screening for major depression in the older hospitalisedpatient with medical illness. *J Am Geriatr Soc* 1988; **36**: 699–706.

68. Yesavage JA, Brink TL. Development and validation of a geriatric depression screening scale: a preliminary report. *J Psychiatr Res* 1983; **17**: 37–49.

69. Adshead F, Cody DD, Pitt B. BASDEC: a novel screening instrument for depression in elderly medical inpatients. *BMJ* 1992; **305**: 397.

70. Evans ME. Development and validation of a screening test for depression in the elderly physically ill. *Int Clin Psychopharmacol* 1993; **8**: 333–36.

71. Schneider L, Plopper M. Geropsychiatry and consultation liaison services. *Am J Psychiatry* 1984; **141**: 721–22.

72. Schuckit MA, Miller PL, Hahlbohm D. Unrecognised psychiatric illness in elderly medical–surgical patients. *J Gerontol* 1975; **30**: 655–60.

73. Ban T. Chronic disease and depression in the geriatric population. *J Clin Psychiatry* 1984; **45**: 18–23.

74. Bazire S. *Psychotropic Drug Directory*. Wiltshire: Mark Allen, 1995.

75. West ED. Electroconvulsive therapy in depression: a double blind controlled trial. *BMJ* 1981; **282**: 355–57.

76. Brandon S, Cowley P, McDonald C *et al*. Electroconvulsive therapy: results in depressive illness from the Leicestershire trial. *BMJ* 1984; **288**: 22–25.

77. Benbow SM. The role of electroconvulsive therapy in the treatment of depressive illness in old age. *Br J Psychiatry* 1989; **155**: 147–52.

78. Wilkinson DG. ECT in the elderly. In Levy R, Howard R, Burns A (eds), *Treatment and Care in Old Age Psychiatry*. Petersfield: Wrightson Biomedical, 1993.

79. Guthrie E. Emotional disorder in chronic illness: psychotherapeutic interventions. *Br J Psychiatry* 1996; **168**: 265–73.

80. Georgotas A, McCue R. The additional benefit of extending an antidepressant trial past seven weeks in the depressed elderly. *Int J Geriatr Psychiatry* 1989; **4**: 191–95.

81. Mayou R, Hawton K, Feldman E. What happens to medical patients with psychiatric disorder? *J Psychosom Res* 1988; **32**: 541–49.

82. Hawton K. The long-term outcome of psychiatric morbidity detected in general medical patients. *J Psychosom Res* 1981; **25**: 237–43.

83. Feldman E, Mayou R, Hawton K *et al*. Psychiatric disorder in medical inpatients. *Q J Med* 1987; **241**: 405–12.

84. Koenig HG, Goli V, Shelp F *et al*. Major depression in hospitalised medically ill older men: documentation, management and outcome. *Int J Geriatr Psychiatry* 1992; **7**: 25–34.

85. Cooper B. Psychiatric disorders among elderly patients admitted tohospital medical wards. *J R Soc Med* 1987; **80**: 13–16.

86. Gordon WF. Elderly depressives, treatment and follow-up. *Can J Psychiatry* 1981; **26**: 110–13.

87. Post F. *The Significance of Affective Symptoms in Old Age*, Chapter X: Conclusions. Maudsley Monograph No. 10. London: Oxford University Press, 1962.

88. Baldwin RC, Jolley DJ. The prognosis of depression in old age. *Br J Psychiatry* 1986; **149**: 574–83.

89. Rabins PV, Harvis K, Koven S. High fatality rates of late life depression associated with cardiovascular disease. *J Affect Disord* 1985; **9**: 165–67.

90. Avery D, Winokur G. Mortality in depressed patients treated with ECT and antidepressants. *Arch Gen Psychiatry* 1976; **33**: 1029–37.

91. Rorsman B, Hagnell O, Lanke J. Mortality and hidden mental disorder in the Lundby study: age-standardised death rates amongmentally ill 'non-patients' in a total population observed during a 25 year period. *Neuropsychobiology* 1983; **10**: 83–89.

92. Gregory RJ, Jimmerson DC, Walto BE *et al*. Pharmacotherapy of depression in the medically ill: directions for future research. *Gen Hosp Psychiatry* 1992; **14**: 36–42.

93. Yates WR, Wesner RB, Thompson R. Organic mood disorder: a valid psychiatry consultation diagnosis. *J Affect Disord* 1991; **22**: 37–42.

94. Burvill PW, Hall WD, Stampfer HG, Emmerson JP. The prognosis of depression in old age. *Br J Psychiatry* 1991; **158**: 64–71.

95. Lloyd GG, Cawley RH. Distress or illness? A study of psychological symptoms after myocardial infarction. *Br J Psychiatry* 1983; **142**: 120–25.

96. Gurland BJ, Cross P. Epidemiology of psychopathology in old age. *Psychiatr Clin N Am* 1982; **5**: 11–25.

97. Gurland BJ, Meyers B. Geriatric psychiatry. In Talbott J, Hales R, Yudofsky S (eds), *A Textbook of Psychiatry*. Washington, DC: American Psychiatric Press, 1987.

98. Cattell H. Suicidal behaviour. In Copeland JRM, Abou-Saleh MT, Blazer DG (eds), *Principles and Practice of Geriatric Psychiatry*, 1st edn. Chichester: Wiley, 1994.

99. Alexopoulos GS, Chester JG. Outcomes of geriatric depression. *Clin Geriatr Med* 1992; **8**: 363–76.

100. Stoudmire A, Thompson TL. Medication non-compliance: systematic approaches to evaluation and intervention. *Gen Hosp Psychiatry* 1983; **5**: 223–39.

101. Rodin GM, Chmara J, Ennis J. Stopping life-sustaining medical treatment: psychiatric considerations in the termination of medical dialysis. *Can J Psychiatry* 1981; **26**: 540–44.

82

Depression After Stroke

Peter Knapp and Allan House

University of Leeds, UK

Stroke patients have high rates of all types of depressive disorder, although estimates of the prevalence of depression within the first month of stroke vary greatly[1,2], according to the type of measure used and the way the sample was derived. A recent systematic review of observational studies suggests that the point prevalence of depression at any time in the first year after stroke is about 33%[3]. The frequency of depression is about the same whether measured soon or later after stroke, although later rates are less certain because of patient attrition in studies. Depression remits in some patients, while in others it persists: one study reported that 50% of those depressed within three weeks of stroke remained depressed one year later[4]. Depression not only affects quality of life: patients with depression after stroke may be at greater risk of mortality[5], cognitive impairment[6] and poorer functional or social recovery[7,8].

There are claims that post-stroke depression is a distinct subtype[9]. There is little unequivocal evidence to support this claim, since psychological and biological symptoms reported by patients are found in depression seen in non-stroke patients[10]. What does appear to be distinctive is the increased prevalence of uncontrollable crying (emotionality) among stroke patients. A small number of patients suffer pathological laughing and crying, a syndrome which is probably neurological in origin, in which emotional expression arises after minor provocation that often appears meaningless[11]. A more common syndrome, emotionalism, is also characterized by increased tearfulness, but is more complex. The emotional episodes are provoked by meaningful stimuli, but the crying is characterized by a lack of warning and control. There appears to be a psychological component to its origin[12]. Emotionalism is associated with an increased risk of depression[13], but patients with emotionalism may be at greater risk of psychological problems not explained by concurrent depression[14,15]. This syndrome is probably under-recognized.

Reaching a diagnosis of depression after stroke can be complicated by the presence of problems such as communicative or cognitive impairment[16]. Patients with expressive communication problems can often be assessed by the careful use of closed questions. The assessment of those with receptive communication problems or significant cognitive impairment is much more complex: a non-language-based assessment of depression shows promise but is insufficiently reliable in its present form for accurate diagnosis[17]. The use of a 'smiley faces' symbol measure has also been shown not to be a reliable screening tool[18]. Screening for depression by the use of questionnaire measures can be quick and easy to do; the main disadvantage is their low positive predictive validity: they identify many false positive cases[19]. A recent study suggests that such pencil and paper screening measures have greater validity when administered twice several weeks apart: patients scoring above the threshold on only one occasion are less likely to have a persistent depression that warrants treatment[20].

The diagnosis of depression by clinical interview might also be confused by facial palsy and a disturbance of speech prosody (rhythm in speech), both of which are relatively common after stroke and which give the patient the appearance of a person with depression[21]. The dexamethasone suppression test is not sufficiently sensitive to be used as a diagnostic tool[22].

The high rate of depression reported in some stroke research has led to the suggestion that the neurological damage is a key factor in its aetiology[23]. As a result, many studies have attempted to link depression after stroke with lesion location. A series of studies proposed, first, that patients with left hemisphere lesions were at greater risk of depression[24], and later, that those with left anterior lesions were at most risk[25,26]. Other researchers[27–29] have not replicated these findings, suggesting that patient sampling and the timing of assessment might explain the differences.

Even if lesion location is associated with greater risk of depression, the context of this relationship is important. First, it is clear that stroke patients with all sorts of lesions can suffer depression[9], so factors other than lesion location must also be at work. Second, stroke location is extremely varied[30], so those with any particular lesion (such as left anterior lesions) will be a minority of patients, making the attributable risk due to any one type of lesion small. Last, although the rate of depression in stroke patients is higher than in age-matched non-stroke controls, it is about the same as in patients with non-neurological disabling illness[21,31], suggesting that non-neurological factors are important. Relevant non-neurological aetiological factors are likely to include the threat of disability and a sense of loss.

That psychosocial factors are likely to be relevant to both the onset and persistence of depression has been illustrated in several studies. For example, one study found that depression at four months after stroke onset was commoner among those with greater disability, those who were divorced and those with higher pre-stroke alcohol intake[28]. Depression is more likely in those patients who perceive their stroke as a greater threat, and in those who have fewer psychological resources or social support to deal with that threat. Patients with previous history of depression or other psychological disorder are also at higher risk of depression after stroke[32].

Principles and Practice of Geriatric Psychiatry, 3rd edn. Edited by Mohammed T. Abou-Saleh, Cornelius Katona and Anand Kumar
© 2011 John Wiley & Sons, Ltd

Patients with depression after stroke might be considered for pharmacological or psychological treatments. A recent systematic review of the treatment trials showed limited beneficial effects of antidepressants, with moderate reduction in symptoms compared to placebo[33]. Trials are generally small with high drop-out rates and inadequate evidence on other outcomes (such as functional recovery or mortality) or adverse events. The evidence for treating emotionalism with antidepressants is rather stronger – both tricyclics and selective serotonin re-uptake inhibitors (SSRIs) have been shown to reduce the frequency of crying episodes[15]. There is no good trial evidence to draw upon in assessing whether psychological interventions are effective in treating depression after stroke[33].

Some services aim to intervene in an attempt to prevent the onset of depression after stroke. There is no evidence to support the use of antidepressants in preventing the onset of depression[34]. Three recently completed studies suggest that brief psychological interventions may be beneficial[34]. Randomized trials of motivational interviewing, care management and problem-solving therapy all showed small but statistically significant benefits. Each needs replication in further trials before these interventions can be recommended for implementation as a matter of routine, although it is encouraging that relatively brief, structured psychological interventions can show benefits. There are disadvantages to psychological management: it may be difficult to implement in patients with significant speech and cognitive impairment[35], and some patients find psychological treatments unacceptable, both before and after the treatment has started.

An unresearched question relates to the best means of structuring interventions. Evidence from other areas suggests that there are substantial benefits to be had when pharmacological and psychological treatments are delivered in an integrated approach according to standard protocols[36], when treatment is tailored to severity of depression and its response to first-line treatment, as in stepped care programmes[37] and when it is delivered in programmes of collaborative care that involve both primary and secondary care specialists[38].

In summary, depression after stroke is common, and its causes are probably multiple – biological, psychological and social – as is the case in other physical illnesses. The evidence for benefit from antidepressant drugs is accruing but remains surprisingly poor, considering their problematic side effects and how widely they are prescribed. The potential for psychological therapies is evident in several studies and its use has been under-evaluated, which is a deficit that needs correcting. The completion of several systematic reviews of intervention trials and prevalence studies has been beneficial for providing evidence for clinicians but, pending the completion of further primary research, clinicians will largely need to rely on evidence from other areas of physical medicine to inform their treatments.

REFERENCES

1. Kotila M, Numminen H, Waltimo O, Kaste M. Depression after stroke: results of the FINSTROKE Study. *Stroke* 1998; **29**: 368–72.
2. Pohjasvaara T, Leppavuori A, Siira I *et al*. Frequency and clinical determinants of poststroke depression. *Stroke* 1998; **29**: 2311–17.
3. Hackett ML, Yapa C, Parag V, Anderson CS. Frequency of depression after stroke: a systematic review of observational studies. *Stroke* 2005; **36**: 1330–40.
4. Wade DT, Leigh-Smith J, Hewer RA. Depressed mood after stroke. A community study of its frequency. *Br J Psychiatry* 1987; **151**: 200–205.
5. Morris PL, Robinson RG, Samuels J. Depression, introversion and mortality following stroke. *Aust N Z J Psychiatry* 1993; **27**: 443–49.
6. House A, Dennis M, Warlow C *et al*. Intellectual impairment after stroke and its relation to mood disorder. *PsycholMed* 1990; **20**: 805–14.
7. Starkstein SE, Parikh RM, Robinson RG. Post-stroke depression and recovery after stroke. *Lancet* 1987; **1**: 743.
8. Feibel JH, Springer CJ. Depression and failure to resume social activities after stroke. *Arch Phys Med Rehabil* 1982; **63**: 276–78.
9. Robinson RG. Neuropsychiatric consequences of stroke. *Annu Rev Med* 1997; **48**: 217–29.
10. House A. Depression associated with stroke. *J Neuropsychiatry Clin Neurosci* 1996; **8**: 453–57.
11. Andersen G. Treatment of uncontrolled crying after stroke. *Drugs Aging* 1995; **6**: 105–11.
12. Allman P, Hope T, Fairburn CG. Crying following stroke: a report on 30 cases. *Gen Hosp Psychiatry* 1992; **14**: 315–21.
13. Calvert T, Knapp P, House A. Psychological associations with emotionalism after stroke. *J Neurol Neurosurg Psychiatry* 1998; **65**: 928–29.
14. Eccles S, House A, Knapp P. Psychological adjustment and self reported coping in stroke survivors with and without emotionalism. *J Neurol Neurosurg Psychiatry* 1999; **67**: 125–26.
15. House AO, Hackett ML, Anderson CS, Horrocks JA. Pharmaceutical interventions for emotionalism after stroke. *Cochrane Database Syst Rev* 2004, Issue 2: CD003690.
16. Spencer KA, Tompkins CA, Schulz R. Assessment of depression in patients with brain pathology: the case of stroke. *Psychol Bull* 1997; **122**: 132–52.
17. Sutcliffe LM, Lincoln NB. The assessment of depression in aphasic stroke patients: the development of the Stroke Aphasic Depression Questionnaire. *Clin Rehabil* 1998; **12**: 506–13.
18. Lee ACK, Tang AW, Yu GKK, Cheung RTF. The smiley as a simple screening tool for depression after stroke: a preliminary study. *Int J Nurs Stud* 2008; **45**: 1042–54.
19. Gilbody SM, House AO, Sheldon TA. Routinely administered questionnaires for depression and anxiety: systematic review. *BMJ* 2001; **322**: 406–409.
20. West R, Hill K, Hewison J, Knapp P, House AO. Psychological disorders after stroke are an important influence on functional outcomes: a prospective cohort study Stroke (in press).
21. House A. Mood disorders after stroke: a review of the evidence. *Int J Geriatr Psychiatry* 1987; **2**: 211–21.
22. Harvey SA, Black KJ. The dexamethasone suppression test for diagnosing depression in stroke patients. *Ann Clin Psychiatry* 1996; **8**: 35–39.
23. Castillo CS, Robinson RG. Depression after stroke. *Curr Opin Psychiatry* 1994; **7**: 87–90.
24. Robinson RG, Lipsey JR, Price TR. Diagnosis and clinical management of post-stroke depression. *Psychosomatics* 1985; **26**: 769–78.
25. Parikh RM, Lipsey JR, Robinson RG, Price TR. Two-year longitudinal study of post-stroke mood disorders: dynamic changes in correlates of depression at one and two years. *Stroke* 1987; **18**: 579–84.

26. Astrom M, Adolfsson R, Asplund K. Major depression in stroke patients. A 3-year longitudinal study. *Stroke* 1993; **24**: 976–82.

27. Andersen G, Vestergaard K, Ingemann-Nielsen M, Lauritzen L. Risk factors for post-stroke depression. *Acta Psychiatr Scand* 1995; **92**: 193–98.

28. Burvill P, Johnson G, Jamrozik K *et al*. Risk factors for post-stroke depression. Int *J Geriatr Psychiatry* 1997; **12**: 219–26.

29. MacHale SM, O'Rourke S, Dennis MS, Wardlaw JM. Depression and its relation to lesion location after stroke. *J Neurol Neurosurg Psychiatry* 1998; **64**: 371–74.

30. Bamford J, Sandercock P, Dennis M *et al*. Classification and natural history of clinically identified subtypes of cerebral infarction. *Lancet* 1991; **337**: 1521–26.

31. Kennedy G, Kelman H, Thomas C. The emergence of depressive symptoms in later life: the importance of declining health and increasing disability. *J Community Health* 1990; **15**: 93–104.

32. Hackett ML, Anderson CS. Predictors of depression after stroke: a systematic review of observational studies. *Stroke* 2005; **36**: 2296–301.

33. Hackett ML, Anderson CS, House AO, Xia J. Interventions for treating depression after stroke. *Cochrane Database Syst Rev* 2008, Issue 4: CD003437.

34. Hackett ML, Anderson CS, House AO, Halteh C. Interventions for preventing depression after stroke. *Cochrane Database Syst Rev* 2008; Issue 3: CD003689.

35. Gainotti G. Emotional, psychological and psychosocial problems of aphasic patients: an introduction. *Aphasiology* 1997; **11**: 635–50.

36. Rush AJ, Fava M, Wismewski SR *et al*. Sequenced treatment alternatives to relieve depression (STAR*D). *Control Clin Trials* 2004; **25**: 119–42.

37. National Institute for Health and Clinical Excellence (NICE). *Depression: Management of Depression in Primary and Secondary Care*. NICE guidance CG23. London: NICE: 2004.

38. Katon W, Von Korff M, Lin E *et al*. The Pathways Study: A randomised trial of collaborative care in patients with diabetes and depression. *Arch Gen Psychiatry* 2004; **61**: 1042–49.

83

Cross-Cultural Variation in the Experience of Depression in Older People in the UK

Vanessa Lawrence[1], Joanna Murray[1], Anthony Klugman[2] and Sube Banerjee[1]

[1]Institute of Psychiatry, King's College London, London, UK
[2]Old Age Psychiatry, South London and Maudsley NHS Foundation Trust, London, UK

INTRODUCTION

Depression is the most common mental disorder in later life, affecting up to 15% of those over 65[1]. Studies focused on the needs of people from minority ethnic groups suggest at least the same high prevalence of depression among south Asian and black Caribbean groups in the UK[2]. It has been suggested that ethnic elders may be more vulnerable to mental illness than the majority population and the term 'triple jeopardy' has been used to describe the combined challenge of racism, ageism and socioeconomic deprivation faced by older people from minority backgrounds[3]. Census data reveal that the proportion of black and minority ethnic individuals over the age of 65 increased from 3% in 1991, to over 8% in 2001. Therefore, it appears inevitable that the prevalence of depression in minority ethnic groups, and the challenges that this presents to health and social services in the UK will rise[2]. It is also of concern that older adults from minority ethnic groups appear to have lower levels of service use compared with the majority population[4].

There are major discontinuities in the management of depression in old age throughout the health and social care system. It is estimated that only 15% of older people with depression receive appropriate treatment from primary or secondary care services[5]. This may be a function of the inherent complexities of the illness with the presentation of depression anything but uniform. From a cross-cultural perspective, there are suggestions that Asian and black Caribbean patients have their psychological problems identified less frequently than their white counterparts[6]. Again, this may in part be explained by the variable ways in which depression is manifested and reported by different ethnic groups[7,8]. The National Service Framework for Older People has explicitly acknowledged that depression is undertreated in older people, and a key aim is to ensure the early recognition and effective management of depression across ethnic groups[9].

BARRIERS ON THE PATHWAY TO CARE

Suggestions of unmet need among ethnic elders[10] require an exploration of the potential barriers and facilitators to service use. Goldberg and Huxley (1980) described a succession of filters in the 'pathway to care' that determine whether people access mental health services[11]. Sufferers Beliefs about the nature of the condition, and what is appropriate help, may act as barriers at each of these stages, influencing whether and from whom to seek help, the idioms for expressing the condition, and the acceptability of various treatments[12]. At present, much of our data on these issues has been derived from studies focused on the needs of working-age adults[13,14]; among older adult research very few studies have examined the experience of depression across ethnic groups. In the United Kingdom, as in most health-care systems, general practitioners (GPs) are the first point of access to health care, directly providing most of the treatment for common mental disorders as well as referral to specialist mental health services. The beliefs of primary care professionals may represent a further barrier in the pathway to care influencing the recognition and management of depression in older patients[7]. Thus, it is important to consider whether the large discrepancies between prevalence, identification and treatment of depression is to be found in the attitudes and behaviour of GPs, their older patients or some combination between the two.

Levkoff and colleagues (1988) hypothesized that the most common reason for older people not to seek help from their GP was that they tended to 'normalize' symptoms of depression and attribute their condition to the ageing process rather than to disease[12]. Attributions of the causes of depression have been found to vary between different ethnic groups[14]. Bhugra (1996) found that south Asian women of all ages had a clear understanding of psychosocial aspects of depression but were not predisposed towards medical models or explanations[15]. Abas (1996) suggested that older Caribbean people construe mental disorders as secondary to other unmet needs (e.g. physical, social, spiritual)[16]. There is also evidence that south Asian and black Caribbean adults may favour self-help strategies for depression rather than seeking professional help[14]. Religious practices (e.g. prayer) have been identified as important ways of coping among minority ethnic groups living in the UK and traditional healers or religious leaders could be considered by these individuals to be a more appropriate and acceptable source of help than Western models of psychiatric care[17]. Alternatively, talking to friends and family may represent the first line of treatment[18]. Certainly, research suggests that south Asian and black Caribbean adults do not always envisage primary care consultations as an appropriate response to depression[13,19]. Negative attitudes towards antidepressants and

Principles and Practice of Geriatric Psychiatry, 3rd edn. Edited by Mohammed T. Abou-Saleh, Cornelius Katona and Anand Kumar
© 2011 John Wiley & Sons, Ltd

mental health services in general, may discourage help seeking within minority ethnic groups[20].

Yet depression is also under-recognized and poorly managed in primary care[5]. It appears that the stigma of mental disorder is keenly felt by older adults and feelings of shame have been cited to explain underreporting of affective symptoms by older patients[28]. Research has pointed to even higher levels of stigma surrounding depression within minority ethnic groups[17,19]. There is evidence that GPs construe presentations by south Asian patients as being dominated by physical rather than psychological complaints[7]. Odell et al. (1997) speculated that a tendency in south Asians to somatise their psychological distress might contribute to low detection rates[8]. However, Bhui and colleagues (2001) commented that the frequent use by GPs of 'somatic' and 'sub-clinical' labels in relation to Punjabi patients suggests that although they did not perceive there to be 'significant psychiatric disorders' they were aware of some emotional disturbance[7]. Comino et al. (2001) reported substantial underdetection of depression by GPs among south Asian patients, though the patients were able to identify common symptoms of anxiety and depression themselves[6]. However, there is accumulating evidence to suggest that the language used to express psychological distress is culturally informed[15,16,21]. Again it is important to emphasize that very few data deal specifically with older people with depression from minority ethnic groups. In order to generate services that are accessible and acceptable to older adults across ethnic groups, service providers need to understand the beliefs that underlie help-seeking behaviour and the likelihood of help being offered and accepted.

A CROSS-CULTURAL QUALTATIVE STUDY OF THE BARRIERS AND FACILITATORS TO CARE

In the light of the gaps in the evidence base identified above, we completed a programme of work to investigate the attitudes, experiences and beliefs of older adults from the three largest ethnic groups in the UK and primary care professionals concerning depression[22-24]. In-depth interviews were conducted with 110 older adults and 30 primary care professionals (see Table 83.1).

The data incorporates the perspective of older adults with depression (both treated and untreated) and the general older population. Each group included black Caribbean, south Asian and white British older adults; this enabled us to compare and contrast attitudes among the two largest minority ethnic groups in the UK with the majority population. A 'case' of depression was defined as a score of 7 or

above on the Hospital Anxiety and Depression Scale (HADS)[25]. Treatment was not limited a priori to pharmacological interventions (i.e. antidepressants) but in the event no participants were receiving psychological treatments alone. We identified participants through seven primary care practices and through day centres and lunch clubs serving the black Caribbean, south Asian and white British communities. Topics for the interview guide were generated from the research literature. We used a vignette describing an older person with symptoms typical of depression as a starting point to enable us to explore the idioms used to express mental distress and attitudes toward mental illness in our sample[18,19,21]. Interviews then explored: what the word depression meant to participants; what participants thought might cause depression; what someone with depression should do, what help might someone with depression need; who should help them and how. The older adults were then asked to give their opinions on a range of treatments and services. Information sheets, consent forms, the HADS and the vignette were available in four Asian languages: Gujarati, Hindi, Punjabi and Urdu. Interviews were conducted in participants' homes, unless they stated a preference to be seen elsewhere, lasted around one hour and were conducted in the participants' preferred language. All were recorded on audio-tape and transcribed verbatim.

In depth individual interviews were conducted with GPs, practice nurses and practice counsellors working in 18 primary care centres in south London. The sample was selected purposively to include professionals working in different settings (single-handed and group practices), serving areas of contrasting socioeconomic and ethnic characteristics. One-third of the participants were recruited from primary care research networks, and two-thirds were selected from information published on local primary care trust websites. Key topics explored in the interviews included: perceptions of the experience and presentation of depression in older people; perceptions of older people's beliefs about depression; cultural differences in the above. Analysis of the data was based on the grounded theory approach[26]. Three members of the research team scrutinized and coded the initial transcripts. Emerging themes were identified and labelled with codes. A constant comparison technique was used to delineate the properties of the codes and to develop categories and subcategories. As the analysis proceeded, we verified and developed existing codes and added new codes where necessary. The researchers compared their coding strategies and any instances of disagreement were discussed and resolved by the wider research team. NVivo qualitative data analysis software was used to process the transcripts. The number of interviews completed in each group

Table 83.1 Number of participants

	Older adults		
	Black Caribbean	South Asian	White British
Total	32	33	45
Treatment status			
Depressed and treated	9	6	15
Depressed and not treated	13	12	12
Not depressed	10	15	18
	Primary care professionals		
	General practitioners	Practice nurses	Practice counsellors
Total	18	7	5

was determined by 'saturation of data', i.e. the point at which no new themes emerged from the interviews.

FINDINGS

The themes to be presented in this chapter emerged from the analysis of: firstly, older adults' perception of the concepts and causation of depression; secondly, older adults' attitudes towards help seeking for depression; and thirdly, primary care professionals' perceptions of the experience and presentation of depression across ethnic groups. The data will be considered in relation to the existing literature.

Older Adults' Concepts and Causation of Depression

The older adults in our study felt that the ageing process had a considerable number of physical, circumstantial and emotional implications that contributed to depression. It has been suggested that there is a propensity among the elderly to 'explain away' depression as a normal part of ageing and that this prevents them seeking help for the condition[12]. However, in our study, an acceptance of the social and ageing precipitants of depression was not incompatible with the concept of depression as an illness. Roughly three-quarters of the black Caribbean elders and two-thirds of the white British participants defined depression in this way. Assigning the label 'illness' appeared to validate and legitimize the experience. Almost half of the white British and black Caribbean participants also viewed depression as a serious condition that was distinct from sadness and grief. Thus, depression was concurrently viewed by these groups as being an understandable, yet dysfunctional, consequence of old age.

It was notable that south Asian participants were least likely to identify depression as an illness or a serious condition and most likely to equate depression with 'normal' feelings of sadness and grief. The apparent incompatibility of these beliefs with the Western biomedical model of depression might make south Asian older adults less likely to seek or accept health services for depression. A further challenge to services exists in the recurring belief that emerged among south Asian and, to a lesser extent, black Caribbean participants that depression stems from a weakness or deficiency in character. This is consistent with previously reported high levels of stigma surrounding depression in these cultures[27]. Research has suggested that fear of being ostracized by peers could act as a deterrent to help seeking within minority communities[17].

The language used to describe depression also emerged as culturally influenced. A large proportion of black Caribbean participants defined depression in terms of feeling low or down, which is consistent with previous findings in younger age groups[28]. The white British participants spoke of variations in mood and feelings of hopelessness with even greater frequency, often employing metaphors of darkness to illustrate their point. The tendency of these groups to describe depression in terms of its emotional impact implies both an ability and willingness to enter into a psychological discourse. Conversely, only a small number of south Asian elders described depression in terms of hopelessness or low mood. Along with Caribbean elders, they frequently defined depression in terms of worry, with emphasis repeatedly being placed on troubles within the mind. Notably, the south Asian participants often articulated this worry in terms of 'thinking too much', a phrase previously identified as a descriptor of mental distress within south Asian younger adults[21].

Differences in attribution were found in the themes emerging from the three ethnic groups. Complaints of loneliness were the focus of the black Caribbean responses, which is consistent with the suggestion that black Caribbean older adults miss the traditional social networks that characterize Caribbean society[29]. As in research in younger adults[14], black Caribbean and white British participants tended to consider mistreatment and abandonment by partners to be a likely cause of depression. Members of the south Asian group related wider family problems to depression, which similarly accords with work in younger age groups[18]. Participants discussed the negative impact of a difficult 'home atmosphere', and they expressed concerns about the discordance in values between their children and themselves. Interestingly, members of the black Caribbean and south Asian groups made very few references to the effects of racism on their emotional well-being, which contrasts with the expressed views of a working-age adult group[14].

Over half of the white British participants cited the death of a spouse as a key cause of depression. Another major cause of unhappiness within the white British group was the feeling that they enjoyed very little contact or support from their family. Increased contact was both longed for and highly valued when received. It seems likely that this absence of family support is related to the predominant role occupied by spouses within the white British group, where loss of the spouse is likely to leave an even greater vacuum in emotional support. A large proportion of white British participants receiving antidepressants attributed their depression to bereavement, suggesting that bereavement may be used to initiate discussion about depression in this group. Research suggests that social problems may be a criterion used by GPs to make a psychiatric diagnosis[30]. In an exploration of the reasons for low treatment rates and high suicide rates in south Asian women, mental health professionals considered it advantageous to have an understanding of the cultural background and reasons why an individual may be experiencing depression[31].

Older Adults' Attitudes towards Help Seeking

Personal responsibility for coping was a recurrent theme. We found consensus across the ethnic groups that the impetus to combat depression must come from the individual. Forcing oneself to get out and engage in activities was identified as the most effective means of self-help. We found less of a focus on cognitive strategies compared with working age adults[14], suggesting that older people tend to adopt a more behavioural approach to tackling the experience of depression. Behavioural strategies that encourage efforts to interact and remain active may provide an acceptable adjunct or alternative to pharmacological or psychotherapeutic interventions. However, it remains a fact that up to one in six older adults are depressed at any one time[1] and public education campaigns must communicate that the nature of depression often necessitates help from others.

There was a tendency among south Asian older adults to identify families as a prominent source of help for depression, which is consistent with research in younger age groups[32]. The black Caribbean group placed less emphasis on the role of the family but stressed the cathartic value of discussing worries and concerns with friends, suggesting a willingness within this group to discuss emotional problems in a candid way. Our results echo the importance and acceptability of religion in helping many black Caribbean people of all ages cope with emotional distress[14,17]. Prayer was allied to the concept of self-help, and it was implied that without a true relationship with God, depression would be difficult to overcome. Seeking informal or formal help might signify insufficient faith in this context. Health-care professionals may need to work closely with religious leaders if they are to challenge these deep-seated beliefs. Fewer south Asian participants cited religion as a coping mechanism, but of those who did, religious worship presented as an enduring and integral part of life. Participants described visiting the temple as a means of sustaining emotional well-being. In contrast to previous research[17,21] no reference was made to traditional healers as a source of help.

Research indicates that younger south Asian people tend not to medicalize emotional distress[21]. This may account for the tendency among the south Asian group within our study to view the nature of depression as incompatible with the GP's role, which they conceived as prescribing medication and making referrals. Promoting the concept of depression as a treatable medical condition might resolve this problem and legitimize help seeking. However, it is also likely to be of value to reassure older adults that it is appropriate to voice concerns about their emotional state in a GP consultation. The black Caribbean group viewed GPs as serving the additional function of listening and discussing what was on their mind. Consequently, they praised GPs for allowing individuals to discuss their worries and concerns, yet were highly critical of instances where GPs spent insufficient time with their patients or appeared to take insufficient interest. Therefore, the belief of the black Caribbean participants that GPs could and should help resulted in polarized positive and negative evaluations. Reservations about seeking help from GPs were similar across the ethnic groups; doctors were too busy and overly reliant on medication as a form of treatment. Others explained that limited GP consultation time forced them to prioritize their physical, rather than their psychological, complaints.

Psychiatrists were generally regarded negatively and many participants were conscious of the stigma attached to this profession. This was especially pronounced within the ethnic minority groups as has been reported in other studies[33]. However, experience of psychiatrists, which tended to be limited to the white British and black Caribbean groups, often predicated the more positive remarks. The idea of counselling was embraced by the black Caribbean group in particular. Their limited experience of counselling paralleled that of other groups, yet their greater enthusiasm possibly reflects the high value they place on confiding in others[33] and being genuinely 'listened to' by professionals[16]. For the south Asian group, their unease at discussing personal matters with strangers appeared to contribute to a negative view of counselling. This mirrors previous research that highlighted the pertinent issue of confidentiality within south Asian communities[18]. Medication was cautiously advocated across the groups. Participants generally felt that certain circumstances dictated its use although there was widespread concern about side effects and dependency.

Primary Care Professionals' Perceptions of Depression in Older People

All but one of the primary care professionals in our study believed that cultural differences in illness beliefs had an important influence on how older adults communicated the experience of depression. This builds upon previous cross-cultural studies of depression that have discussed the ways in which culture can shape expressions of distress[34]. A number of GPs held the view that the Western concept of depression was less recognized in some cultures. Although GPs were reluctant to make generalizations on the basis of ethnicity most admitted that it could be difficult to engage patients from minority ethnic groups in discussions about psychological problems. Professionals were of the opinion that the belief that 'non-medical' problems were

inappropriate or not important enough to warrant medical attention prevented older people from all ethnic groups from talking about psychosocial difficulties in a primary care setting. However, black Caribbean and south Asian older adults were thought to be even less likely than their white British peers to disclose psychological symptoms. Moreover, and in accordance with previous research[7], GPs suggested that there was a propensity among south Asian elders in particular to express psychological distress as physical pain or concerns about heart disease. One GP commented that excessive worry about physical symptoms often masked the presence of depression and that those patients who eventually received a diagnosis usually had more severe and enduring symptoms. As the first point of contact with health care, most GPs were aware there were particular requirements for sensitive exploration of symptoms, interpretation and explanation with all older adults. Some had clear strategies for introducing the concept of depression while keeping within the patient's physical formulation of their problem. Others negotiated a treatment plan or even colluded with the patient by making the requested referral to a specialist for physical tests while initiating treatment for depression. While GPs encountered more somatic presentations of depression, practice nurses and counsellors had more opportunities to identify and explore social difficulties. People with chronic conditions were often in regular contact with the practice nurse and there seemed important possibilities in using these contacts more systematically to identify and treat depression in primary care.

The suggestion that it is a lack of 'psychological-mindedness' that leads to somatic presentation of emotional distress has increasingly been rejected within the literature and research has suggested that bodily complaints may in part indicate the use of somatic metaphors[35]. While many of the primary care professionals in our study believed that there were cultural differences in the type of symptoms presented, others believed the differences lay in the use of language and metaphor rather than the attribution of symptoms. Abas (1996) described a wide range of psychological language used by African-Caribbean elders to convey emotional distress[16]. Indeed expressions used to convey feelings of depression such as 'low spirit' and 'weighed down'[16,28] explicitly reveal low mood. Similarly south Asian patients, although tending to present somatic symptoms, have been shown to articulate their distress in psychological terms[36]. Comino and colleagues (2001) concluded that the tendency of GPs to rely exclusively on Western-based concepts and diagnostic traditions when assessing people from other cultures represented a significant detection barrier[6]. Finally, primary care staff were acutely aware of the stigma of mental disorder and had observed embarrassment, failure and shame among older patients in admitting to feelings of depression. The stigma of mental illness was thought to have more serious consequences in minority ethnic communities with a diagnosis of depression potentially bringing shame upon the family. This represented an important barrier to addressing psychosocial aspects of the illness and gaining the patient's agreement to begin appropriate treatment.

IMPLICATIONS FOR POLICY AND PRACTICE

These data have implications for policy, practice and education. The model used by older adults from all ethnic groups was more akin to a social than a classic biomedical schema. This suggests that the approach clinicians need to take in attempting to engage older people with depression in a therapeutic alliance would benefit from being framed in social as well as physical terms. Enquiries about recent life events and losses could be used to facilitate discussion with older adults about depression. More emphasis in medical training and continuing professional development on how symptom attribution differs across ethnic groups could enable practitioners to frame their questions within an appropriate cultural framework. However, this is only a first step: clinicians need to be able to explain the interaction of the social, psychological and biological elements of causation, thus generating a shared understanding of the value of biological (such as antidepressant medication), as well as social and psychological, interventions. Recent evidence suggests that older adults incorporate medical and experiential knowledge into their model of depression[37]. However, it has also been argued that GPs should explicitly relate diagnosis and treatment options to the individual's social experience of depression if they are to have relevance beyond the clinical context in which the diagnosis is made[37]. Proctor (2008) takes this further, concluding that the acceptability and effectiveness of treatment for depression depends on the practitioners' ability to connect it to other medical and social problems of later life, which the study indicated occupy a higher priority among older adults[38].

There were striking consistencies in the barriers to care described by older people and primary care staff. Primary care professionals and older adults acknowledged that multiple health problems might prompt elderly patients to prioritize physical complaints in order to avoid 'wasting the doctor's time'. GPs considered this to be compounded by the common belief that doctors are there to deal with physical conditions rather than psychological problems. Yet white British and black Caribbean older adults displayed a willingness to disclose emotional difficulties associated with depression, which is an encouraging indication that older adults would respond to discussion with health and social care professionals about their mood. Together these data indicate that practitioners need to provide assurance that disclosure of feelings is appropriate in a medical consultation. Longer appointments might facilitate this process and enable primary care staff to address the mental health needs of older patients as a matter of routine. Practice nurses felt that they were well placed to discuss the implications of life events, family problems and other 'non-medical' crises with older patients. Given the high co-morbidity of depression in later life with physical illness[39], the increasing role of practice nurses in the management of chronic disease may provide a setting to explore psychosocial problems. The pronounced interest in counselling demonstrated by black Caribbean participants highlights the need for greater access to a wider range of treatments. Psychotherapy has been identified as a preferred treatment option among black American older adults and its provision in primary care has been associated with better depression outcomes[40]. Unfortunately, access to talking therapies remains limited among older people in the UK despite assertions that this is an entitlement for all.

The study confirms that the language and metaphors used to describe depression can be culturally influenced. Sensitivity to the 'language of depression' used by different groups (e.g. 'excessive thinking' within the south Asian group) will increase the likelihood of reaching an acceptable diagnosis and treatment plan. An understanding of cultural variation in the expression of mental illness is fundamental to good health care, and this should form a normal part of training for health-care professionals. Ethnic differences in the conceptualization and attributions of depression also highlight the need for practitioners to emphasize, particularly with patients from minority ethnic groups, that depression is not a sign of weakness and that anyone can become depressed. In turn, cultural- and language-specific public education could be directed as modifying public attitudes and understanding of depression not only to reduce stigma, but also to enable self-identification of the disorder. Lastly, the data point towards the need for education concerning the role of psychiatrists, as well as for accurate information regarding the risks of dependency and actual side effects with medication.

REFERENCES

1. Livingston G, Hawkins A, Graham N, Blizard B, Mann AH. The Gospel Oak Study: prevalence rates of dementia, depression and activity limitation among elderly residents in Inner London. *Psychol Med* 1990; **20**: 137–46.
2. McCracken CF, Boneham MA, Copeland JRM, Williams KE, Wilson K, Scott A *et al*. Prevalence of dementia and depression among elderly people in black and ethnic minorities. *Br J Psychiatry* 1997; **171**: 269–73.
3. Rait G, Burns A, Chew C. Age, ethnicity, and mental illness: a triple whammy. *BMJ* 1996; **313**: 1347–8.
4. Boneham MA, Williams KE. Elderly people from ethnic minorities in Liverpool: mental illness, unmet need and barriers to service use. *Health Soc Care Community* 1997; 5: 173–80.
5. Blanchard M, Waterreus A, Mann AH. The nature of depression in older people in Inner London, and the contact with primary care. *Br J Psychiatry* 1994; **164**: 396–402.
6. Comino EJ, Silove D, Manicavasagar V, Harris E, Harris MF. Agreement in symptoms of anxiety and depression between patients and GPs: the influence of ethnicity. *Fam Pract* 2001; **18**: 71–7.
7. Bhui K, Bhugra D, Goldberg D, Dunn G, Desai M. Cultural influences on the prevalence of common mental disorder: general practitioners' assessments and help-seeking among Punjabi and English people visiting their general practitioner. *Psychol Med* 2001; **31**: 815–25.
8. Odell SM, Surtees PG, Wainwright NW, Commander MJ, Sashidharan SP. Determinants of general practitioner recognition of psychological problems in a multi-ethnic inner-city health district. *Br J Psychiatry* 1997; **171**: 537–41.
9. Department of Health. *National Service Framework for Older People*. London: Department of Health, 2001.
10. Ebrahim S. Caring for older people: ethnic elders. *BMJ* 1996; 313: 610–13.
11. Goldberg D, Huxley P. *Mental Illness in the Community: The Pathway to Psychiatric Care*. London: Tavistock Publications, 1980.
12. Levkoff SE, Cleary PD, Wetle T, Besdine RW. Illness behavior in the aged: implications for clinicians. *J Am Geriatr Soc* 1988; **36**: 622–9.
13. Commander MJ, Odell SM, Surtees PG, Sashidharan SP. Care pathways for South Asian and white people with depressive and anxiety disorders in the community. *Soc Psychiatry Psychiatr Epidemiol* 2004; **39**: 259–64.
14. O'Connor W, Nazroo J. *Ethnic Differences in the Context and Experience of Psychiatric illness: A Qualitative Study*. National Centre for Social Research, 2002.
15. Bhugra D. Depression across cultures. *Prim Care Psychiatry* 1996; **2**: 155–65.
16. Abas MA. Depression and anxiety among older Caribbean people in the UK: screening, unmet need and the provision of appropriate services. *Int J Geriatr Psychiatry* 1996; **11**: 377–82.

17. Cinnirella M, Loewenthal KM. Religious and ethnic group influences on the beliefs about mental illnesses: a qualitative study. *Br J Med Psychol* 1999; **72**: 505–24.

18. Bhugra D, Baldwin D, Desai M. Focus groups: implications for primary and cross-cultural psychiatry. *Prim Care Psychiatry* 1997; **3**: 45–50.

19. Marwaha S, Livingston G. Stigma, racism and choice: why do depressed ethnic elders avoid psychiatrists? *J Affect Disord* 2002; **72**: 257–65.

20. Schnittker J. Misgivings of medicine? African Americans' scepticism of psychiatric medication. *J Health Soc Behav* 2003; **44**: 506–24.

21. Fenton S, Sadiq-Sangster A. Culture, relativism and the experience of mental distress: South Asian women in Britain. *Sociol Health Illn* 1996; **18**: 66–85.

22. Lawrence V, Murray J, Banerjee S, Turner S, Sangha K, Byng R *et al*. Concepts and causation of depression: a cross-cultural study of the beliefs of older adults. *Gerontologist* 2006; **46**: 23–32.

23. Lawrence V, Banerjee S, Bhugra D, Sangha K, Turner S, Murray J. Coping with depression in later life: a qualitative study of help seeking in three ethnic groups. *Psychol Med* 2006; **36**: 1375–83.

24. Murray J, Banerjee S, Byng R, Tylee A, Bhugra D, Macdonald A. Primary care professionals' perceptions of depression in older people: a qualitative study. *Soc Sci Med* 2006; **63**: 1363–73.

25. Zigmond AS, Snaith RP. The Hospital Anxiety and Depression Scale. *Acta Psychiatr Scand* 1983; **67**: 361–70.

26. Glaser BG, Strauss AL. *The Discovery of Grounded Theory: Strategies for Qualitative Research*. Chicago: Aldine, 1967.

27. Rack P. *Race, Culture and Mental Disorder*. London: Tavistock, 1982.

28. Mallet R, Bhugra D, Leff J. African-Caribbean perspectives on depression. Paper presented to Royal College of Psychiatrists Defeat Depression consensus meeting, 1994.

29. Stephenson ML. Travelling to the ancestral homelands: the aspirations and experiences of a UK Caribbean community. *Curr Issues Tourism* 2002; **5**: 378–423.

30. Marino S, Bellantuono C, Tansella M. Psychiatric morbidity in general practice in Italy. *Soc Psychiatry Psychiatr Epidemiol* 1990; **25**: 67–72.

31. Burr J. Cultural stereotypes of women from South Asian communities: mental health care professionals' expectation for patterns of suicide and depression. *Soc Sci Med* 2002; **55**: 835–45.

32. Sonuga-Barke E, Mistry M. Mental health of three generations of Asians in Britain: a comparison of Hindus and Muslims in nuclear and extended families. *Br J Clin Psychol* 2000; **34**: 79–81.

33. Priest RG, Vize C, Roberts A, Roberts M, Tylee A. Lay people's attitudes to treatment of depression: results of opinion poll for Defeat Depression Campaign just before its launch. *BMJ* 1996; **313**: 858–9.

34. Kleinman A. Anthropology and psychiatry: the role of culture on cross-cultural research on illness. *Br J Psychiatry* 1987; **151**: 447–54.

35. Mumford DB. Somatization: a transcultural perspective. *Int Rev Psychiatry* 1993; **5**: 231–42.

36. Krause IB. Sinking heart. A Punjabi communication of distress. *Soc Sci Med* 1992; **29**: 563–75.

37. Wittink MN, Dahlberg B, Biruk C, Barg FK. How older adults combine medical and experiential notions of depression. *Qual Health Res* 2008; **18**: 1174–83.

38. Proctor EK, Hasche L, Morrow-Howell N, Shumway M, Snell G. Perceptions about competing psychosocial problems and treatment priorities among older adults with depression. *Psychiatr Serv* 2008; **59**: 670–5.

39. Moussavi S, Chatterji S, Verdes E, Tandon A, Patel V, Ustun B. Depression, chronic diseases and decrements in health: result from the World Health Surveys. *Lancet* 2007; **370**: 851–8.

40. Arean PA, Ayalon L, Hunkeler E, Lin EHB, Tang L, Harpole L *et al*. Improving depression care for older, minority patients in primary care. *Med Care* 2005; **43**: 381–90.

84

Treatment of Late-Life Depression In Community Settings

Carolyn Chew-Graham

School of Community Based Medicine, University of Manchester, UK

EPIDEMIOLOGY

It has been stated that 10–15% of all older people meet the clinical criteria for a diagnosis of depression[1], and major depression is a recurring disorder, with the majority of older patients having a recurrence within three years[2]. Some groups are more at risk of depression: 40% of people in care homes are depressed[3] and the community prevalence of depression in South Asian older people may approach 20%[4].

Older people have the highest suicide rate for women and second highest for men (National Confidential Inquiry into Suicides and Homicides) and is the one age group where rates have not declined. In contrast with young people, self-harm in older people usually signifies mental illness, mostly depression, with high risk of completed suicide[5].

The over-85 population of the United Kingdom will increase by 50% over the next 15 years, from 1.2 million in 2005 to 1.8 million in 2021, compared with a 30% increase in the over-65 population. In just half that time, the older black and minority ethnic (BME) population will increase by up to 170%. This is not purely a change affecting the United Kingdom – ageing is a global issue and in the United States the number of centenarians will rise from 72 000 in 2000 to 834 000 by 2050. (www.grg.org/calment.html). The concept of multiple jeopardy postulates that ethnic elders, by virtue of age, socioeconomic difficulties and minority status are at greater risk of illness, thus in greater need of health services[4].

Co-morbidities or multi-morbidities are the norm in later life. Thus emotional and physical health problems of older people are entwined and manifested in complex co-morbidity[6] and those with a physical disability have five times higher rates of depression. Although there is variation between studies, it has been estimated that up to 26% of people with diabetes also suffer from depression[7] and comparable figures have been reported for coronary heart disease[7].

Being equipped to meet these complex needs is critical in settings like primary care and residential care.

OLDER PEOPLE'S MENTAL HEALTH PROBLEMS IN PRIMARY CARE

Primary care is on the front line in dealing with older people's mental health, supporting families and managing people with complex co-morbidities. Older people consult almost twice as often as other age groups[9] and 22% of older people will have attended their general practitioner (GP) within the last two weeks and 40% may have a mental health problem. In the United Kingdom primary care is a key NHS service provider for care homes, where at least 40% of older people have depression and 50–80% dementia[3].

Depression is under-treated in older people with around 5 out of 6 older people with depression receiving no treatment at all. Only one third of older people with depression discuss their symptoms with their GP and less than half of these will receive adequate treatment[10,11]. Most people with mental health problems are managed in primary care with only 6% of older people with depression receiving specialist mental health care.

MAKING THE DIAGNOSIS

The literature suggests that diagnostic difficulties of depression in later life occur largely in relation to four areas: patient factors, practitioner factors, organizational factors and societal factors.

Patient Factors

Two-thirds of older people with serious depression have symptoms that fit poorly with current classifications of mood disorders. These classifications have been generated to reflect symptoms observed in younger people, and have inherent limitations for diagnosis of depression in older people whose presentation may differ because of ageing, physical illness or both[10]. Thus, older people can present with non-specific symptoms such as malaise, tiredness or insomnia rather than disclosing depressive symptoms[12]. Physical symptoms, in particular pain, are also common and the primary care clinician may feel they represent organic disease. Forgetfulness may also be manifest, leading to concern that the patient has cognitive impairment and early dementia[13]. Older adults may have beliefs that prevent them from seeking help for depression, such as a fear of stigmatization. They may be under the impression that antidepressant medication is addictive[11], or they may misattribute symptoms of major depression for 'old age', ill-health[13] or grief. Ethnic elders in particular do not see psychiatric services as appropriate and believe they are primarily for psychosis and violence. People across cultures often present with

Principles and Practice of Geriatric Psychiatry, 3rd edn. Edited by Mohammed T. Abou-Saleh, Cornelius Katona and Anand Kumar
© 2011 John Wiley & Sons, Ltd

culturally specific idioms of distress. South Asians often describe their distress using terms such as 'sinking heart' or 'gas in abdomen' (*gola*) as a symptom of distress. This may mislead the clinicians, causing them to tend to overlook the psychological distress and focus solely on the physical aspect of the presentation[15].

Practitioner Factors

Primary care practitioners may lack the necessary consultation skills or confidence to correctly diagnose late-life depression. They may be wary of opening a 'Pandora's box' in time-limited consultations and instead collude with the patient in what has been called 'therapeutic nihilism'[14]. In deprived areas primary care physicians have been shown to view depression as a normal response to difficult circumstances, illnesses or life events[16] and depression may be underdiagnosed because of dissatisfaction with the types of treatment that can be offered, especially a lack of availability of psychological interventions[14].

Organizational Factors

The trend in the United Kingdom for mental health services to be 'carved out' from mainstream medical services may disadvantage older depressed people who may have difficulties in attending different sites for mental and physical disorders[17]. New contractual arrangements for primary care provide no new incentives to offer re-configured services for older people with depression[18].

Societal Factors

The barriers described are likely to be particularly difficult for economically poor and minority populations who tend to have more ill-health and are more disabled. The National Service Framework (Older People)[18] had as its first standard the rooting out of age discrimination. However, little is known about the efficacy or implementation of the Framework at Primary Care Trust level. The 2009 Equality Bill[i] will, if enacted, make age-based discrimination in the provision of health and social care illegal for the first time in the United Kingdom. This Framework will be superseded by the New Horizons initiative[ii] which stresses the importance of well-being and resilience, prevention and early intervention. The Framework provides a focus on the mental health of older people.

THE CONSULTATION

Literature suggests that GPs experience difficulties in negotiating the diagnosis of depression with patients, including older people[14]. The Quality and Outcomes Framework (QOF) of the new General Medical Services (GMS) Contract[19] requires that GPs and practice nurses use two screening questions within the previous 15 months with patients with chronic disease in order to increase the detection of depression in patients with diabetes and heart disease:

- 'During the past month, have you often been bothered by feeling down, depressed or hopeless?'

- 'During the past month, have you often been bothered by having little interest or pleasure in doing things?'

A 'yes' to either question is considered a positive test. A 'no' response to both questions makes depression highly unlikely.

It would be logical to consider using these screening questions in consultations with other older people who are also at high risk of depression, for example:

- those with recent (<3 months) major physical illness or hospital admission;
- patients with chronic illness/long-term conditions;
- those in receipt of high levels of home care, including residential care;
- people with recent bereavement;
- socially isolated people;
- people persistently complaining of loneliness; or
- patients complaining of persistent sleep problems.

Little evidence has yet been found, however, for this approach[20].

There is some evidence[21] that a further question 'Is this something you want help with?' increases the usefulness of the screening questions in practice. It is then suggested that an assessment of severity of the depression is made by the GP using a schedule such as PHQ-9[22]. In addition it is vital that the GP explores with the patient ideas and plans for self-harm, and factors preventing the patient from acting on such ideas or plans.

Other authors question the usefulness of such a reductionist approach[23] and emphasize the value of professional judgement over the narrow use of schedules[24].

MANAGEMENT OPTIONS

Most patients with depression are managed in primary care settings, however, a substantial number of patients are not recognized, and those who are diagnosed often do not receive effective treatment[25]. There is, however, a good evidence base for the management of depression in older people. There is evidence to show that there are effective pharmacological treatments[26] but only one in four depressed older people receive effective pharmacological treatment and less than 10% a talking therapy[27] despite the fact that many people express a preference for such treatments[28,29]. Evidence for individual psychosocial interventions is presented in Chapter 87, but will be discussed here in the context of what the primary care practitioner can utilize. While a preventative approach to early prevention and detection of depression in older people is being evaluated and has a growing evidence base[30] most focus has been, and should be, on the treatment of an established, recognized disorder. Exercise is recommended by the NICE guidelines as a treatment for mild to moderate depression[31] but there is only limited evidence for this approach in elderly people[32]. Training in the use of the Internet to increase social support has been shown to reduce complaints of loneliness and depression[33] and there is recent evidence that befriending has a useful function in the management of mild depression in older people[34]. NICE guidelines[31] recommend a stepped care approach for the management of depression, although there is limited evidence for this approach, particularly in elderly people[35], and it is suggested[36] that systematic models of care dedicated to proactively managing depression as a chronic illness are required. The PROSPECT study[37] (Prevention of Suicide in Primary Care Elderly: Collaborative Trial)

---

[i]Government Equalities Office. A fairer future: the Equality Bill and other action to make equality a reality. 2009. www.equalities.gov.uk/pdf/NEWGEO_FairerFuture_may09_acc.pdf

[ii]http://www.dh.gov.uk/en/Healthcare/Mentalhealth/NewHorizons/DH_102135

studied the effect of a depression care manager offering recommendations to GPs according to a guideline and helping patients with adherence to medication. The IMPACT[38,39] study (Improving Mood: Promoting Access to Collaborative Care Treatment) utilized a case manager co-ordinating care and delivering a specific psychosocial intervention (behavioural activation or problem-solving treatment) with or without medication management, and liaising with both the GP and the specialist mental health services. Both studies suggest the effectiveness of such a collaborative care approach which has been shown to be acceptable to family physicians[40] and initial evidence from the United Kingdom[41] is promising. Such a service, however, is not widely commissioned in the United Kingdom as it is recommended by NICE[31] only for people with depression and chronic physical health problems.

It is vital that the GP explores the patient's view of their problem and the options that might be available to them. Thus, if antidepressants are going to be prescribed, a full discussion about these drugs, the time taken to work and the possible side effects are discussed. Similarly, a discussion about the patient's views on talking treatments or psychosocial interventions, what to expect and waiting times is vital. On-going support and review from the GP, accompanied by written information, particularly when antidepressants are prescribed, is important. In addition, the GP has a role in signposting to third sector agencies (if acceptable to the patient) and thus should be familiar with groups and local networks in his or her area.

When treatment is not leading to improvement of the patient's symptoms, it is vital that the GP considers co-morbidities, concurrent prescribing, alcohol excess, continuing loss and loneliness or a diagnosis of vascular depression[42]. At this stage, discussion with and/or referral to an old age psychiatrist is indicated.

CULTURALLY SENSITIVE INTERVENTIONS

Pharmacological and Psychological Interventions

There is little research to support any particular pharmacological therapy being specifically beneficial for ethnic elders. The general considerations about prescribing antidepressants discussed in Chapter 86 should be followed but there is a particular need for detailed explanation about the basis for suggesting medication.

Similarly, there are no culturally-sensitive psychological therapies available but again engaging the patient is critical. Abas and colleagues[43], working in the African-Caribbean community, provide a helpful framework to these issues. Consultation should be carried out with the following characteristics:

- a courteous, respectful and warm manner, along with interest in ethnicity and country of origin;
- flexibility about usual professional boundaries, for example, being prepared to share some experiences that facilitate rapport and acceptance of help;
- not offering false promises;
- offering a copy of written material (appropriately translated);
- comprehensive questions and not assuming that complaints or symptoms will be volunteered;
- acknowledging losses, both recent and chronic, including racism.

Encouraging ethnic elders to attend community and faith-based groups organized by the voluntary sector can often provide much needed social support which they are used to, but which is gradually eroding over time due to acculturation and changing family structure.

Working with the Family

The social stigma of depression causes families to deny, conceal, delay or even fail to seek treatment. This warrants public education within a cultural framework, as well as collaborative efforts by the ethnic community and health care providers. Particularly in ethnic elders from South Asia who still live in extended families it is important to keep the family 'on board'. This may seem difficult, as they may not share the viewpoint with the health provider on depression. So efforts to educate not only the patient, but also carers, becomes all the more important, particularly regarding issues around medication use, side effects and time delay in symptom improvement[44].

DEPRESSION IN RESIDENTIAL HOMES

Depression is prevalent in people in residential care homes yet usually goes undetected. Training care staff to recognize possible symptoms of depression can improve detection[45] and using a collaborative care approach to management is effective in improving outcomes[46]. Evidence suggests that using life review to people newly moved into a residential home, compared with a 'friendly visit', can prevent depression in this group of older people[47]. Other interventions such as social activation, however, have been shown to be ineffective in preventing depression[48]. The usefulness in older studies such as this, when the population in UK residential homes today may be very different to that 20 years ago, is questionable. More recent studies suggest that there are effective interventions that can be implemented in residential homes, such as group reminiscence therapy[49] and introduction of a pet into the home[50]. The role of the GP in detecting depression in elderly people in residential homes has not been evaluated, but is vital and probably limited due to current arrangements for provision of care for this group of people, who are dependent upon paid carers to request contact with their GP. Alternative models of primary care for residential homes may need to be explored.

POLICY IMPLICATIONS

Recent policy initiatives in the United Kingdom represent lost opportunities to invest and develop older people's mental health services through the National Service Framework for Mental Health[51] which excluded older people and the National Service Framework for Older People[18] which had too narrow a focus.

The publication of *Everybody's Business – Integrated Mental Health Services for Older Adults* (CSIP, 2005)[52] helpfully set out the key components of a comprehensive service for older adults with mental health needs. Regrettably though, there has been no additional targeted investment in the United Kingdom to support implementation and in the absence of clear 'must do's', performance indicators or targets, commissioners and providers find it all too easy to disregard or distort what this Department of Health guidance states.

There is a need for education at the public health level to increase community awareness of depression as a legitimate problem to take to the doctor through media campaigns and Age Concern[3], England has been active in this regard. In addition, education of health professionals in the recognition of depression in older people, a skill that requires cultural competence and different problem formulation is important, although educational initiatives alone tend to be ineffective in primary care. It is vital, then, that services commissioned are evidence-based and incorporate effective care pathways and the provision of alternative models of care, such as collaborative care, where appropriate. There needs to be increased availability of psychological services for older people, and the Improving Access to Psychological Services (IAPT)[53] initiative may not fulfil this role, as there is evidence that GPs continue to refer younger rather than older people for talking treatments[54]. In addition, interventions need to be tailored to older people's perspectives and the social rather than the psychological emphasized.

CONCLUSIONS

Depression in older people presents a challenge for the primary care physician or GP, particularly when compounded with a patient of an ethnic minority background, when the GP may not be culturally competent, or a person in a residential home, who may not receive adequate levels of contact with the GP, such that depression remains undiagnosed. There is, however, a good evidence base for the management of late-life depression and evidence that older people would prefer the option of a talking treatment. Thus there is a need for the education of primary care practitioners so that they develop the skills to diagnoses and support people with depression. In addition, the services commissioned need to meet the needs of older people with depression.

ACKNOWLEDGEMENTS

I would like to thank Robert Baldwin (Consultant in Old Age Psychiatry at Manchester Mental Health and Social Care Trust) and Alistair Burns (Professor of Old Age Psychiatry at the University of Manchester) for their ongoing support. In addition, I would like to thank Saadia Aseem, Heather Burroughs, Pam Clarke and Jonathan Lamb, members of the AMP team (www.liv.ac.uk/amp/) for their interest in this area of work.

REFERENCES

1. Beekman A, Copeland JRM, Prince MJ. Review of community prevalence of depression in later life. *Br J Psychiatry* 1999; **17**: 307–11.
2. Reynolds CF, Perel JM, Frank E *et al*. Nortriptyline and interpersonal psychotherapy as maintenance therapies for recurrent major depression. A randomised controlled trial in patients older than 59 years. *JAMA* 1999; **281**: 39–45.
3. Age Concern. *UK Inquiry into Mental Health and Well-Being in Later Life*. Coordinated by Age Concern, 2006.
4. Rait G, Burns A, Chew CA. Old age, ethnicity and mental illness: a triple whammy. (Invited Editorial) *BMJ* 1996; **313**: 1347–48.
5. Alexopoulus A. Depression in the elderly. *Lancet* 2005; **365**: 1961–70.
6. Katon W, Ciechanowski P. Impact of major depression on chronic medical illness. *J Psychosom Res* 2002; **53**: 859–63.
7. Anderson RJ, Freedland KE, Clouse RE, Lustman PJ. The prevalence of comorbid depression in adults with diabetes. *Diabetes Care* 2001; **24**: 1069–78.
8. Katon W, Lin E, Kroenke K. The association of depression and anxiety with medical symptom burden in patients with chronic medical illness. *Gen Hosp Psychiatry* 2007; **29**: 147–55.
9. Craig R, Mindell J (eds). *Health Survey for England 2005: Health of Older People*. Leeds: The Information Centre, 2007.
10. Chew-Graham C, Burns A, Baldwin R. Treating depression in later life: We need to implement the evidence that exists. [Editorial] *BMJ* 2004; **329**: 181–82.
11. Licht-Strunk E, Van Marwijk HWJ, Hoekstra T, Twisk JWR, De Haan M, Beekman ATF. Outcome of depression in later life in primary care: longitudinal cohort study with three years' follow-up. *BMJ* 2009; **338**: 463–66.
12. Rabins P. Barriers to diagnosis and treatment of depression in elderly patients. *Am J Geriatr Psychiatry* 1996; **4**: 79–84.
13. Unützer J, Katon W, Sullivan M, Miranda J. Treating depressed older adults in primary care: narrowing the gap between efficacy and effectiveness. *The Millbank Quarterly* 1999; **77**: 225–56.
14. Burroughs H, Morley, M, Lovell, K, Baldwin R, Burns A, Chew-Graham CA. 'Justifiable depression': How health professionals and patients view late-life depression; a qualitative study. *Fam Pract* 2006; **23**: 369–77.
15. Krause IB. Sinking heart: a Punjabi communication of distress. *Soc Sci Med* 1989; **29**: 563–75.
16. Chew-Graham CA, Mullin S, May CR, Hedley S, Cole H. The management of depression in primary care: another example of the inverse care law? *Fam Pract* 2002; **19**: 632–37.
17. NHS Confederation. *Investing in General Practice – the new General Medical Services Contract*. NHS Confederation, February 2003.
18. Department of Health, *National Service Framework (Older People)*. London: Department of Health, 2001.
19. Department of Health. *Quality and Outcomes Framework. Guidance*. London: Department of Health, 2004.
20. Whooley M, Stone B, Sogikian K. Randomized trial of case-finding for depression in elderly primary care patients. *J Gen Intern Med* 2000; **15**: 293–300.
21. Arroll B, Goodyear-Smith F, Kerse N *et al*. Effect of the addition of a 'help' question to two screening questions on specificity for diagnosis of depression in general practice: diagnostic validity study. *BMJ* 2005; **331**: 884–6A.
22. Kroenke K, Spitzer RL, Williams JB. The PHQ-9: validity of a brief depression severity measure. *J Gen Intern Med* 2001; **16**: 606–13.
23. Dowrick, *Beyond Depression*, 2nd edn. Oxford: Oxford University Press, 2009.
24. Van Weel C, van Weel Baumgarten, van Rijswijk E. Treatment of depression in primary care. Incentivised care is no substitute for professional judgment. *BMJ* 2009; **338**: b934.
25. Kessler D, Lloyd K, Lewis G *et al*. Cross sectional study of symptom attribution and recognition of depression and anxiety in primary care. *BMJ* 1999; **318**: 436–40.
26. Wilson K, Mottram P, Sivanranthan A, Nightingale A. Antidepressant versus placebo for depressed elderly (Cochrane Review). In: *The Cochrane Library*, Issue 2, Oxford: Update Software, 2001.
27. Singleton N, Bumpstead R, O'Brien M, Lee A, Meltzer HY. *Office of National Statistics: Psychiatric Morbidity Among Adults Living in Private Households, 2000*. London: HMSO, 2001.
28. Givens J, Datto C, Ruckdeschel K *et al*. Older patients' aversion to antidepressants: a qualitative study. *J Gen Intern Med* 2006; **21**: 146–51.
29. Areán PA, Alvidrez J, Barrera A, Robinson GS, Hicks S. Would older medical patients use psychological services? *The Gerontologist*, 2002; **42**: 392–98.
30. van't Veer-Tazelaar N, van Marwijk H, van Oppen P *et al*. Prevention of anxiety and depression in the age group of 75 years

and over: a randomised controlled trial testing the feasibility and effectiveness of a generic stepped care programme among elderly community residents at high risk of developing anxiety and depression versus usual care. *BMC Publ Health* 2006; **6**: 186.

31. National Collaborating Centre for Mental Health. NICE clinical guideline 90. *Depression: the treatment and management of depression in adults (partial update of NICE clinical guideline 23)*. http://www.nice.org.uk/nicemedia/live/12329/45888/45888.pdf

32. Singh NA, Clements KM, Fiatarone MA. A randomized controlled trial of progressive resistance training in depressed elders. *J Gerontol A Biol Sci Med Sci* 1997; **52**: M27–35.

33. White H, McConnell E, Clipp E, Branch L, Sloane R, Pieper C, Box T. A randomized controlled trial of the psychosocial impact of providing internet training and access to older adults. *Aging Ment Health* 2002; **6**: 213–21.

34. Mead N, Lester H, Chew-Graham C, Gask L, Bower P. A systematic review and meta-analysis of the effects of befriending on depressive symptoms and distress in the community. *Br J Psychiatry* 2010; **196**: 96–101.

35. Bower P, Gilbody S. Stepped care in psychological therapies: access, effectiveness and efficiency: narrative literature review. *Br J Psychiatry* 2005; **186**: 11–17.

36. Unutzer J. Diagnosis and treatment of older adults with depression in primary care. *Biol Psychiatry* 2002; **52**: 285–92.

37. Bogner HR, Bruse ML, Reynolds CF *et al*. The effect of memory, attention and executive dysfunction on outcomes of depression in a primary care intervention trial: the PROSPECT study. *Int J Geriatr Psychiatry* 2007; **22**: 922–29.

38. Unutzer J, Katon W, Callahan C *et al*. Collaborative care management of late-life depression in the primary care setting: a randomized controlled trial. *JAMA* 2002; **288**: 2836–45.

39. Unutzer J, Katon W, Fan M, Schoenbaum M, Lin E, Della Penna R. Long-term cost effects of collaborative care for late-life depression. *Am J Manag Care* 2008; 14: 95–100.

40. Levine S, Unutzer J, Yip JY *et al*. Physicians' satisfaction with a collaborative disease management program for late-life depression in primary care. *Gen Hosp Psychiatry* 2005; **27**: 383–91.

41. Chew-Graham CA, Lovell K, Roberts C *et al*. A randomised controlled trial to test the feasibility of a collaborative care model for the management of depression in older people. *Br J Geriatr Psychiatry* 2007; **57**: 364–70.

42. Alexopoulos GS, Meyers BS, Young RC *et al*. 'Vascular depression' hypothesis. *Arch Gen Psychiatry* 1997; **54**: 915–22.

43. Abas MA, Phillips C, Carter J, Walter J, Banerjee S, Levy R. Culturally sensitive validation of screening questionnaires for depression in older African-Caribbean people living in south London. *Br J Psychiatry* 1998; **173**: 249–54.

44. Chew-Graham C, Baldwin R, Burns A. *The Integrated Management of Depression in the Elderly*. Cambridge: Cambridge University Press. 2008.

45. Eisses A-MH, Kluiter H, Jongenelis K, Pot AM, Beekman ATF, Ormel J. Care staff training in detection of depression in residential homes for the elderly: randomised trial. *Br J Psychiatry* 2005; **186**: 404–409.

46. Llewellyn-Jones RH, Baikie KA, Smitliers H, Cohen J, Snowdon J, Tennant CC. Multifaceted shared care intervention for late life depression in residential care: randomised controlled trial. *BMJ* 1999; **319**: 676–82.

47. Haight BK, Michel Y, Hendrix S. Life review: preventing despair in newly relocated nursing home residents short- and long-term effects. *Int J Ageing Hum Dev* 1998; **47**: 119–42.

48. Arnetz BB, Theorell T. Psychological, sociological and health behaviour aspects of a long term activation programme for institutionalized elderly people. *Soc Sci Med* 1982; **17**: 449–56.

49. Chao SY, Liu HY, Wu CY *et al*. The effects of group reminiscence therapy on depression, self esteem, and life satisfaction of elderly nursing home residents. *J Nurs Res* 2006; **14**: 36–34.

50. Stasi MF, Amati D, Costa C *et al*. Pet-therapy: a trial for institutionalized frail elderly patients. *Arch Gerontol Geriatrics* 2004; Suppl: 407–12.

51. Department of Health. *National Service Framework for Mental Health: Modern standards and service models*. London: Department of Health, 1999.

52. Care Services Improvement Partnership (2005) National Older People's Mental Health Programme Guidance note. *Everybody's Business, Integrated Mental Health Services For Older People: A Service Development Guide*. www.olderpeoplesmentalhealth.csip.org.uk/silo/files/age-equalityguidance-note-pdf.pdf, accessed 18 June 2008.

53. IAPT. *Improving Access to Psychological Therapies*. www.iapt.nhs.uk, accessed February 2010.

54. Kendrick T, Dowrick C, McBride A *et al*. Management of depression in UK general practice in relation to scores on depression severity questionnaires: Analysis of medical record data. *BMJ* 2009; **338**: b750.

85

Electroconvulsive Therapy (ECT)*

David G. Wilkinson

Moorgreen Hospital, Botley Road, West End, Southampton, UK

Those who decry it in the elderly are sentimental and ill-informed. ECT for suitable patients not only relieves intolerable anguish but saves lives (Pitt, 1974[1]).

Electroconvulsive therapy (ECT) is an important though controversial treatment for certain subgroups of individuals suffering from severe mental disorder. These subgroups consist primarily of patients with severe depressive disorder, catatonia, mania and occasionally certain patients with schizophrenia. In addition, depending on the co-morbidity with medical and/or neurological disorders and on the risk analysis in relation to the necessity to treat, ECT is best seen as a low-risk procedure for some patients and a high-risk one for others. ECT should be administered following valid and informed consent by the patient when appropriate and in adherence to a set of guidelines of administration procedures[2].

Despite continued opposition to its use, ECT remains a fundamental tool in the armamentarium of the psychiatrist treating the severely mentally ill. There have now been thousands of papers and articles published concerning its use and we have a wealth of accumulated wisdom, and yet the controversy continues[3].

In geriatric psychiatry there is no controversy: papers continue to confirm that in the elderly ECT is an effective treatment for severe affective disorders[4-7] and is the treatment of choice in severe delusional depression[8-11]. It is safe, despite the likelihood of multiple system disorders and medications[12]. It is well tolerated, if not always well liked[13], but does sometimes exacerbate confusion. There is no convincing evidence of brain damage or even of lasting memory impairment, particularly if brief pulse right unilateral ECT is used[14]. ECT should be considered in every patient with severe delusional depression who has either failed to respond to other treatments, or who is suffering intolerable distress, or who may die through inanition or dehydration as a result of his/her depression. It is probably for these reasons that ECT continues to be used six to seven times more frequently in the elderly than in their younger counterparts[15]. The fact that in the USA it has also been shown that early use of ECT reduces inpatient costs may have also been an influential factor in its greater use[16].

INDICATIONS

Depressive Disorders

The introduction of ECT for the treatment of severe depressive illness is one of the most dramatic developments in psychiatry. It is widely considered to be the most effective treatment for severe depressive illness compared with all other modalities including the range of pharmacological treatments. Since its introduction in the early 1930s it has undergone important development and improvement with the use of anaesthesia and muscle relaxation which rendered it more safe and acceptable. The recall of ECT in the USA in the 1970s was 'plagued by hostility to the treatment'[17] fuelled by images of barbaric, inhumane and coercive treatment. In contrast to such an approach, many national psychiatric associations and societies have promoted ECT and many countries have introduced guidelines for practice: Australia, Canada, New Zealand, UK and the USA[18]. It is, however, of considerable concern that in many third-world countries, ECT is still used without the benefit and safety of anaesthesia or modern ECT devices[17,19].

The Evidence Base

A recent systematic review and meta-analysis of randomized controlled trials and observational studies of the efficacy and safety of ECT in depressive disorders[20] reported the following findings:

- ECT versus simulated ECT – ECT was significantly more effective than simulated ECT in the reduction of depressive symptoms and no difference in premature discontinuation from treatment for patients receiving ECT and simulated ECT. Patients treated with ECT were better able to retrieve remote memories than those treated with simulated ECT and had more recognition errors immediately after treatment.
- ECT versus pharmacotherapy – treatment with ECT was significantly more effective than pharmacotherapy and discontinuation was significantly lower in the ECT group than in the pharmacotherapy group.
- Bilateral versus unilateral electrode placement – Bilateral ECT was more effective than unilateral ECT in the reduction of depressive symptoms. High-dose unilateral ECT might be as effective as bilateral ECT and causes fewer adverse cognitive effects. Bilateral ECT was associated with impairment in anterograde memory impairment within seven days of the end of the randomized phase of treatment but no long-term cognitive impairment.
- Frequency of ECT – ECT administered once a week, twice and three times a week had similar effects on depressive symptoms and no difference in discontinuation of treatment but more frequent ECT led to more cognitive impairment.
- Dose of electrical stimulus – high-dose ECT led to greater reduction in depressive symptoms, but was associated with more

*Updated by Mohammed T. Abou-Saleh

Principles and Practice of Geriatric Psychiatry, 3rd edn. Edited by Mohammed T. Abou-Saleh, Cornelius Katona and Anand Kumar

impairment in anterograde memory but not in terms of personal memory.

- Stimulus wave form – brief pulse and sine wave ECT were equally effective with some indication that patients receiving brief pulse ECT recovered more quickly and had better recall of word associates learned shortly before the treatment than did those receiving sign wave ECT.

A meta-analysis of the efficacy of ECT in depression deriving from 15 randomized controlled trials (RCTs) showed ECT to be superior to pharmacotherapy and simulated ECT, with the presence of psychotic symptoms predicting better response to ECT[21]. The report found no evidence for a superior speed of action of ECT or for a difference between sine wave and brief pulse stimulation. ECT has been shown to be more effective in delusional than in non-delusional depression[22,23]. A recent Cochrane Review assessed the efficacy and safety of ECT compared to simulated ECT or antidepressants in the depressed elderly[24]. Only three trials could be included and all had methodological shortcomings. The results nonetheless indicated that ECT was more effective than simulated ECT, but the comparative efficacy of unilateral over bilateral ECT and safety could not be assessed adequately.

Older age confers a greater likelihood of achieving a remission with bilateral, dose-titrated, continuation ECT in comparison with continuation pharmacotherapy[25].

The NICE Review[26] of data from 90 randomized controlled trials (RCTs) of ECT in depressive disorders (not specifically in older people) concluded that:

- real ECT (where electric current was applied) is more effective than simulated ECT (no electric current was applied) in the short term;
- bilateral ECT is more effective than unilateral ECT;
- raising the electrical stimulus above the individual's threshold supported the efficacy of unilateral ECT at the expense of increased cognitive impairment.
- ECT was more effective than antidepressants notwithstanding the variable quality of RCTs and the inadequate doses and duration of antidepressants that were used in many of the trials;
- ECT is associated with cognitive impairment, particularly in those who had bilateral ECT or unilateral ECT applied to the dominant hemisphere;
- cognitive function does not last more than six months from the administration of ECT;
- there is no evidence that ECT is associated with greater mortality than that associated with the administration of general anaesthetics. Studies that use brain-scanning techniques showed no evidence that ECT causes brain damage;
- there is no evidence to suggest that the benefits and safety of ECT are age-dependent;
- there are no complications of ECT in pregnancy but the risks should be balanced against refusing antidepressant.

As mentioned studies on the efficacy of ECT, which have largely been conducted on younger patients[8], all emphasize that ECT appears to be more effective than placebo, single-drug therapy and tricyclic/neuroleptic combinations, and that patients with more florid symptoms of recent onset fare best[27–29]. Experience with the elderly would confirm these findings. Indicators of response are perhaps less clear in the elderly, with some authors finding psychomotor disturbance and psychosis a positive predictor of response[11] and others suggesting that patients without these features can also do well[30]. That the classic distinction between neurotic and psychotic depression appears less helpful in this group as a predictor of good response is nothing new. Post[31] in 1976 stressed the practical irrelevance of any subclassification of elderly depressives, as he found that ECT rendered severe psychotic depressives fit for discharge only slightly more often than neurotic depressives. The presenting picture of apparent hysterical illness, hypochondriasis or other apparent neurotic illness may well be caused by an underlying functional psychosis, often depressive in the elderly. More recently, in a study of 163 elderly patients given ECT, it was found that 27% had predominantly neurotic depressive features and yet had a good response to treatment[4]. In fact, in the study by Fraser and Glass[32], psychic anxiety, along with the more expected features of short duration, severity of illness, guilt and agitation, was one of the symptoms correlated with a favourable response to ECT, whereas the typical endogenous features of late insomnia and diurnal variation in mood were not. Older patients with treatment-resistant depression often do respond to ECT, although not as well as non-resistant patients[33]. However, they do respond better to ECT than to SSRIs[29] and Flint[6] found that ECT was significantly superior to tricyclic/neuroleptic combinations, even when the former had been augmented with lithium. A pragmatic consensus would suggest that in the elderly a trial of ECT is indicated in any depressed patient who might otherwise be regarded as a treatment non-responder, and if the illness is severe and of short duration there is likely to be a good response, regardless of the presenting symptoms. If the illness has been present for a long time, it still may respond, particularly if there is a clear history of a recent change for the worse in a patient who had previously maintained a stable personality and had coped normally with the vicissitudes of life. Prolonged or abnormal bereavement reactions with marked depressive features not responding to antidepressants or talking therapies may need to be treated with ECT before psychotherapy or counselling can be effective. ECT may need to be given within a few months of the loss if hopelessness and suicidal ideation suggest a risk to life, and should not be withheld due to the feeling that the patient must work through his/her grief naturally, as he/she may never get that chance.

Continuation Pharmacotherapy after ECT

High relapse rates of depression have been consistently reported after remission with ECT. Five controlled trials have demonstrated the efficacy of continuation treatment with antidepressants and lithium in reducing relapse after remission with ECT[34]. Further RCTs have demonstrated the efficacy of continuation treatment with imipramine and paroxetine in relapse prevention in such patients[35]. Nortriptyline monotherapy and its combination with lithium has also been shown to be superior to placebo over six months in preventing relapses in unipolar depression following remission with ECT[36].

A recent study used a longitudinal, randomized, single-blind design to compare by survival analysis the two-year outcome of two subgroups of elderly patients with psychotic unipolar depression who were ECT (plus nortriptyline) remitters[37]. The mean survival time was significantly longer in the combined ECT plus nortriptyline subgroup than in the nortriptyline subgroup. No differences were observed between treatments with regard to tolerability. The authors advocated the judicious use of combined continuation/maintenance ECT and antidepressant treatment in elderly patients with psychotic unipolar depression who are ECT remitters.

Schizophrenia

Paraphrenia will often respond to ECT[38], although this is more likely if there are obvious depressive symptoms or delusions. A Cochrane Review assessed the evidence for the efficacy of ECT in terms of clinically meaningful benefits in patients with schizophrenia, and whether variations in the practical administration of ECT influences outcome[39]. The Review included 24 trials and 46 reports and showed the following:

- Fewer patients remain unimproved with ECT, with less relapses and earlier discharge than patients treated with placebo or simulated ECT.
- Limited data indicated visual memory impairment with ECT compared with simulated ECT.
- ECT is less beneficial than antipsychotic medication.
- Continuation ECT added to antipsychotics is superior to antipsychotics alone but is associated with more memory impairment.

There is relatively little evidence specific to the use of ECT in older patients with schizophrenia. ECT has been shown to have good short-term effects and be safe in middle-aged and elderly patients with intractable catatonic schizophrenia[40] and in treatment resistant schizophrenia[41].

In schizophrenia, the NICE Review[26] of the data from 25 RCTs indicated that ECT may be effective in acute episodes of certain types of schizophrenia and reduces the occurrence of relapses. However, the results were not conclusive and the design of many of the studies did not reflect current practice. Moreover, there are no RCTs of ECT compared with antipsychotics. Furthermore, studies that include patients with treatment-resistant schizophrenia had not reported the use of clozapine. The Review concluded that ECT alone is not more effective than antipsychotic medication but that the combination of ECT and pharmacotherapy may be more effective than pharmacotherapy alone although the evidence is not conclusive.

ECT is certainly useful in the depressed (and usually elderly) patient with Parkinson's disease, as the motor symptoms will improve as well as the depression, and indeed, some authors advocate ECT as the treatment of choice for certain stages of Parkinson's disease, whether or not depression is a major problem[42,43]. I have given daily ECT with excellent results to a Parkinsonian patient who had developed severe paranoid delusions. His refusal to accept his medication rendered him rigid and immobile with pressure sores, he needed intravenous fluids and nasogastric feeding until he had four treatments, whereupon his physical and emotional improvement was dramatic.

Fogel[27] suggests that ECT might be more readily used in the elderly if we were more objective about its virtues as compared with the severe side effects often associated with neuroleptics, which are quite readily used in the agitated elderly patient. Extrapyramidal effects were usually the limiting factor but are not so noticeable with atypical neuroleptics. However, he postulates that the demented patient who is very agitated and screaming might suffer less indignity and fewer side effects if treated with ECT, rather than tranquillizers, as the patient may have an underlying affective disturbance manifest only by the agitation and negativism that one often sees in this condition.

Mania

Mania is another potential indication for a trial of ECT[44], particularly in the elderly, where neuroleptics may fail to control the symptoms and yet produce unsteadiness, postural hypotension or falls, and lithium may not be tolerated due to toxicity problems.

The NICE Review[26] of four RCTs indicated that ECT may be of benefit in rapid control of mania and catatonia, a suggestion that is supported by the results of observational studies. Overall, however, it concluded that the evidence for the effectiveness of ECT and for the determination of the most appropriate therapeutic strategy is inconclusive. In contrast, a recent literature review of continuation and maintenance ECT in treatment-resistant bipolar disorder reported good evidence for efficacy[45]. ECT is indicated in severe and prolonged mania (excitement, delirium, psychosis, or rapid-cycling manic states), especially when the anti-manic medications (lithium, neuroleptics) have been relatively inefficient[46]. It seems that the NICE Review has been restrictive in the studies it considered and the conclusions drawn from them. It must also be emphasized that the evidence reviewed above is not specific to elderly people.

CONTRAINDICATIONS

There are no absolute contraindications, only relative risks, in which the risks of ECT and associated general anaesthesia are weighed up against the morbidity and mortality of untreated depression. The limiting factor is whether the patient is physically fit for the light anaesthetic that ECT requires. The majority of risk factors are therefore associated with the cardiovascular system. Many people are denied treatment due to irrational caution. For example, pacemakers are not barriers to treatment; the bodily tissues, being highly resistant, prevent the ECT stimulus from reaching the pacemaker. The patient should remain insulated from the ground, however, to prevent the unlikely event of the current leaking to earth and being conducted down the pacemaker wire to the heart. Equally, myocardial infarction is not a contraindication to treatment if the depression is so severe as to threaten life; in less severe cases, an interval (governed by sentiment rather than science) of 4–6 weeks is usually recommended. The risks are greatest during the first 10 days post-infarct, and probably negligible after three months. I have treated a patient with hypothyroidism who had two prosthetic heart valves, was therefore on anticoagulants and had a pacemaker, with no special precautions or untoward effects. Patients with osteoporosis or with recent femoral neck fractures can be treated, provided an adequate muscle relaxant is given. Stroke is certainly not a contraindication, and ECT given as soon as one month after does not present a major risk to patients. There is now a growing body of literature attesting to the usefulness of ECT in treating post-stroke depression[47].

The case of deep venous thrombosis (DVT) is less clear. I have given ECT to a patient who had a DVT in his calf during his depressive illness, once he was adequately anticoagulated. In fact, the risk of pulmonary embolism seems, in my practice, greater in older severely depressed patients who are dehydrated and immobile depressive than in those receiving ECT.

Arterial hypertension is often regarded as a contraindication, as blood pressure is well known to rise during ECT. This can sometimes be controlled and the pressor response avoided by using sublingual nifedipine or short-acting b-blockers shortly before treatment[48]. Chronic glaucoma is another condition in which ECT causes fewer problems than tricyclic antidepressants; in fact, intraocular pressures are said to reduce ECT[49]. Insulin-dependent diabetes is a condition, like Parkinson's disease, which alters during ECT. Insulin requirements may decrease quite substantially during the course of ECT, so more careful monitoring of blood glucose levels is needed. It is also necessary to avoid hyperglycaemia prior to treatment, which may significantly raise the fit threshold, and the timing of ECT administration may need consideration to prevent undue fluctuations in diabetic control.

Transient asystole occasionally occurs, for some reason less frequently in the old-old, but it is not of any long-term clinical consequence and need not prevent further treatments[50,51].

Epileptic patients on anticonvulsants should not stop their medication during ECT, as that might increase the risk of status epilepticus. However, they may need higher than usual electrical dosages to produce an adequate epileptiform response.

It is interesting that the seizure during ECT is invested with great powers of harm compared with epileptic seizures per se, which can of course occur in patients with any disease or at any time and seldom result in death. It seems understandable, then, that a seizure in the controlled conditions of the ECT room is probably even less likely to result in fatality. There is, of course, a mortality rate associated with ECT but, as noted by Fink[52], the treatment rate of 0.002% compares favourably with the rate for anaesthetic induction alone (0.003–0.04%).

ADMINISTRATION

The responses of senior psychiatrists to the process of ECT vary from those who simply prescribe six treatments and leave the administration to the newest recruit, who has often had no training at all, to the surgeon manqué who may overstate the risks and precautions in order to increase the perceived risk of his (or her) job. Clearly, the ideal path lies somewhere between, but nearer the latter than the former! ECT is the only psychiatric treatment in the elderly that involves significant medical intervention with general anaesthesia, and as such, the psychiatrist should have a clear understanding of what he/she is prescribing and regular involvement in its administration. As much attention should be paid to the prescription of ECT as to any other prescription.

A clear decision as to whether bilateral or unilateral electrode placement is wanted should be made; the ECT record sheet should be reviewed to ensure that an adequate convulsive response has occurred without excessive stimulus; treatments should not be in blocks of six, but response should be evaluated after each treatment. Provided that the illness is one with a good prognosis, treatment should be continued until the expected degree of improvement is obtained, whether that is after three or 23 treatments.

There is no evidence that the habit of giving one or two extra ECTs after full recovery is effective in preventing relapse[53]. The decision to give unilateral or bilateral ECT in the elderly is made easier by the fact that high-dose unilateral ECT does seem to produce less confusion, memory loss and headache and appears to be equally effective in many patients[54,55]. However, there is a great deal of discrepancy in the results of comparative studies, possibly due to differences in diagnosis, age and gender, together with variance in the technique of administration of unilateral ECT. The consensus seems to indicate that, for many patients, both treatments are equally effective; some patients require more right unilateral treatments than bilateral to achieve the same result and some patients who do not respond to right unilateral ECT will respond when switched to bilateral treatment. Male gender and older age are also associated with better response to bilateral treatment.

It is my practice to use bilateral treatment initially in very severe psychotic depressives but right unilateral treatment in most other cases, particularly if there is evidence of prior cognitive impairment, switching to bilateral treatment if there is no response after six to eight right unilateral treatments. Brief pulse ECT at a moderately supra-threshold stimulus (which is often only around 275–350 millicoulombs) appears to offer efficacy, with the advantage of much less memory loss and confusion than the modified sine wave stimulus, and should be used in all cases, with a record of dosage received by the patient to ensure adequate technique[56].

There is considerable debate about the necessity to use a dose titration technique to establish seizure threshold prior to treatment, with some viewing this as unnecessary and even detrimental in those patients requiring several non-convulsive stimuli. Adequate seizure response can be measured using interictal EEG monitoring. Some clinicians seem to have developed an excessive interest in stimulus intensity, seizure threshold and seizure duration. It is clear that seizure threshold will increase by about 40% during the course of ECT and the seizure duration will tend to decrease by about one-third. However, while it seems that outcome is not correlated with either seizure duration or threshold for bilateral ECT[57], it may be more important to keep the stimulus intensity above seizure threshold in unilateral treatment[58]. Seizure duration is more difficult to evaluate, as some patients regularly have brisk and brief responses with good results. The use of propofol to induce anaesthesia consistently reduces seizure duration, although apparently without affecting efficacy[59,60]. The use of caffeine prior to treatment to prolong seizure activity has been associated with improved efficacy in some patients[61]. It would seem that, as a rule of thumb, we should aim for a seizure length of around 25 s and any seizure less than 15 s or more than 120 s is likely to adversely affect response[62]. Cumulative seizure duration again seems less interesting now than it once was as a measure of the length of a course of treatment, and clinical response still seems the best measure.

There is no evidence that routine atropine premedication improves cardiac stability or lessens secretions. Theoretically it could cause confusion, but there is no convincing evidence of this either. Glycopyrrolate, which does not cross the blood–brain barrier, may be a better drug to use as a drying agent but is not widely used.

Methohexitone for the induction of anaesthesia at a dosage of 30–50 mg is adequate to ensure sleep without hangover, and muscle relaxation with a suxamethonium dosage of 20–40 mg is enough to modify the convulsion without abolishing all evidence of motor activity. If the minimum amount of anaesthetic is combined with treatment early in the morning, the patient is not required to starve any longer than usual, he/she is less likely to be dehydrated, is less likely to break his/her fast, has less time to become anxious and agitated and will recover quickly enough to enjoy a breakfast with the other patients on the ward. If this routine is combined with regular supervision of treatment by the prescribing psychiatrist, the patient will derive the maximum benefit from each treatment and the course will not be unnecessarily prolonged or ineffective. Outpatient ECT does not appear to be as effective in the elderly, except occasionally as maintenance, and consequently most patients will require admission to a specialist unit, where the effects of ECT combined with the therapeutic milieu will hasten improvement. Familiar staff administering the treatment and a well-designed ECT suite will help reduce anxiety.

MAINTENANCE AND CONTINUATION ECT

In 1990 the American Psychiatric Association task force on ECT defined continued administration of ECT over a six-month period to prevent relapse after induction of remission as continuation ECT (C-ECT); treatment beyond six months was termed maintenance ECT (M-ECT). This was felt to be a viable form of management for selected patients.

Maintenance ECT has been used for many years: a survey of British psychogeriatricians in 1991[63] found that 20% were using it but there is little more than anecdote to support its use in the literature. Such studies as there are consist mainly of case studies and small series of hospitalized patients, all of a 'naturalistic' nature.

In a one-year follow-up of nine elderly patients, continuation treatment, even if discontinued fairly quickly, seemed to confer some lasting advantage in prevention of relapse[64], as did Petrides et al.'s study, looking at 33 courses of C-ECT[65]. The conclusion seemed to be that where patients have responded to acute ECT but previously failed on continuation pharmacotherapy there was compelling evidence for C-ECT and little therapeutic alternative. The four patients in this study[65] who continued with M-ECT remained well and the five who had previously stopped did not. Naturally this result is open to other interpretations, but it does suggest that C-ECT should be considered for those with recurrent depression who respond well to ECT acutely but receive no prophylaxis from pharmacotherapy. The practicalities of using outpatient M-ECT have prevented my using it more. Bringing elderly patients to hospital for outpatient ECT early in the day, from a rural catchment area some distance from the hospital, can be problematic, they soon lose enthusiasm for the treatment and consequently often withdraw consent. This is an issue recently addressed by Kim[66]. However, Schwarz's findings, that rehospitalization rates were reduced by 67% after instituting M-ECT, suggest that we should try and overcome the practical difficulties[67].

The recent NICE update of guidance on the treatment of depression[68] has recommended that further research is urgently required to examine the long-term efficacy and safety of ECT, including its use as a maintenance therapy and its use in particular subgroups who may be at increased risk particularly the elderly. This research should reflect modern techniques and the use of ECT in comparison and in conjunction with the antipsychotic and antidepressant drugs used in current practice.

CONSENT

Popular myths about ECT are always more readily believed than the reality and can be part of what the patient believes they are consenting to. Occasionally patients consent as part of their death wish. I use a video of myself administering ECT to a patient seen before and after treatment, to show anxious or interested relatives and patients; no one having seen it has then declined the treatment. There is one study suggesting that understanding is not enhanced by this method. The issue of informed consent in depressed patients is complex. As I have suggested, many care little and are prepared to do anything their doctor suggests, and patients' recollection of what was explained to them, after the ECT and when the depression has lifted, is often vague. A careful explanation should be made and recorded, and if there are doubts on either side a chance to preview the ECT room or an explanatory video may be helpful. However, it is doubtful whether the explanation of ECT is any less detailed than that of most surgical procedures and most people are willing to consent without seeing a video of the operation in question. Passive acceptance of ECT is often the case in the severely depressed but this should not prevent a full explanation, including consulting relatives if appropriate.

Involuntary ECT should never be given except within the guidelines of the relevant mental health legislation if we are to ensure the availability of ECT as a treatment option in the future. Nevertheless, depression is such a serious and debilitating illness that the chance of a cure through use of ECT should never be denied to a patient whose prognosis is favourable, simply through difficulty in obtaining actual written consent.

ADVERSE EFFECTS

As already mentioned, confusion and memory loss are often regarded as an inevitable corollary of ECT in the elderly, but this is clearly not the case and there are well-conducted studies showing no objective permanent effects on memory, and in fact this often improves as a result of improvement in the depression[32,69,70].

Nevertheless, there is no doubt that some patients who were given bilateral sine wave ECT experienced long-term, even permanent, memory loss, and bland reassurances that this or even brief pulse bilateral ECT will not cause any memory loss is foolish and counterproductive. Some patients given bilateral brief pulse ECT may have amnestic gaps, but can be assured that no lasting effect on memory function, i.e. new learning or intelligence will occur. The situation with right unilateral brief pulse ECT is different, with any subjective memory impairment being transient and undetectable six months later[71,72]. Patients with existing dementia may well show signs of memory impairment, even with unilateral ECT. This may be acceptable in view of the relief from distress and agitation and improvement in behaviour and performance.

The cognitive side effects can be minimized by reducing concomitant medications, particularly benzodiazepines, anticholinergic antidepressants and lithium[73], although a recent study found no problems with the administration of ECT and lithium[74].

Benzodiazepines, given intravenously as the seizure ends, can be of use in controlling emergent delirium, which can last for 15–30 min after treatment and be very difficult to control otherwise.

Dementia per se does not preclude the use of ECT, provided that the co-existing depression is circumscribed. A history of depression before the dementia adds weight to the decision, particularly if there was a good response to ECT previously. Other side effects of treatment, such as headache and dizziness or muscle pain, usually only after the first anaesthetic, are minimal and soon forgotten as the depression lifts.

REPETITIVE TRANSCRANIAL MAGNETIC STIMULATION (rTMS)

Repetitive transcranial magnetic stimulation (rTMS) involves focal stimulation of the superficial layers of the cerebral cortex using a rapidly changing magnetic field applied using an external coil. It does not require anaesthesia and can be performed on an outpatient basis. Treatment with rTMS usually involves daily sessions lasting about 30 min for 2–4 weeks and possibly longer. Its use in the treatment of depression has recently been the subject of NICE Interventional Procedures Guidance IPG 242. A recent meta-analysis for patients with treatment resistant depression which included 24 studies (1092 patients) meeting their inclusion criteria[75] found that active rTMS was significantly superior to sham conditions in producing clinical response, with a risk difference of 17%. However, the pooled response and remission rates were only 25% and 17%, and 9% and

6% for active rTMS and sham conditions, respectively. They concluded that further studies are required before adopting rTMS as a first-line treatment for treatment-resistant depression. The recent NICE update[68] concluded that the efficacy of rTMS depends on higher intensity, greater frequency, bilateral application and/or longer treatment durations and there appears to be no major safety concerns associated with its use.

CONCLUSION

ECT is a valuable and as yet essential tool in the treatment of depression in old age, a disease which untreated carries a significant mortality. It is interesting that in practice elderly patients who have attempted suicide are nearly all offered ECT. This is because those, albeit only very few in number, who have subsequently killed themselves during a depressive illness have all been patients who have either refused ECT or not been given it at the time of their index suicide attempt. However, while there are many compelling arguments for the use of ECT, it is not a universal panacea. ECT, like any potent treatment, should be prescribed with accuracy and its use monitored carefully by those prescribing it.

Depression in the elderly presents with protean manifestations. ECT should be part of an eclectic approach to treatment and as such will continue to relieve distress and save lives.

REFERENCES

1. Pitt B. *Psychogeriatrics*. Edinburgh: Churchill Livingstone, 1974.
2. Abou-Saleh MT, Papakostas Y, Zervas I, Christodoulou, G. The World Psychiatric Association position statement on the use and safety of electroconvulsive therapy. *Science and Care, Bulletin of the WPA Scientific Sections* 2004; **1**: 7–11.
3. Wilkinson DG, Daoud J. The stigma and enigma of ECT. *Int J Geriatr Psychiatry* 1998; **13**: 833–5.
4. Godber C, Rosenvinge H, Wilkinson DG *et al*. Depression in old-age: prognosis after ECT. *Int J Geriatr Psychiatry* 1987; **2**: 19–24.
5. Stroudemire A, Hill CD, Maarquardt M *et al*. Recovery and relapse in geriatric depression after treatment with antidepressants and ECT in a medical–physical population. *Gen Hosp Psychiatry* 1998; **20**(3): 170–4.
6. Flint AJ, Rifat SL. The treatment of psychotic depression in later life: a comparison of pharmacotherapy and ECT. *Int J Geriatr Psychiatry* 1998; **13**(1): 23–8.
7. Williams JH, O'Brian JT, Cullum S. Time course of response to electroconvulsive therapy in elderly depressed subjects. *Int J Geriatr Psychiatry* 1997; **12**(5): 563–6.
8. Johnstone EC, Deakins JF, Lawler P *et al*. The Northwick Park electroconvulsive therapy trial. *Lancet* 1980; **ii**: 1317–20.
9. Baldwin RC. Delusional and non-delusional depression in late life. Evidence of distinct sub-types. *Br J Psychiatry* 1988; **152**: 39–44.
10. Ottoson J. Use and misuse of electroconvulsive treatment. *Biol Psychiatry* 1985; **20**: 933–46.
11. Hickie I, Mason C, Parker G, Brodaty H. Prediction of ECT response; validation of a refined sign-based (CORE) system for defining melancholia. *Br J Psychiatry* 1996; **169**(1): 68–74.
12. Gaspar D, Samarasinghe LA. ECT in psychogeriatric practice – a study of risk factors, indications and outcomes. *Comp Psychiatry* 1982; **23**: 170–5.
13. Hughes J, Barraclough B, Reeve W. Are patients shocked by ECT? *J R Soc Med* 1981; **74**: 283–5.
14. Abrams R. *Electroconvulsive Therapy*. New York: Oxford University Press, 1988.
15. Flint AJ. Electroconvulsive therapy in the elderly. *Curr Opin Psychiatry* 1999; **12**: 481–5.
16. Olfson M, Marcus S, Sackeim HA *et al*. Use of ECT for the inpatient treatment of recurrent major depression. *Am J Psychiatry* 1998; **155**: 22–9.
17. Fink M. ECT has much to offer our patients: it should not be ignored. *World J Biol Psychiatry* 2001; **2**(1): 1–8.
18. Bauer M, Whybrow PC, Angst J, Versiani M, Moller HJ. World Federation of Societies of Biological Psychiatry (WFSBF) Task Force on treatment guidelines for unipolar depressive disorders. *World J Biol Psychiatry* 2002; **3**(2): 69–86.
19. Abou-Saleh MT, Christodoulou G. World Psychiatric Association Position Statement on the ethics of unmodified ECT. *Arab J Psychiatry* 2009; **20**(1): 23–30.
20. The UK ECT Review Group. Efficacy and safety of electroconvulsive therapy in depressive disorder: a systematic review and meta-analysis. *Lancet* 2003; **361**: 799–808.
21. Kho KH, Van Vreeswijk MF, Simpson S, Zwinderman AH. A meta-analysis of electroconvulsive therapy efficacy in depression. *J ECT* 2003; **19**(3): 139–47.
22. Meyers BS, Klimstra SA, Gabriele M, Hamilton M, Kakuma T, Tirumalasetti F, Alexopoulos GS. Continuation treatment of delusional depression in older adults. *Am J Geriatr Psychiatry* 2001; **9**(4): 415–22.
23. Birkenhager TK, Pluijms EM and Lucius SA. ECT response in delusional versus non-delusional depressed inpatients. *J Affect Disord* 2003; **74**(2): 191–5.
24. Van der Wurff FB, Stek ML, Hoogendijk WL, Beekman ATF. Electroconvulsive therapy for the depressed elderly (Cochrane Review). The Cochrane Library, Issue 4, 2003.
25. O'Connor MK, Knapp R, Husain M, Rummans TA, Petrides G, Smith G *et al*. The influence of age on the response of major depression to electroconvulsive therapy: a CORE report. *Am J Geriatr Psychiatry* 2001; **9**(4): 382–90.
26. National Institute for Clinical Excellence. *Guidance on the Use of Electroconvulsive Therapy*, 2003, 1–36.
27. Fogel B. Electroconvulsive therapy in the elderly: a clinical research agenda. *Int J Geriatr Psychiatry* 1988; **3**: 181–90.
28. Kroessler D. Relative efficacy rates for therapies of delusional depression. *Convuls Ther* 1985; **1**: 173–82.
29. Folkerts HW, Michael N, Tolle R *et al*. Electroconvulsive therapy vs. paroxetine in treatment-resistant depression – a randomised study. *Acta Psychiatr Scand* 1997; **96**: 334–42.
30. Sobin C, Prudic J, Devanand DP *et al*. Who responds to electroconvulsive therapy? A comparison of effective and ineffective forms of treatment. *Br J Psychiatry* 1996; **169**(3): 322–8.
31. Post F. The management and nature of depressive illness in late life: a follow-through story. In Gallant D (ed.), *Depression*. New York: Spectrum, 1976.
32. Fraser R, Glass I. Unilateral and bilateral ECT in elderly patients. A comparative study. *Acta Psychiatr Scand* 1980; **62**: 13–31.
33. Prudic J, Haskett RF, Mulsant B *et al*. Resistance to antidepressant medications and short term clinical response to ECT. *Am J Psychiatry* 1996; **153**(8): 985–92.
34. Abou-Saleh MT, Coppen AJ. Continuation therapy with antidepressants after electroconvulsive therapy. *J Psychiatr Res* 1988; **4**(4): 263–8.

35. Lauritzen L, Odgaard K, Clemmesen L, Lunde M, Ohrstrom J, Black C, Bech P. Relapse prevention by means of paroxetine in ECT-treated patients with major depression: a comparison with imipramine and placebo in medium-term continuation therapy. *Acta Psychiatr Scand* 1997; **96**(5): 405–6.

36. Sackeim HA, Haskett RF, Mulsant BH, Thase ME, Mann JJ, Pettinati HM *et al*. Continuation pharmacotherapy in the prevention of relapse following electroconvulsive therapy: a randomized controlled trial. *JAMA* 2001; **285**(10): 1299–307.

37. Navarro V, Gastó C, Torres X, Masana G, Penadés R, Guarch J *et al*. Continuation/maintenance treatment with nortriptyline versus combined nortriptyline and ECT in late-life psychotic depression: a two-year randomized study. *Am J Geriatr Psychiatry* 2008; **16**(6): 498–505.

38. Turek I. Combined use of ECT and psychotropic drugs: antidepressive and antipsychotics. *Comp Psychiatry* 1973; **14**: 495–502.

39. Tharyan P, Adams CE. Electroconvulsive therapy for schizophrenia. *Cochrane Database System Reviews* 2000; **2**: CD000076.

40. Suzuki K, Awata S, Matsuoka H. Short-term effect of ECT in middle-aged and elderly patients with intractable catatonic schizophrenia. *J ECT* 2003; **19**(2): 73–90.

41. Tang WK, Ungvari GS. Efficacy of electroconvulsive therapy in treatment-resistant schizophrenia: a prospective open trial. *Prog Neuropsychopharmacol Biol Psychiatry* 2003; **27**(3): 373–9.

42. Lebensohn Z, Jenkins R. Improvement of Parkinsonism in depressed patients treated with ECT. *Am J Psychiatry* 1975; **132**: 283–5.

43. Douyon R, Sorby M, Klutchko B *et al*. ECT and Parkinson's disease revisited: a naturalistic study. *Am J Psychiatry* 1989; **146**: 1451–5.

44. Black D, Winokur G, Nasrallah A. Treatment of mania: naturalistic study of electroconvulsive therapy versus lithium in 438 patients. *J Clin Psychiatry* 1987; **48**: 132–9.

45. Vaidya NA, Mahableshwarkar AR, Shahid R. Continuation and maintenance ECT in treatment-resistant bipolar disorder. *J ECT* 2003; **19**(1): 10–16.

46. Mukherjee S, Sackeim HA, Schnur DB. Electroconvulsive therapy of acute manic episodes: a review of 50 years' experience. *Am J Psychiatry* 1994; **151**: 169–76.

47. Murray G, Shea V, Conn D. Electroconvulsive therapy for post-stroke depression. *J Clin Psychiatry* 1986; **47**: 258–60.

48. Wells D, Davies G, Rosewarne F. Attenuation of electroconvulsive therapy-induced hypertension with sublingual nifedipine. *Anaes Intens Care* 1989; **17**: 31–3.

49. Kalinowsky L, Hippius H, Klein H. *Biological Treatments in Psychiatry*. New York: Grune and Stratton, 1982.

50. Burd J, Kettl P. The incidence of asystole in electroconvulsive therapy in elderly patients. *Am J Geriat Psychiatry* 1998; **6**(3): 203–11.

51. McCall WV. Asystole in electroconvulsive therapy: Report of four cases. *J Clin Psychiatry* 1996; **57**(5): 199–203.

52. Fink M. *Convulsive Therapy: Theory and Practice*. New York: Raven, 1979.

53. Barton J, Mahta S, Snaith R. The prophylactic value of extra ECT in depressive illness. *Acta Psychiatr Scand* 1973; **49**: 386–92.

54. Weiner R. The role of electroconvulsive therapy in the treatment of depression in the elderly. *J Am Geriatr Soc* 1982; **30**: 701–12.

55. Sackeim HA, Prudic J, Devanand DP *et al*. A prospective, randomized, double-blind comparison of bilateral and right unilateral electroconvulsive therapy at different stimulus intensities. *Arch Gen Psychiatry* 2000; **57**(5): 425–34.

56. McCall WV, Reboussin DM, Weiner RD, Sackeim HA. Titrated moderately suprathreshold vs fixed high-dose right unilateral electroconvulsive therapy: acute antidepressant and cognitive effects. *Arch Gen Psychiatry* 2000; **57**(5): 438–44.

57. Shapira B, Lidsky D, Garfine M, Lever B. Electroconvulsive therapy and resistant depression: clinical implications of seizure threshold. *J Clin Psychiatry* 1996; **57**(1): 32–8.

58. Krystal AD, Coffey CF, Weiner RD *et al*. Changes in seizure threshold over the course of electroconvulsive therapy affect therapeutic response and are detected by vital EEG ratings. *J NeuroPsychiatry Clin Neurosci* 1998; **10**(2): 178–86.

59. Kirkby KC, Beckett WG, Matters RM *et al*. Comparison of propofol and methohexitone in anaesthesia for ECT: effect on seizure duration and outcome. *Aust NZ J Psychiatry* 1995; **29**(2): 229–303.

60. Malsch E, Gratz I, Mani S *et al*. Efficacy of electroconvulsive therapy after propofol and methohexital anesthesia. *Convuls Ther* 1994; **10**(3): 212–19.

61. Kelsey MC, Grossberg GT. Safety and efficiency of caffeine augmented ECT in elderly depressives: a retrospective study. *J Geriatr Psychiatry Neurol* 1995; **8**(3): 168–72.

62. Haas S, Nash K, Lippmann SB. ECT-induced seizure durations. *J Kentucky Med Assoc* 1996; **94**(6): 233–6.

63. Benbow SM. Old age psychiatrists' views on the use of ECT. *Int J Geriatr Psychiatry* 1991; **6**: 317–22.

64. Mirchandani I, Abrams R, Young R, Alexopoulos G. One-year follow-up of continuation convulsive therapy prescribed for depressed elderly patients. *Int J Geriatr Psychiatry* 1994; **9**: 31–6.

65. Petrides G, Dhossche D, Fink M, Francis A. Continuation ECT: relapse prevention in affective disorders. *Convuls Ther* 1994; **10**: 189–94.

66. Kim E, Zisselman M, Pelchat R. Factors affecting compliance with maintenance electroconvulsive therapy: a preliminary study. *Int J Geriatr Psychiatry* 1996; **11**: 473–6.

67. Schwarz T, Loewenstein J, Isenberg K. Maintenance ECT: indications and outcome. *Convuls Ther* 1995; **11**: 14–23.

68. National Institute for Health and Clinical Excellence. Final Draft Depression Update: Final version (October 2009) Depression in Adults: the treatment and management of depression in adults. National Clinical Practice Guideline 90 National Collaborating Centre for Mental Health. At http://www.nice.org.uk/nicemedia/pdf/Depression_Update_FULL_GUIDELINE.pdf.

69. Squire L, Chace P. Memory functions six to nine months after electroconvulsive therapy. *Arch Gen Psychiatry* 1975; **32**: 1557–64.

70. Freeman C, Weeks D, Kendall R. ECT: II: Patients who complain. *Br J Psychiatry* 1980; **137**: 17–25.

71. Weiner R, Rogers H, Davidson J. Effects of stimulus parameters on cognitive side effects. *Ann NY Acad Sci* 1986; **462**: 315–25.

72. Abrams R, Taylor M. A prospective follow-up study of cognitive functions after ECT. *Convuls Ther* 1985; **1**: 4–9.

73. Summers W, Robins E, Reich T. The natural history of acute organic mental syndrome after bilateral electroconvulsive therapy. *Biol Psychiatry* 1979; **14**: 905–12.

74. Jha AK, Stein GS, Fenwick P. Negative interaction between lithium and electroconvulsive therapy – a case-control study. *Br J Psychiatry* 1996; **168**(2): 241–3.

75. Lam RW, Chan P, Wilkins-Ho M, Yatham LN. Repetitive transcranial magnetic stimulation for treatment-resistant depression: a systematic review and meta-analysis. *Can J Psychiatry* 2008; **53**(9): 621–31.

86

Pharmacological Treatment of Depression

Mohammed T. Abou-Saleh[1] and Cornelius Katona[2]

[1]*Division of Mental Health, St George's, University of London, London, UK*
[2]*Hon Professor, Dept Mental Health Sciences, University College London*

INTRODUCTION

Mood disorders are a major public health problem, with poor recognition, diagnosis and treatment despite the availability of reasonably safe, effective, economical treatments and the established effectiveness of continuing educational programmes for care providers[1]. The magnitude of the following problems is greater in the elderly with mood disorders for several reasons: poor recognition for most somatic and cognitive symptoms; increased physical morbidity and disability; and high mortality from suicide and other causes. This situation, however, is balanced by increased recognition that pharmacological treatments are effective and reasonably safe. There is, however, marked variation in rate, stability and direction of recovery with reliable pretreatment predictors of outcome[2]. The usefulness of pharmacological treatment for patients with subsyndromal depression, albeit to a lesser extent than major depressive disorders, has been also investigated[3].

PRETREATMENT CONSIDERATIONS

There are a number of issues to be considered before starting specific pharmacological treatment of mood disorders in the elderly[4]. With advancing age, there are important and clinically significant changes in distribution, metabolism and elimination of these drugs. The age-related increase in volume of distribution results in a longer half-life for all psychotropic drugs. Hepatic drug metabolism decreases with age, also resulting in a prolonged half-life, which may be two to three times longer than in younger patients, and the decrease in renal function with advancing age is particularly relevant with regard to lithium, which also results in two to three times higher plasma levels than those in younger patients on the same daily dose. A recent review[5] emphasized decreases in passive drug absorption, changes in the proportion of body fat (increased) and lean muscle mass (decreased) and the resultant increase in the elimination half-life of (fat-soluble) antidepressants. In addition, changes in binding proteins result in lower free levels of tricyclics but increased free levels of selective serotonin re-uptake inhibitors (SSRIs). Of particular importance, however, has been the study of the inhibitory effects of the SSRIs on the cytochrome p450 enzymes; these pharmacodynamic actions have pharmacokinetic consequences for co-administered drugs, such as tricyclic antidepressants (TCAs), which are dependent on these enzymes for biotransformation. Patients on anticoagulants in particular need close monitoring. The potential of the various SSRIs to cause significant interactions varies considerably; citalopram, escitalopram and sertraline may carry relatively low risk.

To determine the best pharmacological treatment options for individual patients requires careful consideration of a number of clinical factors, which include the following: type of mood disorder; degree of urgency for treatment; previous response to treatment; concurrent medical problems; concurrent drug therapy; risk of overdose; reasonable half-life; dosing flexibility; and affordability[6].

TREATMENT OF DEPRESSION

Older patients with depression can be successfully treated with conventional TCAs, monoamine oxidase inhibitors (MAOIs), SSRIs and atypical antidepressants. TCAs have the major limitations of anticholinergic effects, postural hypotension, excessive daytime sedation and cardiotoxicity in overdose. Their advantages, however, are their established efficacy and low cost. Among the TCAs, the secondary amines desipramine and nortriptyline have more favourable side-effect profiles, with desipramine having the fewest anticholinergic effects and nortriptyline causing the least postural hypotension[6]. The secondary amines also have the advantage of therapeutic drug monitoring, with an established therapeutic window for nortriptyline and a therapeutic plasma level of desipramine. Therapeutic drug monitoring enables the clinician to determine the minimal therapeutic dose and to monitor compliance. Nortriptyline has been well investigated for use in elderly patients, including patients older than 80 years[7] and patients who have had strokes[8].

Among the MAOIs, phenelzine has been shown to be effective in treating elderly patients with depression[9,10], particularly for patients who could not tolerate TCAs and those with resistant depression. Their main limitation is their interaction with tyramine-rich foods, causing hypertensive crisis. For this, they are superseded by moclobemide, a reversible and selective inhibitor of monoamine oxidase type A. Comparative trials in the elderly have established its efficacy compared with imipramine[11], nortriptyline[12] and placebo[13]. Moclobemide also showed benefits on cognitive function in patients who had dementia and co-morbid depressive symptoms[14].

The SSRIs, however, have provided the most important practical advance in the successful and safe management of depression in late life. This group of drugs includes fluoxetine, fluvoxamine, sertraline, paroxetine and citalopram. The SSRIs have replaced tricyclic

Principles and Practice of Geriatric Psychiatry, 3rd edn. Edited by Mohammed T. Abou-Saleh, Cornelius Katona and Anand Kumar

antidepressants as first-line antidepressants for older people as well as for younger adults. More recently, several other antidepressants have become available including bupropion, mirtazapine, another SSRI (escitalopram), and the serotonin and noradrenaline re-uptake inhibitors (SNRIs) venlafaxine and duloxetine[14]. The advantages of SSRIs over TCAs are the absence of anticholinergic effects, orthostatic hypotension and arrhythmia in the side-effect profiles, and their safety in overdose[7]. Comparison of fluoxetine with nortriptyline in in-patients with severe depression and heart disease showed that nortriptyline may be more effective in this population[15]. A meta-analysis of the comparative efficacy and safety of SSRIs and TCAs in elderly patients[16] showed no differences in safety and dropout rates.

A recent meta-analysis[17] of the efficacy of second-generation antidepressants (SSRIs, SNRIs bupropion and mirtazapine) showed response rates of 44% for active drug and 35% for placebo, suggesting only modest efficacy (number needed to treat = 11). A similarly small difference in favour of active drug was found for remission rates (33% vs. 26%). There authors reported marked heterogeneity between studies, with superiority over placebo found for fluoxetine in one of three studies, for paroxetine in two studies, for sertraline and for duloxetine but not for escitalopram or venlafaxine. Results for bupropion showed borderline superiority over placebo in terms of response rate but not in terms of remission. Studies lasting 10 weeks or more were associated with greater superiority for active drug over placebo than studies lasting 6–8 weeks, supporting the traditional view that antidepressant response may take longer to emerge in older people[14].

A similar review of single versus dual action antidepressants in older people included head-to-head comparator trials as well as those with a placebo arm, and continuation as well as acute trials[18]. They concluded that overall, dual action agents 'do not appear to confer any additional benefits in efficacy over single action agents (SSRIs)'. Unlike the meta-analysis reviewed above[17], the primary analysis in this study was by class and they did not examine whether there was heterogeneity between individual studies.

One striking feature of these trials is the relatively low overall response and remission rate for active antidepressant medication. Sneed et al.[19] have carried out a systematic review comparing reported response rates in placebo-controlled and comparator trials of antidepressants in older people. They identified nine comparator trials and seven placebo-controlled trials published since 1985 that met their entry criteria. Response rates were considerably higher (60%) than in the placebo-controlled trials (46%); the odds of being a responder were 1.82 times higher in the comparator trials. Type of trial (placebo-controlled vs. comparator) accounted for 27% of the variation in responder rate. The authors conclude that expectation is an important contributor to outcome in such trials and that concern about possibly being on placebo may lead to a suppression of the antidepressant response[14].

The side-effects profile of SSRIs includes nausea, diarrhoea, insomnia, headaches, agitation, anxiety and sexual dysfunction. The SSRIs also seem to worsen Parkinsonism. As with other antidepressants[20], there have been case reports of hyponatraemia, hypomania and seizures[7]. An important aspect of their use is their drug–drug interactions, and their inhibitory effects on hepatic cytochrome p450 isoenzymes, the route through which many drugs commonly prescribed for elderly people are metabolized[21]. Paroxetine, norfluoxetine and sertraline have clinically important inhibitory effects (in vivo) on cytochrome P2D6, resulting in increased plasma concentrations of co-administered TCAs, such as desipramine, and antipsychotics, such as haloperidol[22]. Sertraline,

however, had a modest effect on plasma nortriptyline levels in depressed elderly patients[23]. Fluoxetine increases plasma levels of co-administered carbamazepine; alprazolam and fluvoxamine increase plasma concentration of co-administered TCAs and antipsychotics by inhibiting cytochrome P1A29. An extensive list of drugs metabolized by various p450 isoenzyme types is provided in the reviews by Catterson et al.[4] and by Rivard[6].

Despite these potential problems, two recent reviews of (SSRIs) in older people[24,25] have found that they are generally well tolerated but that gastrointestinal (GI) problems including nausea are relatively common. Increased risk of GI bleeding is potentially important because older people are in any case at greater risk of such bleeding. SSRI-induced restlessness, sedation and extra-pyramidal movement disorders may also be particularly disabling in older people. SSRI-induced hyponatraemia is increasingly recognized to be common in older people. Older age, female gender, low body weight and co-administration of diuretics are indicators of increased risk. Inappropriate secretion of antidiuretic hormone (mediated by activation of 5HT2 and 5HT1C serotonergic receptors) is a likely mechanism. Serum sodium should be checked frequently in older patients on SSRIs, particularly in the first few months of treatment. Drug interactions involving the cytochrome P450 enzyme system may be clinically relevant in older people. Patients on anticoagulants in particular need close monitoring. The potential of the various SSRIs to cause significant interactions varies considerably; citalopram, escitalopram and sertraline may carry relatively low risk.

In the light of this it is perhaps surprising that a recent Australian study[26] found that although antidepressant use had increased in all age groups and most markedly in the 65+ age group, older people remained the highest users of tricyclic antidepressants whose side effects are well documented as being particularly hazardous in older people. This may, however, reflect the tendency to reuse a previously effective antidepressant for a recurrent episode of depression, and the still frequent use of tricyclics in low dose as hypnotics and analgesics in an older population.

CONTINUATION AND PROPHYLACTIC TREATMENT

Early studies indicated a poor outcome of late-life depression[27], with high relapse, recurrence and chronicity. This view was based on naturalistic observation without monitoring of compliance, adequate dosage and duration of treatment, including prophylactic treatment, and was therefore challenged[28]. Controlled studies of maintenance antidepressant medication, however, showed a relatively good outcome for late-life depression[29]. The Pittsburgh group[30] reported a three-year follow-up study of maintenance treatment with nortriptyline or placebo with or without interpersonal psychotherapy (IPT) and showed that 80% of patients assigned to nortriptyline, with or without IPT, remained in remission. The Pittsburgh group also identified the elderly patients who remained well after placebo-controlled discontinuation of antidepressant medication for a period of one year. Recovery of good subjective sleep quality by early continuation treatment was useful in identifying which remitted elderly depressed patients remained well with monthly IPT after discontinuation of antidepressant medication[31]. A study of the effect of treatment on the two-year course of late-life depression[32] showed a 74% survival rate without relapse. This good outcome was obtained by the use of full-dose antidepressant medication, frequent follow-up and rigorous treatment of relapse.

The US National Institute of Mental Health consensus statement update[33] concluded that the overall evidence supports the recommendation for at least six months of treatment beyond recovery for those with first onset in late life, and for at least 12 months for those with a recurrent illness[34]. Moreover, prophylactic treatment should be of the same type and dosage as that which was successful in the initial acute phase. The consensus statement also concluded that treatment response and long-term outcome for all the patients is generally similar to that observed in younger adults, but the temporal course may be somewhat slower in the elderly and risk of relapse somewhat greater[33].

The effectiveness of the tricyclic antidepressant nortriptyline in reducing relapse and recurrence in older depressed patients at high risk is well established[35]. This study also indicated that interpersonal psychotherapy had an additional preventative effect. More recently Reynolds et al.[36] replicated their findings using the SSRI paroxetine. In this study they did not focus specifically on patients at high risk. They failed to identify any additional benefit from interpersonal psychotherapy. Klysner et al.[37] have shown that continued treatment with citalopram is associated with much lower relapse and recurrence than placebo in patients who remitted on citalopram and were then randomized to citalopram or placebo for the next two years. A similar study by Wilson et al.[38] failed to show superiority for the SSRI sertraline over placebo over two years, but the dropout rate in their study was extremely high. Gorwood et al.[39] examined relapse rates over 24 weeks in older depressed patients who remitted on open-label escitalopram and were then randomized either to continue with escitalopram or to be switched to placebo. Risk of relapse was 4.4 times higher on placebo.

Though co-morbid anxiety does not appear to affect acute response to antidepressants, the secondary analysis of data from a controlled study of paroxetine and interpersonal psychotherapy by Andreescu et al.[40] found that co-morbid anxiety was associated with a slower response and a higher recurrence rate.

Overall the results summarized above provide strong evidence that older people who respond to antidepressants are substantially less likely to experience relapse or recurrence if their antidepressant treatment is continued for up to two years.

The use of lithium in continuation and prophylactic treatment of depression in the elderly has also been recommended[29,41,42], with the use of lower doses/plasma levels[34]. Lithium may be a more favourable prophylactic treatment than antidepressants in recurrent depression with melancholia and in depression with psychotic features (delusional depression), which are particularly common among the elderly, with a tendency to respond less well to antidepressants[28,42]. The other advantage of lithium therapy is the evident decreased mortality, whether from suicide or other causes[43]. A one-year prospective, placebo-controlled study of maintenance lithium in conjunction with cognitive behavioural psychotherapy in elderly depressed patients[44] showed that, although cognitive behavioural psychotherapy reduced depression severity during follow-up, lithium therapy was no better than placebo. This appears to be related to poor compliance, a finding that highlights the serious difficulties in undertaking prophylactic studies in elderly depressed patients.

TREATMENT OF BIPOLAR DISORDER

Elderly patients with late presentation or late-onset mania respond well to standard antimanic treatment with neuroleptics, lithium and anticonvulsants[45]. Neuroleptic treatment is best avoided in the elderly because of its known extrapyramidal side effects, except for floridly psychotic, agitated and behaviourally disturbed patients who need rapid control of symptoms. Lithium remains the treatment of choice, followed by valproic acid[45]. The evidence for the efficacy of lithium in late-life mania is based on retrospective and uncontrolled studies; there have been no controlled studies, and there have been no controlled studies of the efficacy of anticonvulsants in late-life mania. It has been suggested that valproate is a safer alternative treatment to lithium than carbamazepine, whether used as single or adjunct treatment, in elderly manic patients[45]. There are no guidelines regarding the optimal plasma concentration of valproate in relation to efficacy[45].

An evidence-based review of the treatment of mania, mixed state and rapid cycling in younger populations[46] concluded that lithium and divalproex sodium are effective in mania, whereas divalproex sodium and carbamazepine are more effective in mixed states. Divalproex sodium is the drug of choice for rapid cycling disorder. With bipolar depression, lithium is recommended as a first-line treatment and the addition of a second mood stabilizer or a TCA would be an appropriate next step[47].

The guidelines for the continuation and prophylactic treatment of bipolar illness in late life are similar to those advocated for younger patients, except for the notion of high recurrence rates necessitating prophylactic treatment, even after a first-onset manic episode. Lithium remains the medication of choice for prophylaxis[42]. An open naturalistic study of lower doses/plasma–lithium levels[42] showed efficacy in the elderly comparable to that in younger patients at plasma–lithium levels as low as 0.4 mmol/l, with fewer side effects and renal and thyroid adverse effects.

TREATMENT-RESISTANT DEPRESSION

Treatment-resistant depression occurs in one-third of elderly depressed patients[48] and can only be ascertained after adequate recognition, compliance with treatment and effective treatment[49]. It has also been related to cognitive impairment, physical and psychiatric co-morbidity, late onset and presence of melancholic and psychotic features[41]. Moreover, elderly patients with anxious depression are less responsive to nortriptyline than are those without significant anxiety symptoms[50].

Although TCAs[15] and MAOIs[51] have shown efficacy, the SSRIs are specifically advocated[41]. Fluvoxamine has shown efficacy (70% good response) in desipramine non-responders[52,53], and patients who were intolerant of fluoxetine completed a trial of sertraline with a response rate of 76%[54]. Venlafaxine also has long-established efficacy in older people with refractory depression[55].

Combination and augmentation strategies have been advocated[49]. Lithium augmentation in TCA non-responders is effective in 20–65% of cases[56–58]. It is, however, associated with cognitive and/or neurological side effects in 50% of patients[56,57,59,60]. Lithium has been successfully added to SSRIs, notwithstanding the risk of neurotoxicity with an SSRI–lithium combination[49]. Advocated augmentation/combination strategies include TCA/tri-iodo-thyronine, SSRI/TCA, SSRI/anticonvulsants and SSRI/oestrogen (ibid.). Elderly patients requiring adjunctive medication to achieve remission may need continuation of adjunctive medication to remain well and to avoid early relapse[61].

Rajji et al.[5] emphasize the limited evidence base from controlled-clinical trials on optimal strategies where initial antidepressant treatment has failed. They note, however, that remission rates of up to 50% have been reported with a 'switch' to the MAOIs phenelzine[62] or selegiline[63], as well as with sequential augmentation strategies. Augmentation with lithium[64] and with the atypical antipsychotic aripiprazole[65] have also recently been reported to result in useful remission rates in treatment-resistant older people. Most of the studies to date have been small and few are placebo controlled. This is clearly an area where more research is needed.

For refractory bipolar disorders, a review[66] concluded that the safest combination of mood stabilizers is valproate plus lithium. This was also shown in a series of elderly patients with lithium-resistant rapid cycling mania[67].

CONCLUSION

Although there have been impressive advances in the pharmacological treatment of mood disorders in general, there has been a relative paucity of controlled studies in the elderly, particularly in maintenance and prophylaxis. Generalization from the results of studies of younger patients may be inappropriate in view of the significant changes associated with normal ageing and concomitant medical illness, which affect the pharmacokinetics and pharmacodynamics of psychotropic drugs.

Nevertheless, there has been a change of culture. The nihilism that had prevailed in the treatment of mood disorders in late life has been replaced by cautious optimism with regard to the results of controlled trials in naturalistic settings, as well as studies in high-risk groups, including patients with multiple medical conditions and subsyndromal states.

A large majority of elderly patients with depression could be treated successfully with antidepressants, particularly the SSRIs, because of their favourable side-effect profiles and their low toxicity in overdose. The SSRIs, however, challenge the clinician with their clinically significant drug–drug interactions. Patients who improve should receive continuation of prophylactic treatment with the same dose. For mania, lithium remains the optimal treatment, with anticonvulsants, particularly divaloproex, providing a second-line treatment. The efficacy and safety of atypical neuroleptics remain to be evaluated in both acute and long-term management of bipolar illness. There is also hope for those with resistant-mood disorders with the design of augmentation/combination strategies, which require further evaluation.

REFERENCES

1. Patel V, Araya R, Chaterjee S et al. Treatment and prevention of mental disorders in low-income and middle-income countries. *Lancet* 2007; **370**: 991–1005.
2. Dew MA, Reynolds CF III, Houck PR et al. Temporal profiles of the course of depression during treatment. *Arch Gen Psychiatry* 1997; **54**: 1016–24.
3. Tadic A, Helmreich I Mergl R et al. Early improvement is a predictor of treatment outcome in patients with mild major, minor or subsyndromal depression *J Affect Disord* 2010; **120**: 86–93.
4. Catterson ML, Preskorn SH, Martin RM. Pharmacodynamic and pharmacokinetic considerations in geriatric psychopharmacology. *Geriatr Psychiatry* 1997; **20**: 205–19.
5. Rajji TK, Mulsant BH, Lotrich FE, Lokker C and Reynolds CF Use of antidepressants in late-life depression. *Drugs Aging* 2008; **25**(10): 841–53.
6. Rivard MFT. Pharmacotherapy of affective disorders in old age. *Can J Psychiatry* 1997; **42**(suppl 1): 10–18S.
7. Salzman C, Schneider L, Alexopoulos G. Pharmacological treatment of depression in late life. In Bloom F, Kupfer D (eds), *Psychopharmacology: The Fourth General of Progress*. New York: Raven, 1995, 1771–7.
8. Robinson RG, Morris PH, Fedoroff JP. Depression and cerebrovascular disease. *J Clin Psychiatry* 1990; **51**: 26–33.
9. Georgotas A, McCue RE, Hapworth W et al. Comparative efficacy and safety of MAOI vs. TCAs in treating depression in the elderly. *Biol Psychiatry* 1986; **21**: 1155–66.
10. Lazarus LW, Groves L, Gierl B et al. Efficacy of phenelzine in geriatric depression. *Biol Psychiatry* 1986; **21**: 699–701.
11. Pancheri P, Delle CR, Donnini M et al. Effects of moclobemide on depressive symptoms and cognitive performance in a geriatric population: a controlled comparative study vs. imipramine. *Clin Neuropharmacol* 1994; **17**(suppl 1): 58–73S.
12. Nair NP, Amin M, Holm P et al. Moclobemide and nortriptyline in elderly depressed patients: a randomised multicentre trial against placebo. *J Affect Disord* 1995; **33**: 1–9.
13. Roth M, Mountjoy CQ, Amrein R. The International Collaborative Study Group. Moclobemide placebo-controlled trial. *Br J Psychiatry* 1996; **16**: 149–57.
14. Katona C. Current challenges faced by clinicians in managing late-life depression: what can be learnt from the recent evidence base? *Mind Brain*, in press.
15. Roose SP, Glassman AH, Attia E, Woodring S. Comparative efficacy of selective serotonin reuptake inhibitors and tricyclics in the treatment of melancholia. *Am J Psychiatry* 1994; **151**: 1735–9.
16. Mittmann N, Shear NH, Busto VE et al. Comparative evaluation of the efficacy and safety of tricyclic antidepressants and serotonin reuptake inhibitors in the elderly: a meta-analysis. *Clin Invest Med* 1994; **18**: B53.
17. Nelson JC, Delucchi K, Schneider LS. Efficacy of second-generation antidepressants in late-life depression: a meta-analysis of the evidence. *Am J Geriatr Psychiatry* 2008; **16**: 558–67.
18. Mukai Y, Tampi RR. Treatment of depression in the elderly: a review of the recent literature on the efficacy of single- versus dual-action antidepressants. *Clin Ther* 2009; **31**: 945–61.
19. Sneed JR, Rutherford BR, Rindskopf D, Lane DT, Sackeim HA, Roose SP. Design makes a difference: a meta-analysis of antidepressant response rates in placebo-controlled versus comparator trials in late-life depression. *Am J Geriatr Psychiatry* 2008; **16**: 65–73.
20. Spigset O, Hedenmalm K. Hyponatremia in relation to treatment with antidepressants: a survey of reports in the World Health Organization database for spontaneous reporting of adverse drug reactions. *Pharmacotherapy* 1997; **17**: 348–52.
21. Nemeroff CB, DeVane CL, Pollock BG. Newer antidepressants and the cytochrome P450 system. *Am J Psychiatry* 1996; **153**: 311–20.
22. Preskorn SH. Reducing the risk of drug–drug interactions: a goal of rational drug development. *J Clin Psychiatry* 1996; **57**(suppl 1): 3–6S.
23. Solai LK, Mulsant BH, Pollock BG et al. Effect of sertraline on plasma nortriptyline levels in depressed elderly. *J Clin Psychiatry* 1997; **58**: 440–3.
24. Anon. Although adverse effects may occur, selective serotonin reuptake inhibitors are generally well tolerated in the elderly. *Drugs Ther Perspect* 2009; **25**(5): 20–3.

25. Chemali Z, Chahine LM, Fricchione G. The use of selective serotonin reuptake inhibitors in elderly patients. *Harv Rev Psychiatry* 2009; **17**(4): 242–53.

26. Smith AJ, Tett SE. How do different age groups use benzodiazepines and antidepressants: analysis of an Australian database 2003–6. *Drugs Aging* 2009; **26**(2): 113–22.

27. Murphy E. The prognosis of depression and response to antidepressive therapies. *Br J Psychiatry* 1983; **142**: 111–19.

28. Abou–Saleh MT, Coppen A. Classification of depression and response to anti-depressive therapies. *Br J Psychiatry* 1983; **143**: 601–3.

29. Stoudemire A. Recurrence and relapse in geriatric depression: a review of risk factors and prophylactic treatment strategies. *J Neuropsychiat* 1997; **9**: 209–21.

30. Reynolds CF. Treatment of depression in late life. *Am J Med* 1994; **97**(suppl 6A): 39–46S.

31. Reynolds CF III, Frank E, Houck PR *et al*. Which elderly patients with remitted depression remain well with continued interpersonal psychotherapy after discontinuation of antidepressant medication? *Am J Psychiatry* 1997; **154**: 958–62.

32. Flint AJ, Rifat SL. The effect of treatment on the two-year course of late-life depression. *Br J Psychiatry* 1997; **170**: 268–72.

33. Lebowitz BD, Pearson JL, Schneider LS *et al*. Diagnosis and treatment of depression in late life: consensus statement update. *J Am Med Assoc* 1997; **278**: 1186–90.

34. Reynolds CF, Frank E, Perel J *et al*. Maintenance therapies for late life recurrent major depression: research and review circa 1995. *Int Psychogeriat* 1995; **7**(suppl): 27–40.

35. Reynolds CF III, Frank E *et al*. Nortriptyline and interpersonal psychotherapy as maintenance therapies for recurrent major depression: a randomized controlled trial in patients older than 59 years. *JAMA* 1999; **281**(1): 39–45.

36. Reynolds CF III, Dew MA *et al*. Maintenance treatment of major depression in old age. *N Engl J Med* 2006; **354**: 1130–8.

37. Klysner R, Bent-Hansen J, Hansen HL, *et al*. Efficacy of citalopram in the prevention of recurrent depression in elderly patients: placebo-controlled study of maintenance therapy. *Br J Psychiatry* 2002; **181**: 29–35.

38. Wilson KC, Mottram PG, Ashworth L, Abou-Saleh MT. Older community residents with depression: long-term treatment with sertraline. Randomised, double-blind, placebo-controlled study. *Br J Psychiatry* 2003; **182**: 492–7.

39. Gorwood P, Weiller E, Lemming O, Katona C. Escitalopram prevents relapse in older patients with major depressive disorder. *Am J Geriatr Psychiatry* 2007; **15**(7): 581–93.

40. Andreescu C, Lenze EJ, Dew EM, Begley AE. Effect of co-morbid anxiety on treatment response and relapse risk in late–life depression: controlled study. *Br J Psychiatry* 2007; **190**: 344–9.

41. Coppen A, Abou-Saleh MT. Lithium therapy: from clinical trials to practical management. *Acta Psychiatr Scand* 1988; **78**: 759–62.

42. Abou-Saleh MT. Long–term management of affective disorder. In Copeland JRM, Abou-Saleh MT, Blazer DG (eds), *Principles and Practice of Geriatric Psychiatry*, 1st edn. Chichester: Wiley, 1994, 587–96.

43. Coppen A. Depression as a lethal disease: prevention strategies. *J Clin Psychiatry* 1994; **55**(suppl): 37–45.

44. Wilson KCM, Scott M, Abou-Saleh MT *et al*. Long–term effects of cognitive behavioural therapy and lithium therapy on depression in the elderly. *Br J Psychiatry* 1995; **167**: 653–8.

45. Young RC. Bipolar mood disorders in the elderly. *Geriat Psychiatry* 1997; **20**: 121–36.

46. Kusumakar V, Yatham LN, Haslam DRS *et al*. Treatment of mania, mixed state, and rapid cycling. *Can J Psychiatry* 1997; **42**(suppl 2): 79–86S.

47. Yatham LN, Kusumakar V, Parikh SV *et al*. Bipolar depression: treatment options. *Can J Psychiatry* 1997; **42**(suppl 2): 87–91S.

48. Goff DC, Jenike MA. Treatment-resistant depression in the elderly. *J Am Geriat Soc* 1986; **34**: 63–70.

49. Kamholz BA, Mellow AM. Management of treatment resistance in the depressed geriatric patient. *Psychiatry Clin North Am* 1997; **19**: 269–87.

50. Flint AJ, Rifat SL. Anxious depression in elderly patients. Response to antidepressant treatment. *Am J Geriat Psychiatry* 1997; **5**: 107–15.

51. Georgotas A, Friedman E, McCarthy M *et al*. Resistant geriatric depressions and therapeutic response to monoamine oxidase inhibitors. *Biol Psychiatry* 1983; **18**: 195–205.

52. Delgado PL, Price LH, Charney DS, Heninger GR. Efficacy of fluvoxamine in treatment-refractory depression. *J Affect Disord* 1988; **15**: 55–60.

53. White K, Wykoff W, Tynes LL *et al*. Fluvoxamine in the treatment of tricyclic resistant depression. *Psychiatry J Univ Ottawa* 1990; **15**: 156–8.

54. Brown WA, Harrison W. Are patients who are intolerant to one SSRI intolerant to another? *Psychopharmacol Bull* 1992; **28**: 253–6.

55. Nierenberg AA, Feighner JP, Rudolph R *et al*. Venlafaxine for treatment-resistant unipolar depression. *J Clin Psychopharmacol* 1994; **14**: 419–23.

56. Finch EJL, Katona CIE. Lithium augmentation in the treatment of refractory depression in old age. *Int J Geriat Psychiatry* 1989; **4**: 41–6.

57. Flint AJ. Recent developments in geriatric psychopharmacotherapy. *Can J Psychiatry* 1994; **39**(suppl 1): S9–18.

58. Zimmer B, Rosen J, Thornton JE *et al*. Adjunctive lithium carbonate in nortriptyline-resistant elderly depressed patients. *J Clin Psychopharmacol* 1991; **11**: 254–6.

59. Flint AJ, Rifat SL. A prospective study of lithium augmentation in antidepressant-resistant geriatric depression. *J Clin Psychopharmacol* 1994; **14**: 353–6.

60. Lafferman J, Solomon K, Ruskin P. Lithium augmentation for treatment-resistant depression in the elderly. *J Geriat Psychiat Neurol* 1998; **1**: 49–52.

61. Reynolds CF III, Frank E, Perel JM *et al*. High relapse rate after discontinuation of adjunctive medication for elderly patients with recurrent major depression. *Am J Psychiatry* 1996; **153**: 1418–22.

62. Flint AJ, Rifat SL The effect of sequential antidepressant treatment on geriatric depression. *J Affect Disord* 1996; **36**(3–4): 95–105.

63. Sunderland T, Cohen RM, Molchan S *et al*. High-dose selegiline in treatment-resistant older depressive patients *Arch Gen Psychiatry* 1994; **51**(8): 607–15.

64. Kok RM, Vink D, Heeren TJ *et al*. Lithium augmentation compared with phenelzine in treatment-resistant depression in the elderly: an open, randomized, controlled trial. *J Clin Psychiatry* 2007; **68**(8): 1177–85.

65. Freeman MP, Stott AL. Mood stabiliser combinations: a review of safety and efficacy. *Am J Psychiatry* 1998; **155**: 12–21.

66. Rutherford B, Sneed J, Miyazaki M *et al*. An open trial of aripiprazole augmentation for SSRI non-remitters with late life depression. *Int J Geriatr Psychiatry* 2007; **22**(10): 986–91.

67. Schneider AL, Wilcox CS. Divalproate augmentation in lithium resistant rapid cycling mania in four geriatric patients. *J Affect Disord* 1998; **47**: 201–5.

87

Psychotherapy of Depression and Dysthymia

Philip Wilkinson

Department of Psychiatry, University of Oxford, UK

Recent years have seen a steady but slow increase in the application of psychological treatments to manage depression in late life, both as stand-alone treatments and in combination with pharmacotherapy. This stems in part from the large body of evidence supporting the benefits of certain psychological treatments in the management of depressive illness in younger adults[1] and the need to test the benefits with older patients.

There are a number of reasons why psychological treatments warrant investigation in the older population. First, they may help to address the types of psychosocial difficulties often associated with late-life depression such as bereavement, adjustment to chronic disease and loss of autonomy. Second, they may confer benefits in reducing the recurrence of depression, which is a significant problem in older patients. Third, older patients may express a preference for psychological treatment over pharmacological treatment (although this does not necessarily predict their effectiveness)[2]. Finally, neuroimaging data indicate that psychotherapy and pharmacotherapy may target different primary sites of the corticolimbic pathway and may therefore have synergistic effects in the treatment of depression[3].

It cannot be assumed that psychological treatments for depression are as effective in older people as in younger adults. Older people are more likely to have cerebrovascular lesions which are known to be associated with poorer response to physical treatments[4]. Depression beginning in later life is also associated with greater reductions in processing speed and executive dysfunction[5] which could impede response to psychological treatment. Symptom profiles in depressed older people, and therefore the target symptoms of psychotherapy, also differ from those in younger people, with greater motivational deficit and less affective change[6].

This chapter reviews the different psychological therapies that have been developed, and to some extent evaluated, for use with depressed older people. It summarizes the indications and evidence for therapies and ends with a brief discussion of access to therapies and research priorities.

BEHAVIOUR THERAPY AND COGNITIVE BEHAVIOURAL THERAPIES

Behaviour therapy and its related treatments form the largest group of therapies employed in the management of depression. Although their evaluation in older adults is patchy, they offer a number of approaches to helping the depressed older person.

Behaviour Therapy

According to learning theory, depression results from reduced engagement in positively reinforcing behaviours (pleasurable events) and excessive exposure to negative reinforcement (avoidance and negative events)[7]. Behaviour therapy uses an operant conditioning model to reintroduce positive reinforcement, to reduce the time spent on negative events and to overcome avoidance. This model is presented to the patient as a vicious circle that needs breaking, based on diaries of the patient's activity and negative mood. This is then followed by scheduling of positively reinforcing behaviours and monitoring of the effect on mood. It may often be possible for patients to resume their previous activities. However, older people experiencing physical illness and disability may be unable to resume all of their previous activities and may need help in identifying alternatives.

Behavioural approaches to depression were later elaborated by incorporating the patterns of negative thinking that occur in depression, giving rise to cognitive behaviour therapy.

Cognitive Behaviour Therapy (CBT)

According to the cognitive model of depression[8] an individual's underlying beliefs about him- or herself and the world may confer a vulnerability to depression that is then triggered in the face of specific types of event. Faulty information processing in the form of over-generalized negative thoughts shapes behaviour and maintains depressed mood.

The validity of the cognitive model as an explanation for cases of depression arising in late life has been questioned given the evidence for structural causes such as cerebrovascular disease. Another limitation of a vulnerability–diathesis model is that an older person may appear to have held the same beliefs for decades and endured previous negative events without developing depression. However, it has been observed in older patients that certain personal beliefs can be adaptive and functional throughout earlier life but can predispose to depression in response to specific age-related events, such as retirement[9].

Cognitive behaviour therapy for depression begins with behavioural activation but in contrast with behaviour therapy it includes analysis of the thoughts that underlie inactivity. As the following case example illustrates, negative thoughts are then

Principles and Practice of Geriatric Psychiatry, 3rd edn. Edited by Mohammed T. Abou-Saleh, Cornelius Katona and Anand Kumar

addressed through direct verbal challenging and testing them out in specific situations (behavioural experiments), supported by written thought diaries.

CBT Case Example: Mrs Jacobs – a woman with physical problems and depressive illness

Mrs Jacobs was a 78-year-old woman referred for therapy by her general practitioner having developed a depressive illness following a stroke. She had been treated with a course of antidepressants, which had brought about a small improvement although she remained significantly depressed with a 'dread of the future'. She described a loss of confidence and poor concentration and had withdrawn from a number of social activities. She had also noticed a deterioration in her memory, finding it difficult to retain and use new information although this did improve at times when her mood picked up. She had three grown-up children who did not live locally.

Mrs Jacobs had enjoyed a career as a teacher until retiring at the age of 63 years. She had coped with a number of stressful events in her past, such as the loss of her husband, without becoming depressed. Her medical history included hypertension, heart disease and arthritis. Her stroke had occurred after her return from holiday, giving rise to permanent weakness of her right leg. Evaluation by a neurologist, including magnetic resonance imaging, had confirmed the presence of cerebrovascular disease. Fearing further strokes, she became anxious that she would not be able to carry on with her interests which included committee work and trips to the theatre. She feared she would be unable to continue living independently and would have to move to a nursing home. Her therapy goals included being able to manage social events and being able to plan realistically for her future.

In session 1 Mrs Jacobs began to recognize the patterns of thoughts and behaviours which were taking place in her depression. She realized that she had become very conscious of the change in her walking which resulted from her weak leg, thinking that other people were noticing it and commenting on it. This added to her anxiety and caused her to avoid social situations or to go to lengths to check that people were not likely to reject her because of it. These observations were included in a simple formulation and this set the scene for a simple diary of these thoughts and behaviours as they occurred at a committee meeting before session 2. She immediately recognized the biased nature of these thoughts, which brought about some improvement in her mood.

In session 2 Mrs Jacobs was helped to notice the link between her mood, energy and activity. At times she was quite tired with her mind 'in a fog' which caused difficulty organizing activities such as catching up on tasks at home. This led to self-critical thoughts. She expected herself to function as she had before her stroke, discounting any achievements she was now able to make. She was also disappointed by the day-to-day fluctuations in her energy. To illustrate this process she kept a diary between sessions. She was given written information about the link between activity and depression and was asked to begin activity scheduling. This caused her some difficulty as she aimed to complete the activity schedule perfectly, bringing

to attention the high standards she had always set for herself. The exercise also brought to the therapist's attention the extent to which Mrs Jacobs was struggling with mental tasks because of her cognitive slowing. Mrs Jacobs was encouraged to plan things in advance but to allow some flexibility depending on her physical state and external events. She approached larger commitments by breaking them into smaller stages and using more written records. To support these changes she successfully challenged her self-critical thoughts with responses such as 'the list of jobs will never finish, so why blame myself?', 'is it really important to do it now?'. The beliefs underlying Mrs Jacobs's high standards were examined – for example, the belief that 'I must always do everything to the best of my ability' – and she began to accept that getting older allowed her the opportunity to relax her standards and take some rest.

In session 6, Mrs Jacobs was helped to use thought challenging to deal with her fear of rejection by friends. She found questions such as 'What am I afraid might happen?' and 'Am I exaggerating the importance of events?' particularly useful. She recognized a tendency to predict that people would not want her. If others were ambiguous in their behaviour (such as not initiating conversation) it was taken as evidence that they did not want her around. She tested out her thoughts using simple behavioural experiments such as initiating conversation with people and being ready to challenge unhelpful thoughts as they arose. She found that actually putting this into practice was not always easy so she needed to plan the stages in some detail beforehand then complete her thought records and observations soon afterwards. She was successful in reducing the intensity of her thought that she was being rejected from 80% to 5%.

By session 9, Mrs Jacobs was becoming more flexible in her activities and coping better with personal relationships. She was still feeling anxious and low in the mornings. She had hopeless thoughts and although she could challenge these successfully later in the morning, she had difficulty doing this at the time. She therefore developed a list of strategies to cope with depression in the morning such as keeping a reminder by her bed of the challenges to unhelpful thoughts and activities she could engage in rather lying in bed ruminating.

By session 10 Mrs Jacobs's mood was significantly improved. She still reported mild cognitive deficits such as difficulty naming and slower thinking, related to her cerebrovascular disease. She identified unhelpful thoughts about developing Alzheimer's disease or losing control of her life. With the therapist she also identified a distortion in her thinking that having irreversible problems (such as her cerebrovascular disease) meant she had an unmanageable problem. Understanding the physical basis to some of her problems also helped her to challenge her self-critical thoughts. At times of additional stress, such as admission to hospital, she would become anxious and depressed and her fears for the future would recur, but she managed to use thought challenging to handle this (Table 87.1). This also helped her to review the plans she had made in case of further disability in the future, such as financial planning and adding her name to the list for her preferred nursing home. At the end of treatment, Mrs Jacobs made a therapy

'blueprint' which included a summary of what she had done to achieve her improvement and what she would need to do if her problems recurred (Figure 87.1).
Abridged and reproduced with permission from Wilkinson[10], pp. 67–71.

For a detailed description of CBT with older adults, see Laidlaw et al.[11]

Problem-solving Therapy (PST)

Problem-solving therapy is a brief intervention of six to eight sessions that is usually delivered in primary care; it is designed to help depressed patients to take an active approach to tackling their psychosocial problems. PST can be considered a behavioural intervention in that it tackles the avoidance and reduction in pleasurable activities that occur in depression, and as a cognitive intervention in so far as it addresses the negative perceptions that may interfere with finding practical solutions to problems.

Problem-solving therapy involves the following stages: definition of problems; establishing realistic goals; generating, choosing and implementing solutions; and evaluating outcomes. Use of a therapy manual helps patients to practise these skills and to continue their use after therapy has ended. Clearly, older people often face irreversible obstacles such as bereavement or disability, in which case goal setting is an opportunity to regain some sense of control through tackling the consequences and effects of these problems. For instance, a depressed patient unable to drive after a stroke may identify new ways to travel.

Table 87.1 Mrs Jacobs's thought diary

Situation	Emotions	Unhelpful thoughts	Evidence that it's true	Evidence that it's not 100% true	More balanced thought	Feeling now
Planning admission to hospital	Anxiety 60%	'I chan't be able to manage'	My children are too busy to help	If they're busy, they still haven't forgotten me	'It's OK to seek out help'	Anxiety 5%
	Depressed 80%	'I might have to ask for help'	I'm having to make all the arrangements	My neighbour did offer to help	'This is how I feel when I'm under pressure'	Depressed 10%
		'I'm all alone'	People won't ask how I'm getting on	If they don't ask, it doesn't mean they don't care	'Yes, I'm in charge of my life. It's hard work, but it doesn't mean I'm alone in the world'	

Source: Abridged and reproduced with permission from [10], Wilkinson P. (2001) Cognitive behaviour therapy. In: J Hepple, J Pearce & P Wilkinson (Eds), *Psychological Therapies with Older People* (pp. 61–73). Hove: Bruner-Routledge

1. Prioritise my time and don't be too hard on myself if I don't get things done.

2. Watch out for times when I predict the future. Just try to take things as they come.

3. Remember that having to sort things out for myself doesn't mean I am alone in the world.

4. Be aware of future setbacks, e.g. illness, practical problems.

5. If the problems recur do the following:

   - refer to therapy notebook

   - re-read my information on strokes and vascular disease

   - keep thought records

   - if necessary, seek refresher session with therapist

Figure 87.1 Extract from Mrs Jacobs's therapy blueprint
Source: Abridged and reproduced with permission from [10], Wilkinson P. (2001) Cognitive behaviour therapy. In: J Hepple, J Pearce & P Wilkinson (Eds), *Psychological Therapies with Older People* (pp. 61–73). Hove: Bruner-Routledge

Dialectical Behaviour Therapy (DBT)

Dialectical behaviour therapy has been developed to treat younger adults with personality disorder, particularly borderline disorder[12]. Its underlying theory assumes a biological predisposition to increased emotional sensitivity and impaired emotional regulation. It combines individual therapy to tackle self-defeating behaviours, such as self-harm, with group training in emotional regulation and managing interpersonal relationships; these are backed up by telephone coaching from a therapist. Therapy techniques include the use of metaphor and stories (dialectical strategies) and standard cognitive behavioural strategies.

The study of personality and personality disorder in old age is in its infancy and is hampered by a lack of robust longitudinal research[13]. However, there are indications that certain personality traits in older people are associated with recurrent depressive disorder and this has led to the modification of DBT for the treatment of older patients[14]. Self-defeating patterns of behaviour exhibited by older patients and targeted in DBT may include repeated disengagement from treatment.

For a fuller description of DBT with older adults see Cheavens and Lynch[15].

Mindfulness-Based Cognitive Therapy (MBCT)

Mindfulness-based cognitive therapy is used to prevent recurrence of depression. It is derived from both CBT and mindfulness-based stress reduction, an intervention originally developed to reduce distress in patients experiencing chronic pain and illness[16]. Rather than examine the content of thoughts, as in conventional CBT, MBCT teaches patients how to disengage from recurrent patterns of negative thinking by the use of meditation and refocusing on bodily sensations, particularly breathing. Techniques are taught in group classes with the intention that participants will continue to practise meditation and to employ modified techniques in everyday life. As MBCT aims to prevent rumination over insoluble problems, such as ill-health, it has obvious potential in the treatment of older people. Experience suggests that older patients value its educational approach[17].

Efficacy of Cognitive Behavioural Interventions

Despite a significant number of large-scale trials supporting the acute and long-term benefits of CBT in the management of depressive illness in younger adults[1] there have been few large well-powered trials with older participants representative of clinical populations[18]. In one trial[19] 102 adults aged 60 and over with major depressive disorder were treated over three months with CBT alone, the antidepressant desipramine alone, or a combination of the two. The authors concluded that the addition of CBT to desipramine may be of additional benefit in patients with more severe depression. A more recent trial in a UK primary care setting compared CBT with treatment as usual and treatment as usual with talking control[20] in 204 people aged 65 or over with a Geriatric Mental State diagnosis of depression. Based on improvement in Beck Depression Inventory score, CBT was of greater benefit than treatment as usual and talking control.

A Cochrane systematic review of trials of psychological treatments for depression in older adults included five trials comparing therapies from the cognitive behavioural schools with waiting list controls[21]. The cognitive behavioural therapies were found to be significantly more effective than waiting list controls. However, the authors of this review urge caution in generalizing these findings to clinical populations due to the quality of the trials and their clinically unrepresentative patient populations.

Studies of MBCT

The National Institute for Health and Clinical Excellence Depression Guideline[1] recommended MBCT as a maintenance treatment to reduce the likelihood of future relapse for younger adults who have experienced three or more episodes of depression. MBCT may also be more effective than antidepressant medication in reducing overall psychiatric morbidity and improving quality of life[22]. There have been no randomized trials of MBCT with older people, although a descriptive study of 38 older people with recurrent depression showed it to be an acceptable treatment that required minimal modification[23].

IMPACT Trial (Improving Mood, Promoting Access to Collaborative Care Treatment)

In this large multicentre trial in the United States[24], behavioural activation and PST were used as components of a flexible package of treatment for depression alongside patient education, antidepressant treatment and supervision by a depression care manager. Compared with usual primary care treatment (including antidepressants) the collaborative care reduced depressive symptoms and improved rates of remission on the Symptom Check List 90 over two years.

Studies of DBT

There have been two small exploratory randomized controlled trials of DBT in older people. In the first, in which people with major depression received antidepressant medication with or without group skills therapy and telephone coaching, higher rates of remission were found with the combination treatment at six months. The second study was with participants aged 55 and over with major depression and a diagnosis of personality disorder on the Structured Clinical Interview for DSM-IV Personality Disorders and the Inventory of Interpersonal Problems (Personality Disorders) who had not remitted after eight weeks of antidepressant treatment[25]. They were randomized to 24 weeks of either antidepressant medication management alone or medication management plus DBT. Although those receiving the combination achieved remission sooner, there was no difference between groups in overall rates of remission.

INTERPERSONAL PSYCHOTHERAPY (IPT)

Interpersonal psychotherapy is a short-term individual treatment based on the simple principle that whatever its cause, depression inevitably impacts on relationships. It arose from the interpersonal school of psychiatry and under the influence of attachment and life events theories. IPT aims to address one or two interpersonal goals that are identified during a detailed review of the patient's current and recent relationships.

Interpersonal problems are classified into four categories: complicated bereavements, role transitions, interpersonal disputes and interpersonal deficits. With older people the commonest foci are role transition and interpersonal dispute. A role transition may be the loss of a role, such as retirement from work, or the acquisition of a new role such as becoming a carer for a spouse with dementia. A role dispute may occur, for instance, when an older person dealing with ill-health begins to require the practical and emotional support of an adult son or daughter. There is naturally some overlap between these categories: for instance, a complicated bereavement after the death of a spouse implies a role transition to being a single person[26].

Treatment strategies used in IPT begin with education of the patient on the nature of depression and encouragement to temporarily adopt the sick role. This should help to validate the depression as a legitimate health problem which can be important for older people. In the management of bereavement, patients are encouraged to express their feelings associated with their loss and then to build up new relationships. With role transitions, a period of mourning for the old role is encouraged followed by support in adapting to the new role. In interpersonal disputes possible treatment strategies include improving the patient's style of communication before renegotiating the basis of the relationship or seeking its dissolution.

Interpersonal psychotherapy can be used as a short-term acute phase treatment of depression (usually up to 16 sessions) or as a maintenance treatment with sessions more widely spaced over a period of months. The latter allows for a greater number of therapeutic foci to be addressed, including long-standing patterns of interpersonal behaviour that may contribute to recurrence (interpersonal deficits)[27]. In IPT it is generally not intended that the therapeutic relationship become a focus of therapy although in tackling long-term interpersonal deficits it may provide useful insights.

IPT has also been adapted for use with cognitively impaired older people through involvement of caregivers in the delivery of therapy[28].

For a detailed description of IPT with older adults, see Hinrichsen and Clougherty[26].

IPT Case Example: Mr D – I lost my wife and my life

Mr D, a 66-year-old widower and retired lawyer, was brought to treatment by his family. He acknowledged being quite depressed in the aftermath of his wife's death from breast cancer five months earlier. On questioning, he stated that his depression had really begun when he retired from his job to care for her declining health a year and a half earlier. In fact, Mrs D had been fighting breast cancer on and off for eight years, an onslaught that he had described as having gradually taken over their lives. He was distracted from his work, and what he described as a previously warm and close relationship had suffered. 'But why shouldn't I be depressed?' he asked. 'My life is ruined, over.' He reported agitation, rumination, decreased sleep and appetite, a 15 pound weight loss, and passive suicidal ideation, with a sense that he might be reunited with his wife in death. His Hamilton Rating Scale for Depression score was 27.

Mr D reported one prior episode of depression in his early twenties; he had also abused alcohol many years before but denied current use. He reported mild prostatic hypertrophy but was otherwise in good medical condition. He was adamant that he would not take an antidepressant medication.

Given a choice between a role transition based on retirement and complicated bereavement, both therapist and patient agreed to focus for 12 sessions on the latter. Mr D felt guilty that he had let his wife down, believed that he should have cared for her better, and considered her the love of his life, an irreplaceable loss after some 40 years of marriage. The therapist encouraged him to reminisce about what he missed about Mrs D and their marriage. She also noted that Mr D had not discussed his feelings much with his friends and had not really used the available social supports. Mr D stated that many friends and family members had either moved away or died in recent years, and he was not in any case one to talk about his feelings. He had withdrawn and kept to himself from the time of his wife's funeral. The therapist encouraged him to consider building new skills in this area, inasmuch as social supports could provide him with some comfort in his difficult situation.

As therapy continued, Mr D reported that he had begun to attend synagogue for the first time in years and that his rabbi had provided some solace. At the same time, Mr D began to discuss his ambivalent feelings about is wife – how her illness had distracted him from and ultimately ended his career and how she had annoyed him at times despite his wanting to care for her. Although they had had a wonderful marriage, there had (inevitably, his therapist noted) been some problems. He began to discuss these issues with a level of affect, initially apologizing for his tears but gradually relaxing and accepting his feelings. His Hamilton score decreased to 13, and he began to become more socially active.

In the latter part of the 12-week therapy, Mr D returned to the law, conducting pro bono work for senior citizens. He also became active as a volunteer for a local cancer society, raising funds and – somewhat to his surprise – developing new friends. Mr D saw his cancer work as a tribute to his wife. He also re-engaged with his children and other family members. By the end of treatment, his Hamilton Rating Scale for Depression score had fallen to 7. He was proud to have improved 'by myself' without medication. Given his history, Mr D and his therapist agreed to monthly maintenance IPT to help him preserve his gains.

Reproduced by permission of Oxford University Press, Inc. from [29] Weissman MM, Markowitz JC, Klerman GL. (2007) Clinician's quick guide to interpersonal psychotherapy (pp. 108–109). New York: Oxford University Press.

Efficacy of IPT

There is good evidence for the efficacy of IPT as an acute treatment for depression in younger adults[1] but acute phase trials with older people been fewer and smaller (e.g.[30]). The most significant trials of IPT with older people have been in the maintenance phase of treatment; these are reviewed below.

MTLLD I and MTLLD II trials (Maintenance Therapies for Late Life Depression)

These trials examined the effect of IPT with or without antidepressant treatment in participants who had recovered from an episode of depression using a combination of IPT and antidepressant.

In MTLLD I[31] participants were relatively young outpatients (60 years or over) who had suffered at least two episodes of depression.

In maintenance treatment they received nortriptyline alone, drug placebo alone, IPT alone or a combination of both treatments. The combination produced the lowest recurrence rate on the Hamilton Rating Scale for Depression and was superior to drug placebo, IPT alone and possibly to nortriptyline alone although this comparison did not achieve statistical significance. Participants were followed up at monthly intervals for three years (Figure 87.2). Participants aged 70 and over had the highest rate of recurrence in the first year and a secondary analysis suggested that the greatest benefit of combined pharmacotherapy and psychotherapy in reducing recurrence was in this group.

MTLLD II[32] addressed the prevention of recurrence in older patients (70 years or over) (i.e. those potentially at greater risk of recurrence). Participants in this trial had more medical illness than those in MTLLD I; some had cognitive impairment and may have been developing dementia. Half of the participants were in their first episode of depression. They were randomly assigned to paroxetine alone, placebo alone, monthly IPT alone or a combination of paroxetine and IPT; and follow-up was for two years. In contrast to MTLLDI, combined treatment did not produce lower recurrence rates than antidepressant alone and IPT was no more efficacious than drug placebo (Figure 87.3).

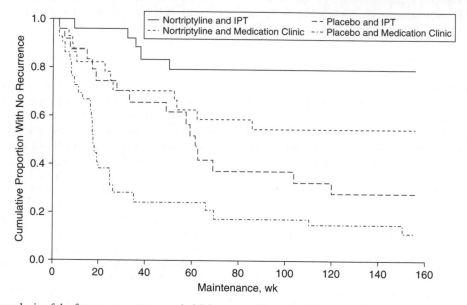

Figure 87.2 Survival analysis of the four treatment groups in Maintenance Therapies for Late Life Depression (MTLLD) I. IPT, interpersonal psychotherapy
Source: Taken with permission from [31] Reynolds *et al*. (1999), *Journal of the American Medical Association*, 281: 42. Copyright © (1999) American Medical Association. All rights reserved

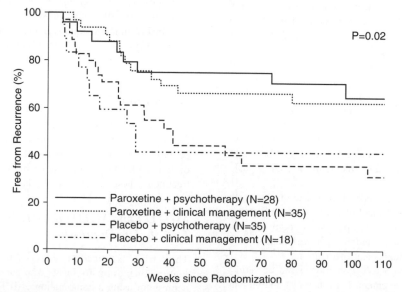

Figure 87.3 Survival analysis of the four treatment groups in MTLLD II
Source: Taken with permission from [32] Reynolds CF *et al*. (2006). Copyright © 2006 Massachusetts Medical Society. All rights reserved

PROSPECT trial (Prevention of Suicide in Primary Care Elderly: Collaborative Trial)

Although this large primary care trial principally studied the reduction in major risk factors for suicide in older people, it gives some indication of the effect on depression of a care management intervention that included IPT[33]. Other components of treatment were antidepressant treatment and support from a depression care manager who also delivered the IPT in both the acute and maintenance phases of treatment. Patients receiving the intervention had a more favourable course of depression and greater rates of remission during a year's follow-up, compared with those receiving usual care.

REMINISCENCE THERAPY AND LIFE REVIEW

Designed specifically for older adults, reminiscence therapy is usually offered in groups in which participants are encouraged to discuss their earlier life experiences with the help of prompts such as photographs, music and everyday objects. Life review, by contrast, is usually an individual therapy offering a more systematic review of the patient's own life experiences.

Efficacy of Reminiscence and Life Review

A number of small, short-term trials have shown positive effect sizes for reminiscence as a treatment for depression, particularly in community-dwelling people; however, a large randomized controlled trial is lacking[34]. In one study, reminiscence and life review appeared less efficacious than problem-solving therapy[35].

USING PSYCHOLOGICAL TREATMENTS IN THE PRIMARY PREVENTION OF DEPRESSION

It is known that the factors that put older people at risk of developing major depression include chronic illness, functional impairment and low-level symptoms of anxiety and depression. For this reason psychological interventions have been developed for those at risk of depression because of a medical disorder or bereavement (selective prevention) or because of having subsyndromal symptoms (indicated interventions). An example of a selective intervention is PST to prevent depression in older people with age-related macular degeneration as evaluated by Rovner et al. in 206 people attending an ophthalmology clinic[36]. This study demonstrated a significant difference in depression levels between intervention and control groups at three months but this was not maintained at six months.

For a summary of prevention trials and a discussion of study design see the review by Cole[37].

PSYCHOLOGICAL TREATMENT OF DYSTHYMIA

Dysthymia indicates a long-standing state of milder depression, especially low mood and is sometimes is accompanied by episodes of major depression. There has been little specific evaluation of psychological treatments for dysthymia, especially with older people, although there is some guidance as to how treatments can be adapted. It is suggested that both CBT and IPT for dysthymia need to take account of the strained relationships and long-term lack of achievement that can accompany it and in IPT the therapeutic focus may need to be the role transition from ill-health to health[29]. It is likely that therapy will take place over a more sustained period with regular maintenance sessions.

OLDER PEOPLE'S ACCESS TO PSYCHOLOGICAL TREATMENTS AND THE NEED FOR FURTHER EVALUATION

Developments in the use of psychological therapies with depressed older people appear not to have significantly influenced provision. In the United States, use of psychotherapy remains uncommon among depressed older people[38] and in the United Kingdom availability has been patchy[39]. The Improving Access to Psychological Therapies programme in the UK[40] has tried to improve uptake through the implementation of a stepped care approach starting with low level interventions such as behavioural activation. Although a key aim of the programme has been to enable working adults to re-enter the workforce it was also intended to improve access for older people. Despite this, older adults have been under-represented in referrals made by general practitioners. Older people appear inclined to take up the offer of psychotherapy, particularly if it presented in an educational format[41].

Availability of therapies may be limited by health care providers. In the United States, for example, Medicare providers may limit the number of therapy sessions or restrict them to certain groups of patients[42]. Therapies that are more straightforward, such as PST, and that can be delivered by non-mental health workers alongside treatment of physical disorders may have more to offer and be more appealing to funders as may brief therapies designed to be delivered in group format[43]. However, before a strong case can be made for an expansion in psychological treatment provision for depressed older people further evaluation of interventions is required. Although the effect sizes in trials with older adults appear to match those with younger people, there remains a paucity of large, robust trials with older adults representative of clinical populations[21,44]. Trials of care management interventions in primary care have been encouraging but these do not measure the specific effects of their psychological treatment components. Indicators of likely response to psychological therapies would help guide decision making and use of resources[45].

REFERENCES

1. NICE (National Institute for Health and Clinical Excellence) Depression: Management of Depression in Primary and Secondary Care, CG23, 2004. http://guidance.nice.org.uk/CG23, accessed February 2010.
2. Gum AM, Arean PA, Hunkeler E et al. Depression treatment preferences in older primary care patients. Gerontologist 2006; 46: 14–22.
3. Peterson TJ. Enhancing the efficacy of antidepressants with psychotherapy. J Psychopharmacol 2006; 20: 19–28.
4. Steffens DC, Conway DR, Dombeck CB et al. Severity of subcortical gray matter hyperintensity predicts ECT response in geriatric depression. J ECT 2001; 17, 45–49.
5. Herrmann L, Goodwin G, Ebmeier K. The cognitive neuropsychology of depression in the elderly. Psychol Med 2008; 37: 1693–702.
6. Prince MJ, Beekman ATF, Deeg DJH. Depression symptoms in late life assessed using the EURO-D scale. Effect of age, gender and marital status in 14 European centres. Br J Psychiatry 1999; 174: 339–45.

7. Lewinsohn PM. A behavioral approach to depression. In Friedman RJ, Katz MM (eds), *The Psychology of Depression: Contemporary theory and research*. Chichester: John Wiley & Sons, Ltd, 1974, 157–76.

8. Beck AT, Rush AJ, Shaw BF *et al. Cognitive Therapy of Depression*. New York: Guilford Press, 1979

9. James IA, Kendell K, Reichelt FK. Conceptualizations of depression in older people: the interaction of positive and negative beliefs. *Behav Cogn Psychother* 1999; **27**: 285–90.

10. Wilkinson P. Cognitive behaviour therapy. In Hepple J, Pearce J, Wilkinson P (eds), *Psychological Therapies with Older People*. Hove: Bruner-Routledge, 2001, 45–75.

11. Laidlaw K, Thompson LW, Dick-Siskin L *et al. Cognitive Behaviour Therapy With Older People*. Chichester: John Wiley & Sons, Ltd, 2003.

12. Binks C, Fenton M, McCarthy L *et al.* Psychological therapies for people with borderline personality disorder. *Cochrane Database Syst Rev* 2006; Issue 1: CD005652.

13. Oppenheimer C. Personality in later life: personality disorder and the effects of illness on personality. In Jacoby R, Oppenheimer C, Dening T, Thomas A (eds), *Oxford Textbook of Old Age Psychiatry*. Oxford: Oxford University Press, 2008, 605–15.

14. Morse JQ, Lynch TR. A preliminary investigation of self-reported personality disorders in late life: prevalence, predictors of depressive severity, and clinical correlates. *Aging Ment Health* 2004; **8**: 307–15.

15. Cheavens JS, Lynch TR. Dialectical behavior therapy for personality disorders in older adults. In Gallagher-Thompson D, Steffen AM, Thompson LW (eds), *Handbook of Behavioral and Cognitive Therapies with Older Adults*. New York: Springer, 2008, 187–99.

16. Segal ZV, Williams JMG, Teasdale JD. *Mindfulness-based Cognitive Therapy for Depression: A New Approach to Preventing Relapse*. New York: Guildford, 2002.

17. Smith A. Clinical uses of mindfulness training for older people. *Behav Cogn Psychother* 2004; **32**: 423–30.

18. Mackin RS, Areán PA. Evidence-based psychotherapeutic interventions for geriatric depression. *Psychiatr Clin N Am* 2005; **28**: 805–20.

19. Thompson LW, Coon DW, Gallagher-Thompson D *et al.* Comparison of desipramine and cognitive/behavioral therapy in the treatment of elderly outpatients with mild-to-moderate depression. *Am J Geriatr Psychiatry* 2001; **9**: 225–40.

20. Serfaty MA, Haworth D, Blanchard M, *et al.* Effectiveness of individual cognitive behavioral therapy for depressed older people in primary care: a randomized controlled trial. *Arch Gen Psychiatry*, 2009; **66(12)**: 1332–40.

21. Wilson K, Mottram PG, Vassilas C. Psychotherapeutic treatments for older depressed people. *Cochrane Database Syst Rev* 2008; Issue 1: CD004853.

22. Kuyken W, Taylor RS, Barrett B *et al.* Mindfulness-based cognitive therapy to prevent relapse in recurrent depression. *J Consult Clin Psychol* 2008; **76**: 966–78.

23. Smith A, Graham L, Senthinathan S. Mindfulness-based cognitive therapy for recurring depression in older people: a qualitative study. *Aging Ment Health* 2007; **11**: 346–57.

24. Hunkeler EM, Katon W, Tang L *et al.* Long term outcomes from the IMPACT randomised trial for depressed elderly patients in primary care. *BMJ* 2006; **332**: 259–62.

25. Lynch TR, Cheavens JS, Cukrowicz KC *et al.* Treatment of older adults with co-morbid personality disorder and depression: a

26. dialectical behavior therapy approach. *Int J Geriatr Psychiatry* 2007; **22**: 131–43.

26. Hinrichsen GA, Clougherty KF. *Interpersonal Psychotherapy for Depressed Older Adults*. Washington DC: American Psychological Association, 2006.

27. Frank E, Frank N, Cornes C *et al.* Interpersonal psychotherapy in the treatment of late-life depression. In Klerman GL, Weissman MM (eds), *New Applications of Interpersonal Psychotherapy*. Arlington, VA: American Psychiatric Publishing, 1993.

28. Miller MD, Richards V, Zuckoff A *et al.* A model for modifying interpersonal psychotherapy (IPT) for depressed elders with cognitive impairment. *Clin Gerontol* 2007; **30**: 1545–2301.

29. Weissman MM, Markowitz JC, Klerman GL. *Clinician's Quick Guide to Interpersonal Psychotherapy*. New York: Oxford University Press, 2007.

30. Sloane RB, Staples FR, Schneider LS. Interpersonal psychotherapy versus nortriptyline for depression in the elderly. In Burrows G, Norman TR, Dennerstein L (eds). *Clinical and Pharmacological Studies in Psychiatric Disorders*. London: John Libbey, 1985, 344–46.

31. Reynolds CF, Frank E, Perel JM *et al.* Nortriptyline and interpersonal psychotheorpy as maintenance therapies for recurrent major depression: a randomized controlled trial in patients older than 59 years. *JAMA* 1999; **281**: 39–45.

32. Reynolds CF, Dew MA, Pollock BG *et al.* Maintenance treatment of major depression in old age. *N Engl J Med* 2006; **354**: 1130–38.

33. Bruce ML, Ten Have TR, Reynolds CF *et al.* Reducing suicidal ideation and depressive symptoms in depressed older primary care patients. A randomized controlled trial. *JAMA* 2004; **291**: 1081–91.

34. Bohlmeijer E, Smit F, Cuijpers P. Effects of reminiscence and life review on late-life depression: a meta-analysis. *Int J Geriatr Psychiatry* 2003; **18**: 1088–94.

35. Arean PA, Perri MG, Nezu AM *et al.* Comparative effectiveness of social problem-solving therapy and reminiscence therapy as treatments for depression in older adults. *J Consult Clin Psychol* 1993; **61**: 1003–10.

36. Rovner B, Casten R, Hegel M *et al.* Preventing depression in age-related macular degeneration. *Arch Gen Psychiatry* 2007; **64**: 886–92.

37. Cole MG. Brief interventions to prevent depression in older subjects: a systematic review of feasibility and effectiveness. *Am J Geriatr Psychiatry* 2008; **16**: 435–43.

38. Wei W, Sambamoorthi U, Olfson M *et al.* Use of psychotherapy for depression in older adults. *Am J Psychiatry* 2005; **162**: 711–17.

39. Evans S. A survey of the provision of psychological treatments to older adults in the NHS. *Psychiatr Bull* 2004; **28**: 411–14.

40. Department of Health. *The IAPT Pathfinders: Achievements and Challenges*, 2008. www.iapt.nhs.uk/2008/01/27/the-iapt-pathfinder-achievements-and-challenges/, accessed 4 February 2010.

41. Areán PA, Alvidrez J, Barrera A *et al.* Would older medical patients use psychological services? *Gerontologist* 2002; **42**: 392–98.

42. Karlin BE, Duffy M. Geriatric mental health policy: impact on service delivery and directions for effecting change. *Prof Psychol Res Pract* 2004; **35**: 509–19.

43. Wilkinson P, Alder N, Juszczak E *et al.* A pilot randomised controlled trial of a brief cognitive behavioural group intervention

to reduce recurrence rates in late life depression. *Int J Geriatr Psychiatry* 2009; **24**: 68–75.

44. Cuijpers P, van Straten A, Smit F *et al*. Is psychotherapy for depression equally effective in younger and older adults? A meta-regression analysis. *Int Psychogeriatr* 2008; **21**: 16–24.

45. Alexopoulos GS. Personalizing the care of geriatric depression. *Am J Geriatr Psychiatry* 2008; **165**: 790–92.

88

Acute Management of Late-Life Depression*

V. Gardner and D.C. Steffens

Department of Psychiatry and Behavioral Sciences, Duke University Medical Center, Durham, NC, USA

The acute management of late-life depression may require hospitalization, both for accurate diagnosis and for effective treatment. Ambulatory management is frequently favoured because of rising hospital costs in a managed care environment. However, the elderly present special challenges that may require that diagnosis and/or treatment be undertaken in a hospital setting. The hospital provides an environment for the monitoring of symptoms for accurate diagnosis and proper personnel for regular and accurate treatment administration. Several factors may interfere with both accurate diagnosis and effective treatment on an ambulatory basis[1], including underlying chronic medical illness, pain, neurodegenerative changes, dementia, adverse life events, inadequate family support, secret self-medication, substance abuse, bereavement, interpersonal conflicts and social isolation of the elderly patient.

Actually, the elderly patient who is cognitively intact may be reliably managed on an ambulatory basis and can be instructed about medication side effects. Similarly, the more impaired elderly patient who has adequate social support for observation and medication management may only need the community support of a visiting psychiatric nurse, assuming one is available. Varying levels of care are also implemented in the hospital environment. Patients may have the usual care of routine monitoring or may have more intense one-to-one monitoring if they are an imminent risk to themselves or others.

As a general rule, the more the physical and psychiatric impairments and the fewer the psychosocial resources, the greater the need to hospitalize for accurate diagnosis and effective treatment. When deciding safe and effective management, the following factors favour hospitalization: poor or unstable physical health, high suicide risk, impaired judgement and reality testing, likelihood of poor compliance, impaired cognitive functioning, lack of social support, and severe anorexia and weight loss.

CO-MORBIDITY OF PHYSICAL ILLNESS: THE INTERFACE OF PRIMARY CARE AND PSYCHIATRY

Accurate diagnosis is a prerequisite for effective treatment. Elderly patients with depression present to their primary care physicians and psychiatrists in a complex manner, and signs and symptoms of physical illness and depression overlap. Even the normal effects of ageing may cause diagnostic difficulties and restrict treatment

options. Many primary care physicians diagnose and treat late-life depression without referral. However, those patients who fail two or three trials with antidepressants, usually selective serotonin reuptake inhibitors (SSRIs) or newer agents, are commonly referred to a psychiatrist for further management. These patients represent a treatment challenge and may require more complex medication regimens. Hospitalization may be necessary to enable close monitoring and minimise risk of self-neglect, suicidality and treatment side effects. Primary care physicians also refer for the following reasons: suicidality, co-morbidity with substance abuse, dementia, anxiety disorder, presence of psychosis (delusions, hallucinations), catatonia, bipolar disorder and inability to tolerate antidepressant treatment[2,3].

Depression is often co-morbid with other physical diseases. Approximately 80% of older adults suffer from at least one chronic health problem[4]. The prevalence of co-morbid depression may be up to 30% in stroke patients, 18% in myocardial infarction patients, 51% in patients with hip fracture and 50% in patients with chronic pain[1]. Existence of an undiagnosed and untreated depression with these illnesses leads to higher disability[5]. The diagnosis of depression in the context of established physical illnesses may be challenging, and the hospital environment provides the necessary monitoring and support staff when complicated medication changes are required. For example, a patient with cardiovascular disease may present with decreased energy and apathy. Determining whether this is caused by a compromised cardiac status, a medication side effect, or is actually a symptom of depression may be difficult without hospitalization, close monitoring and various medication trials.

Formerly, hospitalization was favoured for the initiation of tricyclic antidepressant therapy in elderly patients with unstable cardiac disease. First-line treatment with SSRIs has made this less often necessary, though older people are also vulnerable to adverse effects of SSRIs such as hyponatraemia.

Co-morbid neurological illness is also common in geriatric depression. Patients with depressive symptoms following a cerebrovascular accident also present a diagnostic challenge. There may be communication difficulties or other neurological abnormalities. Depression may be diagnosed only by the report of the nursing staff and family, who observe apathy, irritability, tearfulness and weight loss[7]. Patients with Parkinson's disease may develop an affective illness or psychosis, which may be secondary to treatment with L-dopa or dopaminiergic agonists. Hospitalization may be required for medication changes if outpatient support is inadequate.

*Updated by Mohammed T. Abou-Saleh

Severe anorexia, weight loss and refusal to eat are indications for hospitalization for safe and effective treatment[1,8]. Poor oral intake commonly accompanies severe depression, but it may also result from a variety of medical conditions. For example, individuals with active rheumatoid arthritis may experience insomnia, fatigue and poor appetite equally from their physical illness or an associated depression[9].

SUICIDE RISK AND THE DECISION TO HOSPITALIZE

Suicidality is the most common reason for psychiatric hospitalization. The goals for inpatient treatment are: (i) the preservation of life and safety; (ii) the elimination of suicidal intent and ideation and treatment of underlying disorders; and (iii) the improvement of intrapsychic capabilities, personal factors and psychosocial circumstances to facilitate coping after discharge and decreasing risk of the return of suicidality. However, implementation of these treatment plans is predicted on the initial detection of suicidality.

Careful assessment of suicide risk in depressed older adults is thus vital. The elderly are less likely to have made a prior suicide attempt, but they consistently demonstrate a higher rate of completed suicides[10]. The ratio of attempted to completed suicides decreases with age from 200:1 in young adulthood to 4:1 in the elderly[11]. The higher rate is due primarily to the increased frequency of deaths among older, white males. In 1992, people 65 and older accounted for 13% of the population but almost 20% of suicides. Even though the frequency of suicide has increased among older persons in the United States, the prevalence is not as high as that of other industrialized societies[12].

Recognition of variables such as gender and race may influence management decisions. Risk factors for suicide in late life include increased age, with the highest prevalence of suicide of persons older than 85[10]. Also, being male, white, single, separated or divorced, or widowed are risk factors for suicide. Other risk factors implicated in late-life suicide include: a positive psychiatric history (especially depression and alcohol abuse and dependence); physical illness and functional disability (especially diseases of the central nervous system, malignancies, cardiopulmonary conditions, and urogenital diseases in men); previous suicide attempts; psychological factors (i.e. hopelessness); social factors (stressful life events, e.g. bereavement); and biological susceptibility (dysregulation of the hypothalamic–pituitary–adrenal axis or the serotonin system).

Most older people who commit suicide have seen a primary care provider within 30 days of death[11]. This observation stresses the need for collaborative efforts with primary care physicians and the need to make careful assessment based on risk factors.

A number of assessment guidelines have been developed to aid in the evaluation of potentially suicidal patients. A four-item screen for identification of suicidal ideation among general medical patients was developed by Cooper-Patrick et al.[12]:

1. Have you ever felt that life is not worth living?
2. Have you ever thought of hurting or harming yourself?
3. Have you considered specific methods for harming yourself?
4. Have you ever made a suicide attempt?

This fourfold layered approach to assessment is useful in obtaining the necessary data without disrupting the therapeutic relationship. If the answer to the first or second question is negative, then the enquiries can cease and the older person may be considered at low risk for suicide[10]. This approach has advantages over other assessment tools, which usually suggest one question to be asked to assess suicidal risk.

DELUSIONS AND LATE-LIFE DEPRESSION

Accurate diagnosis and effective treatment of depressed elderly patients with delusions can be hindered by their impairment of reality testing. Their sometimes well-organized and complex delusions may make them distrust medicine and the physician who prescribes it. This disorder is less frequent in the community and more prevalent in the hospital setting[13,14]. Accurate diagnosis is necessary, as some studies have suggested that the depression is more severe[14,15] and it has been associated with suicide[13]. Varying reports also demonstrate decreased cognitive functioning and social functioning among patients with delusional depression[16]. These patients are best treated in the hospital. They cannot be relied upon to take accurate doses of medications. Effective pharmacologic treatment for delusional depression may require combination treatment with antipsychotic medication and antidepressants[15]. ECT remains an effective and relatively safe treatment for the treatment of delusional depression[17–19] and can be performed on an outpatient basis only with adequate social support.

COGNITIVE DYSFUNCTION AND LATE-LIFE DEPRESSION

A full discussion of how depression is distinguished from dementia is given elsewhere in this book. To summarize, diagnosis is difficult because several symptoms of depression and dementia overlap, such as a flattened affect, psychomotor retardation and presence, at times, of delusions[20]. Delusions are reported to occur in up to 40%[13] of Alzheimer's disease patients, although they are described as transient and less organized than in delusional depression[13]. Major depression occurs in over 20% of patients with Alzheimer's disease and vascular dementia[4,21]. This significant co-morbidity may lead to profound disability[22].

The diagnosis of depression in dementia usually requires the input of family members or nursing personnel[23,24]. The patient with cognitive dysfunction and impaired reality testing cannot reliably report symptoms, take medication accurately, or reliably report side effects.

Dementia with depression and behavioural disturbance is frequently too complex to treat on an outpatient basis. These patients may even require involuntary commitment. Aggression may be verbal or physical. Aggression and agitation in dementia may be as high as 50% in the outpatient population[25,26]. The hospital environment is the only setting with constant monitoring to make an accurate diagnosis, contain behaviour and monitor medication.

The reversible cognitive impairment that may accompany depression also increases disability[27]. With treatment, the cognitive impairment usually improves. However, these patients are at higher risk of developing an irreversible dementia in the future[28].

REFERENCES

1. Montano CB. Primary care issues related to the treatment of depression in elderly. *J Clin Psychiatry* 1999; **60**(suppl. 20): 45–51.

2. Mulsant B, Ganguli M. Epidemiology and diagnosis of depression in late life. *J Clin Psychiatry* 1999; **60**(20): 9–14.
3. Unutzer J, Katon W, Sullivan M, Miranda J. Treating depressed older adults in primary care: narrowing the gap between efficacy and effectiveness. *Millbank Q* 1999; **77**: 225–56.
4. Edelstein B, Kalish K *et al*. Assessment of depression and bereavement in older adults. In Lichtenberg P (ed.), *Handbook of Assessment in Clinical Gerontology*. New York: Wiley & Sons Inc., 1999, 11–58.
5. Das Gupta K. Treatment of depression in elderly patients: recent advances. *Arch Fam Med* 1998; **7**(3): 274–80.
6. Roose S, Spatz E. Treatment of depression in patients with heart disease. *J Clin Psychiatry* 1999; **60**(20): 34–37.
7. Mather R. Old age psychiatry in a general hospital. In Jacoby R, Oppenheimer C (eds), *Psychiatry in the Elderly*. New York: Oxford University Press, 1997, 536–73.
8. Joseph S. Practical diagnostic and management guidelines. In Joseph S (ed.), *Symptom Focused Psychiatric Drug Therapy for Managed Care*. Binghamton, NY: Haworth Medical, 1997, 25–45.
9. Baldwin RC. Depressive illness. In Jacoby R, Oppenheimer C (eds), *Psychiatry in the Elderly*. New York: Oxford University Press, 1997, 336–54.
10. Steffens DC, Blazer DG. Suicide in the elderly. In Jacobs DG (ed.), *Guide to Suicide Assessment and Intervention*. San Francisco, CA: Jossey-Bass. 1999, 443–62.
11. Conwell Y. Management of suicidal behavior in the elderly. *Psychiat Clin N Am* 1997; **20**: 667–83.
12. Cooper-Patrick L, Crum RM, Ford DE. Identifying suicidal ideation in general medical patients. *JAMA* 1994; **272**: 1757–62.
13. Meyers BS. Geriatric delusional depression. *Clin Geriatr Med* 1992; **8**: 299–308.
14. O'Brien J, Ames D, Schweitzer I, Desmond P, Coleman P, Tress B. Magnetic resonance imaging and endocrinological differences between delusional and non-delusional depression in the elderly. *Int J Geriatr Psychiatry* 1999; **12**: 211–18.
15. Chiu HF. Antidepressants in the elderly. *Int J Clin Pract* 1997; **51**: 369–74.
16. Blazer DG. Severe episode of depression in late life: the long road to recovery. *Am J Psychiatry* 1996; **153**: 1620–23.
17. Spar JE, LaRue A. Mood disorders: treatment. In Spar JE, LaRue A (eds), *Concise Guide to Geriatric Psychiatry*. Washington DC: American Psychiatric Press, 1990, 65–88.
18. Alexopoulos GS. Affective disorders. In Sadavey J, Lazarus LW, Jarvik LF, Grossberg GT (eds), *Comprehensive Review of Geriatric Psychiatry*, vol. II. Washington DC: American Psychiatric Press, 1996; 563–92.
19. Small GW. Treatment of geriatric depression. *Depress Anxiety* 1998; **8**: 32–42.
20. Reisberg B, Kluger A. Assessing the progression of dementia: diagnostic considerations. In Salzman C (ed.), *Clinical Geriatric Psychopharmacology*. Baltimore, MD: Williams and Wilkins, 1998, 432–62.
21. Newman S. The prevalence of depression in Alzheimer's disease and vascular dementia in a population sample. *J Affect Disord* 1999; **52**: 169–76.
22. Simpson S, Allen H, Tomenson B, Burns A. Neurological correlates of depressive symptoms in Alzheimer's disease and vascular dementia. *J Affect Disord* 1999; **53**: 129–36.
23. Plopper M. Common psychiatric disorders. In Yoshikawa TT (ed.), *Ambulatory Geriatric Care*. St. Louis, MO: Mosby Year Book, 1993, 346–62.
24. Harwood D, Barker WW, Ownby RL, Duara R. Association between premorbid history of depression and current depression in Alzheimer's disease. *J Geriatr Psychiatr Neurol* 1999; **12**: 72–75.
25. Kunick ME, Yudofsky SC, Silver JM, Hales RE. Pharmacologic approach to management of agitation associated with dementia. *J Clin Psychiatry* 1994; **55**: 13–17.
26. Tueth M, Zuberi P. Life-threatening psychiatric emergencies in the elderly: overview. *J Geriatr Psychiatr Neurol* 1999; **12**: 60–66.
27. Katz IR, Miller D *et al*. Diagnosis of late-life depression. In Salzeman C (ed.), *Clinical Geriatric Psychopharmacology*. Baltimore, MD: Williams and Wilkins, 1998, 153–83.
28. Alexopoulos GS, Meyers BS, Young RC, Mattis S, Kakuma T. The course of geriatric depression with reversible dementia: a controlled study. *Am J Psychiatry* 1993; **150**: 1693–99.

89

Bereavement

Robert J. Kastenbaum
Arizona State University at Tempe, Tempe, USA

I have lived longer than the reach of my wildest dreams. Every day is a bonus!
My body's done its job. I've done mine. So! When it's time to go, it's time to go!

Self-reflections of this kind are more common among long-lived people than those who are still making their way towards an as yet unrevealed future. Death is less theoretical, and loss a prominent feature of the lifescape. Advanced age and bereavement are normative circumstances, not psychiatric syndromes. Daily life can present a variety of concerns, such as remembering which medication to take when, fear of falling on icy pavements, and worry about paying bills and continuing to live independently. Bereavement introduces additional concerns. 'Who can I share my day with?' 'Who will do the driving/cooking?' 'Where do I go from here?' These are human rather than geriatric problems.

The psychiatry of bereavement in old age does not assume pathology or need for professional intervention, nor does it assume that all elders respond in the same way. Major research projects find a 'remarkable heterogeneity in older adults' adjustments to loss'[1]. Resilient coping is more common than prolonged distress and dysfunction. Hastily prescribing psychotropic medication for a 'geriatric patient' can become part of the problem, rather than the solution. Instead, we ask, 'Who is this person?' 'What was the nature of this unique relationship that has been ended by death?' 'What does this loss mean to the bereaved person?' – and 'What coping skills and resources can be called upon to make it through?'

A perspective on bereavement in old age can be developed by following the basic sequence of events. We then identify challenges for bereaved elders and those who would offer services to them.

THE PRE-BEREAVEMENT SITUATION

Consider first the situation prior to a bereavement in old age.

1. What was the nature and status of the relationship at this time?

This question should be answered structurally and substantively, e.g. 'He was her older brother; she relied on him for advice and support more than on any other person, including her husband', or 'She was his second wife; he had expected her to look after him – actually, to wait on him hand and foot! – and suddenly he had to be the caring person.' It is useful to explore affective and pragmatic dimensions of the relationship. Was the survivor or the deceased heavily dependent on the other person? Had the relationship been in serious trouble? If so, was this characterized by silent co-existence or stormy disputes? Did the deceased provide most of the couple's link to society? Had the survivor organized his or her life around taking care of the deceased?

An elderly person's response to the death of an adult child or grandchild is too often underestimated[2]. There can be a deep interiorization of grief after the first shock of the loss, followed by an intensified life review. Researchers have documented a 'double pain': their own loss of a grandchild and their anguish over their adult children's grief[3]. There is also often a *disenfranchised grief* situation[4]. Grandparents can be subject to interpersonal signals that they are not fully entitled to mourn the loss. The extent to which grandparents might become isolated in their grief is influenced by their pre-bereavement status in the family. Counselling interventions could include resolving issues that generated intra-family tension prior to the loss. Instead of labelling the problem as 'depression' in the elder, one might instead discover a dysfunctional family pattern that is affecting all the members.

2. How was the prospect of bereavement integrated into the life scenario?

Bereavement in later life most often involves the loss of a sibling or spouse. It is not unusual for elderly people to have floating expectations regarding the loss of people they have known for much of their lives. These cohort peers are at significant risk for death because of their advancing age and accumulated vulnerabilities. Therefore, it will be a sad but not surprising day when their lives come to an end. On the other hand, they have always been around, so it is easy to assume that they will continue to go on and on. A recently bereaved elder might alternate between the more logical and the more habituated-wishful view. Psychologically, the death has been both anticipated and not anticipated.

Anticipatory grief is often a more complex response than usually assumed. Anticipatory grief is similar in many respects to the grief that is experienced after a death[4]. There are affective, cognitive and somatic components, e.g. sadness, obsession, exhaustion etc. It has often been suggested that anticipatory grief helps the survivor to cope with the loss – paid for in advance. Early studies suggested that sudden death has a much more disturbing impact than expected

Principles and Practice of Geriatric Psychiatry, 3rd edn. Edited by Mohammed T. Abou-Saleh, Cornelius Katona and Anand Kumar

death[5]. More recent studies have taken more variables into account and suggest that anticipatory grief does not always cushion the survivor's stress when the loss does occur[1]. Potential caregivers would do well, then, to observe the particulars of the situation carefully, rather than assume that expectation is necessarily ameliorative. (Many elders have told me how they still feel helpless and miserable because they could not do anything to palliate the suffering prior to an expected death.)

Not all deaths are clearly expectable. Fatal accidents (especially falls and motor vehicle) are far more common among people 65 and older than in any other age group. Nevertheless, there is a greater probability the death will have been expectable, if not necessarily expected. Not only does an increasing proportion of deaths occur in old age, but modern health care has lengthened the interval between development of a life-threatening condition and the day of death. The four leading causes of death for elderly people in the USA (heart disease, malignant neoplasms, cerebrovascular disease and respiratory conditions) all involve a long period of living with progressive life-threatening conditions and, therefore, opportunity for both prolonged stress and adaptation to the prospect of death for the patient and significant others.

Physicians and other caregivers have the opportunity to strengthen the survivor's ability to cope with grief by sensitive response to the situation as it exists prior to death. Offering accurate information, suggesting other options and improving the lines of communication within the family are among the ways in which one can help to shape the anticipatory grief period into a source of strength rather than intensified anxiety. The age differential between most caregivers and the elderly bereaved people they are trying to help sometimes interferes with communications, e.g. when elders are patronized and their ability to cope with bad news is underestimated. There is also an underappreciated connection between quality of terminal care and grief recovery. A hospice physician reports that, 'The pain relief we achieve for an old man in his last weeks of life helps his wife to be more of her normal self when he really needs her – and a widow with fewer regrets and nightmares later.'

3. What was the survivor's own health status prior to the bereavement?

This is a particularly useful question to ask with respect to the older bereaved person[6]. The spouse was most frequently the principal family caregiver in the 40 hospices studied by Mor et al.[7] About two thirds of the spouses were above the age of 55 and it was not unusual for the caregivers to be over 75. Elderly caregivers seldom developed new physical problems over the course of the spouse's final illness, but they tended to ignore their own existing conditions. During the first months of bereavement, the survivor's health was sometimes impaired by exacerbation of previous illnesses and impairments. It would be helpful, then, to encourage the spouse and other elderly family members and friends to look after their own health during the pre-bereavement period, and to see that health status is carefully assessed afterward. Symptoms that might appear to be part of an anxious depression syndrome could be related to physical health problems that have not received the attention they deserved.

4. Who else was there and what else was happening?

Strained interpersonal relationships and unanswered questions sometimes increase stress on patient, family and staff. It might be useful to assess the prevailing attitudinal climate. Some bereaved elders report that they felt unwelcome by staff members during their bedside visits.

'I never had a chance to really be with Herman. The nurses thought they owned him.' Others said they were told different things by different people. 'I can understand things if I'm told right. I worry more when I'm not sure what to worry about.' By contrast, some bereaved elders drew comfort and strength from the bedside scene. 'The people from the church were over all the time. They really cared. We were so far from the rest of the family, but they were just like family to us.' 'Miriam seemed so at peace with herself. She whispered to me once, "This is a great place to die. They're all so nice".'

A consultant can make a positive difference by identifying interpersonal issues in the end of life period and encouraging humane and effective approaches.

AT THE TIME OF DEATH

Learning what happened around the time of death can help us understand the bereaved elder's state of mind. Consider, for example, the difference between death at home and in a hospital setting. A terminally ill woman was being looked after at home by her elderly mother, with support from a local hospice service. The mother had accepted her daughter's wish to be allowed to die at home without intubation and other futile procedures. But when the daughter appeared to be actively dying, the mother panicked and called not the hospice but a visiting nurse service. Now, as a survivor, the old woman is haunted by memories of her suctioned, intubated and drugged daughter accusing her with her eyes[8]. In a more frequent scenario, an elderly person will call for assistance from paramedics when his/her spouse appears to have died. But when the paramedic team arrives, the caller may have second thoughts about seeing the spouse's body subjected to resuscitation procedures. Some bereaved elderly persons remain troubled by unanswered questions about whether they did the right thing at the right time.

Knowing only that the death took place in a hospital does not tell us whether supportive nurses encouraged a woman to be with her husband right through to the end and to have time with him afterward – or whether she was made to feel unwelcome and hustled away. Perhaps, again, she had not been notified until some time after the death. The particularities of the final scene can provide either an acceptable conclusion to the story of a marriage or friendship, or torment the survivor with resentment, self-doubt and other disturbing thoughts.

The psychiatrist often has the opportunity to increase the sensitivity of physicians, nurses and caregivers in their communication patterns around the time of death. Survivors may hold on to a word or gesture, either as a cherished or an infuriating/depressing memory. Often one can be helpful simply by validating the survivor-to-be's feelings and offering the opportunity to clarify his/her own thoughts by active listening. The generational differences between bereaved person and psychiatrist can be a source of misunderstanding. An aged widow, for example, might keep feelings bottled up in accordance with the implicit rules that characterized her generation. Patience and encouragement could help her to express and cope with her feelings. It happens the other way, too: caregivers whose own tradition is marked by subdued behaviour and restraint of emotions may not be prepared for families in which intense expressions of grief are expected, even required.

EARLY PHASES OF BEREAVEMENT

The idea that there are fixed 'stages' of either dying or grief has attracted more believers than it deserves. One can select and force observations to fit stage theories, but to what purpose? Individual responses to grief deviate markedly from the models: this is even more common in old age, where uniqueness has been deeply engraved and polished to a high gloss.

It does make sense, though, to differentiate between responses during earlier and later periods subsequent to bereavement. Indicators of a potentially intense, disabling and protracted reaction often appear within a short time. In their classic study, Parkes and Weiss[9] found that those who had the most difficult time coping with the spouse's death tended to smoke and drink more heavily, use tranquillizers and express depressive mood. Other investigators have also found that response to loss within the first few months provides a fairly reliable forecast of long term adjustment. The obvious lesson here is that early-appearing indicators, such as loss of appetite, withdrawal from friends and activities, sleep disturbances and escape into alcohol and drugs (including the hoarding of prescription or over-the-counter elixirs) should be taken seriously. Time alone will not necessarily prove the healer.

Dependency needs often come to the fore when the survivor is experiencing significant difficulties in coping. Counsellors and therapists can be effective in helping survivors to rekindle their sense of competency and autonomy. This is likely to be a step by step progression, in which the therapist may have to play the roles of protector and mentor for some time. The advanced age of the bereaved person does not necessarily stand in the way of therapeutic success. Many people bring positive coping skills and experience into their later years of life, and some continue to participate in mutually rewarding social support networks.

It is not unusual for an elderly person to seem relatively unresponsive to a death. In some situations this is the observer's failure to notice subtle but significant changes. But the lack of a strong overt response is sometimes associated with bereavement overload[10]. Re-activated grief from previous losses can command the person's attention so that there is not enough emotional energy available to respond fully to the most recent death. Survivors of the Holocaust and other disasters have often been burdened in this way.

An upsurge in fear of personal death is also not unusual, especially when it is a sibling who has died[11]. A death that hits that closely to the survivor's own situation can lead to a dysfunctional pattern in which depression and anxiety vie for dominance. Here again, therapists have found it useful to bolster the individual's sense of competence and autonomy, as well as to encourage sharing of the concern.

Abundant if somewhat circumstantial research evidence supports the proposition that enhancing self-esteem can be a powerful hedge against mortal terror[12,13].

LATER PHASES OF BEREAVEMENT

Many senior adults have proven highly resilient after experiencing bereavement. Studies do not invariably find that widows sit around weeping and feeling helpless. The gender dimension is important here. Women outnumber men in the upper age echelons and often show themselves more skilful in providing – and receiving – social support. By contrast, the bereaved older man runs more risk of becoming isolated. In some environments, such as the retirement community with its high density of older women, the widower may be valued and looked after. Nevertheless, there is a major problem of hidden grief among older men, a problem that often persists for years after the loss. Quiet, keeping to himself, expressing little

obvious emotion, the older bereaved man is more likely to be suffering intensely than his female peer, with her greater facility in self-expression and more sensitive support network[1]. Psychiatrists and other caregivers might be well advised to give more attention to the possibility of bereavement – even a remote bereavement – as the underlying factor in a variety of behavioural and somatic problems experienced by older men. Unfortunately, some of the most traumatic bereavements leave the elderly survivor with the most limited social support. This is especially the case with suicide. The high rate of suicide among elderly white men often leaves their spouses and siblings alone with their grief.

A FEW SPECIAL CONSIDERATIONS

First, grief counselling is proving effective for many adults, including those of advanced age, who had been experiencing significant adjustment problems. A false alarm received widespread attention before being revealed as such. A 'finding' that grief counselling is not only ineffective but sometimes harmful was itself found to be without empirical and scholarly credibility[14]. Grief counselling remains a viable option for bereaved people whose personal and interpersonal resources have been temporarily overwhelmed.

Second, bereavement is a status marker in spousal death. The survivor, no longer a husband or wife, tends to be treated in a different way, sometimes as 'the odd one out.' Counsellors can be helpful in supporting the survivor's transition to meaningful new roles, and the restoration of self-confidence.

Third, the 'little deaths' that often accompany the later years of life can both intensify and anticipate grief reactions. The old man may have been mourning the loss of his mobility even before his wife died; the older woman who was relieved of her starring role as a church soloist may have felt abandoned and rejected long before her husband's death.

Fourth, the death of animal companions can lead to authentic grief reactions[15]. The grief syndrome may be similar to what is experienced upon the death of a human companion, although the intensity is less likely to endure as long. Rage joins with grief when an elderly person is placed in a nursing home and then learns that his/her animal companion has been taken to the pound and destroyed.

Fifth, the profile of the senior adult population and the conditions of their lives are continuing to change. Care providers have the challenge of keeping up with these transformations instead of relying on practices and assumptions that might be outdated. Some examples of relevant population trends are:

- More elders are receptive to counselling and becoming acquainted with the internet. Each new generation of elders is bringing enhanced technological background and receptivity to mental health options.
- The burden of Alzheimer's disease is being experienced by an increasing number of elderly family caregivers both during the course of the illness and in the mixed relief and sorrow that occurs in bereavement[16,17]. The increasing scale of caregiver stress and vulnerability presents a challenge that has not yet been fully addressed.
- Population experts see the USA as rapidly becoming 'a majority of minorities'. Familiar ways of life and death have centred on a white Christian majority. Increasing ethnic and racial diversity is bringing a new mix of attitudes and expectations, including care of the dying and mourning and memorialization practices. There are

often attitude divisions within the same family system as tradition contends with response to external influences. Care providers will have their sensitivities tested.

• Life course coherence and continuity were once bolstered by long-time residence in a relatively stable place and by other supports for familiarity, belonging and predictability. Fewer of today's elders are dying from the worlds they knew and which knew them well[18]. The sense of meaning, coherence, and completion is becoming more difficult to achieve both as life nears its end and as the bereaved try to come to terms with their loss. It remains to be seen whether or not mental health specialists will expand their range to include such ongoing changes in the life course.

In a sense, there are no 'little griefs', and there may be no 'getting over' the greatest losses we experience in our lives. But most elderly adults have learned to live with disappointments, limitations and suffering. When bereavement comes, as a rule they do not need drugs, hospitalization and the whole rigmarole of the health care system. To be offered companionship and to see in that companion's eyes that one is still valued and needed is often all that is required for the survivor to get on with life.

REFERENCES

1. Carr D. Factors that influence late-life bereavement: considering data from the Changing Lives of Older Couples study. In Straube MS, Hansson RO, Schut H, Stroebe W (eds), *Handbook of Bereavement Research and Practice*. American Psychological Association, Washington, DC, 2008, 397–416.

2. Hayslip B, Jr, White DL. The grief of grandparents. In Straube MS, Hansson RO, Schut H, Stroebe W (eds), *Handbook of Bereavement Research and Practice*. American Psychological Association, Washington, DC, 2008, 441–60.

3. Nehari M, Grebler D, Toren A. A voice unheard: grandparents' grief over children who died of cancer. *Mortality* 2007; **13**: 66–79.

4. Doka KJ. Disenfranchised grief in historical and cultural perspective. In Straube MS, Hansson RO, Schut H, Stroebe W (eds), *Handbook of Bereavement Research and Practice*. American Psychological Association, Washington, DC, 2008, 223–40.

5. Gilliland G, Fleming S. A comparison of spousal anticipatory grief and conventional grief. *Death Stud* 1998; **22**: 541–70.

6. D'Epinay CJL, Cavalli S, Spini D. The death of a loved one: impact on health and relationships in very old age. *Omega* 2003; **47**: 265–84.

7. Mor V, Greer DS, Kastenbaum R (eds). *The Hospice Experiment*. Baltimore, MD: Johns Hopkins University Press.

8. Kastenbaum R. *The Psychology of Death*, 3rd edn. New York: Springer, 2000.

9. Parkes CM, Weiss RS. *Recovery from Bereavement*. New York: Basic Books, 1983.

10. Kastenbaum R. Death and bereavement in later life. In Kutscher AH (ed.) *Death and Bereavement*. Springfield, CT: Charles C. Thomas, 1969, 28–54.

11. Cicirelli VC. Sibling death and death fear in relation to depressive symptomatology in older adults. *J Gerontol B Psychol Sci Soc Sci* 2009; **64**(1): 24–32.

12. Greenberg J, Solomon S, Pyszcynski T. Terror management theory of self-esteem and cultural worldviews: empirical assessments and conceptual refinements. In Zanna MP (ed.), *Advances in Experimental Social Psychology*, vol. 29. San Diego: Academic Press, 1997, 61–141.

13. Kastenbaum R. Should we manage terror – if we could? *Omega* 2009; **59**(4): 271–304.

14. Larson DG, Hoyt WT. What has become of grief counseling? An evaluation of the empirical foundations of the new pessimism. *Prof Psychol Res Pr* 2007; **38**: 347–55.

15. Weisman AD. Bereavement and companion animals. *Omega* 1990–1991: **22**(4): 22–43.

16. Ballenger JF. *Self, Senility, and Alzheimer's Disease in Modern America: A History*. Baltimore, MD: Johns Hopkins University Press, 2006.

17. Sanders C, Ott CH, Kelger ST, Noonan P. The experience of high levels of grief in caregivers of persons with Alzheimer's disease and related dementia. *Death Stud* 2008; **32**: 495–523.

18. Kastenbaum R. Grieving in contemporary society. In Straube MS, Hansson RO, Schut H, Stroebe W (eds), *Handbook of Bereavement Research and Practice*. American Psychological Association, Washington, DC, 2008, 67–87.

90

Suicidal Behaviour

Brian Draper

School of Psychiatry, University of NSW, Sydney, Australia

Despite an increase in research knowledge about suicidal behaviour in old age, the translation into community understanding and clinical practice still lags. One common misunderstanding is about the rationality of suicide associated with age-related suffering[1]. While much old age suicidal behaviour occurs in this context, that does not mean it is rational. To better understand suicidal behaviour in late life, it is also important to look at the vulnerability factors from early and mid life. This chapter will examine suicidal behaviour from a life cycle perspective and consider a framework for prevention.

Although suicide rates worldwide are highest on average in persons aged over 75 years, being approximately three times higher than in persons under 25 years of age, the pattern is variable, with about one third of countries that report mortality data to the World Health Organization having higher rates in young adults than in older persons[2]. Furthermore, over the past 30 years many countries have reported a decline in suicide rates in older people alongside an increase in suicide rates in youth and young adults[2]. The reasons for this reduction are unclear but may include improved physical health in middle age and old age, better community services for the disabled to enhance independence, greater financial security in later life, marriage and the prescription of antidepressants[1,3].

In contrast, non-fatal suicidal behaviour declines with age in most countries, with the ratio of attempted to completed suicide in old age being estimated to be between 2:1 and 4:1 as compared with 100:1 to 200:1 in young persons[2]. Attempted suicide in old age closely resembles suicide, with high levels of lethal intent, less impulsivity and clinical features that are similar to those found in completed suicide[4,5]. Thus suicidal behaviour in the elderly is more likely to have a fatal outcome. However, there is a recently observed trend for the 'young old' aged 65–75 years to have higher rates of less lethal and more impulsive attempts, a phenomenon described as 'elderly adolescentism'[2]. Rates of indirect self-destructive behaviour in residential care are high, with one study reporting a weekly prevalence of 61% although the extent to which the behaviour could be regarded as intentional or part of a spectrum of suicidal behaviour is unclear[6]. Suicidal ideation in old age has prevalence rates reported between 2.3% and 15.9% in the previous month and lower rates have been reported in individuals aged over 75 years compared with those 'under 55 years of age'[2].

RISK FACTORS FOR SUICIDAL BEHAVIOUR

Risk factors in late life are similar to younger age groups and include demographic characteristics, psychopathology, personality traits, traumatic life events, physical ill health and disability, previous suicidal behaviour, genetic factors and access to lethal means[2]. However, over the age range, factors have different levels of influence, with one psychological autopsy study finding major depression was more likely in suicides aged over 55 years while substance abuse was more likely in suicides aged 21–54 years[7]. Risk factors that are more overtly important in suicidal behaviour in younger people may still convey vulnerability in late life. In a life cycle approach to understanding the development of risk for late life suicidal behaviour, it is important to recognize that some pathways begin early in life. It is often the interaction of distal risk factors with proximal factors that provides the lethal mix.

Demographic Factors

Across the life span, males have approximately a four times higher risk of suicide than females and with advancing age the male to female ratio increases[1]. Females are at higher risk of non-fatal suicidal behaviour, with rates about 1.5 times higher than males, but the rates tend to converge with advancing age[6]. There is some evidence that suicidal behaviour is more common in those who are divorced or widowed[2,4].

There is heterogeneity of suicide rates between countries and ethnicity appears to be a factor, with different suicide rates of ethnic groups within multicultural societies[2]. For example, in Australia suicide rates of older migrants are closely related to suicide rates in their country of origin[8]. Other cross-national research has found elderly suicide rates to be associated with population growth, the elderly dependency ratio and the proportion of elderly in the population[9]. There is also regional variation within countries, with higher rates reported in rural areas of some countries such as Australia[10]. In the United States, cross-state variation is related to macro-social indicators of social integration and aspects of state-level policies[11]. Low socioeconomic status has been found as a risk factor worldwide[1].

Early Life Factors

Genetic factors contribute to suicide risk by mediating transmission of impulsive aggression or neuroticism and neurocognitive deficits[12]. While there has been little research in late life, one study has suggested that an interaction between genetic factors and the physiological effects of ageing might have an important role in violent suicides[13]. Genetic factors also work indirectly by increasing the risk of mood disorders and substance abuse[12].

Principles and Practice of Geriatric Psychiatry, 3rd edn. Edited by Mohammed T. Abou-Saleh, Cornelius Katona and Anand Kumar
© 2011 John Wiley & Sons, Ltd

Childhood adversity, which includes abuse and parental neglect through death, separation and inadequate care, is a well-established risk factor for suicidal behaviour, depression and substance abuse in younger adults[12,14]. There is increasing evidence that childhood adversity influences late life suicidal behaviour and mental disorders too. Higher rates of childhood adversity were found in older persons who attempted suicide compared with controls[15]; childhood physical and sexual abuse was significantly more frequently reported by older persons with a history of suicidal behaviour, mood disorders and alcohol abuse in a large general practice survey[16]; and the risk of attempted suicide and suicide is higher in older Holocaust survivors[1].

Childhood adversity and genetic factors also affect personality development. A number of personality traits have been linked to suicidal behaviour in late life, including inflexibility, anxious, obsessional and 'low openness to experience' (individuals that are comfortable with the familiar and have a constricted range of interests) traits[1,17]. In essence these traits describe an older individual who has difficulty coping with the challenges related to ageing, including failing health, loss of confidants and demanding life events.

Adulthood Factors

It would seem self-evident that the lifestyle followed by an individual as an adult, including their interpersonal relationships and employment, will have some bearing on their health and well-being in late life. For example, involuntary job loss near retirement age has been found to lead to enduring depressive symptoms in individuals with low finances[18].

The links to late life suicidal behaviour are indirect and largely mediated through the impact mid-life lifestyle factors have upon the development of late life risk factors such as physical health and depression. There is increasing evidence that mid-life vascular risk factors such as hypertension, smoking, diabetes and metabolic syndrome, which are associated with lifestyle factors such as diet and exercise, may lead to late life depression, cognitive impairment, and cerebrovascular and cardiovascular disorders[19,20]. Further, a case-control of suicides over age 50 years found that cerebrovascular risk factor scores were significantly higher in suicide cases[21].

Late Life Factors

Psychopathology

Up to 97% of older persons with serious suicidal behaviour have a mental disorder[1,4,5,22]. A review of controlled psychological autopsy studies found that the presence of any Axis I disorder was associated with an elevated risk of suicide in older persons with significant odds ratios ranging from 27.4 to 113.1[22]. Depression is the major independent risk factor across cultures and although the type of depression varies, major depression is the strongest predictor of suicidal behaviour in late life, accounting for about 50% of cases[1,4,5,7,22]. Although many cases are recurrent episodes, first-episode major depression is prominent too[1,4,22]. Other types of depression including dysthymia, minor depression and subsyndromal depression are also important and may have a particular role in older persons with co-morbid chronic physical ill health and disability[1,4]. In the context of recovery from a depressive episode, unremitting hopelessness can increase suicide risk[23].

Other mental disorders are less commonly found in late life suicidal behaviour, though co-morbid disorders are common[1,4,5,22]. Late-life psychoses, including schizophrenia and bipolar disorder, account

for less than 10% of attempted and completed suicides[1,4,5,22]. The role of anxiety disorders is unclear, with some studies finding an increased risk though it seems usually in the context of mixed anxiety/depressive states[1,22]. Alcohol abuse, though less frequently implicated in old age compared to younger suicides, remains a significant factor especially with co-morbid depression[1,4,5]. Personality disorders are less common in suicidal behaviour in late life compared with younger cohorts, being present in 2.5–7% of older suicide attempters[1,5].

Until recently, dementia has not been regarded as a risk factor for suicide. A nationwide longitudinal study from Denmark using register data reported that hospital-diagnosed dementia was associated with an elevated risk of suicide particularly in those aged 50–69 years, where the relative risk was 8.5 in men and 10.8 in women. The risk was higher in the first three months after diagnosis, particularly in men. Controlling for mood disorders reduced but did not eliminate the increased risk. The risk was higher in Alzheimer's disease than in vascular dementia[24]. In some, frontal lobe impairments may lead to impulsive, poorly planned attempts. It is unclear whether insight into the dementing process is a factor that increases the risk of suicidality[1,4].

Previous suicidal behaviour

Compared with younger age groups, a history of suicidal behaviour is less frequent in older persons with suicidal behaviour but follow-up studies of older suicide attempters have found high rates of repetition[1,25]. In the WHO/EURO multicentre study of suicidal behaviour, 13% of older people admitted to hospital after a suicide attempt died by suicide within 12 months and 11% made further attempts[25]. Survivors of suicidal behaviour in old age remain a high risk group and require close monitoring. Observational studies suggest that older suicide attempters are likely to receive specialist mental health management, particularly if they have a diagnosed mood disorder, but treatment studies are lacking[5].

Physical health and disability

While physical ill health is a contributory factor in most cases of late life suicidal behaviour, its precise role is unclear[1]. Some studies have found an independent effect of physical illness that is increased when there are multiple illnesses, while others have found little evidence of a physical illness effect[1,26]. There is a lack of consistency regarding specific illnesses that might increase suicide risk, but chronic pain, breathlessness and functional impairment are frequently reported features[1,26]. These may result in dependence on carers, loss of dignity and the fear of institutionalization that may contribute to demoralization, depression and suicidality. A threshold phenomenon may exist whereby the physically ill may become suicidal with milder degrees of depression[4], or, put another way, physical illnesses may amplify suicide risk in those with premorbid vulnerability[27]. Depression, pain and insomnia have the capacity to temporarily affect judgement by subtly distorting the patient's perceptions in a manner that may convince family, friends and doctor of the 'rationality' of suicide, especially in those with terminal illness, which is present in about 5–10% of older persons with suicidal behaviour. Yet the wish to die usually resolves once these symptoms are treated. Psychological reactions occur, with some people feeling overwhelmed by the knowledge of a serious illness and others convincing themselves that they have cancer, often ignoring reassurances by their doctor[28]. Some physical illnesses, including cancers, thyroid disorders and cerebrovascular disease, can cause severe depression and these might not be detected until after a suicide attempt[4].

Psychosocial factors

In general, disruption of social ties increases suicide risk in old age independent of the presence of mental disorders[22]. As in other age groups, family discord is perhaps the most powerful psychosocial factor[1,22,27]. In many cases the problems are chronic and there is some evidence that males are more vulnerable[1]. It is likely that chronic family discord interacts with physical health issues in situations that include those who are disabled and feel a burden on others, and in caregivers who become severely stressed in caring for a disabled partner, where there is an increased risk of murder/suicide[1]. A range of other life events, particularly those involving loss, including recent bereavement, and financial problems have been implicated in late life suicidal behaviour[1,4,5,27].

Living alone has consistently been identified as a factor and this is often regarded as a proxy for loneliness, social isolation and inadequate social support[1,4,5,22]. Accommodation issues, including fear of nursing home placement and dissatisfaction with living arrangements, are also reported[1,4]. It is unclear whether the suicide rate in nursing homes is different to the general population but the main risk factors of depression and physical disability are the same[1]. Indirect self-destructive behaviour, including refusal to eat, drink or take medications, is common in nursing home residents and while most cases appear to be associated with severe dementia rather than depression with suicidal intent[6], there are likely to be some suicidal individuals.

Biological factors

As with the previously mentioned genetic factors, two other biological factors associated with suicide have not been well studied in late life. Serotonergic neurotransmitter abnormalities have been found to be associated with suicidal behaviour across the age range with low levels of 5-hydroxyindoleactic acid in cerebrospinal fluid[29]. Non-suppression of the dexamethasone suppression test, which is a measure of the hypothalamic–pituitary axis activity in mood disorders, is also predictive of suicide[29].

Other late life biological factors include cerebrovascular disease and Alzheimer's disease. The risks of suicide and suicidal ideation have been reported as higher in Alzheimer's disease than in vascular dementia but studies of Alzheimer's disease neuropathological changes in late life suicide are inconsistent[1]. Interestingly, older subjects with major depression who were apolipoprotein E ε4 (APOE4) carriers had an increased suicide attempt history than depressed subjects who were not APOE4 carriers[30].

Risk factors are unlikely to act independently in most cases but at present our understanding of how identified risk factors interact to determine risk in an individual is limited[1,22]. The motivations that appear to drive the final suicidal act are quite varied and reflect this multiplicity of pathways[28]. In addition, whether an individual has access to a lethal means that is acceptable to them plays a critical role, and this latter factor varies between cultures[1].

STRATEGIES FOR SUICIDE PREVENTION IN LATE LIFE

While an understanding of factors that are associated with suicidal behaviour provides a platform upon which to build prevention strategies, there is very little known about protective factors. There is weak evidence that spirituality and good quality of life may be protective but more research is required[1].

A public health approach to suicide prevention considers three levels of interventions. Universal strategies implement broadly directed initiatives to prevent suicidal behaviour and related morbidity through reducing risk and enhancing protective factors at a population level. Selective strategies target 'high risk' (at a population level) asymptomatic or presymptomatic older persons with distal risk factors for suicide. Indicated strategies focus on individuals with detectable symptoms and/or other proximal risk factors for suicide[1].

Universal Prevention

These strategies should concentrate upon improvement of quality of life and prevention of depression in late life in the general population. A whole of life approach to ageing that addresses key issues such as reduction of childhood adversity, provision of basic health care, reduction of poverty, and promotion of a healthy lifestyle, including diet, exercise, and reduction of substance abuse and smoking is required. The relationship between vascular disease and late-life depression is an obvious focus of health education programmes over the life span. As such, suicide prevention would not be the main focus of the strategy but rather it would be one of the potential outcomes.

Benefits accrue for persons of all ages so programmes that focus on late life issues such as ageism, normal ageing, healthy lifestyle in late life, and stigma of late-life mental disorder are important. It is important to realize that there is still a perception that it is 'normal' for older people to be depressed and that 'nothing can be done' about it, even though the available evidence contradicts this. These negative attitudes can set the tone of society.

Psychosocial strategies that might improve well-being and reduce depression in late life could focus upon encouragement of social interaction through attendance at clubs, connection with family, participation in casual work, becoming a volunteer, and engagement in pleasurable activities such as physical exercise, music, dance, education, travel and sport. For many older people lack of transport thwarts efforts to accomplish these goals so an improved senior's transport strategy would be beneficial. An important study of a community-based programme that targeted the elderly in the rural town of Yuri in Japan involved population strategies including psychoeducation, group activities and self-assessment of depression over an eight-year period. It proved to be effective in reducing the risk of suicide in females but not males[31].

Selective Prevention

The aim of selective prevention is to prevent suicidal behaviour and related morbidity by addressing the specific characteristics that confer high risk. Older persons with a history of depression and/or suicidal behaviour, chronic pain sufferers, and disabled older persons who live alone or with few social supports are some examples.

Education is an important strategy. Asymptomatic older persons with a history of major affective disorder should be educated about warning signs of depression to enable early intervention. Programmes that aim to minimize the effects of disability upon older people by providing services that enhance independent function are of critical importance. This has been the general direction taken in many countries where aged care service delivery has increasingly focused upon maintaining older disabled persons at home. A programme established in the Veneto region of Italy used Tele-Help, a portable device that lets users send alarm signals activating a pre-established network of help and assistance, and Tele-Check, where trained staff members contact each client at least twice a week to offer emotional support and monitor the client's condition through a short, informal interview. At ten-year evaluation, a significantly lower than expected number of suicidal deaths was observed in the users compared to the general population[32]. Another approach is to focus upon the prevention of depression in the elderly with chronic physical co-morbidity. A six-session problem-solving therapy intervention in older patients with age-related macular degeneration led to a 50% reduction of new episodes of major and minor depression at two months after completion of the treatment although the effect had disappeared by six months[33].

The promotion of community groups and religious organizations to contact and support isolated older people should be encouraged. Potential target groups include rural elders, older migrants and carers. Older men are particularly vulnerable to depression and suicide in the year after divorce or death of their spouse and so could be specifically targeted for counselling in primary health care.

Indicated Prevention

The aim of indicated prevention is to identify and treat older persons with detectable symptoms and/or other proximal risk factors for suicide. Recognition of depression and suicide risk by gatekeepers (e.g. general practitioners, clergy, nurses, home care workers, police, ambulance officers, social workers) is an important component. GPs and other physicians have difficulties in the identification, assessment and management of depression and suicide risk in old age. This is accentuated with co-morbid physical illness where there are low levels of recognition, diagnosis and treatment of depression[34].

Studies from around the developed world consistently find that the majority of older suicide victims have been in contact with health professionals, particularly GPs, in the months before death[1]. While communication of suicidal ideation occurs in up to 45% of mental health contacts, it is less likely to occur in GP contacts and with older persons[1]. There is little known about contacts with nurses and other allied health professionals in the context of hospital and community treatment of physical ailments. Hence it is unclear how often health professional contacts in the weeks before suicide represent an opportunity for suicide prevention.

Despite this uncertainty, education of 'at risk' older people and their carers, gatekeepers and health professionals involved in their care is the key. The education needs to be linked to an intervention to improve its effectiveness, with strategies that include the removal of barriers to care, depression screening, and the use of treatment guidelines. A community-based 10-year suicide prevention programme for older people in the Japanese rural town of Joboji with strategies including screening for depression, follow-up with mental health care or psychiatric treatment, and health education on depression found that the relative risks estimated by the age-adjusted odds ratios for both males and females were reduced to almost 25% more than a regional historical trend, with a better response to education for females than for males[35].

One important component of health professional education is the assessment of suicide risk and management of older people at high risk. Even when depression is suspected, the assessment of suicide risk is often missed in older patients. A GP survey using case vignettes of older people with depression found high levels of depression recognition but only 2.4% spontaneously indicated that they would ask about suicidal ideation, which increased to 77% with prompting. The rest either indicated that they thought the patient would communicate suicidal thoughts themselves or that they feared that they might induce suicide by asking directly[36]. Assessment of suicide risk requires the health professional to be attentive, calm and non-threatening; to give the patient space and time to vent; to work in collaboration with the patient; and to use the word suicide without flinching. The use of open-ended questions followed up by specific questions about the nature, timing and context of suicidal thoughts is recommended. The only effective means of identifying those at risk is direct questioning[37]. Deterrents to suicidal behaviour, including religion and fear of upsetting family or friends, need to be determined. Collateral information from family and friends should be obtained as often the family member is aware of suicide risk but will not inform the health professional unless specifically asked[38]. The American Psychiatric Association's 'Practice Guideline for the Assessment and Treatment of Patients with Suicidal Behaviors' states that family and friends can be contacted without the patient's consent if suicidality is suspected[39].

All depressed older persons should be assessed for suicide risk but how often this should be repeated during the course of the illness is unclear. If enquiries about suicide risk are repeated too often therapeutic rapport might be undermined. Many older depressed patients were assessed by GPs to be improving in the weeks before suicide and so suicide risk assessment was not considered[38]. Improvement in depression can be deceptive in terms of suicide risk[1].

In the absence of clinical depression there are some other situations in the context of the older person's life circumstances that might warrant a suicide risk assessment. Persons with late-life psychosis with distressing persecutory symptoms are one example. As noted earlier, suicide risk is increased in older people with obsessional, anxious and low 'openness to experience' personality traits. Such individuals may have a restricted capacity to adapt to change and the various challenges associated with ageing. Recent life stressors, including the diagnosis of cancer or other serious disorders such as Alzheimer's disease or the death of a spouse or a close friend, may be overwhelming. Chronic stressors such as pain, loneliness, complicated grief or severe disability, especially in the absence of adequate social support, are all circumstances that might lead to a suicide attempt in the vulnerable person, especially if there has been a history of previous suicide attempts and in the presence of substance abuse. There are some types of behaviour that might alert the clinician to suicidal preoccupation. These include the giving away of possessions, changing of will, stockpiling of pills and passive indirect self-destructive behaviour such as refusal to eat and medication non-compliance. However, pervasive hopelessness was the most frequently reported observation in one study of the last health professional contact with suicide victims[38].

High-risk management guidelines for older suicidal patients in primary care settings were developed for the Prevention of Suicide in Primary Care Elderly: Collaborative Trial (PROSPECT)[37]. The intensity of the suicidal ideation, clarity of plans and access to means should determine the location of care. Hospitalization is often indicated, particularly when there is severe depression with features of psychosis, agitation, hopelessness, refusal to eat, poor insight, ruminating insomnia or where there is co-morbid substance abuse. Impulsivity, especially in association with impairments of executive function, is another feature that might require short-term hospitalization. Other factors to consider include the lack of social supports, and presence of concurrent medical issues and associated functional impairment that impact upon safe outpatient treatment, a history of poor compliance with treatment, or where the older person appears to have 'given up'[1].

Outcomes of hospitalization related to suicidal behaviour have not been specifically studied. The resolution of suicidal ideation before discharge is paramount and the clinician needs to be aware that the intensity of suicidal thoughts can fluctuate from day to day in the context of major depression[40]. Integration of hospital and post-discharge community care improves the outcomes of older depressed patients through strategies that include having the community nurse get to know the patient before discharge, a pre-discharge home visit to check on functional needs and remove any guns or stockpiled medications, continuity of medical care post-discharge, and members of the multidisciplinary inpatient team having a transitional role to help the older patient and the family settle in at home[1].

Optimal management of the older suicidal patient requires the development of a therapeutic alliance that is often best achieved by ensuring that alleviation of the patient's suffering, whether it be physical, psychological or spiritual, is central to the care being provided. Important components of community treatment include an individualized case management approach with ongoing care (at least weekly until suicidal risk has settled), medication monitoring, and psychoeducation of the patient and carer. Explicit written instructions to the older patient and family about what to do if suicidal thoughts recur and the provision of an emergency contact are required. Avoidance of alcohol and illicit drugs should be stressed[37].

It is beyond the scope of this chapter to discuss treatment of depression in detail but it is essential that effective treatment be provided that not only obtains a response but also achieves remission. The available evidence suggests that electroconvulsive therapy is the most effective treatment for severe depression in late life, particularly when there are psychotic features or with high acute suicide risk. Antidepressant medication remains the cornerstone of effective treatment for major depression even with co-morbid chronic physical illness where effectiveness is reduced and should be maintained for at least two years to prevent relapse. Psychosocial treatments, including the various types of psychotherapy, activity programmes, exercise and supportive therapies, are crucial[34].

Improving the effectiveness of the treatment of depression in primary care can be achieved through collaborations between primary care health professionals and mental health professionals. The collaboration should involve a significant educational and supervisory approach by the mental health professional. An example is provided by the multi-centre PROSPECT study, where a depression health specialist was assigned to assist the primary care physician with guideline management based on an algorithm that included the selective serotonin re-uptake inhibitor (SSRI) antidepressant citalopram and/or interpersonal psychotherapy. Rates of suicidal ideation declined faster in the intervention patients compared with usual care after four months of treatment[41].

There is debate about whether antidepressants reduce the risk of suicide, with naturalistic studies suggesting that the higher rates of antidepressant prescription since the introduction of the SSRIs have been associated with lower suicide rates[1]. Concerns have been raised that SSRIs might increase the risk of suicide in the elderly, particularly violent suicide, in the first month of treatment but the absolute risk is low and probably outweighed by the benefits of treatment[42]. There is stronger evidence that lithium prophylaxis has specific anti-suicide effects apart from its prophylactic efficacy in affective disorders but there are no studies that have specifically examined whether this occurs in old age[1].

CONCLUSION

A life cycle approach is required to obtain a better understanding of suicidal behaviour in late life because the causes are complex and involve factors that arise from the entire lifespan. No single prevention strategy is likely to be successful. A multifaceted, multilayered approach to suicide prevention in old age is required.

REFERENCES

1. De Leo D, Draper B, Krysinska K. Suicidal elderly people in clinical and community settings. Risk factors, treatment, and suicide prevention. In Wasserman D, Wasserman C (eds), *Oxford Textbook of Suicidology and Suicide Prevention. A Global Perspective*. Oxford: Oxford University Press, 2009, 703–19.
2. De Leo D, Krysinska K, Bertolote JM *et al*. Suicidal behaviors on the five continents among the elderly. In Wasserman D, Wasserman C (eds), *Oxford Textbook of Suicidology and Suicide Prevention. A Global Perspective*. Oxford: Oxford University Press, 2009, 693–702.
3. Gunnell D, Middleton N, Whitley E *et al*. Why are suicide rates rising in young men but falling in the elderly? – a time-series analysis of trends in England and Wales 1950–1998. *Soc Sci Med* 2003; **57**: 595–611.
4. Draper B. Attempted suicide in old age. Editorial review. *Int J Geriatr Psychiatry* 1996; **11**: 577–87.
5. Chan J, Draper B, Banerjee S. Deliberate self-harm in older adults: a review of the literature from 1995 to 2004. *Int J Geriatr Psychiatry* 2007; **22**: 720–32.
6. Draper B, Brodaty H, Low L-F *et al*. Self destructive behaviours in nursing home residents. *J Am Geriatr Soc* 2002; **50**: 354–8.
7. Conwell Y, Duberstein PR, Cox C *et al*. Relationships of age and Axis 1 diagnoses in victims of completed suicide: a psychological autopsy study. *Am J Psychiatry* 1996; **153**: 1001–8.
8. Burvill P. Suicide in immigrant populations in Australia: the last four decades. *Synergy* 2000; **winter**: 3.
9. Shah A. The relationship between population growth and elderly suicide rates: a cross-national study. *Int Psychogeriatr* 2009; **21**: 379–83.
10. Morrell S, Taylor R, Slaytor E *et al*. Urban and rural suicide differentials in migrants and the Australian born, NSW Australia. *Soc Sci Med* 1999; **49**: 81–91.
11. Giles-Sims J, Lockhart C. Explaining cross-state differences in elderly suicide rates and identifying state-level public policy responses that reduce rates. *Suicide Life Threat Behav* 2006; **36**: 694–708.
12. Brent DA, Melham N. Familial transmission of suicidal behaviour. *Psychiatr Clin North Am* 2008; **31**: 157–77.
13. Stefulj J, Kubat M, Balija M *et al*. TPH gene polymorphism and aging: indication of combined effects on the predisposition to violent suicide. *Am J Med Genet B Neuropsychiatr Genet* 2006; **141**: 139–41.
14. Arnow BA. Relationships between childhood maltreatment, adult health and psychiatric outcomes, and medical utilization. *J Clin Psychiatry* 2004; **65**(suppl 12): 10–15.
15. Beautrais AL. A case-control study of suicide and attempted suicide in older adults. *Suicide Life Threat Behav* 2002; **32**(1): 1–9.
16. Draper B, Pfaff J, Pirkis J *et al*. The long-term effects of childhood abuse on the quality of life and health of older people:

results from the DEPS-GP Project. *J Am Geriatr Soc* 2008; **56**: 262–71.

17. Duberstein P, Conwell Y, Caine ED. Age differences in the personality traits of suicide completers: preliminary findings from a psychological autopsy study. *Psychiatry* 1994; **57**: 213–24.

18. Gallo WT, Bradley EH, Dubin JA *et al.* The persistence of depressive symptoms in older workers who experience involuntary job loss: results from the health and retirement survey. *J Gerontol B Psychol Sci Soc Sci* 2006; **61**(4): S221–8.

19. Koponen H, Jokelainen J, Keinanen-Kiukaanniemi S *et al.* Metabolic syndrome predisposes to depressive symptoms: a population-based 7-year follow-up study. *J Clin Psychiatry* 2008; **69**(2): 178–82.

20. Flicker L. Vascular factors in geriatric psychiatry: time to take a serious look. *Curr Opin Psychiatry* 2008; **21**: 551–4.

21. Chan SS, Lyness JM, Conwell Y. Do cerebrovascular risk factors confer risk for suicide in later life? A case-control study. *Am J Geriatr Psychiatry* 2007; **15**: 541–4.

22. Conwell Y, Duberstein PR, Caine ED. Risk factors for suicide in later life. *Biol Psychiatry* 2002; **52**: 193–204.

23. Szanto K, Reynolds CF, III, Conwell Y *et al.* High levels of hopelessness persist in geriatric patients with remitted depression and a history of attempted suicide. *J Am Geriatr Soc* 1998; **46**: 1401–6.

24. Erlangsen A, Zarit SH, Conwell Y. Hospital-diagnosed dementia and suicide: a longitudinal study using prospective, nationwide register data. *Am J Geriatr Psychiatry* 2008; **16**: 220–28.

25. De Leo D, Padovani W, Lonnqvist J *et al.* Repetition of suicidal behaviour in elderly Europeans: a prospective longitudinal study. *J Affect Disord* 2002; **72**: 291–5.

26. Juurlink DN, Herrmann N, Szalai JP *et al.* Medical illness and the risk of suicide in the elderly. *Arch Intern Med* 2004; **164**: 1179–84.

27. Duberstein P, Conwell Y, Conner KR *et al.* Suicide at 50 years of age and older: perceived physical illness, family discord and financial strain. *Psychol Med* 2004; **34**: 137–46.

28. Snowdon J, Baume P. A study of suicides of older people in Sydney. *Int J Geriatr Psychiatry* 2002; **16**: 1–9.

29. Mann JJ, Currier D, Stanley B *et al.* Can biological tests assist prediction of suicide in mood disorders? *Int J Neuropsychopharmacology* 2006; **9**: 465–74.

30. Hwang JP, Yang CH, Hong CJ *et al.* Association of APOE genetic polymorphism with cognitive function and suicide history in geriatric depression. *Dement Geriatr Cogn Disord* 2006; **22**: 334–8.

31. Oyama H, Watanabe N, Ono Y *et al.* Community-based suicide prevention through group activity for the elderly successfully reduced the high suicide rate for females. *Psychiatry Clin Neurosci* 2005; **59**: 337–44.

32. De Leo D, Dello Buono M, Dwyer J. Suicide among the elderly: the long-term impact of a telephone support and assessment intervention in northern Italy. *Br J Psychiatry* 2002; **181**: 226–9.

33. Rovner BW, Casten RJ, Hegel MT *et al.* Preventing depression in age-related macular degeneration. *Arch Gen Psychiatry* 2007; **64**: 886–92.

34. Chiu E, Ames D, Draper B, Snowdon J. Depressive disorders in the elderly: a review. In Herrman H, Maj M, Sartorius N (eds), *Depressive Disorders*, 3rd edn. Chichester: Wiley-Blackwell, 2009, 197–257.

35. Oyama H, Koida J, Sakashita T *et al.* Community-based prevention for suicide in elderly by depression screening and follow-up. *Community Ment Health J* 2004; **40**(3): 249–63.

36. Stoppe G, Sandholzer H, Huppertz C *et al.* Family physicians and the risk of suicide in the depressed elderly. *J Affect Disord* 1999; **54**(1–2): 193–8.

37. Brown GK, Bruce ML, Pearson JL. High-risk management guidelines for elderly suicidal patients in primary care settings. *Int J Geriatr Psychiatry* 2001; **16**(6): 593–601.

38. Draper B, Snowdon J, Wyder M. A pilot study of a suicide victim's last contact with a health professional. *Crisis* 2008; **29**: 96–101.

39. Practice guideline for the assessment and treatment of patients with suicidal behaviors. *Am J Psychiatry* 2003; **160**(11 suppl): 1–60.

40. Szanto K, Reynolds CF, III, Frank E *et al.* Suicide in elderly depressed patients. Is active vs passive suicidal ideation a clinically valid distinction? *Am J Geriatr Psychiatry* 1996; **4**: 197–207.

41. Bruce ML, Ten Have TR, Reynolds CF, III *et al.* Reducing suicidal ideation and depressive symptoms in depressed older primary care patients: a randomized controlled trial. *JAMA* 2004; **291**(9): 1081–91.

42. Juurlink DN, Mamdani MM, Kopp A *et al.* The risk of suicide with selective serotonin reuptake inhibitors in the elderly. *Am J Psychiatry* 2006; **16**(5): 813–21.

91

The Assessment of Depressive Syndromes

Adriana P. Hermida and William M. McDonald

Emory University School of Medicine, Atlanta, USA

Among community dwelling older adults, the prevalence of major depression ranges between 1% and 4% with a higher proportion of women meeting criteria for depression with no significant racial or ethnic differences[1]. Although the prevalence of individuals with major depressive disorder may not be as high as for younger subjects[2], high levels of *depressive symptoms* are relatively common in the elderly living in the community, and the number of elders with depression syndromes increases in patients with chronic medical illnesses[1,3,4]. The number of medically ill elders diagnosed with depressive syndromes in long-term care facilities is estimated at 10–15% with up to 35% experiencing significant depressive symptoms[5-7].

The diagnosis of depression in the elderly requires a multidimensional approach and should be undertaken with a clear understanding of the normal ageing process and the psychosocial factors that are unique to the elderly. These aspects of ageing are discussed in Chapter 18. Depression and depressive disorders are often misunderstood by physicians caring for the elderly as well as by the lay public, including family members and, often, the elderly patient. 'Ageism' is the term used to describe the discrimination against people because of their age and nowhere is this more apparent than in the diagnosis and treatment of depressed elders, particularly those with co-morbid medical illnesses. The oft-repeated phrases epitomize this way of thinking 'Why wouldn't they be depressed … they are old?' and 'Of course they are depressed – they live in a nursing home and have cancer'. Underlying this viewpoint is the notion that treating the depressed elderly is futile and a waste of valuable health care resources. Among other factors ageism has been shown to be an important component in the decision as to whether to start drug therapy in elderly patients[8].

A more rational view is to consider the costs of the treatment of depression in comparison with potential treatment benefits, including the cost savings to society of an individual remaining functionally independent in a community setting[9]. In this light the treatment of depression in the elderly has the potential for providing both benefits to the individual and health care savings. Depressive symptoms can lead to accelerated cognitive decline, physical impairment and increased health care costs[10]. Increased service utilization and social morbidity are common in patients with depressive symptoms even when these symptoms are not severe enough to fulfil the criteria for a major psychiatric disorder[11]. Concomitant depression can limit compliance with medical treatments and worsen the cognitive decline

associated with dementia. Further, depression can adversely affect the clinical course of other medical illnesses and increase morbidity and mortality[12,13], and the elderly have the highest suicide rate of any age group[14]. The social and economic consequences of this disorder in the elderly are severe.

Yet the diagnosis and treatment of elderly depressive disorders can be difficult. The elderly are often subject to more adverse side effects from pharmacotherapy, and the diagnosis of depression is complicated by the overlapping symptoms of depression, concomitant medical illnesses and normal ageing[15]. In fact, the elderly often present with more subtle forms of depression (e.g. minor or subsyndromal depressive disorders) that can be difficult to diagnose, yet cause significant disability and make the decision to treat more difficult. Some have argued that elderly depressives should have specific age-appropriate criteria that include these subsyndromal symptoms since the elderly are not easily classified by traditional psychiatric nomenclature[16].

This chapter will review the multiple depressive syndromes in depression and provide guidance on making the correct diagnosis of depression in elderly patients, particularly those with concomitant medical illness. The diagnosis and clinical significance of subsyndromal depressive syndromes will also be outlined in detail. Finally, the appropriate method for taking a history and the basic laboratory tests needed to eliminate common medical conditions that mimic depression as well as the medications that may cause depressive symptoms will also be reviewed.

THE SYNDROME OF LATE-LIFE DEPRESSION

To accurately assess the depressed older adult, the clinician must consider the range of depressive disorders from the more severe major depression to the subsyndromal depressive disorders. Depressive disorders include the mood disorders outlined in the Diagnostic and Statistical Manual of Mental Disorders Version IV (DSM-IV): major depressive disorder, dysthymic disorder, mood disorder due to a general medical condition, substance-induced mood disorder, bipolar disorder, mood disorder not otherwise specified (which include the minor and subsyndromal depression) and adjustment disorder.

Major depression is distinguished from the other mood disorders by the severity and persistence of symptoms, which by definition have lasted for at least two weeks and are associated with significant impairment in an individual's social, occupational or other

Principles and Practice of Geriatric Psychiatry, 3rd edn. Edited by Mohammed T. Abou-Saleh, Cornelius Katona and Anand Kumar
© 2011 John Wiley & Sons, Ltd

important areas of functioning. Symptoms of major depression comprise depressed mood and/or anhedonia and associated neurovegetative and cognitive symptoms, including significant weight loss/weight gain or decreased/increased appetite, insomnia or hypersomnia, psychomotor agitation or retardation, diminished ability to think or concentrate, feelings of worthlessness or excessive inappropriate guilt, and recurrent thoughts of death or suicide.

Specifiers describing the quality of the current episode include melancholic, atypical and catatonic features. *Melancholic* features consist of lack of mood reactivity to pleasurable stimuli, diurnal variation in mood (i.e. depression worse in the morning), early morning awakening, psychomotor retardation or agitation, significant weight loss or anorexia and excessive or inappropriate guilt. A melancholic depression may be associated with specific neuroanatomic changes[17], and may affect response to antidepressants[18-21], electroconvulsive therapy (ECT)[22,23] and psychotherapy[24,25]. *Atypical* features include mood reactivity, increased appetite or weight gain, hypersomnia, leaden paralysis and extreme sensitivity to interpersonal rejection. Atypical depression in the elderly has been shown to respond preferentially to monoamine oxidase inhibitors (MAOIs) although the MAOIs may be more difficult to use in this population[15,26]. The specifier *catatonic features* is appropriate when the clinical picture is characterized by marked psychomotor disturbances that involve motoric immobility, excessive motor activity, extreme negativism, mutism, peculiarities of voluntary movements, echolalia and echopraxia. Motoric immobility can be manifested by cataplexy or stupor. Catatonic states have been found to occur in 5–9% of psychiatric inpatients. Among inpatients, 25–50% of catatonic states occur in association with mood disorders, 10–15% in association with schizophrenia, and the remainder in association with other mental disorders and a wide variety of medical conditions[27].

An additional specifier of major depression in the DSM-IV criteria is a *seasonal pattern*, which is associated with the onset and remission of major depressive episodes at characteristic times of the year. This pattern of onset and remission of episodes must have occurred during the past two years.

In the DSM-IV, depression is subtyped according to whether the mood disturbance is associated with psychotic symptoms. Psychotic symptoms in major depression are more likely to be mood-congruent (i.e. delusions or hallucinations of a depressive nature). Psychotic depression may be more common in late life. Many elderly patients with psychosis develop delusions of poverty, somatic delusions or persecutory ideations[28,29]. Hallucinations of derogatory voices are rare. Known precipitants of psychotic symptoms in the elderly include personal trauma, physical illness and certain medications such as corticosteroids and anti-parkinsonian medications.

Subsyndromal depressions (SSDs) include minor depression, dysthymia and syndromal depression that does not meet the criteria for major depression. SSDs are characterized by depressive symptoms that do not meet full criteria for a major depression but are associated with depressed mood and significant disability[30]. SSD is common and associated with significant impairment in a number of areas of social and occupational functioning and an increased risk of developing syndromal major depression[31,32]. Minor depression is a mood disorder that does not meet full criteria for major depressive disorder but which is associated with at least two depressive symptoms that are sustained for a period of two weeks (although not necessarily every day) without the degree of impairment in major depression. Technically a patient with minor depression would be coded as 'Depression, not otherwise specified' or NOS since minor depression is a research diagnosis. Research, much of it in primary care clinics, supports the

validity of minor depression as a distinct clinical entity[31]. Dysthymic disorder (dysthymia) is defined as a chronic low-grade depression, which lasts for at least two years. Personality styles and the individual's ability to cope with changing life situations may predispose the individual to develop a dysthymic disorder (see Chapter 104) and older adults with changing roles and life conditions may be particularly prone to dysthymia. Additionally, dysthymic disorder may develop secondary to a medical disorder, anxiety disorder or somatization disorder. Dysthymia preceding a major depressive episode has been shown to predict a poor outcome to treatment[33]. Phenomenologically, SSD is the 'grey' zone between syndromal major depression and depressive symptoms. In geriatric psychiatry, depression is often defined as a spectrum rather than a dichotomy. There is increasing evidence that elderly subjects meeting the criteria for SSD have levels of cognitive and functional impairment intermediate between elders who are not depressed and those with major depression[34]. Nevertheless, patients with SSD demonstrate significant disability, are more likely to have persistent depressive symptoms which worsen over a year, be at a higher risk of developing major depression, and benefit from somatic treatments and psychotherapy[25,35]. Clearly, future research is needed to clarify the prevalence and treatment response of SSD in order to target appropriate treatments.

Substance-induced mood disorder is a prominent and persistent disturbance in mood that is judged to be due to the direct physiological effects of a substance such as excessive alcohol use. Alcohol abuse in older adults is common and may go for years misdiagnosed[36]. The elderly are particularly prone to substance-induced mood disorders because of chronic and often excessive use of over-the-counter medications mixed with prescription medications[37,38]. Increasingly the elderly are using herbal medications and often the effects of herbal medications are unknown, particularly in combination with other drugs[39].

The diagnosis of adjustment disorder with depressed mood is appropriate for an elderly patient adjusting to severe changes in lifestyle and the loss of loved ones. In the DSM-IV, the patient is not classified with an adjustment disorder unless his/her reaction is considered maladaptive and the level of impairment is significantly severe, and greater than what would be normally expected. Whether the elderly subject's reaction to these stressors is classified as a disorder is a clinical judgement. Several common life events that may prove to be stressors in the elderly include retirement, financial problems, living in high crime areas, physical illness, the death of a spouse and moving to an institutional setting. Yet older adults also may also be protected from stress as those who survive into old age are more likely to have relatively more socioeconomic security and the benefit of the wisdom that can come with older age[40]. Regardless, the clinician should observe the patient diagnosed with adjustment disorder longitudinally for the development of symptoms of a major depression if the individual's reaction to stress is persistent or severe.

The symptom profile of older patients with depression has also been described as qualitatively distinct from that of younger adults. Depressed elderly patients are more likely to show cognitive changes, somatic symptoms, fatigue and loss of interest as opposed to depressed mood and guilt[41,42]. Other researchers emphasize that these differing presentations are the result of accompanying cognitive changes with ageing and co-morbid medical illness, which are more likely to occur in older depressed patients, and that depressed elderly patients without concomitant medical illnesses have presentations similar to younger subjects[43]. Support for this latter view has been provided by Blazer and his colleagues[44], who compared depressive symptoms in a group of middle-aged (35–50-year-old) and older (60-year-old) inpatients with melancholic depression. The symptom profiles of these patients were markedly similar to the elderly, differing only in their more frequent reporting of weight loss and less frequent suicidal thoughts. Finally, Blazer discusses some of the misconceptions of depression in the elderly, pointing out that, as discussed above, symptomatically there is little difference when compared to adult early-onset depression.

CO-MORBID MEDICAL DISEASE

A variety of medical illnesses are associated with depressive symptoms. Mood disorder due to a general medical condition is a persistent disturbance in mood due to the direct physiological effect of a general medical condition. In the geriatric population the differentiation between mood disorder due to a general medical condition and depression as a psychological reaction to the disability due to the medical illness is challenging.

There are basically two different approaches to defining depression in medically ill patients. The *inclusive approach* counts a symptom if it is present without considering whether it is due to the underlying medical condition. Using the inclusive approach, a patient with Parkinson's disease and insomnia would be counted as having insomnia as a depressive symptom if they stated that they could not fall asleep for two hours regardless of whether they said the insomnia was due to dyskinesias or guilty ruminations. The *aetiological approach* counts a symptom towards a diagnosis of depression only if the rater determines that it is not due to the underlying medical disorder. In the example given above the clinician would try to determine if the insomnia was due to depression or dyskinesias. Clearly this distinction can be difficult, particularly because patients, their families and clinicians tend to discount many depressive symptoms because they are felt to be a symptom of the medical illness.

However, the research in this area would support the use of the inclusive approach as more reliable in diagnosing depression in patients with co-morbid medical illnesses[45] and medical conditions such as post-stroke depression[46]. The inclusive approach is more objective, whereas the aetiological approach is subject to the judgement of the clinician and is inherently less reliable. The danger in using the inclusive approach is a loss of specificity and an over-diagnosis of depression. However, the real danger in evaluating medically ill patients with depression is a loss of sensitivity and missing patients who could potentially benefit from somatic treatments. As described below, co-morbid medical illnesses can have a significant detrimental effect on long-term outcomes and mortality. The available treatments for depression are increasingly better tolerated by the elderly and the risk/benefit ratio favours a modest overtreatment of depressive syndromes in the elderly.

Certain endocrine and vitamin deficiencies, medications and medical conditions are associated with depressive symptoms. Discontinuing the offending medication, and/or correcting the endocrine or vitamin deficiency should be done prior to starting an antidepressant[47]. Other medical conditions, such as Parkinson's disease, multiple sclerosis, pancreatic cancer and stroke, are associated with high rates of co-morbid depression and the depressive episode should be treated while managing the co-morbid medical condition. Again, the clinician should not try to determine if the depression is due to the disability of the medical condition but should treat the depression if the patient meets criteria for the disorder.

Parkinson's disease is illustrative of a neurological condition associated with high rates of depression, overlapping symptoms of depression, and the importance of recognizing and treating co-morbid depression in patients with medical disorders. Co-morbid depression occurs in about 20–30% of patients with Parkinson's disease[48,49]. There is considerable overlap of the symptoms of Parkinson's disease and depression, including flat affect, bradykinesia, fatigue, agitation (in the form of psychomotor agitation or dyskinesias), insomnia and cognitive problems. Yet depression in patients with Parkinson's disease can be accurately diagnosed using the inclusive approach and many depression psychiatric rating scales[50]. Co-morbid depression is not simply a reaction to the medical illness and disability[51]; there is evidence of the underlying neuroanatomic degeneration secondary to Parkinson's disease as a cause of depressive syndromes in Parkinson's disease[52], and the treatment of depression can lead to an improvement in the overall quality of life[53]. The identification and treatment of Parkinson's disease with co-morbid depression is therefore important.

Cerebrovascular disease has been shown to be associated with the development of mood symptoms. Depression is a risk factor for stroke[54] and approximately half of post-stroke depressions will meet criteria for major depression, and the other half will have minor depression[55]. Robinson pioneered the early work in understanding the relationship between lesion location (i.e. subcortical in the left anterior pole) as crucial to the development of depression[56-58] and independent of the amount of physical disability caused by the stroke[59]. Post-stroke depression is associated with a longer recovery time[60] and increased mortality[61], and the treatment of post-stroke depression is associated with improved recovery in activities of daily living, cognition and decreased mortality[62].

Controversy still exists whether a left-sided stroke presents with more depressive and catastrophic responses than right-sided insults, which have been described as lesions with emotional neglect, indifference and even euphoric responses[58,63]. Hama et al.[64] found that the severity of affective depression was associated with left frontal lobe damage whereas apathetic depression was mostly related to basal ganglia damage. However, Robinson's relationship of anatomic lesions to psychiatric symptoms laid the groundwork for understanding the interrelationship of depression and medical disease. The body of evidence in stroke with co-morbid depression also supports the importance of the detection and treatment of depressive syndromes in the long-term course of patients with cerebrovascular disease.

The relationship between dementia and depression is complicated. Over 50% of patients with dementing illnesses such as Alzheimer's disease may also have depressive symptoms, with 20% meeting criteria for a major depressive episode[65]. Depressive symptoms may also precede cognitive decline in community elders[66], and a significant number of individuals with depression and reversible cognitive deficits eventually progress to syndromic dementia[67,68]. The biological markers of Alzheimer's disease are found in patients with major depression, including the genotype apolipoprotein E $\varepsilon 3/\varepsilon 4$ (APOE4)[69], which has been linked to Alzheimer's disease. Additionally, depressed patients with the APOE4 genotype have more hippocampal shape abnormalities than depressed patients without APOE4[70], and individuals with late-onset depression and mild cognitive deficits have significant brain amyloid load in a pattern similar to the pattern found in Alzheimer's disease[71].

Diagnosing depression and initiating appropriate treatment in patients with co-morbid medical disorders is therefore important in long-term outcomes and may have a significant effect on the course of the illness. The diagnosis should be made using the DSM criteria and generally the clinician should not attempt to distinguish if the symptoms are due to depression or to the medical illness (i.e. an 'inclusive' approach).

TAKING A HISTORY FROM THE DEPRESSED OLDER ADULT AND FAMILY

The key elements in the patient's history include evidence of a previous psychiatric illness, especially a major depressive or manic episode, particularly if that episode responded to somatic therapy (e.g. lithium, antidepressants or electroconvulsive therapies). Obtaining pharmacy and other medical records regarding the symptoms, dose and the duration of medication trials can further aid in the assessment of depressed individuals. Major depression is a recurrent illness, with about half of the patients experiencing two or more episodes in their lifetime.

In general the clinician evaluating the depressed older adult should include a knowledgeable informant. Depressed elders tend to discount their depressive symptoms[72] and the DSM criteria have been shown to be reliable in elderly patients with primary depression as well as depression secondary to co-morbid medical conditions such as stroke[62] and Parkinson's disease[50].

In order to distinguish dementia from depression, researchers have relied upon the findings in the family and individual histories, mental status and laboratory examinations[73]. Determining the time of onset of the depressive symptoms and the number of episodes may also be useful, since most dementias are slowly developing, with early evidence of cognitive decline (e.g. the inability to balance a chequebook) being present months to years before the typical form of the disease becomes apparent. In contrast, the course of depressive illness may seem more abrupt. In fact Driscoll et al.[74] found that late-onset, recurrent depression takes longer to respond to treatment than late-onset single-episode depression and is more strongly associated with cognitive and functional impairment.

An accurate family history may also provide valuable diagnostic information, since dementing illnesses (e.g. Huntington's chorea and Alzheimer's disease, particularly the early-onset form) and major depression (especially the early-onset form) have both been demonstrated to have a genetic diathesis. The family history should also include questions about neurological and medical disease, alcohol/drug abuse, anxiety, suicide and psychosis, since these conditions are often associated with concomitant depression.

THE MENTAL STATUS EXAMINATION

The mental status examination and standardized depression rating scales may also aid in determining whether the patient has depression, dementia or (as is often the case) both[75]. The depressed patient approaches the mental status examination with the same lack of interest that is also apparent in other areas of his/her life. The depressed patient may attempt to prematurely terminate the interview or consistently refuse to try to answer questions. On the other hand, the demented patient may be quite concerned about his/her declining cognitive skills and, at the same time, make attempts to cover his/her deficits with confabulation. He/she may use notes and other reminders to keep up with facts and uncovering his/her deficits might be quite distressing. This is in marked contrast to the apathetic attitude of the depressed patient[41]. The depressed inpatient is also more likely to be able to find his/her way around the ward and to keep track of the ward routine and personnel. In contrast, the demented patient will forget meal times and confuse familiar faces. This confusion may often get worse as evening approaches and is incorporated in the well-known clinical syndrome of 'sundowning'.

Apathy can be difficult to distinguish from depression. Apathy is essentially the loss of interest without a loss of pleasure but can be misdiagnosed as depression since it is frequently associated with many of the same symptoms (e.g. disinterest, withdrawal, flat affect). Apathy is associated with dementia and other medical conditions that occur with depression, including stroke[76] and Parkinson's disease[77].

The mental status examination of patients with physical illnesses may show primarily problems with concentration and attention. In more severe cases, evidence of delirium may be present. Delirium is diagnosed when the level of consciousness becomes impaired. In this condition, disorientation and memory impairment may be present along with illusions (which are misinterpretations of environmental stimuli), hallucinations and disturbances in psychomotor activity and the sleep–wake cycle. As opposed to dementia, these symptoms usually evolve over hours and days rather than months and may show a waxing and waning course along with autonomic instability.

A common clinical dilemma occurs in patients who are known to be demented, but in whom the clinician seeks to make an accurate diagnosis of depression. In these patients, the clinician may need to assign more importance to neurovegetative signs, such as weight loss and insomnia, although these same symptoms may occur in non-depressed demented patients if they are too disorganized to prepare a meal or have night-time confusion. Some researchers have pointed to the presence of cognitive symptoms of depression (i.e. depressed mood, anxiety, helplessness, hopelessness and worthlessness) as being more prominent in demented patients, whereas neurovegetative signs are notably absent[78].

Monitoring the patient over time, observing for some overall consistent pattern of depressed mood and affect, is also helpful. Although there is little or no data to support empirical trials of antidepressants, given the relatively low side-effect profile of the newer antidepressants[79,80] (SSRIs; see Chapter 86), many clinicians will often attempt a trial of an antidepressant in these difficult situations in hopes the treatment may improve cognition and function. Methylphenidate has been used to treat depressive symptoms such as fatigue, apathy, lack of energy and decreased concentration in depressed medically ill older adults. Despite the long history of its use due to rapid effect, there is little definitive evidence to support this. A few trials have been conducted. Small sampled double-blind trials suggest that methylphenidate is generally well tolerated and modestly efficacious in medically burdened patients[81]. Caution is advised regarding the possible exacerbation of anxiety, psychosis, arrhythmia and potential interaction with warfarin.

PSYCHOLOGICAL TESTS

Neuropsychological assessment is a useful tool to determine the level of cognitive functioning of a patient at a certain point in time but cannot be used to accurately differentiate depression from dementia, especially during the acute episode of depression. Patients suffering from depression have impairments in visuo-spatial ability, memory, psychomotor slowing, speed of information processing and executive functioning, with the executive deficits being particularly related to late age at onset of first lifetime depressive episode[82]. The demented patient will demonstrate a more global decline, with relatively lower scores on aspects of the testing requiring adaptability and processing of information (e.g. performance IQ) as opposed to rote skills and long-term memory tasks (e.g. verbal IQ). Even though a neuropsychological assessment often does not yield a definitive diagnosis, there are some characteristics in patient behaviour that are important to consider when evaluating an older cognitively impaired patient for depression. The depressed patient will more likely show results that are inconsistent over time and are effort-dependent.

Several other factors in depression have been related to worse performance in cognitive testing, including severe depressive symptoms, severe anxiety, the presence of vegetative symptoms and psychotic symptoms. A recent study by Bhalla *et al.*[83] examined cognitive diagnosis among subjects 65 and older before and after depression treatment response. They found that 48% of remitted depressed subjects had persistent cognitive impairment after effective treatment of depressive symptoms. The same group found that very few depressed individuals went from cognitively impaired to cognitively normal over one year follow-up[84]. It is not clear if depression represents a risk factor for or occurs in the prodromal stage of dementia[83,85], but some studies have reported that late-life depression may be associated with subsequent mild cognitive impairment and dementia including Alzheimer's disease and vascular dementia[86].

Standardized depression scales may yield false positive results in demented patients, particularly if they are heavily weighted for cognitive symptoms such as attention and concentration, which overlap with symptoms of depression. Depression scales that have been specifically designed to grade levels of depression in patients known to be demented include the Cornell Scale for Depression and Dementia (CSDD), the Geriatric Depression Scale (GDS), the Beck Depression Inventory (BDI) and the Montgomery–Asberg Depression Rating Scale (MADRS); all are useful tests that can help aid in evaluation of a depressed older patient[87-89]. Each instrument has advantages and disadvantages. For example, the GDS is a self-report measure with yes or no answers that includes evaluation of subjective experience of cognitive impairment but minimizes somatic symptoms and suicidal ideation. The BDI is also self-report and has many more questions related to the somatic symptoms of depression so medically ill older patients can appear more depressed. The BDI does have an excellent question on suicidal ideation and comes in a short form, which abbreviates the questions without losing validity. The CSDD combines patient reports, interviewer observation and informant report for forming a general opinion, so reliability can be difficult if informants are not given specific instructions on how to answer the questions. The MADRS is observer reported and has been shown to be valid and reliable in a number of clinical settings. All these instruments can aid in the diagnosis but, most importantly, can track the severity of symptoms[90], and many of these rating scales are valid in medical diseases with high rates of co-morbid depression that are common in ageing such as Parkinson's disease[50].

LABORATORY TESTS

The common laboratory tests for depression may lose much of their specificity in demented patients. The dexamethasone suppression test (DST) was shown to be useful in mild dementia of Alzheimer's type in distinguishing depressed from non-depressed patients. However, findings in more severe dementia were less specific[91].

The sleep electroencephalogram, however, does maintain its specificity and is able to distinguish a group of elderly depressed patients from those with dementia[92]. Several biological markers have been associated with depression, such us higher platelet monoamine oxidase activity, platelet alpha2-adrenoreceptors, blunted thyroid stimulating hormone (TSH) response to thyroid releasing hormone (TRH), presence of a variant in a gene coding for a potassium channel, and genetic variation in a kainic acid-type glutamate receptor. Many other potential biological markers of depression have been identified[93].

Any physical illness that can potentially affect the central nervous system (CNS) can present with depressive and dementing symptoms; these illnesses include encephalitis, chronic subdural haematoma and normal pressure hydrocephalus. Depressive symptoms such as fatigue, insomnia, weight loss and concentration problems can occur in other illnesses that do not directly affect the CNS. These illnesses include infectious diseases (e.g. tuberculosis, influenza), cardiovascular disease (e.g. congestive heart failure), endocrine abnormalities (e.g. thyroid disease, diabetes), electrolyte disturbances (e.g. hyponatraemia, hypocalcaemia), and renal and hepatic disease. Cerebrovascular disease has also been linked to depression in the elderly, and both cerebral vascular accidents and periventricular white matter disease are related to depressive symptoms in the elderly[94,95].

MEDICAL WORK-UP

The work-up of medical conditions that present with depressive symptoms in the elderly includes a personal history of medical illness, mental status examination and laboratory tests[13,41,96]. Many of these medical conditions are reversible with proper treatment, and geriatric textbooks emphasize the importance of reversible conditions presenting as dementia in the assessment of demented older adults. However, the occurrence of a reversible dementia is actually quite rare in clinical practice[97]. Nevertheless, a basic laboratory work up is important in the evaluation of depressed older adults, including those with cognitive impairment.

A complete medication history should be obtained. Medication, including the antihypertensive medications such as beta-blockers and centrally acting *a*-methyldopa and reserpine, has been shown to cause depressive symptoms. Medications including steroids, barbiturates and sedatives are also frequent causes of depression in the elderly. Patients at risk should be screened for heavy metals, including lead, arsenic and the organophosphates.

The typical laboratory screening for elderly patients with depressive symptoms is outlined in Table 91.1. Clearly, the medical history and physical examination would influence the laboratory testing that was actually done. The neurological examination should be particularly thorough and include an examination of both subtle (e.g. frontal release signs) and prominent (e.g. reflex changes) signs of neurological dysfunction.

SUMMARY

Depressive symptoms are common in the elderly, whereas the syndrome of a major depressive episode is relatively rare. Regardless, depressive symptoms can have a significant effect on functioning, quality of life and mortality in the elderly. Symptoms of depression can be manifestations of either dementing or medical illnesses, both of which are common in the elderly. Psychosocial factors that are unique to the elderly may be aetiological in the genesis of depressive symptoms, but nevertheless require the clinician to assess each patient fully and treat as appropriate. Successful treatment mandates a detailed history, often with collaboration from the family,

Table 91.1 Laboratory work-up in the depressed elderly patient

Laboratory test	Underlying condition
Complete blood count	Infectious disease
	Encephalitis
	Meningitis
	Sub-acute bacterial endocarditis
	Anaemia
Electrolytes and metabolic panel	Hypokaelemia
	Hyponatraemia
	Diabetes
	Uraemia
B12/folate	Pernicious anaemia
Homocysteine	Vascular disease
25-Hydroxyvitamine D	Vitamin D deficiency
Thyroid panel	Hypo/hyperthyroidism
Liver enzymes	Hepatitis
	Liver cancer
Calcium/phosphorus	Hyperparathyroidism
Guiaic stool	Colon disease
Urinalysis	Infection
	Renal disease
Additional tests	
Electrocardiogram	Particularly patients who complain of fatigue, oedema or shortness of breath, or who are being considered for antidepressant therapy
Electroencephalogram	For patients in delirium, particularly those with a seizure history and when non-convulsive status epilepticus is suspected
Urine drug screen	For lead (exposure to paint), mercury (textile manufacturing), organophosphates and arsenic (insecticides). Also drugs of abuse (e.g. opiates, marijuana etc.)
Human immune deficiency virus (HIV)	Exposure to potentially contaminated blood products (surgery, drug use) or a history of promiscuity or homosexuality
Brain computed tomography	Neoplasia, stroke
Brain magnetic resonance imaging	Particularly to view the posterior brainstem

and a thorough medical evaluation for other co-morbid illnesses that may contribute to the patient's current presentation. The treatment of depressive symptoms in the elderly requires an understanding of both the origin of these symptoms and the proper treatment of the underlying disorder, whether the symptoms are secondary to medical, cognitive or psychosocial factors.

REFERENCES

1. Blazer DG. Depression in late life: review and commentary. *J Gerontol A Biol Sci Med Sci* 2003; **58**(3): 249–65.

2. Blazer D, Hughes DC, George LK. The epidemiology of depression in an elderly community population. *Gerontologist* 1987; **27**(3): 281–7.

3. Blazer DG, 2nd. Controversies in community-based psychiatric epidemiology: let the data speak for themselves. *Arch Gen Psychiatry* 2000; **57**(3): 227–8.

4. Blazer DG. Depression in the elderly. Myths and misconceptions. *Psychiatr Clin North Am* 1997; **20**(1): 111–19.

5. Parmelee PA, Katz IR, Lawton MP. Depression among institutionalized aged: assessment and prevalence estimation. *J Gerontol* 1989; **44**(1): M22–9.

6. Hybels CF, Blazer DG. Epidemiology of late-life mental disorders. *Clin Geriatr Med* 2003; **19**(4): 663–96, v.

7. Alexopoulos GS. Depression in the elderly. *Lancet* 2005; **365**(9475): 1961–70.

8. Dombrower H, Izukawa TA, Veinish SL. Factors affecting access to drug therapy in the elderly. *Drugs Aging* 1998; **13**(4): 303–9.

9. Scharf S, Flamer H, Christophidis N. Age as a basis for healthcare rationing. Arguments against agism. *Drugs Aging* 1996; **9**(6): 399–402.

10. Charney DS, Reynolds CF, 3rd, Lewis L *et al.* Depression and Bipolar Support Alliance consensus statement on the unmet needs in diagnosis and treatment of mood disorders in late life. *Arch Gen Psychiatry* 2003; **60**(7): 664–72.

11. Cui X, Lyness JM, Tang W, Tu X, Conwell Y. Outcomes and predictors of late-life depression trajectories in older primary care patients. *Am J Geriatr Psychiatry* 2008; **16**(5): 406–15.

12. Gebretsadik M, Jayaprabhu S, Grossberg GT. Mood disorders in the elderly. *Med Clin North Am* 2006; **90**(5): 789–805.

13. Unsar S, Sut N. Depression and health status in elderly hospitalized patients with chronic illness. *Arch Gerontol Geriat* 2010; **50**(1): 6–10.

14. Bruce ML, Ten Have TR, Reynolds CF, III *et al.* Reducing suicidal ideation and depressive symptoms in depressed older primary care patients: a randomized controlled trial. *JAMA* 2004; **291**(9): 1081–91.

15. Bressler R, Katz MD. Drug therapy for geriatric depression. *Drugs Aging* 1993; **3**(3): 195–219.

16. Jeste DV, Blazer DG, First M. Aging-related diagnostic variations: need for diagnostic criteria appropriate for elderly psychiatric patients. *Biol Psychiatry* 2005; **58**(4): 265–71.

17. Tupler LA, Krishnan KRR, McDonald WM *et al.* Anatomic location and laterality of MRI signal hyperintensities in late-life depression. *J Psychosom Res* 2002; **53**(2): 665–76.

18. Parker G. Is the diagnosis of melancholia important in shaping clinical management? [see comment]. *Curr Opin Psychiatry* 2007; **20**(3): 197–201; discussion 2–3.

19. Parker G, Roy K, Wilhelm K, Mitchell P. Assessing the comparative effectiveness of antidepressant therapies: a prospective clinical practice study. *J Clin Psychiatry* 2001; **62**(2): 117–25.

20. Marneros A. Is the diagnosis of melancholia important in shaping clinical management? [comment]. *Curr Opin Psychiatry* 2007; **20**(3): 206–7.

21. Taylor MA, Fink M. Restoring melancholia in the classification of mood disorders. *J Affect Disord* 2008; **105**(1–3): 1–14.

22. Janakiramaiah N, Gangadhar BN, Naga Venkatesha Murthy PJ *et al.* Antidepressant efficacy of Sudarshan Kriya Yoga (SKY) in melancholia: a randomized comparison with electroconvulsive therapy (ECT) and imipramine. *J Affect Disord* 2000; **57**(1–3): 255–9.

23. Fink M, Rush AJ, Knapp R et al. DSM melancholic features are unreliable predictors of ECT response: a CORE publication. *J ECT* 2007; **23**(3): 139–46.

24. Brown WA. Treatment response in melancholia. *Acta Psychiatr Scand Suppl* 2007; (433): 125–9.

25. Pinquart M, Duberstein PR, Lyness JM. Treatments for later-life depressive conditions: a meta-analytic comparison of pharmacotherapy and psychotherapy. *Am J Psychiatry* 2006; **163**(9): 1493–501.

26. Lazarus LW, Groves L, Gierl B et al. Efficacy of phenelzine in geriatric depression. *Biol Psychiatry* 1986; **21**(7): 699–701.

27. Fink M, Taylor MA. Catatonia – in 100 words. *Br J Psychiatry* 2009; **194**(4): 325.

28. Kamara TS, Whyte EM, Mulsant BH et al. Does major depressive disorder with somatic delusions constitute a distinct subtype of major depressive disorder with psychotic features? *J Affect Disord* 2009; **112**(1–3): 250–55.

29. Thomas P, Hazif-Thomas C, Pareaud M. [Hypochondriasis and somatisation in elderly]. *Rev Prat* 2008; **58**(18): 1977–81.

30. VanItallie TB. Subsyndromal depression in the elderly: underdiagnosed and undertreated. *Metabolism* 2005; **54**(5 suppl 1): 39–44.

31. Lyness JM. Naturalistic outcomes of minor and subsyndromal depression in older primary care patients. *Int J Geriatr Psychiatry* 2008; **23**(8): 773–81.

32. Lyness JM, Kim J, Tang W et al. The clinical significance of subsyndromal depression in older primary care patients. *Am J Geriatr Psychiatry* 2007; **15**(3): 214–23.

33. Hybels CF, Blazer DG, Steffens DC. Predictors of partial remission in older patients treated for major depression: the role of comorbid dysthymia. *Am J Geriatr Psychiatry* 2005; **13**(8): 713–21.

34. Lyness JM, Heo M, Datto CJ et al. Outcomes of minor and subsyndromal depression among elderly patients in primary care settings. *Ann Intern Med* 2006; **144**(7): 496–504.

35. Lyness JM, Chapman BP, McGriff J, Drayer R, Duberstein PR. One-year outcomes of minor and subsyndromal depression in older primary care patients. *Int Psychogeriatr* 2009; **21**(1): 60–68.

36. Loukissa D. Under diagnosis of alcohol misuse in the older adult population. *Br J Nurs* 2007; **16**(20): 1254–8.

37. Lam A, Bradley G. Use of self-prescribed nonprescription medications and dietary supplements among assisted living facility residents. *J Am Pharm Assoc (2003)* 2006; **46**(5): 574–81.

38. Yoon SL, Schaffer SD. Herbal, prescribed, and over-the-counter drug use in older women: prevalence of drug interactions. *Geriatr Nurs* 2006; **27**(2): 118–29.

39. Bruno JJ, Ellis JJ. Herbal use among US elderly: 2002 National Health Interview Survey. *Ann Pharmacother* 2005; **39**(4): 643–8.

40. Blazer DG, 2nd, Hybels CF. Origins of depression in later life. *Psychol Med* 2005; **35**(9): 1241–52.

41. Fiske A, Wetherell JL, Gatz M. Depression in older adults. *Annu Rev Clin Psychol* 2009; **5**: 363–89.

42. Salzman C, Shader RI. Depression in the elderly. I. Relationship between depression, psychologic defense mechanisms and physical illness. *J Am Geriatr Soc* 1978; **26**(6): 253–60.

43. Himmelhoch JM, Auchenbach R, Fuchs CZ. The dilemma of depression in the elderly. *J Clin Psychiatry* 1982; **43**(9 pt 2): 26–32.

44. Blazer D, Bachar JR, Hughes DC. Major depression with melancholia: a comparison of middle-aged and elderly adults. *J Am Geriatr Soc* 1987; **35**(10): 927–32.

45. Koenig HG, George LK, Peterson BL, Pieper CF. Depression in medically ill hospitalized older adults: prevalence, characteristics, and course of symptoms according to six diagnostic schemes. *Am J Psychiatry* 1997; **154**(10): 1376–83.

46. Fedoroff JP, Starkstein SE, Parikh RM, Price TR, Robinson RG. Are depressive symptoms nonspecific in patients with acute stroke? *Am J Psychiatry* 1991; **148**(9): 1172–6.

47. Kritz Silverstein D, Schultz ST, Palinska LA, Wingard DL, Barrett Connor E. The association of thyroid stimulating hormone levels with cognitive function and depressed mood: the Rancho Bernardo study. *J Nutr Health Aging* 2009; **13**(4): 317–21.

48. Ranoux D. [Depression and Parkinson disease]. *Encephale* 2000; **26**(spec no 3): 22–6.

49. Allain H, Schuck S, Mauduit N. Depression in Parkinson's disease. *Br Med J* 2000; **320**(7245): 1287–8.

50. Schrag A, Barone P, Brown RG et al. Depression rating scales in Parkinson's disease: critique and recommendations. *Mov Disord* 2007; **22**(8): 1077–92.

51. Menza MA, Mark MH. Parkinson's disease and depression: the relationship to disability and personality. *J Neuropsychiatry Clin Neurosci* 1994; **6**(2): 165–9.

52. McDonald WM. Depression. In Factor SA, Weiner W (eds), *Parkinson's Disease: Diagnosis and Clinical Management*, 2nd edn. New York: Demos, 2008, 159–78.

53. Global Parkinson's Disease Survey Steering Committee. Factors impacting on quality of life in Parkinson's disease: results from an international survey. *Mov Disord* 2002; **17**(1): 60–67.

54. Krishnan M, Mast BT, Ficker LJ, Lawhorne L, Lichtenberg PA. The effects of preexisting depression on cerebrovascular health outcomes in geriatric continuing care. *J Gerontol A Biol Sci Med Sci* 2005; **60**(7): 915–19.

55. Robinson RG. Treatment issues in poststroke depression. *Depress Anxiety* 1998; **8**(suppl 1): 85–90.

56. Starkstein SE, Robinson RG, Price TR. Comparison of cortical and subcortical lesions in the production of poststroke mood disorders. *Brain* 1987; **110** (pt 4): 1045–59.

57. Morris PL, Robinson RG, Raphael B, Hopwood MJ. Lesion location and poststroke depression. *J Neuropsychiatry Clin Neurosci* 1996; **8**(4): 399–403.

58. Narushima K, Kosier JT, Robinson RG. A reappraisal of poststroke depression, intra- and inter-hemispheric lesion location using meta-analysis. *J Neuropsychiatry Clin Neurosci* 2003; **15**(4): 422–30.

59. Robinson RG, Starkstein SE. Mood disorders following stroke: new findings and future directions. *J Geriatr Psychiatry* 1989; **22**(1): 1–15.

60. Parikh RM, Lipsey JR, Robinson RG, Price TR. Two-year longitudinal study of post-stroke mood disorders: dynamic changes in correlates of depression at one and two years. *Stroke* 1987; **18**(3): 579–84.

61. Morris PL, Robinson RG, Andrzejewski P, Samuels J, Price TR. Association of depression with 10-year poststroke mortality. *Am J Psychiatry* 1993; **150**(1): 124–9.

62. Robinson RG. Poststroke depression: prevalence, diagnosis, treatment, and disease progression. *Biol Psychiatry* 2003; **54**(3): 376–87.

63. Santos M, Kovari E, Gold G *et al*. The neuroanatomical model of post-stroke depression: towards a change of focus? *J Neurol Sci* 2009; **283**(1–2): 158–62.

64. Hama S, Yamashita H, Shigenobu M *et al*. Post-stroke affective or apathetic depression and lesion location: left frontal lobe and bilateral basal ganglia. *Eur Arch Psychiatry Clin Neurosci* 2007; **257**(3): 149–52.

65. Brown EL, Raue P, Halpert KD, Adams S, Titler MG. Detection of depression in older adults with dementia. *J Gerontol Nurs* 2009; **35**(2): 11–15.

66. Sachs-Ericsson N, Joiner T, Plant EA, Blazer DG. The influence of depression on cognitive decline in community-dwelling elderly persons. *Am J Geriatr Psychiatry* 2005; **13**(5): 402–8.

67. Saez-Fonseca JA, Lee L, Walker Z. Long-term outcome of depressive pseudodementia in the elderly. *J Affect Disord* 2007; **101**(1–3): 123–9.

68. Alexopoulos GS, Meyers BS, Young RC, Mattis S, Kakuma T. The course of geriatric depression with 'reversible dementia': a controlled study. *Am J Psychiatry* 1993; **150**(11): 1693–9.

69. Krishnan KR, Tupler LA, Ritchie JC, Jr *et al*. Apolipoprotein E-epsilon 4 frequency in geriatric depression. *Biol Psychiatry* 1996; **40**(1): 69–71.

70. Qiu A, Taylor WD, Zhao Z *et al*. APOE related hippocampal shape alteration in geriatric depression. *Neuroimage* 2009; **44**(3): 620–26.

71. Butters MA, Klunk WE, Mathis CA *et al*. Imaging Alzheimer pathology in late-life depression with PET and Pittsburgh Compound-B. *Alzheimer Dis Assoc Disord* 2008; **22**(3): 261–8.

72. Alexopoulos GS, Borson S, Cuthbert BN *et al*. Assessment of late life depression. *Biol Psychiatry* 2002; **52**(3): 164–74.

73. Gilles C. [Dementia–depression: how are they related? From depressive pseudodementia to pseudodepression in dementia]. *Rev Med Brux* 1994; **15**(5): 296–9.

74. Driscoll HC, Basinski J, Mulsant BH *et al*. Late-onset major depression: clinical and treatment–response variability. *Int J Geriatr Psychiatry* 2005; **20**(7): 661–7.

75. Müller-Thomsen T, Arlt S, Mann U, Mass R, Ganzer S. Detecting depression in Alzheimer's disease: evaluation of four different scales. *Arch Clin Neuropsychol* 2005; **20**(2): 271–6.

76. Starkstein SE, Fedoroff JP, Price TR, Leiguarda R, Robinson RG. Apathy following cerebrovascular lesions. *Stroke* 1993; **24**(11): 1625–30.

77. Leentjens AF, Dujardin K, Marsh L *et al*. Apathy and anhedonia rating scales in Parkinson's disease: critique and recommendations. *Mov Disord* 2008; **23**(14): 2004–14.

78. Lazarus LW, Newton N, Cohler B, Lesser J, Schweon C. Frequency and presentation of depressive symptoms in patients with primary degenerative dementia. *Am J Psychiatry* 1987; **144**(1): 41–5.

79. Bélicard-Pernot C, Manckoundia P, Ponavoy E, Rouaud O, Pfitzenmeyer P. [Antidepressant use in demented elderly subjects: current data]. *Rev Med Interne* 2009; **30**(11): 947–54.

80. Bains J, Birks JS, Dening TR. The efficacy of antidepressants in the treatment of depression in dementia. *Cochrane Database Syst Rev* 2002; (4): CD003944.

81. Hardy SE. Methylphenidate for the treatment of depressive symptoms, including fatigue and apathy, in medically ill older adults and terminally ill adults. *Am J Geriatr Pharmacother* 2009; **7**(1): 34–59.

82. Lockwood KA, Alexopoulos GS, Kakuma T, Van Gorp WG. Subtypes of cognitive impairment in depressed older adults. *Am J Geriatr Psychiatry* 2000; **8**(3): 201–8.

83. Bhalla RK, Butters MA, Becker JT *et al*. Patterns of mild cognitive impairment after treatment of depression in the elderly. *Am J Geriatr Psychiatry* 2009; **17**(4): 308–16.

84. Bhalla RK, Butters MA, Mulsant BH *et al*. Persistence of neuropsychologic deficits in the remitted state of late-life depression. *Am J Geriatr Psychiatry* 2006; **14**(5): 419–27.

85. Chen P, Ganguli M, Mulsant BH, DeKosky ST. The temporal relationship between depressive symptoms and dementia: a community-based prospective study. *Arch Gen Psychiatry* 1999; **56**(3): 261–6.

86. Jean L, Simard M, van Reekum R, Clarke DE. Differential cognitive impairment in subjects with geriatric depression who will develop Alzheimer's disease and other dementias: a retrospective study. *Int Psychogeriatr*. 2005; **17**(2): 289–301.

87. Beck AT, Ward CH, Mendelson M, Mock J, Erbaugh J. An inventory for measuring depression. *Arch Gen Psychiatry* 1961; **4**: 561–71.

88. Yesavage JA, Brink TL, Rose TL *et al*. Development and validation of a geriatric depression screening scale: a preliminary report. *J Psychiatr Res* 1982; **17**(1): 37–49.

89. Alexopoulos GS, Abrams RC, Young RC, Shamoian CA. Cornell Scale for Depression in Dementia. *Biol Psychiatry* 1988; **23**(3): 271–84.

90. Steffens DC, Otey E, Alexopoulos GS *et al*. Perspectives on depression, mild cognitive impairment, and cognitive decline. *Arch Gen Psychiatry* 2006; **63**(2): 130–38.

91. Hatzinger M, Z'Brun A, Hemmeter U *et al*. Hypothalamic–pituitary–adrenal system function in patients with Alzheimer's disease. *Neurobiol Aging* 1995; **16**(2): 205–9.

92. Reynolds CF, 3rd, Kupfer DJ, Houck PR *et al*. Reliable discrimination of elderly depressed and demented patients by electroencephalographic sleep data. *Arch Gen Psychiatry* 1988; **45**(3): 258–64.

93. Papakostas GI, Fava M. Predictors, moderators, and mediators (correlates) of treatment outcome in major depressive disorder. *Dialogues Clin Neurosci* 2008; **10**(4): 439–51.

94. McDonald WM, Krishnan KR, Doraiswamy PM *et al*. Magnetic resonance findings in patients with early-onset Alzheimer's disease. *Biol Psychiatry* 1991; **29**(8): 799–810.

95. McDonald WM, Krishnan KR, Doraiswamy PM, Blazer DG. Occurrence of subcortical hyperintensities in elderly subjects with mania. *Psychiatry Res* 1991; **40**(4): 211–20.

96. McCusker J, Cole M, Dufouil C *et al*. The prevalence and correlates of major and minor depression in older medical inpatients. *J Am Geriatr Soc* 2005; **53**(8): 1344–53.

97. Ovsiew F. Seeking reversibility and treatability in dementia. *Semin Clin Neuropsychiatry* 2003; **8**(1): 3–11.

92

Mania: Epidemiology and Risk Factors

Susan W. Lehmann

The Johns Hopkins University School of Medicine, Department of Psychiatry and Behavioral Sciences, Baltimore, MD, USA

In recent years there has been increased clinical interest and research regarding the syndrome of mania in the elderly. While it has become clearer that older persons with bipolar disorder are a heterogeneous group, many questions regarding differences between early-onset bipolar disorder and later-onset bipolar disorder remain. Much of the current work in this area has focused on the following: How does bipolar disorder in the elderly differ from that in younger people? Can age of onset be used to distinguish clinically meaningful subtypes of bipolar disorder?

EPIDEMIOLOGY

The manic phase of bipolar affective disorder, or mania, is an uncommon disorder in the elderly although the exact prevalence of bipolar disorder among older adults in the community is uncertain[1]. In the five-site Epidemiologic Catchment Area study of more than 20 000 non-institutionalized individuals, one-month prevalence rates for mania were 0.4–0.8% for 18–44 year olds and 0.2% in the 45- to 64-year-old group. Notably, no cases of mania were identified among people over age 64[2]. In a 12-month prevalence study of 2798 community-dwelling adults age 65 or older in Quebec, 0.6% were found to have had a manic episode[3].

Nevertheless, elderly patients with mania are seen in significant numbers in a variety of clinical settings. In Roth's[4] retrospective review of 464 psychogeriatric patients over age 60 in a long-term hospital, 14 cases were manic, representing 6% of the total number of cases of affective disorder. Two studies of first admissions to British psychiatric hospitals, using Department of Health statistics, found that the number of first admissions with mania either remained steady with age[5] or increased with advancing age[6]. In the USA, other studies in short-stay hospitals have reported that mania accounted for approximately 5% of elderly psychiatric admissions[7–9]. Elderly patients with bipolar disorder have been found to use disproportionately more outpatient mental health and day hospital services than older patients with unipolar major depression[10]. Most studies of elderly manic patients have found more females than males[7–9,11], though men have been reported to have an earlier age of onset[12].

For the majority of elderly bipolar patients, the first episode of affective disorder is usually a depression. Indeed, it is quite common for a first manic episode to occur 10 years or more after an initial depressive episode and to be preceded by multiple depressive episodes over many years[7,13,14]. Generally, elderly patients have been found to have suffered more episodes of depression before a first manic episode and to have had a long gap between an initial depression and a first manic episode than young manic patients[14].

It has been estimated that about 10% of older patients with bipolar disorder experienced onset of illness after age 50[15]. Still, at the present time, there is no agreed-upon standard regarding which age should serve as the dividing line between early- and late-onset bipolar disorder. This uncertainty is compounded by a lack of consensus regarding how to determine age of onset itself. Different criteria have been used among various investigators to identify age of onset of bipolar disorder, including first onset of any mood symptoms, first hospitalization and first time at which the patient met full criteria for the disorder[9].

Several studies have observed bi-modality in age of onset of mania among elderly patients. In these studies, one subgroup of patients was found to have developed bipolar disorder in early life with a mean age in their thirties, and another subgroup developed a first manic episode after age 60[9,14]. A study of first-episode mania presenting for psychiatric treatment over a 35-year period in London found a two-component distribution in age of onset with a peak in early adult life and a smaller peak in mid-life[16]. A bimodal age of onset of bipolar disorder has also been reported by others [17–19] although a tri-modal distribution of age of onset has been proposed as well[20]. While controversy continues regarding how best to define early- and late-onset cases, results from numerous studies support the relevance of distinguishing between early- and late-onset bipolar disorder. Late-onset bipolar patients tend to have had a longer gap between first depression and first mania than early-onset bipolar patients[14] and in one study were more likely to be married or living with a significant other[9]. Elderly bipolar patients with late-onset have been reported to have a more favourable outcome and to be less likely to have rapid cycling compared with elderly patients with early-onset illness[21].

RISK FACTORS

A number of studies have reported that elderly bipolar patients who had an early age of onset were more likely to have had first-degree relatives with affective disorder than late-onset elderly bipolar patients[14,22]. This trend holds across studies that have used ages between 20 and 60 years to divide early and late cases and suggests that genetics plays a greater role in the disease of early-onset bipolar disorder. At the same time, many investigators have reported associations between late-onset mania and cerebrovascular risk factors. In two studies comparing elderly patients with early- and late-onset bipolar disorder, researchers found that patients with late-onset mania had increased vascular risk factors[9,17].

In another recent study of 50 elderly bipolar patients with no known history of stroke or neurological disease, patients with late-onset bipolar disorder had higher stroke risk scores than patients with early-onset illness[19]. In a prospective study of mania in 35 patients over age 60, the elderly mania patients had more cortical atrophy on CT scans than age-matched controls[14]. However, no significant difference in cortical atrophy was found between elderly patients with early- and late-onset mania. In addition, subcortical hyperintensities have been reported on magnetic resonance imaging (MRI) in elderly patients with mania [23]. These hyperintensities are believed to be due to focal loss of brain parenchyma but they do not seem to be specific to elderly patients with mania, since subcortical hyperintensities have also been found in late-onset depression as well as late-onset paranoid disorders[24].

Krauthammer and Klerman[25] proposed criteria for secondary mania that included cases of no prior family history, no past psychiatric history and a definable medical or neurological aetiology. While it is true that organic factors may precipitate mania in some elderly patients, these cases appear to be in the minority. Manic episodes can be caused by such widely prescribed medications as levodopa, procyclidine, pergolide, selegiline and bromocriptine[26]. A variety of steroids have been reported to produce manic syndromes, as have thyroid supplements, and there have been case reports of mania associated with H_2-antagonists, antiarrhythmics, oestrogen and antitubercular agents[27]. In addition, mania can occur in association with systemic infections, such as influenza, Q fever and St. Louis type A encephalitis. Cases of mania secondary to space-occupying lesions, such as meningiomas, subarachnoid haemorrhages and metastases (usually in the non-dominant hemisphere), have also been reported[8]. In these cases, mania usually resolves with removal of the offending pharmacological agent or treatment of the underlying disorder.

More commonly, mania has been reported in elderly patients with cerebrovascular and neurological disorders. A cohort study comparing 50 elderly patients with mania to 50 age- and sex-matched patients with unipolar depression found that 36% of the manic patients had neurological disorders compared with only 8% of the depressed patients[28]. Interestingly, among these neurologically impaired manic patients, 33% had a positive family history of affective disorder in first-degree relatives. A prospective study found that 20% of patients with mania over the age of 60 had a first manic episode closely temporally related to a cerebral organic disorder[14]. Another prospective study of 20 manic patients with onset over age 50 found that 65% developed bipolar disorder after a silent cerebral infarction[29]. In particular, injury to the right hemisphere appears to be strongly associated with the development of mania.

Overall, however, mania following stroke is much less common than depression after a stroke. In one large study of 700 stroke victims only three developed manic syndromes[30]. There have been reports of secondary mania in patients with ischaemic injury to right-sided basal ganglia, orbitofrontal cortex, right basotemporal cortex[31] and right temporoparietal cortex[32]. There have also been two case reports of mania secondary to infarctions in the thalamic and perithalamic areas[33]. It has been hypothesized that these brain areas may be significant because of their connections to the limbic system and the modulation of emotion. Starkstein et al.[34] studied 11 patients who developed mania after stroke and found that eight had lesions involving limbic areas and nine had right hemispheric involvement. These patients also had significantly larger bifrontal and third ventricular brain ratios than matched control patients, indicating pre-existing anterior subcortical atrophy. Moreover, almost half of the patients had family history of affective disorder in a first-degree relative.

Taken together, the current literature on mania in patients with neurological and cerebrovascular disorder underscores that genetic loading is also a factor contributing to the development of mania in these patients. Furthermore, while up to a quarter of elderly manic patients in various studies have been found to have some evidence of concurrent cerebral disease, it is still unclear to what extent these impairments play an aetiological role in the development of mania. If cases in which subjects with a known previous history of affective disorder are excluded, few cases of clear secondary mania are found[8,14,22]. An exception to this is Shulman et al.[28], who felt that 36% of elderly patients they studied who were hospitalized with mania had true secondary mania associated temporally with clearly documented neurological disorders. Still, recent findings that late-onset mania is associated with greater vascular risk factors and greater cerebrovascular disease suggest that medical management of vascular risk factors in older patients with depressive disorders may minimize their vulnerability to developing mania[19].

Mania can occur in the setting of dementia, although it is rare. In a retrospective chart review of 134 patients with Alzheimer's disease 2% were found to have had mania[35], although others have reported higher rates[36]. A recent study of a large Danish cohort found that patients with dementia had an elevated probability of developing mania, depression or a first bipolar episode compared with patients with other chronic illnesses, and this risk remained increased throughout the rest of the patient's life[37].

As in younger patients, stressful life events have been felt by some investigators to precipitate mania in elderly patients. One study that reported on 10 elderly manic patients found that 70% had major changes in lifestyle in the six months preceding onset of mania. Stresses included marital discord and disruption of living arrangements[7].

REFERENCES

1. Sajatovic M. Aging-related issues in bipolar disorder: a health services perspective. *J Geriatr Psychiatry Neurol* 2002; **15**: 128–33.
2. Regier DA, Boyd JH, Burke JD Jr. *et al.* One-month prevalence of mental disorders in the United States. *Arch Gen Psychiatry* 1988; **45**, 977–86.
3. Preville M, Boyer R, Grenier S *et al.* The epidemiology of psychiatric disorders in Quebec's older adult population. *Can J Psychiatry* 2008; **53**: 822–33.
4. Roth M. The natural history of mental disorder in old age. *J Ment Sci* 1955; **101**: 281–301.
5. Eagles JM, Whalley LJ. Ageing and affective disorders: The age at first onset of affective disorders in Scotland. *Br J Psychiatry* 1985; **147**, 180–87.
6. Spicer CC, Hare EH, Slater E. Neurotic and psychotic forms of depressive illness: evidence from age-incidence in a national sample. *Br J Psychiatry* 1973; **123**: 535–41.
7. Yassa R, Nair V, Nastase C *et al.* Prevalence of bipolar disorder in a psychogeriatric population. *J Affect Disord* 1988; **14**: 197–201.
8. Glasser M, Rabins P. Mania in the elderly. *Age Ageing* 1983; **13**: 210–13.

9. Wylie ME, Mulsant BH, Pollock BG *et al.* Age at onset in geriatric bipolar disorder. *Am J Geriatr Psychiatry* 1999; **7**: 77–83.

10. Bartels SJ, Forester B, Miles KM, Joyce T. Mental health service use by elderly patients with bipolar disorder and unipolar major depression. *Am J Geriatr Psychiatry* 2000; **8**: 160–66.

11. Shulman K, Post F. Bipolar affective disorder in old age. *Br J Psychiatry* 1980; **136**, 26–32.

12. Kennedy N, Boydell J, Kalidindi *et al.* Gender differences in incidence and age at onset of mania and bipolar disorder over a 35-year period in Camberwell, England. *Am J Psychiatry* 2005; **162**: 257–62.

13. Snowdon J. A retrospective case-note study of bipolar disorder in old age. *Br J Psychiatry* 1991; **158**: 485–90.

14. Broadhead J, Jacoby R. Mania in older age: a first prospective study. *Int J Geriatr Psychiatry* 1990; **5**: 215–22.

15. Clayton PJ. The prevalence and course of the affective disorders. In: David J, Maas J (eds), *The Affective Disorders*. Washington DC: American Psychiatric Press, 1983, 193–201.

16. Kennedy N, Everitt B, Boydell J *et al.* Incidence and distribution of first-episode mania by age: results from a 35-year study. *Psychol Med* 2005; **35**: 855–63.

17. Cassidy F, Carroll BJ. Vascular risk factors in late onset mania. *Psychol Med* 2002; **32**: 359–62.

18. Lehmann SW, Rabins PV. Factors related to hospitalization in elderly manic patients with early and late-onset bipolar disorder. *Int J Geriatr Psychiatry* 2006; **21**: 1060–64.

19. Subramaniam H, Dennis MS, Byrne EJ. The role of vascular risk factors in late onset bipolar disorder. *Int J Geriatr Psychiatry* 2007; **22**: 733–37.

20. Bellivier F, Golmard JL, Rietschel M *et al.* Age at onset in bipolar I affective disorder: further evidence for three subgroups. *Am J Psychiatry* 2003; **160**: 999–1001.

21. Oostervink F, Boomsma M, Nolen WA *et al.* Bipolar disorder in the elderly; different effects of age and age of onset. *J Affect Disord* 2009; **116**: 176–83.

22. Stone K. Mania in the elderly. *Br J Psychiatry* 1989; **1155**: 220–24.

23. McDonald WM, Krishnan KRR, Doraiswamy PM, Blazer DG. Occurrence of subcortical hyperintensities in elderly subjects with mania. *Psychiatr Res Neuroimag* 1991; **40**: 211–20.

24. Schulman K. Recent developments in the epidemiology, co-morbidity and outcome of mania in older age. *Rev Clin Gerontol* 1996; **6**: 249–54.

25. Krauthammer C, Klerman GL. Secondary mania. *Arch Gen Psychiatry* 1978; **35**: 1333–39.

26. Factor SA, Molho BS, Podskalny GD *et al.* Parkinson's disease: drug-induced psychiatric states. *Behav Neurol Mov Disord* 1995; **65**: 115–38.

27. Ganzini L, Millar SB, Walsh JR. Drug-induced mania in the elderly. *Drugs Aging* 1993; **3**: 428–35.

28. Shulman KI, Tohen M, Satlin A *et al.* Mania compared with unipolar depression in old age. *Am J Psychiatry* 1992; **149**: 341–45.

29. Fujikawa T, Yaamawaki S, Touhouda Y. Silent cerebral infarctions in patients with late-onset mania. *Stroke* 1995; **26**: 946–50.

30. Robinson RG, Staff LB, Price TR. A two-year longitudinal study of mood disorders following stroke: prevalence and duration at six months follow-up. *Br J Psychiatry* 1984; **144**: 256–62.

31. Starkstein SE, Mayberg HS, Berthier ML *et al.* Mania after brain injury: neuroradiological and metabolic findings. *Ann Neurol* 1990; **27**: 652–59.

32. Celik Y, Erdogan E, Tuglu C, Utku U. Letter to the editor: Post-stroke mania in late life due to right temporoparietal infarction. *Psychiatry Clin Neurosci* 2004; **58**: 446–47.

33. Cummings JL, Mendez MF. Secondary mania with focal cerebrovascular lesions. *Am J Psychiatry* 1984; **141**: 1084–87.

34. Starkstein SE Pearlson GD, Boston JB, Robinson RG. Mania after brain injury: a controlled study of causative factors. *Arch Neurol* 1987; **44**, 1069–73.

35. Lyketsos C, Corazzini K, Steele C. Mania in Alzheimer's disease. *I Neuropsychiatry* 1995; **150**: 350–52.

36. Burns A, Jacoby R, Levy R. Psychiatry phenomena in Alzheimer's disease, III: disorders of mood. *Br J Psychiatry* 1992; **157**: 81–86.

37. Nilsson FM, Kessing LV, Sorensen TM *et al.* Enduring increased risk of developing depression and mania in patients with dementia. *J Neurol Neurosurg Psychiatry* 2002; **73**: 40–44.

93

Acute Mania and Bipolar Affective Disorder

M. Sajatovic[1], N. Herrmann[2] and K.I. Shulman[2]

[1]*Case Western Reserve University School of Medicine and University Hospitals Case Medical Center, Cleveland, OH, USA*
[2]*Sunnybrook Health Sciences Centre, Toronto, Ontario, Canada*

INTRODUCTION

The term 'bipolar disorder' includes a wide spectrum of clinical expression ranging from early to very late onset, single to recurrent episodes, manic only to bipolar episodes and mild hypomania to severe mania. However, the defining feature of bipolar disorder has always been evidence of a manic or hypomanic episode. Recent notions have challenged the concept of 'bipolar disorder' to include other perspectives including treatment response and family history[1]. This review of bipolar disorder in later life will focus on features that are unique to older adults including its late age of onset, long-term clinical course and the high prevalence of co-morbidity including cognitive impairment, other psychiatric disorders and neurobiological features. Ultimately, we will attempt to synthesize the determinants of mania in old age and review the implications for assessment and clinical diagnosis before addressing management issues specific to older adults.

EPIDEMIOLOGY

Data on the community incidence and prevalence of mania and bipolar disorder in old age are confounded by a number of methodological concerns. Similar to patients who suffer from paranoid disorders, manic patients are not readily amenable to interview or cooperation with community surveys. Diagnostic uncertainty is also related to the high levels of co-morbidity that cloud the diagnostic horizon[2]. This includes the association with co-morbid medical and neurologic disorders. DSM-IV has categorized this as 'a mood disorder due to a general medical condition' (293.83). The assumption in that classification is that the mood disturbance is a 'direct physiologic consequence of the general medical condition'. However, because of the high levels of neurological and medical co-morbidity, it is difficult to ascertain with any degree of certainty whether this is the case. Further, the historical category of 'secondary mania' implies that cerebral organic factors are responsible for the syndrome[3]. The neurological literature complicates the issue by use of the term 'disinhibition syndrome', the features of which are identical to what is considered mania in the psychiatric literature. All of this conspires to create uncertainty as to the true incidence and prevalence of the disorder. Our best data, however, suggest that the prevalence of mania in the community decreases from a high of 1.4% in young adults to a negligible < 0.1% prevalence of mania in the over-65s[4-7].

Community epidemiological surveys, including the Epidemiologic Catchment Area Study (ECA)[4,8], found a very early age of onset, close to 20 years. However, in studies of mixed-age manic patients, the mean age of onset tends to be slightly higher at 30 years[9,10]. Despite this very early onset of bipolar disorder in the general population, only a relatively small number of elderly bipolar inpatients are known to experience their first manic episode before the age of 40[7,11]. The question 'where have all the young bipolar patients gone?' has not yet been answered.

A number of hypotheses for this phenomenon include the relatively high mortality rate from natural causes and suicide in bipolar patients[7] while the Iowa 500 data suggested evidence of 'burn out' of the disorder over a long-term course[12]. The latter phenomenon has been challenged in recent epidemiological surveys based on the Veterans Affairs database[13]. Outpatient samples may reveal a different pattern compared to hospitalized patients.

In contrast, hospital admission rates show an opposite trend to that of the community prevalence of bipolar illness. For inpatient psychogeriatric units, Yassa *et al.*[14] found a relatively high 'treated prevalence' ranging from 4 to 8%. In Britain, a national survey examining first admission rates for mania showed a modest increase in the extremes of old age[15,16], assuming that this was associated with the increased prevalence of dementia in late life. The development of specialized inpatient units for older adults included significant numbers of individuals with late-life bipolar disorders ranging from 7 to 10 admissions per year[11,14,17]. In Finland, 20% of first admissions with the diagnosis of bipolar disorder occurred after the age of 60[18]. Reconciling the opposing patterns of community prevalence and hospital admission rates has been a challenge. Are the 'bipolar' disorders in late life qualitatively different than those in younger adults or is the higher admission rate in older adults a reflection of increased frailty and the effect of neurological changes?

AGE OF ONSET

Age of onset is an important variable that might help to distinguish the subtypes of mania and reduce the genetic heterogeneity inherent in the bipolar spectrum[19]. Consensus seems to be heading towards a cut-off of age 50 as a distinguishing feature of 'early-' versus 'late-onset' bipolar disorder. Recently Moorhead and Young[20] used a UK psychiatric case registry to determine age of onset retrospectively in bipolar I patients. Those subjects without a family history tended to have later age of onset with a modal age of onset at 49 years, consistent with the studies above. They concluded that non-genetic factors were more relevant in this subgroup and also suggested that age 50 would be a useful cut-off for the early- vs. late-onset designation. It is worth noting that age of onset is significantly influenced by the cut-off used for 'elderly' probands. Most studies use age 60 or 65 as a cut-off for 'geriatric', 'elderly' or 'older adult'.

Studies that have examined the relationship of family history with age of onset in older bipolar probands have shown a wide range of prevalence of psychiatric disorder in first-degree relatives ranging from 24% to 88%[7,11,21-24]. Methodological issues are significant because most of the studies are retrospective in nature and the rigorous use of criteria for positive family history are not consistent in these studies. Nonetheless, a general trend towards a higher rate of family history is evident in those with early age of onset[22,24]. The converse is true in those elderly bipolar probands with a neurological disorder mainly associated with a late onset of bipolar disorder. However, even in the 'neurological subgroup' of older bipolar patients, the prevalence of a positive family history in first-degree relatives remains quite high, at about 30%[7,11,25]. Thus, even in those manic or bipolar patients with evidence of co-morbid neurological lesions, familial vulnerability appears to be a contributory factor.

COURSE OF ILLNESS

Early retrospective studies of bipolar disorder in late life found that about half of all index patients experienced depression as their first mood episode[7,11,22,23]. Moreover, elderly bipolar patients whose first episode was depression (mean age of 50, went on to experience a very long latency (mean of 15 years) before their first manic episode became evident[11,17]. In the subgroup with a latency between first depression and first mania, 25% of this group experienced a latency of at least 25 years and half of this group suffered at least three consecutive depressive episodes before developing a manic episode[7,17,22], begging the question of the pathogenesis of a switch from unipolar depression to bipolarity. The switch mechanism has been attributed in part to the high prevalence of co-morbid neurological disorders and cognitive changes described further below[2], but may also be a function of normal degenerative changes allowing for uncovering of an underlying disposition to bipolarity.

Although little is written about a unipolar mania subtype, Shulman and Tohen[26] found that 12% of their sample met strict criteria for a course of unipolar mania. The criteria included at least three distinct manic episodes without major depression including a minimum period of 10 years follow-up from the time of their first admission for a manic episode. This group also had a relatively earlier age of onset (41 years) compared with a mean of 65 years for a larger group of elderly bipolar patients. However, further study of unipolar manic patients has not been forthcoming.

The long-term outcome of older bipolar patients has primarily been studied retrospectively[11,27,28]. Shulman et al.[11] found a high mortality rate in a cohort of elderly manic inpatients. About half of the manic patients had died at a mean six-year follow-up compared with only 20% of age- and sex-matched patients with depression. Berrios and Bakshi[27] found a poor prognosis in older bipolar patients with limited response to treatment and a higher prevalence of cognitive impairment and cerebrovascular dysfunction associated with persistent disturbances in psychosocial functioning. Dhingra and Rabins[28] observed a significant decline in cognition in their six-year mean follow-up study.

Lehmann and Rabins[29] used a retrospective chart review of patients over the age of 65 to identify factors that contributed to relapse and hospitalization in elderly bipolar patients. They noted a distribution of age of onset consistent with previous findings using a cut-off at about age 45 rather than 50 years for late onset. The early-onset patients tended to be more behaviourally disturbed prior to admission and were less adherent with prescribed psychiatric medications. Relapse and readmissions were very common in elderly manic patients with both early- and late-onset disorders. They emphasized the need for improved medication adherence in order to prevent recurrent episodes and admissions.

PSYCHIATRIC AND MEDICAL CO-MORBIDITY

Two recent studies have focused on the question of psychiatric co-morbidity with late-life bipolar disorders[30,31]. Sajatovic and Kales[32] used the Veterans Affairs database (National Psychosis Registry) to document a lower prevalence of substance abuse in older bipolar patients compared with mixed-age samples who had co-morbid substance abuse of over 60%. A total of 29% of older bipolar patients with a mean age of 70 years experienced either substance abuse, post traumatic stress disorder, other anxiety disorders or dementia[32]. In this study, the anxiety disorders represented 15.2% of the sample, including post-traumatic stress disorder (PTSD) which occurred in 5.4% and other anxiety disorders in 9.8% of this group. Substance abuse was lower than other studies at 8.9% in this sample. Goldstein et al.[30] derived data from the National Epidemiology Survey on Alcohol Related Conditions (NESARC). Eighty-four elderly bipolar patients were identified and were found to have a lifetime and 12-month co-morbid prevalence of alcohol use disorders of 38%. Patients with generalized anxiety disorder had a lifetime prevalence of 20.5% and a 12-month prevalence of 9.5%. Prevalence figures for panic disorder showed a 19% lifetime prevalence and a 12-month prevalence of 11.9%. These studies show a consistently high co-morbidity that appears to be slightly lower than mixed-age and younger samples.

Medical co-morbidity has only recently been examined in bipolar elders[33,34]. Using a prospective sample of elderly bipolar patients, Gildengers et al.[33] undertook to determine the profile of disease burden between elderly patients with major depression compared to those with bipolar disorder. They hypothesized that medical burden would be greater for bipolar patients, particularly in endocrine/metabolic and cardiovascular disease given the association of bipolar disorder with obesity, diabetes mellitus, dyslipidaemia and hypertension. They did not find a significant difference between the depressive and bipolar groups on the Cumulative Illness Rating Scale for Geriatrics (CIRS-G) or body mass index (BMI). However, they did confirm that metabolic disease was higher in the bipolar group. This is consistent with the findings of Subramaniam et al.[34] who conducted a cross-sectional survey of elderly bipolar patients and showed that the late-onset group had higher stroke risk scores compared with the early-onset group of older bipolar patients but did not find any differences in cognitive functioning.

These recent studies confirm concerns that have been identified in a number of previous retrospective studies of late-life bipolar disorder where significant neurological co-morbidity was noted. This literature has consisted primarily of individual case reports and small case series, but showed a tendency for heterogeneous right hemisphere lesions to be associated with mania[35-38]. The findings were consistent with the psychiatric literature that used the term 'secondary mania'[3] and the neurological literature that tended to use the term 'disinhibition syndrome'[39]. The phenomenon of pathological laughing has also been associated with right-sided lesions[40]. Moreover, the right orbital frontal circuit (OFC) has been implicated in the pathogenesis of manic syndromes[41,42]. This hypothesis is based on the observation that normal mood is dependent on the integrity of the frontal, limbic and basal ganglia circuits. Starkstein and Robinson[39] previously suggested that disinhibition syndromes or secondary mania cases are caused by a disruption of connections within the orbital frontal circuits. They note that the frontal lobes modulate motivational and psychomotor behaviour, limbic connections modulate emotions, and the biogenic amine nuclei in the hypothalamus, amygdala and brainstem modulate instinctive behaviours. This may be the neurobiological basis and pathogenesis for the development of mania in later life associated with a higher prevalence of neurological lesions[43].

Braun et al.[44] reviewed a series of published case reports involving focal unilateral cortical lesions, and also found a tendency towards right-sided lesions for what they termed 'mania and pseudomania'. Earlier retrospective studies of mania by Shulman et al.[11] noted a very high association of neurological disorders in the manic group (36%) compared with only 8% in a comparison group of elderly depressives. Moreover, very late-onset mania is strongly associated with neurological co-morbidity as well as high mortality due to cerebrovascular disease[25]. In this retrospective cohort study, 10 out of 14 elderly manic patients had evidence of neurological disorders, primarily due to cerebrovascular disease.

A heterogeneous group of neurological and medical disorders have been associated with secondary mania as reported by case reports including head injuries[45], endocrine conditions[46–48], HIV[49] and epilepsy[37]. However, the majority of case reports of secondary mania are associated with right-sided cerebrovascular lesions[2].

The presence of cerebrovascular disease associated with mania has led to the proposal of a bipolar vascular subtype[38]. Similar to the vascular depression hypothesis of Alexopoulos et al.[50], vascular mania is defined in the context of a finding of cerebrovascular disease based on clinical or neuroimaging findings with further evidence of cognitive impairment. The cohort of elderly manic patients with cerebrovascular disease may fit in the proposed vascular subtype although the hypothesis still needs better data for corroboration. Using a cut-off of 49 years, Wylie[51], found that the late-onset group had more cerebrovascular risk factors which are elaborated on below. Hays et al.[24] also found an increase in vascular co-morbidity in their sample of elderly bipolar patients whose mean age was 74 years. Silent cerebral infarctions were found to occur most commonly in late-onset mania when compared with age- and sex-matched group of depressive patients[52]. The proportion of manic patients over the age of 60 found to have silent cerebral infarctions was greater than 20% with a relatively modest family history in first-degree relatives.

NEUROIMAGING STUDIES

Most studies have focused on the presence of subcortical hyperintensities, decreased cerebral blood flow and evidence of silent cerebral infarctions[2]. The relationship of hyperintensities with risk factors such as hypertension, atherosclerotic heart disease and diabetes mellitus strengthens the relationship of mania to cerebrovascular pathology.

The potential for examining structural brain changes in late-life neuropsychiatric disorders implies that hypothesis-driven theses can now be performed[53]. New methods may be able to help understand the pathophysiology of bipolarity within specific neural circuits. The important side benefits of studying geriatric patients is also the opportunity to integrate MRI with postmortem analysis, thus generating new hypotheses[54].

Braun et al.[55] collected a second series of single-case reports of unilateral lesions involving at least one manic symptom. They assembled a subgroup of 59 clearly defined manic patients, the majority of whom had right hemisphere lesions. However, elation alone without a manic symptom complex was not significantly predicted by lesion side. Rather, the association of right hemisphere lesions with mania is primarily related to disinhibition rather than a shift of mood as a result of the release of left hemisphere influence. This hypothesis is illustrated in a recent case study from Japan in which a 78-year-old woman with major depression developed a right-sided infarction in the middle cerebral artery distribution followed by acute post-stroke mania. Single photon emission computed tomography (SPECT) scan showed a unique pattern of left orbital frontal hyperperfusion with extensive right frontal hypoperfusion. Similar to Braun et al.'s[55] theory, they postulate a functional imbalance within the right and left orbital frontal cortices that result in the development of mania[56].

The examination of cortical atrophy has not been as frequent as that of hyperintensities and silent cerebral infarcts but Beyer et al.[57] found a decreased right caudate volume in older bipolar patients compared with controls related to the duration of illness. This was most pronounced in a late-onset subgroup and points to the role of the caudate in the emotional brain circuitry involving the prefrontal cortex, the amygdala, thalamus and other basal ganglia structures. Another interesting associated finding from Beyer et al.[58] was an increase in left hippocampal volume in elderly bipolar patients. They hypothesized that lithium treatment may have been responsible for this and point to the possible neuroplasticity and cellular resilience in this region of the brain possibly induced by lithium[59].

COGNITIVE IMPAIRMENT

Young et al.[60] conducted a systematic literature review involving seven studies of elderly bipolar patients and also used a cross-sectional sample of 70 bipolar patients who completed the Mini-Mental State Examination (MMSE) and the Mattis Dementia Rating Scale. The literature review identified methodological problems and differences in assessing cognitive function but overall found a pattern of significant cognitive impairment. In their clinical sample, the manic patients had lower scores on the two rating instruments compared to a comparison group. The cognitive scores did not correlate with Young Mania Rating Scale scores and were considered persistent deficits.

Tsai et al.[61] used a retrospective chart review to study cognition in bipolar I patients over the age of 60. The cognitive screening instruments included the clock drawing test, the MMSE and the cognitive ability screening instrument (CASI). Their cut-off for early onset was age 40 and they found that 42% of early-onset euthymic older bipolar patients had impaired cognition. Gildengers et al.[62] studied euthymic older bipolar patients and found that half of this group scored below the mean of the comparison subjects. They concluded that these findings were persistent changes and not associated with an abnormal mood state, similar to the finding of Young et al.[60].

Despite the very significant association of cognitive dysfunction with late-life mania, earlier studies have not been able to establish a clinical course consistent with the development of dementia in this group compared to age-matched controls. However, because of the finding by Alexopoulos et al.[50] that reversible dementia in major depression eventually led to irreversible dementia, this issue remains of concern. Of considerable interest has been the recent finding of neuroprotection associated with lithium treatment[63,64].

Terao et al.[65] conducted a retrospective study of clinical records to show that those patients with a history of lithium exposure as well as current lithium treatment had higher MMSE scores than their comparison subjects. The putative neuroprotective impact of lithium has been postulated to be associated with its ability to decrease the enzyme glycogen synthase kinase-3 (GSK-3) which leads to the accumulation of amyloid-beta proteins and senile plaques, as well as hyperphosphorylated tau and neurofibrillary tangles in Alzheimer's disease.

A number of recent studies have addressed the relationship between cognitive dysfunction and bipolar disorder with similar findings. Schouws et al.[66] studied a small sample of euthymic elderly patients over the age of 60 with onset less than 50 years. A comprehensive neuropsychological test battery found that these euthymic bipolar patients were impaired across a wide range of cognitive domains and were similar to the cognitive dysfunction found in younger bipolar patients. Depp et al.[67] used an outpatient sample and found that bipolar disorder was associated with significant neurocognitive impairment compared to comparison subjects, and that this pattern of impairment was distinct from that found in schizophrenia. They also confirmed that the cognitive deficits in the bipolar group were not related to either the severity or duration of the psychiatric or manic symptoms, but were related to their quality of life. Sajatovic et al.[31] found a co-morbid dementia in 4.5% of their sample of older bipolar patients in the Veterans Affairs database.

Similar to Tsai et al.[61], an Argentinian study[68] used a small sample of euthymic older patients with bipolar disorders to demonstrate that their pattern of cognitive and motor dysfunction was similar to that described in younger euthymic bipolar patients. Psychosocial functioning was correlated with this impairment. Euthymic bipolar elderly patients were also studied by Radanovic et al.[69] who demonstrated language impairment compared to control subjects.

Gunning-Dixon et al.[70], also using a small sample of non-demented manic bipolar patients, showed that their performance on executive functioning was worse than controls as well as comparison depressed subjects. They hypothesized that the executive dysfunction found in this group supported the possibility that specific frontostriatal network dysfunction was associated with late-life bipolar disorder.

Lin et al.[71] used two study cohorts identified in the Taiwan National Health Insurance Research Database. Patients hospitalized with bipolar disorder compared to those undergoing appendectomy had twice the likelihood of developing stroke.

CLINICAL PRESENTATION AND HEALTH SERVICE UTILIZATION

Various studies[13,23] suggest that the presentation of bipolar disorder remains fairly constant across the life span, including the general range of symptoms. There is also a consistently high use of health services by older bipolar patients[13,72]. Subsequent studies including those by Bartels et al.[72] report that elderly bipolar patients have greater severity of symptoms and impairment of community living skills compared with age-matched older adults with unipolar depression. Moreover, they use almost four times the total amount of

mental health services, including hospitalization. Generally, bipolar patients are found to have greater medical co-morbidity, more cognitive impairment and a less robust response to treatment[13,72]. Depp et al.[73] noted that elderly bipolar patients were less likely to use hospital facilities compared to younger bipolar patients, but were more likely to use case management services.

Kessing[74] used a nation-wide psychiatric registry in Denmark to study different diagnostic subtypes of bipolar disorder in patients with late-onset (over 50) and early-onset. He found that those bipolar patients whose first psychiatric hospitalization occurred after the age of 50 tended to present with less psychotic manic episodes and more severe depressions including psychosis compared with younger onset patients.

Beyer et al.[75] examined stressful life events in older bipolar patients. They showed that the number of serious stressful life events in the 12 months prior to a manic episode was no different in older or younger bipolar patients. In general, negative life events were more prevalent in both older and younger bipolar patients compared to a control group. Depp et al.[76] noted that psychotic depressive symptoms as well as cognitive impairment in elderly adults with bipolar disorder contributed to the finding of a lower health-related quality of life and functioning in this sample.

In summary, older adults with new or persistent bipolar disorder are profoundly affected by their illness, resulting in a decrease in their quality of life. Moreover, these disorders represent a significant challenge to geriatric and psychiatric services because of the high levels of morbidity and mortality.

CLINICAL IMPLICATIONS OF A NEW DIAGNOSIS OF BIPOLAR DISORDER IN LATE LIFE

One of the unique features of mania and the switch into bipolarity in late life is the association with heterogeneous brain lesions, predominantly cerebrovascular disease. This suggests that any elderly patient presenting with a manic episode, particularly for the first time late in life, deserves a rigorous neurological workup, especially for evidence of cerebrovascular disease, including brain scanning. Consequently, the management of vascular risk factors becomes an important aspect of the management of this neuropsychiatric disorder and accounts for the high rate of medical co-morbidity and increased use of health services by this subgroup of patients[13,72]. Ruling out other neurological lesions or disorders is particularly important in late-onset cases and those without significant family history.

Our understanding of the determinants of manic illness in old age also point to the significant affective vulnerability in this subgroup manifest by a high familial prevalence of mood disorder in 50–80% of first-degree relatives[11,24]. However, our clinical experience suggests that affective vulnerability is not based solely on genetics but also on the psychological events of early life. Early loss and trauma in childhood and adolescence may very well be significant risk factors for affective vulnerability late in life. As Beyer et al.[75] have shown, stressful events in old age also play a role but are not more prevalent than in younger individuals with bipolar disorder. However, it is the perfect storm of genetics, psychological stressors and the localization of brain lesions to the right hemisphere involving the orbital frontal circuit that may be critical for the manifestation of mania in old age. These findings in older adults with mania and bipolar disorders may help to shed light on the pathogenesis of mania in the much larger mixed-age population of individuals with bipolar disorder. To what extent the management and pharmacological treatment is similar or different in older adult is the focus of the next section of this chapter.

MANAGEMENT OF THE OLDER ADULT WITH BIPOLAR DISORDER

The management of bipolar disorder in the elderly is fraught with multiple challenges (Table 93.1). As noted previously, rates of medical and psychiatric co-morbidity are extremely high in elderly bipolar patients, necessitating caution during arriving at a diagnosis and ordering investigations/laboratory or imaging assessment. A careful history and collaborative history is often required to rule out co-morbid substance abuse and anxiety disorders. The medical history should in particular focus on previous head injury, cerebrovascular disease and related cardiac risk factors. The use of concomitant medications must be documented in order to avoid or manage drug interactions. Baseline laboratory investigations should include a complete blood count (CBC), fasting glucose and lipid profile, liver function, kidney function, thyroid, urinalysis and an ECG. Neuroimaging has generally also been considered an essential component of the baseline investigations for elderly bipolar patients.

The next major challenge facing the clinician is the lack of randomized controlled trials and evidence-based treatment guidelines. At the present time, there is not a single published randomized trial of lithium, valproate, other mood stabilizers, antidepressants, antipsychotics, electroconvulsive therapy (ECT), or psychotherapy conducted with elderly bipolar patients. While there are numerous reviews on the management and pharmacotherapy of late-life bipolar disorders[77-80], none of the popular clinical practice guidelines[81,82] provide evidence-based, specific recommendations for the elderly. Unfortunately, the situation is also unlikely to improve in the near future. A review of the clinical trial registry[83] revealed only four trials recruiting geriatric bipolar patients. Of these four trials, none were placebo-controlled, three were open label, and only one was a randomized trial of lithium vs. valproate that has already been recruiting for several years.

In the absence of specific data, guidelines from adult populations have of necessity been applied to geriatric populations. For example, in a small open-label trial of 31 elderly bipolar patients[84], standardized treatment protocols were applied based on the Systematic Treatment Enhanced Program for Bipolar Disorder (STEP-BD)[85]. The authors concluded that they were successfully able to apply standardized therapy even though most of the patients did not experience sustained recovery. Any adaptation of adult treatment guidelines however must consider age-specific pharmacological issues such as the fact that the elderly generally have a reduced capacity to metabolize drugs, they are more sensitive to adverse effects, and they are more likely to be taking concomitant medications, increasing the risk of drug interactions[86].

Treatment of Acute Mania in Older Adults

First-line therapy for acute mania would include lithium, divalproex (valproic acid), an atypical antipsychotic (olanzapine, risperidone, quetiapine, aripiprazole, ziprasidone) and the combination of lithium or divalproex with an atypical antipsychotic, based on recent evidence-based clinical practice guidelines for bipolar disorder[82]. Second-line therapy would include use of carbamazepine, oxcarbazepine, ECT, and the combination of lithium and divalproex. Clozapine is included under third-line agents in these guidelines. The choice of these agents would be reasonable for elderly bipolar patients as well, taking into consideration dosing and titration appropriate for the elderly.

While other first-line agents are being used more frequently, lithium remains a commonly used mood stabilizer in old age[87]. In fact, in the study of standardized treatment for elderly bipolar patients mentioned previously[84], lithium was the most commonly prescribed treatment used by over 60% of patients. Available data on the use of lithium in elderly manic patients comes from a small number of open-label case series, naturalistic and retrospective studies, which suggest lithium can be used safely and effectively[84,89-92]. Lithium therapy highlights many of the challenges associated with pharmacotherapy in elderly bipolar patients. Lithium is eliminated exclusively by the kidney, and age-related changes such as decreased creatinine clearance and glomerular filtration rate significantly affect lithium pharmacokinetics. In a study of lithium pharmacokinetics, Hardy et al.[93] determined that lithium excretion in the elderly was half the rate of younger patients. The elderly may also be more sensitive to adverse events and toxicity even with lithium serum levels considered 'normal' in adult populations[94-96]. This has led to some controversy regarding appropriate lithium dosages and serum levels for the elderly. Some have recommended serum levels as low as 0.5 mmol/l[97], though others have argued that higher levels are associated with better outcome[92,98]. A review of published studies in the elderly suggested that lithium dosages were 25–50% lower in the elderly with serum levels typically below 0.7 mmol/l[80]. In the study of standardized treatment of geriatric bipolar disorder, the average dose of lithium used was 657 mg per day with an average serum level of 0.67 mmol/l[84].

The potential adverse effects of lithium include a wide range of disturbances involving the central nervous system (CNS), gastrointestinal, kidney, cardiac and endocrine systems. Common CNS effects include lithium-induced tremor, aggravation of parkinsonian symptoms and spontaneous extrapyramidal effects. In an administrative

Table 93.1 Challenges in the management of elderly patients with bipolar disorder

Diagnosis	Multiple psychiatric co-morbidities: dementia, anxiety and substance use disorders are the most likely particular concerns
	Multiple medical co-morbidity: metabolic/endocrine, cardiovascular and neurological diseases are particular concerns
Treatment	Lack of evidence-based treatment guidelines specific to geriatric bipolar disorder
	Age-related changes in drug metabolism
	Reduced tolerance to medication side effects (e.g. falls risk)
	Need to treat medical co-morbidity
	Multiple concomitant medications increase risk of drug interactions
	Age-specific adverse medication affects (e.g. mortality risk associated with antipsychotics)
Service delivery	Issues related to changes in social environment (isolation, communication or transportation difficulties) and treatment adherence
	Intensive service needs – increased need to coordinate care between health care providers, service agencies and/or family
	Projected shortage in specialty care clinicians and available services for geriatric populations

health database study of 2422 elderly new users of lithium, the rate of hospitalization for lithium-induced delirium was 2.5 per 100 person years, not significantly different from the rate of valproate-induced delirium[99]. The risk of lithium-induced hypothyroidism might be greater in elderly patients than that seen in younger populations. For example, in a community study of elderly lithium users, one-third were on thyroid replacement or had elevated levels of thyroid-stimulating hormone[87]. In a study of 1705 new elderly lithium users, 6% were treated for hypothyroidism, about twice the prevalence expected from a mixed-age population[100]. Finally, another major concern related to lithium use in the elderly is the risk of drug–drug interactions. Numerous commonly used concomitant medications can reduce lithium clearance including diuretics, angiotensin-converting enzyme (ACE) inhibitors and some non-steroidal anti-inflammatory drugs[77]. While thiazide diuretics were classically thought to be the drugs of greatest concern, these other agents might be even more problematic. In a population-based nested case–control study with 10 000 elderly lithium users, approximately 4% were hospitalized for lithium toxicity[101]. New use of a loop diuretic (e.g. furosemide) or an ACE-inhibitor independently increased the risk of hospitalization for lithium-induced toxicity by five- to sevenfold.

In the absence of controlled trial data, it is perhaps surprising that new use of valproate therapy for bipolar elders is surpassing that of lithium use. For example, in an administrative database study conducted between 1993 and 2000, new use of lithium carbonate fell consistently while valproic acid use increased, surpassing new lithium prescriptions midway through the observation period[88]. By the end of the observation period, there were almost three new prescriptions for valproate written for every prescription of lithium. While there are no published randomized controlled studies, naturalistic observational studies suggest the use of valproate for acute mania in the elderly is effective and reasonably well tolerated[84,92,102–108]. Dosages have ranged between 250 and 2250 mg per day and serum levels between 25 and 120 µg/ml with about 60% demonstrating some degree of benefit[77].

Based on case reports, valproate appears effective for elderly rapid-cycling bipolar patients as monotherapy[109] or in combination with lithium[110,111]. Successful use of intravenous valproate has also been documented for acutely manic elderly patients who refused oral medications[112]. There are significant dose-dependent changes in valproate pharmacokinetics in the elderly, including prolonged elimination half-life, especially important at higher doses, which might predispose the elderly to toxicity[113,114]. The most frequent adverse events associated with valproate are excessive sedation and gastrointestinal intolerance, though under-recognized and potentially important side effects in the elderly also include thrombocytopenia[115] and hyperammonaemia potentially leading to delirium[116]. In fact, while valproate is often considered a better tolerated, safer alternative to lithium for the elderly, one study found no differences in the rates of hospitalization for delirium comparing valproate to lithium[99]. Valproic acid is also highly protein-bound and a weak inhibitor of cytochrome P450 2D6. As a result, potential drug interactions exist, including drugs such as tricyclic antidepressants, acetylsalicylic acid, warfarin and diazepam[117].

There are no randomized controlled trials of the use of carbamazepine in the elderly and only a small number of naturalistic studies reported[118,119]. Some have raised concerns about the tolerability of carbamazepine in the elderly suggesting that relatively low serum levels (below 9 µg/ml) are necessary to avoid neurotoxicty[98]. Significant potential for important drug interactions may also limit its use in the elderly[117].

There are virtually no published studies on the use of other anticonvulsants such as oxcarbazepine, topiramate and zonisamide for mania in the elderly. One case series of gabapentin therapy in elderly manic patients suggested it was safe and effective[120].

Though typical antipsychotics are not considered first-line agents for mania[82], they are still used frequently in the elderly as adjunctive treatments for bipolar disorder. Typical antipsychotics can cause considerable side effects in the elderly, including anticholinergic effects, orthostatic hypotension and extrapyramidal effects[79]. Rates of incident tardive dyskinesia in the elderly associated with typical antipsychotics are high[121]. In contrast, rates of acute extrapyramidal effects and tardive dyskinesia are very much lower with atypical antipsychotics and as a result they are being used with increasing frequency for elderly manic patients[122]. Atypical antipsychotics also appear to have mood-stabilizing properties that have earned them recognition as first-line therapies for acute mania in evidence-based treatment guidelines[82]. However, in contrast to the numerous randomized controlled trials of atypical antipsychotics in elderly demented patients[123] and a smaller number of studies in elderly schizophrenic patients[124–127], there are no randomized controlled trials of atypical antipsychotics for elderly bipolar patients. While commonly used for mania in the elderly as monotherapy and adjunctive treatments[78], there are remarkably few naturalistic studies and even case series reported in the elderly. In one case series, risperidone was found to be effective for elderly bipolar patients[128] and clozapine has been reported to be effective in a couple of case reports[129,130]. In the case of clozapine, older adults are at greater risk of developing drug-related agranulocytosis compared with younger/mixed-age populations[131].

Besides their well-described metabolic adverse effects, the use of atypical antipsychotics may be associated with specific concerns in the elderly including the risk of cerebrovascular adverse events and mortality[132,133]. Interestingly, despite the obvious increases in weight, glucose intolerance and hyperlipidaemia associated with drugs like clozapine, olanzapine, quetiapine, and to a lesser extent risperidone, neither the randomized controlled trials in the elderly dementia patients, nor population-based studies have suggested a similar concern[133]. Whether this is because the elderly are less susceptible to these effects, or that the lower doses typically used for the elderly mitigate these effects is unclear. Despite the lack of a similar concern from the published data, it is important to note that elderly bipolar patients may have different susceptibility risks compared to dementia patients. Furthermore, it would seem prudent to be particularly cautious in patients who are at high risk for the metabolic consequences of atypical antipsychotics such as those with obesity and pre-existing diabetes and hyperlipidaemia.

With respect to cerebrovascular adverse events, while both risperidone and olanzapine carry black-box warnings for these events based on the randomized controlled trials in elderly dementia patients, it is likely that the other atypical antipsychotics as well as the typicals have similar risks[132]. Similarly, all antipsychotics, both typical and atypical, now carry black-box warnings for an increased risk of mortality based on the randomized controlled trials with dementia patients, as well as population-based observational studies[133]. Taken together, it is unclear whether elderly bipolar patients have similar susceptibility to these serious cardiovascular/elevated mortality adverse events demonstrated in elderly patients with dementia.

Finally, there are no specific data on the use of benzodiazepines, ECT, transcranial magnetic stimulation or psychosocial interventions for elderly manic patients, even though they are clearly being used and have been recommended for the elderly[86].

Treatment of Bipolar Depression in Older Adults

Bipolar depression is a severe and pervasive problem among all individuals with bipolar illness, and mixed-age individuals with bipolar disorder experience depressive symptoms three times more frequently than manic symptoms[134,135]. In addition to greater time duration, disability associated with bipolar depression is disproportionately greater than that associated with bipolar mania[136,137]. Underscoring the malignant effects of dysphoric mood states in bipolar populations, bipolar depression has been reported as a major contributor to completed suicide[138].

An analysis by Depp and colleagues[76] evaluated health-related quality of life among middle-aged and older adults with bipolar disorder, finding that depressive symptoms, along with psychosis and cognitive impairment significantly contribute to reduced quality of life. In depressed bipolar elders, treatments directed at mood dysregulation can alleviate disability[139], and may help avoid 'behavioural disuse atrophy'[140,141].

While the earliest and largest number of prospective randomized controlled bipolar treatment trials have evaluated the anti-manic activity of various drug treatments[142], the most salient issue for individuals with bipolar disorder appears to be efficacy of treatments for bipolar depression. A recent study involving 469 individuals with bipolar disorder found that patients prioritized reduction of depression severity over mania severity[143].

Unfortunately, there are few established treatments for bipolar depression, and the topic area has been severely neglected up until very recently[144]. Commonly utilized drug therapies in mixed-age patients include lithium, the anticonvulsants valproate, lamotrigine and carbamazepine as well as the atypical antipsychotics and combination therapy with antidepressant medications adjunct to mood stabilizers[145,146]. Fountoulakis and Vieta[144] noted that good research-based evidence supported by at least one placebo-controlled trial of 'sufficient' magnitude exists for selected atypical antipsychotic agents (olanzapine, quetiapine both as monotherapy or olanzapine in combination with fluoxetine). A recent International Consensus Group (ICG) suggested that only three monotherapies (lithium, lamotrigine, quetiapine) have first-level evidence for the treatment of acute and long-term bipolar depression[147]. In addition, the use of antidepressants is controversial in bipolar depression because of potential negative consequences (switching, rapid cycling), and the ICG has not supported their general use for bipolar depression[147]. The American Psychiatric Association (APA) guidelines for the treatment of Bipolar Disorder[148] recommend that the use of antidepressant agents in bipolar populations be approached cautiously and parsimoniously.

Uncontrolled and secondary analyses in geriatric bipolar depression suggest a possible role for the traditional mood-stabilizing medication lithium and for lamotrigine[149,150]. In addition, a group of US investigators have recently initiated a preliminary, open-label trial of adjunct lamotrigine therapy in geriatric (age 60 and over) bipolar depressed populations utilizing a geriatric bipolar trials network. Preliminary data from the first seven patients (intention to treat) demonstrated significant reduction in change from baseline Montgomery Asberg Depression Rating (MADRS) scores (baseline mean 28, endpoint last observation carried forward (LOCF) mean 14.7, $P = 0.005$, with good tolerability of lamotrigine by bipolar depressed elders[151].

Some atypical antipsychotic drugs, widely used in mixed-age bipolar populations may also be of benefit in bipolar elders. Sajatovic and Paulsson[152] conducted a secondary analysis of combined results from two eight-week, double-blind, randomized, placebo-controlled studies of quetiapine in fixed doses (300 or 600 mg/day) in the treatment of depressive episodes associated with bipolar I or II disorder[153,154]. The primary efficacy endpoint was MADRS total score change from baseline to week 8. Efficacy populations included 72 adults aged 55–65 years (mean $\pm$ SD 58.4 $\pm$ 2.6 years; $n = 23$, 23 and 26 for quetiapine 300 mg/day, quetiapine 600 mg/day and placebo, respectively) and 906 adults aged 18 to <55 years (mean 35.7 $\pm$ 9.9 years; $n = 304$, 298 and 304, respectively). Illness characteristics, including DSM-IV diagnoses and baseline MADRS and Hamilton Depression Scale (HAM-D) scores were broadly similar between older and younger adults receiving quetiapine or placebo. In older adults, least square mean $\pm$ SE MADRS score decreased 13.4 $\pm$ 2.4 with quetiapine 300 mg/day and 14.2 $\pm$ 2.5 with quetiapine 600 mg/day vs. 8.0 $\pm$ 2.3 with placebo ($P = 0.097$ and 0.057, respectively, vs. placebo). In younger adults, mean MADRS score decreased 16.8 $\pm$ 0.7 and 16.5 $\pm$ 0.7 vs. 11.2 $\pm$ 0.7, respectively ($P < 0.001$, both doses vs. placebo). Quetiapine (both doses) significantly decreased HAM-D and CGI-S scores and increased CGI-I scores relative to placebo in older and younger adults. The most frequent adverse effects associated with quetiapine in older and younger adults were dry mouth, somnolence, sedation and dizziness. Rates of treatment-related withdrawals were similar in older and younger adults.

Aripiprazole, an atypical antipsychotic compound which is approved by the US Food and Drug Administration (FDA) for the treatment of bipolar mania and for the long-term treatment of bipolar disorder was recently prospectively tested in a small sample ($N = 20$) of bipolar older adults[155]. Older bipolar I adults who were suboptimally responsive to their bipolar pharmacological treatments received 12 weeks of open-label aripiprazole added on to existing mood stabilizer[156]. Aripiprazole was initiated at 5 mg daily and increased as tolerated. Efficacy outcomes included psychopathology scores (Young Mania Rating Scale (YMRS), HAM-D), extrapyramidal symptom assessments, and level of functioning measurement (Global Assessment Scale (GAS)). Mean age of the sample was 59.6 years, range 50–83 years. The majority of individuals had bipolar depression. Individuals had significant reductions in HAM-D and YMRS scores. There were also significant improvements in the GAS. Mean daily dose of aripiprazole was 10.26 mg/day SD $\pm$ 4.9, range 5–20 mg/day. Overall, aripiprazole was efficacious and relatively well tolerated. Of particular note, aripiprazole therapy was associated with improvements in bipolar depression in this older population. While atypical antipsychotics offer potential promise in treating geriatric bipolar depression, this must be tempered by concerns regarding antipsychotic drugs in elders discussed above.

While the role of antidepressant agents to treat bipolar depression in mixed-age populations is controversial due to concerns regarding manic switching, mixed episodes and rapid cycling[148,144], preliminary data in geriatric bipolar depression suggest that antidepressants can have beneficial effects on selected health outcomes. One analysis found decreased rates of hospitalization for manic/mixed episodes during a 5135 person-years follow-up study of antidepressant use among older adults with bipolar disorder[156]. Another report suggested that older bipolar adults with a recent history of suicide attempts were less likely to have received treatment with mood stabilizers and antidepressants compared to older bipolar individuals with no recent history of suicide attempts[157]. Finally, ECT must be mentioned as an efficacious and well-tolerated somatic therapy for bipolar depressed elderly individuals[158].

Maintenance Treatment of Bipolar Disorder in Older Adults

Maintenance or longer term treatments for geriatric bipolar disorder are minimally presented in the psychiatric literature. A recent retrospective analysis of elders with unipolar depression and elders with bipolar disorder compared each patient to his or her own clinical course before and after lithium treatment[159]. In this analysis lithium maintenance significantly reduced the probability of relapse and recurrence, suicidal behaviour, and severity of mood disturbance[159].

A secondary analysis of older adults (age 55 and older) from two placebo-controlled, double-blind bipolar maintenance treatment studies compared patients randomized to treatment with lamotrigine, lithium or placebo for up to 18 months[160]. The primary endpoint was time-to-intervention for any mood episode; secondary measures included time-to-intervention for depression and mania/hypomania/mixed mood. The group of 638 patients included 98 older adults. Mean age of the older adult sample was 61 years (± SD 6.0, range 55–82 years). In the group of older adults, lamotrigine, but not lithium, significantly delayed time-to-intervention for any mood episode compared with placebo. Lamotrigine also significantly delayed time-to-intervention for a depressive episode compared with lithium and placebo. Lithium did significantly better than lamotrigine for time-to-intervention for mania. Side effects for both lamotrigine and lithium were generally mild to moderate in severity including similar rates of skin rash (3% for lamotrigine, 5% for lithium). Lamotrigine and lithium daily doses were 240 mg/day and 750 mg/day, respectively.

Elderly and young adults from the Systematic Treatment Enhancement Program for Bipolar Disorder (STEP-BD) were compared on prescription patterns and recovery status[161]. STEP-BD was a multicentre National Institute of Mental Health (NIMH)-funded project designed to evaluate the longitudinal outcome of patients with bipolar disorder that involved extensive assessment across multiple domains including demographic data, diagnosis, symptom severity, treatment and clinical status. Patients achieved 'recovered' status when they experienced eight consecutive weeks without significant symptoms. Treatment regimes and doses were compared between younger participants ($N = 3364$) 20–59 years old, and older participants 60 and above ($N = 246$). Of the 3615 STEP BD patients, 67.6% ($N = 2442$) achieved a recovered status – 78.5% ($N = 193$) of older patients vs. 66.8% of the younger patients. On average, participants who reached a recovered status took 2.05 medications with no difference between age groups. Lithium was prescribed to 37.8% of younger patients vs. 29.5% of older patients. Younger and older patients differed significantly on dosages prescribed of lithium, valproate and risperidone (lower dose for elderly). Significant reduction in lithium dosing was observed among individuals aged 50 and older although 42.1% of recovered bipolar elders achieved recovery with lithium alone compared with only 21.3% of the younger cohort. Thus, while recovery is achievable in the elderly, more than one medication is generally needed regardless of age.

Psychotherapy may improve illness self-management in bipolar elders. For example, McBride and Bauer[162] have suggested that older adults with bipolar disorder appear to benefit from psychosocial interventions that assist in managing both mental illness and ageing-related issues. A manual-based medical care model (BCM) developed by Kilbourne and colleagues[163] appears feasible for implementation in bipolar older adult populations. The BCM includes sessions on bipolar symptom patient self-management, use of nurse-run coordination/management, and dissemination of guidelines to care providers on cardiovascular disease risk in bipolar elders[163]. Given the generally substantial medical co-morbidity seen in elderly bipolar patients, integrated therapies that address both bipolar and medical conditions are likely to be critical in order for optimal outcomes.

Emerging evidence suggests a possible neuroprotective/neurotrophic of maintenance lithium treatment[164–166]. As noted above, lithium has been found to inhibit glycogen synthase kinase-3, which is a key enzyme in the metabolism of amyloid precursor protein and in the phosphorylation of tau protein involved in the pathogenesis of Alzheimer's disease[59,144,167]. A cross-sectional, case–control study from Brazil found that long-term lithium treatment reduced the prevalence of Alzheimer's disease in elderly patients with bipolar disorder to levels consistent with those seen in the general population[166]. Similarly, results from a nation-wide Danish register-based study suggest that maintenance lithium treatment may be associated with a reduced rate of dementia[164]. In addition, in bipolar elders (mean age 66.0 ± 9.7 years), brain lithium levels and N-acetylaspartate (NAA), a marker of neuronal integrity, seems to be positively associated on magnetic resonance spectroscopy[165].

Adherence to Treatment

It has been demonstrated that nearly 1 in 2 individuals with bipolar disorder is non-adherent with prescribed medications[168,169]. Age, marital status, gender, educational level, and psychiatric co-morbidity, in particular substance abuse, have all been reported to be related to treatment non-adherence[168,170,171]. One study[172] evaluated antipsychotic medication adherence among older (age 60 and older) vs. younger individuals with bipolar disorder using a large Veterans Affairs case registry ($N = 73\,964$). Medication adherence was evaluated using pharmacy refill patterns. Among older adults, 61.0% ($N = 3350$) were fully adherent, while 19% ($N = 1043$) were partially adherent and 20% ($N = 1098$) were non-adherent. Among younger adults, 49.5% ($N = 10\,644$) were fully adherent, while 21.8% ($N = 4680$) were partially adherent, and 28.7% ($N = 6170$) were non-adherent. In both groups, co-morbid substance abuse and homelessness were predictors of bipolar medication non-adherence.

Additional studies in populations prescribed mood-stabilizing medications note that patient knowledge of mood stabilizers correlates negatively with age, whereas sex and duration of treatment seem unrelated to knowledge[74,173]. Older individuals on mood stabilizers have been found to have more negative views on the doctor–patient relationship and more negative views on mood stabilizers in general[74] compared to younger patients. While non-adherent rates in bipolar elders can be substantial, it is possible that adherence behaviours could be modified via intensive efforts at improving illness and medication knowledge as well as approaches that improve the doctor–patient relationship.

CONCLUSIONS

While the literature on late-life bipolarity has increased in recent years, there remain numerous and important gaps in the published data on the neurobiology, epidemiology, phenomenology and evidence base of treatment of geriatric bipolar affective disorder. This knowledge deficit limits our ability to fully understand and anticipate future healthcare requirements or to plan an optimal care-system.

Older adults with bipolar illness often experience substantial symptomotology, impaired physical and psychosocial functioning, and utilize extensive health care resources. More research is critically needed to understand expected illness trajectory, relationship to cognitive status and treatments that optimize all levels of health and functioning.

There is very limited evidence to support specific biologic or psychosocial interventions for either acute or longer term care of older adults with bipolar disorder. The current literature, based mainly on retrospective analyses or small sample and mixed-age studies, suggests that medication treatments for bipolar elders will generally require modification in dosing and titration, and should be guided by medical burden/frailty as well as the presence of medications that are co-prescribed for medical illnesses. Elderly patients with bipolar illness may be prone to specific drug-related side effects such as renal failure or extrapyramidal symptoms, and when side effects occur, the sequelae may lead to marked disability (for example, a fall leading to hip fracture). Family members and/or caregivers should be involved in treatment planning if at all possible, and clinicians need to be alert to the important issues of ageing-related reduced ability to metabolize/clear psychotropic drugs, treatment adherence and the development of medication intolerance that may develop over time. The ageing process will also often require modifications in psychosocial treatments for bipolar illness. Finally, bipolar elders will generally require close clinical monitoring, flexibility on the part of treatment providers, and utilization of available supports such as ancillary care staff and family.

REFERENCES

1. Phelps J, Angst J, Katzow J, *et al.* Validity and utility of bipolar spectrum models. *Bipolar Disord* 2008; **10**: 179–93.
2. Shulman KI, Herrmann N. Manic syndromes in old age. In Jacoby R, Oppenheimer C, Dening T *et al.* (eds), *The Oxford Textbook of Old Age Psychiatry*, 4th edn. Oxford: Oxford University Press, 2008.
3. Krauthammer C, Klerman GL. Secondary mania: manic syndromes associated with antecedent physical illness or drugs. *Arch Gen Psychiatry* 1978; **35**: 1333–39.
4. Weissman MM, Bruce ML, Leak PJ *et al.* Affective disorders. In Robins LN, Regier DA, (eds.) *Psychiatric Disorders in America: The Epidemiologic Catchment Area Study*. New York: Free Press, 1991.
5. Tsuang MT. Suicide in schizophrenics, manics, depressives, and surgical controls. A comparison with general population suicide mortality. *Arch Gen Psychiatry* 1978; **35**: 153–55.
6. Weeke A, Vaeth M. Excess mortality of bipolar and unipolar manic-depressive patients. *J Affect Disord* 1986; **11**: 227–34.
7. Snowdon J. A retrospective case-note study of bipolar disorder in old age. *Br J Psychiatry* 1991; **158**: 485–90.
8. Kessler RC, Rubinow DR, Holmes C *et al.* The epidemiology of DSM-III-R bipolar I disorder in a general population survey. *Psychol Med* 1997; **27**: 1079–89.
9. Goodwin FK, Jamison KR. *Manic-Depressive Illness*. New York: Oxford University Press, 1990.
10. Tohen M, Waternaux CM, Tsuang MT. Outcome in mania. A 4-year prospective follow-up of 75 patients utilizing survival analysis. *Arch Gen Psychiatry* 1990; **47**: 1106–11.
11. Shulman KI, Tohen M, Satlin A *et al.* Mania compared with unipolar depression in old age. *Am J Psychiatry* 1992; **149**: 341–45.
12. Winokur G. The Iowa 500: heterogeneity and course in manic-depressive illness (bipolar). *Compr Psychiatry* 1975; **16**: 125–31.
13. Sajatovic M, Blow FC, Ignacio RV *et al.* Age-related modifiers of clinical presentation and health service use among veterans with bipolar disorder. *Psychiatr Serv* 2004; **55**: 1014–21.
14. Yassa R, Nair V, Nastase C *et al.* Prevalence of bipolar disorder in a psychogeriatric population. *J Affect Disord* 1988; **14**: 197–201.
15. Eagles JM, Whalley LJ. Ageing and affective disorders: the age at first onset of affective disorders in Scotland, 1969–1978. *Br J Psychiatry* 1985; **147**: 180–87.
16. Spicer CC, Hare EH, Slater E. Neurotic and psychotic forms of depressive illness: evidence from age-incidence in a national sample. *Br J Psychiatry* 1973; **123**: 535–41.
17. Shulman K, Post F. Bipolar affective disorder in old age. *Br J Psychiatry* 1980; **136**: 26–32.
18. Rasanen P, Tiihonen J, Hakko H. The incidence and onset-age of hospitalized bipolar affective disorder in Finland. *J Affect Disord* 1998; **48**: 63–68.
19. Leboyer M, Henry C, Paillere-Martinot ML *et al.* Age at onset in bipolar affective disorders: a review. *Bipolar Disord* 2005; **7**: 111–18.
20. Moorhead SR, Young AH. Evidence for a late onset bipolar-I disorder sub-group from 50 years. *J Affect Disord* 2003; **73**: 271–77.
21. Glasser M, Rabins P. Mania in the elderly. *Age Ageing* 1984; **13**: 210–13.
22. Stone K. Mania in the elderly. *Br J Psychiatry* 1989; **155**: 220–24.
23. Broadhead J, Jacoby R. Mania in old age: A first prospective study. *Int J Geriatr Psychiatry* 1990; **5**: 215.
24. Hays JC, Krishnan KR, George LK *et al.* Age of first onset of bipolar disorder: demographic, family history, and psychosocial correlates. *Depress Anxiety* 1998; **7**: 76–82.
25. Tohen M, Shulman KI, Satlin A. First-episode mania in late life. *Am J Psychiatry* 1994; **151**: 130–32.
26. Shulman KI, Tohen M. Unipolar mania reconsidered: evidence from an elderly cohort. *Br J Psychiatry* 1994; **164**: 547–49.
27. Berrios GE, Bakshi N. Manic and depressive symptoms in the elderly: their relationships to treatment outcome, cognition and motor symptoms. *Psychopathology* 1991; **24**: 31–38.
28. Dhingra U, Rabins PV. Mania in the elderly: a 5–7 year follow-up. *J Am Geriatr Soc* 1991; **39**: 581–83.
29. Lehmann SW, Rabins PV. Factors related to hospitalization in elderly manic patients with early and late-onset bipolar disorder. *Int J Geriatr Psychiatry* 2006; **21**: 1060–64.
30. Goldstein BI, Herrmann N, Shulman KI. Comorbidity in bipolar disorder among the elderly: results from an epidemiological community sample. *Am J Psychiatry* 2006; **163**: 319–21.
31. Sajatovic M, Blow FC, Ignacio RV. Psychiatric comorbidity in older adults with bipolar disorder. *Int J Geriatr Psychiatry* 2006; **21**: 582–87.
32. Sajatovic M, Kales HC. Diagnosis and management of bipolar disorder with comorbid anxiety in the elderly. *J Clin Psychiatry* 2006; **67**(suppl 1): 21–27.

33. Gildengers AG, Whyte EM, Drayer RA *et al*. Medical burden in late-life bipolar and major depressive disorders. *Am J Geriatr Psychiatry* 2008; **16**: 194–200.

34. Subramaniam H, Dennis MS, Byrne J. The role of vascular risk factors in late onset bipolar disorder. *Int J Geriatr Psychiatry* 2007; **22**: 733–37.

35. Starkstein SE, Mayberg HS, Berthier ML *et al*. Mania after brain injury: neuroradiological and metabolic findings. *Ann Neurol* 1990; **27**: 652–59.

36. Strakowski SM, MeElroy SL, Keck PW, Jr. *et al*. The co-occurrence of mania with medical and other psychiatric disorders. *Int J Psychiatry Med* 1994; **24**: 305–28.

37. Carroll BT, Goforth HW, Kennedy JC *et al*. Mania due to general medical conditions: frequency, treatment, and cost. *Int J Psychiatry Med* 1996; **26**: 5–13.

38. Steffens DC, Krishnan KR. Structural neuroimaging and mood disorders: recent findings, implications for classification, and future directions. *Biol Psychiatry* 1998; **43**: 705–12.

39. Starkstein SE, Robinson RG. Mechanism of disinhibition after brain lesions. *J Nerv Ment Dis* 1997; **185**: 108–14.

40. Sackeim HA, Greenberg MS, Weiman AL *et al*. Hemispheric asymmetry in the expression of positive and negative emotions. Neurologic evidence. *Arch Neurol* 1982; **39**: 210–18.

41. Pearlson GD. Structural and functional brain changes in bipolar disorder: a selective review. *Schizophr Res* 1999; **39**: 133–40; discussion 162.

42. Zald DH, Kim SW. Anatomy and function of the orbital frontal cortex, I: anatomy, neurocircuitry; and obsessive-compulsive disorder. *J Neuropsychiatry Clin Neurosci* 1996; **8**: 125–38.

43. Shulman KI. Disinhibition syndromes, secondary mania and bipolar disorder in old age. *J Affect Disord* 1997; **46**: 175–82.

44. Braun CM, Larocque C, Daigneault S *et al*. Mania, pseudo-mania, depression, and pseudodepression resulting from focal unilateral cortical lesions. *Neuropsychiatry Neuropsychol Behav Neurol* 1999; **12**: 35–51.

45. Jorge RE, Robinson RG, Starkstein SE *et al*. Secondary mania following traumatic brain injury. *Am J Psychiatry* 1993; **150**: 916–21.

46. Sweet RA. Case of craniopharyngioma in late life. *J Neuropsychiatry Clin Neurosci* 1990; **2**: 464–65.

47. Lee S, Chow CC, Wing YK *et al*. Mania secondary to thyrotoxicosis. *Br J Psychiatry* 1991; **159**: 712–13.

48. Ur E, Turner TH, Goodwin TJ *et al*. Mania in association with hydrocortisone replacement for Addison's disease. *Postgrad Med J* 1992; **68**: 41–43.

49. Lyketsos CG, Hanson AL, Fishman M *et al*. Manic syndrome early and late in the course of HIV. *Am J Psychiatry* 1993; **150**: 326–27.

50. Alexopoulos GS, Meyers BS, Young RC *et al*. The course of geriatric depression with 'reversible dementia': a controlled study. *Am J Psychiatry* 1993; **150**: 1693–99.

51. Wylie ME, Mulsant BH, Pollock BG *et al*. Age at onset in geriatric bipolar disorder. Effects on clinical presentation and treatment outcomes in an inpatient sample. *Am J Geriatr Psychiatry* 1999; **7**: 77–83.

52. Fujikawa T, Yamawaki S, Touhouda Y. Silent cerebral infarctions in patients with late-onset mania. *Stroke* 1995; **26**: 946–49.

53. Smith GS, Eyler LT. Structural neuroimaging in geriatric psychiatry. *Am J Geriatr Psychiatry* 2006; **14**: 809–11.

54. Rajkowska G, Miguel-Hidalgo JJ, Dubey P *et al*. Prominent reduction in pyramidal neurons density in the orbitofrontal cortex of elderly depressed patients. *Biol Psychiatry* 2005; **58**: 297–306.

55. Braun CM, Daigneault R, Gaudelet S *et al*. Diagnostic and Statistical Manual of Mental Disorders, Fourth Edition symptoms of mania: which one(s) result(s) more often from right than left hemisphere lesions? *Compr Psychiatry* 2008; **49**: 441–59.

56. Mimura M, Nakagome K, Hirashima N *et al*. Left frontotemporal hyperperfusion in a patient with post-stroke mania. *Psychiatry Res* 2005; **139**: 263–67.

57. Beyer JL, Kuchibhatla M, Payne M *et al*. Caudate volume measurement in older adults with bipolar disorder. *Int J Geriatr Psychiatry* 2004; **19**: 109–14.

58. Beyer JL, Kuchibhatla M, Payne ME *et al*. Hippocampal volume measurement in older adults with bipolar disorder. *Am J Geriatr Psychiatry* 2004b; **12**: 613–20.

59. Manji HK, Duman RS. Impairments of neuroplasticity and cellular resilience in severe mood disorders: implications for the development of novel therapeutics. *Psychopharmacol Bull* 2001; **35**: 5–49.

60. Young RC, Murphy CF, Heo M *et al*. Cognitive impairment in bipolar disorder in old age: literature review and findings in manic patients. *J Affect Disord* 2006; **92**: 125–31.

61. Tsai SY, Lee HC, Chen CC *et al*. Cognitive impairment in later life in patients with early-onset bipolar disorder. *Bipolar Disord* 2007; **9**: 868–75.

62. Gildengers AG, Butters MA, Seligman K *et al*. Cognitive functioning in late-life bipolar disorder. *Am J Psychiatry* 2004; **161**: 736–38.

63. Kessing LV, Nilsson FM. Increased risk of developing dementia in patients with major affective disorders compared to patients with other medical illnesses. *J Affect Disord* 2003; **73**: 261–69.

64. Nunes PV, Forlenza OV, Gattaz WF. Lithium and risk for Alzheimer's disease in elderly patients with bipolar disorder. *Br J Psychiatry* 2007; **190**: 359–60.

65. Terao T, Nakano H, Inoue Y *et al*. Lithium and dementia: a preliminary study. *Prog Neuropsychopharmacol Biol Psychiatry* 2006; **30**: 1125–28.

66. Schouws SN, Zoeteman JB, Comijs HC *et al*. Cognitive functioning in elderly patients with early onset bipolar disorder. *Int J Geriatr Psychiatry* 2007; **22**: 856–61.

67. Depp CA, Moore DJ, Sitzer D *et al*. Neurocognitive impairment in middle-aged and older adults with bipolar disorder: comparison to schizophrenia and normal comparison subjects. *J Affect Disord* 2007; **101**: 201–209.

68. D. Martino, A. Igoa, E. Marengo, M. Scápola, E. Ais, S. Strejilevich. Cognitive and motor features in elderly people with bipolar disorder. *J. Affect Disord*. 2008; **105**: 291–95.

69. Radanovic M, Nunes PV, Gattaz WF *et al*. Language impairment in euthymic, elderly patients with bipolar disorder but no dementia. *Int Psychogeriatr* 2008; **20**: 687–96.

70. Gunning-Dixon FM, Murphy CF, Alexopoulos GS *et al*. Executive dysfunction in elderly bipolar manic patients. *Am J Geriatr Psychiatry* 2008; **16**: 506–12.

71. Lin H-C, Tsai S-Y, Lee H-C. Increased risk of developing stroke among patients with bipolar disorder after an acute mood episode: a six-year follow-up study. *J Affect Disord*. 2007; **100**: 49–54.

72. Bartels SJ, Forester B, Miles KM *et al*. Mental health service use by elderly patients with bipolar disorder and unipolar major depression. *Am J Geriatr Psychiatry* 2000; **8**: 160–66.

73. Depp CA, Lindamer LA, Folsom DP *et al*. Differences in clinical features and mental health service use in bipolar disorder across the lifespan. *Am J Geriatr Psychiatry* 2005; **13**: 290–98.

74. Kessing LV. Diagnostic subtypes of bipolar disorder in older versus younger adults. *Bipolar Disord* 2006; **8**: 56–64.

75. Beyer JL, Kuchibhatla M, Cassidy F *et al*. Stressful life events in older bipolar patients. *Int J Geriatr Psychiatry* 2008; **23**: 1271–75.

76. Depp CA, Davis CE, Mittal D *et al*. Health-related quality of life and functioning of middle-aged and elderly adults with bipolar disorder. *J Clin Psychiatry* 2006; **67**: 215–21.

77. Shulman KI, Herrmann N. The nature and management of mania in old age. *Psychiatr Clin North Am* 1999; **22**: 649–65.

78. Young RC, Gyulai L, Mulsant BH *et al*. Pharmacotherapy of bipolar disorder in old age: review and recommendations. *Am J Geriatr Psychiatry* 2004; **12**: 342–57.

79. Sajatovic M, Madhusoodanan S, Coconcea N. Managing bipolar disorder in the elderly: defining the role of the newer agents. *Drugs Aging* 2005; **22**: 39–54.

80. Aziz R, Lorberg B, Tampi RR: Treatments for late-life bipolar disorder. *Am J Geriatr Pharmacother* 2006; **4**: 347–64.

81. American Psychiatric Association. *APA Practice Guidelines for the Treatment of Patients with Bipolar Disorder*. Washington, DC: American Psychiatric Association, 2002.

82. Yatham LN, Kennedy SH, O'Donovan C *et al*. Canadian Network for Mood and Anxiety Treatments (CANMAT) guidelines for the management of patients with bipolar disorder: update 2007. *Bipolar Disord* 2006; **8**: 721–39.

83. National Institutes of Health. www.clinicaltrials.gov, 2009.

84. Gildengers AG, Mulsant BH, Begley AE *et al*. A pilot study of standardized treatment in geriatric bipolar disorder. *Am J Geriatr Psychiatry* 2005; **13**: 319–23.

85. Sachs GS, Thase ME, Otto MW *et al*. Rationale, design, and methods of the systematic treatment enhancement program for bipolar disorder (STEP-BD). *Biol Psychiatry* 2003; **53**: 1028–42.

86. Sajatovic M. Treatment of bipolar disorder in older adults. *Int J Geriatr Psychiatry* 2002; **17**: 865–73.

87. Head L, Dening T. Lithium in the over-65s: who is taking it and who is monitoring it? A survey of older adults on lithium in the Cambridge Mental Health Services catchment area. *Int J Geriatr Psychiatry* 1998; **13**: 164–71.

88. Shulman KI, Rochon P, Sykora K *et al*. Changing prescription patterns for lithium and valproic acid in old age: shifting practice without evidence. *BMJ* 2003; **326**: 960–61.

89. Van der Velde CD. Effectiveness of lithium carbonate in the treatment of manic-depressive illness. *Am J Psychiatry* 1970; **127**: 345–51.

90. Himmelhoch JM, Neil JF, May SJ *et al*. Age, dementia, dyskinesias, and lithium response. *Am J Psychiatry* 1980; **137**: 941–45.

91. Schaffer CB, Garvey MJ. Use of lithium in acutely manic elderly patients. *Clin Gerontology* 1984; **3**: 58–60.

92. Chen ST, Altshuler LL, Melnyk KA *et al*. Efficacy of lithium vs. valproate in the treatment of mania in the elderly: a retrospective study. *J Clin Psychiatry* 1999; **60**: 181–86.

93. Hardy BG, Shulman KI, Mackenzie SE *et al*. Pharmacokinetics of lithium in the elderly. *J Clin Psychopharmacol* 1987; **7**: 153–58.

94. Roose SP, Bone S, Haidorfer C *et al*. Lithium treatment in older patients. *Am J Psychiatry* 1979; **136**: 843–44.

95. Murray N, Hopwood S, Balfour DJ *et al*. The influence of age on lithium efficacy and side-effects in out-patients. *Psychol Med* 1983; **13**: 53–60.

96. Sproule BA, Hardy BG, Shulman KI. Differential pharmacokinetics of lithium in elderly patients. *Drugs Aging* 2000; **16**: 165–77.

97. Shulman KI, Mackenzie S, Hardy B. The clinical use of lithium carbonate in old age: a review. *Prog Neuropsychopharmacol Biol Psychiatry* 1987; **11**: 159–64.

98. Young RC. Treatment of geriatric mania. In Shulman KI, Tohen M, Kutcher SP (eds), *Mood Disorders Across the Life Span*. New York: Wiley-Liss, 1996.

99. Shulman KI, Sykora K, Gill S *et al*. Incidence of delirium in older adults newly prescribed lithium or valproate: a population-based cohort study. *J Clin Psychiatry* 2005; **66**: 424–27.

100. Shulman KI, Sykora K, Gill SS *et al*. New thyroxine treatment in older adults beginning lithium therapy: implications for clinical practice. *Am J Geriatr Psychiatry* 2005; **13**: 299–304.

101. Juurlink DN, Mamdani MM, Kopp A *et al*. Drug-induced lithium toxicity in the elderly: a population-based study. *J Am Geriatr Soc* 2004; **52**: 794–98.

102. McFarland BH, Miller MR, Straumfjord AA. Valproate use in the older manic patient. *J Clin Psychiatry* 1990; **51**: 479–81.

103. Risinger RC, Risby ED, Risch SC. Safety and efficacy of divalproex sodium in elderly bipolar patients. *J Clin Psychiatry* 1994; **55**: 215.

104. Kando JC, Tohen M, Castillo J *et al*. The use of valproate in an elderly population with affective symptoms. *J Clin Psychiatry* 1996; **57**: 238–40.

105. Noaghiul S, Narayan M, Nelson JC. Divalproex treatment of mania in elderly patients. *Am J Geriatr Psychiatry* 1998; **6**: 257–62.

106. Mordecai DJ, Sheikh JI, Glick ID. Divalproex for the treatment of geriatric bipolar disorder. *Int J Geriatr Psychiatry* 1999; **14**: 494–96.

107. Niedermier JA, Nasrallah HA. Clinical correlates of response to valproate in geriatric inpatients. *Ann Clin Psychiatry* 1998; **10**: 165–68.

108. Puryear LJ, Kunik ME, Workman R, Jr. Tolerability of divalproex sodium in elderly psychiatric patients with mixed diagnoses. *J Geriatr Psychiatry Neurol* 1995; **8**: 234–37.

109. Gnam W, Flint AJ. New onset rapid cycling bipolar disorder in an 87 year old woman. *Can J Psychiatry* 1993; **38**: 324–26.

110. Schneider AL, Wilcox CS. Divalproate augmentation in lithium-resistant rapid cycling mania in four geriatric patients. *J Affect Disord* 1998; **47**: 201–205.

111. Goldberg JF, Sacks MH, Kocsis JH. Low-dose lithium augmentation of divalproex in geriatric mania. *J Clin Psychiatry* 2000; **61**: 304.

112. Regenold WT, Prasad M. Uses of intravenous valproate in geriatric psychiatry. *Am J Geriatr Psychiatry* 2001; **9**: 306–308.

113. Felix S, Sproule BA, Hardy BG *et al*. Dose-related pharmacokinetics and pharmacodynamics of valproate in the elderly. *J Clin Psychopharmacol* 2003; **23**: 471–78.

114. Bryson SM, Verma N, Scott PJ *et al.* Pharmacokinetics of valproic acid in young and elderly subjects. *Br J Clin Pharmacol* 1983; **16**: 104–105.

115. Trannel TJ, Ahmed I, Goebert D. Occurrence of thrombocytopenia in psychiatric patients taking valproate. *Am J Psychiatry* 2001; **158**: 128–30.

116. Beyenburg S, Back C, Diederich N, *et al.* Is valproate encephalopathy under-recognized in older people? A case series. *Age Ageing* 2007; **36**: 344–46.

117. Janicak PG. The relevance of clinical pharmacokinetics and therapeutic drug monitoring: anticonvulsant mood stabilizers and antipsychotics. *J Clin Psychiatry* 1993; **54**(suppl: 35–41): discussion 55–36.

118. Kellner MB, Neher F. A first episode of mania after age 80. *Can J Psychiatry* 1991; **36**: 607–608.

119. Schneier HA, Kahn D. Selective response to carbamazepine in a case of organic mood disorder. *J Clin Psychiatry* 1990; **51**: 485.

120. Sethi MA, Mehta R, Devanand DP. Gabapentin in geriatric mania. *J Geriatr Psychiatry Neurol* 2003; **16**: 117–120.

121. Jeste DV. Tardive dyskinesia rates with atypical antipsychotics in older adults. *J Clin Psychiatry* 2004; **65**(suppl 9): 21–24.

122. Jeste DV, Lacro JP, Bailey A *et al.* Lower incidence of tardive dyskinesia with risperidone compared with haloperidol in older patients. *J Am Geriatr Soc* 1999; **47**: 716–19.

123. Herrmann N, Lanctot KL. Pharmacological management of neuropsychiatric symptoms of Alzheimer disease. *Can J Psychiatry* 2007; **52**: 630–46.

124. Howanitz E, Pardo M, Smelson DA *et al.* The efficacy and safety of clozapine versus chlorpromazine in geriatric schizophrenia. *J Clin Psychiatry* 1999; **60**: 41–44.

125. Tzimos A, Samokhvalov V, Kramer M *et al.* Safety and tolerability of oral paliperidone extended-release tablets in elderly patients with schizophrenia: a double-blind, placebo-controlled study with six-month open-label extension. *Am J Geriatr Psychiatry* 2008; **16**: 31–43.

126. Barak Y, Shamir E, Zemishlani H *et al.* Olanzapine vs. haloperidol in the treatment of elderly chronic schizophrenia patients. *Prog Neuropsychopharmacol Biol Psychiatry* 2002; **26**: 1199–202.

127. Jeste DV, Barak Y, Madhusoodanan S *et al.* International multisite double-blind trial of the atypical antipsychotics risperidone and olanzapine: 175 elderly patients with chronic schizophrenia. *Am J Geriatr Psychiatry* 2003; **11**: 638–47.

128. Madhusoodanan S, Brenner R, Araujo L *et al.* Efficacy of risperidone treatment for psychoses associated with schizophrenia, schizoaffective disorder, bipolar disorder, or senile dementia in 11 geriatric patients: a case series. *J Clin Psychiatry* 1995; **56**: 514–18.

129. Shulman RW, Singh A, Shulman KI. Treatment of elderly institutionalized bipolar patients with clozapine. *Psychopharmacol Bull* 1997; **33**: 113–18.

130. Frye MA, Altshuler LL, Bitran JA. Clozapine in rapid cycling bipolar disorder. *J Clin Psychopharmacol* 1996; **16**: 87–90.

131. Gareri P, De Fazio P, Russo E *et al.* The safety of clozapine in the elderly. *Expert Opin Drug Saf* 2008; **7**: 525–538.

132. Herrmann N, Lanctot KL. Do atypical antipsychotics cause stroke? *CNS Drugs* 2005; **19**: 91–103.

133. Herrmann N, Lanctot KL. Atypical antipsychotics for neuropsychiatric symptoms of dementia: malignant or maligned? *Drug Saf* 2006; **29**: 833–43.

134. Judd LL, Akiskal HS, Schettler PJ *et al.* The long-term natural history of the weekly symptomatic status of bipolar I disorder. *Arch Gen Psychiatry* 2002; **59**: 530–37.

135. Kupka RW, Altshuler LL, Nolen WA *et al.* Three times more days depressed than manic or hypomanic in both bipolar I and bipolar II disorder. *Bipolar Disord* 2007; **9**: 531–35.

136. Post RM, Denicoff KD, Leverich GS *et al.* Morbidity in 258 bipolar outpatients followed for 1 year with daily prospective ratings on the NIMH life chart method. *J Clin Psychiatry* 2003; **64**: 680–90.

137. Judd LL, Akiskal HS, Schettler PJ *et al.* Psychosocial disability in the course of bipolar I and II disorders: a prospective, comparative, longitudinal study. *Arch Gen Psychiatry* 2005; **62**: 1322–30.

138. Vieta E, Benabarre A, Colom F *et al.* Suicidal behavior in bipolar I and bipolar II disorder. *J Nerv Ment Disord* 1997; **185**: 407–409.

139. Klausner EJ, Clarkin JF, Lieberman S *et al.* Late-life depression and functional disability: the role of goal-focused group psychotherapy. *Int J Geriatr Psychiatry* 1998; **13**: 707–16.

140. Alexopoulos GS, Vrontou C, Kakuma T *et al.* *Disability in Geriatric Depression*. Washington, DC: American Psychiatric Association, 1995.

141. Lehman AF, Alexopoulos GS, Goldman H *et al.* Mental Disorders and disability. Time to re-evaluate the relationship. In Kupfer DJ, First MB, Regier DA. (eds), *Research Agenda for DSM-V*. Washington, DC: American Psychiatric Association, 2002, 201–218.

142. Smith LA, Cornelius V, Warnock A, *et al.* Pharmacological interventions for acute bipolar mania: a systematic review of randomized placebo-controlled trials. *Bipolar Disord* 2007; **9**: 551–560

143. Johnson FR, Ozdemir S, Manjunath R *et al.* Factors that affect adherence to bipolar disorder treatments: a stated-preference approach. *Med Care* 2007; **45**: 545–52.

144. Fountoulakis KN, Vieta E. Treatment of bipolar disorder: a systematic review of avialable data and clinical perspectives. *Int J Neuropsychopharmacol* 2008; **11**: 999–1029.

145. Gijsman HJ, Geddes JR, Rendell JM *et al.* Antidepressants for bipolar depression: a systematic review of randomized, controlled trials. *Am J Psychiatry* 2004; **161**: 1537–547.

146. Fontoulakis KN, Vieta E, Bouras C *et al.* A systematic review of existing data on long-term lithium therapy: neuroprotective or neurotoxic? *Int J Neuropsychopharmacol* 2008; **11**: 269–87.

147. Kaspar S, Calabrese J, Johnson G *et al.* International Consensus Group on the evidence-based pharmacologic treatment of bipolar I and II depression. *J Clin Psychiatry* 2008; **69**: 1632–46.

148. American Psychiatric Association (APA). Practice guideline for the treatment of patients with bipolar disorder (Revision). *Am J Psychiatry* 2002; **159**(4 suppl): 1–50.

149. Young RC, Gyulai L, Mulsant BH *et al.* Pharmacotherapy of bipolar disorder in old age: review and recommendations. *Am J Geriatr Psychiatry* 2004; **12**: 342–57.

150. Aziz R, Lorber B, Tampi RR. Treatments for late-life bipolar disorder. *Am J Geriatr Pharmacother* 2006; **4**: 347–64.

151. Sajatovic M. Advances in late-life bipolar disorder treatment. Paper presented at the American Association of Geriatric Psychiatry (AAGP) Annual Meeting. Honolulu, Hawaii, March 7, 2009.

152. Sajatovic M, Paulsson B. Quetiapine for the treatment of depressive episodes in adults aged 55 to 65 years with bipolar

disorder. New research poster. AAGP Annual Meeting, New Orleans, Louisiana, March 2007.

153. Calabrese J, Keck PE Jr, Macfadden W *et al*. A randomized, double-blind, placebo-controlled trial of quetiapine in the treatment of bipolar I or II depression. *Am J Psychiatry* 2005; **162**: 1351–60.

154. Thase ME, Macfadden W, Weisler RH *et al*. Efficacy of quetiapine monotherapy in bipolar I and II depression: a double-blind, placebo-controlled study (the BOLDER II study). *J Clin Psychopharmacol* 2006; **26**: 600–609.

155. Sajatovic M, Coconcea N, Ignacio RV *et al*. Aripiprazole therapy in 20 older adults with bipolar disorder: A 12-week, open label trial. *J Clin Psychiatry* 2008; **69**: 41–46.

156. Schaffer A, Mamdani M, Levitt A, Hermann N. Effect of antidepressant use on admissions to hospital among elderly bipolar patients. *Int J Geriatr Psychiatry* 2006; **13**: 275–80.

157. Aizenberg D, Olmer A, Barak Y. Suicide attempts amongst elderly bipolar patients. *J Affect Disord* 2006; **91**: 91–94.

158. Van der Wurff FB, Stek ML, Hoogendijk WJG *et al*. The efficacy and safety of ECT in depressed older adults, a literature review. *Int J Geriatr Psychiatry* 2003; **18**: 894–904.

159. Lepkifker E, Iancu I, Horesh N *et al*. Lithium therapy for unipolar and bipolar depression among the middle-aged and older adult patient subpopulation. *Depress Anxiety* 2006; **24**: 571–76.

160. Sajatovic M, Gyulai L, Calabrese JR *et al*. Maintenance treatment outcomes in older patients with bipolar I disorder. *Am J Geriatr Psychiatry* 2005; **13**: 305–11.

161. Al Jurdi RK, Marangell LB, Petersen NJ *et al*. Prescription patterns of psychotropic medications in elderly compared with younger participants who achieved a 'recovered' status in the systematic treatment enhancement program for bipolar disorder. *Am J Geriatr Psychiatry* 2008; **16**: 922–33.

162. McBride L, Bauer MS. Psychosocial interventions for older adults with bipolar disorder. In Sajatovic M, Blow F (eds), *Bipolar Disorders in Later Life*. Baltimore, MD: Johns Hopkins Press, 2007.

163. Kilbourne AM, Post EP, Nossek A *et al*. Improving medical and psychiatric outcomes among individuals with bipolar disorder: a randomized controlled trial. *Psychiatr Serv* 2008; **59**: 760–68.

164. Kessing LV, Søndergaard L, Forman JL, Andersen PK. Lithium treatment and risk of dementia. *Arch Gen Psychiatry* 2008; **65**: 1331–35.

165. Forester PB, Fin CT, Berlow YA *et al*. Grain lithium, N-acetyl aspartate and myo-inosital levels in older adults with bipolar disorder treated with lithium: a lithium-7 and proton magnetic resonance spectroscopy study. *Bipolar Disord* 2008; **10**: 691–700.

166. Nunes PV, Forlenza OV, Gattaz WF. Lithium and risk for Alzheimer's disease in elderly patients with bipolar disorder. *Br J Psychiatry* 2007; **190**: 359–60.

167. Caccamo A, Oddo S, Tran LX *et al*. Lithium reduces tau phosphorylation but not A beta or working memory deficits in a transgenic model with both plaques and tangles. *Am J Pathol* 2007; **170**: 1669–75.

168. Lingam R, Scott J. Treatment non-adherence in affective disorders. *Acta Psychiatr Scand* 2002; **105**: 164–72.

169. Perlick DA. Medication non-adherence in BPD: A patient-centered review of research findings. *Clin Approaches Bipolar Disord* 2004; **3**: 54–56.

170. Berk M, Berk L, Castle D. A collaborative approach to the treatment alliance in BPD. *Bipolar Disord* 2004; **6**: 504–18.

171. Aagaard J, Vestergaard P, Maarbjerg K. Adherence to lithium prophylaxis: II. Multivariate analysis of clinical, social, and psychosocial predictors of nonadherence. *Pharmacopsychiatry* 1988; **21**: 166–70.

172. Sajatovic M, Blow FC, Kales HC *et al*. Age comparison of treatment adherence with antipsychotic medications among individuals with bipolar disorder. *Int J Geriatr Psychiatry* 2007; **22**: 992–98.

173. Schaub RT, Berghoefer A, Muller-Oerlinghausen B. What do patients in a lithium outpatient clinic know about lithium therapy? *J Psychiatry Neurosci* 2001; **26**: 319–24.

Schizophrenic Disorders and Mood-Incongruent Paranoid States

Late-Life Psychotic Disorders: Nosology and Classification

Nicole M. Lanouette, Lisa T. Eyler and Dilip V. Jeste

University of California, San Diego, La Jolla, CA, USA

With the 5th edition of the Diagnostic and Statistical Manual of Mental Disorders (DSM-V) and 11th edition of the International Classification of Diseases (ICD-11) currently under development, it is timely to review the history of the nomenclature of psychiatric disorders. The notion that mental disorders could occur in particular periods of life, such as old age, first appeared only in the latter half of the nineteenth century[1]. During this short history, there has been great inconsistency regarding the nosology and classification of late-life mental disorders, particularly psychotic disorders.

There are two groups of adults with late-life non-affective psychotic disorders. The first includes individuals who are now older, but whose psychotic illness (e.g. schizophrenia, delusional disorder) emerged early in life. Debates about the classification of these patients are the same as those for younger adults (e.g. degree of overlap between psychosis and affective disorders, issues of duration and course), and there is general consensus that these patients should retain their original diagnosis into old age unless symptoms change dramatically enough to warrant a different diagnosis. The second group of patients includes those with new onset of non-affective psychosis late in life. In the majority of these cases, psychosis is secondary to a general medical condition such as dementia. As there has been little controversy about how to classify these 'organic' psychoses in the elderly, this group is not discussed in the present chapter. In contrast, there has been extensive debate about how to classify late-onset, non-affective, non-organic psychoses. The history of the nosology of this group is replete with overlapping terms, inconsistent age cut-offs, multiple definitions of the same nomenclature, and different methods of conceptualizing similar disorders. In an effort to bring greater consistency to the field, experts in late-life psychotic disorders from 12 countries convened in 1998 and produced an international consensus statement[2]. This statement presented an agreed-upon set of terms to describe late-life psychotic disorders, and recommended that late-onset schizophrenia (LOS, with onset of symptoms after age 40) be designated a formal subtype of schizophrenia. However, neither the ICD-10[3] nor the DSM-IV-TR[4] incorporated this recommendation, continuing the debate over how to best categorize late-onset psychotic disorders.

EARLY HISTORY

Kraepelin was one of the first clinical researchers to recognize that non-affective psychoses could arise in middle age or later in life. Although the term 'dementia praecox', with its inherent emphasis on an early age of onset, would seem to exclude late-onset cases, Kraepelin himself reported that one-third of his patients had symptom onset after age 30[5]. Kraepelin also studied a group of patients he described as suffering from 'paraphrenia'. This term had been used earlier by Guislain as a synonym for the syndrome of 'folly'[6], and was used by Kraepelin to characterize a group of patients with minimal volitional and affective disturbance, prominent paranoia and a relatively preserved personality. While some of the subgroups of paraphrenia he described had a relatively later age of onset, Kraepelin did not consider paraphrenia to be exclusively a late onset disorder. Furthermore, follow-up studies of these patients showed that they did not differ greatly from those classified as dementia praecox[7,8]. Thus, many of Kraepelin's followers ultimately came to believe that dementia praecox and paraphrenia were the same disorder and that this disorder could arise early or late in life.

Other clinician investigators working during this time, however, felt that psychotic disorders arising for the first time in late life should be classified separately. The history of these classifications has been thoroughly reviewed[9]. Gaupp[10] distinguished between dementia praecox and a disorder diagnosed for the first time in postmenopausal women that was characterized by depressive agitation, resulting in 'mental weakness'. Stransky[11] used the term 'dementia tardiva' to describe late-onset dementia praecox. Some authors emphasized the prevalence of paranoid symptoms among those with onset of psychosis late in life by using terms such as 'paranoia chronica'[12] or 'involutional paranoia'[13]. Following this tradition, Albrecht's[14] classification of late-onset psychotic patients distinguished between patients with paranoid symptoms and little personality disturbance ('presenile paraphrenia') and those with 'depressive madness resulting in imbecility'. The latter category seemed somewhat similar to a late-onset form of dementia praecox. Others who described syndromes of late-onset dementia

Principles and Practice of Geriatric Psychiatry, 3rd edn. Edited by Mohammed T. Abou-Saleh, Cornelius Katona and Anand Kumar
© 2011 John Wiley & Sons, Ltd

praecox used the terms 'involutional paraphrenia'[15], 'stiffening involutional psychosis'[16] and 'paraphrenia'[17]. Unfortunately, the use of 'paraphrenia' to indicate an age of onset distinction led to a great deal of later confusion. Some psychiatrists employed the term to indicate a separate phenomenology independent of age of onset (much like Kraepelin's original use; e.g. Leonhard[18]), while others used that diagnosis to encompass most late-onset psychoses.

1940–1970

Using his father's term for dementia praecox, 'schizophrenia', Manfred Bleuler[19] described individuals with 'late-onset schizophrenia' as those with onset after age 40 exhibiting symptoms similar to those with an earlier onset of the disorder and no evidence of brain disease. Very few of these patients had onset after the age of 60. This classification was adopted by most subsequent German authors[9].

In the UK during this period, however, the classification of late-onset psychotic disorders took a somewhat different path. Studying a group of patients with onset after age 60, Roth and Morrissey[20] described a syndrome of paranoid delusions and hallucinations in the context of preserved intellect, personality and affect. Because of the phenomenological similarity to Kraepelin's 'paraphrenia' and due to its late onset, Roth and colleagues termed this disorder 'late paraphrenia'[21,22], a name that was designed to encompass all late-onset, non-affective, non-organic psychoses in which paranoid symptoms were prominent. Thus, the term was both broader than late-onset schizophrenia, in that it encompassed late-onset delusional disorder, and more restrictive, in that it did not include non-paranoid forms of late-onset psychosis. Post[23] developed a different descriptive system. He divided late-onset (after age 50) psychoses into paranoid hallucinosis, schizophreniform syndrome, and schizophrenic syndrome. Based on a three-year follow-up, however, he concluded that these three diseases were actually a continuum of the same disorder with slightly different symptom profiles.

European debates and developments were slow to influence the classification system used in the USA. The first Diagnostic and Statistical Manual of Mental Disorders (DSM-I)[24] used the term 'involutional psychotic reaction', which encompassed both paranoid ideation and depression in older patients. This amalgam of affective and psychotic symptoms in the elderly was split in the second edition (DSM-II)[25] in favour of 'involutional paranoid state (involutional paraphrenia)' and 'involutional melancholia'. The former disorder, like Roth's late paraphrenia, was characterized by 'delusion formation with onset in the involutional period. The absence of conspicuous thought disorders typical of schizophrenia distinguishes it from that group'[25]. Schizophrenia could be diagnosed in individuals with any age of onset.

1970–PRESENT

As European psychiatrists began to study patients with late paraphrenia more systematically, new classification systems in the USA were restricting the diagnosis of late-onset psychosis. One of the five Feighner Research Criteria[26] for schizophrenia was age of onset before age 40. In the third edition of the DSM (DSM-III)[27], a diagnosis of schizophrenia could not be made if the onset of symptoms was after age 45. Late-onset psychosis that involved persistent persecutory delusions with prominent hallucinations could be given a diagnosis of 'paranoid disorder'. This classification system was in

stark contrast to both earlier RDC (research diagnostic criteria)[28] and to the ninth version of the International Classification of Diseases (ICD-9)[29], neither of which imposed age-of-onset restrictions for schizophrenia. The ICD-9 also allowed for a diagnosis of paraphrenia at any age. The revised version of DSM-III (DSM-III-R)[30] rectified the omission of late-onset schizophrenia by providing a separate diagnostic category for those diagnosed with schizophrenia after age 45. In the most recent versions of the DSM (DSM-IV-TR)[4] and the ICD (ICD-10)[3], no special categories exist for late-onset psychoses, although schizophrenia may be diagnosed at any age.

TOWARD A CONSENSUS

It is clear from this historical review that there has been little consensus regarding the classification of late-onset, non-affective, non-organic psychoses. Two opposing lines of thought have pulled the terminology in different directions. On the one hand, some authors have preferred to emphasize the similarity of late-onset psychoses to the corresponding early onset disorders. This has resulted either in the use of terms such as 'late-onset schizophrenia' and 'late-onset delusional disorder' or has prompted a move toward ignoring age of onset altogether in classification (e.g. DSM-IV-TR[4], ICD-10[3]). On the other hand, some members of the psychiatry community (mainly in Europe) have preferred to emphasize differences between the phenomenology of late- and early onset psychosis and thus have tended to use distinct terminology, such as 'paraphrenia' or 'late paraphrenia'[31].

Thus, questions remain about which terminology would optimally serve the clinical and research communities. These questions have become particularly timely with the development of DSM-V[32,33] and ICD-11. There are at least two overlapping issues to consider. First, how similar or different are the late-onset, non-affective, non-organic psychoses from early onset disorders? If late-onset patients are no different from early onset patients in terms of demography, phenomenology, aetiological factors, prognosis and treatment, then it would be redundant to classify them in a separate category. If, however, such features differ between early onset and late-onset individuals, then it would seem important to preserve a distinct diagnostic category in order to encourage further research and allow for optimal prognostic evaluation and treatment. The magnitude or extent of the differences between early-and late-onset individuals should also influence the terminology chosen for the diagnostic categorization. If a majority of critical clinical features are shared with an early onset disorder, then it would make sense to adopt a term such as 'late-onset schizophrenia'. If the extent of differences is sufficiently large, a separate term would be warranted. A second issue to consider in determining the best classification scheme is what age of onset should be called 'late'. Most of the American studies of late-onset, non-affective, non-organic psychosis have included patients with onset after age 45 and generally before age 65. In addition, among the patients in Bleuler's late-onset schizophrenia studies, only 4% had an onset after age 60[9]. In contrast, most studies of late paraphrenia have been conducted with patients whose onset was after age 65. Differences in age of onset between late-onset schizophrenia and late paraphrenia studies may help to explain some of the diagnostic confusions that have persisted.

Only relatively recently has the weight of evidence become sufficiently great in the field of late-life psychoses to allow for adequate consideration of these issues. In 1998, the International Late-Onset Schizophrenia Group met to present reviews of published data on

Table 94.1 Comparison of typical-onset (age 15–40) schizophrenia, middle-age-onset (age 41–65) schizophrenia and very-late-onset (age ≥ 65) schizophrenia-like psychosis

	Typical onset	Middle-age onset	Very late onset
Female : male ratio	0.6 : 1	2 : 1	up to 8 : 1
Poor premorbid functioning	++	+	−
Family history of schizophrenia	++	++	−
Sensory deficits	−	−	+
Negative symptoms	+++	++	−
Thought disorder	+++	+++	−
Structural brain abnormalities (strokes, tumours)	−	−	+
Antipsychotic dose	+++	++	+
Tardive dyskinesia risk	+	+	++

+, presence; −, absence; number of symbols indicates degree of presence.

late-onset, non-affective, non-organic psychosis and to develop a consensus statement regarding diagnostic categories[2]. The statement recognizes two illness classifications: late-onset (onset after the age of 40 years) schizophrenia and a very-late onset (onset after age 60) schizophrenia-like psychosis. Thus, the group determined that it was important to recognize a diagnostic distinction based on age of onset, due to differences between late- and early onset patients, but that the disorders were not sufficiently different to warrant a separate nomenclature. In addition, the group felt that a further distinction was warranted within late-onset patients between those with onset in middle age and those with very late onset, based on major differences between these groups.

The similarities and differences among early onset schizophrenia, late-onset schizophrenia and very-late-onset schizophrenia-like psychosis are summarized in Table 94.1. There are many areas of similarity between both late-onset groups and early onset schizophrenia, such as symptoms[34–36], family history[35], brain imaging findings[37–39], and nature of cognitive impairments[38]. The decision to retain the word 'schizophrenia' in the nomenclature of both disorders was driven by these strong similarities. However, while the nature of cognitive impairments and symptoms are similar, late-onset patients typically show less severe cognitive impairment compared to early onset patients[35,40], and a recent study found late-onset patients had less severe overall psychopathology[41]. On the other hand, the consensus statement's distinction between those with middle-age-onset and old-age-onset psychoses was motivated by epidemiological, aetiological and symptom differences between these two groups. Very-late-onset schizophrenia-like psychosis is different from both early- and late-onset schizophrenia, in that these cases tend to be associated with sensory impairment and social isolation[22], although these may be consequences rather than causes of these disorders[42]. Patients with very-late-onset schizophrenia are also less likely to exhibit formal thought disorder, negative symptoms[35,43] and a wide range of cognitive biases[44], but are more likely to have visual hallucinations[28,37,45] and have less familial aggregation of schizophrenia[46]. A recent magnetic resonance diffusion tensor imaging study of frontal cortex white matter connections found no structural differences between normal controls and patients with onset of psychosis after age 60[47]. It should be emphasized that the members of the International Late-Onset Schizophrenia Group were not unanimous in their support of the particular age cut-offs given in the consensus statement and also felt that the proposed nomenclature was not an end but a beginning of future research into this important topic. Their proposed groupings have

been at least partially supported by subsequent research[41], but more investigations are needed.

Late-onset schizoaffective disorder and late-onset delusional disorder are not specifically addressed in the consensus statement. Late-onset schizoaffective disorder appears to share a majority of critical clinical and demographic features with late-onset schizophrenia[48]. Thus, late-onset schizoaffective disorder appears to be a subgroup of late-onset schizophrenia in which mood symptoms are also present. Late-onset delusional disorder, by contrast, can be distinguished from late-onset schizophrenia by a unique preoccupation with non-bizarre delusions in the context of preserved affective and personality functioning in other domains[49]. In addition, treatment of these individuals may be more challenging than in schizophrenia due to a difficulty in establishing rapport with therapists[50]. Cognitive function, however, is somewhat more preserved in older patients with delusional disorder than in those with schizophrenia[50]. Unfortunately, there is a lack of research comparing early- and late-onset delusional disorder.

Further research is needed to clarify the classification of late-onset psychotic disorders. Specifically, longitudinal follow-up studies are necessary to determine whether the course of illness is different in the three groups of patients and how the course of late-onset disorders compares to that of early onset syndromes. The consensus classification provided a framework for these investigations, although it remains to be seen how those guidelines will be incorporated in DSM-V and ICD-11. In summary, despite a tumultuous history, the future for research and clinical work in late-onset psychotic disorders appears to be on firmer footing.

ACKNOWLEDGEMENTS

This work was supported, in part, by the National Institute of Mental Health Grants MH080002 and MH019934 and by the Department of Veterans Affairs.

REFERENCES

1. Berrios GE. Late-onset mental disorders: a conceptual history. In Marneros A (ed.), *Late-Onset Mental Disorders: The Potsdam Conference*. London: Gaskell, 1999, 1–23.
2. Howard R, Rabins PV, Seeman MV, Jeste DV, the International Late-Onset Schizophrenia Group. Late-onset schizophrenia and very-late-onset schizophrenia-like psychosis: an international consensus. *Am J Psychiatry* 2000; **157**: 172–8.

3. World Health Organization. *ICD-10. The International Statistical Classification of Diseases and Related Health Problems*, vol. 1, 2. Washington, DC: American Psychiatric Press, 1991.

4. American Psychiatric Association. *Diagnostic and Statistical Manual of Mental Disorders, Fourth Edition, Text Revision*. Washington, DC: American Psychiatric Association, 2000.

5. Kraepelin E. *Dementia Praecox and Paraphrenia*. Chicago: Chicago Medical Book, 1919.

6. Campbell RJ. *Psychiatry Dictionary*. New York: Oxford University Press, 1996.

7. Mayer W. On paraphrenic psychoses (in German). *Z Gesamte Neurol Psychiatr* 1921; **71**: 187–206.

8. Mayer-Gross W. Die Schizophrenie (IV. Die Klinik. V. Erkennung und Differential Diagnose). In Bumke O (ed.), *Handbuch der Geiskrankheiten*. Berlin: Springer, 1932, 293–578.

9. Reicher-Rossler A. Late onset schizophrenia; the German concept and literature. In Howard R, Rabins PV, Castle DJ (eds), *Late Onset Schizophrenia*. Basel, Switzerland: Wrightson Biomedical Publishing Ltd, 1999, 3–16.

10. Gaupp R. Depression des hoheren Lebensalters. *Munch Med Wochenschr* 1905; **52**: 1531–7.

11. Stransky E. Dementia tardiva. *Mschr Psychiatr* 1906; **18**: 1–38.

12. Berger H. Klinische Beitrage zur Paranoiafrage. *Mschr Psychiatr* 1913; **34**: 181–229.

13. Kleist K. Die Involutionsparanoia. *Allg Z Psychiatr* 1913; **70**: 1–134.

14. Albrecht H. Die funktionellen Psychosen des Ruckbildungsalters. *Z Neurol Psychiatr* 1914; **22**: 306–44.

15. Serko A. Die Involutionsparaphrenie. *Mschr Psychiatr* 1919; **45**: 245–86.

16. Medow W. Eine Gruppe depressiver Psychosen des Ruckbildungsalters mit ungunstiger Prognose. *Arch Psychiatry* 1922; **64**: 480–506.

17. Kolle K. *Die primare Verrucktheit:psychopathologische, Klinische und genealogische Untersuchungen*. Leipzig: Theime, 1931.

18. Leonhard K. *Aufteilung der endogenen Psychosen*. Berlin: Akademie, 1957.

19. Bleuler M. Late schizophrenic clinical pictures. *Fortschr Neurol Psychiatr* 1943; **15**: 259–90.

20. Roth M, Morrissey JD. Problems in the diagnosis and classification of mental disorder in old age: with a study of case material. *J Ment Sci* 1952; **98**: 66–80.

21. Roth M. The natural history of mental disorder in old age. *J Ment Sci* 1955; **101**: 281–301.

22. Kay DWK, Roth M. Environmental and hereditary factors in the schizophrenias of old age ("late paraphrenia") and their bearing on the general problem of causation in schizophrenia. *J Ment Sci* 1961; **107**: 649–86.

23. Post F. *Persistent Persecutory States of the Elderly*. London: Pergamon Press, 1966.

24. American Psychiatric Association. *Diagnostic and Statistical Manual of Mental Disorders, First Edition*. Washington, DC: American Psychiatric Press, 1952.

25. American Psychiatric Association. *Diagnostic and Statistical Manual of Mental Disorders, Second Edition*. Washington, DC: American Psychiatric Press, 1968.

26. Feighner JP, Robins E, Guze SB *et al*. Diagnostic criteria for use in psychiatric research. *Arch Gen Psychiatry* 1972; **26**: 57–63.

27. American Psychiatric Association. *Diagnostic and Statistical Manual of Mental Disorders, Third Edition*. Washington, DC: American Psychiatric Press, 1980.

28. Spitzer RL, Endicott J, Robins E. *Research Diagnostic Criteria for a Selected Group of Functional Disorders*. New York: New York State Psychiatric Institute, 1978.

29. World Health Organization. *ICD-9. The International Statistical Classification of Diseases and Related Health Problems*. Washington, DC: American Psychiatric Press, 1978.

30. American Psychiatric Association. *Diagnostic and Statistical Manual of Mental Disorders, Third Edition-Revised*. Washington, DC: American Psychiatric Press, 1987.

31. Howard R, Rabins P. Late paraphrenia revisited. *Br J Psychiatry* 1997; **171**: 406–8.

32. Regier DA, Narrow WE, Kuhl EA, Kupfer DJ. The conceptual development of DSM-V. *Am J Psychiatry* 2009; **166**: 645–50.

33. Kupfer DJ, Kuhl EA, Regier DA. Research for improving diagnostic systems: consideration of factors related to later life development. *Am J Geriatr Psychiatry* 2009; **17**: 355–8.

34. Howard R, Castle D, Wessely S, Murray RM. A comparative study of 470 cases of early and late-onset schizophrenia. *Brit J Psychiatry* 1993; **163**: 352–7.

35. Jeste DV, Symonds LL, Harris MJ *et al*. Non-dementia non-praecox dementia praecox? Late-onset schizophrenia. *Am J Geriatr Psychiatry* 1997; **5**: 302–17.

36. Pearlson GD, Kreger L, Rabins RV *et al*. A chart review study of late-onset and early-onset schizophrenia. *Am J Psychiatry* 1989; **146**: 1568–74.

37. Howard RJ, Almeida O, Levy R *et al*. Quantitative magnetic resonance imaging volumetry distinguishes delusional disorder from late-onset schizophrenia. *J Clin Psychiatry* 1999; **60**: 874–82.

38. Jeste DV, McAdams LA, Palmer BW *et al*. Relationship of neuropsychological and MRI measures with age of onset of schizophrenia. *Acta Psychiatr Scand* 1998; **98**: 156–64.

39. Pearlson GD, Tune LE, Wong DF *et al*. Quantitative D_2 dopamine receptor PET and structural MRI changes in late onset schizophrenia. *Schizophr Bull* 1993; **19**: 783–95.

40. Rajji TK, Ismail Z, Mulsant BH. Age at onset and cognition in schizophrenia: a meta-analysis. *Br J Psychiatry* 2009; **195**: 286–93.

41. Girard C, Simard M. Clinical characterization of late- and very late-onset first psychotic episode in psychiatric inpatients. *Am J Geriatr Psychiatry* 2008; **16**: 478–87.

42. Prager S, Jeste DV. Sensory impairment in late-life schizophrenia. *Schizophr Bull* 1993; **19**: 755–72.

43. Sato T, Bottlender R, Schroter A, Moller HJ. Psychopathology of early-onset versus late-onset schizophrenia revisited: an observation of 473 neuroleptic-naive patients before and after first-admission treatments. *Schizophr Res* 2004; **67**: 175–83.

44. Moore R, Blackwood N, Corcoran R *et al*. Misunderstanding the intentions of others: an exploratory study of the cognitive aetiology of persecutory delusions in very late-onset schizophrenia-like psychosis. *Am J Geriatr Psychiatry* 2006; **14**: 410–18.

45. Rabins PV, Pauker S, Thomas J. Can schizophrenia begin after age 44? *Compr Psychiatry* 1984; **25**: 290–3.

46. Howard R, Graham C, Sham P *et al*. A controlled family study of late-onset non-affective psychosis (late paraphrenia). *Br J Psychiatry* 1997; **170**: 511–14.

47. Jones DK, Catani M, Pierpaoli C *et al*. A diffusion tensor magnetic resonance imaging study of frontal cortex connections in very-late-onset schizophrenia-like psychosis. *Am J Geriatr Psychiatry* 2005; **13**: 1092–9.

48. Evans JD, Heaton RK, Paulsen J *et al.* Schizoaffective disorder: a form of schizophrenia or affective disorder. *Br J Psychiatry* 1994; **165**: 474–80.

49. American Psychiatric Association. *Diagnostic and Statistical Manual of Mental Disorders, Fourth Edition*. Washington, DC: American Psychiatric Association, 1994.

50. Evans JD, Paulsen JS, Harris MJ, Heaton RK, Jeste DV. A clinical and neuropsychological comparison of delusional disorder and schizophrenia. *J Neuropsychiat Clin Neurosci* 1996; **8**: 281–6.

95

Schizophrenic Disorder and Mood-Incongruent Paranoid States: Epidemiology and Course

Cynthia D. Fields and Peter V. Rabins

Department of Psychiatry and Behavioral Sciences, Johns Hopkins School of Medicine, Baltimore, USA

OVERVIEW OF SCHIZOPHRENIA AND RELATED DISORDERS

Schizophrenia is a psychotic illness characterized by positive symptoms (hallucinations, delusions, disorganized speech with thought disorder, and disorganized behaviour), negative symptoms (inexpressive or 'flat' affect, poverty of speech, inability to initiate activity) and progressive impairment of social and occupational functioning. Typically, schizophrenia begins in late adolescence or early adulthood and follows a chronic course. Age of onset is, on average, 10 years earlier in males than in females. Recovery to baseline personality and social functioning is rare. The Diagnostic and Statistical Manual of Mental Disorders, fourth edition, text revision (DSM-IV-TR) requires that symptoms be present for six months as a means of ensuring chronicity. To qualify for a diagnosis of schizophrenia, symptoms cannot be due to a primary mood disorder, such as major depression or bipolar disorder, cognitive impairment, including delirium, an acute medical condition or the effects of a substance.

Less commonly, schizophrenia can begin in middle or late life. Summing up the epidemiological studies, Harris and Jeste concluded that almost one quarter of schizophrenia patients had onset of illness after the age of 40[1]. In addition, late-onset psychotic symptoms, such as hallucinations and delusions, can be seen in a variety of disorders, ranging from delirium to bipolar disorder. Schizophrenia should be distinguished from delusional disorder, which tends to begin in mid-life and is characterized by the presence of non-bizarre, fixed, false beliefs. In delusional disorder, hallucinations, when present, are not prominent, and psychosocial functioning is not markedly impaired. Several subtypes of this disorder exist, with persecutory delusions being the most common in the elderly.

EARLY-ONSET VERSUS LATE-ONSET DISORDERS

It remains unclear whether early-onset and late-onset schizophrenias (EOS and LOS, respectively) are distinct disorders. Both EOS and LOS are characterized by the presence of positive symptoms, particularly systematized delusions. In late-onset cases delusions most often are of the persecutory or partition type, with partition delusions being almost unique to that group. Partition delusions refer to the belief that persons or forces (such as gas or electricity), usually of a threatening nature, are operating or entering the home through the walls, ceilings, floors or doors, attempting to interfere. Hallucinations can also be seen in both EOS and LOS. Multimodal hallucinations (i.e. auditory, visual, sensory, gustatory and tactile) are characteristic of the late-onset group[2], while early-onset cases typically have auditory hallucinations only. Schneiderian first-rank symptoms, e.g. hearing a running commentary or two or more voices conversing, can be seen in both groups[3].

Important differences between early- and late-onset cases include infrequent formal thought disorder and fewer negative symptoms, such as affective flattening, in late-onset cases, as well as better premorbid functioning, including better occupational and marital histories. Mental functioning and personality remain relatively well preserved in late-onset cases. Jeste *et al.* compared three groups – younger persons with EOS, older persons with EOS, and LOS – and found a similar overall pattern of neuropsychological impairment, but with some slight differences favouring the late-onset group[4]. Likewise, a recent review by Rajji and Mulsant compared older patients with EOS versus LOS and found them to be equally cognitively impaired, exhibiting deficits in executive functioning, visuo-spatial ability and verbal fluency[5]. Both groups respond well to neuroleptics but later onset cases have a more favourable short-term prognosis than those with onset before 40. In spite of the many similarities, the preservation of personality and lack of deterioration in function lead some experts to challenge the inclusion of later onset cases in the traditional definition of schizophrenia.

INTERPRETATION OF EPIDEMIOLOGICAL DATA

Epidemiological studies of schizophrenia and associated disorders in the elderly face several challenges. First, terminology has changed over time. In 1912 Emil Kraepelin introduced the term 'paraphrenia' to describe a condition characterized by schizophrenia-like delusions and hallucinations not associated with mood disorder, but in the last edition of his text book classified such individuals as having schizophrenia because the course of their illness followed that disease. Roth later revived and modified the phrase 'late paraphrenia' to describe a late-life-onset disorder characterized by prominent paranoid delusions but an absence of social and functional deterioration[6].

Principles and Practice of Geriatric Psychiatry, 3rd edn. Edited by Mohammed T. Abou-Saleh, Cornelius Katona and Anand Kumar
© 2011 John Wiley & Sons, Ltd

Second, diagnostic criteria pertaining to age cut-offs have changed over time. Prior to DSM-III-R, schizophrenia could not be diagnosed in individuals who had onset of symptoms after age 44. Beginning with DSM-III-R, onset after 44 was allowed but cut-offs for what could be defined as 'late-onset' schizophrenia have varied. More recently, a consensus statement proposed by an international group of experts in the field defined late-onset schizophrenia as arising after 40 years of age and very-late-onset schizophrenia-like psychosis (VLOSLP)as arising after 60 years of age[7].

Methodological challenges are a third reason why estimates of the incidence and prevalence of schizophrenic illness in late life vary widely. For example, suspicious individuals are more likely to refuse to participate in population-based surveys and this is compounded by the likelihood that such individuals are socially isolated. Furthermore, individuals with cognitive impairment are often excluded from studies in both community and institutional settings, resulting in an underestimate of the true incidence and prevalence of psychosis in the elderly. Finally, since the prevalence of psychotic disorders is much lower than that of cognitive or affective disorders, misattribution of psychotic symptoms to these other disorders is likely.

INCIDENCE AND PREVALENCE OF PSYCHOTIC DISORDERS

Methodological challenges aside, the incidence and prevalence of psychotic disorders in late life are rather low. Data from community samples suggests that the prevalence of schizophrenia is 1% or less in older age groups, regardless of age of onset. The Epidemiologic Catchment Area Study[8], a large multisite community survey in the United States conducted in the early 1980s, estimated the prevalence of schizophrenia in the community to be 0.6% in the age group 45–64 years, and 0.2% in the 65 and over age group using DSM-III criteria. These rates were approximately one-half that of the younger age groups. Almost twenty years later, Copeland et al. sampled general practitioner lists in the UK and found similarly low rates of DSM-III-R schizophrenia (0.12%) and delusional disorder (0.04%) in the 65+ age group[9]. Copeland's group also reported on incidence, with 3.0 new cases of schizophrenia and 15.6 cases of delusional disorder having developed per 100 000 per year.

In a recent large study of the prevalence of psychotic disorders in the Finnish population, Perala et al. reported DSM-IV schizophrenia in 1.15% of 45–54 year-olds, 0.86% of 55–64 year-olds and 0.92% of those aged 65 and over. Almost 0.5% of the 65 and over age group met criteria for delusional disorder, whereas delusional disorder was not found in persons under age 45[10]. It is important to note that Perala et al.'s use of multiple sources of information, including case notes, may have resulted in higher prevalence estimates. Incidence estimates primarily come from clinical samples and suggest that the development of schizophrenia in late life is rare.

In 1975 Kay used first-admission data from England and Wales to assess the incidence of LOS and found the rates of schizophrenic illness (broadly defined) in ages 65+ to be 10–15 and 20–25 per 100 000 per year in men and women, respectively[11]. These estimates were similar to those reported years later by Holden, with an estimated annual incidence of VLOSLP between 17 and 24 per 100 000 population[12]. The incidence of LOS was reported in another Camberwell study to be 12.6 per 100 000, half that for the under 25 age group. Conversely, van Os et al., using first-admission data, found that, over the age of 60, the annual incidence of schizophrenia-like psychosis increased by 11% with each 5-year increase in age[13].

INCIDENCE AND PREVALENCE OF SINGLE PSYCHOTIC SYMPTOMS

The prevalence of psychotic symptoms in the elderly in disorders other than LOS and VLOSLP is high. For example, estimates of the point prevalence of isolated persecutory or paranoid ideation in the general elderly population are between 4% and 6%, while the incidence of auditory hallucinations and delusions in community-dwelling elderly has been estimated at 6.0% over a period of 3.6 years. Tien's analysis of ECA data showed a general rise in the incidence of hallucinations, including auditory, visual and somatic, with advanced age, especially after about age 65 or 70[14]. Visual hallucinations have been shown to be significantly associated with visual impairment in the elderly. The label Charles Bonnet syndrome is applied to isolated vivid visual hallucinations seen in the setting of ocular pathology, in which insight is at least partially retained. Among non-demented 85-year-olds in Sweden, Ostling and Skoog reported the prevalence of hallucinations as 6.9%; 5.5% had delusions and 6.9% had paranoid ideation not of delusional proportions[15]. Similarly high prevalence estimates were also found in a later sample of non-demented 95-year-olds[16]. As noted above, these high rates are likely due, at least in part, to the use of multiple sources of information, such as key informants and medical records, rather than a reliance on examination by researchers alone. In a related study, Ostling's group also reported a cumulative incidence of first-onset psychotic symptoms at almost 20% in non-demented elderly who survive until age 85.

RISK FACTORS SEEN IN ASSOCIATION WITH LOS AND VLOSLP

The most prominent risk factor associated with late-onset schizophrenia is female gender, with the ratio of women to men being approximately 7:1. Incidence curves for men and women also differ, with early-onset cases developing on average one decade later in women. Hearing loss and ocular pathology also appear to be risk factors. In a review of 27 studies of sensory impairment in psychotic patients, a significant association was found between hearing impairment and late-onset schizophrenia or paranoid disorder[17]. Premorbid schizoid and paranoid personality traits are further risk factors that predispose to the development of schizophrenia. Because very-late-onset cases often live alone, social isolation is thought to play a role. In general, family history of psychotic disorder is less common than in early-onset cases, although the evidence for genetic factors is inconsistent. Some studies have found no increased prevalence of schizophrenia in the first-degree relatives of late-onset schizophrenic probands, while others have determined the risk to be intermediate between that of the general population and earlier-onset cases. Some immigrant populations have also been shown to have significantly higher rates of VLOSLP than indigenous elders.

LONGITUDINAL COURSE AND LATER DEVELOPMENT OF DEMENTIA

Not much is known about the long-term course of schizophrenia in the elderly because most longitudinal studies provide data for only several years. The Vermont Longitudinal Study[18] is exceptional in that it prospectively followed a large cohort of chronic patients, most of whom had been diagnosed with DSM-I schizophrenia at a young age, for over thirty years after their release from the state hospital. Harding found that one third to one half of these patients did not have the expected deterioration and actually showed functional improvement. In the second part of this study[19], Harding *et al.* reassessed the patients and found that almost one half of those who retrospectively met criteria for DSM-III schizophrenia at their index hospitalization had no symptoms (either positive or negative) at follow-up. Harding's studies demonstrate the heterogeneity of functioning at outcome, even when more stringent diagnostic criteria for schizophrenia are used.

Outcomes related to the development of dementia have been of particular interest. In 1955, Roth published the results from his landmark study of a group of 'late paraphrenia' patients, in which only 1 out of 45 patients (i.e. 2%) went on to develop dementia after 3–4½ years of observation[6]. Many years later, using Roth's criteria, Holden found higher rates, reporting that 13 out of 37 (i.e. 35%) patients with late paraphrenia progressed to dementia within 3 years of follow-up[12]. Overall, most studies of LOS and VLOSLP have shown that cognitive deficits are relatively stable over time and that these disorders are not precursors to the development of dementia[20]. It has been reported that hallucinations, especially visual, but not delusions, predict the later development of dementia[21]. Korner *et al.* recently studied the Danish nationwide registers of all hospital in- and outpatients making first-ever contact with late ($\geq$ 40 years of age) or very-late ($\geq$ 60 years) schizophrenia or osteoarthritis during an eight-year period[22]. Over twenty thousand individuals were identified and followed to a first diagnosis of dementia. Korner's group demonstrated that, when compared to patients with osteoarthritis, patients with late as well as very-late first-contact schizophrenia have a three times higher risk of subsequently getting a first diagnosis of dementia.

REFERENCES

1. Harris MJ, Jeste DV. Late-onset schizophrenia: an overview. *Schizophr Bull* 1988; **14**(1): 39–55.
2. Pearlson GD, Kreger L, Rabins PV *et al.* A chart review study of late-onset and early-onset schizophrenia. *Am J Psychiatry* 1989; **146**(12): 1568–74.
3. Rabins P, Pauker S, Thomas J. Can schizophrenia begin after age 44? *Compr Psychiatry* 1984; **25**(3): 290–93.
4. Jeste DV, Symonds LL, Harris MJ *et al.* Nondementia nonpraecox dementia praecox? Late-onset schizophrenia. *Am J Geriatr Psychiatry* 1997; **5**(4): 302–17.
5. Rajji TK, Mulsant BH. Nature and course of cognitive function in late-life schizophrenia: a systematic review. *Schizophr Res* 2008; **102**(1–3): 122–40.
6. Roth M. The natural history of mental disorder in old age. *J Ment Sci* 1955; **101**(423): 281–301.
7. Howard R, Rabins PV, Seeman MV, Jeste DV. Late-onset schizophrenia and very-late-onset schizophrenia-like psychosis: an international consensus. The International Late-Onset Schizophrenia Group. *Am J Psychiatry* 2000; **157**(2): 172–8.
8. Robins LN, Regier DA. *Psychiatric Disorders in America: The Epidemiologic Catchment Area Study*. New York: Free Press, 1991.
9. Copeland JR, Dewey ME, Scott A *et al.* Schizophrenia and delusional disorder in older age: community prevalence, incidence, comorbidity, and outcome. *Schizophr Bull* 1998; **24**(1): 153–61.
10. Perala J, Suvisaari J, Saarni SI *et al.* Lifetime prevalence of psychotic and bipolar I disorders in a general population. *Arch Gen Psychiatry* 2007; **64**(1): 19–28.
11. Kay DW. Schizophrenia and schizophrenia-like states in the elderly. *Br J Psychiatry* 1975; (spec no 9): 18–24.
12. Holden NL. Late paraphrenia or the paraphrenias? A descriptive study with a 10-year follow-up. *Br J Psychiatry* 1987; **150**: 635–9.
13. Van Os J, Howard R, Takei N, Murray R. Increasing age is a risk factor for psychosis in the elderly. *Soc Psychiatry Psychiatr Epidemiol* 1995; **30**(4): 161–4.
14. Tien AY. Distributions of hallucinations in the population. *Soc Psychiatry Psychiatr Epidemiol* 1991; **26**(6): 287–92.
15. Ostling S, Skoog I. Psychotic symptoms and paranoid ideation in a nondemented population-based sample of the very old. *Arch Gen Psychiatry* 2002; **59**(1): 53–9.
16. Ostling S, Borjesson-Hanson A, Skoog I. Psychotic symptoms and paranoid ideation in a population-based sample of 95-year-olds. *Am J Geriatr Psychiatry* 2007; **15**(12): 999–1004.
17. Prager S, Jeste DV. Sensory impairment in late-life schizophrenia. *Schizophr Bull* 1993; **19**(4): 755–72.
18. Harding CM, Brooks GW, Ashikaga T, Strauss JS, Breier A. The Vermont Longitudinal Study of persons with severe mental illness, I: Methodology, study sample, and overall status 32 years later. *Am J Psychiatry* 1987; **144**(6): 718–26.
19. Harding CM, Brooks GW, Ashikaga T, Strauss JS, Breier A. The Vermont Longitudinal Study of persons with severe mental illness, II: Long-term outcome of subjects who retrospectively met DSM-III criteria for schizophrenia. *Am J Psychiatry* 1987; **144**(6): 727–35.
20. Rabins PV, Lavrisha M. Long-term follow-up and phenomenologic differences distinguish among late-onset schizophrenia, late-life depression, and progressive dementia. *Am J Geriatr Psychiatry* 2003; **11**(6): 589–94.
21. Ostling S, Palsson SP, Skoog I. The incidence of first-onset psychotic symptoms and paranoid ideation in a representative population sample followed from age 70–90 years. Relation to mortality and later development of dementia. *Int J Geriatr Psychiatry* 2007; **22**(6): 520–28.
22. Korner A, Lopez AG, Lauritzen L, Andersen PK, Kessing LV. Late and very-late first-contact schizophrenia and the risk of dementia – a nationwide register based study. *Int J Geriatr Psychiatry* 2009; **24**(1): 61–7.

96

Clinical Assessment and Differential Diagnosis

David N. Anderson

Mossley Hill Hospital, Liverpool, UK

The schizophrenias of late life, previously called late paraphrenia[1] and paranoid states in old age, present fascinating, complex, biopsychosocial problems that span the whole of psychiatry and medicine. The characteristics and associations of schizophrenia with onset in later life have been summarized by an international consensus group[2]. These conditions usually present with paranoid ideation, most commonly persecutory in nature, with or without other schizophrenia-like symptoms.

The central abnormality implied by the term 'paranoid' is a morbid distortion of beliefs, but not all distorted beliefs are delusions and not all elderly people expressing them are mentally ill. Many aspects of old age increase vulnerability, exposing elderly people to abuse and victimization, and a thoughtful appreciation of this situation is needed when assessing the paranoid elderly patient. Furthermore, not all patients with delusions have schizophrenia[3] and the first aim of assessment will be to clarify the nature of paranoid symptoms and consider a differential diagnosis. In most cases a diagnosis will be clear from the detailed historical account of symptoms and their course, abnormalities of mental state and simple physical investigations. Assessment must, then, evaluate the individual's level of functioning, independence, vulnerability, social and family support, and physical health, which will all be of relevance to aetiology and management. The assessment will aim to consider patients and their symptoms within the wider context of their social environment, and physical and psychological limitations. It is, therefore, necessary to have knowledge of premorbid personality, lifestyle, life experience and cultural background, remembering that young and older generations have important cultural differences.

Ideally, the assessment will take place in the patient's home, when environment may be maximally appreciated. Home assessment provides a more complete picture of the patient's circumstances and helps put the problem into a living context. Commonly, paranoid ideas in old age relate to the patient's immediate, local environment and people within it. Herbert and Jacobson[4] used the term 'partition delusions' to describe the belief that things were happening just the other side of the wall, floor or ceiling. Post[5] found that paranoid symptoms often temporarily disappeared when the patient was removed from the hostile environment, which can give a misleading impression of their nature and a reason to avoid admission to hospital when it will become difficult to gauge response to treatment.

The floridly deluded and hallucinated patient is easily recognized, but in old age paranoid ideation may be almost plausible when complaints of being abused, victimized, stolen from or manipulated are

Table 96.1 Differential diagnosis

Delirium
Dementia
Organic delusional/hallucinatory disorder, secondary to physical illness or drugs
Late-onset schizophrenia
Delusional disorder
Depression
Mania
Schizoaffective disorder
Paranoid personality disorder
Factual (basis in fact)
Sensory impairment

not beyond the bounds of possibility. Trying to establish the validity of such claims requires observation and information from a variety of sources.

We need, first, to consider the differential diagnosis of paranoid symptoms (Table 96.1) and how clinical assessment helps to differentiate diagnostic categories before discussing the process of assessment in more detail.

DIFFERENTIAL DIAGNOSIS

The point prevalence of paranoid ideas in the general elderly population is 4–6%[6-8]. A population-based study from Sweden found 8% of non-demented 70-year olds developed first-onset psychotic symptoms during a 20-year follow-up and of those surviving to age 85 the cumulative incidence was 20%[9]. These were most commonly visual hallucinations and persecutory delusions. The more common conditions will be reviewed briefly from the perspective of clinical differentiation, although for detailed consideration reference should be made to the relevant chapters.

Delirium (Acute Confusion)

The history is short, usually days or a few weeks, and the onset rapid. A structured assessment, using validated instruments, of 100 people with delirium (17% also had dementia) found 50% experienced perceptual disturbances and hallucinations and 31% delusions[10]. These are typically poorly organized, fluctuating and variable in content, while hallucinations most commonly occur in the visual modality and can be vivid and complex. Other features of delirium will normally be present.

Alcohol intoxication and withdrawal from alcohol, benzodiazepines and barbiturates may all cause paranoid delirium, and withdrawal syndromes should be particularly considered when psychosis develops shortly after a hospital admission.

Dementia (Chronic Confusion)

Ballinger et al.[11] found delusions and hallucinations in 38% and 34%, respectively, of 100 dementia admissions. Another study of 178 Alzheimer's patients revealed persecutory ideation (20%), delusions (16%) and hallucinations (17%) to be common[12]. Fifty per cent of patients with multi-infarct dementia may have delusions at some time[13]. Paulsen et al.[14] reported a cumulative incidence for hallucinations and delusions of 51% over four years for people with probable Alzheimer's disease. The clinical course of diffuse Lewy body disease is particularly characterized by psychotic symptoms, and visual hallucination is a defining characaterisic[15]. In this case the hallucinations may precede other evidence of the disorder.

The manifestations of progressive, global, cognitive impairment will usually be present, although dementia may present with paranoid symptoms that can be indistinguishable from functional illness[16]. Paranoid ideas are frequently related to cognitive deficits, especially memory, leading to accusations of theft or problems arising from perceptual difficulties and misidentification[12]. Like delirium, these fluctuate and may be ferociously denied, or forgotten, at interview, although the theme and content remain fairly consistent.

Depression

If depression is of delusional proportions, biological and characteristic depressive symptoms are usually marked. Delusions and hallucinations, occurring in all sensory modalities, are normally mood-congruent but incongruent symptoms occur and may be difficult to distinguish from those of primary paranoid disorders.

Kay et al.[17] suggested six historical variables that help distinguish affective and paranoid psychoses: life events and family history of affective illness favoured an affective diagnosis, while low social class, few surviving children and social deafness favoured paranoid disorder. Premorbid personality proved the best discriminator, with paranoid patients being solitary, shy, touchy, suspicious and emotionally aloof, and patients with affective disorders reporting subjective ratings of high premorbid anxiety.

Mania

Traditional teaching suggested that mania in old age was both rare and atypical in presentation. Broadhead and Jacoby's[18] prospective study found that young and older-onset patients were clinically very similar. The onset of mania in old age is more common than once thought[19] and the majority of patients will have a history of affective disorder, some 50% having had three or more depressive episodes, with a latency of 15–17 years from first depression to mania[18-21].

Organic Delusional/Hallucinatory Disorder

Paranoid hallucinatory disorders have been associated with a variety of organic conditions[3,8,22-25] and pharmacological agents[3,26,27]. The symptoms may be typical of functional disorders[28] and the diagnosis depends on establishing a clear aetiological link and temporal relationships between a physical disorder or drug and mental disturbance. As Kay put it, 'Had the organic diagnosis not been reached independently of the psychiatric symptomatology, most of the cases would have been regarded as, indubitably, schizophrenic'[28].

The more common causes encountered in clinical practice include hypothyroidism, intra- and extracerebral tumours, epilepsy and cerebrovascular disease, and pharmacological agents such as psychostimulants, anti-parkinsonian and dopaminergic drugs, and steroids.

Possibly the most common is the psychosis of Parkinson's disease. This may be seen in the presence or absence of dementia complicating Parkinson's disease, and psychotic symptoms may occur at any stage. Up to 50% of people may develop psychotic symptoms and 30% experience visual hallucinations within the first five years[29,30]. Visual hallucinations are most common though auditory hallucination and delusions can occur.

Paranoid Personality Disorder

This is necessarily a life-long problem, which must be demonstrable from early adulthood. It is characterized by a sensitive and defensive attitude that causes people to feel they are victims of life and interpret events in a self-referential way. The effects of ageing and the vicissitudes of later life may accentuate these traits and, if dementia or functional illness supervenes, will colour the symptomatology.

Late-onset Schizophrenia

The development of ICD-10[31] and DSM-IV[32] saw the disappearance of age-defined categories of schizophrenia. This reflects the evidence that the symptoms are essentially the same regardless of age, certainly positive symptoms. It is estimated that 23.5% develops after age 40[33], and first admission data suggests the annual incidence of schizophrenia-like psychosis increases by 11% for every five-year period for people over the age of 60[34].

Though positive symptoms are similar regardless of age, negative symptoms are much less common with onset after age 60, when visual hallucination may be more common[2].

Familial risk and genetic contributions to aetiology decline with increasing age of onset. With onset over age 60, the association is weak but associations with sensory impairment, particularly deafness, and social isolation are more evident. These differences led an international consensus to recommend the nomenclature of late onset to refer to onset after age 40 and very late onset after age 60[2]. The preponderance of females in the very-late-onset group appears to be consistent, and very-late-onset cases seem more likely to have premorbid paranoid or schizoid traits though not amounting to personality disorder. Later onset is typically associated with better premorbid educational, occupational and psychosocial functioning than early onset[2].

However, prevalence and gender ratio have been shown to vary in a study of first contacts with onset after age 60 in migrant populations in London[35,36].

Roth and Kay[37] provide a thoughtful discussion of the apparent similarities and differences of the associated features of late- and early-onset schizophrenia.

Delusional Disorders

These are conditions characterized by a persistent, circumscribed delusional theme, and if hallucinations occur they are not prominent.

They are defined by their delusional content, which may be erotic, jealous, hypochondriacal, persecutory or grandiose. These conditions have not been the subject of systematic study in old age, when they are thought to be relatively rare[26]. Onset is usually in middle age but as patients normally function well outside their particular delusion and symptoms frequently persist, they may present in old age. Unlike late-onset schizophrenia, delusional disorder seems not to be associated with premorbid paranoid personality or deafness[38], although querulent paranoia has been related to deviant personality structure[39].

Familially they appear unrelated to affective or schizophrenic illnesses[40,41]. Howard *et al.*[42] found dilatation of lateral and third ventricle volumes by magnetic resonance imaging (MRI) to be more a feature of delusional disorder than schizophrenia in old age, as defined by ICD-10 criteria.

A small retrospective study comparing paraphrenia (schizophrenia of late onset) with paranoia (delusional disorder of late onset) found cerebral infarction on CT brain scan to be a feature of paranoia rather than paraphrenia. Furthermore, social isolation and being unmarried were not features of paranoiacs with cerebral infarction, suggesting separate groups defined by organic or social associations. Response to antipsychotic drugs was worse for paranoia[43].

ASSESSMENT

Interview

Interviewing paranoid elderly people may be complicated by deafness, speech problems or visual handicap, so time and patience are essential. An informant history is mandatory and often several sources may be required.

It is crucial to establish the interview situation, explain its purpose, allay anxieties and put patients at their ease. Many patients will be anxious and fearful. The patients should decide whether they prefer to be seen in private or with a confidant(e) as another's presence may equally inhibit or encourage the disclosure of sensitive material. For similar reasons an informant may wish to speak privately though discussions should never appear clandestine.

Deafness and communication problems should be openly acknowledged, hearing aids worn and working, and extraneous noise eliminated, otherwise false impressions of cognitive state may be formed. If a patient is seen in a hospital setting, insist on a separate, quiet interview room, otherwise conversation will be inhibited and information lost. Posture and attitude convey sincerity, concern and how seriously problems are considered. The patient needs to form a trusting relationship, and a respectful, honest but never patronizing approach is normally accepted. A sympathetic hand can reassure and encourage an anxious or fearful patient.

The importance of establishing a positive therapeutic relationship at this early stage cannot be overstated, as it can have far-reaching effects, not only for the openness of discussion but also for future compliance and prognosis.

History

The nature of psychotic symptoms, their form, content and course must be detailed. Late-onset schizophrenia may develop insidiously over months or a year or more, delusional depression over weeks or a few months, delirium over days and dementia over one to two years. The intensity of paranoid ideas and their effect on behaviour

assist diagnosis and the evaluation of risk. Associated symptoms, particularly affective and cognitive, should then be elicited.

Current and past medical problems and their temporal relationship to the onset of paranoid symptoms must be clearly established, including visual or auditory failure. Aetiologically significant hearing loss in very-late-onset schizophrenia is typically of long duration, severe and due to bilateral middle ear disease, often originating in early life. Details of prescribed and non-prescribed drugs, dosages and recent alterations are essential.

Previous episodes of mental disorder should be confirmed from medical records, when past diagnoses and response to treatment may quickly clarify a diagnostic dilemma. Careful enquiry might uncover past episodes of untreated, self-limiting illness, and changes in behaviour may date the onset of current problems.

Premorbid personality and behaviour are important because departures from these in old age usually signify the onset of a morbid process. Forty to fifty per cent of late-onset schizophrenics have schizoid or paranoid premorbid traits[2,3] and the diagnosis of personality disorder depends on establishing a life-long attitude. Brenes Jette and Winnett[44] emphasized the interaction of narcissistic personality traits and the psychosocial consequences of ageing in their psychodynamic formulation of late-onset paranoid disorder.

The genetic loading of schizophrenia in old age is less marked than with younger patients but a positive family history may be found. Odd behaviour or suicide among family members may be discovered when formal psychiatric treatment is absent.

Current social circumstances and recent change are of relevance to aetiology and management. The schizophrenias of late life are particularly associated with social isolation, but rarely with precipitating life events. Paranoid patients frequently have poor socioeconomic status and multiple difficulties[6], and social support has prognostic implications. Enquiring about alcohol and drug abuse must not be avoided for fear of offending a respectable elderly person. The elderly are not without vice and may be less inclined to confess it.

Mental State Examination

The detailed psychopathology of these conditions is described elsewhere and only points relevant to the process of mental state examination in this context will be mentioned here.

It is important to ensure that the patient understands the terminology used to elicit abnormal experiences and that a common language is being used. Eliciting paranoid and psychotic symptoms can be difficult, but with tact and careful choice of words most patients will participate in an exchange of ideas about their experiences. This must be an unthreatening process for the patient and it is unwise to challenge or trivialize complaints at an early stage. A neutral position is advisable until a firm relationship is established, when complaints may be gradually reframed so that they can be viewed by the patient as problems that can be relieved, rather than unchangeable realities that are not amenable to therapeutic intervention. Suggesting that 'it's all imagination' will be considered insulting and the patient's confidence will be lost.

Perceptual disturbance, thought process and content, mood and cognitive function are areas of particular focus.

Insight is rarely retained and patients may not volunteer experiences if they interpret questions as purely an enquiry into the state of their health. Patients have limited ability to accept the presence of illness or recognize psychiatric experiences as pathological[45]. Needless to say, the mental state examination must be thorough.

Physical Examination

A complete physical examination should be performed routinely, with particular emphasis on neurological status and sensory function. The association between sensory impairment and very-late-onset schizophrenia makes attention to this area important, and remediable conditions may be found. Visual impairment, particularly due to cataracts, is often found in association with delusions and deafness[46], and visual hallucinations may be as much to do with ocular pathology as psychiatric diagnosis[47]. A particular form of acute, elaborate visual hallucinosis, the Charles Bonnet syndrome, is usually related to eye disease or cerebral organic disorder[48]. Simple clinical interview and self-reporting underestimate sensory impairment, and more detailed ophthalmic and audiometric examination may be necessary. A simple battery of laboratory investigations is required for all patients, including haematology, biochemistry, thyroid function, urinalysis and chest radiography.

Advanced neuroradiological techniques promise much for the future but have limited clinical application at the present time. Some authors recommend the routine use of computed tomography (CT) and magnetic resonance imaging (MRI).

Structural cerebral abnormalities, including increased ventricular size and volume reduction in various brain areas, are found in schizophrenia regardless of age at onset[2] and deep white matter hyperintensities in depression of late onset[49]. They appear to bear little relationship to clinical state or outcome in the schizophrenia-like disorders[50,51] but in mood disorder may indicate relative treatment resistance and associated executive dysfunction[52]. Structural imaging is important for excluding conditions like space-occupying lesions.

Functional imaging also shows abnormalities in schizophrenia and depression[2,52].

In dementia neuroimaging has diagnostic significance and has become a routine procedure. MRI is recommended in all cases of dementia[53] and single photon emission computed tomography (SPECT) has considerable diagnostic power in dementia associated with Lewy bodies and Parkinson's disease[54-56].

Psychometric testing may provide a useful baseline measure that can be serially repeated when the possibility of dementia arises. Psychometric testing certainly reveals cognitive deficits in late-onset schizophrenic patients, particularly affecting frontal lobe and memory function[2]. These rarely signify dementia and are more like the deficits found with early-onset schizophrenia than Alzheimer's disease. They do not correlate with severity of psychosis or other clinical parameters. However, it appears that late-onset schizophrenia or psychotic symptoms, particularly visual hallucinations, do predict an increased risk of dementia[9,57].

CONCLUSION

Most patients with late-onset schizophrenia, delusional disorders, dementia and psychotic symptoms will be adequately and preferably managed from home. The need to admit to hospital seems to have declined[58] and may be determined more by social and physical factors or treatment compliance as degree of psychopathology. This is unlikely to be the case for conditions like delirium or psychotic mood disorder, which are often life threatening. For the patient requiring more than outpatient treatment, a day hospital can provide more intensive assessment of mental state, physical health and functional level.

The multifactorial contributions from ageing, physical disability, sensory impairment and social factors demand a multi-professional approach and all relevant disciplines must be available and involved. The evaluation of these conditions requires clinical skill, rigorous attention to detail and a holistic approach. The accuracy of diagnosis and success of management will depend on the quality of initial assessment and if diagnostic doubts exist, treatment should be postponed until the situation becomes clear. Occasionally a diagnostic trial of treatment will be justified.

The paranoid disorders of old age are stimulating, complex, challenging clinical problems that encompass the breadth of psychiatry, medicine and social sciences in their assessment and management.

REFERENCES

1. Kay DWK, Roth M. Environmental and hereditary factors in the schizophrenias of old age (late paraphrenia) and their bearing on the general problems of causation in schizophrenia. *J Ment Sci* 1961; **107**: 649–86.
2. Howard R, Rabins PV, Seeman MV *et al.* Late-onset and very-late-onset schizophrenia-like psychosis: an international consensus. The International Late-Onset Schizophrenia Group. *Am J Psychiatry* 2000; **157**: 172–8
3. Manschreck TC, Petri M. The paranoid syndrome. *Lancet* 1978; **ii**: 251–3.
4. Herbert ME, Jacobson S. Late paraphrenia. *Br J Psychiatry* 1967; **113**: 461–9.
5. Post F. *Persistent Persecutory States of the Elderly*. Oxford: Pergamon, 1966.
6. Christenson R, Blazer D. Epidemiology of persecutory ideation in an elderly population in the community. *Am J Psychiatry* 1984; **141**: 1088–91.
7. Henderson AS, Korten AE, Levings C *et al.* Psychotic symptoms in the elderly: a prospective study in a population sample. *Int J Geriatr Psychiatry* 1998; **13**: 484–92.
8. Forsell Y, Henderson AS. Epidemiology of paranoid symptoms in an elderly population. *Br J Psychiatry* 1998; **172**: 429–32.
9. Ostling S, Palsson SP, Skoog I. The incidence of first onset psychotic symptoms and paranoid ideation in a representative population sample followed from age 70–90 year. Relation to mortality and later development of dementia. *Int J Geriatr Psychiatry* 2007; **22**: 520–28.
10. Meagher DJ, Moran M, Raju B *et al.* Phenomenology of delirium. Assessment of 100 adult cases using standardised measures. *Br J Psychiatry* 2007; **190**: 135–41.
11. Ballinger BR, Reid AH, Heather BB. *Br J Psychiatry* 1982; **140**: 257–62.
12. Burns A, Jacoby R, Levy R. Psychiatric phenomena in Alzheimer's disease. I. Disorders of thought content. II. Disorders of perception. *Br J Psychiatry* 1990; **157**: 72–81.
13. Cummings JL, Miller B, Hill MA, Neshkes R. Neuropsychiatric aspects of multi-infarct dementia and dementia of the Alzheimer type. *Arch Neurol* 1987; **44**: 389–93.
14. Paulsen JS, Salmon DP, Thal LJ *et al.* Incidence and risk factors for hallucinations and delusions in patients with probable AD. *Neurology* 2000; **54**: 1965–71.
15. McKeith IG, Dickson DW, Lowe J *et al.* Diagosis and management of dementia with Lewy bodies: third report of the DLB consortium. *Neuology* 2005; **65**: 1863–72.
16. Holden NL. Late paraphrenia or the paraphrenias? A descriptive study with a 10 year follow-up. *Br J Psychiatry* 1987; **150**: 635–9.

17. Kay DWK, Cooper AF, Garside RF, Roth M. The differentiation of paranoid from affective psychoses by patients' premorbid characteristics. *Br J Psychiatry* 1976; **129**: 207–15.

18. Broadhead J, Jacoby R. Mania in old age: a first prospective study. *Int J Geriatr Psychiatry* 1990; **5**: 215–22.

19. Eagles JM, Whalley LJ. Ageing and affective disorders: the age at first onset of affective disorders in Scotland, 1969–1978. *Br J Psychiatry* 1985; **147**: 180–87.

20. Shulman K, Post F. Bipolar affective disorder in old age. *Br J Psychiatry* 1980; **136**: 26–32.

21. Stone K. Mania in the elderly. *Br J Psychiatry* 1989; **155**: 220–24.

22. Davison K, Bagley CR. Schizophrenia-like psychoses associated with organic disorders of the central nervous system: a review of the literature. In Herrington RN (ed.), *Current Problems in Neuropsychiatry*, British Journal of Psychiatry special publication no. 4. Ashford: Headley Brothers, 1969, 113–84.

23. Miller BL, Benson DF, Cummings JL, Neshkes R. Late life paraphrenia: an organic delusional syndrome. *J Clin Psychiatry* 1986; **47**: 204–7.

24. Dupon RM, Munro Cullum C, Jeste DV. Post-stroke depression and psychosis. *Psychiatr Clin North Am* 1988; **11**: 133–49.

25. Galasko D, Kwo-On-Yuen PF, Thal L. Intracranial mass lesions associated with late onset psychosis and depression. *Psychiatr Clin North Am* 1988; **11**: 151–66.

26. Stoudemire A, Riether AM. Evaluation and treatment of paranoid syndromes in the elderly: a review. *Gen Hosp Psychiatry* 1987; **9**: 267–74.

27. Wood KA, Harris MJ, Morreale A, Rizos AL. Drug induced psychosis and depression in the elderly. *Psychiatr Clin North Am* 1988; **11**: 167–93.

28. Kay DWK, Late paraphrenia and its bearing on the aetiology of schizophrenia. *Acta Psychiatr Scand* 1963; **39**: 156–69.

29. Fenelon G, Mahieux F, Huon R *et al.* Hallucinations in Parkinson's disease: prevalence, phenomenology and risk factors. *Brain* 2000; **123**: 733–45.

30. Graham JM, Grunewald RA, Sagar HJ. Hallucinations in idiopathic Parkinson's disease. *J Neurol Neurosurg Psychiatry* 1997; **63**: 434–40.

31. World Health Organization. *The ICD 10 Classification of Mental and Behavioural Disorders*. Geneva: World Health Organization, 1992.

32. American Psychiatric Association. *Diagnostic and Statistical Manual of Mental Disorders*, 4th edn. Washington, DC: American Psychiatric Association, 1994.

33. Harris MJ, Jeste DV. Late onset schizophrenia: an overview. *Schizophr Bull* 1988; **14**: 39–45.

34. van Os J, Howard R, Takei N *et al.* Increasing age is a risk factor for psychosis in the elderly. *Soc Psychiatry Psychiatr Epidemiol* 1995; **30**: 161–4.

35. Mitter PR, Krishnan S, Bell P *et al.* The effect of ethnicity and gender on first-contact rates for schizophrenia-like psychosis in Bangladeshi, Black and White elders in Tower Hamlets, London. *Int J Geriatr Psychiatry* 2004; **19**: 286–90.

36. Mitter PR, Reeves S, Romero-Rubiales F *et al.* Migrant status, age and social isolation in very late-onset schizophrenia-like psychosis. *Int J Geriatr Psychiatry* 2005; **20**: 1046–51.

37. Roth M, Kay DWK. Late paraphrenia: a variant of schizophrenia manifest in late life or an organic clinical syndrome? A review of recent evidence. *Int J Geriatr Psychiatry* 1998; **13**: 775–84.

38. Watt JAG. Hearing and premorbid personality in paranoid states. *Am J Psychiatry* 1985; **142**: 1453–5.

39. Astrup C. Querulent paranoia: a follow-up. *Neuropsychobiology* 1984; **11**: 149–54.

40. Winokur G. Delusional disorder (paranoia). *Compr Psychiatry* 1977; **18**: 511–21.

41. Watt JAG. The relationship of paranoid states to schizophrenia. *Am J Psychiatry* 1985; **142**: 1456–8.

42. Howard RJ, Almeida O, Levy R *et al.* Quantitative magnetic resonance imaging volumetry distinguishes delusional disorder from late-onset schizophrenia. *Br J Psychiatry* 1994; **165**: 474–80.

43. Flint AJ, Rifat SL, Eastwood MR. Late-onset paranoia: distinct from paraphrenia? *Int J Geriatr Psychiatry* 1991; **6**: 103–9.

44. Brenes Jette CC, Winnett RL. Late-onset paranoid disorder. *Am J Orthopsychiatry* 1987; **57**: 485–94.

45. Almeida OP, Levy R, Howard RJ, David AS. Insight and paranoid disorders in late life (late paraphrenia). *Int J Geriatr Psychiatry* 1996; **11**: 653–8.

46. Cooper AF, Porter R. Visual acuity and ocular pathology in the paranoid and affective psychoses of later life. *J Psychosom Res* 1976; **20**: 107–14.

47. Berrios GE, Brook P. Visual hallucination and sensory delusions in the elderly. *Br J Psychiatry* 1984; **144**: 662–4.

48. Damas-Mora J, Skelton-Robinson M, Jenner FA. The Charles Bonnet syndrome in perspective. *Psychol Med* 1982; **12**: 251–61.

49. Teodorczuk A, O'Brien JT, Firbank MJ *et al.* White matter changes and late life depressive symptoms. Longitudinal study. *Br J Psychiatry* 2007; **191**: 212–17.

50. Hymas N, Nagulb M, Levy R. Late paraphrenia: a follow up study. *Int J Geriatr Psychiatry* 1989; **4**: 23–9.

51. Burns A, Carrick J, Ames D *et al.* The cerebral cortical appearance in late paraphrenia. *Int J Geriatr Psychiatry* 1989; **4**: 31–4.

52. Alexopoulos GS. Depression in the elderly. *Lancet* 2005; **365**: 1961–70.

53. National Institute for Health and Clinical Excellence, and Social Care Institute for Excellence. *Dementia: Supporting People with Dementia and Their Carers in Health and Social Care*, NICE clinical guideline 42. London: NICE/SCIE, 2006.

54. O'Brien JT, McKeith IG, Walker Z *et al.* Diagnostic accuracy of 123I-FP-CIT SPECT in possible dementia with Lewy bodies. *Br J Psychiatry* 2009; **194**: 34–9.

55. National Institute for Health and Clinical Excellence. *Parkinson's Disease: National Clinical Guideline for Diagnosis and Management in Primary and Secondary Care*. London: Royal College of Physicians, 2006.

56. Walker Z, Jaros E, Walker RWH *et al.* Dementia with Lewy bodies: a comparison of clinical diagnosis, FP-CIT single photo emission computed tomography imaging and autopsy. *J Neurol Neurosurg Psychiatry* 2007; **78**: 1176–81.

57. Korner A, Lopez AG, Lauritzen L *et al.* Late and very-late first-contact schizophrenia and the risk of dementia – a nationwide register based study. *Int J Geriatr Psychiatry* 2009; **24**: 61–7.

58. Christie AB, Wood ERM. Further change in the pattern of mental illness in the elderly. *Br J Psychiatry* 1990; **157**: 228–31.

97

Treatment of Late-Life Psychosis

Peter Connelly and Neil Prentice

Murray Royal Hospital, Perth, UK

The treatment of late-life psychosis raises a considerable number of practical and ethical issues. People with this diagnosis are likely to have developed the prodrome of their illness over a significant period of time, often measured in years, during which they might have been considered to be 'eccentric' by the general public and by health and social service professionals. Reeves et al.[1] found an average duration of three years of formal symptoms prior to presentation to specialist services. Compared to people with affective disorders, historical data[2] would suggest that they are more likely to live alone and more likely to suffer hearing loss or other sensory impairment. A significant number[3] will have evidence of a premorbid paranoid personality, with associated poor interpersonal relationships, hypochondriasis, which may have alienated them from primary care services, and depressive symptoms, which inhibit their ability to initiate help-seeking behaviour. Although it is important to avoid stereotypes, and to recognize that people with psychosis in late life tend to have more family contact than younger adults with schizophrenia[4], the description of a typical case in the key study by Kay et al.[5] of a shy, reserved, touchy, suspicious person with difficulty in maintaining or establishing relationships and less likely to display sympathy towards their peers, may lead to individuals with late-life psychosis becoming intensely socially isolated with little in the way of external input during the development of their delusions, at a point where some rationalization of developing beliefs might have helped to prevent them becoming chronically established.

ETHICAL ISSUES

Although there is a fundamental need to protect the health and safety of individuals with late-life psychosis and that of their perceived persecutors – who are often neighbours or relatives – immediate recourse to emergency mental health legislation may undermine the potential to develop a therapeutic relationship in which the necessary challenges to their delusional thinking can take place. The elderly person with a well-developed and long-standing delusional system is unlikely to accept that it is they who are suffering from an illness. Much more likely they will be of the view that some intervention is required to deal with the people who are causing them problems. Patients who are intensely frightened at the thought of others being able to get into their house, despite often elaborate security systems, may well be willing to consider a change of location or temporary admission to hospital, but in many cases the only option will be to try to treat people with late-life psychosis in their existing environ-

ment. Legislation may well become necessary if there is evidence of severe self-neglect, violence or other offending behaviour towards those involved in their delusions or their property.

Persuading the patient with chronic delusions or hallucinations to take antipsychotic drugs can be problematic. Such patients will see no logic in the view that were they to take a drug it would somehow change the behaviour of people in the next block of flats. Suggesting that someone takes an antipsychotic as a way of 'protecting their body' while professionals have the opportunity to get to work on their persecutors to try to reduce the frequency or intensity of their alleged toxic behaviour can be seen as coercive and out of keeping with existing legislation on mental capacity, yet such an explanation may be readily understandable to a patient who has taken steps to protect the fabric of their property from toxic waves or sprays and is in keeping with the non-confrontational exploration of beliefs necessary to try to build cooperation. People who are fearful may accept that antipsychotics or antidepressants may have a role in reducing anxiety and agree to take medication but even with this explanation an ethical debate will continue. Although there does not appear to be specific literature on this topic, it may be surprising to find that whatever explanation has been given to the patient about antipsychotics, compliance with treatment can be surprisingly good.

DRUG THERAPY

While antipsychotics are used extensively in older patients to treat a variety of symptoms, including psychotic symptoms as features of behavioural and psychological symptoms in dementia, much of their use in treating late-life psychosis is inferred from studies of treatment for psychosis in younger patients. This is particularly problematic since older patients are more likely to suffer from major physical illness as a co-morbid feature, and a number of studies have drawn into focus concerns about the over-use of antipsychotic medication, particularly in nursing homes[6], and excess mortality associated with antipsychotic prescribing in the elderly[7].

While the majority of people with late-life psychotic symptoms will have hallucinations and delusions from delirium secondary to a physical cause, as a behavioural and psychological symptom of dementia, or indeed as part of an affective illness, those with schizophrenia or other late-life psychosis comprise 0.1–0.5% of the population over the age of 65[8]. Of all people over the age of 65 with schizophrenia, the majority will have developed their illness prior to age 45[9]. While there are benefits from extrapolating data derived from adults

Principles and Practice of Geriatric Psychiatry, 3rd edn. Edited by Mohammed T. Abou-Saleh, Cornelius Katona and Anand Kumar
© 2011 John Wiley & Sons, Ltd

under 65, in the absence of large multicentre double-blind placebo-controlled studies into treatment of late-life psychosis, there are a number of problems associated with this approach. Primarily the difficulties fall into areas including metabolic side effects, increased risk of extrapyramidal side effects and movement disorder, and the problems of polypharmacy, co-morbid major physical illness and pharmacokinetic changes associated with ageing.

Typical antipsychotics have been used extensively in treating older people with psychosis despite the fact that their high affinity for dopamine D2 receptors is associated with increasing extrapyramidal side effects in older people[10]. In addition these medications tend to be sedating and associated with quite marked anticholinergic side effects, which can cause additional confusion and disorientation in patients with mild cognitive impairment or dementia. By contrast, atypical antipsychotics are associated with less in the way of significant side effects in older people[11] and less hospitalization by comparison to typicals[12]. Both olanzapine and quetiapine are associated with a lower incidence of extrapyramidal side effects than typical antipsychotics[13], though sedation can be problematic and there are additional issues in relation to olanzapine and increased risk of diabetes[14]. Risperidone has been used extensively principally because of the low incidence of sedation or anticholinergic side effects. Clozapine has been used extensively in younger patients, though hypersalivation, neutropaenia and increased risk of agranulocytosis, particularly in older patients, limit its use[15]. Much of the evidence for efficacy of antipsychotics in late-onset psychosis consists of case reports and open studies though these are at times conflicting and there is not clear evidence to suggest that atypical antipsychotics are any more effective in this group of patients. However, compliance is better[16].

In the absence of robust double-blind placebo-controlled data for meta-analysis, guidelines for management of late-onset psychosis focus primarily on the expert consensus approach. Focusing on the management of schizophrenia, the use of atypical antipsychotics is clearly favoured, with 93% of experts rating risperidone as first-line treatment in this group of patients, perhaps because of its low incidence of anticholinergic or sedative side effects. While quetiapine and olanzapine were also rated as first-line treatments by 67% of experts and aripiprazole by 60%, the doses recommended in this group of patients were higher than the treatment doses used in psychosis in dementia[17].

A recent study of attitudes to antipsychotic prescribing in Australian specialists working within old age psychiatry identified a preference for the use of atypical antipsychotics as opposed to typical antipsychotics in an elderly population although no clear preference for any individual atypical antipsychotic was apparent[18]. The principal reasons for this centred on the impression that not only were atypical antipsychotics less likely to be associated with adverse events, particularly in an elderly population who were more likely to be suffering from co-morbid physical conditions, but they were also perceived as being clinically more effective than typical antipsychotics. This was supported by clinical global impression of change data within the clinicians' own patient groups, where 33% of patients with schizophrenia were rated as having improved from moderately ill to mildly ill while on atypical antipsychotics. This is similar to rates of reduction in PANSS[19] total score for elderly patients with psychotic illness treated with amisulpride and risperidone[20] though a more recent open label study of amisulpride treatment for very-late-onset schizophrenia-like psychosis showed significant improvement over a variety of measures and 46.6% reduction in PANSS total score[21].

Taking into account the likelihood of co-morbid physical or psychiatric symptoms in elderly patients and the altered pharmacodynamics and pharmacokinetics of older people, the limited evidence available suggests that treatment with atypical antipsychotic medication may be useful. Although there are recent concerns in relation to increased cerebrovascular risk in older patients with dementia treated with atypical antipsychotic medication[22] and also concerns in relation to excess mortality associated with these drugs[7], their cautious utilization continues to be appropriate in the absence of any clear alternative treatments.

The use of depot medication may not lead to additional advantages. Reeves et al.[1] found that treatment response was not increased by the use of depot and concluded that regular contact with a community psychiatric nurse, an intervention likely to increase social exposure, may be as important in maintaining treatment response.

COGNITIVE BEHAVIOURAL THERAPY

The most common types of delusions are those of reference, control or hypochondriasis[23]. Partition delusions[24] are also over-represented in the late-life onset group. A detailed description of cognitive models and cognitive behavioural interventions lies outwith the scope of this chapter, but an understanding of the development of delusions comes from cognitive behavioural work with younger adults. Cognitive models have been used to explain delusion formation and maintenance[25]. Similar errors in attribution have been proposed as mechanisms leading to hallucinations[26], although some exploratory work to examine the cognitive aetiology of delusions in people with late-life psychosis[27,28] suggests that the wider range of cognitive distortions described in younger adults with schizophrenia may not be as pertinent in older people.

Bentall et al.[29] describe the development of persecutory thinking as a way of the person protecting themselves from perceived assaults on their self-esteem by allowing them to attribute negative events to external causes. Since many patients with late-life onset psychoses have a history of such attribution during most of their adult life, it is easy to understand the continuum of a person feeling that others are in some way hostile towards them, through the development of more eccentric beliefs with associated social withdrawal and finally explicit persecutory delusions in an intensely isolated individual. Protective behaviours become increasingly explicit and the picture of a chronically isolated, elderly lady sitting in a cold, dark house, unheated because she believes the neighbours are stealing her electricity through some tenuously understandable process, and covering surfaces of her furniture or cooking utensils with silver foil to prevent the effects of toxic spray used by the same neighbours will not be unfamiliar to clinicians treating this group of people.

Although techniques were first described by Beck in 1952[30], cognitive behavioural therapy (CBT) studies in people with psychosis began to appear more frequently in the early 1990s. The literature is well reviewed by Rathod et al.[31], who conclude that CBT has emerged as an effective adjuvant to antipsychotic medication in the treatment of schizophrenia. However, the guidelines of the National Institute for Health and Clinical Excellence in the UK[32] concluded that CBT may improve depressive symptoms but is unlikely to improve psychotic symptoms. Enlarging on this, a detailed review by Wykes et al.[33] suggested a clear relationship between the methodological quality of CBT studies and the effect size that they report, with better quality studies reporting a lower effect size.

Fewer CBT studies specifically report outcome with respect to delusions and hallucinations. Of these, fewer still involve a randomized design and report results with standard deviations. Durham et al.[34] is one of these few and they report no benefit for CBT over supportive psychotherapy in these domains. CBT was associated with a greater number of people achieving a 25% improvement in the overall PANSS score but with a relatively high number needed to treat of 13. No patient in this study was aged over 65 and only 2 (of 66) had delusional disorder. The review of long-term outcomes by Durham et al.[35] found a reduction of symptom severity when used for anxiety but not psychosis. McCulloch et al.[27] suggested that people with late-onset psychosis had no evidence of either overt depression or low self-esteem, so a different form of psychological approach may be required. Drawing conclusions about the effectiveness of CBT in late-life onset psychosis would be best done through quality research rather than extrapolation from younger people but limited benefits at best are likely to result. The improvement in socialization that may occur through engagement in CBT programmes may be at least as helpful[31].

There are few studies looking at interventions in middle or late life. Patterson et al.[36] described benefits in the field of everyday living skills among older Latino patients attending a specialized clinic in the USA, such as improved use of public transportation, but no significant change in psychopathology was noted in this pilot study. Granholm et al.[37] explored the effect of cognitive behavioural social skills training in a randomized controlled trial over 24 weeks. Again, social functioning was improved, though benefits in achieving greater insight into psychotic symptoms were not significant overall and were lost after a further six months follow-up[38]. Repetition of the programme led to no additional benefits[37], though social improvements were maintained at follow-up[38].

OTHER NON-PHARMACOLOGICAL INTERVENTIONS

A search of the Cochrane Database of Systematic Reviews reveals many interventions that have been tested in randomized controlled trials in people with schizophrenia. The list includes art therapy, music therapy, compliance therapy, assertive community treatment, distraction techniques, drama therapy and exercise. Of all the studies reviewed in these areas, virtually none include people over 65. The effects reported are influenced by the inconsistency of the data in many areas and it is difficult to recommend any of these be used routinely when dealing with someone with late-life psychosis.

One Chinese study[39] of a family psychoeducational programme included people up to 80 years old, but the number over 65 is not reported and would be very small. It is possible that group may have consisted of people with affective disorder rather than schizophrenia. The improvement in families of their understanding of the patient's illness and an improved problem-solving approach led to better treatment compliance by patients and less inappropriate care delivered by families. Although the culture in China is very different from Western society, these lessons are equally pertinent when considering how to maximize the effectiveness of mental health team input. The area of non-pharmacological interventions for late-life psychosis is likely to prove to be a fruitful ground for research.

UNMET NEED

There has been very little systematic research into the needs of older people with psychoses, especially the generation who have aged in

an era where, in the UK at least, the emphasis on care provision in the community has been more common than dependence on long stay care.

McNulty et al.[40] interviewed 58 people over 65 with a mean of 75 years, 54 of whom had schizophrenia and 2 delusional disorder. They found a total of 152 'needs' in that population, i.e. a problem requiring action for which a suitable intervention exists but which has not been given a recent adequate trial. Of these 56 lay in the social field, with an absence of social life and accommodation problems being uppermost. This group found a considerable level of cognitive impairment among their population, with a mean Mini-Mental State Examination (MMSE) score[41] of 20/30 among their participants. This is considerably lower than a more recent London-based study[42], which found a mean MMSE score of 26.5 among its 77 participants. That group also found social activity, day care and housing among the needs unmet because of lack of service, although unmet needs because of patient refusal of social activity or day care was almost four times higher.

The higher prevalence of cognitive impairment in the former study may reflect the level of deprivation in their population, although a high level of young-onset dementia[43,44] and cerebrovascular disease[45] has also been described in the same geographical region. Services managing people with late-life psychoses should, however, be aware of the possibility of concurrent cognitive impairment, which may have detrimental effects on emotion, motivation and daily living skills, as well as further impairment of reasoning and judgement. This may complicate discussions about potential changes of accommodation, and capacity-based legislation may require to be used.

REHOUSING

The delusions experienced by people with late-life onset psychoses are often highly circumscribed and tend to be local to their present accommodation. However, although there is a plethora of literature which relates to how people hospitalized because of psychoses adapt to community living following discharge[46], there appears to be none which examines the effect of rehousing people in alternative accommodation in the community. In fact a systematic review of the health effects of housing improvement[47] found little evidence linking housing and health, and Blackman et al.[48] found that people over 50 had disappointing health improvement results when moved because of medical priority although this group was less likely than younger people to be rehoused on medical grounds.

LONELINESS

Among the consequences of chronic isolation resulting from late-life psychosis is the presence of loneliness. This may have adverse effects on physical health, particularly higher blood pressure, poor sleep and poor cognition[49]. The importance of regular physical health checks, in people who may have disengaged with health services over long periods of time, cannot be over-emphasized.

VIOLENCE

The traditional view that older people are rarely perpetrators of violence is somewhat dispelled by the Healthcare Commission National Audit of Violence 2006–2007[50], which found that more nurses on older people's inpatient wards reported that they had been physically assaulted than in services for adults of working age. Although the risk of physical assault was greatest in services for people with organic disorders, more than half of the nursing staff on functional units had been assaulted.

Staff may be aware of the risk of potential assault when dealing with a delusional person at home and be careful about how they challenge the delusional beliefs. However, as Taylor[51] points out, relatives and friends may be much more blunt in their challenges and be at increased risk of violence. It may be necessary to include advice to the carer when formulating any treatment plan. This may include training relatives or friends in how to discuss delusional beliefs without exposing themselves to potential violence.

CONCLUSION

The treatment of older people with psychosis is an area in which high-quality research is limited. A clearer understanding of the needs of these people is required urgently. Up to one fifth of non-demented older people who survive to age 85 develop first-onset psychotic symptoms[52] and 2.4% of 95-year-olds meet operational criteria for schizophrenia[53]. An increased number of people with these disorders is inevitable.

As with younger adults, the use of drugs alone is insufficient to achieve stability. The place of psychological therapies is yet to be fully established and the need for an evidence base for both pharmacological and non-pharmacological interventions needs to be expanded. Reduction of social isolation and helping family members cope with the constant expression of delusional material will both help engagement with treatment. Attention to physical care and unmet social needs is vital. Realistically, the goal of treatment is to maintain people in the community and reduce the impact of symptoms. Long-term follow-up of the effects of relocation on individuals would help professionals decide on the risk and benefits of such a move.

REFERENCES

1. Reeves S, Stewart R, Howard R. Service contact and psychopathology in very-late-onset schizophrenia-like psychosis: the effects of gender and ethnicity. *Int J Geriatr Psychiatry* 2002; **17**(5): 473–9.
2. Kay DWK, Roth M. Environmental and hereditary factors in the schizophrenias of old age (late paraphrenias) and their bearing on the general problem of causation in schizophrenia. *J Ment Sci* 1961; **107**: 649–86.
3. Bergmann K. Psychiatric aspects of personality in late life. In Jacoby R, Oppenheimer C (eds), *Psychiatry in the Elderly*, 3rd edn. Avon: Bath Press, 2002, 722–43.
4. Semple SJ, Patterson TL, Shaw WS et al. The social networks of older schizophrenia patients. Clinical Research Center on Late Life Psychosis Research Group. *Int Psychogeriatrics* 1997; **9**(1): 81–94.
5. Kay D, Cooper A, Garside R, Roth M. The differentiation of paranoid from affective psychoses by patients' premorbid characteristics. *Br J Psychiatry* 1976; **129**: 207–15.
6. McGrath AM, Jackson GA. Survey of neuroleptic prescribing in residents of nursing homes in Glasgow. *Br Med J* 1996; **312**(7031): 611–12.
7. Schneider LS, Dagerman KS, Insel P. Risk of death with atypical antipsychotic drug treatment for dementia: meta-analysis of randomized placebo-controlled trials. *JAMA* 2005; **294**(15): 1934–43.
8. Howard R, Rabins PV, Seeman MV, Jeste DV. Late-onset schizophrenia and very-late-onset schizophrenia-like psychosis: an international consensus. *Am J Psychiatry* 2000; **157**(2): 172–8.
9. Harris A, Jeste D. Late onset schizophrenia: an overview. *Schizophr Bull* 1998; **14**: 39–55.
10. Masand P. Clinical effectiveness of atypical antipsychotics in elderly patients with psychosis. *Eur Neuropsychopharmacol* 2004; **14**(suppl 4): S461–9.
11. Neil W, Curran S, Wattis J. Antipsychotic prescribing in older people. *Age Ageing* 2003; **32**(5): 475–83.
12. Aparasu RR, Jano E, Johnson ML, Chen H. Hospitalization risk associated with typical and atypical antipsychotic use in community-dwelling elderly patients. *Am J Geriatr Pharmacother* 2008; **6**(4): 198–204.
13. Gareri P, De Fazio P, De Fazio S et al. Adverse effects of atypical antipsychotics in the elderly: a review. *Drugs Aging* 2006; **23**(12): 937–56.
14. Koro CE, Fedder DO, L'Italien GJ et al. Assessment of independent effect of olanzapine and risperidone on risk of diabetes among patients with schizophrenia: population based nested case-control study. *Br Med J* 2002; **325**(7358): 243–5.
15. Sajatovic M, Madhusoodanan S, Buckley P. Schizophrenia in the elderly: guidelines for management. *CNS Drugs* 2000; **13**(2): 103–15.
16. Dolder CR, Lacro JP, Dunn LB, Jeste DV. Antipsychotic medication adherence: is there a difference between typical and atypical agents? *Am J Psychiatry* 2002; **159**(1): 103–8.
17. Alexopoulos GS, Streim J, Carpenter D, Docherty JP, Expert Consensus Panel for Using Antipsychotic Drugs in Older Patients. Using antipsychotic agents in older patients. *J Clin Psychiatry* 2004; **65**(suppl 2): 5–99.
18. Tiller J, Ames D, Brodaty H et al. Antipsychotic use in the elderly: what doctors say they do, and what they do. *Aust J Ageing* 2008; **27**(3): 134–42.
19. Kay SR, Fiszbein A, Opler LA. The Positive and Negative Syndrome Scale (PANSS) for schizophrenia. *Schizophrenia Bull* 1987; **13**: 261–76.
20. Moller HJ, Riedel M, Eich FX, for the Amielderly Study Group. A six-week, double-blind, randomized trial comparing the safety and efficacy of amisulpiride and risperidone in elderly patients with schizophrenia. *Eur Neuropsychopharmacol* 2005; **15**(suppl 3): 511.
21. Psarros P, Theleritis CG, Paparrigopoulos TJ, Politis AM, Papadimitriou GN. Amisulpiride for the treatment of very-late-onset schizophrenia-like psychosis. *Int J Geriatr Psychiatry* 2009; **24**: 518–22.
22. Medicines and Healthcare Products Regulatory Authority. *Pharmacovigilance Working Party Public Assessment Report on Antipsychotics and Cerebrovascular Accident*, 2006. At www.mhra.gov.uk/home/groups/pl-p/documents/websiteresources/con2024914.pdf, accessed 1 May 2009.
23. Howard R, Almeida O, Levy R. Phenomenology, demography and diagnosis in late paraphrenia. *Psychol Med* 1994; **24**(2): 397–410.

24. Howard R, Castle D, O'Brien J et al. Permeable walls, floors, ceilings and doors: partition delusions in late paraphrenia. *Int J Geriatr Psychiatry* 1992; **7**(10): 719–24.

25. Garety PA, Kuipers E, Fowler D, Freeman D, Bebbington PE. A cognitive model of the positive symptoms of psychosis. *Psychol Med* 2001; **31**(2): 189–95.

26. Bentall R. The illusion of reality: a review and integration of psychological research on hallucinations. *Psychol Bull* 1990; **107**(1): 82–95.

27. McCulloch Y, Clare L, Howard R, Peters E. Psychological processes underlying delusional thinking in late-onset psychosis: a preliminary investigation. *Int J Geriatr Psychiatry* 2006; **21**(8): 768–77.

28. Moore R, Blackwood N, Corcoran R et al. Misunderstanding the intentions of others: an exploratory study of the cognitive etiology of persecutory delusions in very late-onset schizophrenia-like psychosis. *Am J Geriatr Psychiatry* 2006; **14**(5): 410–18.

29. Bentall RP, Corcoran R, Howard R, Blackwood N, Kinderman P. Persecutory delusions: a review and theoretical integration. *Clin Psychol Rev* 2001; **21**(8): 1143–92.

30. Beck AT. Successful outpatient psychotherapy of a chronic schizophrenic with a delusion based on borrowed guilt. *Psychiatry* 1952; **15**: 305–12.

31. Rathod S, Kingdon D, Weiden P, Turkington D. Cognitive-behavioral therapy for medication-resistant schizophrenia: a review. *J Psychiatr Pract* 2008; **14**(1): 22–33.

32. National Institute for Health and Clinical Excellence. *Core Interventions in the Treatment and Management of Schizophrenia in Primary and Secondary Care (Update)*, National Clinical Practice Guideline no. 82, 2009. At www.nice.org.uk/nicemedia/pdf/CG82FullGuideline.pdf, accessed 3 Apr 2009.

33. Wykes T, Steel C, Everitt B, Tarrier N. Cognitive behavior therapy for schizophrenia: effect sizes, clinical models, and methodological rigor. *Schizophr Bull* 2008; **34**(3): 523–37.

34. Durham RC, Guthrie M, Morton RV et al. Tayside–Fife clinical trial of cognitive-behavioural therapy for medication-resistant psychotic symptoms. Results to 3-month follow-up. *Br J Psychiatry* 2003; **182**: 303–11.

35. Durham RC, Chambers JA, Power KG et al. Long-term outcome of cognitive behaviour therapy clinical trials in central Scotland. *Health Technol Assess* 2005; **9**(42): 1–174.

36. Patterson TL, Bucardo J, McKibbin CL et al. Development and pilot testing of a new psychosocial intervention for older Latinos with chronic psychosis. *Schizophr Bull* 2005; **31**(4): 922–30.

37. Granholm E, McQuaid JR, McClure FS et al. A randomized, controlled trial of cognitive behavioral social skills training for middle-aged and older outpatients with chronic schizophrenia. *Am J Psychiatry* 2005; **162**(3): 520–29.

38. Granholm E, McQuaid JR, McClure FS et al. Randomized controlled trial of cognitive behavioral social skills training for older

39. Xiang M, Ran M, Li S. A controlled evaluation of psychoeducational family intervention in a rural Chinese community. *Br J Psychiatry* 1994; **165**(4): 544–8.

40. McNulty SV, Duncan L, Semple M, Jackson GA, Pelosi AJ. Care needs of elderly people with schizophrenia. Assessment of an epidemiologically defined cohort in Scotland. *Br J Psychiatry* 2003; **182**: 241–7.

41. Folstein MF, Folstein SE, McHugh PR. 'Mini-mental state': a practical method for grading the cognitive state of patients for the clinician. *J Psychiatr Res* 1975; **12**(3): 189–98.

42. Abdul-Hamid WK, Lewis-Cole K, Holloway F, Silverman M. Older people with enduring mental illness: a needs assessment tool. *Psychiatr Bull* 2009; **33**: 91–5.

43. Whalley LJ, Thomas BM, McGonigal G et al. Epidemiology of presenile Alzheimer's disease in Scotland (1974–88): I. Non-random geographical variation. *Br J Psychiatry* 1995; **167**(6): 728–31.

44. Whalley LJ, Thomas BM, Starr JM. Epidemiology of presenile Alzheimer's disease in Scotland (1974–88): II. Exposures to possible risk factors. *Br J Psychiatry* 1995; **167**(6): 732–8.

45. Starr JM, Thomas B, Whalley LJ. Population risk factors for hospitalization for stroke in Scotland. *Int J Epidemiol* 1996; **25**(2): 276–81.

46. Holloway F. The RDP Cane Hill Closure Research Project: an overview. *J Ment Health* 1994; **3**(3): 401–11.

47. Thomson H, Petticrew M, Morrison D. Health effects of housing improvement: systematic review of intervention studies. *Br Med J* 2001; **323**(7306): 187–90.

48. Blackman T, Anderson J, Pye P. Change in adult health following medical priority rehousing: a longitudinal study *J Pub Health Med* 2003; **25**(1): 22–8.

49. Luanaigh CO, Lawlor BA. Loneliness and the health of older people. *Int J Geriatr Psychiatry* 2008; **23**(12): 1213–21.

50. Royal College of Psychiatrists' Centre for Quality Improvement. *Healthcare Commission National Audit of Violence 2006–7 Final Report – Older People's Services*. London: Royal College of Psychiatrists, 2008.

51. Taylor PJ. Delusional disorder and delusions: is there a risk of violence in social interactions about the core symptom? *Behav Sci Law* 2006; **24**(3): 313–31.

52. Ostling S, Palsson SP, Skoog I. The incidence of first-onset psychotic symptoms and paranoid ideation in a representative population sample followed from age 70–90 years. Relation to mortality and later development of dementia. *Int J Geriatr Psychiatry* 2007; **22**(6): 520–28.

53. Ostling S, Borjesson-Hanson A, Skoog I. Psychotic symptoms and paranoid ideation in a population-based sample of 95-year-olds. *Am J Geriatr Psychiat* 2007; **15**(12): 999–1004.

people with schizophrenia: 12-month follow-up. *J Clin Psychiatry* 2007; **68**(5): 730–37.

Neuroses (Anxiety Disorders)

98

Nosology and Classification of Neurotic Disorders

David Bienenfeld

Department of Psychiatry, Wright State University Boonshoft School of Medicine, Dayton, OH, USA

INTRODUCTION

The grouping of a variety of psychopathological entities under the heading of 'neurotic disorders' represents the current attempt to solve a nosological tangle dating back further than the time of Sigmund Freud. The contemporary categorization is controversial and less than satisfying to many. A brief look at its historical roots offers some explanation of the sense behind the current ICD-10 and DSM-IV structures.

HISTORY OF THE CLASSIFICATION OF THE NEUROSES

It was Hippolyte-Marie Bernheim who introduced the term 'psychoneurosis' for hysteria and allied conditions. Freud, who studied with Bernheim, differentiated the 'actual neuroses' (including neurasthenia, anxiety neurosis and hypochondria) from the psychoneuroses. The latter category included not only the 'transference neuroses', such as hysteria and obsessive neurosis, but also the psychoses (paraphrenia, schizophrenia, paranoia and manic depression), perversions and neurotic character. Both types of neurosis were related to sexual disturbance; the actual neuroses were direct somatic consequences of a noxious physical influence resulting from misdirected sexual energy; the psychoneuroses were caused by unconscious conflict between instinctual and counter-instinctual forces[1]. Although Freud's thinking on the precise nature of the mental aetiology of the psychoneuroses changed over the years from about 1894 to 1906, he remained consistent in his stance that the psychoneuroses were defined by their aetiology rather than by their phenomenology[2]. Eventually, the psychoses were classified independently, consistent with the views of Kraepelin.

In 1952, the American Psychiatric Association published the first Diagnostic and Statistical Manual of Mental Disorders (DSM-I). It identified the subtypes of psychoneurotic disorders as anxiety, dissociative, conversion, phobic, obsessive-compulsive and depressive reactions[3]. By the mid-1960s, the major diagnostic schemata, ICD-8 and DSM-II, codified the selection of the descriptive framework for identifying the neuroses. Anxiety was seen as the chief characteristic, whether felt and expressed directly or diverted unconsciously into other symptoms. The neuroses were also grouped by severity; they were more specifically symptomatic than the personality disorders, but entailed no gross distortion or impairment of reality testing, as in the psychoses. Categories included in the 300-code section were anxiety, hysterical, phobic, obsessive-compulsive, depressive, neurasthenic, depersonalization and hypochondriacal neuroses. Transient situational disturbances constituted their own category (code 307)[4].

The descriptive focus was emphasized in ICD-9 with the substitution of the term 'neurotic disorders' for 'neuroses', although the categorization was not significantly modified[5]. In 1980, the American Psychiatric Association published the DSM-III[6], which took a substantial leap towards atheoretical descriptive diagnosis by adopting empirically validated criteria based on research diagnostic criteria. One of the most controversial changes was the elimination of the entire class of neuroses. The neurotic disorders were included in the affective, anxiety, somatoform, dissociative and psychosexual disorders[7]. The grouping by severity was abandoned in favour of clusters based on similarity of features. The diagnostic entities retained numerical codes compatible with ICD-9 and ICD-9-CM.

The other revolutionary change introduced with DSM-III was the use of a multiaxial system for diagnosis. Under this scheme, personality disorders, which often predispose individuals to the development of specific neurotic (and other) syndromes, were relegated to a separate and parallel Axis II. The 1987 revision, DSM-III-R, changed some names and criteria but retained the same hierarchy of the neurotic disorders and the same multiaxial formula[8]. DSM-IV, published in 1994, was a more substantive revision overall than DSM-III-R, with only a few changes relevant to the neurotic disorders. The diagnosis of Acute Stress Disorder was added for compatibility with ICD-10. Dissociative Identity Disorder was added to Axis I to replace Multiple Personality Disorder, which was removed from Axis II. Simple Phobia was renamed Specific Phobia for compatibility with ICD-10[9].

Neurotic Disorders in ICD-10 and DSM-IV

The creators of ICD-10 were faced with a formidable challenge, as this version, unlike its nine predecessors, was to be designed as the last of the series to be scheduled for regular revisions[10]. It therefore had to contain a format that would allow for flexibility in minor revisions while establishing a more permanent structure than versions 1–9. While following the lead of the phenomenological school in separating out a major category for mood disorders that includes both psychotic and neurotic levels of severity, it retains the major classification of neurotic disorders, including somatoform disorders and stress-related disorders[11]. This grouping solves the objection that the term 'neurosis' groups together entities which could be better classified, e.g. by placing neurotic types of depression together with other mood disorders, rather than with anxiety disorders. It does, however, retain the historical commonality that traces to Freud's original stress on the aetiological similarity of the psychoneuroses, acknowledging the current state of scientific knowledge that is, at best, ambiguous concerning the aetiology of these disorders[12,13].

Table 98.1 compares the relative positions of the neurotic disorders in ICD-10 and Axis I of DSM-IV. The alphanumeric organization of the International Classification requires the constraint of all mental disorders to 10 major categories. DSM-IV, under no such limitation, separates out anxiety, somatoform and dissociative disorders but keeps them within the same gradient of severity between mood disorders and sexual disorders. Adjustment disorders are removed to a position implying less severity, as well as an implied direction that higher ranking diagnoses are to be made or eliminated first. Personality disorders, of course, are assigned to Axis II.

Under the category of the neurotic disorders, the international and American systems differ in their organization, as outlined in Table 98.2. DSM-IV groups the phobic disorders, obsessive compulsive disorder, post-traumatic stress disorder and generalized anxiety disorder together as anxiety disorders. ICD-10 separates phobic disorders, anxiety disorders and obsessive compulsive disorders. Post-traumatic stress disorders are classified with adjustment disorders. Both schemes separate dissociative and somatoform disorders. ICD-10 groups conversion disorder with dissociative states, consistent with the historical, aetiologically based classification of the hysterias. DSM-IV combines it with the somatoform disorders, based on their phenomenological similarities. ICD-10 retains the diagnosis of neurasthenia; while DSMIII- R refers the clinician to dysthymia, categorized unequivocally as a mood disorder, DSM-IV eliminates the term entirely[8,9,11].

DIAGNOSTIC FEATURES OF NEUROTIC DISORDERS

While each of the major categories of neurotic disorders is described in the chapters that follow, the clinical features of the seven ICD-10 groupings are presented here for overview and comparison[11].

Phobic disorders are a set of disorders in which anxiety is invoked only, or predominantly, by well-defined situations that are not in themselves dangerous. By definition, the object of the fear is external to the individual, so that fears of bodily processes are more appropriately relegated to the category of somatoform disorders. The feared objects are characteristically avoided, and anticipatory anxiety is common.

Other anxiety disorders are those in which anxiety is the major symptom but which are not restricted to specific situations. They include panic disorder, generalized anxiety disorder, and mixed anxiety and depressive disorder. The latter is reserved for cases where symptoms of both are present, neither is predominant, and the depression is not severe enough to be classified under mild depressive disorder.

Obsessive-compulsive disorder is characterized by recurrent obsessional thoughts or compulsive acts, or both. These thoughts and acts are subjectively distressing. Subjective anxiety is usually present and depressive features are common.

Reactions to severe stress and adjustment disorders represent a unique category, in that the component disorders are identified on the grounds of both symptomatology and causation. In these disorders, anxiety follows an exceptionally stressful life event or a significant life change. While psychosocial stressors may precipitate a wide variety of psychiatric syndromes, they are elsewhere neither necessary nor sufficient to explain the occurrence and form of the disorder. The stress and adjustment disorders, however, are seen as arising as a direct consequence of the trauma or life change.

Dissociative disorder is a group of entities that share a partial or complete loss of the normal integration between memory of the past, awareness of identity and immediate sensations, and control of

Table 98.1 Relative positions of neurotic disorders in the diagnostic schemata

ICD 10	DSM-IV
F0 Organic mental disorders	Disorders usually first evident in infancy, childhood or adolescence
F1 Mental and behavioural disorders due to psychoactive substance uses	Delirium; dementia and amnestic and other cognitive disorders
F2 Schizophrenia, schizotypal states and delusional disorders	Mental disorders due to a general medical condition not elsewhere classified
F3 Mood disorders	Substance-related disorders
F4 NEUROTIC, STRESS-RELATED AND SOMATOFORM DISORDERS	Schizophrenia and other psychotic disorders
F5 Behavioral syndromes and mental disorders associated with physiological dysfunction and hormonal changes	Mood disorders
F6 Abnormalities of adult personality and behaviour	ANXIETY DISORDERS
F7 Mental retardation	SOMATOFORM DISORDERS
F8 Developmental disorders	DISSOCIATIVE DISORDERS
F9 Behavioural and emotional disorders with onset usually occurring in childhood or adolescence	Factitious disorders
	Sexual and gender identity disorders
	Eating disorders
	Sleep disorders
	Impulse-control disorders not elsewhere classified

Table 98.2 Classification of neurotic disorders

ICD-10	DSM-IV
F40 *Phobic disorder*	*Anxiety disorders*
40.0 Agoraphobia	300.21 Panic disorder with agoraphobia
.00 Without panic disorder	300.01 Panic disorder without agoraphobia
.01 With panic disorder	300.22 Agoraphobia without history of panic disorder
40.1 Social phobias	300.29 Specific phobia
40.2 Specific (isolated) phobias	300.23 Social phobia
F41 *Other anxiety disorders*	300.3 Obsessive-compulsive disorder
41.0 Panic disorder	309.89 Post-traumatic stress disorder
41.1 Generalized anxiety disorder	308.3 Acute stress disorder
41.2 Mixed anxiety and depressive disorder	300.02 Generalized anxiety disorder
F42 *Obsessive-compulsive disorder*	*Somatoform disorders*
42.0 Predominantly obsessional thoughts	300.81 Somatization disorder
42.1 Predominantly compulsive acts	300.11 Conversion disorder
F43 *Reaction to severe stress and adjustment disorders*	307 Pain disorder
43.0 Acute stress reaction	300.7 Hypochondriasis
43.1 Post-traumatic stress disorder	300.7 Body dysmorphic disorder
43.2 Adjustment disorder	*Dissociative disorders*
.20 Brief depressive reaction	300.12 Dissociative amnesia
.21 Prolonged depressive reaction	300.13 Dissociative fugue
.22 With predominant disturbance of other emotions	300.14 Dissociative identity disorder
.23 With predominant disturbance of conduct	300.6 Depersonalization disorder
.24 With mixed disturbance of emotions and conduct	*Adjustment disorder*
F44 *Dissociative and conversion disorder*	309.0 With depressed mood
44.0 Psychogenic amnesia	309.24 With anxiety
44.1 Psychogenic fugue	309.40 With mixed disturbances of emotions and conduct
44.2 Psychogenic stupor	309.28 With mixed anxiety and depressed mood
44.3 Trance and possession states	309.3 With disturbance of conduct
44.4 Psychogenic movement disorders	
44.5 Psychogenic convulsions	
44.6 Psychogenic anaesthesia and sensory loss	
F45 *Somatoform disorders*	
45.0 Multiple somatization disorder	
45.1 Undifferentiated somatoform disorder	
45.2 Hypochondriacal syndrome	
45.3 Psychogenic autonomic dysfunction	
45.4 Psychogenic pain	
F48 *Other neurotic disorders*	
48.0 Neurasthenia	
48.1 Depersonalization–derealization syndrome	

bodily movements. It is presumed that, in these disorders, the ability to exert conscious and selective control over memory, sensation or bodily function is impaired.

Somatoform disorders are those in which physical symptoms are repeatedly presented with requests for investigation or treatment, in spite of the absence of physical findings to substantiate the perception. Compared with patients who suffer from psychogenic movement or sensory disorders, those with somatoform disorders will demand attention and usually resent physicians who fail to believe in the physical nature of their illnesses. Even when the onset of symptoms is temporally related to a stressful life event, or when external manifestations of depression or anxiety are obvious to others, these patients will frequently resist speculation about psychological causation.

Other neurotic disorders feature two clinical entities, neurasthenia and depersonalization–derealization syndrome. The former,

recalling the pre-Freudian nomenclature, is a controversial category in contemporary psychiatry. Its main feature is fatigue, which may occur upon either mental or physical exercise. The diagnosis is to be made only after depressive and anxiety disorders have been ruled out. Depersonalization–derealization syndrome is a rare disorder in which the patient feels that his/her own mental activity, body or surroundings are changed in quality so as to be unreal or remote. This phenomenon is more commonly observed as a feature of depression, phobias, obsessive-compulsive disorder and some psychoses.

Special Considerations in Geriatric Patients

Anxiety, both as a symptom and as a disorder, is common among the elderly, but not remarkably more or less so than at other ages. The nature of worry and its clinical manifestations, however, change with increasing age. The intricate relationships among psychosocial stress, physical illness, depression and anxiety in late life make the recognition, diagnosis and classification of neurotic disorders in the elderly quite complex[14–16].

The clinician can usually compare the fears and concerns of a younger patient against those of his/her own peers and arrive at a credible assessment of whether or not the anxieties are pathological. The aged, however, have different fears; they worry about physical illness, crime, institutionalization, financial disaster, senility and physical dependency. It is often hard for the younger physician to determine whether the subjective interpretation of events, or the anticipation of future events, is in the realm of clinical anxiety or constitutes adaptive concern. Anxiety results from feelings of vulnerability, and the elderly are truly vulnerable in many ways. It is no easy task to diagnose agoraphobia in an 80-year-old person whose fear of crime in her neighbourhood may exceed its statistical likelihood. The clinician walks a fine line between pathologizing a healthy response and failing to recognize neurotic dysfunction[14].

Physical illnesses with psychiatric manifestations increase in prevalence with age, as does the need to take medications with emotional or behavioural side effects. Emphysema, for example, may produce features indistinguishable from those of panic disorder. Hyperthyroidism is commonly accompanied by symptoms resembling those of generalized anxiety disorder. Further, the guiding symptom profiles for the underlying disorders may be absent or muted in the ageing person. 'Silent myocardial infarction' and afebrile pneumonia are fairly common. Finally, the elderly consume significantly more medication than do younger people and exhibit psychiatric side effects at lower doses and serum levels. Bronchodilators may produce the symptoms of many anxiety states; recommended doses of over-the- counter medications for sleep or colds may induce presentations resembling dissociative states[16].

As could be expected, the diagnosis of somatoform disorders and hypochondriasis is particularly complicated in the elderly. Somatic complaints are common. To some extent, the somatic presentation of emotional disorders is a sociocultural cohort phenomenon. The generation of people over 70 in the 2000s, for example, grew up in the 1940s and earlier. At that time, words such as 'depression' and 'anxiety' were not commonplace parts of everyday conversation. Emotional introspection was not culturally normative. Thus, the older person who complains today of having 'butterflies in my stomach' may be aware of the physical concomitants of anxiety, but not of the emotional state underlying it. The clinician must 'translate' somatically phrased complaints to help determine the affective condition. Furthermore, the increase in prevalence of almost all physical illnesses with age confounds the determination of pathological perception and behaviour, necessary for making diagnoses of somatoform disorders. Both DSM-IV and ICD-10 leave room for a subjective judgement of whether the presence of physical symptoms is sufficient to explain the intensity of the patient's response. There are no objective grounds for deciding when a complaint of abdominal pain constitutes a somatoform disorder in a person with concurrent emphysema, arthritis and congestive heart failure[14,17].

While the delineation of the diagnosis and treatment of post-traumatic stress disorder (PTSD) followed the societal impact of returning Vietnam War veterans, the syndrome is not uncommon in older individuals. The trauma may have been a different war (Second World War or Korea), a natural disaster or a personal event such as physical assault. Symptoms may occur early and continue for decades. In many cases, symptoms may not even be manifest until many years after the traumatic event. Often, the symptoms of delayed PTSD are precipitated by a psychologically reminiscent contemporary event; a concentration camp survivor may not experience stress-related symptoms overtly until becoming widowed and being institutionalized half a century later[14,15].

SUMMARY

The current classification of neurotic disorders is the most recent step in the evolution of the nosological understanding of a diverse group of syndromes. The ICD-10 grouping represents a compromise between the phenomenological grouping of neurotic conditions on a scale of severity between healthy and psychotic function, and the aetiological clustering of disorders presumed to arise from internal conflicts and vulnerabilities to external stressors. The ambiguities inherent in this system reflect the incomplete state of knowledge about the aetiologies of the constituent conditions. The North American schema of DSM-IV sets aside questions of aetiology, except in the case of adjustment disorders, and relies on ostensibly atheoretical phenomenological criteria. Although the diagnostic criteria are technically independent of the age of the patient in both systems, ageing affects the presentation of many of these disorders and makes clinical diagnosis challenging. The multiple biological and social stressors of late life blur the distinction between 'normal' and 'pathological' responses to these threats. Physical illnesses, which increase in frequency with ageing, may produce clinical symptoms easily mistaken for neurotic anxiety. The prevalence of somatic pathology forces subjective judgements about the presence of somatoform and conversion disorders. Chronic and delayed stress reactions are clinically distinct from the acute forms seen in younger individuals. The lack of clarity in the classification of these disorders, however, is probably less a manifestation of the shortcomings of the nosological systems than a reflection of the complicated function of the human mind. The neurotic disorders, as well as current science can determine, are a product not of brain disease but of human response to a complicated and stressful world. Simplicity in their nosology would belie the challenges they pose to patients and clinicians.

REFERENCES

1. Gray M. *Neuroses: A Comprehensive and Critical Review*. New York: Van Nostrand Reinhold, 1978, 1–32.
2. Brenner C. *An Elementary Textbook of Psychoanalysis*. Garden City: Doubleday, 1973, 171–92.
3. American Psychiatric Association. *Diagnostic and Statistical Manual of Mental Disorders (DSM-I)*. Washington, DC: American Psychiatric Association, 1952.
4. American Psychiatric Association. Diagnostic and Statistical Manual of Mental Disorders, 2nd edn (DSM-II). Washington, DC: American Psychiatric Association, 1968.
5. World Health Organization. *Manual of the International Statistical Classification of Diseases, Injuries, and Causes of Death*, 9th revision. Geneva: World Health Organization, 1977.
6. American Psychiatric Association. *Diagnostic and Statistical Manual of Mental Disorders*, 3rd edn (DSM-III). Washington, DC: American Psychiatric Association, 1980.
7. Spitzer RL. Introduction. In *Diagnostic and Statistical Manual of Mental Disorders*, 3rd edn (DSM-III). Washington, DC: American Psychiatric Association, 1980, 1–12.
8. American Psychiatric Association. *Diagnostic and Statistical Manual of Mental Disorders*, 3rd edn, Revised (DSM-III-R). Washington, DC: American Psychiatric Association, 1987.

9. American Psychiatric Association. *Diagnostic and Statistical Manual of Mental Disorders*, 4th edn (DSM-IV). Washington, DC: American Psychiatric Association, 1994.

10. Sartorius N. International perspectives of psychiatric classification. *Br J Psychiatry* 1988; **152**(1): 9–14.

11. World Health Organization. *Tenth Revision of the International Classification of Diseases, Chapter V(F): Mental and Behavioural Disorders* (Draft, revision 4). Geneva: World Health Organization, 1987.

12. Freeman CP. In Kendell RE, Zeally AK (eds), *Neurotic Disorders in Companion to Psychiatric Studies*, 4th edn. Edinburgh: Churchill Livingstone, 1988, 374–406.

13. Cooper JE. The structure and presentation of contemporary psychiatric classifications with special reference to ICD-9 and -10. *Br J Psychiatry* 1988; **152**(1): 21–8.

14. Ruskin PE. In Bienenfeld D (ed.), *Anxiety and Somatoform Disorders in Verwoerdt's Clinical Geropsychiatry*, 3rd edn. Baltimore, MD: Williams and Wilkins, 1990, 137–50.

15. Flint AJ. Anxiety disorders in later life: from epidemiology to treatment. *Am J Geriatr Psychiatry* 2007; **15**(8): 635–8.

16. Brenes GA, Penninx BWJH. Judd PH, Rockwell E, Sewell DD, Wetherell JL. Anxiety, depression and disability across the lifespan. *Aging Ment Health* 2008; **12**(1): 158–63.

17. Blazer D. Hypochondriasis and other somatoform disorders. In Blazer D (ed.), *Emotional Problems in Later Life*. New York: Springer, 1998, 123–42.

99

The Epidemiology of Depression and Anxiety

Robert Stewart[1] and James Lindesay[2]

[1]Section of Epidemiology, Institute of Psychiatry, King's College London, London, UK
[2]Department of Health Sciences, University of Leicester, Leicester, UK

GENERAL CONSIDERATIONS

Depression and anxiety are common and important disorders in later life. Before reviewing their epidemiology, it is important to consider some issues around research in old age, to the extent that these impinge on research findings.

What is Old Age?

Research in 'older people' often arbitrarily focuses on people aged 65 years and over, that is, above the usual retirement age in Western nations. This '65+' range includes very varied populations: those within a decade after retirement who can reasonably expect to be in good health, through to more advanced decades where physical and mental decline become much more common and where profound social changes are more frequent, such as bereavement and challenges to independent living. The '65+' cut-off already has little social meaning in many nations and will become steadily less relevant as retirement ages become more flexible in the West. For anxiety and depression, at least two age-group targets may be more appropriate. Retirement itself is a major life-event and may exert a substantial impact on later health; for example, whether the retirement was planned, the retiree's earlier attitude to financial planning and the resources they have put aside, their ability to find alternative occupation, and the quality of interpersonal relationships as life becomes more home centred. Research around this life-transition should have a broader age focus that includes the decade or more leading up to retirement, in order to understand better what happens afterwards. At the other extreme, more 'traditional' late-life research into the impact of physical ill health and social stressors should shift its focus towards older age groups where these have highest salience.

Constructs of Anxiety and Depressive Disorders

Anxiety and depression are applied to mental states where there are no clearly identifiable boundaries between normality and abnormality. The way in which a syndrome is defined is an important consideration. Instruments which define case-level symptoms in a broad and inclusive way will give rise to higher prevalence estimates than those which define in a more selective manner. More restricted syndromes have a higher individual impact, but more 'mild' cases may have a stronger societal impact, because of their substantially higher prevalence. Restrictive criteria are often favoured by researchers because it is easier to achieve comparability between studies. However, they frequently encompass only a small proportion of cases seen routinely by clinical services and underestimate substantially the syndrome's wider impact. It is best not to view one approach as 'better' or 'worse' than another; they are merely different, and these differences should be taken into account when between-study comparisons are made.

Underlying Dimensions

Hypertension is an artificial category applied to a known physiological parameter (blood pressure), and it is likely that the same can be said for anxiety and depression. However, the underlying parameters are much less well understood, may not be unitary, and may not perfectly reflect traditional 'diagnosis' constructs. Criteria for depression as a diagnosis do not simply reflect the pervasiveness of depressed mood but also take into account its manifestations (tearfulness, anhedonia etc.) as well as the presence of other symptoms (e.g. appetite disturbance, insomnia), the quality of other symptoms (e.g. early morning wakening rather than initial insomnia), the manifestation of the overall syndrome (e.g. duration, pervasiveness, diurnal fluctuation) and the degree to which this affects daily life. The concept of the 'syndrome' is core to psychiatric nosology. However, a substantial part of this lies in tradition rather than empirical evidence, and it may be preferable for research to clarify underlying symptoms before assuming the validity of syndromes. For example, the EURO-D instrument generates two underlying dimensions (motivation and affective distress) which have different correlates (lower motivation associated with increased age, affective distress associated with female gender[1]). It is not yet established whether these findings apply beyond this instrument; however, they at least suggest that a more flexible attitude is needed towards categories and dimensions.

Are Anxiety and Depression Different Disorders?

Although anxiety and depression have traditionally been defined as separate conditions, this tradition has evolved in secondary and tertiary care settings. In community samples of any age group, mixed syndromes predominate. Furthermore, the impact of common mental

Principles and Practice of Geriatric Psychiatry, 3rd edn. Edited by Mohammed T. Abou-Saleh, Cornelius Katona and Anand Kumar

disorders appears to depend principally on the number of symptoms rather than whether they are anxious or depressive[2]. An exception to this is mortality as an outcome, where U-shaped associations with anxiety symptom load have been found compared to more linear associations with number of depressive symptoms[3], which may reflect differences in health service access and use. For example, delay in breast cancer presentation was found to be positively associated with previous depressive disorder but negatively associated with previous phobic disorder[4]. In this chapter, we shall consider depressive and anxiety disorders separately for the most part, but limitations in this approach should be borne in mind.

EPIDEMIOLOGY AND COURSE OF DEPRESSION: PREVALENCE, INCIDENCE AND OUTCOME

'Depression' as a diagnosis generally requires persistent low mood which is accompanied by other symptoms (such as disturbance of sleep and appetite), and which is causing significant distress and/or disablement. However, mood states vary across a spectrum of normality to abnormality and the prevalence of depression (i.e. how common it is in a given population) depends substantially on the cut-off severity applied. As discussed earlier, severe depressive syndromes have a high individual impact but are rare, while milder syndromes have a lower individual impact but affect many more people.

Prevalence studies using more restrictive criteria include the Epidemiologic Catchment Area (ECA) surveys in five areas of the USA, in which the Diagnostic Interview Schedule (DIS) was administered, and which found major depression in 0.4% of men and 1.4% of women aged 65 years and over[5]. Other estimates include those from the Cache County Study in Utah, also using the DIS, finding major depression in 2.7% of men and 4.4% of women aged 65 years and over[6], as well as a survey in the Netherlands finding major depression in 2.0% of residents aged 65 years and over[7].

An alternative approach has sought to define 'depression of clinical significance'; that is, a syndrome severity which would warrant clinical intervention. This construct in older people tends to be found 5–10-times more commonly than major depression, with prevalence ranging from 10 to 20% in most studies. These include studies which have measured 'clinically significant depressive symptoms' using brief instruments such as the Centre for Epidemiologic Studies Depression scale (CES-D); for example 16% and 9% of older residents scoring at case level (16+) in two US studies[8,9]. A more diagnostic approach is taken by the structured Geriatric Mental State (GMS) interview schedule with its accompanying AGECAT computerized diagnostic algorithm[10,11], which has probably the most wide international use including the EURODEP collaboration of late-life depression surveys in Western Europe[12], the UK Medical Research Council Cognitive Function and Ageing Study[13] and the 10/66 surveys of older people in low- and middle-income countries[14]. The EURO-D instrument was derived from the GMS and has been applied to EURODEP data[1,12,15] as well as used more recently in the Study of Health and Retirement in Europe (SHARE) surveys[16,17]. Principal findings from the EURODEP collaboration were GMS depression prevalence ranging from 8.8% (Iceland) to 23.6% (Munich) with a weighted average of 12.3% in total: 14.1% in women and 8.6% in men[12]. The SHARE surveys using the EURO-D reported lowest prevalence in Denmark (18.1%) and Germany (18.8%) and highest prevalence in the three Western Mediterranean sites – France (33.3%), Italy (33.7%) and Spain (36.8%). These differences largely persisted following

standardization for demographic profiles[17]. Prevalence estimates for similar definitions of late-life depression in other world regions have been broadly comparable – for example a 14.8% prevalence of depressed mood in a meta-analysis of studies in China[18]. In three Latin American sites (Peru, Mexico and Venezuela) of the 10/66 population-based survey programme, prevalence ranges were 1.3–2.8% for DSM-IV major depression, 4.5–5.1% for ICD-10 depressive episode, 30.0–35.9% for GMS-AGECAT 'clinically significant' depression, and 26.1–31.2% for EURO-D caseness[19].

Prevalence of depression is a product of both new cases arising (incidence) and duration of case-level disorder. A higher prevalence in one site or group compared to another may be because of higher incidence or delayed recovery. For late-life depression it could also be accounted for by delayed case mortality, although mortality has been found to be higher in older people with depression[20]. Incidence of late-life depression has been less commonly measured. Major depression incidence was 0.15% per year in the ECA studies and, in a Swedish cohort, 0.12% per year in men and 0.30% in women[21]. One-year incidence of a broader depression syndrome (17% baseline prevalence) in the north London Gospel Oak study was 12%[22], and 2.5 year incidence in Korea using the GMS (baseline prevalence 14%) was also 12%[23]. Persistence of depression in the Gospel Oak cohort after a one-year interval was 63%[22]. However, two-point surveys give relatively crude information on clinical course. Incidence is underestimated (because depression episodes in the intervening period which have recovered by the follow-up point will be missed), and persistence is over-estimated (since some of those with depression at both times may have had an intervening period of recovery).

The course of depression, a classically fluctuating condition, is therefore poorly represented by binary concepts such as 'incidence' and 'maintenance', particularly in two-wave studies. An alternative approach has described clinical course in a more qualitative manner. The Longitudinal Ageing Study of Amsterdam investigated the six-year outcome of depression defined both by the CES-D and DIS. Only 14% of episodes were found to be short lived. Remission occurred in 23%, an unfavourable but fluctuating course was followed by 44%, and a severe, chronic course by 33%[24]. These are similar to findings from a very early study of late-life depression where, over six years, 31% recovered, 28% had one or more relapse, 23% had a partial recovery and 17% remained depressed[25]. In another early study with a one-year follow-up, 35% had a good recovery, 48% had had a recurrence or continuation of the syndrome, 3% had developed dementia, and 14% had died[26]. In a more recent review of depression prognosis, no clinically significant differences were found in response to pharmacotherapy or ECT by older/younger age of onset, although older people had a higher risk of future episodes. Medical co-morbidity was a potential confounder, being more common in older people and associated with a worse prognosis. Older people with early onset depression had a larger number of previous episodes, which also contributed to a worse prognosis[27].

AETIOLOGY OF DEPRESSION

Age

The prevalence of depressive disorders increases from young to mid-adult age groups, often followed by a fall in prevalence for older people within a decade of the retirement age[28]. However, studies that have focused upon depressive symptoms and broader depressive syndromes indicate either an increase in their frequency, or stability with increasing age[29]. Blazer concluded that, if a symptom factor structure was examined, there were no age, race or gender differences in scores[21]. Where positive associations between age and depression prevalence are found, the high prevalence of physical and social stressors in these more advanced age groups is most likely to be responsible. The exclusion, in DSM diagnostic criteria[30], of symptoms that are considered to be primarily attributable to bereavement and physical illness may account in part for the apparent lower prevalence of thus-defined depressive disorders in older people. The expression of depression may also be qualitatively different in older people: for example, a higher age of onset for melancholic symptoms such as non-interaction, psychomotor retardation, and agitation[31], concurring with the positive association between increased age and diminished motivation in the EURO-D scale, both in EURODEP[1] and SHARE centres[17].

Cross-sectional associations with age may reflect birth cohort effects as well as chronological age, but these have been poorly captured to date. On the one hand, rapid improvements in health and economic prosperity for the 'young elderly' (e.g. 65–75 years) have been a particular feature of demographic ageing. On the other hand, there may be a reduction in 'stoicism' and 'resilience' as well as possible differences in willingness to admit to depressive symptoms. Birth cohort differences can only really be evaluated by repeated surveys covering the same population using similar measurements and case definitions; data which have not so far been available for late-life depression.

As well as the age distribution, some research has attempted to estimate the age of onset of late-life depression; that is, the proportion which occurs as new episodes. For example, an Australian study estimated that 52% of cases had their onset at age 60 or above[32], while a US study of people receiving home care estimated that 71% of those who were depressed were experiencing their first episode[33]. However, this approach depends on accurate recall of previous episodes, an assumption which is questioned by a prospective study in Sweden of people who had been hospitalized 25 years earlier for major depression. Of those traced, only 50% recalled sufficient details for diagnostic criteria to be applied and 30% did not recall the episode at all[34]. Recollections of more mild forms of depression are likely to be substantially more inaccurate.

Gender and Marital Status

Higher prevalence of depression is usually found in women compared to men, but this difference is substantially less than that found in younger age groups[35]. The EURODEP consortium[1] reported an excess of depression symptoms in older women in 13 out of 14 European centres. This association was consistently modified by marital status, with marriage being protective for men but associated with higher risk for women. These findings are consistent with the observation from several studies that married older men cite their wife as their main confidant, whereas women more often cite a friend outside the home, and with the association between married status and relatively low mortality or good health being stronger for men than for women.

Social Support/Activity

A consistent finding has been the salience to mood and morale in older people of contact with friends, in particular intimate and confiding relationships. While older people typically receive instrumental support from spouses and relatives, they value friends for the companionship and emotional support which they can provide. However, this generalization does not take into account the fact that some individuals may prefer a relatively isolated existence and find higher levels of social contact stressful. In the longitudinal Gospel Oak study, no contact with friends was the only social support variable prospectively associated with the onset of depression[22]. In this study, lack of social support and social participation were associated with maintenance rather than onset of depression, and the same has been found in a prospective French study where both social activity and disablement were associated with CES-D depressive symptoms at baseline but, for those with case-level symptoms at baseline, only higher levels of social activity predicted a reduction in symptoms at follow-up[36]. Physical health, age and gender may modify or explain to some extent the association between social support and late-life depression. There are large gender differences in late-life social support, with women typically having more supportive and extensive networks of friends than men. These may deteriorate following bereavement. Social engagement, such as visiting friends, is impaired by disability, indicating complex relationships between these exposures.

Social Adversity and Life Events

Many surveys find associations between late-life depression and relative disadvantage in income; poverty, for example, was one of the top five correlates of late-life depression along with disability, illness, isolation and bereavement[37]. These are highly correlated characteristics, and it will always be difficult to determine the effect of one independent of the others. At least some of the effect of poverty may be confounded by and/or mediated through physical health. Environmental measures have received less attention, although one study found that worse quality of the internal home environment was an independent predictor of incident depression one year later[38], particularly for cohabiting residents. Poverty, isolation and poor housing represent chronic stressors. The importance of acute stressors has also been investigated, with most studies finding some association[39,40] although varying in exposure and outcome measurement. Specific life events may have particular salience, such as bereavement, threats to health and interpersonal conflicts[41,42]. In British residents aged 16–74 years, associations between recent life events and common mental disorder increased in strength from early to midlife and then decreased in the oldest (65–74 year) group. Lifetime events suggesting adverse childhood exposures, however, remained strongly associated with mental disorder[43]. In younger people, early adversity is believed to act as a vulnerability factor, increasing the risk of depression in the presence of a life event[44], but this was not found in the British survey.

The Inter-Relationship between Depression and Chronic Non-Communicable Diseases

Worse physical health may be an acute or chronic stressor. However, depression is also a risk factor for worse physical health. A large part of the relationship between worse physical health and depression is mediated through higher disability levels reflecting loss of function[45]. In Gospel Oak, handicap was the most important risk factor for incident depression, with a population attributable risk fraction of 0.78[22]. However, as discussed above, the association appears to be with onset rather than with maintenance[22,36]. Three studies have suggested an interaction between disablement and social support, with the strongest effect of disablement in those with the least social support[45-48].

The 'vascular depression' hypothesis

Evidence for disorder-specific risk of depression (beyond what would be expected through disability) is fairly scant. Possibly the strongest candidate is stroke, where depression occurs very commonly[49] and where this association frequently remains robust to adjustment for disability[50,51]. However, associations with specific arterial territory involvement have not been consistent[52], and it is quite possible that there are additional personal impacts of stroke which account for the high risk of depression, rather than cerebral damage. Incidence of depression is also increased after myocardial infarction (15–30% major depression), principally in the first month[53]. However, associations with conventional risk factors for cardiovascular disease have been absent or accounted for by disability[50,51,54], and a recent study found that vascular disorders (compared to non-vascular disorders), while specifically related to cognitive impairment, showed no specificity as correlates of mental disorder[55]. The concept of 'vascular depression'[56] therefore appears to have little epidemiological support, although may still apply to the more rare and severe (and/or treatment resistant) syndromes seen in secondary care.

Depression, mortality and cardiovascular outcomes

There is substantial excess all-cause mortality associated with mental disorder. Depression, studied most extensively, is associated with an approximately 70% increased risk[57]. In a French study of late-life depression, associations with mortality varied by gender with mortality predicted by symptom severity and previous antidepressant use in men, but in women only by severe untreated depression[20]. Associations with mortality may be mediated by disability, but not apparently by cardiovascular disease, cardiovascular risk factors or antidepressant use. There is strong evidence for associations between depression and outcomes such as angina, non-fatal and fatal myocardial infarction[58], as well as stroke[59]; in many studies after 10 years or more, ruling out depression induced by preclinical cardiovascular disease as an explanation. The associations are, surprisingly, independent of vascular risk factors such as obesity, smoking and hypertension. A prospective neuroimaging study found that depression also predicted worsening of white matter hyperintensities[60].

Co-morbid depression is a consistent and independent predictor of adverse outcomes after non-fatal myocardial infarction, such as recurrent coronary heart disease (CHD) events, CHD mortality, and all-cause mortality[58]; explained partly by poor adherence to prophylactic behaviour and lifestyle changes. Post-stroke depression is also associated with worse functional outcomes[61] and substantially higher mortality[62].

Depression and dementia

Dementia and depression have strong interrelationships in older people. Depression occurs commonly in people with dementia, and late-life depression is also a predictor of dementia[63], although it has not been clarified whether this is because depression is a risk factor or an early symptom. Common risk factors may also operate and interact over a long period. These could include cardiovascular risk factors,

cerebrovascular disease and social isolation or deprivation (predisposing to cognitive decline, and impacting negatively on access to health and social care).

Recent research strongly supports an overarching model, in which it is the disability and restriction in social participation associated with any chronic health condition that most parsimoniously explains the increased risk for late-life depression. This finding, highlighted in the UK Gospel Oak study, has been subsequently confirmed in several other cohorts.

Genetic Factors

Gene–environment interactions have attracted increasing interest for depression, with several studies finding that stressful life events are stronger risk factors in the presence of a risk allele of the serotonin transporter (*5HTLPR*) gene[64]. This was replicated for stressful life events and GMS-defined depression in an elderly sample in Korea, with brain derived neurotrophic factor (*BDNF*) also implicated[23]. Similar interactions have also been found in this sample for other environmental stressors such as number of chronic disorders with *5HTTLPR*[65], and incident stroke with *BDNF*[66] which, taken together, suggest that gene–environment interactions may persist into later life. However, the interaction between stressful life events and *5HTTLPR* genotype could not be replicated for CES-D caseness in an older French population[67].

THE EPIDEMIOLOGY OF ANXIETY

Anxiety symptoms and disorders are also common in elderly populations, particularly those suffering with chronic physical illness. Like depression, they are distressing and disabling, and associated with increased mortality. However, they remain under-diagnosed and under-treated in both primary and secondary care. However, there is still uncertainty about the nature of anxiety in late life and its relationship with other disorders, such as depression and dementia.

The Nature of Anxiety in Old Age

As with depression, the experience and phenomenology of anxiety in old age may differ from that in young adulthood, and these differences may make identification difficult, in both clinical and research settings. Most instruments and diagnostic criteria were developed and validated in young populations, and may under-diagnose anxiety in older adults[68,69]. Attributing physical symptoms to anxiety can be problematic in late life, particularly with co-morbid physical illness[70,71], and 'somatization' of distress[68]. Psychological and cognitive components may also differ; for example, worry appears to be less common in late life and more strongly associated with mental disorder[72]. Severity and duration of anxiety symptoms may also alter with increasing age. Anxiety disorders might be less severe in late life because of reduced reactivity to stress, 'healthy survivor' cohort effects and better coping skills born of greater maturity and experience[73]. If so, then diagnostic severity thresholds defined for younger adults may not be appropriate for elderly individuals.

The Prevalence of Anxiety in Old Age

In a recent review by Bryant *et al.*[74], a systematic database search was carried out for articles published between 1980 and 2007 reporting data on anxiety disorders or symptoms in community or clinical populations, in subjects aged 60 years and above. A total of 49 articles met their criteria, reporting results from a wide range of North American and European epidemiological studies; however, heterogeneity precluded formal meta-analysis.

This review found wide variation in the estimated prevalence of anxiety and its disorders. A few studies reported the prevalence of anxiety symptoms, which ranged from 15% (two or more symptoms on HSC[75]) to 52.3% (one or more symptoms on GMS[76]). Regarding anxiety disorders, overall prevalence rate ranged from 1.2% (GMS-AGECAT[77]) to 14% (DSM-IV[78]). The prevalence of phobic disorders ranged from 1.4% (GMS-AGECAT[77]) to 25.6% (PDS[79]), with specific phobia the most common phobic disorder, and social phobia the least common. Generalized anxiety disorder (GAD) prevalence ranged from 1.3% (CIDI[80]) to 7.1% (HSC[81]) and, overall, was the commonest anxiety disorder reported. Prevalence data on the less common anxiety disorders in old age are much more limited. The Longitudinal Aging Study in Amsterdam reported six-month prevalence of 0.9% for case-level PTSD and 13.1% for sub-threshold PTSD[82]. The episodic nature of panic attacks and panic disorder render them difficult to capture in cross-sectional surveys, so it is not surprising that very low prevalence has been found of 1% or less.

In clinical studies, data are limited, but overall the results are again very variable, with anxiety symptoms ranging from 15% (geriatric hospital, GMS-AGECAT[83]) to 56% (general hospital, GMS-AGECAT[84]), and anxiety disorders from 1% (general hospital, GMS-AGECAT[84]) to 24% (primary care, CIDI-SF[85]).

While some of the differences in the reported prevalence rates may reflect genuine differences between populations, Bryant et al.[74] conclude that much is due to conceptual and methodological differences between studies. As with depression, a key factor is variation in the level of severity that is used to define a case. Studies using GMS-AGECAT demonstrate this: typically, they report quite high prevalence for sub-cases but very low prevalence for cases, indicating a high threshold. Another important factor is the application of different diagnostic rules. Instruments and diagnostic algorithms applying hierarchical rules exclude cases of anxiety co-occurring with other disorders such as depression and dementia (e.g. GMS-AGECAT, DIS-DSM-III) and, not surprisingly, identify far fewer cases of anxiety disorder than measures that do not operate such rules. The magnitude of this effect in relation to phobic disorders is shown by Lindesay and Banerjee[79], who applied different diagnostic criteria to the same population; a hierarchical system (GMS-AGECAT) yielded a prevalence of 3.6% as against 25.6% when a non-hierarchical system (PDS) was used. This problem is most pronounced in elderly populations, where there is extensive co-morbidity between depression and anxiety, particularly GAD[86–88]. Indeed, the extent of this co-morbidity has led some to question the utility of depression and GAD as distinct diagnoses, and propose instead a dimensional construct[89–91].

To what extent do the prevalence rates of anxiety disorders change with increasing age? A number of epidemiological studies have examined prevalence across the adult age-range, but findings have been heterogeneous. In the US ECA study, the prevalence of anxiety disorders generally declined with increasing age, although this was less pronounced for some categories, such as phobic disorder. In the UK National Survey of Psychiatric Morbidity, the prevalence of GAD peaked in 50s and declined thereafter. Few studies report data on the very oldest age groups, but there is some suggestion that rates of anxiety may increase in extreme old age. However, most findings are drawn from cross-sectional data which must be interpreted with caution. Although it is possible that vulnerability diminishes with

age, findings may also be the result of excess mortality associated with anxiety, or birth cohort differences[92]. Measurement validity may also vary, with risk of under-diagnosis in elderly subjects[93].

Evidence regarding the incidence rates of anxiety in older age groups is still sparse. In studies that have looked retrospectively at age of onset, such as the ECA, most of the cases of GAD had their onset prior to the age of 65 years[94]. In a three-year follow-up of the Liverpool survey using GMS-AGECAT[95], the estimated incidence rate of neurotic disorders overall was 0.44% per year; the limitations of two-point surveys to determine incidence discussed above should be noted, however.

Risk Factors for Anxiety in Old Age

Factors influencing the risk of developing an episode of anxiety may be classed as premorbid vulnerability factors, those that trigger the onset of a particular episode (destabilization), and those that determine the duration of the episode (restitution)[96]. It is likely that the exposure to and impact of specific risk factors will change over the lifespan, with some, for example chronic physical ill health and disability, having more effect in old age compared to young adulthood, and vice versa. However, ageing per se does not appear to be a risk factor for anxiety[97]; indeed, it may be protective[98]. Vink et al.[99] reviewed studies of factors associated with anxiety and depression in elderly subjects published between 1995 and 2005. The number of studies of risk factors for anxiety, either alone or with depression, was limited compared to the number examining depression alone. Heterogeneity between the studies was also high and no formal meta-analysis was attempted. Risk factors were classified as biological, psychological or social. The principal biological risk factors associated with anxiety disorders in cross-sectional studies were: number of chronic health problems, poor self-perceived health, and functional limitation[91,100]. Evidence from the few longitudinal studies was limited, with only poor self-perceived health and sensory deprivations emerging as predictors of anxiety symptoms[82,101]. The psychological risk factors for anxiety identified in both cross-sectional and longitudinal studies were: external locus of control and neuroticism, poor coping strategies, and psychopathology[82,91,100]. Not many studies have examined social risk factors for anxiety in late life in any detail. Social demographic associations such as female gender and lower educational level are reported[91,97,98], and the size and quality of social network has been identified in some studies[82,97,102]. The evidence base for social risk factors for depression is larger, and there are some differences. In comparative studies, infrequent social contacts, childlessness, adverse life events and low income were associated with anxiety only, whereas small social network size and being unmarried were associated with depression. Regarding life events, depression seems to be associated more with losses, and anxiety with threats and trauma. Overall, however, the risk profile for anxiety and depression and for symptoms and disorders appear very similar, supporting the dimensional rather than categorical modelling of these conditions[99].

CONCLUSIONS

While there are many commonalities in the epidemiology of depression and anxiety across the adult lifespan, there are also some important differences due to the effects of ageing, survival and changes in the physical and social environment. These point to the need for some different interventions for older adults, aimed at increasing social engagement and reducing the impact of physical disability, if these disorders are to be effectively prevented.

REFERENCES

1. Prince MJ, Beekman ATF, Deeg DJH *et al.* Depression symptoms in late-life assessed using the EURO-D scale. *Br J Psychiatry* 1999; **174**: 339–45.
2. Das-Munshi J, Goldberg D, Bebbington PE *et al.* Public health significance of mixed anxiety and depression: beyond current classification. *Br J Psychiatry* 2008; **192**: 171–7.
3. Mykletun A, Bjerkeset O, Overland S *et al.* Levels of anxiety and depression as predictors of mortality: The HUNT study. *Br J Psychiatry* 2009; **195**: 118–25.
4. Desai MM, Bruce ML, Kasl SV. The effects of major depression and phobia on stage at diagnosis of breast cancer. *Int J Psychiatry Med* 1999; **29**: 29–45.
5. Weissman M, Bruce M, Leaf P *et al.* Affective disorders. In Regier DA, Robins LN (eds), *Psychiatric Disorders in America.* New York: The Free Press, 1991, 53–80.
6. Steffens D, Skook I, Norton MC. Prevalence of depression and its treatment in an elderly population: the Cache County study. *Arch Gen Psychiatry* 2000; **57**: 601–7.
7. Beekman A, Deeg D, van Tilberg T *et al.* Major and minor depression in later life: a study of prevalence and risk factors. *J Affect Disord* 1995; **36**: 65–75.
8. Berkman LF, Berkman CS, Kasl S *et al.* Depressive symptoms in relation to physical health and functioning in the elderly. *Am J Epidemiol* 1986; **124**: 372–88.
9. Blazer D, Burchett B, Service C *et al.* The association of age and depression among the elderly: an epidemiologic exploration. *J Gerontol* 1991; **46**: M210–15.
10. Copeland JRM, Kelleher MJ, Kellet JM *et al.* A semi-structured clinical interview for the assessment of diagnosis and mental state in the elderly: the Geriatric Mental State Schedule. *Psychol Med* 1976; **6**: 439–49.
11. Copeland JRM, Dewey ME, Griffith-Jones HM. A computerised psychiatric diagnostic system and case nomenclature for elderly subjects: GMS and AGECAT. *Psychol Med* 1986; **16**: 89–99.
12. Copeland JR, Beekman AT, Braam AW *et al.* Depression among older people in Europe: the EURODEP studies. *World Psychiatry* 2004; **3**: 45–49.
13. McDougall FA, Kvaal K, Matthews FE *et al.* Prevalence of depression in older people in England and Wales: the MRC CFA Study. *Psychol Med* 2007; **37**: 1787–95.
14. Prince M, Ferri CP, Acosta D *et al.* The protocols for the 10/66 Dementia Research Group population-based research programme. *BMC Public Health* 2007; **7**: 165.
15. Copeland JRM, Beekman ATF, Dewey ME *et al.* Depression in Europe. Geographical distribution among older people. *Br J Psychiatry* 1999; **174**: 312–21.
16. Castro-Costa E, Dewey M, Stewart R *et al.* Ascertaining late-life depressive symptoms in Europe: an evaluation of the survey version of the EURO-D scale in 10 nations. The SHARE project. *Int J Methods Psychiatr Res* 2008; **17**: 12–29.
17. Castro-Costa E, Dewey M, Stewart R *et al.* Prevalence of depressive symptoms and syndromes in later life in ten European countries: the SHARE study. *Br J Psychiatry* 2007; **191**: 393–401.
18. Chen R, Copeland JRM, Wei L. A meta-analysis of epidemiological studies in depression of older people in the People's Republic of China. *Int J Geriatr Psychiatry* 1999; **14**: 821–30.
19. Guerra M, Ferri CP, Sosa AL *et al.* Late-life depression in Peru, Mexico and Venezuela - the 10/66 population based study. *Br J Psychiatry* 2009; **195**: 510–5.
20. Ryan J, Carriere I, Ritchie K *et al.* Late-life depression and mortality: the influence of gender and antidepressant use. *Br J Psychiatry* 2008; **192**: 12–18.
21. Blazer DG. Depression in late life: review and commentary. *J Gerontol A Biol Sci Med Sci* 2003; **58A**: M249–65.
22. Prince MJ, Harwood RH, Thomas A *et al.* A prospective population-based cohort study of the effects of disablement and social milieu on the onset and maintenance of late-life depression. The Gospel Oak Project VII. *Psychol Med* 1998; **28**: 337–50.
23. Kim J-M, Stewart R, Kim S-W *et al.* Interactions between life stressors and susceptibility genes (5-HTTLPR and BDNF) on depression in Korean elders. *Biol Psychiatry* 2007; **62**: 423–8.
24. Beekman ATF, Geerlings SW, Deeg DJH *et al.* The natural history of late-life depression. A 6-year prospective study in the community. *Arch Gen Psychiatry* 2002; **59**: 605–11.
25. Post F. *The Significance of Affective Symptoms at Old Age.* Oxford: Oxford University Press, 1962.
26. Murphy E. The prognosis of depression in old age. *Br J Psychiatry* 1983; **142**: 111–19.
27. Mitchell AJ, Subramaniam H. Prognosis of depression in old age compared to middle age: a systematic review of comparative studies. *Am J Psychiatry* 2005; **162**: 1588–1601.
28. Evans O, Singleton N, Meltzer H *et al. The Mental Health of Older People.* London: HMSO, 2003.
29. Tannock C, Katona C. Minor depression in the aged. Concepts, prevalence and optimal management. *Drugs Aging* 1995; **6**: 278–92.
30. American Psychiatric Association. *Diagnostic and Statistical Manual of Mental Disorders, Fourth Edition.* Washington, DC: American Psychiatric Association, 1994.
31. Parker G, Roy K, Hadzi-Pavlovic D *et al.* The differential impact of age on the phenomenology of melancholia. *Psychol Med* 2001; **31**: 1231–6.
32. Brodaty H, Luscombe G, Parker G *et al.* Early and late onset depression in old age: different aetiologies, same phenomenology. *J Affect Disord* 2001; **66**: 225–36.
33. Bruce ML, McAvay GJ, Raue PJ *et al.* Major depression in elderly home health care patients. *Am J Psychiatry* 2002; **159**: 1367–74.
34. Andrews G, Anstey K, Brodaty H *et al.* Recall of depressive episode 25 years previously. *Psychol Med* 1999; **29**: 787–91.
35. Djernes JK. Prevalence and predictors of depression in populations of elderly: a review. *Acta Psychiatr Scand* 2006; **113**: 372–87.
36. Isaac V, Stewart R, Artero S, Ancelin ML, Ritchie K. Social activity and improvement in depressive symptoms in older people: a prospective community cohort study. *Am J Geriatr Psychiatry* 2009; **17**: 688–96.
37. Kennedy GJ, Kelman HR, Thomas C *et al.* Hierarchy of characteristics associated with depressive symptoms in an urban elderly sample. *Am J Psychiatry* 1989; **146**: 220–25.
38. Stewart R, Prince MJ, Harwood RH *et al.* Quality of accommodation and risk of depression. An analysis of prospective data

from the Gospel Oak Project. *Int J Geriatr Psychiatry* 2002; **17**: 1091–8.

39. Cervilla JA, Prince MJ. Cognitive impairment and social distress as different pathways to depression in the elderly: a cross-sectional study. *Int J Geriatr Psychiatry* 1997; **12**: 995–1000.

40. Brilman EI, Ormel J. Life events, difficulties and onset of depressive episodes in late life. *Psychol Med* 2001; **31**: 859–69.

41. Murphy E. Social origins of depression in old age. *Br J Psychiatry* 1982; **141**: 135–42.

42. Devenand DP, Kim MK, Paykina N *et al.* Adverse life events in elderly patients with major depression or dysthymic disorder and in healthy-control subjects. *Am J Geriatr Psychiatry* 2002; **10**: 265–74.

43. Jordanova V, Stewart R, Goldberg D *et al.* Age variation in life events and their relationship with common mental disorders in a national survey population. *Soc Psychiatry Psychiatr Epidemiol* 2007; **42**: 611–16.

44. Hammen C, Henry R, Daley S. Depression and sensitization to stressors among young women as a function of childhood adversity. *J Consult Clin Psychol* 2000; **68**: 782–7.

45. Prince MJ, Harwood RH, Blizard RA *et al.* Impairment, disability and handicap as risk factors for depression in old age. The Gospel Oak Project V. *Psychol Med* 1997; **27**: 311–21.

46. Beekman AT, Penninx BW, Deeg DJ *et al.* Depression and physical health in later life: results from the Longitudinal Aging Study Amsterdam (LASA). *J Affect Disord* 1997; **46**: 219–31.

47. Schoevers RA, Beekman AT, Deeg DJ *et al.* Risk factors for depression in later life; results of a prospective community based study (AMSTEL). *J Affect Disord* 2000; **59**: 127–37.

48. Prince MJ, Harwood RH, Blizard RA *et al.* Social support deficits, loneliness and life events as risk factors for depression in old age. The Gospel Oak Project VI. *Psychol Med* 1997; **27**: 323–32.

49. Pohjasvaara T, Leppavuori A, Siira I *et al.* Frequency and clinical determinants of poststroke depression. *Stroke* 1998; **29**: 2311–17.

50. Stewart R, Prince M, Richards M *et al.* Stroke, vascular risk factors and depression. A cross sectional study in a UK Caribbean-born population. *Br J Psychiatry* 2001; **178**: 23–8.

51. Kim J-M, Stewart R, Shin I-S *et al.* Vascular disease/risk and late life depression in a Korean community population. *Br J Psychiatry* 2004; **185**: 102–7.

52. Carson AJ, MacHale S, Allen K *et al.* Depression after stroke and lesion location: a systematic review. *Lancet* 2000; **356**: 122–6.

53. Strik JJ, Lousberg R, Cheriex EC *et al.* One year cumulative incidence of depression following myocardial infarction and impact on cardiac outcome. *J Psychosom Res* 2004; **56**: 59–66.

54. Kim J-M, Stewart R, Kim S-W *et al.* Vascular risk factors and incident late-life depression in a Korean population. *Br J Psychiatry* 2006; **189**: 26–30.

55. Begum A, Tsopelas C, Lindesay J *et al.* Cognitive function and common mental disorders in older people with vascular and non-vascular disorders. A national survey. *Int J Geriatr Psychiatry* 2009; **24**: 701–8.

56. Alexopoulos GS, Meyers BS, Young RC *et al.* 'Vascular depression' hypothesis. *Arch Gen Psychiatry* 1997; **54**: 915–22.

57. Saz P, Dewey ME. Depression, depressive symptoms and mortality in persons aged 65 and over living in the community:

a systematic review of the literature. *Int J Geriatr Psychiatry* 2001; **16**: 622–30.

58. Hemingway H, Marmot M. Psychosocial factors in the aetiology and prognosis of coronary heart disease: systematic review of prospective cohort studies. *Br Med J* 1999; **318**: 1460–67.

59. Larson SL, Owens PL, Ford D *et al.* Depressive disorder, dysthymia, and risk of stroke. Thirteen-year follow-up from the Baltimore Epidemiologic Catchment Area Study. *Stroke* 2001; **32**: 1979–83.

60. Godin O, Dufouil C, Maillard P *et al.* White matter lesions as a predictor of depression in the elderly: the 3C-Dijon study. *Biol Psychiatry* 2008; **63**: 663–9.

61. Parikh RM, Robinson RG, Lipsey JR *et al.* The impact of post-stroke depression on recovery in activities of daily living over a 2-year follow-up. *Arch Neurol* 1990; **47**: 785–9.

62. Morris PL, Robinson RG, Andrzejewski P *et al.* Association of depression with 10-year poststroke mortality. *Am J Psychiatry* 1993; **150**: 124–9.

63. Devenand DP, Sano M, Tang MX *et al.* Depressed mood and the incidence of Alzheimer's disease in the elderly living in the community. *Arch Gen Psychiatry* 1996; **53**: 175–82.

64. Caspi A, Sugden K, Moffitt TE *et al.* Influence of life stress on depression: moderation by a polymorphism in the 5-HTT gene. *Science* 2003; **301**: 386–9.

65. Kim J-M, Stewart R, Kim S-W *et al.* Modification by two genes of associations between general somatic health and incident depressive syndrome in older people. *Psychosom Med* 2009; **71**: 286–91.

66. Kim J-M, Stewart R, Kim S-W *et al.* BDNF genotype potentially modifying the association between incident stroke and depression. *Neurobiol Aging* 2008; **29**: 789–92.

67. Power T, Stewart R, Ancelin M-L *et al.* 5-HTTLPR genotype, stressful life events and late-life depression: No evidence of interaction in a French population. *Neurobiol Aging*, in press.

68. Flint A. Anxiety and its disorders in late life: moving the field forward. *Am J Geriatr Psychiatry* 2005; **17**: 117–23.

69. Palmer B, Jeste D, Sheikh J. Anxiety disorders in the elderly: DSM-IV and other barriers to diagnosis and treatment. *J Affect Disord* 1997; **46**: 183–90.

70. Wijeratne C, Hickie I. Somatic distress syndromes in later life: the need for paradigm change. *Psychol Med* 2001; **31**: 72–82.

71. Jeste D, Blazer DG, First M. Aging-related diagnostic variations: need for diagnostic criteria appropriate for elderly psychiatric patients. *Biol Psychiatry* 2005; **58**: 265–71.

72. Lindesay J, Baillon S, Brugha T *et al.* Worry content across the lifespan: an analysis of 16- to 74-year-old participants in the British National Survey of Psychiatric Morbidity. *Psychol Med* 2007; **36**: 1625–33.

73. McCrae R, Costa P, Ostendorf F *et al.* Nature over nurture: temperament, personality and life span development. *J Pers Soc Psychol* 2000; **78**: 173–86.

74. Bryant C, Jackson H, Ames D. The prevalence of anxiety in older adults: methodological issues and a review of the literature. *J Affect Disord* 2008; **109**: 233–50.

75. Mehta K, Simonsick E, Penninx B *et al.* Prevalence and correlates of anxiety symptoms in well-functioning older adults: findings from the Health Aging and Body Composition Study. *J Am Geriatr Soc* 2003; **51**: 499–504.

76. Schaub RT, Linden M. Anxiety and anxiety disorders in the old and very old – results from the Berlin Aging Study. *Compr Psychiatry* 2000; **41**: 48–54.

77. Copeland J, Gurland B, Dewey M *et al*. Is there more dementia, depression and neurosis in New York? A comparative study of the elderly in New York and London using the computer diagnosis AGECAT. *Br J Psychiatry* 1987; **151**: 466–73.

78. Ritchie K, Artero S, Beluche I. Prevalence of DSM-IV disorder in the French elderly population. *Br J Psychiatry* 2004; **184**: 147–52.

79. Lindesay J, Banerjee S. Phobic disorder in the elderly: a comparison of three diagnostic systems. *Int J Geriatr Psychiatry* 1993; **8**: 387–93.

80. Hunt C, Issakidis C, Andrews G. DSM-IV Generalised Anxiety Disorder in the Australian National Survey of Mental Health and Well-being. *Psychol Med* 2002; **32**: 649–59.

81. Uhlenhuth E, Balter M, Mellinger G *et al*. Symptom checklist syndromes in the general population: correlations with psychotropic drug use. *Arch Gen Psychiatry* 1983; **40**: 1167–73.

82. van Zelst W, de Beurs A, Beekman A *et al*. Prevalence and risk factors of posttraumatic stress disorder in older adults. *Psychother Psychosom* 2003; **72**: 333–42.

83. Ames D, Flynn E, Harrigan S. Prevalence of psychiatric disorders among in-patients in an acute geriatric hospital. *Aust J Ageing* 1994; **13**: 8–11.

84. Ames D, Tuckwell V. Psychiatric disorders among elderly patients in a general hospital. *Med J Aust* 1994; **160**: 671–5.

85. Tolin D, Robinson J, Gaztambide S *et al*. Anxiety disorders in older Puerto Rican primary care patients. *Am J Geriatr Psychiatry* 2005; **13**: 150–6.

86. Lindesay J, Briggs K, Murphy E. The Guy's/Age Concern Survey: prevalence rates of cognitive impairment, depression and anxiety in an urban elderly community. *Br J Psychiatry* 1989; **155**: 317–29.

87. Manela M, Katona C, Livingston G. How common are the anxiety disorders in old age? *Int J Geriatr Psychiatry* 1996; **11**: 65–70.

88. Jeste D, Hays J, Steffens D. Clinical correlates of anxious depression among elderly patients with depression. *J Affect Disord* 2006; **90**: 37–41.

89. Tyrer P. The division of neurosis: a failed classification. *J R Soc Med* 1990; **83**: 614–16.

90. Lindesay J. Introduction: The concept of neurosis. In Lindesay J (ed.), *Neurotic Disorders in the Elderly*. Oxford: Oxford University Press, 1995, 1–11.

91. Schoevers R, Beekman A, Deeg D *et al*. Comorbidities and risk patterns of depression, generalised anxiety disorder and mixed anxiety-depression in later life: results from the Longitudinal Aging Study Amsterdam. *Int J Geriatr Psychiatry* 2003; **18**: 994–1001.

92. Klerman GL. The current age of youthful melancholia: evidence for increase in depression among adolescents and young adults. *Br J Psychiatry* 1988; **152**: 4–14.

93. O'Connor D. Do older Australians truly have low rates of anxiety and depression? A critique of the 1997 National Survey of Mental Health and Wellbeing. *Aust N Z J Psychiatry* 2006; **40**: 623–31.

94. Blazer DG, Hughes D, George LK *et al*. Generalised anxiety disorder. In Robins LN, Regier DA (eds), *Psychiatric Disorders in America. The Epidemiological Study*. New York: Free Press, 1990, 180–203.

95. Larkin BA, Copeland JRM, Dewey M *et al*. The natural history of neurotic disorders in an elderly urban population: findings from the Liverpool longitudinal study of continuing health in the community. *Br J Psychiatry* 1992; **160**: 681–6.

96. Goldberg D, Huxley P. *Common Mental Disorders: A Bio-Social Model*. London: Tavistock/Routledge, 1992.

97. Beekman AT, Bremmer MA, Deeg DJ *et al*. Anxiety disorders in later life: a report from the Longitudinal Aging Study Amsterdam. *Int J Geriatr Psychiatry* 1998; **13**: 717–26.

98. Heun R, Papassotiropoulos A, Ptok U. Subthreshold depressive and anxiety disorders in the elderly. *Eur Psychiatry* 2000; **15**: 173–82.

99. Vink D, Aartsen MJ, Schovers RA. Risk factors for anxiety and depression in the elderly: A review. *J Affect Disord* 2008; **106**: 29–44.

100. Beekman AT, de Beurs E, van Balkom AJ *et al*. Anxiety and depression in later life: co-occurrence and communality of risk factors. *Am J Psychiatry* 2000; **157**: 89–95.

101. de Beurs E, Beekman A, Geerlings S *et al*. On becoming depressed or anxious in late life: Similar vulnerability factors but different effects of stressful life events. *Br J Psychiatry* 2001; **179**: 426–31.

102. Forsell Y. Predictors for depression, anxiety and psychotic symptoms in a very elderly population: data from a 3-year follow-up study. *Soc Psychiatry Psychiatr Epidemiol* 2000; **35**: 259–63.

100

Psychopharmacological Treatment of Anxiety

John L. Beyer

Duke University Medical Center, Durham, NC, USA

INTRODUCTION

Though the prevalence of anxiety disorders declines with age (a finding consistent with most other mental disorders), anxiety disorders remain the most common psychiatric illness in the elderly[1]. An estimated 10–20% of older adults experience clinically significant symptoms of anxiety[2]. Unfortunately, many individuals may never seek treatment, or their anxiety may not be recognized. The result has been a significant under treatment of a very treatable illness.

There are no 'perfect' anxiolytic medications for treating the elderly[3,4]. Medications may vary in effectiveness or have problems with side effects. Further, there are significant gaps in the literature about best treatment practices, which makes evidence-based decisions difficult[5]. Therefore, we will first review general considerations about treating anxiety in the elderly before reviewing current pharmacological options. Classes of medications rather than specific recommendations for each anxiety disorder will be reviewed since research has not clarified primary treatments for most anxiety disorders in the elderly. Finally, guidelines for the evaluation and selection of pharmacological treatments are suggested.

GENERAL CONSIDERATIONS

Recognition of Anxiety

Despite the ubiquity of anxiety, either as a disorder or a symptom, recognition is not always apparent. This is especially true in treating the elderly patient. Elders often are less willing to discuss 'anxiety', but may report 'anxiety-equivalent' symptoms and physical illnesses. Thus a patient may deny feeling 'anxious', but admit to feeling 'jittery', 'sick', 'uneasy', 'flustered', 'restless', 'ill', 'achy' or 'bad'. Alternatively, the patient may deny having anxiety, but report having physical symptoms, such as 'heart pain', 'insomnia' or 'indigestion'. These complaints may obscure the true diagnosis or complicate another. The physician must therefore be sensitive, not reactive, to the presenting complaint.

Differential Diagnosis

The DSM-IV-TR has identified 12 types of anxiety disorders (Table 100.1). They are based on a cluster of symptoms with a characteristic course and treatment. Anxiety may present as a primary disorder (such as panic disorder, generalized anxiety disorder,

obsessive-compulsive disorder etc.) or as a symptom of another disorder. For example, many common medical disorders (like chronic obstructive pulmonary disease, coronary artery disease, early dementia) or common prescription and non-prescription medications (especially caffeine-containing products, cold and flu medications, alcohol or nicotine withdrawal, and certain herbal remedies) may cause anxiety (see Table 100.2). Finally, environmental and social stressors common to late life, such as bereavement, relocation or hospitalization may also cause anxiety. Thus, differentiating the source or sources of anxiety may be difficult.

When to Treat

When considering the treatment of anxiety in older adults, it is important to remember that anxiety is an adaptive emotion that occurs as a normal consequence of stressful experiences[6]. Stressful life events that frequently occur with age, such as loneliness, fear of isolation, diminished sensory abilities, diminished physical abilities, increased incidence of illness, financial limitations, and the prospect of dying, often generate considerable amounts of anxiety[7]. While anxiety may be a normal response to life events, it may also become maladaptive, meeting criteria for one of the 12 anxiety disorders. The decision to treat the anxious older patient with medication depends on the severity of the anxiety and the degree to which it interferes with the patient's functioning[8,9]. This frequently is seen in decreased coping skills, worsening of cognitive function, exacerbation of physical illnesses, or even a breakdown in support systems[10]. Therefore, the first task is to assess the impact of the anxiety symptoms on social and emotional functioning or the severity of a co-existing physical illness.

Challenge of Treatment

Research in the treatment of anxiety disorders for elderly patients is limited. A National Institute of Mental Health Workshop on Late-Life Anxiety[5] noted three significant research gaps: (i) little consensus on the 'best' approach to measure and count anxiety symptoms, syndromes, or disorders in late life; (ii) insufficient numbers of studies that examine anxiety among older adults; and (iii) limited knowledge of the differences in 'early' and 'later' onset of various anxiety disorders. These limitations become especially significant when making treatment recommendations for elderly anxiety patients. There are very few controlled clinical trials of medication or psychosocial interventions for anxiety disorders in the elderly[4]. Most recommendations

Principles and Practice of Geriatric Psychiatry, 3rd edn. Edited by Mohammed T. Abou-Saleh, Cornelius Katona and Anand Kumar
© 2011 John Wiley & Sons, Ltd

Table 100.1 DSM-IV anxiety disorders

Panic disorder without agoraphobia
Panic disorder with agoraphobia
Agoraphobia without a history of panic disorder
Specific phobia
Social phobia
Obsessive-compulsive disorder
Posttraumatic stress disorder
Acute stress disorder
Generalized anxiety disorder
Anxiety disorder due to ... *[a general medical condition]*
Substance-induced anxiety disorder
Anxiety disorder, NOS

Table 100.2 Medical disorders associated with anxiety as a symptom

Cardiopulmonary
  Asthma
  Chronic obstructive pulmonary disease
  Hypoxic states
  Angina pectoris
  Mitral valve prolapse
  Cardiac arrhythmias
  Congestive heart failure
  Cerebral arteriosclerosis
  Hypertension
  Pulmonary embolism
Neurologic
  Partial complex seizures
  Early dementia
  Delirium
  Post-concussion syndrome
  Cerebral neoplasm
  Huntington's disease
  Multiple sclerosis
  Vestibular dysfunction
Endocrine
  Carcinoid syndrome
  Cushing's syndrome
  Hypoglycaemia; hyperinsulinism
  Hypo- or hyperthyroidism
  Hypo- or hyperparathyroidism
  Menopause
  Pheochromocytoma
  Premenstrual syndrome
Medications
  Anticholinergic medications
  Caffeine
  Cocaine
  Steroids
  Sympathomimetics
  Alcohol
  Narcotics
  Sedative hypnotics

are usually based on case reports or open-label studies in the elderly, or extrapolated from the clinical studies of younger mixed-age adult populations and personal clinical experience. For the most part, there is little reason to doubt the applicability of the studies to the elderly patient, yet the clinician should be aware of the limitations of the research, and sensitive to the developing research in this area.

Special Adaptations for the Elderly Patient

Before prescribing anti-anxiety medicines for the elderly, the physician should also be aware of the several age-related physiological changes that may alter drug pharmacokinetics and contribute to increased risk of adverse reactions (see also Chapter 10). These include changes in drug absorption, drug distribution, protein binding, cardiac output, hepatic metabolism and renal clearance[11-13]. In addition, changes in neurotransmitter and receptor function in the central nervous system (CNS) may make a patient more sensitive to psychotropic drugs[14]. In general, the usual starting dose of psychotropic drugs for elderly patients is roughly one-half of the starting dose for younger adult patients.

PSYCHOPHARMACOLOGICAL DRUGS

Over the past century, a variety of agents have been used for the treatment of anxiety and anxiety disorders, with varying degrees of success. These include antidepressants, antihistamines, antipsychotics, benzodiazepines, beta-blockers and buspirone. Despite the multiple medicines available, Zimmer and Gershon's (1991) conclusion[15] that the 'ideal geriatric anxiolytic' has yet to be developed still holds true today. Therefore, effective treatment for excessive anxiety is especially dependent upon a thoughtful, accurate assessment of the patient, as well as a thorough knowledge of the patient's medication history, medical problems and social support/stress.

BENZODIAZEPINES

Since the 1960s, the benzodiazepines have been the mainstay of drug treatment for patients with situational anxiety, generalized anxiety disorder, and panic disorder[16]. They are also frequently prescribed for insomnia, relaxation prior to medical procedures, seizure disorders or 'agitation'. However, in the last two decades, increased attention has been given to the prescription pattern of benzodiazepines in the elderly. In the recent past, benzodiazepines were prescribed at a much higher rate among elderly patients

than that of the general population[17,18]. The percentage of use has declined, especially since the introduction of the SSRIs; however, benzodiazepines remain extensively used in the elderly.

Benzodiazepines are usually classified in two groups based primarily on their length of action: anxiolytics and sedative-hypnotics. Currently, seven benzodiazepines are available for the treatment of anxiety. Listed in their order of introduction, they are chlordiazepoxide, diazepam, oxazepam, clorazepate, lorazepam, alprazolam and clonazepam[19]. The most common sedative-hypnotics are triazolam, temazepam and flurazepam. Table 100.3 lists the currently available benzodiazepines and their individual characteristics.

Pharmacokinetics

Each benzodiazepine follows one of two biotransformative pathways: oxidation or glucuronide conjugation. Oxidative transformation occurs slowly, contributing to a longer half-life and producing many active metabolites. Conjugative transformation usually occurs

Table 100.3 Commonly used benzodiazepines in the elderly

Generic name	Trade name	Onset of action	Indication	Half-life (h)	Metabolism	Active metabolites	Geriatric dose (mg/day)	Route of administration
Short to intermediate half-life								
Triazolam	Halcion	Fast	Hypnotic	2–5	Conjugation	None	0.125–0.5	Oral
Oxazepam	Serax	Intermediate to slow	Anxiolytic	5–15	Conjugation	None	5–30	Oral
Alprazolam	Xanax	Intermediate	Anxiolytic	6–15	Oxidation	Yes	0.125–3.0	Oral
Lorazepam	Ativan	Intermediate	Anxiolytic	10–20	Conjugation	None	0.5–3.0	Oral, IV, IM
Temazepam	Restoril	Intermediate to slow	Hypnotic	12–24	Conjugation	None	15–30	Oral
Long half-life								
Chlordiazepoxide	Librium	Intermediate	Anxiolytic	8–30	Oxidation	Yes	5–30	Oral, IV, IM
Diazepam	Valium	Fastest	Anxiolytic	26–53	Oxidation	Yes	2–10	Oral, IV, IM
Clorazepate	Tranxene	Fast	Anxiolytic	30–200	Oxidation	Yes	7.5–15	Oral
Clonazepam	Klonopin	Intermediate	Anxiolytic	30–40	Oxidation	Yes	0.25–3.0	Oral
Flurazepam	Dalmane	Fast	Hypnotic	64–150	Oxidation	Yes	15	Oral

more rapidly and the metabolic products are pharmacologically inactive. As a general rule, benzodiazepines that are inactivated by conjugation are less likely to interact with other medications. For example, cimetidine has been found to inhibit the metabolism of benzodiazepines that require oxidation, but not benzodiazepines inactivated by conjugation. Table 100.4 lists several important drug interactions with benzodiazepines.

When used for their sedative properties in the elderly, effects of ultra-short, short and intermediate half-life benzodiazepines do not extend to the next day[20]. Ultra-short benzodiazepines are generally used to treat insomnia rather than daytime anxiety. However, they can cause rebound insomnia after abrupt discontinuation. Safety concerns about triazolam (i.e. after being noted to cause confusion, agitation and hallucinations) have led to its ban in several European countries[18]. Benzodiazepines with long half-lives can significantly contribute to increased risk of falls and hip fracture in elderly patients[21].

The onset of action after a single dose is primarily dependent upon the drug's absorption rate. Most benzodiazepines are highly lipophilic. Benzodiazepines that are more lipid soluble have a faster

Table 100.4 Drug interactions with the benzodiazepines

Drug	Effect
Alcohol	Increased CNS sedation
Neuroleptics	Increased CNS sedation
Narcotics	Increased CNS sedation
Antihistamines	Increased CNS sedation
MAO inhibitors	Increased CNS sedation
Cimetidine	Increased elimination half-life and decreased clearance of alprazolam, diazepam and chlordiazepoxide
Isoniazid	Decreased metabolism of diazepam
Rifampicin	Increased metabolism of diazepam
Antacids	Decreased absorption of clorazepate and chlordiazepoxide
Digoxin	Increased digoxin levels
Levodopa	Decreased control of parkinsonism by levodopa
Fluvoxamine	Increased levels of alprazolam

onset of action because they are absorbed and diffused into central synapses more rapidly[22,23]. This rapid onset of action can produce euphoria and thereby enhance abuse potential.

Efficacy

Although benzodiazepines have been shown to be effective in younger populations, systematic studies in the elderly are lacking. Benzodiazepines are effective for generalized anxiety disorder (GAD). Clonazepam has been shown to be effective for social phobia. Clonazepam and alprazolam are effective in panic disorder. Efficacy and use in posttraumatic stress disorder (PTSD) is limited. A paradoxical reaction has been documented when some patients with PTSD are treated with benzodiazepines. None of the benzodiazepines appear effective for obsessive-compulsive disorder. Of note, though short-term efficacy has been well documented, there are no data on long-term results.

Dependence and Withdrawal

True physiological dependence, resulting in a withdrawal and abstinence syndrome, develops for benzodiazepines usually after three to four months of daily use[14]. Withdrawal symptoms are likely to be more severe with abrupt discontinued therapy, and with patients receiving short half-life benzodiazepines, or higher daily doses. The symptoms of withdrawal include tachycardia, orthostasis, intention tremors, diaphoresis, hyper-reflexia, anxiety, insomnia, nightmares, malaise, anorexia, headache, muscle pain and twitching, tinnitus, hyperacusis, photophobia, metallic taste, strange smells and, in more severe cases, hyperthermia, nausea, vomiting, delirium, seizures and psychosis.

Side Effects

Adverse drug reactions with benzodiazepines are almost twice as common in patients over the age of 70 years compared with those aged 40 years or less[24]. Benzodiazepines have a greater effect on the central nervous system of the elderly than younger patients[8,12,13]. The most common side effect is a dose-dependent dampening of central nervous system activity. The resulting symptoms include fatigue, drowsiness, muscle weakness, blurred vision, nystagmus and (of special concern in the elderly) impaired psychomotor and cognitive performance that may lead to falls and fractures[12,25,26]. The impairment of motor coordination causes drivers taking benzodiazepines to be five-times more likely to be involved in a serious road accident[27]. Cognitive impairment can be severe enough to present as a pseudodementia in susceptible elderly patients. The risks of side effects appear to persist or worsen with chronic treatment[28], making the risk/benefit ratio for benzodiazepines appear unfavourable in the long-term treatment of anxiety disorders in the elderly[6].

Benzodiazepines may also cause a paradoxical reaction of restlessness, confusion, irritability and even aggression. Outbursts of anger in elderly patients receiving benzodiazepines may indicate the need to consider an alternative medicine. Benzodiazepines may cause mild respiratory depression in patients with chronic obstructive lung disease. Mixing benzodiazepines with other CNS depressants such as alcohol can lead to severe intoxication or (potentially lethal) respiratory depression.

Selection

In general, benzodiazepines are equivalent in terms of overall efficacy[29]. The selection of a particular benzodiazepine is primarily based upon the patient's particular problem and the medication properties (route of metabolism, length of half-life, onset of action and presence of active metabolites)[30]. In general, the following guidelines should be considered when using a benzodiazepine:

1. Benzodiazepines which undergo conjugation (e.g. temazepam, lorazepam, oxazepam) have no active metabolites and their pharmacokinetics are not significantly changed by the ageing process[12]. They are probably the wisest choice for elderly patients with impaired hepatic function.
2. Short (but not ultra-short) half-life drugs are preferable to long half-life medications since they appear less likely to increase the risk for hip fractures[21].
3. Accumulation of benzodiazepines is directly related to the amount of fat. Therefore, the thin or medically frail patients may be at increased risk.
4. Avoid benzodiazepine use in patients dependent on alcohol or other drugs.
5. Begin with lower doses and titrate upwards gradually. ('Start low and go slow.')
6. Try to limit the length of use to three to four months. Taper benzodiazepines over a four to eight week period.
7. Evidence suggests that early anxiolytic benefits from benzodiazepines improve overall compliance to antidepressant treatments in older patients[31].

BUSPIRONE

Buspirone is a novel anti-anxiety medicine whose mechanism of action is probably related to its high affinity for the serotonin type 5-HT$_{1A}$ receptor, which causes reduced serotonergic activity. In addition, it enhances brain dopaminergic and noradrenergic activity[32,33].

Efficacy

Buspirone was shown to be effective in the treatment of generalized anxiety disorder (GAD) in the elderly in a small (40 patient)

and short (four week) double-blind study[34]. It is well tolerated and as effective as the benzodiazepines for GAD[35-37]; however, buspirone does not appear effective in the treatment of panic disorder[38]. Some researchers suggest that buspirone may be helpful in mixed anxiety/depression symptoms. It may also be effective as an adjunct treatment for obsessive-compulsive disorder. Its use in posttraumatic stress disorder and social phobia appears to be limited.

Administration

Therapeutic doses of buspirone range from 20 to 60 mg daily. Because of its short half-life, buspirone is usually given three times a day. Further, as opposed to benzodiazepines, the anxiolytic effect of buspirone may not become apparent for one to three weeks. Some researchers have also suggested that the efficacy of buspirone may be reduced in patients who have previously been treated with benzodiazepines[39].

Side Effects

Buspirone is usually very well tolerated, but potential side effects may include nausea, headache, nervousness, dizziness, lightheadedness and fatigue. Unlike the benzodiazepines, buspirone does not appear to cause psychomotor impairment, dependence, withdrawal or abuse[40]. Further, it does not interact with alcohol and other sedative drugs. Therefore, it may be of particular value in the treatment of patients unable to tolerate the sedative effects of benzodiazepines[41], or patients with a history of substance abuse.

ANTIDEPRESSANTS

Tricyclic Antidepressants

Efficacy

Tricyclic antidepressants (TCAs) have been shown to be effective in treating mixed anxiety-depression states, panic disorder, and generalized anxiety disorder in the elderly[42-45]. In the general adult population, TCAs are frequently used in posttraumatic stress disorder, and clomipramine has been approved by the FDA to treat obsessive-compulsive disorder. However, the overall use of TCAs has decreased as other options (especially the SSRIs) have become available. This is primarily due to the significant side effects TCAs have at therapeutic doses, which also increases the risk to physically ill patients and potentiates toxicity in overdose. Further, like all other medications used for the treatment of anxiety (except the benzodiazepines), TCAs usually require several weeks to show maximal benefit. Despite their shortcomings, tricyclic antidepressants remain an alternative treatment for generalized anxiety disorder[46].

Side effects

Common side effects may be mediated by alpha-adrenergic blockade, anticholinergic effects and antihistaminergic effects. The alpha-adrenergic blockade of TCAs may cause significant orthostatic hypotension or cardiac conduction irregularities. The elderly are particularly susceptible to injury from orthostatic falls. Patients with complete heart block should not be given TCAs because these medications can cause a prolonged QRS complex. Trazodone, a heterocyclic antidepressant, is sometimes used as a sedative or in the treatment of agitation for demented patients, but the side effects of postural hypotension may limit its use[20].

Anticholinergic side effects of TCAs are dry mouth, blurred vision, constipation, urinary retention and confusion or even psychosis. This may be particularly significant in patients with Alzheimer's disease or other disorders which impair memory. The major antihistaminergic effect is sedation.

Guidelines for use

Imipramine and amitriptyline have long been established in the adult population for use in various anxiety disorders. However, their tertiary amine structure tends to cause increased anticholinergic, adrenergic and sedative side effects. The secondary amines, nortriptyline and desipramine, are preferred for use in the elderly due to their less intense side effects. In general, anxiety disorders appear to respond at doses lower than those used in mood disorders. A baseline EKG is highly recommended prior to starting therapy since TCAs can cause a prolonged QRS complex.

Monoamine Oxidase Inhibitors (MAOIs)

Monoamine oxidase inhibitors have been effective in treating mixed anxiety-depression and panic disorder but not pure generalized anxiety[43,44]. MAOIs are rarely used now because of their potential side effects (especially the drug/diet interactions) and the wider availability of newer antidepressant choices. Phenelzine and tranylcypromine are the best MAOI choice for the elderly in the United States[9]. Interestingly, phenelzine was found to be more effective in the elderly than in younger patients[43], and just as well tolerated as nortriptyline[47]. The starting dose is 15 mg daily in the morning, increasing by 15 mg every few days to an average dose of 45–60 mg[48].

Orthostatic hypotension is a frequent side effect of MAOIs; however, the major concern is the possibility of an acute hypertensive crisis due to the drug and dietary interactions.

Selective Serotonin Re-Uptake Inhibitors (SSRIs)

Efficacy

The introduction of selective serotonin re-uptake inhibitors has transformed the treatment of both depression and anxiety in the adult population. Seven SSRIs are now available for use in the US: fluoxetine, sertraline, paroxetine, paroxetine CR (controlled release), fluvoxamine, citalopram and escitalopram. Since their introduction, certain SSRIs have obtained indications for the treatment of not only depression, but also panic disorder, bulimia, obsessive-compulsive disorder and social phobia. They have also been shown to be effective for use in posttraumatic stress disorder and generalized anxiety disorder. Surprisingly, there has still been little research into the use of SSRIs for the treatment of anxiety disorders in the elderly. Fluoxetine has been shown to be effective in treatment of elderly depressed patients with agitation[20]. Fluvoxamine was found to be effective in a sample of elderly patients with a mixture of anxiety disorders (mostly GAD)[49], though near-maximal doses of fluvoxamine were needed to achieve remission. A study of 60 elderly patients with anxiety disorders (primarily GAD) found citalopram to be effective, with improvements noted through the first 20 weeks of treatment[50]. Fluvoxamine and fluoxetine have been shown to be

effective in clinical trials for obsessive-compulsive disorder that have included some elderly patients[51,52]. Case studies have shown sertraline, paroxetine, venlafaxine, fluoxetine and fluvoxamine effective in social phobias and anxiety[53–56].

Side effects

All SSRIs can cause gastrointestinal effects (nausea and diarrhoea), sexual arousal and performance changes, and a decrease in appetite and weight. The nausea and diarrhoea are usually dose dependent and resolve for most patients within the first week of treatment. An increasing concern has been SSRI-associated weight gain seen with extended use. Paroxetine has been noted to have some anticholinergic activity that may be more apparent in elderly, sensitive patients. A significant potential side effect of SSRIs includes a tendency to stimulate patients, causing tremor and jitteriness.

Guidelines for use

SSRIs have now become the first line treatment for most anxiety disorders. Some researchers have found that an initial use of benzodiazepine augmentation improves overall compliance with treatment[31] without an increased risk of falls[6]. Smith and colleagues[57] have recommended that SSRIs which have shorter half-lives and are less activating, such as paroxetine or sertraline, be used preferentially to fluoxetine. However, it should be noted that fluoxetine has been shown to be effective in treating anxiety symptoms associated with depression.

Newer Antidepressants

Venlafaxine, an SNRI (serotonin-norepinephrine re-uptake inhibitor), is approved for the treatment of generalized anxiety disorder in adults. A retrospective analysis of elderly subjects in the phase III studies for venlafaxine ER (extended release) found a 25% greater response rate than placebo (similar to that observed in younger adults)[58]. Older subjects had a lower rate of side effects than younger subjects, though the side effect-related discontinuation rate was the same (15%). Overall, the side effect profile of venlafaxine is similar to the SSRIs. Small elevations in blood pressure may be seen at dosages above 200 mg/day.

Nefazodone may be a useful antidepressant for depressed elderly patients who have concomitant anxiety symptoms[20]. It has an acceptable level of daytime sedation for the elderly[59], but minimal anticholinergic and other side effects. Its more moderate serotonin re-uptake inhibition may make it less likely to create agitation than the SSRIs[60]. Nefazodone does inhibit P-450 isoenzymes and is contraindicated for use with terfenadine, astemizole and cisapride. It will also increase the plasma levels of alprazolam, midazolam and triazolam.

Mirtazapine, a noradrenergic and specific serotonergic antidepressant (NaSSA) has shown beneficial effects on the concomitant symptoms of anxiety and sleep disturbances in depression trials[61]. It has few anticholinergic, adrenergic and serotonin-related adverse effects, but can be very sedating due to the antihistaminergic effects. There are no current data on its effectiveness in the elderly.

BETA-BLOCKERS

The usefulness of beta-blockers for treatment of anxiety in the elderly is unclear since the data for the elderly are restricted to clinical case reports[30]. Beta-blocking agents have been shown to be specifically beneficial in younger patients with predominantly somatic symptoms associated with generalized anxiety or anxiety related to stressful situations[62]. They may also have potential use in the treatment of aggression and agitation in patients with organic brain disease[63]. Although beta-blockers decrease autonomically mediated symptoms such as diaphoresis, palpitation, tremor and gastrointestinal upset, they usually do not reduce the inner subjective effects[3,7].

Propranolol in small doses (such as 5–10 mg one to four times a day) may be effective in elderly patients[20]. These drugs should not be used in patients with chronic obstructive pulmonary disease, congestive heart failure, heart block, insulin-dependent diabetes, severe renal disease or peripheral vascular disease.

ANTIHISTAMINES

Sedating antihistamines such as hydroxyzine and diphenhydramine hydrochloride are sometimes useful for anxiety or insomnia in the elderly. They have been rarely recommended because they are less effective than benzodiazepines, and their anticholinergic side effects outweigh their weak anxiolytic effects[3]. They may be used in patients with mild symptoms, in severe chronic obstructive pulmonary disease, in patients with substance misuse, or in patients for whom more traditional drugs are not effective[64]. However, physicians must be aware that the elderly patient is much more susceptible to their anticholinergic properties, which may cause blurred vision, tachycardia, dry mouth, urinary urgency, constipation, restlessness, hallucinations and confusion.

GENERAL GUIDELINES

Despite the limited data on treatment of anxiety disorders in the elderly, the clinician can successfully treat patients with a conservative and thoughtful use of medications. The following guidelines have been adapted from Small (1997)[20]:

1. Conduct a complete psychiatric evaluation. Listen specifically for expression of anxiety. Does this patient have anxiety that significantly affects their quality of life or functioning?
2. Consider the full differential diagnosis. Does the pattern of anxiety identify itself as a formal anxiety disorder, or as a symptom of another psychiatric or medical disorder? Geriatric psychiatry has been called the specialty of co-morbidity. There may be several potential aetiologies for anxiety symptoms that should be considered before initiating treatment.
3. Consider non-pharmacologic treatments first. Education and reassurance are invaluable in the treatment of anxiety, and may themselves be adequate treatments. Specifically address social stressors and evaluate the effectiveness of the support systems. Attention to family caregivers may facilitate the positive response to other treatment. Remember, the ability to benefit from therapy is not based on age.
4. Minimize polypharmacy. In the elderly population (especially those in the nursing care facilities), the use of multiple medications is the rule rather than the exception. Most clinicians stress the importance of reviewing the medication list for potential areas of reduction, prior to adding new treatments. Reducing the number of medications may actually treat the anxiety symptoms[20].

5. When selecting an anxiolytic, consider the full presentation rather than just the anxiety when choosing an initial medication. For example, use an antidepressant if depressive symptoms are apparent. Avoid anticholinergic medications in patients with dementia. Avoid benzodiazepines when the patient's ability to ambulate is compromised.
6. Presently, treatment recommendations for elderly with anxiety disorders are similar to those in younger patients. In general, SSRIs and venlafaxine are considered first line pharmacotherapy for anxiety disorders in the elderly[6].
7. As far as possible, make medication changes one at a time in order to clarify whether a complaint results from a medication side effect or an underlying illness.
8. 'Start low and go slow.' Most medications are started at lower doses than those used for younger adults, but it is generally necessary to increase to usual therapeutic doses.

REFERENCES

1. Blazer DG, George LK, Hughes DC. The epidemiology of anxiety disorders: an age comparison. In Salzman C, Lebowitz BD (eds), *Anxiety in the Elderly: Treatment and Research*. New York: Springer, 1991, 17–30.
2. Hocking LB, Koenig HG. Anxiety in medically ill older patients: a review and update. *Int J Psychiatry Med* 1995; **25**: 221–38.
3. Barbee JG, McLaulin JB. Anxiety disorders: diagnosis and pharmacotherapy in the elderly. *Psychiatric Annal* 1990; **20**: 439–45.
4. Krasucki C, Howard R, Mann A. Anxiety and its treatment in the elderly. *Int Psychogeriatr* 1998; **11**(1): 25–45.
5. Pearson JL. Summary of a National Institute of Mental Health workshop on late-life anxiety. *Psychopharmacol Bull* 1998; **34**(2): 127–38.
6. Lenze EJ, Shear MK, Mulsant BH, Reynolds CF. Anxiety disorders in late life: an evolving picture. *CNS Spectr* 2002; **7**(11): 805–10.
7. Shader RI, Greenblatt DJ. Management of anxiety in the elderly: the balance between therapeutic and adverse effects. *J Clin Psychiatry* 1982; **43**: 8–18.
8. Salzman C. Pharmacologic treatment of the anxious elderly patient. In Salzman C, Lebowitz BD (eds), *Anxiety in the Elderly: Treatment and Research*. New York: Springer, 1991, 149–73.
9. Schneider L. Overview of generalized anxiety disorder in the elderly. *J Clin Psychiatry* 1996; **57**(Suppl 7): 34–45.
10. Watkins LL, Grossman P, Krishnan R, Blumenthal JA. Anxiety reduces baroreflex cardiac control in older adults with major depression. *Psychosom Med* 1999; **61**(3): 334–40.
11. Jenike MA. Anxiety disorders of old age. In *Geriatric Psychiatry and Psychopharmacology, a Clinical Approach*. 1989, 248–71.
12. Thompson TL II, Moran MG, Nies AS. Psychotropic drug use in the elderly. *N Engl J Med* 1983; **308**: 134–8.
13. Ouslander JG. Drug therapy in the elderly. *Ann Intern Med* 1981; **95**: 711–22.
14. Salzman C. Practical considerations in the pharmacologic treatment of depression and anxiety in the elderly. *J Clin Psychiatry* 1990; **51**(Suppl 1): 40–3.
15. Zimmer B, Gershon S. The ideal late life anxiolytic. In Salzman C, Lebowitz BD (eds), *Anxiety in the Elderly: Treatment and Research*. New York: Springer, 1991, 277–303.

16. Hayes PE, Dommisse CS. Current concepts in clinical therapeutics: anxiety disorders, part 1. *Clin Pharmacy* 1987; **6**(2): 140–7.

17. American Psychiatric Association. *Benzodiazepine Dependence, Toxicity, and Abuse*. Washinton, DC: American Psychiatric Association, 1990.

18. Shorr RI, Robin DW. Rational use of benzodiazepines in the elderly. *Drugs Aging* 1994; **4**: 9–20.

19. Baldessarini RJ. Drugs and the treatment of psychiatric disorders. In AG Gilman, TW Rall, AS Nies, P Taylor (Eds) Goodman and Gilman's. *The Pharmacological basis of Therapeutics*, 8th Edn. Pergamon, New York, 1990; 383–485.

20. Small GW. Recognizing and treating anxiety in the elderly. *J Clin Psychiatry* 1997; **58** (Suppl 3): 41–7.

21. Ray WA, Griffin MR, Downey W. Benzodiazepines of long and short elimination half-life and the risk of hip fracture. *JAMA* 1989; **262**: 3303–6.

22. Dubovsky SL. Generalized anxiety disorder: New concepts and psychopharmacologic therapies. *J Clin Psychiatry* 1990; **51**(Suppl 1): 3–10.

23. Greenblatt DJ, Shader RI, Abernethy DR. Current status of benzodiazepines, part 1. *N Engl J Med* 1983; **309**: 354–8.

24. Boston Collaborative Drug Surveillance Program. Clinical depression of the central nervous system due to diazepam and chlordiazepoxide in relation to cigarette smoking and age. *N Engl J Med* 1973; **288**(6): 277–80.

25. Pomara N, Stanley B, Block R *et al*. Adverse effects of single therapeutic doses of diazepam on performance in normal geriatric subjects: relationships to plasma concentrations. *Psychopharmacology* 1984; **27**: 273–81.

26. Nikaido AM, Ellinwood EH Jr, Heatherly DG, Dubow D. Differential CNS effects of diazepam in elderly adults. *Pharmacol Biochem Behav* 1987; **27**: 273–81.

27. Skegg DCG, Richards SM, Doll R *et al*. Minor tranquilizers and road accidents. *Br Med J* 1979; **1**(6168): 917–19.

28. Pomara N, Tun H, DaSilva D *et al*. The acute and chronic performance effects of alprazolam and lorazepam in the elderly: relationship to duration of treatment and self-rated sedation. *Psychopharmacol Bull* 1998; **34**: 139–53.

29. Gershon S, Eison AS. Anxiolytic profiles. *J Clin Psychiatry* 1983; **44**(11Pt 2): 45–57.

30. Sadavoy J, LeClair JK. Treatment of anxiety disorders in late life. *Can J Psychiatry* 1997; **42**(Suppl 1): 28S–34S.

31. Buysse DJ, Reynolds CF, Houck PR, Begley A, Kupfer DJ. Does adjunctive lorazepam impair the antidepressant response to nortriptyline in elderly depressed patients? *Sleep Res* 1996; **25**: 153.

32. Eison AS, Temple DL Jr. Buspirone: review of its pharmacology and current perspectives on its mechanism of action. *Am J Med* 1986; **80**(Suppl 3B): 1–9.

33. Goa KL, Ward A. Buspirone: a preliminary review of its pharmacologic properties and therapeutic efficacy as an anxiolytic. *Drugs* 1986; **32**: 114–29.

34. Bohm C, Robinson DS, Gammans RE *et al*. Buspirone therapy in anxious elderly patients: a controlled clinical trial. *J Clin Psychopharmocol* 1990; **10**(Suppl 3): 47S–51S.

35. Napoleillo MJ. An interim multicentre report on 677 anxious geriatric out-patients treated with buspirone. *Br J Clin Pract* 1986; **40**: 71–3.

36. Singh AN, Beer M. A dose range finding study of buspirone in geriatric patients with symptoms of anxiety. *J Clin Psychopharmacol* 1988; **8**: 67–8.

37. Robinson D, Napoliello MJ, Schenk J. The safety and usefulness of buspirone as an anxiolytic drug in elderly versus young patients. *Clin Ther* 1988; **10**(6): 740–6.

38. Sheehan DV, Raj AB, Sheehan KH, Soto S. Is buspirone effective for panic disorder? *J Clin Psychopharmacol* 1990; **10**(1): 3–11.

39. Schweizer E, Rickels K, Lucki I. Resistance to the anti-anxiety effect of buspirone inpatients with a history of benzodiazepine use. *N Engl J Med* 1986; **314**: 719–20.

40. Banazak DA. Anxiety disorders in elderly patients. *J Am Board Fam Pract* 1997; **10**(4): 280–9.

41. Steinberg JR. Anxiety in elderly patients. A comparison of azapirones and benzodiazepines. *Drugs Aging* 1994; **5**(5): 335–45.

42. Rifken A, Klein DF, Dillon D, Levitt M. Blockade by imipramine or desipramine of panic induced sodium lactate. *Am J Psychiatry* 1981; **138**: 676–7.

43. Crook T. Diagnosis and treatment of mixed anxiety-depression in the elderly. *J Clin Psychiatry* 1982; **43**(9): 35–43.

44. Hershey LA, Kim KY. Diagnosis and treatment of anxiety in the elderly. *Ration Drug Ther* 1988; **22**(3): 1–6.

45. Hoehn-Saric R, McLeod DR, Zimmerli WD. Differential effects of alprazolam and imipramine in generalized anxiety disorder: somatic vs. psychic symptoms. *J Clin Psychiatry* 1988; **49**: 293–301.

46. Rickels K, Downing R, Schweizer E *et al*. Antidepressants for the treatment of generalized anxiety disorder: a placebo-controlled comparison of imipramine, trazodone, and diazepam. *Arch Gen Psychiatry* 1993; **50**: 884–95.

47. Georgotas A, McCue RE, Hapworth W *et al*. Comparative efficacy and safety of MAOIs vs TCAs in treating depression in the elderly. *Biol Psychiatry* 1986; **21**: 1155–66.

48. Fyer AJ, Sandberg D. Pharmacologic treatment of panic disorder. In Francis AJ, Hales RE (eds), *Review of Psychiatry*. Washington, DC: American Psychiatric Press, 1988, 88–120.

49. Wylie ME, Miller MD, Shear MK *et al*. Fluvoxamine pharmacotherapy of anxiety disorders in later life: preliminary open-trial data and a review of the literature. *J Geriatr Psychiatry Neurol* 2000; **12**: 43–8.

50. Blank S, Lenze EJ, Mulsant BH *et al*. Outcomes of late-life anxiety disorders during 32 weeks of citalopram treatment. *J Clin Psychiatry* 2006; **67**(3): 468–72.

51. Feighner JP, Boyer WF, Meredith CH, Hendrickson G. An overview of fluoxetine in geriatric depression. *Br J Psychiatry* 1988; **3**: 105–8.

52. Perse TL, Greist JH, Jefferson JW, Rosenfield R, Dar R. Fluvoxamine treatment of obsessive-compulsive disorder. *Am J Psychiatry* 1987; **144**: 1543–8.

53. Katzelnick DJ, Greist JH, Jefferson JW, Kobak KA. Sertraline in social phobia: a controlled pilot study. *Neuropsychopharmacol* 1994; **10**(Suppl 35): 260S.

54. Kelsey JE. Venlafaxine in social phobia. *Psychopharmacol Bull* 1995; **31**: 767–71.

55. Van Ameringen M, Mancini C, Streiner DL. Fluoxetine efficacy in social phobia. *J Clin Psychiatry* 1993; **54**: 27–32.

56. van Vliet IM, den Boer JA, Westenberg HG. Psychopharmacological treatment of social phobia: a double-blind placebo controlled study with fluvoxamine. *Psychopharmacology Berl* 1994; **115**: 128–34.

57. Smith SL, Sherrill KA, Colenda CC. Assessing and treating anxiety in elderly persons. *Psychiatr Serv* 1995; **46**(1): 36–42.

58. Katz IR, Reynolds CF, Alexopooulos GS, Hackett D. Venlafaxine ER as a treatment for generalized anxiety disorder in older adults: pooled analysis of five randomized placebo-controlled clinical trials. *J Am Geriatr Soc* 2002; **50**: 18–24.

59. van Laar MW, van Willigenburg AP, Volkerts ER. Acute and subchronic effects of nefazodone and imipramine on highway driving, cognitive functions, and daytime sleepiness in healthy adult and elderly subjects. *J Clin Psychopharmacol* 1995; **15**: 30–40.

60. Fawcett J, Marcus RN, Anton SF *et al*. Response of anxiety and agitation symptoms during nefazodone treatment of major depression. *J Clin Psychiatry* 1995; **37**: 713–38.

61. Kasper S, Przschek-Rieder N, Tauscher J, Wolf R. A risk-benefit assessment of mirtazapine in the treatment of depression. *Drug Saf* 1997; **17**(4): 251–64.

62. Peet M. The treatment of anxiety with beta-blocking drugs. *Postgrad med J* 1988; **64**(Suppl 2): 45–9.

63. Greendyke R, Kanter D, Schuster D *et al*. Propranolol treatment of assaultive patients with organic brain disease: A double blind cross-over, placebo-controlled study. *J Nerv Ment Dis* 1986; **174**: 290–4.

64. Rickels K. Nonbenzodiazepine anxiolytics: clinical usefulness. *J Clin Psychiatry* 1983; **44**(11): 38–43.

101

Obsessive-Compulsive Disorder

James Lindesay

Department of Health Sciences, University of Leicester, Leicester, UK

Although obsessive-compulsive disorder (OCD) is known to occur in old age, studies are few and information is limited. This may be because it is often not perceived as a disorder of late life. The mean age of onset of the condition is 20–25 years[1–3] and it is unusual for OCD to have its first onset after the age of 50 years. However, OCD can become a chronic disorder; as a recent 40-year follow-up study has shown, while most patients improve to some extent, less than half show complete or partial recovery[4]. A significant proportion of cases persist into old age, at which point they may present to services for the first time. It is important, therefore, that old age psychiatrists are aware of this disorder and of its management.

CLINICAL FEATURES

Diagnostic Criteria

OCD is characterized by intrusive, persistent obsessive thoughts, images or impulses and/or compulsive behaviours that are a significant source of distress, or interfere with the patient's personal or social functioning. The current diagnostic criteria, as set out in DSM-IV[5] and ICD-10[6], apply to all patients, irrespective of age. The limited evidence available indicates that the clinical features of OCD in elderly patients are very similar to those of younger adults. In their comparative study, Kohn *et al.*[7] found that concerns about symmetry, need-to-know and counting rituals were less common in elderly patients, and hand-washing and fear of having sinned were more common, but otherwise there were few differences in clinical features compared with younger OCD patients. Extreme ego-syntonic religiosity has been proposed as a variant of OCD that may be more common in older patients[8].

Differential Diagnosis

Unpleasant, intrusive thoughts and abnormal stereotyped behaviours occur in other mental disorders, and OCD is not diagnosed if their content is exclusively related to another disorder, for example guilty preoccupations in depression, worries in generalized anxiety, concern with illness in hypochondriasis, weight control in anorexia or avoidance in phobic disorders[5]. It should be borne in mind that conditions such as depression, generalized anxiety and substance abuse may be co-morbid with OCD. In elderly patients, increased anxious orderliness may be a prodrome of dementia; however, this behaviour is not resisted or associated with the tension that occurs in OCD. The compulsive behaviours of OCD resemble the stereotyped behaviours that occur in certain other disorders, such as Tourette's syndrome, Sydenham's chorea, encephalitis and partial complex seizures. Tourette's syndrome and OCD commonly co-occur[9], and patients with OCD may have a history of Sydenham's chorea in childhood[10]. There is currently some debate as to whether conditions such as OCD, body dysmorphic disorder, trichotillomania and hypochondriasis might form an obsessive-compulsive 'spectrum of disorders'.

Despite its similar name, obsessional personality disorder is quite distinct from OCD. It is characterized not by obsessions and compulsions, but by a preoccupation with orderliness, perfection and control dating back to early adulthood[5]. Individuals who are unable to discard personal possessions may present as the so-called 'senile squalor' syndrome after a lifetime of accumulating rubbish. This syndrome overlaps both obsessional personality disorder and OCD[11].

Not all patients with OCD have insight into the irrationality and inappropriateness of their obsessions and compulsions. If the obsessional thoughts are held with delusional intensity, an additional diagnosis of delusional disorder may be warranted. The ruminative delusions and stereotypies of schizophrenia are usually not ego-dystonic, and therefore would not be regarded as OCD[5].

Clinical Assessment

An effective treatment plan for OCD requires a detailed clinical assessment. What exactly are the main problems? What, if anything, exacerbates or improves the symptoms? How long has the condition been present, and how has it evolved since its onset? What treatments, if any, have been tried in the past? What other symptoms or disorders are present? Any concomitant depression, mania, psychosis or alcohol dependency will require specific management before behavioural treatments for OCD can be effective. If the patient is cognitively impaired, this will have implications for the choice of treatment; for example, some behavioural strategies will not work if information cannot be retained or recalled. In elderly patients with OCD of recent onset, it is important to investigate carefully for any underlying cerebral disease. Late-onset cases are associated with frontal dysfunction[12], which may be caused by a variety of focal and generalized disorders, including cerebrovascular disease, tumours and primary neurodegenerative dementias. Late-onset OCD may also be the result of external factors, such as adverse life events and exposure to trauma, that weaken an elderly individual's resistance to long-standing subclinical obsessionality[13].

Principles and Practice of Geriatric Psychiatry, 3rd edn. Edited by Mohammed T. Abou-Saleh, Cornelius Katona and Anand Kumar
© 2011 John Wiley & Sons, Ltd

EPIDEMIOLOGY

Most of our knowledge about the epidemiology of OCD in old age derives from the US National Institute for Mental Health (NIMH) Epidemiologic Catchment Area (ECA) Program. Overall, the one-year prevalence for those aged 65 years and older was 0.85% (men 0.75%, women 0.93%), as opposed to 1.65% for the sample as a whole[14]. A more detailed analysis of the elderly population at the Eastern Baltimore site found prevalence rates of 1.3% for those aged 65–74 years and 0.6% in those aged 75+[15]. Following the second wave of the ECA, annual incidence rates were estimated. In males aged 65+, the incidence rate of OCD was one-third of that for males of all ages, but in females there was a non-significant upturn in the incidence rate after age 65[16]. In common with a number of other psychiatric disorders, the lifetime prevalence of OCD decreased with age in this study. The reason for this is unclear, but it may be the result of cohort effects, differential mortality or age-specific differences in symptom ascertainment and recall. A rather higher overall one-year prevalence rate of 1.5% in over-65-year-olds has been reported in a more recent community study in Quebec, greater than that found for major depression (1.1%)[17].

AETIOLOGY

OCD is familial; it occurs in 40–50% of parents, 19–39% of siblings and 16% of children of probands with the disorder[18]. Just what is inherited is not clear; other anxiety disorders are also more common in the families of OCD probands[19]. At least part of this familiality is due to genes, and most of the studies that have been carried out have focused on candidate genes in the serotonergic and dopaminergic neuronal pathways[20]. However, to date most of these studies have been too small to establish linkage with an acceptable level of significance, and apart from the glutamate transporter gene, there has been no replication of findings. It is not known how the expression of any genetic susceptibility to OCD may vary across the life span.

Most of the evidence from clinical, neuropsychological and neuroimaging studies implicates the basal ganglia and their connections with the thalamus and the cerebral cortex in the aetiology of OCD[21]. Specifically, it has been proposed that there are structural and functional abnormalities in a neuronal circuit involving the orbitofrontal cortex, the basal ganglia, the substantia nigra and the ventrolateral pallidum[22]. Recent developments in imaging, such as voxel-based morphometry and multivoxel analyses have confirmed abnormality of the orbitofrontal-striatal areas in OCD, but indicate that other regions such as the dorsolateral and ventrolateral pre-frontal and parietal areas are also involved[23]. The specific response of OCD to serotonin (5-HT) re-uptake-inhibiting drugs (see below) suggests that serotonergic neuronal systems are involved, directly or indirectly. In the cognitive behavioural model of OCD, obsessions and compulsions result from pathological, anxiety-provoking over-control of normal intrusive cognitions[24].

TREATMENT

There are no randomized, controlled trials of treatment of OCD in elderly patients. Accordingly, the guidelines that follow are based upon case reports and extrapolations from studies in younger adults[25]. The current evidence-based UK NICE Guideline on OCD recommends a stepped care approach, with low-intensity psychological treatment for mildly impaired patients, and more intensive psychological treatment or pharmacotherapy for the more severely impaired, or those who fail to respond to low-intensity treatment[26]. This document also outlines some useful principles underlying the effective care of this group of patients.

Non-Pharmacological Treatments

Behavioural therapy, in the form of exposure and response prevention (ERP), is well described as an effective intervention for OCD in younger adults[27]. This involves exposing the patient to the feared situation, and helping him/her to resist the urge to perform the compulsive behaviours that would normally follow this exposure[28]. ERP is least effective in those who have obsessional thoughts and covert rituals unaccompanied by compulsive behaviour. In these patients, a cognitive approach directed at modifying the misinterpretation of intrusive thoughts is more appropriate[29]. A recent systematic review of randomized trials of psychological treatments for OCD in comparison with treatment as usual has concluded that treatments based on cognitive behavioural models are effective in younger adults, although larger studies with longer periods of follow-up are still needed[30]. Another systematic review has found that group cognitive behaviour therapy for OCD is effective in comparison with several control conditions, although it is not yet clear how this compares with individual treatment formats[31]. There are a number of case reports of effective behavioural interventions in elderly OCD patients[24,32–35], which suggest that it is reasonable to extrapolate the available evidence from randomized, controlled trials involving younger adults. It should be borne in mind, however, that most of the case reports are difficult to interpret because of the concomitant administration of medication, although in the case described by Calamari et al.[35], significant improvement following ERP was maintained without medication at eight-month follow-up.

Sigmund Freud originally proposed that obsessional symptoms were a regression to a pre-genital anal–sadistic phase of development. However, despite this and subsequent psychodynamic formulations of the disorder, there is no evidence that psychodynamic psychotherapy is an effective treatment for OCD at any age.

Pharmacological Treatments

Studies in younger adults indicate that 30–60% of patients with OCD show improvement on appropriate medication, and that drug treatments appear to be more effective for obsessional thoughts than for compulsive behaviours. In practice, drug treatment and behavioural therapy are often given in combination, and there is some evidence that this is an effective strategy[36].

The theory that OCD is a disorder of serotoninergic function is based upon the empirical observation that it can be effectively treated by drugs that inhibit serotonin re-uptake. Clomipramine is the most extensively studied drug treatment for OCD, and its effectiveness has been established in a number of double-blind, placebo-controlled trials in younger adults[37]. However, its lack of receptor sensitivity means that it has significant anticholinergic and antihistaminergic side effects that limit its usefulness in elderly patients[38]. In this age group, the current drug of first choice is one of the specific serotonin re-uptake inhibitors (SSRIs). Fluoxetine, paroxetine, fluvoxamine and escitalopram are currently licensed in the UK for the treatment of OCD, although none of the trials supporting this indication specifically involved elderly patients. A systematic review of trials of SSRI drugs for OCD in comparison with placebo has concluded that they are effective, at least in the short term, and that there are some differences between the different SSRIs with respect to their adverse effects[39]. The effective dose for the treatment of OCD with these drugs tends to be higher than that required to treat depression, and the time taken to respond is typically much longer: 10–18 weeks. Studies suggest that long-term therapy is required, as discontinuation of medication leads to relapse of symptoms[40].

There is little evidence for the effectiveness of other drug treatments in OCD. There are some case reports suggesting that monoamine oxidase inhibitors (MAOIs) may be useful in patients with concomitant panic or severe anxiety. Anxiolytic drugs may also help with the anxiety associated with OCD, but do not appear to have any effect on the core symptoms. A possible exception is buspirone, which may augment the effect of fluoxetine[41,42]. A recent meta-analysis of randomized, controlled trials supports the use of antipsychotic drugs in combination with an SSRI in patients resistant to first-line drug treatment[43]; the best evidence is for haloperidol and risperidone. Several other drugs, including carbamazepine, gabapentin, memantine and mirtazapine have been reported to be effective in combination with SSRIs in small uncontrolled studies. Lithium augmentation of fluoxetine has also been reported as effective in one elderly case[44].

Physical Treatments

There is very little evidence to suggest that ECT is effective in the treatment of OCD in patients who are not also depressed[45]. Similarly, the therapeutic potential of transcranial magnetic stimulation in this disorder has yet to be demonstrated[46]. Some good results have been reported for stereotactic neurosurgical procedures in patients with severe and treatment-refractory illness, including elderly subjects[25], but since negative outcomes are rarely described, this evidence is difficult to interpret.

CONCLUSIONS

OCD may present for the first time in old age, and many elderly patients with chronic illness will not have been exposed to the full range of pharmacological and cognitive behavioural interventions that are now available. It is important that old age psychiatry services are aware of these treatments and develop some experience in their delivery. There is some evidence that they are effective in elderly patients, but further research is needed. Patients with a new onset of OCD in late life need careful assessment to exclude underlying organic brain disease.

REFERENCES

1. Rachman SJ, Hodgson RJ. *Obsessions and Compulsions*. Englewood Cliffs, NJ: Prentice Hall, 1980.
2. Thyer BA, Parrish RT, Curtis GC et al. Ages of onset of DSM-III anxiety disorders. *Comp Psychiat* 1985; **26**: 113–22.
3. Rasmussen SA, Eisen JL. Epidemiology and clinical features of obsessive-compulsive disorder. In Jenike MA, Baer L, Minichiello WE (eds), *Obsessive Compulsive Disorders: Theory and Management*. Littleton, MA: PSG Publishing, 1990, 10–27.
4. Skoog G, Skoog I. A 40-year follow-up of patients with obsessive-compulsive disorder. *Arch Gen Psych* 1999; **56**: 131–2.
5. American Psychiatric Association. *Diagnostic and Statistical Manual of Mental Disorders. Fourth Edition*. Washington, DC: American Psychiatric Association, 1994.
6. World Health Organization. *International Classification of Diseases (10th Revision)*. Geneva: World Health Organization, 1992.
7. Kohn R, Westlake RJ, Rasmussen SA et al. Clinical features of obsessive-compulsive disorder in elderly patients. *Am J Geriat Psychiat* 1997; **5**: 211–15.
8. Fallon BA, Liebowitz MR, Hollander E et al. The pharmacotherapy of moral or religious scrupulosity. *J Clin Psychiat* 1990; **51**: 517–21.
9. Pauls D, Leckman J. The inheritance of Gilles de la Tourette's syndrome and associated behaviours: evidence for autosomal dominant transmission. *N Engl J Med* 1986; **315**: 993.
10. Swedo S, Rapaport J, Cheslow D et al. High prevalence of obsessive compulsive disorder symptoms in patients with Sydenham's chorea. *Am J Psychiat* 1989; **146**: 46–9.
11. Pertusa A, Fullana MA, Singh S et al. Compulsive hoarding: OCD symptom, distinct clinical syndrome, or both? *Am J Psychiatry* 2008; **165**: 1289–98.
12. Philpot MP, Banerjee S. Obsessive-compulsive disorder in the elderly. *Behav Neurol* 1998; **11**: 117–21.
13. Colvin C, Boddington SJA. Behaviour therapy for obsessive compulsive disorder in a 78-year-old woman. *Int J Geriat Psychiat* 1997; **12**: 488–91.
14. Karno M, Golding JM. Obsessive-compulsive disorder. In Robins LN, Regier DA (eds), *Psychiatric Disorders in America*. New York: Free Press, 1991, 204–19.
15. Kramer M, German PS, Anthony J et al. Patterns of mental disorders among the elderly residents of Eastern Baltimore. *J Am Geriat Soc* 1985; **33**: 236–45.
16. Eaton WW, Kramer M, Anthony J et al. The incidence of specific DIS/DSM-III mental disorders: data from the NIMH Epidemiologic Catchment Area program. *Acta Psychiat Scand* 1989; **67**: 414–28.
17. Préville M, Boyer R, Grenier S et al. The epidemiology of psychiatric disorders in Quebec's older adult population. *Can J Psychiatry* 2008; **53**: 822–32.
18. Marks IM. Genetics of fear and anxiety disorders. *Br J Psychiat* 1986; **149**: 406–18.
19. Black DW, Noyes R, Goldstein RB, Blim N. A family study of obsessive-compulsive disorder. *Arch Gen Psychiat* 1992; **49**: 362–8.
20. Pauls DL. The genetics of obsessive compulsive disorder: a review of the evidence. *Am J Med Genet C Semin Med Genet* 2008; **148**: 133–9.
21. Piggott TA, Myers KR, Williams DA. Obsessive-compulsive disorder: a neuropsychiatric perspective. In Rapee RM (ed.), *Current Controversies in the Anxiety Disorders*. New York: Guilford, 1996, 134–60.
22. Insel TR. Neurobiology of obsessive compulsive disorder: a review. *Int Clin Psychopharmacol* 1992; **7**(Suppl 1): 31–3.
23. Menzies L, Chamberlain SR, Laird AR et al. Integrating evidence from neuroimaging and neuropsychological studies of obsessive-compulsive disorder: the orbitofronto-striatal model revisited. *Neurosci Biobehav Rev* 2008; **32**: 525–49.
24. Salkovskis PM. Cognitive-behavioural approaches to the understanding of obsessional problems. In Rapee RM (ed.), *Current Controversies in the Anxiety Disorders*. New York: Guilford, 1996, 103–33.

25. Jenike MA, Baer L, Minichiello WE. *Obsessive Compulsive Disorders: Theory and Management*, 2nd edn. Chicago, IL: Year-book Medical Publishers, 1990.

26. National Collaborating Centre for Mental Health. *Clinical Guideline 31: Obsessive-Compulsive Disorder: Core Interventions in the Treatment of Obsessive-Compulsive Disorder and Body Dysmorphic Disorder*. National Institute for Health and Clinical Excellence. At www.nice.org.uk/nicemedia/pdf/cg031niceguideline.pdf, accessed 22 Feb 2010.

27. Marks IM, Lelliot P, Basoglu M, Noshirvani H. Clomipramine, self-exposure and therapist aided exposure for obsessive-compulsive rituals: I. *Br J Psychiat* 1988; **136**: 1–25.

28. Salkovskis PM, Kirk J. Obsessional disorders. In Hawton K, Salkovskis PM, Kirk J, Clark DM (eds), *Cognitive Behaviour Therapy for Psychiatric Problems: A Practical Guide*. Oxford: Oxford University Press, 1989, 129–68.

29. Salkovskis PM, Warwick HMC. Cognitive therapy of obsessive compulsive disorder: treating treatment failures. *Behav Psychother* 1985; **13**: 243–55.

30. Gava I, Barbui C, Aguglia E *et al*. Psychological treatments versus treatment as usual for obsessive compulsive disorder (OCD). *Cochrane Database Syst Rev* 2007; **18**: CD005333.

31. Jónsson H, Hougaard E. Group cognitive behavioural therapy for obsessive-compulsive disorder: a systematic review and meta-analysis. *Acta Psychiatr Scand* 2009; **119**: 98–106.

32. Rowen VC, Holborn SW, Walker JR, Siddiqui AR. A rapid multi-component treatment for an obsessive-compulsive disorder. *J Behav Ther Exp Psychiat* 1984; **15**: 347–52.

33. Junginger J, Ditto B. Multitreatment of obsessive compulsive checking in a geriatric patient. *Behav Modif* 1984, **8**: 379–90.

34. Austin LS, Zealberg JJ, Lydiard RB. Three cases of pharmacotherapy of obsessive-compulsive disorder in the elderly. *J Nerv Ment Dis* 1991; **179**: 634–5.

35. Calamari JE, Faber SD, Hitsman BL, Poppe CJ. Treatment of obsessive-compulsive disorder in the elderly: a review and case example. *J Behav Ther Exp Psychiat* 1994; **25**: 95–104.

36. Simpson HB, Foa EB, Liebowitz MR *et al*. A randomized, controlled trial of cognitive-behavioral therapy for augmenting pharmacotherapy in obsessive-compulsive disorder. *Am J Psychiatry* 2008; **165**: 621–30.

37. Thoren P, Asberg M, Cronholm B *et al*. Clomipramine treatment of obsessive-compulsive disorder: a clinical controlled trial. *Arch Gen Psychiat* 1980; **37**: 1281.

38. Jackson CW. Obsessive-compulsive disorder in elderly patients. *Drugs Aging* 1995; **7**: 438–48.

39. Soomro GM, Altman D, Rajagopal S, Oakley-Browne M. Selective serotonin re-uptake inhibitors (SSRIs) versus placebo for obsessive-compulsive disorder (OCD). *Cochrane Database Syst Rev* 2008; **23**: CD001765.

40. Fineberg NA, Tonnoir B, Lemming O, Stein DJ. Escitalopram prevents relapse of obsessive-compulsive disorder. *Eur Neuropsychopharmacol* 2007; **17**: 430–9.

41. Markovitz PJ, Stagno SJ, Calabrese JR. Buspirone augmentation of fluoxetine in obsessive-compulsive disorder. Abstract no. 379, Biological Psychiatry Annual Meeting, 1989, San Francisco, CA.

42. Jenike MA, Baer L, Ballantine HT *et al*. Cingulotomy for refractory obsessive-compulsive disorder: a long-term follow-up of 33 patients. *Arch Gen Psychiat* 1991; **48**: 548–55.

43. Skapinakis P, Papatheodorou T, Mavreas V. Antipsychotic augmentation of serotonergic antidepressants in treatment-resistant obsessive-compulsive disorder: a meta-analysis of the randomized controlled trials. *Eur Neuropsychopharmacol* 2007; **1**: 79–93.

44. Bajulaiye R, Addonizio G. Obsessive compulsive disorder arising in a 75-year-old woman. *Int J Geriat Psychiat* 1992; **7**: 139–42.

45. Mellman LA, Grossman JM. Successful treatment of obsessive-compulsive disorder with ECT. *Am J Psychiat* 1984; **141**: 596–7.

46. Martin JL, Barbanoj MJ, Sacristán M. Transcranial magnetic stimulation for the treatment of obsessive-compulsive disorder. *Cochrane Database Syst Rev* 2003; **3**: CD003387.

102

Somatoform Disorders and Unexplained Physical Symptoms

Bart Sheehan

Health Sciences Research Institute, Warwick Medical School, Coventry, UK

HISTORY

Mysterious physical symptoms of uncertain origin have been noted as long as medical matters have been written about. Early explanations of mysterious symptoms involved the abnormal movement or function of the womb, hence the origin of the term hysteria from the Greek word *hysterikos*. Such explanations may now seem absurd, but were influential till at least the seventeenth century, when Sydenham first wrote of hypochondriasis (a male condition) and hysteria (a female equivalent). Sydenham described the two conditions as alike 'as one egg is to another'. He recognized that psychological disturbance was primary, that symptoms were changeable and that these conditions cause great diagnostic difficulty. Over the next 200 years, acceptance of a psychological origin for some ill-defined physical symptoms grew, along with the concept of a group of psychological illnesses called neuroses.

Interest in these ill-defined symptoms really accelerated with the popularization of Sigmund Freud's early ideas about unconscious conflicts and psychological disturbance. Freud was struck by Charcot's demonstrations in Paris of hysterical physical symptoms. He developed the idea that unconscious conflicts were manifest as physical symptoms, as a form of defence mechanism. After the First World War, no-one who had seen the victims of 'shell-shock' could doubt the ability of psychological trauma to cause physical symptoms.

Proponents of psychoanalytic ideas developed terms like somatization and psychosomatic illnesses. As the influence of these ideas eventually waned after the Second World War, clinicians became less focused on aetiology and more on careful description of patients with persistent troublesome physical symptoms. By 1980, when DSM-III was published, the term hysteria was dropped. Somatization disorder, in which multiple physical symptoms persist over years, with no organic explanation, and hypochondriasis, in which patients dread a particular disease and cannot be reassured despite investigation, became the prototypical somatoform disorders. Thus, Sydenham's observations from 300 years previously were confirmed in modern medicine.

MODERN TERMINOLOGY

Both DSM-IV and ICD-10 have categories of somatoform disorders. Both include core somatization disorder and hypochondriacal disorder, and a handful of other disorders like conversion disorder and body dysmorphic disorder (DSM-IV), Somatoform autonomic disorder (ICD-10) and persistent pain disorders (both classifications).

Clinicians dealing with older patients are likely to mainly encounter less differentiated admixtures of unexplained symptoms and hypochondriacal beliefs. The diagnostic categories in DSM-IV are unlikely to be especially helpful when faced with a persistently complaining patient who is likely also to have at least one organic illness. The term 'medically unexplained symptoms' is sometimes used to cover the wider range of patient presentations. This term avoids diagnostic confusion and can sometimes be useful in the presence of real physical illness.

CLINICAL PRESENTATIONS

Case 1

Mr W is a 76-year-old man admitted with worsening depression to a psychiatric ward. In the last two weeks he has become increasing preoccupied with his bowels, plaguing his primary care doctor for consultations. He is now convinced that his bowels have stopped working due to 'a blockage ... cancer or something'. He is reluctant to eat or drink and feels that any treatment is futile. Examination and investigation shows mild constipation but no evidence of any other organic lesion. Reassurance is ineffective. He eventually requires intravenous rehydration and ECT. He begins to improve after about a week, initially saying 'I am not so sure', then later 'I suppose I was worrying too much'. He regains much of the weight he had lost and is discharged home after seven weeks in hospital.

Principles and Practice of Geriatric Psychiatry, 3rd edn. Edited by Mohammed T. Abou-Saleh, Cornelius Katona and Anand Kumar
© 2011 John Wiley & Sons, Ltd

A case of severe depressive disorder with psychotic features (hypochondriacal and nihilistic delusions). Rapid improvement in physical complaints noted with definitive treatment of underlying psychiatric disorder.

Case 2

Mrs K is a 64-year-old woman who is referred to psychiatric services for the fifth time in her life. She is well known to primary care as a frequent attender and for the last three years has seen her general practitioner at least once a week. She complains of multiple symptoms including pain in the head, back and limbs, abdominal discomfort, bloating and frequency of bowel motions, blurred vision, dry mouth, urinary frequency, some shortness of breath and chest pain, and is 'unable to settle at night'. She has had multiple referrals to secondary care over 40 years. Investigations by gynaecology, general surgery, cardiology and gastroenterology have been negative but did not help. She does not feel taken seriously and is 'fed up with doctors ... the whole time they just try to get rid of me'. She has mild depression but is very reluctant to see a psychiatrist or counsellor. The psychiatrist writes 'No sign of formal mental illness' and discharges the patient back to the general practitioner.

A probable case of somatization disorder. Psychiatry is unhelpful here, maintaining the disorder by rejecting the validity of the complaint and offering nothing helpful to the GP.

Case 3

Mrs T, a 76-year-old widow, presents to her GP with abdominal pain. This has come on in the last three weeks. There are no findings on examination and she has no significant medical or surgical history. Her husband died about six years ago. She becomes tearful during the consultation and says she is 'desperately worried' that the marriage of her only daughter is in trouble. This daughter is her main social support. She thinks she may not see her grandchildren again for some time. She agrees that stress makes the pain worse, and agrees that the family situation is stressful. She comes back to see the GP after two weeks. The pain has lessened, though she is still worried. She has told her daughter of her worry, and been reassured that she will not lose contact with any family members.

Illustrates how mild physical symptoms may follow psychological distress, and how watchful waiting and a sympathetic approach may be associated with improvement and no unnecessary referrals.

EPIDEMIOLOGY

While strictly defined somatoform disorders are relatively rare at all ages, somatoform presentations are very common. In all cultures, somatized symptoms are probably the most common way for depressive disorders to present in primary care. In secondary care, psychological distress and outright somatoform disorders have both been consistently linked with frequent attendance, high costs and chronicity of presentations.

Good-quality evidence on the prevalence and incidence of these presentations among older people is lacking. Somatoform presentations are often defined in loose or confusing ways, or highly selected populations may be sampled. Some studies define somatoform presentations as strict classical presentations with a primary hypochondriacal or somatization disorder, others are rates of ill-defined somatic symptoms. Prospective studies which follow somatoform presentations among older people are especially rare.

Community Samples

Surveys among community samples of older people have tended to show very low prevalence (0.0–3.9%) of strictly defined hypochondriacal or somatization disorders. A consistent finding in studies comparing younger with older people is that older people are no more preoccupied with physical health than younger people. This counters a widespread stereotype of older people concentrating introspectively on physical health.

Primary Care Samples

In older UK primary care patients[1], 5% were reported to have hypochondriacal neurosis, but many more had at least a few somatoform symptoms (unexplained symptoms). In the same study, primary care physicians were asked about the likely origins of the older patients' physical symptoms. A third were rated as having physical symptoms that were equally or mainly of psychological origin. A careful Italian primary care study[2] showed a similar figure of 8.1% having a primary somatoform disorder.

General Hospital Samples

Rates of somatoform disorders, or unexplained physical presentations, in secondary care have consistently been shown to be high. The few studies which have included secondary care patients from across the age range have shown very similar rates between young and old. Unsurprisingly, older hypochondriacal patients at general hospital settings do have higher rates of other true organic illnesses.

Psychiatric Samples

Most interest has been in the prevalence of somatoform presentations among older people with depression. Older patients with either anxiety disorders or depressive disorders have been consistently shown to commonly present with somatized physical symptoms, and these presentations are more common than among younger patients with depressive and anxiety disorders. Unexplained physical symptoms among frail older people are more strongly associated with depressed mood than with the burden of 'real' physical illness. This is an important clinical point: the presence of unexplained symptoms should trigger consideration of psychiatric as well as physical illness.

AETIOLOGY

Many theories about the origins of somatoform presentations have been advanced. Some, like the ancient view that such symptoms arose from uterine causes, are now dismissed due to modern understanding of anatomy and physiology. Others, including the influential psychoanalytic view that somatization arose from the 'conversion' of unacceptable unconscious mental conflicts, have been highly influential but difficult to examine in scientific study. Modern theories on aetiology have three key themes:

1. Somatoform presentations as manifestations of other psychiatric disorders – Somatoform presentations are undoubtedly found most frequently among people with higher rates of psychiatric disorder, especially depressive disorder.
2. Somatoform presentations as reflecting a stable, internal personality style – Research has shown that neurotic personality styles are much more common among somatizers. It is common when dealing with chronic severe somatizers to note the early appearance of unexplained physical symptoms and persistent pattern of medical help-seeking. In some cases this may be related to early maternal loss, abuse or other trauma. People who have a tendency to negative self-evaluation and to somatosensory amplification (a tendency to interpret normal physical symptoms as aversive) are much more likely to report physical symptoms to a health professional.
3. Somatoform presentations reflecting a social construct (i.e. an understandable reaction to the medical system or societal norms that a person lives in). It is widely held that somatoform presentations are more common in non-western cultures. The largest international study of somatization[3] reported rates of somatization in primary care in 14 centres. Somatization was found commonly in all centres and especially so as a means of presentation of psychiatric disorder. Only South American centres showed higher rates; even here, rates of depressive disorder were as common among those presenting somatically. Another possibility is that somatoform presentations are encouraged by the medical or social system people live in. Somatizing patients consume large amounts of resources, and early recognition of the problem, fewer prescriptions and fewer hospital referrals are associated with better outcomes.

Among older people, the strongest aetiological link has been with depressive illness. While some older people are simply chronic somatoform presenters grown old, new somatoform presentations remain common in old age. Depressive disorders are the most common association, with certain symptoms including fatigue, dizziness, weakness, pain and heavy feelings in the limbs among the symptoms most commonly reported. Moreover, the association with depressive illness is independent of that with physical disorder. Among older people, the traditional concept of 'masked depression' has held up better than many other theories of the origins of somatoform presentations.

OUTCOMES

Most studies at any age indicate that somatoform disorders will tend to persist if they are severe and outcomes also depend on the medical response to the initial presentation. The clinical context is important; mild somatoform presentations in primary care may be transient though the style of presentation, that is, the tendency to present with physical symptoms when emotionally distressed, tends to persist. Among patients with clear-cut severe somatoform disorders in secondary care, persistence is part of the diagnostic criteria.

Patients have often had a very persistent course with 10–20 years of relentless presentations despite multiple investigations and failed reassurance. Such patients are difficult to treat, but may greatly trouble health professionals.

Among older patients, few studies have followed somatoform presentations prospectively. Among UK older primary care patients, a prospective study[1] found that severe cases of full somatoform disorders tended to remit, but vague or unexplained physical symptoms were highly persistent at nine-month follow-up. The attribution of physical symptoms to a physical cause was also highly stable over time. These findings are somewhat contrary to reports among younger people. Somatized symptoms were prospectively associated with frequent attendance in primary care. Though research is limited, it is fair to assume that among older patients, milder somatoform presentations use significant amounts of primary care time and are likely to persist. More severe somatoform presentations, especially when secondary to depressive disorder, may be likely to respond to treatment.

TREATMENT

Specific Treatment of Somatoform Disorders

Many controlled trials have been carried out among patients with somatoform disorders. The most frequently evaluated interventions have been cognitive behavioural therapy (CBT) and antidepressant medication. These interventions have been subject to systematic review[4]. This review specified the somatoform disorders addressed, including both pure somatization disorder and lower threshold disorders. Of good-quality trials of CBT, 11 of 13 studies showed benefit above control treatment, while among studies of antidepressant medication, 4 of 5 trials showed benefit. Of those trials addressing health care resource use, 10 of 11 studies showed cost reductions for the intervention group. The author concluded that the best evidence was for CBT. The cognitive behavioural model requires highly trained and skilled therapists and represents a challenge among older patients. Problems may include inadequate provision of psychological therapy for older people and the fact that these patients are likely to have admixtures of somatoform symptoms as well as symptoms from organic illness. A further challenge is to find ways to amend CBT to integrate its use into primary care. No intervention studies have been carried out among older patients with somatoform disorders.

Studies among Patients with Psychiatric Disorders

Studying somatoform presentations among older patients being treated for depressive or anxiety disorders tends to show improvement in somatoform presentations over time. Those trials of antidepressant medication that have examined which symptoms predict positive outcomes tend to consistently show that hypochondriacal or somatization symptoms predict a poorer outcome, though those clinicians with experience of treating severe hypochondriasis among people with depression will be aware that severe hypochondriasis does resolve along with other psychotic symptoms.

AN APPROACH TO MANAGEMENT OF MEDICALLY UNEXPLAINED SYMPTOMS IN OLDER PEOPLE

This approach draws on what is known to be effective among younger people with somatization. Older people have a high prevalence of physical illness so a commonsense approach to management of new or uncharacteristic physical symptoms must be taken. It may be easier for medically qualified staff to tolerate uncertainty with such patients.

Is There a Physical Illness?

Is it being adequately dealt with?

In the majority of cases the patient will be adequately investigated and treated before somatization is considered.

Is There a Psychiatric Illness?

In depressive disorder, the low mood and biological symptoms such as poor sleep, weight loss, poor appetite, poor concentration and retardation/agitation usually precede the physical complaints. Patients usually admit to gloomy introspection and are likely to admit to depression rather than reject such suggestions.

Is it being adequately treated?

Antidepressant medication will usually resolve depression, with resolution of somatized symptoms.

Do Medically Unexplained Symptoms Need Independent Treatment?

If both physical and psychiatric illness is being reasonably dealt with, but unexplained symptoms are persisting and causing distress, then a positive and structured response is needed.

• Stop investigations and hospital referrals. Explain that investigations are not helping but as a clinician you believe the patients' symptoms and will continue to monitor them.

• Schedule regular appointments with the patient. The patient should be seen regularly but not necessarily frequently. This means they do not need to report symptoms in order to be seen and may reduce demands for appointments at short notice.

• Explain that investigations have shown no condition that they cannot recover from. This allows the prospect of recovery to be available, maintaining hope.

• Use cognitive behavioural techniques. Identify dysfunctional beliefs ('headaches usually mean brain tumour', 'muscle aches mean exercise has damaged the muscle fibres') and dysfunctional behaviours ('I will stay in bed all weekend to give my muscles a chance to recover').

• Identify positive thinking and behaviour strategies. For example, demonstrate that holding a book in an outstretched hand causes pain – to show effect of muscle tension. Exercise increases blood flow and fitness of muscle fibres. Schedule increasing levels of activity and record symptoms in fatigue diary.

REFERENCES

1. Sheehan B, Bass C, Briggs R, Jacoby, R. Somatization among older primary care attenders. *Psychol Med* 2003; **33**: 867–77.
2. Balestrieri M, Marcon G, Samani F *et al*. Mental disorders associated with benzodiazepine use among older primary care attenders. *Soc Psychiatry Psychiatr Epidemiol* 2005; **40**: 308–15.
3. Gureje, O, Simon, GE, Ustun, TB, Goldberg, DP. Somatization in cross-cultural perspective: A World Health Organization study in primary care. *Am J Psychiatry* 1997; **154**: 989–95.
4. Kroenke, K. Efficacy of treatment for somatoform disorders: a review of randomized controlled trials. *Psychosom Med* 2007; **69**: 881–88.

103

Other Neurotic Disorders

Jerome J. Schulte, C. Michael Hendricks and David Bienenfeld

Department of Psychiatry Wright State University, Boonshoft School of Medicine, OH, USA

REACTION TO SEVERE STRESS AND ADJUSTMENT DISORDERS

Before the Second World War it was generally held that psychiatric patients were constitutionally different from 'normals'. During the War it was observed that previously asymptomatic individuals experiencing unusual environmental stress sometimes suffered from transient psychiatric difficulties. This observation led to a reclassification of psychiatric disorders to allow for behavioural and emotional symptoms in people who would return to their premorbid state with the removal of the unusual environmental precipitant[1]. DSM-I and ICD-6 classified these transient difficulties as 'gross stress reaction' and 'adult situational reaction'; DSM-II and ICD-8 classified them as 'transient situational disturbances'. ICD-9 introduced the categories of 'acute reaction to stress' and 'adjustment disorder'. ICD-10 defines 'acute stress reaction', 'post-traumatic stress disorder' and 'adjustment disorder'; although DSM-III-R recognized only the latter two of these, DSM-IV-TR recognizes all three[2].

ACUTE STRESS REACTION

Clinical Features

According to ICD-10, acute stress reaction is a transient disturbance occurring in persons without apparent mental disorder, in response to exceptional physical and/or mental stress and subsiding in hours or days. The diagnosis should not be made for an exacerbation of symptoms of a diagnosable psychiatric disorder already present, except for accentuation of personality traits. Previous history of another psychiatric disorder does not invalidate this diagnosis. An immediate, clear connection between the stressor and the onset of symptoms should be seen.

Symptoms of this disorder show a mixed and changing picture, with no one symptom predominating for long. They appear within minutes of the stress and resolve rapidly when the stressor is removed or, if the stress remains, symptoms decrease after 24–48 hours and are minimal after three days. Typical symptoms include an initial state of 'daze', constriction of consciousness, narrowing of attention, decreased comprehension of stimuli and disorientation. Withdrawal, agitation or overactivity may follow. Autonomic signs of panic (tachycardia, sweating, flushing) are common. Amnesia for the traumatic present may also be present. In the elderly, organic factors and life stage events can be predisposing factors to acute stress reaction[3]. The multiple bereavements that are not uncommon in late life can be the precipitants for acute stress reaction. However, recent data do suggest the older population may tolerate acute stress better than the younger and middle-aged[4].

DSM-IV differs somewhat from ICD-10 in its diagnostic classification of acute stress disorder. Unlike ICD-10, which requires that symptoms appear within minutes of the stress and diminish to minimal intensity after three days, DSM-IV requires symptoms to last a minimum of two days and allows for persistence up to four weeks. DSM-IV also includes dissociative symptoms not included under ICD-10: a subjective sense of numbing, detachment or absence of emotional responsiveness; derealization and depersonalization. Another DSM-IV requirement is that the traumatic event is persistently re-experienced in at least one of the following ways: recurrent images, thoughts, dreams, illusions, flashback episodes, or a sense of reliving the experience; or distress on exposure to reminders of the traumatic event. DSM-IV also requires marked avoidance of stimuli that arouse recollections of the trauma[5].

Differential Diagnosis

The differential diagnosis includes post-traumatic stress disorder (PTSD) and adjustment disorder. PTSD (see below) occurs after a latency period of weeks or longer, while the symptoms of acute stress reaction begin immediately after the traumatic event. The repetitive, intrusive imagery characteristic of PTSD is not usually a feature of the ICD-10 diagnosis of acute stress reaction. DSM-IV, however, does include repetitive intrusive imagery among the features of acute stress disorder. If psychotic symptoms follow an extreme stress, acute (brief) psychotic disorder should be considered. Adjustment disorders are less severe, and longer lasting, than acute stress reactions. Events that precipitate adjustment disorders are also less intense than those responsible for acute stress reactions.

Therapy

By definition, the symptoms of acute stress reaction are time-limited and will resolve without specific therapeutic intervention. Treatment may be requested, however, for intolerable tension or insomnia. For tension, short-term use of benzodiazepines with simple metabolic pathways and short half-lives, such as lorazepam or oxazepam, are safest in the elderly. For insomnia, temazepam or

Principles and Practice of Geriatric Psychiatry, 3rd edn. Edited by Mohammed T. Abou-Saleh, Cornelius Katona and Anand Kumar
© 2011 John Wiley & Sons, Ltd

the non-benzodiazepine sedative hypnotic zolpidem[6] are justified. Families and patients may be reassured that the acute response does not indicate a psychotic decompensation, and that the prognosis for rapid recovery is favourable. Acutely, and in the aftermath of the traumatic event, it is useful to help the patient gain mastery over the trauma[7] by using a brief treatment model, consisting of fostering abreaction and integration of the event as quickly as possible, with the expectation that the trauma victim will return to full functioning. Abreaction can be fostered through individual or group psychotherapy[8].

POST-TRAUMATIC STRESS DISORDER

Post-traumatic stress disorder (PTSD) first appeared in DSM-III but was based on older concepts tied to the history of warfare. Da Costa wrote of 'irritable heart' following the American Civil War. In the First World War the disorder was known as 'shell shock'. Early twentieth century psychoanalytic theory called it 'traumatic neurosis' and in the Second World War it was known as 'traumatic war neurosis' or 'combat neurosis.' In DSM-I it was renamed 'gross stress reaction', a reaction to great stress in a normal personality. During the relatively peaceful time between the Second World War and the Vietnam War, the category was omitted from DSM-II[9]. ICD-9 defined catastrophic stress and combat fatigue as two diagnoses under the category of acute reaction to stress. DSM-III defined intrusive re-experience of the trauma, together with emotional numbing, as the central features of PTSD. DSM-III-R placed more emphasis on the avoidance of stimuli associated with the trauma and less on numbing.

DSM-IV changed the definition of the trauma to an event where a person experienced, witnessed or was confronted with threatened death or serious injury or threat to physical integrity of self or others. Here, the response to the trauma involves intense fear, helplessness or horror. Also, where DSM-III-R required either numbing or avoidance behaviour, DSM-IV requires both[5]. ICD-10 criteria more closely resemble those of DSM-III, highlighting the restriction of emotional responsiveness. In ICD-10 the late chronic sequelae of devastating stress (i.e. those manifesting decades after the stressful experience) should be classified under enduring personality change after catastrophic experience[3].

Clinical Features

The prevalence rate of PTSD in the elderly is about 1%[10-12]. The ICD-10 diagnosis of PTSD requires evidence of trauma, or a response to a stressful event or situation of exceptionally threatening or catastrophic nature, likely to cause pervasive distress in anyone. The central symptoms are repetitive and intrusive recollections (flashbacks) or re-enactment of the event in memories, daytime imagery or dreams. The onset follows the trauma with a latency period of a few weeks to months (rarely exceeding six months).

There may also be a sense of 'numbness' and emotional blunting, and avoidance of activities and situations reminiscent of trauma. Anxiety, depression, suicidal ideation and insomnia are also common in many PTSD patients, particularly with advancing age[9]. PTSD is also associated with alcohol and drug abuse, possibly reflecting attempts to cope with PTSD symptoms. Dissociative symptoms, commonly described in younger PTSD victims, become less prevalent with increasing age[13,14]. However, psychotic symptoms tend to be more common in older PTSD patients[15].

It remains a subject of debate what factors, if any, predispose individuals to the development of the post-traumatic stress syndrome. Some traumas, particularly the concentration camp experience, are so severe that symptoms are almost universal in survivors. Because retrospective assessment of function before the traumatic event is always coloured by the response to the event, correlations are difficult to draw and empirical analyses have been inconclusive[16]. Certain personality traits (e.g. compulsive, asthenic), neurotic illness, and a history of adverse events in early childhood[10] may all lower the threshold for manifestation of the disorder[3]. PTSD can also develop from bereavement. One study surveyed surviving spouses two months after their spouses' deaths and found that 10% of those whose spouses died after a chronic illness met criteria for PTSD; 9% of those whose spouses died unexpectedly met PTSD criteria; and 36% of those whose spouses died from 'unnatural' causes (suicide or accident) had PTSD[17]. Other late life events, including falls, stroke, myocardial infarction and breast cancer, have also been shown to put the elderly at increased risk of developing PTSD[18-21].

Although PTSD symptoms can persist for many years, with increased frequency of symptoms towards the end of life[22], the typical course is one of fluctuating symptoms[23]. One study, examining current PTSD symptoms in elderly Second World War and Korean War prisoners of war (POWs), suggested that severity of exposure to trauma and lack of post-military social support were moderately predictive of PTSD. In this study, 53% of POWs met criteria for lifetime PTSD, with 29% meeting criteria for current PTSD, but for those POWs most severely traumatized, the lifetime PTSD rates were 83%, with current PTSD at 59%[24].

There are two types of PTSD to which the elderly seem susceptible: delayed-onset PTSD and chronic PTSD. In delayed-onset PTSD, patients may exhibit signs of the disorder decades after the trauma, and in chronic PTSD symptoms have been persistent since the time of the trauma. Delayed-onset PTSD may be a reactivation of remote PTSD earlier in life. A typical pattern is the onset of symptoms after initial exposure, a gradual decline in symptoms over several decades, followed by a reemergence in late life[25]. In some elderly Second World War veterans, media coverage commemorating the 50th anniversary of the end of the War triggered PTSD symptoms[26]. Commonly, guilt, distorted memory, emotional numbing, estrangement and feelings of detachment are seen[27]. Patients in this group can present with physical symptoms of cardiovascular, gastrointestinal and musculoskeletal diseases[16].

In general, the onset of severe symptoms can be linked to a profound recent life event, such as death of a wife, job retirement or loss of physical integrity from illness[27]. Most often, the contemporary precipitant reawakens emotions and perceptions from the original trauma. Holocaust survivors and POWs have been noted to begin displaying symptoms of PTSD after admission to nursing homes, where they re-experience a loss of freedom and autonomy. Second World War veterans found the loss of physical integrity due to somatic illness particularly upsetting, since it evoked memories of a traumatic period when their physical integrity was in jeopardy[14].

Differential Diagnosis

Although adjustment disorders also occur in response to life events, these events are in the normal range of human experience, unlike the extraordinary traumas responsible for PTSD. Specific features of numbing and flashbacks do not occur, and adjustment disorders, by definition, do not last more than six months. Acute stress reaction is characterized by a more variable clinical picture that resolves within days. Whether PTSD is predicted by acute stress reactions remains unclear[28]. While anxiety and depression are common features of PTSD, generalized anxiety disorder and phobic disorder have anxiety as a more specific and central symptom. Major depression is marked by deep and persistent mood disturbance, usually with loss of reactivity; dysthymia results in chronic, indolent dysphoria. None of these disorders includes the specific symptom of intrusive recollections.

Therapy

The signs and symptoms of PTSD include distorted expectations and perceptions, mood disturbances, psychophysiological symptoms and social withdrawal. Thus, common sense dictates, and empirical data confirm, that multimodal treatment is most advisable[11,29]. Psychosocial intervention and pharmacotherapy each has its place. Historically, dynamic psychotherapy has been a useful approach, but recent treatment guidelines support exposure-based psychotherapies as the most evidence-based form of treatment for PTSD[29]. Antidepressants can offer symptomatic relief by diminishing dysphoria, intrusive thoughts, insomnia and nightmares[30]. In particular, selective serotonin re-uptake inhibitors (SSRIs) have been shown to be effective pharmacotherapeutic treatment for PTSD, especially in reducing avoidant symptoms[31-37].

Other second-generation antidepressants do show promise in the management of PTSD but sufficient evidence is lacking at this time[35]. Prazosin, an alpha-1 adrenergic receptor antagonist, has been shown to be helpful with the sleep disturbance and nightmares of PTSD, but should be used with caution in the elderly because of the risk of orthostatic hypotension, particularly in combination with other medications that may lower blood pressure[29,38]. Beta-adrenergic blocking agents have been used in younger PTSD patients for relief of symptoms of autonomic arousal, tremors and startle reactions[39]. Older patients, however, are less likely to display a clinical profile of hyperarousal, and are more susceptible to the cardiovascular complications and organic mood disorders associated with adrenergic blockade. There are case reports of positive results using atypical antipsychotics as augmenting agents when added to SSRIs for treatment of refractory PTSD[35,40]. However, this class of medications must be used with caution in the older population given current concerns of increased mortality in older demented patients. Conversely, benzodiazepines do not appear to be a helpful treatment for PTSD[35] and should be avoided as much as possible in ageing individuals since they can cause paradoxical excitation and frequently induce subtle cognitive impairment[41]. Similarly, divalproex (valproate) has been demonstrated to be ineffective as monotherapy for PTSD in older veterans[42].

ADJUSTMENT DISORDER

The diagnosis of adjustment disorder refers to a state of subjective distress or emotional disturbance, interfering with social functioning or performance, arising in a period of adaptation to a significant life change or subsequent to a stressful life event. It is assumed that the condition would not have arisen without the stressor. According to DSM-IV, onset is within three months of the stressor. The duration of symptoms should not exceed six months, except in the case where the stressor is chronic (e.g. a chronic general medical condition) or the stressor has enduring consequences (e.g. the financial and emotional difficulties resulting from a divorce)[5]. ICD-10 describes onset as arising in the period of adaptation to the stressor[3].

Clinical Features

Symptoms of adjustment disorder may include: depressed mood, anxiety, worry, impairment in performance of daily routines and inability to cope or plan ahead. Adjustment disorders can be specified as brief depressive reaction, prolonged depressive reaction, adjustment disorder with predominant disturbance of other emotions, adjustment disorder with predominant disturbance of conduct, or adjustment disorder with mixed disturbance of emotions and conduct. The precipitating events for adjustment disorders can affect social network or values, and may involve the individual, his group or community. Common events causing such symptoms in older patients include physical illness or injury, placement in a nursing home and retirement[43]. The events, while subjectively profoundly meaningful, are of considerably smaller magnitude than those precipitating acute stress reaction and PTSD. Individual predisposition and vulnerability to these stressful life events thus plays a greater role in the occurrence of adjustment disorders. Poor pre-stressor social and co-existing physical problems[44], current dementia[45] and a history of a past psychiatric disorder[46] all increase vulnerability to adjustment disorders. However, while these premorbid risk factors are frequently observed, they do not appear essential. In a recent large study of elderly veterans with no recent psychiatric history admitted to medical/surgical units, adjustment disorder was diagnosed in over 20% of the patients post discharge[47].

Therapy

The cornerstone of treatment for adjustment disorders is focal psychotherapy, although it appears that antidepressants may be of value in the successful management of adjustment disorders in some outpatient settings that often lack ready access to psychotherapy[50]. Based on a psychodynamic understanding of emotions and behaviour, focal therapy identifies the most specific nidus of current distress and views it in the context of the patient's core conflicts or deficits. The therapy is of relatively brief duration, usually 6–20 sessions. The major techniques employed are clarification and confrontation[48]. Quite frequently, the precipitating event can be framed as a narcissistic threat or injury. In psychotherapy, the patient will come to view the therapist as a self-object, looking for restoration of the self-esteem provided by the lost function, role or friend. The therapist helps restore the wholeness of self by allowing the patient to modify his or her expectations of him- or herself and environment[49].

DISSOCIATIVE AND CONVERSION DISORDERS

In the last three decades of the nineteenth century, dissociation was studied extensively by Janet and conversion by Freud. DSM-I incorporated the concepts of dissociation and conversion into its classification scheme. Conversion reaction was assigned to hysterical neurosis, and amnesia was placed in the category of dissociative reaction. In DSM-II they were united under the heading of hysterical neurosis, but divided into conversion type and dissociative type. In DSM-III, DSM-III-R and DSM-IV the two conditions were renamed and separated once again. Hysteria, conversion type, became conversion disorder and was assigned to somatoform disorders. Hysteria, dissociative type, was expanded into the dissociative disorders[51]. ICD-10, however, continues to contain both under the heading of dissociative disorders.

Dissociative Amnesia

Dissociative amnesia is characterized by loss of memory, usually of important recent events, that is too great to be explained by ordinary forgetfulness or fatigue; and amnesia, either partial or complete, for recent events that are of a traumatic or stressful nature. The amnesia is usually partial and selective. The extent and completeness of the amnesia varies from day to day and between inquirers, but a persistent common core cannot be recalled in the waking state. Complete, generalized amnesia is rare and is usually part of a dissociative fugue. Affective states in amnesia are varied but severe depression is rare.

Perplexity, distress and varying degrees of attention-seeking behaviour may be evident, but calm acceptance is also sometimes striking. Purposeless local wandering may occur, but is rarely accompanied by self-neglect and rarely lasts more than a day or two. Often in dissociative amnesia, new learning is preserved[52]. Disturbing external circumstances causing despair or anxiety may predispose an individual, but a single event is usually at the centre of the syndrome.

As a rule, dissociative amnesia becomes less prominent with age and is uncommon in the elderly[53,54]. However, it has been seen in First World War combat soldiers[55] and soldiers in other conflicts. In most patients the amnesia is short-lived, 75% of cases lasting between 24 hours and 5 days[56]. Its features resemble those of more frequently observed disorders. Organic amnesia is usually anterograde[52]. In postconcussional syndromes there may be a combination of hysterical and organic amnesia that can be difficult to untangle. In dementia, memory loss is seen in the context of global cognitive impairment, which is stable over a period of weeks to months. The syndrome of pseudodementia also features variable memory impairment, but affective disturbance, usually severe depression, is evident[57].

Dissociative Fugue

Fugue exhibits all the features of dissociative amnesia, plus an apparently purposeful journey away from home or place of work during which self-care is maintained. A new identity is assumed and organized travel may be undertaken to places previously known and of possible emotional significance. Although there is retrograde amnesia during the fugue, behaviour during fugue is normal. A severe precipitating stress is almost universal as a precipitant of dissociative fugue. Times of marital discord, financial difficulty, major role change or personal loss may precede the fugue. Depressed mood is frequently present before fugue symptoms are displayed[52]. Fugue is rare in elderly people. Because its features, with the exception of travel, are identical to those of dissociative amnesia, it has been proposed that the two disorders be considered as one.

Treatment

Therapy for dissociative amnesia and that for dissociative fugue are virtually identical. Patients usually seek treatment after the amnesic period has ended. They desire help in recovering memory of events during the fugue. Hypnosis[58], benzodiazepines[59] and short-acting barbiturates have been used to reconstitute repressed memories,

although typically they return spontaneously. Psychodynamic psychotherapy has been used to facilitate resolution of conflicts that lead to fugue states. This treatment may decrease the vulnerability of the patient to dissociate in future times of stress[60].

DISSOCIATIVE DISORDERS OF MOVEMENT AND SENSATION (CONVERSION DISORDERS)

In conversion disorder, there is a loss or alteration in movements or sensations (usually cuteneous) in a patient presenting as having a physical disorder. No somatic condition can be found, however, that explains the symptoms. Instead, the symptoms represent the patient's concept of the physical disorder, which may be at variance with physiological or anatomical principles. Here, mental state and social situation suggest that disability resulting from the loss of function is helping the patient to escape an unpleasant conflict, or helps the patient to express dependency or resentment indirectly. Conflicts may be evident to others, but the patient often denies their presence and attributes distress to the physical symptoms or the resulting disability.

In making the diagnosis it is essential that: (i) evidence of a physical disorder is absent and (ii) sufficient knowledge of the psychological and social setting and personal relationships of the patient allows a convincing formulation of the reasons for the disorder.

Predisposing factors to conversion disorder are premorbid abnormalities of personal relationships, childhood sexual abuse[61], and personality disturbance, with histrionic personality being the most common[62]. Also, close relatives or friends may have suffered from physical illness with symptoms resembling the patient's. A few patients establish a repetitive pattern of reaction to stress by production of these disorders, which can continue into middle and old age[3].

The most important differential diagnosis is the group of somatoform disorders (although DSM-IV classifies conversion disorder as a somatoform disorder instead of a dissociative disorder). In the latter, the patient's presentation centers around persistent requests for medical attention and pervasive concern with the perceived medical disorder; patients with conversion disorder are much more likely to take their presumed illnesses in stride. Conversion disorders generally begin in adolescence and young adulthood, and occur in single or recurrent episodes with substantial remission. Somatoform disorders may not increase in prevalence with increasing age, but they tend to assume the quality of a pervasive character style with little remission.

Most conversion disorders remit with non-specific, supportive interventions. Hypnosis[63], anxiolytics and behavioural relaxation exercises may be helpful. Also, psychotherapy aimed at helping the patient recognize and cope with the psychosocial stress that provoked the symptom can be impressively beneficial if the patient can be engaged in a cooperative alliance of therapeutic curiosity. The prognosis of conversion disorder is generally good, since conversion symptoms are of short duration with abrupt onset and resolution. A few become chronic, and some recur, most commonly when the precipitating stress is chronic or recurrent, when there is other psychopathology or when there is marked secondary gain.

NEURASTHENIA (FATIGUE SYNDROME)

Historical Perspective

George Beard introduced the term 'neurasthenia' in 1869. He viewed neurasthenia as a physical illness caused by loss of nerve strength. Janet differentiated psychasthenia from neurasthenia. Freud similarly separated anxiety neurosis, a 'psychoneurosis', from neurasthenia, an 'actual neurosis' he attributed to misdirected libidinal energy. In the First World War, the syndrome was defined by the term 'shell shock'; in the Second World War, 'operational fatigue'. Although it remains in ICD-10, the diagnosis of neurasthenia was deleted from DSM-III and replaced by dysthymia. In the United States the symptom cluster known as chronic fatigue syndrome is almost identical to the current ICD classification of neurasthenia[64-66].

Clinical Features

Neurasthenia is characterized by persistent, distressing complaints of fatigue after mental effort, or complaints of bodily weakness and exhaustion after minimal physical effort, along with at least two of the following: muscular aches and pains, dizziness, tension headaches, sleep disturbance, inability to relax, irritability or dyspepsia. If autonomic or depressive symptoms are present, they cannot be sufficiently persistent and severe to fulfil the criteria for any more specific disorder[3]. Premorbid fatigue may be the single most reliable predictor of the development of neurasthenia[67].

Differential Diagnosis

Differential diagnosis includes primarily major depression and somatoform disorders. In the elderly it is especially important to rule out depression, since somatic complaints and fatigue are common presentations of depressive disorders in late life. Physical symptoms with no demonstrable organic pathology are the essential features of somatoform disorders. However, these complaints do not include the specific physical symptoms of fatigue or exhaustion found in neurasthenia.

Therapy

Specific treatment for neurasthenia has not been established. Given the high likelihood, particularly in old age, that the neurasthenic picture is a manifestation of a mood disorder, treatment with antidepressant medication and psychotherapy, as for depressive conditions, is generally warranted[68].

REFERENCES

1. Ginsberg GL. Adjustment and impulse control disorders. In Kaplan HI, Sadock BJ (eds), *Comprehensive Textbook of Psychiatry*, vol. IV. Baltimore, MD: Williams and Wilkins, 1985, 1097–105.
2. Katzman JW, Tomori O. Adjustment disorders. In Sadock BJ, Sadock VA (eds), *Comprehensive Textbook of Psychiatry*, 8th edn. Philadelphia, PA: Lippincott Williams and Wilkins, 2005, 2055–56.
3. World Health Organization. Mental and behavioural disorders. *Tenth Revision of the International Classification of Diseases and Related Health Problems (ICD-10)*, chapter V. Geneva: World Health Organization, 2006.
4. Cohen M. Acute stress disorder in older, middle-aged and younger adults in reaction to the second Lebanon war. *Int J Geriatr Psychiatry* 2008; **23**: 34–40.
5. American Psychiatric Association. *Diagnostic and Statistical Manual of Mental Disorders*, 4th edition text revision (DSM-IV-TR). Washington, DC: American Psychiatric Association, 2000.
6. Stoudemire A. Epidemiology and psychopharmacology of anxiety in medical patients. *J Clin Psychiatry* 1996; **57**(suppl 7): 64–72.
7. Pasnau RO, Fawzy FI. Stress and psychiatry. In Kaplan HI, Sadock BJ (eds), *Comprehensive Textbook of Psychiatry*, vol. V. Baltimore, MD: Williams and Wilkins, 1989, 1231–39.
8. Davidson JR. Post-traumatic stress disorder and acute stress disorder. In Kaplan HI, Sadock BJ (eds), *Comprehensive Textbook of Psychiatry*, vol. VI. Baltimore, MD: Williams and Wilkins, 1995, 1227–36.
9. McCartney JR, Severson K. Sexual violence, post-traumatic stress disorder and dementia. *J Am Geriatr Soc* 1997; **45**: 76–78.
10. van Zelst WH, de Beurs E, Beekman AT *et al*. Prevalence and risk factors of posttraumatic stress disorder in older adults. *Psychother Psychosom* 2003, **72**: 333–42.
11. Charles E, Garand L, Ducrocq F, Clement JP. Post-traumatic stress in the elderly. *Psychol Neuropsychiatr Vieil* 2005; **3**: 291–300.
12. Spitzer C, Barnow S, Volzke H, John U, Freyberger HJ, Grabe HJ. Trauma and posttraumatic stress disorder in the elderly: findings from a German community study. *J Clin Psychiatry* 2008; **69**: 693–700.
13. Davidson J, Kudler H. Symptom and co-morbidity patterns in World War II and Vietnam veterans with posttraumatic stress disorder. *Compr Psychiatry* 1990; **3**: 162–70.
14. Lipton M, Schaffer W. Physical symptoms related to post-traumatic stress disorder in an ageing population. *Military Med* 1988; **156**: 316.
15. Bowing G, Schmidt KU, Juckel G, Schroder SG. Psychosis in elderly post-traumatic stress disorder patients. *Nervenarzt* 2008; **79**: 73–79.
16. Kinzie DJ. Post-traumatic stress disorder. In Kaplan HI, Sadock BJ (eds), *Comprehensive Textbook of Psychiatry*, vol. V. Baltimore, MD: Williams and Wilkins, 1989, 1000–1008.
17. Zisook S, Chentsova-Dutton Y, Shuchter SR. PTSD following bereavement. *Ann Clin Psychiatry* 1998; **10**: 157–63.
18. Chung MC, McKee KJ, Austin C *et al*. Posttraumatic stress disorder in older people after a fall. *Int J Geriatr Psychiatry* 2009; **24**: 955–64.
19. Sembi S, Tarrier N, O'Neill P *et al*. Does post-traumatic stress disorder occur after stroke: a preliminary study. *Int J Geriatr Psychiatry* 1988; **13**: 315–22.
20. Chung MC, Berger Z, Jones R, Rudd H. Posttraumatic stress disorder and general health problems following myocardial infarction (Post-MI PTSD) among older patients: the role of personality. *Int J Geriatr Psychiatry* 2006; **21**: 1163–74.
21. Green BL, Rowland JH, Krupnick JL *et al*. Prevalence of post-traumatic stress disorder in women with breast cancer. *Psychosomatics* 1998; **39**: 102–11.
22. Hamilton JD, Workman RH. Persistence of combat-related post-traumatic stress symptoms for 75 years. *J Traum Stress* 1998; **11**: 763–68.
23. Tennant C, Fairley MJ, Dent OF *et al*. Declining prevalence of psychiatric disorder in older former prisoners of war. *J Nerv Ment Dis* 1997; **185**: 686–89.
24. Engdahl B, Dikel TN, Eberly R, Blank A. Posttraumatic stress disorder in a community group of former prisoners of war: a normative response to severe trauma. *Am J Psychiatry* 1997; **154**: 1576–81.

25. Port CL, Engdahl B, Frazier P. A longitudinal and retrospective study of PTSD among older prisoners of war. *Am J Psychiatry* 2001; **158**: 1474–79.

26. Hilton C. Media triggers of post-traumatic stress disorder 50 years after the Second World War. *Int J Geriatr Psychiatry* 1997; **12**: 862–67.

27. Lipton M, Schaffer W. Post-traumatic stress disorder in the older veteran. *Military Med* 1986; **151**: 522–24.

28. Mellman TA, David D, Bustamante V *et al.* Predictors of post-traumatic stress disorder following severe injury. *Depress Anxiety* 2001; **14**: 226–31.

29. Benedek DM, Friedman MJ, Zatzick D, Ursano RJ. Guideline Watch (March 2009): Practice guideline for the treatment of patients with acute stress disorder and posttraumatic stress disorder. *APA Practice Guidelines* 2009, 1–2.

30. Falcon S, Ryan C, Chamberlain K *et al.* Tricyclics: possible treatment for post-traumatic stress disorder. *J Clin Psychiatry* 1985; **46**: 385–88.

31. Schwartz AC, Rothbaum BO. Review of sertraline in post-traumatic stress disorder. *Exp Opin Pharmacother* 2002; **3**: 1489–99.

32. Martonyi F, Brown EB, Zhang H *et al.* Fluoxetine versus placebo in posttraumatic stress disorder. *J Clin Psychiatry* 2002; **63**: 199–206.

33. Tucker P, Zaninelli R, Yehuda R *et al.* Paroxetine in the treatment of chronic posttraumatic stress disorder: results of a placebo-controlled, flexible-dosage trial. *J Clin Psychiatry* 2001; **62**: 860–68.

34. Marshall RD, Lewis-Fernandez R, Blanco C *et al.* A controlled trial of paroxetine for chronic PTSD, dissociation, and interpersonal problems in mostly minority adults. *Depress Anxiety* 2007, **24**: 77–84.

35. American Psychiatric Association. Treatment of Patients With Acute Stress Disorder and Posttraumatic Stress Disorder. *APA Practice Guidelines* 2004, chapter V: 1–14.

36. Sadavoy J. Survivors: a review of the late-life effects of prior psychological trauma. *Am J Geriatr Psychiatry* 1997; **5**: 287–301.

37. Davidson J, Roth S, Neewman E. Treatment of post-traumatic stress disorder with fluoxetine. *J Traum Stress* 1991; **4**: 419–23.

38. Raskind MA, Peskind ER, Hoff DJ *et al.* A parallel group placebo controlled study of prazosin for trauma nightmares and sleep disturbance in combat veterans with post-traumatic stress disorder. *Biol Psychiatry* 2007; **61**: 928–34.

39. Van der Kolk BA. Psychopharmacologic issues in posttraumatic stress disorder. *Hosp Commun Psychiatry* 1983; **34**: 683–91.

40. Sattar SP, Ucci B, Grant K *et al.* Quetiapine therapy for posttraumatic stress disorder. *Ann Pharmacother* 2002; **36**: 1875–78.

41. Salzman C. Principles of psychopharmacology. In Bienenfeld D (ed.), *Verwoerdt's Clinical Geropsychiatry*, 3rd edn. Baltimore, MD: Williams and Wilkins, 1990, 234–49.

42. Davis LL, Davidson JR, Ward LC *et al.* Divalproex in the treatment of posttraumatic stress disorder: a randomized, double-blind, placebo-controlled trial in a veteran population. *J Clin Psychopharmacol* 2008; **28**: 84–88.

43. Tang WK, Ungvari GS, Chiu HF *et al.* Psychiatric morbidity in first time stroke patients in Hong Kong: a pilot study in a rehabilitation unit. *Aust N Z J Psychiatry* 2002; **36**: 544–49.

44. Lazaro L, Marcos T, Valdes M. Affective disorders, social support, and health status in geriatric patients in a general hospital. *Gen Hosp Psychiatry* 1995; **17**: 299–304.

45. Orrell M, Bebbington P. Life events and senile dementia: affective symptoms. *Br J Psychiatry* 1995; **166**: 613–20.

46. Oxman TE, Barrett JE, Freeman DH, Manheimer E. Frequency and correlates of adjustment disorder related to cardiac surgery in older patients. *Psychosomatics* 1994; **35**: 557–68.

47. Gerson S, Mistry R, Bastani R *et al.* Symptoms of depression and anxiety (MHI) following acute medical/surgical hospitalization and post-discharge psychiatric diagnoses (DSM) in 839 geriatric US veterans. *Int J Geriatr Psychiatry* 2004; **19**: 1155–67.

48. Wheeler BG, Bienenfeld D. Principles of individual psychotherapy. In Bienenfeld D (ed.), *Verwoerdt's Clinical Geropsychiatry*, 3rd edn. Baltimore, MD: Williams and Wilkins, 1990, 204–22.

49. Lazarus LW. Self-psychology: its application to brief psychotherapy with the elderly. *J Geriatr Psychiatry* 1988; **21**: 109–25.

50. Hameed U, Schwartz TL, Malhotra K *et al.* Antidepressant treatment in the primary care office: outcomes for adjustment disorder versus major depression. *Ann Clin Psychiatry* 2005; **17**: 77–81.

51. Nemiah JC. Dissociative disorders. In Kaplan HI, Sadock BJ (eds), *Comprehensive Textbook of Psychiatry*, vol. IV. Baltimore, MD: Williams and Wilkins, 1985, 942–57.

52. Kopelman MD. Amnesia: organic and psychogenic. *Br J Psychiatry* 1987; **150**: 428–42.

53. Labinsky E, Blair W, Yehuda R. Longitudinal assessment of dissociation in Holocaust survivors with and without PTSD and nonexposed aged Jewish adults. *Ann N Y Acad Sci* 2006; **1071**: 459–62.

54. Merckelbach H, Dekkers T, Wessel I, Roefs A. Dissociative symptoms and amnesia in Dutch concentration camp survivors. *Compr Psychiatry* 2003; **44**: 65–69.

55. Van der Hart O, Brown P, Graafland M. Trauma-induced dissociative amnesia in World War I combat soldiers. *Aust NZ J Psychiatry* 1999; **33**: 37–46.

56. Coons PM. The dissociative disorders: rarely considered and underdiagnosed. *Psychiatr Clin N Am* 1998; **21**: 637–48.

57. Wells CE. Pseudodementia. *Am J Psychiatry* 1979; **136**: 895–900.

58. Jasper FJ. Working with dissociative fugue in a general psychotherapy practice: a cautionary tale. *Am J Clin Hypn* 2003; **45**: 311–22.

59. Ilechukwu ST, Henry T. Amytal interview using intravenous lorazepam in a patient with dissociative fugue. *Gen Hosp Psychiatry* 2006; **28**(6): 544–45.

60. Reither AM, Stoudemire A. Psychogenic fugue states: a review. *South Med J* 1988; **81**: 568–71.

61. Roelofs K, Keijsers GP, Hoogduin KA *et al.* Childhood abuse in patients with conversion disorder. *Am J Psychiatry* 2002; **159**: 1908–13.

62. Kuloglu M, Atmaca M, Tezcan E *et al.* Sociodemographic and clinical characteristics of patients with conversion disorder in Eastern Turkey. *Soc Psychiatry Psychiatr Epidemiol* 2003; **38**: 88–93.

63. Moene FC, Spinhoven P, Hoogduin KA, van Dyck R. A randomized controlled clinical trial of a hypnosis-based treatment for patients with conversion disorder, motor type. *Int J Clin Exp Hypn* 2003; **51**: 29–50.

64. Greenberg DB. Neurasthenia in the 1980s. *Psychosomatics* 1990; **31**: 129–37.

65. Fukuda K, Straus SE, Hickie I *et al.* The chronic fatigue syndrome: comprehensive approach to its definition and study. *Ann Intern Med* 1994; **121**: 953–59.

66. Demitrack MA. Chronic fatigue syndrome and fibromyalgia: dilemmas in diagnosis and clinical management. *Psychiatr Clin N Am* 1998; **21**: 671–92.

67. Lawrie SM, Manders DN, Geddes JR, Pelosi AJ. A population-based incidence study of chronic fatigue. *Psychol Med* 1997; **27**: 343–53.

68. Stubhaug B, Lie SA, Ursin H, Eriksen HR. Cognitive-behavioural therapy v. mirtazapine for chronic fatigue and neurasthenia: randomized placebo-controlled trial. *Br J Psychiatry* 2008; **192**: 217–23.

Part H

Personality Disorders

104

Personality Disorders: Description, Aetiology, and Epidemiology

Victor Molinari[1] and Daniel L. Segal[2]

[1]University of South Florida, Tampa, FL, USA
[2]University of Colorado at Colorado Springs, Colorado Springs, CO, USA

According to the Diagnostic and Statistical Manual of Mental Disorders, 4th edition, text revision (DSM-IV-TR)[1], 'A Personality Disorder is an enduring pattern of inner experience and behaviour that deviates markedly from the expectations of the individual's culture, is pervasive and inflexible, has an onset in adolescence or early adulthood, is stable over time, and leads to distress or impairment' (p. 685). Also included in the definition of personality disorder is that the traits have to be rigid, maladaptive and pervasive across a broad range of situations rather than expectable reactions to particular life experiences or a normal part of a developmental stage. An important caveat in the DSM-IV-TR is that, although the definition of personality disorder requires an onset no later than early adulthood, it is often the case that a person with a personality disorder may not be diagnosed or treated until later life.

One possible explanation for this caveat is that the individual with personality disorder may have presented clinically with the more obvious signs of an Axis I clinical disorder such as anxiety, depression, disordered eating or substance abuse, whereas the underlying personality disorder features may not have been examined as closely. Another important factor is that in some cases, personality traits can be adaptive at one phase of life but become maladaptive at a later developmental phase. For example, an extremely aloof, reserved and emotionally detached man may have functioned successfully in the occupational sphere by choosing a job requiring little social interaction (e.g. a computer programmer who writes code at home). He managed to live alone and had little use for others during much of his adult life. Imagine the discomfort and distress he would face, however, if in later life he becomes physically frail and debilitated and out of medical necessity is re-located to a nursing home where he is forced to cope with the presence of medical professionals, caregivers and other residents. In this case, it would be only after the person has failed to adjust to his new living situation that his personality traits would be viewed as dysfunctional (and a personality disorder diagnosis given). Thus, the *context* in which personality traits are expressed is an extremely important concept in determining their relative usefulness or hindrance across the lifespan.

Personality disorder in older adults is an important area of study for a number of reasons. First, since personality disorder affects the way an older adult copes with life, individuals with specific personality disorders may be less able to successfully negotiate age-related losses (e.g. a histrionic person who has relied on her physical attractiveness and sexual provocativeness to garner attention for herself may feel neglected as she ages and loses some of her seductiveness; an obsessive–compulsive individual may feel out of control because he feels his medical problems reduce his control over his body; a dependent person may lose his main source of support due to the death of a spouse, siblings, adult children etc.) or the interpersonal compromises necessary for peaceful institutional living (e.g. anger episodes erupt when the interpersonal needs of a borderline or narcissistic person are not immediately met). Second, personality disorder can influence the presentation of Axis I symptomatology, frequently generating complicated diagnostic and assessment dilemmas. For example, disruptive behaviour in the nursing home may camouflage the fact that the person is suffering from a depression that is exacerbating premorbid antisocial personality features. Third, just as for young adults, the presence of personality disorder warrants modification of treatment strategies and prognosis for those with co-morbid Axis I disorders in certain geriatric settings.

In recent years, there has been an ever-expanding body of knowledge about personality disorder in older adults. Notably, there has even been the publication of two books solely devoted to personality disorder in older adults[2,3]. However, as we shall see, there remain many unanswered questions spawned by thorny conceptual and methodological quandaries in this controversial area. This chapter will summarize what is known about the aetiology, diagnosis, epidemiology and prognosis of personality disorder in older adults.

AETIOLOGY

Because personality disorders and personality disorder features begin relatively early in life and have a generally persisting impact across the lifespan, it can be assumed that the aetiology of personality disorders includes psychosocial and biological factors[3]. Concerning personality disorder among older adults, it is helpful to focus on dimensional aspects of personality as well as the categorical diagnosis of personality disorder.

Principles and Practice of Geriatric Psychiatry, 3rd edn. Edited by Mohammed T. Abou-Saleh, Cornelius Katona and Anand Kumar

Psychosocial Factors

Freud noted the importance of Axis II traits in the aetiology of Axis I symptoms. He embedded the idea of personality within his psychosexual schema regarding oral, anal, oedipal, latency and genital stages. Inborn temperamental traits combine with parental influences in these early developmental periods to shape an individual's personality. How early figures react to the growing child's bio-psycho-social needs forges a rigid template that is operative throughout the person's life, and reflects whether the person will satisfy his or her intrapsychic and interpersonal needs in an adaptive manner or in an exaggerated repetitious fashion. Acute symptomatology erupts when current stressors intersect with the psychosocial dynamics and interpersonal sensitivities laid out in early childhood forming this hard bedrock of personality traits. Working from this grand model, Freud erroneously concluded that by the age of 40 personality patterns were invariably set, and advised psychoanalysts to spend their time with younger analysands.

Erik Erikson[4] enhanced the Freudian framework to include three stages of adulthood that were yoked to specific life challenges. Those in young adulthood are faced with the crisis of deciding on a career and achieving intimacy; those in middle adulthood raise their family, maintain a career and hopefully become generative; those in late adulthood are confronted with preparing for death, gaining wisdom and achieving ego integrity. Unfortunately, the heuristic value of these conceptualizations has not been realized because limited research has been conducted to validate these stages.

Coming from a more empirical tradition, Costa and McCrae[5] conducted both cross-sectional and longitudinal research with their well-validated NEO Personality Inventory (which measures five broad lexically derived personality factors of neuroticism, extraversion, openness, agreeableness and conscientiousness) and concluded that there is general continuity of personality across the life span. However, other researchers have argued that Costa and McCrae's five-factor model tends to minimize personality change in adulthood, particularly with respect to environmental factors[6]. Indeed, in his 50-year follow-up study of Harvard undergraduates, Vaillant[7] discovered that significant change can occur for certain individuals, related either to specific negative or positive adult life events (e.g. alcoholism; supportive spouse). Consistent with these formulations, Identity Process Theory[8] postulates that older adults tend first to assimilate and (if assimilation is non-successful) then to accommodate discrepant experiences to maintain self-esteem via a consistent sense of self. Those with rigid understandings of themselves that characterize personality disorders may be less able to employ these more mature coping mechanisms and negotiate the vagaries of ageing. From this conceptual basis, too much or too little stability in personality as we age may become maladaptive.

Finally, a well-researched cognitive model of psychopathology suggests that personality disorders may be characterized by cognitive distortions which are derived from biases in information processing and dysfunctional schema or core beliefs that influence people's perceptions and thoughts at the conscious level[9]. Examples of cognitive distortions include all-or-none thinking (seeing personal qualities or situations in absolutist 'black and white' terms, and failing to see shades of grey), catastrophizing (perceiving negative events as intolerable calamities, commonly referred to as 'making mountains out of molehills'), magnification and minimization (exaggerating the importance of negative characteristics and experiences while discounting the importance of positive characteristics and experiences) and personalization (assuming one is the cause of an event when other factors are also responsible). Schemas are often expressed as unconditional evaluations about the self and others. Some examples include beliefs that: 'I am incompetent', 'I am defective', 'I am unlovable', 'I am special', 'Others are hurtful and not to be trusted', 'Others need to take care of me', and 'Others must love and admire me'. Schemas are generally thought to be formed early in life but to persist if no conscious effort is made to identify, examine and challenge them.

Some examples of cognitive distortions and schema relevant to specific personality disorders include:

- an individual with paranoid personality disorder is prone to habitually and chronically perceive others as deceitful, abusive and threatening;
- an individual with borderline personality disorder is prone to sort people into categories of either 'all good' or 'all bad';
- an individual with obsessive–compulsive personality disorder tends to be a slave to the belief that he or she must be perfect and always in control;
- an individual with dependent personality disorder sees him- or herself as weak, incompetent and inadequate, requiring constant reassurance, nurturance and direction.

Whereas a few studies have attempted to validate the specific relationships between core beliefs and personality disorder pathology[10], notably lacking are studies that specifically examine these relationships in older adult samples.

Genetic Factors

A growing literature base has focused on the genetic factors that contribute to personality disorders. In a study of 483 adult twin pairs, Jang et al.[11] found a median heritability of 0.44 for 66 of 69 personality disorder facet traits. Similar data were reported by Coolidge et al.[12] who found a median heritability coefficient of 0.75 for 12 specific personality disorders in their sample of 112 child twin pairs. Interestingly, Jang et al.[13] found in their cross-sectional twin study that genetic contributions to personality disorder traits actually increase with age. Torgersen et al.[14] used a structured interview to diagnose the full range of personality disorders, finding an overall heritability estimate of .60. Finally, a very recent study with a large sample of young adult Norwegian twins found one genetic factor reflecting a broad vulnerability to personality disorder pathology and negative emotionality whereas two other genetic factors more specifically reflected high impulsivity/low agreeableness and introversion[15]. In summary, there is clear evidence of heritability for some personality disorders but much that remains unexamined. Perhaps the best conclusion from this data is that heritable traits play a significant role in the formation of personality disorders but heritability alone does not directly cause an individual to develop a specific personality disorder.

DIAGNOSIS

The diagnosis of personality disorders is known to be particularly challenging across the lifespan. Specifically, in adulthood, it is generally difficult to distinguish one personality disorder from another[16]. Later life adds further complications to diagnosis. There are, for instance, problems in obtaining a reliable diagnosis and, at present, there is no 'gold standard' of diagnosis for personality disorder in older adults. Molinari *et al.*[17] studied geropsychiatric inpatients with depression, and found general discordance between patient self-report, family informant ratings, social worker evaluations and consensus case conference categorical diagnosis of personality disorder. It appears that there are varied perceptions of an individual's personality, all of which should be taken into account for a comprehensive evaluation of Axis II pathology.

Personality disorder is commonly seen in practice settings yet seldom formally identified. Mental health professionals are loathe to diagnose it, particularly in old age, due to concerns over pejorative bias, pessimistic beliefs about the prospects of therapeutic change for personality disorder pathology, managed care reimbursement biases, and focus on medical or Axis I pathology (particularly cognitive impairment) in old age. Often the patient with personality disorder presents in a demanding, blaming manner with an inappropriate, rigid interpersonal stance and limited insight. Unfortunately these same features are sometimes erroneously interpreted as part of the natural ageing process[18]. Perhaps it is most important to recognize that 'either/or' thinking is often incorrect in the diagnosis of older adults. Comorbidity is the rule rather than the exception, with research consistently finding that older adults with depression also may have longstanding maladaptive personality disorder traits[18-20].

Another factor that impacts identification and diagnosis of personality disorders in later life is that, in some cases, there is an emergence of personality disorder symptoms that were 'hidden' earlier in life[3]. For example, consider a highly dependent woman who was supported by a caring, perhaps dominating, spouse who did not mind making all of the decisions for the couple and essentially took care of his wife throughout much of their adult lives. It would not be until she struggled to take care of herself after becoming a widow that the extent of her 'disorder' would become recognized and perhaps diagnosed. A final diagnostic challenge is that the sets of diagnostic criteria do not fit older adults as well as they do younger adults[3]. In an empirical investigation of potential age-bias using item analysis, Balsis *et al.*[21] found evidence of age-bias in 29% of the criteria for seven personality disorders. In this study, some diagnostic criteria were differentially endorsed by younger and older adults with equivalent personality disorder pathology, suggesting a bias.

EPIDEMIOLOGY

Some early anecdotal reports suggested that personality characteristics become uniformly less harsh with age[22,23]. Other clinicians working with older adults believed that the 'high-energy' personality disorders (e.g. Cluster B) mellow whereas the 'low-energy' personality disorders (e.g. Cluster C) may be aggravated by the ageing process[24-26]. DSM-IV-TR[1] states that 'Some personality disorders tend to become less obvious or remit with age, whereas this appears to be less true for some other types' (p. 688). Early research yielded wide variability in personality disorder prevalence rates due to inadequate definitions of personality disorder, non-standardized measures and different samples of older adults. With the employment of better diagnostic criteria, some consistent findings have emerged. This section on epidemiology will therefore largely focus on studies using standardized measures, and will be divided into community, institutional, outpatient and depression studies.

Community Settings

In community settings, two studies[23,27] compared young and older adults utilizing the Coolidge Axis II Inventory. Coolidge *et al.*[23] found a greater need for organization and more restricted affect in older adults, whereas Segal *et al.*[27] found that older adults were significantly higher on obsessive–compulsive and schizoid personality disorder, but lower on the antisocial, borderline, histrionic, narcissistic and paranoid scales. Ames and Molinari[28] used the Structured Interview for Disorders of Personality scale (SIDP-R) and detected a trend of less personality disorder in older adults, with significantly fewer older adults meeting the criteria for more than one personality disorder. Cohen *et al.*[29] used the Structured Psychiatric Examination and found that individuals 55 years old and older were less likely (6.6% vs. 10.5%) to have personality disorder, due to a threefold decrease of Cluster B personality disorder in older adults. These data documenting personality 'mellowing' in older adult community samples are in stark contrast to the results of a study by Segal *et al.*[30], who found that a high number (63%) of community-dwelling older adults surveyed at a senior center met personality disorder criteria by self-report. However, this study used a measure known to be overly sensitive to personality disorder pathology, and the cognitive status of the participants was also not taken into account.

Institutional Settings

Early personality disorder prevalence rates in nursing home settings were reported to be 12–15%[31,32], whereas for geropsychiatric inpatients, personality disorder estimates were more variable (7–58%). In a large sample of hospitalized male veterans, Molinari *et al.*[33] conducted a cross-sectional investigation of personality changes across different age groups for those clinically diagnosed with personality disorder. Older adults with personality disorder were more responsible and less impulsive, paranoid, energetic and antisocial than young adults diagnosed with personality disorder. Kunik *et al.*[34] studied 547 older psychiatric inpatients, and found that a consensus case conference diagnosis of personality disorder varied widely, depending upon the specific co-morbid Axis I diagnosis (e.g. 6% for patients with an organic mental disorder, but 24% for those with depression). Only a few studies of geropsychiatric institutionalized patients utilized standardized instruments. Molinari *et al.*[35] used the SIDP-R and found that older adults had personality disorder rates similar to those of a young adult comparison sample; however, older adults were less likely to meet criteria for more than one personality disorder, and clinical diagnoses yielded fewer personality disorders than the SIDP-R. Likewise, Coolidge *et al.*[36] used the Coolidge Axis II Inventory and found similarly high personality disorder rates among young (66%) and old (58%) chronically mentally ill patients, but the younger group was more likely to be specifically diagnosed with antisocial, borderline, and schizotypal personality disorder. Finally, among older inpatient veterans, Kenan *et al.*[37] found a 55% personality disorder prevalence rate.

Outpatient Settings

The findings from the lone study conducted with a structured personality disorder scale in a geropsychiatric outpatient setting are consistent with the latter inpatient studies. Molinari and Marmion[38] found that older adults were less likely to meet the criteria for more than one personality disorder than younger adults, and clinical diagnosis again yielded fewer personality disorders than the SIDP-R.

Depression

One area of intense study has been the relationship between personality disorder and depression in older adults. Kunik *et al.*[20] studied 154 depressed older inpatients and identified 24% with co-morbid personality disorder, whereas Molinari and Marmion[39] determined that 63% of depressed geropsychiatric outpatients met personality disorder criteria. Thompson et al.[40] found that 33% of depressed older adults who were being treated with psychotherapy in a geropsychiatric outpatient clinic met personality disorder criteria. In a study investigating the relationship between personality disorder and functioning in acutely depressed older psychiatric patients, Axis II pathology was found to be associated with greater disability and more impaired social and interpersonal functioning[41]. In their review of the literature on personality disorder in older adults, Agronin and Maletta[42] posit that personality disorder in late life may be intrinsically related to Axis I pathology, particularly major depressive disorder.

Summary of Epidemiological Studies

In an attempt to lend clarity to the burgeoning literature on personality disorder in older adults, Abrams and Horowitz[43] conducted a meta-analysis of the most methodologically sophisticated epidemiological studies. They inferred a personality disorder prevalence rate of 10% (with a range of 6–33%) for those over the age of 50, and concluded that research neither substantiates nor disconfirms an age effect. However, these authors remark that the bulk of the evidence supports, at least for certain personality disorders, a decline in frequency and intensity with age. The cause for this decline is one of the most controversial and debated topics in the literature on personality disorder in older adults. Four main reasons have been postulated.

First, there is a general mellowing of the 'high-energy' Cluster B personality disorders due to biological (reduced testosterone in males) and developmental changes (those with personality disorder finally master a single interpersonal strategy to manage stresses). This accounts for the consistent result that older adults are less likely to meet the criteria for more than one personality disorder, and is also supported by the study of Segal et al.[27], who discovered lower levels of dysfunctional dispositional coping styles among older adults compared with younger adults.

Second, the decline in 'high-energy' personality disorder relates to the greater mortality rates of those with Cluster B personality disorder in their younger years. Older adults with personality disorder are thereby a selective sample of less extreme personality disorder 'survivors'. Third, personality disorder is generally under-diagnosed, particularly in older adults, where cognitive and medical causes are emphasized or personality disturbance (avoidance, dependency, emotional lability) is viewed as normal[44].

Fourth, the decline in personality disorder with age is a methodological artefact, since some DSM criteria are age-insensitive. For example, occupational and vocational impairment are often irrelevant to older adults. From this point of view, there really is no true decline in personality disorder rates with age, just a change in form that is inadequately assessed. These so-called 'geriatric variants'[45] reflect the more subclinical, non-specific or age-relevant personality disorder traits that account for personality disorder NOS (not otherwise specified) to be diagnosed with particular high frequency in older adults. These formulations are consistent with the theory of heterotypic continuity[46] which proposes that core psychological constructs remain constant, but that they are manifested in different ways throughout the life cycle (e.g. failure to conform to social norms may be reflected by repeated fights in younger individuals with antisocial personality disorder, but by repeated rule infractions in long-term care settings by older adults with antisocial personality disorder). The construction of a new geriatric nosology has been proposed to accommodate the late life changes in Axis II pathology[42,43,45]. Such re-classification will need to: (i) reconsider the diagnostic requirement that maladaptive personality disorder behaviour be rooted so early in young adulthood; (ii) routinely address Axis II pathology in the context of more acute Axis I symptomatology; and (iii) integrate age-related developmental, medical (Axis III) and psychosocial/environmental stressors (Axis IV) with Axis II manifestations[42].

PROGNOSIS

Unfortunately, only a few seemingly contradictory studies have investigated the prognosis of personality disorder in late life. In two separate studies of geropsychiatric outpatients, personality disorder was found to be a poor prognostic sign for the psychotherapeutic treatment of depression[40,47]. However, Molinari[48] examined the one-year relapse rates for 100 male geropsychiatric inpatients and found no significant differences for those diagnosed with and without personality disorder. Consistent with the finding of Kunik and colleagues[20] that personality disorder diagnosis had no impact on the acute response of inpatient treatment for depression with older adults, no differences were found in relapse rates for a subgroup of depressed inpatients with and without personality disorder[48]. It appears that in inpatient geropsychiatric settings, Axis I symptomatology overrides Axis II pathology as an outcome predictor, probably related to the complex combination of medical, cognitive and psychiatric symptoms often observed in those older patients needing acute care. More generally, the prognosis for older adults with personality disorder is highly variable and contextualized. Some adults with personality disorder clearly mature with advanced age, some seem to deteriorate in the face of challenges associated with ageing (e.g. loss of prestige, reduced physical stamina and attractiveness, increased need for assistance from others) and yet the third pattern is the unabated continuity of similar levels of dysfunctional behaviours from younger life to later life[3].

SUMMARY

1. There are psychosocial and genetic determinants of personality disorder in older adults.
2. The assessment of personality disorder in older adults is challenging, especially due to the presence of Axis I and Axis III co-morbidities.
3. There are poor concordance rates of personality disorder diagnosis between clinical examination, structured interviews and self-reports, suggesting the need for data collection from a variety of sources.
4. There may be an age-related mellowing of the 'high-energy' personality characteristics of individuals with personality disorder, and/or there are 'geriatric variants' of personality disorder not tapped by DSM.
5. There is a positive association between depression and personality disorder diagnosis.
6. Identifying personality disorder in older adults may be more useful prognostically in outpatient settings, where the Axis I symptomatology is less severe.
7. DSM-V must do a better job of accommodating late life changes in personality disorder presentation.

Although age-related changes in personality disorder expression may be in the less volatile and impulsive direction, novel geriatric manifestations still can create a significant burden in stressful caregiving contexts for family members, friends, health care professionals and administrators of institutions attempting to support a flawed and vulnerable older adult. Future empirical research guided by conceptual advances in psychodynamic, self/identity, cognitive and life span developmental theories of personality that address the interrelationship of genetic, biological, psychological and social variables promises to yield exciting progress in the creation of gero-specific assessment instruments and treatment protocols for personality disorder in older adults.

REFERENCES

1. American Psychiatric Association. *Diagnostic and Statistical Manual of Mental Disorders, 4th edition, text revision*. Washington, DC: APA, 2000.

2. Rosowsky E, Abrams L, Zweig R (eds). *Personality Disorders in Older Adults: Emerging Issues in Diagnosis and Treatment*. Mahwah, NJ: Erlbaum, 1999.

3. Segal DL, Coolidge FL, Rosowsky E. *Personality Disorders and Older Adults: Diagnosis, Assessment, and Treatment*. Hoboken, NJ: John Wiley and Sons Inc., 2006.

4. Erikson EH. The life cycle. *International Encyclopedia of the Social Sciences*. New York: Macmillan, 1968.

5. Costa PT Jr., McCrae RR. Looking backward: Changes in the mean levels of personality traits from 80 to 12. In Cervone D, Mischel M (eds), *Advances in Personality Science*. New York: Guilford, 2002, 219–37.

6. Roberts BW, Walton KE. Personality traits change in adulthood: Reply to Costa and McCrae (2006). *Psychol Bull* 2006; **132**: 29–32.

7. Vaillant GE. *Aging Well*. Boston: Little, Brown, and Company, 2002.

8. Whitbourne SK. *The Aging Individual: Physical and Psychological Perspectives*. New York: Springer, 1996.

9. Beck AT, Freeman A, Davis DD, Associates. *Cognitive Therapy of Personality Disorders*, 2nd edn, New York: Guilford, 2004.

10. Arntz A, Dreessen L, Schouten E, Weertman A. Beliefs in personality disorders: A test with the personality disorder belief questionnaire. *Behav Res Ther* 2004; **42**: 1215–25.

11. Jang KL, Livesley WJ, Vernon PA, Jackson DN. Heritability of personality disorder traits: A twin study. *Acta Psychiatr Scand* 1996; **94**: 438–44.

12. Coolidge FL, Thede LL, Jang KL. Heritability of personality disorders in childhood: a preliminary investigation. *J Personal Disord* 2001; **15**, 33–40.

13. Jang KL, Livesley WJ, Vernon PA. The genetic basis of personality at different ages: A cross-sectional twin study. *Personal Individual Diff* 1996; **21**: 299–301.

14. Torgersen S, Lygren S, Øien PA *et al.* A twin study of personality disorders. *Compr Psychiatr* 2000; **41**: 416–25.

15. Kendler KS, Aggen SH, Czajkowski N *et al.* The structure of genetic and environmental risk factors for *DSM-IV* personality disorders: A multivariate twin study. *Arch Gen Psychiatr* 2008; **65**: 1438–46.

16. Coolidge FL, Segal, DL. Evolution of the personality disorder diagnosis in the Diagnostic and Statistical Manual of Mental Disorders. *Clin Psychol Rev* 1998; **18**: 585–99.

17. Molinari V, Kunik M, Mulsant B, Rifai H. The relationship between patient, informant, social worker, and consensus diagnoses of personality disorders in elderly depressed inpatients. *Am J Geriatr Psychiatry* 1998; **6**: 136–44.

18. Sibert T, Swartz M. Aetiology and genetics. In Copeland JRM, Abou-Saleh MT, Blazer D (eds). *Principles and Practice of Geriatric Psychiatry*. New York: Wiley, 1994, 771–82.

19. Abrams RC, Alexopoulos GS, Young RC. Geriatric depression and DSM-III-R personality disorder criteria. *J Am Geriatr Soc* 1987; **35**: 383–86.

20. Kunik ME, Mulsant BH, Rifai AH *et al.* Personality disorders in elderly inpatients with major depression. *Am J Geriatr Psychiatry* 1993; **1**: 38–45.

21. Balsis S, Gleason MEJ, Woods CM, Oltmanns TF. An item response theory analysis of DSM-IV personality disorder criteria across younger and older age groups. *Psychol Aging* 2007; **22**: 171–85.

22. Hyer L, Harrison W. Late life personality model: diagnosis and treatment. In Brink TL (ed.), *Clinical Gerontology: A Guide to Assessment and Treatment*. New York: Haworth, 1986, 399–415.

23. Coolidge FL, Burns EM, Nathan JH, Mull CE. Personality disorders in the elderly. *Clin Gerontol* 1992; **12**: 41–55.

24. Verwoerdt A. *Clinical Geropsychiatry*. Baltimore, MD: Williams & Wilkins, 1976.

25. Sadavoy J, Fogel B. Personality disorders in old age. In Birren J, Sloane RB, Cohen G (eds), *Handbook of Mental Health and Aging*. San Diego, CA: Academic Press, 1992, 433–62.

26. Tyrer P, Seivewright H. Studies of outcome. In Tyrer P (ed.), *Personality Disorders: Diagnosis, Management and Course*. London. Wright, 1988, 119–36.

27. Segal DL, Hook JN, Coolidge FL. Personality dysfunction, coping styles, and clinical symptoms in younger and older adults. *J Clin Geropsychol* 2001; **7**: 201–12.

28. Ames A, Molinari V. Prevalence of personality disorders in community-living elderly. *J Geriatr Psychiatry Neurol* 1994; **7**: 189–94.

29. Cohen BJ, Nestadt G, Samuels JF *et al.* Personality disorders in late life: a community study. *Br J Psychiatry* 1994; **165**: 493–99.

30. Segal DL, Hersen M, Kabacoff RI *et al.* Personality disorders and depression in community-dwelling older adults. *J Ment Health Aging* 1998; **4**: 171–82.

31. Teeter RB, Garetz FK, Miller WR, Heiland WF. Psychiatric disturbances of aged patients in skilled nursing homes. *Am J Psychiatry* 1976; **133**: 1430–34.

32. Margo JL, Robinson JR, Corea S. Referrals to a psychiatric service from old people's homes. *Br J Psychiatry* 1988; **136**: 396–401.

33. Molinari V, Kunik M, Snow-Turek L *et al.* Age-related differences in inpatients with personality disorder: a cross-sectional study. *J Clin Geropsychol* 1999; **5**: 191–202.

34. Kunik ME, Mulsant BH, Rifai AH *et al.* Diagnostic rate of comorbid PD in elderly psychiatric inpatients. *Am J Psychiatry* 1993; **151**: 603–605.

35. Molinari V, Ames A, Essa M. Prevalence of personality disorders in two geropsychiatric inpatient units. *J Geriatr Psychiatry Neurol* 1994; **7**: 209–15.

36. Coolidge FL, Segal D, Pointer JC *et al.* Personality disorders in older inpatients with chronic mental illness. *J Clin Geropsychol* 2000; **6**: 63–71.

37. Kenan MM, Kendjelic EM, Molinari VA *et al*. Age-related differences in the frequency of personality disorders among inpatient veterans. *Int J Geriatr Psychiatry* 2000; **15**: 831–37.
38. Molinari V, Marmion J. Personality disorders in geropsychiatric outpatients. *Psychol Rep* 1993; **73**: 256–58.
39. Molinari V, Marmion J. The relationship between affective disorders and Axis II diagnoses in geropsychiatric patients. *J Geriatr Psychiatry Neurol* 1995; **8**: 61–65.
40. Thompson LW, Gallagher D, Czirr R. Personality disorder and outcome in the treatment of late-life depression. *J Geriatr Psychiatry* 1988; **21**: 133–46.
41. Abrams RC, Spielman LA, Alexopoulos GS, Klausner E. Personality disorder symptoms and functioning in elderly depressed patients. *Am J Geriatr Psychiatry* 1998; **6**: 24–30.
42. Agronin ME, Maletta G. Personality disorders in late life: understanding and overcoming the gap in research. *Am J Geriatr Psychiatry* 2000; **8**: 4–18.
43. Abrams RC, Horowitz SV. Personality disorders after age 50: a meta-analysis. *J Personality Disord* 1996; **10**: 271–81.
44. Segal DL, Coolidge FL. Personality disorders. In Bellack AS, Hersen M (eds), *Comprehensive Clinical Psychology: Clinical Geropsychology*, vol. 7. New York: Pergamon, 1998, 267–89.
45. Rosowsky E, Gurian B. Impact of borderline personality disorder in late life on systems of care. *Hosp Commun Psychiatry* 1992; **43**: 386–89.
46. Kagan, J. The three faces of continuity in human development. In Goslin DA (ed.), *Handbook of Socialization Theory and Research*. Chicago: Rand McNally, 1969, 53–65.
47. Vine RG, Steingart AB. Personality disorder in the elderly depressed. *Can J Psychiatry* 1994; **39**: 392–98.
48. Molinari V. Personality disorders and relapse rates among geropsychiatric inpatients. *Clin Gerontol* 1994; **14**: 49–52.

105

Diagnostic and Treatment Issues Regarding Personality Disorder in Older Adults

Richard A. Zweig[1] and Dana Scherr Parchi[2]

[1]*Ferkauf Graduate School of Yeshiva University, Bronx, NY, USA*
[2]*The Child and Family Institute at St Luke's and Roosevelt Hospitals, New York, NY, USA*

A growing body of epidemiological and observational studies support the notion that personality disorder is highly prevalent in community and clinical samples of adults and older adults (see Chapter 104) and that personality disorder moderates the presentation, course and outcome of Axis I disorders in both younger[1,2] and older adults[3-5]. The potential import of such findings for prevention and treatment cannot be overstated; recent findings, for example, suggest that personality pathology in the elderly may be a risk factor for coronary heart disease[6] and late-life suicidal behavior[7]. Even normative variations in personality appear to play a salient role, as inter-individual differences in personality have been linked to outcomes such as physical and psychological well-being, functional ability and longevity in older adults[8,9]. Yet, much personality pathology remains undetected and undertreated in clinical settings.

It is likely that efforts to translate these findings to practice settings have been hampered by differing conceptual models and methods (e.g. dimensional versus categorical)[10] as well as myriad obstacles to the assessment of personality pathology in the elderly[11]. Additionally, the lack of appropriate detection and treatment of personality disorder exacts a heavy cost, as personality disorders have been associated with long-term functional impairment[12] and a doubling of treatment expenses[13]. In this chapter, we review methods and measures for assessing personality pathology, describe obstacles to accurate detection, and delineate some common challenges in the differential diagnosis of personality pathology from other late-life disorders. We also discuss the psychotherapeutic and pharmacological management and treatment of these disorders.

DETECTION OF PERSONALITY PATHOLOGY

Methods and measures for detecting personality pathology have advanced considerably in the past four decades, such that an array of structured clinical interviews, multiscale self-report inventories and other measures have been developed and refined for this purpose[14,15]. Most current measures are derived from categorical or dimensional models of personality. Broadly speaking, measures based upon a categorical model tend to adhere closely to the American Psychiatric Association's Diagnostic and Statistical Manual of Mental Disorders, fourth edition, text revision (DSM-IV-TR) constructs of personality disorder[16], and determine presence/absence of personality disorder based upon whether an individual meets or exceeds DSM thresholds for each personality disorder type and manifests significant functional impairment or distress, in a manner analogous to the diagnostic assessment of Axis I syndromes. Measures of this type, such as the Structured Interview for DSM-IV Personality (SIDP-IV)[17] and the International Personality Disorders Examination (IPDE)[18], are more reliable than unstructured interviews, allow for the use of informant data to control for biased reporting of symptoms, and incorporate clinician judgement as to whether personality disorder symptoms are maladaptive, pervasive and inflexible across situations and contexts. Dimensional measures of personality (e.g. NEO-PI-R)[19] are derived from models that view personality disorder typologies as extreme variants of normative personality traits (e.g. neuroticism/emotional stability; introversion/extraversion; compliance/antagonism). Such measures, which typically rely on a patient's self-report of inner experiences and behaviours, allow for a more heterogeneous picture of patients' personality traits, and rely less on clinician inference, but vary in their accordance with DSM criteria for personality disorder.

Recent trends favour a dimensional approach to assessments of personality pathology, as flaws in the current categorical model of personality disorder, including arbitrary diagnostic thresholds with limited empirical support, high co-occurrence of personality disorder typologies, and inadequate coverage of diverse presentations of personality disorder in practice settings, appear insurmountable[10]. Moreover, recent research suggests that select dimensional personality traits (e.g. neuroticism, agreeableness) independently predict remission in adults with borderline personality disorder (BPD)[20], adding incremental validity to efforts to assess for personality pathology.

BARRIERS TO DETECTION OF PERSONALITY DISORDER IN OLDER ADULTS

Avoidance of Disclosure

Personality disorder may be undetected or inaccurately assessed due to difficulties engaging in the personality assessment process on the part of patients and clinicians, and due to limitations in applying current measures and constructs for this purpose. Specifically, many older adults grew up in an age when it was not acceptable

Principles and Practice of Geriatric Psychiatry, 3rd edn. Edited by Mohammed T. Abou-Saleh, Cornelius Katona and Anand Kumar

to openly talk about discordant feelings or interpersonal conflicts. Perceived stigma may impede inquiry into deviant inner experiences or behaviours, and would also make it unlikely that an older adult would have received a previous personality disorder diagnosis of which they can inform their current physician[21]. In a complementary manner, some clinicians adhere to the erroneous belief that older adults simply do not have personality disorders[14]. In addition, personality disorders may increase risk for developing Axis I disorders and it is often for this subsequent condition that patients seek professional help. Axis I conditions may be easier to recognize and accept, for both the clinician and patient, and are therefore often deemed the focus of diagnoses and treatment.

Assessment Measures

The structured interview is often considered an ideal assessment tool for diagnoses of personality disorder, but is subject to biases and inaccuracies when assessing older adults. As longitudinal evidence is required for a diagnosis of personality disorder, older adults may be asked to recount events and trends from 30–50 years before, and it is often doubtful that such information is valid or reliable[21]. Furthermore, measures of personality disorder cannot fully account for the potential influences of current psychological states, medical or neurological problems, situational or environmental contexts, or sociocultural roles on reporting of current symptoms or behavioural patterns[21]. Self-report inventories face similar vulnerabilities[14,15], and must be supplemented by a practitioner's clinical judgement.

Diagnostic Criteria

DSM-IV criteria for many personality disorders may not be generalizable to experiences and behaviours displayed by older adults. For example, symptoms of personality disorder such as increased dependency, social withdrawal, or rigid and moralistic thinking may be misinterpreted by clinicians as part of the natural ageing process and therefore may not enable discrimination between normal and pathological behaviour. In a large epidemiological survey which compared younger and older adults with equivalent levels of personality disorder pathology, an item analysis found evidence for age bias in two thirds of personality disorder criteria sets[22,23]. Difficulties determining when impairment in social and occupational functioning is significant enough to warrant a diagnosis of personality disorder may also impede diagnosis. In the lives of older adults, where retirement and smaller social circles are common, this may not be an accurate measure of impairment[14,21]. Finally, discrete behaviours upon which inferences as to personality are based may be more fallible in older adulthood. As individuals age, changing physical and developmental capabilities may limit their repertoire of behaviour, and thus the likelihood that behaviours are completely representative of their inner character. In this context it may be dangerous to rely on a solely behavioural framework for diagnoses[11,24].

DOES THE AGEING PROCESS ALTER PERSONALITY PATHOLOGY?

One of the most prominent barriers to accurate detection of personality disorder pathology is uncertainty as to whether and how age-related biopsychosocial changes affect the phenomenology of personality disorder, and a definitive answer remains elusive. Tyrer

and Sievewright[25] suggested that personality disorders can be divided into mature and immature types, in which the mature types, such as obsessive–compulsive, paranoid, schizoid and schizotypal, remain stable with age. In contrast, the more dramatic disorders, termed immature (borderline, narcissistic, histrionic), are hypothesized to decrease in intensity with age.

Empirical studies of normal personality find evidence for both stability and change over the life span. Major personality traits, such as those represented in the five-factor model (FFM) of personality (neuroticism, extraversion, openness, agreeableness and conscientiousness) have a prominent genetic basis, appear universal across cultures, and demonstrate substantial stability over the life course[10,26,27]. Hence, one might expect that maladjusted individuals with personality disorder tend to remain so as they age. However, a recent meta-analysis of 92 longitudinal studies of reports of personality traits over the life span found that 'people tend to become more socially dominant, conscientious, and emotionally stable through midlife' (p. 21)[28], suggesting a positive maturational effect for most adults likely linked to age-graded roles (e.g. work, marriage, parenthood). Personality processes, such as emotion regulation, also display favourable age-related changes in cross-sectional studies of younger and older adults[29,30]. Such findings are in accord with case series reports and cross-sectional studies of late life personality disorder[31], and suggest that normative, maturational effects may favourably modify the phenomenology of personality disorder in older adults, especially in areas such as affect regulation and impulsivity.

Longitudinal studies of personality disorder are limited, but extant research provides further insight into stability and change in the phenomenology of personality disorder over the life span. McGlashan[32] performed a longitudinal study on inpatients diagnosed with BPD, unipolar depression, or schizophrenia. He obtained follow-up data for over 288 participants (mean age of 47) at an average of 15 years after discharge (range 2–32 years). Compared to the other groups, the BPD group displayed the highest level of global functioning at follow-up, particularly in those conducted 10–19 years after discharge compared to subsequent follow-ups. Instrumental and global functioning increased for participants with BPD, whereas their interpersonal relationships often remained problematic or non-existent. McGlashan speculated that as patients with personality disorder age and lose employment capabilities, earlier improvements in instrumental functioning become less relevant and the lack of close relationships becomes more significant, potentially resulting in diminished functioning later in the life span. Similarly, a 16- to 45-year longitudinal follow-up of male inpatients diagnosed with antisocial personality disorder (ASPD) found that over half had improved or remitted, but that many also had enduring problems with occupational performance, interpersonal discord and social isolation[33].

Perry[34] reviewed 26 longitudinal studies on personality disorders, with the majority focusing on BPD. At an average follow-up of 8.7 years, only 57% of BPD patients continued to meet diagnostic criteria. This relationship was reportedly linear, with approximately 3.7% of borderline cases remitting each year. A more recent 10-year follow-up study of inpatients with BPD found that 88% achieved remission (many within 2 years), and that symptoms such as impulsivity were likely to resolve, while chronic dysphoria and interpersonal symptoms persisted[20,35].

In sum, investigations into the temporal stability of personality traits, disorders and processes find evidence for substantial continuity, particularly for major traits and for interpersonal functioning, but also for favourable change in select areas, such as emotion regulation and impulsivity. Although we are unaware of studies that follow personality disorder into older adulthood, such findings suggest shifts in the phenotypic expression of personality disorder, and provide further empirical support for recommendations that clinicians consider possible attenuation and exacerbation of personality disorder traits and symptoms over the life span, apply time course criteria flexibly, and appreciate the salience of subsyndromal presentations of personality disorder in late life[11,24].

CHALLENGES IN THE DIFFERENTIAL DIAGNOSIS OF PERSONALITY DISORDER IN LATE LIFE

In addition to the barriers described above, clinicians who work with older adults face added diagnostic challenges, as personality disorder is often embedded in a complex matrix of age-related changes in cognitive and physical health, functional ability, interpersonal roles, and coping resources and behaviours. Although co-morbidity is the rule rather than the exception in geriatric practice, the DSM-IV-TR 'General Criteria for Personality Disorder'[16] require that manifestations of personality disorder be disentangled from major psychiatric syndromes, medical and neurological disorders, situational behaviours or coping styles, and social/cultural roles. Among the most vexing issues are difficulties differentiating personality disorder from (i) an unremitted Axis I disorder; (ii) context-dependent roles and behaviours; (iii) subtle neurocognitive impairment; or (iv) a difficult doctor–patient relationship.

Personality Disorder Versus Unremitted Axis I Disorder

In practice settings an older person's long-standing and unremitted Axis I pathology, especially if associated with features of irritability, negativism and caregiver exhaustion, is often attributed to personality pathology. Although personality pathology is correlated with poorer treatment outcomes and persisting decreases in functioning in older depressed samples[3–5], it is not a 'diagnosis of exclusion' and such a conclusion may confuse personality disorder with illness duration and/or treatment responsiveness. This challenge may be addressed through careful application of the general diagnostic criteria for personality disorder, supplemented by dimensional personality measures and informant reports, with special attention to temporal relationships between the onset of Axis I and Axis II symptoms. If core features of personality disorder persist following maximal treatment of Axis I syndromes with combination therapies, a definitive diagnosis of personality disorder may be warranted.

Personality Disorder Versus Context-Dependent Roles and Behaviours

Older adults confronted with significant, ongoing life stressors such as serious medical illness (e.g. becoming disabled), interpersonal loss or role transition (e.g. becoming a caregiver), or the need to navigate a novel social environment (e.g. long-term care setting) may exhibit behaviours that mimic aspects of personality pathology. For example, confronted with medical problems or physical limitations, some elderly may express their distress somatically as if to manipulate the responses of caregivers; others may become antagonistic and demanding; still others may regress to a child-like dependency. Although significant psychosocial stressors may lead underlying personality disorder features to emerge[24], it is often the case that such behaviours are context-dependent, or only loosely tied to personality traits rather than disorders. A longitudinal history, supplemented by informant data and dimensional measures of personality, may help clarify whether personality disorder symptoms and behaviours preceded the change in life context, thus meriting a diagnosis of personality disorder.

Personality Disorder Versus Subtle Neurocognitive Impairment

Neurological disorders such as Alzheimer's disease, Parkinson's disease, and vascular and frontotemporal dementias are common in late life, and both their characteristic features and associated behavioural manifestations are well recognized. Recent evidence suggests that personality changes (such as increased egocentricity, emotional lability, rigidity or apathy) may represent early or prodromal manifestations of dementia[36]. Further, neuroscience research affirms that impairment of discrete brain regions often manifests as personality changes: orbital frontal lobe dysfunction is associated with reduced empathy and disinhibition; dorsolateral frontal lobe impairment is related to impaired initiation, planning and social awareness; parietal and temporal lobe insults are associated with misperception of the emotional context of speech[74]. Personality manifestations that are prominent, have insidious onset or long duration, and overshadow evidence of neurocognitive impairment (which may be subtle) may be mistaken for personality disorder. When such personality features are the consequence of a medical condition, result in functional impairment and are not attributable to a diagnosis of dementia, delirium or another Axis I disorder, they are best described in DSM-IV-TR nosology as 'Personality Change Due To ... (a general medical condition)'[16]. A careful historical review of the temporal relationship between medical or neurocognitive and personality symptoms, assisted by a neuropsychological evaluation or diagnostic neuroimaging may clarify this differential diagnosis.

Personality Disorder Versus a Difficult Doctor–Patient Relationship

Patients who are especially challenging to treat due to prominent mood states such as irritability/hostility or fearfulness/mistrust, who deny emotional distress or express this through somatic complaints, or whose interpersonal behaviour violates 'expected rules' of the doctor–patient relationship are often experienced as difficult by their clinicians. Although clinicians' emotional experiences may signal the presence of a patient with personality disorder, difficulty experienced in the doctor–patient relationship can also occur in the context of somatization disorder and other Axis I disorders[37,38]. Hence clinicians' emotional experiences provide important data, but may be non-specific regarding presence/absence of personality disorder. For purposes of differential diagnosis, such data might best be evaluated alongside informant information, clinical history and other assessment approaches described above.

One might expect that the above challenges would result in many false positive diagnoses of personality disorder in late life, but more commonly, behavioural problems that mimic personality disorder are informally and erroneously attributed to 'personality' in much the same way that ambiguous medical problems are ascribed to 'ageing'. Both practices may serve to reduce clinicians' discomfort with diagnostic uncertainty or other dissonant experiences, but can also result in failure to detect or properly manage an underlying, potentially treatable condition.

MANAGEMENT AND TREATMENT OF PERSONALITY DISORDER IN OLDER ADULTS

Progress in the development of strategies to manage and treat personality disorder has been slow, and evidence-based guidelines regarding the treatment of personality disorder in older adults currently do not exist. Hence clinicians engaged in the psychotherapeutic or pharmacological treatment of older adults with personality disorder often extrapolate from treatment models developed for younger adults. Generally, approaches for managing late-life personality disorder are based on the following premises: (i) evidence-based treatments for Axis I disorders require augmentation when personality pathology is present; (ii) standardized psychotherapeutic treatments developed to target aspects of personality disorder in adults are more effective than usual care; (iii) initial studies suggest that older adults may also benefit from these targeted treatments; (iv) guidance regarding the treatment of personality disorder in late life may be derived from common ingredients of effective approaches, extant research and clinical observations.

Studies of depressed younger or older adults provided with standardized brief treatments demonstrate that those with co-morbid personality disorder achieve less favourable outcomes[4,39]. Importantly, these data do not suggest that depressed older adults with co-morbid personality disorder cannot derive some benefit from treatment for Axis I conditions[40], but they underscore that those with personality disorder are at higher risk of slower treatment response or adverse outcomes[5]. The presence of a personality disorder may interfere with the success and efficacy of such treatments in a variety of ways: long-standing maladaptive interpersonal patterns can pose challenges to forming a working therapeutic alliance; patients may be unwittingly invested in their symptoms and reluctant to get better for fear that secondary gains (attention, sympathy, intimacy) of illness may be lost; other aspects of the patient's life may be so chaotic that treatment adherence is difficult; or a patient may act out in offensive or self-destructive ways, causing the clinician to decrease their commitment to and optimism about treatment.

Empirical studies of psychotherapeutic approaches developed for the treatment of personality disorder in adults demonstrate promising findings. Dialectical behaviour therapy (DBT), schema-focused therapy, transference-based psychotherapy, and interpersonal group therapy have displayed efficacy in treating characteristic maladaptive coping styles and behaviours common to BPD in adults[41–43]. Preliminary findings suggest that at least some of these models may have utility in treating depressed elderly with co-morbid personality disorder. In a recent trial, older adults with chronic depression and co-morbid personality disorder demonstrated improved remission rates when antidepressant treatment was combined with an adapted form of DBT. Those offered combined treatment also showed reduced interpersonal sensitivity and aggression, although it is unclear if other components of personality disorder were ameliorated[44].

Since effective approaches to treating personality disorder appear to share common ingredients, Livesley has argued for an integrative, common factors therapeutic approach[1,45]. Such an approach would combine treatment modalities (psychotherapeutic and psychopharmacologic; individual and group psychotherapies) and techniques (behavioural, cognitive and psychodynamic) and maximally draw upon common factors found to be effective across treatments as part of an intensive, long-term intervention. Although this model has yet to be validated for older adults, it is consistent with models, emerging research and clinical reports regarding the treatment of late-life personality disorder[31,44,46–50].

PSYCHOTHERAPEUTIC MANAGEMENT: BASIC PRINCIPLES

Collaborative Multimodal Treatment, Managing Crises and Ensuring Safety

Effective treatment approaches for personality disorder tend to utilize a collaborative multimodal approach, in which clinicians of different disciplines combine treatment interventions to help the patient. Since older adults with personality disorders are likely to experience functional impairment in multiple areas (health, mood, social functioning), a multimodal approach in which the person may receive individual and group therapy, pharmacotherapy, medical attention for health concerns and case management is often ideal.

As with any psychiatric illness, the utmost priority in the treatment of patients with personality disorder is ensuring the patient's safety. Older adults with personality disorder may be prone to act in impulsive and self-destructive ways, arousing clinicians' concerns regarding their potential for self-harm or suicidal behaviour. A collaborative and cohesive treatment approach, often including all treatment team members and enlisting the patient's family or significant others to ensure safety, may assist to defuse such crises. This approach can also help clinicians evaluate the patient's need for hospitalization, closely monitor symptoms, and modify treatment parameters as needed.

Treatment Parameters

Effective psychopharmacological or psychotherapeutic treatment of individuals with personality disorder requires that clinicians attend carefully to treatment parameters such as session frequency and duration, availability of clinicians during non-treatment hours, policies regarding confidentiality and consent, and the respective roles and responsibilities of the patient and team members. Individuals with personality disorders may be more likely to cross boundaries with clinicians, or in some cases, encourage clinicians to cross boundaries for them. When clinicians find themselves stepping outside their normal repertoire of behaviour for a patient, whether in a positive or negative way (avoiding sessions, letting the session go overtime, doing tasks for patients that one would expect other patients to do for themselves, having intrusive thoughts or fears about a patient), this can reflect an enactment of the patient's interpersonal problems. When a clinician conceptualizes such boundary disturbances in a therapeutic manner (i.e. this person crosses boundaries because it is likely that someone crossed boundaries inappropriately with them in the past), it may be easier for the clinician to intervene using a combination of empathic clarification and limit-setting approaches, while maintaining a therapeutic alliance with the patient.

A common clinical occurrence when working with individuals with personality disorder is the propensity for the patient to split the treatment team. Splitting describes a tendency to engage in dichotomous thinking, such as categorizing people or experiences as all good or all bad, often evoking responses that appear to confirm this polarized and distorted perspective. When splitting does happen, it is of utmost importance that the treatment team recognizes it, retains solidarity and acts towards the patient as a unified front, especially in regard to treatment parameters, expectations regarding the patient's responsibilities in the treatment, and consequences regarding a failure to meet these expectations.

Patients with personality disorder may be especially prone to acting out or becoming more symptomatic when there is a transition regarding the treatment team. Whether prompted by a clinician's departure or the patient's need for a different level of care, such personnel changes may be interpreted implicitly as rejection or abandonment, and it is essential that transitions be handled with sensitivity and increased alertness regarding safety issues. Anticipatory discussions of these transitions permit an exploration of how the patient perceives them, and a respectful and empathic response by the clinician may serve to diminish the chance of exacerbated symptoms or maladaptive behaviours. An interdisciplinary treatment team of providers may also serve to offer some constancy during such times.

Therapeutic Relationship and Treatment Alliance

Some of the most effective treatments for people with personality disorders are those that highlight the importance of the therapeutic relationship. For example, dialectical behaviour therapy, schema-focused therapy, transference-based psychotherapy and interpersonal group therapy all include a focus upon emotion regulation and the recognition of maladaptive interpersonal patterns, with special attention to how these problems may affect the therapeutic alliance. Several of these models, tested primarily in adults with BPD, suggest that clinicians assist patients to recognize and expect the emergence of underlying insecurities that would normally rupture the therapeutic process. For example, when conflicts in therapy arise, the clinician may enquire about past relationships in which the person had a similar experience or felt the same way. Clarifying similarities and differences between experiences of current and past relationships, and recognizing and correcting cognitive distortions about relationships, can be beneficial. During this process, as individuals with personality disorder come to recognize and label their own underlying emotions and experiences, they tend to engage less in acting out unacknowledged affective states, prompting interpersonal relationships to improve.

Since maladaptive interpersonal behaviours are core aspects of personality disorder, clinicians often find it difficult to form and maintain the alliance that is needed as a foundation of treatment. Clinicians challenged by this ongoing struggle may find it helpful to keep the aetiological factors of personality disorder, such as early trauma or aversive psychosocial experiences, in mind. Without understanding the underlying issues which often drive patients with personality disorder to act in offensive or self-destructive ways, clinicians are bound to be put off and frustrated by such patients, and it is likely that a clinician's instinctive defensive or avoidant response may reinforce the patient's pathological beliefs and interpersonal patterns. Thus, clinicians need to draw on their reservoir of knowledge to understand the underlying motivations for such behaviour so as not to contribute to its negative effects. Accordingly, a useful clinical guideline to keep in mind when treating individuals with personality disorders is to respond to underlying anxieties rather than maladaptive coping styles or defences. If one conceptualizes an individual's personality disorder in terms of an underlying vulnerability (e.g. sensitivity to issues of abandonment, loss of control, rejection etc.), one may be better able to respond to these insecurities as opposed to the maladaptive behaviours they can inspire. When the clinician can maintain a therapeutic stance (often putting their own ego and pride aside) and respond to the patient by acknowledging and validating fears, they are more likely to be able to successfully set limits, break interpersonal patterns, and provide patients with a new experience that can lead to real change.

PSYCHOPHARMACOLOGICAL MANAGEMENT

As mentioned above, psychopharmacological intervention is often an important component of a multimodal integrative approach to the treatment of personality disorder, and both theoretical and practical rationales may be presented for pharmacotherapy for late-life personality disorder. First, there is evidence that neurochemical abnormalities (e.g. serotonergic dysfunction) mediate the relationship between adverse genetic or environmental diatheses (e.g. temperament) and manifestations of personality pathology (e.g. impulsive aggression; suicidal and compulsive behaviours)[51]. Similarly, there is some evidence that dimensions of personality pathology (e.g. affective dysregulation, cognitive-perceptual dysfunction, impulse dyscontrol) may share common psychobiological substrates with Axis I disorders, and thus targeted pharmacotherapies might address neurotransmitter systems linked to these underlying substrates[49,52]. A second, practical rationale for adjunctive pharmacotherapy is that personality disorder is often associated with Axis I disorders, brief destabilizing symptoms such as agitation or psychotic-like experiences, and behavioural crises, in which cases pharmacotherapy can be employed to manage acute symptoms, restore emotion regulation and reduce overall functional impairment.

Controlled studies find that psychopharmacological interventions have some effectiveness in treating circumscribed symptoms related to personality disorder, but research has been limited to three personality disorder types (borderline, schizotypal and antisocial personality disorder) and has only been conducted in young adult samples[31]. Studies of patients with BPD have found that atypical antipsychotic, anti-epileptic, and SSRI or SNRI medications effectively treat symptoms of cognitive-perceptual disturbance, mood instability and negative emotionality or aggression, respectively[51]. However, a review of forty randomized controlled trials of pharmacotherapy for adults with personality disorder (borderline, schizotypal and antisocial types) cautioned that although useful, psychotropic medications tend to only induce partial improvement in circumscribed areas[53].

A general framework for psychopharmacologic management of older adults with personality disorder augments general principles of geriatric psychopharmacology with an understanding of both the potential goals and challenges of managing symptoms in the context of late-life personality disorder. Once the best possible diagnostic formulation is reached, clinicians are advised to review with the patient all medications and remedies currently in use, and to attend to possible medication interactions[49]. The presence of co-morbid medical illnesses, cognitive impairment and other factors that may affect adherence should be identified. Even when target symptoms and goals are identified and agreed upon, it is important that both clinician and patient recognize that pharmacotherapy will not cure the personality disorder, and so the potential benefits and risks of treatment should be carefully reviewed and documented. In regard to specific agents, recent reviews suggest that SSRIs be used as first-line interventions for low mood as well as suicidal, aggressive or obsessional behaviours, and that mood stabilizers be considered to control affective fluctuations, which may occur in the context of cluster B and C personality disorders. Atypical antipsychotic medications may be helpful when psychotic-like symptoms are present, or in cluster A personality disorders. All reviews emphasize the prescribing clinician's need to carefully attend to the doctor–patient relationship, as a tenuous alliance and medication misuse or non-adherence are common in work with patients with personality disorders[11,31,53,54].

CONCLUSIONS

Personality and personality pathology exert profound effects on psychological well-being in older adults, yet are often underdetected and undertreated. Barriers to effective diagnostic assessment include the limitations of current measures, the differing phenomenology of late-life personality disorder and problems in differential diagnosis. Current findings favour a two-step, multimethod assessment approach in which presence/absence of personality disorder is first identified according to DSM-IV 'General Criteria for Personality Disorder'[16] and then supplemented by collaterally informed semistructured interviews, and dimensionally-based personality self-report measures to characterize personality disorder type[45]. Longitudinal assessment may be required to fully sort out personality disorder from Axis I disorders, subtle neurocognitive impairment, context-dependent behaviours, or other causes of difficult doctor–patient relationships.

Although randomized controlled trials of the treatment of late-life personality disorder are rare, recent findings in young adults suggest that components of personality disorder are amenable to targeted psychotherapies and pharmacotherapies. An integrative approach that combines treatment modalities and the common therapeutic ingredients of efficacious approaches may offer the best hope for the management and treatment of late-life personality disorder.

REFERENCES

1. Livesley WJ. *Handbook of Personality Disorders: Theory, Research, and Treatment*. New York: Guilford, 2001.
2. Zweig RA, Hillman J. Personality disorders in adults: a review. In Rosowsky E, Abrams R, Zweig R (eds), *Personality Disorders in Older Adults: Emerging Issues in Diagnosis and Treatment*. Mahwah, NJ: Lawrence Erlbaum, 1999, 31–53.
3. Abrams RC, Alexopoulos GS, Spielman LA *et al.* Personality disorder symptoms predict declines in global functioning and quality of life in elderly depressed patients. *Am J Geriatr Psychiatry* 2001; **9**(1): 67–71.
4. Gradman T, Thompson L, Gallagher-Thompson D. Personality disorders and treatment outcome. In Rosowsky E, Abrams R, Zweig R (eds), *Personality Disorders in Older Adults: Emerging Issues in Diagnosis and Treatment*. Mahwah, NJ: Lawrence Erlbaum, 1999, 69–94.
5. Morse JG, Pilkonis P, Houck PR *et al.* Impact of cluster C personality disorders on outcomes of acute and maintenance treatment for late life depression. *Am J Geriatr Psychiatry* 2005; **13**: 808–14.
6. Pietrzak RH, Wagner JA, Petry NM. DSM-IV personality disorders and coronary heart disease in older adults: results from the National Epidemiologic Survey on Alcohol and Related Conditions. *J Gerontol B Psychol Sci Soc Sci* 2007; **62**: P295–9.
7. Heisel M, Links PS, Conn D, van Reekum R, Flett GL. Narcissistic personality and vulnerability to late life suicidality. *Am J Geriatr Psychiatry* 2007; **15**(9): 734–41.
8. Hooker K, McAdams DP. Personality reconsidered: a new agenda for aging research. *J Gerontol B Psychol Sci Soc Sci* 2003; **58**: 296–304.
9. Widiger TA, Seidlitz L. Personality, psychopathology, and aging. *J Res Pers* 2002; **36**: 335–62.
10. Widiger TA, Trull TJ. Plate tectonics in the classification of personality disorder: shifting to a dimensional model. *Am Psychol* 2007; **62**: 71–83.
11. Abrams RC. Personality disorders in the elderly: a flagging field of inquiry. *Int J Geriatr Psychiatry* 2006; **21**: 1013–17.
12. Weissman M. The epidemiology of personality disorders: a 1990 update. *J Pers Disord* 1993; **7**(suppl): 44–62.
13. Rendu A, Moran P, Patel A, Knapp M, Mann A. Economic impact of personality disorders in UK primary care attenders. *Br J Psychiatry* 2002; **181**: 62–6.
14. Segal DS, Hersen M, Van Hasselt VB, Silberman CS, Roth, L. Diagnosis and assessment of personality disorders in older adults: a critical review. *J Pers Disord* 1996; **10**: 384–99.
15. Zweig RA. Personality disorder in older adults: assessment challenges and strategies. *Prof Psychol Res Pr* 2008; **39**: 298–305.
16. American Psychiatric Association. *Diagnostic and Statistical Manual of Mental Disorders*, 4th edn, text revision. Washington, DC: American Psychiatric Association, 2000.
17. Pfohl B, Blum N, Zimmerman M. *Structured Interview for DSM-IV Personality (SIDP-IV)*. Iowa City: University of Iowa, 1995.
18. World Health Organization. *The International Personality Disorder Examination (IPDE) DSM-IV Module*. Washington, DC: American Psychiatric Association Press, 1995.
19. Costa PT, McCrae RR. *Revised NEO Personality Inventory (NEO-PI-R) and NEO Five-factor Inventory (NEO-FFI) Professional Manual*. Odessa, FL: Psychological Assessment Resources, 1992.
20. Zanarini MC, Frankenberg FR, Hennen J, Reich D, Silk K. Prediction of the 10-year course of borderline personality disorder. *Am J Psychiatry* 2006; **163**: 827–32.
21. Agronin M, Maletta, G. Personality disorders in late life: understanding and overcoming the gap in research. *Am J Geriatr Psychiatry* 2000; **8**: 4–18.
22. Balsis S, Gleason ME, Woods CM, Oltmanns TF. An item response theory analysis of DSM-IV personality disorder criteria across younger and older age groups. *Psychol Aging* 2007; **22**: 171–85.
23. Balsis S, Woods CM, Gleason MEJ, Oltmanns TF. Overdiagnosis and underdiagnosis of personality disorders in older adults. *Am J Geriatr Psychiatry* 2007; **15**: 742–53.
24. Sadavoy J, Fogel B. Personality disorder in old age. In Birren JE, Sloane RB, Cohen GD (eds), *Handbook of Mental Health and Aging*, 2nd edn. San Diego, CA: Academic Press, 1992, 433–62.
25. Tyrer P, Sievewright H. Studies of outcome. In Tyrer P (ed.) *Personality Disorders: Diagnosis, Management, and Course*. London: Wright, 1988, 119–36.
26. Costa PT, McCrae RR. Personality in adulthood: a six-year longitudinal study of self-reports and spouse ratings on the NEO Personality Inventory. *J Pers Soc Psychol* 1988; **54**: 853–63.
27. Widiger TA, Simonsen E, Krueger R, Livesley WJ, Verheul R. Personality disorder research agenda for the DSM-V. *J Pers Disord* 2005; **19**: 315–38.
28. Roberts BW, Walton KE, Viechtbauer W. Patterns in mean-level change in personality traits across the life course: a meta-analysis of longitudinal studies. *Psychol Bull* 2006; **132**: 1–25.
29. Carstensen LL. Social and emotional patterns in adulthood: support for socio-emotional selectivity theory. *Psychol Aging* 1992; **7**: 331–8.
30. Magai C, Passman V. The interpersonal basis of emotional behavior and emotion regulation in adulthood. *Annu Rev Geriatr Gerontol* 1997; **17**: 104–37.
31. Zweig RA, Agronin ME. Personality disorders in late life. In Agronin M, Maletta G (eds), *Principles and Practice of Geriatric*

Psychiatry. Philadelphia, PA: Lippincott, Williams & Wilkins, 2006, 449–69.

32. McGlashan TH. The Chestnut Lodge follow-up study, III: Long-term outcome of borderline personalities. *Arch Gen Psychiatry* 1986; **43**: 20–30.

33. Black DW, Baumgard CH, Bell SE. A 16- to 45-year followup of 71 men with antisocial personality disorder. *Compr Psychiatry* 1995; **36**: 130–40.

34. Perry JC. Longitudinal studies of personality disorders. *J Pers Disord* 1993; **7**(suppl): 63–85.

35. Zanarini MC, Frankenberg FR, Reich D *et al*. The subsyndromal phenomenology of borderline personality disorder: a 10-year follow-up study. *Am J Psychiatry* 2007; **164**: 929–35.

36. Balsis S, Carpenter B, Storandt M. Personality change precedes clinical diagnosis of dementia of the Alzheimer type. *J Geront B Psychol Sci Soc Sci* 2005; **60**: 98–101.

37. Hahn SR. The difficult doctor patient relationship questionnaire. In Maruish ME (ed.), *Handbook of Psychological Assessment in Primary Care Settings*. Mahwah, NJ: Lawrence Erlbaum, 2000, 653–83.

38. Hahn SR, Kroenke K, Spitzer RL *et al*. The difficult patient: prevalence, psychopathology, and functional impairment. *J Gen Intern Med* 1996; **11**: 1–8.

39. Farmer R, Nelson-Grey RO. Personality disorders and depression: hypothetical relations, empirical findings, and methodological considerations. *Clin Psychol Rev* 1990; **10**: 453–76.

40. Thompson L, Gallagher D, Czirr R. Personality disorder and outcome in the treatment of late-life depression. *J Geriatr Psychiatry* 1988; **21**: 133–46.

41. Clarkin J, Levy KN, Lenzenwweger MF, Kernberg O. Evaluating three treatments for borderline personality disorder: a multiwave study. *Am J Psychiatry* 2007; **164**: 922–8.

42. Giesen-Bloo J, van Dyck R, Spinhoven P *et al*. Outpatient psychotherapy for borderline personality disorder: randomized trial of schema-focused therapy vs. transference-focused psychotherapy. *Arch Gen Psychiatry* 2006; **63**: 649–58.

43. Leichsenring F, Leibing E. The effectiveness of psychodynamic therapy and cognitive behavior therapy in the treatment of personality disorders: a meta-analysis. *Am J Psychiatry* 2003; **160**: 1223–32.

44. Lynch TR, Cheavens JS, Cukrowicz KC *et al*. Treatment of older adults with co-morbid personality disorder and depression: a dialectical behavior therapy approach. *Int J Geriatr Psychiatry* 2007; **22**: 131–43.

45. Livesley WJ. *Practical Management of Personality Disorder*. New York: Guilford, 2003.

46. Sadavoy J. Character disorders in the elderly: an overview. In Sadavoy J, Leszcz M (eds), *Treating the Elderly with Psychotherapy: The Scope for Change in Later Life*. Madison, CT: International Universities Press, 1987, 175–229.

47. Sadavoy J. The effect of personality disorder on axis I disorders in the elderly. In Duffy M (ed.), *Handbook of Counseling and Psychotherapy with Older Adults*. New York: John Wiley & Sons, 1999, 397–413.

48. Agronin M. Personality disorders. In Jeste D, Friedman J (ed.), *Psychiatry for Neurologists*. Totowa, NJ: Humana Press, 2005, 105–21.

49. De Leo D, Scocco P, Meneghel G. Pharmacological and psychotherapeutic treatment of personality disorders in the elderly. *Int Psychogeriatrics* 1999; **11**: 191–206.

50. Segal DL, Coolidge FL, Rosowsky, E. *Personality Disorders and Older Adults: Diagnosis, Assessment, and Treatment*. Hoboken, NJ: John Wiley & Sons, 2006.

51. Markovitz PJ. Recent trends in the pharmacotherapy of personality disorders. *J Per Dis* 2004; **18**: 90–101.

52. Grossman, R. Pharmacotherapy of personality disorders. In Magnavita JJ (ed.), *Handbook of Personality Disorders: Theory and Practice*. Hoboken, NJ: John Wiley & Sons, 2004, 331–55.

53. Triebwasser J, Siever LJ. Pharmacotherapy of personality disorders. *J Ment Health* 2007; **16**: 5–50.

54. Agronin M. Pharmacologic treatment of personality disorders in late life. In Rosowsky E, Abrams RC, Zweig RA (eds), *Personality Disorders in Older Adults: Emerging Issues in Diagnosis and Treatment*. Mahwah, NJ: Lawrence Erlbaum, 1999, 229–54.

Part I

Mental and Behavioural Disorders Due to Psychoactive Substances

106

Alcohol Abuse and Treatment in the Elderly

Helen H. Kyomen[1] and Benjamin Liptzin[2]

[1]McLean Hospital, Belmont, MA and Harvard Medical School, Boston, MA, USA
[2]Department of Psychiatry, Baystate Medical Center, Springfield,
MA and Tufts University School of Medicine, Boston, MA, USA

INTRODUCTION

Alcohol abuse in the elderly involves the persistent and intended use of ethyl alcohol despite problems caused by its use[1,2]. It is often overlooked, as elderly with alcohol abuse may present with non-specific concerns such as confusion, mood lability, depression, anxiety, unusual behaviour, self-neglect, falls, injuries, diarrhoea, malnutrition, myopathy, incontinence, hypothermia[3-5] and motor vehicle accidents[6]. However, as these conditions are evaluated, signs of the characteristic addictive use of ethyl alcohol may be uncovered with: (i) tolerance; (ii) withdrawal symptoms; (iii) loss of control of use; (iv) social decline; and (v) mental and physical decline[2]. Late-life alcoholism is a substantial problem. In a recent population representative study which included 4236 non-institutionalized elderly, at-risk alcohol use was described by 13% of men and 8% of women, and binge drinking was reported by over 14% of men and 3% of women[7]. In another recent study of 24 863 elderly primary clinic patients, 21.5% were moderate drinkers, 4.1% were at-risk drinkers and 4.5% were heavy or binge drinkers[8].

EFFECTS OF ALCOHOL IN THE ELDERLY

Older people are at greater risk and more vulnerable to the toxic effects of alcohol for two main reasons.

1. The elderly have a decreased volume of distribution due to decreased muscle mass, a greater proportion of fat and a smaller water compartment. These all result in a higher blood alcohol level than in a younger adult for the same amount of alcohol consumed[9,10]. In a younger person, larger amounts of alcohol consumption may be necessary before detrimental effects from alcohol abuse become grossly evident. A susceptible elderly person may reach this threshold for hazardous use of alcohol after drinking relatively less.
2. The general decrease in the capacity to withstand stress and maintain homeostasis as well as a higher risk for medical illness and disability in elderly people may hinder adaptation to the noxious effects of alcohol and magnify the consequences of alcohol abuse in the elderly[11].

The interaction of these two main factors places the elderly alcohol-using person at greater risk for multiple impairments resulting from the use of alcohol.

There are many possible detrimental effects from alcohol abuse in the elderly. Among them are the following:

1. Driving ability can be adversely affected with the consumption of minimal amounts of alcohol. In some elderly, relatively small amounts of alcohol can exacerbate or lead to confusion, visuospatial impairment, problem-solving deficits, motor impairment[12] and motor vehicle accidents[6].
2. Cognitive impairments suggesting dementia may be caused by alcohol abuse. Though some cognitive impairment can result from even social drinking, chronic consumption of higher doses of alcohol has been shown to cause marked cognitive deficits with associated cortical atrophy and ventricular dilatation on brain scan[12].
3. Elderly alcoholics have a higher prevalence of alcohol-related medical conditions than the elderly population at large. Such conditions include alcoholic liver disease, alcoholic cardiomyopathy, hypertension, chronic obstructive pulmonary disease, neurological diseases (including cognitive disorders and peripheral neuropathy), malnutrition, osteopenia, psoriasis, peptic ulcer disease and various cancers[9,12,13].
4. Alcohol use can adversely affect the elimination of some drugs and add to the toxicity of others. This places an elderly person with medical illness or disability who is taking prescription medication at great risk for having subtherapeutic or adverse effects from the medication[14,15]. The magnitude of this problem is evident when one considers that the elderly are the largest per capita prescription drug users[16] and the most at risk for medication associated adverse events[17].
5. The depressant effects of alcohol on the central nervous system may mimic or contribute to depression in the elderly. Some elderly with depressed mood may resort to drinking in order to 'self-medicate' themselves. This may alleviate the depressive symptoms initially, but later lead to an increase in depression, anxiety, sleep disturbances and impotence[18,19].

Principles and Practice of Geriatric Psychiatry, 3rd edn. Edited by Mohammed T. Abou-Saleh, Cornelius Katona and Anand Kumar
© 2011 John Wiley & Sons, Ltd

6. Alcohol can contribute to malnutrition in the elderly. Malnutrition can result from the interaction of the following factors[20,21]:
   (a) Food intake can be hindered if the elderly alcoholic develops depressed mood, becomes apathetic and experiences loss of appetite. If the elderly alcoholic's impaired ambulation or driving results in a reduced capacity to obtain food, or if limited financial resources are used to purchase alcohol instead of food, dietary intake may be restricted further.
   (b) The effect of alcohol on the gastrointestinal tract is to produce malabsorption of fats, fat-soluble vitamins, calcium, magnesium, iron and zinc. The active transport of B vitamins is also impaired.
   (c) Alcohol can contribute to increased losses of magnesium, phosphate, potassium and zinc through the urine. If vomiting and diarrhoea occur, there may be increased loss of sodium, potassium and chloride.
   (d) Alcohol use increases the requirements for folate and pyridoxine.
7. Alcohol use contributes to accidents and injuries that may lead to fractures or subdural hematomas[3,6,22].
8. Heavy use of alcohol is associated with greater mortality[23-25].
9. Alcoholism can disrupt the elderly alcoholic's family structure and cohesiveness, and may even lead to family violence. This can result in dysfunctional family relationships, with consequent increased difficulty in treatment of the alcohol-related problems.

Despite the many unfavourable effects of alcohol abuse in the elderly, researchers have also reported positive aspects of alcohol use. Light to moderate alcohol consumption has been associated with decreased mortality risk[24,25], reduced risk of substantial functional health decline[26], better cognitive health and well-being[27,28], improved bone mineral density[29] and, in elderly coronary patients, elevated high-density lipoprotein cholesterol[30].

CHARACTERISTICS OF ELDERLY ALCOHOL ABUSERS

Elderly alcohol abusers differ from younger alcohol abusers in a number of ways. Alcohol abuse in the elderly is often associated with clusters of stressors such as job retirement, widowhood, the deaths of close friends and relatives, medical illness and disability in oneself and one's peers, and perceived loss of meaningful roles or functions. Some authors consider late-onset alcoholism to be associated with tension reduction, where alcohol is used to regulate stress. However, the extent to which alcohol abuse in the elderly is precipitated by stress is unclear. Some researchers have found little or unexpected change in alcohol consumption or drinking behaviour due to life stressors[31,32].

The time of onset of alcohol abuse may also significantly differentiate the younger alcoholic from the older one[10,33,34]. The early-onset alcoholics have a greater amount of psychopathology and family history of alcoholism than the late-onset alcoholics. The early-onset alcoholics are characterized by being male relatives of alcoholic men with histories of violence with and without alcohol, legal problems due to alcohol use and illegal substance abuse. The late-onset alcoholics are characterized by having isolated alcohol-induced problems with health, marital relationships, or self-care, and much reduced histories of arrests, violence or other substance abuse. Many elderly with alcohol problems fall into the late-onset alcoholic group. These findings suggest that the aetiology and predisposition of a person to an alcohol use disorder may differ by onset age. If this is so, the

treatments and interventions for an alcohol use disorder may also differ with age of onset and need to be individualized accordingly.

Individual feelings towards alcohol use are affected by exposure to cultural and historical attitudes[35]. For example, the experience of the American elderly alcoholic may differ from that of younger alcoholics in that the elderly alcoholic and his peers may have been exposed to the turmoil of the Prohibition era[36]. The moral issues highlighted in this historical period may influence the willingness that some elderly may have in recognizing and accepting a diagnosis of and treatment for alcoholism. In some retirement communities, evening cocktails are a part of the social routine, leading some individuals to increase their prior alcohol consumption.

THE RECOGNITION OF ALCOHOL ABUSE IN THE ELDERLY

Alcohol abuse in the elderly often comes to the attention of health professionals through presentation with a non-specific medical or psychiatric symptom, such as self-neglect, falls, confusion, emotional lability, depression, unusual behaviour, injuries, diarrhoea, malnutrition, myopathy, incontinence or hypothermia. In cases where alcohol abuse is suspected, alcohol dependence must be considered. Alcohol dependence is suggested when there is: (i) tolerance; (ii) withdrawal symptoms; (iii) loss of control of use; (iv) social decline; and (v) mental and physical decline[2,37].

Tolerance to alcohol may be assessed by establishing a reliable history of the patient's drinking pattern. Corroboration from family members and others close to the patient may be crucial. Tolerance is suggested if the patient exhibits a quantity and frequency of drinking which is increased over his baseline pattern of drinking. A patient with tolerance to alcohol will require a greater quantity of alcohol to achieve the same amount of inebriation that a lower quantity had been able to achieve previously. Tolerance is strongly suggested if there has been at least a 50% increase in the amount of alcohol required to attain a given effect[2,37].

Withdrawal symptoms occur when a patient who is physically dependent on alcohol experiences a rapid decrease in blood alcohol concentration. In an older person, the onset of withdrawal may be delayed by days after drinking cessation, and the duration of withdrawal may be prolonged[37,38]. Symptoms of the alcohol withdrawal syndrome stem from autonomic hyperactivity and include tachycardia with a pulse of greater than 110 beats per minute, tachypnea, hypertension, low-grade fever, sweating, nausea, vomiting, hand tremors and increased anxiety. In some cases, the patient may develop seizures or delirium tremens with confusion, agitation and visual or tactile hallucinations. An elderly patient undergoing withdrawal may experience one or all of these symptoms[37,38].

Loss of control means that the patient is no longer able to consistently choose the amount of alcohol consumed in a given situation[37]. The patient may also experience blackouts, and behave and feel in unpredictable ways.

Social decline in the elderly alcoholic is assessed from a baseline of age-appropriate behaviours[2,37,38]. Many elderly people no longer hold a steady job, do not drive or hold a driver's license, and have lost many of their close friends and associates with whom they used to socialize. Thus, it may not be as appropriate to assess for social decline by investigating these areas of the elderly patient's life as it would be in a younger patient. However, it is relevant and revealing to ask elderly people if they are in contact with their children or grandchildren, and to what extent. It is also useful to find out whether the patient's relatives express any concern about the patient's alcohol use. Investigating the patient's functioning with respect to hobbies or other enjoyed activities can also be useful.

Physical, psychological and laboratory findings may also uncover problems with alcohol use[37–39]. Addictive alcohol use can lead to malnutrition, gastrointestinal upset and bleeding, delirium, falls, depression, hypertension and neglect of self. Recurrent diseases of the stomach, pancreas or liver may also be caused by excessive alcohol abuse. These medical conditions often bring the elderly alcoholic to clinical attention. Laboratory results of macrocytosis, elevated mean corpuscular volume and increased liver enzyme levels, especially gamma glutamyl transpeptidase, may correlate with alcohol abuse in the elderly. Carbohydrate-deficient transferrin is approved by the Food and Drug Administration (FDA) as a clinical diagnostic test for identifying heavy alcohol use[39]. Blood alcohol levels, and urine or breath tests for alcohol, may be used to confirm alcohol intoxication.

Assessment of tolerance, withdrawal, loss of control, social decline and mental and physical decline are useful clinical parameters to recognize and diagnose alcohol addiction. Several screening instruments have been devised to help clinicians recognize alcoholism. These scales typically assess the quantity and frequency of drinking, social and legal problems resulting from alcohol abuse, health problems related to excessive alcohol use, symptoms of addictive drinking and/or self-recognition of alcohol-related problems[40,41]. Three screening instruments that are commonly used with the elderly are the CAGE screen[42], the Short Michigan Alcoholism Screening Test-Geriatric Version (S-MAST-G)[43] and the Alcohol Use Disorders Identification Test (AUDIT)[44].

The CAGE screen is the most widely used. 'CAGE' is a mnemonic for the questions: Have you ever felt a need to Cut down on drinking? Have you ever felt Annoyed by others enquiring about your drinking? Have you ever felt Guilty about drinking? Do you ever use alcohol for an Eye-opener? If two or more of these questions are answered positively, a need for more extensive evaluation for alcohol abuse is indicated. The validity of the CAGE screen for alcoholism in the elderly has been examined empirically[42].

A more detailed screen is the 10-item S-MAST-G[43] or the original 24-item MAST-G[45]. The S-MAST-G was developed for screening older adults in various settings and has excellent psychometric characteristics. Scores of ≥2 on the S-MAST-G or of ≥5 on the MAST-G are indicative of possible problems with alcohol.

The AUDIT[44] emphasizes the identification of harmful drinking and need for current treatment. It was validated in a sample of non-elderly adults and is composed of two parts: a 10-item AUDIT Core Questionnaire and an 8-item AUDIT Clinical Procedure. The AUDIT Core Questionnaire includes specific questions about the quantity and frequency of drinking and can be incorporated into a general interview or medical history. In the original study sample, all alcoholics scored ≥9 on the AUDIT Core Questionnaire. The AUDIT Clinical Procedure complements the AUDIT Core Questionnaire and includes questions about clinical signs associated with harmful drinking, such as fractures, tremors and hepatic abnormalities. The AUDIT Clinical Procedure may be especially helpful in evaluating patients who underestimate their alcohol-related problems. A short version of the AUDIT, the AUDIT-C[46], is a 3-item screen composed of the alcohol consumption questions of the AUDIT. The AUDIT-C has been reported to be a valid primary care screen for heavy drinking and/or current alcohol abuse/dependence. Various versions of the AUDIT have been used widely, but for older adults, the overall accuracy is low and multiple screening methods are recommended[47,48].

THE TREATMENT OF ALCOHOL ABUSE IN THE ELDERLY

In acutely intoxicated patients, a thorough evaluation for and treatment of other co-existing medical or psychiatric problems must be initiated at the same time as the patient is being detoxified. Providing adequate nutrition and hydration is especially important in the elderly alcoholic due to increased nutritional problems and impaired thirst mechanisms in the elderly. Benzodiazepines are generally avoided in most elderly due to their potential for causing delirium. However, if significant withdrawal symptoms occur, benzodiazepines should be administered according to assessments of alcohol withdrawal severity[38,49]. Withdrawal severity may be evaluated using the revised Clinical Institute Withdrawal Assessment Scale for Alcohol (CIWA-Ar)[50] and taking sequential vital sign measurements. Elderly patients may experience a delayed onset of and more severe withdrawal from alcohol and require higher doses of benzodiazepines than younger patients[38]. In general, detoxification using a symptom-triggered regimen with benzodiazepines with a shorter half-life is recommended in the elderly. Longer acting benzodiazepines may allow a smoother course of withdrawal but may cause more sedation in elderly patients[38]. They may also cause ataxia which can lead to falls. Non benzodiazepine GABAergic medications are considered to be potential agents to treat alcohol withdrawal[51], but their effectiveness in elderly patients is unclear. There is anecdotal experience for trying an anticonvulsant such as divalproex to prevent withdrawal seizures.

Once the elderly alcoholic patient is detoxified, adequate relapse prevention and rehabilitative treatment is crucial for the patient to maintain sobriety. The elderly alcoholic must first come to an acceptance of the alcohol abuse problem. Family members or others who are close to the patient may intervene to help the patient break through the denial regarding alcohol abuse seen in many alcohol abusers. Family members may also be instrumental in motivating the patient to stop drinking. Patient and family education about the effects of alcohol must be provided, and the need to abstain from alcohol must be stressed. Although light-to-moderate drinking has been reported to be health promoting [24–30], abstinence may be the healthiest goal for those who are unable to drink normally, tend to lose control of their drinking, or lose control of themselves when drinking. Early intervention includes brief alcohol counselling (BAC) to patients and family which encompasses expressions of concern, feedback associating the patient's drinking with health issues and explicit advice to reduce drinking[52]. Age-specific relapse prevention and rehabilitative programmes may improve treatment participation and completion[53]. A behavioural and self-management treatment module has resulted in marked success in treating alcohol-use problems in the elderly[53]. This module educates the elderly alcoholic about drinking behaviour, the acquisition of self-management skills and the reestablishment of social networks.

The elderly alcoholic patient's recovery and rehabilitation is an ongoing process. The patient needs to learn to readjust to life without alcohol. The patient's family and close relatives and friends can help him in this endeavour by supporting sobriety in the patient and incorporating the non-drinking patient into their lives without the presence of alcohol. Family members may have been 'enabling' the patient to drink, and they need to be made aware of these patterns of behaviour and change them through family education and family therapy. Sometimes, even when relatives are aware of the harmful effects of alcohol, they still provide alcohol if the patient insists. If the elderly alcohol abuser is a parent and the enablers are his children, the role reversal that is inherent in the children's setting limits on their parents may make this task especially difficult. Group therapy may help the patient adjust to a non-alcoholic lifestyle. In this setting, he can develop non-alcohol-related social skills and learn to bond with others in safe surroundings, free of the context of alcohol. If elderly alcoholics can be treated in age-specific groups, they may remain in treatment significantly longer and be more likely to complete treatment than those treated in mixed-age groups[53]. Involvement in Alcoholics Anonymous with people with whom the patient feels comfortable and can consider his peers is important, especially if he has no close relatives or friends. The relationships with others that can be formed in these settings can provide a replacement for the alcohol to which he was bonded previously. Family involvement with the patient in Alcoholics Anonymous and in other affiliated groups such as Alanon, Alateen or Alatot is important, as alcoholism adversely affects family members who also need support, education and treatment.

Use of alcohol-deterrent medication such as disulfiram or anticraving medication such as naltrexone may serve as adjunctive treatments. Disulfiram is infrequently used in the elderly due to concerns about adverse effects. Naltrexone was approved by the FDA for the treatment of alcohol dependence, based on efficacy studies with middle-aged patients with alcohol dependence[54,55]. It seems to be well tolerated in many elderly. A study in older veterans aged 50–70 found that treatment with naltrexone 50 mg/day resulted in decreased rates of relapse to heavy drinking, but no improvement in total abstinence[56]. These drugs may help motivated alcohol abusers reduce the quantity of alcohol used or the number of drinking days. However, these medications generally are not effective unless prescribed and monitored as part of an overall, multidisciplinary treatment and relapse prevention plan. Acamprosate has anti-craving therapeutic effects and also has been FDA approved for the treatment of alcohol dependence. It seems to be well tolerated by elderly, but there are no clinical trials focusing on its use in elderly[52].

The cultural aspects of alcohol abuse intervention are also worthy of consideration. In instituting any type of treatment or intervention, it is important to consider the context of the problem that is being addressed and the context into which the treatment or intervention will be instituted. The consumption of alcohol can take on a variety of cultural meanings. To some groups, ethanol is a food or is associated with religious rituals. For others, it is a means to relax and calm one's nerves. For still others, alcohol is considered to be a sinful intoxicant used by those of weak moral fibre. To intervene most effectively with an aged person for whom alcohol consumption has become a problem, it is important to understand what meaning the use of the alcohol has for him as an individual, a family member and as part of the greater society, including his cultural group. The contextual meaning of the change in alcohol use must likewise be considered. To understand these contextual meanings most effectively, the clinician must be aware of what his inherent assumptions may be about these contextual meanings and try not to confound with his own biases, his understanding of the situation. Members of the patient's contextual and cultural groups may be very helpful in providing meaningful insights into these understandings. Once these cultural factors are understood, interventions to reduce the problematic alcohol consumption to the desired outcome of abstinence or, perhaps, of less harmful alcohol use can be creatively formulated and instituted more effectively and efficiently.

CONCLUSION

In summary, alcohol abuse in the elderly is a significant problem that needs to be addressed aggressively. Recognition and diagnosis of alcohol abuse may be more difficult in the elderly. The biological and psychosocial losses and decline that are often used to identify alcoholism in younger people can occur in many elderly who do not abuse alcohol. The clinical presentation of an elderly alcoholic is often with a medical condition that may be masked by other medical diagnoses. For these reasons, the clinician must be especially alert to the possible presence of alcohol abuse in this age group. If alcohol abuse is identified, the clinician must then be prepared to direct or initiate treatment in a culturally appropriate, sensitive, flexible and creative manner that is geared to the elderly individual and his family and significant others.

REFERENCES

1. Blazer DG, Wu LT. The epidemiology of substance use and disorders among middle aged and elderly community adults: national survey on drug use and health. *Am J Geriatr Psychiatry* 2009; **17**: 237–45.
2. American Psychiatric Association. *Diagnostic and Statistical Manual of Mental Disorders*, 4th edn, text revision. Washington, DC: American Psychiatric Association, 2000.
3. Fink A, Hays RD, Moore AA, Beck JC. Alcohol-related problems in older persons. *Arch Intern Med* 1996; **156**: 1150–6.
4. Sattar SP, Padala PR, McArthur-Miller D, Roccaforte WH, Wengel SP, Burke WJ. Impact of problem alcohol use on patient behavior and caregiver burden in a geriatric assessment clinic. *J Geriatr Psychiatry Neurol* 2007; **20**: 120–7.
5. Moos RH, Schutte KK, Brennan PL, Moos BS. Older adults' alcohol consumption and late-life drinking problems: a 20-year perspective. *Addiction* 2009; **104**: 1293–302.
6. Sorock GS, Chen LH, Gonzalgo SR, Baker SP. Alcohol-drinking history and fatal injury in older adults. *Alcohol* 2006; **40**: 193–9.
7. Blazer DG, Wu L. The epidemiology of at-risk and binge drinking among middle-aged and elderly community adults: national survey on drug use and health. *Am J Psychiatry* 2009 (doi: 10.1176/appi.ajp.2009.09010016).
8. Kirchner JE, Zubritsky C, Cody M, Coakley E, Chen H, Ware JH *et al.* Alcohol consumption among older adults in primary care. *J Gen Intern Med* 2007; **22**: 92–7.
9. Vestal RE, McGuire EA, Tobin JD, Andres R, Norris AH, Mezey E. Aging and ethanol metabolism. *Clin Pharmacol Ther* 1977; **21**: 343–54.
10. Dufour M, Fuller RK. Alcohol in the elderly. *Annu Rev Med* 1995; **46**: 123–32.
11. Kalant H, Gomberg E, Hegedius A, Zucker R. Pharmacological interactions of aging and alcohol. In Gomberg E, Hegedius A, Zucker R (eds), Bethesda: National Institutes of Health. *Alcohol Problems and Aging* (vol. NIAAA Research Monograph no. 33, Publication no. 98-4163), 1998, 99–116.
12. Oscar-Berman M, Marinkovic K. Alcohol: effects on neurobehavioral functions and the brain. *Neuropsychol Rev* 2007; **17**: 239–57.
13. Dar K. Alcohol use disorders in elderly people: fact or fiction? *Adv Psychiatr Treat* 2006; **12**: 173–81.
14. Pringle KE, Ahern FM, Heller DA, Gold CH, Brown TV. Potential for alcohol and prescription drug interactions in older people. *J Am Geriatr Soc* 2005; **53**: 1930–6.

15. Moore AA, Whiteman EJ, Ward KT. Risks of combined alcohol/medication use in older adults. *Am J Geriatr Pharmacother* 2007; **5**: 64–74.

16. Catlin A, Cowan C, Hartman M, Heffler S, National Health Expenditure Accounts Team. National health spending in 2006: a year of change for prescription drugs. *Health Aff* 2008; **27**: 14–29.

17. Gurwitz JH, Field TS, Harrold LR, Rothschild J, Debellis K, Seger AC *et al*. Incidence and preventability of adverse drug events among older persons in the ambulatory setting. *JAMA* 2003; **289**(9): 1107–16.

18. Aira M, Hartikainen S, Sulkava R. Drinking alcohol for medicinal purposes by people aged over 75: a community-based interview study. *Fam Pract* 2008; **25**: 445–9.

19. Gum AM, Cheavens JS. Psychiatric comorbidity and depression in older adults. *Curr Psychiatry Rep* 2008; **10**: 23–9.

20. Manari AP, Preedy VR, Peters TJ. Nutritional intake of hazardous drinkers and dependent alcoholics in the UK. *Addict Biol* 2003; **8**: 201–10.

21. Vanderkroft D, Collins CE, Fitzgerald M, Lewis S, Capra S. Minimising undernutrition in the older patient. *Int J Evid Based Health* 2007; **5**: 56–136

22. Reid MC, Boutros NN, O'Connor PG, Cadariu A, Concato J. The health-related effects of alcohol use in older persons: a systematic review. *Subst Abus* 2002; **23**: 149–64.

23. Pearl R. Alcohol and mortality. In Starling E (ed.), *The Action of Alcohol on Man*. London: Longmans, 1923, 213–86.

24. Di Castelnuovo A, Costanzo S, Bagnardi V, Donati MB, Iacoviello L, de Gaetano G. Alcohol dosing and total mortality in men and women: an updated meta-analysis of 34 prospective studies. *Arch Intern Med* 2006; **166**: 2437–45.

25. Lee SJ, Sudore RL, Williams BA, Lindquist K, Chen HL, Covinsky KE. Functional limitations, socioeconomic status, and all-cause mortality in moderate alcohol drinkers. *J Am Geriatr Soc* 2009; **57**: 955–62.

26. Chen LY. Alcohol consumption and health status in older adults. *J Aging Health* 2009; **21**: 824–47.

27. Lang I, Wallace RB, Huppert FA, Melzer D. Moderate alcohol consumption in older adults is associated with better cognition and well-being than abstinence. *Age Ageing* 2007; **36**: 256–61.

28. Chan AM, von Muhlen D, Kritz-Silverstein D, Barrett-Connor E. Regular alcohol consumption is associated with increasing quality of life and mood in older men and women: the Rancho Bernardo study. *Maturitas* 2009; **62**: 294–300.

29. Tucker KL, Jugdaohsingh R, Powell JJ, Qiao N, Hannan MT, Sripanyakorn S *et al*. Effects of beer, wine, and liquor intakes on bone mineral density in older men and women. *Am J Clin Nutr* 2009; **89**: 1188–96.

30. de Jong HJI, de Goede J, Griep LMO, Geleijnse JM. Alcohol consumption and blood lipids in elderly coronary patients. *Metabolism* 2008; **57**: 1286–92.

31. Welte JW, Mirand AL. Drinking, problem drinking and life stressors in the elderly general population. *J Stud Alcohol* 1995; **56**: 67–73.

32. Veenstra MY, Lemmens PH, Friesema IH, Garretsen HF, Knottnerus JA, Zwietering PJ. A literature overview of the relationship between life-events and alcohol use in the genereal population. *Alcohol Alcohol* 2006; **41**: 455–63.

33. Irwin M, Schuckit M, Smith T. Clinical importance of age of onset in type 1 and type 2 primary alcoholics. *Arch Gen Psychiatry* 1990; **47**: 320–4.

34. Liberto JG, Oslin DW. Early versus late onset of alcoholism in the elderly. *Int J Addict* 1995; **30**: 1799–818.

35. Gomberg ES. Treatment for alcohol-related problems: special populations: research opportunities. *Recent Dev Alcohol* 2003; **16**: 313–33.

36. Blocker JS Jr. Did prohibition really work? Alcohol prohibition as a public health innovation. *Am J Public Health* 2006; **96**: 233–43.

37. Beresford TP. What is addiction, what is alcoholism? *Liver Transpl* 2007; **13**: S55–S58.

38. Menninger JA. Assessment and treatment of alcoholism and substance-related disorders in the elderly. *Bull Menninger Clin* 2002; **66**: 166–83.

39. Das SK, Dhanya L, Vasudevan DM. Biomarkers of alcoholism: an updated review. *Scand J Clin Lab Invest* 2007; **68**: 81–92.

40. Graham K. Identifying and measuring alcohol abuse among the elderly: serious problems with existing instrumentation. *J Stud Alcohol* 1986; **47**: 322–6.

41. O'Connell H, Chin AV, Hamiton F, Cunningham C, Walsh JB, Coakley D, Lawlor BA. A systematic review of the utility of self-report alcohol screening instruments in the elderly. *Int J Geriatr Psychiatry* 2004; **19**: 1074–86.

42. Buchsbaum DG, Buchanan RG, Welsh J, Centor RM, Schnoll SH. Screening for drinking disorders in the elderly using the CAGE questionnaire. *J Am Geriatr Soc* 1992; **40**: 662–5.

43. Blow FC, Gillespie BW, Barry KL, Mudd SA, Hill EM. Brief screening for alcohol problems in elderly populations using the Short Michigan Alcoholism Screening Test-Geriatric Version (SMAST-G). *Alcohol Clin Exp Res* 1998; **22**: 131A.

44. Bohn MJ, Babor TF, Kranzler HR. The Alcohol Use Disorders Identification Test (AUDIT). validation of a screening instrument for use in medical settings. *J Stud Alcohol* 1995; **56**: 423–32.

45. Blow FC, Brower KJ, Schulenberg JE, Demo-Dananberg LM, Young JP, Beresford TP. The Michigan Alcoholism Screening Test-Geriatric Version (MAST G): a new elderly-specific screening instrument. *Alcohol Clin Exp Res* 1992; **16**: 372.

46. Bush K, Kivlahan DR, McDonell MB, Fihn SD, Bradley KA. The AUDIT alcohol consumption questions (AUDIT-C): an effective brief screening test for problem drinking. *Arch Intern Med* 1998; **158**: 1789–95.

47. Reid MC, Tinetti ME, O'Connor PG, Kosten TR, Concato J. Measuring alcohol consumption among older adults: a comparison of available methods. *Am J Addiction* 2003; **12**: 211–19.

48. Reinert DF, Allen JP. The Alcohol Use Disorders Identification Test: an update of research findings. *Alcohol Clin Exp Res* 2007; **31**: 185–99.

49. McKeon A, Frye MA, Delanty N. The alcohol withdrawal syndrome. *J Neurol Neurosurg Psychiatry* 2008; **79**: 854–62.

50. Sullivan JT, Sykora K, Schneiderman J, Naranjo CA, Sellers EM. Assessment of alcohol withdrawal: the revised Clinical Institute Withdrawal Assessment for Alcohol scale (CIWA-Ar). *Br J Addiction* 1989; **84**: 1353–7.

51. Leggio L, Kenna GA, Swift RM. New developments for the pharmacological treatment of alcohol withdrawal syndrome: a focus on non-benzodiazepine GABAergic medications. *Prog Neuropsychopharmacol Biol Psychiatry* 2008; **32**: 1106–17.

52. Oslin DW. Evidence-based treatment of geriatric substance abuse. *Psychiatr Clin N Am* 2005; **28**: 897–911.

53. Kofoed LL, Tolson RL, Atkinson RM, Toth RL, Turner JA. Treatment compliance of older alcoholics: an elder specific

approach is superior to 'mainstreaming'. *J Stud Alcohol* 1987; **48**: 47–51.

54. Volpicelli JR, Alterman AI, Hayashida M, O'Brien CP. Naltrexone in the treatment of alcohol dependence. *Arch Gen Psychiatry* 1992; **49**: 876–80.

55. O'Malley SS, Jaffe AJ, Chang G, Schottenfeld RS, Meyer RE, Rounsaville B. Naltrexone and coping skills therapy for alcohol dependence: a controlled study. *Arch Gen Psychiatry* 1992; **49**: 881–7.

56. Oslin D, Liberto JG, O'Brien J, Krois S, Norbeck J. Naltrexone as an adjunctive treatment for older patients with alcohol dependence. *Am J Geriatr Psychiatry* 1997; **5**: 324–32.

107

Epidemiology of Alcohol Problems and Drinking Patterns

Celia F. Hybels and Dan G. Blazer

Department of Psychiatry and Behavioral Sciences, Center for the Study of Aging and Human Development, Duke University Medical Center, Durham, NC, USA

Alcohol use in excess of recommended limits is an important clinical issue for older adults. This chapter begins by summarizing the epidemiology of alcohol use disorders. Some older adults, however, fail to meet criteria for alcohol abuse or dependence yet engage in heavy drinking. The chapter continues with a discussion of patterns of alcohol use and problem drinking as well as the factors and outcomes associated with alcohol problems in this population. Issues of detection and co-morbidity are also addressed.

PREVALENCE OF ALCOHOL USE DISORDERS

Over the past decade, large community-based epidemiologic studies have provided new information concerning the prevalence of alcohol use disorders in the general population. In the National Comorbidity Survey Replication (NCS-R), conducted in the USA between 2001 and 2003 with a representative sample of 9282 adults, the lifetime prevalence of DSM-IV alcohol abuse disorder was 13.2%, a lifetime prevalence similar to that of major depression, specific phobia and social phobia, and therefore one of the more common lifetime psychiatric disorders. The lifetime prevalence of alcohol abuse disorder among those 60 years or older was 6.2%, lower than that observed for those aged 45–59 years (14.0%), 30–44 years (16.3%) and 18–29 years (14.3%). The lifetime prevalence of alcohol dependence was not as high as that of alcohol abuse, and among those aged 60 or older was 2.2%[1]. Although higher estimates were reported from the 2001–2002 National Epidemiologic Survey of Alcohol and Related Conditions (NESARC) in the USA (the lifetime prevalence of any alcohol use disorder was 16.1% among those aged 65 or older), younger or middle-aged adults were still 2.5 to 3.5-times more likely to have a lifetime alcohol use disorder than those aged 65+[2]. These estimates are similar to those obtained in the landmark Epidemiologic Catchment Area (ECA) surveys where the lifetime prevalence of alcohol abuse/dependence was 13.52% among older males compared to 26–28% among males aged 18–44. The lifetime prevalence among older females was 1.49%[3].

Similar to lifetime estimates, the current prevalence of alcohol use disorders has been shown in cross-sectional studies to decline with age. In the NESARC, the 12-month prevalence of DSM-IV alcohol abuse was 7.0% among those aged 18–29, 6.0% among those 30–44, 3.5% among those 45–64 and 1.2% among those aged 65+. A similar decline was observed for alcohol dependence with a 12-month prevalence of 9.2% among those aged 18–29 and 0.2% among those aged 65+[2]. These estimates are in agreement with the 12-month prevalence of any alcohol use disorder in the ECA among those aged 55+ (2.6–2.8%)[4]. One-month prevalence estimates of any alcohol use disorder among those aged 65+ in the ECA were 1.8% in males and 0.3% in females[5].

The prevalence in clinical samples of older adults can be higher. In one sample of 2405 patients aged 60+ seen in the emergency department, the prevalence of any current alcohol use disorder was 5.3%. The disorders occurred more frequently among men. Compared to older patients without disorders, those with alcohol use disorders were more likely to be homeless, live alone, be divorced or be never married. The most common alcohol-induced disorders were alcohol intoxication and alcohol-induced mood disorders. Falls and delirium were frequent emergency admission circumstances in the elderly drinkers[6].

While the proportion of older adults with defined alcohol use disorders may be low in comparison to younger adults, alcohol consumption at any level may potentially be problematic in this age group due to increased sensitivity to alcohol[7]. Because of decreased lean body mass and smaller volume of distribution, higher peak ethanol concentrations per dose are found in older compared to younger adults[8]. Also, even in small amounts, alcohol may exacerbate or mask symptoms of illness. Finally, many older adults are users of both prescription and over-the-counter medications that may interact with alcohol[7]. In a study of 700 persons aged 75+ from Finland, the prevalence of alcohol consumption was 44%. However, 86.9% of the alcohol drinkers used medications on a daily basis and 87.8% used medications as needed, including medications known to interact with alcohol[9]. In another study, 19% of older adults who used alcohol-interactive drugs also reported concomitant alcohol use[10]. These factors suggest alcohol use in older adults, especially in excess of recommended limits, may have adverse consequences. The number of older adults is projected to increase significantly over the next few decades as the post-Second World War generation ages, bringing a higher lifetime prevalence of alcohol disorders. This could potentially result in higher numbers of older adults with alcohol-related problems[11].

Defining recommended limits given these age-related issues can be difficult. Chermack et al. examined the relationship between alcohol consumption patterns and the presence of DSM-III-R alcohol symptoms among 443 current drinkers aged 55+, and found that both average daily consumption and days of heavy drinking in the past year independently predicted symptom status. Consumption levels for men and women were only different for symptomatic drinkers. The authors reported that their results supported the recommendation that moderate consumption levels should be lower for older than for younger adults, and the recommendation not to exceed one drink/day to reduce the risk of symptoms[12].

PREVALENCE OF ALCOHOL USE

Alcohol use declines with age. In the 2001–2002 NESARC, 45.1% of the participants aged 65+ reported that they had consumed one or more drinks in the past year, compared to 64.3% among those 45–64, 72.9% among those 25–44 and 70.8% among those 18–24. Among those aged 65+, 28.5% reported former alcohol use and 26.4% reported lifetime abstinence. Among older adults, the prevalence of current drinkers was 48.3% among Whites, 23.4% among Blacks, 37.9% among American Indians/Alaskan Natives, 32.7% among Asian/Pacific Islanders, and 36.6% among Hispanics. Among current drinkers aged 65+, 64.3% were classified as light drinkers, 20.7% as moderate drinkers and 13.9% as heavy drinkers. A total of 58.0% of older adults with excellent/very good self-perceived health were current drinkers compared to 29.1% of those who rated their health as fair/poor[13].

This decline in alcohol use by age is also observed among the oldest old. Ruchlin examined the prevalence of alcohol consumption in adults aged 55+ and found 46% had consumed alcohol in the past year, with a continuous decline across age groups, from 52.9% of those aged 55–64 categorized as current drinkers compared to 24.7% of those aged 85+. A total of 17% of the sample reported that they had consumed alcohol every day in the past two weeks. In controlled regression analyses, more people aged 65–74 drank every day, compared to those 55–64 (odds ratio = 1.36), but people aged 75+ drank less than those aged 55–64. Males and Whites used alcohol more frequently and were more likely to be heavy drinkers than females and non-Whites. The lower one's perceived health status, the lower the odds of drinking every day. Believing excessive drinking increased the chances of getting cirrhosis of the liver decreased the odds of moderate and heavy drinking[14].

There are various explanations as to why the prevalence of alcohol use is lower in older adults. Selective survival may be a factor, in that persons who drink may be less likely to survive to older ages. Cohort effects are also possible. Persons who grew up before the Second World War may have had lower alcohol use throughout their lives. In the NESARC, the proportion of lifetime abstainers was highest in the 65+ age group (26.4 vs. 13.7% among those aged 25–44 years)[13]. Studies have also shown that some older adults decrease their use as they grow older. Busby et al. investigated alcohol use in a community-based sample of adults aged 70+ in New Zealand. Both frequency and quantity of intake decreased with age. A total of 60.1% of the men and 30.3% of the women said they drank less compared to middle age, while 7.4% of the men and 11.1% of the women said they drank more. The main reasons cited for decreased

use of alcohol were change in health and fewer social opportunities, with reasons cited for increased intake being more time and money[15].

Adams et al. followed a cohort of 270 healthy community-dwelling adults aged 60+ over seven years. At baseline, the investigators found a decline in percentage of drinkers with increasing age. In the seven-year follow-up, there was a 2% per year decline in the percentage of subjects consuming any alcohol, but the mean alcohol intake did not change for those who continued to drink, except among heavy drinkers, suggesting an age-related decline rather than a cohort effect[16]. A study from Denmark of adults aged 50–74 interviewed at five time points between 1987 and 2005 reported that the unadjusted probability of heavy drinking declined with age but increased by calendar year and year of birth for both men and women[17].

Using data from four time points over 20 years, Karlamangla et al. found evidence for age and period effects for heavy drinking but not cohort effects across all age groups. The prevalence of heavy drinking decreased with increasing age, an age effect, and also tracked declines in USA per capita alcohol consumption, a period effect. The prevalence of heavy drinking in specified age groups did not differ by birth year[18]. Cohort effects have been noted across all age groups, however, for beverage-specific consumption, with adults born before 1940 more likely to drink spirits than those born after 1940, and elevated beer consumption among those born between 1946 and 1965[19]. In the NESARC, beverage preference among current drinkers aged 65+ was coolers (long drinks with ice, 1.3%), beer (23.6%), wine (31.1%), liquor (14.2%) and no preference (29.7%). Preference for beer was lower and preference for wine and liquor was higher compared to other age groups[13].

While the NESARC reported that less than half of older adults in the USA had consumed any alcohol in the previous year, regional studies have shown much variation. In a sample of 270 healthy men and women aged 65–89 living in the Southwestern USA, 48% of the participants reported in their three-day diet record that they had consumed alcohol, with 66% reporting they had consumed alcohol at least monthly[20]. The prevalence of alcohol use reported from the Established Populations for Epidemiologic Studies of the Elderly (EPESE) studies of persons aged 65+ varied by site. In East Boston, 70.5% of the sample drank alcohol in the past year and 54.7% had used alcohol in the past month. Similar findings were reported from New Haven, where 65.8% had used alcohol in the past year and 51.9% in the past month. The proportions were lower in Iowa and North Carolina. In the Iowa sample, 46.3% had used alcohol in the past year, while 31.2% had done so in the past month. In the North Carolina EPESE, 37.4% had consumed alcohol in the past year and 24.6% in the past month[21,22].

Samples from clinical populations have also found a range of alcohol use among older adults. Saunders et al. reported, among men and women aged 65+ randomly selected from patient rosters, that 10.5% admitted to drinking more or less every day (17.7% men and 6.1% women). At the three-year follow-up, one-fifth of the participants were regular drinkers, drinking at least on one occasion per week[23]. In a sample of 539 medical admissions aged 65+, the prevalence of alcohol abuse was 7.8%. An additional 29.7% of the sample who were neither abstainers nor occasional drinkers or alcohol abusers drank regularly: 43% of the men and 16% of the women[24].

PREVALENCE OF HEAVY DRINKING

Heavy drinking in older adults has been documented in research studies in various ways. In the EPESE baseline studies, the percentage of persons who drank two or more ounces of absolute alcohol per day in the previous month was 8.4% in East Boston, 6.6% in New Haven, 5.4% in Iowa and 7.2% in North Carolina[21,22]. Goodwin et al. found in their sample from the Southwestern USA that 17% of the drinkers drank more than 30 g alcohol per day on average[20]. In a study of older Medicare beneficiaries, 9% reported exceeding recommended drinking limits. The prevalence was higher in men (16%) than women (4%). Exceeding limits was defined as monthly use exceeding 30 drinks per typical month, or consuming four or more drinks a day in a typical month[25]. In a report from the 2004 Behavioral Risk Factor Surveillance System (BRFSS), the prevalence of binge drinking decreased with age, from 27.4% among those aged 18–24 to 3.7% among those aged 65+. However, among binge drinkers, those aged 65+ reported the highest average number of binge drinking episodes during the previous month. The number of drinks consumed during the most recent binge episode decreased with age, from 9.8 among those aged 18–24 to 6.4 among those aged 65+[26].

The prevalence of heavy alcohol use among drinkers has also been reported. In the NESARC, daily limits across all age groups were defined as 5+ drinks per day for men and 4+ for women. A total of 3.9% of older drinkers reported excess drinking 1–11 times in the previous year, and 6.1% reported excess consumption 12+ times in the past year. Weekly limits were defined as 14 drinks per week for men and 7 per week for women. A total of 13.9% of the older drinkers exceeded the weekly or both daily and weekly limits during the previous year[13]. Saunders et al. found that 19.5% of the men and 19.6% of the women who were regular drinkers were exceeding sensible limits[23].

The prevalence of heavy drinking in clinical samples is similar. Adams et al. screened 5065 primary care patients aged 60+ and found that 15% of the men and 12% of the women regularly drank in excess; 9% of the men and 2% of the women reported regularly consuming more than 21 drinks per week[27]. Iliffe et al. studied 241 patients aged 75+ from general practice and found that 51% of the men and 22% of the women reported using alcohol in the past three months. Among drinkers, 3.6% of the men admitted consuming more than 21 units and 3.2% of the women more than 14 units of alcohol per week. Weekly alcohol consumption was not associated with age, cognitive impairment, depression, falls or inpatient or outpatient care[28]. Callahan and Tierney found the prevalence of CAGE[29]-defined alcoholism was 10.6% among primary care patients aged 60+. Patients with alcoholism were more likely to be younger, have fewer years of education, and be male, Black, smokers and malnourished[30]. In another sample of adults aged 65–103 years selected from primary care, 70% reported no alcohol consumption during the past year. A total of 21.5% were moderate drinkers, 4.1% were at-risk drinkers and 4.5% were heavy or binge drinkers[31].

Bristow and Clare interviewed 650 medical and geriatric admissions over age 65 and found 9% of the men but few of the women drank in excess of recommended safety limits. Another 10% had drunk heavily over the age of 65 but cut down because of medical, social, financial or other reasons. Compared to the non-drinkers and light drinkers, the heavy drinkers were more likely to smoke, to be unmarried and to have some impairment of mobility[32]. In a similar sample of hospital patients aged 65+, 54% reported no alcohol consumption and 9% screened positive for alcohol problems (17% among male and 2.5% among female patients). Seven percent of the patients were discharged with an alcohol-related diagnosis[33].

IDENTIFICATION OF PROBLEM DRINKING

Clinicians may have difficulty detecting and diagnosing alcohol problems in older adults for a number of reasons. Screening instruments used in younger populations to detect problem drinking may not be as reliable for older adults[34,35]. Adams et al. compared responses to a beverage-specific self-administered questionnaire about the quantity and frequency of alcohol use and episodes of binge drinking to the widely used CAGE questionnaire (Cut down, Annoyed by criticism, Guilty about drinking, Eye-opener drinks)[29] in 5065 primary care patients age 60+, and found the CAGE performed poorly in detecting heavy or binge drinkers[27]. Many of the screening instruments enquire about frequency and quantity of alcohol use, but even small amounts may be problematic for older adults with chronic health conditions and in combination with certain medications. Criteria for alcoholism often include problems with social and/or occupational functioning. However, older adults are less likely to be married or employed, and therefore less likely to report marital or job problems. Older drinkers may also be less likely to cause public disturbances resulting in legal problems[36].

Clinicians may be reluctant to enquire about alcohol use out of embarrassment or because the patient doesn't fit the stereotype of an alcoholic. They may also fail to diagnose alcohol problems because symptoms of alcohol misuse may be similar to symptoms of ageing such as cognitive difficulties[37]. Adams et al. screened patients 65+ seen in the emergency department for alcoholism. Using their criteria of either CAGE-positive or self-reported drinking problems and alcohol use within the past year, they found the current prevalence of alcohol abuse was 14%, with a high prevalence (22%) among those presenting with gastrointestinal problems. Physicians, however, detected only 21% of current alcohol abusers[38]. In a study from primary care, only 41.6% of older patients who screened positive for alcoholism had a diagnosis of alcoholism recorded in their medical record[30]. In a study where all new admissions to the medical service were screened for alcoholism using the CAGE and the Short Michigan Alcohol Screening Test (SMAST)[39], the prevalence of alcoholism was 27% in patents under 60 and 21% among patients aged 60+. These age differences were not significant. However, 60% of screen-positive younger patients were identified as having alcoholism by their house officers compared to only 37% of those aged 60+. Older patients with alcoholism were less likely to be diagnosed if they were White, female, or had completed high school. Even when diagnosed, older patients with alcoholism were less likely than younger patients to be referred for treatment[40].

Another identification problem is establishing what constitutes excessive drinking in older adults. Moos et al. compared several guidelines defining excessive drinking in a sample of 1291 older adults. Depending on the criteria used, 23 to 50% of the women and 29 to 45% of the men engaged in potentially unsafe drinking patterns. The number of drinks per week and per day was associated with alcohol use problems. The authors concluded that safe alcohol consumption levels should not necessarily be higher for men[41]. The National Institute on Alcohol Abuse and Alcoholism (NIAAA) and the Center for Substance Abuse Treatment Improvement protocol recommends that persons aged 65+ consume no more than one standard drink per day or seven drinks per week. Also, they should not consume more than four standard drinks on a given day[7].

In a study of community-dwelling older adults from New Zealand, the prevalence of hazardous alcohol consumption was 9.9%, and the lifetime prevalence of DSM-IV alcohol dependence was 24.8%. None of the physicians identified by the participants, however, had diagnosed alcohol problems in the past year, and only 4% reported a history of alcohol problems. The adults with hazardous patterns of alcohol use were twice as likely to be hospitalized but less likely to have seen their physician in the past year[42].

FACTORS ASSOCIATED WITH ALCOHOL USE

In general, older adults who consume alcohol are more likely to be male, be married, and have higher income and years of education, have a good social life and have fewer health conditions[13,20,43]. Older drinkers are also more likely to be current or former smokers[13]. Goodwin et al. found no differences in social support between elderly drinkers and non-drinkers, and no relationship between alcohol intake and emotional status. They also reported that those older adults who consumed alcohol performed better on cognitive functioning tests, but no relationship was found between past alcohol consumption and present cognitive performance[20].

A somewhat different profile emerges for older adults with drinking problems. Heavy drinking has been shown to be associated with male gender, younger age, being unmarried, fewer years of education, smoking, depressive symptoms, impairment in cognitive functioning and poor self-rated health[25,30,32,44,45]. While some studies have shown an association between alcoholism and functional limitations[32,45], Mangion et al. found that men aged 65+ classified as alcohol abusers were more independently mobile than those not abusing alcohol, suggesting greater physical fitness[24]. As another example of conflicting results, in a sample of Medicare beneficiaries, unhealthy drinking patterns were associated with higher education and income and better health status[25].

In a study of 209 patients selected from a geriatric inpatient ward in France, 54.5% of the patients had consumed alcohol in the past month and 52% consumed at least once per week. A total of 9% of the patients (3% of the women and 18% of the men) met criteria for DSM-IV alcohol dependence. In a comparison between those with and without alcohol dependence, those with the disorder were more likely to be younger, male, to consume alcohol at least one day a week, consume alcohol alone, to begin to drink in the morning, to have more drinking days per week, to more often consume >5 drinks on one occasion, be treated with benzodiazepines, and be dependent on nicotine[46].

In a study of adults aged 70–75 in Italy, higher self-reported alcohol consumption was associated with: male gender; better mood, daily function and somatic health; not living alone and being married; while CAGE-detected alcoholism was associated with male gender, poorer cognitive function and income dissatisfaction. There was not much overlap between the groups[47]. Mirand and Welte studied the relationship between health-oriented lifestyle and heavy drinking among older adults in Erie County, New York, and reported that the prevalence of heavy drinking was 6%. Heavy drinking was positively associated with being male, having suburban residency and currently smoking, and negatively associated with socioeconomic status, rural residency and degree of health orientation. Age and level of active lifestyle were not related to drinking[48].

Changes in alcohol use have also been studied. Moos et al. followed a cohort of adults aged 55–65 for 10 years and found overall that health-related problems increased and alcohol consumption and drinking problems declined over the follow-up interval. Medical conditions, physical symptoms, medication use and acute health events predicted a higher likelihood of abstinence and less frequent and lower alcohol consumption. Increased health problems predicted

reduced alcohol consumption but more drinking problems[49]. Pereira and Sloan examined the relationship between the experience of life events and changes in alcohol consumption using four waves of the Health and Retirement Study. Alcohol consumption did not change for the majority of older adults (68%) over the six years. Hospitalization and onset of a chronic illness were associated with a decrease in consumption, while widowhood was associated with a short-term increase in drinking. Onset of retirement was associated with increased drinking. Getting married or divorced was associated with both increases and decreases in drinking[50].

ONSET OF PROBLEM DRINKING

In research focusing on the age of onset among elderly problem drinkers, two groups have emerged. There are older adults who have had problems with alcohol for most of their adult life and have survived to old age, generally referred to as 'early-onset' problem drinkers. There are also older adults who may or may not have consumed alcohol earlier in their lives, but who do not become problem drinkers until later in their adult life, a group referred to as 'late-onset' problem drinkers.

Atkinson et al. studied the age of onset among 132 men aged 60+ admitted into an outpatient treatment programme and found onset after age 60 in 15% of the sample and in 29% of the sample aged 65+. Later-onset alcohol problems were milder, associated with less family alcoholism and associated with greater psychological stability. Treatment variables were better predictors of outcome than age of onset[51]. In a similar sample of patients admitted to an alcoholism treatment programme, late-onset alcoholism was present in 39% of the men and 46% of the women. Few differences were noted between the two groups[52].

Symptom presentation may differ by age of onset. In a study of 268 patients on an alcohol detoxification ward in Germany, alcohol dependence was diagnosed in 94.1% of those with an earlier onset but in only 62.2% among those with a later onset. Those with late onset were less likely than those with a younger onset to report a strong desire to drink alcohol, impaired capacity to control drinking, and preoccupation with drinking[53].

Brennan and Moos reported that late-middle-aged problem drinkers reported more negative life events, chronic stressors and social resource deficits than did non-problem drinkers. Among problem drinkers, those with late onset consumed less alcohol, reported fewer alcohol-related problems, functioned better and had fewer stressors than early-onset problem drinkers[54,55].

Age of onset may differ by gender. Brennan et al. found that women with drinking problems consumed less alcohol, had fewer drinking problems, and reported more recent onset of drinking problems than did male problem drinkers. The female problem drinkers also used more psychoactive medications, were more depressed and were less likely to seek treatment[56]. Osterling and Berglund examined gender differences in age of onset among older first-time admitted alcoholics in Sweden across two time periods. During the period 1978–1982, they found that age of onset of problem drinking occurred significantly later in females compared to males. One decade later, during the period 1988–1992, sex ratios indicated a significant convergence in age of onset for female patients to that of males[57].

Moos et al. followed a cohort of problem drinkers aged 55–65 for one year. Remitted problem drinkers were those who did not experience any problems in the follow-up period. Late-onset drinkers were more likely to remit during the year. At baseline, the to-be remitted problem drinkers consumed less alcohol, reported fewer drinking problems, had friends who approved less of their drinking, and were likely to seek help from a mental health practitioner[58].

OUTCOMES ASSOCIATED WITH ALCOHOL USE

The relationship between alcohol use and physical health is not straightforward. In cross-sectional studies, patients with alcoholism have an increased likelihood of some chronic diseases and decreased likelihood of others. Callahan and Tierney reported that patients with alcoholism were less likely to have a diagnosis of hypertension, arthritis or diabetes, and more likely to have obstructive lung diseases, injuries and gout[30]. Hurt et al. described 216 older inpatients treated for alcoholism. The frequency of serious medical disorders among this group was higher than what would be expected for the overall population aged 65+. Hypertension was less frequent among these patients, but alcoholic liver disease, chronic obstructive pulmonary disease, peptic ulcer disease and psoriasis were more prevalent among the alcoholic group compared to the population at large. The frequencies of ischaemic heart disease, cerebrovascular disease and diabetes were about the same as what would be found in an older population[52].

In longitudinal studies, moderate alcohol use in older adults has been shown to decrease the risk of stroke[59], heart failure[60–62] and incident diabetes[63]. It is not clear whether there is a true protective effect of alcohol or whether older adults who consume alcohol are already in better health. In the Framingham Study, alcohol consumption was not associated with stroke across all age groups, but alcohol intake among those aged 60–69 was associated with a lower risk of stroke. In addition, former drinking of 12 or more grams of alcohol per day was associated with 2.4-times higher risk of stroke among men[64]. Drinking in excess has been associated with adverse health outcomes as well as protective effects. For example, heavy consumption of alcohol may be associated with an increased risk of stroke[59]. In the Cardiovascular Health Study, however, consumption of 14 or more drinks per week was associated with a reduced risk of coronary heart disease[65]. In the NESARC, women aged 65 or older who consumed alcohol had better self-perceived health, improved cardiovascular health and lower rates of hospitalizations. No associations for men were significant[66]. Older adults particularly those with pre-existing drinking problems may use alcohol to manage pain. Older men with drinking problems who used alcohol to manage pain had more health problems and injuries while female problem drinkers who used alcohol for pain had more drinking problems three years later[67].

Studies have also shown that alcohol problems in older adults are associated with psychiatric co-morbidity. Saunders et al. reported that 44% of men aged 65 or older with a history of heavy drinking were given current psychiatric diagnoses, compared with 12% of the men without a history of heavy drinking. The most common diagnoses were depression and dementia. The association between drinking history and current psychiatric morbidity was not explained by current drinking habits[68]. The prevalence of alcohol use is three- to four-times greater among depressed older adults compared to those who are non-depressed. Among older adults with major depression, the prevalence of an alcohol use disorder is 15–30%. Depression can put the older adult at risk for alcohol problems, and alcohol use disorders can be a risk factor for late-life depression[69].

Increased hospitalizations have also been linked with alcohol use in the elderly. Callahan and Tierney reported that older patients with alcoholism were more likely to be hospitalized within the year following the interview, compared to those without alcoholism (21.5% vs. 16.9%)[30]. Using 1989 hospital claims data, the prevalence of alcohol-related hospitalizations among persons age 65+ in the USA was 54.7 per 10 000 population for men and 14.8 per 10 000 for women, a proportion similar to that seen for myocardial infarction[70].

The relationship between alcohol use and mortality is also complex. In a study from Finland, drinking had an independent protective effect on 10-year mortality among older adults. Mortality was lowest among frequent and occasional drinkers, second lowest among abstainers, and highest among ex-drinkers. In analyses controlling for variables such as chronic disease and smoking, frequent drinkers had a reduced risk compared with abstainers[71]. Paganini-Hill et al. studied changes in alcohol intake over 23 years in a sample of residents of a California retirement community. Those who drank 2+ drinks per day had a 15% reduced risk of death. Stable drinkers also had a reduced risk compared to non-stable drinkers. Women who quit drinking had an increased risk of death, suggesting persons who quit may do so for reasons that affect mortality[72]. In a community-based longitudinal Australian study of women 70–75 years old at baseline, women who did not consume alcohol or drank rarely were more likely to die compared to women in the low-intake category[73].

In contrast to moderate drinking, alcoholism has been linked to increased mortality. In a sample of elderly male veterans from primary care clinics at Veteran Administration medical centres, where the prevalence of alcohol use can be higher than in the general older population, 48% of the veterans reported drinking in the past year. Half of the drinkers and non-drinkers screened positive for problem drinking. Overall health status and survival were better in drinkers compared to non-drinkers, but worse in those who screened positive for problem drinking compared to those who screened negative[74]. Callahan and Tierney found that patients with alcoholism were more likely to die within two years than those without evidence of alcoholism; 10.6% compared to 6.3%, controlling for age, gender, race, education and smoking history[30]. Hurt et al. followed a sample of inpatients treated for alcoholism for an average of 5.2 years. A total of 32% had died by follow-up. Of those who died, 47% of the deaths could be attributed to the patient's alcoholism[52]. In the Canadian Study of Health and Aging, alcohol abuse was associated with short-term mortality[75]. In a retrospective case control study of 1735 older people that died of falls, motor vehicle crashes or death by suicide and 13 381 controls, having 12+ drinks in the past year was associated with an increased risk of fatal injury[76]. Finally, at-risk drinking was associated with increased 20-year mortality in men when 'at-risk' was determined by the amount of alcohol consumed in the presence of relevant co-morbidities (e.g. an illness or medication use)[77].

Heavy drinking has also been shown to be associated with impairments in physical function. In a study of 161 primary care patients aged 60+, 16% of the patients consumed 8–14 drinks, and 22% had more than 14 drinks per week. Forty two percent of the sample (33% of the men and 51% of the women) reported binge drinking (four or more drinks on one occasion for men and three or more for women) in the past year. Compared to those having fewer than 7 drinks per week, those consuming more than 14 drinks per week were more likely to have impairments in instrumental activities of daily living (IADLs) and advanced activities of daily living (ADLs). Those having 7–14 drinks per week were more likely to have impairments in IADLs but not ADLs. Binge drinkers were more likely to have impairments in IADLs[78].

Other studies have reported different findings. Using data from the Health and Retirement Study in the United States and the English

Longitudinal Study of Ageing, samples of adults aged 65+ followed from four to five years, Lang *et al.* reported that 10.8% of US men, 28.6% of English men, 2.9% of US women and 10.3% of English women drank above USA recommended limits for this age group. Functional outcomes did not differ between those who drank >0–1 drink per day and those who drank >1–2 drinks per day[79]. Karla-mangla *et al.* found that light to moderate drinking was associated with a decreased risk of incident disability compared with abstention. Disability risk decreased with light to moderate drinking among men and women with good or better self-reported health, but not among those with fair or worse self-rated health[80]. La Croix *et al.* found, by following three of the EPESE cohorts for four years, that older adults who did not consume alcohol had an increased risk of losing mobility, defined as the ability to climb up and down stairs and walk half a mile, compared to those with small to moderate amounts of alcohol consumption[81].

The relationship between alcohol consumption and cognitive performance has received considerable attention in this population. In the Honolulu-Asia Aging Study, non-drinkers and heavy drinkers had poorer scores on cognitive functioning tests compared to those who consumed 1–60 ounces (28.4–1701 g) of alcohol per month[82]. A protective effect has also been reported from longitudinal studies. In the Cardiovascular Health Study, older adults who consumed one to six drinks weekly had a lower risk of incident dementia compared to those who abstained[83]. In a study of adults aged 75+ from Sweden, light to moderate drinking was associated with a decreased risk of six-year incident dementia and Alzheimer's disease compared with non-drinking[84]. In a two-year study of older adults in China, light to moderate drinking was associated with a lower risk of dementia compared to non-drinking, while excessive drinking was associated with a higher risk of dementia[85]. In the Canadian Study of Health and Aging, the occurrence of all types of dementia except probable Alzheimer's disease was higher in those older adults with definite or questionable alcohol abuse[75]. Other studies have not found an association between drinking and incident cognitive impairment[86]. A study from China reported among older adults with mild cognitive impairment that those with light to moderate alcohol consumption had a decreased risk of transition to dementia over two years when compared to abstainers or heavy drinkers. Heavy drinkers with mild cognitive impairment had a higher risk compared to those with light to moderate use and abstainers[87]. Researchers from the Italian Longitudinal Study on Aging reported that older adults with mild cognitive impairment who were moderate drinkers had a lower rate of progression to dementia than abstainers. Older adults with mild cognitive impairment and higher levels of drinking, however, did not have a higher rate of progression to dementia compared to abstainers. Incidence of mild cognitive impairment was not associated with any level of drinking compared to abstainers[88].

In the NESARC, only 3.54% of current drinkers aged 65+ with an alcohol use disorder in the past year and 1% of older adults classified as heavy drinkers received any alcohol treatment in the past year[13]. Long-term remission among older untreated problem drinkers followed for 10 years was predicted by being female, having a recent onset of drinking problems, having fewer and less severe drinking problems, having friends who approved less of drinking, and drinking less and less frequently at baseline. Long-term remitted problem drinkers attained levels of functioning and life context similar to those of lifetime non-problem drinkers, but remitted problem drinkers continued to report more incipient drinking problems, depressive symptoms, health and financial stressors, psychoactive

medication use, less social support and dependence on avoidance coping strategies compared to lifetime non-problem drinkers[89].

SUMMARY

Alcohol use, including drinking in excess, among older adults is prevalent, particularly among males. Because of interactions with chronic disease and prescribed medications, the use of alcohol among older adults is an important health concern. Given the higher prevalence of alcohol use disorders among middle-aged adults, the numbers of older adults with alcohol-related problems is expected to increase in future generations. Screening and questioning for alcohol problems should be routine. Drinking within recommended guidelines could potentially decrease the proportion of alcohol-related illness, hospitalizations and mortality seen in this population.

REFERENCES

1. Kessler RC, Berglund P, Demler O *et al.* Lifetime prevalence and age-of-onset distributions of DSM-IV disorders in the National Comorbidity Survey Replication. *Arch Gen Psychiatry* 2005; **62**: 593–602.
2. Hasin DS, Stinson FS, Ogburn E *et al.* Prevalence, correlates, disability, and comorbidity of DSM-IV alcohol abuse and dependence in the United States: results from the National Epidemiologic Survey on Alcohol and Related Conditions. *Arch Gen Psychiatry* 2007; **64**: 830–42.
3. Helzer JE, Burnam A, McEvoy LT. Alcohol abuse and dependence. In Robins LN, Regier DA (eds), *Psychiatric Disorders in America: The Epidemiologic Catchment Area Study*. New York: Macmillan, 1991, 81–115.
4. Narrow WE, Rae DS, Robins LN *et al.* Revised prevalence estimates of mental disorders in the United States. *Arch Gen Psychiatry* 2002; **59**: 115–23.
5. Regier DA, Boyd JH, Burke JD *et al.* One-month prevalence of mental disorders in the United States. *Arch Gen Psychiatry* 1988; **45**: 977–86.
6. Onen S-H, Onen F, Mangeon J-P *et al.* Alcohol abuse and dependence in elderly emergency department patients. *Arch Gerontol Geriatr* 2005; **41**: 191–200.
7. Oslin DW. Late-life alcoholism. *Am J Geriatr Psychiatry* 2004; **12**: 571–83.
8. Vestal RE, McGuire EA, Tobin JD *et al.* Aging and ethanol metabolism. *Clin Pharmacol Ther* 1977; **21**: 343–54.
9. Aira M, Hartikainen S, Sulkava R. Community prevalence of alcohol use and concomitant use of medication – a source of possible risk in the elderly aged 75 and older? *Int J Geriatr Psychiatry* 2005; **20**: 680–5.
10. Pringle KE, Ahern FM, Heller DA *et al.* Potential for alcohol and prescription drug interactions in older people. *J Am Geriatr Soc* 2005; **53**: 1930–6.
11. Patterson TL, Jeste DV. The potential impact of the baby-boom generation on substance abuse among elderly persons. *Psychiatr Serv* 1999; **50**: 1184–8.
12. Chermack ST, Blow FC, Hill EM *et al.* The relationship between alcohol symptoms and consumption among older drinkers. *Alcohol Clin Exp Res* 1996; **20**: 1153–8.
13. National Institute on Alcohol Abuse and Alcoholism. *Alcohol Use and Alcohol Use Disorders in the United States: Main Findings from the 2001–2002 National Epidemiologic Survey*

on *Alcohol and Related Conditions (NESARC)*. Bethesda, MD: National Institutes of Health, 2006.

14. Ruchlin HS. Prevalence and correlates of alcohol use among older adults. *Prev Med* 1997; **26**: 651–7.

15. Busby WJ, Campbell AJ, Borrie MJ *et al.* Alcohol use in a community-based sample of subjects aged 70 years and older. *J Am Geriatr Soc* 1988; **36**: 301–5.

16. Adams WL, Garry PJ, Rhyne R *et al.* Alcohol intake in the healthy elderly: Changes with age in a cross-sectional and longitudinal study. *J Am Geriatr Soc* 1990; **38**: 211–16.

17. Bjork C, Thygesen LC, Vinther-Larsen M *et al.* Time trends in heavy drinking among middle-aged and older adults in Denmark. *Alcohol Clin Exp Res* 2008; **32**: 120–7.

18. Karlamangla A, Zhou K, Rueben D *et al.* Longitudinal trajectories of heavy drinking in adults in the United States of America. *Addiction* 2006; **101**: 91–9.

19. Kerr WC, Greenfield TK, Bond J *et al.* Age, period and cohort influences on beer, wine and spirits consumption trends in the US National Alcohol Surveys. *Addiction* 2004; **99**: 1111–20.

20. Goodwin JS, Sanchez CJ, Thomas P *et al.* Alcohol intake in a healthy elderly population. *Am J Public Health* 1987; **77**: 173–7.

21. Cornoni-Huntley J, Brock D, Ostfeld A *et al. Established Populations for Epidemiologic Studies of the Elderly: Resource Data Book*, NIH publication no. 86-2443. Bethesda, MD: National Institutes of Health, 1986.

22. Cornoni-Huntley J, Blazer DG, Lafferty ME *et al. Established Populations for Epidemiologic Studies of the Elderly: Resource Data Book Volume II*, NIH publication no. 90-495. Washington, DC: National Institutes of Health, 1990.

23. Saunders PA, Copeland JRM, Dewey ME *et al.* Alcohol use and abuse in the elderly: findings from the Liverpool Longitudinal Study of Continuing Health in the Community. *Int J Geriatr Psychiatry* 1989; **4**: 103–8.

24. Mangion DM, Platt JS, Syam V. Alcohol and acute medical admission of elderly people. *Age Ageing* 1992; **21**: 362–7.

25. Merrick EL, Horgan CM, Hodgkin D *et al.* Unhealthy drinking patterns in older adults: prevalence and associated characteristics. *J Am Geriatr Soc* 2008; **56**: 214–23.

26. Centers for Disease Control and Prevention (CDC). Sociodemographic differences in binge drinking among adults – 14 states, 2004. *MMWR Morb Mortal Wkly Rep* 2009; **58**: 301–4.

27. Adams WL, Barry KL, Fleming MF. Screening for problem drinking in older primary care patients. *J Am Med Assoc* 1996; **276**: 1964–7.

28. Iliffe S, Haines A, Booroff A *et al.* Alcohol consumption by elderly people: a general practice survey. *Age Ageing* 1991; **20**: 120–3.

29. Mayfield D, McLeod G, Hall P. The CAGE questionnaire: validation of a new alcoholism screening instrument. *Am J Psychiatry* 1974; **131**: 1121–3.

30. Callahan CM, Tierney WM. Health services use and mortality among older primary care patients with alcoholism. *J Am Geriatr Soc* 1995; **43**: 1378–83.

31. Kirchner JE, Zubritsky C, Cody M *et al.* Alcohol consumption among older adults in primary care. *J Gen Intern Med* 2007; **22**: 92–7.

32. Bristow MF, Clare AW. Prevalence and characteristics of at-risk drinkers among elderly acute medical in-patients. *Br J Addict* 1992; **87**: 291–4.

33. Ganry O, Joly J-P, Queval M-P *et al.* Prevalence of alcohol problems among elderly patients in a university hospital. *Addiction* 2000; **95**: 107–13.

34. Beullens J, Aertgeerts B. Screening for alcohol abuse and dependence in older people using DSM criteria: a review. *Aging Ment Health* 2004; **8**: 76–82.

35. O'Connell H, Chin AV, Hamilton F *et al.* A systematic review of the utility of self-report alcohol screening instruments in the elderly. *Int J Geriatr Psychiatry* 2004; **19**: 1074–86.

36. O'Connell H, Chin A-V, Cunningham C *et al.* Alcohol use disorders in elderly people – redefining an age old problem in old age. *BMJ* 2003; **327**: 664–7.

37. Sorocco KH, Ferrell SW. Alcohol use among older adults. *J Gen Psychol* 2006; **133**: 453–67.

38. Adams WL, Magruder-Habib K, Trued S *et al.* Alcohol abuse in elderly emergency department patients. *J Am Geriatr Soc* 1992; **40**: 1236–40.

39. Selzer ML, Vinokur A, Rooijen L. A self-administered Short Michigan Alcoholism Screening Test (SMAST). *J Stud Alcohol* 1975; **36**: 117.

40. Curtis JR, Geller G, Stokes EJ *et al.* Characteristics, diagnosis, and treatment of alcoholism in elderly patients. *J Am Geriatr Soc* 1989; **37**: 310–16.

41. Moos RH, Brennan PL, Schutte KK *et al.* High-risk alcohol consumption and late-life alcohol use problems. *Am J Public Health* 2004; **94**: 1985–91.

42. Khan N, Davis P, Wilkinson TJ *et al.* Drinking patterns among older people in the community: hidden from medical attention? *N Z Med J* 2002; **115**: 72–5.

43. Hajat S, Haines A, Bulpitt C *et al.* Patterns and determinants of alcohol consumption in people aged 75 years and older: results from the MRC trial of assessment and management of older people in the community. *Age Ageing* 2004; **33**: 170–7.

44. Finlayson RE, Hurt RD, Davis LJ *et al.* Alcoholism in elderly persons: a study of the psychiatric and psychosocial features of 216 inpatients. *Mayo Clin Proc* 1988; **63**: 761–8.

45. St John PD, Montgomery PR, Tyas SL. Alcohol misuse, gender and depressive symptoms in community-dwelling seniors. *Int J Geriatr Psychiatry* 2009; **24**: 369–75.

46. Lejoyeux M, Delaroque F, McLoughlin M *et al.* Alcohol dependence among elderly French inpatients. *Am J Geriatr Psychiatry* 2003; **11**: 360–4.

47. Geroldi C, Rozzini R, Frisoni GB *et al.* Assessment of alcohol consumption and alcoholism in the elderly. *Alcohol* 1994; **11**: 513–16.

48. Mirand AL, Welte JW. Alcohol consumption among the elderly in a general population, Erie County, New York. *Am J Public Health* 1996; **86**: 978–84.

49. Moos RH, Brennan PL, Schutte KK *et al.* Older adults' health and changes in late-life drinking patterns. *Aging Ment Health* 2005; **9**: 49–59.

50. Perreira KM, Sloan FA. Life events and alcohol consumption among mature adults: a longitudinal analysis. *J Stud Alcohol* 2001; **62**: 501–8.

51. Atkinson RM, Tolson RL, Turner JA. Late versus early onset problem drinking in older men. *Alcohol Clin Exp Res* 1990; **14**: 574–9.

52. Hurt RD, Finlayson RE, Morse RM *et al.* Alcoholism in elderly persons: medical aspects and prognosis of 216 inpatients. *Mayo Clin Proc* 1988; **63**: 753–60.

53. Wetterling T, Veltrup C, John U *et al*. Late onset alcoholism. *Eur Psychiatry* 2003; **18**: 112–18.

54. Brennan PL, Moos RH. Life stressors, social resources, and late-life problem drinking. *Psychol Aging* 1990; **5**: 491–501.

55. Brennan PL, Moos RH. Functioning, life context, and help-seeking among late-onset problem drinkers: comparisons with nonproblem and early-onset problem drinkers. *Br J Addict* 1991; **86**: 1139–50.

56. Brennan PL, Moos RH, Kim JY. Gender differences in the individual characteristics and life contexts of late-middle-aged and older problem drinkers. *Addiction* 1993; **88**: 781–90.

57. Osterling A, Berglund M. Elderly first time admitted alcoholics: a descriptive study on gender differences in a clinical population. *Alcohol Clin Exp Res* 1994; **18**: 1317–21.

58. Moos RH, Brennan PL, Moos BS. Short-term processes of remission and nonremission among late-life problem drinkers. *Alcohol Clin Exp Res* 1991; **15**: 948–55.

59. Sacco RL, Elkind M, Boden-Albala B *et al*. The protective effect of moderate alcohol consumption on ischemic stroke. *J Am Med Assoc* 1999; **281**: 53–60.

60. Bryson CL, Mukamal KJ, Mittleman MA *et al*. The association of alcohol consumption and incident heart failure. *J Am Coll Cardiol* 2006; **48**: 305–11.

61. Djousse L, Gaziano JM. Alcohol consumption and risk of heart failure in the Physicians' Health Study I. *Circulation* 2007; **115**: 34–9.

62. Abramson JL, Williams SA, Krumholz HM *et al*. Moderate alcohol consumption and risk of heart failure among older persons. *J Am Med Assoc* 2001; **285**: 1971–7.

63. Djousse L, Biggs ML, Mukamal KJ *et al*. Alcohol consumption and Type 2 diabetes among older adults: the Cardiovascular Health Study. *Obesity* 2007; **15**: 1758–65.

64. Djousse L, Ellison RC, Beiser A *et al*. Alcohol consumption and risk of ischemic stroke: the Framingham Study. *Stroke* 2002; **33**: 907–12.

65. Mukamal KJ, Chung H, Jenny NS *et al*. Alcohol consumption and the risk of coronary heart disease in older adults: the Cardiovascular Health Study. *J Am Geriatr Soc* 2006; **54**: 30–7.

66. Balsa AI, Homer JF, Fleming MF *et al*. Alcohol consumption and health among elders. *Gerontologist* 2008; **48**: 622–36.

67. Brennan PL, Schutte KK, Moos RH. Pain and use of alcohol to manage pain: prevalence and 3-year outcomes among older problem and non-problem drinkers. *Addiction* 2005; **100**: 777–86.

68. Saunders PA, Copeland JRM, Dewey ME *et al*. Heavy drinking as a risk factor for depression and dementia in elderly men: findings from the Liverpool Longitudinal Community Study. *Br J Psychiatry* 1991; **159**: 213–16.

69. Devanand DP. Comorbid psychiatric disorders in late life depression. *Biol Psychiatry* 2002; **52**: 236–42.

70. Adams WL, Yuan Z, Barboriak JJ *et al*. Alcohol-related hospitalizations of elderly people: prevalence and geographic variation in the United States. *J Am Med Assoc* 1993; **270**: 1222–5.

71. Tolvanen E, Seppa K, Lintonen T *et al*. Old people, alcohol use and mortality: a ten-year prospective study. *Aging Clin Exp Res* 2005; **17**: 426–33.

72. Paganini-Hill A, Kawas CH, Corrada MM. Type of alcohol consumed, changes in intake over time and mortality: the Leisure World Cohort Study. *Age Ageing* 2007; **36**: 203–9.

73. Byles J, Young A, Furuya H *et al*. A drink to healthy aging: the association between older women's use of alcohol and their health-related quality of life. *J Am Geriatr Soc* 2006; **54**: 1341–7.

74. Bridevaux IP, Bradley KA, Bryson CL *et al*. Alcohol screening results in elderly male veterans: association with health status and mortality. *J Am Geriatr Soc* 2004; **52**: 1510–17.

75. Thomas VS, Rockwood KJ. Alcohol abuse, cognitive impairment, and mortality among older people. *J Am Geriatr Soc* 2001; **49**: 415–20.

76. Sorock GS, Chen LH, Gonzalgo SR *et al*. Alcohol-drinking history and fatal injury in older adults. *Alcohol* 2006; **40**: 193–9.

77. Moore AA, Giuli L, Gould R *et al*. Alcohol use, comorbidity, and mortality. *J Am Geriatr Soc* 2006; **54**: 757–62.

78. Moore AA, Endo JO, Carter MK. Is there a relationship between excessive drinking and functional impairment in older persons? *J Am Geriatr Soc* 2003; **51**: 44–9.

79. Lang I, Guralnick J, Wallace RB *et al*. What level of alcohol consumption is hazardous for older people? Functioning and mortality in U.S. and English national cohorts. *J Am Geriatr Soc* 2007; **55**: 49–57.

80. Karlamangla AS, Sarkisian CA, Kado DM *et al*. Light to moderate alcohol consumption and disability: variable benefits by health status. *Am J Epidemiol* 2009; **169**: 96–104.

81. LaCroix AZ, Guralnick JM, Berkman LF *et al*. Maintaining mobility in late life: II. Smoking, alcohol consumption, physical activity, and body mass index. *Am J Epidemiol* 1993; **137**: 858–69.

82. Galanis DJ, Joseph C, Masaki KH *et al*. A longitudinal study of drinking and cognitive performance in elderly Japanese American men: the Honolulu-Asia Aging Study. *Am J Public Health* 2000; **90**: 1254–9.

83. Mukamal KJ, Kuller LH, Fitzpatrick AL *et al*. Prospective study of alcohol consumption and risk of dementia in older adults. *J Am Med Assoc* 2003; **289**: 1405–13.

84. Huang W, Qiu C, Winblad B *et al*. Alcohol consumption and incidence of dementia in a community sample aged 75 years and older. *J Clin Epidemiol* 2002; **55**: 959–64.

85. Deng J, Zhou DHD, Li J *et al*. A 2-year follow-up study of alcohol consumption and risk of dementia. *Clin Neurol Neurosurg* 2006; **108**: 378–83.

86. Cervilla JA, Prince M, Mann A. Smoking, drinking, and incident cognitive impairment: a cohort community based study included in the Gospel Oak project. *J Neurol Neurosurg Psychiatry* 2000; **68**: 622–6.

87. Xu G, Liu X, Yin Q *et al*. Alcohol consumption and transition of mild cognitive impairment to dementia. *Psychiatry Clin Neurosci* 2009; **63**: 43–9.

88. Solfrizzi V, D'Introno A, Colacicco AM *et al*. Alcohol consumption, mild cognitive impairment, and progression to dementia. *Neurology* 2007; **68**: 1790–9.

89. Schutte KK, Byrne FE, Brennan PL *et al*. Successful remission of late-life drinking problems: a 10-year follow-up. *J Stud Alcohol* 2001; **62**: 322–34.

108

Drug Misuse in the Elderly

Martin M. Schmidt and Mohammed T. Abou-Saleh

Division of Mental Health, St George's University of London, London, UK

Substance misuse occurs mainly in young adults, with most research focusing on this group. Several factors, however, suggest a growing trend towards substance misuse in the elderly. Increasing age is associated with chronic illnesses and multiple medications, with the attendant risk of dependence. There is also evidence to support a growing trend to increased alcohol consumption in the over-65s, while a generation of lifetime drug users are now entering old age[1]. Along with the increase in ageing of European and North American populations, the number of older adults requiring treatment for substance misuse is predicted to double between 2001 and 2020[2]. The need for age-appropriate treatment interventions has never been greater.

USE, ABUSE AND HARMFUL USE

When considering drug use among the elderly it is helpful to consider substances of misuse in three broad categories: medications, both prescribed and non-prescribed; socially sanctioned psychoactive substances; and illicit substances. Self-evidently this will differ between countries due to religious, cultural and legal differences[3]. Some of the consequences of drug misuse are determined by the status of the drug rather than its physical effects. Difficulties in obtaining a drug supply and financing that use may account for as much harm as the physical effects of the drugs themselves in younger adults. Among the elderly, drugs from the medicines category are overrepresented in cases of misuse when compared to other age groups[4]. This reflects the increased access to medicines among this group, allied to the physical and social barriers that make accessing other drugs harder for this group. This chapter will focus on drug misusers who display 'harmful use'. This is defined as 'a pattern of psychoactive drug use that causes damage to health, either mental or physical'[5]. This definition allows consideration of individuals suffering damage as a result of drug use, irrespective of the nature or the source of the drug of abuse. It excludes cases where omission of a psychoactive medication may be harmful, e.g. in cases of underuse of antidepressants.

Harmful use may be related to a single episode of drug misuse resulting in harm, such as a fall while intoxicated. More often it is a chronic condition associated with a dependence syndrome. 'Dependence syndrome' describes the cluster of cognitive, behavioural and physical phenomena that are observed when use of a substance becomes a greater priority for the individual than other previously more valued activities. It is characterized by:

- a compulsion to take the substance;
- difficulties in controlling the substance use in terms of timing and levels of use;
- withdrawal symptoms on discontinuation of the substance, with relief of these symptoms on reinstatement of use;
- tolerance or neuroadaptation, where increasing amounts of the substance are required to achieve effects previously possible at lower doses;
- progressive neglect of alternative activities, due to prioritization of drug-related behaviour;
- persistent use of the substance in spite of evidence of harmful consequences.

Presence of three or more of the above features simultaneously in the past year supports a definite diagnosis of dependence syndrome, using World Health Organization criteria[6].

PHARMACOKINETICS

Ageing is associated with a series of physiological changes that significantly alter the fraction of an ingested drug available for a psychoactive effect. Drug absorption shows little variation with age, despite changes in gastrointestinal motility and acidity, reduced absorption surface and slowed gastric emptying. However, once absorbed, the volume of distribution in an elderly subject is likely to have changed.

Ageing results in an increase in percentage body fat and a fall in total body water. Hydrophilic drugs, such as alcohol, are distributed in body water, such that with increasing age the volume of distribution falls and the peak concentration for a given dose may rise by 20%[7], resulting in lower levels of intake giving the same intoxicant effect. Conversely, lipophilic drugs, such as benzodiazepines and other psychotropics, that are stored in fatty tissue will remain in the body for longer but at lower peak concentrations. A fall in plasma albumin in old age results in increased bioavailability of protein-bound drugs, such as warfarin and diazepam.

Drug elimination occurs primarily through direct excretion or metabolism. Both routes are reduced in the elderly. Glomerular filtration rates fall steadily in old age, leading to the accumulation of renally excreted drugs. This may be compounded by renal damage due to drug misuse, e.g. analgesic abuse[8]. Hepatic metabolism is impaired due to a loss of liver mass and a reduced blood flow, which may also be compounded by toxic drug effects. The efficiency

Principles and Practice of Geriatric Psychiatry, 3rd edn. Edited by Mohammed T. Abou-Saleh, Cornelius Katona and Anand Kumar
© 2011 John Wiley & Sons, Ltd

of microsomal oxidation also falls with age, leading to reduced drug excretion of hepatically metabolized drugs[9]. The combination of these effects may greatly alter pharmacokinetics in the elderly. For example the half-life of diazepam in the very elderly has been shown to be over 3 days, compared with 20 h in a younger subject[10].

Multiple drug use complicates the pharmacokinetics of a substance, due to competition for binding sites and metabolic pathways. Polypharmacy may have different effects, depending on whether it is acute or chronic. Alcohol will inhibit microsomal enzyme activity in acute use, while prolonged administration will induce the same enzymes. Hence, alcohol will acutely raise concentrations of benzodiazepines, while lowering them if used chronically[11].

Pharmacodynamics also alter in the elderly. Sensitivity to drugs, particularly those acting on the central nervous system, tends to increase, while drug receptor populations also change with increased age. The particular effects of age-related brain changes on the reward effects of abused substances is currently difficult to predict[12].

As a consequence of all these variables, the extrapolation of a drug's effects in the elderly, based on observation in younger adults, is foolhardy.

CONCLUSION

The terms 'old age' and 'substance misuse' are both terms that have a wide range of meaning to different readers. The current literature is based primarily upon chronological age banding of individuals, as opposed to banding by overall health, possibly a more valid measure. Definitions of substance misuse are similarly varied. Often in transgenerational studies, definitions of caseness are set at a level to prevent false-positive reports for younger adults. In older age groups, where less of a substance may have a greater effect, there is the possibility of missing cases if such standards are applied.

PREVALENCE AND CORRELATES

The elderly may display harmful use of any psychoactive substance. However, access to a potential substance of abuse is key to determining what an individual may misuse. Alcohol is obtainable with ease in most industrialized nations and is a socially acceptable and accessible psychoactive drug. Sedatives, hypnotics and analgesics are easily accessible through prescription and consequently, along with alcohol, are responsible for the majority of cases of harmful use. Over-the-counter medication is also easily obtained and may be misused. Illicit drugs are usually only available in potentially dangerous environments from individuals who may pose a significant risk to vulnerable older adults. Illicit drug use is therefore not commonly observed in the elderly, but numbers are on the rise[13]. Shah and Fountain identified the following as factors associated with illicit drug use in the elderly: male gender, 'young old' age group, belonging to the post-war cohort, African American ethnicity, prior convictions, diagnosis of mental illness or alcohol misuse, serious medical illness and past history of substance misuse with onset before age of 30[14].

BENZODIAZEPINES

Benzodiazepines replaced barbiturates as the mainstay of pharmacological interventions in both anxiety and sleep disturbance. Benzodiazepines accumulate more readily in the elderly due to changes in body composition, leading to a greater volume of distribution for lipophilic drugs[10]. Chronic use may contribute to toxic effects, including cognitive impairment, poor attention and anterograde amnesia, cerebellar signs such as ataxia, dysarthria, tremor, impaired coordination and drowsiness[15]. Increased falls and hip fractures are associated with benzodiazepine use in the elderly[16] while withdrawal may be accompanied by rebound insomnia, agitation, convulsions and an acute confusional state. If benzodiazepines are required for the elderly then short-acting drugs (i.e. with half-life less than 24 hours) at the lowest effective dose may be used for a short duration[17]. There is no 'safe' period of use but tolerance and dependence levels increase with prolonged use[18].

Prevalence of Benzodiazepine Use

Establishing levels of benzodiazepine among the elderly is problematic. National prescription audits can reflect trends in use but are unhelpful when considering particular population subgroups.

Following the publication of guidance for the appropriate use of benzodiazepines by the UK Committee on Safety of Medicines (CSM) in 1988[19], prescribing of benzodiazepines has fallen dramatically. In England and Wales prescriptions have fallen by 32% from 1987 to 1996[20], while prescribing of benzodiazepines by general practitioners in England has fallen from 15.8 million prescriptions in 1992 to 12.7 million in 2002[21]. Of concern, however, is that 30% of prescriptions were for long-term treatment and 56% of prescriptions for the three most commonly prescribed benzodiazepines were issued to patients over the age of 65[21]. More recent trends for England show a relatively stable annual prescription rate of 10 million items for hypnotics; however, Z drugs (zopiclone, zolpidem, zaleplon) appear to be responsible for a larger proportion of prescriptions, rising from 33% in 2001 to 44% in 2004[22].

A community follow-up study of 5 000 over-65s in Liverpool[23] revealed that 10% were using benzodiazepines on first assessment and that of these some 70% were taking a benzodiazepine two years later. A further four-year follow-up revealed that 69% of these were still on benzodiazepines. Women were twice as likely to be taking a benzodiazepine as men at any stage in the study. In the USA, a study found 6.3% of a large sample of over-65s used a hypnotic, one third of these daily and nine tenths for at least a year[24]. Five-year follow-up found 46.6% still using hypnotics, but with a switch away from barbiturates and longer-acting benzodiazepines towards short-acting ones[25].

Use of benzodiazepines in institutional samples has traditionally been higher and associated with female gender, greater age, bereavement and poor health[26]. Chronic benzodiazepine use in older adults' nursing homes has been associated with depression, sleep disturbances and demand for medication[27]. In the USA a study found that one quarter of nursing home residents were prescribed a benzodiazepine and nearly 10% of all residents had chronic benzodiazepine use[27]. Studies from other countries reveal similarly high levels of benzodiazepine use among institutionalized older adults[28].

The level of morbidity among institutional residents is likely to be higher than community-dwelling elders. While chronic pain may require treatment with dependence-inducing medication, there are few indications for long-term benzodiazepine use. It has been argued that the regular use of benzodiazepines in institutions is a form of behavioural control, used more for the benefit of staff and others than these users. In many cases, the individual may be incapable of giving valid consent to taking such medication. The use of medication in such circumstances may be considered benzodiazepine misuse by some and as elder abuse by others[29].

Correlates

Psychiatric morbidity

Significantly high rates of psychiatric disorder have been described among elderly benzodiazepine users[30]. Among elders using short-acting benzodiazepines as hypnotics, one third reach caseness for depression, while a further third have a diagnosable anxiety disorder. Among users of anxiolytic benzodiazepines, half are depressed and one fifth are anxious in spite of treatment. As with alcohol misusers, one third of elders requiring inpatient treatment for benzodiazepine misuse are of late onset, while two thirds have graduated from misusing benzodiazepines or other drugs while younger[31]. The incidence of co-morbid alcohol abuse has not been consistently shown to be significantly greater among benzodiazepine misusers[31]. However, more recent research suggests that a prior history of alcoholism may predispose to later benzodiazepine misuse in the elderly[32]. An all-age study found that DSM-III-R Axis I co-morbidity existed in all cases of a sample of benzodiazepine-dependent users in Spain[33]. The commonest diagnoses were insomnia, anxiety disorders and affective disorders. Obsessive–compulsive, histrionic and dependent personality disorders were found in half of the cases and physical problems in one third of the cases.

Gender and age

Benzodiazepine use is over-represented among women of all ages. The likelihood of use of a benzodiazepine increases with age. There is little evidence that this gender divide narrows on reaching old age. Legislative approaches and prescribing guidelines have made some inroads into the over-representation of prescribing to the elderly[34]. Increasing public awareness of the side effects of benzodiazepines and an increase in advocacy services for the elderly are likely to have a similar effect.

OTHER PRESCRIBED AND OVER-THE-COUNTER MEDICATION

The elderly routinely receive a wide variety of medications, the majority of which may be misused. One quarter of prescription drugs sold in the United States are used by the elderly often for conditions such as chronic pain, insomnia and anxiety[35]. Ten per cent of over-64s are on prescribed analgesics at any one time, with at least an equal number using over-the-counter medication. Edwards and Salib[36] found 3% of a community sample of over-65s to have been using mild opiate analgesics for a period of at least a year; 40% of this group were deemed to fulfil the criteria for dependence. In addition to the dependence caused by these drugs, physical harm may also result, e.g. nephropathy may be caused by the use of paracetamol, salicylates and pyrazole derivatives, while renal impairment occurs with non-steroidal anti-inflammatory drug use[37]. Chronic nephropathy may also be caused by the excessive ingestion of analgesic mixtures combining two or more antipyretic analgesics, along with codeine or caffeine (both independently capable of causing addiction). Such acute and chronic effects are more likely among the elderly, where relative drug levels are higher and less biological reserve exists. Similar physical complications may arise from the misuse of other medications, the commonest being laxatives and cough mixtures.

ILLICIT DRUG MISUSE

Little is known about levels of illicit drug use among the over-65s, although the general perception is that it has been less of a problem than the misuse of prescribed medication. Overall the prevalence of illicit drug use in the elderly is low compared to younger people[14].

In the Epidemiological Catchment Area Study (ECA), only 0.1% of elders met the criteria for drug abuse for an illicit substance in the previous month. Lifetime prevalence was 1.6% for over-65s[38]. Figures from the 2005 and 2006 National Survey on Drug Use and Health found similar low rates in the elderly along with higher rates in the middle aged, lending further evidence to the suggestion that prevalence rates may rise in the elderly as the younger cohort ages[39]. Current predictions are that the number of older adults requiring substance abuse treatment in the USA will increase from 1.2 million in 2000 to 4.4 million in 2020[13].

The 2007/8 British crime survey reported the following in 55–59 year olds: 17.9% had used illicit drugs at some point in the past, 1.7% had used in the last year, and 0.9%, in the last month[40]. No figures were available for older age groups because respondents over 59 were not asked about illicit drug use. The decision to omit drug use questions in this age group was based on previous surveys which showed a lifetime prevalence of less than 1% for people aged 60 and over[14].

In the UK, few cases of illicit drug use among the over-65s have found their way into the literature; one exception is a series of seven elderly reported to have initiated injecting heroin in later life. They attributed their behaviour to a combination of loneliness and depression[41].

In the USA, in a study of a Veterans Administration old age psychiatry inpatient facility, 3% of the patients were found to have a primary drug misuse disorder involving prescribed medication, while 1% were addicted to illicit substances[32]. Also in the USA, attendance at methadone maintenance clinics by the elderly is reported to be rising, although over-60s still form 2% of those attending[4]. Similarly, a number of elders are reported to continue their use of cannabis into late life[42]. Anecdotal evidence also points to some individuals initiating the use of cannabis in later life in a search for its reputed therapeutic benefit in conditions such as multiple sclerosis.

On balance, it appears that illicit drug use is less of a problem in the elderly than the abuse of legally sanctioned drugs.

POLYSUBSTANCE MISUSE

The elderly have access to a variety of drugs of misuse. In many cases they may misuse one drug without misusing others. This is often the case with prescribed medication, where one medication is overused while compliance with the prescription is maintained for the others. Where non-prescribed substances become involved, the possibility of abuse of more than one substance is elevated. Finlayson and Davis[30] found 15% of over-65s requiring inpatient detoxification from alcohol were also dependent upon a second substance, usually a hypnotic, anxiolytic or analgesic. The phenomenon of cross-tolerance must also be considered. Psychoactive substances may have a cumulative effect, due to either a shared outcome effect or to different drugs acting as interchangeable substitutes for one another (cross-tolerance). Cross-tolerance exists within each class of drug, such that the clinician should always consider the total benzodiazepine or opioid dose, using class-specific equivalence charts[43]. Cross-tolerance for some drugs may also occur outside of the class, most notably for alcohol and benzodiazepines. While this phenomenon is widely exploited for detoxification, failure to consider the clinical possibility may lead to overlooking cases of dependence.

CONCLUSION

Alcohol and prescribed medication remain the most prevalent substances misused by the elderly. There is little clear evidence of great changes in individuals' addictive behaviour patterns with increasing age. However, a convincing body of evidence points towards a relative and absolute increase in older adults requiring specialist treatment for illicit drug use in the future.

TREATMENT

Treatment of substance misuse is a multistage process involving the integrated use of physical, psychological and social interventions. These interventions should, where possible, run concurrently as opposed to consecutively and must be provided in a form that is acceptable to the individual and sensitive to the specific needs of the elderly[44]. Among this client group, individuals rarely present complaining directly of a substance misuse disorder but may present with associated physical problems. The first step of treatment is the identification of cases. This requires clinical observation allied to sensitive yet persistent enquiry. The routine use of standardized screening tools may help to focus clinical impression more accurately. Once potential candidates for treatment have been identified, their attitude towards their substance misuse requires examination. Exploration of the risks and a discussion of potential avenues for change may help to establish or reinforce the motivation to change. Drugs that cause significant physical dependence may necessitate detoxification regimens, while co-morbid conditions such as depression that perpetuate the disorder need to be adequately treated. Social issues, such as housing and a social network that is comprised mainly of substance misusers, may perpetuate the problem and need to be examined for opportunities to change. The individual requires psychological rehabilitation to address the issues that may have contributed to the uncontrolled use of substances and to provide future coping strategies to prevent a relapse into substance misuse.

DETECTION

Self-presentation by elders may be limited by a number of factors[45,46]. Practical issues, such as accessibility of treatment centres to disabled individuals, large-print information sources for the visually impaired and the availability of domiciliary treatment, are fundamental. Elders may not realize that they are ill, or may not realize that the medical profession identifies substance misuse as an illness and will offer help. Traditional forms of service promotion may fail to reach the elderly, while a service staffed by young professionals may seem intimidating or inappropriate for someone much older, particularly if his/her substance misuse is associated with a high degree of shame. If self-presentation is unlikely, then the number of professional caregiver contacts that the elderly have provides a further opportunity for education about the problem and

potential sources of help. This resource appears underdeveloped at present, with a need for better training for carers in identification of at-risk individuals and in appropriate actions once misusers are identified[47].

Currently, evidence suggests that carers are often unaware of sources of help and frequently are in collusion with alcohol misuse, citing reasons such as the elder 'has not got long to live' or that 'it's his only pleasure'[47]. Studies have found that many agencies providing care for the elderly have no written policy to guide their employees when encountering a client with an alcohol problem. Greenwood[48] argues that substance misusers, and the elderly in particular, suffer as the result of stigmatization, as their disorder is perceived as self-inflicted. This stigma may be reflected in a clinician's reluctance to become involved by acknowledging the problem. For other carers, their own previous experiences with elderly substance misusers, both professional and personal, may lead to attempts to justify the behaviour, resulting in a similar loss of objectivity.

BENZODIAZEPINE USE DETECTION

Prevention and early recognition form the basis of management of benzodiazepine misuse. Appropriate prescribing of sedatives for time-limited periods should be accompanied with vigilance for drug-seeking behaviour. Such behaviour includes early requests for repeat prescriptions or requests for increased doses. The elderly may also receive medication from multiple sources, particularly where they are under the care of prescribing hospital specialists as well as their primary prescribers. Careful exchange of clinical information is vital in such settings. For those abusing over-the-counter medication, chance presentation or the intervention of a pharmacist presents the best hope of detection. The Severity of Dependence Scale has been validated as a screening tool for benzodiazepine dependence[49]. It consists of five questions, referring to the past month:

1. Did you think your use of tranquillizers was out of control?
2. Did the prospect of missing a dose make you anxious or worried?
3. Did you worry about your use of tranquillizers?
4. Did you wish you could stop?
5. How difficult would you find it to stop or go without your tranquillizers?

Each of the items is scored on a four-point scale (Items 1–4: 0 = never/almost never, 1 = sometimes, 2 = often, 3 = always/nearly always. Item 5: 0 = not difficult, 1 = quite difficult, 2 = very difficult, 3 = impossible). A total score of 6 or more indicates problematic use, with a specificity of 94.2% and sensitivity of 97.9%[49].

Urine screening provides a reliable means of establishing the presence or absence of drug metabolites, but its clinical utility can be limited by the unacceptability of the test to many who may be offended by the suggestion that they have a substance misuse problem. In addition, urine screening is usually qualitative rather than quantitative. For those abusing a prescribed drug, the mere presence or absence of the drug is clinically uninformative. With these considerations in mind, the need for dependence-inducing drug prescriptions should be regularly reviewed and co-morbid contributory conditions, such as depression, should be actively treated. Changes in legislation on prescribing practice may reduce the opportunity for drug misuse[34].

INITIATING TREATMENT

There is no published data about the level of uptake of offers of help once elders abusing substances are identified. However, elders do achieve equivalent or better results than younger adults when they do enter treatment[2]. Motivational interviewing and education as to the risks of alcohol use, along with the benefits of even a small reduction in levels of alcohol intake, may persuade some elders to change. Unfortunately, the pessimistic attitudes held by many professionals and carers towards the likelihood of successful resolution of the problem are frequently also held by the individual too. A fatalistic resignation to a life of substance misuse is often reported, particularly by long-term users, while more recent-onset users may express greater motivation for treatment[50].

Once long-term use of benzodiazepines is established, dose reduction can be difficult to achieve. Withdrawal insomnia and rebound anxiety make patient motivation difficult to achieve. Where abstinence is desired, a conversion to a longer-acting benzodiazepine and a gradual reduction in dosage over the course of months is advisable[43]. Rapid detoxification is associated with breakthrough withdrawal symptoms and may be complicated by convulsions. If a rapid withdrawal is necessary, it is best conducted in an inpatient setting if severe dependency is suspected. As with alcohol, the withdrawal period for the elderly is more likely to be complicated by confusion than in younger adults. Longer term prescribing of benzodiazepines should adhere to the following general principles: clear indication of benzodiazepine dependence, clear intermediate treatment goals, regular review and methods to prevent diversion[51].

Psychological techniques, such as relaxation training and educative initiatives in the areas of sleep hygiene and correct medication use, may also prove valuable. Cormack et al.[52] demonstrated that writing to benzodiazepine users in primary care urging them to reduce their medication use resulted in a fall in total use by one third over the next six months. Treatment of other forms of drug misuse in the elderly is under-researched. Misuse of analgesics may require formal detoxification if opioids are involved or physical dependence has developed. More often the patient requires information to allow him/her to make an informed choice about drug use and an alternative form of treatment for his/her condition. Still less information is available on the treatment of illicit drug use in the elderly although several key publications argue for age-appropriate services to be formed[2,44]. These services should pay particular attention to co-morbid health problems and should provide basic-level medical services[2]. Severe or complex health problems should be identified and referred to appropriate specialist services.

PSYCHOLOGICAL INTERVENTIONS

Once a patient is detoxified, rehabilitation is necessary to address the issues behind his/her substance use and to foster coping strategies for the future. Few studies have examined the particular needs of the elderly in a rehabilitation setting and have mostly focused on alcohol. Janik and Dunham report on comparative outcomes for over 3 000 over-60-year-olds and younger entrants into alcohol treatment programmes[53]. Outcomes after six months showed no differences between the groups.

Psychological programmes designed specifically with the elderly in mind may be more appropriate for consideration. Some success has been claimed for models encouraging the development of social networks with self-management skills[54]. Kofoed et al.[55], in a small study, reported that retention in outpatient treatment of older adults was greater in an age-specific treatment group that focused on socialization and minimal confrontation (a mainstay of many programmes), compared with older patients in a mixed-age treatment group. At one-year follow-up the effect was lost.

Variations of the Alcoholics Anonymous 12-step model tailored to the needs of elders have been reported in the USA, with varying degrees of success[56]. Models low on confrontation, traditionally regarded as fundamental to overcoming denial on the part of the patient, appear to be supported by the work of Kashner et al.[57], who found that one-year follow-up of elders in a confrontational programme revealed half the levels of abstinence as compared with a group in a programme where self-esteem, tolerance and peer relationships were promoted.

Behavioural approaches, including cue identification and avoidance, have also been reported to be of clinical benefit[54]. A programme focusing on cognitive techniques, such as cognitive restructuring, assertion training and self-monitoring of drinking, resulted in 75% of those completing the programme sticking to their treatment goals at one-year follow-up.

The evidence suggests that a range of therapeutic techniques may be beneficial for the elderly and that local provision may depend upon the skills available to the treating agency. It is suggested that even if an elders-only therapeutic programme is not available, a better therapeutic outcome may occur from a more homogeneous group, where the opportunity for identification and vicarious learning is enhanced.

Even fewer age-specific studies are available to guide the clinician in the provision of aftercare to the elderly non-alcoholic drug user. An avoidance of drugs that have a dependence potential is advisable if practical. Adequate rehabilitation and continuing support of the individual are indicated. This may be provided through generic old age psychiatry services or through specialist drug services, depending upon which service appears best able to cater for the specific needs of the user. The choice of service provider should reflect the lifestyle of the patient, as opposed to being a decision based solely on chronological as opposed to biological age. Further services may also be available in the form of mutual support groups similar to those available for alcohol. The adoption of a cognitively based programme low on confrontation and designed to foster strong social support appears optimal, as shown in work in the field of alcohol.

CONCLUSION

Substance misuse and old age psychiatry have long been unpopular choices for specialization. Both fields are known for providing challenging patients with differing priorities to those of the clinician. Research in either field is hampered by the difficulty in obtaining reliable clinical data on conditions for which few empirical measures exist. The field of old age substance misuse has suffered to some extent in clinical practice, where patients do not fit neatly into either service and are welcomed by neither. It is, however, clear that there exists a significant morbidity due to drug use in the elderly. The problem may be iatrogenic and autogenic in origin. Increased life expectancy and the cohort effect of generations of recreational drug users reaching old age are likely to intensify the problem. Adequate research to identify at-risk individuals and the provision of appropriate and accessible treatment services for the elderly drug misuser remain the major challenges to health care providers.

REFERENCES

1. Patterson TL, Jeste DV. The potential impact of the baby-boom generation on substance abuse among elderly persons. *Psychiatr Serv* 1999; **50**(9): 1184–8.
2. European Monitoring Centre for Drugs and Drug Addiction. *Substance Use among Older Adults: A Neglected Problem*. Luxembourg: Office for Official Publications of the European Communities, 2008, 1–4.
3. Murphy JT, Harwood A, Götz M, House AO. Prescribing alcohol in a general hospital: 'not everything in black and white makes sense'. *J R Coll Physicians Lond* 1998; **32**(4): 358–9.
4. Pascarelli EF. Drug abuse and the elderly. In Lowinson JH, Ruiz P (eds), *Substance Abuse: Clinical Problems and Perspectives*. Baltimore, MD: Williams & Wilkins, 1981, 752–7.
5. United Nations International Drug Control Programme. *World Drug Report*. Oxford: Oxford University Press, 1997.
6. World Health Organization. *The ICD-10 Classification of Mental and Behavioural Disorders: Clinical Descriptions and Diagnostic Guidelines*. Geneva: World Health Organization, 1992.
7. Dunne FJ, Schipperheijn JAM. Alcohol and the elderly. *Br Med J* 1989; **298**(6689): 1660–61.
8. Ghodse AH. Substance misuse leading to renal damage. *Prescr J* 1993; (33): 151–3.
9. Sheehan O, Feely J. Prescribing considerations in elderly patients. *Prescriber* 1999; **10**: 75–82.
10. Klotz U, Avant GR, Hoyumpa A, Schenker S, Wilkinson GR. The effects of age and liver disease on the disposition and elimination of diazepam in adult man. *J Clin Invest* 1975; **55**(2): 347–59.
11. Lisi DM. Alcoholism in the elderly. *Arch Intern Med* 1997; **157**(2): 242–3.
12. Dowling GJ, Weiss SRB, Condon TP. Drugs of abuse and the aging brain. *Neuropsychopharmacology* 2008; **33**(2): 209–18.
13. Gfroerer J, Penne M, Pemberton M, Folsom R. Substance abuse treatment need among older adults in 2020: the impact of the aging baby-boom cohort. *Drug Alcohol Depend* 2003; **69**(2): 127–35.
14. Shah A, Fountain J. Illicit drug use and problematic use in the elderly: is there a case for concern? *Int Psychogeriatr* 2008; **20**(6): 1081–9.
15. World Health Organization. *Programme on Substance Abuse. Rational Use of Benzodiazepines*. Geneva: World Health Organization, 1996.
16. McCree DH. The appropriate use of sedatives and hypnotics in geriatric insomnia. *Am Pharmacol* 1989; **NS29**(5): 49–53.
17. Fick DM, Cooper JW, Wade WE *et al*. Updating the Beers criteria for potentially inappropriate medication use in older adults: results of a US consensus panel of experts. *Arch Intern Med* 2003; **163**(22): 2716–24.
18. Grantham P. Benzodiazepine abuse. *Br J Hosp Med* 1987; **37**(4): 292–3, 296–300.
19. CSM/MCA. Benzodiazepines, dependence and withdrawal symptoms. *Curr Probl* 1988; (21): 1–2.
20. Milburn A. House of Commons Written Answers, 6 May 1998. At www.publications.parliament.uk/pa/cm199798/cmhansrd/vo980506/text/80506w12.htm#80506w12.html_sbhd4, accessed 9 Feb 2010.
21. Department of Health. *Benzodiazepines warning*. CMO's update 37, 2004. At www.dh.gov.uk/dr_consum_dh/groups/dh_digitalassets/@dh/@en/documents/digitalasset/dh_4070176.pdf, accessed 9 Feb 2010.
22. National Health Service. Benzodiazepines and newer hypnotics. *MeReC Bull* 2005; (5): 17–20.
23. Taylor S, McCracken CF, Wilson KC, Copeland JR. Extent and appropriateness of benzodiazepine use. Results from an elderly urban community. *Br J Psychiatry* 1998; **173**(5): 433–8.
24. Stewart RB, May FE, Hale WE, Marks RG. Psychotropic drug use in an ambulatory elderly population. *Gerontology* 1982; **28**(5): 328–35.
25. Stewart RB, May FE, Moore MT, Hale WE. Changing patterns of psychotropic drug use in the elderly: a five-year update. *Ann Pharmacother* 1989; **23**(7): 610–13.
26. Morgan K. Sedative-hypnotic drug use and ageing. *Arch Gerontol Geriatr* 1983; **2**(3): 181–99.
27. Svarstad BL, Mount JK. Effects of residents' depression, sleep, and demand for medication on benzodiazepine use in nursing homes. *Psychiatr Serv* 2002; **53**(9): 1159–65.
28. Opedal K, Schjøtt J, Eide E. Use of hypnotics among patients in geriatric institutions. *Int J Geriatr Psychiatry* 1998; **13**(12): 846–51.
29. Pillemer K. Maltreatment of patients in nursing homes: overview and research agenda. *J Health Soc Behav* 1988; **29**(3): 227–38.
30. Finlayson RE, Davis LJ, Jr. Prescription drug dependence in the elderly population: demographic and clinical features of 100 inpatients. *Mayo Clin Proc* 1994; **69**(12): 1137–45.
31. Van Balkom A, Beekman ATF, De Beurs E. Comorbidity of the anxiety disorders in a community-based older population in the Netherlands. *Acta Psychiatr Scand* 2000; **101**(1): 37–45.
32. Edgell RC, Kunik ME, Molinari VA, Hale D, Orengo CA. Nonalcohol-related use disorders in geropsychiatric patients. *J Geriatr Psychiatry Neurol* 2000; **13**(1): 33–7.
33. Martínez-Cano H, de Iceta Ibáñez de Gauna M, Vela-Bueno A, Wittchen HU. DSM-III-R co-morbidity in benzodiazepine dependence. *Addiction* 1999; **94**(1): 97–107.
34. Brahams D. Benzodiazepine overprescribing: successful initiative in New York State. *Lancet* 1990; **336**(8727): 1372–3.
35. Culberson JW, Ziska M. Prescription drug misuse/abuse in the elderly. *Geriatrics* 2008; **63**(9): 22–31.
36. Edwards I, Salib E. 'Silent dependence syndrome' in old age ...! *Int J Geriatr Psychiatry* 1999; **14**(1): 72–4.
37. Elseviers MM, De Broe ME. Analgesic abuse in the elderly: renal sequelae and management. *Drugs Aging* 1998; **12**(5): 391–400.
38. Regier DA, Farmer ME, Rae DS *et al*. One-month prevalence of mental disorders in the United States and sociodemographic characteristics: the Epidemiologic Catchment Area study. *Acta Psychiatr Scand* 1993; **88**: 35–47.
39. Blazer DG, Wu LT. The epidemiology of substance use and disorders among middle aged and elderly community adults: national survey on drug use and health. *Am J Geriatr Psychiatry* 2009; **17**(3): 237–45.
40. Hoare J, Flatley J. Drug misuse declared: findings from the 2007/2008 British Crime Survey England and Wales. *Home Office Stat Bull* 2008; **18**(13/08).
41. Frances J. Pain killer. *Comm Care* 1994; (Dec): 15–21.
42. Solomon K, Manepalli J, Ireland GA, Mahon GM. Alcoholism and prescription drug abuse in the elderly: St. Louis University grand rounds. *J Am Geriatr Soc* 1993; **41**(1): 57–69.
43. Taylor D, Paton C, Kerwin R. *The Maudsley Prescribing Guidelines*, 9th edn. London: Informa Healthcare; 2007.

44. Crome I, Bloor R. Older substance misusers still deserve better treatment interventions – an update (part 3). *Rev Clin Gerontol* 2006; **16**(1): 45–57.

45. Ward M, Goodman C. *Alcohol Problems in Old Age*. Birmingham: Staccato, 1995.

46. Wesson J. *The Vintage Years: Older People and Alcohol*. Birmingham: Aquarius, 1992.

47. Herring R, Thom B. The role of home carers: findings from a study of alcohol and older people. *Health Care Later Life* 1998; **3**(3): 199–211.

48. Greenwood J. Stigma: substance misuse in older people. *Geriatr Med* 2000; **30**(4): 43–9.

49. Cuevas CDL, Sanz EJ, Padilla J, Berenguer JC. The Severity of Dependence Scale (SDS) as screening test for benzodiazepine dependence: SDS validation study. *Addiction* 2000; **95**(2): 245–50.

50. Schonfeld L, Dupree LW. Alcohol abuse among older adults. *Rev Clin Gerontol* 1994; **52**(4): 217–25.

51. Department of Health. *Drug Misuse and Dependence: UK Guidelines on Clinical Management*. London: Department of Health, 2007.

52. Cormack MA, Sweeney KG, Hughes-Jones H, Foot GA. Evaluation of an easy, cost-effective strategy for cutting benzodiazepine use in general practice. *Br J Gen Pract* 1994; **44**(378): 5–8.

53. Janik SW, Dunham RG. A nationwide examination of the need for specific alcoholism treatment programs for the elderly. *J Stud Alcohol* 1983; **44**(2): 307–17.

54. Dupree LW, Broskowski H, Schonfeld L. The gerontology alcohol project: a behavioral treatment program for elderly alcohol abusers. *Gerontologist* 1984; **24**(5): 510–16.

55. Kofoed LL, Tolson RL, Atkinson RM, Toth RL, Turner JA. Treatment compliance of older alcoholics: an elder-specific approach is superior to 'mainstreaming.' *J Stud Alcohol* 1987; **48**(1): 47–51.

56. Schonfeld L, Dupree LW. Antecedents of drinking for early- and late-onset elderly alcohol abusers. *J Stud Alcohol* 1991; **52**(6): 587–92.

57. Kashner TM, Rodell DE, Ogden SR, Guggenheim FG, Karson CN. Outcomes and costs of two VA inpatient treatment programs for older alcoholic patients. *Psychiatr Serv* 1992; **43**(10): 985–9.

Learning and Behavioural Studies

109

Old Age and Learning Disability

Oyepeju Raji and Asim Naeem

St George's University of London, London, UK

INTRODUCTION

In England and Wales approximately 2.5% of the population have learning disabilities, of which 1.2 million are at the mild end of the spectrum[1]. While the mortality rate for people with learning disabilities is higher compared with the general population[2], improved standards of care, more positive lifestyles and attitudes to treatment for serious illnesses have contributed to increased longevity. Mean life expectancy is estimated to be 74 years, 67 years and 58 years for those with mild, moderate and severe learning disabilities, respectively[3]. This has made the issue of age-related illnesses within this population group highly relevant.

MENTAL ILLNESS IN OLDER ADULTS WITH LEARNING DISABILITIES

Mental illness is common among adults with learning disabilities. Cooper's epidemiological study[4] comparing the prevalence rates of psychiatric disorder among older (≥65 years) and younger (20–65 years) adults with learning disabilities found significantly higher rates among the elderly cohort (68.7% compared with 47.9%). This was mainly accounted for by the higher point prevalence rates for dementia, generalized anxiety disorder and depression in the older cohort groups. While the ageing process can bring about a similar increased vulnerability to mental illness as seen in the general population, additional risk factors apply for people with learning disabilities. These include: the detrimental effect of pre-existing brain damage; co-morbid physical illnesses like epilepsy; specific psychiatric or behaviour disorders associated with genetic risk factors; low self-esteem which may be related to frequent placement breakdowns, past exploitation, neglect or abuse; and the complications of learned maladaptive behaviours such as self-injurious head injury.

Mental illness may go unrecognized due to a number of barriers in the pathways to health care. Service barriers can include the lack of specialist services or the lack of expertise in mainstream services, complex appointment systems that largely presume reading ability, and inaccessible health-care delivery. Problems with the doctor–user interface include communication difficulties, 'power imbalance' exacerbating the suggestibility of the person with learning disability, capacity issues and the complexities of atypical clinical presentations. Diagnostic overshadowing (assuming that any changes in behaviour or presentation are due to the learning disability, rather than a co-morbid illness) remains one of the major barriers preventing people with learning disabilities from accessing adequate health care[5]. User–carer barriers include pre-existing cognitive impairments making it difficult to obtain an accurate timeline of symptoms, the effects of past negative experiences of health-care delivery and the failure of carers to recognize symptoms. Older people with learning disabilities from ethnic minority groups may have particular problems accessing appropriate services[6].

DEMENTIA IN OLDER ADULTS WITH LEARNING DISABILITIES

The rates of dementia in older people with learning disabilities are four times higher than in the general population[7]. However, these high rates cannot be attributed just to those with Down syndrome and Alzheimer's disease. Strydom *et al.*'s epidemiological survey[8] of dementia in older adults (aged ≥60 years) with learning disabilities, but without Down syndrome, has confirmed this. Alzheimer's disease was found to be the most common sub-type, but the prevalence rates (8.6%) were almost three times higher than expected. While vascular dementia is the second commonest sub-type in the general population, Lewy body and frontotemporal dementias were found to be commoner in the older learning disabled population. Vascular dementia had a prevalence rate of 2.7%. Explanations for these increased prevalence rates include the effects of poorly controlled epilepsy or other physical illnesses, the detrimental effects of brain damage during birth and early life, and genetic risk factors[9].

Diagnosing dementia in people with learning disabilities can be difficult due to the wide range of pre-existing baseline cognitive, functional and behavioural impairments. Individuals are more likely to present with the behavioural and psychological symptoms of dementia, or with atypical symptoms such as unexplained seizures. Greater emphasis should be placed on personality and behavioural changes, in association with functional change, as diagnostic indicators[9]. Diagnostic difficulties can also result from altered social or communication skills making it difficult to identify subjective symptoms (psychosocial masking/intellectual distortion), and from diagnostic overshadowing[10].

Good collateral information from the person's carers is essential. The exacerbation of pre-existing deficits ('baseline exaggeration') may only be detected in day-care environments, where the person has more demands placed upon them.

Principles and Practice of Geriatric Psychiatry, 3rd edn. Edited by Mohammed T. Abou-Saleh, Cornelius Katona and Anand Kumar
© 2011 John Wiley & Sons, Ltd

Table 109.1 Differential diagnoses of dementia: what are the causes of cognitive, behavioural or psychological decline in an older person with learning disability?

Causes	Examples
Medical	*Physical*
	Hypothyroidism
	Recurrent urinary/respiratory tract infections
	Deteriorating epilepsy
	Anaemia
	Persistent or intermittent constipation
	Visual impairments (e.g. cataracts)
	Hearing impairments (including ear wax)
	Medication side effects (e.g. beta-blockers, anticonvulsants)
	Psychiatric
	Dementia
	Normal age-related decline
	Depression
	Anxiety-related disorders (e.g. worsening obsessive-compulsive disorder or phobias)
	Psychotropic medication side effects
Psychological	Bereavement-like response to loss events (e.g. death of a family member/carer/friend; care staff/friends moving; day centre closure)
	Environmental re-triggering of past traumatic events
Social	Changes in staffing/layout/structure/routine at home/day activities, within the context of autism
	Physical/sexual/other abuse

A detailed history and clinical examination, incorporating the 'medical-psychological-social model' can help exclude 'pseudo-dementia' symptoms (Table 109.1). While the clinical domains affected in Alzheimer's disease in older adults with learning disabilities are similar to those in the general elderly population, their presentation can be different (Table 109.2).

The Mini Mental State Examination is not valid for use in people with learning disabilities, but there are a number of alternative observer-rated scales available. Examples include the Dementia Scale for Down Syndrome (DSDS), the Dementia Questionnaire for Persons with Mental Retardation (DMR), and the Modified Cambridge Examination for Mental Disorders of the Elderly informant interview[11].

Medical investigations should be focused on excluding the differential diagnoses of dementia. A full blood count, B12/folate levels, ESR or CRP, urea/electrolytes, blood glucose/calcium levels, liver function/thyroid function tests and urinalysis should be done. A baseline ECG (to exclude bradycardic conduction deficits) can be helpful if anticholinesterase treatment is being considered. Neuroimaging should be used to help support a clinical diagnosis, as people with learning disabilities can have baseline frontotemporal abnormalities. Within the context of dementia, people with Down syndrome may develop more significant atrophy in the frontal and temporal lobes[12], hippocampus and amygdala[13].

Management should be based upon pharmacological and non-pharmacological interventions within the context of broad, multidisciplinary 'bio-psycho-social' approaches. Affected individuals can often be maintained in their existing environment[10] with additional support or adaptations. If the person needs to be moved into residential care, significant issues arise as to the suitability of mainstream dementia homes with significantly older people[6].

A number of studies have reported on the efficacy and safety of using acetylcholinesterase inhibitors (especially donepezil) in older people with learning disabilities[14,15]. Antidementia drug treatment can be initiated by the learning disabilities psychiatrist[16]. Associated behavioural and psychological symptoms that fail to respond to non-pharmacological measures may require treatment with an antidepressant, anxiolytic or antipsychotic medication. Persistent seizures may require anticonvulsant treatment. Non-pharmacological interventions such as reality orientation using a life-story photo book, art/music therapies and aromatherapy are of most use in people with learning disabilities.

As with the general population, the prognosis for dementia is generally poor, and the average duration of dementia is generally shorter.

ALZHEIMER'S DISEASE IN OLDER ADULTS WITH DOWN SYNDROME

While neuropathological studies have consistently revealed the evidence of neuritic plaques and intracellular neurofibrillary tangles in nearly all adults with Down syndrome over the age of 40 years[17], not all develop Alzheimer's disease. However, there is a marked exponential rise of Alzheimer's disease in adults with Down syndrome from 30 to 59 years of age, with prevalence rates rising from 2.0% (30–39 years age) to 36.1% (50–59 years age)[18]. For adults with Down syndrome living beyond 60 years of age, approximately three in four will have Alzheimer's disease. The mean age range of onset of the clinical manifestations of Alzheimer's disease is 50–55 years, with the rate of deterioration increasing with age. There are no clear relationships between the level of learning disability and risk of dementia or age of onset of dementia[19].

Neuropathological factors that may explain the increased risk of dementia include the over-expression of the amyloid precursor protein gene, the influence of apolipoprotein E alleles, genetic risk factors, the detrimental oxidative effect of increased superoxide dimutase activity in the brain, the earlier loss of the neuroprotective effects of oestrogen in women, and the effects of atypical karyotypes.

Compared to the general population, executive dysfunction (frontal lobe) symptoms such as social withdrawal, diminished initiative and pervasive slowness are common at an early stage of dementia in people with Down syndrome[20]. Isolated impairments in verbal/long-term memory and visuospatial construction deficits, without significant impairment in other areas of functioning, are more likely to indicate normal age-related decline.

The Dementia Screening Questionnaire for Individuals with Intellectual Disabilities (DSQIID)[21] is a reliable, observer-rated screening questionnaire for use in older people with Down syndrome. It allows the screening out of pre-morbid behaviours, with only changes in behaviour (or new behaviours) positively scored.

PHYSICAL ILLNESS IN OLDER ADULTS WITH LEARNING DISABILITIES

Older people with learning disabilities have health-care needs associated with ageing, and higher rates of respiratory disorders, arthritis, hypertension, urinary incontinence, immobility, hearing impairment and cerebrovascular disease[22].

Table 109.2 Clinical presentation of Alzheimer's disease in older people with learning disabilities

Clinical domain	Examples of symptoms and signs
Memory	Forgetfulness of recent events, e.g. content of meals/day activities (episodic memory impairment)
	Forgetfulness of future planned outings/activities
	Forgetting location of recently placed objects (spatial memory impairment)
	Geographical disorientation (e.g. unable to find their way around their own home/neighbourhood)
	Forgetting names of/failing to recognize familiar people (semantic memory impairment)
	Loss of previously learned skills, e.g. making a cup of tea or dialling a phone (procedural memory impairment)
Abstract reasoning skills (judgement, planning and organization)	No longer selecting appropriate clothing for planned activities/routines, or putting on clothes back to front
	Decline in shopping skills
	Difficulty following more than one instruction at a time
	Decline in ability to dress/feed self, or brush teeth (apraxia)
	Decline in reading (alexia), writing (agraphia) or language skills (aphasia)
	Using common everyday objects inappropriately (agnosia), e.g. combing hair with toothbrush
	Being unable to distinguish between day and night
Mood	Low mood/decreased energy/loss of interest/apathy
	Emotional lability (e.g. unexplained tearfulness)
	Overactivity/restlessness/poor concentration
	Irritability/anxiety
	Sleep changes (insomnia or hypersomnia)
Social behaviours	Increased dependence on others
	Personality changes, e.g. aggression/disinhibition, pervasive slowness
	Obsessional slowness/repetitiveness in completing tasks
	Social isolation
	Fear of stairs, kerbs or uneven surfaces
	'Covering up' of memory loss (e.g. saying 'sorry' to tasks they cannot do)
Perceptions	Auditory, visual or tactile hallucinations
Neurological	Gait disturbance/decreased mobility/falls
	Bradykinesia-like slowness in movements
	Seizures (early in Down syndrome)
	Dysphasia
	Dystonia/myoclonus/pathological reflexes
	Urinary incontinence

Hearing problems might further compound already poor communication skills and can be caused by structural abnormalities, neural damage or impacted earwax. People with learning disabilities also have a higher prevalence of sight problems, which may be acquired as they get older, or be as a result of brain damage or cerebral visual impairment[22]. The prevalence of ocular health problems ranges from 25% (in the mildly disabled) to 60% (in the profoundly disabled)[23].

Prevalence rates of epilepsy are considerably higher in people with learning disabilities compared to the general population (16.1% vs. 0.4–1%)[2]. Individuals often have complex seizure types and patterns.

People with learning disabilities have higher levels of oesophageal, stomach and gall-bladder cancers, but lower rates of lung, prostate, breast and cervical cancers.

An increased risk of respiratory tract infections in people with learning disabilities can be caused by aspiration or reflux due to swallowing difficulties. Levels of obesity are higher in people with learning disabilities because of poor diet, lack of physical exercise and difficulty understanding health promotion information, which can increase the likelihood of heart disease, stroke and type II diabetes mellitus. Many people with learning disabilities have high levels of *Helicobacter pylori* which may require testing and treatment throughout life[22].

Certain syndromes that cause learning disabilities are particularly associated with an increased risk of specific morbidity. Down syndrome is associated with increased risks of congenital heart problems, respiratory disease, a poor immune system, eye disorders, lymphoblastic leukaemia, coeliac disease and hypothyroidism. People with fragile-X syndrome have increased connective tissue disease and cardiac abnormalities. Prader–Willi syndrome has an associated risk of obesity-related pathology.

AGEING AND SOCIAL NEEDS OF PEOPLE WITH LEARNING DISABILITIES

Most long-stay hospitals have now closed, with individuals moving to community residential provision motivated by the philosophy of 'normalization'. In England, national policy requires local authorities to offer person-centred planning to all people with learning disabilities, alongside regularly updated health action plans[1]. Staff roles and training now focus on social inclusion, choice, independence and rights.

People with learning disabilities experience low employment and fewer meaningful relationships, as daily activities are usually only provided as part of a package of care. Placements often experience a high staff turnover resulting in carers having an incomplete knowledge of the individual. Many older adults may have been raised in institutions. Younger adults are more likely to have been raised within caring families in the wider community, with better lifestyles and opportunities that may have been denied to their seniors[4].

With good planning, people may stay in their own home funded through the personalization agenda. Accommodation and support varies from minimal to total. People with milder learning disabilities might live by themselves or semi-independently with some structured support each day. Those who need greater levels of support may live in housing managed by private or voluntary organizations, or by health and social services.

SERVICES FOR OLDER ADULTS WITH LEARNING DISABILITIES

Being elderly and having learning disabilities can make people vulnerable to 'double discrimination', as services for both groups tend to be underfunded. Debate exists whether to use mainstream older people's psychiatric services (which may lack neurodevelopmental expertise), to continue with existing learning disability services, or to develop specific specialist services. National policies advocate that people with learning disabilities should be able to access mainstream health services where appropriate, and specialist community learning disability teams (CLDTs) can promote this by providing specialist advice and support to their mainstream colleagues. Some CLDTs operate a life-span approach, but the majority work with people from age 16 or 18 with no exit age. However, such teams need to develop additional skills with regard to age-associated disorders.

Older people with learning disabilities face additional difficulties in primary care settings. Primary care physicians list lack of awareness of conditions specific to learning disabilities as among the top five barriers to care[24]. Strategic health facilitator posts tackle some of these issues by ensuring that people with learning disabilities are offered health screening, and that health promotion materials are accessible to them.

PALLIATIVE CARE ISSUES FOR PEOPLE WITH LEARNING DISABILITIES

Mainstream palliative care services need to be responsive to the needs of people with learning disabilities, as the combination of problems identifying symptoms and diagnostic overshadowing can result in the late presentation of illness at a stage when there is already advanced disease and severe symptomatology[25]. Many people with learning disabilities can be surrounded by a 'conspiracy of silence', where information about the illness and impending death is not shared with them[26]. Carers of people with learning disabilities may equate palliative care with hospice care, triggering unpleasant memories of largely institutional care. Educating well-meaning care staff and family members of the positive role of services in supporting the dying person in the community (within their home) can help alleviate these fears.

Effective end-of-life care requires close collaboration between learning disability services, palliative care teams, carers (including family members, who may highlight important religious or cultural issues) and other medical services.

CONCLUSION

People with learning disabilities share the general experiences and difficulties of becoming old with the rest of the population. Their increasing life span brings about important challenges in view of additional risk factors, increased prevalence rates, co-morbidity and atypical presentations of mental and physical illnesses. There is need for more research, education and training, alongside collaboration between services, to inform service developments. Person-centred approaches take into account an individual's life experiences, clinical needs and the support mechanisms needed for their immediate carers and family. Psychiatrists can act as drivers of positive health outcomes by facilitating access to appropriate pathways to care. Commissioners of older people's and learning disability services need to take these factors into account for future planning.

REFERENCES

1. Department of Health. *Valuing People: A New Strategy for Learning Disability for the 21st Century*. London: Stationery Office, 2001.
2. Morgan C, Baxter H, Kerr M. Prevalence of epilepsy and associated health service utilisation and mortality among patients with intellectual disability. *Am J Ment Retard* 2003; **108**: 293–300.
3. Bittles A, Petterson BA, Sullivan SG *et al*. The influence of intellectual disability on life expectancy. *J Gerontol* 2002; **57A**: 470–2.
4. Cooper SA. Epidemiology of psychiatric disorders in elderly compared with younger adults with learning disabilities. *Br J Psychiatry* 1997; **170**: 375–80.
5. Ali A, Hassiotis A. Illness in people with intellectual disabilities. *BMJ* 2008; **336**: 570–1.
6. Hubert J, Hollins S. Working with elderly carers of people with learning disabilities and planning for the future. *Adv Psychiatry Treat* 2000; **6**: 41–8.
7. Cooper SA. High prevalence of dementia among people with learning disabilities not attributed to Down syndrome. *Psychol Med* 1997; **27**: 606–16.
8. Strydom A, Livingstone G, King M *et al*. Prevalence of dementia in intellectual disability using different diagnostic criteria. *Br J Psychiatry* 2007; **191**: 150–7.
9. Holland AJ. Ageing and learning disability. *Br J Psychiatry* 2000; **176**: 26–31.
10. Stanton LR, Coetzee RH. Down syndrome and dementia. *Adv Psychiatry Treat* 2004; **10**: 50–8.
11. Ball SL, Holland AJ, Huppert FA *et al*. The modified CAMDEX informant interview is a valid and reliable tool for use in the diagnosis of dementia in adults with Down syndrome. *J Intellect Disabil Res* 2004; **48**: 611–20.
12. Lawlor BA, McCarron M, Wilson G *et al*. Temporal lobe-orientated CT scanning and dementia in Down syndrome. *Int J Geriatr Psychiatry* 2001; **16**: 427–9.

13. Aylward EH, Li Q, Honeycutt NA *et al*. MRI volumes of the hippocampus and amygdala in adults with Down syndrome with and without dementia. *Am J Psychiatry* 1999; **156**: 564–8.

14. Prasher VP, Huxley A, Haque MS. A 24-week, double-blind, placebo-controlled trial of donepezil in patients with Down syndrome and Alzheimer's disease. Pilot study. *Int J Geriatr Psychiatry* 2002; **17**: 270–8.

15. Prasher VP, Adams C, Holder R *et al*. Long term safety and efficacy of donepezil in the treatment of dementia in Alzheimer's disease in adults with Down syndrome: open label study. *Int J Geriatr Psychiatry* 2003; **18**: 549–51.

16. National Institute for Health and Clinical Excellence. *Donepezil, galantamine, rivastigmine (review) and memantine for the treatment of Alzheimer's disease (amended)*. London: NICE, 2007.

17. Mann DMA. Alzheimer's disease and Down syndrome. *Histopathology* 1988; **13**: 125–37.

18. Prasher VP. Age-specific prevalence, thyroid dysfunction and depressive symptomatology in adults with Down syndrome and dementia. *Int J Geriatr Psychiatry* 1995; **10**: 25–31.

19. Holland AJ, Hon J, Huppert FA *et al*. Population-based study of the prevalence and presentation of dementia in adults with Down syndrome. *Br J Psychiatry* 1998; **172**: 493–8.

20. Deb S, Hare M, Prior L. Symptoms of dementia among adults with Down syndrome: a qualitative study. *J Intellect Disabil Res* 2007; **51**: 726–39.

21. Deb S, Hare M, Prior L *et al*. Dementia Screening Questionnaire for Individuals with Intellectual Disabilities. *Br J Psychiatry* 2007; **190**: 440–4.

22. Hardy S, Woodward P, Woolard P *et al*. *Meeting the Health Needs of People with Learning Disabilities: Guidance for Nursing Staff*. London: Royal College of Nursing, 2007.

23. McCulloch D, Sludden P, McKeon K. Vision care requirements among intellectually disabled adults. *J Intellect Disabil Res* 1996; **40**: 140–50.

24. Lennox N, Diggens J, Ugoni A. The general practice care of people with intellectual disability: barriers and solutions. *J Intellect Disabil Res* 1997; **41**: 380–90.

25. Tuffrey-Wijne I, Hogg J, Curtis L. End-of-life and palliative care for people with intellectual disabilities who have cancer or other life-limiting illness: a review of the literature and available resources. *J Appl Res Intellect* 2007; **20**: 331–44.

26. Tuffrey-Wijne I, Bernal J, Jones A *et al*. People with intellectual disabilities and their need for cancer information. *Eur J Oncol Nursing* 2006; **10**: 106–16.

110

The Elderly Offender

Graeme A. Yorston

St Andrew's Hospital, Northampton, UK

The elderly are far more likely to be the victims of crime than the perpetrators, but a small number of older people do commit crimes, and this group is important for a number of reasons. First, the mental disorders of late life may lead previously law abiding people to act out of character and behave in a dangerous and distressing manner. Second, the criminal justice system is less sensitive to the ways in which mental disorders can present in older adults, with the result that they may go undetected, and, third, the needs of older mentally disordered offenders are often difficult to meet in existing prisons and secure hospitals, leaving them vulnerable, an easy target for physical aggression and with little chance of moving on because of inadequately developed risk management strategies and care pathways.

A question which most researchers in this field have posed is the age at which an offender should be deemed 'elderly'. Prison studies, particularly in the US, often include everyone over the age of 40! Others have used 45, 50 or 60 but relatively few the more traditional 65 cut-off. People who have had hard lives, no stable employment or relationships, several terms in prison, a history of drug or alcohol use, and patchy health care often appear much older than their peers who have led more conventionally prosocial lives, with the result that many are starting to look and feel old in their forties and fifties. There is a strong case, therefore, for using a lower age limit for research purposes, but all figures based on chronological age are arbitrary, and what is more important in the clinical assessment of an individual is *biological age*, as it is this that will largely determine their needs.

OFFENCE TYPES

Despite an ageing population, statistical data from the UK and US show the number of convictions of people over the age of 60 has been remarkably stable over the past 12 years[1,2]. Broadly speaking, the elderly account for around 1% of recorded crime, though this figure varies considerably for the type of crime.

Sexual Offences

Sexually inappropriate behaviour in dementia is a familiar problem to all old age psychiatrists. Most of this behaviour is mild in severity and does not reach the attention of the police or criminal justice system. Older adults can and do commit more serious sex crimes, however, and account for approximately 1% of convictions for these offences in the UK, with broadly comparable figures from other countries.

The proportion of older adults is rather higher for those convicted of sexual offences against children, and a number of possible explanations for this have been proposed, including the greater ease by which children may be dominated by someone of declining physical strength, the degree of trust afforded grandparental figures, ready access to grandchildren, and regression to childhood fantasy objects. The proportion of older sex offenders with suspected or proven organic psychiatric diagnoses varies in published case series from 0% to 60%[3-5]. Other diagnoses reported in the literature include antisocial personality disorder, alcoholism, learning disability, depression and schizophrenia. Though research has consistently shown that older adults are capable of committing the most serious violent penetrative offences, there has been a tendency to minimize the seriousness of offending by this group in the past[6]. Several studies have shown lower rates of recidivism for older offenders[7-9], but some of these failed to account for the reduced time at risk of re-offending of elderly men, and the fact that, as a group, older sex offenders tend to commit less serious offences which have lower recidivism rates. It should also be borne in mind that the lower recidivism rate is of little help in assessing risk in individual cases, which should be approached in a structured manner. The potential for serious harm should never be underestimated on the basis of age alone.

Homicide

There have been few psychiatric studies of elderly homicide offenders, though the individual case study literature is much richer. Rollin[10] described a typical case of a 71-year-old man with a history of depressive illness who battered his wife to death after becoming convinced that she was beginning to fail in health and was too proud to allow herself to be looked after by anyone else should anything happen to him. Large homicide case series often include a small number of elderly cases: in Gillies' classic series of 400 homicides in Scotland[11], there were only three men over the age of 65 and the oldest woman was 54. Unlike the majority of people accused of homicide, who were considered mentally normal (82%), all three of the over-65s were psychotic at the time of the offence.

In a comparison of older and younger homicide and attempted homicide suspects in Canada[12], much lower rates of previous convictions and past hospitalization for mental illness were found in the elderly group. Half of the elderly group had psychotic diagnoses, with none found in those under the age of 30; 19% of the elderly group had an organic mental disorder, with none in the younger group;

Principles and Practice of Geriatric Psychiatry, 3rd edn. Edited by Mohammed T. Abou-Saleh, Cornelius Katona and Anand Kumar

50% had alcohol problems (31% in the younger group); and only 13% had antisocial personality disorder (compared to 68% of the younger group). Surprisingly, though, fewer of the elderly group were found not guilty by reason of insanity (19% compared to 30%). This finding contrasts with sentencing data from Scotland in the 1990s, which showed that elderly homicides were more likely to be given hospital disposals than younger offenders and far less likely to be given life sentences (F. Thorne, personal communication).

Forensic pathologist Bernard Knight[13] coined the term *Darby and Joan syndrome* for elderly couple homicides which occurred in apparently close, loving relationships, in contrast to younger partner homicides which typically occurred against a background of infidelity, jealousy and money disputes, fuelled by alcohol or drugs. He cited the case of a woman in her seventies who killed her husband with repeated brutal blows to the back of his head with a heavy metal object while he was sitting watching television. No rational explanation for the act could be obtained. Knight commented on the extreme brutality used in elderly couple homicides and cited two cases of octogenarian men who killed their elderly wives with hammers – one of whom rained down 37 blows on his wife's head, resulting in multiple compound fractures of her skull. He also commented on the presence of *bizarre postmortem bondage* in many of the cases he was involved with, describing how a man trussed his wife up in a chair with twine and cord after killing her and then bound her face with towels and cloths secured by more twine.

Though the psychiatric literature emphasizes the differences between elderly homicide offenders and younger homicides, criminological data from US studies show that though elderly homicide rates vary between different US states, they are correlated with the non-elderly rates, which are themselves strongly correlated with urbanization and poverty, suggesting that the same societal pressures influence young and old alike[14]. Other US studies have shown that the elderly are more likely to kill family members, to use firearms and to carry out the offence in the home[15,16]. The majority of elderly homicides are committed by men, but in a study of coroner's office and county prosecutor files of 179 homicides by the over-60s in Cincinnati and Detroit[17] it was found that women accounted for 18% of cases. There have been no systematic studies of elderly women homicides, however, though there are a number of brief case descriptions[18,19].

Homicide–Suicide

A number of studies have demonstrated that homicide followed by suicide is commoner in older adults[20]. It usually occurs in a spousal relationship, and depression and alcohol problems are common. One study showed a mean age difference of 18 years between perpetrators and victims along with prominent histories of discord, violence and separation. There are published case studies of homicide–suicides that have no history of conflict, however: for example, an 82-year-old man who shot his frail 84-year-old wife and then himself after becoming unable to provide care for her after he suffered a myocardial infarction[21]. In such cases it can be difficult to distinguish between homicide–suicide cases and suicide pacts.

Non-Fatal Violence

Minor aggression in elderly dementia sufferers is common, with up to 90% displaying some sort of aggression during the course of the illness[22]. Most is not serious and relatively easily managed, in

contrast to the type of behaviour described in an Australian case series of fourteen older adults accused of attempted homicide[23,24]. The only one who succeeded in killing his victim in this series was a 68-year-old man who shot his neighbour with a shotgun.

Arson

There is no published literature on arson by the elderly. Clinical experience suggests that pyromaniacs, fascinated by fire and fire services, do not typically present in old age, but such individuals, many of whom have spent years in secure hospital or prison, may live on to old age and develop a neurodegenerative disorder. Such cases present extraordinary difficulties for psychiatric and social services, and the criminal justice system, which often struggle to balance the risk to others and individual vulnerability issues. It is not clear how risk to others from arson, or indeed sexual or violent offending, changes with the progression of a dementing illness, and so care generally has to be provided in an environment where risks can be managed through relational and procedural security measures. What appears to be more common in old age is the emergence of a pattern of setting small fires, often within residential homes. Though many of these fires cause little actual damage, because of the potentially devastating consequences, all fires in elderly care settings have to be taken seriously. As few old age psychiatrists have much experience of assessing fire setters, referral for a forensic psychiatric assessment is recommended. Arson in the elderly has been linked with personality disorder, psychosis, dementia and previously unrecognized learning disability.

Acquisitive Offending

Shoplifting is the commonest offence of late life, but most cases of acquisitive offending never come to the attention of old age psychiatrists. Anecdotally there is said to be an association with depressive illness, but there have been few studies on this topic. The shame of being arrested for shoplifting can have disastrous consequences for individuals with no previous criminal history, and the case of Lady Isobel Barnett, a British television personality who committed suicide four days after being convicted of stealing a can of tuna and carton of cream in 1980, is well known[25].

Drug- and Alcohol-Related Crime

For people born in the 1940s or before, drug use was uncommon when they were going through their period of highest risk; however, this is not the case for those born in the following decade, and old age psychiatry services are now beginning to see people with active drug problems, something that was almost unheard of previously. At present drugs do not present major problems in UK older adult secure hospital services, unlike services for younger patients, but this is likely to change over the coming years. Alcohol is being increasingly recognized as a problem in older adults[26] and alcohol problems are common among older men in prison in the US[27]. When this is linked to offending behaviour it has serious implications for risk management. The assessment of older offenders with a history of alcohol abuse is further complicated by the possibility of alcohol-related cognitive impairment.

DIAGNOSTIC CONSIDERATIONS

All of the mental disorders that occur in late life can lead to criminal behaviour; for the overwhelming majority of individuals, changes in behaviour as a result of mental disorder are recognized as such and dealt with by medical services. Sometimes, however, the behaviour can be so sudden and so severe that health services are not involved until after an offence has been committed. In these circumstances it is important that the individual receives an assessment by a clinician familiar with the psychiatry of old age.

Delirium

Metabolic and other causes of delirium, superimposed on the early stages of dementia or a pre-existing depressive illness, can lead to fatal aggression. Some of the bizarre, apparently motiveless homicides described above and many from my own experience have been the result of delirium, often occurring as a side effect of medication, including steroids, anti-parkinsonian medication and the anticholinergic effects of first-generation antidepressants.

Dementia

There are isolated case reports of crime associated with dementia, but given that it is so common, it is surprising that there are not more and that it has not been more systematically studied. Experience suggests that individuals with more than a mild degree of dementia are easily identified as such and not dealt with by the criminal justice system. This is not the case for those with very early dementia, or in cases of frontotemporal dementia with a well-preserved social façade. Dementia can present with a change in behaviour: either the emergence of new behaviours that were not present at all previously, or a change in the type, frequency and character of existing behaviour. Old age psychiatrists are familiar with the evaluation of such issues by taking careful histories from carers and relatives, but forensic psychiatrists are generally more used to assessing individuals through detailed mental state examinations, which may reveal little in early dementia. In a study of referrals to a regional medium secure unit in England, it was found that forensic psychiatrists did not routinely use standardized rating scales for the assessment of cognitive functioning[28]. For these reasons individuals presenting with offending behaviour for the first time in old age ideally need assessment by clinicians with experience of both specialties, or if none are available, by clinicians from each specialty working closely together.

Psychosis

Unlike the psychosis of younger adults in which schizophrenia is the diagnosis most commonly associated with serious aggression and homicide[29], homicidal psychosis in the elderly is more commonly depressive in nature and characterized by nihilistic delusions, and it is often the spouse of the perpetrator who is the victim. The mindset is often that one or both of the couple are ill, leading to worries of how one would cope without the other, and the conclusion that they would both be better off dead. In such cases, the depression can be relatively mild on the surface and be missed by those looking for the entire gamut of symptoms, but careful enquiry about worries and preoccupations and changes in habit can be revealing. In a study of elderly men in English prisons in the 1990s[30], it was estimated that there were up to 50 older men in the UK prison system at any one time suffering from a depressive illness with psychotic symptoms severe enough to be in need of urgent transfer to hospital.

Developmental Disability

Asperger's syndrome, previously unrecognized, can present for the first time in late life and be associated with serious offending. This is commonly due to decompensation because of a change in routine by going into a residential home or through the loss of a supportive relationship, often a very old parent. Making developmental disability diagnoses in the absence of a reliable informant is difficult, however, and can be complicated further if a neurodegenerative disorder is suspected as well.

Personality Disorder

By definition, personality disorders cannot begin in old age, but what may happen is that a change in circumstances reveals a personality that has been disordered throughout life but compensated for by some means, often a spouse or other significant relationship. At retirement of one party or the other, or at the death of a partner, or entry into a care home, personality issues previously hidden within the family can emerge. These may simply cause annoyance or minor distress or be associated with criminal damage, fire setting or violence.

THE ELDERLY IN THE CRIMINAL JUSTICE SYSTEM

Arrest

Anecdotal evidence suggests the police may be reluctant to get involved in offences committed by elderly people with obvious mental health difficulties. This is particularly noticeable if either the perpetrator or victim suffers from dementia, presumably because of difficulties in obtaining evidence. This can lead to very serious offences being inadequately investigated, which then makes risk assessment almost impossible. A study of a special police project in one region in England in 1990[31] showed that of 367 consecutive arrestees aged 60 or over, less than 10% were prosecuted. The remainder were cautioned if they admitted guilt, or were subject to no further action. Nearly two thirds of the arrests had been for shoplifting, in most cases of grocery items of small value. There were 15 arrests for violence, most of which was not serious, and 11 arrests for indecent assault. Police referred the arrestees to their primary care physician or to the police doctor more often than to any other agency. Though only 50 arrestees agreed to have research interviews, nearly one third of these were identified as 'psychiatric cases'.

Trial

All jurisdictions have rules on fitness to plead and fitness to stand trial. For older adults mental health issues must be considered along with physical health and perceptual issues. Is the defendant able to see and hear adequately? Do they need shorter court sessions because of fatigability? Do they need extra toilet breaks or different seating? All these questions need to be addressed when assessing an older adult. However, the main question to be answered in determining fitness to plead in the majority of cases is whether the defendant is able to follow the course of the proceedings in court. The answer to this can be very obvious for someone with severe dementia, or in someone with relatively mild or well-managed mental health problems, but in many cases of mild to moderate dementia, the issue is far from clear. Standard cognitive testing in such cases can be helpful but in serious cases fuller neuropsychological evaluation is recommended, which should include tests of malingering and suggestibility.

Prison

The number of older people in prison has risen sharply over the past 20 years: in England and Wales, there were 365 sentenced prisoners aged 60 and over in 1990[32]. By 2007, this figure had increased sixfold to 2 192, and older prisoners now make up 2.9% of the total prison population[33]. In the US the number of older inmates showed a similar increase, tripling between 1990 and 2001, and their proportion in the total prison population doubled (from 4.0% to 8.2%)[34]. These increases appear to be due largely to changes in sentencing by the courts. 'Three strikes and out' sentences were first introduced in the US in 1993, and in the UK in 1998, with the result that recidivist violent offenders in particular remain in prison well into old age, such that many US states have been obliged to develop nursing home wings for older prisoners and the UK prison service is having to take seriously the needs of older inmates.

In the UK, much of the prison estate is old and difficult to adapt to meet the needs of older adults. Prison regimes can appear harsh and inflexible, as they are primarily concerned with the maintenance of security and discipline, and not with meeting health care needs. The result is that older prisoners can be extremely vulnerable and they are not uncommonly on the receiving end of serious aggression, despite the often very caring attitude of the majority of younger prisoners. Special units for older prisoners began to appear in the US in the 1970s, and a body of qualitative research showed that older prisoners, generally, though not always, preferred being in these units away from the noise and aggression of younger inmates[35]. In a study of sentenced older male prisoners in England and Wales high levels of psychiatric and physical morbidity were found[30,36]. In total, 53% had a psychiatric diagnosis, most commonly personality disorder and depressive neurosis, but 5% had a psychotic illness. In contrast to studies of younger prisoners, in which schizophrenia is the commonest psychotic illness, depressive psychosis was found to be the most common in older prisoners, yet only 12% of those diagnosed with depression were on antidepressants. Somewhat surprisingly, only two cases of dementia were found, but the sample of prisons included in the study contained few lifer units, in which cases of dementia are more common.

It is known that younger prisoners have worse physical health than age-matched controls. There is also evidence that such ill health continues into old age, with the elderly having more physical health problems than younger inmates and age-matched community living elders. A recent US study[28] highlighted the importance of thorough physical evaluation of older men coming in to prison to ensure they benefited from secondary preventive treatment for cerebrovascular disease and other common physical health problems. The study also showed that sexually transmitted disease (STD) is common among older prisoners. Clinicians unfamiliar with working with the elderly often assume that older people are sexually inactive, and do not ask about the possibility of STDs. Older prisoners should have access to primary and secondary care physicians who are familiar with the latest research and guidance on health promotion in this age group.

Women

The number of older women in prison has risen sharply over the past ten years. Many of these are long-term prisoners, though there are some who have committed serious offences for the first time in late life. It is likely that they have at least the same prevalence of mental health problems, if not greater, than their younger peers. But as numbers are small, little formal research has been carried out. In a sociological study of older women prisoners in the UK, it was found that there were a number of older women from ethnic minorities who suffered the double isolation of being different because of their age and different because of their culture[37].

Psychiatric Services

In the past it was very difficult for older patients to access specialist secure psychiatric services, particularly in the UK. Only 1% of those newly admitted to high and medium secure beds in England and Wales between 1988 and 1994 were over 60[38]. The conclusion drawn was that this was because people of such age were regarded as unsuitable for existing UK forensic services, mainly because of concerns about their potential vulnerability to aggression from younger patients. A number of studies have shown that older adults make up between 1% and 3% of referrals to forensic mental health services in the UK and Sweden[39–41]. There have been several descriptive studies of the elderly in high security, but these mainly focused on diagnostic issues[42–44]. In a more recent study at Broadmoor high security hospital in England the heterogeneity of older mentally disordered offenders in terms of diagnosis, assessed needs and expressed preferences was highlighted[45]. Despite there being a ward specifically for older vulnerable patients, the 16 patients over the age of 65 identified in the study were spread across 9 different wards in the hospital. Some authors have proposed 'streamlining' older offenders to make their care more cost-effective[27], but if the findings of the Broadmoor study are replicated then it would appear that streamlining will be very difficult. Older patients have some similarities one with another, because of their age, but the range of problems they present and their needs appear to be just as diverse as those of younger patients. It would be wrong to confine them all together solely on grounds of chronological age. This important issue emerged in some of the earlier qualitative work in prisons when it was found that not all older inmates wanted to be housed together; some liked the hustle and bustle and felt they enjoyed a high status in mixed age units because of their age and life experience[46].

Care homes for older adults often cope with high levels of minor physical aggression and sexually disinhibited behaviour[47]. However, they are not equipped to deal with more serious aggression or predatory sexual behaviour. The understanding of risk issues and how to assess and manage them is often highly sophisticated for the common behavioural problems of dementia, but for behaviour driven by antisocial personality traits it is usually lacking. This means there is a lack of suitable facilities for older offenders who have been assessed and require ongoing nursing care in an environment that is also able to manage their risky behaviour. In the UK specialist hospital units have been set up for those who require inpatient assessment and treatment, but a lack of suitable places to discharge patients to once they have been stabilized, though not necessarily to a state where the risks they pose to others have been substantially reduced, means that many remain in hospital for longer than would otherwise be necessary. Most offenders with established dementia will be unfit to plead or stand trial, and, if violence has been serious, will require further care and supervision in a hospital unit specially designed to meet their mental and physical health care needs with just sufficient security to ensure public protection.

TREATMENT ISSUES

The most important consideration in the treatment of the mental health problems of elderly offenders is location. For less serious offenders, normal treatment by their community mental health team in conjunction with their general practitioner is appropriate. For those in custody, treatment by a visiting psychiatrist and prison in-reach team may be sufficient, but for others assessment and treatment in hospital will be required. For some of these it may be appropriate for an old age psychiatrist to manage the case within their own service with advice from the local forensic psychiatric team, but in some cases the individual may need treatment in secure hospital. The ethos and treatment philosophy of specialist secure units for older adults should ideally be a synthesis of older adult and forensic psychiatric service models, modified and adapted to ensure that security is maintained without unnecessary levels of physical security. They should aim to be comfortable and homely without compromising safety. Staff training is paramount: a well-intentioned but infantilizing approach is likely to be robustly rejected by patients unused to *fluffy nurses* – a pejorative term used by patients to describe staff who are unfamiliar with forensic issues. Equally, a harsh and emotionless approach with an over-reliance on physical restraint is unlikely to meet the needs of individuals who may spend the rest of their lives on a particular ward and have no social contacts outside the ward team and co-patients. Pharmacological treatments are no different for elderly offenders with mental health problems than for their community peers, but the risk/benefit balance is tilted more towards drug treatment than would be the case in standard old age psychiatric practice. Despite all the safety concerns about using antipsychotic medication in dementia[48], there would be few who would argue against a trial of medication in an individual displaying thousands of aggressive acts per month in whom all other treatments have proved ineffective. Antipsychotics in schizophrenia tend to be used at doses more typical of working age adult services than old age services and occasionally there is justification for a trial of high dose antipsychotic medication providing safety guidelines are followed. Anti-libidinal medication can be useful in the treatment of sexual offenders with personality disorders and organic mental health problems though the evidence base for this is still very limited.

RISK ASSESSMENT

The unstructured clinical assessment that was the cornerstone of forensic psychiatric practice a generation ago has been largely replaced by a range of actuarial and structured clinical assessment tools backed up by a substantial body of research. The problem of using these tools is that none has been validated in the elderly, and many tend to focus on past behaviour or negative characteristics. There is a potential for misuse of actuarial tools that predict future risk as their positive predictive value depends on the base rate of offending in the population, which is of course much lower in the elderly than in younger adults on whom the instruments were developed. In the absence of instruments designed for the elderly, the use of structured clinical risk assessment tools such as the HCR-20[49] for physical violence and Risk of Sexual Violence Protocol (RSVP)[50] for sexual violence is recommended to ensure a systematic approach to the gathering of risk information.

PREVENTION

A number of studies in the US have shown that the elderly, being less physically able, make greater use of firearms than younger violent offenders[15,16,27]. Access to guns is much more restricted in the UK, yet older homicide offenders still manage to find weapons of sufficient lethality without too much difficulty. The weapon of choice for such incidents is usually a blunt object, and I have dealt with homicide cases by older adults involving repeated blows to the head with a ceramic fruit bowl, a club hammer, a walking stick, a pair of long handled garden loppers, an antique flat iron, a stone in a sock and decapitation with a saw. Restricting access to conventional weapons is unlikely to affect the rate of these domestic homicides in the UK because the victims are generally of similar age and may be quite frail, and almost any household implement can be made into a lethal weapon given sufficient will and a little physical strength. A far better preventive strategy would be to focus efforts on delivering good quality psychiatric care to all older people with mental health problems, and increasing the skills of primary care physicians for early identification of depression. Other priorities will include persisting with efforts to help those with alcohol problems and routinely asking patients and carers about physical aggression and sexually inappropriate behaviour.

REFERENCES

1. *Home Office Statistical Bulletin*. Criminal Statistics 2005 (England and Wales). At www.homeoffice.gov.uk/rds/pdfs06/hosb1906.pdf, accessed 25 Aug 2009.
2. Federal Bureau of Investigation. Uniform Crime Reports 1995–2007. At www.fbi.gov/ucr/ucr.htm accessed 25 Aug 2009.
3. Clark C, Mezey G. Elderly sex offenders against children: a descriptive study of child sex abusers over the age of 65. *J Forens Psychiatry Psychol* 1997; **8**: 357–69.
4. Hucker SJ, Ben-Aron MH. Elderly sex offenders. In Langevin R (ed.), *Erotic Preference, Gender Identity and Aggression in Men: New Research Studies*. Hillsdale, NJ: Lawrence Erlbaum, 1985, 211–23.
5. Rayel MG. Elderly sexual offenders admitted to a maximum security forensic hospital. *J Forens Sci* 2000; **45**: 1190–92.
6. Whiskin FE. The geriatric sex offender. *Geriatrics* 1967; **22**: 168–72.
7. Fazel S, Sjöstedt G, Långström N, Grann M. Risk factors for criminal recidivism in older sexual offenders. *Sex Abuse* 2006; **18**: 159–67.
8. Hanson K. Recidivism and age: follow-up data from 4673 offenders. *J interpers Violence* 2002; **17**: 1046–62.
9. Barbaree H, Blanchard R, Langton C. The development of sexual aggression through the life span: the effect of age on sexual arousal and recidivism among sex offenders. *Ann N Y Acad Sci* 2003; **989**: 59–71.
10. Rollin HR. Deviant behaviour in relation to mental disorder. *Proc R Soc Med* 1973; **66**: 99–104.
11. Gillies H. Homicide in the west of Scotland. *Br J Psychiatry* 1976; **128**: 105–27.
12. Hucker SJ, Ben-Aron MH. Violent elderly offenders – a comparative study. In Wilbanks W, Kim PKH (eds), *Elderly Criminals*. Lanham, MD: University Press of America, 1984, 69–81.
13. Knight B. Geriatric homicide – or the Darby and Joan syndrome. *Geriatr Med* 1983; **13**: 297–300.

14. Willbanks W. The elderly offender: relative frequency and patterns of offenses. *Int J Aging Human Dev* 1984–1985; **20**: 269–81.

15. Kratcoski PC, Walker DB. Homicide among the elderly: analysis of the victim/assailant relationship. In McCarthy B, Langworthy R (eds), *Older Offenders: Perspectives in Criminology and Criminal Justice*. New York: Praeger, 1988, 63–75.

16. Goetting A. Patterns of homicide among the elderly. *Violence Vict* 1992; **7**: 203–15.

17. Kratcoski PC. Circumstances surrounding homicide by older offenders. *Crim Just Behav* 1990; **17**: 420–30.

18. Epstein LJ, Mills C, Simon A. Antisocial behaviour of the elderly. *Compr Psychiatry* 1970; **11**: 36–42.

19. Vartiainen H, Hakola P. Homicides in residential homes: the price of savings in mental health services? *J Forens Psychiatry* 1994; **5**: 421–5.

20. Cohen D, Llorente M, Eisdorfer C. Homicide–suicide in older persons. *Am J Psychiatry* 1998; **155**: 390–96.

21. Berman AL. Dyadic death: a typology. *Suicide Life Threat Behav* 1996; **26**: 342–50.

22. Patel V, Hope RA. A rating scale for aggressive behaviour in the elderly – the RAGE. *Psychol Med* 1992; **22**: 211–21.

23. Ticehurst SB, Ryan MG, Hughes F. Homicidal behaviour in elderly patients admitted to a psychiatric hospital. *Dementia* 1992; **3**: 86–90.

24. Ticehurst SB, Gale IG, Rosenberg SJ. Homicide and attempted homicide by patients suffering from dementia; two case reports. *Aust N Z J Psychiatry* 1994; **28**: 136–40.

25. Gallagher J. *Isobel Barnett: Portrait of a Lady*. London: Methuen, 1982.

26. Sorocco KH, Ferrell SW. Alcohol among older adults. *J Gen Psychol* 2006; **133**: 453–67.

27. Lewis CF, Fields C, Rainey E. A study of geriatric evaluees: who are the violent elderly? *J Am Acad Psychiatry Law* 2006; **34**: 324–332.

28. Curtice M, Parker J, Wismayer F, Tomison A. The elderly offender: an 11 year survey of referrals to a regional forensic psychiatry service. *J Forens Psychiatry Psychol* 2003; **14**: 253–65.

29. *National Confidential Inquiry into Suicide and Homicide by People with Mental Illness*, Annual Report, England and Wales, 2009. Manchester: University of Manchester. At www.medicine.manchester.ac.uk/psychiatry/research/suicide/prevention/nci/inquiryannualreports/AnnualReportJuly2009.pdf, accessed 9 Feb 2010.

30. Fazel S, Hope T, O'Donnell I, Jacoby R. Hidden psychiatric morbidity in elderly prisoners. *Br J Psychiatry* 2001; **179**: 535–9.

31. Needham-Bennett H, Parrott J, Macdonald AJD. Psychiatric disorder and policing the elderly offender. *Crim Behav Ment Health* 1996; **6**: 241–52.

32. Howse K. *Growing Old in Prison: A Scoping Study on Older Prisoners*. London, Prison Reform Trust, 2003.

33. HM Inspectorate of Prisons. *Older Prisoners in England and Wales: A Follow-up to the 2004 Thematic Review*. London: HM Inspectorate of Prisons, 2008.

34. Aday RH. *Aging Prisoners: Crisis in American Corrections*. Westport, CT: Praeger, 2003.

35. Bachand DJ. The elderly offender: an exploratory study with implications for continuing education of law enforcement personnel. Doctoral Thesis, University of Michigan, Ann Arbor, 1984.

36. Fazel S, Hope T, O'Donnell I, Jacoby R. Health of elderly male prisoners: worse than the general population, worse than younger prisoners. *Age Ageing* 2001; **30**: 403–7.

37. Wahidin, A. *Older Women and the Criminal Justice System: Running Out of Time*. London: Jessica Kingsley, 2004.

38. Coid J, Fazel S, Kahtan N. Elderly patients admitted to secure forensic psychiatry services. *J Forens Psychiatry* 2002; **13**: 416–27.

39. Tomar R, Treasaden I, Shah A. Is there a case for a specialist forensic psychiatry service for the elderly? *Int J Geriatr Psychiatry* 2005; **20**: 51–6.

40. Fazel S, Grann M. Older criminals: a descriptive study of psychiatrically examined offenders in Sweden. *Int J Geriatr Psychiatry* 2002; **17**: 907–13.

41. McLeod C, Yorston G, Gibb R. Referrals of older adults to forensic and psychiatric intensive care services: a retrospective case-note study in Scotland. *Br J Forens Pract* 2008; **10**: 36–40.

42. Farragher B, O'Connor A. Forensic psychiatry and elderly people: a retrospective. *Med Sci Law* 1995; **35**: 269–73.

43. Wong MTH, Lumsden J, Fenton GW, Fenwick PBC. Elderly offenders in a maximum security mental hospital. *Aggress Behav* 1995; **21**: 321–4.

44. Rayel MG. Clinical and demographic characteristics of elderly offenders at a maximum security forensic hospital. *J Forens Sci* 2000; **45**: 1193–6.

45. Yorston G, Taylor PJ. Older patients in an English high security hospital: a qualitative study of the experiences and attitudes of patients aged 60 and over and their care staff in Broadmoor Hospital. *J Forens Psychiatry Psychol* 2009; **20**: 255–67.

46. Goetting A. The elderly in prison: issues and perspectives. *J Res Crime Delinq* 1983; **20**: 291–309.

47. Talerico KA, Evans LK, Strumpf NE. Mental health correlates of aggression in nursing home residents with dementia. *Gerontologist* 2002; **42**: 169–77.

48. Haw C, Yorston G, Stubbs J. Guidelines on antipsychotics for dementia – are we losing our minds? *Psychiatr Bull* 2009; **33**: 57–60.

49. Webster CD, Douglas KS, Eaves D, Hart SD. *HCR-20: Assessing Risk for Violence*. Burnaby, British Columbia: Mental Health, Law, and Policy Institute, Simon Fraser University, 1997.

50. Hart S, Kropp R, Laws R et al. *The Risk for Sexual Violence Protocol (RSVP)*. Mental Health, Law and Policy Institute, Simon Fraser University, Pacific Psychological Assessment Corporation and British Columbia Institute against Family Violence, 2003.

111

Sleep and Ageing: Disorders and Management

Helen Chiu[1] and Joshua Tsoh[2]

[1]Department of Psychiatry, The Chinese University of Hong Kong, Shatin, New Territories, Hong Kong
[2]Prince of Wales Hospital, Shatin, New Territories, Hong Kong

INTRODUCTION

Sleep changes significantly across the human lifespan, and sleep disturbances are particularly prevalent in older populations[1-12]. Epidemiological studies around the world have reported that the prevalence of insomnia symptoms increases with age and reaches around 50% in the elderly (readers can refer to Ohayon, 2002[9], for a review). A representative study by Foley et al. on over 9000 participants aged 65 or older in three US communities reveals that over 54% of the subjects had one or more sleep complaints most of the time; the number of complaints rises with age, and the odds for women to have difficulty falling asleep are almost 50% higher than for men[5]. Upon longitudinal examination, insomnia emerges with an annual incidence rate of at least 5% among the seniors who did not have insomnia at baseline[6].

Apart from being a major source of vexation to the elderly and their caregivers, persistent sleep disruptions are associated with poorer mental and physical health, elevated fall incidents, worse cognitive and functional performance, lower quality of life, earlier institutionalization and greater mortality over time[12].

To formulate evidence-based solutions to meet this public health challenge, clinicians should examine and understand the interplay of clinical factors, which include physiological changes in sleep architecture with ageing, sleep disorders that are more prevalent among the elderly (e.g. sleep disordered breathing (SDB), restless legs syndrome (RLS), rapid eye movement sleep behavioural disorder (RSBD)), and sleep modulating effects from physical and mental disorders, medications, undesirable sleep habits and environmental factors that are more common in later life.

INSOMNIA

Insomnia is the most common clinical sleep complaint; it can refer to difficulties initiating or maintaining sleep, waking up too early or an inability to obtain sleep that is of adequate duration or perceived as restorative. However, not all individuals with symptoms of insomnia are dissatisfied with their sleep or face daytime consequences[9]. A diagnosis of insomnia as a disorder according to the International Classification of Sleep Disorders (ICSD) criteria[13] would require the concomitant presence of persistent sleep difficulty, daytime impairment and adequate sleep opportunity.

In a review of 13 representative epidemiological studies from around the world (involving 33 000 non-institutionalized elderly)[9], Ohayon finds that the prevalence of insomnia symptoms varied vastly (9 to 65%) according to criteria differences, but the figures are consistently higher in females. Two studies have examined insomnia as a disorder (Chiu et al., 1999[14]; Ohayon and Vecchierini, 2002[15]), in which cases the prevalence is comparable, and significantly more female than male elders suffer from insomnia (around 16 to 18% and 9 to 12%, respectively).

The high rate of insomnia in the elderly might be related to physiological ageing of the structures involved in homeostatic and circadian rhythm mechanisms, secondary to medical and psychosocial conditions that abound in late life, or a combination of these factors[1-4,8-12].

Sleep Architectural Changes with Physiological Ageing

The suprachiasmatic nucleus (SCN) in the hypothalamus is the biological 'master clock' that controls the circadian rhythms of physiological processes including sleep, body temperature and endocrine output in a roughly 24-hour cycle[16]. Its endogenous periodicity is entrained by external zeitgebers ('time-givers'), most notably environmental light, through the retinohypothalamic tract (RHT)[16]. Its rhythmicity is also affected by a number of interlocking feedback mechanisms, including pineal secretion of melatonin (a hormone causing drowsiness and lower body temperature), which peaks in the middle of the night[16]. Current evidence shows that sleep is initiated upon reciprocal inhibition of cholinergic, noradrenergic and serotonergic arousal systems in the brain stem by the ventral lateral preoptic (VLPO) area of the anterior hypothalamus, which is in turn influenced by circadian signals from the SCN. Once sleep begins, an ultradian oscillator in the mesopontine junction of the brain stem controls the regular alternation of non-rapid eye movement (NREM) and REM phases of sleep, which usually occur four to five times per night[16]. NREM sleep is divided into four progressively deeper stages (I, II, III and IV), is characterized by slow waves on an electroencephalogram (EEG), and predominates in the early part of sleep. REM sleep, on the other hand, is characterized by an active EEG pattern, REM clusters on the electrooculography (EOG), and muscle atonia. REM sleep is more pronounced in the latter cycles of sleep as NREM sleep becomes concomitantly shallower.

Principles and Practice of Geriatric Psychiatry, 3rd edn. Edited by Mohammed T. Abou-Saleh, Cornelius Katona and Anand Kumar

With ageing there is a physiological change in the circadian cycle at all levels; it has been observed that reduction in SCN cell numbers/neuronal activity[3] and melatonin secretion occurs with advancing age[17]. The responsiveness of the circadian clock and pineal melatonin secretion to zeitgebers also diminishes, along with age-related decline in sensitivity to light in the visual structures[3]. The aged circadian system is also less adaptive to changes; difficulty adjusting to shift-work and jet lag are more common in middle-aged persons than in their younger counterparts[3]. Furthermore, along with other circadian physiological processes, phase-advances in sleep have consistently been observed[3]. Circadian amplitudes might also become less pronounced; the sleep of older individuals is often punctuated by periods of wakefulness, and they are also more easily aroused from sleep by environmental stimuli[2,3,18]. Napping is generally more common; recent studies show that naps do not necessarily have a negative impact on the nocturnal sleep architecture[1–3,18–20].

In terms of sleep polysomnographical findings, Ohayon et al. reported, in a meta-analysis on 2400 healthy, non-institutionalized individuals aged 19 to 102 years from the US and Europe[8], that there is a decrease in total sleep time (TST), sleep efficiency (SE), percentage of slow wave sleep (SWS; stages III and IV of NREM sleep) and REM sleep across the adult life span; on the other hand, an increase in stages I and II sleep, and wake after sleep onset (WASO) take place. Age-related differences in sleep and REM latencies are not pronounced; gender differences are modest.

It is, however, noteworthy that most of the stated age-related changes have taken place *already* in younger adulthood. When the sleep of older adults (aged 60 or older) in particular is examined, apart from the SE, which declines mildly, no clear changes in the sleep macroarchitecture are found with advancing age[8].

These polysomnographical findings suggested that the normal sleep macrostructural changes with physiological ageing in later life are (probably with the exception of advanced sleep phase disorder) largely not accountable for the prevailing epidemiological findings of a rising rate of insomnia with age in the elderly, especially among older women.

Other Causes for Insomnia with Ageing

The Foley et al. cohort study of 9000 community-dwelling elders in the US found that advancing age was not associated with insomnia after adjusting for differences in health status[5]. Upon follow-up three years later, 93% of persons with incident insomnia in this interval were found to have risk factors including chronic physical disease, depressed mood, physical disability, poor perceived health, widowhood and use of sedatives, while improved self-perceived health was associated with remission of the 2000 survivors with chronic insomnia at baseline. The authors concluded that the incidence of insomnia in the elderly is not related to the ageing process *per se* but to other risk factors, a finding echoed by epidemiological studies on insomnia disorder subsequently conducted in populations from China and from France[9,14,15].

Recent studies have confirmed that incidences of secondary insomnia far outnumber those of primary insomnia disorder in the older population[9,12,21]. Particularly common clinical conditions leading to secondary insomnia in late life include neuropsychiatric degeneration (e.g. Alzheimer's disease or Parkinson's disease), a number of age-related sleep disorders (SDB, RLS and RSBD), psychiatric illnesses (especially depressive and anxiety disorders, alcohol dependence) and other medical disorders (particularly those affecting the musculoskeletal, cardiovascular, gastrointestinal, pulmonary and genitourinary systems, malignancies, painful conditions, and the drugs used to treat them)[9,12,21].

Interested readers can refer to Barczi and Juergens, 2006[21] and Garcia, 2008[22] for two extensive reviews on the relations between prevalent medical disorders and insomnia in the elderly. It should be noted that 'co-morbid insomnia' is the term currently preferred over 'secondary insomnia' when the causative relationships are not clearly proven[23]. The specific conditions of SDB, RLS, RSBD and sleep disorders related to dementia will be discussed in separate sections in this chapter.

Evaluation of Insomnia Disorder

A carefully taken sleep history is important; Lichstein et al. recommend a multidimensional approach to exploring contributory factors to insomnia in the (i) circadian; (ii) psychiatric; (iii) pharmacologic; (iv) medical or neurological; and (v) psychophysiological reactivity (like subclinical anxiety and physiological tension) and negative conditioning (e.g. from poor sleep hygiene, or performance anxiety related to frequent insomnia) domains[4]. Along with a relevant physical examination, the primary condition(s) leading to insomnia should first be elucidated and treated where present. Routine investigation with polysomnography (PSG) is not recommended for insomnia disorder by the American Academy of Sleep Medicine except when there is diagnostic uncertainty (covert cases of RLS, SDB or RSBD are more common with advanced age) or prior treatment failure[4,24].

Non-Pharmacological Treatment of Insomnia Disorder

Psychological and behavioural interventions are effective in the treatment of insomnia in older adults, and in the treatment of insomnia among chronic hypnotic users[25]. They are most commonly cognitive behavioural therapies that comprise a combination of relaxation exercises, stimulus control (e.g. limiting bedroom use for sleep), sleep restriction, sleep compression (gradual reduction of time in bed) and cognitive therapy that counters excessive worries about sleep, and education on sleep hygiene. The positive effects are most pronounced on measures of SE, WASO and sleep onset latency (SOL)[4]. Interested readers can refer to Lichstein et al.[4] for a detailed review on the results from clinical trials of each cognitive behavioural therapy (CBT) technique. The role of light therapy in insomnia disorder needs to be further elucidated[26].

Pharmacological Treatment of Insomnia Disorder

In general, agents with a short half-life (thus less hangover/daytime sedation), a low dependence potential and a low propensity for disrupting normal sleep architecture are preferred. The newer benzodiazepine agonists including zolpidem, zopiclone, eszopiclone and zaleplon have all been found to be generally safe for short-term use in older adults. Zopiclone might be associated with a mild increase in SWS. For a comprehensive review, readers can refer to Salzman[27].

Complementary and Alternative Medicine for Insomnia Disorder

The use of complementary and alternative medicine approaches for sleep disturbances in older adults is widespread. Thus far there is evidence of the efficacy of melatonin in treatment of circadian rhythm disorders, but its effect is less conclusive in primary and secondary insomnias. Mind–body exercises like meditation, yoga, and Tai Chi showed promising results in open trials; their roles require further evaluation[28].

RAPID EYE MOVEMENT SLEEP BEHAVIOUR DISORDER (RSBD OR RBD)

First described by Schenck *et al.* in 1986[29], RSBD is now understood to be a parasomnia characterized by abnormal behaviours during REM sleep that cause sleep disruption and/or injury. It is a male-predominant disorder that usually emerges after the fifth decade, although any age group can be affected[13]. The data concerning its prevalence are scant; it was estimated to be 0.5% among the UK general population by a phone survey[30] and determined to be around 0.4% in a two-phase study on community-dwelling Chinese elders[31]. It could take an acute form upon REM rebound state (like withdrawal from alcohol or hypnotics) or be precipitated by intake of different antidepressants (except bupropion)[29]. More commonly, RSBD takes an idiopathic, chronic form which follows a progressively worsening course[29].

Patients with RSBD have dream-enactment behaviours during the REM stage of their sleep; they might talk, shout aloud, walk, kick or punch their bed partners, or fall out of bed[13,32–35]; in clinical series studying US and Chinese populations, about 30 to 50% of patients injure themselves; about 60% hurt their bed partners[32,34]. The patients often can recall their dreams, which are vivid and contain a high degree of violent/aggressive content that is usually out of keeping with the patient's normal behavioural patterns[36].

Moreover, features suggestive of early synucleinopathy including deficit pattern in brain perfusion scans[37] and abnormal cardiac autonomic regulation (likely from a loss of cardiac sympathetic terminals) on cardiac ^{123}I-metaiodobenzylguanidine (MIBG) scintigraphy[38–40] have been reported in patients with idiopathic RSBD. In fact, RSBD also occurs with disproportionately greater frequency in synucleinopathies like multiple system atrophy, Parkinson's disease and dementia with Lewy bodies compared to other neurodegenerative disorders. RSBD has been conceptualized as a manifestation of evolving synucleinopathies[41].

Diagnosis of RSBD is by clinical history, supplemented by video-polysomnographic study[42]. Electromyogram (EMG) during REM sleep reveals an excess of muscle tone or phasic EMG twitch activities[13]. Differential diagnoses include sleep-walking, night terrors, nightmares, nocturnal seizures, obstructive sleep apnoea, posttraumatic stress disorder, dissociative states and nocturnal confusional states[33].

High treatment efficacy (close to 90%) with clonazepam has been found in international studies. Protective measures against injuries during sleep might also be necessary, indicating the importance of the early recognition and management of RSBD[32–35].

SLEEP-RELATED MOVEMENT DISORDERS

Sleep-related movement disorders are characterized by stereotyped movements that disturb the sleep of the affected individual and, not uncommonly, their bed partners as well.

Restless legs syndrome (RLS) involves complex movements in the lower limbs to relieve the unpleasant local dysaesthesia (usually a deep-seated sensation described as 'creeping, crawling', 'pins and needles', 'tearing' and even 'burning' or 'electric-current-like'), which usually take place at night, begin or worsen when the patient is restful and relaxed and are not better explained by another medical disorder[12,13,43,44]. Low awareness and misdiagnosis of RLS are very common[44], which add to already significant distress and impairment from sleep disruption. Differential diagnoses include neuropathy, arthritic conditions, or vascular insufficiency in lower limbs, and leg cramps; RLS is distinguished by its high circadian rhythmicity (peak symptoms from midnight to 3 a.m.) and absence of local signs related to the mentioned disorder. Akathisia from antipsychotics is another differential diagnosis; apart from the drug history, features of akathisia are less focal than RLS[44].

The patho-mechanism for primary RLS is largely unknown. Subnormal dopamine neurotransmission has been implicated. Currently the only FDA-approved medication for RLS is the dopamine agonist ropinirole[43] (although, in suitable cases, other dopamine agonists might be considered, according to the practice guidelines of the American Academy of Sleep Medicine[45]). Low ferritin levels in adult RLS patients have also been reported in a number of studies involving blood tests, neuroimaging and cerebrospinal fluid examination, although the relationship in older individuals appeared less consistent[43]. Secondary RLS has been recognized in uraemia and pregnancy[13]. Some argued that wandering behaviours in demented individuals might be related to unrecognized RLS[46]. Therefore, drugs used to treat neuropsychiatric symptoms of dementia (e.g. antipsychotics and some antidepressants) might potentially aggravate the condition.

A related condition is *periodic limb movements in sleep (PLMS)* which involves clusters of stereotyped, repeated, non-epileptiform leg jerks (typically involving dorsiflexion of the anterior tibilis muscle, although the movement might involve the hip, or be confined to the toe) taking place at 20–40 second intervals over the course of sleep, with each jerk causing a brief awakening that could be captured on PSG; a diagnosis is made when there are at least five kicks per hour of sleep[12,43]. The prevalence of PLMS in the elderly is estimated to be relatively high, at 45%[12]. It is found in 80–90% of patients with RLS, and is also very common in other primary sleep disorders[13,43].

PLMS usually occurs in NREM sleep[13]. Typically, the patient is unaware of the limb movement or the frequent arousals, and might not report sleep dissatisfaction. Usually no treatment is required in such cases. The ICSD criteria require PLMS features occurring in conjunction with clinical sleep disturbance and/or complaint of daytime fatigue for a diagnosis of *periodic limb movement disorder (PLMD)* to be made[13]. Drug treatment with dopamine agonists might also be considered in such cases[45], along with judicious elimination of drugs (serotonin-specific re-uptake inhibitors (SSRIs), antipsychotics etc.) that might worsen the condition in applicable cases[43].

An epidemiological study involving 18 980 adult subjects who were 15 to 100 years old (representative of the general population of five European countries) revealed that the prevalence of RLS, but not PLMD, significantly increased with age. The prevalence of ICSD-based diagnoses of PLMD in older age groups (60 or over) was 3–4% and that of RLS was 8–9%. Risk factors for both disorders include female sex, musculoskeletal disease, heart disease, SDB, cataplexy, intense physical activity close to bedtime and the presence of a mental disorder. Factors solely associated with RLS are advanced age, obesity, hypertension, drinking at least three alcoholic beverages per day, smoking more than 20 cigarettes per day and the use of SSRIs. Factors specific to PLMD include shift-work, coffee intake, use of hypnotics and the presence of stress[47].

SLEEP-RELATED BREATHING DISORDERS

Sleep-disordered breathing (SDB) is characterized by apnoeas (complete cessation of airflow lasting 10 seconds or more), hypopnoeas (reduction of airflow of 10 seconds or longer, accompanied by an oxygen saturation decreased by 3–4% or more) on sleep PSG[48]. The number of apnoeas and hypopnoeas per hour of sleep is called the *apnoea-hypopnoea index (AHI)*. Apnoeas and hypopnoeas during sleep leads to repeated arousals and hypoxaemia during sleep, and the *respiratory disturbance index (RDI)* refers to the number of apnoeas, hypopnoeas and the respiratory effort-related arousals per hour of sleep[49]. In general, an AHI from 5 to 19 is referred to as mild obstructive sleep apnoea (OSA), an AHI from 20 to 29 as moderate, and 30 and above as severe OSA. When the AHI is 5 or greater and coupled with excessive daytime sleepiness (EDS) the patient is considered to have the OSA syndrome (OSAS)[49].

Symptomatically, OSAS manifests as loud snoring and daytime somnolence; associated features include headache, insomnia, apnoea and excessive movements observed during sleep, and nocturia and dry mouth on waking. In addition to sleep fragmentation, patients show decreased SWS and SE on PSG[11]. Complications including elevated cardiovascular morbidities (hypertension, strokes, worsened cardiac functions) and mortalities, and cognitive impairments, especially in the domains of attention and vigilance, executive function, visuospatial learning and motor performance[49]. There are two main types of sleep apnoea: obstructive and central; the former is more common.

The prevalence of SDB rises with age: in middle-aged adults (aged 30–60), the figures for OSA (with AHI 5 or over) are 9% for females and 24% for males; and those for OSAS are 2% and 4%, respectively. In adults aged over 60, the prevalence of OSA is reported to be around 38–62%; there is also a stepwise increase in the prevalence of SDB with each decade of life in old age, which might be due to an increase in central events (readers can refer to Norman and Loredo, 2008[49] for a review).

It remains unresolved, however, as to whether the clinical significance of SDB in the elderly diminishes as compared to that in their younger counterparts. The association between SDB and body mass index (BMI) and reports of snoring also decrease with ageing[11,12]. Before further studies are available to cast light on the issue, elderly patients with symptomatic apnoeas or possible cardiovascular and cognitive complications should be treated as younger individuals would be treated. The mainstay of treatment is continuous positive airway pressure (CPAP) during sleep, which provides continuous air pressure, acting as a pneumatic splint to maintain patency of the upper airway. There is evidence that SDB complications might also reverse with this treatment[49]. General measures including weight reduction, and the avoidance of alcohol and sedative medications should also be undertaken.

Compliance to CPAP could be a problem. Alternative options include oral appliance therapy (in elderly persons with full or nearly full dentition), and an array of surgeries designed to improve airflow in the upper airway. There is, however, scant evidence to support the clinical efficacy of these two alternatives in older adults[49].

SLEEP DISTURBANCES IN DEMENTIA

Sleep disturbances are common in patients with dementia[12]; among patients with Alzheimer's disease (AD) in clinic- and community-based samples, the prevalence varies between 24 and 44%[50-52], and is a major cause of caregiver distress and institutionalization[12,53].

Characteristic changes include significant sleep fragmentation, reduced SWS and REM sleep, decreased SE and TST, reversal of circadian rhythm, EDS and daytime napping, and 'sundowning' (a nocturnal exacerbation of disruptive behaviour or agitation)[12,53]. Poor sleep in AD might, in turn, worsen cognitive function[53].

Causes of sleep disturbances in AD occur at multiple levels. Intrinsically, accelerated degeneration of the SCN and decreased pineal melatonin secretion might cause circadian rhythm disruptions. Degeneration of the cholinergic neurons in the nucleus basalis of Meynert and pedunculopontine tegmental and laterodorsal tegmental nuclei and noradrenergic neurons of the brainstem may account for decreased REM sleep in AD patients, and predispose them to RSBD[12,52-54]. Degeneration of the brainstem respiratory neurons and those in the supramedullary respiratory pathways may heighten risk for SDB in AD; in fact, the *APOE*4* genotype might be a predisposing factor for SDB in the general population[53].

Extrinsic factors might include reduced bright light, diminished daytime activities and increased noise in the environment, especially in group residential facilities. General medical conditions affecting the cardiovascular and respiratory systems and medications might also have negative effects on sleep; for example, cholinesterase inhibitors for dementia might cause vivid dreams and insomnia[12,52-54].

Treatment for sleep problems in dementia should likewise be multimodal. Techniques to counter circadian rhythm disturbances may include structured daytime social and physical activities, restriction of time in bed, and bright light, especially in the morning and evening[12,52-55]. Hypnotics and antipsychotics are often used, although they are more commonly associated with adverse effects like sedation, parkinsonism or orthostatic hypotension and, for a number of antipsychotics, an elevated risk for stroke[56]. Results from randomized controlled trials of melatonin are thus far conflicting[57]. On the other hand, proper identification and treatment of SDB and depression in AD might improve sleep quality and reduce agitation[53,58].

CONCLUSIONS AND FUTURE DIRECTIONS

The management of sleep disorders in the elderly is a major public health challenge, given the rapid growth of the older population in most nations, the high prevalence of sleep complaints and variety of sleep disorders in this phase of life, the plethora of co-morbid clinical conditions and environmental factors that are associated with insomnia in seniors, and their greater susceptibility to the side effects of sedative medications in general.

As reviewed in this chapter, current evidence suggests that insomnia is not an inevitable effect of physiological ageing and the corresponding changes in sleep architecture. Given the fact that sleep disturbances are common in the elderly and that many of the underlying causes are reversible, sleep assessment should be a habitual part of their comprehensive clinical evaluation, with the sleep symptoms compared against a carefully taken history of physical and psychiatric conditions, medications, sleep habits and activity schedules, lifestyle changes and residential conditions. Standard sleep questionnaires in indicated cases (e.g. the Pittsburgh Sleep Quality Index) might facilitate the multidimensional evaluation of sleep quality and disturbances. Investigations should be arranged to rule out co-morbid medical conditions, and sleep polysomnography is indicated for cases in which specific sleep disorders like RLS, SDB, or RSBD are suspected (readers can refer to Misra and Malow, 2008[59] for a review).

Future directions for sleep research on the elderly may include longitudinal outcome of insomnia and specific sleep disorders, and further elucidation of the roles of light therapy, enriched activity schedules, complementary medicine and other measures that might potentially enhance the quality of sleep.

REFERENCES

1. Espiritu JR. Aging-related sleep changes. *Clin Geriatr Med* 2008; **24**: 1–14.

2. Vitiello MV. Sleep in normal aging. In Ancoli-Israel S (ed.), *Sleep Medicine Clinics*. New York: Elsevier, 2006, 171–6.

3. Naylor E, Zee PC. Circadian rhythm alterations with aging. In Ancoli-Israel S (ed.), *Sleep Medicine Clinics*. New York: Elsevier, 2006, 187–96.

4. Lichstein KL, Stone KC, Nau SD *et al*. Insomnia in the elderly. In Ancoli-Israel S (ed.), *Sleep Medicine Clinics*. New York: Elsevier, 2006, 221–30.

5. Foley DJ, Monjan AA, Brown SL *et al*. Sleep complaints among elderly persons: an epidemiologic study of three communities. *Sleep* 1995; **18**: 425–32.

6. Foley DJ, Monjan A, Simonsick EM *et al*. Incidence and remission of insomnia among elderly adults: an epidemiologic study of 6,800 persons over three years. *Sleep* 1999; **22**(Suppl): S366–72.

7. Foley D, Ancoli-Israel S, Britz P *et al*. Sleep disturbances and chronic disease in older adults: results of the 2003 National Sleep Foundation Sleep in America Survey. *J Psychosom Res* 2004; **56**: 497–502.

8. Ohayon MM, Carskadon MA, Guilleminault C *et al*. Meta-analysis of quantitative sleep parameters from childhood to old age in healthy individuals: developing normative sleep values across the human lifespan. *Sleep* 2004; **27**: 1255–73.

9. Ohayon MM. Epidemiology of insomnia: what we know and what we still need to learn. *Sleep Med Rev* 2002; **6**: 97–111.

10. Ohayon MM. Interactions between sleep normative data and sociocultural characteristics in the elderly. *J Psychosom Res* 2004; **56**: 479–86.

11. Redline S, Kirchner HL, Quan SF *et al*. The effects of age, sex, ethnicity, and sleep-disordered breathing on sleep architecture. *Arch Intern Med* 2004; **164**: 406–18.

12. Ancoli-Israel S, Ayalon L. Diagnosis and treatment of sleep disorders in older adults. *Am J Geriatr Psychiatry* 2006; **14**: 95–103.

13. American Academy of Sleep Medicine. *International Classification of Sleep Disorders*, 2nd edn. Westchester, IL: American Academy of Sleep Medicine, 2005.

14. Chiu HF, Leung T, Lam LC *et al*. Sleep problems in Chinese elderly in Hong Kong. *Sleep* 1999; **22**: 717–26.

15. Ohayon MM, Vecchierini MF. Daytime sleepiness and cognitive impairment in the elderly population. *Arch Intern Med* 2002; **162**(2): 201–8.

16. Pace-Schott EF, Hobson JA. The neurobiology of sleep: genetics, cellular physiology and subcortical networks. *Nat Rev Neurosci* 2002; **3**(8): 591–605.

17. Pandi-Perumal SR, Zisapel N, Srinivasan V *et al*. Melatonin and sleep in aging population. *Exp Gerontol* 2005; **40**: 911–25.

18. Martin JL, Ancoli-Israel S. Napping in older adults. In Ancoli-Israel S (ed.), *Sleep Medicine Clinics*. New York: Elsevier, 2006, 177–86.

19. Monk TH, Buysse DJ, Carrier J *et al*. Effects of afternoon "siesta" naps on sleep, alertness, performance, and circadian rhythms in the elderly. *Sleep* 2001; **24**: 680–7.

20. Campbell SS, Murphy PJ, Stauble TN. Effects of a nap on nighttime sleep and waking function in older subjects. *J Am Geriatr Soc* 2005; **53**: 48–53.

21. Barczi SR, Juergens TM. Comorbidities: psychiatric, medical, medications and substances. In Ancoli-Israel S (ed.), *Sleep Medicine Clinics*. New York: Elsevier, 2006, 231–46.

22. Garcia AD. The effect of chronic disorders on sleep in the elderly. *Clin Geriatr Med* 2008; **24**: 27–38.

23. State-of-the-Science Panel. National Institutes of Health State of the Science Conference statement on manifestations and management of chronic insomnia in adults, June 13–15, 2005. *Sleep* 2005; **28**(9): 1049–57.

24. Littner M, Hirshkowitz M, Kramer M. Practice parameters for the use of polysomnography in the evaluation of insomnia. Standards of Practice Committee of the American Sleep Disorders Association. *Sleep* 1995; **18**: 55–7.

25. Morgenthaler T, Kramer M, Alessi C *et al*. Practice parameters for the psychological and behavioral treatment of insomnia: an update. An American academy of sleep medicine report. *Sleep* 2006; **29**: 1415–19.

26. Gammack JK. Light therapy for insomnia in older adults. *Clin Geriatr Med* 2008; **24**: 139–49.

27. Salzman C. Pharmacologic treatment of disturbed sleep in the elderly. *Harv Rev Psychiatry* 2008; **16**: 271–8.

28. Gooneratne NS. Complementary and alternative medicine for sleep disturbances in older adults. *Clin Geriatr Med* 2008; **24**: 121–38.

29. Schenck CH, Bundlie SR, Ettinger MG *et al*. Chronic behavioral disorders of human REM sleep: a new category of parasomnia. *Sleep* 1986; **9**: 293–308.

30. Ohayon MM, Caulet M, Priest RG. Violent behavior during sleep. *J Clin Psychiatry* 1997; **58**: 369–76.

31. Chiu HF, Wing YK, Lam LC *et al*. Sleep-related injury in the elderly – an epidemiological study in Hong Kong. *Sleep* 2000; **23**: 513–17.

32. Wing YK, Lam SP, Li SX *et al*. REM sleep behaviour disorder in Hong Kong Chinese: clinical outcome and gender comparison. *J Neurol Neurosurg Psychiatry* 2008; **79**: 1415–16.

33. Chiu HF, Wing YK. REM sleep behaviour disorder: an overview. *Int J Clin Pract* 1997; **51**: 451–4.

34. Olson EJ, Boeve BF, Silber MH. Rapid eye movement sleep behaviour disorder: demographic, clinical and laboratory findings in 93 cases. *Brain* 2000; **123**(Pt 2): 331–9.

35. Sforza E, Krieger J, Petiau C. REM sleep behavior disorder: clinical and physiopathological findings. *Sleep Med Rev* 1997; **1**(1): 57–69.

36. Fantini ML, Corona A, Clerici S *et al*. Aggressive dream content without daytime aggressiveness in REM sleep behavior disorder. *Neurology* 2005; **65**: 1010–15.

37. Mazza S, Soucy JP, Gravel P *et al*. Assessing whole brain perfusion changes in patients with REM sleep behavior disorder. *Neurology* 2006; **67**: 1618–22.

38. Miyamoto T, Miyamoto M, Inoue Y *et al*. Reduced cardiac 123I-MIBG scintigraphy in idiopathic REM sleep behavior disorder. *Neurology* 2006; **67**: 2236–8.

39. Miyamoto T, Miyamoto M, Suzuki K *et al*. 123I-MIBG cardiac scintigraphy provides clues to the underlying neurodegenerative

disorder in idiopathic REM sleep behavior disorder. *Sleep* 2008; **31**: 717–23.

40. Lanfranchi PA, Fradette L, Gagnon JF, Colombo R, Montplaisir J. Cardiac autonomic regulation during sleep in idiopathic REM sleep behavior disorder. *Sleep* 2007; **30**: 1019–25.

41. Boeve BF, Silber MH, Ferman TJ *et al*. Association of REM sleep behavior disorder and neurodegenerative disease may reflect an underlying synucleinopathy. *Mov Disord* 2001; **16**: 622–30.

42. Zhang J, Lam SP, Ho CK *et al*. Diagnosis of REM sleep behavior disorder by video-polysomnographic study: is one night enough? *Sleep* 2008; **31**: 1179–85.

43. Bliwise DL. Periodic leg movements in sleep and restless legs syndrome: considerations in geriatrics. In Ancoli-Israel S (ed.), *Sleep Medicine Clinics*. New York: Elsevier, 2006, 263–72.

44. Spiegelhalder K, Hornyak M. Restless legs syndrome in older adults. *Clin Geriatr Med* 2008; **24**: 167–80.

45. Littner MR, Kushida C, Anderson WM *et al*. Practice parameters for the dopaminergic treatment of restless legs syndrome and periodic limb movement disorder. *Sleep* 2004; **27**(3): 557–9.

46. Allen RP, Picchietti D, Hening WA *et al*. Restless legs syndrome: diagnostic criteria, special considerations, and epidemiology. A report from the restless legs syndrome diagnosis and epidemiology workshop at the National Institutes of Health. *Sleep Med* 2003; **4**(2): 101–19.

47. Ohayon MM, Roth T. Prevalence of restless legs syndrome and periodic limb movement disorder in the general population. *J Psychosom Res* 2002; **53**(1): 547–54.

48. Stone KL, Redline S. Sleep-related breathing disorders in the elderly. In Ancoli-Israel S (ed.), *Sleep Medicine Clinics*. New York: Elsevier, 2006, 247–62.

49. Norman D, Loredo JS. Obstructive sleep apnea in older adults. *Clin Geriatr Med* 2008; **24**: 151–65.

50. McCurry SM, Logsdon RG, Teri L *et al*. Characteristics of sleep disturbance in community-dwelling Alzheimer's disease patients. *J Geriatr Psychiatry Neurol* 1999; **12**: 53–9.

51. Moran M, Lynch CA, Walsh C *et al*. Sleep disturbance in mild to moderate Alzheimer's disease. *Sleep Med* 2005; **6**: 347–52.

52. Vitiello MV, Borson S. Sleep disturbances in patients with Alzheimer's disease: epidemiology, pathophysiology and treatment. *CNS Drugs* 2001; **15**: 777–96.

53. Avidan AY. Sleep and neurologic problems in the elderly. In Ancoli-Israel S (ed.), *Sleep Medicine Clinics*. New York: Elsevier, 2006, 273–92.

54. Paniagua MA, Paniagua EW. The demented elder with insomnia. *Clin Geriatr Med* 2008; **24**: 69–81, vii.

55. Deschenes CL, McCurry SM. Current treatments for sleep disturbances in individuals with dementia. *Curr Psychiatry Rep* 2009; **11**: 20–6.

56. Douglas IJ, Smeeth L. Exposure to antipsychotics and risk of stroke: self controlled case series study. *BMJ* 2008; **337**: a1227.

57. Serfaty M, Kennell-Webb S, Warner J *et al*. Double blind randomised placebo controlled trial of low dose melatonin for sleep disorders in dementia. *Int J Geriatr Psychiatry* 2002; **17**: 1120–7.

58. Erkinjuntti T, Partinen M, Sulkava R *et al*. Sleep apnea in multiinfarct dementia and Alzheimer's disease. *Sleep* 1987; **10**: 419–25.

59. Misra S, Malow BA. Evaluation of sleep disturbances in older adults. *Clin Geriatr Med* 2008; **24**: 15–26.

112

Sexual Disorders

Walter Pierre Bouman

Mental Health Services for Older People, University Hospital, Nottingham, UK

INTRODUCTION

Sexuality is an essential part of any person and expressing it is a basic human need and right of all individuals, including older people. Although sexual functioning and frequency decrease with age[1-3], a significant proportion of older people remain sexually active well into advanced old age and many older people continue to enjoy their sex lives. In fact, several cross-sectional studies have shown that sexual satisfaction does not decline with age[4,5], and the role and value of sexual activity and intimacy remain important quality of life issues to older people[5,6].

Older people can experience sexual problems for all the same reasons as their younger counterparts. Sex research in older women and men emphasizes the widespread prevalence of sexual difficulties[7-9], which are strongly correlated with physical and mental health and with satisfaction in the intimate relationship[10-12].

Should a person or a couple wish to continue but experience sexual difficulties they deserve the same access to treatment as younger people. Furthermore, prevention of sexual difficulties in older people should be encouraged, including appropriate counselling before genital surgery[13], during chronic medical care and after acute medical events such as a myocardial infarction or cerebrovascular accident[14] and the provision of advice on safe sex practices.

HORMONAL CHANGES AND AGEING

In healthy men, testosterone production remains relatively stable until the fifth decade and then decreases slowly over the remainder of the man's life at a rate of about 1.0% per year[15]. It is probably mainly a result of testicular ageing, although a rise in sex hormone-binding globulin (SHBG) and testosterone-binding, a relative failure of the hypothalamo-pituitary axis to drive the testes, and a decline in the level of sensitivity of testosterone receptors in the brain also contribute. The decline in circulating testosterone occurring in older men is responsible for the decrease in desire, but not erectile function, although clinically it may be difficult to distinguish reliably between the two complaints[16].

In women, the most prominent biochemical markers of sexual maturation and senescence are the age-related changes in the level of oestrogen and testosterone. The structural integrity of the female genitalia is predominantly maintained by oestrogen. Vaginal dryness and atrophy, dyspareunia and urinary tract symptoms suggest a lack of oestrogen which is more prevalent following the menopause[17].

In healthy women testosterone levels decline markedly until the fourth decade with stable levels during the menopause transition. Testosterone levels then increase slowly over the rest of the life span[18].

AGE-RELATED CHANGES AND SEXUAL RESPONSE

Master and Johnson's[19] landmark research in the physiology of sexual responses have provided important information regarding sexuality and ageing, although their sample size was small. In both sexes, as one ages, the speed and intensity of the various vasocongestive responses to sexual stimulation tend to be reduced. In men all responses are slower and less intense from nipple and penile erection to rectal orgasmic contractions. An erection takes longer to develop and usually requires more direct tactile stimulation. The period of sustaining an erection gets shorter.

Ejaculation becomes less powerful with fewer contractions and seminal fluid volume is reduced. The point of ejaculatory inevitability becomes more difficult to recognize. Resolution following orgasm is rapid, with loss of erection occurring within seconds and the refractory period is markedly longer in comparison to younger men, sometimes extending to more than a day. In women the responses parallel those of the male. Increased time is required to become sexually aroused and vaginal lubrication is slower and less marked. Orgasms tend to be less intense and there is an increased need for stimulation to become orgasmic. There is no change in the ability to have orgasms, although multiple orgasms are less likely to occur. Resolution is more rapid.

Many older people are unaware of the normal age-related changes in sexual response that accompany ageing and are perplexed or put off by changes in their own or their partner's sexual response. If not appreciated, these changes are easily misinterpreted as sexual dysfunction. Explicit information about changes in sexual physiology with ageing can help eliminate false expectations and can permit modification in longstanding sexual practices that may have become counterproductive. Couples can be advised, for example, not to delay sexual exchange until late at night when tiredness or sleepiness may be great but, rather, to schedule their sexual encounters at a time of greater energy and alertness.

Similarly, increased manual or oral stimulation of the penis may be necessary to achieve an adequate erection for intercourse and may augment the effects of pharmacological therapy[20]. The female partner is often unaware of this important physiological change in her partner, and may misattribute his lack of erection to sexual disinterest or her loss of sexual attractiveness to her partner[21].

Many older couples indicate they would enjoy greater sexual experimentation in their relationship, even though many have minimal experience of foreplay or non-intercourse forms of sexual stimulation[22]. While the overall decline of the sexual responses may seem gloomy and unpleasant, this process tends to develop extremely gradually, allowing an individual or a couple to adjust to a less intense, but not necessarily less enjoyable form of sexual activity.

EFFECTS OF ILLNESS AND MEDICATION ON SEXUALITY

One of the most frequent reasons given by older people for stopping sexual activity is the onset of illness; this may operate through a number of different mechanisms. Physical illness may generate unfounded anxieties about the risks of sexual activity (as in heart disease or stroke); it may make intercourse difficult, exhausting or painful (as in respiratory disease, arthritis and (sexually transmitted) infection); or it may impair responsiveness of the sexual organs (as in diabetes mellitus or peripheral vascular disease).

Illness may further undermine self-confidence and the feeling of attractiveness (as in mutilating operations such as mastectomy or colostomy), and it may have a direct effect in reducing sexual desire (as in depression, chronic renal or hepatic failure, and Parkinson's disease). Older people in general are more likely to suffer from a variety of chronic diseases which may impact on their sexual function[23]. They also commonly undergo surgery, which may influence sexual function, either because of psychological sequelae or as a result of organic damage[16].

If illness has reduced the capacity to respond to sexual stimulation, and this is something a couple cannot understand or discuss, then they cannot resolve this difficulty. In a relationship where the assumption was that the man always takes the active role in sexual exchange, his partner may be quite unused to stroking his penis as part of their preparation for intercourse, and may find it difficult to help him if this is what he requires. Similarly, if there is a transition from an equal partnership to one of caregiver and patient due to severe illness the latter may lose the self-esteem which reassures him that he is still contributing to the relationship; or the caring partner may think it unkind and selfish to make demands on the sexual responsiveness of the one who is ill. Particularly if there is a lack of communication around sexual issues, sexual relationship changes may never be adequately worked out. But even simple actions can have far-reaching effects, such as when a couple decide they should sleep apart so as to give the ill partner a better night's rest, resulting in a potential reduction of closeness and intimacy.

Furthermore, a substantial proportion of older people take medication, and often there is considerable polypharmacy. The list of drugs that can interfere with sexual function is extensive and the most widely prescribed drugs are mentioned[24,25] (Table 112.1).

Where drug-induced sexual dysfunction is suspected, discontinuing the suspected medication or substituting with a different agent can usually resolve the question.

Occasionally medication can enhance (or overstimulate) sexual function, which has been described with trazodone[26,27] and L-dopa[28].

Table 112.1 Drugs associated with sexual dysfunction[24,25]

Anticonvulsants
Antidepressants
Antihypertensives
Antipsychotics
Benzodiazepines
Chemotherapeutic agents
Digoxin
Diuretics
H_2 recepter blockers
Illegal substances ('street' drugs)
Lipid-lowering agents
Lithium
Opioids

SEXUAL PROBLEMS AND AGEING

Generally, the complaints in older people differ little from those of younger people who seek help for their sexual problems; they may have psychological or physical origins, or both. Fear of poor performance, lack of, or diminished sexual desire, difficulty becoming sexually aroused either physically or psychologically, difficulty maintaining an erection, difficulty achieving orgasm, and pain or discomfort with sexual activity, especially during intercourse, as well as a lack of opportunities for sexual encounters are among the most common of the complaints that older people present with[21,29,30].

Sexual dysfunction may also arise simply from a lack of information about the normal age-related changes in sexual physiology. A slower onset of erectile function, or a reduced need to ejaculate, may be interpreted by the man as the onset of impotence, or by the woman as a sign of declining interest in her; and their fearful or offended reactions may then aggravate the difficulty. Similarly, a reduced vaginal lubrication response may cause pain and discomfort during intercourse, leading the woman to avoid further sexual intimacy, which may be interpreted by the man as a rejection of the love he wants to express.

In addition to these problems, older people may mourn or regret changes in their body – its size, shape and firmness may differ significantly from the past. They may complain, as well, about the changing body of their partner, the reduction in, or loss of, passion and attention given to emotional and sexual intimacy, sexual boredom, jealousy of younger potential rivals and changes in sexual urgency or intensity. Menopause, surgery and various losses, both psychological and physical, can exacerbate these complaints.

Despite prevailing preconceptions, many older people are willing and open to address their sexual difficulties. Research suggests that if sex was a source of pleasure and gratification during early and middle adulthood, it will probably continue to be an important source of life satisfaction as one grows older[31]. On the other hand, it must be acknowledged that there remain many older people who grew up in fundamental and traditional households in which sexually proscriptive values and beliefs persist. For these individuals, sex is sanctioned primarily for procreation; sexual behaviours other than intercourse, such as oral–genital sex, are considered unnatural; sexual relations outside marriage are forbidden; and masturbation is sinful. For such individuals, the opportunity to 'retire' from an active sexual life may be ardently anticipated and easily accepted.

SEXUAL DISORDER IN OLDER MEN

Erectile Dysfunction

Erectile dysfunction is the persistent or recurrent inability to attain, or to maintain until completion of the sexual activity, an adequate erection. It is the most common sexual disorder in older men and may be the first harbinger of cardiovascular disease[32]. The increase in the prevalence of erectile dysfunction in ageing men is well documented. The Massachusetts Male Aging Study surveyed 1290 men ranging in age from 40 to 70 years from the Boston area[28]. A definite relationship was found between age and the probability of erectile dysfunction, such that the probability of severe erectile dysfunction tripled from 5.1% to 15% in men between 40 and 70 years, and the probability of moderate erectile dysfunction doubled from 17% to 34%.

The oral phosphodiesterase type 5 (PDE5) inhibitors, which include sildenafil (Viagra), tadalafil (Cialis) and vardenafil (Levitra), have significantly improved the treatment of erectile dysfunction[33]. A concomitant essential part of first-line treatment for erectile dysfunction is the modification of risk factors, which include ischaemic heart disease, hypertension, diabetes mellitus, dyslipidaemia, depression, cigarette smoking, use of recreational or medically indicated drugs and alcohol misuse; this is vital in order to improve erectile function and the patient's response to treatment.

Despite the safety, efficacy and tolerability of PDE5 inhibitors, 30–35% of patients fail to respond[34]. Educating patients on the correct use of these drugs can increase efficacy[35]. Other treatment options include a vacuum constriction device[36], intracavernosal[37] and intraurethral[38] administration of alprostadil, psychosexual counselling, androgen replacement and penile prosthesis implantation. Despite the growing clinical evidence that combination treatment may be successful in men for whom monotherapy fails, research is lacking to establish the benefits, optimal dosage, possible adverse effects and acceptability to patients of these treatments.

Hypoactive Sexual Desire

Hypoactive sexual desire is described as a deficiency or absence of sexual fantasies and desire for sexual activity and can be caused by organic and psychosocial factors. It is considered a disorder if it causes significant distress or relationship problems. It is not an uncommon condition in older men although objective epidemiological data are lacking.

Schiavi[16] found a prevalence as high as 17% in a highly selected sample of 236 men with a mean age of 65.7 years although the vast majority also had a diagnosis of erectile dysfunction. As sexual desire is androgen-dependent its loss can be caused by deficient androgenic stimulation. This may result from decreased testosterone secretion or increased production of sex hormone-binding proteins, causing decreased circulating free testosterone. The diagnosis of hypogonadism in older men can be difficult where there is a discrepancy between symptoms and endocrine assay results[39], so specialist advice is usually required.

Any therapeutic trial of androgen treatment must be preceded by exclusion of prostate cancer. A common psychosocial cause for loss of sexual desire in a long-term relationship is habituation and routine[11]. Couples should be encouraged to bring variety into their sexual script to prevent or overcome this problem. Depression should also be considered as a cause for loss of sexual desire.

Ejaculation Disorders

Premature ejaculation can prompt an older man to seek treatment, but it is a rare presentation at this age compared to younger men[40]. It may have been a life-long problem with the man presenting for consultation when he finds himself in a new sexual relationship. Alternatively, and more commonly premature ejaculation occurs for the first time as a reflection of the man's feeling of erectile insecurity – he ejaculates quickly before he loses his erection. Treatment should then focus on improving erectile function. Rarely, the onset of premature ejaculation may result from neurological or prostatic disease, and clinical examination is therefore necessary.

In the absence of controlled research data, clinical experience suggests that cognitive behavioural approaches to premature ejaculation such as the stop–start and squeeze techniques[41] are usually ineffective in older men. Treatment with serotonergic antidepressants are highly effective[42], but side effects can be troublesome. Currently these drugs are not licensed to treat premature ejaculation.

More frequent than premature ejaculation is delayed or failed ejaculation, which troubles many older men. This may be a reflection of ageing but can also result from inadequate stimulation. Reduced force of ejaculation, a decrease in the volume of ejaculate and decreased ejaculatory sensation are common age-related effects. Regular pelvic floor exercises may improve ejaculatory sensation.

SEXUAL DISORDER IN OLDER WOMEN

Hypoactive Sexual Desire

Desire problems are the most common sexual problem of older women. A recent nationally representative probability sample of community-dwelling persons 57–85 years of age from households across the United States yielded a prevalence rate of 43%, closely followed by 39% of the sample complaining of arousal difficulties[3]. The majority of studies investigating sexual desire in this population report similar findings[43] – a reduction in sexual thoughts or fantasy as well as a reduction in sexual intercourse. As in men, the age-related decrease in sexual desire is caused by a variety of factors including the age, health, sexual desire and sexual problems of both the woman and her partner, relationship satisfaction, the woman's past level of sexual satisfaction, sexual comfort and sexual interest, medication affecting sexual response that either she or her partner is taking, and finally, the effects of the hormonal changes following the menopause. Although a reduction or lack of desire is common in older women, it does not signal the end of sexual pleasure.

Sexual Arousal Disorder

As with reduced (hypoactive) sexual desire, changes in sexual arousal are also caused by many factors in addition to the postmenopausal hormonal changes. More than a decade ago Goldstein et al.[44] showed that arousal difficulties in older women may be exacerbated or caused by atherosclerotic vascular disease, which results in delayed vaginal engorgement, diminished vaginal lubrication, pain or discomfort with intercourse, and decreased vaginal and clitoral sensations and orgasm. Since then the use of vasoactive drugs has been evaluated by many pharmaceutical companies as a means of enhancing sexual arousal in women, but to date no treatment has been approved.

Dyspareunia

Dyspareunia is described as recurrent or persistent pain associated with sexual intercourse. It is probably one of the most common sexual complaints of older women seeking gynaecological consultation[45]. Pain that occurs in the absence of any infection or inflammation may indicate insufficient vaginal lubrication or incomplete arousal, so that the inner part of the vagina does not expand to make space for penetration. Lubricants and topical low-dose oestrogen treatment are available, if indicated. Alternatively, vulvodynia, which causes exquisite pain to the touch could be present, and this would require gynaecological assessment and possibly medication.

Orgasmic Difficulties

Some women experience changes in their orgasm with ageing, notably changes in the duration of orgasm, the ease and reliability of orgasm, and the number of uterine and vaginal contractions which accompany orgasm. Women who have lost their uterus and/or ovaries may have greater difficulty becoming sexually aroused and orgasmic because the uterus may contribute to arousal and orgasmic contractions. On the other hand the clitoris can be quite effective in providing erotic sensations and the ability to remain multi-orgasmic continues[21].

COMMON SEXUAL PROBLEMS IN COUPLES

A number of common sexual difficulties may come up during consultation which can be helped by relatively simple advice and education. They include (i) when to restart sexual intercourse after a myocardial infarction or cerebrovascular accident; (ii) identifying different positions and different timing for analgesic medication for intercourse when arthritis or pain is a problem; and (iii) how long to wait before resuming sexual activity and how much activity to attempt after surgery. It should be pointed out that weakness may hinder usual sexual activity and 'going slow' may be the optimum approach. Concrete examples, such as 'if you can walk a flight of stairs without shortness of breath, you can resume intercourse' may be helpful.

With patients or partners who have undergone mutilative surgery, mastectomy or ostomies, it is important to address fears of causing pain and the need to respond to fears of rejection because of drastic changes in body image. The healthy partner may be reluctant to discuss feelings of revulsion or contagion[46].

If intercourse is no longer a possibility, masturbation should be discussed as another source of self-pleasuring and as an appropriate activity to enhance individual or couple-pleasuring activities. Depending upon the individual's religious and cultural background, masturbation may not be perceived as an appropriate or comfortable option. If this is not the case, discussing the subject, and giving implicit permission, may be all that is needed to enable the couple to begin engaging in sexual exchange again.

CONCLUSION

What are the implications for clinical practice of this chapter? Physicians and other health care staff are generally known to feel embarrassed and to lack confidence in their ability to take an appropriate sexual history. This is particularly so when the patients' personal characteristics (such as their gender, age and sexual orientation) differ from their own[47]. This may especially disadvantage older people who are already assumed to be invisible and post sexual by society. Such people may be even less likely than most to approach health care staff with sexual problems and concerns, although research shows that most people hope that their physician will approach them[48].

Given that sex plays and increasingly important role in the lives of older women and men clinicians should ask – and be trained to ask – every patient, regardless of age, 'Are you experiencing any sexual problems or concerns?' The principles of taking a sexual history are not altered by the age of the patient[49]. Clinical competency in discussing sexual issues in an open and non-judgemental manner, and the level of training received in dealing with sexuality, is a major factor in determining how sexual problems present or whether they are presented at all.

One can only speculate on the number of patients who set out to seek advice for their sexual difficulty, but fail because of the discouraging response from the clinician involved. Although clinicians may feel awkward and unskilled, the very willingness to discuss sexual problems offers the patient an opportunity that society rarely provides. Physicians in particular are not only well placed to normalize and affirm the value of fulfilling sexual relations for the well-being of the older patient, but also have a responsibility to ensure that their sexual concerns and problems are appropriately and adequately addressed and managed.

REFERENCES

1. Cain V, Johannes C, Avis N, Mohr B, Schocken M, Skurnick J, Ory M. Sexual functioning and practices in a multi-ethnic study of midlife women: Baseline results from SWAN. *J Sex Res* 2003; **40**: 266–76.
2. Araujo AB, Mohr BA, McKinlay JB. Changes in sexual function in middle-aged and older men: Longitudinal data from the Massachusetts Male Aging Study. *J Am Geriatr Soc* 2004; **52**: 1502–509.
3. Lindau ST, Schumm LP, Laumann EO, Levinson W, O'Muircheartaigh CA, Waite LJ. A study of sexuality and health among older adults in the United States. *N Engl J Med* 2007; **357**: 762–64.
4. Schiavi RC, Mandeli J, Schreiner-Engel P. Sexual satisfaction in healthy ageing men. *J Sex Marital Ther* 1994; **20**: 3–13.
5. Beckman N, Waern M, Gustafson D, Skoog I. Secular trends in self reported sexual activity and satisfaction in Swedish 70 year olds: cross sectional survey of four populations, 1971 2001. *BMJ* 2008; **337**: 151–54.
6. Gott M. *Sexuality, Sexual Health and Ageing*. Maidenhead, Berkshire: Open University Press, 2005.
7. Laumann EO, Paik A, Rosen RC. Sexual dysfunction in the United States: Prevalence and predictors. *JAMA* 1999; **281**: 537–44.
8. Nicolosi A, Buvat J, Glasser DB, Hartmann U, Laumann EO, Gingell C. Sexual behaviour, sexual dysfunctions and related help seeking patterns in middle-aged and elderly Europeans: the global study of sexual attitudes and behaviours. *World J Urol* 2006; **24**: 423–28.
9. Parish WL, Laumann EO, Pan S, Hao Y. Sexual dysfunctions in urban China: A population-based national survey of men and women. *J Sex Med* 2007; **4**: 1559–74.
10. DeLamater J. Sexual desire in later life. *J Sex Res* 2005; **42**: 138–49.
11. Bitzer J, Platano G, Tschudin S, Alder J. Sexual counseling in elderly couples. *J Sex Med* 2008; **5**: 2027–43.

12. Laumann EO, Das A, Waite LJ. Sexual dysfunction among older adults: Prevalence and risk factors from a nationally representative U.S. probability sample of men and women 57–85 years of age. *J Sex Med* 2008; **5**: 2300–11.

13. Lawton FG, Hacker NF. Sex and the elderly. *BMJ* 1989; **299**: 1279.

14. Rees J, Wilcox, JR, Cuddihy RA. Psychology in rehabilitation of older adults. *Rev Clin Gerontol* 2002; **12**: 343–56.

15. Gray A, Feldman HA, McKinlay JB, Longcope C. Age, disease, and changing sex hormone levels in middle-aged men: results of the Massachusetts male ageing study. *J Clin Endocrinol Metab* 1991; **73**: 1016–25.

16. Schiavi RC. *Aging and Male Sexuality*. Cambridge: Cambridge University Press, 1999.

17. Bancroft J. *Human Sexuality and its Problems*, 3rd edn. Edinburgh: Churchill Livingstone, 2009.

18. Morley JE. Testosterone and behaviour. *Clin Geriatr Med* 2003; **19**: 605–16.

19. Masters WH, Johnson VE. *Human Sexual Response*. Boston: Little Brown, 1966.

20. Rosen RC. Reproductive health problems in ageing men. *Lancet*, 2005; **366**: 183–85.

21. Leiblum SR (ed.) *Principles and Practice of Sex Therapy*, 4th edn. New York: Guilford Press, 2007.

22. Perelman MA. Psychosocial evaluation and combination treatment of men with erectile dysfunction. *Urol Clin N Am* 2005; **32**: 441–45.

23. Morley JE, Tariq SH. Sexuality and disease. *Clin Geriatr Med* 2003; **19**: 563–73.

24. Thomas DR. Medication and sexual function. *Clin Geriatr Med* 2003; **19**: 553–62.

25. Taylor D, Paton C, Kerwin R. *The South London and Maudsley NHS Trust & Oxleas NHS Trust Prescribing Guidelines*, 9th edn. London: Taylor & Francis, 2007.

26. Garbell N. Increased libido in women receiving trazodone. *Am J Psychiatry* 1986; **143**: 781–82.

27. Sullivan G. Increased libido in three men treated with trazodone. *J Clin Psychiatry* 1988; **49**: 202–203.

28. Uitti RJ, Tanner CM, Rajput AH, Goetz CG, Klawans HL, Thiessen B. Hypersexuality with antiparkinsonian therapy. *Clin Neuropharmacol* 1989; **12**: 375–83.

29. Bretschneider JG, McCoy, NL. Sexual interest and behavior in healthy 80- to 102-year-olds. *Arch Sex Behav* 1988; **17**: 109–29.

30. Feldman HA, Goldstein I, Hatzichristou DG, Krane RJ, McKinlay JB. Impotence and its medical and psychosocial correlates: results of the Massachusetts male ageing study. *J Urol* 1994; **151**: 54–61.

31. George LK, Weiler SJ. Sexuality in middle and later life; the effects of age,cohort and gender. *Arch Gen Psychiatry* 1981; **38**: 919–23.

32. Thompson IM, Tangen CM, Goodman PJ, Probstfield JL, Moinpour CM, Coltman CA. Erectile dysfunction and subsequent cardiovascular disease. *JAMA* 2005; **294**: 2996–3002.

33. Salonia A, Briganti A, Montorsi P *et al*. Safety and tolerability of oral erectile dysfunction treatments in the elderly. *Drugs Aging* 2005; **22**: 323–38.

34. McMahon CN, Smith CJ, Shabsigh R. Treating erectile dysfunction when PDE5 inhibitors fail. *BMJ* 2006; **332**: 589–92.

35. Atiemo HO, Szostak MJ, Sklar GN. Salvage of sildenafil failures referred from primary care physicians. *J Urol* 2003; **170**: 2356–58.

36. Turner LA, Althof SE, Levine SB, Kursh E, Bodner D, Resnick M. Treating erectile dysfunction with external vacuum device: Impact upon sexual, psychological and marital functioning. *J Urol* 1990; **144**: 79–82.

37. Linet OI, Ogrine FG. Efficacy and safety of intracavernosal alprostadil in men with erectile dysfunction. *N Engl J Med* 1996; **334**: 873–77.

38. Padma-Nathan H, Hellstrom WJG, Kaiser FE *et al*. Treatment of men with erectile dysfunction with transurethral alprostadil. *N Engl J Med* 1997; **336**: 1–7.

39. Wang C, Nieschlag E, Swerdloff R *et al*. Investigation, treatment, and monitoring of late-onset hypogonadism in males: ISA, ISSAM, EAU, EAA, and ASA recommendations. *Eur Urol* 2009; **55**: 121–30.

40. Montorsi F. Prevalence of premature ejaculation: a global and regional perspective. *J Sex Med* 2005; **2**(suppl 2): 96–102.

41. Zilbergeld B. *The New Male Sexuality*. New York: Bantam Books, 1999.

42. Waldinger MD, Zwinderman AH, Schweitzer DH, Olivier B. Relevance of methodological design for the interpretation of efficacy of drug treatment of premature ejaculation: a systematic review and meta-analysis. *Int J Impot Res* 2004; **16**: 369–81.

43. Laumann EO, Nicolosi A, Glasser DB *et al*. for the GSSAB Investigators' Group. Sexual problems among women and men aged 40–80 y: prevalence and correlates identified in the Global Study of Sexual Attitudes and Behaviors. *Int J Impot Res* 2005; **17**: 39–57.

44. Goldstein I, Lue TF, Padma-Natham H, Rosen R, Steers WD, Wicker PA. Oral sildenafil in the treatment of erectile dysfunction. *N Engl J Med* 1998; **338**: 1397–404.

45. Bachmann G, Leiblum S, Grill J. Sexuality in sexagenarian women. *Maturitas* 1989; **13**: 45–50.

46. Szwabo PA. Counseling about sexuality in the older person. *Clin Geriatr Med* 2003; **19**: 595–604.

47. Maurice WL. *Sexual Medicine in Primary Care*. St Louis: Mosby, 1999.

48. Metz M, Seifert MH. Differences in men's and women's sexual health needs and expectations of physicians. *Can J Hum Sex* 1993; **2**: 53–59.

49. Tomlinson J. ABC of sexual health: taking a sexual history. *BMJ* 1998; **317**: 1573–76.

Part K

Cultural Differences, Service Provision and Training in Old Age Psychiatry

113

Assessing Mental Health in Different Cultures

Rob Butler[1], Sati Sembhi[1] and Melanie Abas[2]

[1]Suffolk Mental Health Partnership NHS Trust, St Clement's Hospital, Ipswich, Suffolk, UK
[2]Institute of Psychiatry, Kings College London, London, UK

INTRODUCTION

Assessing older people from different cultures requires a broad set of skills. Older people have acquired a wealth of life experience and knowledge. Clinicians need to understand how this and culture shapes their presentation and symptoms of mental disorders. Clinicians also need to be aware of their own cultural identity and to have some knowledge about customs and religions in different countries. Assessing older people includes asking about life history, social and family circumstances, and preferences for service delivery. This chapter offers an overview of how cultural competence can help with the clinical assessment. It includes some specific pointers for assessing depression, psychosis and dementia. It is worth noting that, due to a range of barriers, many older people from different cultures have poor access to psychiatric care and face a 'triple jeopardy' of disadvantage in terms of age, ethnicity and socioeconomic deprivation[1-3].

CULTURAL COMPETENCE

Culture is a network of knowledge, meanings, ideas and social rules shared by a group, often referred to as an ethnic group, who may also share geographical origins, religion and language. Culture will affect how illness is understood, the presentation of symptoms, and expectations regarding treatment and treatment choice[4]. The culture of the clinician will often differ to some extent from that of the patient[5]. The clinical setting in which treatment occurs has its own culture, which in turn influences the clinical relationship. Cultural competence means having an awareness of all three dimensions – that is, the culture of the older person, the culture of the clinician and the cultural setting – even when these are not obvious[4]. A culturally competent clinician can recognize the diversity of viewpoints, is willing to seek background cultural information from other members of the ethnic group or experts, and is flexible in approaching the doctor–patient relationship[4]. It should be appreciated that, in today's multicultural world, many people move between or within different cultures, and so it is important to avoid making assumptions about a patient's background which can lead to ethnic stereotyping[6]. Awareness of one's own culture and of potentially strong feelings about another's culture is important. Respectful enquiry and a desire

to learn about other lifestyles is the only way to engage with a patient's lived experience of ethnicity and its role in determining what is important for them. One consequence of cultural differences is that occasionally a patient may interpret a well-intentioned enquiry as intrusive or stigmatizing[6]. The Explanatory Models Approach is a method of understanding symptoms without making cultural assumptions[6]. The following questions form the basis of a discussion which explores the patient's experience and perception of illness:

What do you call this problem?
What do you believe is the cause of this problem?
What course do you expect it to take? How serious is it?
What do you think this problem does inside your body?
How does it affect your body and your mind?
What do you fear most about this condition?
What do you fear most about the treatment?

ASSESSMENT

The patient should be asked early on about his or her background and, for migrants, his or her place of origin, experience of migration and existence in the new setting. The clinician will sometimes need to work hard to develop rapport and trust. Within reasonable professional boundaries, the clinician should be willing to respond to any questions about him or herself. For example, with older Jamaican migrants, making 'a connection' with the doctor has been found to facilitate the assessment and acceptance of care[7]. The power imbalance in the patient–doctor relationship may evoke feelings of mistrust, particularly when the patient has been subject to discrimination. The clinician should be willing to discuss issues such as racism and social needs. It is helpful to show sensitivity, but not to neglect important areas on 'cultural' grounds (e.g. alcohol consumption in the case of Muslims). Ideas that appear persecutory must be explored and may reflect an appropriate response to injustice. History-taking should include use of traditional medicines and complementary treatments. Enquiries about spirituality may reveal deeply held views which are important for the patient to follow as part of recovery. Attitudes to death, widowhood and care homes may vary considerably. Consultation may be needed with a wide circle of people from the relevant culture.

Principles and Practice of Geriatric Psychiatry, 3rd edn. Edited by Mohammed T. Abou-Saleh, Cornelius Katona and Anand Kumar
© 2011 John Wiley & Sons, Ltd

FAMILY AND CARERS

Assessment will naturally include family and carers' roles and needs. The levels of caregiver stress, burden and depression vary across cultures. The use of prayer, faith or religion may be used as a coping mechanism. There may be a difference between generations in adapting to a new culture, for example because of fewer opportunities for older people to learn a new language or make social contacts at work. This may exaggerate differences between generations. Many groups, including refugees, may not have family support in their adopted country.

COMMUNICATION

Requiring patients to speak in a non-native language can distort the clinical picture. Language barriers can be reduced by employing an ethnically close bilingual worker. Alternatively, you can use a competent interpreting and advocacy service, preferably with individuals with experience in the mental health field. Some local services and national bodies, such as the Royal College of Psychiatrists in the UK, keep lists of psychiatrists who can speak different languages.

Using interpreters is a skill, and training is available for the effective use of such services. Before they begin, the clinician and interpreter should discuss their expectations of each other and of how the interview should proceed. It should be confirmed whether the interpreter's role will be confined to translating or will extend to advising on non-verbal communication and cultural appropriateness. The clinician should be aware that even though an interpreter may be from the same country as the patient, differences in class, gender, religion, tribal group and so on may limit their ability to accurately interpret their culture. Idioms and jokes should be avoided. The patient should be addressed in the second person. Clear, concise language should be used and interpreters given manageable chunks to translate. Sometimes, word-for-word translation will be needed rather than the interpreter's summary. The interpreter should be able to give an indication of language use and structure to aid assessment of formal thought disorder. The assessment will be more time-consuming and tiring for the patient, possibly requiring more than one session. Misunderstandings and miscommunications may occur even with trained clinical interpreters, often because information is skewed to fit the interpreter's or clinician's viewpoint[8].

Aspects of non-verbal communication differ, such as avoidance of direct eye-to-eye contact in some Asian and Pacific cultures. Many cultures do not shake hands. There are differences in expression, gesticulation, speech patterns and communication styles. In some cultures, saying 'yes' may not indicate an affirmative response but be a mark of respect or deference to the doctor. There may be taboo subjects, such as the discussion of death in some Asian cultures.

CONFIDENTIALITY

In cultures with an individual focus, the expectation is that the patient is assessed alone and confidentiality between patient and clinician maintained. However, in cultures where the social group is more dominant, family members may expect to play a full role in the assessment, and have access to all information. Equally, the family might have strong views about topics they do not want disclosed to the older person. Taking the time to talk this through will usually help in finding a compromise. It is important to explain where the information you collect will be stored and who will have access to

it. Third-party information should be identified in case the privacy of the informant is infringed.

ASSESSMENT TOOLS

Most screening instruments, assessment tools and diagnostic schedules have been developed within a certain cultural setting. This means that they may lack validity if applied without modification to people from different cultures. The clinician is likely to need more time and perhaps a wider set of informants to assess psychiatric history and symptoms, in order to ensure diagnostic accuracy. Some specific examples of instruments for depression, functional psychosis and dementia are given below. A research tool developed for use in one culture will likely need to be adapted and translated, and then undergo reassessment for reliability and validity, before being used in a different culture[9,10].

DIFFERENT PRESENTATIONS OF EMOTIONAL DISTRESS

People from all cultures experience both somatic and psychological symptoms when emotionally distressed. One reason for a more somatic presentation may be that this is considered a more appropriate focus for medical consultation by some cultures. Secondly, there may be a continuum of experience and interpretation, with the more 'somatizing' culture at one end and the more 'psychologizing' at the other[11]. Finally, a large number of 'somatic' complaints are actually metaphors for mental distress. Many of these relate to heart discomfort (e.g. a heart that is 'sinking' or 'uncomfortable') and to abdominal sensation[12]. Culture-bound syndromes often represent cultural explanations for recognizable mental disorders[13]. For example, dhat, a belief that semen is leaking from the body in urine, is a complaint in India. It may be a presenting feature, and is used as an explanation for weakness due to depression or organic disease.

DEPRESSION

There has been much debate about the existence of depression as a universal cross-cultural category[11]. However, it is reasonably well established that depressive disorders exist across cultures and are very strongly related to local constructs[12]. While there are similarities in the cross-cultural expression and experience of depression, there are also differences. For example, depressed older Jamaicans and African Americans may describe feeling 'low', 'bad' or 'fed-up'[7], or they may have multiple somatic symptoms, or they may present metaphors for psychological distress. Some cultures emphasize their explanation (e.g. social or spiritual) for their symptoms. Depression in old age may be more difficult to recognize because symptoms such as poor concentration or lack of interest can mimic dementia, and carers may perceive them as an inevitable part of ageing. The validity of screening scales may vary; for example, a lower cut-off point for the Geriatric Depression Scale has been recommended for older African Caribbeans[14]. The prevalence of depressive symptoms and probable depression in older people varies across Europe and appears not to simply reflect differences in age, gender, education or cognitive function[15]. Depression at community level also appears to be highly correlated with anxiety[16]. As a result, it is important to enquire about the *full* range of affective and other symptoms; and a wide definition of mood disorders is likely to be most useful in the clinical setting. Cultures vary in the acceptability of suicide, ranging from a belief that it is an acceptable way to avoid dishonour to a belief that it is never acceptable and is always a sin. Islam forbids self-killing; the Muslim person who expresses the wish that God 'takes back' his life may be indicating he has suicidal thoughts which must be taken seriously.

PSYCHOSIS

Psychotic symptoms and signs are similar in form across a wide variety of settings[17]. However, the content of delusions and hallucinations will be influenced by culture. Also, the patient's and family's explanation for the illness will depend on their cultural framework[18]. For example, someone from Zambia who upholds traditional explanatory models may explain schizophrenia in the same way as they might explain a stroke, depression or a burglary – as being due to bewitchment or to having angered a spirit. An apparently unusual idea, such as believing oneself to be bewitched, is only a delusion if it is out of keeping with the beliefs of others in the same culture. This can be explored by asking someone with appropriate knowledge. If faced with the patient alone, the clinician should ask how he or she came to believe this, and if others close to him or her agree. If a traditional healer told him or her so, and his or her peers agree, then it is at least likely that this is a culturally sanctioned belief. Another error is to assume that a belief is culturally normal when it is actually abnormal.

DEMENTIA

The prevalence of dementia is increasing worldwide as populations grow and people live longer. New tools are being validated across countries[10,19]. However, dementia is frequently unrecognized or misunderstood, and some languages lack wording for such impairment. Diagnostic criteria for dementia require the demonstration of cognitive impairment of sufficient severity to interfere with activities of daily living. Cultures vary in the extent to which they expect older people to take responsibility for aspects of daily living, such as domestic activities. Also, physical impairment is more common in socially disadvantaged people and will be difficult to distinguish from that due to dementia, requiring greater emphasis on physical examination and tests. Many cognitive tests include items affected by education and may have little relevance in certain cultures (e.g. 'take 7 from 100'). Bilingual immigrants often lose their adopted language quicker than their native one, leading to a possible overestimation of impairment. When testing those unfamiliar with such approaches, the clinician should be courteous and encouraging without 'helping', and give explicit instructions and some dummy tasks to allay anxiety. Rather than doggedly adhering to the original version of instruments, it is appropriate either to make rational adaptations or to develop new instruments. Novel adaptations will, of course, require translation, back-translation and retesting[9]. The Community Screening Instrument for Dementia[9] combines culture-fair cognitive testing with a structured informant interview. Fully operationalized criteria appear to improve measurement of dementia in cross-cultural research[19].

CONCLUSION

Training in cultural psychiatry needs to form an integral part of mental health training for clinicians[20]. Rather than regarding the acquisition of cultural competence as useful only in rare and exotic situations, it should be seen as an extension of good clinical skills. In the UK, the Royal College of Psychiatrists has developed a Race Equality Action Plan that emphasizes the importance of cultural capability in core training and education[21]. Clinicians are keen to acquire skills in the assessment and delivery of care to people from different cultures, and they should receive regular training in cultural capability, awareness, appropriateness and sensitivity to improve their knowledge, skills and attitudes[22].

REFERENCES

1. Bhugra D, Lippett R, Cole E. Pathways into care: an explanation of the factors that may affect minority ethnic groups. In Bhugra D, Bahl V (eds), *Ethnicity: An Agenda for Mental Health*. London: Royal College of Psychiatrists, 1999, 29–39.
2. Oommen G, Bashford J, Shah A. Ageing, ethnicity and psychiatric services. *Psychiatr Bull R Coll Psychiatr* 2009; **33**: 30–4
3. Rait G, Burns A, Chew C. Age ethnicity and mental illness: a triple whammy. *BMJ* 1996; **313**: 1347.
4. Tseng W, Streltzer J (eds). *Cultural Competence in Clinical Psychiatry*. Washington, DC: Springer, 2004.
5. Laugharne R. Evidence-based medicine, user involvement and the post-modern paradigm. *Psychiatr Bull R Coll Psychiatr* 1999; **23**: 641–3.
6. Kleinman A, Benson P. Anthropology in the clinic: the problem of cultural competency and how to fix it. *PLoS Med* 2006; **3**: e294.
7. Abas M, Phillips C, Richards M *et al*. Initial development of the new culture specific screen for emotional distress in older Caribbean people. *Int J Geriatr Psychiatry* 1996; **12**: 1097–103.
8. Elderkin-Thompson V, Silver RC, Waitzkin H. When nurses double as interpreters: a study of Spanish-speaking patients in a U.S. primary care setting. *Soc Sci Med* 2001; **52**: 1343–58.
9. Hall K, Ogunniyi AO, Hendrie H *et al*. A cross-cultural community-based study of dementias: methods and performances of the survey instrument in Indianapolis, USA, and Ibadan, Nigeria. *Int J Methods Psychiatr Res* 1996; **6**: 129–42.
10. Prince M, Acosta D, Chiu H *et al*. Dementia diagnosis in developing countries: a cross-cultural validation study. *Lancet* 2003; **361**: 909–17.
11. Kleinman A. Anthropology and psychiatry. *Br J Psychiatry* 1987; **151**: 447–54.
12. Abas M, Broadhead J. Depression and anxiety amongst women in an urban setting in Zimbabwe. *Psychol Med* 1997; **27**: 59–71.
13. Rack P. *Race, Culture and Mental Disorder*. London: Tavistock, 1982.
14. Abas M, Phillips C, Carter J *et al*. Culturally sensitive validation of screening questionnaires for depression in older Africa-Caribbean people living in South London. *Br J Psychiatry* 1998; **173**: 249–54.
15. Castro-Costa E, Dewey M, Stewart R *et al*. Prevalence of depressive symptoms and syndromes in later life in ten European countries: the SHARE study. *Br J Psychiatry* 2007; **191**: 393–401.
16. Jacob K, Everitt B, Patel V. The comparison of latent variable models of non-psychosis morbidity in four culturally different populations. *Psychol Med* 1998; **28**: 145–52.
17. World Health Organization. *The International Pilot Study of Schizophrenia*, vol. 1. Geneva: WHO, 1973.

18. Faberga H. Psychiatric stigma in non-Western societies. *Compr Psychiatry* 1991; **32**: 534–51.

19. Prince MJ, de Rodriguez JL, Noriega L *et al*. The 10/66 Dementia Research Group's fully operationalised DSM-IV dementia computerized diagnostic algorithm, compared with the 10/66 dementia algorithm and a clinician diagnosis: a population validation study. *BMC Public Health* 2008; **8**: 219

20. Kirmayer LJ, Rousseau C, Guzder J *et al*. Training clinicians in cultural psychiatry: a Canadian perspective. *Acad Psychiatry* 2008; **32**: 313–19.

21. Royal College of Psychiatrists. *Race Equality Action Plan*. London: Royal College of Psychiatrists, 2007.

22. Department of Health. *Delivering Race Equality in Mental Health Care: An Action Plan for Reform Inside and Outside Services and the Government's Response to the Independent Inquiry into the Death of David Bennett*. DH, 2004. Available at www.dh.gov.uk.

114

The Cross-Cultural Epidemiology of Mental Illness in Old Age

Martin Prince

*Centre for Global Mental Health, Department of Health Service and Population Research,
Institute of Psychiatry, King's College London, UK*

BACKGROUND

Discussion of the mental health of 'older people' most often focuses on those aged 65 years and over – that is, above the most frequent, statutory retirement age in Western nations[1]. This is arbitrary and culture-specific, and for research in low- and middle-income countries (LMIC) the cut-point is often set at 60 years. According to the Global Burden of Disease report, neuropsychiatric disorders account for 13.5% of the global burden of disease, and 27.5% of that attributable to non-communicable diseases (NCD)[2], while for those aged 60 years the proportion is smaller – 7.4% of the global burden of disease and 8.3% of that arising from non communicable diseases. While the prevalence of dementia rises sharply in later life, doubling with every five-year increase of age, that of depression is, perhaps, a little lower than among younger adults. Many people with chronic severe psychosis do not survive into old age, and there is a small incidence of late-onset psychosis. However, mental ill health in later life poses particular challenges for public health. Health profiles among older people, particularly the oldest old, are somewhat distinct, with mental ill health often complicated by co-morbidity with chronic physical and cognitive disorders, a combination that is particularly strongly associated with disability and dependency. Beyond the challenges of living with chronic disease and disability, further obstacles to the maintenance of good mental health into late life include retirement (loss of occupational role, status and income) and a shrinking social network (loss of spouses, siblings and friends through bereavement)[1].

Older people, their health and social welfare, have for too long been under-prioritized in global public health policy. This is now changing with increasing recognition, over the past 20 years, of their growing importance in LMIC[3]. Demographic ageing is proceeding more rapidly than first anticipated in all world regions, particularly China, India and Latin America[4]. The proportion of older people increases as mortality falls and life expectancy increases. Population growth slows as fertility declines to replacement levels. In the 30 years up to 2020 the oldest sector of the population will have increased by 200% in LMIC as compared to 68% in the developed world[5]. By 2020, two-thirds of all those over 60 will be living in LMIC[6], where, in the accompanying health transition, non-communicable diseases assume a progressively greater significance. NCDs are already the leading cause of death in all world regions apart from sub-Saharan Africa. Of the 35 million deaths in 2005 from NCDs, 80% will have been in LMIC[7]. This is partly because most of the world's older people live in these regions. However, changing lifestyles and patterns of risk exposure also contribute. Among the NCDs, dementia and depression in older people have only fairly recently begun to be given the attention that they deserve in population-based research in LMIC. The purpose of this chapter is to describe the contribution of this research to our understanding of the epidemiology of these disorders, to contextualize these findings with what has been observed in high-income countries (HIC), and to describe some of the methodological challenges to be overcome in conducting this research in varied cultural settings.

DEPRESSION IN LATE-LIFE

'Depression', as a diagnosis applied in clinical settings, generally requires persistent and pervasive low mood and/or loss of pleasure, accompanied by other characteristic symptoms (including guilt, sleep and appetite disturbance), sufficient to cause significant distress and disability[8]. However, mood states do not fall naturally into discrete categories, but instead represent a spectrum from normality through increasing degrees of morbidity. As with any 'cut-off' applied to an underlying continuum (e.g. hypertension), the prevalence of the disorder depends substantially on the threshold that is selected. Severe depressive disorders have a high individual impact on those affected, but are rare. Milder syndromes have a lower individual impact but, given their higher prevalence, may have a substantially greater public health impact.

The Cross-Cultural Validity of the Assessment and Diagnosis of Late-Life Depression

There is reasonably strong evidence to support the cross-cultural validity of measurement of depression among older people. This has been most extensively studied with respect to the 12-item EURO-D depression symptom scale, which has been shown to have a similar factor structure in 14 European sites[9], as well as in India, China and Latin America[10]. Measurement invariance was later formally established for the EURO-D across 10 European countries in the SHARE study, using confirmatory factor analysis to confirm a common factor structure and Mokken analysis to confirm a common hierarchical relationship between items[11]. The subsequent demonstration of higher levels of EURO-D depression symptoms among older people in three countries sharing a 'Latin' ethno-lingual heritage; France, Spain and Italy; after standardizing for age, sex, education and cognitive function suggested a possible role of culture in determining risk[12]. In terms of clinical diagnostic assessments of depression, the strongest evidence for cross-cultural validity exists for the Geriatric Mental State and its AGECAT algorithm, probably the most widely used such assessment internationally[13]. The instrument has been validated against most major diagnostic systems, but primarily only in HIC settings[13]. As part of the 10/66 Dementia Research Group's pilot studies in 26 centres in Latin America, India, China, Nigeria and Russia, its Stage 1 AGECAT depression algorithm was found to have sensitivity varying between 89% and 100% by region against a criterion of MADRS score of 18[10]. Specificity was difficult to establish, since depression was not formally excluded from the control groups, whose main purpose was to validate the dementia component of the algorithm. Nevertheless, the prevalence of AGECAT depression was negligible in these groups other than in Latin American sites[10]. The AGECAT depression algorithm was subsequently validated in Hefei City, China, where there was a diagnostic agreement of 83.6% and a Kappa of 0.67 against Chinese psychiatrists' independent gold standard diagnostic evaluation[14].

In the absence of qualitative research demonstrating the ecological validity of late-life depression as a pathological construct, the evidence for the cross-cultural validity of the commonly used ICD-10 and DSM-IV clinical diagnostic criteria among older people in LMIC is limited mainly to concurrent validation, that is from observations of cross-sectional associations with disability and impaired quality of life. In Nigeria[15] and Brazil[16], depression diagnosed was associated with high levels of social disability and impaired quality of life. In Mexico, Peru and Venezuela, high levels of disability were also identified in those with sub-syndromal depression identified with the EURO-D scale, suggesting a considerable prevalence (an additional 23–24%) of clinically significant disorder beyond the established diagnostic boundaries[17]. More research is needed to determine if these findings are typical of less developed regions in general.

The Prevalence of Late-Life Depression

The prevalence of late-life depression has been extensively studied in developed countries in the European, North America and Asia Pacific regions[18,19]. The main influence on prevalence is the criterion used to make the diagnosis[20]. According to rigorous research diagnostic criteria such as the *Diagnostic and Statistical Manual of Mental Disorders, Fourth Edition (DSM-IV)* major depression and the *International Classification of Diseases, Tenth Edition (ICD-10)* depressive episode late-life depression is uncommon with a weighted mean prevalence of only 1.8%; when all those with clinically relevant symptoms are included, the weighted mean prevalence rises to 13.3%[18]. The relative lack of epidemiological data from LMIC is particularly striking – in the two systematic reviews, all of the 34 publications covering the period 1989–96[18] and the 122 papers covering the period 1993–2004[19] described research carried out in high-income countries. Recently published prevalence studies from Nigeria, Brazil, Latin America and China have helped to redress this imbalance. Two publications report

an exceptionally high prevalence of DSM-IV major depression in Nigeria (7.1%)[15] and of ICD-10 depressive episode in Brazil (19.2%)[16]. The 10/66 Dementia Research Group has also recently reported on the prevalence of ICD-10 and DSM-IV depression in three Latin American countries, Mexico, Peru and Venezuela, which in these settings was closer to that reported in HIC, the prevalence of DSM-IV depression varying between 1.3 and 2.8% and that of ICD-10 depression between 4.5 and 5.1%[17]. Conversely, the prevalence of GMS/AGECAT depression in Hefei City, China, was only 2.2%, roughly five times lower than in European studies using the same assessment and case definition[14]. The prevalence in a rural village in Anhui province was slightly higher, at 6.0%[21].

In the few studies in LMIC to have examined this issue, treatment of clinically significant depression seems to be severely suboptimal – in the 10/66 Latin American studies only 24.1% of those in urban Peru with a current ICD-10 depressive episode, 18.8% in rural Peru, 11.8% in urban Mexico, 4.4% in rural Mexico and 19.6% in Venezuela reported ever having received in-patient or out-patient treatment for depression[17]: In Nigeria, only 37% of lifetime cases had received any treatment[15].

Sociodemographic Correlates of Late-Life Depression

The few studies to have assessed prevalence of depressive disorders across the adult age range suggest an increase from young to mid-adult age groups, followed by a fall in prevalence for older people within a decade of the retirement age[22,23]. A striking trend in the opposite direction has been observed in Nigeria, the authors speculating that lack of social protection for older people may have contributed to their much higher prevalence of DSM-IV major depressive disorder.[15] Studies from HIC that have focused upon depressive symptoms and broader depressive syndromes also indicate either an increase in their frequency[24] or stability with increasing age[25]. The exclusion, in some diagnostic criteria, of symptoms thought to be attributable to bereavement and physical illness may account in part for the apparent lower prevalence of depressive disorders in older people. In European studies, the prevalence of late-life depression is consistently higher in women compared to men[12,24], but the gender difference tends to be smaller than that found in mid-life. In European studies, the effect of gender is consistently modified by marital status, with marriage being protective for men but associated with higher risk among women[24]. A higher prevalence of late-life depressive disorder among women is also a consistent finding in studies in LMIC, replicated in Brazil[16], Nigeria[15] and the 10/66 Dementia Research Group Latin American studies[17]. However, in the 10/66 studies the association with female gender was entirely confounded by socioeconomic status and physical impairment, both of which were more common in women – a similar finding was reported in the SABE studies in six Latin American cities, although depression in that study was defined by a cutpoint on the Geriatric Depression Scale rather than a clinical diagnosis[26].

There have been many reports from cross-sectional community surveys, from a variety of cultures, of associations between late-life depression and socioeconomic disadvantage, for example with respect to educational level, occupational social class and income[19]. These are highly correlated variables, and it is difficult to determine the effect of one independent of the others. Reverse causality is possible – those whose adult life has been scarred by depression may experience lifelong occupational and economic disadvantage. Findings from LMIC are currently inconsistent – suggestive trends in the direction of an association between socioeconomic disadvantage and depression were observed, rather inconsistently, in the five sites in the three 10/66 Latin American countries[17]. Level of education seemed to be more relevant than income or wealth. Food insecurity was strongly associated with depression in Mexico, with non-significant trends in Peru and Venezuela. Depression in Hefei City, China was also positively associated with economic disadvantage[14]. Unusually, in Nigeria, an association was observed in the opposite direction, with the highest prevalence of depression among older people with the highest economic status[15].

The Aetiology of Late-Life Depression

To date there have been no prospective studies of potential aetiologic factors for late-life depression in LMIC. There have, however, been a large number of well-designed cohort studies carried out in Europe and North America, the findings from which have been subject to systematic review[19,27] and quantitative meta-analysis[27]. There is strong and fairly consistent evidence to support an increased risk for incident depression associated with female gender, disability, prior depression, bereavement and sleep disturbance. Disability is probably the most salient of these factors. Prospective studies in older adults have consistently indicated a very strong association between disability at baseline and the subsequent onset of depression[28-32]. In one of these studies[31] the population attributable fraction was as high as 0.69. In general, the level of disability associated with a health condition, rather than the nature of the pathology mediates the risk for depression[31,33,34]. Stroke may be an exception as some studies show persistence of associations with depression after adjustment for disability[35]. Three population-based studies have suggested an interaction between disability and social support, with the strongest effect of disability in those with the least social support[31,32,36]. However, there is also strong evidence for causal pathways leading from depression to the progression or emergence of disability[37,38]. Cross-sectional data from the 10/66 studies in Mexico, Peru and Venezuela also support a strong association between limiting physical impairments and depression, with a past history of depression being the other consistently observed association[17].

One of the more consistent findings from previous Western research is the apparent salience of contact with friends, in particular intimate, confiding relationships to mood and morale in older people. While older people typically receive instrumental support from spouses and relatives, they value friends for companionship and emotional support. In the longitudinal Gospel Oak study, no contact with friends was the only social support variable prospectively associated with the onset of depression[31]. The social environment for older people is affected by the ageing process. Social networks deteriorate with increasing age consequent upon bereavement. Social engagement, such as visiting friends, is impaired in those with disability. Women typically have more supportive and extensive networks of friends than men. Married older men cite their wife as their main confidant, whereas women more often cite a friend outside the home. There have been few such studies conducted in other cultural settings, but in a cross-sectional study in Cuba, social networks, mainly centred around children and extended families, were associated with fewer depressive symptoms in both older men and women[39].

DEMENTIA

Dementia is a syndrome due to disease of the brain, usually chronic and progressive, in which there is disturbance of multiple higher cortical functions, including memory, learning, orientation, language, comprehension and judgement. Diagnosis is on the basis of decline in cognitive function and independent living skills. There are many underlying causes. Alzheimer's disease, vascular dementia, dementia with Lewy bodies and frontotemporal dementia are the commonest. Mixed pathologies may be the norm. Studies in developed countries have consistently reported Alzheimer's disease (AD) to be more prevalent than vascular dementia (VaD)[40]. Early surveys from South-East and East Asian countries provided an exception with an equal distribution of AD and VaD[40]. More recent research suggests this situation has now reversed[41,42]. This may be due to increasing longevity and better physical health: AD, whose onset is in general later than VaD, increases as the number of very old people increases; while better physical health reduces the number of stroke sufferers and thus the number with VaD[41]. This change also affects the gender balance among dementia sufferers, increasing the number of females and reducing the number of males. Some rare causes of dementia (subdural haematoma, normal pressure hydrocephalus, hypercalcaemia and deficiencies of thyroid hormone, vitamin B12 and folic acid) may be treated effectively – these may, theoretically, be overrepresented in LMIC, but their contribution particularly in young onset cases has yet to be investigated.

The Validity of Dementia Diagnosis Across Cultures

The validity of the construct of dementia in less-developed settings is supported by three qualitative studies in India. The features of dementia were widely recognized, and named[43-45]. However, there was no awareness of dementia as an organic brain syndrome, or medical condition. Rather, it was perceived as a normal, anticipated part of ageing. The consequences are little help seeking from formal medical care services[44], no structured training on the recognition and management of dementia at any level of the health service, and no constituency to advocate for more responsive dementia care services[45]. Behavioural and psychological symptoms of dementia (BPSD) can lead to stigma and blame attaching to the carers as well as the person with dementia[46]. In India, likely causes were cited as 'neglect by family members, abuse, tension and lack of love'[44], and carers tended to misinterpret BPSD as deliberate misbehaviour[45].

The validity of methods used in cross-cultural research is fundamental to the success of the enterprise. Without this, informative cross-cultural comparisons are impossible. Many potential obstacles needed to be overcome[47]. Those with little or no education may appear to 'fail' on cognitive screening tests even in the absence of cognitive impairment or decline. The task may be unfamiliar to them, or the information requested irrelevant. Tasks involving literacy, numeracy or drawing are particularly problematic, but in practice any cognitive item for which the probability of a correct response is strongly influenced by education will tend to be biased. Culture, including language, may also influence the salience and feasibility of cognitive items, and their relative difficulty. Cultural influences, as we shall see, may also impact on the assessment of social or occupational disability, since the normal roles of older people may vary considerably between cultures.

The history of cross-cultural research in dementia is characterized by careful attention to the applicability and validity of the measures employed. In the 1990s, the National Institute of Aging funded US–Nigeria and US–India studies developed[48] or adapted[49,50] cognitive tests to render them suitable and normed for the cultural setting, and also developed culture-specific assessments of functional impairment[51]. In the wake of these efforts, the 10/66 Dementia Research Group carried out pilot studies in 26 centres from 16 LAMIC in Latin America and the Caribbean, Africa, India, Russia, China and SE Asia, demonstrating the feasibility and validity of a one-phase culture and education-fair diagnostic protocol for population-based research[52]. The Geriatric Mental State (a structured clinical interview assessing dementia, depression and psychosis syndromes)[53], the Community Screening Instrument for Dementia (a cognitive test, and informant interview for evidence of intellectual and functional decline, used in the US–Nigeria study)[48] and the modified CERAD 10-word list-learning task (used in the US–India study) each independently predicted dementia diagnosis[49]. A probabilistic algorithm derived in one-half of the sample from all four of these elements performed better than any of them individually; applied to the other half of the sample it identified 94% of dementia cases with false positive rates of 15%, 3% and 6% in the depression, high education and low education groups[52]. This algorithm (the 10/66 Dementia Diagnosis) was 'education-fair' in that the false positive rate among those with low levels of education was low, and 'culture-fair' in that equivalent validity was established for a wide variety of countries, languages and cultures. It therefore provides a sound basis for dementia diagnosis in clinical and population-based research.

The prevalence of DSM-IV dementia was strikingly low in the US–Nigeria and US–India studies[54,55]. The validity of this criterion, developed in the USA, had not been established in LMIC settings. In the 10/66 Dementia Research Group studies, a computerized application of the DSM-IV criterion was devised and validated[56]. The relative concurrent and predictive validity of the two diagnostic approaches, 10/66 Dementia and DSM-IV dementia, could thus be compared. In the Cuban 10/66 population-based study, the 10/66 dementia diagnosis agreed better with Cuban clinician diagnoses than did the DSM-IV computerized algorithm, which missed many recent onset and mild cases[56]. An essential feature of the dementia syndrome is that it is a progressive neurodegenerative disorder; the principal rationale for an early diagnosis is that it alerts the person concerned and their family to the probability of future deterioration. The 10/66 Dementia Research Group confirmed the predictive validity of their diagnosis in the population-based study sample in Chennai, South India, identifying a high mortality rate, and greater cognitive and functional decline over three years among 10/66 dementia cases and those with cognitive impairment but no dementia[57]. There was also clear evidence of clinical progression and increasing needs for care among the large majority of 10/66 dementia cases. The strong predictive validity of the 10/66 dementia diagnosis was consistent with a lack of sensitivity of the DSM-IV criterion to mild to moderate cases, and, thus, with the notion that it may underestimate prevalence in less developed regions[57].

The Prevalence and Incidence of Dementia

Dementia is largely a disease of older persons; only 2% of cases are to be found in those aged under 65 years. After this the prevalence doubles with every five-year increment in age. The EURODEM meta-analysis of European population-based studies from the 1990s used data from 11 studies carried out in eight European countries[58]. Prevalence was consistent across sites; the pooled prevalence for males and females is shown in Table 114.1.

The annual incidence rates reported in the EURODEM meta-analysis[59] are roughly one-quarter of the point prevalence

Table 114.1 EURODEM meta-analysis of European population-based studies: pooled prevalence for males and females

Age groups	Annual incidence per 100 (68)		Prevalence (%) (67)	
	Males	Females	Males	Females
60–64	0.2	0.2	0.4	0.4
65–69	0.2	0.3	1.6	1.0
70–74	0.6	0.5	2.9	3.1
75–79	1.4	1.8	5.6	6.0
80–84	2.8	3.4	11.0	12.6
85–89	3.9	5.4	12.8	20.2
90+	4.0	8.2	22.1	30.8

(Table 114.1), suggesting an average disease duration (from onset to death) of four years. Clinical studies have suggested a duration of five to seven years from diagnosis. A recent meta-analysis[60] of the age-specific incidence of all dementias was based on data from 23 published studies. The incidence of both dementia and AD rose exponentially up to 90 years, with no sign of levelling off. The incidence rates for VaD varied greatly from study to study, but the trend was also for an exponential rise with age. While there was no sex difference in dementia incidence, for the oldest old the incidence of AD was higher in women, and for the younger old the incidence of VaD was higher in men.

In LMIC there is more uncertainty as to the frequency of dementia, with few studies and widely varying estimates[47]. Early onset cases are again rare, although this may be changing in those world regions where HIV/AIDS is endemic. In 2004, Alzheimer's Disease International convened a panel of international experts to review the global evidence on the prevalence of dementia, and to estimate the prevalence of dementia in each world region, the current numbers of people affected, and the projected increases over time (Lancet/ADI estimates). A tendency previously noted for age-specific prevalence to be lower in LMIC than in the developed north[47,54,55] was supported by the consensus judgement of the expert panel[61]. Differences in survival could only be part of the explanation, as estimates of incidence in some studies[62,63] were also much lower than those reported in the West. Differences in levels of exposure to environmental risk factors may also have contributed, with low levels of cardiovascular risk[64] and hypolipidaemia[65,66] in some developing countries suggested as explanations. Other potential risk exposures will be more prevalent in LMIC, for example anaemia associated with AD in rural India[67]. High infant mortality may contribute to population differences in dementia frequency; constitutional and genetic factors that confer survival advantage in early years may protect against neurodegeneration or delay its clinical manifestations. It seems plausible that as patterns of morbidity and mortality converge with those of the developed West, then dementia prevalence in LMIC will do likewise[68]. While studies of secular trends in Sweden, 1947 to 1952[69] and in the US, 1975 to 1980[70], suggested no change in the prevalence of dementia over time, it is possible that age-specific prevalence of dementia in HIC might fall in the future because of reduced incidence linked to improvements in cardiovascular health or rise, due to reduction in mortality among those with dementia.

However, the Lancet/ADI estimates were described as 'provisional', given that prevalence data were lacking in many world regions, and patchy in others, with few studies and widely varying estimates[61]. Coverage was good in Europe, North America and in developed Asia-Pacific countries: South Korea, Japan, Taiwan and Australia. Several studies have been published from India and China, but estimates were too few and/or too variable to provide a consistent overview for these huge countries. There was a particular dearth of published epidemiological studies in Latin America[71-73], Africa[54], Russia, the Middle East and Indonesia. Therefore, there was a strong reliance upon the consensus judgement of the international panel of experts for LMIC.

The 10/66 Dementia Research Group prevalence studies

The 10/66 Dementia Research Group subsequently completed its population-based surveys (2003–7) of dementia prevalence and impact in 12 sites in eight LMIC (India, China, Cuba, Dominican Republic, Brazil, Venezuela, Mexico and Peru)[74-79], with a second wave of surveys underway in Puerto Rico, Sri Lanka and South Africa. Cross-sectional comprehensive one-phase surveys were conducted of all residents aged 65 and over of geographically defined catchment areas in each site with a sample size of 2000–3000 in each country. The net result is a unique resource of directly comparable data on over 20 000 older adults from three continents. All studies used the same cross-culturally validated assessments (dementia diagnosis and subtypes, other mental and physical health, anthropometry, demographics, extensive non-communicable disease risk factor questionnaires, disability, health service utilization, care arrangements and caregiver strain). The prevalence of DSM-IV dementia varied widely, from less than 1% in the least developed sites (India and rural Peru) to 6.4% in Cuba[75]. 10/66 dementia prevalence was higher than that of DSM-IV dementia, and more consistent across sites, varying between 5.6% and 11.7%[75]. The discrepancy was explained by the observation that informants in the least developed sites, particularly India, were less likely to report cognitive decline and social impairment (an essential criterion for DSM-IV dementia diagnosis) even in the presence of objective memory impairment[75]. Levels of disability were similar for 10/66 dementia cases regardless of whether or not they were confirmed by the DSM-IV dementia algorithm[75]. After standardizing for age and sex, DSM-IV prevalence was similar in the urban Latin American sites to that in Europe, but in China the prevalence was only one-half, and in India and rural Latin America one-quarter or less of the European prevalence. The group concluded that the DSM-IV dementia criterion is likely to have underestimated dementia prevalence, particularly in regions with low awareness of this emerging public health problem. There are several possible explanations for the discrepancy between objective cognitive impairment and informant reports[75].

1. The high levels of instrumental support routinely provided to all older people may mean that objective cognitive impairment may be less likely to lead to noticeable impairment in the performance of normal social roles, particularly in the early stages of dementia. More attention may need to be given to developing culturally relevant assessments to detect the consequences of early intellectual decline.
2. A culture of respect to elders making it difficult for informants to disclose report decline (supported by the finding of lower informant report scores for heads of household and male participants[75]).
3. Low awareness of dementia may mean that decline is attributed to 'normal ageing'[44,45] and hence not worthy of mention given the implicit focus of the assessments upon abnormality.

The World Alzheimer Report – new estimates of global prevalence of dementia

Since the Lancet/ADI estimates were published, the global evidence base has expanded considerably. There have been new studies from Spain[80,81], Italy[82] and the USA[83]. The exciting development, however, has been an explosion of studies from LMIC, and other regions and groups previously underrepresented in the literature. These included 10/66 Dementia Research Group studies in Brazil, Cuba, Dominican Republic, Peru, Mexico, Venezuela, India and China[75,76], and further new prevalence studies from, Brazil[84], Peru[85], Cuba[86], Venezuela[87], China[88], Korea[89], India[90], Thailand[91], Australia (indigenous people[92]), Guam[93], Poland[94] and Turkey[95]. The leaders of the Lancet/ADI review were commissioned in 2008 to assist the World Health Organization in updating the Global Burden of Disease (GBD) estimates, by conducting fully systematic reviews of the prevalence and incidence of dementia, and associated mortality, in 21 GBD world regions. This provided an ideal opportunity to revisit the literature, and to assess the extent to which it was possible, in some or all regions, to summarize the evidence on the prevalence of dementia by quantitative meta-analysis of the available data, rather than relying on expert consensus. Findings from this exercise were published in Alzheimer's Disease International's World Alzheimer Report[96].

The systematic review identified 147 prevalence studies worldwide since 1980. A recent marked increase in the number of studies from LMIC was accompanied by a sharp decline in research in high income countries. In many of these countries, the evidence base is fast becoming out of date. When compared with the earlier Lancet/ADI consensus, after age standardization to the Western European population structure, the new estimates of dementia prevalence for all those aged 60 years and over were higher for three regions – Western Europe (7.29% vs. 5.92%), South Asia (5.65% vs. 3.40%) and Latin America (8.50% vs. 7.25%). Those for East Asia were lower (4.98% vs. 6.46%). However, in comparison with the much greater heterogeneity seen in the Lancet/ADI estimates, regional estimates had generally converged (Figure 114.1). While there was a four-fold variation in prevalence overall, from 2.07% (sub-Saharan Africa, West) to 8.50% (Latin America), most of the standardized prevalences lay in a band between 5% and 7%. The major source of variation was clearly the very low estimated prevalence for the four sub-Saharan African regions.

When regional prevalence estimates were applied to population estimates, it was calculated that there were 35.6 million people with dementia worldwide in 2010, the numbers nearly doubling every 20 years, to 65.7 million in 2030 and 115.4 million in 2050. These figures for global prevalence were approximately 10% higher than the earlier Lancet/ADI estimates. In 2010, 58% of all people with dementia worldwide lived in LMIC, rising to 71% by 2050. Proportionate increases over the next 20 years in the number of people with dementia will be much steeper in low- and middle- compared with high-income countries (see Figure 114.2). The World Alzheimer Report forecast a 40% increase in numbers in Europe, 63% in North America, 77% in the southern Latin American cone and 89% in the developed Asia-Pacific countries. These figures are to be compared with 117% growth in East Asia, 107% in South Asia, 134–146% in the rest of Latin America, and 125% in North Africa and the Middle East.

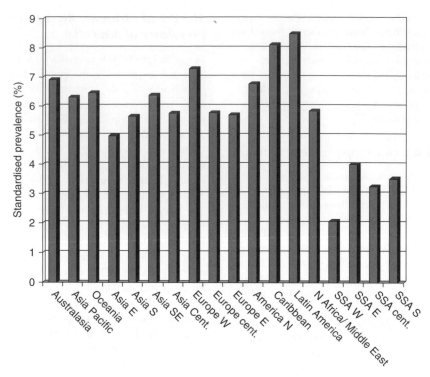

Figure 114.1   The prevalence of dementia in different Global Burden of Disease world regions, after standardizing for age (SSA = Sub-Saharan Africa)
Source: World Alzheimer Report 2009[96]

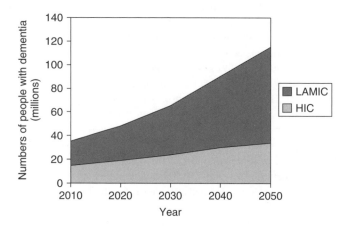

Figure 114.2   Projected increases (2010–50) in the number of people with dementia worldwide, broken down by country income status
Source: World Alzheimer Report 2009[96]

The Impact of Dementia

Worldwide, surprisingly few epidemiological studies of dementia have gone beyond reporting on prevalence, incidence and aetiology of dementia. The impact of dementia upon the individual, the family and society has been little studied. In the Global Burden of Disease report, dementia was accorded a higher disability weight than almost any other condition and contributed 11.2% of all years lived with disability among people aged 60 and over; more than stroke (9.5%), musculoskeletal disorders (8.9%), cardiovascular disease (5.0%) and

all forms of cancer (2.4%). The global economic cost of dementia was recently estimated at US$317 billion, 77% attributable to HIC where costly long-term care services are widely available[97]. In HIC, as the disease progresses, formal sector care costs increase and institutionalization is the main cost driver. Informal (family) care is more important in resource poor countries, accounting for 56% of costs in LIC and 42% in MIC, compared with just 31% in HIC[97]. According to the 10/66 Dementia Research Group pilot study in 26 LMIC centres, levels of carer strain were as high as those typically seen in European studies. In addition, care giving in LMIC often leads to substantial economic disadvantage[98]. A high proportion of carers had to cut back on their paid work, and paid carers were also common[98]. Compensatory benefits for carers and disability pensions for people with dementia were practically non-existent[98,99].

The 10/66 Dementia Research studied the relative contribution of chronic physical, mental and cognitive disorders (common physical impairments, depression, dementia, hypertension, diabetes, heart disease, stroke, chronic obstructive pulmonary disease and arthritis) to disability, in the baseline phase of its population-based studies in Latin America, China and India[99]. Contrary to the Global Burden of Disease report, which cites blindness and deafness as the two leading contributors to years lived with disability among older people in LMIC, dementia made much the largest contribution to disability, with a median population attributable fraction of 25.5% (range across sites 19.3–43.5%). Other substantial contributors were limb impairment (11.7%, 5.6–34.0%), stroke (11.5%, 2–21.2%), arthritis (9.9%, 2.8–35.0%), depression (8.3%, 0.5–22.9%), eyesight (5.7%, 0–17.6%) and gastrointestinal impairments (5.1%, 0–23.2%). These findings suggest that chronic diseases of the brain and mind deserve greater prioritization. Aside from disability, they lead to dependency and present stressful, complex long-term challenges to carers. Societal costs are enormous[97]. Evidence from population-based research on ageing and dementia from LMIC should help to stimulate a wider debate about older people's health and social care needs, and how they should be met[100].

The Aetiology of Dementia

Currently most of the evidence from population-based studies on the aetiology of dementia comes from HIC, since the few incidence studies conducted in LMIC gathered data on a very limited range of potential risk exposures at baseline[63,101].

Genetic and environmental factors

The rare early-onset form of AD is highly heritable, and single-gene mutations at one of three loci (beta amyloid precursor protein, presenilin1 and presenilin2) account for the majority of cases. Late-onset AD is a multi-factorial disorder. The apolipoprotein E (*apoE*) gene polymorphisms account for up to 50% of the population attributable fraction, the e4 allele being enriched among AD cases[102,103]. The association between APOE e4 and dementia has been observed in population-based[102,103] studies in India, China and Latin America. However, the association seems to be attenuated among those with African ancestry[104,105] and no association was observed among older Nigerians[106]. Modest concordance rates among monozygotic twins for dementia diagnosis suggest a substantial environmental influence[107]. Evidence from cross-sectional and case-control studies suggest associations between AD and limited education[108], and head injury[109,120], which, however, are only partly supported by prospective studies[111]. Depression is a risk factor in short-term prospective studies, but this may be because depression is an early presenting symptom, rather than depression being a cause of dementia[112].

Dementia, cardiovascular risk factors and cardiovascular disease

The health transition currently underway in many LMIC will see an epidemic of cardiovascular disease (CVD). Latin America exemplifies the third stage of health transition. As life expectancy improves, and high fat diets, cigarette smoking and sedentary lifestyles become more common, so CVDs have maximum public health salience – more so than in stage 2 regions (China and India) where risk exposure is not yet so elevated, and than in stage 4 regions (Europe) where public health measures have led to reduced exposure to cardiovascular risk factors (CVRF)[113]. This is a matter of concern with respect to dementia in LMIC, given that recent research from developed countries suggests that vascular disease predisposes to AD as well as to vascular dementia[114]. While there has been no research to date on associations with dementia in LMIC, the INTERHEART cross-national case-control study suggests that risk factors for coronary heart disease operate equivalently in all world regions, including Latin America and China[115]. Despite occasional negative findings from large prospective studies[116,117], the accumulated evidence from HIC for a causal role for CVRF and CVD in the aetiology of dementia and AD is very strong. In short[118-120] and longer latency[121,122] incidence studies, smoking increases the risk for Alzheimer's disease. Diabetes

is also a risk factor[123], and in longer term cohort studies, midlife hypertension[124,125] and hypercholesterolemia[125] are associated with AD onset in later life. Aggregated cardiovascular risk indices incorporating hypertension, diabetes, hypercholesterolaemia and smoking incrementally increase risk for dementia incidence whether exposure is measured in midlife[121] or a few years before dementia onset[120]. Recent studies report associations between metabolic syndrome and incident cognitive decline[126], and insulin resistance and impaired executive function[127]. This has led to the hypothesis that atherosclerosis and AD are convergent disease processes[128], with some common pathophysiological and aetiological factors (APOE e4 polymorphism, hypercholesterolaemia, hypertension, hyperhomocysteinaemia, diabetes, metabolic syndrome, smoking, systemic inflammation, increased fat intake and obesity).

Nutritional factors

In LMIC, dietary deficiencies, particularly of micronutrients, are widespread and strongly linked to poverty. Deficiencies of folate and vitamin B_{12} are of particular interest given their consequences; anaemia, neuropathy, hyperhomocysteinaemia[129], increased risk of stroke and IHD[130]. Vitamin B_{12} deficiency is strikingly prevalent (>40%) across Latin America[131-133], linked to gastrointestinal infections and diets deficient in meat and dairy produce[131]. Folate deficiency is endemic in those living in poverty[132], and after economic crisis[133]. Diets deficient in legumes may have contributed. Micronutrient deficiency is probably more prevalent in the elderly but there are few data on this age group[131]. Research on micronutrients and dementia in developed countries has focused upon antioxidants[134] with less attention towards deficiencies in vitamin B_{12} and folate, which result in hyperhomocysteinaemia; only four small incidence studies[135-138], all underpowered and with inconsistent findings. Two out of three studies testing for an effect of folate were positive[135,136], in one case independent of homocysteine[135]. B_{12} was associated in only one out of four studies[136].

Iodine deficiency has also been a major public health problem in most Latin American countries[139]. Iodized salt is now generally available but iodine content is poorly regulated[139]. The prevalence of sub-clinical hypothyroidism was as high as 16.1% in post-menopausal Brazilian women[140]. Overt hypothyroidism is a potentially reversible cause of dementia. Sub-clinical hypothyroidism (raised TSH levels with normal T4) is more prevalent, affecting up to 20% of older people in developed countries. It is associated with elevated total cholesterol and progression to overt hypothyroid disease, possibly also CVD[141]. It was strongly associated with risk for dementia in one cross-sectional study[142]. Conversely, a small incidence study reported a strong association with sub-clinical hyperthyroidism (low TSH)[143].

Opportunities for prevention

Currently, efforts to prevent and control the coming epidemic of cardiovascular and other chronic non-communicable diseases in LMIC are in their infancy[144]. Advocated measures include the implementation of tobacco-free policies, taxation of tobacco products, comprehensive bans on advertising of tobacco products, salt reduction through voluntary agreements with the food industry, and combination drug therapy for individuals at high risk of CVD[144]. The detection and control of hypertension, hyperlipidaemia, diabetes and metabolic syndrome is poorly implemented by overstretched primary care services that struggle to cope with the double burden of historic priorities (maternal, child and communicable diseases) and the rising tide of chronic disease in adults. Health systems are not trained, equipped or structured to deal with the latter. Given the strong evidence for CVD and CVRF as risk factors for dementia, the success or otherwise of these initiatives should in principle have an important effect on the future prevalence and incidence of dementia in LMIC[61]. Against this, is the disappointing evidence from prevention trials. One trial of antihypertensive agents has reported a protective effect on dementia[145], but four others did not find effects on cognitive function in primary analyses[146-149]. Three large trials of cholesterol lowering agents have also failed to find effects on cognitive function[150,151]. A randomized controlled trial of HRT in post-menopausal women indicated, against expectation, that women randomized to HRT had nearly double the risk of going on to develop dementia in the short follow-up period[152].

CONCLUSION

Major advances have been made in our understanding of the cross-cultural validity of measurement and diagnosis of late-life depression and dementia. The prevalence of late-life depression meeting clinical diagnostic criteria has been found to be higher than the norm for developed Western countries in some but not all LMIC studies. Depression is consistently associated with high levels of disability and is considerably undertreated. Early indications are that patterns of risk association also seem to be somewhat different. With a large recent growth in the evidence base, the prevalence of dementia among older people living in LMIC, originally reported to be much lower than that in HIC, now seems to be quite similar worldwide. The possible exception is Sub-Saharan Africa, but the low prevalence of dementia seen in the one good quality study yet to have been conducted in that region[54] needs to be confirmed by more research. Possible similarities or differences in the risk factor profile for dementia across cultures, and between HIC and LMIC have attracted much attention[105], but very little is known due to the lack of informative incidence studies in LMIC. The incidence phase of the 10/66 Dementia Research group's population-based studies in Latin America and China, due to be completed in 2010, will go some of the way to redressing this imbalance[74]. Aside from prevention of disease and promotion of healthy functioning, there is an urgent need to strengthen the ability of community health services to deliver evidence-based mental health care for older people. This should be done in an integrated way, within an overarching chronic disease management framework. More research is needed, into the epidemiology of late-life mental disorder (particularly their aetiology), into the effectiveness of high-risk prevention strategies for late-life depression and interventions for depression and dementia[153].

REFERENCES

1. Prince MJ. Mental health promotion and prevention across the lifespan – old age. In Petersen I, Bhana A, Flisher AJ, Swartz L, Richter L (eds), *Promoting Mental Health in Scarce-Resource Contexts. Emerging Evidence and Practice*. Cape Town: HSRC Press, 2010.
2. Prince MJ, Patel V, Saxena S, Maj M, Maselko J, Phillips MR *et al.* No health without mental health. *Lancet* 2007; **370**(9590): 859–77.
3. Kalache A. Ageing is a third world problem too. *Int J Geriatr Psychiatry* 1991; **6**: 617–18.
4. United Nations. *World Population Prospects: The 2002 Revision – Highlights*. New York: United Nations, 2003.
5. Harvard School of Public Health. *The Global Burden of Disease. A Comprehensive Assessment of Mortality and Disability from Diseases, Injuries and Risk Factors in 1990 and Projected to 2020*. Cambridge, MA: Harvard University Press, 1996.
6. Prince MJ. The need for research on dementia in developing countries. *Tropical Med Health* 1997; **2**: 993–1000.
7. Fuster V, Voute J. MDGs: chronic diseases are not on the agenda. *Lancet* 2005; **366**(9496): 1512–14.
8. American Psychiatric Association. *Diagnostic and Statistical Manual of Mental Disorders*, 4th edn. Washington, DC: American Psychiatric Association, 1994.
9. Prince MJ, Reischies F, Beekman ATF, Fuhrer R, Hooijer C, Kivela S *et al.* The development of the EURO-D scale – A European Union initiative to compare symptoms of depression in 14 European centres. *Br J Psychiatry* 1999; **174**: 330–8.
10. Prince M, Acosta D, Chiu H, Copeland J, Dewey M, Scazufca M *et al.* Effects of education and culture on the validity of the Geriatric Mental State and its AGECAT algorithm. *Br J Psychiatry* 2004; **185**: 429–36.
11. Castro-Costa E, Dewey M, Stewart R, Banerjee S, Huppert F, Mendonca-Lima C *et al.* Ascertaining late-life depressive symptoms in Europe: an evaluation of the survey version of the EURO-D scale in 10 nations. The SHARE project. *Int J Methods Psychiatr Res* 2008; **17**(1): 12–29.
12. Castro-Costa E, Dewey M, Stewart R, Banerjee S, Huppert F, Mendonca-Lima C *et al.* Prevalence of depressive symptoms and syndromes in later life in 10 European countries. The SHARE study. *Br J Psychiatry* 2007; **191**: 393–401.
13. Copeland JR, Prince M, Wilson KC, Dewey ME, Payne J, Gurland B. The Geriatric Mental State Examination in the 21st century. *Int J Geriatr Psychiatry* 2002; **17**(8): 729–32.
14. Chen R, Hu Z, Qin X, Xu X, Copeland JR. A community-based study of depression in older people in Hefei, China – the GMS-AGECAT prevalence, case validation and socio-economic correlates. *Int J Geriatr Psychiatry* 2004; **19**(5): 407–13.
15. Gureje O, Kola L, Afolabi E. Epidemiology of major depressive disorder in elderly Nigerians in the Ibadan Study of Ageing: a community-based survey. *Lancet* 2007; **370**(9591): 957–64.
16. Costa E, Barreto SM, Uchoa E, Firmo JO, Lima-Costa MF, Prince M. Prevalence of International Classification of Diseases, 10th Revision common mental disorders in the elderly in a Brazilian community: The Bambui Health Ageing Study. *Am J Geriatr Psychiatry* 2007; **15**(1): 17–27.
17. Guerra M, Ferri CP, Sosa AL, Salas A, Gaona C, Gonzales V *et al.* Late-life depression in Peru, Mexico and Venezuela: the 10/66 population-based study. *Br J Psychiatry* 2009; **195**(6): 510–15.
18. Beekman ATF, Copeland JRM, Prince MJ. Review of community prevalence of depression in later life. *Br J Psychiatry* 1999; **174**: 307–11.
19. Djernes JK. Prevalence and predictors of depression in populations of elderly: a review. *Acta Psychiatr Scand* 2006; **113**: 372–87.
20. Beekman A. A Review of the Literature. Depression in Later Life: Studies in the Community. PhD thesis, Vrije University, Amsterdam, 1996.

21. Chen R, Wei L, Hu Z, Qin X, Copeland JR, Hemingway H. Depression in older people in rural China. *Arch Intern Med* 2005; **165**(17): 2019–25.

22. Evans O, Singleton N, Meltzer H, Stewart R, Prince M. *The Mental Health of Older People*. London: HMSO, 2003.

23. Weissman MM, Leaf PJ, Tischler GL, Blazer DG, Karno M, Bruce ML et al. Affective disorders in five United States communities [published erratum appears in *Psychol Med* 1988; **18**(3): following 792]. *Psychol Med* 1988; **18**: 141–53.

24. Prince M, Beekman A, Fuhrer R, Hooijer C, Kivela S, Lawlor B et al. Depression symptoms in late-life assessed using the EURO-D scale. Effect of age, gender and marital status in 14 European centres. *Br J Psychiatry* 1999; **174**: 339–45.

25. Tannock C, Katona C. Minor depression in the aged. Concepts, prevalence and optimal management. *Drugs Aging* 1995; **6**: 278–92.

26. Alvarado BE, Zunzunegui MV, Beland F, Sicotte M, Tellechea L. Social and gender inequalities in depressive symptoms among urban older adults of Latin America and the Caribbean. *J Gerontol B Psychol Sci Soc Sci* 2007; **62**(4): S226–36.

27. Cole MG, Dendukuri N. Risk factors for depression among elderly community subjects: a systematic review and meta-analysis. *Am J Psychiatry* 2003; **160**(6): 1147–56.

28. Phifer JF, Murrell SA. Etiologic factors in the onset of depressive symptoms in older adults. *J Abnorm Psychol* 1986; **95**(3): 282–91.

29. Kennedy G, Kelman H, Thomas C. The emergency of depressive symptoms in late life: the importance of declining health and increasing disability. *J Community Health* 1990; **15**(2): 93–104.

30. Beekman AT, Deeg DJ, Smit JH, van TW. Predicting the course of depression in the older population: results from a community-based study in the Netherlands. *J Affect Disord* 1995; **34**(1): 41–9.

31. Prince MJ, Harwood RH, Thomas A, Mann AH. A prospective population-based cohort study of the effects of disablement and social milieu on the onset and maintenance of late-life depression. The Gospel Oak Project VII. *Psychol Med* 1998; **28**(2): 337–50.

32. Schoevers RA, Beekman AT, Deeg DJ, Geerlings MI, Jonker C, van TW. Risk factors for depression in later life: results of a prospective community based study (AMSTEL). *J Affect Disord* 2000; **59**(2): 127–37.

33. Ormel J, Kempen GI, Penninx BW, Brilman EI, Beekman AT, van SE. Chronic medical conditions and mental health in older people: disability and psychosocial resources mediate specific mental health effects. *Psychol Med* 1997; **27**(5): 1065–77.

34. Broe GA, Jorm AF, Creasey H, Grayson D, Edelbrock D, Waite LM et al. Impact of chronic systemic and neurological disorders on disability, depression and life satisfaction [erratum appears in *Int J Geriatr Psychiatry* 1999; **14**(6): 497–8]. *Int J Geriatr Psychiatry* 1998; **13**(10): 667–73.

35. Stewart R, Prince M, Mann A, Richards M, Brayne C. Stroke, vascular risk factors and depression: cross-sectional study in a UK Caribbean-born population. *Br J Psychiatry* 2001; **178**(1): 23–8.

36. Beekman AT, Penninx BW, Deeg DJ, Ormel J, Braam AW, van TW. Depression and physical health in later life: results from the Longitudinal Aging Study Amsterdam (LASA). *J Affect Disord* 1997; **46**(3): 219–31.

37. Bruce ML. Psychosocial risk factors for depressive disorders in late life. *Biol Psychiatry* 2002; **52**(3): 175–84.

38. Penninx BW, Deeg DJ, van Eijk JT, Beekman AT, Guralnik JM. Changes in depression and physical decline in older adults: a longitudinal perspective. *J Affect Disord* 2000; **61**(1–2): 1–12.

39. Sicotte M, Alvarado BE, Leon EM, Zunzunegui MV. Social networks and depressive symptoms among elderly women and men in Havana, Cuba. *Aging Ment Health* 2008; **12**(2): 193–201.

40. Roman GC. Facts, myths, and controversies in vascular dementia. *J Neurol Sci* 2004; **226**(1–2): 49–52.

41. Suh GH, Shah A. A review of the epidemiological transition in dementia – cross-national comparisons of the indices related to Alzheimer's disease and vascular dementia. *Acta Psychiatr Scand* 2001; **104**(1): 4–11.

42. Dong MJ, Peng B, Lin XT, Zhao J, Zhou YR, Wang RH. The prevalence of dementia in the People's Republic of China: a systematic analysis of 1980–2004 studies. *Age Ageing* 2007; **36**(6): 619–24.

43. Cohen L. Toward an anthropology of senility: anger, weakness, and Alzheimer's in Banaras, India *Med Anthropol Q* 1995; **9**(3): 314–34.

44. Patel V, Prince M. Ageing and mental health in a developing country: who cares? Qualitative studies from Goa, India. *Psychol Med* 2001; **31**(1): 29–38.

45. Shaji KS, Smitha K, Praveen Lal K, Prince M. Caregivers of patients with Alzheimer's disease: a qualitative study from the Indian 10/66 Dementia Research Network. *Int J Geriatr Psychiatry* 2002; **18**: 1–6.

46. Ferri CP, Ames D, Prince M. Behavioral and psychological symptoms of dementia in developing countries, *Int Psychogeriatr* 2004; **16**(4): 441–59.

47. The 10/66 Dementia Research Group. Methodological issues in population-based research into dementia in developing countries. A position paper from the 10/66 Dementia Research Group. *Int J Geriatr Psychiatry* 2000; **15**: 21–30.

48. Hall KS, Hendrie HH, Brittain HM, Norton JA, Rodgers DD, Prince CS et al. The development of a dementia screeing interview in two distinct languages. *Int J Methods Psychiatric Res* 1993; **3**: 1–28.

49. Ganguli M, Chandra V, Gilby JE, Ratcliff G, Sharma SD, Pandav R et al. Cognitive test performance in a community-based nondemented elderly sample in rural India: the Indo–U.S. Cross-National Dementia Epidemiology Study. *Int Psychogeriatr* 1996; **8**(4): 507–24.

50. Ganguli M, Ratcliff G, Chandra V, Sharma S, Gilby J, Pandav R et al. A Hindi version of the MMSE: the development of a cognitive screening instrument for a largely illiterate rural elderly population in India. *Int J Geriatr Psychiatry* 1995; **10**: 367–77.

51. Hendrie HC, Lane KA, Ogunniyi A, Baiyewu O, Gureje O, Evans R et al. The development of a semi-structured home interview (CHIF) to directly assess function in cognitively impaired elderly people in two cultures. *Int Psychogeriatr* 2006; **18**(4): 653–66.

52. Prince M, Acosta D, Chiu H, Scazufca M, Varghese M. Dementia diagnosis in developing countries: a cross-cultural validation study. *Lancet* 2003; **361**(9361): 909–17.

53. Copeland JRM, Dewey ME, Griffith-Jones HM. A computerised psychiatric diagnostic system and case nomenclature for

elderly subjects: GMS and AGECAT. *Psychol Med* 1986; **16**: 89–99.

54. Hendrie HC, Osuntokun BO, Hall KS, Ogunniyi AO, Hui SL, Unverzagt FW *et al.* Prevalence of Alzheimer's disease and dementia in two communities: Nigerian Africans and African Americans. *Am J Psychiatry* 1995; **152**: 1485–92.

55. Chandra V, Ganguli M, Pandav R, Johnston J, Belle S, DeKosky ST. Prevalence of Alzheimer's disease and other dementias in rural India. The Indo–US study. *Neurology* 1998; **51**: 1000–8.

56. Prince MJ, de Rodriguez JL, Noriega L, Lopez A, Acosta D, Albanese E *et al.* The 10/66 Dementia Research Group's fully operationalised DSM-IV dementia computerized diagnostic algorithm, compared with the 10/66 dementia algorithm and a clinician diagnosis: a population validation study. *BMC Public Health* in press. 2008 Jun 24; 8:219.

57. Jotheeswaran AT, Williams JD, Prince MJ. The predictive validity of the 10/66 Dementia diagnosis in Chennai, India: A 3-Year Follow-up Study of Cases Identified at Baseline. *Alzheimer Dis Assoc Disord*. 2010 May 13. [Epub ahead of print].

58. Lobo A, Launer LJ, Fratiglioni L, Andersen K, Di Carlo A, Breteler MM. Prevalence of dementia and major subtypes in Europe: a collaborative study of population-based cohorts. Neurologic diseases in the elderly research group. *Neurology* 2000; **54**(11 Suppl 5): S4–9.

59. Fratiglioni L, Launer LJ, Andersen K, Breteler MM, Copeland JR, Dartigues JF *et al.* Incidence of dementia and major subtypes in Europe: a collaborative study of population-based cohorts. Neurologic diseases in the elderly research group. *Neurology* 2000; **54**(11 Suppl 5): S10–15.

60. Jorm AF, Jolley D. The incidence of dementia: a meta-analysis. *Neurology* 1998; **51**(3): 728–33.

61. Ferri CP, Prince M, Brayne C, Brodaty H, Fratiglioni L, Ganguli M *et al.* Global prevalence of dementia: a Delphi consensus study. *Lancet* 2005; **366**(9503): 2112–7.

62. Hendrie HC, Ogunniyi A, Hall KS, Baiyewu O, Unverzagt FW, Gureje O *et al.* Incidence of dementia and Alzheimer disease in 2 communities: Yoruba residing in Ibadan, Nigeria, and African Americans residing in Indianapolis, Indiana. *JAMA* 2001; **285**(6): 739–47.

63. Chandra V, Pandav R, Dodge HH, Johnston JM, Belle SH, DeKosky ST *et al.* Incidence of Alzheimer's disease in a rural community in India: the Indo-US study. *Neurology* 2001; **57**(6): 985–9.

64. Hendrie HC, Hall KS, Ogunniyi A, Gao S. Alzheimer's disease, genes, and environment: the value of international studies. *Can J Psychiatry* 2004; **49**(2): 92–9.

65. Breteler MM, Bots ML, Ott A, Hofman A. Risk factors for vascular disease and dementia. *Haemostasis* 1998; **28**(3–4): 167–73.

66. Chandra V, Pandav R. Gene–environment interaction in Alzheimer's disease: a potential role for cholesterol. *Neuroepidemiology* 1998; **17**, 225–32.

67. Pandav RS, Chandra V, Dodge HH, DeKosky ST, Ganguli M. Hemoglobin levels and Alzheimer disease: an epidemiologic study in India. *Am J Geriatr Psychiatry* 2004; **12**(5): 523–6.

68. McGee MA, Brayne C. The impact on prevalence of dementia in the oldest age groups of differential mortality patterns: a deterministic approach. *Int J Epidemiol* 1998; **27**(1): 87–90.

69. Rorsman B, Hagnell O, Lanke J. Prevalence and incidence of senile and multi-infarct dementia in the Lundby Study: a comparison between the time periods 1947–1957 and 1957–1972. *Neuropsychobiology* 1986; **15**: 122–9.

70. Kokmen E, Chandra V, Schoenberg BS. Trends in incidence of dementing illness in Rochester, Minnesota, in three quinquennial periods, 1960–1974. *Neurology* 1988; **38**: 975–80.

71. Herrera E Jr, Caramelli P, Silveira AS, Nitrini R. Epidemiologic survey of dementia in a community-dwelling Brazilian population. *Alzheimer Disease Associated Disord* 2002; **16**(2): 103–8.

72. Nitrini R, Caramelli P, Herrera E Jr, Bahia VS, Caixeta LF, Radanovic M *et al.* Incidence of dementia in a community-dwelling Brazilian population. *Alzheimer Disease Associated Disord* 2004; **18**(4). 241–6.

73. Rosselli D, Ardila A, Pradilla G, Morillo L, Bautista L, Rey O *et al.* The Mini-Mental State Examination as a selected diagnostic test for dementia: a Colombian population study. GENECO. *Rev Neurol* 2000; **30**(5): 428–32.

74. Prince M, Ferri CP, Acosta D, Albanese E, Arizaga R, Dewey M *et al.* The protocols for the 10/66 Dementia Research Group population-based research programme. *BMC Public Health* 2007; **7**(1): 165.

75. Llibre RJ, Ferri CP, Acosta D, Guerra M, Huang Y, Jacob KS *et al.* Prevalence of dementia in Latin America, India, and China: a population-based cross-sectional survey. *Lancet* 2008; **372**(9637): 464–74.

76. Scazufca M, Menezes PR, Vallada HP, Crepaldi AL, Pastor-Valero M, Coutinho LM *et al.* High prevalence of dementia among older adults from poor socioeconomic backgrounds in Sao Paulo, Brazil. *Int Psychogeriatr* 2008; **20**(2): 394–405.

77. Llibre RJ, Valhuerdi A, Sanchez II, Reyna C, Guerra MA, Copeland JR *et al.* The prevalence, correlates and impact of dementia in Cuba. A 10/66 group population-based survey. *Neuroepidemiology* 2008; **31**(4): 243–51.

78. Acosta D, Rottbeck R, Rodriguez G, Ferri CP, Prince MJ. The epidemiology of dependency among urban-dwelling older people in the Dominican Republic: a cross-sectional survey. *BMC Public Health* 2008; **8**(1): 285.

79. Jacob KS, Kumar PS, Gayathri K, Abraham S, Prince MJ. The diagnosis of dementia in the community. *Int Psychogeriatr* 2007; **19**(4): 669–78.

80. Lobo A, Saz P, Marcos G, Dia JL, De-la-Camara C, Ventura T *et al.* Prevalence of dementia in a southern European population in two different time periods: the ZARADEMP Project. *Acta Psychiatr Scand* 2007; **116**(4): 299–307.

81. Fernandez M, Castro-Flores J, Perez-de las HS, Mandaluniz-Lekumberri A, Gordejuela M, Zarranz J. Prevalence of dementia in the elderly aged above 65 in a district in the Basque Country. *Rev Neurol* 2008; **46**(2): 89–96.

82. Francesconi P, Roti L, Casotto V, Lauretani F, Lamponi M, Bandinelli S *et al.* Prevalence of dementia in Tuscany: results from four population-based epidemiological studies. *Epidemiol Prev* 2006; **30**(4–5): 237–44.

83. Plassman BL, Langa KM, Fisher GG, Heeringa SG, Weir DR, Ofstedal MB *et al.* Prevalence of dementia in the United States: the aging, demographics, and memory study. *Neuroepidemiology* 2007; **29**(1–2): 125–32.

84. Bottino CM, Azevedo D, Jr., Tatsch M, Hototian SR, Moscoso MA, Folquitto J *et al.* Estimate of dementia prevalence in a

community sample from Sao Paulo, Brazil. *Dement Geriatr Cogn Disord* 2008; **26**(4): 291–9.

85. Custodio N. *Prevalencia de demencia en una comunidad urbana de Lima: Un estudio puerta a puerta*. Santo Domingo, Republica Dominicana, XII Congreso Panamericano de Neurologia, 2007.

86. Llibre JJ, Fernandez Y, Marcheco B, Contreras N, López AM, Ote M. Prevalence of dementia and Alzheimer's disease in a Havana municipality: a community-based study among elderly residents. *MEDICC Rev* 2009; **11**(2): 29–35.

87. Molero AE, Pino-Ramirez G, Maestre GE. High prevalence of dementia in a Caribbean population. *Neuroepidemiology* 2007; **29**(1–2): 107–12.

88. Zhang ZX, Zahner GE, Roman GC, Liu XH, Wu CB, Hong Z *et al*. Socio-demographic variation of dementia subtypes in china: Methodology and results of a prevalence study in Beijing, Chengdu, Shanghai, and Xian. *Neuroepidemiology* 2006; **27**(4): 177–87.

89. Jhoo JH, Kim KW, Huh Y, Lee SB, Park JH, Lee JJ *et al*. Prevalence of dementia and its subtypes in an elderly urban Korean population: results from the Korean Longitudinal Study on Health and Aging (KLoSHA). *Dement Geriatr Cogn Disord* 2008; **26**(3): 270–6.

90. Shaji S, Bose S, Verghese A. Prevalence of dementia in an urban population in Kerala, India. *Br J Psychiatry* 2005; **186**: 136–40.

91. Wangtongkum S, Sucharitkul P, Silprasert N, Inthrachak R. Prevalence of dementia among population age over 45 years in Chiang Mai, Thailand *J Med Assoc Thai* 2008; **91**(11): 1685–90.

92. Smith K, Flicker L, Lautenschlager NT, Almeida OP, Atkinson D, Dwyer A *et al*. High prevalence of dementia and cognitive impairment in indigenous Australians. *Neurology* 2008; **71**(19): 1470–3.

93. Galasko D, Salmon D, Gamst A, Olichney J, Thal LJ, Silbert L *et al*. Prevalence of dementia in Chamorros on Guam: relationship to age, gender, education, and APOE. *Neurology* 2007; **68**(21): 1772–81.

94. Bdzan LB, Turczynski J, Szabert K. Prevalence of dementia in a rural population. *Psychiatr Pol* 2007; **41**(2): 181–8.

95. Gurvit H, Emre M, Tinaz S, Bilgic B, Hanagasi H, Sahin H *et al*. The prevalence of dementia in an urban Turkish population. *Am J Alzheimers Dis Other Demen* 2008; **23**(1): 67–76.

96. Alzheimer's Disease International. *World Alzheimer Report 2009*. London: Alzheimer's Disease International, 2009.

97. Wimo A, Winblad B, Jonsson L. An estimate of the total worldwide societal costs of dementia in 2005. *Alzheimer's Dementia* 2007; **3**: 81–91.

98. 10/66 Dementia Research Group. Care arrangements for people with dementia in developing countries. *Int J Geriatr Psychiatry* 2004; **19**(2): 170–7.

99. Sousa RM, Ferri CP, Acosta D, Albanese E, Guerra M, Huang Y *et al*. Contribution of chronic diseases to disability in elderly people in countries with low and middle incomes: a 10/66 Dementia Research Group population-based survey. *Lancet* 2009; **374**(9704): 1821–30.

100. Prince M, Acosta D, Albanese E, Arizaga R, Ferri CP, Guerra M *et al*. Ageing and dementia in low and middle income countries-Using research to engage with public and policy makers. *Int Rev Psychiatry* 2008; **20**(4): 332–43.

101. Ogunniyi A, Hall KS, Gureje O, Baiyewu O, Gao S, Unverzagt FW *et al*. Risk factors for incident Alzheimer's disease in African Americans and Yoruba. *Metab Brain Dis* 2006; **21**(2–3): 235–40.

102. Saunders AM, Strittmatter WJ, Schmechel D, St George-Hyslop PH, Pericak-Vance MA, Joo SH *et al*. Association of apolipoprotein E allele e4 with late-onset familial and sporadic Alzheimer's disease. *Neurology* 1993; **43**: 1467–72.

103. Nalbantoglu J, Gilfix BM, Bertrand P, Robitaille Y, Gauthier S, Rosenblatt DS *et al*. Predictive value of apolipoprotein E genotyping in Alzheimer's disease: results of an autopsy series and an analysis of several combined studies. *Ann Neurol* 1994; **36**(6): 889–95.

104. Farrer LA, Cupples LA, Haines JL, Hyman B, Kukull WA, Mayeux R *et al*. Effects of age, sex, and ethnicity on the association between apolipoprotein E genotype and Alzheimer disease. A meta-analysis. APOE and Alzheimer Disease Meta Analysis Consortium. *JAMA* 1997; **278**(16): 1349–56.

105. Kalaria RN, Maestre GE, Arizaga R, Friedland RP, Galasko D, Hall K *et al*. Alzheimer's disease and vascular dementia in developing countries: prevalence, management, and risk factors. *Lancet Neurol* 2008; **7**(9): 812–26.

106. Gureje O, Ogunniyi A, Baiyewu O, Price B, Unverzagt FW, Evans RM *et al*. APOE epsilon4 is not associated with Alzheimer's disease in elderly Nigerians. *Ann Neurol* 2006; **59**(1): 182–5.

107. Breitner JC, Welsh KA, Gau BA, McDonald WM, Steffens DC, Saunders AM *et al*. Alzheimer's disease in the National Academy of Sciences-National Research Council Registry of Aging Twin Veterans. III. Detection of cases, longitudinal results, and observations on twin concordance. *Arch Neurol* 1995; **52**(8): 763–71.

108. Ott A, Breteler MM, van Harskamp F, Claus JJ, van der Cammen TJ, Grobbee DE *et al*. Prevalence of Alzheimer's disease and vascular dementia: association with education. The Rotterdam study. *BMJ* 1995; **310**(6985): 970–3.

109. Mortimer JA, van Duijn CM, Chandra V, Fratiglioni L, Graves AB, Heyman A *et al*. Head trauma as a risk factor for Alzheimer's disease: a collaborative re-analysis of case-control studies. EURODEM Risk Factors Research Group. *Int J Epidemiol* 1991; **20**(Suppl 2): S28–35.

110. Mayeux R, Ottman R, Maestre G, Ngai C, Tang MX, Ginsberg H *et al*. Synergistic effects of traumatic head injury and apolipoprotein-epsilon 4 in patients with Alzheimer's disease. *Neurology* 1995; **45**(3Pt 1): 555–7.

111. Stern Y, Gurland B, Tatemichi TK, Tang MX, Wilder D, Mayeux R. Influence of education and occupation on the incidence of Alzheimer's disease. *JAMA* 1994; **271**(13): 1004–10.

112. Devanand DP, Sano M, Tang MX, Taylor S, Gurland BJ, Wilder D *et al*. Depressed mood and the incidence of Alzheimer's disease in the elderly living in the community. *Arch Gen Psychiatry* 1996; **53**(2): 175–82.

113. Yusuf S, Reddy S, Ounpuu S, Anand S. Global burden of cardiovascular diseases: part I: general considerations, the epidemiologic transition, risk factors, and impact of urbanization. *Circulation* 2001; **104**(22): 2746–53.

114. Hofman A, Ott A, Breteler MMB, Bots ML, Slooter AJC, van Harskamp F *et al*. Atherosclerosis, apolipoprotein E, and prevalence of dementia and Alzheimer's disease in the Rotterdam Study. *Lancet* 1997; **349**: 151–4.

115. Yusuf S, Hawken S, Ounpuu S, Dans T, Avezum A, Lanas F *et al*. Effect of potentially modifiable risk factors associated with myocardial infarction in 52 countries (the INTERHEART study): case-control study. *Lancet* 2004; **364**(9438): 937–52.

116. Yip AG, Brayne C, Matthews FE. Risk factors for incident dementia in England and Wales: The Medical Research Council Cognitive Function and Ageing Study. A population-based nested case-control study. *Age Ageing* 2006; **13**.

117. Bursi F, Rocca WA, Killian JM, Weston SA, Knopman DS, Jacobsen SJ *et al*. Heart disease and dementia: a population-based study. *Am J Epidemiol* 2006; **163**(2): 135–41.

118. Ott A, Slooter AJC, Hofman A, van Harskamp F, Witteman JCM, Van Broeckhoven C *et al*. Smoking and risk of dementia and Alzheimer's disease in a population-based cohort study: the Rotterdam Study. *Lancet* 1998; **351**: 1841–3.

119. Juan D, Zhou DH, Li J, Wang JY, Gao C, Chen M. A 2-year follow-up study of cigarette smoking and risk of dementia. *Eur J Neurol* 2004; **11**(4): 277–82.

120. Luchsinger JA, Reitz C, Honig LS, Tang MX, Shea S, Mayeux R. Aggregation of vascular risk factors and risk of incident Alzheimer disease. *Neurology* 2005; **65**(4): 545–51.

121. Tyas SL, White LR, Petrovitch H, Webster RG, Foley DJ, Heimovitz HK *et al*. Mid-life smoking and late-life dementia: the Honolulu-Asia Aging Study. *Neurobiol Aging* 2003; **24**(4): 589–96.

122. Whitmer RA, Sidney S, Selby J, Johnston SC, Yaffe K. Midlife cardiovascular risk factors and risk of dementia in late life. *Neurology* 2005; **64**(2): 277–81.

123. Ott A, Stolk RP, van HF, Pols HA, Hofman A, Breteler MM. Diabetes mellitus and the risk of dementia: The Rotterdam Study. *Neurology* 1999; **53**(9): 1937–42.

124. Skoog I, Lernfelt B, Landahl S, Palmertz B, Andreasson LA, Nilsson L *et al*. 15-year longitudinal study of blood pressure and dementia. *Lancet* 1996; **347**(9009): 1141–5.

125. Kivipelto M, Helkala EL, Laakso MP, Hanninen T, Hallikainen M, Alhainen K *et al*. Midlife vascular risk factors and Alzheimer's disease in later life: longitudinal, population based study. *BMJ* 2001; **322**(7300): 1447–51.

126. Yaffe K, Kanaya A, Lindquist K, Simonsick EM, Harris T, Shorr RI *et al*. The metabolic syndrome, inflammation, and risk of cognitive decline. *JAMA* 2004; **292**(18): 2237–42.

127. Abbatecola AM, Paolisso G, Lamponi M, Bandinelli S, Lauretani F, Launer L *et al*. Insulin resistance and executive dysfunction in older persons. *J Am Geriatr Soc* 2004; **52**(10): 1713–18.

128. Casserly I, Topol E. Convergence of atherosclerosis and Alzheimer's disease: inflammation, cholesterol, and misfolded proteins. *Lancet* 2004; **363**(9415): 1139–46.

129. Selhub J, Jacques PF, Wilson PW, Rush D, Rosenberg IH. Vitamin status and intake as primary determinants of homocysteinemia in an elderly population. *JAMA* 1993; **270**(22): 2693–8.

130. Robinson K, Arheart K, Refsum H, Brattstrom L, Boers G, Ueland P *et al*. Low circulating folate and vitamin B6 concentrations: risk factors for stroke, peripheral vascular disease, and coronary artery disease. European COMAC Group. *Circulation* 1998; **97**(5): 437–43.

131. Allen LH. Folate and vitamin B12 status in the Americas. *Nutr Rev* 2004; **62**(6Pt 2): S29–33.

132. Garcia-Casal MN, Osorio C, Landaeta M, Leets I, Matus P, Fazzino F *et al*. High prevalence of folic acid and vitamin B12 deficiencies in infants, children, adolescents and pregnant women in Venezuela. *Eur J Clin Nutr* 2005; **59**(9): 1064–70.

133. Arnaud J, Fleites-Mestre P, Chassagne M, Verdura T, Garcia G, I, Hernandez-Fernandez T *et al*. Vitamin B intake and status in healthy Havanan men, 2 years after the Cuban neuropathy epidemic. *Br J Nutr* 2001; **85**(6): 741–8.

134. Luchsinger JA, Mayeux R. Dietary factors and Alzheimer's disease. *Lancet Neurol* 2004; **3**(10): 579–87.

135. Ravaglia G, Forti P, Maioli F, Martelli M, Servadei L, Brunetti N *et al*. Homocysteine and folate as risk factors for dementia and Alzheimer disease. *Am J Clin Nutr* 2005; **82**(3): 636–43.

136. Wang HX, Wahlin A, Basun H, Fastbom J, Winblad B, Fratiglioni L. Vitamin B(12) and folate in relation to the development of Alzheimer's disease. *Neurology* 2001; **56**(9): 1188–94.

137. Seshadri S, Beiser A, Selhub J, Jacques PF, Rosenberg IH, D'Agostino RB *et al*. Plasma homocysteine as a risk factor for dementia and Alzheimer's disease. *N Engl J Med* 2002; **346**(7): 476–83.

138. Crystal HA, Ortof E, Frishman WH, Gruber A, Hershman D, Aronson M. Serum vitamin B12 levels and incidence of dementia in a healthy elderly population: a report from the Bronx Longitudinal Aging Study. *J Am Geriatr Soc* 1994; **42**(9): 933–6.

139. Pretell EA, Delange F, Hostalek U, Corigliano S, Barreda L, Higa AM *et al*. Iodine nutrition improves in Latin America. *Thyroid* 2004; **14**(8): 590–9.

140. Petri Nahas EA, Nahas-Neto J, Ferreira Santos PEM, Ferreira da Silva Mazeto GM, Dalben I, Pontes A *et al*. Prevalence of subclinical hypothyroidism and its effects on lipidic profile and bone mineral density in postmenopausal women. *Revista Brasileirade Ginecologia e Obstetrica* 2005; **27**(8).

141. Surks MI, Ortiz E, Daniels GH, Sawin CT, Col NF, Cobin RH *et al*. Subclinical thyroid disease: scientific review and guidelines for diagnosis and management. *JAMA* 2004; **291**(2): 228–38.

142. Ganguli M, Burmeister LA, Seaberg EC, Belle S, DeKosky ST. Association between dementia and elevated TSH: a community-based study. *Biol Psychiatry* 1996; **40**(8): 714–25.

143. Kalmijn S, Mehta KM, Pols HA, Hofman A, Drexhage HA, Breteler MM. Subclinical hyperthyroidism and the risk of dementia. The Rotterdam study. *Clin Endocrinol* 2000; **53**(6): 733–7.

144. Epping-Jordan JE, Galea G, Tukuitonga C, Beaglehole R. Preventing chronic diseases: taking stepwise action. *Lancet* 2005; **366**(9497): 1667–71.

145. Forette F, Seux M-L, Staessen JA, Thijs L, Birkenhager WH, Babarskiene M-R *et al*. Prevention of dementia in randomised double-blind placebo-controlled systolic hypertension in Europe (Syst-Eur) trial. *Lancet* 1998; **352**: 1347–51.

146. Prince MJ, Bird AS, Blizard RA, Mann AH. Is the cognitive function of older patients affected by antihypertensive treatment? Results from 54 months of the Medical Research Council's treatment trial of hypertension in older adults. *BMJ* 1996; **312**: 801–4.

147. Starr JM, Whalley LJ, Deary IJ. The effects of antihypertensive treatment on cognitive function: results from the HOPE study. *J Am Geriatr Soc* 1996; **44**: 411–15.

148. Lithell H, Hansson L, Skoog I, Elmfeldt D, Hofman A, Olofsson B *et al*. The Study on Cognition and Prognosis in the Elderly (SCOPE): principal results of a randomized double-blind intervention trial. *J Hypertension* 2003; **21**: 875–86.

149. Tzourio C, Anderson C, Chapman N, Woodward M, Neal B, MacMahon S *et al*. Effects of blood pressure lowering with perindopril and indapamide therapy on dementia and cognitive decline in patients with cerebrovascular disease. *Arch Internal Med* 2003; **163**: 1069–75.

150. Santanello NC, Barber BL, Applegate WB, Elam J, Curtis C, Hunninghake DB *et al*. Effect of pharmacologic lipid lowering on health-related quality of life in older persons: results from the Cholesterol Reduction in Seniors Program (CRISP) Pilot Study. *J Am Geriatr Soc* 1997; **45**: 8–14.

151. Heart Protection Study Collaborative Group. MRC/BHF Heart Protection Study of cholesterol lowering with simvastatin in 20,536 high-risk individuals: a randomised placebo-controlled trial. *Lancet* 2002; **360**: 7–22.

152. Shumaker SA, Legault C, Kuller L, Rapp SR, Thal L, Lane DS *et al*. Conjugated equine estrogens and incidence of probable dementia and mild cognitive impairment in postmenopausal women: Women's Health Initiative Memory Study. *JAMA* 2004; **291**(24): 2947–58.

153. Prince MJ, Acosta D, Castro-Costa E, Jackson J, Shaji KS. Packages of care for dementia in low- and middle-income countries. *PLoS Med* 2009; **6**(11): e1000176.

115

Mental Illness in the Elderly in South Asia

Vikram Patel[1] and K. S. Shaji[2]

[1]London School of Hygiene and Tropical Medicine (UK) and Sangath (India), Sangath Centre, Goa, India
[2]Government Medical College, Thrissur, Kerala, India

South Asia will house over 100 million older people by 2020[1]. This chapter describes mental health problems that affect elders, focusing on the two commonest conditions: dementia and depression. The chapter will first review the epidemiology of these disorders and then consider the implications for care and policies in the region. While the scope of our chapter is intended to address the entire South Asian region, we note that as most of the research on mental illness in the elderly has been carried out in India, much of our discussion will pertain specifically to India.

DEMENTIA

Prevalence studies from the region have indicated a lower prevalence of dementia when compared to developed countries. However, there are wide variations in reported rates, ranging from 1.4% to 4.4%[2-7]. One study reported an incidence of Alzheimer's disease (AD) of 3.24 per 1000 person-years for those aged 65 years[8]. Dementia incidence is predicted to increase in the developing world in tandem with the ageing population and the increasing burden of vascular risk factors[9]. It is estimated that there are already about 1.5 million people with dementia in India and this number is likely to increase dramatically in the next four decades[1]. The major causes of dementia in the region are AD and vascular dementia. One study from Kerala reported that vascular dementia was more common than AD in a rural community sample[6]. A cross-national study compared *APOE*4*–AD epidemiological associations in India and the United States. Frequency of *APOE*4* was significantly lower ($p < 0.001$) in India. Correspondingly, the frequency of probable or possible AD was also lower in the Indian samples[10]. However, although there was a very low prevalence of AD in the Indian sample, the association of *APOE*4* with AD was of similar strength in Indian and US samples.

A challenge for the diagnosis of dementia, which relies heavily on interview-based examination, is the cultural and educational factors such as illiteracy. Several efforts have been made to improve the detection and diagnosis of dementia in this context. Screening questionnaires such as the Mini-Mental State Examination have been translated and validated for use in a North Indian population[11]. A scale for activities of daily living has also been developed by the same investigators[12]. In an epidemiological survey with a largely illiterate sample of 5126 individuals aged 55 and older in the rural community of Ballabgarh in northern India, the Hindi version of the MMSE, a neuropsychological battery, and the Everyday Abilities Scale for India (EASI) had sensitivities of 81.3%, 81.3% and 62.5%, respectively, with specificities of 60.2%, 74.5% and 89.7%, respectively. The combination of all three was 93.8% sensitive and 41.8% specific[13]. An advantage of the EASI was that it could also be administered to informants of subjects who were cognitively not testable. In this largely illiterate community, with a low prevalence of dementia, the combination of cognitive tests and a functional ability questionnaire had substantial value for population screening.

The 10/66 Dementia Research Group interviewed 2885 persons aged 60 and over in 25 centres, including several in India, China and South East Asia. The sample included 729 people with dementia, and three groups free of dementia; 702 with depression, 694 normals with high education and 760 normals with low education. Experienced local clinicians diagnosed dementia and depression. The Geriatric Mental State, the Community Screening Instrument for Dementia and the modified CERAD 10 word list-learning task were then administered by an interviewer, masked to case status. Each measure independently predicted dementia diagnosis. An algorithm derived from all three performed better than any individually and identified 94% of dementia cases with false positive rates of 15%, 3% and 6% in the depression, high education and low education groups. The algorithm developed and tested in this study provides a sound basis for culture and education-fair dementia diagnosis in clinical and population-based research in India[14].

Dementia remains a largely hidden problem in India. People do not differentiate between normal ageing and phenomena that are secondary to conditions like dementia[15]. Even when it is identified, it does not lead to caregivers receiving practical advice or longer-term support[16]. Given the low awareness about mental disorders in elders, there is a need to develop culturally sensitive methods for identification of probable cases. Shaji *et al.* have described a simple, cost-effective method of training community health workers to identify dementia in Kerala[17]. After two and a half hours of formal training, local community health workers in rural Kerala were asked to identify possible cases of dementia from the community they served. Diagnoses were then verified by a senior local psychiatrist with clinical and research interests in old age psychiatry. This method was found to have a positive predictive value of 64.7%. Later in this chapter, we will review the evidence on the burden of dementia, services for people with dementia, and innovative new strategies for addressing the needs of families affected by dementia.

Principles and Practice of Geriatric Psychiatry, 3rd edn. Edited by Mohammed T. Abou-Saleh, Cornelius Katona and Anand Kumar
© 2011 John Wiley & Sons, Ltd

DEPRESSION

There are a growing number of epidemiological studies of depression or common mental disorders (a broad diagnostic term which encompasses mood and anxiety disorders) in elders in the region, which have sampled general populations and clinical populations. Prevalence rates vary even more widely than those for dementia: rates in a community sample of elders vary from 6% in South India[18] to over 50% in rural West Bengal[19]. Median prevalence rates tend to be higher in clinical populations[20-23]. One of the largest recent population-based studies was carried out with 1000 participants aged over 65 years from Kaniyambadi block, Vellore, India[24]. The prevalence of depression (ICD-10) within the previous one month was 12.7% (95% CI 10.64–14.76%).

The common presenting complaints are tiredness, sleep complaints, aches, tingling numbness in the hands, and palpitations[25]. The hallmark cognitive feature is anhedonia or loss of interest. Suicidal feelings and agitation are also common[18]. The suicide rate is nearly twice as high in the 50+ age group (12/100 000) as compared to the national average (7/100 000). Co-morbidity with physical ill health is common; by some estimates, more than 90% of elders with a psychiatric disorder also have some physical disorder[18]. Risk factors for depression include female gender, low education, poverty, social isolation, chronic diseases such as diabetes, and family discord[20,21,23-26]. Nuclear family structures, in particular, appear to be associated with a higher risk[20]. The latter is on the rise as a result of the breakdown of traditional community structures as a result of the massive migration of younger productive members of families to urban areas and reduced economic activity in rural areas[15]. Older women face a triple jeopardy: that of being old, of being women, and of being poor. Elders living in rural areas may represent another risk group because rural areas lack resources, and with agriculture being the main occupation, there is neither income security nor any systematic provision for old age[27]. One outcome study was carried out with a sample of patients attending psychiatry services of a tertiary care hospital in India. After 12 months, only 28% of patients had recovered. Factors predicting good outcomes were shorter duration of episode and living in a joint family system[28].

Help-seeking is not uncommon for somatic complaints associated with depression. However, the commonest treatments in primary care are symptomatic. Thus, benzodiazepines for insomnia and vitamins and 'tonics' for tiredness are among the commonest prescriptions for common mental disorders in general health care, while antidepressants or psychotherapy are rarely offered[29]. Detection rates are very low, but there is good evidence that short screening questionnaires can considerably improve detection rates in primary care[30]. One study evaluated the sensitivity and specificity of a two-question screen to identify depression and common mental disorders in the elderly, against the gold standard criterion of a structured diagnostic interview. The two-question screen has a sensitivity of 93.8% and specificity of 48.2%[31]. There are no specific treatment studies for older people with depression in the region, but it would be reasonable to expect that the considerable treatment evidence on the care of depression in general in developing countries would also apply to older people[32].

CARE ARRANGEMENTS FOR THE ELDERLY WITH MENTAL DISORDERS

Ancient Indian scriptures advocate the preparation for old age by adopting the disengagement theory. Respect towards elders and the concept of obligation towards parents forms part of the cultural value system[33]. In contemporary Indian society, however, the position and status of the elderly and the care and protection they traditionally enjoyed have been undermined by several factors. Urbanization, migration, the break-up of the joint family system, growing individualism, the change in the role of women from being full-time carers, and increased dependency status of the elderly are some of the prominent factors. There have been changes in terms of education, aspirations and values, and the allocation of resources to different members of the family. Often the family has been unable to meet the financial, social, psychological, medical, recreational and welfare needs of the elderly[27]. Care has often been conditional upon the child's expectation of inheriting the parent's property[15]. Care for those with dependency needs was almost entirely family based, with little or no formal services. Not surprisingly, fear for the future, and in particular 'dependency anxiety' was commonplace among older persons[15].

Formal care arrangements for elders, for example in the public health sector, are scarce. Indeed, geriatric medicine as a special area of health care is not available in most medical colleges or hospitals in the region. The number of residential places for elders with severe mental disorders such as dementia is very low and inequitably distributed. There are no accurate estimates for the treatment gap for dementia in India in general, but a rough estimate is that this gap exceeds 90% in most parts of the country, with the exception of urban areas and the two southern states of Kerala and Tamil Nadu[34]. Studies by the 10/66 Dementia Research Network in Goa and Chennai examined the impact of care giving for elders[35]. Carers of people with dementia spent a significantly longer time providing care than did carers and co-residents of depressed persons and controls. The highest proportion of time was spent in communicating, supervising, and helping with eating and toileting. Levels of carer strain were notably higher among carers of people with dementia. They were 16-times more likely to have a common mental disorder than carers or co-residents of controls, and twice as likely as carers or co-residents of people with depression. Economic strain was indicated by the high proportion of caregivers of people with dementia who had given up work to provide care, coupled with the increased likelihood that the family had to meet relatively high health care costs. This was explained by the increased propensity for people with dementia to use expensive private medical care services rather than free or low cost government services.

There are several major barriers to closing this treatment gap, including the low levels of awareness about dementia and depression as medical disorders; however, the most significant barrier is the very low human resource capacity for the care of people with mental disorders. This scarcity of resources is true for all mental disorders across the continuum of life and has been systematically documented in the recent *Lancet* series on Global Mental Health[36]. South Asia lacks the economic and human capital to achieve widespread coverage of specialist services; furthermore, specialist services tend to focus almost entirely on medical interventions, which have only a limited role in the long-term care of people with mental disorders, especially dementia. In view of the above, those responsible for service development for families of older people with mental disorders should keep in mind that the service should be home based, address the diverse medical and psychosocial health needs of the affected persons and their caregivers and be provided at a cost that the family can afford (and therefore use public and low-cost service providers).

Thus, the challenge for South Asia is to develop culturally appropriate interventions that can be delivered within existing resources, such as supporting families in their role as caregivers.

A randomized controlled trial has recently been completed in two *talukas* of Goa, evaluating the benefits of a low-cost, home-based intervention aimed at supporting families affected by dementia[37]. The intervention was delivered by a community team and each team comprised two full-time Home Care Advisors (HCAs), a part-time local psychiatrist from the public health services and a part-time lay counsellor. The minimum requirements for being a HCA were knowledge of the local language, being literate, preferably having passed higher secondary school, and being motivated to be involved in the community care of older people. The specific components of the intervention carried out by the HCA were: basic education about dementia; education about common behaviour problems and how they can be managed; support to the caregiver, for example for an elderly caregiver living alone with the patient, in activities of daily living; referral to psychiatrists or the family doctor when behaviour problems are severe and warrant medication intervention; networking of families to enable the formation of support groups; and advice regarding existing government schemes for elders. The HCA applied a flexible home-care programme tailored to the needs of the individual and the family. The HCA were supported, and supervised, by the two part-time specialists. The intervention demonstrated a significant impact in reducing the caregiver burden, mental stress and distress due to the behavioural and psychological symptoms of dementia.

It is important to note that mental illness is seldom an isolated event among elderly people; thus, co-morbidity with other mental illnesses and physical health problems is typically the rule[19,27]. The most common problems include deficits of vision and hearing, hypertension, diabetes mellitus, cardiovascular disorders and osteoarthritis. Thus, an ideal model of care for mental disorders in older people must fully address their physical health needs as well. There is a need to raise awareness about mental disorders in late life in the community and among health professionals, and to improve access to appropriate health care for the elderly with mental illness. Health education should aim to educate health workers and the community to recognize the common symptoms of mental disorders and, in particular, to stress that depression and dementia are real disorders and not just the natural consequences of ageing. Caregiver strain has not been acknowledged; instead, a near mythical strength is attributed to the abilities of families to cope. This distracts from the need for a rational debate regarding the future balance between informal family support and formal care services, and hinders evidence-based policymaking. We suggest prioritizing home-based support for elderly persons with dementia and their carers. Collaboration is required with non-governmental organizations (such as the Alzheimer's and Related Disorders Society of India) that are pioneering programmes to empower the elderly and support families with a mentally ill elder and provide health care sensitive to their needs. Working with the existing manpower and health and social service infrastructure is likely to be more successful in meeting the mental health needs of elders in South Asia than developing specialized psychogeriatric services throughout the country.

REFERENCES

1. Ferri CP, Prince M, Brayne C *et al*. Global prevalence of dementia: a Delphi consensus study. *Lancet* 2005; **366**(9503): 2112–7.
2. Chandra V, Ganguli M, Pandav R *et al*. Prevalence of Alzheimer's disease and other dementias in rural India: the Indo-US study. *Neurology* 1998; **51**(4): 1000–8.
3. Vas CJ, Pinto C, Panikker D *et al*. Prevalence of dementia in an urban Indian population. *Int Psychogeriatr* 2001; **13**(4): 439–50.
4. Rajkumar S, Kumar S. Prevalence of dementia in the community – a rural–urban comparison from Madras, India. *Aust J Ageing* 1996; **15**: 9–13.
5. Rajkumar S, Kumar S, Thara R. Prevalence of dementia in a rural setting: a report from India. *Int J Geriatr Psychiatry* 1997; **12**(7): 702–7.
6. Shaji S, Promodu K, Abraham T, Roy KJ, Verghese A. An epidemiological study of dementia in a rural community in Kerala, India. *Br J Psychiatry* 1996; **168**(6): 745–9.
7. Shaji S, Bose S, Verghese A. Prevalence of dementia in an urban population in Kerala, India. *Br J Psychiatry* 2005; **186**: 136–40.
8. Chandra V, Pandav R, Dodge HH *et al*. Incidence of Alzheimer's disease in a rural community in India: the Indo-US study. *Neurology* 2001; **57**(6): 985–9.
9. Kalaria RN, Maestre GE, Arizaga R *et al*. Alzheimer's disease and vascular dementia in developing countries: prevalence, management, and risk factors. *Lancet Neurol* 2008; **7**(9): 812–26.
10. Ganguli M, Chandra V, Kamboh MI *et al*. Apolipoprotein E polymorphism and Alzheimer disease: the Indo-US Cross-National Dementia Study. *Arch Neurol* 2000; **57**(6): 824–30.
11. Ganguli M, Ratcliff G, Chandra V *et al*. A Hindi version of the MMSE: the development of a cognitive screening instrument for a largely illiterate rural elderly population in India. *Int J Geriatr Psychiatry* 1995; **10**: 367–77.
12. Fillenbaum GG, Chandra V, Ganguli M *et al*. Development of an activities of daily living scale to screen for dementia in an illiterate rural population in India. *Age Ageing* 1999; **28**: 161–8.
13. Pandav R, Fillenbaum GG, Ratcliff G, Dodge HH, Ganguli M. Sensitivity and specificity of cognitive and functional screening instruments for dementia: the Indo-U.S. Dementia Epidemiology Study. *J Am Geriatr Soc* 2002; **50**: 554–6.
14. Prince M, Acosta D, Chiu H, Scazufca M, Varghese M. Dementia diagnosis in developing countries: a cross-cultural validation study. *Lancet* 2003; **361**(9361): 909–17.
15. Patel V, Prince M. Ageing and mental health in developing countries: who cares? Qualitative studies from Goa, India. *Psychol Med* 2001; **31**: 29–38.
16. Shaji KS, Smitha K, Lal KP, Prince MJ. Caregivers of people with Alzheimer's disease: a qualitative study from the Indian 10/66 Dementia Research Network. *Int J Geriatr Psychiatry* 2003; **18**(1): 1–6.
17. Shaji KS, Arun Kishore NR, Lal KP, Prince M. Revealing a hidden problem. An evaluation of a community dementia case-finding program from the Indian 10/66 dementia research network. *Int J Geriatr Psychiatry* 2002; **17**(3): 222–5.
18. Venkoba Rao A. Psychiatry of old age in India. *Int Rev Psychiatry* 1993; **5**: 165–70.
19. Nandi PS, Banerjee G, Mukherjee SP, Nandi S, Nandi DN. A study of psychiatric morbidity of the elderly population of a rural community in West Bengal. *Indian J Psychiatry* 1997; **39**: 122–9.
20. Taqui AM, Itrat A, Qidwai W, Qadri Z. Depression in the elderly: does family system play a role? A cross-sectional study. *BMC Psychiatry* 2007; **7**: 57.

21. Ganatra HA, Zafar SN, Qidwai W, Rozi S. Prevalence and predictors of depression among an elderly population of Pakistan. *Aging Ment Health* 2008; **12**(3): 349–56.

22. Khattri JB, Nepal MK. Study of depression among geriatric population in Nepal. *Nepal Med Coll J* 2006; **8**(4): 220–3.

23. Prakash O, Gupta LN, Singh VB, Singhal AK, Verma KK. Profile of psychiatric disorders and life events in medically ill elderly: experiences from geriatric clinic in Northern India. *Int J Geriatr Psychiatry* 2007; **22**(11): 1101–5.

24. Rajkumar AP, Thangadurai P, Senthilkumar P *et al.* Nature, prevalence and factors associated with depression among the elderly in a rural south Indian community. *Int Psychogeriatr* 2009; **26**: 1–7.

25. Jain RK, Aras RY. Depression in geriatric population in urban slums of Mumbai. *Indian J Public Health* 2007; **51**(2): 112–3.

26. Ganguli M, Dube S, Johnston JM *et al.* Depressive symptoms, cognitive impairment and functional impairment in a rural elderly population in India: a Hindi version of the Geriatric Depression Scale(GDS-H). *Int J Geriatr Psychiatry* 1999; **14**: 807–20.

27. Varghese M, Patel V. The graying of India. In Agarwal S, Goel D, Salhan R, Ichhpujani R, Shrivastava S (eds), *Mental Health: An Indian Perspective 1946-2000*. New Delhi: Elsevier, 2004, 240–8.

28. Jhingan HP, Sagar R, Pandey RM. Prognosis of late-onset depression in the elderly: a study from India. *Int Psychogeriatr* 2001; **13**(1): 51–61.

29. Patel V, Pereira J, Coutinho L *et al.* Poverty, psychological disorder and disability in primary care attenders in Goa, India. *Br J Psychiatry* 1998; **172**: 533–5.

30. Patel V, Araya R, Chowdhary N *et al.* Detecting common mental disorders in primary care in India: a comparison of five screening questionnaires. *Psychol Med* 2008; **38**(2): 221–8.

31. Biswas SS, Gupta R, Vanjare HA *et al.* Depression in the elderly in Vellore, South India: the use of a two-question screen. *Int Psychogeriatr* 2009; **13**: 1–3.

32. Patel V, Simon G, Chowdhary N, Kaaya S, Araya R. Packages of care for depression in low- and middle-income countries. *PLoS Med* 2009; **6**: e1000159.

33. Venkoba Rao A. Mental health and ageing in India. *Indian J Psychiatry* 1993; **23**: 11–20.

34. Dias A, Patel V. Closing the treatment gap for dementia in India. *Indian J Psychiatry* 2009; **51**(Suppl): S93–7.

35. Dias A, Samuel R, Patel V *et al.* The impact associated with caring for a person with dementia: a report from the 10/66 Dementia Research Group's Indian network. *Int J Geriatr Psychiatry* 2004; **19**(2): 182–4.

36. Saxena S, Thornicroft G, Knapp M, Whiteford H. Resources for mental health; scarcity, inequity, and inefficiency. *Lancet* 2007; **370**(9590): 878–89.

37. Dias A, Dewey ME, D'Souza J *et al.* The effectiveness of a home care program for supporting caregivers of persons with dementia in developing countries: a randomised controlled trial from Goa, India. *PLoS ONE* 2008; **3**(6): e2333.

116

Dementia and Depression in Africa

Olusegun Baiyewu

Department of Psychiatry, College of Medicine, University of Ibadan, Ibadan, Nigeria

INTRODUCTION

In 2001 it was projected that about 7% of Africans would be aged 60 years and over in the year 2002[1]. Although the emphasis of health care in Africa is on preventable and communicable diseases in children and nursing mothers, as over 50% of the population is under 18 years of age, it has been estimated that the number of people aged 60 years and older in Africa will increase over the next few years. It thus becomes increasingly important that chronic illnesses associated with old age are considered. In this category are dementia and depression. In the last decade, a few studies have been carried out in Africa on dementia and depression; although the quantity of research on older person is small, significant advancements have been made.

Depression

One of the earliest community surveys on depression in the elderly in Africa was the study by Ben-Arie *et al.*[2], but since the 1990s there have been a number of research reports on old age depression in Africa[3–6]. These studies were done in various locations, rural, urban and a combination of both and the prevalence rates varied depending on the methodology. For example, studies in which screening questionnaires alone are used tend to have higher rates, in the range of 20%, while those that have second-stage clinical diagnosis have rates ranging from 5 to 8%. A theme that emerges in all studies is that populations with high levels of depression correlate with low levels of education and low income.

Some hospital-based studies have looked at depression and other psychiatric disorders in clinic attendees[7], and in patients admitted to non-psychiatric facilities[8,9]. In these groups, high level of medical co-morbidity is a regular finding, though relationship between medical co-morbidity and depression is not often established. Another issue is that depression is often not recognized and neither is it treated[5]. Interaction between depression and chronic medical illnesses, such as heart failure, stroke and cancer, need further research. Intervention and outcome studies are also lacking.

Dementia

The flagship of dementia research in Africa is the Indianapolis–Ibadan Dementia Research Project, which has been ongoing since 1992. This group has reported prevalence and incidence rates for dementia and Alzheimer's disease in Ibadan and Indianapolis and found that rates for both conditions were lower in Ibadan elders than in African Americans in Indianapolis[10,11]. One important issue in assessment of cognitive functioning is that many questionnaires used in Western countries need modification when used in developing countries as the elders often have low education levels and have been involved in low occupational pursuits all their life. For example the Mini Mental State Examination (MMSE)[12] has both a ceiling and a floor effect due to education. In contrast, a screening questionnaire like the Community Screening Interview for Dementia (CSI-'D')[13] has little education or culture effect and has been used in disparate populations. Another questionnaire developed by the group is Stick Design[14], which resolves the graphomotor function difficulties experienced by people with little education when asked to carry out a constructional praxis test.

In this group of studies risk factors for poor cognitive functioning identified include age and female gender, but the most important risk factor for Alzheimer's disease, apolipoprotein E4, is not related to either dementia or Alzheimer's disease in Nigerians[15,16]. A similar report from East Africa also found that ApoE4 is not related to Alzheimer's disease[17].

A study from Egypt, however, reported a prevalence of 4.5% based on DSM-IV diagnosis[18]. This is close to the 5% often reported in Euro-American studies.

A study of mortality in the Indianapolis–Ibadan group showed increased mortality in Ibadan generally and a higher though non-significant rate in demented subjects when the two sites were compared[19]. While this might be a reflection of poor health delivery service to the residents of Ibadan, it is important to note that mortality associated with dementia is not significantly different. Studies on behavioural and psychological symptoms in dementia (BPSD) have shown that the pattern of presentation is probably not different from that observed in other regions of the world. BPSD is related to cognitive and functional impairment and in Western societies, BPSD is one of the most important reasons for nursing home placement. Even though nursing homes are unpopular in Africa, there is evidence that caregivers of demented subjects who have BPSD experience considerable distress[20]. A small study of nursing home residents indicated that about 48% of the residents had dementia and 17% depression[21], rates that are not too different from those reported in Western societies. Nursing homes, however, need further study.

There is some controversy about why prevalence of dementia reported in Africa and some developing countries is so low. One argument is that the elders in these countries are shielded from activities of daily life in the multi-generational living arrangements they tend to have; it is possible that mild dementia may be missed[22]. While that is so, it is possible that prevalence of dementia may be truly different. Differential mortality rates may affect the prevalence of dementia. Elders in developing countries are generally likely to have shorter life spans because of the poor health care available; but factors such as the lower level of cholesterol and other cardiovascular risk factors may also affect the prevalence of dementia. In a community survey of elderly residents, cholesterol and triglycerides were higher in Indianapolis residents compared with those from Ibadan[23].

COGNITIVE IMPAIRMENT

The border area between normality and dementia is often referred to as mild cognitive impairment (MCI)[24] or cognitive impairment no dementia (CIND)[25]. People with MCI or CIND have a higher rate of conversion to dementia compared with normal individuals. Although they have problems associated with memory which is about 1.5 standard deviation below the norm, they have little or no functional impairment.

Little or no information is available on MCI or CIND in Africans. Baiyewu et al.[26] reported a lower rate of conversion to dementia in Nigerians and it has been noted that conversion to dementia or Alzheimer's disease is not related to the presence of ApoE4, as is observed in many studies in Western society.

TREATMENT

Health care delivery in Africa is generally poor, this is more so for the elderly. There are very few specialized care facilities for the elderly. Elderly persons find it difficult to use general adult clinics in hospitals unless they have knowledgeable relatives or caregivers ready to take care of their needs. The situation is worse for mental health. Gureje et al.[5] observed that many of the depressed elderly persons they studied in the community had never received treatment. Anti-dementia drugs are not available in many African countries. To the best of the knowledge of the present author there has been only one study in which patients from South Africa were included as part of a multicentre drug trial study on dementia covering five countries[27]. Despite this, Ferri et al.[28] have estimated a 82% increase in the number of people with dementia in Africa between the years 2001 and 2020.

It could be argued that there are also non-pharmacological treatment options for dementia, but even these are not available in many African countries. The goal for the future is to raise awareness of these problems among policy makers so that they can be addressed.

REFERENCES

1. United Nations Organization. *World Population Prospects: the 2000 Revision*. New York: United Nations, 2001.
2. Ben-Aire O, Swartz L, Dickman BJ. Depression in elderly living in the community. Its presentation and features. *Br J Psychiatry* 1987; **150**: 169–74.
3. Uwakwe R. The pattern of psychiatric disorders among the aged in a selected community in Nigeria. *Int J Geriatr Psychiatry* 2000; **15**: 355–62.
4. Mogga S, Prince M, Alem A et al. Outcome of major depression in Ethiopia population based study. *Br J Psychiatry* 2006; **189**: 241–46.
5. Gureje O, Kola L, Afolabi E. Epidemiology of major depressive disorders in elderly Nigerians in the Ibadan Study of Ageing. A community based sample. *Lancet* 2007; **370**: 957–64.
6. Baiyewu O, Smith-Gamble V, Lane KA et al. Prevalence estimates of depression in elderly community-dwelling African American in Indianapolis and Yoruba in Ibadan, Nigeria. *Int Psychogeriatrics* 2007; **19**: 679–89.
7. Sokoya OO, Baiyewu O. Geriatric depression in Nigerian primary care attendees. *Int J Geriatr Psychiatry* 2003; **18**: 506–10.
8. Uwakwe R. Psychiatric morbidity in elderly patients admitted to non-psychiatric wards in a general/teaching hospital in Nigeria. *Int J Geriatr Psychiatry* 2000; **15**: 346–54.
9. Nakasujja N, Musisi S, Walugembe J, Wallace D. Psychiatric disorders among the elderly in non-psychiatric wards in an African setting. *Int Psychogeriatrics* 2007; **19**: 691–704.
10. Hendrie HC, Osuntokun BO, Hall KS et al. Prevalence of Alzheimer's Disease and dementia in two communities: Nigerian Africans and African Americans. *Am J Psychiatry* 1996; **152**: 1485–92.
11. Hendrie HC, Ogunniyi AO, Hall KS et al. The incidence of dementia in two communities, Yoruba residing in Ibadan, Nigeria, and African Americans in Indianapolis, USA. *JAMA* 2001; **285**: 739–47.
12. Folstein MF, Folstein SE, McHugh PR. 'Mini-Mental State': a practical method for grading the cognitive state of patients for the clinician. *J Psychiatr Res* 1975; **12**: 189–98.
13. Hall KS, Gao S, Emsley CL, Ogunniyi AO, Morgan O, Hendrie HC. Community screening interview for dementia(CSI-'D') performance in five disparate study sites. *Int J Geriatr Psychiatry* 2000; **15**: 521–31.
14. Baiyewu O, Unverzagt. FW, Lane KA et al. Stick design test: a new measure of visuoconstructional ability. *J Int Neuropsychol Soc* 2005; **11**: 598–605.
15. Osuntokun BO, Sahota A, Ogunniyi AO et al. Lack of association between the e4 Allele of dimentia and Alzheimer disease in a community study of elderly Nigerians. *Ann Neurol* 1995; **38**: 463–65.
16. Gureje O, Ogunniyi A, Baiyewu O et al. APOE epsilon4 is not associated with Alzheimer's disease in elderly Nigerians. *Ann Neurol* 2006; **59**. 182–85.
17. Kalaria RN, Ogengo JA, Patel NB et al. Evaluation of risk factors for Alzheimer's disease in elderly east Africans. *Brain Res Bull* 1997; **44**: 573–77.
18. Farrag A, Farwiz HM, Khedr EH, Mahfouz RM, Omran SM. Prevalence of Alzheimer's disease and other dementing disorders: Assiut-Upper Egypt study. *Dement Geriatr Cogn Disord* 1998; **9**: 323–28.
19. Perkins AJ, Hui SL, Ogunniyi A et al. Risk of mortality for dementia in a developing country: the Yoruba in Nigeria. *Int J Geriatr Psychiatry* 2002; **17**: 566–73.
20. Baiyewu O, Smith-Gamble V, Akinbiyi A et al. Behavioral and caregiver reaction of dementia as measured by NPI in Nigerian community residents. *Int Psychogeriatr* 2003; **15**: 399–409.
21. Baiyewu O, Adeyemi JD, Ogunniyi AO. Psychiatric disorders in Nigerian nursing home residents. *Int J Geriatr Psychiatry* 1997; **12**: 1146–50.
22. Rodriguez JJL, Ferri CP, Acosta D et al. prevalence of dementia in Latin America, India and China: a population based cross-sectional survey. *Lancet* 2008; **372**: 464–74.

23. Deeg A, Baiyewu O, Gao S *et al.* A comparison of cardiovascular disease risk factor biomakers in African Americans and Yoruba Nigerians. *Ethnicity Dis* **2008**; 18: 427–33.

24. Petersen RC. Conceptual overview. In Petersen RC (ed.), *Mild Cognitive Impairment: Aging to Alzheimer's Disease*. New York, Oxford University Press, 2007.

25. Graham JE, Rockwood K, Beattie BL *et al.* Prevalence and severity of.cognitive impairement with and without dementia in an elderly population. *Lancet* 1997; **349**: 1793–96.

26. Baiyewu O, Unverzagt FW, Ogunniyi AO *et al.* Cognitive impairment in community-dwelling older Nigerians: clinical correlates and stability of diagnosis. *Eur J Neurol* 2002; **9**: 573–80.

27. Rockwood K, Mitzer J, Truyen L, Wessel T, Wilkinson D. Effect of a flexible galantamine dose in Alzheimer's disease: a randomised controlled trial. *J Neurol Neurosurgery Psychiatry* 2001; **71**: 589–95.

28. Ferri CP, Prince M, Brayne C *et al.* Global prevalence of dementia:a Delphi consensus study. *Lancet* 2005; **360**: 2112–17.

117

Dementia and Depression in China

Helen Chiu and Cindy Tam

The Chinese University of Hong Kong, Shantin, Hong Kong

According to data from the World Health Organization, 11% of China's 1.3 billion people were above the age of 60 in 2006. Life expectancy in China was 72 years for males and 75 years for females in 2006. The percentage of citizens over the age of 65 is projected to triple by 2050, from 8% of the population in 2006 to 24% in 2050, for a total of 322 million. China has 32 provinces and 2 special administrative regions (Hong Kong and Macau) and 56 ethnic groups. It has diverse geographic characteristics and demographic features, including dialects, customs and diet, which vary widely across the country.

DEMENTIA IN CHINA

Prevalence of Dementia

The number of people suffering from dementia in China was estimated to be 5 million in 2001, and it has been projected that there will be a more than 300% increase in this number by 2040[1].

Since 1980, a number of epidemiological surveys of dementia using standardized instruments and diagnostic criteria have been carried out. However, only a few of these studies have been published in international journals. Dementia prevalence estimates vary widely within China. This variation may be related to differences in population structure, genetics and lifestyle in the country's various regions, but it may also be due to different mortality rates of dementia and to methodological differences between studies. Chiu and Zhang reviewed 16 studies carried out between 1980 and 1999 and found the prevalence rates of dementia to range from 0.46% to 7.0%[2]. Dong *et al.* performed a meta-analysis of 25 Chinese studies that were conducted between 1980 and 2004 and comprised a total population of more than 76 000. They estimated that the overall prevalence of dementia in China was 2.8% in people aged 60 or above[3]. Alzheimer's disease and vascular dementia were found to be the most common types of dementia, with the prevalence rate of the former reported to be 1.6% and that of the latter to be 0.8%. Both reviews[2,3] found the rates of dementia, particularly that of Alzheimer's disease, to be lower than those reported in Western developed countries. In addition, Dong *et al.*[3] found that the prevalence of Alzheimer's disease increased significantly from 1980 to 2004, and reported that the gap in the prevalence of dementia between China and Western countries has been decreasing.

Several epidemiological surveys that examined the prevalence of dementia in different regions of China using larger samples were published in international journals between 2004 and 2008[4-8]. The initial screening for these surveys was usually performed using the Chinese version of the Mini-Mental State Examination, with diagnoses confirmed through neuropsychological assessment and clinical interviews. The results of some of these studies are presented in Table 117.1. A recent large-scale survey reported that the prevalence rates of Alzheimer's disease and vascular dementia were 3.5% and 1.1%, respectively. Greater prevalence of dementia was apparent in the northern regions compared with the south, but no difference was found between urban and rural Chinese residents[4,9]. The burden of Alzheimer's disease and vascular dementia was not distributed equally among all regions and sociodemographic groups. Significant north–south variation was observed for both Alzheimer's disease and vascular dementia, but was more pronounced for the latter than the former. In both crude and age-adjusted associations, the prevalence odds of vascular dementia were approximately double in northern areas relative to southern areas. He *et al.* reported that the northern cities of China have a threefold higher incidence of stroke compared to southern cities, a fact that may be associated with different exposures to such risk factors as hypertension, a diet high in salt, and heavy alcohol and cigarette consumption[10]. In addition to this north–south variation, Zhang *et al.* also observed an east–west difference in the prevalence of dementia. Western China is less developed than the east, and life expectancy is also lower in the former. Thus, the lower prevalence rate of dementia in the western part of China may reflect a higher case fatality rate following Alzheimer's disease onset in the younger age groups or fewer persons at risk of Alzheimer's disease surviving until the period of onset[9].

Incidence of Dementia

Studies on the incidence of dementia in China are scarce. Li *et al.* examined 1 090 elderly aged 60 or above in Beijing using the DSM-III criteria in a study that lasted from 1986 to 1989[11]. The annual incidence rate of dementia was 0.6%. A similar cohort study was conducted in the same urban district of Beijing from 1997 to 1999[6]. In this study, 1 593 elderly aged 60 or above were examined using the DSM-IV criteria. The annual incidence rate was 0.9%, which was

Principles and Practice of Geriatric Psychiatry, 3rd edn. Edited by Mohammed T. Abou-Saleh, Cornelius Katona and Anand Kumar
© 2011 John Wiley & Sons, Ltd

Table 117.1 Prevalence of dementia in China

Study	Location	Urban/rural	Sample size	Age	Prevalence (%)
Zhang et al.[4]	Beijing, Xi'an, Shanghai and Chengdu	Urban and rural	34 807 (aged ≥55)	≥65	3.5 (AD) 1.1 (VaD)
Zhou et al.[5]	Linxin	Rural	16 095	≥50	1.83 (AD)
Li et al.[6]	Beijing	Urban	1 593	≥60	2.5
Rodriguez et al.[7]	Xicheng, Beijing	Urban	1 160	≥65	DSM-IV dementia:
	Daxing	Rural	1 002		3.1 (urban) 2.0 (rural) 10/66 dementia: 8.0 (urban) 4.8 (rural)
Lam et al.[8]	Hong Kong	Urban	6 100	≥70	8.99 (mild dementia)

AD, Alzheimer's disease; VaD, vascular dementia.

significantly higher than that reported 10 years earlier. Zhang et al. examined 1 970 elderly aged 65 or above in Shanghai in 1987 and followed them up for five years[12]. They reported an annual dementia incidence rate of 1.15%. Qu et al. surveyed 2 197 elderly in Xi'an in 1998 and 2001[13]. The annual incidence rate of dementia was found to be 0.89% among the elderly aged 65 or above. Of particular interest is the common finding that the incidence rate of dementia was higher in the illiterate groups in these studies.

Treatment

Guidelines for the treatment of dementia have been published recently. These guidelines cover the pharmacological and non-pharmacological treatment of cognitive and neuropsychiatric symptoms in dementia. In a section on potential drug treatments, acetylcholinesterase inhibitors (AChEIs) and memantine are listed along with other drugs, such as antioxidants and vasodilators. In clinical practice, huperzine A is used much more often in the treatment of dementia in China than other AchEIs, such as donepezil or rivastigmine, as it is covered by the National Drug Catalogue (China) and is inexpensive. It is an alkaloid isolated from the Chinese herb *Huperzia serrata*, and it is a reversible inhibitor of acetylcholinesterase. Randomized controlled trials in China have reported huperzine A to have some success in improving general cognitive functioning for patients with Alzheimer's disease[14]. The other cholinesterase inhibitors and memantine are not consistently covered by the National Drug Catalogue.

The drugs used in the treatment of neuropsychiatric symptoms include AChEIs, antipsychotics, antidepressants, anxiolytics and mood stabilizing agents. The US Food and Drug Administration (FDA) warning of increased adverse cardiovascular events with the use of atypical antipsychotics in dementia is mentioned in the Chinese guidelines. Such non-pharmacological treatments as reminiscence therapy, validation therapy, reality orientation and behavioural modification are also recommended. These guidelines emphasize the comprehensive assessment of the needs of both patients and their caregivers, as well as a multidisciplinary management approach.

Although not mentioned in the national treatment guidelines for dementia, numerous Chinese medicinal formulations have long been used for the treatment of insomnia and memory deficits. Some of the herbs used in these formulations, such as *Ginkgo biloba* and the

root of *Salvia miltiorrhiza* have been reported to exhibit cholinergic activities relevant to the treatment of Alzheimer's disease. In addition to these herbal agents, acupuncture has also been used in the treatment of dementia in China.

Access to Treatment

Zhang et al. found that about half of patients with dementia are classified as normally ageing and that only one fifth have adequate access to diagnostic assessment[9]. A low degree of public awareness, under-diagnosis and under-treatment are common hurdles to dementia care in China, which is similar to the case in other developing countries.

In general, patients with dementia are managed by traditional Chinese practitioners or primary care doctors, but their training may be inadequate. Those in urban areas may be managed by neurologists or psychiatrists, but there is no well-established referral system to specialist care yet in place. In Hong Kong, in contrast, psychogeriatric and geriatric services are well established, and these services play the main role in the medical care of patients with dementia.

Care of Dementia in China

The family has traditionally played a central role in support for the elderly in China. 'Filial piety' is a strongly held cultural norm that assumes that the care of older people with dementia will be provided primarily by the family. In recent years, however, the breakdown of the extended family, urbanization and the movement of young people to other cities for work have led to the weakening of family support for dementia sufferers. At the same time, community support and residential care facilities remain very limited in China and are particularly scarce in rural areas. All of these factors influence the pattern of care for dementia sufferers and create challenges for dementia care. In Hong Kong, in contrast, non-governmental organizations play a substantial role in providing community facilities and residential care for the elderly with dementia.

An organization called Alzheimer's Disease China was established in 2001 and is a member of Alzheimer's Disease International. In Hong Kong, the Alzheimer's Disease Association was set up in 1995, and the Hong Kong Psychogeriatric Association was established in 1998. Among their objectives are the facilitation of training, public awareness and advocacy for dementia.

DEPRESSION IN CHINA

Prevalence of Depression

Depression is one of the most common psychiatric disorders in the elderly population. Very few studies on the prevalence of this mood disorder have been carried out among the elderly in China. In 1999, Chen et al. conducted a meta-analysis of 10 epidemiological studies of the prevalence of geriatric depression in 13 565 subjects in China[15]. The pooled prevalence of depression was 3.86%, whereas that of depressive mood was 14.81%. The results reported in published Chinese studies vary, which may be due to methodological issues, non-standardized assessments and/or different definitions of depression.

The prevalence rates of geriatric depression in five recent epidemiological studies of major depression published in international journals from 2000 to 2008 are presented in Table 117.2. These studies adopted standardized instruments, and generally found lower rates than those reported in Western countries. The results of the Chinese studies can be interpreted in a number of ways. They may indicate a genuine rarity of depression. Indeed, some factors may protect the Chinese from depression, including such coping mechanisms as quiescence and stoicism, family and cultural support systems, and a traditional cultural belief in fatalism[21]. The lower prevalence rates may also be due to a lower level of reportage of depressive symptoms or the existence of 'depressive-equivalent' conditions. For instance, neurasthenia is a more generic label applied to wide-ranging symptoms, including somatic symptoms (such as insomnia, fatigue and dizziness), cognitive symptoms (such as poor memory and unpleasant thoughts) and emotional symptoms (such as excitability and nervousness), in addition to any depressive symptoms. Chinese patients and psychiatrists seem to prefer such a label to the psychiatric label of 'depression'[22]. Even in the 1990s, neurasthenia remained a more common diagnosis in Chinese patients than in other populations.

The elderly in rural areas seem more likely to suffer from depression than city dwellers[15,20]. The relatively lower socioeconomic status of the rural elderly, as well as a poorer health care system and fewer social activities compared to their urban counterparts may increase the risk[20].

Treatment of Depression

Of the subjects with geriatric depression interviewed by Ma et al., 25.2% received some type of treatment, with only 4.7% seeking treatment from mental health professionals[20]. This low rate of help-seeking behaviour may be explained by the following: (i) many Chinese people do not believe that depression is a treatable psychiatric disorder; (ii) stigmatization and discrimination prevent psychiatric patients from using mental health services in China; and (iii) the country offers inadequate access to community-based psychiatric services.

Treatment guidelines for depression have recently been published. Various types of antidepressants, including tricyclic antidepressants (TCA), selective serotonin re-uptake inhibitors (SSRI) and serotonin norepinephrine re-uptake inhibitors (SNRI), are available. The guidelines recommend the use of the newer antidepressants for geriatric depression, SSRI in particular, because they have less pronounced side effects and are safer for people with cardiovascular diseases. Modified electroconvulsive therapy was introduced to China only in recent years, and it is now recommended for the treatment of severe or treatment-resistant depression. Psychotherapy is briefly mentioned in these guidelines, but is not widely practised for depression. It is noteworthy that cognitive behavioural therapy training has only begun in recent years. Although not mentioned in the guidelines, acupuncture and traditional Chinese medicine have long been used to treat insomnia associated with depression.

ELDERLY SUICIDE IN CHINA

The suicide rate among the elderly is higher than that among the general population in China, which is similar to the pattern in many countries. What is unique in China is the fivefold difference between the urban and rural rates for suicide among the elderly[23]. The rates of suicide among elderly rural residents of China, particularly for women, are among the highest reported in any country. Between 1995 and 1999, the suicide rates of elderly rural and urban residents aged 60–84 were 82.8 and 16.7 per 100 000, respectively[23]. Wei et al.[24] studied 304 elderly suicides using psychological autopsy and found that 64.8% suffered from mental illness and 40.5% from depression. The most common method of suicide for this population is pesticide ingestion, followed by hanging[24]. Insecticides are readily available in rural areas, and emergency medical care in these areas is relatively limited. Moreover, the elderly in rural areas have limited access to health care in general and are offered little social and financial assistance. These factors may contribute to the higher suicide rates of the rural elderly compared with their urban counterparts. However, it is interesting to note that the prevalence of depression in older Chinese

Table 117.2 Prevalence of geriatric depression in China

Study	Location	Sample/age	Diagnosis/instrument	Prevalence (%)
Chen et al.[16]	Hefei (urban)	1 736 age ≥65	GMS-AGECAT	2.2 (point prevalence)
Chen et al.[17]	Yingshang (rural)	1 600 age ≥60	GMS-AGECAT	6.0 (point prevalence)
Lee et al.[18]	Beijing and Shanghai (urban)	547 age ≥65	DSM-IV/CIDI	2.6 (lifetime prevalence of major depressive disorder)
Lu et al.[19]	Kunming (urban and rural)	(5 033 age ≥15 in the survey)	DSM-IV/CIDI	3.63 for those aged ≥65 (lifetime prevalence of major depressive disorder)
				2.09 (12-month prevalence)
Ma et al. (2008)[20]	Beijing (urban and rural)	1 601 age ≥60	DSM-IV/CIDI	7.83 (lifetime prevalence of major depressive disorder)
				4.33 (12-month prevalence)
				8.42 (12-month prevalence in rural sample)
				2.55 (12-month prevalence in urban sample)

residents of rural areas remains low, although the suicide rate is high. The exact reason for this discrepancy remains unclear.

In the special administrative region of Hong Kong, the suicide rate is also relatively high among the elderly, at 50 per 100 000/year for those aged 75 or above. Chiu et al. investigated suicide among elderly Chinese in Hong Kong using psychological autopsy[25]. They found that 86% of those who had committed suicide had a psychiatric problem prior to doing so and that 53% had suffered from major depression, which is consistent with findings reported in Western countries.

CONCLUSION

Both dementia and depression are important and prevalent disorders in the elderly population. Although the reported prevalence rates of both syndromes are lower than those in Western countries, an enormous number of people are affected, given the sheer size of the population. As China's population is ageing rapidly, the country will face exponentially increasing demand for care for those elderly who suffer from these disorders. Mental health services for the elderly in China remain in the early stage of development. More epidemiological studies and clinical research are needed to guide the future development of such services and care.

REFERENCES

1. Ferri CP, Prince M, Brayne C, Brodaty H et al. Global prevalence of dementia: a Delphi consensus study. *Lancet* 2005; **366**(9503): 2112–17.
2. Chiu, HFK, Zhang MY. Dementia research in China. *Int J Geriatr Psychiatry* 2000; **15**: 947–53.
3. Dong MJ, Peng B, Lin XT et al. The prevalence of dementia in the People's Republic of China: a systematic analysis of 1980–2004 studies. *Age Ageing* 2007; **36**: 619–24.
4. Zhang ZX, Zahner GE, Roman GC et al. Dementia subtypes in China: prevalence in Beijing, Xian, Shanghai and Chengdu. *Arch Neurol* 2005; **62**: 447–53.
5. Zhou DF, Wu CS, Qi H et al. Prevalence of dementia in rural China: impact of age, gender and education. *Acta Neurol Scand* 2006; **114**: 273–80.
6. Li S, Yan F, Li G et al. Is the dementia rate increasing in Beijing? Prevalence and incidence of dementia 10 years later in an urban elderly population. *Acta Psychiatr Scand* 2007; **115**: 73–9.
7. Rodriguez JJL, Ferri CP, Acosta D et al. The prevalence of dementia in Latin America, India and China. A 10/66 Dementia Research Group population-based survey. *Lancet* 2008; **372**: 464–74.
8. Lam LCW, Tam CWC, Lui VWC et al. Prevalence of very mild and mild dementia in community dwelling Chinese older persons in Hong Kong. *Int Psychogeriatrics* 2008; **20**(1): 135–48.

9. Zhang ZX, Zahner GE, Roman GC et al. Socio-demographic variation of dementia subtypes in China: methodology and results of a prevalence study in Beijing, Chengdu, Shanghai and Xian. *Neuroepidemiology* 2006; **27**: 177–87.
10. He J, Klag MJ, Wu Z et al. Stroke in the People's Republic of China. II. Meta-analysis of hypertension and risk of stroke. *Stroke* 1995; **26**: 2228–32.
11. Li G, Shen YC, Chen CH et al. A three-year follow-up study of age related dementia in an urban area of Beijing. *Acta Psychiatr Scand* 1991; **83**: 99–104.
12. Zhang M, Katzman R, Yu E et al. A preliminary analysis of incidence of dementia in Shanghai, China. *Psychiatry Clin Neurosci* 1998; **52**(suppl): S291–4.
13. Qu QM, Qiao J, Han JF et al. The incidence of dementia among elderly people in Xi'an, China. *Zhonghua Liu Xing Bing Xue Za Zhi* 2005; **26**(7): 529–32.
14. Li J, Wu HM, Zhou RL et al. Huperzine A for Alzheimer's disease. *Cochrane Database Syst Rev* 2008; **2**: CD005592.
15. Chen R, Copeland JRM, Wei L. A meta-analysis of epidemiological studies in depression of older people in the People's Republic of China. *Int J Geriatr Psychiatry* 1999; **14**: 821–30.
16. Chen R, Hu Z, Qin X et al. A community-based study of depression in older people in Hefei, China: the GMS-AGECAT prevalence, case validation and socio-economic correlates. *Int J Geriatr Psychiatry* 2004; **19**: 407–13.
17. Chen, R, Wei L, Hu A et al. Depression in older people in rural China. *Arch Intern Med* 2005; **165**: 2019–25.
18. Lee S, Tsang A, Huang YQ et al. The epidemiology of depression in metropolitan China. *Psychol Med* 2009; **39**: 735–47.
19. Lu J, Ruan Ye, Huang Y et al. Major depression in Kunming: prevalence, correlates and co-morbidity in a south-western city of China. *J Affect Disord* 2008; **111**: 221–6.
20. Ma X, Xiang YT, Li SR et al. Prevalence and sociodemographic correlates of depression in an elderly population living with family members in Beijing, China. *Psychol Med* 2008; **38**: 1723–30.
21. Parker G, Gladstone G, Chee KT. Depression in the planet's largest ethnic group: the Chinese. *Am J Psychiatry* 2001; **158**: 857–64.
22. Lee S, Kleinman A. Are somatoform disorders changing with time? The case of neurasthenia in China. *Psychosom Med* 2007; **69**: 846–9.
23. Phillips MR, Li X, Zhang Y. Suicide rates in China, 1995–99. *Lancet* 2002; **359**: 835–40.
24. Wei LW, Xue TW, Phillips MR et al. [Psychological autopsy of Chinese elderly and adolescent suicides]. *J Clin Psychol Med* 2005; **15**(5): 305–306 (in Chinese).
25. Chiu HFK, Yip PSF, Chi I et al. Elderly suicide in Hong Kong – a case-controlled psychological autopsy study. *Acta Psychiatr Scand* 2004; **109**: 209–305.

118

Spirituality and Mental Illness in Old Age

Susan Mary Benbow[1] and David Jolley[2]

[1]Centre for Ageing and Mental Health, Staffordshire University, Stafford, UK
[2]Personal Social Services Research Unit, Manchester University, Manchester, UK

CONTEXT: SPIRITUALITY, FAITH AND RELIGION

Spirituality is an important concept and often regarded as intrinsic to mental health: the Health Education Authority includes it within its definition of mental health· 'the emotional and spiritual resilience which enables us to enjoy life and to survive pain, disappointment and sadness. It is a positive sense of well-being and an underlying belief in our own, and others', dignity and worth'[1].

Nevertheless spirituality is difficult to pin down, and its differentiation from (and relation to) religious faith is a matter of debate. The Church of England Archbishops' Council with the National Institute for Mental Health in England (NIMHE)[2] has defined it as: 'A quality that goes beyond religious affiliation: that strives for inspiration, reverence, awe, meaning and purpose, even in those who do not believe in God'. Thus spirituality can be independent of religious faith, or, as Paul Wilson[3] writes, 'Spirituality is the searching for the meaning of life. Religion is one way of conducting the search'. Much of the literature relates health to religious belief and practice rather than spirituality as such and only now are we beginning to tease out how spirituality and faith interact.

As a concept, spirituality is sometimes criticized as free-floating and nebulous, although it has gained acceptability and respectability in Western societies, where adherence to faith or religion is sometimes regarded with suspicion, or as primitive, old-fashioned or outdated. On a global level there is massive commitment to religious faiths[4,5]. Numbers of adherents to Islam continue to grow, and though there has been a decline in active belief and church going within the nominally Christian countries of the West, the number of Christians worldwide is sustained or growing[6]. Population movements mean that most countries are now home to communities of many faiths. Thus an understanding of the research evidence concerning the relationships between spirituality, religion and health is essential for health care practitioners. In addition, it is important to be aware of the influence of spiritual and religious beliefs on the perception and interpretation of symptoms by patients and their families. Beliefs will also modify views on the acceptability or appropriateness of interventions intended to be therapeutic.

Health is often divided into six dimensions: physical, mental, emotional, social, environmental and spiritual[7]. The first five are accepted routinely as significant in the understanding, aetiology and management of health/illness. Spirituality is the dimension that has been neglected in Western professional health care theory, research and practice during the twentieth century, with health care staff taking little account of patients' perspectives regarding their experience of health/illness. Recent years have seen a return to interest in alternative views of life and a corresponding increase in study and research in this area. At a basic biological level, George et al.[8] demonstrated an association between spiritual beliefs and enhanced immunity, while, within the realms of clinical psychiatry and behaviour, Strawbridge et al.[9] found that strong spiritual beliefs were associated with a reduced risk of suicide. The Royal College of Psychiatrists has established a Special Interest Group on spirituality[10]. The evidence is such that the National Institute for Health and Clinical Excellence's (NICE) guidance on the supportive and palliative care of adults with cancer[11] recommends provision of spiritual support services, and the NIMHE Guiding Statement on Recovery[12] includes consideration of spirituality as intrinsic to holistic treatment.

Why should strong spiritual beliefs be associated with better health outcomes? Could it simply relate to the social support provided by membership of a faith community? Is it possible that interest in spirituality/membership of a faith community is independently linked with better health? Or are there specific aspects of a faith (such as prayer or worship) that carry additional advantages to health? Is it the case that, as Andrew Sims writes, 'one of the best kept secrets of modern epidemiological medicine is the effect that religious belief and practice have upon outcome from both physical and mental disorders'?[13]

Chronic illness (whether physical or mental) is likely to be an area where the relationship between spirituality and health assumes particular importance. How does spirituality impact on long-term illness and coping? What effect does long-term illness itself have on spirituality and faith? How does chronic illness affect membership of a faith community? What of the families and carers of those living with long-term physical and/or mental illness? As yet we cannot answer these questions, but there is evidence which hints at possible answers. The evidence divides into qualitative (often personal accounts of living with a chronic illness, e.g. Robert Davis's account of changes in his faith and understanding while living with Alzheimer's disease[14]) and quantitative. Researchers are exploring this area, measuring associations using instruments such as Hill and Hood's Measures of Religiosity[15], which records 126 different measures of religion, faith, belief and spirituality, and the Royal Free Interviews for Religious and Spiritual Beliefs[16,17].

Principles and Practice of Geriatric Psychiatry, 3rd edn. Edited by Mohammed T. Abou-Saleh, Cornelius Katona and Anand Kumar

DEMENTIA AND SPIRITUALITY

Katsuno[18] studied 23 people with mild dementia attending a day centre in the United States, using both qualitative and quantitative measures, and found a positive correlation between strength of spirituality and quality of life. Religion was reported to be important in the everyday lives of 19 of the group. One main theme, 'Faith in God', and six related categories were identified: beliefs, support from God, sense of meaning in life, private activities, public activities, and changes arising from dementia. Katsuno argues from her sample that it is an individual's intrinsic religiosity, rather than the social support they receive from a faith community, which influences their quality of life.

We used the Royal Free Interview for Religious and Spiritual Beliefs: self-report version[19] in a memory clinic population in the West Midlands[20] to start to explore the following issues:

- How are spirituality and faith affected by dementia?
- How are spirituality and faith affected by caring for someone with dementia?
- How do religious communities view dementia and respond to its presence within their membership?
- How is the experience of dementia modified for patient and carer by their spirituality and faith?
- Are there opportunities for strengthening spirituality and faith and/or improving life for patients and carers in this situation?

A group of people attending a memory clinic in the West Midlands and their carers completed the Royal Free questionnaire and in additional semi-structured interviews were carried out with patients, carers and local faith leaders. The patients were mainly women living with Alzheimer's disease and they described themselves predominantly as Christian. They scored a mean of 24 on the Mini-Mental State Examination[21]. Our main conclusions were as follows: patients with dementia are interested in, and able to talk about, issues of faith and spirituality; the spectrum of their beliefs is similar to that of their main carers; the strength of their beliefs is at least as strong as their carers; and satisfaction with life and carer stress (as measured by the General Health Questionnaire[22]) appear to be independent of strength of spiritual belief in this population. Both patients and carers ranked the personal components of spirituality most highly: for carers, coping came highest ('do you believe in a spiritual power which helps you cope with events which occur in your life?'), and for patients' strength of belief ('how strongly do you hold to your spiritual/religious view of life?'). Both patients and carers considered practices associated with their beliefs to be very important.

What of people with more advanced dementia? Some formulations argue that as dementia progresses and erodes the individual's abilities, memory traces and emotional repertoire, their spiritual identity is lost to a primitive chaotic biological base. Others say that if you know the person well, their spirit remains available for contact, and, indeed, that their spirituality becomes more evident and precious[23,24]. Meeting spiritual needs is certainly accepted as part of supportive and palliative care in dementia as in other terminal conditions[11] and is anticipated in residential care, which pre-dates death for many people[25,26]. Lawrence[27] argues that 'spiritual matters remain pervasively in the background' as dementia progresses and that staff need to employ non-verbal methods and devote time to connecting with the spiritual needs of people with dementia. Families and carers who have sustained intense involvement through this final stage will take time to adjust to the transition to life without their relative after the latter's death. Their experience of communication may continue and the mode, manner and completeness of resolution will be influenced by their established beliefs[28,29].

DEPRESSIVE DISORDERS, PSYCHOSIS AND SPIRITUALITY

It is widely accepted that spiritual beliefs and religious practices can have positive effects on health and well-being in general. Lawler-Row and Elliott[30] reported an investigation of the role of religious activity and spirituality in the health and well-being of older adults and found that people with higher levels of existential well-being had lower scores on depression. It is said that people with a spiritual or religious affiliation are up to 40% less likely to get depressed than people who do not have such affiliation; an increased commitment to religion has been linked with lower levels of depression in medically ill hospital patients; and religious/spiritual commitment is associated with lower levels of substance abuse[2]. Koenig[31] studied older medical inpatients with major and minor depression and found that they were less religiously involved then non-depressed patients and that greater severity of depression was associated with lower intrinsic religiosity, less involvement in reading scripture and prayer, and lower religious attendance.

Ceramidas[32] has described a qualitative study of depression and Christian faith in later life. Those participants who had what is described as a 'closer relationship with God' found comfort and strength in the practice of their faith but did not experience their churches as safe places to disclose their depression, fearing stigma and rejection.

Suicide has been regarded as a sin by most major religions, and attracted strong religious sanctions in the past, although views have moderated over recent years. Depression with suicidal ideation is therefore strongly influenced by spiritual/religious beliefs and different communities respond to it in different ways. This can be particularly challenging in large multi-ethnic multi-faith cities[33].

THE SPIRITUAL NEEDS OF SERVICE USERS

Kitwood and Bredin[34] introduced the term 'personhood' and defined it as 'a standing or status bestowed on one human being by others in the context of relationship and social being. It implies recognition, respect and trust.' They went on to describe the main psychological needs of a person with dementia as attachment, comfort, identity, occupation and inclusion. These ideas were developed in the context of Kitwood's work with people with dementia, particularly in institutional settings, but the concepts can be applied more widely. Kitwood came from a faith background, but later preferred a non-religious vision and interpretation of spiritual life which could be turned into operational therapeutic activities[35,36]. In this he was a leader from whom followers are gaining strength and guidance in sensitizing services to the deeper needs of patients and families. This has additional benefits for care professionals, but makes additional demands on them.

There are practical ways in which staff can support the spiritual needs of service users[37]. First, it is essential to take time to discover something about the personal beliefs and family culture that have informed the individual's life to this point. This may be achieved by a one-to-one interview, but may be more complete with the assistance of family and friends. Just to talk about things with a sympathetic, non-judgmental listener will be helpful. From this it may be possible to identify contacts, tracts, music or other resources that can be used for spiritual nourishment within a care setting. Alternatively, outside settings may be identified whose ambience brings meaning and sustenance. Faith, hope and compassion are contributory components of clinical care[38] and inevitably impact on the two-way relationship between service user and care provider. This means that carers who are open to the dimension of spirituality and faith in their work with patients require some sophistication in understanding the origins and limits of their own spirituality and how this may be used to strengthen and support their work. It is important to be aware that their own beliefs may be threatened (or be threatening) when exposed to new and different views and value sets. Thus there is need for support and supervision with reflection and growth from experiences gained. 'Do-it-yourself' is not a safe option for carers or those they care for. Addressing this issue is a task for every organization offering care to dependent and vulnerable people, and a complex matter that is rarely approached comprehensively.

Wallace[39] has described the development of guidelines to support staff working with people with dementia, and recently Gilbert[40] has produced guidelines on spirituality for staff in acute mental health services.

Post and colleagues[41] have addressed ethical aspects of attending to spiritual and religious aspects of a patient's experience. They consider the relationship between physician and patient, and the professional boundary between physician and chaplain, and note that patients' spiritual needs should be respected by those who aim to maximize therapeutic efficacy.

There are important ways in which faith communities can support people who have mental health problems[2]. For individuals who have active membership of an organization, this will include maintaining the continuity of established social contacts and allowing them opportunities for shared prayer, worship and rituals as well as pastoral care. Others, who have known a faith but fallen out of regular contact, may find the experience of illness acts as a trigger to reconsider their thoughts and beliefs. Still others may have had little or no contact with a faith community, but begin to wonder from their disability or distress, whether there is more to be learned. These are situations when hospital or health care chaplains can be helpful, but the first approach may come via a friend or family member to a local church or other faith centre. It is possible that what begins as a challenge from the threats that illnesses carry can become a source of unplanned enlightenment and positive growth. Faith communities are known to provide support and comfort in times of illness, loss and bereavement – but there is the possibility of much more[42].

THE SPIRITUAL NEEDS OF MENTAL HEALTH SERVICE STAFF

An area of potential difficulty is the possible dissonance between the spirituality and religious beliefs of service users and the staff who are supporting and treating them. The first step in dealing with this is to acknowledge it and then to provide information, education and support in reflective supervision so that unspoken fears and conflicts can be uncovered and examined.

Differences may be based, in part, on the generation gap between staff and the older people they are caring for. In all societies, older people are more taken up with spiritual/faith matters than younger people[43]. Older people have a role in maintaining traditions that were operative in their earlier years and will carry the culture of those times into the present. In addition, maturation takes place with accumulating years and the eventual approach of the end of life,

bringing increased interest in matters of the mind and spirit, and less preoccupation with the pleasures of flesh.

But there are other factors, for paid carers are quite often drawn from a race, religion, country of origin, social stratum and language that set them apart from those they are caring for[44]. Within a staff group, there may be wide variation of experience and belief. This may be spread unevenly between those providing hands-on care and those with management responsibilities, and there can be hazards associated with cliques and groupings.

Such differences are inescapable features of the fabric of care: awareness of their potential to impact adversely on the quality of care is essential and needs to be built into education, training and reflective practice. One useful tool in this work is Cecchin et al.'s concept of 'prejudice'[45]. Prejudice is conceived as meaning 'any pre-existing thought that contributes to one's view, perceptions of, and actions in a therapeutic encounter'. Encouragingly, they argue that, when identified and confronted, prejudices can be construed creatively and usefully: 'any meeting of prejudices can create change'.

This change requires that, rather than one party attempting to impose the 'correct' view on any other, there is openness and negotiation between professional carers and those they care for. However, this runs counter to the power paradigm deemed usual within the staff–patient relationship. Involvement with, and respect for, family, friends and faith leader of the older person in discussions and care planning adds to complexity but also to the potential richness of care and health outcomes.

PAST, PRESENT AND FUTURE

There is evidence that people living with a mental disorder, including dementia, have spiritual needs which must be addressed in order to promote well-being and quality of life, that religious practices provide coping resources for people, and that their personal spirituality offers a source of comfort and strength for individuals[46]. Newitt[47] argues that people without religious faith also benefit from approaches that address aspects of spirituality. This is a tricky area, for there is no easily accessible formula or accepted approach when seeking to engage spirituality outside the rites of a faith. The Royal Free studies have found that high spirituality outside a faith carries a poor prognosis for health outcomes (M. King, personal communication), which is an interesting insight, but considering how it might be dealt with in practice is challenging.

There is much to be learned, but we have made considerable progress in giving back respect to spiritual and faith dimensions of individuals, families and communities. Perhaps health and social care professionals will now recognize the need to join more closely with colleagues who have expertise in matters of the faith and spirituality of service users and their families in order to improve both health services and health for older people with mental health problems in the future.

REFERENCES

1. Health Education Authority. *Mental Health Promotion: A Quality Framework*. London: Health Education Authority, 1997.
2. Church of England: Archbishops' Council and National Institute for Mental Health in England. *Promoting Mental Health: A Resource for Spiritual and Pastoral Care*. London: Mentality, 2004. At www.cofe.anglican.org/info/socialpublic/homeaffairs/mentalhealth/parishresource.pdf, accessed 2 Jun 2009.

3. Wilson P. Remembering God: worship and Alzheimer's disease, MPhil thesis. Faculty of Arts, Department of Religion and Theology, University of Manchester, 1997.

4. *Atlas of World Religions*. Englewood Cliffs, NJ: Prentice Hall, 2005.

5. Ausloos M, Petroni F. Statistical dynamics of religions and adherents. *Europhys Lett* 2007; **77**: 38002. At http://arxiv.org/PS_cache/physics/pdf/0612/0612032v1.pdf, accessed 2 Jun 2009.

6. Brierley P. *Future Church: A Global Analysis of the Christian Community to the Year 2010*. London: Monarch, 1998.

7. Edlin G, Golanty E, McCormack Brown K. *Essentials of Health and Wellness*. Sudbury: Jones and Barlett, 1999.

8. George LK, Larson DB, Koenig HG. Spirituality and health: state of the evidence. *J Soc Clin Psychol* 2000; **19**: 102–16.

9. Strawbridge W, Shema S, Cohen R, Kaplan G. Religious attendance increases survival by improving and maintaining good health behaviours, mental health and well being. *Ann Behav Med* 2001; **23**: 68–74.

10. Dein S. Working with patients with religious beliefs. *Adv Psychiatr Treat* 2004; **10**: 287–93.

11. National Institute for Health and Clinical Excellence. *Supportive and Palliative Care. Improving Supportive and Palliative Care for Adults with Cancer*, 2004. At www.nice.org.uk/guidance/index.jsp?action=byID&o=10893, accessed 2 Jun 2009.

12. National Institute for Mental Health England. *NIMHE Guiding Statement on Recovery*, 2005. At www.psychminded.co.uk/news/news2005/feb05/nimherecovstatement.pdf, accessed 2 Jun 2009.

13. Sims A. Epidemiological medicine's best kept secret? Invited commentary on: Working with patients with religious beliefs. *Adv Psychiatr Treat* 2004; **10**(4): 294–5.

14. Davis R. *My Journey into Alzheimer's Disease*. Carol Stream, IL: Tyndale House, 1989.

15. Hill PC, Hood RW (eds). *Measures of Religiosity*. Birmingham, AL: Religious Education Press, 1999.

16. King M, Speck P. The Royal Free Interview for Religious and Spiritual Beliefs: development and standardization. *Psychol Med* 1995; **25**: 1125–34.

17. King M, Jones L, Barnes K *et al.* Measuring spiritual belief: development and standardisation of a Beliefs and Values Scale. *Psychol Med* 2006; **36**: 417–25.

18. Katsuno T. Personal spirituality of persons with early-stage dementia. *Dementia* 2003; **2**(3): 313–35.

19. King M, Speck P, Thomas A. The Royal Free Interview for Spiritual and Religious beliefs: development and validation of a self-report version. *Psychol Med* 2001; **31**: 1015–23.

20. Jolley D, Benbow SM, Grizzell M *et al.* Spirituality and dementia. *Dementia* in press.

21. Folstein M, Folstein S, McHugh P. Mini Mental State: a practical way of grading the cognitive state of patients for the clinician. *J Psychiatr Res* 1975; **12**: 189–98.

22. Goldberg D, Hillier V. A scaled version of the GHQ. *Psychol Med* 1979; **9**: 139–45.

23. MacKinlay E. *Spiritual Growth and Care in the Fourth Age of Life*. London: Jessica Kingsley, 2006.

24. Morris B. Declining moments, 2004. At www.poynton.com/barbara/PDFs/Stern_essay_for_web.pdf, accessed 2 Jun 2009.

25. Department of Health/Care Services Improvement Partnership. *Everybody's Business. Integrated Mental Health Services for Older Adults: A Service Development Guide*, 2005. At www.mentalhealthequalities.org.uk/our-work/later-life/everybodys-business.html, accessed 2 Jun 2009.

26. Keene J, Hope T, Fairburn C, Jacoby R. Death and dementia. *Int J Geriatr Psychiatry* 2001; **16**: 969–74.

27. Lawrence RM. Aspects of spirituality in dementia care: when clinicians tune in to silence. *Dementia* 2003; **2**: 393–402.

28. Shamy E. *A Guide to the Spiritual Dimension of Care for People with Alzheimer's Disease and Related Dementia*. London: Jessica Kingsley, 2003.

29. Goldsmith M. *In a Strange Land: People with Dementia and the Local Church*. Southwell: 4M, 2004.

30. Lawler-Row KA, Elliott J. The role of religious activity and spirituality in the health and well-being of older adults. *J Health Psychol* 2009; **14**: 43–52.

31. Koenig HG. Religion and depression in older medical inpatients. *Am J Geriatr Psychiatry* 2007; **15**: 282–91.

32. Ceramidas D. 'Who is God in the Pit of Ashes?': the interplay of faith and depression in later life. In MacKinlay E (ed.), *Ageing, Disability and Spirituality*. London: Jessica Kingsley, 2008, 163–81.

33. Tadros G, Jolley D. The stigma of suicide. *Br J Psychiatry* 2001; **179**: 178.

34. Kitwood T, Bredin K. Towards a theory of dementia care, personhood and well-being. *Ageing Soc* 1992; **12**: 269–87.

35. Kitwood T. *Dementia Reconsidered*. Maidenhead: Open University Press, 1997.

36. Downs M, Bowers B. *Excellence in Dementia Care: Principles and Practice*. Maidenhead: Open University Press, 2008.

37. Mental Health Foundation. *Making Space for Spirituality. How to Support Service Users*, 2007. At www.mentalhealth.org.uk/information/mental-health-a-z/spirituality/making-space-for-spirituality, accessed 2 Jun 2009.

38. Culliford L. Spirituality and clinical care. *Br Med J* 2002; **325**: 1434–5.

39. Wallace D. Spiritual care and the person with dementia: the development of guidelines to support staff working with people with dementia. *Dementia* 2003; **2**: 422–6.

40. Gilbert P. Guidelines on spirituality for staff in acute care services. At www.mentalhealthequalities.org.uk/silo/files/guidelines-on-spirituality-for-staff-in-acute-care-services-.pdf, accessed 2 Jun 2009.

41. Post SG, Puchalski CM, Larson DB. Physicians and patient spirituality: professional boundaries, competency, and ethics. *Ann Intern Med* 2008; **132**: 578–83.

42. Age Concern and the Mental Health Foundation. *Promoting Mental Health and Well-Being in Later Life. A First Report from the UK Inquiry into Mental Health and Well-Being in Later Life*, 2006. At www.ageconcern.org.uk/AgeConcern/report_mentalhealthandwellbeing.asp, accessed 2 Jun 2009.

43. McFadden SH. Religion and wellbeing in aging persons in an aging society. *J Soc Issues* 1995; **51**: 161–75.

44. Montoro-Rodriguez J. The role of conflict resolution styles on nursing staff morale, burnout and job satisfaction in long-term care. *J Aging Health* 2006; **18**(3): 385–406.

45. Cecchin G, Lane G, Ray WA. *The Cybernetics of Prejudices in the Practice of Psychotherapy*. London: Karnac, 1994.

46. Stuckey JC, Gwyther LP. Dementia, religion and spirituality. *Dementia* 2003; **2**: 291–6.

47. Newitt M. Personal view. Hospital chaplaincy services are not only for religious patients. *Br Med J* 2009; **338**: 893.

119

Development of Health and Social Services in the UK from the Twentieth Century Onwards

John P. Wattis

Centre for Health and Social Care Research, University of Huddersfield, Huddersfield, UK

IMPERIAL BEGINNINGS: THE POOR LAW AND THE ASYLUM

In Britain, the twentieth century dawned in a blaze of imperial glory. By the beginning of the twenty-first century, the world, including health and social services, had changed beyond recognition. In the year 1900, UK public health measures were rudimentary and confined largely to the establishment (in 1848) of sanitary authorities with medical officers of health to oversee sewers and water supplies. The poor law was still in force and poor law institutions were made deliberately unpleasant. This followed the principle of 'lesser eligibility', set out in 1834, which stated that those receiving poor law assistance should not be as 'eligible' (well provided for) as an 'independent labourer of the lowest class'[1]. For the poor sick this had been ameliorated, to some extent, by the setting up of poor law infirmaries in 1868, but there was still a vast gulf between these institutions and the voluntary hospitals, which were supported by rich philanthropists. Retirement pensions, even retirement itself, were things of the future and there was an association between poverty, ill health and old age which was recognized by an 1895 Royal Commission on the aged poor. Despite over 50 years of the National Health Service (NHS), the association between poverty, ill health and old age is maintained to this day.

Until the middle of the twentieth century, mentally ill people were still incarcerated in large county asylums. In 1808, partly as a response to the appalling conditions in some private 'madhouses', local magistrates had been given the power to set up asylums, and in 1845 this provision had been made mandatory. In recent years we have seen a return to the private sector for some aspects of health and social care provision for people with mental health problems.

From 1900 onwards, developments have been influenced by major world events, political philosophy, public opinion and the power of pressure groups. The Boer War, starting in 1899, revealed the poor physical fitness and ill health of many young men. Improvements in midwifery and child care were soon legislated for, with school meals starting in 1906 and the notification of live births, health visiting and the school medical service soon following. In 1908 the first national scheme for old age pensions was set up to try to alleviate poverty among old people. It was non-contributory and means tested. Initially, recipients also had to be 'of good character'!

The Royal Commission on the Poor Laws and the Relief of Distress in 1909 considered most of the issues of domiciliary and hospital medical care. A minority report condemned the poor law institutions as a public scandal, with the infirmaries understaffed and lacking skilled medical input[2]. Out of hospital, the poor law doctors had no contact with local authority public health services, the voluntary dispensaries were overcrowded and ineffective and the medical clubs, financed by workers' subscriptions, underpaid their doctors and did not cater for the chronic sick or dependants. The writers of this report dismissed the idea of a medical insurance system.

Yet, in 1911, the establishment of such a system marked an important development in the evolution of general practice in the UK. The medical profession fought for, and won, independence and capitation fees rather than a salaried service, and administration by insurance-based panels rather than local authorities[3]. Higher income groups, families and hospital care were excluded but the scheme was nevertheless a qualified success.

THE MINISTRY OF HEALTH: BETWEEN THE WARS

In 1918 the Ministry of Health for England and Wales was formed and the minister quickly appointed a consultative council, which in 1920 produced a report described by Pater[2] as 'nothing less than the outline of a national health service' (p. 7). Their scheme might well have avoided some of the split between general practitioners and hospital doctors that has been one of the problems of the NHS as it was eventually implemented.

Control of the workhouses passed to local authorities in 1930, the beginning of the end for the poor law. After a post-war cash crisis, the voluntary hospitals continued, becoming more specialized in acute care and leaving the chronic sick and infectious diseases to the local authorities. A number of reports pressed for a more coordinated hospital system and for universal health insurance. Knowledge was advancing. In 1935, Warren[4,5] began her work in developing geriatric medicine and, a few years later, pioneers began to write of the issues concerning old people with mental illness[6-8].

Before the Second World War, the Emergency Medical Service (EMS) was set up to cope with expected severe civilian casualties from the bombing of cities. On the declaration of war, 140 000

Principles and Practice of Geriatric Psychiatry, 3rd edn. Edited by Mohammed T. Abou-Saleh, Cornelius Katona and Anand Kumar

people, many of them elderly, were discharged from hospital over two days[9]. The EMS also coordinated the work of the voluntary and local authority hospitals, providing the framework for the future NHS Regional Hospital Boards. Physicians and surgeons from the elitist voluntary hospitals came face to face with the conditions of the former poor law institutions.

THE POST-WAR NATIONAL HEALTH SERVICE

The last of the series of British Medical Association (BMA) reports pressing for reform in 1942 coincided with the Beveridge report and was followed in 1944 by the NHS White Paper, enacted in 1946 and effective in 1948.

The National Health Service, as then set up, was tripartite. Primary care services – general practitioners, opticians, dentists and pharmacists – were answerable to local executive committees; maternity, child welfare, health visiting, health education, immunization and ambulances remained the responsibility of the local authority; and hospitals were administered by Regional Hospital Boards with teaching hospitals retaining boards of governors directly answerable to the Ministry of Health. One of the assumptions when the NHS was set up was that increasing health in the population would cause health expenditure to level off. It never did, and in 1956 the Guillebaud Committee, appointed to find ways of avoiding a rising charge upon the exchequer, concluded that there was no evidence of inefficiency or extravagance in the NHS. In fact, the committee was concerned about a lack of capital expenditure (a concern again of relevance more recently). In 1962, this problem was addressed in the Hospital Plan.

Meanwhile, in the mental health field, the idea of community care was gaining ground. Tinker[10] attributed this to five factors. First, there was a general dissatisfaction with institutional care and a search for alternatives. Some of the experiments in the 'therapeutic community' work of the Second World War[11] had challenged the accepted authoritarian culture of the mental hospital. In addition, the advent of electroconvulsive therapy (ECT), antipsychotics and effective antidepressants facilitated the move away from custodial care to medical treatment at home or in ordinary hospitals. Next, there were beginning to be practical problems in running residential establishments, including staff recruitment. Then there was concern about the cost of institutional care and, finally, a recognition that mentally ill people were entitled to live in as normal a way as permitted by modern treatments. The 1959 Mental Health Act liberalized the treatment of mentally ill people and opened the way for a move away from the old psychiatric hospitals to the new concept of psychiatric units attached to the district general hospitals of the 1962 Hospital Plan.

The large institutions were, in any case, rocked by a series of scandals about the mistreatment of patients. This resulted in the establishment of the Hospital Advisory Service (later the Health Advisory Service), effectively an inspectorate to monitor standards and spread good practice.

In general practice, a financial allowance for practices in deprived areas combined with other factors to promote the rapid development of local health centres and group practices from the mid 1960s. Local authorities produced their own health and welfare plans but there was poor coordination with the hospital authorities and the general practitioners' executive committees. Within the local authorities, the Seebohm report (1968) was followed by the Social Services Act, which required the setting up of social services departments. The Department of Health and Social Security was created in 1968 by the amalgamation of the Ministries of Health and Social Security, a merger that lasted for some 20 years.

REFORMS

In 1974, for the first time since its inception, the NHS itself was reorganized. The chief elements of this reorganization were the separation out of health and social services functions (now in the process of being reversed in children's services at least!), the integration of all health functions under one management and the establishment of area health authorities, generally coterminous with local authorities, to facilitate joint planning. Community Health Councils were also created to represent the views of consumers. Unfortunately, the reformed service did not work well. There were too many layers of responsibility, and taking decisions seemed to be delayed while information and responsibility were passed up and down the tree. There was an increase in clerical and administrative staff without a corresponding increase in managerial efficiency. During this period, important government reports were produced, including *Better Services for the Mentally Ill*[12] and *A Happier Old Age*[13].

In 1982 the Area Health Authorities were abolished and new district health authorities combined the functions of the old areas and districts. In some areas, coterminosity with local government was lost. A new government was determined to cut public expenditure, and the rate of growth of the NHS slowed. Following the Griffiths report[14], a general management structure was established within the NHS, and Family Practitioner Committees became independent. Government payment for continuing care was channelled to the private sector, and social services and hospital provision for this group of patients/residents was either reduced or failed to keep pace with demographic changes[15].

Psychiatric services were coping with the implementation of the 1983 Mental Health Act (MHA), which set up time-consuming quasi-judicial procedures for reviewing patients who were detained in hospital under compulsory orders. The new Act also set up a Mental Health Act Commission to review treatment of detained patients and to advise on certain types of treatment. This Act was revised in 2007 to incorporate a number of changes, including broadening the categories of those who could apply for admission under the MHA and of those who could be responsible for their care under the Act. Generally, in combination with the Mental Capacity Act, the new legislation has improved patients' rights under law, but at the expense of increasing bureaucracy.

MARKET FORCES AND COMPETITION: A RADICAL DEPARTURE?

Then came the most radical reform of the NHS attempted to that date, a reform not just of the service but of the basic philosophy of 'service' underlying it. Some suspected that it was the beginning of the end for the National Health Service. The political theory was that nationalized industries were subject to 'producer capture' and that the workers tended to run the service in their own interest rather than that of the 'customers'. Competition and 'market forces' were seen as the remedy. The 1990 National Health Service and Community Care Act introduced the concept of an 'Internal Market'. The new health authorities became planners and purchasers of health care at 'arm's length' from the providers, which were initially directly managed units (DMUs), and became semi-independent Trusts. The health authorities were provided with a budget for the local population and placed contracts for care with Trusts or the private and voluntary sector in order to obtain the best 'value for money'. Quality was, at least in theory, specified in the contract, and monitored.

Competition and other features of business life were 'introduced' into the NHS, not least by setting up groups of 'fundholding' general practitioners, who were enabled to make their own contracts for secondary care. In fact, doctors, health care workers, general practices and hospitals have always competed on reputation, but money was the new incentive. Some of the changes were potentially positive, such as the setting up of Trust Boards to manage local services and an emphasis on sound financial regulation through corporate governance. Unfortunately, the bottom line was very clearly financial and in many cases clinical services were sacrificed to balance the books.

These proposals were pushed through in the teeth of strong opposition from staff and groups representing the consumer. Honigsbaum[16] analysed the situation in 1990 and concluded that if patient care suffered, then 'the nation may decide that the restraints imposed are not worth the savings they produce. Today, as in 1911 and 1948, it is the public interest that will predominate'. The medical profession were largely excluded from the plans for this reorganization. Klein concluded that, if a new political settlement were not reached between the government and the profession, it seemed unlikely that the NHS would survive long into the twenty-first century[17].

A NEW NHS?

In fact, perhaps partly because of public dissatisfaction with what was happening to the NHS, the government was not re-elected, and a radical reforming Labour government came to power. From here, developments in the constituent parts of the UK became more dissociated. This account mainly follows what happened in England, since to follow all the differences following devolution would require more space than is available. The engines of privatization and the internal market were (temporarily) reversed and new reforms introduced. In December 1997 a White Paper, *The New NHS: Modern, Dependable*[18] outlined a comprehensive new vision for the NHS. Two of the main planks of the new policy were the setting up of primary care groups (PCGs) to replace the fundholding/non-fundholding split, and the introduction of comprehensive quality controls to ensure high standards and equity in access across the country. PCGs were local groupings of general practices, involved in the commissioning of local community and secondary services. In a further reform, they became Primary Care Trusts (PCTs), providing community services and commissioning secondary services. More recently still, the concept was developed of 'Care Trusts' which could provide primary care and some secondary services, such as mental health services. The 'Quality Framework' involved a three-layer approach[19]. *Clear standards of service*, set by National Service Frameworks (NSFs), and a National Institute for Clinical Excellence (now National Institute for *Health* and Clinical Excellence, but still known by the acronym NICE), which evaluated new treatments in terms of cost–benefit as well as the safety and efficacy demanded for licensing. The NSF for Older People was published in 2001[20]. The first of eight standards was 'rooting out age discrimination'. The seventh concerned mental health and included NICE guidelines for antidementia drugs (since revised to restrict use to those with moderate Alzheimer's disease). The new NSF made it clear that standards in the Mental Health NSF already published applied to older people. Local delivery of services was to be made dependable by a combination of lifelong learning[21] linked to professional self-regulation and clinical governance. *Clinical governance*[22] placed obligations on chief executives of NHS Trusts to make arrangements to monitor and continuously improve the quality of health care their organizations provided. This was underpinned by the *national monitoring* of standards involving a National Performance Framework, an inspectorate (the Commission for Health Improvement, renamed the Healthcare Commission and renamed and reorganized again in April 2009 as the Care Quality Commission) and a National Patient and User Survey. This ambitious vision set a massive agenda for change and demanded radical shifts in the management and clinical cultures of the NHS[23]. These well-intentioned reforms have been accompanied by a plethora of central guidance, much of it driven by a philosophy of competition and performance management that does not sit well with the complicated needs of patients and the real motivators of human behaviour. The emphasis on control and performance management clashes with the self-determination model that is rightly increasingly popular when it comes to service users and medical education[24].

PCGs initially resulted in a much greater influence for general practitioners and other primary care workers in the commissioning of secondary services. In the move to PCTs, PCGs were merged and grew, effectively to replace the former District Health Authorities (DHAs). They now have a board structure with executive and non executive directors, analogous to the boards of existing secondary care Trusts. The strategic role of the former DHAs has been taken over by new Strategic Health Authorities (SHAs) covering areas even larger than the former Regional Health Authorities (RHAs). In England and Wales, 'standalone' Mental Health Trusts or Care Trusts have become the normal providers of mental health care. In smaller towns, a mixture of specialist Trusts covering wide geographical areas and of direct provision through PCTs remains. The provider Trusts have been encouraged to become 'Foundation' Trusts with yet another monitoring body (imaginatively called 'Monitor') overseeing the process. There was something of a scandal when a Trust preparing for Foundation status let its guard down on clinical quality and saw a significant increase in mortality rates. Shortly after Monitor cleared it to become a Foundation Trust, the Healthcare Commission was called in to investigate Mid Staffordshire NHS Foundation Trust and found serious failings. So far nobody at the Department of Health has publicly acknowledged that the pace of change and the New NHS structures might be causing damage.

The doctrine of 'commissioner–provider split', embodied in the new slogan 'World Class Commissioning', means that the mental health services as part of PCTs in England are unlikely to persist. For old age psychiatry, most current arrangements mean that the managerial separation between old age psychiatry and geriatric medicine continues. Unless imaginative and pragmatic solutions are found, this could result in many demarcation problems. However, a new culture of collaboration rather than competition could make all the difference (if not strangled at birth by political doctrine).

The *funding* of the NHS is probably even more important than its organization in determining the future of health care in the UK. It was the squeeze on NHS development in the 1980s that provoked the medical profession to campaign for more development money. In the light of international comparisons, both of spending on health care and the age structure of the population, this campaign seemed fully justified. Earlier reorganizations increased management costs and reduced the morale of many in the NHS. In the last 10 years there has been a marked increase in investment in the NHS. The controversial

Private Finance Initiative (PFI – rebadged as Public–Private Partnership, PPP) has continued to be a main strand of funding because it limits the Public Sector Borrowing Requirement. There is concern that PFI/PPP will result in a reduction in bed numbers and diversion of money away from services to support repayments to private providers in respect of capital developments; this is especially a risk if investment in the NHS slows down.

The government has recognized the need to train more doctors, nurses and other health care workers but, despite considerable investment, workforce planning is still problematic as demonstrated by the debacle in 2007/8 over the failed introduction of 'run through' training for doctors.

The direct reforms of the NHS were accompanied by a Royal Commission to review long-term care. The report of this Commission[25] controversially suggested that the personal care and residential elements of continuing care should be separately funded. It recommended that personal care should be paid for from general taxation, while living and housing expenses should continue to be means tested and subject to co-payment. The government did not make a positive response to this.

WHAT NEXT?

The 'Next Stage Review' of the NHS was commissioned in 2007 and published in 2008[26]. There are many recommendations and supporting documents available on the Department of Health website (www.dh.gov.uk). The review incorporates visions from each of the new Strategic Health Authorities and combines an emphasis on preventative medicine ('helping people lead healthy lives') and quality with a vision of partnership and local clinical leadership. Already there are signs that some of the good ideas are being slowly strangled by bureaucracy. If there is anything to learn from the last 10 years it is that too much ill-considered change produces a churning of management staff that reduces efficiency, and that too many central targets distort provision towards that which is politically fashionable or easy to measure (e.g. surgical waiting lists). At the same time, the pace of change and emphasis on 'top-down' performance management reduces the responsible autonomy we need to encourage for staff and service users alike. As this chapter goes to press a new UK government has just been elected which professes support for the NHS and a strong distaste for excessive bureaucracy and central control. We can expect more change.

REFERENCES

1. Brocklehurst JC. *Textbook of Geriatric Medicine and Gerontology*. Edinburgh: Churchill Livingstone, 1978, 747.
2. Pater JE. *The Making of the National Health Service*. London: King Edward's Hospital Fund for London, 1981, 2–4, 7.
3. Ham C. *Health Policy in Britain*, 6th edn. London: Palgrave Macmillan, 2009, 10–11.
4. Warren MW. A case for treating chronic sick in blocks in a general hospital. *Br Med J* 1943; **1**: 822–3.
5. Warren MW. Care of the chronic aged sick. *Lancet* 1946; **1**: 841–3.
6. Post F. Some problems arising from a study of mental patients over the age of 60 years. *J Ment Sci* 1944; **90**: 554–65.
7. Lewis A. Ageing and senility: a major problem of psychiatry. *J Ment Sci* 1946; **92**: 150–70.
8. Affleck J. Psychiatric disorders among the chronic sick in hospital. *J Ment Sci* 1948; **94**: 33–5.
9. Means R, Smith R. *The Development of Welfare Services for Elderly People*. London: Croom Helm, 1985, 25.
10. Tinker A *The Elderly in Modern Society*. London: Longman, 1984, 37–8.
11. Martin DV. *Adventure in Psychiatry*, London: Cassirer, 1974.
12. Department of Health and Social Security. *Better Services for the Mentally Ill*. London: HMSO, 1975.
13. Department of Health and Social Security. *A Happier Old Age*. London: HMSO, 1978.
14. Department of Health and Social Security. *NHS Management Inquiry* ("The Griffiths Report"). London: HMSO, 1983.
15. Grundy E, Arie T. The falling rate of provision of residential care for the elderly. *Br Med J* 1982; **284**: 799–802.
16. Honigsbaum F. The evolution of the NHS. *Br Med J* 1990; **301**: 694–9.
17. Klein R. The state and the profession: the politics of the double bed. *Br Med J* 1990; **301**: 700–2.
18. Department of Health. *The New NHS: Modern, Dependable*. Cm3807. London: The Stationery Office, 1997.
19. Department of Health. *A First Class Service: Quality in the New NHS*. London: Department of Health, 1998.
20. Department of Health. *National Service Framework for Older People*. London: Department of Health, 2001.
21. Wattis J, McGinnis P. Clinical governance and continuing professional development. *Adv Psychiat Treat* 1999; **5**: 233–9.
22. Department of Health. *Clinical Governance: Quality in the New NHS*. London: Department of Health, 1999, 1–25.
23. Wattis J, McGinnis P. Clinical governance: making it work. *Clin Manage* 1999; **8**: 12–18.
24. Williams G, Deci E. The importance of supporting autonomy in medical education. *Ann Intern Med* 1998; **129**: 303–8.
25. The Royal Commission on Long-term Care. *With Respect to Old Age: A Report*. London: The Stationery Office, 1999.
26. Professor the Lord Darzi of Denham. *High Quality Care for All: The NHS Next Stage Review Final Report*. London: Department of Health, 2009. Available at www.dh.gov.uk.

120

The Pattern of Psychogeriatric Services

John P. Wattis

Centre for Health and Social Care Research, University of Huddersfield, Huddersfield, UK

HISTORICAL BACKGROUND

The roots of the National Health Service (NHS) and the development of psychogeriatric services in the UK are discussed in Chapter 119. The evolution of psychogeriatric services has been guided by professional knowledge and opinion, by the politics of the health and social services, by financial constraints and, occasionally, by public opinion. From the inception of the NHS, which effectively antedated the beginning of provision of specialist psychogeriatric services, until the 1990s there was a consensus about how developments in services should occur in response to changing demography and epidemiology as well as advances in medical knowledge. This consensus was shattered in the UK by the imposition of the ideology of 'market forces'. Much long-stay hospital accommodation was effectively 'privatized' by decisions to support patients in private nursing and residential homes from state funds and to close down as many long-stay NHS beds as possible. The ideology of market forces was also applied to local authority provision of community care. Since April 1991, psychiatric patients with social needs have been subject to a 'care-planning procedure' in which all parties, including social services, have to agree. In April 1993 the full implementation of the Community Care Act made local social services departments responsible for purchasing continuing nursing and residential home care, largely from the private sector and with a limited budget.

In the late 1990s, a government came to power that did not appear to share the vision of market forces as the best way to regulate the NHS. However, the internal market has crept back in England under the guise of 'world class commissioning' and 'contestability', and the NHS remains a 'political football'. Political devolution of health care arrangements has also resulted in different patterns of service development in England, Wales, Scotland and Northern Ireland. One can no longer write about 'UK' psychiatric services as a whole and this text mostly follows the situation in England. The professional consensus about how services should develop has been replaced by a centralized pattern of decision making and the important decisions, made at the inception of the specialty of old age psychiatry in the UK, about providing a comprehensive service for all severe mental illness in old age, whether organic or functional, have been disregarded in some areas.

THEORETICAL BASIS FOR PSYCHOGERIATRIC SERVICES

The pioneers of specialist psychiatric services for old people were motivated by the increasing need for psychiatric services for the age group, consequent upon increased life expectancy, the growing knowledge base about psychiatric disorders among old people, and the success of geriatric medicine. The special needs of older people were not always recognized by the generic services. Diagnostic problems included the differential diagnosis of dementia, the association of apparent cognitive impairment with some cases of depressive illness, and the non-specific presentation of disease in old people. The multiple pathology suffered by old people led to a need for new patterns of multidisciplinary working and for close liaison with physicians in geriatric medicine and social services[1-3]. As in the early days of geriatric medicine, assessment and treatment in the community were emphasized not only because of 'blocked beds' but also because a more realistic picture of the patient's health problems usually emerged. More recently, advances in psychosocial care[4], interest in the spiritual needs of old people[5] and the advent of new classes of antidepressant, antipsychotic and antidementia drugs (discussed elsewhere in this volume) have all had their impact on the organization and delivery of psychiatric services.

CARE OR TREATMENT: PRIMARY OR SECONDARY?

One of the key theoretical issues for the future development of community services is likely to be the distinction between care and treatment. 'Care' is a word with many connotations. Some are positive but, in the medical world at least, some are negative. For example, 'care' is seen as what is provided when there is no possibility of effective treatment, as in the 'prescription' of 'tender loving care' for the terminally ill person. 'Care' tends to be relegated to untrained (although not necessarily unskilled) workers employed by social care agencies and commissioned by social services departments, whereas 'treatment' is the province of highly trained personnel employed by the Health Service. The move to 'Care in the Community' has served to reclassify older mentally ill people, especially those with dementia, as not needing medical treatment. Thus long-term care of people

---

Principles and Practice of Geriatric Psychiatry, 3rd edn. Edited by Mohammed T. Abou-Saleh, Cornelius Katona and Anand Kumar

with severe dementia, once shared by psychogeriatric and geriatric services within the NHS, is now provided in private institutions and is 'means tested', reducing the burden on the state but increasing the burden on afflicted families.

This situation is further complicated by the tendency of some health planners to equate primary care with *low cost and community care*, and secondary care with *high cost and hospital care*. Old age psychiatry services straddle the hospital–community divide and provide essentially secondary services, largely in a community setting. The new term, 'intermediate care', describes well some of these community services, but some who use the term believe that community psychiatric nursing services should be part of 'primary care', when in old age they work most effectively as part of secondary community care. Certainly, with the increasing prevalence of dementia, it is essential that primary care services and general hospital services become more proficient in recognizing and managing these conditions appropriately.

KEY COMPONENTS OF PSYCHOGERIATRIC SERVICES

Catchment Area and Comprehensiveness

Until recently, virtually all psychogeriatric services in the UK worked to a defined geographical catchment area, and the vast majority aimed to provide a comprehensive psychiatric service to all people over the age of 65 years[6,7]. Many services are now also trying to provide for people with early-onset dementia, although often without any dedicated resources[7]. In some areas, managers are seeking to save money by closing specialist wards for old people with functional mental illness and diverting those who need inpatient care onto wards designed for working age adults. Some old age psychiatrists feel they are being pushed towards developing 'dementia only' services.

The Multidisciplinary Team

For some this is an outmoded concept, for others an ideal that cannot be obtained, but for many psychogeriatricians it is an essential context for all their endeavours. Most multidisciplinary teams for the elderly incorporate *community nurses*, a *social worker*, one or more *occupational therapists*, a *physiotherapist* and often a *psychologist*. Various patterns of working have evolved and been described but they have in common an attempt to involve all disciplines in formulating treatment plans for the patient. In parts of England, there continue to be problems in fully integrating social workers and psychologists into such teams.

Home Assessment

This lies at the heart of most psychogeriatric services. Until the last few years, around two-thirds of referrals were seen at home by a doctor, one-fifth by other members of the team and one-tenth in outpatient clinics[6,7]. Just over 1 in 10 were seen as liaison referrals, although in some services this rose to a quarter or even one-third, perhaps partly depending on the admission policies of local geriatric services. Less than 1 in 20 were admitted direct without prior assessment. Patterns described as 'New Ways of Working' have now spread from working age adult psychiatry to old age. Generally this involves new referrals being assessed at home by various members of the team, and the senior medical staff tend to see people in the outpatient department after a preliminary assessment by another member of

the team (often a community psychiatric nurse). This has reduced the burden of new assessments falling on psychiatrists, and the impact on the quality of initial assessments has yet to be evaluated.

Community Treatment

Historically, the rate of acute admissions was only one-third of the rate of referrals, reflecting the fact that most home assessments do not result in admission but in treatment in the community. Home visits by community nurses are probably the commonest form of treatment in the community, although home visits by doctors and other members of the multidisciplinary team also play an important part. The rate of acute admission is probably reducing further as acute inpatient beds are closed.

Day Hospitals

In 1985, there were about 1.2 day hospital places per 1000 elderly people, and this had not changed significantly by the mid 1990s. Some services and Health Regions had relatively more and others less. The use of day hospitals varied from area to area, depending on the resource availability locally. The old government guidelines overestimated the need for dementia places. In many but not all cases of dementia, the need is for *care* rather than *treatment* and so a proportion of this day provision can be provided by social services or voluntary agencies. Here, however, issues will have to be addressed as to what kind of care is of most benefit to older people with dementia and their relatives, neighbours and friends. Elderly people with functional illness often have problems with psychiatric or psychological management that demand the *treatment* resources of a true day hospital or the more recently developed home treatment services. In the last five years there has been strong central pressure to close day treatment facilities, in some cases replacing them with home treatment teams.

Acute Inpatient Beds

The national rate of provision in 1985 was around 1 per 1000 elderly served, and again did not vary much over the next 10 years. In recent years there appears to have been a further reduction in acute beds. The reducing numbers may be insufficient to cope with the increasing demands caused by demographic changes and the loss of long-stay beds. Ultimately this depends on the community services available, since there is potential for considerable 'marginal shift' between community and inpatient resources. One study showed that around a quarter of acute psychiatric beds for all age groups were occupied by elderly people with depressive illness, and in many areas anecdotal evidence suggests that a greater proportion of acute psychiatric beds is being used for functional illness, principally depression. As with day hospital places, it appears that the old guidelines may have overestimated the needs for dementia assessment beds and underestimated the needs for patients with depressive illness and other functional illnesses. Because of the high prevalence of physical illnesses in mentally ill old people, it is recommended that acute beds should be on or adjacent to a general hospital site. Some services are now beginning to differentiate the assessment and management of behavioural problems in demented people, which can be carried out in the community or in community-based units, from the management of patients with depression, who often have major associated physical illness or disability (and may need ECT) and are therefore better managed on an acute hospital site. The same may apply to atypical dementia patients requiring high levels of investigation or to patients with dementia and delirium. This last group may be best helped on geriatric medical wards.

Long-Stay Beds

The provision in 1985 was around 3.4 beds per 1000 elderly. Since then a large number of beds have been closed, with patients discharged to the private sector, where developments have been funded through the social security budget and means-tested contributions from patients and their families. In 1996 the number had reduced to around 1.1 beds per 1000 elderly. Since provision was largely (but not exclusively) for those with severe dementia, whose main need is for care rather than treatment, this development appears to demand a cautious welcome. Patients are generally being cared for in smaller units. However, there must be reservations. The smaller units are harder to inspect and they are not necessarily in the patients' communities of origin, since planning permission and housing costs enter into the commercial equation. They are subject to capricious changes in the market, including government refusal to pay the 'going rate'. They are not under specialist medical management and there is some evidence that this management may be one of the factors that reduces the rate of decline in demented elderly people (a factor which, if confirmed, might also have relevance in the day care setting). The switch to private care has been engineered for political reasons and its impact is yet to be fully assessed. Some psychogeriatric services have retained a proportion of their long-stay beds for rehabilitation and respite care. A survey of old age psychiatrists[8] showed the majority in favour of around 1.5 long-stay (including respite) beds per 1000 elderly in community NHS units, with national rather than local eligibility criteria. The use of such beds for respite care to support carers in the community is now well established, and there is a potential for developing community units as centres of excellence for dementia care and education, as well as bases for multidisciplinary community teams.

GUIDELINES

The first guidelines for provision of psychiatric services for old people came in a Department of Health circular in 1972[9]. The government White Paper, *Better Services for the Mentally Ill*[10], in 1975, suggested that services for old people should often be provided by a psychiatrist with 'a special interest', and incorporated guidelines for bed and day hospital provision for the 'elderly severely mentally infirm'. Subsequently, the Royal College of Psychiatrists produced guidelines intended to help College representatives reviewing job descriptions for new or replacement consultants. These were endorsed by the Health Advisory Service in its report, *The Rising Tide*[11], and by the joint Royal College of Physicians and Psychiatrists report, *Care of Elderly People with Mental Illness*[12]. The second joint report[13] adopted a more multidisciplinary approach and described the different types of mental illness in old age as well as appealing for equity and 'national reference frameworks', which corresponded closely to the concept of 'National Service Frameworks' introduced by the new government[14]. Since the turn of the century there has been a plethora of government guidance, especially on dementia, culminating in the National Dementia Strategy[15]. Unfortunately, despite their excellence in many respects, none come near to specifying resources

to be deployed even in the surrogate way of the old 'bed norms'. Further, many old age psychiatrists fear that the needs of older people with functional mental illness, especially depression, are being sidelined.

Reality and Guidelines

Although, in the UK, old age psychiatry has been recognized as a specialty by the Department of Health for many years, we are still awaiting the collection of routine statistics. Initial manpower statistics appeared to be grossly inaccurate. The most comprehensive data available are from the 1985 survey, updated by the 1996 survey, which unfortunately did not achieve such wide coverage. There are also now agreed international standards for old age psychiatry services[16], and an international survey has established that basic levels of service exist in 12 countries worldwide[17].

SPECIALIST SERVICES OR NOT?

In view of the documented rapid expansion of services over the years, this question may seem superfluous. However, it was possible, as a result of the 1985 survey, to compare services where psychogeriatricians worked half-time or more in the specialty, with those where the consultant commitment to the elderly was less than half-time[18]. Specialist services had generally higher staffing ratios (with the exception of non-consultant medical staff), a higher proportion of acute beds on general hospital sites and a greater proportion of long-stay beds within the area served. These last two could be regarded as surrogate indicators of quality of care. In addition, the specialist psychiatrists were more likely to look after all mental illness in old age (the pattern of service recommended by the Royal College Faculty for the Psychiatry of Old Age). They were also reported to be more likely to engage in teaching and to show an interest in research in the specialty.

CONCLUSION

Readers wishing to see a more comprehensive narrative of the early development of old age psychiatry in the UK are referred to a historical study hosted by the Glasgow University website: www.gla.ac.uk/media/media_107314_en.pdf. Psychogeriatrics has 'come of age' in the UK. Provision, although geographically patchy and relatively under-resourced, still provides one model for future developments. This model, fostered in the National Health Service with its principles of equality of access, payment from general taxation and central planning, survived the major changes of the 1990 'reforms'. However, centrally directed changes, under the regime of equity and quality proposed by the last UK government, appear to be sometimes having perverse effects and introducing greater (and perhaps inappropriate) variability. Old age psychiatrists need to show leadership in these times of rapid change, and governments need to furnish adequate resources and ensure national standards, both in terms of quality and quantity of provision.

REFERENCES

1. Arie T. Morale and planning of psychogeriatric services. *Br Med J* 1971; **3**: 166–70.
2. Arie T, Dunn T. A "do-it-yourself" psychiatric-geriatric joint patient unit. *Lancet* 1973; **2**: 1313–16.

3. Royal College of Psychiatrists, British Geriatric Society. Guidelines for collaboration between geriatric physicians and psychiatrists in the care of the elderly. *Bull R Coll Psychiat* 1979; **11**: 168–9.

4. Kitwood T. *Dementia Reconsidered: the Person Comes First*. Buckingham: Open University Press, 1997.

5. Koenig HG. *Aging and God*. Binghampton, NY: Howarth Pastoral, 1994.

6. Wattis JP. Geographical variations in the provision of psychiatric services for old people. *Age Ageing* 1988; **17**: 171–80.

7. Wattis J, Macdonald A, Newton P. Old age psychiatry: a specialty in transition – results of the 1996 survey. *Psychiat Bull* 1999; **23**: 331–5.

8. Wattis J, Macdonald A, Newton R. Old age psychiatrists' views on continuing inpatient care. *Psychiat Bull* 1998; **22**: 621–4.

9. Department of Health and Social Security. *Services for Mental Illness Related to Old Age*, HM(72)71. London: DHSS, 1972.

10. Department of Health and Social Security. *Better Services for the Mentally Ill*. London: DHSS, 1975.

11. National Health Service. *The Rising Tide: Developing Services for Mental Illness in Old Age*. Sutton, Surrey: NHS Health Advisory Service, 1982.

12. Royal College of Physicians of London, Royal College of Psychiatrists. *Care of Elderly People with Mental Illness: Specialist Services and Medical Training*. London: Royal College of Psychiatrists and Royal College of Physicians of London, 1989.

13. Royal College of Psychiatrists, Royal College of Physicians of London. *Care of Older People with Mental Illness*, Council Report CR69. London: Royal College of Psychiatrists and Royal College of Physicians of London, 1999.

14. Department of Health. *A First Class Service: Quality in the New NHS*. London: Department of Health, 1998.

15. Department of Health, *Living Well with Dementia: A National Dementia Strategy*. London: Department of Health, 2009.

16. World Health Organization, World Psychiatric Association. *Organization of Care in Psychiatry of the Elderly*. Geneva: WHO, 1997.

17. Reifler BV, Cohen W. Practice of geriatric psychiatry and mental health services for the elderly: results of an international survey. *Int Psychogeriatr* 1998; **10**: 351–7.

18. Wattis JP. A comparison of specialised and non-specialised psychiatric services for old people. *Int J Geriatr Psychiatry* 1989; **4**: 59–62.

121

The Multidisciplinary Team and Day Care Provision

Martin Orrell[1] and Kunle Ashaye[2]

[1]Department of Mental Health Sciences, University College London, London, UK
[2]Mental Health Unit, Lister Hospital, Stevenage, Hertfordshire, UK

THE MULTIDISCIPLINARY TEAM

The multidisciplinary team assessments and treatment of older people with mental health problems enables a holistic approach to care for and meet the complex health and social needs this group of patients may present with. The concept of the multidisciplinary team has been described as a group of members of different professions whose working skills, when combined for the needs of the patient, aim to exceed in quality the simple summation of their individual abilities[1]. In describing features of a successful multidisciplinary team, Rosenvinge included communication within the team; high quality leadership; maintaining audit activities to help maintain and improve service delivery and management; and maintenance of morale of team members[1]. Multidisciplinary team members may include psychiatrists, mental health nurses, occupational therapists, social workers, clinical psychologists, physiotherapists, speech and language therapists, pharmacists and support workers. Improving multidisciplinary assessments to promote health and social care of community-dwelling frail older people has become an important issue for policy makers throughout the developed world[2]. In England, the introduction of the Single Assessment Process was to help multidisciplinary team members target the complex needs of older people, and may help identify appropriate team members or specialists to help meet those needs; however, in many areas it has not been effectively implemented[3]. It has, however, led to an increase in multidisciplinary assessments[2]. Multidisciplinary teams are found in various settings in mental health services for older people, such as community mental health teams, day hospitals and day centres, along with newer services like the Assertive Outreach Teams and Crisis Assessment and Treatment Teams.

THE ROLE OF DAY HOSPITALS

Day services available to older people with mental health problems include day centres and day hospitals. Psychiatric day hospitals for older people tend to be managed and provided through health services and run by multidisciplinary teams consisting of the various mental health professionals. Day centres tend to be managed and funded through local authorities, social services or voluntary organizations with fewer or no health professionals. The first psychiatric day hospitals were opened in the Soviet Union in the 1930s, probably as a result of inpatient bed shortages, and by the early 1950s many had been opened worldwide in developed psychiatric services[4]. In the United Kingdom, the first psychiatric day hospital was the Marlborough Day Hospital in London, opened in 1946[5]. Other psychiatric day care services for older people followed, with dramatic increases in the 1960s and 1970s[6]. The main factor in the growth of day hospitals was attributed to the development of new psychiatric treatments such as neuroleptics. They enabled the mentally ill to be treated in day hospitals, providing a high level of care during the day, but returning to their homes each evening.

The development of effective community support systems is essential for the successful shift from inpatient to community care for mental health services. The identified needs of severely mental ill individuals in the community include medication monitoring and therapy; psychosocial treatment, day and vocational activities; supported and supervised residential services[7]. Day hospitals with their various functions are ideally placed to play a significant role in assessment and community care.

The psychiatric day hospital provides short- and medium-term care to the mentally ill, with the option of receiving at times intensive psychiatric care without hospitalization. In the 1970s, a fully integrated psychiatric service for older people was described by Donovan et al. (1971) to include a day hospital serving four functions[8]. These functions were:

1. The outpatient investigation and treatment of older patients with physical and psychiatric disorders.
2. The continued observation of patients discharged from hospital.
3. To prevent deterioration from self neglect, loneliness or apathy.
4. To offer respite to carers, hence delaying or preventing inpatient admission.

Holloway (1988) described four main functions of day hospitals for mentally ill persons[9]. They are similar to those above and include:

1. An alternative to admission for people who are acutely ill and cannot be maintained as outpatients.
2. A service for support and monitoring in the often difficult transition between a stay in an inpatient ward and life at home.
3. A source of long-term structure and support for those with chronic handicaps, preferably in a friendly, low pressure environment.
4. A site for relatively brief, intensive therapy for people with personality difficulties, severe neurotic illnesses or in need of short-term focused rehabilitation.

Principles and Practice of Geriatric Psychiatry, 3rd edn. Edited by Mohammed T. Abou-Saleh, Cornelius Katona and Anand Kumar

In recognition of their important place in the care of older people, guidelines for current service provision for older people with mental health problems have included the provision of day hospital places[10,11].

For older people, Corcoran et al. (1994) described two objectives of the day hospitals established in Ireland as being[12]:

1. To provide acute psychiatric treatment, thereby functioning as an alternative to admission for patients of over 65 years with functional psychiatric illness.
2. To treat patients with behavioural disturbances associated with dementia.

These objectives are similar to those described above for generic psychiatric day hospitals, though the distribution of diagnoses is different[8,9]. This is especially so in the case of persons with dementia, who are more likely to be found in a day hospital for older people than in a generic psychiatric day hospital. With such varied clientele, outcome and needs in various day hospitals will depend to a large extent on the type of patients being served, and available resources. One benefit of the above-listed functions taking place in day hospitals is that attenders are not taken away from home into hospital, but return home each day. This ensures that routines which may be difficult to re-establish after a long stay in hospital are less disrupted, other than due to illness, and so probably reduces the risk of institutionalization. Furthermore, reports obtained from home, by relatives and carers, give day hospital staff an extra tool in monitoring progress of attenders. For patients with cognitive impairment, maintaining them at home while attending the day hospital is likely to reduce problems of disorientation, resulting from movement into new environments like inpatient wards, as day hospital patients return to the familiar surroundings of their homes each day.

Shah and Ames (1994) described potential functions of an old age psychiatry day hospital as including: assessment, treatment, rehabilitation, long-term support, development of social networks and support of carers[13]. According to Rosenvinge (1994), characteristics of older patients' needs most likely to be met in a psychiatric day hospital can be grouped into functional and organic illnesses[14]. They include:

1. Assessment and management of acute functional illness.
2. Maintenance treatment of high-risk or vulnerable patients.
3. Continuation of treatment of discharged inpatients.
4. Assessment and management of patients suffering from dementia.
5. Provision of long-term support for those with severe dementia.
6. Treatment possibilities in dementia, such as advances in drug treatments requiring close supervision.

These characteristic needs are likely to be found in a wide variety of patients who are likely to benefit from day hospital care.

EVALUATION OF DAY SERVICES

Woods and Phanjoo (1991), in a retrospective study of day hospital patients with dementia, observed the outcome of care after three years[15]. Circumstances of discharges were classified into planned and unplanned. Of the 145 discharges, 65 (45%) were unplanned, with reasons ranging from emergency admission in 14 (9%), to death or physical illness in 40 (28%) and refusal to attend in 11 (8%) patients. Of the planned discharges from the day hospital, only 11

(8%) were discharges to the community, with the remaining 69 (48%) transferred to long-term care in hospital or nursing\residential homes. Though not a randomized controlled study, the authors suggested that outside factors, such as the presence or absence of spouses or others who have taken on the role of carers affected outcome among day hospital attenders. Day hospital patients with spouses were observed to be less likely be admitted to residential or nursing homes than those without spouses. Reasons that they proposed to account for the differences were that the patients with dementia remained longer with their spouses, and that when care was required, the severity of problems presented with at the time would require long-term hospital care rather than placement in residential or nursing homes. The findings of their study would suggest that it is essential that day hospital studies take into consideration such external factors as living spouses, carers and social support networks of patients.

In a study reviewing the impact of closure of a geriatric day hospital, following closure due to staff industrial action, Bhattacharyya et al. (1980) found few ill effects on patients over a six week period[16]. Ratings of mobility, self care, continence, mental state and need for services such as general practitioner, 'meals on wheels', day care or home help revealed minimal differences before and during the day hospital closure. Of the 55 patients in the study, most had cerebrovascular disorders, arthropathy and/or cardiovascular disorders, and only 9 patients had problems with dementia or depression.

In a similar study in older patients with mental health problems, Rolleston and Ball (1994) observed the impact of a two week closure of a psychiatric day hospital[17]. Data on well-being of patients and their carers were collected over eight weeks, to include three weeks prior to closure, two weeks of day hospital closure and three weeks following re-opening of the day hospital. They used two brief questionnaires, designed for patients and their main caregivers respectively, asking whether they felt the same, better or worse than usual, during the preceding week. They found a trend towards decline in well-being during the day hospital closure, which returned to pre-closure levels for both carers and patients on re-opening the day hospital. These findings would suggest that the day hospital was of benefit to both carers and patients. However, this study suffers from the arguments against many day hospital studies, in that they are not randomized controlled studies, hence no consideration is taken for confounding variables, such as the festive season during which closure took place, compliance with medication and/or the social network available to replace the day hospital over the same period.

Corcoran et al. (1994) noted that day hospital treatment enabled the older people with functional illnesses to be treated in the community with low usage of beds, and provided short/medium-term care for patients with dementia who had little support from statutory services[12]. They reviewed all regular attenders of two day hospitals over a three-year period, in which 139 (59%) patients had an organic disorder, mainly dementia, and 98 (41%) patients had a functional disorder, with the most common diagnosis being depression. There was a low uptake of community services at the time of day hospital admission, despite the relatively high level of dependency, especially among patients with dementia. During the course of the study, the uptake in community services, such as meals on wheels, home help and day care, doubled. The average length of admission was five months for those with functional disorders and eight months for those with dementia. Of those patients with functional disorders, 71% were managed effectively through the day hospital and community psychiatric nursing visits, while 25% of them required inpatient care, of which two-thirds were for deterioration in physical health. In the case of those patients with organic disorders, 88 (63%) entered into residential care, on average about eight months after initial referral to the day hospitals. In 20% of patients with dementia, the day hospitals served as a long-term supportive facility, with average attendance of 18 months among this group of patients with severe dementia. This study highlights the benefits of day hospital care in older persons with both functional and organic disorders, though it can be argued that the lack of a control group or comparison with any alternative form of care weakens its findings. The authors themselves acknowledge the importance of an increased range of support services in the community for day hospital attenders.

Johansson and Gustafson (1996) observed that the old age psychiatry day hospitals offered flexible and effective care, especially in supporting people with dementia at home[18]. The most frequent psychiatric symptoms that they observed among the day hospital attenders included delirium, anxiety, sleep disturbances and depressed mood.

Kitchen et al. (2002), in a study evaluating care provided through day hospitals, revealed insufficient clinical disciplines in terms of lack of psychiatrists, occupational therapists and psychologists in several day hospitals[19]. The physical environments were often unsuitable, highlighting the need for purpose-built or adapted day hospitals for older people.

COMPARING DAY HOSPITALS AND DAY CENTRES

Day hospitals, being a health resource, are often located on or close to hospital sites, whereas day centres run by local authorities are more community based, often closer to the clients they serve. Eagles and Warrington (2002) suggested that day centres could carry out similar roles to the day hospitals, as attendees had similar characteristics across both settings, such as severity of dementia, dependency and the range of behaviour problems[20]. They further argued that unless the benefits of mental health staff in day care were demonstrated, resources would be focused on using cheaper untrained staff in day hospitals.

Furness et al. (2000) compared the characteristics and unmet needs of 129 older people attending day hospitals and day centres[21]. The day centres had a higher proportion of people with cognitive impairment, while day hospital attendees had increased behavioural problems and psychotic symptoms. There were similar high levels of high satisfaction expressed by carers of both groups. Collier and Baldwin (1999) found that day hospital patients presented with more behaviour problems than those attending day centres[22]. Though considerable research has been carried out comparing day centres and day hospitals, it has been suggested that they form part of a continuum. Day hospitals, with the various health professionals, can offer the short-term care required for patients with acute and increasing mental and physical health problems who need ongoing multidisciplinary team assessments, review of medication and psychological treatments. Day centres with more untrained staff should have the long-term goals of ongoing social care support and daytime respite for carers for relatively stable patients with enduring mental health problems.

DAY HOSPITAL VERSUS COMMUNITY MENTAL HEALTH TEAMS: THE DEBATE

The lack of adequate scientific data concerning the effectiveness of day hospitals has led to both an enthusiasm for newer service models and, contrastingly, the more conservative approach of leaving the day hospitals as they are. According to Howard (1995), in favour of day hospitals for older people is the fact that carer support by day hospitals has been endorsed by the National Institute of Social Work[23]. Most psychiatrists with access to day hospitals find that they can be used to prevent inpatient admission and facilitate early discharge from wards. Howard mentions that day hospitals may increase carer strain, caused by preparing patients to attend day hospitals and disruption of normal routines. Other arguments include that there is no evidence that day hospital attendance delays or prevents admission of patients with dementia to acute or continuing care placements.

Ball (1993) reviewed the future of day care in old age psychiatry, in which day hospitals undertook a wide range of activities, ranging from acute management of functionally ill to long-term management of patients with dementia[24]. He noted that high levels of distress and depression were found among carers of patients with dementia and this could be relieved by attendance at a day hospital. Though claiming that models exist to examine the effectiveness and efficiency in day hospitals, he failed to give any examples, except to propose that their days may be limited with the coming of community teams working with small local units. To the present date, no randomized controlled trial of the two services in older people with mental health problems as been undertaken.

Day hospitals and day centres provide not only social contact for the elderly mentally ill, and support over crisis periods, but the former also provide treatment in the community. It is argued, however, that these are roles that community mental health teams could also be able to undertake. The community teams working with small local units would be able to target specialist care at groups of patients in need of support, and guidance to those carers providing for their ordinary needs[25].

The day hospital is no longer uniformly or unreservedly accepted as an essential service component in old age psychiatry[23]. Despite the wide use of day hospitals in old age psychiatry, debates still continue over the effectiveness of day hospital care, as it has not been well researched[6,26]. Fasey (1994), in arguing against day hospitals, highlighted the expenses, which included transport, capital investments and highly trained staff[6]. He questioned whether there could be a better and more cost-effective way of delivering the same service. An example he gave was the use of day centres with professional staff providing support and training to less skilled day centre staff. It was further noted that the stated aims of day care, such as delaying or preventing admission of persons with dementia and decreasing carer burden with daytime respite were not achieved[15,27,28]. However, 10 of the 155 day hospital patients with dementia followed up by Woods and Phanjoo (1991) were still attending after three years, indicating that day hospitals can serve long-term needs of patients and their carers[15]. Diesfeldt (1992) undertook a retrospective, longitudinal study of older people with dementia, involving a day care centre rather than a day hospital[27]. Over the five-year period of the study, 150 (67%) of the 224 patients admitted to day care died. At time of admission, 148 lived in the community, but by the fifth year, only 9 (4%) patients still lived in the community and 65 were in long-term care residential/nursing homes. This study highlighted the well-known fact that dementia is associated with increasing dependency and mortality. However, the outcome of day care is difficult to identify, in light of the fact that it was a retrospective, longitudinal, descriptive study rather than a randomized controlled one.

Hassall et al. (1972) and Arie (1978) have highlighted problems with day hospitals, including the fact that a high proportion of day hospital attenders had been inpatients[29,30]. This implies that the day hospital failed to serve as an alternative to inpatient care, and is further supported by the findings of Greene and Timbury (1979) that significant numbers of day hospital attenders were admitted to long-stay care six months later[31]. In this latter study, most of these patients who went on to long-term care in a residential\nursing home or hospital had dementia and had been admitted because of their families' inability to cope, and their admission to day hospital was for, on average, six months.

Despite doubts about the usefulness of day hospitals, Corcoran et al. (1994) indicated that 71% of patients with functional disorders were managed effectively in the community with a combination of day hospital care and visits by nurses[12]. They also observed that day hospital attendance enabled thorough assessment and treatment, ensuring that only those with illnesses who could not manage in the community with maximum support were transferred into residential care.

The focus of shifting psychiatric care to the community, coupled with poor scientific evidence of day hospital care effectiveness, has resulted in support for community mental health teams in place of day hospitals[23]. In evaluating the multidisciplinary approach of community mental health teams to psychiatric diagnoses in the elderly, Collighan et al. (1993) noted a high degree of accuracy when compared to independent formal assessments and consensus diagnoses by research psychiatrists[32]. A total of 378 new referrals to a community mental health team for older people were assessed independently by the team and research psychiatrists. The research assessment consisted of a structured psychiatric interview, full medical and psychiatric history, physical examination and routine blood investigations. Level of agreement between team and research diagnoses was between 90% and 99%. This finding suggests that community multidisciplinary team assessments are at least no worse that those done by psychiatrists, and possibly more likely to flag up problems in non-clinical areas like housing and social support.

Community mental heath teams, like day hospitals, are staffed by nurses, occupational therapist, psychologists, psychiatrists and social workers[33]. The teams are said to provide care that is less focused on a hospital or institution setting[34]. However, it is uncertain whether they lead to benefit for seriously mentally ill people, their carers and society, with respect to how they function or behave[35]. Lives of carers, especially relatives of persons with severe mental health problems, may be disrupted by the high degree of dependency and uncertainty that care involves. The profile of mental health is frequently raised in the media when there is an untoward event involving persons with mental health problems heightening the negative attitude and fear of the public at large. Some of the problems of community mental health teams, and possibly day hospitals too, emanate from this, in that people frequently do not want mental health resources near their homes, or make relocation and employment of persons with mental health problems more difficult.

A review of the literature on the use of community mental health teams in the care of older people does not indicate a marked difference in outcome from day hospital care. In a follow-up study of older people with mental health problems, referred to four community mental health teams, Bedford et al. (1996) reviewed outcome after six months of referral to the teams[36]. They noted a poor outcome in patients with dementia, in that, over the six-month period, 22 of the 63 patients with dementia moved from living at home into institutional care settings and 11 (17%) had died. A recent systematic review of the literature by Hoe et al. (2005) found the evidence for the effectiveness of day hospital care for older people with mental health problems increasing[37]. It was observed that the day hospitals were effective in meeting the needs of patients.

THE FUTURE: INNOVATIVE DAY CARE AND DAY SERVICES

The National Service Framework for Older People is an essential component of the UK government's plan to develop health and social services[38,39]. Key components include care of people with dementia and depression; range of community- and hospital-based services that should be made available; emphasis on the need for integrated, joined-up care and highlighting of the need for specialist mental health services to provide outreach. These requirements are likely to lead to more integrated day services, involving health authority, local authority and voluntary agency jointly run day services, with outreach day care available in the community rather than residing on hospital sites. It has been observed that, despite the introduction of the National Service Framework for Older People, there are substantial variations in service provisions[40]. This may lead to the continued differences observed in day care provision as well.

Some recent innovative practices in day care have included the fast-track day hospitals providing rapid assessment and treatment of behavioural problems in dementia[41], and Alzheimer's cafés, run jointly between statutory and voluntary services providing support to carers of patients with dementia. Crisis Intervention teams, more commonly placed in Adult Psychiatry, are becoming more accessible to older patients, and dementia care multidisciplinary teams offering intensive dementia care at home are being established, preventing hospital admissions. These developments may lead to less reliance on day care.

The Meeting Centres Support Program (MCSP) integrates different types of support for persons with dementia and their carers. The programme focuses on persons with mild or moderate dementia living in the community, and their carers. It is offered by a small professional staff (2 or 3 professionals for 15 people with dementia and 15 carers) in social cultural community centres in the neighbourhood, which is why it is called the Meeting Centre Support Program. Studies comparing MCSP to routine day care have found the programme to be more effective in influencing the feeling of competence of carers, and appeared to delay nursing home placement, along with a positive effect on behaviour and depressed mood[42,43]. In a later study, aside from delay in institutionalization, MCSP proved more effective in decreasing psychological and psychosomatic symptoms in carers of people with dementia than routine day care[44].

In England, the drive towards creating more capable teams and new ways of working in multidisciplinary teams is leading to changing responsibilities and roles of various disciplines[45]. Other team members are expected to carry out psychiatric assessments, prescribe and be the responsible clinician, which were once considered the traditional roles of the psychiatrists. This may lead to a different picture of staff and skill mix in multidisciplinary teams in various settings such as in day care services and community mental health teams.

With the expected rise in elderly population, governments are going to look more closely at various innovative cost-efficient means of delivering health care. It is likely to lead to even more demands to assess the effectiveness of day care services and the need to make day care more efficient and accessible. A comprehensive and flexible mental health service is likely to best serve and meet the changing needs of older people with mental health problems. The delivery of such care through multidisciplinary teams available in such settings as community mental health services, day hospitals and day centres will ensure the adaptability to meet varying needs of this group of patients.

REFERENCES

1. Rosenvinge H. The multidisciplinary teams. In Copeland JRM, Abou-Saleh MT, Blazer DG (eds), *The Principles and Practice of Geriatric Psychiatry*, 1st edn. Chichester: John Wiley & Sons, Ltd, 1994, 887–95.

2. Sutcliffe C, Hughes J, Abendstern M, Clarkson P, Challis D. Developing multidisciplinary assessment – exploring the evidence from a social care perspective. *Int J Geriatr Psychiatry* 2008; **23**: 1297–1305.

3. Department of Health. *Guidance on the Single Assessment Process for Older People*, HSC 2002/001, LAC (2002)1. London: Department of Health, 2002.

4. Marshall M, Crowther R, Almaraz-Serrano AM *et al*. Day hospital versus admission for acute psychiatric disorders. *Cochrane Database Syst Rev* 2003; **1**: CD004026. DOI. 10.1002/14651858.CD004026.

5. Farndale J. *The Day Hospital Movement in Great Britain*. Oxford: Pergamon, 1961.

6. Fasey C. The day hospital in old age psychiatry: the case against. *Int J Geriatr Psychiatry* 1994; **9**: 519–23.

7. Ford J, Young D, Perez BC *et al*. Needs assessment for persons with severe mental illness: what services are needed for successful community living? *Community Ment Health J* 1992, **28**(6): 491–504.

8. Donovan JF, Williams IEI, Wilson TS. A fully integrated psychogeriatric service. In Kay DWK, Walk A (eds), *Recent Developments in Psychogeriatrics*. Ashford: Headley Brothers Ltd, 1971, 113–25.

9. Holloway F. Day care and community support. In Lavender A, Holloway F (eds), *Community Care in Practice*. Chichester: John Wiley & Sons, Ltd, 1988, 161–86.

10. Royal College of Physicians of London, Royal College of Psychiatrists. *Care of Elderly People with Mental Illness: Specialist Services and Medical Training*. London: Royal College of Psychiatrists and Royal College of Physicians of London, 1989.

11. Department of Health. *A Handbook on the Mental Health of Older People*. London: Department of Health, 1997.

12. Corcoran E, Guerandel A, Wrigley M. The day hospital in psychiatry of old age – what difference does it make? *Ir J Psychol Med* 1994; **11**(3): 110–15.

13. Shah A, Ames D. Planning and developing psychogeriatric services. *Int Rev Psychiatry* 1994; **6**: 15–27.

14. Rosenvinge HP. The role of the psychogeriatric day hospital. A consensus document. *Psychiatr Bull R Coll Psychiatr* 1994; **18**, 733–6.

15. Woods JP, Phanjoo AL. A follow-up of psychogeriatric day hospital patients with dementia. *Int J Geriatr Psychiatry* 1991; **6**: 183–8.

16. Bhattacharyya BK, Isherwood J, Sutcliffe RLG. Survey of elderly day hospital patients during a period of industrial action. *Age Ageing* 1980; **9**(2): 106–11.

17. Rolleston M, Ball C. Evaluating the effects of brief day hospital closure. *Int J Geriatr Psychiatry* 1994; **9**(1): 51–3.

18. Johansson A, Gustafson L. Psychiatric symptoms in patients treated in a psychogeriatric day hospital. *Int Psychogeriatr* 1996; **8**(4): 645–58.

19. Kitchen G, Reynolds T, Ashaye K *et al*. A comparison of methods for the evaluation of mental health day hospitals for older people. *J Mental Health* 2002; **11**(6): 667–75.

20. Eagles JM, Warrington J. Day care. In Copeland JRM, Abou-Saleh MT, Blazer DG (eds), *The Principles and Practice of Geriatric Psychiatry*, 2nd edn. Chichester: John Wiley & Sons, Ltd, 2002, 681–3.

21. Furness L, Simpson R, Chakrabarti S *et al*. A comparison of elderly day care and day hospital attenders in Leicestershire: patient profile, carer stress and unmet needs. *Aging Ment Health* 2000; **4**: 326–31.

22. Collier EH, Baldwin RC. The Day Hospital Debate – a contribution. *Int J Geriatr Psychiatry* 1999; **4**: 587–91.

23. Howard R. The place of day hospitals in old age psychiatry. *Curr Opin Psychiatry* 1995; **8**: 240–1.

24. Ball C. The future of day care in old age psychiatry. *Psychiatr Bull R Coll Psychiatr* 1993; **17**: 427–8.

25. Murphy E. Community mental health services: a vision for the future. *Br J Psychiatry* 1991; **302**: 1064–5.

26. Howard R. Day hospitals: The case in favour. *Int J Geriatr Psychiatry* 1994; **9**: 525–9.

27. Diesfeldt H. Psychogeriatric day care outcome: a five year follow-up. *Int J Geriatr Psychiatry* 1992; **7**: 673–9.

28. Berry GL, Zarit SH, Rabatin VX. Caregiver activity on respite and nonrespite days: a comparison of two service approaches. *Gerontologist* 1991; **31**(6): 830–5.

29. Hassall C, Gath D, Cross KW. Psychiatric day care in Birmingham. *Br J Prev Soc Med* 1972; **2**: 112–18.

30. Arie T. Day care in geriatric psychiatry. *Age Ageing* 1978; **8**(Suppl): 87–91.

31. Greene JG, Timbury GC. A geriatric day hospital service: a five year review. *Age Ageing* 1979; **8**: 49–53.

32. Collighan G, Macdonald A, Herzberg J *et al*. An evaluation of the multidisciplinary approach to psychiatric diagnoses in elderly people. *Br Med J* 1993; **306**: 821–4.

33. Tyrer P, Coid J, Simmonds S, Joseph P, Marriott S. Community mental health teams (CMHTs) for people with severe mental illnesses and disordered personality. *Cochrane Database Syst Rev* 1998; **4**: CD000270. DOI: 10.1002/14651858.CD000270.

34. Merson S, Tyrer P, Onyett S *et al*. Early intervention in psychiatric emergencies: a controlled clinical trial. *Lancet* 1992; **339**: 1311–14.

35. Dowell DA, Ciarlo JA. Overview of the community mental health centres program from an evaluation perspective. *Am J Psychiatry* 1993; **19**: 95–125.

36. Bedford S, Melzer D, Dening T *et al*. What becomes of people with dementia referred to community psychogeriatric teams? *Int J Geriatr Psychiatry* 1996; **11**: 1051–6.

37. Hoe J, Ashaye K, Orrell M. Don't seize the day hospital! Recent research on the effectiveness of day hospitals for older people with mental health problems. *Int J Geriatr Psychiatry* 2005; **20**: 694–8.

38. Department of Health. *The NHS Plan: A Plan for Investment. A Plan for Reform*. London: The Stationery Office, 2000.

39. Department of Health. *National Service Framework for Older People*. London: Department of Health, 2001.

40. Tucker S, Baldwin R, Hughes J et al. Old age mental health services in England: implementing the National Service Framework for Older People. Int J Geriatr Psychiatry 2007; 22: 211–17.

41. Law E, Prentice N, Connelly P. The fast track day hospital maintaining clinical improvement in community setting. Int J Geriatr Psychiatry 2008; 3: 109–10.

42. Droes RM, Breebaart E, Melland FJ et al. Effect of Meeting Centres Support Program on feelings of competence of family carers and delay of institutionalisation of people with dementia. Aging Ment Health 2004; 8: 201–11.

43. Dröes RM, Melland F, Schmitz M, van Tilburg W. Effect of combined support for people with dementia and carers versus regular day care on behaviour and mood of persons with dementia: results from a multi-centre implementation study. Int J Geriatr Psychiatry 2004; 19: 673–84.

44. Dröes RM, Melland F, Schmitz M, van Tilburg W. Effect of the Meeting Centres Support Program on informal carers of people with dementia: results from a multi-centre study. Aging Ment Health 2006; 10: 112–24.

45. Royal College of Psychiatrists, National Institute for Mental Health in England. New Ways of Working for Psychiatrists: Enhancing Effective Person Centred Services through New Ways of Working in Multidisciplinary and Multi-Agency Contexts. London: Department of Health, 2005.

122

NHS Continuing Care

Clive Ballard[1], Ramilgan Chitramohan[2], Zunera Khan[1] and Jean Beh[1]

[1]King's College London, London, UK
[2]Birmingham and Solihull Mental Health Foundation Trust, Heartlands Hospital, Birmingham, UK

BACKGROUND

All health and care systems have to address the difficult problem of providing appropriate treatment and care for people with severe dementia, who often have a complex combination of needs. This usually requires a variety of service provision options tailored to the needs of particular individuals and their families, which may include domiciliary support models, private care home and nursing home facilities and directly run National Health Service (NHS) nursing homes and NHS continuing care facilities. Within the UK system, services for people with dementia who have the highest level and greatest complexity of need are provided within the framework of 'NHS continuing care'. This has been technically defined as care for an individual whose treatment needs can only be met by NHS provision, usually meaning 24-hour specialist nurse input, with continuous overview supervision by an NHS specialist consultant. Depending on the needs of particular individuals and the service models in operation in different localities, this can be provided through intense NHS support for people in their own homes, through provision in private nursing homes with additional NHS support or through directly NHS-managed NHS continuing care units. Traditionally, these 'NHS units' were hospital wards, but the service provision has become more flexible, and the continuing care units are now more frequently stand-alone units, run by the NHS, but located in community settings.

This chapter is very much a personal view of the authors, highlighting the context of NHS continuing care and the key elements which the authors believe are essential to enable people to 'live well' with severe and complex dementia.

UK LEGAL STATUS OF NHS CONTINUING CARE

Various legal challenges have enabled refinement of the system and the models of care. Importantly, people who need NHS continuing care, whatever the setting in which that care is provided, receive the care free of charge. This is of course in complete contrast to care provision within the nursing homes, for which people contribute substantially to their financial cost using a means-tested formula[1]. It has, however, been clarified that NHS hospital trusts are obliged to provide adequate NHS continuing care provision in some form. This has led to several major changes in practice:

1. A widespread review of continuing care provision within individual organizations, and an increased flexibility of that provision, which by and large has been helpful and appears to have reduced the widespread dismantling of NHS continuing care provision that was previously occurring as part of achieving 'cost efficiencies'.
2. Setting up of review panels to consider all individuals referred for NHS continuing care to ensure that those individuals have sufficiently complex needs to require NHS continuing care rather than an alternative form of care such as that provided by private sector nursing homes.
3. Ongoing review of people receiving NHS continuing care to ensure that their level of need continues to meet the criteria for this type of care provision. This is a marked departure from the traditional philosophy, which was that NHS care provision was a 'home for life', and a change to a model where the expectation is that most individuals will achieve a reduction in the complexity of their needs as part of the treatment and care that they receive, enabling their needs to then be met within a private sector care facility.

The Alzheimer's Society presented a comprehensive review of the definitions, framework and criteria for costings in 2007, and updated in 2008 to include new legal precedence[1].

CONTINUING CARE NHS MODELS

Traditionally, NHS continuing care has been provided in dedicated inpatient ward environments. These wards still exist in some NHS settings but are poorly designed for the provision of care for people with severe dementia and often concurrent behavioural and psychological symptoms of dementia (BPSD). There are usually a limited number of private rooms, with dormitory facilities that make it difficult to respect privacy and dignity and to meet the needs of individual patients. In addition, the environments are not designed specifically for people with dementia, are often in a poor state of repair, are rarely 'homely' and infrequently have access to outside space. As a result, many NHS organizations have now either built or leased smaller, purpose-built units in a community setting, or set up contracts with private sector providers to offer NHS continuing care beds with an agreed level of NHS support. Although the provision of

Principles and Practice of Geriatric Psychiatry, 3rd edn. Edited by Mohammed T. Abou-Saleh, Cornelius Katona and Anand Kumar
© 2011 John Wiley & Sons, Ltd

better designed, more homely facilities is likely to be an advantage, there has been limited evaluation of either model.

WHICH PATIENTS ARE PLACED IN NHS CONTINUING CARE

The proportion of people residing in care facilities who have dementia has consistently increased over the last 20 years, with most reports over the last decade indicating that at least two-thirds of care home residents have dementia, even though only a quarter of care home beds are registered specifically for people with this level of need[2,3]. As a consequence, there has also been some blurring of boundaries between different types of care provision with respect to the needs of the individuals for whom they cater. For example, the proportion of people with dementia in nursing homes and specially register beds is not substantially different from that in 'ordinary care homes'[2-4]. There also appears to be a similar blurring of boundaries between the specialist nursing homes and NHS continuing care, with a similar proportion of people with a similar severity of dementia and comparable high levels of BPSD in both settings[4]. This possibly suggests that some people are being placed in private sector care homes when their level of need may require NHS continuing care, either within a dedicated unit or by providing much more substantial NHS support to enable the effective care of those individuals.

WHAT IS THE QUALITY OF CARE IN NHS CONTINUING CARE ENVIRONMENTS

There is an absence of published audit data or randomized controlled trials to provide a meaningful evaluation of usual NHS continuing care or novel models of care provision. An audit of 17 care facilities across the UK conducted in 2001 included 10 private sector residential or nursing homes and 7 NHS continuing care units[5]. Disappointingly, based upon daytime evaluation of well-being and activities, a similar pattern of impoverished daytime activities and poor overall well-being was evident in both care settings, and there was no evidence that NHS continuing care offered improved activities, well-being or quality of life for care recipients.

This does not reflect our anecdotal experience of clinical practice, and it will be increasingly important for more widespread evaluation of care using standardized approaches to measure overall quality of care provision, to enable benchmarking against the best care services and to enable continual improvement of professional practice and the quality of treatment and care provided.

Additional information is available from studies examining the transfer of people to different care environments when NHS continuing care facilities have closed. The primary outcome measure in these studies has tended to be mortality rates[6] rather than wider health outcomes, and the effects of relocation on older people with dementia are not straightforward, with conflicting findings reported in different studies. For example, some authors such as Robertson et al.[7] reported that disruption associated with the move was associated with higher mortality among residents after the move, while others found no increase in mortality or health problems[8]. However, two consistent findings did emerge from the literature relating to the relocation of older people with mental health needs. Firstly, that the moving of patients and staff together ('en bloc') minimizes disruption associated with the relocation. Secondly, that an individualized and comprehensive preparation programme is vital in maximizing the holistic outcome for the resident.

In a more recent report examining relocation of an NHS continuing care unit within the South London and Maudsley NHS trust, 23 residents from an NHS continuing care facility were relocated, 9 residents underwent individual transfers over a 12-month period and 14 were transferred 'en bloc' to a new unit[9]. The baseline assessments included an assessment of quality of life, which indicated 'adequate coping' and suggested considerably better quality of life than had previously been reported among people with complex mental health problems residing in long-term care[10].

Importantly, the group of residents who were moved individually to new accommodation showed a significant decline in behavioural disturbance (as measured by the Neuropsychiatric Inventory), while the group who moved together to the new unit showed no change. This unexpected finding may be explained by the fact that considerable effort was taken to re-accommodate residents to locations of their and their relatives' choice. Those residents who moved away to new units were often situated much closer to their relatives, which may have provided greater opportunities for social interaction. This in turn may have had a positive impact on residents' behaviours. This does indicate that successful transfer of individual patients from NHS continuing care to other care environments can be achieved with careful planning and assessment[9].

Several studies have evaluated more specific models of providing NHS continuing care, such as the *domus* model. 'Domus care' is provided in small units based in the community, operating with core 'person centred' principles and a 'rites-based philosophy' that the domus is the person's home. Evaluation of this model has demonstrated advantages over traditional NHS continuing care settings[11]. In particular, BPSD and communication skills improved significantly among residents, although providing this type of care was twice as expensive as traditional models. While it is encouraging that good quality care can result in improvements in well-being and communication, it is unclear whether this is a specific feature of the domus model, related to better staffing ratios or an example of what can be achieved by motivated staff in a well designed environment. As a proof of concept it is, however, extremely important, as it demonstrates that it is possible to provide high quality care that meets the needs of these individuals.

The recent change in NHS continuing care to focus on 'rehabilitation' to reduce the level of need and enable transfer to other settings such as private nursing home facilities is contrary to the 'domus philosophy', and is likely to result in significant changes in care practice and the style of treatment and care. Further evaluations will be needed to determine whether this has a positive or negative impact on people with dementia living in these environments.

WHAT IS NEEDED TO PROVIDE TOP QUALITY NHS CARE

Provision of high-quality NHS continuing care for people with dementia requires a highly skilled group of staff, a well-designed, purpose-built environment and excellent links with other medical, social care and palliative care teams to provide a physical and social environment that can meet a broad range of need. Key areas include basic activities of daily living (ADLs), social needs, BPSD, transfer, mobility and reduction of falls risk, management of pain and concurrent physical health needs, feeding, skin care, other needs related to end-of-life issues, working with families and understanding the legal framework within which this care must operate.

UNDERSTANDING OF RELEVANT LEGAL FRAMEWORKS

The majority if not all of the people in NHS continuing care settings will lack capacity to make decisions regarding their medical treatment or long-term care. Many such individuals can be looked after in these settings under the general provisions of the Mental Capacity Act 2005 in the best interest of these individuals so long as their care regime is not considered to deprive them of their liberties[12]. Those whose care regime is so restrictive as to amount to deprivation of liberty will come under the new Deprivation of Liberty safeguards which can authorise detention in the individual's best interests for up to 12 months after 6 assessments (the main issues are highlighted by Behan in a Department of Health Document, 2007)[12].

Some individuals may initially be admitted to an NHS continuing care unit under the auspices of the Mental Health Act (see[13] for more detailed guidance on the 2007 Act), or such an order may be applied at some point during an individual's care. These are mainly patients who object to being looked after in such settings.

Specific decisions regarding resuscitation and other end-of-life treatment issues are complex and fall under various legal frameworks. Staff working within this sector therefore would need to understand a complex network of legal frameworks, and how to work within these frameworks to achieve a level of treatment and care that meets the best interests of the individual patient. At an organizational level this requires excellent training and processes, and at a unit management level requires excellent operationalization of these processes so that they contribute to, rather than hinder, good quality treatment and care.

SUPPORTING BASIC ACTIVITIES OF DAILY LIVING

Most people with dementia of a severity sufficient to require residence in a care home or NHS continuing care setting will require at least some assistance with basic self care, usually requiring help, prompting or supervision for washing, dressing and going to the toilet. The opportunities and skills to engage in other more complex activities such as cooking, making tea and activities outside the care facility such as shopping are likely to be limited by safety concerns, the organization of the care setting and the skills of the individual. With well-thought-through care plans and an appropriate level of assistance and supervision it is, however, possible to enable many individuals to take part in a limited number of more 'general' activities as part of supporting social needs (see subsequent section). In NHS continuing care settings this will vary hugely between different individuals depending upon the balance of complex needs. Some patients will have very severe dementia, while others may have dementia of moderate severity with additional BPSD and/or physical health care needs. A full assessment of every individual is therefore essential, working to the principle of maximizing people's abilities and competencies. Assessment tools like the Pool Activity Level[14] and the person's life story work[15,16] will inform the care planning process. As part of this assessment, detailed personalized care plans should be developed, outlining skills which it is important to enable people to continue using, self care activities which can be partly completed by the individual with appropriate prompting and help, and self care activities which need to be undertaken for the individual. In the latter circumstance it is also important to plan the support with self care in such a way as to maximize the opportunities it creates for normal social interaction, to minimize anxiety and distress, to make the assistance less challenging for the individual and

reduce the likelihood or impact of BPSD (see subsequent section). Supporting an individual's basic activities of daily living is vital and requires good care planning, but would not on it's own constitute a level of need requiring NHS continuous care. When ADL needs are linked closely to other needs such as BPSD, skin care and feeding, the complexity of the 'need', and the skills needed to meet the 'need' effectively increase substantially.

Case Example

Mr Bell, a 65-year-old gentleman, was fully dependent on staff for all his needs. He was also bed bound. Whenever staff attended to his personal care, they would come out of his room exhausted and complaining that he was resistive and aggressive and it was 'a fight' caring for his needs.

But when Mary (staff member) attended to his personal care, she did not have the same experience. She would call him by his preferred name David, and explain to him step by step what she was going to do for him. She would inform him that she was going to wash his face before applying the wet flannel. She would also ask if he could relax his arm while she tried to take off the sleeve of his shirt. After much explanation and time taken with David in carrying out his personal care, Mary and her colleague would feel happy that they managed David's personal care without much struggle. David too looked comfortable sitting up in bed.

MEETING SOCIAL NEEDS

As part of statutory and regulatory frameworks and in developing care standards, the social needs of residents in care homes and NHS continuing care environments have been rather neglected. This is a major oversight as it is fundamental to everyone's well-being, and something which needs to be a key part of the care planning for every individual. People all have a large social need, which is frequently unmet in care settings. At as gross level, this is well evidenced by the fact that, based upon large studies of Dementia Care Mapping[17], people spend less than 15% of their daytime period engaged in social interaction or any other positive or enjoyable activity[5].

Often, the knee-jerk reflex to addressing social needs is to organize 'activities', usually games (e.g. bingo, a quiz), dancing/singing/music or an opportunity for reminiscence. In itself, if well planned, this type of activity can be very positive for residents who enjoy these types of event, but thought does need to be given to individual choice and to the development of more personalized care plans for every individual. It is rarely possible for 'Care home wide' activities to be undertaken more than a few times a week, and therefore, although a positive contribution to social need, they are generally a small contribution.

Talking to an individual, their families and friends to build up a life book, which includes details of their hobbies, interests, usual household activities and occupation, is an excellent way of learning more about each individual, developing material for reminiscence and for identifying specific individualized activities which may be beneficial or enjoyable for a particular person. A care plan can then be developed to create opportunities for specific activities that can be safely undertaken with the right level of support. Several excellent research studies have shown the value of enhancing individualized care planning and individualized activities to improve well-being and reduce agitation[18,19].

Case Example

Ethel, an 80-year-old lady, would shout and scream every afternoon. The staff would play the same music (1950s songs); two of the residents would sing the songs, but Ethel would continue to shout loudly. Janet (staff) approached Ethel and asked her what was troubling her; Ethel just replied 'I am bored'. Janet asked her what she would like to do; Ethel replied 'push me around'. Ethel was chair bound and when she was well, she enjoyed going out for walks. Janet pushed Ethel's chair around the unit, into the garden and around the corridors of the unit. While Ethel was going round the unit and into the garden, Janet talked to her about the plants, flowers and pictures on the wall. Ethel would respond with 'that is lovely' or 'push the chair faster'. All the time Ethel was travelling around the unit, she stopped shouting and spoke quietly to Janet.

In addition, it is important to think about the environment: organizing chairs in a way that facilitates conversation; availability of 'coffee rooms'; providing a choice of television and radio programmes which is not over-loud or intrusive to other residents; providing interesting reading materials and objects for people to enjoy and which can facilitate conversation and reminiscence; providing adequate and interesting indoor and outdoor space to enable people to walk about in a safe and enjoyable way.

In people with very severe dementia, it is possible but more difficult to meet social needs. Again it relies on an individualized assessment, but often people may be more responsive to one-to-one interaction. Sometimes conversation or music may be perceived positively, but for many individuals touch is the most beneficial interaction – holding an individuals hand or an aromatherapy massage may, for example, give the greatest benefit.

Staff need to be encouraged to take steps toward positive risk taking when caring for a person with dementia. This will allow more creative approaches to care for people with dementia if staff are supported by management. Care that is collaboratively planned and managed by a multidisciplinary team after discussions with the person with dementia and their family will ensure that care provided is person centred.

Case Example: Individual Care Plan

John, a 70-year-old gentleman, used to be a dancing instructor. He would often walk up and down the corridor with his head bowed low. Staff had to listen very carefully to what he was saying, at times it was clear but, most times, his speech was muddled. But when staff offered to dance with him down the corridor, he would hold his head up a little, held good eye contact with the staff and, with a smile on his face, danced down the corridor.

MANAGEMENT AND PREVENTION OF BEHAVIOURAL AND PSYCHOLOGICAL SYMPTOMS OF DEMENTIA (BPSD)

Approximately 80% of individuals in NHS continuing care experience BPSD at any one time[5], and probably all individuals experience at least one of these symptoms longitudinally[20]. BPSD are almost always present and severe at the point of admission to NHS continuing care, and are the usually part of the complex need for which NHS continuing care is considered necessary for a particular individual. Aggression and restlessness are the most frequent symptoms, occurring in 60% or more of residents[5], but delusions and shouting are also frequent and problematic, while other less frequently occurring problems, such as sexual disinhibition and concurrent bipolar disorder, can be extremely challenging.

One of the advantages of working in a continuing care setting is that it affords a 'protected environment' with a skilled multidisciplinary work force, which allows time to conduct a detailed assessment and plan interventions carefully. A broad multidisciplinary clinical assessment can therefore be undertaken to inform any changes in treatment. As in any setting, the assessment includes screening for physical health problems such as infection, pain or dehydration, which are common, and often precipitate BPSD. A comprehensive review of pharmacological treatments may identify therapies exacerbating depression, other BPSD or confusion[21]. Visual and auditory impairment can also precipitate BPSD[22], and should be treated when possible. These principles are outlined in more detail by Lyketsos and colleagues (2006)[23]. A careful psychiatric assessment is also important, as specific psychiatric symptoms such as florid delusions or depression may be underlying or contributing to the presentation of other behavioural symptoms such as aggression or agitation. In parallel, a detailed assessment can be undertaken of the frequency and severity of any presenting BPSD and any associated risks to the individual, to other residents or to staff. An approach such as an Antecedent Behaviour Consequence diary can be used to clarify the pattern of occurrence and to identify triggers and re-inforcers.

The strength of this approach is that it provides an overall assessment of the situation, and allows medical, psychiatric and environmental precipitants to be targeted through specific treatments or care plans. It also provides an assessment of risk, which enables the team to carefully balance the risks and benefits of different treatment approaches, including the information to make a carefully weighted decision regarding whether pharmacological treatment is necessary. The assessment also provides the opportunity to get to know the individual and build up a 'life story' and develop a better understanding of the person's preferences by talking to the individual, their family and friends. This enables their needs to be met more effectively, improves communication and interpersonal relationships between the person and the staff, engages the family and provides important information for the development of care plans and for specific non-pharmacological interventions for BPSD. Again, an advantage of a continuing care environment in this situation is that the multi-skilled staff group and NHS medical/psychiatric support means that a less invasive option can often be implemented as a first-line strategy, as detrimental outcomes can be rapidly contained and management plans can be revised quickly. In practice, the most frequent practical management problem is physical aggression occurring when an individual is being assisted with personal care. In our experience, with a careful ABC (antecedent behaviour consequence) assessment, good interpersonal skills and a well-thought-through care plan, it is usually but not always possible to successfully manage and improve the symptoms and the 'personal care experience' for the person and the staff without recourse to pharmacological intervention. If pharmacological interventions are necessary, best practice guidelines appropriate for all individuals with dementia should be applied[24]. This is not discussed in detail here as the same principles apply to the management of dementia in general (for a review of evidence see[21]), but the principles should include limiting the use of atypical antipsychotics to short-term prescribing (up to 6–12 weeks) for serious management problems in most situations; the judicious use of other pharmacological interventions when appropriate, and the use of care and caution to limit multiple prescribing[21,24,25].

Case Example

Peter, a resident in a continuing care unit, was screaming whenever he was awake. The staff could see that he was distressed, but he was unable to communicate his reasons for his distress. The doctor prescribed antipsychotics to reduce his distress but the screaming continued. After much multidisciplinary discussion, it was decided to discontinue all medications except analgesia and to spend more individual time with Peter. The screaming stopped and Peter's distress was reduced to a minimum. To this day, we do not know whether the side effects of the medication were causing Peter's distress or the increased time spent with Peter alleviated his distress. The staff became more aware of the importance of observing for side effects of medication, especially for people who have difficulties in communicating verbally.

Paul, a resident in a continuing care unit, kept coming in to the staff office, especially at meeting times. This was disruptive to the staff as they had to stop their meeting to answer Paul's questions and requests for help. Reading through Paul's life story, the staff realized that he used to work as an administrator. The staff decided to make space for a table and chair in a corner of the dayroom. They left some paper and pens on the table. They informed Paul that the space was for him to do some work if he so wished to do. Paul sat at the table and wrote on the paper, occasionally he would go into the office but, most times, he would sit at his table writing or tidying up papers.

MAINTAINING MOBILITY AND MINIMIZING FALLS

Many individuals with moderately severe or severe dementia begin to lose independent mobility and even ability to mobilize with assistance. As mobility problems progress, even transferring from bed to a chair can be problematic. Mobility problems are likely to present even greater challenges in patients with motor disability related to vascular dementia and stroke or with other physical health problems impacting on the locomotor system, such as severe arthritis. Even in individuals who are able to mobilize, falls are a major clinical problem. Fifty percent of people with Alzheimer's disease fall over a three-year period, and fractures are extremely common[26,27].

There are, hence, a number of important challenges to maximize mobility and minimize fall risk. The importance of a multidisciplinary team is immediately evident. Good access to physiotherapy, consultation/liaison from Geriatric Medicine, robust assessment procedures and good quality person-centred care planning, focusing

specifically on mobility needs, are all essential components. The assessment and care planning procedures will need to determine the level of support needed to enable walking and transfer, such as appropriate walking aids, assistance from staff and a programme to maximize skills, for instance ensure adequate time spent walking to maintain strength, specific exercises to help maintain strength and balance. These types of programmes are clearly beneficial among older people without cognitive impairment[28], although the evidence is less clear in the context of dementia[29]. Nevertheless, this probably is good practice, and will have concurrent benefits such as maintaining muscle strength and improving mood.

A careful assessment of fall risk needs to be undertaken for all individuals. Where possible, person-centred exercise and mobility programmes can then be developed which maximize benefits but reduce risk, for instance supervision needed when walking in outside spaces, or vigilance to ensure assistance during all walking. The assessment may also highlight the need for a more specific physiotherapy evaluation or a medical assessment of specific risks, for example syncopy; or additional measures to reduce risk such as protective underwear, well-fitting footwear, good lighting, corrected vision with spectacles and clear pathways.

For individuals who are unable to mobilize, but can weight bear to transfer from bed to a chair, similar vigilance is required in completing an assessment, an evaluation of risk and a care plan to promote maintenance of skills using practice and exercises. Maintaining the ability to weight bear and avoiding the need for a hoist is a major factor in maintaining some independence and is therefore a very important clinical objective.

Given the severity and complexity of problems in these individuals, even with the best practice and care, disability is progressive and many individuals will eventually lose their ability to weight bear. Under such circumstances a hoist will be needed to transfer a person from a bed to a chair or from a wheelchair to a sitting chair, both important to enable social interaction and to protect skin. Being transferred using a hoist can, however, be a frightening experience. Safely operating different hoists appropriate to the needs of the individual requires practical skills, but excellent interpersonal verbal and non-verbal communications to prevent and reduce fear and anxiety are also critical.

ASSESSMENT AND TREATMENT OF PAIN

Pain can be very difficult to assess in people with severe dementia, but has a massive impact on the quality of life of an individual and contributes to the emergence of other problems such as BPSD. Jiska Cohen-Mansfield and colleagues[30] have recently reported a series of studies developing clinical instruments to assess pain, and demonstrating clear benefits in behaviour and mood with the implementation of appropriate analgesia based upon these assessments. In clinical practice these instruments are an excellent and practical tool. Assessing pain also relies on a detailed knowledge of the individual. As a rule of thumb, if there is a possible indication of pain, or a physical ailment which is likely to be causing pain, our usual practice is to err on the side of providing analgesia, but in the context of careful evaluation of benefits.

ADDRESSING PHYSICAL HEALTH NEEDS

Many individuals living in continuing care environments have vascular dementia, providing the additional challenges of managing disabilities and providing rehabilitation for stroke-related impairments, and providing optimal medical management of related cardiovascular disease and vascular risk factors. For example, there is accumulating evidence that good control of blood pressure, lipids/cholesterol and diabetes significantly reduces the progression of disability and cognitive impairment (e.g. PROGRESS 2001[31]). This again emphasises the need for multidisciplinary working and the importance of open access to geriatric medicine expertise and specialist clinics as appropriate for specific individuals.

More generally, many individuals with dementia in NHS continuing care have concurrent physical illnesses as part of the complexity leading to their placement in this type of facility. High quality treatment and management of these conditions may be important in stabilizing cognitive decline, but is definitely critical in reducing additional disability, minimizing associated pain and discomfort and maximizing quality of life.

Many individuals are on multiple pharmacological treatments, many of which are not well tolerated in people with dementia or which may impact upon cognitive function. Ongoing review of medication is therefore also a key part of good management. The National Service Framework recommends three-monthly medication reviews[32]. For people in NHS continuing care settings, informal medication review should probably happen more frequently, but a more formal three-monthly review is also good practice.

NUTRITION AND FEEDING

Maintaining good nutrition is an important part of maintaining health and well-being. In particular, minimizing weight loss is a key objective, and good nutrition will help to prevent skin breakdown and the development of ulcers. In addition, food is a major source of pleasure to most people and it is a potential opportunity to provide people with some pleasure and enjoyment. Food tastes often change with advancing dementia, and a preference for sweet food types is common. Many people also, however, continue to appreciate food consistent with their own culture, and occasional 'themed' meals may give an opportunity for group participation and other related activities.

Poor appetite or reduced food intake are common problems which need careful assessment and specific personalized care plans. Reduced appetite may be related to depression, physical illness or altered food preferences, all of which can be addressed if identified. Some patients may develop marked restlessness, sometimes of a severity which makes it difficult to encourage people to sit and eat meals or to drink adequately. Again this needs careful assessment to exclude bipolar illness or other specific causes, and may require specific pharmacological or non-pharmacological interventions.

As dementia progresses, a substantial proportion of individuals lose the ability to feed themselves. With a good care plan that assesses level of ability, people can be enabled to continue feeding. For example, providing just one implement of cutlery if coordination of more than one item is challenging, or the provision of finger foods. If diet is changed in this way, it is important to still think about the nutritional value and taste of the food. The Alzheimer's Society has provided a series of booklets which addresses these issues comprehensively[2,3].

Either because of very severe dementia or as a result of concurrent cerebrovascular disease, some individuals will lose or partially lose their swallowing reflex or their ability to coordinate swallowing. Under these circumstances, aspiration of food is a major health risk. In individuals where there is any level of concern, it is important that a careful assessment of swallowing is carried out. Often a specific care plan, such as having meals in a fully upright position, having a 'soft diet' and thickening drinks, will be sufficient to enable meals to be taken safely. In some circumstances, where even these measures are not sufficient to enable food to be taken orally, difficult decisions need to be made in conjunction with family members regarding alternative feeding methods and/or end-of-life care.

OPTIMAL SKIN CARE

Vulnerability of skin to 'break down', and the prevention and treatment of ulcers in pressure areas represent an enormous clinical challenge in the clinical care of people with severe dementia in continuing care settings, particularly in people with limited or no independent mobility, spending a substantial proportion of the day sitting or lying down. Nursing staff require expertise in prophylactic skin care, and access to specialist nurses when ulcers develop and need to be treated. Specialist beds and mattresses are needed for some individuals, together with a breadth of clinical expertise encompassing use of mattresses, management protocols and care plans and the use of appropriate dressings. In addition, the management of related pain/discomfort and infection is important.

END-OF-LIFE ISSUES

Although this may change to some extent as NHS continuing care evolves, and is no longer 'a home for life' for all residents, currently the majority of individuals receiving treatment and care in these settings will die within NHS continuing care facilities. There are many advantages to this, in particular that the staff know the individual and their family well, and understand the needs of the individual and the family members, and the person is cared for in a familiar and comfortable environment. End-of-life issues therefore need to be tackled proactively, so that the wishes of the individual and of the family can be met as far as possible with respect to resuscitation, other medical treatment issues and key care decisions. In addition, the staff group needs to be familiar with and have access to expert advice regarding best practice management protocols to manage pain, distress, discomfort and dehydration in terminal care situations, and to provide support as appropriate to family members.

Working with families: family members continue to be a vital part of people's lives even when they have severe dementia and are residing in NHS continuing care environments. As part of the initial assessment when people are first placed in NHS continuing care, the family can provide key information to confirm the past medical and past psychiatric history, and even more importantly are able to convey an understanding of an individuals personality, background, likes and dislikes, hobbies, occupation and other important considerations such as religious and cultural issues and how important they are as part of someone's life. This enables a 'life book' to be developed and enriches the opportunities to develop better, more personalized care plans that are better suited to meet people's social, cultural and spiritual needs.

Many family members feel disengaged when an individual moves into continuing care or a nursing home. It is important to break down those barriers and to enable people to play an ongoing and active part in the care and support of the individual with dementia, and to help the family, where appropriate, contribute to the implementation of care plans to meet social needs. It is also important to help the person with dementia to continue to feel that they are an important and contributing member of the family, for which links to all generations of the family can be very helpful.

Particularly when advanced directives are not in place, families also play a vital role in the best practice meetings to make key medical and care decisions.

CONCLUSIONS

Providing good quality care to people with complex needs and severe dementia is difficult and requires a multidisciplinary, multi-skilled team with excellent access to appropriate specialist services. Often NHS continuing care has been seen as a low priority, and investment in team development and skills has not always been at the forefront of service planning. As illustrated by specialist models and pockets of excellence, it is possible to meet the needs and enable a good quality of life for even the individuals with the most severe dementia and complex concurrent problems.

Applying the principles of the ten essential shared capabilities for the mental health work force in dementia care will promote care that is truly person centred[33].

REFERENCES

1. Alzheimer's Society. *When Does the NHS Pay for Continuing Care? Guidance on Eligibility for Continuing NHS Health Care Funding in England and How to Appeal if it is Not Awarded*. London: Alzheimer's Society, 2007 (supplement published 2008).

2. Alzheimer's Society. *Dementia Care in Care Homes*. London: Alzheimer's Society, 2007.

3. Alzheimer's Society. *Food for Thought; Finger Food Ideas*, booklet 325. York: Alzheimer's Society, 2008.

4. Margallo-Lana M, Swann A, O'Brien J et al. Prevalence and pharmacological management of behavioural and psychological symptoms amongst dementia sufferers living in care environments. *Int J Geriatr Psychiatry* 2001; **16**: 39–44.

5. Ballard C, Fossey J, Chithramohan R et al. Quality of care in private sector and NHS facilities for people with dementia: cross sectional survey. *BMJ* 2001; **323**: 426–7.

6. Schultz R, Brenner G. Relocation of the aged: a review and theoretical analysis. *J Gerontol* 1977; **32**: 323–33.

7. Robertson C, Warrington J, Eagles JM et al. Relocation mortality in dementia: the effects of a new hospital. *Int J Geriatr Psychiatry* 1993; **8**: 521–5.

8. McAuslane L, Sperlinger D. The effects of relocation on elderly people with dementia and their nursing staff. *Int J Geriatr Psychiatry* 1994; **9**: 981–4.

9. Boddington S, Beh J, Nash J et al. Relocation of a continuing care unit: description of a model and lessons learned. *J Dementia Care*. In Press.

10. Blau TH. Quality of life, social indicators, and criteria of change. *Prof Psychol* 1977; **11**: 464–73.

11. Lindesay J, Briggs K, Lawes M et al. The domus philosophy: a comparative evaluation of a new approach to residential care for the demented elderly. *Int J Geriatr Psychiatry* 1991; **6**: 727–36.

12. Behan D. *Deprivation of Liberty Safeguards and Mental Capacity Act 2005 Local Implementation Networks*, 2007. At www.dh.gov.uk/en/Publicationsandstatistics/Lettersandcirculars/Dearcolleagueletters/DH_080714, accessed 2 Mar 2010.

13. Department of Health. *Mental Health Act 2007 – Overview*, 2008. At www.dh.gov.uk/en/Healthcare/Mentalhealth/DH_078743, accessed 1 Oct 2008.

14. Pool J. *The Pool Activity Level (PAL) Instrument for Occupational Profiling*. London: Jessica Kingsley Publishers, 2008.

15. Murphy C. It Started with a Seashell: Life Story Work and People with Dementia. Stirling: Dementia Services Development Centre, 1994.

16. National Audit Office. *Improving Services and Support for People with Dementia*. London: National Audit Office, 2007.

17. Kitwood T, Bredin K. A new approach to the evaluation of dementia care. *J Adv Health Nursing Care* 1992; **1**: 1–20.

18. Chenoweth L, King MT, Jeon YH et al. Caring for Aged Dementia Care Resident Study (CADRES) of person-centred care, dementia-care mapping, and usual care in dementia: a cluster-randomised trial. *Lancet Neurol* 2009; **8**: 317–25.

19. Cohen-Mansfield J, Libin A, Marx MS et al. Nonpharmacological treatment of agitation: a controlled trial of systematic individualized intervention. *J Gerontol A Biol Sci Med Sci* 2007; **62**: 908–16.

20. Ballard CG, Margallo-Lana M, Fossey J et al. A 1-year follow-up study of behavioral and psychological symptoms in dementia among people in care environments. *J Clin Psychiatry* 2001; **62**: 631–6.

21. Ballard CG, Gauthier S, Cummings JL et al. Management of agitation and aggression associated with Alzheimer disease. *Nat Rev Neurol* 2009; **5**: 245–55.

22. Chapman FM, Dickinson J, McKeith I et al. Association among visual hallucinations, visual acuity, and specific eye pathologies in Alzheimer's disease: treatment implications. *Am J Psychiatry* 1999; **156**: 1983–5.

23. Lyketsos CG, Colenda CC, Beck C et al. Position statement of the American Association for Geriatric Psychiatry regarding principles of care for patients with dementia due to Alzheimer disease. *Am J Geriatr Psychiatry* 2006; **14**: 561–72.

24. Jeste DV, Blazer D, Casey D et al. ACNP White Paper: update on use of antipsychotic drugs in elderly persons with dementia. *Neuropsychopharmacology* 2008; **33**: 957–70.

25. National Institute for Health and Clinical Excellence/Social Care Institute for Excellence. *Dementia: The NICE-SCIE Guideline on Supporting People with Dementia and Their Carers in Health and Social Care*. London: National Collaborating Centre for Mental Health, 2007.

26. Tinetti ME, Speechley M, Ginter SF et al. Risk factors for falls among elderly persons living in the community. *N Engl J Med* 1988; **319**: 1701–7.

27. Van Dijk PTM, Meulenberg OGRM, Van De Sande IIJ et al. Falls in dementia patients. *Gerontologist* 1993; **33**: 200–4.

28. Buchner DM, Cress ME, Wagner EH et al. The Seattle FICSIT/MoveIt study: the effect of exercise on gait and balance in older adults. *J Am Geriatr Soc* 1993; **41**: 321–5.

29. Shaw FE, Bond J, Richardson DA et al. Multifactorial intervention after a fall in older people with cognitive impairment and dementia presenting to the accident and emergency department: randomised controlled trial. *BMJ* 2003; **326**: 73.

30. Cohen-Mansfield J, Lipson S. The utility of pain assessment for analgesic use in persons with dementia. *Pain* 2008; **134**: 16–23.

31. PROGRESS Collaborative Group. Randomised trial of a perindopril-based blood-pressure lowering regimen among 6105 individuals with previous stroke or transient ischaemic attack. *Lancet* 2001; **358**: 1033–41.

32. Department of Health. *National Service Framework for Older People*. London: Department of Health, 2001.

33. Hope, R. *The Ten Essential Shared Capabilities – A Framework for the Whole of the Mental Health Workforce*. London: Department of Health, 2004.

123

Overview of Law, Ethics and Mental Health in Old Age

Julian C. Hughes

*Northumbria Healthcare NHS Foundation Trust and Institute for Ageing and Health,
Newcastle University, UK*

INTRODUCTION

An overview should clarify how things fit together. Where there is a high degree of complexity, however, this might not be possible; or, at least, it might require some digging to unearth the connections. I am going to suggest that what we have to look for in law and ethics is coherence in terms of our patterns of practice. In addition, I wish to point to the notion of the person as being in some sense fundamental.

MORALS AND PRACTICE

Consequentialism and Deontology

Consequentialism suggests that whether an action is good or right depends on its consequences. The best-known consequentialist theory is utilitarianism, which states that actions are right insofar as they maximize happiness or pleasure and minimize the opposite[1]. If, for instance, it seems likely that Mrs Jones will kill herself because of her depression and we have good grounds to believe that she will enjoy her life again if she were to receive appropriate treatment, then treating her would seem to be the ethically right thing to do, even against her wishes. But this depends upon a careful assessment, because although compulsory treatment would seem to maximize happiness, such treatment must not be so unpleasant or upsetting as to cause her permanent discontent.

We can see immediately, therefore, how complicated things might become in pushing forward this argument. What if, for instance, it could be known for certain that Mrs Jones would never be happy again? Should she then be left untreated or at least not treated against her will? A legal issue, about her ability to make decisions for herself, arises and reflects the Law's emphasis on the rights of competent persons to control what happens to their bodies under normal circumstances. Generally speaking, it is only when a person is not 'of sound mind' that others are allowed and required to make decisions on the person's behalf.

To return to the case of Mrs Jones, just as utilitarians might argue that it is best to have a rule that people like Mrs Jones should be treated because this is more likely to maximize happiness (i.e. rule utilitarianism, as opposed to a focus on particular and individual acts, which is called act utilitarianism) so too we could more simply argue that we have a duty (*deon*) to treat Mrs Jones. We quite often speak of a duty of care, for instance, which carries with it the idea that this is something we must do – and the difference between this and utilitarianism is shown by the fact that we add 'whatever the outcome'. In deontology the consequences are not the main issue. What is at stake is how people should behave as rational agents in the world. Given some of our typical concerns as human beings – that we should have a basic level of certain sorts of good (warmth, clothing, food) – it can be argued in deontological mode that there is a duty, for those who are able, to provide these goods to people who lack them. Duties are sometimes thought of as being corollaries of rights. Hence, if a person has a right to be told the truth about his condition, we have a duty to be honest with him. A right to basic standards of care carries with it a duty to provide such care. A right to privacy entails a duty not to invade the person's privacy, to confidentiality a duty to maintain confidences.

Four Principles

In clinical ethics it has become commonplace, partly in order to avoid the complexity of the arguments that emerge in discussions of consequentialism and deontology, to use the four principles of medical ethics[2]. These provide an easy way to access the relevant arguments in connection with health care decisions. Autonomy, often regarded as the main principle, stresses self-rule: the person with dementia should still be able to make decisions for him- or herself. But the second and third principles, beneficence and non-maleficence, stress the need for carers to seek to do good for those they care for and to avoid them coming to harm. So, at some point, doing good for the person with dementia may involve taking over certain decisions in order to avoid harm. Perhaps, because of cognitive impairment, the person's money now needs to be controlled by someone else to avoid financial abuse. Finally, the principle of justice stresses the need to treat people fairly. So resources to help people with dementia should be distributed evenly, or at least in a fair manner (albeit what is considered fair in one political system may not be considered fair elsewhere).

The principles of medical ethics give us a framework within which to discuss moral dilemmas. One of the complaints about these principles, however, is that they do not give us a way to decide between them. Perhaps someone thinks Mrs Jones should be left to make her own decisions about whether or not she commits suicide (i.e. her autonomy should be respected), while someone else feels that compulsory treatment would do her good (i.e. beneficence) and avoid her coming to unnecessary harm (i.e. non-maleficence). The difficulty of deciding between principles seems intractable.

Ethics of Care

In response to the messiness of moral decision-making in the real world, a new approach to ethics has emerged from practice[3]. Whereas the more traditional theories stress calculations of pleasure, rules and principles (they also seem to hold out the possibility of *definitive* answers), the newer approach stresses context and the nature of our relationships within contexts of care. The move from rules to relationships has been regarded as a key feature of feminist ethics. But there have been several such approaches – communicative ethics, narrative ethics, hermeneutic ethics, situation ethics – all of which stress the importance of person-to-person interactions and the nature of our interdependency[1,3]. For any given situation the key elements in deciding the right thing to do will be the nature of the communication, the way in which the stories of those concerned (the actors) interact, the meaning of the events viewed from different perspectives with different interpretations, and so forth. This can lead to the conclusion that there are no definite answers in ethics, because (for any given case) we shall always be told that it depends on the details of the context and the perspective. But, to my mind, this is too relativist, as if anything goes and nothing can be called right or wrong. Rather than say that no 'definite' answers can be given, I should rather say that the answers are not 'definitive' in the sense that they are not final and unconditional. They are revisable and open to new interpretation.

Casuistry

Being open to appeal in the light of new evidence is the approach of casuistry, which considers matters case by case, where the factual details of the case must be understood and those making decisions must immerse themselves in them, but where cases are then compared to sentinel or paradigm cases, where decisions have already been made[4]. Appeal is then made to appropriate moral principles to explain the important moral distinctions between cases, but it is always left open that decisions might be revised in the light of alternative information. Thus, the casuistic process underpins law, allowing a development of legal thought in response to new cases, but with reference to established principles. The same holds for clinical decisions, which tend to be (at one and the same time) both practical and ethical. As with other types of care ethics, casuistry pays attention to the fine-grained details of individual circumstances, which will have a determining effect on our judgements about what might seem either right or wrong in a given case.

Virtue Theory

Virtue ethics draws on a long tradition going back to Aristotle and is based on the idea that the right or good thing is that which the virtuous person would do[5]. Hence, in the case of Mrs Jones, it would be appropriate to look towards those we consider to be good (in the sense of virtuous) in order to decide matters. Although virtue ethics is a well-established ethical theory, it has much in common with the ideas that come from the ethics of care. This is partly because the very notion of 'care' reflects important virtues – compassion or charity – that lie at the heart of clinical practice. In addition, it would not be a virtuous thing to make an ethical decision in a particular instance without being aware of the details of the case.

Some people complain that making a decision about who is virtuous is just too subjective: we might differ in our opinions. This is true, but the fundamental claim of virtue theory is that there are features of the world on which we can agree, even if there is potential disagreement about how these considerations apply in particular cases. Thus, we can agree that we do well as human beings, we 'flourish', if we are brave, compassionate, honest, trustworthy, just and so on. We would not, after all, usually seek advice from someone whom we regarded as cowardly, malicious, dishonest or untrustworthy. In particular, we would want them to be prudent or to show practical wisdom, one of the other virtues highlighted by Aristotle, so that they had a good grasp of the ends at which we should be aiming in our clinical decisions and of how to achieve those ends. We might want to argue about whether a particular decision is just and compassionate, and we need practical wisdom to decide when, for example, to be brave; but in all such cases we are then arguing about the virtues and about what it might be to flourish as a human being. In a sense, then, virtue ethics stresses neither consequences, nor rules or duties, but what we *become* by what we do.

We shall do the right thing for Mrs Jones if we approach her with compassion, with empathic understanding; but we may be required to show steadfastness, to insist she is treated against her wishes on the grounds of our experience (or practical knowledge), which suggests that people with even severe depressions can be helped and that it is certainly worth trying to do so. Similarly, the person with dementia may require a good deal of honesty and integrity to be shown towards him in order that he might comply with decisions being made about his care. It may be that the manner of our dealings with those we care for is crucial and this also falls under the description of the virtues: we can do things in a way that shows basic human charity, or we can behave crassly.

Patterns of Practice

How does all of this come together in terms of our day to day actions and decisions? We do not, after all, routinely consider ourselves to be making ethical decisions. The emphasis on care and virtue ethics, however, helps to underscore the important point that clinical decisions are by their nature ethical: we cannot escape the reach of values in what we do, even in the case of making a diagnosis. An especially good example of this is making a diagnosis of mild cognitive impairment (MCI), which might seem like a benign activity, but is underpinned by a raft of value judgements and ethical concerns[6]. Hence, we should look at our normal patterns of practice since these provide evidence of our values and presumptions[3,7].

Does this mean, however, that just any old patterns of practice will do? On my view the clear imperative is that our patterns of practice should show both internal and external coherence[7]. Internal coherence relies on casuistry: does this decision in these particular circumstances cohere with similar decisions I have made in the past and, if not, what are the morally different aspects of the case that allow me to make the different decision? External coherence is based on acknowledgement of the virtues: does this decision square with the virtues? In other words, can I demonstrate that this is the sort of decision someone would have to make in order to flourish or do well as a human being? In the next section, we shall gesture at how this might work in particular cases.

ETHICS AND THE PERSON

There is, however, one final plank to put into place, which concerns our notion of personhood.

Person-Centred Ethics

Since the seminal work of Tom Kitwood[8], the notion of person-centredness has become ubiquitous in dementia care. This is a broad notion that is, in fact, co-terminous with a number of other types of care: patient-, family-, relationship- and client-centred care all share a number of characterizing themes. They all emphasize: respect for individuality and values, attention to meaning, social context and relationships, an inclusive model of health and well-being, the importance of lay knowledge, the idea of shared responsibility, communication, respect for autonomy and the notion of the professional as a person[9]. Person-centred care, therefore, suggests a broad conception of the person, one that allows and encourages a holistic view, that sees the person as situated in a variety of fields (biological, psychological, social, spiritual, legal, cultural, historical and so forth) and also as an embodied agent: neither simply a disembodied spirit, nor just physical matter[10]. This is the broad view of the person that should underpin our thoughts about our patterns of practice. In occupying this place, it underpins the notion of person-centred ethics too; that is, an approach to ethics that places decisions and actions in the context of the person, where this context is drawn broadly. Some examples should help to make this plain.

Case Study 1

Mr Phipps lives alone and develops the delusion that he is being watched because a neighbour thinks he is a paedophile. He believes there is a conspiracy to kill him by poisoning his food. So he'll only eat food if he can be absolutely sure of its source. He becomes socially withdrawn and gradually loses weight. A decision will have to be made about when to intervene because he will not comply with medication or outside help, although he does not object to seeing health professionals.

The broad notion of person-centred ethics supports the view that Mr Phipps should be taken seriously. He needs to feel he has the support of those who want to help him. They must try to understand how he acquired his odd beliefs. It might be there is a way to pacify his concerns, partly by understanding his social and cultural background. But carers must take seriously his physical and mental health needs too. They will have to be aware that at some stage his physical health will be compromised by his behaviour and so compulsory treatment may become an option. In judging their practices with respect to Mr Phipps, health care workers should be considering the need to approach him with compassion, honesty and integrity. Without these virtues, their practice will not demonstrate external coherence. They might consider, too, how their

management of Mr Phipps coheres with their management of similar cases. Why have they not yet used compulsory powers to enforce treatment as they have done before? Well, perhaps it is because Mr Phipps continues to eat so that his physical condition is not yet as precarious. Or perhaps they feel that they are slowly but surely establishing rapport–not achieved in former cases–which might negate the need for compulsory treatment. Thus, person-centredness and an approach that considers practice in terms of internal and external coherence provides room for a thorough account of the ethical justification for the actions taken, but always against the background possibility that things might need to be re-evaluated, either because of a change in Mr Phipps's state, or because of an alteration in the context that surrounds him.

In many places risk assessment has become the preoccupation of health care managers to the detriment of overall clinical care.

Case Study 2

Mrs Hayward has a moderate to severe Alzheimer's dementia and her family has taken the unhappy decision that she needs to be looked after in a private nursing home. She settles into the home quite quickly and soon becomes very friendly with a man, who also has dementia, whom she refers to as her husband (who had died six years previously). She frequently directs him into her bedroom and one day the staff find him there in a state of undress. A risk assessment concludes that she is at risk of being sexually assaulted by the man, so – since he does not have family whereas Mrs Hayward's have complained – he is moved to a different wing of the home.

This might seem like a perfectly reasonable solution to a potentially difficult situation and one that many health care professionals might endorse. However, it is important that we know the details of the case before we can make this judgement. From the mere outline of the story we do not yet know the thoughts of the main actors in this narrative. Even in the moderate to severe stages we know that people with dementia are able to convey meaning and present them-*selves* precisely as persons[11]. We need to take this person-centred view. On the same ground, we need to consider the value of the relationship for both Mrs Hayward and her friend. Even when people with dementia cannot make choices based on full recollection of their past values or wishes, they can still be valuers[12]. But this potentially sexual relationship is not the only relationship in which Mrs Hayward is situated, for the feelings of her family are not completely irrelevant to our estimation of what is right and wrong. They know more of her history, of her previous beliefs and wishes, all of which must be relevant. It is noteworthy that all of this takes us a long way from mere 'risk assessment', which should now be seen in the context of a fuller approach to the person as a whole.

Having taken a broad and detailed view of Mrs Hayward's standing as a person in this particular context, we can then attempt to judge the decision to move her friend against both similar decisions we might have made in the past and against the broader canvas of the virtues. We need, at least (even if the answer will be negative), to ask whether there might have been a more compassionate or prudent way to deal with the problem. The legal framework for such a decision would be to assess the capacity or competence of those involved to make this particular decision and, if it is deemed they lack capacity, a decision should be made in the person's best interests. But the point has to be made repeatedly that this does not mean assessing her best *medical* interests, it means taking a broad view, which reflects the broad nature of our standing as persons in worldly contexts.

ETHICS AND RESEARCH

Making decisions for others and doing what is best for them are issues that come to the fore in connection with research. Many people lack capacity to consent to participate in research and research is often unlikely to benefit the person individually. This has led, therefore, to a good deal of consideration of the use of surrogates to make decisions for people who are incompetent. Some have also argued that advance directives might be useful as a way to record a person's competent wishes. A surrogate is usually approached to find out what the person is likely to have thought about entering research. And it is usually regarded as good practice to try to seek the person's assent even if they cannot give full consent[13].

For people who lack capacity to consent, research should only be on the condition that affects them. This reflects the principle derived from the philosopher Kant, that people should always be treated as 'ends in themselves' and never as mere means. If the person cannot consent, there should either be some likelihood of benefit, or any harm should be (according to the Mental Capacity Act that covers these matters in England and Wales) 'negligible'. Once again, however, judgements will need to be made about what is appropriate and in keeping with standard and acceptable patterns of practice. The requirement that ethical approval should be sought from an established research ethics committee is one way in which patterns of good practice can be assured.

CONCLUSION

This brief overview has attempted to show the connections that hold together ethics and law in connection with mental health care for older people. What we see are patterns of practice that derive their strength from their coherence. In one direction this points towards the internal coherence of our decisions and actions one with another, where differences need to be justified in terms of established moral precepts. In the other direction we are impelled towards the virtues, where our actions must cohere with those inner dispositions (the virtues) that help to define what would constitute a flourishing human life. Underpinning our understanding of our practices, however, is a broad and complex notion of personhood, which provides the context in which we make decisions.

This framework, it can be argued, forms the basis of a moral and legal approach to health care. It is especially pertinent to the health care of older people, where mental ill health increases the person's vulnerability.

This is most distinctly seen, perhaps, as the person approaches death. When palliative care becomes appropriate, our patterns of practice must tend towards an acceptance of the concrete realities of the situation and life should not be prolonged; but neither should it be shortened. For this would rock the basis of our established social and legal practices, predicated on respect for the dignity of the human person broadly conceived, which prohibit the taking of innocent human lives.

REFERENCES

1. Ashcroft RE, Dawson A, Draper H, McMillan JR (eds). *Principles of Health Care Ethics*, 2nd edn. Chichester: John Wiley & Sons, 2007.
2. Beauchamp TL, Childress JF. *Principles of Biomedical Ethics*, 5th edn. Oxford: Oxford University Press, 2001.
3. Hughes JC, Baldwin C. *Ethical Issues in Dementia Care: Making Difficult Decisions*. London: Jessica Kingsley, 2006.
4. Murray TH. Medical ethics, moral philosophy and moral tradition. In Fulford, KWM, Gillett G, Soskice JM (eds), *Medicine and Moral Reasoning*. Cambridge: Cambridge University Press, 1994, 91–105.
5. Hursthouse R. *On Virtue Ethics*. Oxford: Oxford University Press, 1999.
6. Moreira T, Hughes JC, Kirkwood T, May C, McKeith I, Bond J. What explains variations in the clinical use of mild cognitive impairment (MCI) as a diagnostic category? *Int Psychogeriatr* 2008; **20**: 697–709.
7. Hughes JC. Patterns of practice: a useful notion in medical ethics? *J Ethics Ment Health* 2006; **1**: 1–5.
8. Baldwin C, Capstick A (eds). *Tom Kitwood on Dementia: A Reader and Critical Commentary*. New York: McGraw-Hill; Maidenhead, Berks: Open University Press, 2007.
9. Hughes JC, Bamford C, May C. Types of centredness in health care: themes and concepts. *Med Health Care Philos* 2008; **11**: 455–63.
10. Hughes JC. Views of the person with dementia. *J Med Ethics* 2001; **27**: 86–91.
11. Sabat SR. *The Experience of Alzheimer's Disease: Life Through a Tangled Veil*. Oxford; Blackwell, 2001.
12. Jaworska A. Respecting the margins of agency: Alzheimer's patients and the capacity to value. *Philos Public Affairs* 1999; **28**: 105–38.
13. Hughes JC, Haimes E, Summerville L, Davies K, Collerton J, Kirkwood T. Consenting older adults: research as a virtuous relationship. In Corrigan O, Liddell K, McMillan J, Richards M, Weijer C (eds), *The Limits of Consent – A Socio-Ethical Approach to Human Subject Research in Medicine*. Oxford: Oxford University Press, 2009, 133–49.

124

The US System of Geriatric Mental Health Care: Financing and Future Challenges

Stephen J. Bartels

Dartmouth Centers for Health and Aging, Dartmouth Medical School, Lebanon, NH, USA

INTRODUCTION

The ageing of the 'baby boomer' generation will result in nearly 15 million older adults with mental illness by 2030, dramatically challenging the nation's capacity to adequately serve this population[1]. Further compounding this challenge is a fragmented mental health service delivery system for older adults, a paucity of providers trained in geriatrics and insufficient financing of mental health services under Medicare and Medicaid[2,3]. Major financing and regulatory policy reforms are necessary to provide older adults with the array of services they need.

This overview of the US mental health services delivery system for older adults reflects the assumption that 'form follows finance'. In this chapter, we provide an analysis of the major issues pertaining to mental health policy and ageing, with a focus on: (a) financing geriatric mental health services and (b) future policy directions and challenges.

FINANCING GERIATRIC MENTAL HEALTH SERVICES

Medicare and Medicaid are the primary financiers of the US system of geriatric mental health services. Structured into the delivery of Medicare and Medicaid services are several key components including: (a) Medicare beneficiaries and expenditures; (b) Medicare's benefit design including fee-for-service and managed care arrangements; (c) the emergence of managed Medicare, the Balanced Budget Act of 1997 and Medicare Part C; (d) Medicare Part D prescription drug coverage; (e) dually eligible Medicaid and Medicare beneficiaries; and (f) Medicaid beneficiaries and expenditures. The following sections provide an overview of each area including historical context and current issues.

Medicare Beneficiaries and Expenditures

Medicare is a federally funded health insurance programme. It was enacted in 1965 under President Johnson to cover health care for the elderly. Medicare benefits expanded in 1972 to include coverage of the disabled and individuals with chronic renal failure. Approximately 95% of older Americans receive Medicare health insurance[4]. Medicare comprises the second largest social insurance programme in the United States after social security[5]. In 2008 Medicare expenditures amounted to $468 billion and covered 45.2 million Americans, including 37.8 million individuals aged 65 years and older[6].

Medicare's Benefit Design for Mental Health Services: Fee-for-Service and Managed Care Arrangements

Medicare consists of four components (Parts A, B, C and D). This section reviews the four components of Medicare along with legislation enacted to restore parity in the administration of Medicare mental health benefits.

The fee-for-service (FFS) Medicare insurance programme covering health services is composed of two components (Part A and B). Part A, typically referred to as Hospital Insurance, covers inpatient psychiatric hospital care (up to 190 days lifetime maximum) and partial hospitalization[7]. Part A also covers hospice and home health-care services. Part B, or Medical Insurance, covers medically necessary physician and related ancillary services.

Medicare reimbursement policies have historically posed challenges for older adults and disabled persons seeking outpatient mental health services. Prior to the mid-1980s, Medicare payment policies supported reimbursement for acute inpatient care while restricting payments for outpatient services[8]. Restrictions on outpatient services included a $500 annual cap for outpatient psychotherapy, in conjunction with requiring a 50% co-payment. The Omnibus Budget Reconciliation Act of 1987 (OBRA-87) increased the $500 cap for psychotherapy reimbursement to $2200, yet retained the 50% co-payment. OBRA-87 also exempted medical evaluation and management of psychotropic medications from an annual cap. Subsequently, the Omnibus Budget Reconciliation Act of 1989 (OBRA-89) eliminated the annual cap on psychotherapy, yet retained the 50% co-payment[9]. Sustaining the discriminatory policy of a 50% co-payment for psychotherapy services set the stage for the Stark–Wellstone Medicare Mental Health Modernization Act of 2001 aimed at achieving mental health parity. This act was essential to the future development and enactment of legislation that restored parity in the delivery of mental health services.

In honor of the late Senator Paul Wellstone, the Wellstone–Domenici Mental Health Parity and Addiction Act (MHPAEA) was enacted in October 2008. MHPAEA required equal coverage for mental health and physical health care in group health plans by 2010. According to MHPAEA, equal coverage includes annual and lifetime limits, deductibles, co-payments, number of visits and other similar coverage requirements[10]. Although MHPAEA does not apply to Medicare beneficiaries, it does apply to Medicaid managed care health plans. Medicaid beneficiaries have access to mental health and substance abuse services at parity with other medical benefits[11].

Enactment of the Medicare Improvements for Patients and Providers Act (MIPPA) of 2008 restored parity in the delivery of mental health services to Medicare beneficiaries. Prior to MIPPA, Medicare beneficiaries were subject to a 50% co-payment for outpatient mental health services (but only 20% for medical services). Following enactment of MIPPA, co-payments for mental health services will be reduced to 45% in 2010, 40% in 2012, 35% in 2013, finally reaching parity with medical co-payments of 20% in 2014[11]. This legislation represents a major step towards eliminating the barriers that older adults face in accessing mental health services.

The Emergence of Managed Medicare, The Balanced Budget Act of 1997 and Medicare Part C

Managed care programmes were developed to control the escalating costs of delivering quality care to Medicare beneficiaries. This section provides an overview of managed care and legislation aimed at controlling Medicare expenditures. This section also includes a review of Medicare Part C.

The Balanced Budget Act (BBA-97) of 1997 made significant changes in the payment methodology to Medicare Risk Contracting (MRC) plans. Medicare Part C also introduced managed care alternatives to fee-for-service Medicare. In addition, Medicare Part C, or 'Medicare + Choice', expanded Medicare to health maintenance organizations, preferred provider organizations, provider sponsored organizations, religious fraternal benefit plans, private fee-for-service plans, point-of-service plans, PACE (Programs of All-Inclusive Care for the Elderly) and medical savings plans[12]. However, due to the Plans' inability to manage payments to providers, in addition to modest increases in Medicare plan payments, many providers left the programme. The result spurred an increase in premiums with a reduction in benefits[13]. New legislation became necessary to restore Medicare Part C and patient choice.

In 2003, President Bush signed into law the Medicare Prescription Drug, Improvement and Modernization Act (MMA) (Pub. L. 108-173). MMA expanded the role of private health plans through prescription drug plans and renamed Medicare + Choice to 'Medicare Advantage'[13]. The enactment of MMA enabled Medicare beneficiaries to choose from a variety of health plan options, including regional preferred provider organizations (PPO), health maintenance organizations (HMO), Medicare Special Needs Plans, Medical Savings Accounts (MSAs) and traditional fee-for-service (FFS) Medicare. The legislation also included a prescription drug benefit that allowed beneficiaries to choose among competing prescription drug plans. Although many Medicare Advantage plans offer mental health coverage to beneficiaries (coverage typically consists of a maximum of 20 outpatient visits and 30 hospital days per calendar year), most plans do not cover chronic mental illness in their standard benefit package. Despite the original intent of containing costs through competition by private insurance plans, Medicare Advantage has been characterized as government subsidization of health insurance companies at higher than average costs. In 2009, Medicare Advantage Plans have come under scrutiny by the Obama Administration as a potential source of savings[14].

Medicare Part D Prescription Drug Coverage

The major impact of MMA was the introduction of Medicare Part D and the provision of a prescription drug benefit under fee-for-service Medicare. The implementation of Medicare Part D was meant to protect beneficiaries from the increasing cost of drug expenditures and to reduce costs associated with the underuse of medications[15]. In this section the implementation of Medicare Part D is reviewed along with suggested strategies to improve the delivery of prescription coverage to beneficiaries.

The introduction of Medicare Part D was largely welcomed as a means to address a longstanding lack of coverage for prescribed medications, yet presented specific challenges in covering psychiatric medications. Approximately 25% of Medicare beneficiaries are treated with psychiatric medications[16] that are prescribed on a long-term basis. Some insurers, in an attempt to manage costs, initially provided Part D formularies with restrictions to discourage individuals with psychiatric disorders from enrolling in plans. Despite Part D guidelines intended to ensure patient access to prescribed medications, administrative tactics prohibited some beneficiaries from obtaining medication. Tactics included limited formularies, extensive use of prior authorization and step therapy requirements. Part D plans also included the preferred use of less costly medications, although many were inappropriate for older adults according to Beer's criteria[17].

Despite the welcome coverage of medication prescriptions, clinical providers experienced significant administrative burden with the implementation of Medicare Part D. For example, with some plans, every hour of direct patient care resulted in approximately an hour of administrative time[18]. Additionally, some psychiatrists reported making medication decisions based on whether exceptions or appeals would need to be pursued. Some also avoided patients whose care would entail higher administrative costs. These unintended consequences associated with the administrative burden of Medicare Part D have been cited as potential sources of compromised quality of care for some patients with psychiatric illness, an already vulnerable group[18].

Recent changes have been implemented to improve the administration of Part D. According to a 2009 Medpac-funded report the minimum cost for specialty tiered drugs was raised to $600 a month. Since long-term users of specialty tiered drugs reach the maximum relatively quickly, they also qualify for catastrophic coverage. Federal reinsurance limits the beneficiary's expense by paying 80% of costs once they qualify for catastrophic coverage[19]. Finally, the recently passed health-care reform legislation will result in removing the "donut hole" gap for covering costs of medications in excess of $2,830 and up to $4,550 by the year 2020.

Dually Eligible Medicaid and Medicare Beneficiaries

Some older adults are eligible for both Medicare and Medicaid benefits. This population of individuals is referred to as 'dually eligible'. This section provides an overview of the dually eligible population including estimates of expenditures for individuals with serious mental illness (SMI) (including schizophrenia, bipolar disorder and treatment refractory depression).

Many dually eligible beneficiaries are over the age of 65, have significant disabilities and often have fewer financial resources than the average Medicare beneficiary. According to a 2008 report by MedPac, dually eligible beneficiaries account for a disproportionate amount of Medicare spending. Dually eligible beneficiaries account for 16% of Medicare beneficiaries and 25% of Medicare spending. Medicare spends 1.8 times more on dually eligible beneficiaries as compared to non-dually eligible beneficiaries. According to MedPac, $6212 is spent per non-dually eligible beneficiary while $10 994 is spent per dually eligible beneficiary. An assessment of total spending (including Medicare, Medicaid, supplemental insurance, and out of pocket spending) on dually eligible beneficiaries averaged about $23 554 per person in 2005. This amount is more than twice the amount of other Medicare beneficiaries[20]. Similarly, the dually eligible beneficiaries comprise a major portion (42%) of Medicaid spending[21].

A 2003 study of Medicaid and Medicare dually eligible expenditures indicated that the highest per capita spending was on older beneficiaries with schizophrenia. According to this report, dually eligible beneficiaries age 65 and older with depression cost roughly $27 850, while beneficiaries with dementia and schizophrenia cost $39 154. Conversely, beneficiaries in this age cohort without mental illness generated a per capita cost of $10 898. Per capita spending by diagnosis increases with age. This study indicates a greater service need and cost for dually eligible older adults (age 65 and older) with mental illness[22].

Medicaid Beneficiaries and Expenditures

While Medicare covers a portion of health-care expenditures for the elderly, the Medicaid programme also provides additional benefits and services to some older adults. This section provides an overview of this joint federal–state Medicaid programme which represents one of the largest public health-care insurers in the United States. Medicaid delivers health-care services to poor, blind or disabled individuals, including individuals with serious mental illness. People with SMI may also be covered by Medicaid. Total Medicaid expenditures in 2007 were $333.2 billion. In 2007 57% of Medicaid expenditures were federally financed (190.6 billion), while 43% (142.6 billion) were financed by state funding[23]. By mid-2007, 61.9 million people (one in every five people in the US) were enrolled in Medicaid. Spending on individual beneficiaries averaged an estimated $6120 in 2007. Although older adults and disabled people represent less than a third of Medicaid enrollees, almost three-quarters of the Medicaid budget is expended on this population of beneficiaries[21]. Adults 65 and older covered by Medicaid averaged $14 058 per beneficiary, while disabled persons averaged $14 858 per beneficiary[23].

A considerable amount of Medicaid spending is dedicated to long-term care services in a variety of settings. In 2006, approximately one-third of Medicaid expenditures were for long-term care, including care in nursing homes, as well as home and community-based services (HCBS)[24]. Although nursing home care for adults is an area that Medicaid is required to cover, states may choose whether or not to cover alternative models of community-based long-term care services such as PACE or services for older adults in mental institutions[21]. Medicaid is also accountable for a significant share of the cost of mental health services. In 2001 Medicaid payments comprised more than one-quarter of all mental health expenditures, including both private and public payers. No other payer, including Medicare, spent more on mental health services[25].

Variability in the structure and design of the Medicaid programme limits generalizations that apply to the entire system of care. Many states differ with respect to eligibility criteria (particularly with the dually eligible Medicare–Medicaid population), breadth of coverage for inpatient and outpatient mental health services, prescription coverage, arrangement of co-payments, pre-authorization guidelines for inpatient and outpatient services, and managed care options. A common attribute of most Medicaid programmes, however, is a 20–30% reduction in reimbursement rates for procedures and services relative to the standard fee-for-service charges[26].

Each state is provided the opportunity to administer Medicaid benefits in novel ways through the implementation of 1115(a) waivers or demonstration projects. The Secretary of Health and Human Services, via Section 1115(a), may approve demonstration projects that are time limited to test and evaluate entrepreneurial approaches to delivering and financing health care. According to the Centers for Medicaid and Medicare Services (CMS), many states use Section 1115(a) waivers to implement Medicaid. Various project areas include designing state-based models for eligibility determination, administration, delivery systems, coverage and benefits, quality assurance, access, systems support, financing issues, implementation time frames and evaluation. Demonstration projects typically last for five years and may be renewed for an additional period of time. Also, demonstration projects must remain 'budget neutral', meaning projects cannot cost the federal government more to implement the project than it would cost without the waiver[27].

FUTURE CHALLENGES IN MENTAL HEALTH POLICY AND AGEING

Over the past three decades policy and legislative endeavours have shaped the current financing and delivery system for older adults with mental illness. There are numerous future challenges in mental health policy that will require targeted efforts to meet the needs of an ageing America. Among the most pressing include: (a) Medicare's impending insolvency and health-care reform; (b) implementing integrated mental and physical health care and a true 'medical home'; (c) the changing landscape of long-term care on the increasing need for home and community-based options; (d) the ageing of the population with serious mental illness (SMI); (e) addressing the workforce gap in geriatric providers; and (f) bridging the gap between research, practice and policy.

Medicare's Impending Insolvency and Health Care Reform

According to a 2009 federal report, Medicare will be insolvent by 2017[6]. At the current growth in expenditures, Medicare and Medicaid are predicted to consume 15% of the gross domestic product (GDP) by 2040[28]. Part of the challenge of financing Medicare is directly associated with the demographic realities of an ageing US population.

Older age is associated with increasing episodes of acute medical care (including hospitalizations, surgical procedures and home health care). Older adults constitute a group that have a high risk for needing intensive and expensive services, resulting in 'adverse selection' for individuals with high insurance premium costs. For example, insurance plans (such as Medicare) that primarily target older adults are much more likely to selectively attract patients who present a higher financial risk, and less likely to have the capacity to spread the risk over healthier beneficiaries who are less costly. In addition, older adults disproportionately represent beneficiaries with low incomes. Approximately one-quarter of older adults are at or near the poverty level, including 16% living in poverty and an additional 9% living between poverty and 125% of the poverty level[29]. Finally, the shifting demographic profile associated with the 'greying of America' is resulting in growing numbers of adults reaching retirement age, at the same time that there are proportionately fewer younger adults paying into the Medicare trust fund through employment contributions. When Medicare was enacted in 1965, there were approximately 18.2 older adults for every 100 working age adults. This 'old-age dependency ratio' is projected to climb to 20.9 in 2010, 27.0 in 2020, 34.9 in 2030 and potentially increase to 42.1 older dependents for every 100 workers in 2080[30].

In addition to demographic realities, the predicted insolvency of Medicare is also due to escalating health-care expenditures. Current reform efforts identify regional variations in spending that account for higher costs without better health outcomes. For example, from 1992 to 2006 Medicare spending (adjusted for inflation) grew 3.5% annually. By comparison, spending in Miami, Florida rose by 5%, contrasted with a 2.3% increase in Medicare spending in Salem, Oregon. Similarly, 2007 per capita Medicare spending averaged $12 100 in Manhattan, New York, compared to $6 700 in Minneapolis, Minnesota (31). Higher cost regions are generally associated with fewer primary care physicians, greater numbers of specialists, more spending on discretionary procedures, greater use of intensive care units in the last six months of life and poorer health outcomes[32]. *The Dartmouth Atlas of Healthcare* estimates that reducing annual per capita growth in spending from the current national average of 3.5% to 2.4% would result in a savings of $1.42 trillion, leaving Medicare with a positive balance of $758 billion in 2023 in contrast to the predicted $660 billion deficit[31].

Accountable Care Organizations (health-care systems that are rewarded for high-quality care and lower expenditures) have been proposed in the recently passed health-care reform legislation as one example of a potential model for achieving savings and improving care. However, the structure, financing and role of mental health care in plans for health-care reform will need to be identified to ensure compliance and the delivery of effective care.

Integrated Mental and Physical Health Care and the 'Medical Home'

Conventional mental health services have been organized and financed by 'carving out' care into separate settings, providers and financing that is distinct from general medical care. This separation has been promoted as a means to support the integrity and financing of specialty mental health care. However, it also has been identified as a potential barrier to holistic care that incorporates the interaction of physical and mental health in overall outcomes. Collaborative models of physical and mental health treatment have been proven to result in improved outcomes in primary care[33], home health care[34] and long-term care[35]. Older adults with depression who receive integrated care not only have lower aggregate health-care costs over several years of follow-up[36], but also indicate signs of improved survival, quality of life and patient satisfaction[2]. Studies have also shown that patients with substance abuse related medical conditions who receive integrated care have reduced hospitalizations, inpatient stays, emergency room use and medical costs[37].

A historical barrier to integrating mental and physical healthcare has been the lack of appropriate financing mechanisms. Prior to 1 January 2008, only physicians were permitted to use Current Procedural Terminology (CPT) billing codes that indicated time spent conferring with providers from other disciplines regarding patient care. New CPT codes permit psychologists and other non-physician providers to bill for integrated team conferences[11]. The next step needed in reforming billing is to allow for same-day billing of mental and physical health services 'incident to' a single primary care provider. This change will enable individuals to access physical and mental health care that is integrated, concurrent, co-located and simultaneously addresses the needs and preferences of the whole person.

'Medical home' is a term first coined by the American Academy of Pediatrics in 1967. In a medical home responsibility for care and the coordination of services is in the hands of the patient, family members, a personal medical provider and a medical team. The teams are formed according to patient needs and may include specialists, nurses, social workers, care managers, dieticians, pharmacists, occupational therapists and the community[38]. Key attributes of the medical home include: (a) the use of evidence-based practice and clinical outcome tools to guide joint decision making; (b) an organized process of care coordinated under a single primary care provider that incorporates principles of the Chronic Care Model (CCM); (c) development of an integrated plan of care that connects patients and families to a team of support; and (d) delivery of advanced care through multiple venues including face-to-face, email and telephone communications[38]. Research suggests that medical homes have a significant impact on societal health as they improve medical standards, patient experiences and outcomes[38]. The use of medical homes in the delivery of integrated care may further improve outcomes for older adults with SMI. Policy makers will need to promote greater integration of mental health in primary health care and inclusion of mental health providers in the development of primary care delivery modelled on the concept of a 'medical home'.

The Changing Landscape of Long-Term Care: Home and Community-Based Options

The Olmstead decision enacted by the Supreme Court in 1999 regulated federal policy regarding the inappropriate and unnecessary placement of individuals with disabilities into institutions[39]. States were required to assess thousands of individuals living in psychiatric institutions and nursing homes to conclude whether they could receive care in a community-based setting[40]. However, the lack of community-based residential options for older adults with serious mental disorders is a barrier to complying with the Olmstead mandate[41].

The increasing demand for alternatives to nursing homes is demonstrated by the development of continuing care communities, assisted living facilities, home health-care options and community-based ageing network services. Despite the growing demand for home and community-based services (HCBS), occupancy rates at nursing home facilities have remained constant between 2002–7, and 73% of long-term care Medicaid dollars went to nursing home facilities in 2007[42]. Medicaid spending on HCBS was reported at $17 billion for older and disabled persons while nursing home spending totaled $47 billion. However, the proportion of Medicaid expenditures for HCBS versus nursing homes varies considerably by state. For example, in 2007 New Mexico spent 61% of its Medicaid long-term care budget on HCBS. In contrast Tennessee spent only 1% of the Medicaid long-term care budget on HCBS[42]. Overall, Medicaid spending on HCBS has increased by 68% over the past five years as the number of older and disabled individuals receiving HCBS services has increased to 1.4 million in 2005[42]. The growing demand for HCBS substantially exceeds budgeted resources for home and community-based long-term care alternatives. For example, an estimated 90 000 people were on waitlists for HCBS waiver programmes in 2007[42].

To accommodate the future needs and preferences of older adults, health-care reform will need to shift financial incentives away from supporting nursing homes as preferred long-term care settings to provide incentives for developing an array of HCBS options. In order to be successful these policy initiatives will also need to include financing for integrated mental health services within home and community-based services.

The Ageing of the Population with Serious Mental Illness

The ageing of the population of persons with SMI is challenging state-supported services across the nation to develop and finance an array of services aimed at older adults with schizophrenia, schizoaffective disorder, bipolar disorder and treatment refractory depression. Per capita combined Medicaid and Medicare expenditures for disorders such as schizophrenia in older adults (age 65–74) are over 3.5 times greater than expenditures for dually eligible Medicaid and Medicare beneficiaries receiving services for a medical diagnosis only (without a co-occurring psychiatric disorder)[43]. One of the primary drivers of higher expenditures is the association of SMI with higher rates of institution-based long-term care. Nearly two-thirds of older adults with SMI are hospitalized or admitted to a nursing home annually. Middle-aged and older adults with schizophrenia are three times more likely to be admitted to a nursing home than adults without SMI[44]. Medicaid beneficiaries with schizophrenia are admitted to nursing homes nearly 13 years earlier than other Medicaid beneficiaries (age 65 versus age 78)[45]. Finally, adults with SMI have a 25–30-year shorter lifespan than the general population, presenting a dramatic health disparity associated with the need for improved health care and attention to prevention and health promotion as a core component of quality mental health services[46].

Effective interventions exist for older adults with SMI[47]. A reorganization of the mental health services system must take into account the leading factors attributed to high rates of institutionalization among the SMI population including: poor social skills and supports; high medical co-morbidity; and inadequate independent living skills. Mental health services that include age-appropriate psychosocial rehabilitation combined with physical care are likely to reduce health disparities and address the needs of older adults with SMI[48]. New integrated models of care for older adults with SMI will need to be developed and implemented that attend to the combined need for psychosocial rehabilitation and health care addressing the needs of the 'whole person'[47,49].

Addressing the Workforce Gap in Geriatric Providers

As the population ages, current demographic projections for the number of older adults with mental health problems or cognitive impairment indicate that the system of health care will become increasingly unable to deliver effective services to this population[50]. Conversely, projected declines in health-care providers with expertise in geriatrics will pose a serious challenge. For instance, over half of geriatric psychiatry fellowship slots went unfilled in 2006[51]. Recently, the Institute of Medicine (IOM) released a report that underscores the issue of a serious shortfall in the geriatric health-care provider workforce[2]. The American Association of Geriatric Psychiatry (AAGP) has suggested a follow-up study to advocate for loan forgiveness legislation, funding for the Geriatric Health Professions Program, and reform of Medicare to enhance mental health coverage[50].

Several legislative initiatives have been proposed to begin to address the shortfall in the workforce of geriatric health providers. In March 2009, the 'Geriatricians Loan Forgiveness Act' (H.R. 1457) was referred to the House Committee for review[52]. The Act would classify each year a person is enrolled in a geriatric training programme as a year of obligated service under the National Health Service Corp Loan Repayment Program guidelines. Individuals are entitled to repayment of $35 000 in educational loans. Another loan repayment bill, the 'Caring for an Aging America Act of 2008' (S. 2708) would include loan forgiveness as well as other incentives to attract and retain geriatric care providers into the workforce. At the time of this update both bills are under review.

Bridging the Gap Between Research, Practice and Policy

The gap between what we know regarding effective mental health treatment and the services currently offered by health-care providers constitutes a major challenge in improving the effectiveness and efficiency of health care[53,54]. Although a significant array of evidence-based practices (EBPs) are effective in the prevention and treatment of mental disorders[55,56], research has shown that it takes more than a decade to implement findings into the delivery of care[57].

Current initiatives from the National Institute of Mental Health (NIMH), the Substance Abuse and Mental Health Services Administration (SAMHSA) and the Administration on Aging (AoA) are focused on multiplying the availability and use of EBPs[58]. NIMH and SAMHSA have partnered to promote and support the use of evidence-based services in state mental health systems. These strategies and others must continue to expand in order to reduce barriers to implementing EBPs for older adults. Possible areas of focus include increased emphasis on interventions that are designed for use in real-world settings by real-world providers, development of financing options and incentives, improved educational opportunities for health and social service providers and improved understanding of effective dissemination and implementation strategies.

SUMMARY AND CONCLUSION

This chapter summarizes the major components of the Medicare and Medicaid programmes for older adults in the United States with attention to the delivery of mental health services. The most substantial changes to improving the delivery of mental health care to older adults have occurred through the implementation of recent legislation and programming including: (a) the Wellstone–Domenici Mental Health Parity and Addiction Act of 2008; (b) the Balanced Budget Act of 1997, and the Medicare Prescription Drug, Improvement and Modernization Act of 2003; (c) the implementation of Medicare Part D and the provision of prescription drug coverage to older adults; (d) the provision of coverage to beneficiaries dually eligible for Medicaid and Medicare benefits; and (e) the provision of long-term care to older adults through Medicaid, and 1115(a) waivers and demonstration projects aimed at encouraging novel home and community-based Medicaid services.

While the enactment of legislation and programmes have enhanced Medicare and Medicaid services for older adults with SMI, the system still faces many challenges. In order to improve the mental health services that older adults receive, attention must be paid to addressing: (a) Medicare's impending insolvency; (b) integrated care and the 'medical home'; (c) the changing landscape of long-term care with attention to home and community-based options; (d) the ageing of older adults with SMI; (e) the workforce gap in geriatric providers; and (f) the gap between research, practice and policy. Timely and thoughtful attention to each of these issues will not only improve the delivery of mental health care that older adults receive, but may also reduce the current administrative and economic burdens associated with the delivery care. Addressing the future challenges of an ageing America will require innovative approaches to organizing, delivering and financing mental health services as a core component of general health care for older adults.

REFERENCES

1. Jeste DV, Alexopoulos GS, Bartels SJ, Cummings JL, Gallo JJ, Gottlieb GL *et al*. Consensus statement on the upcoming crisis in geriatric mental health: research agenda for the next 2 decades. *Arch Gen Psychiatry* 1999; **56**: 848–53.
2. Institute of Medicine (US), Committee on the Future Health Care Workforce for Older Americans. Retooling for an aging America building the health care workforce, 2008. At http://books.nap.edu/openbook.php?record_id=12089.
3. Bartels SJ, Lebowitz BD, Reynolds CF, Bruce ML, Halpain M, Faison WE *et al*. A model for developing the pipeline of early career geriatric mental health researchers: outcomes and implications for other fields. *Acad Med* 2010; **85**: 26–35.
4. Hoffman ED, Klees BS, Curtis CA. *Brief Summaries of Medicare and Medicaid Title XVIII and Title XIX of the Social Security Act* Centers for Medicare & Medicaid Services, Department of Health and Human Services, 2007.
5. Centers for Medicare and Medicaid Services. *Trustees Report and Trust Fund Overview*. At www.cms.hhs.gov/ReportsTrustFunds, accessed 15 June 2009.
6. The Boards of Trustees, Federal Hospital Insurance and Federal Supplementary Medical Insurance Trust Funds. *2009 Annual Report of the Boards of Trustees of the Federal Hospital Insurance and Federal Supplementary Medical Insurance Trust Funds*, 2009.
7. Centers for Medicare and Medicaid Services. *Your Medicare Benefits*. CMS Publication Number 10116, August 2008.
8. Bartels SJ, Colenda CC. Mental health services for Alzheimer's disease. Current trends in reimbursement and public policy, and the future under managed care. *Am J Geriatr Psychiatry* 1998; **6**: S85–100.
9. Rosenbach ML, Ammering CJ. Trends in Medicare Part B mental health utilization and expenditures: 1987–92. *Health Care Financ Rev* 1997; **18**: 19–42.
10. Centers for Medicare and Medicaid Services. Health Insurance Reform for Consumers: The Mental Health Parity Act, 2009. At www.cms.hhs.gov/healthinsreformforconsume/04_thementalhealthparityact.asp, accessed 14 June 2009.
11. American Psychological Association Presidential Task Force on Integrated Care for an Aging Population. *Blueprint for Change: Achieving Integrated Health Care for an Aging Population*, 2008. At www.apa.org/pi/aging/blueprint.html, accessed 14 June 2009.
12. Geriatrics P. Medicare managed mental health care: a looming crisis. *Psychiatr Serv* 2005; **56**: 795–7.
13. Biles B, Dallek G, Nicholas LH. Medicare advantage: deja vu all over again? *Health Aff (Millwood)* 2004; Suppl Web Exclusives: W4-586-97.
14. DoBias M. Fee-for-service punching bag. As the Obama administration sets out to reform healthcare, Medicare advantage is one of the first and most prominent targets. *Mod Health* 2009; **39**: 6–7.
15. Pauly MV. The new Medicare drug benefit: much ado about little? *LDI Issue Brief* 2004; **9**: 1–6.
16. Rosenberg JM. Overview of Medicare Part D prescription drug benefit: potential implications for patients with psychotic disorders. *Am J Health Syst Pharm* 2007; **64**: S18–23; quiz S24–5.
17. American Society of Consultant Pharmacists. *Letter to CMS from ASCP and Five Other Health Professional Organizations about Medicare Part D and Long-Term Care – Formulary Restrictions and Cost-Management Tools, 2006*. At www.asccp.com/medicarerx/upload/LTSignOnLetter.pdf, accessed 14 June 2009.
18. Wilk JE, West JC, Rae DS, Rubio-Stipec M, Chen JJ, Regier DA. Medicare Part D prescription drug benefits and administrative burden in the care of dually eligible psychiatric patients. *Psychiatr Serv* 2008; **59**: 34–9.
19. Hargrave E, Hoadley J, Merrell K. *Drugs on Specialty Tiers in Part D*, 2009. No. 09-1.
20. MedPac. *A Data Book: Healthcare Spending and the Medicare Program – Dual Eligible Beneficiaries*, 2008.
21. Henderson TM, Wilhide S. Medicaid: overview and policy issues. *Am Fam Physician* 2005. At www.aafp.org/.../aafp.../policy/.../medicaid-overview.../stateadvocacy_MedicaidOverviewandPolicyIssues.pdf.
22. Bartels SJ, Clark RE, Peacock WJ, Dums AR, Pratt SI. Medicare and Medicaid costs for schizophrenia patients by age cohort compared with costs for depression, dementia, and medically ill patients. *Am J Geriatr Psychiatry* 2003; **11**: 648–57.
23. Truffer CJ, Klemm JD, Hoffman ED, Wolfe CJ. *2008 Actuarial Report on the Financial Outlook for Medicaid*, 2008.
24. ASPE. *Residential Care and Assisted Living Compendium. 2007*, 2007.
25. Mark TL, Buck JA. Components of spending for Medicaid Mental Health Services, 2001. *Psychiatr Serv* 2005; **56**: 648.
26. Bartels SJ, Levine KJ, Shea D. Community-based long-term care for older persons with severe and persistent mental illness in an era of managed care. *Psychiatr Serv* 1999; **50**: 1189–97.
27. Centers for Medicare and Medicaid Services. *Research and Demonstration Projects – 1115*, 2005. At www.cms.hhs.gov/MedicaidStWaivProgDemoPGI/03_Research&DemonstrationProjects-Section1115.asp, accessed 14 June 2009.
28. Executive Office of the President Council of Economic Advisers. *The Economic Case for Health Care Reform*, 2009.
29. MedPac. *A Data Book: Healthcare Spending and the Medicare Program – Medicare Beneficiary Demographics*, 2008.
30. The Board of Trustees, Federal Old-Age and Survivors Insurance and Federal Disability Insurance Trust Funds. *The 2006 Annual Report of the Board of Trustees of the Federal Old-Age and Survivors Insurance and Federal Disability Insurance Trust Funds*, 2006; 26–267.
31. Fisher ES, Bynum JP, Skinner JS. Slowing the growth of health care costs – lessons from regional variation. *N Engl J Med* 2009; **360**: 849–52.
32. Wennberg JE, Fisher ES, Goodman DC, Skinner JS. Tracking the care of patients with severe chronic illness. *The Dartmouth Atlas of Health Care*, 2008.
33. Unutzer J, Schoenbaum M, Druss BG, Katon WJ. Transforming mental health care at the interface with general medicine: report for the presidents commission. *Psychiatr Serv* 2006; **57**: 37–47.

34. Bruce ML. Mental health services in home healthcare: opportunities and challenges. *Generations – J Am Soc Aging* 2002; **26**: 78–82.

35. Bartels SJ, Moak GS, Dums AR. Models of mental health services in nursing homes: a review of the literature. *Psychiatr Serv* 2002; **53**: 1390–6.

36. Unutzer J, Katon WJ, Fan MY, Schoenbaum MC, Lin EH, Della Penna RD *et al.* Long-term cost effects of collaborative care for late-life depression. *Am J Manag Care* 2008; **14**: 95–100.

37. Parthasarathy S, Mertens J, Moore C, Weisner C. Utilization and cost impact of integrating substance abuse treatment and primary care. *Med Care* 2003; **41**: 357–67.

38. Barr M, Ginsburg J. *The Advanced Medical Home: A Patient-Centered, Physician-Guided Model of Health Care*. Philadelphia: American College of Physicians, 2006.

39. Williams L. Long-term care after Olmstead v. L.C.: will the potential of the ADA's integration mandate be achieved? *J Contemp Health Law Policy* 2000; **17**: 205–39.

40. National Council for Community Behavioral Healthcare. Olmstead: Department of Health and Human Services Urges Implementation of Olmstead, 2000.

41. Bartels SJ, Van Citters AD. Community-based alternatives for older adults with serious mental illness: the Olmstead decision and deinstitutionalization of nursing homes. *Ethics Law Aging Rev* 2005; **11**: 3–22.

42. Houser A, Fox-Grage W, Gibson MJ. *Across the States: Profiles of Long Term Care and Independent Living*. Washington, DC: AARP Public Policy Institute, 2009.

43. Bartels SJ, Clark RE, Peacock WJ, Dums AR, Pratt SI. Medicare and Medicaid costs for schizophrenia patients by age cohort compared with costs for depression, dementia, and medically ill patients. *Am J Geriatr Psychiatry* 2003; **11**: 648–57.

44. Bartels SJ, Forester B, Miles KM, Joyce T. Mental health service use by elderly patients with bipolar disorder and unipolar major depression. *Am J Geriatr Psychiatry* 2000; **8**: 160–6.

45. Andrews A, Bartels SJ, Xie H, Peacock WJ. Increased risk of nursing home admission among middle aged and older adults with schizophrenia. *Am J Geriatr Psychiatry* 2009; **17**: 697–705.

46. Colton CW, Manderscheid RW. Congruencies in increased mortality rates, years of potential life lost, and causes of death among public mental health clients in eight states. *Prev Chronic Dis* 2006; **3**: A42.

47. Pratt SI, Van Citters AD, Mueser KT. Psychosocial rehabilitation in older adults with serious mental illness: a review of the research literature and recommendations for development of rehabilitative approaches. *Am J Psych Rehab* 2008; **11**: 7–40.

48. Pratt SI, Bartels SJ, Mueser KT, Forester B. Helping older people experience success: an integrated model of psychosocial rehabilitation and health care management for older adults with serious mental illness. *Am J Psych Rehab* 2008; **11**: 41–60.

49. Bartels SJ. Caring for the whole person: integrated health care for older adults with severe mental illness and medical comorbidity. *J Am Geriatr Soc* 2004; **52**: S249–57.

50. Caring for our seniors, US Senate. How can we support those on the frontlines? Hearing before the Special Committee on Aging. 2008.

51. Association of Directors of Geriatric Academic Programs. Fellows in Geriatric Medicine and Geriatric Psychiatry Programs. Training and Practice Update, 2007; **5**(2).

52. Washington Watch. H.R. 1457, The Geriatrics Loan Forgiveness Act of 2009. At http://www.washingtonwatch.com/bills/show/111_HR_1457.html#toc1, accessed 14 June 2009.

53. Institute of Medicine. *Improving the Quality of Health Care for Mental and Substance-Use Conditions: Quality Chasm Series*. New York: National Academies Press, 2006.

54. Bartels SJ. Improving system of care for older adults with mental illness in the United States. Findings and recommendations for the President's New Freedom Commission on Mental Health. *Am J Geriatr Psychiatry* 2003; **11**: 486–97.

55. Bartels SJ, Drake RE. Evidence-based geriatric psychiatry: an overview. *Psych Clin North Am* 2005; **28**: 763–84, vii.

56. Blow FC, Bartels SJ, Brockmann LM. Evidence-based practices for preventing substance abuse and mental health problems in older adults. At www.samhsa.gov/OlderAdultsTAC/SA_MH_%20AmongOlderAdultsfinal102105.pdf, accessed 14 June 2009.

57. Lenfant C. Clinical research to clinical practice – lost in translation? *N Engl J Med* 2003; **349**: 868–74.

58. Substance Abuse and Mental Health Services Administration. *Transforming Mental Health Care in America – The Federal Action Agenda: First Steps*. At: www.samhsa.gov/Federalactionagenda/NFC_execsum.aspx, accessed 14 June 2009.

125

Geriatric Psychiatric Outpatient Care: The Private Practice Model in the USA

Elliott M. Stein[1] and Gary S. Moak[2]

[1]*Jewish Home of San Francisco San Francisco, CA, USA*
[2]*University of Massachusetts Medical School, Worcester, MA, USA*

In the USA, ambulatory or outpatient psychiatric care of individuals in later life is provided in a variety of public and private office settings. These include publicly financed community mental health centres, hospital-sponsored or university-sponsored outpatient clinics or services, the offices of psychiatrists (and other mental health professionals) in private practice, health maintenance organizations (HMOs, both privately and government-funded; the governmentally sponsored ones are now called Medicare Advantage plans) and others. This chapter will focus on practical aspects of providing psychiatric treatment to older Americans in office-based psychiatric private practices. We will not discuss the details of treatment in these settings, but rather the 'mechanics' of the process.

An important focus of community-based psychiatric ambulatory care is the need to create relationships with other community services and providers of care and assistance. This provides both a framework and a means by which many of the services are provided. Some of the barriers and obstacles to care will also be reviewed.

In providing community-based ambulatory care, the psychiatrists must have a comprehensive and patient-centred focus, following the patient to provide whatever psychiatric treatments are needed in whatever setting. While there are some geriatric psychiatrists who limit their activities to specific treatment locations, such as in offices or in-hospital programmes, this type of care may require the patient to be seen and treated sequentially in many places and circumstances.

INFLUENCES ON PRIVATE PRACTICE

For the purposes of this chapter, we will define private practitioners as independently employed or self-employed psychiatrists who work alone or in small groups. These practitioners provide treatment to patients who individually seek their help, and who pay for services received, primarily with Medicare health insurance benefits. Notwithstanding the current and ongoing, large-scale reorganization occurring in the American health care system, private practice remains a widespread model of medical practice in the USA. In many ways it has served as a starting point for the pattern of care provided in the other settings mentioned above. Many of the techniques discussed below are applicable to other models of treatment. Older patients seek care from private practitioners or other mental health providers with varying degrees of utilization and satisfaction[1,2].

Private practices are essentially private businesses, typically started, owned and operated by the individuals providing and/or supervising the clinical services provided. They may be small businesses, comprised of a single individual or several associated people, or they may be larger groupings of multiple people joined together to provide psychiatric/psychological treatment, or be part of a large medical multi-specialty affiliation. Such groups may grow to include dozens, or even hundreds of providers, becoming large businesses in the process. This chapter will focus on the smaller entities which are more typical and more common, although there are market forces which are encouraging practitioners to join together in larger groups to achieve both economies of scale, and to better negotiate with third-party payers of services, and other caregiving entities.

The private practice of medicine in the USA has evolved as a cottage industry within a historically unsystematized, free-enterprise, fee-for-service climate. Changing lifestyle preferences and demographics among young physicians are having some impact on this pattern. From its inception in 1965, the Medicare system had a built-in prejudice against the provision of outpatient psychiatric services. There was a discriminatory 50% patient co-payment requirement for all psychiatric treatment services delivered outside of an acute care hospital setting (unlike all other covered medical services, for which the patient co-payment is 20%)[3]. In 2008, this co-payment requirement was addressed by a new law which will gradually phase out the discrimination over a several year period until 2014, when there will be parity between payments for physical and psychiatric treatment[4]. This limitation on Medicare insurance coverage had constrained provision of these services to the elderly. Over the past 10–15 years, however, much greater influence has been felt from a multitude of other outside forces, at times impeding geriatric psychiatry practice[3,5], but in some cases expanding it. These forces (to list a few) include: efforts by the federal government to rein in Medicare spending[6,7]; the penetration of health maintenance organizations (HMOs) into Medicare; the advent of federal nursing home reform regulations; the growing presence of health care agency accrediting

Principles and Practice of Geriatric Psychiatry, 3rd edn. Edited by Mohammed T. Abou-Saleh, Cornelius Katona and Anand Kumar
© 2011 John Wiley & Sons, Ltd

bodies, such as the Joint Commission for the Accreditation of Health-care Organizations (JCAHO) and the National Council of Quality Assurance (NCQA); the creation by the American Board of Psychiatry and Neurology of subspecialty board examinations in geriatric psychiatry; social attitudes (e.g. public attitudes about medical care and doctors, as well as about mental illness and psychiatric care); the influences of physician attitudes[8] and medical malpractice litigation[9]; the availability of newer psychopharmacologic agents (including their increased acceptance by the public and their increased utilization by primary care physicians); patient finances; and folklore and 'common sense' of both the professional and the general population. Geography also is a factor, as there is significant regional variation among practitioners and communities in different areas of the country, as well as variations in payment rates and public (Medicare/Medicaid) and private (HMOs and other managed care companies) monitoring and regulation. Some geriatric psychiatry practices have adopted the use of physician extenders, such as nurse practitioners or physician assistants, to enhance the scope of treatment options. Adaptation of geriatric assessment and treatment principles has been slow, for the most part, in private general and psychiatric medical practice. Nevertheless, successful practitioners need a working knowledge of these forces in order to function. As a field which is now well into its adolescence in the USA, there are a growing number of examples of psychogeriatric care models that have proven generally applicable. In fact, the fee-for-service system in the USA has thus far been a relative failure in geriatrics, since it has not incorporated many of the accepted principles of geriatric care[10]. Some varying approaches have been tried by practitioners, but most still follow the above-noted model. The incursion of managed care HMOs into the Medicare system held out promise to change this state of affairs. HMOs, in theory, employ methodologies such as integrated delivery systems, screening, prevention and case management that are ideally suited to geriatrics[11]. Their track record has been disappointing, however, and their approach to managing mental health care has been largely ineffective for the elderly. Managed care companies often 'carve out' the management of mental health services by subcontracting it to managed behavioural health care companies with specialized expertise in mental health benefits management[12]. Such companies rarely have any expertise in geriatrics, and do not appreciate its differences from general adult psychiatry[13]. These companies have often ageist attitudes built into their coverage utilization guidelines, and inappropriately limit treatment or completely deny it, especially involving members with Alzheimer's disease, which they do not view as a covered psychiatric disorder. To the extent that managed care has penetrated Medicare, this practice has made the practice of geriatric psychiatry more difficult, as the seniors enrolled in these plans typically may only receive services from health care providers who are contracted with them. This limits their access to care which might otherwise be available.

PRIVATE PRACTICE AS A BUSINESS

Another important factor in discussing this type of psychiatric practice is the previously mentioned idea that geriatric psychiatry is a business. As such, the patients are to be considered as customers. Furthermore, at times, other physicians, and additional referring sources, may also be regarded as customers. As such, it behoves the psychiatrist to organize the practice and to provide services in ways that answer the needs of these customers. The psychiatrist may help the patient to define these needs, provide information about them, alter them or aid them in various ways. The psychiatrist may need to refuse patients' requests when professional judgment dictates this. American consumers, especially the adult children of geriatric patients, are becoming more and more concerned about the availability of health care, its costs, its efficacy and its risks. At the same time they are becoming more educated and aware of health care issues and, due in large measure to the availability of health-related information from the internet, and other mass media sources, more knowledgeable about treatment options and risks, although this knowledge may be of variable accuracy. If the psychiatrist does not do a good job or does not adequately address at least some of the patient's needs (and/or their adult child's needs), the psychiatrist may lose that patient's business. The interaction between them, therefore, has aspects of an exchange of service for payment. Providing a comprehensive service, as mentioned above, is often very satisfying and helpful to patients. At the same time, the business opportunities for income are maximized. In a community-based private practice, people are often referred to the individual doctor, rather than to a hospital, a university or a public clinic where they may be assigned a doctor. Patients may be referred because of the doctor's quality of service, reputation or relationships with the referring party. These qualities therefore become significant aspects of the psychiatrist's success in business as well as clinical practice.

Important factors in satisfying the patient/customer include:

1. Cost: reasonable fees and/or helpfulness and knowledgeability in filling out insurance claims. Acceptance of the patient's insurance coverage in payment for the services.
2. Accessibility: convenient and comfortable office location and surroundings. The psychiatrist may decide to provide more services in more locations.
3. Availability: the availability of the psychiatrist to go to the patient if needed (e.g. to consult at a medical hospital if the patient is admitted by another physician for a physical ailment, or to see the patient at home, in a nursing home, or an assisted living facility) is very important. The convenience of the geriatric psychiatrist going to where the patient lives, rather than the patient coming to the doctor's office, is very attractive to family or caregivers responsible for transportation. Because of the time and effort, as well as the distraction from other activities, the viability of this form of practice, in private practice, depends upon the numbers of people who may need services in that area or location; sometimes arrangements can be made with facilities that ensure an adequate volume of patient visits for each trip to the facility.
4. Scheduling: flexibility to see patients at convenient times without excessively long delays in scheduling appointments. This is crucial, since many frail patients are brought by their adult children, who may work.
5. Communications: the ability to contact the psychiatrist quickly and easily at need (e.g. by telephone by the patient and, when appropriate, by the patient's family). This includes the willingness of the psychiatrist to return such phone calls quickly, and the friendliness and accuracy of the psychiatrist's secretary or answering service. It also includes the ability and willingness of the psychiatrist to speak to the patient (and family) about his/her symptoms, illnesses and treatments in a clear and patient manner.
6. Concern: the feeling that the therapist has a genuine interest and concern for the patient. This feeling of concern extends to the patient's interactions with the office staff. This is an especially vital factor for the older population[14].

7. Confidence: patients and involved family members need to feel that the psychiatrist knows what the patient's problem is and has an idea about what can be done. The doctor does not need to provide definite answers, but must indicate a grasp of the situation and some ideas for an approach to it. This helps to provide a structure to what is often a strange and frightening experience. Empathy with the patient's distress is very helpful in this, as is reassurance to the patient that his/hers is not the worst case the doctor has ever seen (a common fantasy).

8. Understanding: A related skill is being aware of and addressing, when needed, those concerns, preconceptions, prejudices, fears, needs, worries and expectations which may interfere with the provision of services to the identified patient; these can be the patient's feelings or those of the family member(s) involved. They may include fears of being controlled, a bias against doctors, psychiatrists, medications or hospitals, belief that the patient's problematic behaviour is wilful, concerns of financial worries, caregiver stress or the feeling that coming for help is a sign of weakness or failure, the presence of partial information, such as information gleaned from pharmaceutical advertising, news reports about medications, or the neighbour's experience with a particular drug, or the expectation that the doctor has an easy answer to the problem.

There are only limited data available on income and workload for geriatric psychiatrists as a group. For all psychiatrists, 1998 median annual gross income was $171 490 (a 3.5% increase from 1997), and annual net income was $118 630 (a 4.33% increase from 1997). This was the second lowest income of the 20 largest specialties (above general practitioners) surveyed by Medical Economics that year. The rate of inflation in the year 1997–1998 was 1.6%. Comparable 1998 income data for all US physicians show an annual gross income of $256 290 (down 0.7% from 1997) and a net income of $163 940 (up 2.2%); for non-surgical specialties, the gross income was $227 300 (up 1.7%) and the net income was $147 140 (up 2.4%)[15]. When these data are compared to the median annual net income for psychiatrists in the USA in 1989, which was $103 570 (the fourth lowest of 15 office-based specialties surveyed that year; the only doctors who made less were general practitioners, family physicians and paediatricians)[16], we find that the income of psychiatrists had risen 14.5% in that period. The median net income for all fields of medicine rose just under 25% during the same period, while the cumulative inflation rate added up to 35%.

Although most American psychiatrists see few or no geriatric patients, this trend is changing somewhat. There were over 5400 out of the over 36 000 members of the American Psychiatric Association who expressed an interest in geriatrics during their 1997–1998 Professional Activities (Biographical) Survey (unpublished data, courtesy of the American Psychiatric Association, 2000). The membership of the American Association for Geriatric Psychiatry has grown to over 2000 (unpublished data, courtesy of the American Association for Geriatric Psychiatry, 2009), and interest among general psychiatrists continues to increase. In 1991, the American Board of Psychiatry and Neurology first administered a Board Certifying subspecialty examination in geriatric psychiatry. As of December, 2008, there were 2953 individuals who have passed this examination (data courtesy of the American Board of Psychiatry and Neurology, www.abpn.com/cert_statistics.htm, 2009).

In 1996, 18% of American general psychiatrists had geriatric caseloads exceeding 20% of their practices[17]. Overall, in this 1996 survey of 970 responders, an average of 14.0–17.7% of their psychiatric patients were aged 65+, compared to 8.4% found in a 1987 study[18]. When psychiatrists who provide a higher proportion of geriatric services (more than 20% of their case load – HGPs) were compared to those who were low-volume providers with the elderly (less than 20% of their workload – LGPs), it was found that the HGPs spent proportionally less time in their offices (although still spending most of their time there), more time in hospitals and significantly more time in nursing homes, than LGPs[17].

In 2002, the National Survey of Psychiatric Practice[19] found the proportion of HGPs had increased to 26.0% of respondents, and 28.1% of respondent members of the American Psychiatric Association (a 55% increase from the 1996 survey). Of the HGPs, 31% were Board Certified in Geriatric Psychiatry. These geriatric psychiatrists saw approximately three-times as many geriatric patients and five-times as many patients with dementia as the non-HGP generalist psychiatrists. Nonetheless, most did not have exclusive geriatric practices. Of note is the finding of a wide range of annual incomes among the respondents.

The 2008 report of the Institute of Medicine highlighted the existing and future shortfall of geriatric medical care providers, including geriatric psychiatrists[19,20]. At that time there was calculated to be one Board certified geriatric psychiatrist for every 11 372 older Americans, and that, by 2030, if training programmes continued at their current rates, there would be only one for every 20 195 older Americans[21].

A significant impediment to the collection of data on the work done by geriatric psychiatrists and the income generated by this work has been the inability to differentiate those individuals who provide services to the older population from the work of other psychiatrists. The Medicare system has not differentiated general psychiatrists from geriatric specialists. In May, 2009, the Centers for Medicare and Medicaid Services (CMS), the United States federal agency which administers the Medicare programme, approved the creation of a specialty identification code for Geriatric Psychiatry (personal communication, American Association for Geriatric Psychiatry, 2009), as a recognized specialty, beginning in April, 2010. Individuals who choose to do so, may register with Medicare as having a subspecialty in this area. This will allow information to be collected as to the work load, diagnosis and treatment provision and income generated by these practitioners.

There may be changes in the future, but currently there are relatively low numbers of psychiatrists with a specific interest in treating the elderly. When the medical and general communities know that a particular psychiatrist is a geriatric specialist, there is usually no shortage of patients needing these services. However, at the time of this writing, the economic downturn in the United States along with the projections of future medical costs, together with the current governmental motivation to make changes in the nation's health care system, make uncertain the nature and form that medical care, and specifically geriatric psychiatry care, will take.

OFFICE PLANNING AND DESIGN[22,23]

Establishing a practice to treat older patients requires some attention be paid to the setting in which such treatment will occur and to factors that might act as barriers to treatment. Offices that can only be reached by climbing stairs, or those with varying levels into which one must step up or down, are difficult and potentially hazardous. Long corridors that must be traversed are similarly problematic. Chairs should be available that are sturdy and have armrests and firm seats, high enough for ease in sitting or rising. They should be upholstered with waterproof and stain-resistant fabrics. Adequate lighting, readable signs and patient information literature should be planned with poor vision in mind. Interesting, recent magazines and a television in the waiting areas should be available for patients, and those who accompany and wait for them. Area carpets, spring-hinged doors and other possible hazards should also be considered. Toilet facilities and drinking water should be in reasonable proximity.

Mobility and transportation problems are another potential obstacle to treatment. Selection of an office location in a rural community, or in an area with poor public transportation or poor handicapped access may be factors. Convenient parking, especially in crowded urban areas, is necessary. Treatment may be interrupted during the winter months if the cold interferes with the patients' ability to get to the office. Some communities have senior transportation services, which will take people with limited mobility to physicians if reservations are made 24–48 hours in advance. Some hospitals may transport patients to and from the hospital or to physicians' offices located in adjoined buildings. Offices may also be located in senior retirement buildings or communities. Some senior living facilities will bring people to doctor's offices or medical centres. Clear signage on the exterior of the building and in the lobby areas and corridors will help the older patient find you.

THE BEGINNING OF THE RELATIONSHIP

Older patients seek out, are referred to or are brought to the psychiatrist's office for care. An initial 'gatekeeper' function may occur by means of enquiries (usually by telephone) into the reasons for the request to be seen, the age of the prospective patient, the referring source, the status of insurance coverage or other financial information. Such enquiries may lead a particular practitioner who prefers to specialize in geriatrics to decline to accept an adolescent as a patient, or to suggest that a patient being seen by another psychiatrist first discusses the idea of transferring with the current therapist, or to refer the patient to a geriatric psychiatrist in a geographically more convenient location.

A prospective patient, once given an appointment, should be told about additional information the psychiatrist would like to have available at the time of the first visit (e.g. the names of the patient's other treating physicians, current medications being taken, information about past psychiatrists, psychiatric medications, hospitalizations, past and current medical conditions). If the referring source is a physician, family member or a member of the staff of a senior-living facility, information from them as to the nature of the problem may be requested.

THE RANGE OF SERVICES

Among the most important services a psychogeriatric specialist can provide are diagnostic services. Too often, inadequate or erroneous evaluation leads to inadequate or erroneous treatment. A knowledge of physiology, psychology and the illnesses of late life, a comprehensive approach to history taking, assessment and testing and the ability to formulate an appropriate treatment plan form the basis of a unique contribution by geriatric specialists[24,25]. In fact, the ability to provide such a comprehensive evaluation and treatment perspective may be a primary reason why patients and referral sources seek the assistance of a geriatric psychiatrist.

An important aspect of the coordinated treatment plan is the collection of past information. With the patient's permission,

contact is established with the patient's family, other physicians and therapists. To the extent possible, past records, diagnoses, psychological testing reports, doctors' treatments, psychotherapy records, laboratory and radiological reports are requested and reviewed. While not revealing confidential information, these contacts also benefit the patient by making the patient's other physician(s) and support system aware of your activities with the patient. This increases the likelihood that you will be notified of future problems that may occur and that other medical treatments will be coordinated with you by other physicians. In the absence of such relationships, physicians may call a different psychiatrist to provide treatment, due to lack of awareness of your involvement.

As has been reviewed elsewhere[23,26,27], including sections of this volume, older individuals can be suitable candidates for many of the therapeutic modalities provided to younger patients, including individual, group and family psychotherapies, which utilize insight-orientated, cognitive, behavioural and other techniques. Some approaches, such as reminiscence or life-review therapy[28], have more specific applicability to the ageing person. Modification of family therapy may be necessary, for example to address the role of adult children in assisting in the care of a demented or otherwise impaired parent.

Psychopharmacologic treatment of the elderly often requires alteration in the selection, dosing and scheduling of medication because of changes in absorption, distribution, metabolism, receptor sensitivity and excretion[29,30]. Once again, the geriatric psychiatrist may be sought out in recognition of this expertise by the patient and others involved in the patient's care. Pharmacoeconomic trends in the USA create additional conflicts for geriatric psychiatrists in private practice. Pharmaceutical costs are escalating rapidly in the USA compared to many other countries. Patients may have coverage under a Medicare Part D prescription drug plan, a voluntary federal programme begun in 2006. These plans are designed and administered by a number of private corporate entities. There are limitations and restrictions in expenditures and available drugs under these plans[31,32]. For example, benzodiazepines and barbiturates were not covered under the plans. The exclusion of these medications was changed in the 2008 Medicare legislation and will be available for prescription beginning in 2013. Treatment options may be limited by restrictive formularies designed with cost containment in mind, but often with limited consideration of the greater sensitivity of elderly plan members to medication side effects. Nursing homes have also adopted formularies to contain their costs, even in the absence of significant managed care penetration. Consultant pharmacists are employed by the homes to monitor physician prescribing, with respect not only to federal regulations but also to formulary requirements. Psychiatrists in private practice are thus often under pressure to prescribe less costly drugs or to run the risk of receiving fewer referrals from primary care physicians or nursing homes.

Sometimes assistance provided may be primarily educational, such as telling the patient or his/her family about the nature of the ageing process or the symptoms, prognosis and treatment of an illness. Treatment may be primarily informational, directing patients and carers to appropriate senior housing, services for the blind or hearing-impaired, continuing education programmes or volunteer work. At times treatment may be directive, for instance telling a patient to get a physical examination, buy a hearing aid or give up driving, or telling a family member to seek the assistance of respite services to provide some relief in caring for a cognitively impaired person, or to advise that the parent or sibling should no longer live alone. The community-based psychiatrist must develop expert knowledge of the available community resources, as well as relationships with the providers of them.

The initial psychiatric diagnostic evaluation of the patient also is the time of the patient's actual evaluation of the doctor. The practitioner must address the overt and covert concerns, the anxieties and fantasies about the nature of geriatric psychiatry, the reasons why the patient is there and the treatments that will be instituted. Although these anxieties are not unique to this model, the need to address them is. Unlike treatment limited to one location or modality or situation, this relationship will be multifactorial and ongoing. Furthermore, a privately operating care provider is likely to represent an entry contact point into mental health care. If the patient and the associated significant family members are not put at ease, their questions answered and concerns addressed, the contact may quickly end.

Older patients are often novices regarding mental illness and its treatment. They are often fearful of being thought 'crazy' or of being 'put away'. Structuring the beginning of the initial interview can help relieve their anxiety. You may start with 5–10 minutes of specific questions, such as address, age, date of birth, concrete information on marriages, children, parents, siblings, education, employment, interests and so on. This can also give you a lot of information in a short time, helping to give a more complete picture of the patient. Simultaneously, you are assessing aspects of mental status and memory.

Treatment of the older patient includes the time when the patient is away from the office. The patient is helped when assured of the doctor's continued interest and care. This can often be achieved using relatively simple techniques: (i) providing specific information tells the patient that you know what is going to happen, for example 'This medicine is going to take two to three weeks to build up in your system. You may experience some side effects during that period but you will not experience the benefit for two to three weeks. You need to be patient during that time'; (ii) assuring access and inviting communication, for instance 'My telephone number is a 24-hour number. If you have any problems or need to reach me, you can call any time'. Patients rarely do call outside of office hours after being told this, but they feel very reassured; (iii) specific instructions for behaviour and for contacts; for instance, instead of saying, 'Call me if you have any problems', saying 'Call me next Tuesday' assures the patient that you want to hear from him/her. It also reduces the number of calls he/she might otherwise make before next Tuesday.

FAMILY INVOLVEMENT

Families are often interested and involved in the psychiatric care of elders. Relatives and friends can be important sources of information to the doctor. Interactions may include mediation and other interventions into the family system, reinterpretation and re-framing of past and present events, support, reassurance and education. Attention to family issues is especially important in treatment of patients with dementing disorders[33,34].

Because of the increased interrelationships and involvements some families have in an older patient's status and treatment, it is often vital to maintain contact and a positive rapport with the family. Also, patients will often request this. Conversely, when family members feel unnecessarily excluded or denied access to information, they can influence or disrupt the treatment entirely. This is not to imply that therapeutic confidentiality is not maintained; families generally understand this. They do, however, want to know that appropriate help is being provided. Such reassurance can have a positive therapeutic effect on the patient, as a reflection of the family's confidence in the doctor. It can also have the practical influence/effect of helping

to keep the patient in treatment. Differing opinions among relatives may also be a source of potential disruption of the treatment. Patients will often give permission, or even request the doctor to speak to family members. Sometimes family involvement is necessary, such as in ensuring compliance with medications or appointments, or in providing observations of behaviour or of problems which the patient may not report.

In situations where there are no immediate relatives, non-kinship support networks become increasingly important[35]. The therapist may at times utilize the assistance of family surrogates in gathering information and in helping the patient. Where such networks are weak or absent, assisting the patient in their creation can be of great benefit.

RELATIONSHIPS WITH OTHER PHYSICIANS

In the absence of the formalized organization of a university environment or the planned hierarchy of a hospital or corporate structure, the geriatric psychiatrist in private practice must create or seek out relationships with other practitioners. This can be done through involvement in professional societies, participation in the activities of the community's hospitals and through non-medical social contacts. Eventually, further relationships will also be created by patients who seek psychiatric services and request that contact be established with their other treating physicians. Collegial relationships thus created can provide advice and assistance, help in monitoring the status of patients between visits to the psychiatrist and provide sources of referrals for new patients.

As noted previously, private practitioners may also consider other physicians as customers. They are often the ones who initiate, refer or make the appointments for their patients. They do this in the expectation that their patient's needs will be met. They may also feel that, by doing so, they relieve themselves of the burden of caring for that aspect of the patient's condition, therefore making their jobs a little easier.

RELATIONSHIPS WITH OTHER PSYCHIATRISTS

As with other physicians in general, private practitioners must create a network of relationships with other psychiatrists in the area, both near and far. Those at some distance, or whose special areas of interest or expertise differ, can be sources of referrals. Other psychiatrists may receive enquiries or have patients referred to them whom they are unable to treat; they may then direct them to you. Psychiatrists who practice in closer proximity may also be sources of new patient referrals, especially when their treatment interests vary from yours. Furthermore, a certain percentage of patients, especially those with chronic or recurring illness, may be 'doctor-shoppers' and spontaneously, or by referral, change from one practitioner to another over a period of time. Developing good rapport with other local psychiatrists helps in providing better care to these patients by sharing understanding of their needs, pathology and past successful treatments and by helping to avoid duplication of previously attempted unsuccessful treatments.

Formal or informal groupings of private psychiatrists may gather for continuing education and study, to help with supervision, second opinions or 'risk-management' of difficult cases, or to share tasks, such as psychiatric coverage for a local hospital's emergency room. When a private practitioner takes a break, to go on vacation or to a conference, it may be one or more of these local psychiatrists who may help to provide coverage for patient care, who is asked to be available to take care of emergencies or to provide ongoing services to patients who are hospitalized at the time. Such coverage may be done reciprocally as a courtesy for mutual benefit, or may be by formal arrangement.

RELATIONSHIPS WITH OTHER PROFESSIONALS

Other professional care providers with whom privately practicing geriatric psychiatrists and their patients come into contact include psychologists, social workers, nurses, speech therapists, occupational therapists, private care managers, hospital administrators and the operators of day treatment programmes, and senior activity centres, nursing homes, assisted-living and independent living facilities, and other residential settings where seniors reside. Knowledge of these and other community resources is essential for the geriatric psychiatrist. At times the best treatment offered to a patient may be a referral to one of them. Needless to say, each of these can provide valuable services. As they get to know the geriatric psychiatrist, they can also be valuable resources; for example, they can be excellent sources of information about a patient's status and functioning when the patient is not in the doctor's office. They may allow the psychiatrist to provide more and better service to patients by helping to monitor, care for and carry out treatments with the patient. They can alert the doctor when problems are developing, often earlier than the patient might have, and can assist in the management of a crisis by supporting and reassuring the patient. These individuals are sources of referral to the practitioner. They will also speak to others in the community of their experiences and contacts with the practitioner. This is an important facet of how a professional reputation is made.

PROFESSIONAL ORGANIZATIONS

Working alone or in small group practices can be isolating. Involvement in local, regional, national and international professional organizations is yet another important aspect of private practice. These may be specific psychogeriatric, or psychiatric societies, or they may be medical or interdisciplinary. These associations provide mutual support, education and professional validation, and well as being additional avenues for networking and encouraging referrals of new patients.

RELATIONS WITH HOSPITALS

Each psychiatric programme within a hospital can have its own rules, regulations, standards, patterns of practice and pattern of relations with community-based practitioners. Some hospital facilities employ psychiatrists on staff; others may not. Some programmes are organized more in accord with the direction given by the hospital and the hospital-based staff. Others encourage more involvement in programme planning by the community staff physicians. Some facilities are sites for training programmes and have psychiatric residents and Fellows who provide services. There are some geriatric facilities within free-standing psychiatric hospitals and others that are geriatric units within medical hospitals; some are located in private, for-profit hospitals, or in non-profit or public or charitably funded institutions, or in university-affiliated programmes. While the rules, staffing patterns and required paper forms may vary from hospital to hospital, these variations are, for the most part, not so onerous as to be unworkable or impossible to deal with for the community-based

practitioner. In some of these settings, the community-based practitioner may be able to influence the nature of the hospital's policies and treatment programme by participation in psychiatric departmental meetings and activities.

The differences among hospitals require some flexibility on the part of the doctor, but also may allow the possibility of tailoring referrals to the hospital most appropriate to the patient. For a variety of reasons, different hospital units acquire different patient populations and characteristics. Some programmes are age segregated, with specifically designated geriatric psychiatry wards. Others are age integrated, with younger and older patients sharing and participating in the treatment programme together. Some programmes may be more suitable for cognitively intact, physically healthy older people suffering from affective or anxiety disorders or relationship dysfunctions. Others may be more focused on evaluation and treatment of problems associated with dementia or delirium.

THE POSSIBILITY OF INPATIENT HOSPITAL TREATMENT[36]

At the time of the initial visit or at some subsequent time in the course of the treatment of an older patient, the psychiatrist may recommend inpatient hospital treatment. The process begins with an assessment of whether the hospitalization is something that would be beneficial and therapeutic but non-emergent, or is an urgently needed admission due to imminent danger to the patient or others. Immediately after this decision, the psychiatrist must decide whether the patient is capable of consenting to this plan. Depending upon the hospitals and resources available in the community, these assessments may lead to a decision to use a particular inpatient facility. For example, there may be one that can admit people on an involuntary basis, or care for people who are potentially suicidal or aggressive. Similar choices may result from the ability of a specific hospital's psychiatric ward to care for elderly patients who have concurrent severe medical problems, or who are wanderers, or who need the hospital's specific therapeutic approach. Other factors that affect the choice of inpatient service include locations of past hospitalizations, the hospitals used by the patient's other treating physicians, proximity to the patient and the patient's family to allow for visitation and, importantly, whether a particular hospital has a room available for the patient at the time it is needed, and whether the admission can or cannot be delayed until a bed becomes available. In some cases, where room is not available locally or at the time needed or where local facilities are not appropriate, referral for hospitalization may have to be made to a psychiatrist or facility elsewhere.

In the United States, at this time, there are multiple providers of health care insurance for the elderly. These include the Federal and State governments and a variety of private health insurance companies and managed care organizations (MCOs). Some health plans, especially the MCOs, may have contractual agreements with particular hospitals to provide care; this may dictate which hospital may be used for the individual's inpatient care.

ADMISSION TO HOSPITALS

Various hospitals and psychiatric facilities within hospitals may have different procedures for arranging admissions. Typically, the psychiatrist or his staff communicate with a designated person or office to make the reservation for admission. Information that must be provided at this point varies, but usually consists of the patient's name, age, insurance information and admitting diagnosis. Some facilities may also wish to have information regarding the geriatric patient's ability to function in activities of daily living, mobility, signs and symptoms of the patient that warrant admission, a preliminary treatment plan, or the likelihood of the patient being a danger to self or others.

When the patient is admitted, each hospital's usual procedure begins. Administrators and nurses fill out forms. The patient is shown to a room, belongings are put away and the staff make the patient acquainted with the facility and programme of activities. At about the same time, the private psychiatrist is notified that the patient has arrived. If not already given, initial orders are requested. When the psychiatrist is not available to come to the hospital immediately, orders might be given by telephone to the ward nurse, addressing such needs as diet, monitoring of vital signs, laboratory tests, ward therapies and medications to be started and so on.

IN-HOSPITAL TREATMENT[36,37]

In-hospital treatments for the elderly can include the full spectrum of therapeutic approaches devised for psychiatric patients in general, although these might vary depending upon the resources and philosophy of the facility and the specific instructions of the doctor. The psychiatrist may personally provide individual psychotherapy, family therapy, psychotherapeutic medication management, electroconvulsive therapy, or other treatments, as well as ongoing diagnostic evaluation. At times the community psychiatrist may not provide all of the therapeutic services, and may seek the assistance of other professionals, such as utilizing a psychologist to provide psychotherapies. Many older patients also benefit from group, occupational, recreational and ward milieu therapies, physical therapy, speech therapy or reality-orientation/memory-stimulating techniques. The community psychiatrist may not be directly involved in these treatments; the hospital's staff members provide them as part of the hospital's programme and report back to the doctor regarding the patient's progress. Nurses, social workers and other staff members also inform the psychiatrist about the patient's status, symptoms, behaviour and reactions to treatment as observed during the day. Coordination, mutual understanding of achievable goals, cooperation and respect between the psychiatrist and the hospital administration and staff facilitate the psychiatrist's functioning and the treatment of the patient. It is vital that a good working relationship be achieved. If it is not, the doctor and the treatment can be undermined in numerous ways.

Working in the hospital requires flexibility on the part of doctors and staff. The staff must accommodate to various physicians and their styles of treatment. The doctors must adapt to the hospital and its programme, including its staffing pattern, its treatment approach and its physical plant. Patients may be seen at times under less than ideal conditions, including differing circumstances, locations, times and schedules (e.g. seeing a patient in a semiprivate room, planning hospital rounds to not conflict with group therapy programmes, visiting patients only to find that they are in physical therapy or getting X-rays).

POST-HOSPITAL TREATMENT

Planning for hospital follow-up begins during the hospital stay. The physician can direct the social service worker regarding possible directions and options for such problems as living situation changes, needs for at-home services, assistance or care, possible

adult congregate-living facility or nursing home placement[38]. The social worker can investigate these and coordinate planning with the physician, patient and patient's family. Other post-discharge options the doctor can order include visiting nurses, physical therapy and other home health treatments or referral to a senior day centre or a partial hospitalization day programme[39,40]. The patient's needs, desires, finances and therapeutic considerations (including the options for follow-up treatment with the psychiatrist) are important factors in these choices. Similarly, the available, involved members of the family may have opinions or suggestions. They may also direct the psychiatrist's attention towards additional problems or issues they feel are significant.

An important part of discharge planning is the re-engagement of the patient in outpatient treatment in the psychiatrist's office. An appointment can be given at the time of discharge, or the patient may be instructed to make an appointment within a specified period of time. The psychiatrist makes certain that needed hospital records, including discharge summary, list of discharge medications, copies of laboratory and radiograph reports and medical consultation reports, are sent to the office. This enhances completeness and continuity of care. Use of electronic or computerized medical records, where available, can enhance this process.

In addition to other usual psychotherapeutic issues that can be discussed in the post-hospital treatment, it is important to include a review of the patient's reactions to the hospital, the symptoms that necessitated the admission and the patient's progress there. Also, it is important to watch for post-hospital regressions and symptom recurrences, as the patient returns to his/her usual surroundings or to a new environment. Medication compliance and monitoring is another post-discharge task that requires attention, especially if the medication is new, if it is causing some side effects or if it requires special care in its use (e.g. special diet or times of administration).

POST-HOSPITAL TREATMENT IN OTHER SETTINGS

As the American health care system has evolved, many patients who in years past were treated in hospitals for longer periods of time are now felt to have improved sufficiently as to no longer warrant an inpatient level of care, and are therefore discharged back in to the community or to facilities while still in need of some ongoing treatment. Others may be in need of treatment but are deemed suitable for the sub-acute level of care provided in a skilled or long-term nursing facility. This may also be done in an out-patient hospital or partial hospital programme, where the person receives some therapeutic services during the day and returns to his or her usual residence at night.

CONCLUSION

Community-based ambulatory psychiatric care is an evolving treatment area in the USA. Economic, political, medical and demographic forces are all having an impact on the provision of care. While aspects of the treatment of younger adults in the community are being applied to the care of seniors, modifications are important in order to more fully address the special problems and needs of this population.

REFERENCES

1. Stein SR, Linn MW, Edelstein J, Stein EM. Elderly patient's satisfaction with care under HMO vs. private systems. *South Med J* 1989; **82**(12): 3–8.

2. Thomas C, Kelman HR. Health services use among elderly under alternative health services delivery systems. *J Commun Health* 1990; **152**: 77–92.

3. Kyomen HH, Gottlieb GL. Financial issues. In Sadovoy J, Jarvik LF, Grossberg GT, Meyers BS (eds), *Comprehensive Textbook of Geriatric Psychiatry*, 3rd edn. New York: W.W. Norton and Company, 2004, 1207–38.

4. Public Law No. 110-275. *Medicare Improvements for Patients and Providers Act of 2008*.

5. Goldman HH. Financing the mental health system. *Psychiatr Ann* 1987; **17**(9): 580–5.

6. Goldman HH, Cohen GD, Davis M. Expanded Medicare outpatient coverage for Alzheimer's disease and related disorders. *Hosp Community Psychiatry* 1985; **36**: 939–42.

7. Hsiao WC, Braun P, Becker E *et al. A National Study of Resource-Based Relative Value Scales for Physician Services. Final Report*. Boston: Department of Health Policy and Management, Harvard School of Public Health, 1988, 27–43.

8. Ford C, Sbordone R. Attitudes of psychiatrists toward elderly patients. *Am J Psychiatry* 1980; **137**: 571–5.

9. Klein JL, Macbeth JE, Nonek J. *Legal Issues in the Private Practice of Psychiatry*. Washington, DC: American Psychiatric Press, 1984.

10. Lachs MS, Ruchlin HS. Is managed care good or bad for geriatric medicine? *J Am Geriatr Soc* 1997; **45**: 1123–7.

11. Lachs MS, Wagner EH. The promise and performance of HMOs in improving outcomes in older adults. *J Am Geriatr Soc* 1996; **44**: 1251–7.

12. Bartels SJ, Colenda CC. Mental health services for Alzheimer's disease. Current trends in reimbursement and public policy, and the future under managed care. *Am J Geriatr Psychiatry* 1998; **6**: 85–100.

13. Bachman SS. Managed mental health care for elders: the role of the carve-out. *Publ Policy Aging Rep* 1998; **9**: 14–16.

14. Logsdon L. *Establishing a Psychiatric Private Practice*. Washington, DC: American Psychiatric Press, 1985.

15. Goldberg J. Doctor's earnings: you call this progress? *Med Econ* 1999; **18**: 172.

16. Clark L. Pressure grows on psychiatrists' earnings. *Med Econ* 1991; **68**(7): 60–70.

17. Colenda CC, Pincus H, Tanielian TL *et al*. Update of geriatric psychiatry practices among American psychiatrists. *Am J Geriatr Psychiatry* 1999; **7**: 279–88.

18. Loran LM, Taintor Z, Mirza M. Patient characteristics and treatment modalities. In Koran LM (ed.), *The Nation's Psychiatrists*. Washington, DC: American Psychiatric Association, 1987, 109.

19. Colenda CC, Wilk JE, West JC. The geriatric psychiatry workforce in 2002, analysis from the 2002 national survey of psychiatric practice. *Am J Geriatr Psychiatry* 2005; **13**(9): 756–65.

20. Committee on the Future Health Care Workforce for Older Americans, Institute of Medicine. *Retooling for an Aging America: Building the Health Care Workforce*. Washington, DC: National Academies Press, 2008, Chapter 4, 123–98.

21. Association of Directors of Geriatric Academic Programs. Fellows in geriatric medicine and geriatric psychiatry programs. *Training and Practice Update* 2007; **5**(2): 1–7.

22. Stein EM. Some practical considerations in the private practice of psychogeriatrics. *Clin Gerontol* 1983; **2**(1): 56–8.

23. Stein EM. Geriatric psychiatry in office and clinic. *J Appl Gerontol* 1983; **2**: 102–11.

24. Blazer D. The psychiatric interview of the geriatric patient. In Busse EW, Blazer D (eds), *Geriatric Psychiatry*. Washington, DC: American Psychiatric Press, 1989, 263–84.

25. Blazer D, Busse EW, Craighead WE, Evans D. Use of the laboratory in the diagnostic workup of the older adult. In Busse EW, Blazer D (eds), *Geriatric Psychiatry*. Washington, DC: American Psychiatric Press, 1989, 285–312.

26. Lazarus L. Psychotherapy. In Busse EW, Blazer D (eds), *The Ambulatory Care Setting in Geriatric Psychiatry*. Washington, DC: American Psychiatric Press, 1989, 567–91.

27. Nemiroff RA, Colarusso CA. *The Race Against Time – Psychotherapy and Psychoanalysis in the Second Half of Life*. New York: Plenum, 1985.

28. Butler RN, Lewis MI. *Aging and Mental Health: Positive Psychosocial Approaches*. St Louis, MO: C.V. Mosby, 1973.

29. Young RC, Meyers BS. Psychopharmacology. In Sadovoy J, Lazarus LW, Jarvik LF (eds), *Comprehensive Reviews of Geriatric Psychiatry*. Washington, DC: American Psychiatric Press, 1991, 435–68.

30. Davidson J. The pharmacologic treatment of psychiatric disorders. In Busse EW, Blazer D (eds), *The Elderly in Geriatric Psychiatry*. Washington, DC: American Psychiatric Press, 1989, 515–42.

31. Wikipedia. *Medicare Part D*. At http://en.wikipedia.org/wiki/Medicare_Part_D, accessed 3 Mar 2010.

32. US Department of Health and Human Services. *Medicare: Prescription Drug Coverage*. At www.medicare.gov/pdphome.asp, accessed 3 Mar 2010.

33. Cohen D, Eisdorfer C. *The Loss of Self*. New York: Norton, 1986.

34. Mace NL, Rabins PV. *The 36 HourDay*. Baltimore, MD: Johns Hopkins University Press, 1981.

35. Stein EM. Normal aging – psychological and social cultural aspects. In Lazarus W (ed.), *Essentials of Geriatric Psychiatry*. New York: Springer, 1988, 1–24.

36. Whanger AD. Inpatient treatment of the older psychiatric patient. In Busse EW, Blazer D (eds), *Geriatric Psychiatry*. Washington, DC: American Psychiatric Press, 1989, 593–634.

37. Tourigny-Rivard MF. Acute care inpatient treatment. In Sadovoy J, Lazarus LW, Jarvik LF (eds), *Comprehensive Review of Geriatric Psychiatry*. Washington, DC: American Psychiatric Press, 1991, 583–602.

38. Curlik SM, Frazier D, Katz IR. Psychiatric aspects of long-term care. In Sadovoy J, Lazarus LW, Jarvik LF (eds), *Comprehensive Review of Geriatric Psychiatry*. Washington, DC: American Psychiatric Press, 1991, 547–64.

39. Rosie JS. Partial hospitalization: a review of recent literature. *Hosp Commun Psychiatry* 1987; **38**(12): 1291–9.

40. Steingart A. Day programs. In Sadovoy J, Lazarus LW, Jarvik LF (eds), *Comprehensive Review of Geriatric Psychiatry*. Washington, DC: American Psychiatric Press, 1991, 603–12.

126

The Medical Psychiatry Inpatient Unit

Maria I. Lapid and Teresa A. Rummans

Mayo Clinic College of Medicine, Mayo Clinic Rochester, Rochester, USA

Medical psychiatry inpatient units are specialized units designed to provide care to patients with concurrently active psychiatric and medical illnesses. These units focus on the integration of medical and psychiatric care and emphasize a disease model of psychopathology[1]. Two important distinctions of medical psychiatry units from traditional inpatient psychiatric units are: (i) the patient population; and (ii) the capacity to safely manage concurrent medical and psychiatric illnesses that cannot be safely handled on a homogeneous unit alone.

The patient population in a medical psychiatric unit by definition has both active psychiatric and medical illnesses. These co-morbid conditions can co-exist independently, result from a medical illness that causes or contributes to a psychiatric disorder, result from a psychiatric illness that causes or contributes to a medical disorder, or result from a psychiatric illness that requires psychotropic medication with potential to produce medical illnesses[2].

The clinical focus and the organization of medical psychiatry units across the country vary widely. Operations of the units occur either primarily in psychiatric departments or in medical departments, and rarely are they units with combined administrative ownership[3]. However, the existence of a medical psychiatry unit, along with its structural organization and model of care, is based on several factors. Overall institutional need is one factor. Access to medical beds in a general hospital can be impaired by length of stay if patients have co-morbid psychiatric conditions. Transferring these patients to a different specialized environment improves the access for medical patients who do not have psychiatric co-morbidity. Another factor is improving the overall clinical care of patients in the hospital. Patients with acute and/or severe psychiatric conditions can be managed better on a combined unit, rather than leaving patients on medical floors or transferring them to traditional psychiatric units, as medical psychiatry units have greater capability for handling both problems concurrently rather than sequentially. Additionally, many of the medical psychiatry units are more capable of dealing with geriatric issues since there is a growing number of geriatric patients with combined medical illness who also require special environments. As a result, medical psychiatry units that focus on geriatric care will become increasingly important as the United States population ages. This chapter will review the general administrative, clinical, educational and research aspects of medical psychiatry inpatient units. Much of the material is based on our own institutional model of a medical psychiatry inpatient unit within a psychiatric hospital, as empirical published data regarding these units are limited.

ADMINISTRATION

Some medical psychiatry units are based in academic medical centres with full-time faculty, while others are found in private hospitals available to physicians of any specialty (psychiatry, family practice, internal medicine and neurology) with admitting privileges. There are also medical psychiatry units in state hospitals for patients with chronic mental illnesses[4]. There are four types of medical psychiatry units based on level of acuity of medical and psychiatric illness[5]. Type I units primarily provide psychiatric care with a low level of medical acuity. Type II units include general medicine or medical subspecialty units associated with a psychiatric liaison service and provide low levels of psychiatric care to those admitted to the general medical setting. Type III and Type IV units provide care for patients with concurrent and more severe medical and psychiatric problems in a unified setting. Type III units provide care to patients with low to high psychiatric acuity, and medium medical acuity (e.g. a non-compliant, poorly controlled diabetic with borderline personality disorder; a hyponatraemic, agitated schizophrenic patient with primary polydipsia; or a depressed renal failure patient refusing dialysis). Type IV provides care to patients with low to high psychiatric acuity, and medium to high medical acuity (e.g. a patient with chronic factitious disorder/borderline personality disorder who injected him/herself with stool water and is septic; or a delirious patient with a pulmonary embolus; or a ketoacidotic borderline/anorectic/bulimic diabetic patient)[6].

Physical Structure/Layout

The physical environment of a medical psychiatry unit is designed to accommodate patients with medical needs, cognitive impairment, functional impairment and sensory deficits such as hearing or visual impairments. It should also provide safety for those with severe behavioural disturbances in the context of delirium, dementia or other psychiatric illness. Ideally, a medical psychiatry unit is a locked unit, with restricted and secure access for safety and to prevent wandering or elopement. Each bedroom and bathroom should have wall oxygen, an emergency cord and call light. For fall precautions, every bed should have a bed alarm and thin, soft padded strips on the floor to minimize impact of fall and fall-related injuries (these are commercially available). All doors, hallways and the entire unit should be handicap and wheelchair accessible,

Principles and Practice of Geriatric Psychiatry, 3rd edn. Edited by Mohammed T. Abou-Saleh, Cornelius Katona and Anand Kumar
© 2011 John Wiley & Sons, Ltd

with handrails, grab bars and safe flooring. A special tub or shower room is designed to keep patients warm, comfortable and safe while showering or bathing. Transfer equipment such as Hoyer lifts enable safe patient transfers with less risk of injury to patients (i.e. falls) and staff (i.e. back injury).

Medical psychiatry units have the capability to access and obtain essential diagnostic work-up required in evaluation of organic causes, including imaging, electroencephalography, electrocardiogram and other laboratories, procedures and tests. Other important distinctions of a medical psychiatry unit from other general psychiatry units include the capability to provide intravenous fluids and drug therapy, nutritional support such as total parenteral nutrition and feeding tubes, surgical wound and drain care, intravenous access and care of peripheral and central lines, oxygen support, dialysis and isolation[1]. Medical complications arising from electroconvulsive therapy (ECT) can also be managed on a medical psychiatry unit.

Overall, a medical psychiatry unit provides an environment that is pleasant and accommodating to a patient population with high levels of psychiatric and medical acuity, but at the same time has the essential elements that facilitate the rendering of appropriate medical and surgical services.

Admission Criteria

The focus of care of each medical psychiatry unit across the country is diverse, including elderly, neuropsychiatric or behaviourally disturbed patients, substance abuse, eating disorders, chronic pain, schizophrenia and even patients as young as 13 years old[4,7,8]. Similarly, there is a wide variation in sources of referral, including the general hospital, long-term care facilities (nursing homes, assisted living facilities, memory care units), emergency rooms, outpatient clinics, direct referral from community providers, and tertiary referrals.

Medical psychiatry units maintain a distinctive patient population by virtue of admission criteria[9]. Admission criteria are necessary to ensure that the specialty of the medical psychiatry unit best matches the medical psychiatric problems that require treatment. Criteria for admission specify age, acuity of psychiatric and medical illness, acuity of nursing care, skilled care needs, and other factors. Patients without any concurrent medical illness, or with medical illnesses that are chronic and stable and do not require active intervention, are commonly excluded. Those whose high acuity level of medical illness that exceed the capacity of a medical psychiatry unit to safely manage them on the unit are best admitted to medical surgical services, with the consultation liaison service providing psychiatric care appropriately. Patients with severe behavioural problems should be excluded if there is no available staffing or if the physical environment is inadequate to handle the behaviours. Admissions for psychosocial reasons, in particular severe dispositional problems unlikely to be resolved even with effective psychiatric treatment, should not be accepted[1]. A waiting list for admission to the unit should be maintained, and priority given to patients from other psychiatric units within the facility, and those from medical and surgical units in the general hospital.

Despite implementation of admission criteria or a priority system, some admission decisions can still be difficult. It is helpful to have a team (typically a physician and/or an advanced level nurse) review all referrals for admission to ensure compliance to admission criteria and to make gatekeeping decisions. Hospital administration should support the medical director's authority to decline inappropriate admissions. Inappropriate admissions are not unexpected, even with admission criteria in place. One study that examined admissions to a medical psychiatry unit that required transfer to medical-surgical units within 48 hours of admission due to acute changes in medical conditions noted that the acute changes occurred after admission and were not foreseeable, although more vigilant screening for pulmonary, cardiovascular, electrolyte and infectious disorders was recommended[10]. When inappropriate admissions do occur, mechanisms should be in place to correct the problem, such as facilitating transfers to a more appropriate unit.

The Multidisciplinary Treatment Team

A medical model of diagnosis and treatment is practised in a medical psychiatry unit, because the patients are not only psychiatrically but also medically ill. A multidisciplinary treatment team is necessary in order to address the complex needs of this patient population. Similar to other psychiatric inpatient settings, a medical psychiatry unit utilizes a multidisciplinary treatment team to directly provide comprehensive care to patients in a biopsychosocial model. However, medical psychiatric treatment teams have more experience and expertise in providing care for medically compromised and elderly patients with psychiatric problems. One possible model would comprise a physician trained in medicine and psychiatry, or another would be two physicians, one being a psychiatrist and one being an internist. If the model is a single physician, this person should be trained with subspecialty in psychosomatic medicine, geriatric psychiatry, neuropsychiatry, or combined internal medicine and psychiatry. If the model involves a second physician, preferably an internist with specialty training in geriatric medicine, that physician is dedicated to the medical psychiatry unit daily to provide initial and follow-up consultations, to help evaluate and manage acute and chronic medical conditions, urgent or emergent situations, and to conduct medical examinations for clearance for ECT or other procedures.

Psychiatrists commonly lead the multidisciplinary treatment team. It is important for the psychiatrist team leader to have sound medical knowledge of the various aspects of psychiatric interventions (psychotherapy, pharmacotherapy, ECT, behaviour modification etc.), efficiently coordinate patients' care, communicate effectively, and successfully handle or resolve conflicts within or outside the team.

The other core members of the treatment team include nurses, social workers, pharmacists, therapists and chaplains. The nursing staff is one of the most important factors in the successful operation of a high-level acuity medical psychiatry unit[5]. Medical psychiatry nurses should have particularly strong medical/surgical nursing skills. In fact, hiring medical/surgical nurses and training them in the care of psychiatric patients is often preferable. Social workers coordinate placement and liaison with community agencies, meet and provide support to family members, conduct family therapy, and perform a thorough psychosocial assessment. Pharmacists assist with proper medication administration, advising the treatment team of drug interactions, monitoring drug levels and medication reconciliation. Recreational therapists organize and coordinate aspects of the clinical programming related to leisure and recreational activities. Physical therapists are available to provide gait assessment, manage deconditioning, conduct exercise regimens for strengthening, and help improve deconditioning and mobility of patients. Occupational therapists serve many functions. They provide relaxation training and stress management training to reduce anxiety. They conduct safety and cognitive evaluations to help determine disposition planning.

They evaluate patients for activities of daily living (ADLs) and help with improvement of ADLs. Chaplains help assess spiritual needs and concerns, provide spiritual support to patients and lead spirituality groups.

While the psychiatric treatment team is the team that provides the primary care, other services and disciplines are consulted as appropriate. Psychologists provide consultation with personality assessment, neurocognitive assessment and recommendations for behavioural therapy. Other medical or surgical services readily provide consultation and assist management of specific problems.

Unit Operations

Teamwork between a physician medical director and nurse manager is essential in successfully operating a medical psychiatry unit. A medical director in a medical psychiatry unit balances the unit's need to fill beds with the need to screen for appropriate admissions, integrates medical psychiatric care, advocates for high quality of care, addresses financial and regulatory issues, and respects psychosocial and biomedical dimensions of care[11]. Both the medical director and the nurse manager lead a multidisciplinary service committee, comprised of representatives from other disciplines in the unit (nurse, social worker, recreational therapist, other allied health staff), which meets regularly to review operations and clinical issues, hear staff input or concerns, review new rules and regulations or systems changes, resolve conflicts between staff, review unit performance and satisfaction surveys, and discuss other administrative and clinical issues pertinent to the unit.

The costs of operating a medical psychiatry unit are high, and financial issues are significant. There are constant pressures to reduce costs and shorten hospital stays, but at the same time taking care of more medically ill patients increases costs and the amount of staffing requirements and nursing time. This in turn has led to patients with more psychiatric and medical acuity that paradoxically increases the cost, making many medical psychiatry units less viable long-term. Therefore, partnerships must exist to underwrite the up-front costs of care of these patients. This will be beneficial in the long term as it will reduce re-admission rates to medical-surgical hospitals and overall expense of care for patients with co-morbid medical and psychiatric problems. Additionally, medical psychiatry units can decrease the cost of care by shortening hospital stays in the medical-surgical hospital, reducing disability in patients by having the psychiatric co-morbidity in medical patients addressed, delivering better aftercare, and ultimately helping patients become more functional.

Clinical Programming

While medical psychiatry patients receive psychopharmacologic and somatic/biological treatment for their psychiatric illnesses, psychotherapeutic interventions are equally important and should be structured and tailored to the needs of the medical psychiatry patient. An example of how clinical programming can be structured during the day in a medical psychiatry unit is shown in Figure 126.1. Group activities are led by non-physicians, typically nursing or allied health staff. All aspects of the clinical programming are flexible to accommodate various levels of cognitive functioning as well as the physical limitations that are common among medical psychiatry patients.

Different types of group therapy are available, including psychotherapeutic (grief, support, problem solving, cognitive behavioural, reminiscence, spirituality) and psychoeducational (mood disorders in particular depression and anxiety, chemical dependence, coping skills, ECT, proper use of medications), as well as other kinds of therapy (occupational therapy: relaxation, stress management, time management, optimization of ADLs; physical therapy: gait assessment, conditioning, strengthening, mobility, transfers; and recreational therapy: crafts, games, socialization, and other recreational or leisure activities). Family members can be included in some activities. Individual therapy or counselling is available as needed. Community organizations such as a National Alliance for the Mentally Ill (NAMI) family group may be available for families to attend within the psychiatric hospital. Other forms of intervention include modified exercise, music therapy, pet therapy, and other sensory activities such as a sensory room available for use for those who need de-stimulation in a quiet and relaxing environment.

DAILY SCHEDULE—MEDICAL PSYCHIATRIC PROGRAM

Time	Monday	Tuesday	Wednesday	Thursday	Friday	Saturday	Sunday
8:00 am	Breakfast	Breakfast	Breakfast	Breakfast	Breakfast	Breakfast	Breakfast
8:00–10:00 am	Daily Planning Morning Cares Team Rounds	Daily Planning Morning Cares Team Rounds	Daily Planning Morning Cares Team Rounds	Daily Planning Morning Cares Team Rounds	Daily Planning Morning Cares Team Rounds	Daily Planning Morning Cares Team Rounds	Daily Planning Morning Cares Team Rounds
10:00–11:00 am	RT*	Leisure Discussion	RT	Leisure Discussion	RT	Free time of Family Time	Church
11:30–12:00 pm	Free Time	Music Therapy	Free Time	Music Therapy	Free Time	Sittercize	Free Time
12:00–1:15 pm	Lunch	Lunch	Lunch	Lunch	Lunch	Lunch	Lunch
1:15–2:15 pm	Support Group	Support Group	Support Group	Support Group	Support Group	Support Group	Family Support Group
2:30–3:30 pm	RT/Sensory	Sensory	RT/Sensory	Spirituality	RT/Sensory	Sensory	Sensory
3:30–4:30 pm	Walk/Rest	Walk/Rest	Walk/Rest	Walk/Rest	Walk/Rest	Walk/Rest	Walk/Rest
4:30–5:15 pm	Free Time/Rest	Free Time/Rest	Free Time/Rest	Free Time/Rest	Free Time/Rest	Free Time/Rest	Free Time/Rest
5:15–6:00 pm	Dinner	Dinner	Dinner	Dinner	Dinner	Dinner	Dinner
6:00–7:00 pm	Education Group	Education Group	Education Group	Education Group	Education Group	Education Group	Education Group
7:00–7:30 pm	Social Group	Social Group	Social Group	Social Group	Social Group	Social Group	Social Group
7:30–8:30 pm	Provide Relaxing Environment	Provide Relaxing Environment	Provide Relaxing Environment	Provide Relaxing Environment	Provide Relaxing Environment	Movie and Popcorn	Movie and Snack

* RT - Recreational Therapy

Figure 126.1 Daily clinical programming

Factors that Influence Length of Stay and Re-admissions

Many important factors influence the length of hospital stay and re-admission to a medical psychiatry unit. One study examined factors associated with frequent admissions to a university-based acute geriatric psychiatric inpatient unit by dichotomizing patients into single versus multiple admissions, and found that the majority of re-admissions occurred within the first three months following discharge; and that being single, male and having bipolar disorder were significant predictors of rehospitalization[12]. Another study looking at predictors of psychiatric rehospitalization specifically among elderly patients found that re-admission was more likely for diagnoses of schizophrenia, bipolar disorder, depression and substance abuse[13]. The same study found re-admission to be different for mood disorders and non-mood disorders, with very short hospitalizations being associated with increased risk of rehospitalization among persons with a mood disorder. Often treatments can adversely impact length of stay and re-admission. ECT and many psychopharmacological agents are risk factors for falls in a psychogeriatric unit, increasing the length of stay. A similar but more recent study found several factors associated with longer lengths of stay among geriatric psychiatric units[14]. These factors include ECT and its unavailability on weekends; higher positive symptom scores on brief psychiatric rating scales following psychopharmacology complications; multiple prior psychiatric hospitalizations; court proceedings; consultation delays; and placement issues.

CLINICAL ISSUES

Overlap among the geropsychiatric, general medical psychiatry and neuropsychiatric patient population is more common than not. Geriatric psychiatry inpatient units are dedicated to serving patients who are 65 years and older, who have severe psychiatric illnesses that require psychiatric hospitalization. They may or may not have concurrent medical illnesses or high acuity. General medical psychiatry inpatients are adults of any age who require psychiatric hospitalization for acute psychiatric problems, with concurrent active medical problem or problems that need intensive medical care that cannot be safely managed on a general psychiatric inpatient unit. Neuropsychiatry inpatient units provide acute psychiatric care primarily to patients with dementia or active neurological problems that directly contribute to the psychiatric problem. Patients in a medical psychiatry unit are typically geriatric in age and have both co-morbid medical and neurological conditions (see Figure 126.2).

Common Conditions Treated in a Medical Psychiatry Unit

The conditions common to all three patient populations (i.e. geropsychiatric, neuropsychiatric and medical psychiatric) are organic mental disorders (delirium, dementia), mood disorders (depressive and bipolar disorders) and common chronic medical problems. Psychiatrically, depression is the most common condition seen in a medical psychiatry unit. Depression often complicates medical illnesses through medication interactions, side effects or non-compliance. Often, symptoms of depression mimic medical illness and pose diagnostic challenges. Sorting out these issues is a benefit on a medical psychiatric inpatient treatment unit. Untreated depression results in increasing rates of suicide, which is already a significant problem for the geriatric medically ill population. A study of psychogeriatric inpatient suicides in Australia found that

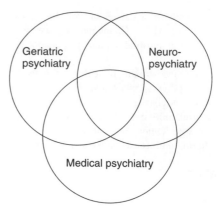

Figure 126.2 Overlap between geriatric psychiatry, medical psychiatry and neuropsychiatry patient populations

compared to younger inpatient suicides, they are more likely to have depression and more alcohol misuse in pre-admission and intra-admissions suicidal ideation[15].

A survey of 11 academic medical psychiatry units reported that mood disorders and organic mental disorders were the most common conditions seen[16]. Other psychiatric diagnoses include schizophrenia, personality disorders, anxiety disorders, somatoform disorders, pain syndromes, drug and alcohol abuse/detoxification and eating disorders. These diagnoses are similar to those in traditional psychiatric units. The most common medical concerns were neurological and cardiovascular. However, most medical psychiatry units that treat older patients have a high prevalence of cardiovascular and respiratory issues.

Other medical psychiatry problems managed on medical psychiatry units include delirium, dementia and behavioural complications; psychiatric manifestations of neurological disorders such as stroke, epilepsy, Parkinson's disease and head trauma; medically complicated eating disorders; chronic pain; paroxysmal behavioural disorders of unknown aetiology; factitious illness; somatoform disorders; and physical illness combined with a complex family of psychosocial problems that interfere with the patient's ability to cooperate with necessary medical treatment[1].

Inpatient Evaluation and Management in a Medical Psychiatry Unit

A comprehensive and thorough evaluation of all active psychiatric and medical problems is the goal in the inpatient medical psychiatry setting, which leads to a similarly comprehensive treatment and management of concurrent psychiatric and medical issues in a unified setting. A multidisciplinary approach is essential in order to meet the complex needs of medical psychiatry patients. The highly supervised and structured environment in an inpatient setting allows care providers to closely assess and monitor a person's psychiatric and medical status, including mood, behaviour, thought process, appetite, sleep patterns, level of physical functioning, vitals signs and other physical parameters. It is possible to see fluctuations in any of these areas in such a closely monitored environment. Members of the treatment team have more time to obtain collateral information regarding a patient's history and recent events leading to hospitalization from family members, friends, local physicians or other care providers.

Diagnostic evaluation is efficiently completed, including laboratories, imaging and other appropriate medical and surgical tests. Because of medical co-morbidities in this psychiatric population, baseline electrocardiogram, complete blood count, electrolytes, glucose, liver function tests, renal function tests and thyroid stimulating hormone should be standard. Other tests should be ordered according to a patient's active symptoms. Medical consultations from dedicated internists (details above under 'Multidisciplinary Treatment Team') are standard, and other consultations from medical and surgical specialties are also easily available and accessible. Care conferences, treatment planning and discharge planning are held in the inpatient unit in a coordinated manner with input from all sides, including patients, families and treatment team.

All modalities of psychiatric treatment are available in the inpatient unit, including psychopharmacologic agents, biologic treatments such as ECT and psychotherapeutic interventions. Because of the frequently more complex discharge needs of medical psychiatric and geriatric patients as dictated by their clinical and psychosocial needs, intensive social work involvement is essential for effective discharge and aftercare planning. Family support throughout hospitalization, and even immediately post-discharge, is commonly provided.

EDUCATION

The medical psychiatry unit is a rich training ground for medical students, residents, fellows and students of other specialties and disciplines. From a medical student perspective, rotations in the medical psychiatry unit allow them to grasp the concepts of mind–body connection and also realize that psychiatry is indeed a medical specialty. Psychiatric residents gain competence in the management of patients who are very ill and have very complicated medical and psychiatric co-morbidities. Other students who rotate on medical psychiatry units include fellows in geriatric psychiatry, psychosomatic medicine and geriatric medicine; residents in neurology or internal medicine; and students from other disciplines, such as nursing, pharmacy, chaplain services and recreation therapy.

RESEARCH

Many issues can be explored more comprehensively on a medical psychiatry inpatient unit to allow us to provide a better value of care for such patients with these co-morbid conditions. The three most pressing issues that should be explored on a medical psychiatry inpatient unit are: (i) research on the interface among medicine and psychiatry, neurology and psychiatry, and geriatrics; (ii) research on treatment outcomes in this patient population to determine which treatments work well and which do not; and (iii) research on the cost effectiveness of providing dual treatment concurrent care rather than separate, fragmented sequential care.

SUMMARY

Medical psychiatry units serve a unique role in the care of the complicated patients who have both psychiatric and medical problems. In addition to clinical care, medical psychiatry units educate medical students to recognize the common interactions between these problems and geriatric patients. Residents and other physicians learn to integrate, rather than fragment, care in order to provide the best patient outcomes. Determining how the medical psychiatry unit can improve value and the overall cost of care is essential for viability.

ACKNOWLEDGMENT

The authors gratefully acknowledge Linda K. Smith, RN, our medical psychiatry unit nurse manager who provided valuable information regarding unit operations.

REFERENCES

1. Stoudemire A, Fogel BS. Organization and development of combined medical-psychiatric units: Part 1. *Psychosomatics* 1986; **27**(5): 341–5.
2. Young LD, Harsch HH. Inpatient unit for combined physical and psychiatric disorders. *Psychosomatics* 1986; **27**(1): 53–60.
3. Fogel BS, Stoudemire A, Houpt JL. Contrasting models for combined medical and psychiatric inpatient treatment. *Am J Psychiatry* 1985; **142**(9): 1085–9.
4. Kathol RG. Medical psychiatry units: the wave of the future [comment]. *Gen Hosp Psychiatry* 1994; **16**(1): 1–3.
5. Kathol RG, Harsch HH, Hall RC *et al*. Categorization of types of medical/psychiatry units based on level of acuity. *Psychosomatics* 1992; **33**(4): 376–86.
6. Kathol RG, Harsch HH, Hall RC *et al*. Quality assurance in a setting designed to care for patients with combined medical and psychiatric disease. *Psychosomatics* 1992; **33**(4): 387–96.
7. Goodman B. Combined psychiatric-medical inpatient units: the Mount Sinai model. *Psychosomatics* 1985; **26**(3): 179–82.
8. Porello PT, Madsen L, Futterman A *et al*. Description of a geriatric medical/psychiatry unit in a small community general hospital. *J Ment Health Adm* 1995; **22**(1): 38–48.
9. Folks D, Kinney FC. The medical psychiatry inpatient unit. In Copeland J, Abou-Saleh M, Blazer D (eds), *Principles and Practice of Geriatric Psychiatry*, 2nd edn. Chichester: John Wiley & Sons, 2002, 709–12.
10. Passov V, Rundell JR. Analysis of transfers from a medical-psychiatry inpatient unit to a medical-surgical unit within 48 hours of admission. *Psychosomatics* 2008; **49**(6): 535–7.
11. Fogel BS, Stoudemire A. Organization and development of combined medical-psychiatric units: Part 2. *Psychosomatics* 1986; **27**(6): 417–20.
12. Woo BK, Golshan S, Allen EC *et al*. Factors associated with frequent admissions to an acute geriatric psychiatric inpatient unit. *J Geriatr Psychiatry Neurol* 2006; **19**(4): 226–30.
13. Prince JD, Akincigil A, Kalay E *et al*. Psychiatric rehospitalization among elderly persons in the United States. *Psychiatr Serv* 2008; **59**(9): 1038–45.
14. Blank K, Hixon L, Gruman C *et al*. Determinants of geropsychiatric inpatient length of stay. *Psychiatr Q* 2005; **76**(2): 195–212.
15. Shah A, Ganesvaran T. Psychogeriatric inpatient suicides in Australia. *Int J Geriatr Psychiatry* 1997; **12**(1): 15–19.
16. Harsch HH, Koran LM, Young LD. A profile of academic medical-psychiatric units. *Gen Hosp Psychiatry* 1991; **13**(5): 291–5.

127

Psychiatric Services in Long-Term Care

Marc E. Agronin[1], Stephen M. Scheinthal[2] and Ashok J. Bharucha[3]

[1]*Miami Jewish Health Systems, Miami, and University of Miami Miller School of Medicine, Miami, FL, USA*
[2]*Geriatric Behavioral Health, New Jersey Institute for Successful Aging, University of Medicine and Dentistry of New Jersey – School of Osteopathic Medicine, Stratford, NJ, USA*
[3]*Robert Young Center, Iowa Health System Moline, IL, USA*

As the percentage of individuals living into their 70s and older continues to increase dramatically across most developed countries in the world, there has been a corresponding increase in the number of individuals living in long-term care (LTC) facilities. In the United States alone there are approximately 1.43 million residents living in nearly 16 000 nursing homes, and over 1 million residents in over 35 000 assisted living facilities (ALFs)[1]. Psychiatric illness represents one major reason for individuals needing the structure and assistance of an LTC facility. Epidemiological surveys indicate that at least two-thirds of all residents suffer from one or more psychiatric conditions, usually dementia, depression, delirium and/or behavioural disturbances[2]. A survey of LTC nursing directors in six states identified not only a pressing need for psychiatric services in general, but also highlighted the need for specific help with non-pharmacological approaches to resident management[3]. All of these figures suggest that competent, skilled provision of mental health services is fundamental to the well-being of these residents. As a result, there is a critical need for geriatric-trained psychiatrists and other mental health specialists to work in these settings. In addition, the myriad regulations that the psychiatrist must understand in caring for patients in a facility is constantly expanding. This chapter will review the potential roles of the geriatric psychiatrist, key clinical issues and the important regulations that guide practice in LTC. Although the regulations cited are specific to the United States, they represent approaches to quality of care that are relevant to international LTC settings.

ROLES

The main role of the geriatric-trained psychiatrist in any LTC setting is to provide psychiatric consultations and follow-up care for residents. These consultations are warranted by the presence of psychiatric illness, by regulations that stipulate routine psychiatric surveillance of residents and monitoring of psychotropic medications, and by the need for risk management for situations in which potentially dangerous behaviours present. In addition, the psychiatrist may play roles in administration, education, clinical oversight and research. A summary of all potential roles can be found in Table 127.1.

Although it is rare for a psychiatrist to serve as the actual medical director of a facility, it should be clear from Table 127.1 that his or

Table 127.1 The roles of the psychiatrist in LTC settings

- Provide psychiatric evaluation and follow-up for residents
- Provide crisis management for residents (e.g. for suicidal, assaultive, abusive and homicidal behaviours)
- Initiate and oversee voluntary and involuntary hospitalizations
- Provide liaison for relevant mental health issues to administrators, social workers, MDS coordinators, risk managers, and other caregiving staff
- Communicate with family and other caregivers regarding resident mental health issues
- Conduct forensic evaluations of decision-making capacity
- Provide oversight for the use of psychotropic medications
- Maintain adherence to state/federal/national regulations
- Educate staff about psychiatric issues
- Administer or lead a mental health team
- Supervise ancillary mental health trainees and staff
- Participate in facility committees: medical staff, pharmacy and therapeutics, ethics etc.
- Assist the primary medical team in facilitating communication of complex medical, psychosocial, and safety issues with clients and their families
- Assist with end-of-life care decisions
- Conduct research studies
- Manage mental health programmes (group therapy, intensive outpatient programmes, memory centres etc.)

her multifaceted roles go well beyond being merely a consultant. In fact, the psychiatrist's deep immersion in the LTC milieu is critical to his or her understanding of the day-to-day dynamics of institutional care that impinge upon the well-being of residents.

The psychiatric consultant is also a key player in risk management. From the perspective of any facility, many situations that involve potential threats of harm to residents or that have the potential to incur substantial liability inevitably involve psychiatric conditions or the effects of psychotropic medications. Several of these circumstances are listed in Table 127.2.

One of the most critical roles of the consultant is to provide oversight for the use of psychotropic medications. As will be discussed

Principles and Practice of Geriatric Psychiatry, 3rd edn. Edited by Mohammed T. Abou-Saleh, Cornelius Katona and Anand Kumar
© 2011 John Wiley & Sons, Ltd

Table 127.2 Psychiatric issues that increase the risk of harm and liability

- Poor safety awareness (wandering off from units, handling inappropriate objects, walking with unsteady gait)
- Suicidal threats, gestures or attempts
- Indirect life-threatening behaviours (e.g. refusing to eat, take medications or submit to life-sustaining tests or treatments)
- Physically aggressive/assaultive behaviours towards other residents and/or staff
- Sexually abusive behaviours
- Homicidal threats
- Risk of falling due to psychotropic medications (e.g. benzodiazepines, antipsychotics, sedative-hypnotics)
- Risk of severe psychotropic medication side effects, especially those related to antipsychotics (e.g. diabetes, severe weight gain, tardive dyskinesia, stroke, cardiac conduction delays and death)

Table 127.3 Optimizing education and communication

- Staff in-sevices on Alzheimer's disease and other dementia types, depression and suicidality, anxiety disorders, behavioural disturbances, sexuality, sleep disorders, psychotropic medications and non-pharmacological management techniques
- Lectures to family and friends of residents on mental health issues
- Routine phone contact with caregivers regarding resident status
- Write educational articles for LTC facility publications and websites, and for local media
- Speak to community organizations that interface with the facility (e.g. guardianship associations, Alzheimer's Association)
- Sponsor memory and depression screenings at the facility or in the community

Table 127.4 Epidemiology of major psychiatric conditions in nursing homes[a]

Diagnosis	Community prevalence (%)	Nursing home prevalence (%)
Major depression	2–4	15
Depressive disorders	10–15	30–47
Anxiety disorders	11	20
Anxiety symptoms	20	40
Dementia (all types, ages 65+)	25	50–67
Schizophrenia	< 1	6

[a] Note: these figures are rounded off and based on approximate ranges from four sources[8–11].

later in the chapter, the use of nearly all psychotropic medications requires clear documentation of the diagnostic indication, implementation of concomitant behavioural strategies, judicious dosing and mandatory attempts at dose reductions for conditions that naturally have symptomatic remission.

Another important role for the psychiatrist is to educate LTC staff about common psychiatric symptoms and diagnoses, and how to initiate referrals and provide clinical data, recognize medication side effects and deal with behavioural disturbances. Any employee of an LTC facility has the potential to recognize psychiatric illness, ranging from nurses, aides, dieticians, therapists and social workers who provide hands-on care, to administrators who deal with complaints and crises, to kitchen and custodial staff who may form bonds with residents and notice early changes in behaviour. Thus, all of these individuals need access to the psychiatrist as well as training in the recognition and management of common psychiatric symptoms.

Communication with family members and other caregivers is one of the most critical and yet often neglected roles of the psychiatric consultant. Not only can these caregivers provide some of the most detailed and accurate clinical information, but they often aide the implementation of treatment plans, from encouraging residents to take medications and participate in activities, to simply providing essential care and companionship[4]. Working in partnership with caregivers helps to reduce caregiver burden that otherwise takes a toll in terms of their mental and physical health[5], and makes the LTC facility feel more like a community and less like an institution[6]. Ideal doctor–caregiver communication also serves a primary role in risk management for the facility, since it can mitigate feelings of anger, alienation and confusion when unfortunate events such as injuries occur – ultimately reducing litigiousness. In fact, such communication can engender realistic expectations of care in the LTC setting and even anticipate certain problems before they erupt. Several ways to optimize education and communication between the psychiatrist, staff and caregivers are listed in Table 127.3.

CLINICAL ISSUES

The entire spectrum of psychiatric diagnoses seen in geriatric patients is present in LTC settings, and requires the same approaches to diagnosis and treatment as in any other setting. One challenge for the psychiatric consultant is that there does tend to be greater medical and psychiatric co-morbidity in residents suffering from either acute delirium or chronic dementia – or both. There is also a greater concentration of psychiatric disorders including depression, dementia, anxiety disorders and schizophrenia compared to the community (see Table 127.4). Many of the same stigmas that limit adequate psychiatric care for elderly in the community will also apply in LTC, such as viewing depression or cognitive impairment as 'normal' in late life, or assuming that older personalities are more rigid, stubborn and treatment resistant[7]. All of these assumptions are incorrect and can prove discriminatory. Complicating the effects of these ageist views is the shortage of geriatric psychiatrists to consult in LTC settings, and the discriminatory reimbursement rates that have historically penalized psychiatric diagnosis (now being reversed by recent US federal legislation).

On the other hand, individuals with psychiatric impairment living in LTC settings have a much greater chance of being evaluated in a timely manner due to mandated regulations. Medication adherence can be better monitored, and supportive staff and therapeutic activities are all on site. Thus, many of the barriers to treatment in the community, such as lack of transportation or timely access to mental health clinicians, do not exist in LTC settings.

The first and most fundamental trigger of psychiatric decompensation in LTC is the transfer to the facility itself. Whether they are coming from a long-standing home or an inpatient ward at a hospital, most new admissions have faced a recent medical or psychiatric stress or crisis and are no longer able to live alone. The psychological impact of the reason for admission and the unfamiliarity of the setting and its rules can be upsetting, especially for individuals who do not like living with others or have set routines that are now being disrupted. The psychiatric consultant must be attuned to the symptomatic manifestations of this stress, found in anxious and depressed moods, anger, agitation, resistance to care, disruptions in sleep and

Table 127.5 Recognition and treatment of adjustment reactions to LTC placement

STEP 1	Review profile and history of resident prior to arrival to anticipate unique needs and challenges (e.g. resident has complicated psychotropic regimen that should be reviewed and monitored from the moment of arrival)
STEP 2	Educate staff to recognize manifestations of difficult adjustment: nervousness, anger, sadness, social withdrawal, agitation, insomnia, anorexia, exaggerated physical complaints, resistance to care, poor rehabilitation
STEP 3	Develop admission procedures for social workers and nursing staff to collect basic psychiatric history as well as to screen for cognitive impairment and depression in order to identify individuals who need early intervention. Staff should be proactive about talking to primary care physicians or the medical director to write orders for psychiatric consultations
STEP 4	Obtain information about residents' interests and needs in order to best provide care and therapeutic activities. Ask family members to provide photos, room decorations, radios, televisions etc. in order to make the new room feel familiar and comfortable
STEP 5	Provide individual and group counselling for adjustment issues
STEP 6	Promote early and aggressive intervention for new psychiatric symptoms or the exacerbation of previous disorders

appetite, exaggerated somatic complaints, poor rehabilitation, and even failure to thrive. Although previous psychiatric history may be a key guide to diagnosis and treatment, the adjustment reaction itself must be addressed. Several ways to recognize and ameliorate this adjustment are listed in Table 127.5.

In general, the diagnosis and treatment of psychiatric disorders in older patients will be similar regardless of whether they live in the community or in an LTC setting. There are, however, a number of clinical features that are unique to LTC settings, summarized in Table 127.6.

The psychiatric consultant often has to work with family members and other caregivers who may be dealing with their own emotional issues over having a loved one in the facility. Strong feelings of guilt, grief and anger are sometimes displaced onto staff members, resulting in conflicts over care issues. Often these conflicts stem from unrealistic expectations of what institutions can provide and how quickly they can do it. In other situations the family or caregivers themselves suffer from psychiatric disorders that limit or distort their interactions with staff. A general rule of thumb is for the consultant to identify the next-of-kin or legally authorized representative of the patient and then communicate early on in order to obtain history and discuss the diagnosis and treatment plan. A team approach can help to optimize care and provide a consistent approach with difficult caregivers. Consultants need to avoid engaging in defensive or passive–aggressive approaches with these caregivers, such as not answering phone calls or arguing over treatment issues, since they will only worsen the situation and lead to further conflict.

In thinking about the provision of psychiatric services in LTC, an obvious question is: what is known about the models of mental health services delivery and the relative effectiveness of such models? A

seminal review of the literature by Bartels, Moak and Dums (2002)[12] identified three relatively distinct models that merit mention: (i) a psychiatrist-centred model, (ii) a psychiatric-nurse-centred model, and (iii) a multidisciplinary team-based approach. The approximately 20 reports that examined these three models, however, were noted to suffer from serious methodological limitations, including (in the vast majority of cases) non-experimental designs, small sample sizes, lack of control groups and outcome measures that may not have been ideally situated to capture the model's effectiveness. Nonetheless, a few broad pragmatic themes emerged that appear to be relevant to clinical practice in LTC settings. Firstly, preliminary evidence indicates that nursing home personnel prefer regularly scheduled psychiatric visits with timely (and medically necessary) maintenance treatment follow-up[3]. Secondly, interdisciplinary, multidimensional approaches appear to be favoured over solo consultations. And finally, innovative approaches that integrate education and training with consultation, and offer hands-on advice about behavioural management in addition to neuropsychiatric diagnostic work-up and treatment planning are considered optimal.

REGULATIONS

For the last two decades, psychiatric care in LTC settings has been under increasing scrutiny from US state and federal governments. This scrutiny began in the 1980s when concern about the inappropriate use of psychotropic medications and physical restraints resulted in the adoption of Nursing Home Reform Amendments in the 1987 US Federal Budget Act, known as the Omnibus Budget Reconciliation Act of 1987 or OBRA '87. Final OBRA regulations came into effect in 1991[13]. OBRA '87 represented the biggest change in Medicare regulations since the programme was created in 1965. One mandate was the reduction and/or elimination of both physical and chemical restraints in nursing homes. Much of the drive to reduce the use of psychotropic medications came from the realization that many of them have potentially serious adverse effects, particularly extrapyramidal symptoms, tardive dyskinesia and neuroleptic malignant syndrome associated with antipsychotic agents.

The philosophy of OBRA is that judicious dosing and frequent attempts at dose reduction will prevent unnecessary use, reduce the frequency and intensity of adverse effects, and promote better surveillance and safety in LTC settings. The implementation of OBRA guidelines and their enforcement through routine surveys has resulted over time in up to a 50% overall decrease in chemical and physical restraints accompanied by a significant increase in the use of behavioural interventions[14,15]. Despite the enactment of these guidelines, however, documented physical restraint usage remains as high as 61% in some facilities[16]. Psychiatrists who work in LTC settings in the USA must understand OBRA guidelines in their entirety and be able to ensure their maintenance in order to optimize psychiatric care and avoid citations from routine surveys. A summary of these responsibilities can be found in Table 127.7.

Prior to an admission to a nursing home in the United States, state licensing agencies (under the authority of the OBRA regulations) must conduct a Preadmission Screening and Annual Resident Reviews or PASARR in order to prevent admission of people with developmental disabilities or severe, chronic mental illness. The PASARR regulation was set in motion in January of 1993. The PASARR screen needs to be conducted independently of a facility, and should be completed annually. To date, however, outcome studies of the PASARR programme have documented poor compliance

Table 127.6 Common psychiatric diagnoses and issues relevant to LTC settings

Diagnosis	Relevant issues
Major depression and depressive disorders	• Suicidal behaviours (may be indirect life-threatening behaviours) • Apathy that interferes with daily functioning • Failure to thrive (with weight loss, malnutrition, dehydration, and complication of co-morbid medical issues)
Alzheimer's disease and other dementias	• Disruptive and/or dangerous behaviours • Psychosis (delusions, hallucinations) • Postural and gait instability and risk of falls • Bladder and bowel incontinence • Risk of aspiration and pneumonia • Sensitivity to centrally active medications
Anxiety disorders	• Phobia of falling may limit ambulation and participation in physical therapy • Compulsive behaviours are frustrated by institutional schedules and lack of privacy • Panic attacks may involve physical and verbal agitation
Schizophrenia and other psychotic disorders	• Disruptive and/or dangerous behaviours based on paranoid, grandiose or bizarre delusions • Suicidality • Risks of antipsychotic side effects • Health and safety risks from excess tobacco use • Lack of appropriately structured therapeutic activities
Personality disorders	• Staff and family burnout due to excess demands and emotional and behavioural crises • Suicidal and homicidal behaviours • Loss of functioning and deconditioning due to excess dependency needs • Non-adherence with institutional rules, medications, and other treatments • Litigiousness

Table 127.7 A summary of the psychiatrist's responsibilities under OBRA '87 Interpretive Guidelines (USA only)

- Become familiar with OBRA Guidelines, including the use of the MDS and RAPs
- Be familiar with Beers criteria which list medications to be avoided since they involve a high potential for adverse outcomes
- Promptly provide comprehensive psychiatric evaluation for requested individuals in order to document: (i) current symptoms, (ii) diagnosis, (iii) potential causes, (iv) use of behavioural interventions, (v) justification for psychotropic and/or physical restraint usage
- Document required diagnoses and stay within OBRA designated dosing ranges when prescribing benzodiazepines, other sedative-hypnotics and antipsychotic agents (unless the rationale for higher doses is documented)
- For sleeping pills, daily use should be for less than 10 days unless a gradual dose reduction has been unsuccessful (and attempted at least 3 times within a 6-month period)
- For antipsychotics, benzodiazepines and sedative-hypnotics, consider and document a gradual dose reduction at least twice within a year (approximately every 6 months)
- For antidepressant medications, document appropriate diagnosis and attempts at gradual dose reduction if there is complete lack of efficacy or long-term symptomatic stability
- Attend regular psychotropic medication meetings at the facility with nursing staff and the consulting pharmacist to review psychotropic drug use and adherence to OBRA guidelines

with recommendations for alternative placement as well as with the implementation of new mental health services[15,17]. These findings highlight yet again the critical role of the psychiatrist in identifying residents in need of mental health services, as well as investigating (both from a clinical as well as research standpoint) care processes that may facilitate implementation of the PASARR mandate.

Upon admission, nursing homes must conduct a comprehensive assessment of each resident's needs and functional capacity and then repeat this yearly using a standardized instrument called the Resident Assessment Instrument (RAI). Two major parts of the RAI include the minimum data set (MDS), which collects a spectrum of relevant resident-specific information on needs and function, and resident assessment protocols (RAPs) which are triggered by certain MDS data, and help clinical staff conduct more detailed evaluations of problems such as mood and behavioural disturbances. Quality indicators (QIs) and Quality measures (QMs) are derived from MDS data and used as rough grading measures for the nursing home (and are even posted for public review on the website of the Center for Medicare and Medicaid Services or CMS). QIs specific to psychiatric care include items that report the prevalence of behavioural symptoms affecting others, symptoms of depression (especially without antidepressant therapy), cognitive impairment, the use of other psychotropic medications, and restraint usage. It is worth noting that the greatest unresolved controversies regarding the validity of the MDS items centres upon the behavioural symptoms, suggesting a need for expert psychiatric evaluation, rather than relying upon clinical assessment by routine staff alone[18].

Psychiatric Consultation

The psychiatric consultant needs to be acutely aware when practicing in LTC facilities (and to a lesser extent in ALFs) that these are highly regulated environments with regular surveys by state, federal and other accreditation organizations. In his or her varied roles, the consultant contributes critical services and oversight that can maintain adherence to key regulations, such as OBRA, and prevent citations for not meeting state regulations. In addition, the consultant must be able to work closely with the medical director, administrator, director of nursing, risk manager, social workers and unit managers to ensure that everyone is 'on the same page' and functioning as a team. These interactions become particularly critical when working with residents with severe behavioural disturbances that pose a risk of harm to self or others, and help to ensure that proper channels of communication are maintained with distressed families.

CMS regulations are very strict as to who may provide psychiatric care in a nursing home. In addition to psychiatrists, clinical nurse specialists with psychiatric training are also allowed to use psychiatric consultative codes and psychotherapy codes, but the regulations for geriatric nurse practitioners are more restrictive. A consult must have a signed order by a physician, typically the primary provider, and the need should be supported by nursing notes. The order should then reflect the specific reason and not simply state 'psychiatric consult requested'. Pre-printed orders and family requests are not sufficient for a consultation because they do not necessarily support medical necessity. Verbal orders are permitted but should be the exception and not the rule. In addition, there should be documentation in the physician's notes as to why a consult is required. The bottom line is that a psychiatric consultation is neither automatic nor at the discretion of non-clinical staff, but must have a specific, documented justification and order.

Psychotropic Drug Reviews

As noted above and in Table 127.1, a primary role of the psychiatrist in LTC facilities is to prescribe and monitor psychotropic medications. The need for clear documentation on diagnosis, rationale for

Table 127.8   OBRA Interpretive Guidelines for specific psychotropics[13]

Short and long-acting benzodiazepines and other anxiolytic/sedative drugs

- Other possible reasons for resident's distress have been considered and ruled out
- The resident meets criteria for one of the following DSM-IV diagnoses: generalized anxiety disorder, organic mental syndrome (delirium, dementia, or amnesic and other cognitive disorders), panic disorder, symptomatic anxiety due to another disorder
- Use is equal to or less than the maximum recommended daily dose
- Daily use at any dose is less than 4 consecutive months, unless an attempt at gradual dose reduction is unsuccessful
- A gradual dose reduction should be attempted at least twice within 1 year
- Long-acting benzodiazepines should only used after an attempt to use a short-acting agent has failed
- Exceptions to the rule for long-acting benzodiazepines: withdrawal from short-acting agent, diazepam for neuromuscular syndromes, clonazepam for bipolar disorder, tardive dyskinesia, nocturnal myoclonus, or seizure disorders

Drugs used for sleep induction

- Other possible reasons for resident's insomnia have been considered and ruled out
- Use is equal to or less than the maximum recommended daily dose
- Daily use at any dose is less than 10 consecutive days, unless an attempt at dose reduction is unsuccessful
- A gradual dose reduction should be attempted at least 3 times within a 6-month period

Antipsychotic drugs

- The resident meets criteria for one of the following DSM-IV diagnoses: schizophrenia or other acute or chronic psychotic disorder, Tourette's disorder, Huntington's disease, organic mental syndromes (delirium and dementia) with associated psychotic and/or agitated behaviours that are documented and that pose a risk of harm to self or others or interfere with staff's ability to provide care
- Use is equal to or less than the maximum recommended daily dose
- prn use discouraged unless a quick taper is being conducted
- A gradual dose reduction should be attempted at least twice within 1 year
- Close monitoring for tardive dyskinesia, postural hypotension, cognitive and behavioural impairment, akathisia, parkinsonism and metabolic disturbances (weight gain, hyperlipidaemia, hyperglycaemia)
- Inappropriate indications: wandering, fidgeting/restlessness/nervousness, insomnia, anxiety, uncooperativeness, unsociability, impaired memory, depression, poor self-care and agitation that does not pose a danger to self and others
- Exceptions to the rule for attempted dose reductions are for chronic psychotic disorders and bipolar disorder

Table 127.9 Drugs and drug–diagnosis combinations with high potential for adverse outcomes based on Beers criteria

* Tricyclic antidepressants (amitriptyline and doxepin)
* Use of tricyclic antidepressants in residents with cardiac arrhythmias
* Use of sedative-hypnotics in residents with chronic obstructive pulmonary disease
* Use of antidepressants with anticholinergic properties in residents with benign prostatic hypertrophy

use, appropriate dosing, behavioural management and attempts at gradual dose reduction has been emphasized. The failure to provide this documentation can not only lead to citations for the facility, but on a broader level can create jeopardy for the psychiatrist in terms of reimbursement for services. Lack of compliance with CMS regulation in terms of medical necessity of the visit and the use of the correct procedural code can lead to hefty fines.

In terms of actual prescribing, OBRA guidelines provide specific lists of regulated medications, conditions that justify their use, and maximum recommended daily doses. Although all of these details are too numerous to list, a condensed list can be found in Table 127.8.

Original OBRA '87 guidelines covered benzodiazepines, other sedative-hypnotic medications and antipsychotic agents. More recent revisions by CMS under Guideline F-329 consider *any* drug as unnecessary if it is being given under any of the following conditions: (i) excessive dose, (ii) duplicate therapy, (iii) a prolonged period of time without justification, (iv) without adequate monitoring, (v) without adequate indications, or (vi) in the presence of adverse consequences. Although each of these requirements seems rooted in common sense and is associated with good clinical practice, their implications are perhaps greatest with respect to the widespread use of antidepressants, antipsychotics, and mood stabilizers in LTC. Whereas in the past a psychiatrist might have routinely considered antipsychotic tapers while maintaining long-standing use of antidepressants, now both classes of medication might be in line for gradual dose reductions (GDRs) if the clinical need for prolonged use is not documented and justified.

Another important set of regulations first promulgated by the geriatrician Mark Beers, and later incorporated into OBRA guidelines, is known as the *Beers criteria*, and is composed of a list of drugs and drug–diagnosis combinations that incur a high risk of adverse outcomes in individuals over the age of 65 years[19,20]. In general, these high-risk situations should be avoided or only used with explicit justification and close monitoring. Beers criteria most relevant to psychiatric practice are listed in Table 127.9.

REFERENCES

1. Gillespie SM, Katz PR. An overview of residents, care providers, and regulation of medical practice in the long-term-care continuum. In Reichman WE, Katz PR (eds), *Psychiatry in Long-Term Care*. Oxford: Oxford University Press, 2009, 449–64.
2. Gruber-Baldini AL, Day H, Magaziner J. Epidemiology of psychiatric conditions in nursing homes. In Reichman WE, Katz PR (eds), *Psychiatry in Long-Term Care*. Oxford: Oxford University Press, 2009, 3–16.
3. Reichman WE, Coyne AC, Borson S *et al*. Psychiatric consultation in the nursing home: a survey of six states. *Am J Geriatr Psychiatry* 1998; **6**(4): 320–7.
4. Bluestein D, Latham Bach P. Working with families in long-term care. *J Am Med Dir Assoc* 2007; **8**(4): 265–70.
5. Etters L, Goodall D, Harrison BE. Caregiver burden among dementia patient caregivers: a review of the literature. *J Am Acad Nurse Pract* 2008; **20**(8): 423–8.
6. Verbeek H, van Rossum E, Zwakhalen SM *et al*. Small, homelike environments for older people with dementia: a literature review. *Int Psychogeriatr* 2009; **21**(2): 252–64.
7. Parker VA, Miyake Geron S. Cultural competence in nursing homes: issues and implications for education. *Gerontol Geriatr Educ* 2007; **28**(2): 37–54.
8. Gurland BJ. Epidemiology of psychiatric disorders. In Sadavoy J, Jarvik LF, Grossberg GT, Meyers BS (eds), *Comprehensive Textbook of Geriatric Psychiatry*, 3rd edn. New York: W.W. Norton & Company, 2004, 3–38.
9. Bharucha AJ, Borson S. Mood disorders. In Reichman WE, Katz PR (eds), *Psychiatry in Long-Term Care*. Oxford: Oxford University Press, 2009, 67–128.
10. Walaszek A, Howell T, Anxiety disorders. In Reichman WE, Katz PR (eds), *Psychiatry in Long-Term Care*. Oxford: Oxford University Press, 2009, 129–48.
11. Savla GN, DelaPena-Murphy J, Sewell DD, Kim DS, Jeste DV. Schizophrenia and other psychotic disorders. In Reichman WE, Katz PR (eds), *Psychiatry in Long-Term Care*. Oxford: Oxford University Press, 2009, 149–68.
12. Bartels SJ, Moak GS, Dums AR. Models of mental health services in nursing homes: a review of the literature. *Psychiatr Serv* 2002; **53**(11): 1390–6.
13. Federal Register 56(187): 48865–921. *Medicare and Medicaid. Requirements for Long-Term Care Facilities, Final Regulations*. Health Care Financing Administration, 1991.
14. Siegler EL, Caezuti E, Maislin G *et al*. Effects of a restraint reduction intervention and OBRA '87 regulations on psychotropic drug use in nursing homes. *J Am Ger Society* 1997; **45**(7): 791–6.
15. Snowden M, Roy-Byrne P. Mental illness and nursing home reform: OBRA-87 ten years later. Omnibus Budget Reconciliation Act. *Psychiatric Serv* 1998; **49**(2): 229–33.
16. Hamers JP, Gulpers MJ, Strik W. Use of physical restraints with cognitively impaired nursing home residents. *J Adv Nurs* 2004; **45**(3): 246–51.
17. Linkins KW, Lucca AM, Housman M, Smith SA. Use of PASRR programs to assess serious mental illness and service access in nursing homes. *Psychiatr Serv* 2006; **57**(3): 325–32.
18. Bharucha AJ, Vasilescu M, Dew MA *et al*. Prevalence of behavioral symptoms: comparison of the minimum data set assessments with research instruments. *J Am Med Dir Assoc* 2008; **9**(4): 244–50.
19. Beers MH, Ouslander JG, Fingold SF *et al*. Inappropriate medication prescribing in skilled nursing facilities. *Ann Int Med* 1992; **117**(8): 354–60.
20. Beers MH. Explicit criteria for determining potentially inappropriate medication use in the elderly: an update. *Ann Int Med* 1997; **157**(14): 1531–6.

Geriatric Psychiatry Care in the Private Psychiatric Hospital Setting

Brent P. Forester[1], Robert Kohn[2], Susan Kim[1] and Thomas Idiculla[1]

[1]McLean Hospital, Harvard University Belmont, MA, USA
[2]The Miriam Hospital, Brown University Providence, RI, USA

INTRODUCTION

The private psychiatric hospital offers an opportunity to deliver specialized treatment to geriatric patients across a continuum of care. The types of psychiatric services offered in these hospitals vary, but may include a dedicated geriatric psychiatry inpatient unit, partial hospital programmes that can accommodate the needs of older patients transitioning out of the acute psychiatric setting or requiring more intensive outpatient treatment, and outpatient services that include memory diagnostic clinics. Private psychiatric hospitals offer unique challenges to providing the appropriate medical care often needed for older adults with complex neuropsychiatric disorders. Most private psychiatric hospitals are not geographically proximate or integrated into the general medical hospital setting. Consequently, they are more limited in the acuity of medical care provided. This chapter will review models of geriatric psychiatry care in the private psychiatric hospital setting, examine the limited literature available on this topic, and describe an analysis of diagnosis and treatment trends over the past 15 years in two private psychiatric hospitals: McLean Hospital and Butler Hospital.

INPATIENT GERIATRIC PSYCHIATRY TREATMENT IN THE PRIVATE PSYCHIATRIC HOSPITAL

Most of the literature describing inpatient geriatric psychiatric treatment does not specifically examine inpatient units in private psychiatric hospitals. However, a review of what we know about inpatient geriatric psychiatry treatment will help provide a useful background for more specific diagnosis and treatment trends in the private hospital setting. Research conducted in New Zealand has shown that treatment in an acute geriatric psychiatry inpatient unit is effective and beneficial. This outcome study found that those with 'functional disorders' showed improvement in behaviour and symptoms, while those with 'organic disorders' had improvement in functional impairment, behaviour and symptoms[1]. Furthermore, there are clinical advantages to having a sub-specialized geriatric psychiatry unit. A retrospective chart review revealed that the specialized geriatric psychiatry unit offered more thorough and dedicated care to their geriatric patients compared to the general psychiatry unit[2]. This study revealed that significantly greater percentages of older inpatients treated on the geriatric psychiatry unit received 'complete organic medical workups, structured cognitive assessment, ageing-sensitive aftercare referral, and monitoring of psychopharmacological side effects and blood levels' than patients on a general psychiatry unit.

Physical Structure of the Inpatient Unit

The physical structure of the geriatric unit is designed to accommodate both the emotional and physical needs of the patients. These units are designed to provide a therapeutic milieu that limits restrictions on the geriatric patient. Adaptations that may not be appropriate or considered safe for a general psychiatric unit (e.g. handrails and grab bars) are made for a specialized geriatric psychiatric unit. Other adaptations include: low beds and over-bed tables, walk out showers, whirlpool tubs, enlarged signs and posters, appropriate furniture (such as seating with arms that enhances independent standing), call lights, personal alarms, non-slip and cushioned flooring, large day rooms with space to wander safely, a designated area for those who yell to limit the disruption of the rest of the unit, wheelchair and walker accessibility, bright lighting, calendars in rooms, and large clocks in rooms. These units may even have fish tanks and other visually stimulating additions. Light and pet therapy, which has been shown to improve 'psychopathological status' and 'perception of quality of life' in cognitively unimpaired elderly subjects[3], may be readily available.

Sub-specialized geriatric units might offer amenities that are specific to the unique needs of geriatric patients such as large signs, colour coordination and enlarged room numbers which aid patients in confronting problems with loss of orientation[4]. Private geriatric psychiatry units may create a home-like ambiance which is associated with 'improved intellectual and emotional well-being, enhanced social interaction, reduced agitation, reduced trespassing and exit seeking and improved functionality of older adults with dementia and other mental illnesses'[4].

Specialized Dementia Units

Private psychiatric hospitals that do offer designated dementia units are able to address needs specific to patients with dementia. For example, such units may utilize decreased auditory and visual stimulation, which has been shown to reduce agitation and aggression levels among demented patients[5]. A number of studies support the efficacy of environmental interventions to successfully manage the prevalent behavioural complications of dementia[4]. Factors to consider include providing patients with dementia-appropriate sensory stimulation and safety measures. Sensory overstimulation may exacerbate problems with distraction, agitation, concentration and confusion[4]. Alternatively, deprivation of sensory stimulation may have negative effects on patients with dementia[4].

Designing a separate unit for patients with dementia may also afford the opportunity to create group treatment programming that is more specific to the needs of cognitively impaired individuals. Although some hospitals may offer a distinct dementia unit for those who are cognitively intact, many units include both those with cognitive disorders and primary affective or psychotic disorders. This requires that the treatment team be versatile in addressing the needs of the unit as the population mix changes.

The Multidisciplinary Team

The inpatient geriatric psychiatry unit utilizes a multidisciplinary team that focuses on respecting the patient and their culture. This team includes the geriatric psychiatrist, the nurses, mental health workers or clinical nurse assistants, an internist preferably specialized in geriatric medicine, a clinical pharmacist, neuropsychologist, social worker, occupational and physical therapists and activity support staff. The geriatric psychiatrist is often the treatment team leader and the medical director, with administrative responsibilities that may include screening admission referrals, managing length of stay and handling personnel training and supervision. The geriatric psychiatrist initiates the appropriate neuropsychiatric work-up, including referral to subspecialists in neurology, geriatric medicine, neuropsychology, physical medicine and rehabilitation, and physical and occupational therapy. The geriatric psychiatry inpatient unit nurse must be comfortable with patients who may require total ADL (activity of daily living) care. The nurse needs to demonstrate flexible skills that enable her to assume the role of a medical nurse while providing traditional psychiatric nursing interventions, including supportive therapy for those who are cognitively intact. The neuropsychologist conducts neurocognitive testing to assist with differential diagnosis of cognitive disorders for patients referred by the geriatric psychiatrist. In addition, the neuropsychologist may assist in developing behavioural treatment recommendations, including implementation of individualized behavioural plans.

Managing Medical Co-morbidity in the Free-Standing, Private Psychiatric Hospital

Any inpatient unit in a private psychiatry hospital (and non-general medical hospital) setting is limited in the management of individuals who are severely medically compromised. Many of these units have a dedicated internal medicine specialist who is an integral member of the treatment team and will round daily and monitor individual medical issues including hydration status, treatment of co-morbid infectious disease (pneumonia, UTI, diarrhoea) and management of chronic medical issues such as diabetes and hypertension. Daily laboratory monitoring or the use of intravenous fluids or antibiotics may be required. The coordination of care with the medical team is essential to allow for a rapid and appropriate assessment of the patient with a suspected delirium. One of the most challenging aspects of this coordination of care is being able to differentiate the medical issues that can be effectively managed on-site and those that require a transfer-out to a local general medical hospital setting for diagnosis and management. In general, the development of a diagnosis of delirium in a hospitalized older adult is a medical emergency, and underlying causes need to be determined and treated in a timely manner. If the aetiology of the delirium is unknown or if there are changes in an individual's vital signs or EKG, a referral to a general medical hospital setting is initiated for further acute medical work-up and treatment.

The Role of the Social Worker

The social worker on a geriatric psychiatry unit has an expanded, multilayered role, but primarily serves to educate families and coordinate post-discharge care with families and community referral sources. The social worker often provides supportive therapy directly to the patient or family. Focused interventions include helping families recognize and manage caregiver stress, feelings of grief related to illness in loved ones, and guilty preoccupation regarding decisions of long-term care placement. Some of the social worker's responsibilities include: advocating for the family while planning for assisted living or nursing home placements, assisting families in arranging financial planning, and managing legal issues related to substituted decision making and guardianship. Social workers will also advocate for and coordinate hospice care after discharge when medically appropriate. The social worker must also be intimately familiar and liaise with community agencies, homecare and nursing agencies and protective services, as well as guardians and attorneys. Although the primary goal of the social worker on the geriatric psychiatry unit is to ascertain that each patient is placed at the appropriate level of care, this must be completed under increasingly time-pressured circumstances in which hospital administration goals and family wishes are often in direct conflict.

The Occupational Therapist

The occupational therapist works with patients on the unit to continuously assess physical and cognitive needs. The occupational therapist examines gait, mobility, motor skills, use of adaptive equipment and independence with activities of daily living (ADLs), including transfers. These assessments are performed throughout the hospitalization, as medications and inactivity may adversely affect gait. Functional independence may be assessed with the structured Occupational Therapy Evaluation of Performance and Support (OTEPS)[6] or the Kohlman Evaluation of Living Skills (KELS)[7], which evaluate mobility, self-care, instrumental ADLs, safety, medication management, financial management, and meal planning and preparation. The occupational therapist functional assessment assists in providing an appropriate disposition for the patients based on their level of function. Furthermore, the occupational therapist will try to create an atmosphere on the inpatient unit that permits inclusiveness of all patients, adjusted for their cognitive level.

The Clinical Neuropsychologist

Neuropsychologists also play a critical role on the geriatric psychiatry inpatient unit, assisting with cognitive assessment, diagnosis and coordinated treatment planning. Examining the relative degree of change in cognitive performance from previous visits can be a very useful guide in understanding the aetiology of cognitive dysfunction and developing discharge planning options. Neuropsychologists may help guide implementation of appropriate group therapy activities with the cognitively impaired patient, and assist caregivers with decisions regarding the level of restriction that should be allotted to a patient. Decisions may also involve matters regarding administration of medication and discharge location[8].

Inpatient Group Therapy Interventions

The daily schedule on the geriatric psychiatry unit is structured with activities planned throughout the day. Patients will be evaluated individually with the psychiatrist and may receive individualized and family therapy with the psychiatrist, nursing staff and/or social worker. Patients are encouraged to participate in group activities regardless of cognitive capacity. Examples of group activities include task-oriented groups or craft activity groups involving patient-centred tasks, groups focusing on spiritual needs of patients, and sensory-oriented groups designed to examine gross motor activities in an environment to help calm patients (e.g. music). An end-of-the-day focus group may include relaxation exercises designed to teach the more cognitively intact patients about sleep hygiene, muscle relaxation and deep breathing.

The geriatric inpatient unit may also have distinct groups modified to address certain needs that are specific to patients with dementia. Memory groups are not only effective in addressing cognitive issues, but also the agitation and aggressive behavioural components that accompany memory loss in dementia. An individual inpatient treatment programme for geriatric patients with dementia and dysfunctional behaviours was found to be effective in improving the agitation and aggressive behaviours of patients with dementia while 'preserving or enhancing cognitive and functional abilities'[5]. Distinct dementia groups may provide therapies, such as morning bright light therapy, which has been shown to be effective in normalizing irregular sleeping behaviours among demented patients by increasing total nocturnal sleep and reducing sleep time in the afternoon[9].

Multi-sensory Behavioural Therapy

'Snoezelen' units, originating in the Netherlands in the 1970s, were developed to provide a multi-sensory experience that promotes the stimulation of all senses and does not rely on verbal interaction. Individuals may choose specific aromas, sounds, colours, tactile experiences and tastes, all of which promote relaxation. 'Snoezelen' units can be large enough to permit sufficient space for individuals who like to wander, thereby reducing intrusion into another patient's personal space. Some units promote stimulation of the senses by being connected to an outdoor area where patients may freely walk within a fenced-in space when the season is appropriate.

Multi-sensory behavioural therapy in single-blinded studies showed a modest reduction in agitation and apathy, and improved ADLs compared with standard psychiatric inpatient treatment alone[10]. Other studies with dementia patients carried out in nursing homes have been negative[11,12], or showed modest improvement in mood and well-being.

The Geriatric Neuropsychiatry Unit at McLean Hospital works exclusively with the dementia population. The unit has a dedicated sensory stimulation room with equipment such as a sound machine, a soft-toned lamp, a weighted blanket, a sand tray and a lighted ball which may be used with supervision in an effort to reduce levels of stress and agitation. A recent pilot study demonstrated the efficacy of a sensory-based intervention for individuals with dementia and associated behavioural disturbances. Interestingly, psychotropic drug administration did not improve the response to this intervention[13].

The Patient Population

Data from Medicare inpatient hospitalizations from 1990 to 1991 found that 19% of patients with a primary psychiatric diagnosis were treated in the psychiatric hospital compared to general hospital psychiatric units or general hospital non-psychiatric units[14]. Those with schizophrenia, bipolar disorder and major depression were most likely to receive inpatient treatment in a psychiatric hospital, while those with anxiety and substance-related disorders were less likely to be treated in a psychiatric hospital. However, the population mix in geriatric psychiatric inpatient units has been changing over the past several decades. One study examining admissions data from 1988 through 1998 found that recent admissions were more likely to have a primary diagnosis of dementia and to present with agitation or psychosis[15]. In 1988, over 60% of admissions had a diagnosis of affective disorder, which was reduced to 34% by 1998. Over this 10-year time period, the admitted patients were older, took more medications on discharge, had shorter lengths of stay, and were less likely to be discharged home.

Several studies have examined factors that result in re-hospitalization among elderly psychiatric patients. These studies have suggested that co-morbid depression and dementia, substance dependence, short lengths of stays, social isolation, maladaptive family systems, being single, co-morbid physical and mental health problems, male gender and bipolar disorder are all potential factors that may increase the risk of re-hospitalization[16].

Length of Stay

Length of stay (LOS) is frequently longer for geriatric patients compared to younger hospitalized individuals. A study conducted at the Institute of Living, where the average length of stay in 2001 was 14.1 days, revealed that 12% of the patients had a length of stay of over 26 days[17]. Factors contributing to an increased length of stay included receiving electroconvulsive therapy (ECT), not performing electroconvulsive therapy on weekends, being more impaired based on the Brief Psychiatric Rating Scale positive symptom scale, falling, pharmacological complications, multiple prior psychiatric hospitalizations, requiring court proceedings to continue treatment, and delays in consultations. Diagnosis and demographic factors did not appear to play a role in length of stay.

In a review of the determinants of LOS on the Geriatric Neuropsychiatry Inpatient Unit at McLean Hospital in 2007, factors associated with an increased length of stay included older age, aggressive or sexual behaviour, need for guardianship and ECT treatment. Furthermore, neither diagnosis on admission nor discharge location contributed to LOS.

The length of stay is longer in the private psychiatric hospital setting, as compared to the general hospital psychiatric unit for elderly patients[14]. Interestingly, the cost for care in the private psychiatric hospital may be lower possibly due to less medical co-morbidity[14].

GERIATRIC PSYCHIATRY INPATIENT ADMISSION PATTERNS: BUTLER HOSPITAL AND MCLEAN HOSPITAL, 1994–2008

We examined admission patterns for 1994–2008 to geriatric psychiatry inpatient units at two private psychiatric hospitals, Butler Hospital in Providence, Rhode Island and McLean Hospital in Belmont, Massachusetts. Butler and McLean Hospitals had a similar age distribution of patients: ages 65–75 (45.1%, 38.9%), 76–85 (39.9%, 44.6%), and over the age of 85 (15.0%, 16.5%). Since 1995 there has been a decline in admitting individuals between the ages of 65 and 75 years, and a steady rise in the other two age groups (Figure 128.1). The decline in those aged 65–75 was more dramatic for Butler Hospital, possibly due to McLean Hospital also having a dedicated dementia unit. Overall, more women than men are hospitalized: 67.8% and 64.4% were females, for Butler Hospital and McLean Hospital, respectively. The female-to-male ratio increased with age for both hospitals, with the 65–75 age group averaging 64.8% and 63.4% women; the 75–85 group averaging 69.7% and 63.0%, and the over 85 group averaging 71.7% and 70.4%. The most common discharge diagnosis for Butler Hospital across all age groups was dementia, followed by substance use disorder and depressive disorders; while for McLean Hospital the most common discharge diagnoses across all groups were dementia, depressive disorders and bipolar disorder. However, diagnosis varied by age group (Table 128.1).

The average length of stay from 1994 to 2008 was 13.4 days; 13.7 days for females and 12.8 days for males for Butler Hospital. McLean Hospital had a longer length of stay: 20.1 days; 20.6 days for females and 19.3 days for males. For Butler Hospital there was little evidence of a significant decrease in length of stay over time. At McLean Hospital there was an overall decrease in length of stay. However, this decrease in the length of stay was not dramatic. For instance, in 1994 the length of stay was 19.4 days and in 2008 it was 17.7 days; there was a peak in 2000 of 25.7 days.

Overall, 37.5% of patients at Butler Hospital and 33.7% of patients at McLean Hospital are discharged from the inpatient unit to a nursing facility, with increasing age related to more frequent nursing home placement. A quarter (24.1% and 25.5%) of those aged 65–75 are discharged to a nursing facility; while 44.6% and 36.3% of those aged 76–85, and 58.8% and 45.8% of those over 85 are sent to a

nursing home from Butler Hospital's and McLean Hospital's geriatric psychiatry units, respectively.

GERIATRIC PARTIAL HOSPITAL PROGRAMMES

The private psychiatric hospital offers an opportunity to have a continuum of care for elderly patients from the inpatient programme to partial or day hospital and outpatient services. One goal for providing geriatric patients with intensive outpatient services is to reduce readmission rates, thereby reducing total costs incurred for the patient and the hospital. Whether such programmes achieve such fiscal savings remains unknown. Private psychiatric hospitals struggle with the conflicting tension between keeping the inpatient census full while also making efforts to reduce inpatient LOS. Older adults with mood and psychotic disorders generally experience recurrent acute exacerbations, which require more intensive interventions. The partial hospital programme may serve to avoid or delay inpatient admission and allow for a more successful transition back to independent community living. Partial hospital programmes may be designed specifically for the geriatric patient or have tracks within the adult partial programme that would be appropriate for the older patient depending on their cognitive capabilities. These programmes typically are Monday through Friday for one or two weeks, and act as a bridge to outpatient care.

Such a programme would have geriatric patients with limited cognitive impairment participating in a general programme that may emphasize cognitive therapy, group therapy, problem-solving therapy and psychoeducation. Problem-solving therapy has demonstrated effectiveness in reducing severity of depression in older patients as measured by the Geriatric Depression Scale and the Hamilton Rating Scale for Depression[18].

However, those who cannot benefit from groups that demand a greater degree of cognitive functioning are best served in a more support-oriented track. Such a track typically has a shorter day and consists of smaller groups, less detailed psychoeducation and more concrete activities such as art therapy, an occupation therapy task group and nutrition teaching. Group therapy in the cognitively compromised track would focus more on daily goals and planning pleasurable activities.

The elderly patient who is cognitively intact would participate in higher-functioning groups such as cognitive behavioural therapy, mindfulness, assertiveness, psychoeducation and behavioural

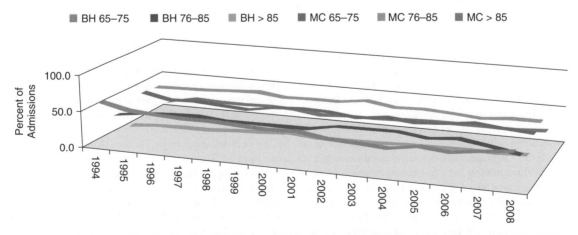

Figure 128.1   Inpatient admissions from Butler Hospital (BH) and McLean Hospital (MC) by age group from 1994 to 2008

PRINCIPLES AND PRACTICE OF GERIATRIC PSYCHIATRY

Table 128.1 Discharge diagnosis (as % of all discharges) by age group for Butler Hospital and McLean Hospital from 1994 to 2008 (based on Butler Hospital ($N = 7213$) and McLean Hospital ($N = 7896$) discharge diagnosis)

	Butler Hospital				McLean Hospital			
	1994–1998	1999–2003	2004–2008	Total	1994–1998	1999–2003	2004–2008	Total
Age 65–75								
Adjustment disorders	1.6	0.8	0.6	0.9	0.7	0.1	0.3	0.4
Anxiety disorders	12.5	10.8	7.0	9.3	1.5	0.9	1.0	1.1
Bipolar disorders	7.2	2.4	1.7	3.0	15.7	18.3	21.3	18.3
Dementia	23.7	29.4	19.2	23.2	26.4	24.7	20.5	23.9
Depressive disorders	20.4	13.7	13.0	14.7	28.0	35.9	35.6	33.0
Non-affective psychosis	4.6	4.3	4.6	4.5	18.2	16.6	17.3	17.4
Substance use disorders	19.3	29.4	36.5	30.8	1.9	2.0	1.6	1.8
Other disorders	12.8	9.5	17.6	13.6	7.8	1.4	2.5	4.0
Age 76–85								
Adjustment disorders	1.4	0.2	0.3	0.4	0.5	0.4	0.2	0.4
Anxiety disorders	11.0	7.7	7.1	8.0	0.4	1.1	0.7	0.7
Bipolar disorders	3.4	2.0	3.3	2.9	6.0	11.2	9.1	8.6
Dementia	31.6	47.8	49.2	45.5	53.2	48.2	46.7	49.6
Depressive disorders	20.3	20.0	11.4	15.7	25.9	29.4	29.6	28.1
Non-affective psychosis	4.8	5.2	3.7	4.4	7.2	5.6	8.0	6.9
Substance use disorders	14.4	9.9	13.0	12.3	1.6	1.5	0.5	1.2
Other disorders	13.0	7.2	12.0	10.7	5.3	2.6	5.2	4.3
Age > 85								
Adjustment disorders	1.7	1.6	0.6	1.1	0.4	1.2	0.2	0.5
Anxiety disorders	6.8	5.5	6.5	6.2	0.2	0.0	0.7	0.3
Bipolar disorders	8.5	1.1	1.9	2.3	2.4	2.9	3.6	2.9
Dementia	33.9	47.3	62.0	54.3	67.2	65.2	65.1	65.9
Depressive disorders	28.8	20.3	11.7	16.3	22.7	25.5	24.0	23.9
Non-affective psychosis	0.0	4.4	4.0	3.7	1.8	3.2	1.8	2.2
Substance use disorders	8.5	8.2	2.2	4.8	1.4	0.3	0.0	0.6
Other disorders	11.9	11.5	11.1	11.3	3.8	1.8	4.7	3.6
Age > 65								
Adjustment disorders	1.5	0.7	0.5	0.7	0.6	0.4	0.2	0.4
Anxiety disorders	11.5	8.9	7.0	8.4	0.8	0.8	0.8	0.8
Bipolar disorders	5.9	2.1	2.3	2.9	9.0	12.8	13.0	11.5
Dementia	27.4	38.8	36.7	35.7	45.4	41.4	39.5	42.3
Depressive disorders	21.0	17.0	12.2	15.3	26.1	31.4	31.0	29.3
Non-affective psychosis	4.4	4.7	4.2	4.4	10.4	9.6	10.6	10.2
Substance use disorders	16.6	19.0	22.6	20.4	1.7	1.5	0.9	1.4
Other disorders	11.6	8.9	14.5	12.3	5.9	1.9	4.0	4.2

activation groups. Table 128.2 illustrates a typical partial hospital schedule using various tracts depending on the level of functioning of the patient. A cognitively impaired partial hospital track may be appropriate for those with mild cognitive impairment or dementia, but adult day care in the community setting may be more helpful for individuals with moderate to severe dementia.

There are a number of financial issues specific to the United States that must be considered when developing a partial hospital programme for the elderly. Medicare requires careful documentation of medical necessity for the initiation and continuation of group therapy interventions in partial hospital programmes. In addition, medications are not covered in partial hospital programmes under Medicare; therefore, the patient is responsible for purchasing and bringing daytime medication to the programme. Importantly, transportation is not covered by insurance and may be a limiting factor.

The partial hospital programme is appropriate for those who can benefit from structure and support. The programme allows for family education and interventions for dealing with conflicts, while also providing support and an opportunity for intensive psychopharmacological management. The partial hospital programme also permits the staff to observe an individual's daily functioning and diurnal changes in behaviour.

Examining data from Butler Hospital and McLean Hospital provides an illustration of the types of patients treated in a partial hospital programme. Between the years 1994 and 2008, the Butler Hospital partial hospital programme had 887 admissions for patients aged 65 and older. The McLean partial hospital programme is considerably larger and had 2702 admissions during that period of time. The majority (77.6% Butler Hospital; 58.0% McLean Hospital) of individuals were between the ages of 65 and 75, while

Table 128.2 An example of a partial hospital schedule for geriatric patients who cognitively cannot participate in a traditional cognitive behavioural therapy-focused programme

Time	Monday	Tuesday	Wednesday	Thursday	Friday
9:30 a.m.[a]	Arrival and individual appointments	Arrival and individual appointments	Arrival and individual appointments	Arrival and individual appointments	Arrival and individual appointments
10:00 a.m.	Goal setting	Goal setting	Goal setting	Goal setting	Goal setting
11:00 a.m.	Focus group	Focus group	Focus group	Focus group	Focus group
11:45 a.m.	Lunch	Lunch	Lunch	Lunch	Lunch
1:00 p.m.	Medication education	Wellness group	Anger management	Spirituality or substance support or task group	Mindfulness or task group
2:00 p.m.	Nutrition or task group	Behavioural activation or task group	Relapse prevention	Sleep education	Leisure skills
3:00 p.m.	End of the day check in	End of the day check in	End of the day check in	End of the day check in	End of the day check in
3:15 p.m.	Medication distribution	Medication distribution	Medication distribution	Medication distribution	Medication distribution

[a] Geriatric patients in this track arrive later at the partial hospital programme than those in the traditional cognitive behavioural tracks. For those who are not cognitively able to manage specific groups, as noted in the schedule task groups are provided as an alternative.

only 2.1% and 6.0% of the admissions were over the age of 85, respectively. The majority of those in the partial hospital programme were females: 62.5% Butler Hospital and 74.8% McLean Hospital. The most common discharge diagnoses for Butler Hospital were depressive disorders, 23.6%; anxiety disorders, 22.8%; substance use disorders, 17.6%; and dementia, 12.2%; whereas McLean Hospital's programme was more focused on depressive disorders, specifically, accounting for 81.9% of discharge diagnoses compared with only 5.7% for bipolar disorder, 8.2% for non-affective psychosis, 8.3% for mild cognitive impairment and 2.7% for dementia.

A cross between the time-limited partial hospital and the outpatient geriatric psychiatry clinic where patients are seen for 15 minutes to an hour on an as-needed basis, is the enhanced outpatient treatment programme. McLean Hospital provides an example of such a programme that was initiated in 2008. The SAGE (or Seniors Aging Gracefully Everyday) programme is now utilized as a step down from inpatient care, or used to prevent the need for hospitalization. The SAGE programme is geared toward those with major depression, bipolar disorder, anxiety disorders and psychotic disorders. Patients attend the programme two to five days weekly for about four hours per day. Individual and group psychotherapy along with psychopharmacological assessment and management are available services. Such a programme typically offers cognitive behavioural therapy, illness education, coping skills, family counselling and community-resource need assessment.

SPECIALTY GERIATRIC PSYCHIATRY PROGRAMMES

The private psychiatric hospitals often have substance abuse treatment programmes, which may offer an opportunity to provide treatment specific for the geriatric population. For instance, Butler Hospital has a weekly group therapy session open to the elderly population. The rationale for this group is that a number of geriatric patients feel intimidated among younger substance users in Alcoholics

Anonymous, and an age-specific group provides them with a more secure environment to promote abstinence.

Memory disorders clinics, directed by either a geriatric psychiatrist or a behavioural neurologist, are also common in the private psychiatric hospital setting. These clinics often are multidisciplinary and include neuropsychology and occupational therapy. The memory clinic primarily focuses on providing diagnostic services and consultation to referring medical professionals. The clinic also provides treatment and follow-up services including the use of medications, counselling for patients and families, and assistance with locating and using community-based resources. Most of these clinics also actively conduct research and may offer patients an opportunity to participate in trials with commercially unavailable medications.

CONCLUSION

There are both challenges and opportunities for the care of older adults with neuropsychiatric disorders in the private psychiatric hospital setting. Foremost among the opportunities is a vertical system of care that integrates traditional inpatient geriatric psychiatry treatment with a range of outpatient services including partial hospital programming and specialty mood and memory disorders clinics. Multidisciplinary teams help provide inpatients with a full range of specialty medical and psychiatric, neurological, neuropsychological, physical and occupational therapy and social work services. Over the past 15 years, trends at two prominent private psychiatric hospitals indicate a shorter inpatient length of stay for both centres, and varying prevalence rates of dementia, affective and psychotic disorders. In addition to the financial hurdles associated with providing geriatric psychiatry care in the private psychiatric hospital setting, are the challenges of managing medically complex inpatients with both neuropsychiatric conditions and medical co-morbidities. Nevertheless, private psychiatric hospitals in the United States remain an important resource for older individuals and their families struggling with mood disturbances, psychosis, behavioural disinhibition syndromes and cognitive impairment.

REFERENCES

1. Cheung G, Strachan J. Routine 'Health of the Nation Outcome Scales for elderly people' (HoNOS65+) collection in an acute pyschogeriatric inpatient unit in New Zealand. *N Z Med J* 2007; **120**: U2660.

2. Yazgan IC, Greenwald BS, Kremen NJ, Strach J, Kramer-Ginsberg E. Geriatric psychiatry versus general psychiatry inpatient treatment of the elderly. *Am J Psychiatry* 2004; **16**: 352–5.

3. Colombo G, Buono MD, Roberta KS, Raviola R, De Leo D. Pet therapy and institutionalized elderly: a study on 144 cognitively unimpaired subjects. *Arch Gerontol Geriatr* 2006; **42**: 207–16.

4. Day K, Carreon D, Stump C. The therapeutic design of environments for people with dementia: a review of the empirical research. *Gerontologist* 2000; **40**: 397–416.

5. Holm A, Michel M, Stern G *et al*. The outcomes of an inpatient treatment program for geriatric patients with dementia and dysfunctional behaviors. *Gerontologist* 1999; **39**: 668–76.

6. Nadler JD, Richardson ED, Malloy PF *et al*. The ability of the Dementia Rating Scale to predict everyday functioning. *Arch Clin Neuropsychol* 1993; **8**: 449–60.

7. Kohlman-Thompson L. *The Kohlman Evaluation of Living Skills*, 3rd edn. Rockville, MD: American Occupational Therapy Association, 1992.

8. Fogel BS, Kroessler D. Treating late-life depression on a medical-psychiatric unit. *Hosp Community Psychiatry* 1987; **38**: 829–31.

9. Mishima K, Okawa M, Hishikawa Y *et al*. Morning bright light therapy for sleep and behavior disorders in elderly patients with dementia. *Acta Psychiatr Scand* 2009; **89**: 1–7.

10. Staal JA, Sacks A, Matheis R *et al*. The effects of Snoezelen (multi-sensory behavior therapy) and psychiatric care on agitation, apathy, and activities of daily living in dementia patients on a short term geriatric psychiatric inpatient unit. *Int J Psychiatry Med* 2007; **37**: 357–70.

11. Baillon S, van Diepen E, Prettyman R *et al*. A comparison of the effects of Snoezelen and reminiscence therapy on the agitated behavior of patients with dementia. *Int J Geriatr Psychiatry* 2004; **19**: 1047–52.

12. Baker R, Holloway J, Holtkamp CC *et al*. Effects of multi-sensory stimulation for people with dementia. *J Adv Nurs* 2003; **43**: 465–77.

13. Knight M, Adkison L, Kovach JS. A comparison of multisensory and traditional interventions on inpatient psychiatry and geriatric neuropsychiatry units. *J Psychosoc Nurs Ment Health Serv* 2010; **48**: 24–31.

14. Ettner SL, Hermann RC. Inpatient psychiatric treatment of elderly Medicare beneficiaries. *Psychiatr Serv* 1998; **49**: 1173–9.

15. Weintraub D, Mazour I. Clinical and demographic changes over ten years on a psychogeriatric inpatient unit. *Ann Clin Psychiatry* 2000; **12**: 227–231.

16. Woo BK, Golshan S, Allen EC *et al*. Factors associated with frequent admissions to an acute geriatric psychiatric inpatient unit. *J Geriatr Psychiatry Neurol* 2006; **19**: 226–30.

17. Blank K, Hixon L, Gruman C *et al*. Determinants of geropsychiatric inpatient length of stay. *Psychiatr Q* 2005; **76**: 195–212.

18. Arean PA, Perri MG, Nezu AM *et al*. Comparative effectiveness of social problem-solving therapy and reminiscence therapy as treatments for depression in older adults. *J Consult Clin Psychol* 1993; **61**: 1003–10.

129

Liaison with Medical and Surgical Teams

David N. Anderson

*Mersey Care NHS Trust, Older People's Mental Health Services, Sir Douglas Crawford Unit,
Mossley Hill Hospital, Liverpool, UK*

'My own experience suggests that the proportion of geriatric referrals is growing and that a liaison psychiatrist increasingly acts as a part-time geropsychiatrist, yet one without the benefit of appropriate training and expertise'[1].

This was said by one of the founding fathers of liaison (general hospital) psychiatry. It demonstrates how the mental health needs of older people admitted to general hospitals is increasing and has been for some time. Global demographic change is becoming a major challenge for all nations of the world. Because ageing is associated with increased health problems and multi-morbidity[2], this will be reflected in hospital populations. Because physical morbidity increases the chance of psychiatric morbidity, this will be reflected in greater need for liaison psychiatry services with expertise in older people's problems.

In most parts of the world, mental health of older people is not a distinct speciality. In the UK, where older people's mental health has become a separate speciality, there had been no consideration of the needs of older people admitted to general hospitals until the Royal College of Psychiatrists published the first national guideline on the development of specialist older people's liaison services[3]. This has stimulated great interest, and these services are now recommended in national guidance from government and professional bodies[4-6].

In the UK, two thirds of National Health Service beds are occupied by people over the age of 64 years[7], and up to 60% of this age group admitted to general hospitals may have or acquire a mental disorder during an admission[3]. Furthermore, this mental disorder will be an independent predictor of poor outcome by increasing mortality, length of hospital stay and loss of independent function, and reducing the prospect of a return to independent living[3]. This morbidity has been shown to increase subsequent health care utilization and cost[8] and readmission to hospital[9].

This adverse effect remains apparent some time after hospital discharge, with increased mortality being evident two years later[10], nine years later for depression[11] and still doubled three years later with delirium[12].

In the UK, liaison psychiatry has been a developed speciality for adults under age 65, but older people received mental health attention by the inferior process of consultation[13]. Consultation is a reactive process where patients are seen on a case-by-case basis, frequently by inexperienced medical staff working independently of the general care team; a single opinion is given and the patient referred again if problems fail to resolve. Liaison is proactive, integrated with general hospital care and based on collaborative working (Table 129.1). The superiority of liaison has been shown in controlled trials and by systematic review (Table 129.2).

The desire by clinicians to move to a liaison approach is clear[14]. This change is supported by accumulating evidence that addressing older people's mental health in general hospitals improves the outcome for patients and the efficiency and effectiveness of general hospitals. How this can be achieved for the more common conditions is briefly discussed in this chapter.

PREVALENCE AND INCIDENCE

Systematic review of the literature finds that the most common disorders are dementia, delirium and depression, which together will account for about 80% of the psychiatric morbidity (Table 129.3). All three are substantially more common in general hospitals than found in the community, and all conditions combined are 3–4-times more common. Rates vary with hospital departments, being particularly high in medical and orthopaedics. There is very little known about rates in emergency departments.

Each of the three major disorders creates different problems and a different focus of approach, discussed later.

DETECTION

Despite mental disorder being so common, detection by general care teams is poor. The diagnosis of delirium is missed in 32–67% of cases[15], and cognitive impairment in over half[16]. A meta-analysis of older medical admissions reported a median detection rate for depression of 10%[17]. In England, a national report found that only 41% of people with dementia had any form of mental assessment recorded[18].

General care teams have difficulty understanding the concept of syndromes, and their response to mental disturbance is, predominantly, a reaction to symptoms. Consequently, crying, not eating, and thoughts of death are synonymous with depression, and any cognitive errors with dementia. Jackson and Baldwin[19] reported how nurses on medical wards recognize symptoms of depression rather than the syndrome. A small qualitative study in the USA found that 75% of general nurses could not distinguish dementia from delirium, despite 75% saying that they had received formal education on the subject or had attended a conference about confusion in the elderly[20].

Principles and Practice of Geriatric Psychiatry, 3rd edn. Edited by Mohammed T. Abou-Saleh, Cornelius Katona and Anand Kumar

Table 129.1 Characteristics of liaison and consultation services

Consultation	Liaison
Reactive	Proactive
Limited resources	More labour intensive
Isolated input	Collaborative
Low priority	High priority
Little impact	Developmental
	Education and training
Slow response	Rapid response
Little review	Frequent review
	Improve quality of referrals
	Improve adherence of recommendations
	Change practice and attitudes
Mental health separate from general services	Mental health integrated with general services
Mental health physically distant from acute care	Mental health physically part of acute care

Table 129.2 Benefits of liaison compared to consultation

Quicker response
Increase referrals and quality of referral
Increased specialist assessments
Improved diagnostic concordance between referrer and assessment
Better adherence with treatment recommendations
Reduced length of admission
More return to independent living
Reduced readmission
Reduced health care utilization
Reduced cost
High patient satisfaction

Table 129.3 Average period prevalence of psychiatric morbidity (%)

Dementia	31
Depression	29
Delirium	20 (50% incident)
Cognitive impairment	22
Anxiety	8
Schizophrenia	0.4
Alcoholism	3

A further example, and one which emphasizes the importance of syndrome diagnosis, is a report on older people referred to a liaison service with depression when 40% were found to be suffering from delirium[21]. Depressive symptoms were as common in the delirious patients as those diagnosed with depression, 50% expressing a wish to die, 25% suicidal thoughts and the majority thoughts of worthlessness and guilt.

But, detection in an acute hospital with serious physical co-morbidity can be difficult. Particularly so for depression, when key biological symptoms like fatigue, loss of appetite, weight and sleep can arise from physical or psychological illness, and evaluating loss of motivation and worry in people seriously physically ill is difficult.

A diagnostic approach to depression based on DSM-III-R[22] criteria, counting all symptoms regardless of their origin (inclusive) or excluding any symptom that could arise from physical illness (exclusive), produces a variation in prevalence of 27 to 46%[23]. The exclusive approach had high specificity for severe and persistent major depression, but missed 49% of major depressions identified by the high-sensitivity inclusive approach, almost 60% of whom continued to experience symptoms of depression weeks after discharge. Furthermore, these findings are based on structured psychiatric interviews, and unstructured clinical impressions are less reliable.

Interpreting cognitive function can be similarly difficult. Is a person's cognitive performance poor simply because they feel ill or too tired to attend? What is the significance of disorientation to day and date when a person has spent weeks or months in hospital or has been very ill?

It is partly for these reasons that mental health liaison teams are needed to develop expertise working in this environment. Assessment and diagnostic instruments do not solve this problem as they also need to be interpreted and few are validated for use with physically ill people. In untrained hands these tools can be dangerous, lead to false conclusions and the mistaken belief that a quick tick-box approach can replace the history and mental state examination.

Routine screening for cognitive impairment and depression has been suggested, but the benefit and method remain uncertain. A screening instrument would need high sensitivity (like the inclusive approach for depression described above) but would yield false positives, while a diagnostic instrument would require high specificity (like the exclusive approach for depression above), but risks missing many people with the disorder who would benefit from treatment.

A systematic review of screening for depression and anxiety in non-psychiatric settings concluded that the routine administration of psychiatric questionnaires with feedback to clinicians does not improve the detection of emotional disorders or patient outcome; although, those with high scores may benefit[24]. Studies of the systematic detection and multidisciplinary treatment of delirium or depression in medical inpatients have, so far, been unable to demonstrate superiority over usual medical care[25,26]. The systematic detection and treatment of delirium has shown small benefits for older surgical patients[27].

The exception is the use of clinical prediction rules to identify older people at risk of developing delirium, and this is discussed later under delirium.

EDUCATION AND TRAINING

The limitations of general care teams discussed above highlights the need for education and training, and suggest that whatever training is currently employed seems to have little effect. Teaching and training is core business for liaison teams and there is evidence that the introduction of liaison services into general hospitals is associated with changes in referral that might be taken to indicate a more informed change of behaviour[28]. And so, it is likely that their presence, in itself and by clinical contacts, has an educative effect.

However, the best way to deliver more formal training to general care teams remains uncertain. Principles of adult learning which may be usefully incorporated into educational programmes include timely and relevant information based on participant identification of learning needs and integration of new information into existing knowledge base(s) with time for consolidation and appropriate non-judgemental feedback to the individual[29].

Case-based discussions that bring immediate relevance, supervision that reinforces knowledge and skills, and audit to evaluate change will be important to effective education. Care pathways can be helpful. This might suggest that an approach which focuses on the needs of specific departments and specialities involving complete clinical teams could be more effective than random teaching sessions for hospital staff and particular professional groups. The circumstances and subject matter should dictate the approach.

Whatever the approach, training time must be built into job plans and the resourcing of liaison teams. The time needed is always underestimated, and when clinical staff are under pressure, training will be relegated to low priority. In one audit of a nurse-led liaison service, 7.5% of time was spent directly on formal education and 33% giving guidance, advice and making recommendations to ward staff[30].

Delivery to large hospitals, including night staff, with staff who move through in training, is difficult and a perpetual process. Incorporating mental health into established teaching programmes will give it credence and importance. The presence of liaison teams in general hospitals offers the prospect of mental health being absorbed into the culture of the hospital and not seen as a separate activity just provided by mental health services. The importance of improving the mental health knowledge and skills of general care teams cannot be overestimated because the vast majority of older people admitted to general hospitals with mental health needs will not be seen by specialist liaison teams. The management of non-referred cases will be the ultimate measure of how successfully liaison services have changed the general hospital's response to mental health.

INTERVENTIONS

Delirium

Delirium is the most common non-specific presentation of physical illness among older people and the most common new condition in the hospitalized elderly. It will complicate 5–10% of routine surgery. Delirium present at the time of admission is referred to as prevalent delirium, and that beginning in hospital as incident delirium. The distinction is important when discussing prevention, as 30–40% of incident delirium may be hospital acquired and preventable. Rates of delirium will vary between hospital departments, being highest with the most ill patients (Intensive Care), higher with emergency than elective surgery and higher with more complex conditions.

It is a cause of death, prolonged admission, loss of independent function, high cost and is associated with an increased risk of hospital-acquired complications including incontinence, falls, pressure sores and infection. Estimates from the USA suggest that it affects more than 2.3 million older people each year, is responsible for more than 17.5 million inpatient days and costs over $4 billion (1994 dollars) each year[31].

Furthermore, it is now clear that not all delirium resolves, and cognitive impairment persists 12 months after a medical admission when 15% still meet the diagnostic criteria for delirium[32]. Patients developing delirium during a medical admission are twice as likely to have died, and six-times more likely to have acquired a diagnosis of dementia three years later[12]. Reversibility seems crucial for outcome. A prospective study of older medical patients found that the 6 and 12 month outcome for delirious people who survive and recover was no different to no-delirium groups in relation to cognition, function or institutional status[33].

Once established, the treatment is that of the underlying condition, with supportive care and management of behavioural and psychotic symptoms[34]. There is a theoretical basis to developing pharmacological prophylaxis and treatment with cholinesterase inhibitors[35,36] and

manipulation of the immune system[37], but small controlled trials of the former have failed to demonstrate efficacy.

There is compelling evidence for interventions which prevent incident delirium that is closely linked to processes of care. Clinical prediction rules have been described for medical, non-cardiac thoracic surgery and elective orthopaedic populations[38–40]. These enable people at risk to be identified on admission to hospital and preventative care strategies employed to reduce delirium risk. Because delirium mostly develops within the first seven days of admission or surgery, this approach can concentrate on that period[41].

The most developed prevention approach arose from studies of older medical patients, identifying the strongest independent predisposing and precipitating factors that predict incident delirium[42,43]. These large studies found the relative risk was 9.5-times greater for people with a high-risk predisposing profile, and 8.9-times greater for those with a high-risk precipitant profile, than those with low risk.

This formed the basis of a controlled trial of a preventative intervention involving 852 older medical inpatients, employing a multi-component intervention strategy (The Elder Life Program). The subjects were identified on admission as being intermediate or high risk, and in the intervention arm the incidence of delirium was 34% lower than usual care. The intervention group experienced significantly lower total days with delirium, lower total number of episodes, improved cognitive function in those already cognitively impaired and lower use of sleep medications[44].

This intervention was shown to be cost effective for intermediate risk (72% of subjects) but not high risk. Cost of the intervention was offset by savings accrued from treatment intensity, including nursing and diagnostic procedures[31].

A randomized controlled trial of 126 older people admitted with hip fracture employed a similar structured prevention strategy of proactive geriatric consultation and protocol of care. The incidence of delirium was 36% lower in the intervention group, with 58% less severe delirium. Number needed to treat was 5.6[45]. Reducing the severity of delirium is important, as increased severity is associated with increased mortality, loss of function and institutionalization[46,47]. Sub-syndromal delirium is also associated with worse outcome compared to no delirium, and equivalent to mild delirium[47].

Though the protocols were different in the medical and surgical studies, they were essentially proactive high-quality medical and nursing care. It has been said that incident delirium is a sign of hospitals failing older people[48].

Dementia

Dementia increases the risk of delirium five-fold, and recognizing delirium superimposed on dementia is particularly difficult[20]. It is, however, very important because delirium is a common presentation of acute physical illness in people with dementia, with no localizing signs. As a general rule, any person with dementia in hospital who shows a sudden change of behaviour, function or mental state should trigger the possibility of delirium. There is no evidence, at present, to indicate any particular approach to the treatment of delirium in those with chronic cognitive impairment, and standard protocols of care apply[49].

People with dementia are highly susceptible to environmental change. Lying in bed, not given the opportunity to maintain their personal care skills, and disruption of familiar routines exposes them to a loss of independent function quickly. They take longer to recover, and cognitive impairment hampers their ability to benefit from rehabilitation.

A cross-sectional regional audit in England found that people with dementia were more likely to be in acute hospitals than any other health care beds, and 68% of those no longer required acute hospital care[18]. In a study of elderly hip fractures, over 70% of cases had not been diagnosed before admission[50].

Consequently, there are multiple reasons why the presence of dementia has to be identified at the time of admission, and general care teams need to recognize the significance this has for management and eventual discharge. Care plans have to take account of the effect of their cognitive impairment and the added risks it creates. All too often, it is only when a person is considered medically fit for discharge that any thought is given to their cognitive function and planning that should have occurred much earlier. A person with dementia is five-times more likely to develop delirium and then suffer the consequential effects on outcome[27].

A randomized, controlled trial of intensive multidisciplinary rehabilitation after hip fracture surgery achieved a reduced length of stay for those with mild or moderate dementia in the intervention arm. Those with mild dementia were as successful returning to independent living as those without dementia[51]. There was no benefit for length of stay or independent living for people with severe dementia, and the mild or moderate group from the intervention arm were more likely to be living independently three months after discharge.

The National Institute for Health and Clinical Excellence[5] recommend that every suspected case of dementia in general hospitals has a specialist assessment and there should be specialist older people's liaison teams available for treatment and training.

Depression

All forms of depression are seen in a general hospital, where presentations are more varied and more difficult to diagnose. Preoperative anxiety and depression are associated with an increased risk of postoperative complications, and usually linked to worries about surgery or the disease. These often resolve following successful surgery. Unfortunately, depression accompanying a medical admission has a poor prognosis[17].

Physical illness and disability increase the risk of depression greatly. Depression in older age increases mortality from natural causes[52] and independently increases six-month readmission after discharge[9]. Up to 50% of people with depression in the general hospital have a disorder present before admission. The course of depression after discharge from a medical admission remains very stable, and a 12-month prospective study of older medical patients failed to find any effect of antidepressants[53]. The more severe course was predicted by higher initial Hamilton Depression Rating Scale score, depressive core symptoms lasting six months, and female sex.

The evidence base for effective treatment is poor in general, and with important co-morbidities. Antidepressants, in general, are better than placebo or usual care in the presence of physical illness, with very respectable number needed to treat or harm; although, this Cochrane review included all adult ages[54]. Antidepressants are also effective for depression in older people, but this Cochrane review comments on how few trials include people with physical illness[55].

Large, placebo-controlled trials have shown the superiority of selective serotonin re-uptake inhibitors after myocardial infarction for severe or recurrent depression, and confirm their safety[56]. This class of antidepressant may reduce the risk of further fatal and non-fatal ischaemic events, possibly by virtue of an effect on platelet coagulability[57].

The evidence for treatment effectiveness in Parkinson's disease, stroke or with chronic obstructive pulmonary disease (COPD) is largely absent[58-61]. There is emerging evidence that older people with COPD may be particularly difficult to engage in antidepressant treatment, but case management with a problem-solving behavioural approach is promising[60]. The differing nature of presentation and outcome of depression with these co-morbidities creates challenging questions about the very nature of these disorders and whether they represent the same condition.

The only randomized, placebo-controlled trial of antidepressants in older people in a general hospital involved medical patients who were quite seriously ill[62]. The protocol purposefully kept exclusion criteria to a minimum, but the study was underpowered. Fluoxetine was superior to placebo, though not a statistically significant difference, and side effects no more likely with active treatment. Despite evidence supporting the safety of selective serotonin re-uptake inhibitors, and some benefit, less than 50% of depressed medical patients and 25% of depressed older hip fracture patients receive antidepressants[17,45].

One controlled study has shown the superiority of interpersonal counselling for older people with mild depression six months after a medical admission[63]. Two prospective randomized controlled trials of older people depressed during a medical admission employed the intervention of an older people's liaison nurse. Though improvement was not statistically significant, possibly due to being underpowered, both showed more symptom improvement with intervention than usual care[64,65], and improved quality of life[65].

Self Harm

Self harm is much more common among younger adults and only 2–3% of cases presenting to general hospitals will involve older people. However, with older people the risk of completed suicide is higher; older people show greater suicidal intent than younger people, and the profile of older people who self harm is similar to that of older people who die by suicide, with 60–90% depressed[66,67]. In a small study of consecutive older medical admissions, 36% expressed suicidal ideas, with 19% still having these thoughts six months later[68]. About one-third of older people with self harm presenting to a general hospital will have a history of previous self harm[69].

Following self harm there is a 66-fold increased risk of suicide in the first year, which increases with age[67], and over 20 years a 49-fold increase of suicide and 33-times increase of open verdicts with older people[70].

Suicide in people with dementia is relatively uncommon, but risk may be difficult to detect. A study of nine years of recorded suicides to the National Confidential Inquiry into Suicide and Homicide by People with Mental Illness found only 1% associated with dementia[71]. This only reports suicides occurring within 12 months of contact with mental health services in England and Wales. It found younger people with dementia over represented (over 20%) and fewer of the typical risk factors for suicide; particularly: history of self harm, psychiatric admissions or noted psychiatric symptoms, and more likely to have a diagnosis in excess of 12 months.

All older people presenting with self harm or suicidal thinking must be assessed by a specialist service.

Somatoform Disorder

This includes somatization and hypochondriasis and is now often referred to as medically unexplained symptoms. These presentations of physical symptoms thought to have psychological origins are common in medical and surgical departments, though much less common with older people. In addition, the development of a mental disorder, particularly depression in later life, may cause exacerbation of symptoms from a long-term condition. If late onset, this last is more common, and most patients will have physical illness or disability even when attribution of the physical symptoms to the known disorders may be difficult.

There is little information about these conditions in general hospital populations and only a limited amount from studies in other health care settings. These conditions can lead to costly investigations and interventions and impair quality of life[72].

In a prospective study of elderly primary care attenders, somatization was found in 5% and associated with depression, physical illness and low perceived social support[73]. It was commonly transient, even though 13.6% had a somatizing attributional style which was quite stable. Frequent attenders were characterized by high rates of depression (28.3%), psychological distress associated with physical symptoms and perceived lack of social support (40%).

Antidepressants and cognitive behaviour therapy have been shown to be effective[74]. Improving perceived social support is likely to be helpful. Treatment should only follow thorough medical investigation.

LIAISON SERVICES

Working in a general hospital environment creates different problems and questions for mental health practitioners than outpatient or community practice. Mental health practitioners will need greater knowledge of acute physical illness and how this changes the meaning of mental disturbance. General hospitals are not designed to cater for mental disorder, and the environment can contribute to the problem and will limit the way in which mental health is both assessed and managed. To acquire the necessary expertise requires that the liaison specialist's time is committed to working in this field. This is discussed by Anderson and Ooman[75].

Though the development of these services for older people is relatively new, there is accumulating evidence of their value and effectiveness. The principle functions are to work collaboratively with general care teams, provide a rapid response, manage complex conditions, improve the detection and understanding of mental health, and deliver training to general care teams that will improve their skills in mental health assessment and management[3].

By improving the treatment of mental disorder they contribute to greater efficiency of general hospitals. A systematic review has shown that the introduction of a specialist liaison service has a significant benefit on health savings[76]. A summary of benefits reported from controlled trails is shown in Table 129.2.

It also seems to be the case that admission to a general hospital is a common first presentation of mental disorder for older people. Holmes[50] found that over 70% of older people with dementia admitted with hip fracture were not previously diagnosed. An analysis of 2760 referrals to a specialist liaison service for older people in the UK showed that 68.2% were not under the care of mental health services, though 20% had been, and 62% of mood disorder cases represented a new-onset disorder (unpublished data: Anderson D, Nortcliffe M, Dechenne S et al. Characteristics of a nurse-led liaison mental health service for older people: the Liverpool Dataset Project).

Several models of service delivery have been described[3] but the essential elements for a service to be most effective are:

- multidisciplinary team
- based in the general hospital
- dedicated to hospital liaison
- strong links with mental health services
- good information system.

Psychiatric morbidity varies between departments, being generally higher in medical and orthopaedic wards. Complex medical co-morbidity, the acute presentation of physical illness and the strong association between cognitive impairment and falls characterise these populations. A liaison service would expect 70% of referrals to come from medical specialities and the referral rate per admitted case is higher from medicine than surgery. The composition of the hospital and presence of very specialist departments will impact on the work of liaison services. Surprisingly little is known about the morbidity in accident and emergency departments. There is evidence that the rate of referral of older people and the average age of those referred has been increasing for at least three decades.

A large series of referrals over a five-year period found the most common reasons for referral to be cognitive assessment (42.8%), depression or anxiety (19.3%) and behaviour disorder (6%) (unpublished data: Anderson D, Nortcliffe M, Dechenne S et al. Characteristics of a nurse-led liaison mental health service for older people: the Liverpool Dataset Project). This generally accords with findings from smaller studies. The most common diagnoses from this series, as expected, were dementia (35%), mood disorder (17%) and delirium (11%). Dementia was more likely to be of vascular type than reported in community services, and 43% of delirium occurred in the context of dementia.

About half the referrals only required a single assessment, and the most common recommendations were for behaviour management (30%), further investigation or assessment (27.1%), medication prescribing (14%) and discharge planning (12.6%). In this series, 66.3% were discharged to their original place of residence and 19.4% to care homes; 8.4% required transfer to a mental health inpatient unit and 8.6% to a community outpatient mental health service.

CONCLUSION

The psychiatric co-morbidity of older people admitted to general hospitals is high, and admission is a common means by which mental disorder of older people comes to the attention of the health care system. General care teams have serious limitations in their ability to detect, diagnose and manage mental disorder. Two-thirds of this morbidity is mild and uncomplicated and will need to be recognized and managed more effectively by general care teams.

The development of specialist liaison services for older people brings an opportunity to improve the outcome for patients and the efficiency of general hospitals. These teams bring the skill and expertise necessary to manage complex co-morbidity, and provide training and education that general care teams require. This developing subspeciality will become increasingly important in ageing populations and is a vehicle for improving the quality of care.

REFERENCES

1. Lipowski ZJ. The need to integrate liaison psychiatry with geropsychiatry. *Am J Psychiatry* 1983; **140**: 1003–5.
2. Fortin M. Multimorbidity's many challenges; time to focus on the needs of this vulnerable and growing population. *BMJ* 2007; **334**: 1016–17.

3. Royal College of Psychiatrists. *Who Cares Wins. Improving the Outcome for Older People Admitted to the General Hospital: Guidelines for the Development of Liaison Mental Health Services for Older People*. London: Royal College of Psychiatrists, 2005.

4. Department of Health. *A New Ambition for Old Age: Next Steps in Implementing the National Service Framework for Older People*. London: Stationery Office, 2006.

5. National Institute for Health and Clinical Excellence, Social Care Institute for Excellence. *Dementia: Supporting People with Dementia and Their Carers in Health and Social Care*, NICE clinical guideline 42. London: NICE, 2006.

6. Department of Health. *Living Well with Dementia: A National Dementia Strategy*. London: Department of Health, 2009.

7. Department of Health. *National Service Framework for Older People*. London: Stationery Office, 2001.

8. Kominski G, Andersen R, Bastani R et al. UPBEAT: the impact of a psychogeriatric intervention in VA medical centers. Unified psychogeriatric biopsychosocial evaluation and treatment. *Med Care* 2001; **39**: 500–12.

9. Wilson K, Mottram P, Hussein M. Survival in the community of the very old depressed discharged from medical inpatient care. *Int J Geriatr Psychiatry* 2007; **22**: 974–89.

10. Nightingale S, Holmes J, Mason J et al. Psychiatric illness and mortality after hip fracture. *Lancet* 2001; **357**: 1264–5.

11. Koenig HG, George LK, Larson DB et al. Depressive symptoms and nine year survival of 1001 male veterans hospitalized with medical illness. *Am J Geriatr Psychiatry* 1999; **7**: 124–31.

12. Rockwood K, Cosway S, Carver D et al. The risk of dementia and death after delirium. *Age Ageing* 1999; **28**: 551–6.

13. Anderson D, Holmes J. Liaison psychiatry for older people – an overlooked opportunity. *Age Ageing* 2005; **34**: 205–7.

14. Holmes J, Bentley K, Cameron I. A UK survey of psychiatric services for older people in general hospitals. *Int J Geriatr Psychiatry* 2003; **18**: 716–21.

15. Inouye SK. The dilemma of delirium: clinical and research controversies regarding diagnosis and evaluation of delirium in hospitalised elderly medical inpatients. *Am J Med* 1994; **97**: 278–87.

16. Harwood DMJ, Hope T, Jacoby R. Cognitive impairment in medical inpatients: II; do physicians miss cognitive impairment. *Age Ageing* 1997; **26**: 37–9.

17. Cole MG, Bellavance F. Depression in elderly medical inpatients: a meta-analysis of outcomes. *Can Med Ass J* 1997; **157**: 1055–60.

18. National Audit Office. *Improving Services and Support for People with Dementia*. London: Stationery Office, 2007.

19. Jackson R, Baldwin B. Detecting depression in elderly medically ill patients: the use of the Geriatric Depression Scale compared with medical and nursing observations. *Age Ageing* 1993; **22**: 340–53.

20. Fick D, Foreman M. Consequences of not recognizing delirium superimposed on dementia in hospitalized elderly individuals. *J Gerontol Nurs* 2000; **26**: 30–40.

21. Farrell KR, Ganzini L. Misdiagnosing delirium as depression in medically ill elderly patients. *Arch Int Med* 1995; **155**: 2459–65.

22. American Psychiatric Association. *Diagnostic and Statistical Manual of Mental Disorders, Third Edition Revised*. Washington, DC: American Psychiatric Association, 1987.

23. Koenig HG, George LK, Peterson BL, Pieper CF. Depression in medically ill hospitalized older adults: prevalence, characteristics and course of symptoms according to six diagnostic schemes. *Am J Psychiatry* 1997; **154**: 1376–83.

24. Gilbody SM, House AO, Sheldon TA. Routinely administered questionnaires for depression and anxiety: systematic review. *Br Med J* 2001; **322**: 406–9.

25. Cole MG, McCusker J, Bellavance F et al. Systematic detection and multidisciplinary care of delirium in older medical inpatients: a randomized trial. *Can Med Ass J* 2002; **167**: 753–60.

26. Cole MG, McCusker J, Elie M et al. Systematic detection and multidisciplinary care of depression in older medical inpatients: a randomized trial. *Can Med Ass J* 2006; **174**: 38–44.

27. Cole MG. Delirium in elderly patients. *Am J Geriatr Psychiatry* 2004; **12**: 7–21.

28. Draper B. The effectiveness of old age psychiatry services. *Int J Geriatr Psychiatry* 2000; **15**: 687–703.

29. Rockwood K. Educational interventions for delirium. *Dem Geriatr Cog Dis* 1999; **10**: 426–9.

30. Sharroch J, Happell B. The psychiatric consultation nurse: thriving in a general hospital setting. *Int J Men Health Nursing* 2002; **11**: 24–33.

31. Rizzo JR, Bogardus ST, Leo-Summers L et al. Multicomponent targeted intervention to prevent delirium in hospitalized older patients. What is the economic value? *Med Care* 2001; **39**: 740–52.

32. McCusker J, Cole M, Dendukuri N et al. The course of delirium in medical inpatients: a prospective study. *J Gen Int Med* 2003; **18**: 696–704.

33. Cole MG, You Y, McCusker J et al. The 6 and 12 month outcomes of older medical inpatients who recover from delirium. *Int J Geriatr Psychiatry* 2008; **23**: 301–7.

34. British Geriatrics Society, Royal College of Physicians. *The Prevention, Diagnosis and Management of Delirium in Older People. National Guidelines*. Concise guidance to good practice series, no. 6. London: RCP, 2006.

35. Liptzin B, Laki A, Garb JL et al. Donepezil in the prevention and treatment of post surgical delirium. *Am J Geriatr Psychiatry* 2005; **13**: 1100–6.

36. Sampson EL, Raven PR, Ndhlovu PN et al. A randomized double blind placebo controlled trial of donepezil hydrochloride (Aricept) for reducing the incidence of postoperative delirium after elective hip replacement. *Int J Geriatr Psychiatry* 2007; **22**: 343–9.

37. Wilson KCM, Broadhurst C, Diver M et al. Plasma insulin growth factor-1 and incident delirium in older people. *Int J Geriatr Psychiatry* 2005; **20**: 154–9.

38. Inouye SK. Prevention of delirium in hospitalized older patients: risk factors and targeted intervention strategies. *Ann Med* 2000; **32**: 257–63.

39. Marcantonio ER, Goldman L, Mangione CM et al. A clinical prediction rule for delirium after elective noncardiac surgery. *JAMA* 1994; **271**: 134–9.

40. Fisher BW, Flowerdew G. A simple model for predicting postoperative delirium in older patients undergoing elective orthopaedic surgery. *J Am Geriatr Soc* 1995; **43**: 175–8.

41. Anderson D. Preventing delirium in older people. *Br Med Bull* 2005; **73**: 1–10.

42. Inouye SK, Viscoli CM, Horwitz RI et al. A predictive model for delirium in hospitalized elderly medical patients based on admission characteristics. *Ann Int Med* 1993; **119**: 474–81.

43. Inouye SK, Charpentier PA. Precipitating factors for delirium in hospitalized elderly persons. *JAMA* 1996; **273**: 852–7.

44. Inouye SK, Bogardus ST, Charpentier PA *et al.* A multicomponent intervention to prevent delirium in hospitalized older patients. *N Engl J Med* 1999; **340**: 669–76.

45. Marcantonio ER, Flacker JM, Wright RJ *et al.* Reducing delirium after hip fracture: a randomised trial. *J Am Geriatr Soc* 2001; **49**: 1327–34.

46. McCusker J, Coole M, Abrahamovich M *et al.* Delirium predicts 12 month mortality. *Arch Int Med* 2002; **162**: 457–63.

47. Marcantonio E, Ta T, Duthie E *et al.* Delirium severity and psychomotor types: their relationship with outcome after hip fracture. *J Am Geriatr Soc* 2002; **50**: 850–7.

48. Inouye SK, Schlesinger MJ, Lydon TJ *et al.* Delirium: a symptom of how hospital care is failing older persons and a window to improve quality of hospital care. *Am J Med* 1999; **106**: 565–73.

49. Britton A, Russell R. Multidisciplinary team interventions for delirium in patients with chronic cognitive impairment. *Cochrane Database Syst Rev* 2001; **1**: CD000395.

50. Holmes J. The detection of psychiatric factors predicting the outcome in elderly hip fracture patients. MD Thesis. Research School of Medicine, University of Leeds, 1999.

51. Huusko TM, Karppi P, Avikainen H *et al.* Randomised clinically controlled trial of intensive rehabilitation in patients with hip fracture: a subgroup analysis of patients with dementia. *Br Med J* 2000; **321**: 1107–11.

52. Ryan J, Carriere I, Ritchie K *et al.* Late life depression and mortality: influence of gender and antidepressant use. *Br J Psychiatry* 2008; **192**: 12–18.

53. McCusker J, Cole M, Ciapi A *et al.* Twelve month course of depressive symptoms in older medical inpatients. *Int J Geriatr Psychiatry* 2007; **22**: 411–7.

54. Gill D, Hatcher S. Antidepressants for depression in medical illness. *Cochrane Database Syst Rev* 2000; **4**: CD001312. DOI: 10.1002/14651858.CD001312.pub2.

55. Wilson K, Mottram PG, Sivananthan A, Nightingale A. Antidepressants versus placebo for the depressed elderly. Cochrane Database Syst Rev 2001; **1**: CD000561. DOI: 10.1002/14651858.CD000561.

56. Glassman AH, O'Connor CM, Califf RM *et al.* Sertraline treatment of major depression in patients with acute MI or unstable angina. *JAMA* 2002; **288**: 701–9.

57. Writing Committee for the ENRICHD Investigators. Effects of treating depression and low perceived social support on clinical events after myocardial infarction. *JAMA* 2003; **289**: 3106–116.

58. The National Collaborating Centre for Chronic Conditions. Parkinson's Disease: National Clinical Guideline for Diagnosis and Management in Primary and Secondary Care. London: Royal College of Physicians, 2006.

59. Hackett ML, Anderson CS, House AO. Interventions for treating depression after stroke. *Cochrane Database Syst Rev* 2004; **3**: CD003437. DOI: 10.1002/14651858.CD003437.pub2.

60. Sirey JA, Raue PJ, Alexopoulos GS. An intervention to improve depression care in older adults with COPD. *Int J Geriatr Psychiatry* 2007; **22**: 154–9.

61. Menza M, Dobkin RD, Marin H *et al.* A controlled trial of antidepressants in patients with Parkinson's disease and depression. *Neurology* 2009; **72**: 886–92.

62. Evans M, Hammond M, Wilson K *et al.* Placebo controlled treatment trial of depression in elderly physically ill patients. *Int J Geriatr Psychiatry* 1997; **12**: 817–24.

63. Mossey JM, Knott KA, Higgins M *et al.* Effectiveness of psychological intervention, interpersonal counseling, for sub-dysthymic depression in medically ill elderly. *J Gerontol* 1996; **51**: 172–8.

64. Baldwin R, Pratt H, Goring H *et al.* Does a nurse led mental health liaison service reduce psychiatric morbidity in acute general medical wards? *Age Ageing* 2004; **33**: 472–8.

65. Cullum S, Tucker S, Todd C *et al.* Effectiveness of liaison psychiatric nursing in older medical inpatients with depression: a randomized controlled trial. *Age Ageing* 2007; **36**: 436–42.

66. Conwell Y, Duberstein OR, Cox C *et al.* Relationship of age and axis 1 diagnoses in victims of completed suicide: a psychological autopsy study. *Am J Psychiatry* 1996; **153**: 1001–8.

67. Hawton K, Zahl D, Weatherall R. Suicide following deliberate self harm: long term follow up of patients who presented to a general hospital. *Br J Psychiatry* 2003; **182**: 537–42.

68. Shah A, Hoxey K, Mayadunne V. Suicidal ideation in acutely medically ill inpatients: prevalence, correlates and longitudinal stability. *Int J Geriatr Psychiatry* 2000; **15**: 162–9.

69. Lamprecht HC, Pakrasi S, Gash A *et al.* Deliberate self harm in older people revisited. *Int J Geriatr Psychiatry* 2005; **20**: 1090–6.

70. Hawton K, Harriss L. Deliberate self harm in people aged 60 years and over: characteristics and outcome of a 20 year cohort. *Int J Geriatr Psychiatry* 2006; **21**: 572–81.

71. Purandare N, Oude Voshaar RC, Rodway C *et al.* Suicide in dementia: 9 year national clinical survey in England and Wales. *Br J Psychiatry* 2009; **194**: 175–80.

72. Sheehan B, Bass C, Briggs R *et al.* Somatisation among older primary care attenders. *Psychol Med* 2003; **33**: 867–77.

73. Sheehan B, Lall R, Bass C. Does somatisation influence quality of life among older primary care attenders? *Int J Geriatr Psychiatry* 2005; **20**: 967–72.

74. Drayer RA, Mulsant BH, Lenze EJ *et al.* Somatic symptoms of depression in elderly patients with medical comorbidities. *Int J Geriatr Psychiatry* 2005; **20**: 973–82.

75. Anderson D, Ooman S. Liaison psychiatry for older people. In Guthrie E, Temple M, Kapur N (eds), *Seminars in Liaison Psychiatry*. London: Gaskell Press, 2010 (In Press).

76. Draper B, Low L-F. What is the effectiveness of acute hospital treatment of older people with mental disorders. *Int Psychogeriatrics* 2005; **17**: 539–56.

130

Rehabilitation

Rob Jones

Mental Health Services for Older People Directorate and Nottingham University Section of Old Age Psychiatry, Queen's Medical Centre, Nottingham, UK

INTRODUCTION

In one sense the broad principles of rehabilitation seem well and securely established. But in another sense they seem to be rediscovered anew by succeeding generations, with sometimes wise old concepts seeming to come newly dressed as fresh approaches. In England up to 70% of acute hospital beds are occupied by older people, a theme familiar to most ageing societies, focusing attention on how to promote recovery more rapidly and ensure it can be sustained, not least with older people with mental health problems.

Rehabilitation of the older person with psychiatric disorder means restoring and maintaining the highest possible level of psychological, physical and social function despite the disabling effects of illness. More broadly it also means preventing unnecessary handicap associated with illness, preventing unnecessary handicap secondary to maladaptive responses to illness and combating the deadening effects of low expectations for older people among professionals, patients, families and society in general. Managing chronic disease and disability is the greatest challenge to modern medicine. Within this, rehabilitation of many older people with psychiatric disorder looms large – although, of course, many old people with psychiatric disorder respond well to 'curative' therapy and require little rehabilitation.

In fact, rehabilitation has always been a fundamental and inseparable part of old age psychiatry (as of all psychiatry). Perhaps for this reason, as with rehabilitation in geriatric medicine[1,2], little writing in the way of conclusive evaluation or substantial trials has addressed the topic specifically. Some particular techniques, such as psychological approaches with the cognitively impaired, have been well described[3,4], but little evaluated[5], and evaluative research is much needed here.

SPECIAL PROBLEMS WITH PSYCHIATRIC DISORDER IN THE OLDER PERSON

'Old age' may span 40 years or more, posing quite different rehabilitation problems; but the most major challenge is the very frail, the old old. In this group multiple disability is prominent, easily complicated by polypharmacy, and physical and mental ill health interact in complex ways. With this vulnerable population, disentangling the respective influences of ageing, previous personality and current ill

health can be exacting. Two thirds of the UK's disabled population are older people and the true extent of handicap due to psychiatric disorder is probably still not established.

With depression especially there may be restriction of physical activity, threatening physical capacity and health. Depression associated with stroke disorder[6] or with Parkinson's disease[7] particularly illustrates both the connection between physical and psychiatric problems and the importance of physiotherapy and occupational therapy in psychiatric rehabilitation.

Physical factors are frequently of great importance in dementia. A quiescent individual may become delirious and disturbed at night through heart failure, obstructive airways disease or even the uncomfortable effects of severe constipation. Settling such problems may transform the reality of care for a carer and seeking out such therapeutic opportunities is an important part of rehabilitation. Similarly, in dementia physiotherapy and occupational therapy to promote and maintain the best possible physical capacity are key elements. Advice and practical aid to carers, such as with lifting and handling the physically disabled person with dementia, can be crucial.

A judicious mixture of the 'therapeutic' (curative) and the 'prosthetic' (supportive) approaches, sagely described over two decades ago by an eminent wise voice in geriatric medicine[8,9], is very necessary in old age psychiatry. While much functional psychiatric disorder and delirium can be 'cured', and this must be the aim, most older people with dementia need some degree of supportive care at some stage. The poor financial and housing state of many older people, together with the lack of children or spouses to help as carers for many of the old old, are further complicating factors. Maximizing 'participation' despite psychiatric disorder needs to be a major goal: maintaining as far as possible a role in the family, social contact, a range of activities and minimization of loss of autonomy or institutionalization. This requires an approach which embraces psychiatric, medical, rehabilitation, nursing and social perspectives. Vigorously pursing active prevention of disability or of reduced participation as a consequence of psychiatric disorder is a vital part of rehabilitation.

SPECIAL PRINCIPLES IN REHABILITATION OF THE OLDER PERSON WITH PSYCHIATRIC DISORDER

Table 130.1 summarizes the principles. The home must be the focus of attention. This is where problems have arisen and where they

Principles and Practice of Geriatric Psychiatry, 3rd edn. Edited by Mohammed T. Abou-Saleh, Cornelius Katona and Anand Kumar
© 2011 John Wiley & Sons, Ltd

Table 130.1 Principles of rehabilitation for the older person with psychiatric disorder

Focus on the home
Ensure comprehensive assessment
Encourage normal function
Treat the treatable
Analyse disabilities and chart progress
Clarify team goals with patient and carers early
Clarify team goals with support workers early
Teach what can be relearned
Adapt the adaptable
Coordinate support and follow-up
Promote flexibility and ingenuity
Promote realistic optimism
Promote participation and autonomy

will need to be overcome. Planning for rehabilitation should begin at the earliest moment; an initial assessment at home by a senior psychiatrist, or other experienced team member, is invaluable – even if 'home' by now is an institution in the community. Home is also where the carers, and often any social services support staff involved, may readily be found. It is where they will need to work with solutions. This contrasts with standard medical rehabilitation where traditionally often no such opportunities for outreach have existed.

Frequently, further assessment by, say, an occupational therapist, physiotherapist or another specialist team member may be necessary – and this can perhaps also be arranged at home. But avoiding disruptive admission should not be at the cost of really meeting assessment needs. The day hospital or a community-based therapy resource centre and their teams may often be useful to complete such assessments. They (or a day centre specially supported with outreach expertise) may be settings where important rehabilitation efforts can be made.

Effectively supporting the carers with people at home is essential for rehabilitation. In the UK, Admiral Nurses are a good example – specially trained mental health nurses who work all the time in the community with people with dementia and their carers.

Poor function or morbidity should never be accepted as immutable, and, still less, as normal. Assessment should aim at a thorough understanding of social, physical and psychological function as well as the previous pattern of personality and lifestyle. From this, diagnoses and specific treatment for the treatable should follow. But also analysis should show the extent of disability, how it is mediated and how it may be overcome. Problems should be clearly recorded, with proposed solutions and with regular review of progress, and with this it is useful to use standardized assessments, such as the Bristol Activities of Daily Living Scale (BADL)[10], and a standardized framework, such as the International Classification of Functioning, Disability and Health (ICF)[11]. From the earliest moment, independent function and improvement should be sensitively encouraged, especially with hospitalized patients.

As early as possible, the agreed goals of rehabilitative efforts need to be clarified with the patient, with the relatives/carers, with the whole rehabilitation team and with any support workers needed in the community. Education, guidance and a rehabilitative 'demonstration' may well be necessary to resolve conflicting views on the prospects for progress. Carers may need therapy or rehabilitation in their own right. Almost always the support of carers is essential, though some stoutly independent patients manage well without this.

A prognosis-based plan is useful. This means assessing: what are the problems and what are their causes? Prognostication will follow: will these get better or worse? To what degree? Over how long a period? From this a plan can flow consistent with what seem the most major likely developments of a problematic nature, over a foreseeable time scale and taking account of what is most remediable.

Sometimes disability strongly distorts the previously stable power and dominance pattern in the family, first noted in classic work[12] but reiterated in evolving family therapy work[13], so that, for instance, a forceful mother becomes dependent on a passive daughter. Relationships are always important and such phenomena can strongly influence outcome. They need to be understood and often complex ambivalence worked through[14]. Such factors are frequently important when carers seem reluctant to resume caring[14,15] and need to be carefully teased out when juggling with the various elements of risk and risk minimization involved in supporting a vulnerable person at home[15]. The patient's 'crutch is not made of wood but of some other person's tolerance or patience'[16].

An agreed balance should be sought between the needs of carers and the patient's right and desire for continued comparative independence despite significant disability – bearing in mind the team's prime responsibility to the patient.

In effect, carers should be 'recruited' as rehabilitation therapists' 'aids'. But often they will need practical help and advice on rehabilitation techniques, and, always, the reassurance of the services' continuing availability for support and sensitive expert response. This is less easy both to offer and in practice as services increasingly become, as in recent years, driven towards short-term involvement and a short-term perspective.

Similar considerations apply with any support staff necessary to help the patient at home – principally social services staff in the UK. Their early involvement and integration into the assessment and rehabilitation process can be logistically difficult but generally is most effective. Again, a longer term perspective and continuity are invaluable.

Good teamwork is of the essence. Clarity and consistency within the multidisciplinary specialist team are essential. Nurses and therapists, for instance, must communicate well, each complementing and enhancing the other's approach.

Specialist and general practitioner must be in accord. The specialist team must carry the confidence of those who will work with the patient outside hospital. (Table 130.2 lists many of the team members and resources requiring coordination for rehabilitation – inevitably there is great overlap.)

Clear goals should be set, in accord with those of the patient and carers, and clearly understood by all[15,17–20]. This is much easier said than done with the vulnerable frail older person; but vitally important is good communication.

Patients are taught what they can learn or relearn but often only modification of domestic equipment, provision of aids or modifications of the home will overcome their disability. More often still problems are only overcome through support services – home-delivered meals or a home help/community care assistant – coming into the home. Ingenuity and diplomacy may be needed with an old person reluctant to accept such necessary support. The great majority of support is provided by relatives/carers and supporting the supporters is the main task. This may require a day hospital or community venue for therapy, day care centre or respite admissions. Maintaining confidence that there will be reliable and appropriate care interventions and responses by the service is vital. Such confidence and such a reality become harder to maintain as there

Table 130.2 People and facilities to aid rehabilitation of the older person with psychiatric disorder

	Specialist psychiatric team	Social services and local authority services	Primary care team
People	Psychiatrists	Social workers	General practitioners
	Hospital specialist nurses	Domiciliary services manager	Practice nurse
	Community psychiatric nurses/Admiral nurses	Home help/community care assistants	District nurse
	Physiotherapist	Meals on wheels	Health visitor
	Occupational therapist (OT)	Community OT	Specialist community nurse
	Clinical psychologist	Support to voluntary sector	Specialist community health support teams
	Social worker	Sitter services	
	Ready access to geriatricians	Carers groups	
	(Speech therapist – sometimes)	Preferably multiagency specialist home support team	
	(Dietician – sometimes)		
	Carers groups		
Facilities	Assessment ward	Luncheon club (often voluntary)	Health centre
	Nursing home	Day centres (often voluntary)	
	Day hospital	Long stay and short stay residential care and nursing homes	
	Outpatients	Housing adaptation	
	Longer stay and respite care facilities	Sheltered and super-sheltered housing	

is more pressure on services to be short term in their outlook and activity.

At some stage with hospital patients, except in the most grossly deteriorated person, a home assessment is advisable with an occupational therapist or physiotherapist, or both, and perhaps with other team members.

Hospital-based staff can be too pessimistic and, allowed to function in her familiar environment, even a person with quite significant dementia can sometimes perform surprisingly well. Often serial home assessments are helpful with increasing challenge, leading to overnight stays. Also, failure initially to manage satisfactorily should not preclude the possibility of later improvement with further therapy or support.

A model of how a person-centred multi-agency specialist home support team for people with dementia and their carers works to achieve valued results has been quoted in the National Dementia Strategy[20] and evaluated in pilot form[21]. This highlights many of the issues arising when striving for a more bespoke, individual approach.

Above all, rehabilitation with older people requires flexibility allied to a realistic but constructively optimistic approach. Innovation and ingenuity are frequently necessary. The complex interaction between physical, social and psychological factors in older patients is further complicated by the likelihood that circumstances, especially perhaps physical health, may change dramatically; this demands a flexible response. The solution, carefully constructed and successful on one day, may need major change on the next as the situation radically alters. For this reason rehabilitation with older people is rarely completely finished, and 'maintenance' measures are often necessary. Careful planning of continuing care, follow-up and continuing availability as problems arise are essential features. The strength and determination of patients, relatives and support staff are considerably bolstered by the knowledge that this approach is backing them up[15,20,21].

REHABILITATION AND LONG STAY CARE

Many patients, especially among those with dementia, despite support end up requiring long-term care but rehabilitation must remain a strong theme. Eventually, multiply disabled people, particularly with dementia, are likely to require 24-hour care. They may often exhibit both difficult, disturbed behaviour and the need for heavy physical care. Providing the best quality of life, given often quite limited resources, is the aim and a major strategy is preventing unnecessary dependency and promoting the maximum retention of function. With descriptions[22–25] of the care of such patients in various settings, a frequent theme has been the availability of skilled and expert staff from the multidisciplinary team to help maintain good function. Evaluation of such long-term care programmes has proved complex and difficult[22,23].

Earlier concerns expressed in the UK that such disabled patients would be excluded from hospital long stay care, largely seemingly for funding reasons, in favour of publicly funded and means-tested placements in private residential or nursing home care[26–28] have been superseded by this reality. In the USA (and many other countries) long-term care of older people has long been provided largely in the private or charitable sector. But in the USA the Omnibus Budget Reconciliation Act (OBRA Act)[29] requires nursing homes to ascertain and meet any needs for therapy and treatment. In the UK the fear is that the drive previously striven for in the best hospital care to provide a good quality of life can be replaced in private and independent care homes by a desire for a quiet life, leading to residents showing unwarranted passivity and dependency, possibly resulting from unnecessary tranquillizing medication[30-32]. Financial constraints could make this more acceptable than the patient's exercise of individuality, movement and self-expression.

Reports of high levels of depression in homes for older people[33-35] emphasize the worry about effective rehabilitation and care for older people with chronic psychiatric disorder. Any institution providing shelter is at risk of providing a relatively impoverished environment[16,22,23] and undue restriction of independence.

Bennett[16] called unnecessary social inactivity and dependence the psychiatric equivalent of contractures. Hospitals (and social services) and care home settings have provided much good practice. Accounts of good long stay care for people with dementia emphasize the invaluable input of occupational therapy, physiotherapy and person-centred approaches[2,36,37]. Sensibly ensuring activity in a structured day and enriching the environment with, for example, music therapy, art therapy, drama therapy or other stimulatory approaches[20] are important wherever the setting (p. 58). Emerging innovative work in Nottingham, logged as commissioned research[38], is usefully looking at the ethnography of the nursing teams in various health settings providing care for people with dementia and how this relates to staff well-being as they strive to deliver quality person-centred care. Preliminary results very much support the theme of the National Dementia Strategy[20].

Community Psychiatric Nurse (CPN) support (indeed, availability of all the specialist team to give support) to such homes is both feasible and helpful, and should be developed[39]. But concern remains about how to monitor effectively and maintain standards in private and all long stay care, especially with people with dementia, epitomized by Objective 10 of the National Dementia Strategy[20]. Ultimately good care here depends on the commitment of sufficient appropriately trained staff to help disabled old people experience to the full their remaining scope for independence and capacity for joy.

NEUROREHABILITATION AND COGNITIVE STIMULATION APPROACHES WITH PEOPLE WITH DEMENTIA

Considerable focus has been placed in recent years on psychological and individual training approaches that help to maximize or maintain function in older people, especially those with dementia, despite the challenge of pathological ageing[4]. Cognitive stimulation therapy has shown promise and much can be achieved by practical and individual approaches exploiting the older person's continuing good function and tendency to adapt most successfully to coping in his/her own individual environment. While work in this area has been promising and should be encouraged[40], the Cochrane Database shows a limited evidence base[5].

DEVELOPING THEMES WITH REHABILITATION IN THE OLDER PERSON

A dominating theme is the need for a more person-centred, individual, bespoke approach, particularly to the older person with dementia, especially when working to support individuals with dementia and their carers at home. Each person with dementia/carer dyad has its own specific problems requiring a bespoke individually tailored solution[21]. Task-centred care, one size fits all, designed to suit the needs of the service provider, will not do.

The emphasis with support of this clientele at home needs to be different from the normal rehabilitation aim of restoration of function.

Here rehabilitation instead seeks to maintain maximum autonomy and participation by the individual despite deterioration. This means flexibly and individually working to promote continuing participatory activity in some form, rather than simply restoring function (no longer possible) or replacing function[41]. Supporting individuals in participating in making cups of tea is preferable to doing it for them when they can no longer relearn this skill. There is considerable challenge here to the standard rehabilitation approach, which focuses on recovering or relearning lost function. The standard rehabilitation approach fits ill with supporting chronic neurodegenerative disease.

Considerable attention in various health fields, including in psychiatry, especially in general adult psychiatry, has focused over the past decade on early and concentrated intervention into the home, often via special teams to give special support[42]. The hospital at home scheme in geriatric medicine has been an example in one area, and assertive outreach schemes, perhaps in tandem with crisis resolution teams, have been another. One emphasis here has been prevention of hospitalization but necessarily emphasis has also been needed on promoting recovery and good function. Linked to this has been promoting earlier discharge from hospital, either with a move to a less acute facility but with an intensive rehabilitative input and/or intensive rehabilitative input into the home following earlier discharge. In the UK intermediate care, with this short intensive input, has been the name applied to this approach. Such approaches and teams have been defined as very short term in their intervention (usually a maximum of six weeks)[43-46]. While the supportive rehabilitative effort has been welcome, there has been a danger of lack of overall coordination and continuity of care for patients and families. Compartmentalized services can fail to link optimally for the patient's benefit across the divides between teams. In the UK such tendencies have arguably been exacerbated by short-termism in funding with performance target management requiring quick discharge. Chronic and degenerative health problems (especially mental health problems in older people) can be especially sensitive to perverse incentives here. They do not fit in well with such short-term approaches. With hospital discharge the fear has been expressed that the target of recovery may have been replaced with 'fit for discharge to a care home'. Again, such difficulties would be avoided more easily by having the dominant focus on individual bespoke outcomes and person-centred care, respecting autonomy[21,41].

With such major interaction in this population between physical health and mental health (and with each commonly interacting with other issues), there is a great need for collaboration between geriatric medicine and old age psychiatry. The area of liaison between these specialties is a prominent theme. More broadly, there is a need for spreading of the knowledge and expertise of old age psychiatry into all physical health care settings that may deal with older people with mental health problems[47]. The area of how older people with medical crises and mental health problems fare in the general hospital is a major issue and concern in the UK. Particular dissatisfaction with this area has been expressed especially by the carers of people with dementia, meriting highlighting in the UK government's National Dementia Strategy[20] and by NICE/SCIE[19]. It is clear that improved collaboration and improved working by such services could impact beneficially in a considerable way on such rehabilitation here.

In terms of service organization, in the UK there seems to have been quite a restriction on and even a move away from the use of old age psychiatry day hospitals with older people. This seems potentially detrimental to rehabilitation approaches. Some of this has been accompanied by spreading mental health expertise more widely into day centres but the main emphasis appears, unfortunately, to have been on cost cutting in specialist services. Good, expert, readily and locally accessible assessment and therapeutic ambulatory facilities on a day or sessional basis remain an essential component necessary for proper rehabilitation approaches with this patient population.

Another service area concerns people termed 'graduates' in the UK – these are people who have developed mental health problems earlier in life and with whom these have endured into old age, beyond 65 years. Many of these people need considerable psychiatric rehabilitation expertise and support. Arguments arise as to who should care for them. The answer is that there should be no age discrimination[48] and that people of any age should receive the service and expertise they need regardless of their age. This may mean them staying with services which predominately deal with younger people or may mean an older person with dementia receiving help from an old age service[49]. It is essential that services plan and agree together the appropriate care for the individuals concerned, so that people do not fall between the 'gap'.

Antidementia drugs (cholinesterase inhibitors) merit mention and should be a part of a broader rehabilitative approach. There is great hope, and some accumulating evidence, that these will have a prophylactic and preventative effect with mild cognitive impairment, such that 'conversion' to Alzheimer's disease is delayed or prevented, with encouraging evidence also in mild/moderate Alzheimer's[50,51]. Neurorehabilitation may usefully come into play with this approach.

The UK National Dementia Strategy[20] emphasizes 'living well with dementia', advocating that with proper information, support and attitudes people with dementia can experience a good quality of life. It lays great emphasis on changing attitudes more positively, educating widely with accurate information and thereby raising expectations so that a good quality of life becomes both expected and the norm. In a tacit way, perhaps, this plays into the rehabilitation approach of maintaining participation and autonomy despite the threat of cognitive decline.

In the UK a new strongly pursued theme in social care involves individuals managing and commissioning their own supportive social services. Known as self-directed care[52], and well used in the USA, this process directly awards individual budgets to clients who have been appropriately assessed, to purchase services as they wish, within some limits. This is being piloted also now in some health care settings. Clearly this is relevant to rehabilitation work and the scheme has been seemingly well demonstrated with younger physically disabled people. Again, a rehabilitation approach focusing on individual answers, promoting participation and autonomy, seems relevant. However, older, frailer, multiply disabled people with mental health problems and possibly inadequate mental capacity may be more vulnerable to exploitation with such a system or unable or just disinclined properly to grapple with it. Such fears arise more prominently with a multi-provider, private provider and market dominated system, towards which the UK has moved significantly, especially with a perceived weakening of the regulating inspecting systems, as exemplified by concerns in the case of the Mid-Staffordshire NHS Foundation Trust[53]. Good advice, availability of brokers and strong, effective regulation are greatly needed with such an approach.

The theme of supporting vulnerable older people at home, particularly people with dementia, raises consideration of the use of 'extra care housing' and the usefulness of assistive technology approaches[54,55]. Both, especially perhaps the latter, must increasingly loom large in most societies around the world in rehabilitation and support approaches for the rising population of older people with mental health problems.

Living at home, with such helpful support, contrasts, particularly for people with dementia, with the experience of living in an institutional care home, which is less good. The UK Alzheimer's Society[25] sadly reported people there having 'little to do' with 'little interaction' and very limited time devoted to them individually by staff. Another study[37] in a similar vein found very uncomfortable depersonalized experiences for people living in such care homes.

ATTITUDES

Adverse feelings about older people have been noted by many[37,56,57]. Commentators have addressed helpful and unhelpful attitudes in health professionals of all kinds, including especially doctors[58-60]. Modern medical education is inculcating a better knowledge base for tomorrow's doctors and also better attitudes[61]. The educational potential of old age psychiatry services, not least exploiting the educational opportunity afforded by rehabilitation (and other concerns) with the most disabled, has been described and remains valid[62]. Not only medical students[57], but all varieties of medical and other professional staff concerned with older people with mental health problems, and also carers and lay audiences, benefit from this educational effort. Public education especially is vital in engendering constructive attitudes in society, on which ultimately will depend all efforts towards care in the community and the political will to provide decent services. These efforts and seeking better intergenerational empathy and understanding should never cease.

CONCLUSIONS

Rehabilitation of older people with psychiatric disorder means restoring/maintaining the best level of psychological, physical and social function despite the disabling effects of illness: preventing unnecessary handicap accompanying illness, unnecessary handicap secondary to maladaptive responses to illness and combating the deadening effects of low expectations with older people. Managing chronic disease and disability is the greatest challenge to modern medicine, within which rehabilitation of many older people with psychiatric disorder looms large – a fundamental and inseparable part of old age psychiatry using a judicious mixture of the 'therapeutic' (curative) and the 'prosthetic' (supportive) approaches.

In summary:

- focus on home
- ensure comprehensive multidisciplinary assessment
- encourage normal function
- treat the treatable
- analyse disabilities, chart progress
- clarify team goals with patient and carers early
- clarify team goals with support workers early
- promote realistic relearning
- adapt the adaptable
- coordinate support and follow-up
- encourage flexibility and ingenuity
- promote realistic optimism, participation and autonomy.

REFERENCES

1. Nocon A, Baldwin S. *Effective Practice in Rehabilitation: The Evidence of Systematic Reviews*. London: King's Fund, 1992.

2. Forster A, Lambley R, Hardy J *et al*. Rehabilitation for older people in long-term care. *Cochrane Database Syst Rev* 2009; (1): CD004294.

3. Holden U, Woods RT. *Positive Approaches to Dementia Care*, 3rd edn. Edinburgh: Churchill Livingstone, 1995.

4. Stuss DT, Winocur G, Robertson IH (eds). *Cognitive Neurorehabilitation*. Cambridge: Cambridge University Press, 2009.

5. Clare L, Woods B. Cognitive rehabilitation and cognitive training for early-stage Alzheimer's disease and vascular dementia. *Cochrane Database Syst Rev* 2003; (4): CD003260.

6. Williams LS. Depression and stroke: cause or consequence? *Sem Neurol* 2005; **25**(4), 396–409.

7. Miyasaki JM, Shannon K, Voon V *et al*. Practice parameter: evaluation and treatment of depression, psychosis, and dementia in Parkinson disease (an evidence-based review). *Neurology* 2006; **66**: 996–1002.

8. Evans JG. Commentary: curing is caring. *Age Ageing* 1989; **18**(4): 217–18.

9. Evans JG. High hopes for geriatrics. *J R Coll Physicians* 1994; **28**: 392–3.

10. Bucks RS, Haworth J. Review: Bristol Activities of Daily Living Scale: a critical evaluation. *Expert Rev Neurother* 2002; **2**(5): 669–76.

11. Rauch A, Cieza A, Stucki G. How to apply the International Classification of Functioning, Disability and Health (ICF) for rehabilitation management in clinical practice. *Eur J Phys Rehabil Med* 2008; **44**: 329–42.

12. Bergmann K. Neurosis and personality disorder in old age. In Isaacs AD, Post F (eds), *Studies in Geriatric Psychiatry*. Chichester: John Wiley & Sons, 1978, 41–76.

13. Benbow SM, Marriott A, Morley M, Walsh S. Family therapy and dementia: review and clinical experience. *Int J Geriatr Psychiatry* 1994; **8**(9): 717–25.

14. Curtis EA, Dixon MS. Family therapy and systemic practice with older people: where are we now? *J Fam Ther* 2005; **27**(1): 43–64.

15. Wattis JP, Curran S. *Practical Psychiatry of Old Age*, 4th edn. London: Radcliffe, 2006.

16. Bennett DH. The mentally ill. In Mattingly S (ed.), *Rehabilitation Today*, 2nd edn. London: Update, 1981, 119–22.

17. Department of Health. *Better Services for Vulnerable People*, EL (97) 62, CI (97) 24. London: Department of Health, 1997.

18. Health and Social Care Joint Unit and Change Agents Team. *Discharge from Hospital: Pathway, Process and Practice*. London: Department of Health, 2003.

19. National Institute for Health and Clinical Excellence, and Social Care Institute for Excellence. *Dementia: Supporting People with Dementia and Their Carers in Health and Social Care*, NICE clinical guideline 42. London: NICE/SCIE, 2006.

20. Department of Health. *Living Well with Dementia: A National Dementia Strategy*. London: Department of Health, 2009.

21. Rothera I, Jones RG, Harwood R *et al*. An evaluation of a specialist multiagency home support service for older people with dementia using qualitative methods. *Int J Geriatr Psychiatry* 2007; **23**(1): 65–72.

22. Kane RA, Kane RL. *Long-Term Care*. New York: Springer, 1987.

23. Kane RL. Strategies for improving chronic illness care: some issues for the NHS. *Aging Health* 2007; **3**(3): 333–42.

24. National Audit Office. *Improving Services and Support for People with Dementia*. London: The Stationery Office, 2007.

25. Alzheimer's Society. *Home from Home*. London: Alzheimer's Society, 2008.

26. Shah A, Phongsathorn V, George C *et al*. Physical dependency and dementia in the NHS continuing care wards and contracted NHS beds in voluntary nursing homes. *Int J Geriatr Psychiatry* 1994; **9**: 229–32.

27. Wattis J, Fairbairn A. Towards a consensus on continuing care for older adults with psychiatric disorder. *Int J Geriatr Psychiatry* 1996; **11**: 163–8.

28. Turrell AR, Castleden CM, Freestone B. Long stay care and the NHS: discontinuities between policy and practice. *Br Med J* 1998; **317**: 942–4.

29. National Mental Health Association. *Summary of the 1987 Omnibus Budget Reconciliation Act (OBRA)*. Washington, DC: NMHA, 1988.

30. McGrath M, Jackson GA. Survey of neuroleptic prescribing in residents of nursing homes in Glasgow. *Br Med J* 1996; **312**: 611–12.

31. Thacker S, Jones R. Neuroleptic prescribing to the community elderly in Nottingham. *Int J Geriatr Psychiatry* 1997; **12**: 833–7.

32. Thacker S, Jones R. Use of neuroleptics in dementia – a review of recent concerns. *Res Pract Alzheimers Dis* 1998; **1**(suppl): 363–72.

33. Snowdon J. The epidemiology of affective disorders in old age. In Chiu E, Ames D (eds), *Functional Psychiatric Disorders of the Elderly*. Cambridge: Cambridge University Press, 2006.

34. Dening T, Bains J. Mental health services for residents of care homes. *Age Ageing* 2004; **33**(1): 1–2.

35. Ames D, Depression in nursing and residential homes. In Chiu E, Ames D (eds), *Functional Psychiatric Disorders of the Elderly*. Cambridge: Cambridge University Press, 2006.

36. Kitwood T. *Dementia Reconsidered: The Person Comes First*. Buckingham: Open University Press, 1997.

37. Commission for Social Care Inspection. *See Me, Not Just the Dementia: Understanding People's Experience of Living in a Care Home*. London: CSCI, 2008.

38. Schneider J. Inpatient care for people with dementia: implications for person-centred practice, SDO/222 Commissioned Project. At www.sdo.nihr.ac.uk/projdetails.php?ref=08-1819-222, accessed 11 Feb 2010.

39. Fossey J, Ballard C, Juszczak E *et al*. Effect of enhanced psychosocial care on antipsychotic use in nursing home residents with severe dementia: cluster randomized trial. *Br Med J* 2006; **332**: 756–61.

40. Clare L, Woods RT. Cognitive training and cognitive rehabilitation for people with early-stage Alzheimer's disease: a review. *Neuropsychol Rehabil* 2004; **14**(4): 385–401.

41. Gladman JR, Jones RG, Radford K, Walker E, Rothera I. Person-centred dementia services are feasible, but can they be sustained? *Age Ageing* 2007; **36**: 171–6.

42. Smyth MG, Hoult J. The home treatment enigma. *Br Med J* 2000; **320**: 305–8.

43. Corrado OJ. Hospital-at-home. *Age Ageing* 2001; **30**(suppl 3): 11–14.

44. Melis RJF, Olde Rikkert MGM, Parker SG *et al*. What is intermediate care? *Br Med J* 2004; **329**: 360–61.

45. Leff B, Burton L, Mader S *et al*. Hospital at home: feasibility and outcomes of a program to provide hospital-level care at home for acutely ill older patients. *Ann Inter Med* 2005; **143**: 11.

46. Shepperd S, Iliffe S. Hospital at home versus in-patient hospital care. *Cochrane Database Syst Rev* 2005; (3): CD000356.

47. Department of Health/Care Services Improvement Partnership. *Everybody's Business. Integrated Mental Health Services for Older Adults: A Service Development Guide*, 2005. At www.mentalhealthequalities.org.uk/our-work/later-life/everybodys-business.html, accessed 2 Jun 2009.

48. Department of Health. *National Service Framework for Older People*. London: Department of Health, 2001.

49. Royal College of Psychiatrists. *The Interface between General and Community Psychiatry and Old Age Psychiatry Services: Report of a Working Group*, 2004. At www.rcpsych.ac.uk/pdf/Interface.pdf, accessed 11 Feb 2010.

50. Grossberg GT, Manes F, Allegri R *et al.* A multinational, randomized, double-blind, placebo-controlled trial of memantine extended-release capsule in patients with moderate to severe Alzheimer's disease. *Ann Neurol* 2008; **64**(S12): S41–2.

51. Porsteinsson AP, Grossberg GT, Mintzer J, Olin JT, for the Memantine MEM-MD-12 Study Group. Memantine treatment in patients with mild to moderate Alzheimer's disease already receiving a cholinesterase inhibitor: a randomized, double-blind, placebo-controlled trial. *Curr Alzheimer Res* 2008; **5**: 83–9.

52. Department of Health, Care Services Improvement Partnership. *Self Directed Support: A Briefing*, 2007. At www.dhcarenetworks.org.uk/_library/Resources/ICN/Self_directed_support_brief_Feb_2007.pdf, accessed 11 Feb 2010.

53. Lister S. Health 'super-regulator' CQC orders 21 hospital trusts to clean up, *The Times* 3 Apr 2009. At www.timesonline.co.uk/tol/life_and_style/health/article6024921.ece, accessed 11 Feb 2009.

54. Vallely S, Evans S, Fear T, Means R. *Opening Doors to Independence: A Longitudinal Study Exploring the Contribution of Extra Care Housing to the Care and Support of Older People*. London: Housing Corporation and Housing 21, 2006.

55. Woolham J. *The Effectiveness of Assistive Technology in Supporting the Independence of People with Dementia: The Safe at Home Project*. London: Hawker, 2005.

56. Smith CW, Wattis JP. Medical students' attitudes to old people and career preferences: the case of Nottingham Medical School. *Med Educ* 1989; **23**: 81–5.

57. Lothian K, Philp I. Maintaining the dignity and autonomy of older people in the healthcare setting. *Br Med J* 2001; **322**: 668–70.

58. Lui NL, Wong CH. Junior doctors' attitudes towards older adults and its correlates in a tertiary-care public hospital. *Ann Acad Med Singapore* 2009; **38**: 125–9.

59. Duthie J, Donaghy M. The beliefs and attitudes of physiotherapy students in Scotland toward older people. *Phys Occup Ther Geriatr* 2009; **27**(3): 245–66.

60. Hughes NJ, Soiza RL, Chua M *et al.* Medical student attitudes toward older people and willingness to consider a career in geriatric medicine. *J Am Geriatr Soc* 2008; **56**(2): 334–8.

61. General Medical Council. *Tomorrow's Doctors*, 2009. At www.gmc-uk.org/education/undergraduate/tomorrows_doctors_2009.asp, accessed 11 Feb 2010.

62. Arie T, Jones R, Smith C. The educational potential of psychogeriatric services. In Arie T (ed.), *Recent Advances in Psychogeriatrics*, vol 1. Edinburgh: Churchill Livingstone, 1985, 197–208.

131

Anaesthetics and Mental State

Andrew Moore Severn[1] and David Gwyn Seymour[2]

[1]*Royal Lancaster Infirmary, Lancaster, UK*
[2]*Medicine for the Elderly, University of Aberdeen, Aberdeen, UK*

INTRODUCTION

Modern surgery and anaesthesia have transformed the lives of millions of older people. However, while the great majority of these will emerge without any long-term cognitive sequelae, absolute guarantees cannot be given. Anaesthesia is a complicated process in which many drugs are administered synchronously in combinations that allow for considerable individual preferences. It is not surprising that unravelling the mental state side effects is a complicated task. The task of assessing which drugs may contribute to a specific change in mental state is also complicated by the physiological response to surgery, and the 'stress', physical and mental, experienced by an elderly patient undergoing elective or emergency surgery.

It is over 50 years since Bedford[1] wrote about 18 elderly patients who had 'never been the same' after surgery and anaesthesia, and concluded that 'operations on elderly people should be confined to unequivocally necessary cases'. While there have been major advances in our understanding of postoperative cognitive dysfunction and the methodology used to investigate it, many questions remain to be answered. Although new drugs and monitoring techniques have supplanted those used in Bedford's day, much of the practice and process of modern general anaesthesia would be recognizable to him. Indeed, the birth of modern anaesthesia was heralded by the introduction of curare, a skeletal muscle relaxant, some 13 years before the Bedford paper.

General anaesthesia requires hypnosis and suppression of motor and autonomic reflexes: until 1942 this was achieved by using a single agent, such as diethyl ether, in high concentrations. Modern anaesthesia, by contrast, involves combinations of agents, in smaller doses, and the use of specific agents to suppress reflex activity, so called 'balanced anaesthesia'. In this way the complications associated with large doses of single agents, such as cardiovascular depression and prolonged coma, are avoided. There has also been a realization of the potential and social acceptability of local anaesthesia. 'Balanced anaesthesia' in today's anaesthetic practice may include a combination of an epidural infusion of local anaesthetic with opioids to provide segmental reflex suppression and a 'light' general anaesthetic to provide a suitably controlled environment for the theatre team and patient.

Local anaesthesia without the concurrent use of general anaesthesia, whether by peripheral nerve block, or by a more substantial spinal or epidural block (collectively referred to as 'regional anaesthesia') is not the panacea for prevention of mental state changes that some might suppose. While it is true that the great 'unknown' – the reversible coma – of general anaesthesia is avoided, the metabolic consequences of all but the simplest of operations outlast the duration of the block and exert a humoral effect on the brain. Furthermore, an operation performed under regional anaesthetic may be conducted under sedation, which in itself may have consequences for postoperative mental state changes.

Admission to hospital for major surgery can be considered a 'major life event', accompanied as such events are by anxiety and other changes in mental health status. The factors that contribute to delirium in older patients in hospital are well known[2] but acute surgical wards rarely provide the environment in which these factors can be managed. For example, devices such as urinary catheters and bed restraints, known to be factors that exacerbate delirium, are used as part of routine surgical practice on many wards, arguably as much for the convenience of hospital staff as for the individual benefit to patients.

In an attempt to bring some structure to the complexity of the subject, it will be considered under the following headings:

- The state of current knowledge of the clinical syndromes of delirium and postoperative cognitive dysfunction
- Mechanisms of anaesthesia and possible interactions with neural pathways involved in higher cortical functions.

In regard to the second heading, mention will also be made of the hypothesis that, in conditions of limited 'cerebral reserve', anaesthetic agents might act on the fragile brains of older patients to accelerate or unmask latent changes of dementia.

DELIRIUM

Classic descriptions of the mental changes that can follow general anaesthesia describe 'emergence delirium' (on immediate awakening from anaesthesia) and 'interval delirium' (occurring in the first few postoperative days). Modern anaesthesia, with its attention to matters such as intensive supervision and pain control by specialist staff in the immediate postoperative period, has almost entirely consigned emergence delirium to history in the case of adults, although publications continue to appear in the field of paediatric anaesthesia. It

Principles and Practice of Geriatric Psychiatry, 3rd edn. Edited by Mohammed T. Abou-Saleh, Cornelius Katona and Anand Kumar

Table 131.1 Risk factors for delirium in a group of patients aged 50 and over undergoing non-cardiac surgery

Age over 70
Alcohol abuse
Poor cognitive status
Poor functional status
Serum electrolyte/glucose disturbances
Thoracic surgery
Aneurysm surgery

Source: Marcantonio *et al.*[5]

Table 131.2 The European Test Battery used in the ISPOCD studies (see text and Table 131.3 for details)

Verbal learning test
Concept shifting test
Stroop colour word interference test
Letter boxes test
Broadbent Cognitive Failure Questionnaire
Zung Depression Score Questionnaire

(The Geriatric Depression Scale is used in ISPOCD2 studies)

is of note that sub-anaesthetic doses of barbiturates have historically had a role in the psychotherapeutic modality known as abreaction.

Emergence delirium aside, postoperative delirium remains a problem. The causes of postoperative delirium, as in delirium in other settings, include acute illness, drugs and drug withdrawal[2-5]. Estimates of the incidence of postoperative delirium in the over-65s range between 7% and 50%, depending on the definitions used and the clinical circumstances[2-5]. The incidence tends to rise with age, the urgency of surgery, the use of sedative and anticholinergic drugs and the degree of preoperative cognitive impairment. Factors (such as sepsis) that favour the development of delirium in a non-surgical situation may also be of relevance postoperatively. Inouye and coworkers have made a major contribution to our understanding of delirium in both medical and surgical situations, by introducing the concept of an interplay between one or more *predisposing* factors (such as age, dementia, co-morbidity and multisensory impairment) and one or more *precipitating* factors (such as acute sepsis, hypoxia, metabolic derangement, or sedating or anticholinergic drugs)[6]. Thus patients who are highly vulnerable because of significant predisposing factors such as dementia or physical frailty might need only a minor precipitating factor to develop delirium, whereas a more robust patient with few or no predisposing factors would require a more major precipitant. O'Keeffe and Chonchubhair[4] concluded that, in at least 90% of cases of delirium following general surgery, it is postoperative medical or surgical complications that are to blame, which implies that the appearance of delirium should lead to a diligent search for underlying physical medical problems. The increased incidence of postoperative delirium with age is likely to be due to age-associated predisposing and precipitating factors rather than direct pharmacological effects arising from age-related differences in the actions of anaesthetic agents[7].

Recent advances in the study of postoperative delirium have included attempts to standardize definitions[4] and a large study in the USA by Marcantonio *et al.*[5], which aimed to develop a clinical prediction rule based on the outcome of 1 341 patients aged 50 and over having major non-cardiac surgery. The latter authors found seven preoperative factors (see Table 131.1) that had an independent relationship with postoperative delirium. When the anaesthetic records of patients who had become delirious were compared with those of patients who had not, certain drugs, notably pethidine and long-acting benzodiazepines, appeared to confer an increased risk of delirium[7].

POSTOPERATIVE COGNITIVE DYSFUNCTION

The widest interpretation of a 'changed mental state' following surgery and/or anaesthesia could embrace many conditions, ranging from mild subjective alterations in concentration or mood at one extreme to major psychosis or coma at the other. For purposes of detailed study, it is helpful to consider a much narrower definition of postoperative cognitive dysfunction (POCD). Indeed, such has been the influence of the work of Moller, Cluitmans, Rasmussen and other colleagues in the International Study of Postoperative Cognitive Dysfunction (ISPOCD) Group[8] that their definition has monopolized the use of the term POCD. A key feature of ISPOCD studies has been the use of the European psychometric test battery (EUPT battery; see Table 131.2), which has been designed as a sensitive and standardized research tool for the detection of postoperative neuropsychological deficits and which can be administered over a 45-minute period. The definition of POCD has been reached by comparing changes in the normalized (Z) scores of individual patients with age-matched controls who were not undergoing surgery, who were studied at the same time intervals[8,9]. Such an approach has allowed sound epidemiological evidence to be gathered and hypothetical risk factors to be investigated and it has also given us useful information about the time course of mental state changes. However, studies to date have told us little about the precise mechanisms of cognitive decline or the determinants of severity in individual cases, and have largely been confined to those with normal cognitive function prior to surgery.

The first ISPOCD study (ISCPOD1) collected data between 1994 and 1996 on 1 218 patients aged 60+ who were undergoing major non-cardiac surgery in 13 hospitals in 8 European countries and the USA[8]. This was a major undertaking, which was intended to answer many of the questions about early and late postoperative cognitive dysfunction in older people that had been raised in the literature over the previous 30 years. As summarized in Table 131.3 and described below, this landmark study has spawned a series of important follow-up studies using the same methodology.

ISPOCD1[8] was particularly concerned to test the hypothesis that hypoxaemia and/or hypotension were causative factors in POCD. Accordingly, oxygen saturation was measured by continuous pulse oximetry before surgery, throughout the day of surgery, and for the next three nights. Similarly, blood pressure was recorded by oscillometry during the operation and every 30 min for the rest of the operative day and night. Patients received general anaesthesia but no restriction was placed on the type of anaesthetic or surgical technique, which conformed to local practice in the study centres. In order to avoid the cerebral vasoconstrictor effects of hypocapnia, normocapnia (as assessed by extrapolation from analysis of the end-tidal CO_2 concentration of the exhaled gas mixture) was a requirement.

Analysis of the data from ISPOCD1 showed that 25.8% of patients had POCD seven days after surgery and that 9.9% of all patients still had evidence of POCD on the repeat neuropsychological tests carried out at three months (corresponding values for controls were 3.4% and

Table 131.3 Studies that have used methods developed by the ISPOCD group to define post-operative cognitive dysfunction following non-cardiac surgery. All studies used pre- and postoperative cognitive testing with a standard test battery (see text and Table 131.2). Standardized (Z) scores were constructed and POCD was defined as described in the text and reference[9]. Most studies also included measures of depression, self-assessed cognitive function and activities of daily living. All patients underwent major surgery, except for those in Canet et al.[10]. Postoperative cognitive testing was carried out at approximately 1 week and 3 months in all studies, but Abildstrom et al.[11] also followed a subset of the ISPOCD1 patients for 1 to 2 years. Exclusions (see ISPOCD1) include a Mini-Mental State test of 23 or less, certain medications, and a number of medical conditions

Reference	Age; no. of subjects; other details of study	Cognitive findings in subjects (S) and controls (C) (95% confidence intervals in brackets)		Other comments and conclusions
		At 1 week or hospital discharge	At 3 months, unless specified	
ISPOCD1 (Moller et al.[8])	Age 60+ N = 1218 Controls: age-matched non-operated UK volunteers (N = 176)	S: 25.8% (23.1–28.5) C: 3.4% (1.3–7.8) $P < 0.0001$	S: 9.9% (8.1–12.0) C: 2.8% (0.9–6.5) $P = 0.0037$	The only major risk factor for POCD at 3 months was age. At 3 months, 39 out of 532 patients (7%) aged 60–69 and 52 out of 378 patients (14%) aged 70 and over had POCD; hypoxia, hypotension and depression were *not* correlated with POCD at 1 week or at 3 months
Abildstrom et al.[11]	Age 60–86 N = 376 (47 controls) 1–2 year follow-up of subset from ISPOCD1		**NB: 1–2 year follow-up** S: 10.4% (7.2–13.7) C: 10.6% (1.8–19.4) P = not significant	Differences in POCD between subjects and controls could not be demonstrated after 1–2 years (but note wide confidence intervals due to small numbers of controls)
Johnson et al.[12]	Age 40–60 (i.e. middle-aged) N = 508 (183 controls)	S: 19.2% (15.7–23.1) C: 4.0% (1.6–8.0) $P = 0.001$	S: 6.2% (4.1–8.9) C: 4.1% (1.7–8.4) $P = 0.33$	While one in five middle-aged patients had evidence of POCD at week 1, by 3 months their rate of POCD was not significantly different from that of non-operated controls. Note that 29% of patients at 3 months reported *subjective* symptoms of impaired cognitive function but this was associated with markers of depression rather than with the objective criteria for POCD
Rasmussen et al.[13]	Age 61–87 N = 128 randomized to GA or RA	GA: 19.7% (14.3–26.1) RA: 12.5% (8.0–18.3) $P = 0.06$	GA: 14.3% (9.5–20.4) RA: 13.9% (9.0–20.2) $P = 0.93$	Results for GA vs. RA were reported on an 'intention to treat' basis, but 10–15% of subjects did not receive the allocated method of anaesthesia. A *per protocol* analysis showed no difference at 3 months, but at 1 week $P = 0.04$
Canet et al.[10]	Age 61–80 N = 372 *Minor* surgery cases only	S: 6.8% (4.3–10.1) (cf. 25.8% for major surgery and 3.4% for controls in ISPOCD1) P = N.S. between S and C	S: 6.6% (4.1–10.0) (cf. 9.9% for major surgery and 2.8% for controls in ISPOCD1) P = N.S. between S and C	On logistic regression, age over 70 and inpatient (vs. outpatient) treatment were predictive of POCD at 1 week but not at 3 months

Table 131.3 (*continued*)

Reference	Age; no. of subjects; other details of study	Cognitive findings in subjects (S) and controls (C) (95% confidence intervals in brackets)		Other comments and conclusions
		At 1 week or hospital discharge	At 3 months, unless specified	
Monk *et al.*[14]	Three age groups: 'young', 18 – 39 $N = 331$ (64 controls) 'middle-aged', 40–59 $N = 378$ (62 controls) 'elderly', 60+ $N = 355$ (56 controls)	Age 18–39: S: 36.6% (31.3–41.8) C: 4.1% (0.9–11.5) Age 40–59: S: 30.4% (25.7–37.1) C: 2.8% (0.3–9.6) Age 60+: S: 41.4% (36.2–46.7) C: 5.1% (1.1–11.2) *Statistical tests* $P = 0.01$ for elderly S vs. middle-aged S $P < 0.001$ for S vs. C, in all three age groups	Age 18–39: S: 5.7% (3.0–8.5) C: 6.3% (1.7–15.2) Age 40–59: S: 5.6% (3.2–8.1) C: 4.8% (1.0–13.5) Age 60+: S: 12.7% (8.9–16.4) C: 1.8% (0.0–9.6) *Statistical tests* $P = 0.001$ for elderly S vs. other two groups $P < 0.001$ for S vs. C, in elderly group only	Independent risk factors for POCD at 3 months were age, lower educational level, a history of previous cerebral vascular accident with no residual impairment, and POCD at 1 week. Deaths within a year of surgery: patients who had POCD at both 1 week and 3 months were more likely to die in the first year after surgery ($P = 0.02$)

GA, general anaesthesia; RA, regional anaesthesia; N.S., not significant.
Source: Modified with permission from Seymour DG and Severn A[15]. Copyright (2009) The British Geriatrics Society.

2.8%). Contrary to expectations, no relationship was found between perioperative hypoxaemia and/or hypotension and the development of 'early' (one week after surgery) or 'late' (three months after surgery) POCD. Indeed, despite analyses of the effects of more than 25 other clinical parameters, only age showed a statistically significant correlation with late POCD. Age was also positively correlated with early POCD, as were duration of anaesthesia, a lesser level of education, a second operation, postoperative infections and respiratory complications. The overall conclusion of the ISPOCD1 investigators was that their study had demonstrated a measurable degree of postoperative cognitive change in a minority of older patients three months after surgery (in about 10% of patients vs. about 3% of non-operated controls) and that the risk increased with age. However, the expected relationship between hypoxaemia and/or hypotension and POCD did not emerge. It was also disappointing that, despite a large number of statistical analyses, the study failed to find any specific risk factors for late POCD that were amenable to therapeutic or preventive intervention. In addition, the hope that the study would give better insight into the pathophysiology of POCD was not fulfilled.

Several well-designed 'ISPOCD2' studies using the basic ISPOCD1 design (Table 131.3) have also failed to identify the major factors contributing to POCD. For example, Rasmussen and colleagues[13] were unable to demonstrate any long-term cognitive benefit of regional anaesthesia over general anaesthesia for major surgery, thus apparently exonerating the drugs and processes of general anaesthesia in the development of the syndrome. As to whether there are any markers of brain damage that might correlate with the appearance of POCD, the answer is inconclusive: markers such as neuron specific enolase (NSE) and S-100 protein fail to correlate with severity of the syndrome. However, for cardiac surgery, different pathological mechanisms may apply as the brain is subjected to a different sort of insult from the process of cardiopulmonary bypass. Rasmussen *et al.*[16] noted that for a cohort

of patients undergoing cardiac surgery the incidence of POCD at 1 week and 23 months was 38.7% and 13.8%, respectively, but found that some 10% of the original sample were so confused that they could not be tested at 1 week, and a further 15% dropped out of subsequent testing. Rises in plasma concentrations of NSE correlated with the syndrome of POCD. Significantly, the largest single rise in the series was noted in one of the patients who was too confused to be tested at 7 days.

A major practical disadvantage of the ISPOCD methodology is that it requires a baseline preoperative assessment, which limits its application to elective surgical procedures. However, the advantage of the approach over earlier studies that simply looked at postoperative cognitive status is that it is not open to the suggestion that some or all of the cognitive impairment observed postoperatively had been present but unobserved preoperatively. For reasons of space, Table 131.3 is limited to studies that have used the ISPOCD technique, but a list of influential 'pre-ISPOCD' studies was given in the previous edition of the present textbook[17].

By design, the ISPOCD studies to date have excluded patients with preoperative Mini-Mental State Examination (MMSE) scores of 23 or less. This was a pragmatic decision because such patients were thought likely to have difficultly in completing the preoperative cognitive test battery. However, this means that a systematic study using ISPOCD techniques in patients who were cognitively impaired prior to surgery has not been carried out, even though theoretical considerations and the clinical experience of anaesthetists and others would suggest that it is this group of patients who are likely to have the highest incidence of short- and long-term POCD[2]. Silverstein *et al.*[18] reanalysed some of the earlier ISPOCD data by dividing patients into a lower (1.5 SD below controls on the ISPOCD battery) and a higher cognitive group but, as stated above, all patients had MMSEs of 24 or more. They found no evidence that those in the lower cognitive group preoperatively had an increased incidence of POCD.

While it is good clinical practice for a simple cognitive test to be recorded in all older people prior to surgery, tests such as the MMSE are blunt instruments that may miss minor degrees of cognitive impairment. The question then has to be asked whether the detection of an unexplained POCD represents a new disease or an unmasking of a previously latent problem. We do not have accurate data about the incidence of long-term cognitive decline in patients who already have a degree of preoperative impairment. If the ISPOCD battery is too complicated a tool to assess such patients then perhaps a simplified battery needs to be employed. However, there would be additional problems of gaining informed consent for studies that set out to study the effects of surgery and anaesthesia in patients with a degree of preoperative dementia. At the other end of the spectrum, some individuals who *subjectively* report impaired concentration after surgery may not be classified as having POCD by the standard ISPOCD method, which might indicate that it is insufficiently sensitive in some situations.

It is not easy to summarize the evidence from Table 131.3 and other literature into a form that can give guidance to individual older people who fear subtle changes in postoperative cognitive function. In a recent Commentary[15] we have attempted to stimulate discussion on this topic with a fictitious scenario of a cognitively well-preserved patient of 75 who is considering whether or not to undergo elective hip surgery for osteoarthritis. We drew three broad conclusions from the data contained in the studies in Table 131.3:

1. If we accept the ISPOCD criteria, POCD one week after major non-cardiac surgery carried out under general anaesthesia is surprisingly common in all age groups. While the incidence in the over-60s was estimated at 19.7–41.4% compared with 3–5% in controls[8,13,14], similar incidences were reported in the 40–60 age group[12,14], and even in those aged 18–39[14].
2. Unlike the situation for POCD at one week, the incidence of POCD at three months appears to be positively associated with advanced age. Thus, in the under-60s, the incidence of POCD three months after surgery was around 5% in both patients and controls[12,14]. However, in the over-60s, POCD incidence at three months was 9.9–14.3%[8,13,14], which was significantly higher than the 1.8–2.8% rates found in controls. Very elderly patients are under-represented in the ISPOCD studies, but in ISPOCD1 those aged 70–79 had twice the rate of POCD of those aged 60–69 (14% vs. 7%)[8].
3. Our ability to draw firm conclusions about POCD beyond three months is limited by lack of long-term follow-up data. However, using a subset of ISPOCD1, Abildstrom et al.[11] reported that 10.4% of the over-60s fulfilled the criteria for POCD 1–2 years after surgery. While this was the same as the rate found in non-operated controls (10.6%), only 47 of the latter were available, so confidence intervals were wide. The link between POCD and death has also been mentioned by two studies. Monk et al.[14] reported an association between POCD at three months and mortality at one year. Steinmetz et al.[19] followed up a cohort of ISPOCD patients for a median of 8.5 years and linked the presence of POCD at three months with increased rates of mortality: the hazard ratio (adjusted for age, gender and cancer) was 1.63 ($p < 0.01$). Visual inspection of the survival curves[19] suggests that the main difference between the mortality rates in the two groups occurred between two and four years after surgery and anaesthesia.

The above three conclusions come with the caveat that some patients who report *subjective* cognitive impairment three months after surgery are classified as normal under the standardized POCD definition used in the above studies. A possible explanation is that some of these patients are depressed rather than cognitively impaired[12], but there is also the possibility that subtle cognitive effects are being missed by the ISPOCD psychometric battery. For example, Hanning[20] cited a case of a patient who needed to take early retirement despite being classified as 'normal' on ISPOCD criteria. It should also be noted that the extent of individual disability and distress caused by different levels of POCD has so far attracted little research attention, although Price et al.[21] have recently explored the effects of impaired memory and/or executive function on activities of daily living. One of the most interesting conclusions from the ISPOCD work relates to the difference between outpatient (day stay) and inpatient minor surgery and appears to support the practice of day stay surgery in the over-70s as a way of reducing POCD at one week[10].

MECHANISMS OF ANAESTHESIA AND POSSIBLE INTERACTIONS WITH NEURAL PATHWAYS INVOLVED IN HIGHER CORTICAL FUNCTIONS

Xie et al.[22] and Inouye[2] have explored the hypothesis that the same mechanisms might cause postoperative delirium and dementia and that anaesthetic agents might sometimes be involved in such mechanisms. The popular scientific press has reported this hypothesis under the alarming headline 'Alzheimer's alert over anaesthetics'[23], although Xie et al. have been quick to point out that sweeping clinical conclusions should not been drawn from 'test tube' studies[24]. Indeed, in their refutation of the more extreme extrapolations, Xie and colleagues have stated, 'The available epidemiological evidence shows no association between Alzheimer's disease and previous surgery requiring anaesthesia. If elderly patients put off necessary surgery for fear that the anaesthetic will harm them, they may place themselves at higher risk of disease or death than any small cognitive effect caused by surgery and anaesthesia'.

The tenets of the hypothetical arguments of Inouye and Xie et al.[2,22] are:

1. There may be common mechanisms underlying delirium (a common postoperative complication) and dementia, as they share several pathophysiological features such as decreased cerebral metabolism, cholinergic deficiency and inflammation. However, a causal relationship has yet to be proved.
2. The two characteristic histological features of Alzheimer's disease are plaques (containing amyloid) and neurofibrillary tangles (containing tau protein). Certain anaesthetic agents can trigger changes of oligomerization of beta-amyloid protein (Abeta) and apoptosis in animal models and cell culture[25]. The halogenated ether isoflurane can induce apoptosis in cell culture, a process which can be inhibited by Congo Red, an agent which is known to inhibit Abeta production[22]. Halothane, a halogenated hydrocarbon has been shown to increase the oligomerization of Abeta amyloid peptide *in vitro*[26].
3. Cholinergic mechanisms are known to play a part in delirium and dementia. It is of considerable interest, though not surprising given the importance of the cholinergic system in maintaining consciousness, that the cholinergic system is a site of binding of

anaesthetic drugs. Thus, Fodale et al.[27] describe nicotinic receptor binding and inhibition by the three volatile inhalational agents in current use in the developed world (isoflurane, sevoflurane and desflurane), and muscarinic blockade by intravenous barbiturates. A discussion of the role of the cholinergic system in the pathophysiology of dementing diseases is outside the scope of this chapter. However, as the types of receptors that mediate anaesthesia appear very similar to the types of receptors that decline in patients with Alzheimer's disease, then it is conceivable that anaesthesia might worsen or hasten the dementing process or unmask latent dementia. In finishing this discussion it is worth noting that acetyl-cholinesterase inhibitors, administered to patients without dementia, do not reduce the incidence of delirium after elective hip replacement[28].

The review by Culley et al.[25] summarized the field up to 2007 and included more laboratory evidence that anaesthetics could alter the metabolism of amyloid protein. It also mentioned the theoretical possibility that tau proteins, contained in the neurofibrillary tangles of the brains of people with Alzheimer's disease, might also be affected. Two recent papers have indeed reported the effects of anaesthesia on tau proteins in animal experiments[29,30] although the study of Planel et al.[29] in mice described the process as being associated with a severe hypothermia occurring under anaesthesia, rather than being specific to any particular anaesthetic (and was avoidable with proper attention to temperature control). The degree of hypothermia observed by Planel et al.[29] was far more than the hypothermia occurring in ordinary anaesthetic practice, with the notable exception of cardiopulmonary bypass. This is of interest as cardiac surgery tends to have higher rates of cognitive impairment than non-cardiac surgery. While this difference has usually been attributed entirely to the direct physical effects of the cardiopulmonary bypass apparatus, the cognitive effects of hypothermia should perhaps be considered as a possible confounder in future studies, with particular attention to the effect of the process on tau production.

As far as patients, relatives and health care personnel are concerned, the major unanswered question is whether the various phenomena discussed in the previous three paragraphs are of clinical relevance. Do certain anaesthetic agents have the potential of triggering the process that leads to the evolution of a degenerative brain disease?

When one considers the history of the development of anaesthetic drugs, the possibility of an uncommon but potentially serious side effect involving long-term cognitive function cannot be dismissed out of hand. The number of potential anaesthetic drugs is enormous – there are huge numbers of variants and isomers of organic compounds such as ethers and alkanes. Volatile inhalational anaesthetics evolved from 1846 by a matter of trial and error with the emphasis, naturally, being on their immediate anaesthetic properties and the lack of any short-term side effects. While many compounds were rejected early on for reasons of toxicity, more subtle toxic effects continued to bedevil clinical experience with these drugs for years after their introduction. Today's volatile inhalational anaesthetic agents, the halogenated ethers sevoflurane, desflurane and isoflurane, derive historically from the original discovery of the anaesthetic properties of diethyl ether. Another class, obsolete in the developed world, comprises the halogenated hydrocarbons. Halothane was the most prominent example of this class, and it was a major advance when introduced in 1950, because of its inert properties, but the association with an idiosyncratic reaction leading to

hepatotoxicity led to its obsolescence. An early halogenated ether, enflurane, became obsolete because of fluoride-induced nephrotoxicity.

Conventional classic models of the mechanism of action of general anaesthetics considered that all the inhalational agents worked in a similar way by a purely physical mechanism, the potency of agents correlating with the physical property known as the oil/water partition coefficient. Techniques such as magnetic resonance spectroscopy demonstrated that lipid-soluble molecules with anaesthetic properties interpose themselves into the cell membrane, increasing fluidity of the membrane and interfering with ion channel function. Given the clear correlation between potency and lipid solubility, the key strategy in pharmaceutical development has been finding a molecule whose effects, in terms of rapid changes of anaesthetic depth, could be most easily manipulated by the anaesthetist. For this purpose the physical property of blood/gas solubility coefficient has consistently been shown to be *the* property determining clinical usefulness. Modern anaesthesia is more predictable and safer because of this development, and older patients have benefited at least as much as the young in this respect. Patients regain consciousness and regain protective reflexes within minutes and can go home within hours. As a consequence they are spared prolonged hypoxia, hypotension and hostile ward environments – factors that we know predispose to delirium. Physical models also give the impression that changes induced by the addition of an agent, in this case an anaesthetic agent, are completely reversible. But the classic physical models of action fail to explain the significant pharmacodynamic differences between volatile agents. To explain these, mechanisms such as differential ion channel blockade are useful. For example, for a given depth of anaesthesia, isoflurane causes more vasodilatation than halothane, and this is an important clinical difference. It is against this background of action – specific ion channel or receptor blockade – that theories on the comparative neurotoxicity of general anaesthetics are being tested.

The link between the *in vitro* studies mentioned above, the theory of interference with the cholinergic system, and the possibility of a dementing process being triggered by a single exposure to anaesthesia in clinically relevant concentrations, is of course tenuous. The Food and Drug Administration (FDA) in the US has judged that it is inappropriate at the present time to make any recommendations about specific anaesthetic agents[25] but this remains a very emotive area, as any search of the internet using the keywords 'anesthesia' (or anaesthesia) and 'dementia' will testify. Suffice for the moment to notice that there is fundamental clinical and laboratory work still to be done, and that this is an area where collaboration between anaesthetists and mental health specialists should be particularly rewarding.

REFERENCES

1. Bedford PD. Adverse cerebral effects of anaesthesia on old people. *Lancet* 1955; **269**(6884): 259–63.
2. Inouye S. Delirium in older persons. *N Engl J Med* 2006; **354**: 1157–65.
3. Lipowski ZJ. *Delirium: Acute Confusional States*. New York: Oxford University Press, 1990.
4. O'Keeffe ST, Chonchubhair AN. Postoperative delirium in the elderly. *Br J Anaesth* 1994; **73**: 673–87.
5. Marcantonio ER, Goldman L, Mangione CM *et al.* A clinical prediction rule for delirium after elective noncardiac surgery. *JAMA* 1994; **271**: 134–9.

6. Inouye SK, Charpentier PA. Precipitating factors for delirium in hospitalized elderly persons, predictive model and interrelationship with baseline vulnerability. *JAMA* 1996; **275**: 852–7.

7. Marcantonio ER, Juarez G, Goldman L *et al.* The relationship of postoperative delirium with psychoactive medications. *JAMA* 1994; **272**: 1518–22.

8. Moller JT, Cluitmans P, Rasmussen LS *et al.* Long-term postoperative cognitive dysfunction in the elderly ISPOCD1 study. ISPOCD investigators. International Study of Post-Operative Cognitive Dysfunction. *Lancet* 1998; **351**(9106): 857–61. Plus erratum in *Lancet* 1998, **351**(9117): 1742.

9. Rasmussen LS, Larsen K, Houx P *et al.* The assessment of postoperative cognitive function. *Acta Anaesthesiol Scand* 2001; **45**(3): 275–89.

10. Canet J, Raeder J, Rasmussen LS *et al.* Cognitive dysfunction after minor surgery in the elderly. *Acta Anaesthesiol Scand* 2003; **47**: 1204–10.

11. Abildstrom H, Rasmussen LS, Rentowl P *et al.* Cognitive dysfunction 1–2 years after non-cardiac surgery in the elderly. *Acta Anaesthesiol Scand* 2000; **44**: 1246–51.

12. Johnson T, Monk T, Rasmussen LS *et al.* Postoperative cognitive dysfunction in middle-aged patients. *Anesthesiology* 2002; **96**: 1351–7.

13. Rasmussen LS, Johnson T, Kuipers HM *et al.* Does anaesthesia cause postoperative cognitive dysfunction? A randomised study of regional versus general anaesthesia in 438 elderly patients. *Acta Anaesthesiol Scand* 2003; **47**: 260–66.

14. Monk TG, Weldon BC, Garvan CW *et al.* Predictors of cognitive dysfunction after major noncardiac surgery. *Anesthesiology* 2008; **108**: 18–30.

15. Seymour DG, Severn AM. Cognitive dysfunction after surgery and anaesthesia, what can we tell the grandparents? *Age Ageing* 2009; **38**: 147–50.

16. Rasmussen LS, Christiansen M, Hansen PB, Moller JT. Do blood levels of neuron specific enolase and S-100 protein reflect cognitive dysfunction after coronary artery bypass? *Acta Anaesthesiol Scand* 1999; **43**: 495–500.

17. Seymour DG. Anaesthetics and mental state. In Copeland JRM, Abou-Saleh MT, Blazer DG (eds), *Principles and Practice of Geriatric Psychiatry*, 2nd edn. Chichester: John Wiley & Sons, 2002, 743–8.

18. Silverstein JH, Steinmetz J, Reicenberg A, Harvey PD, Rasmussen LS. Postoperative cognitive dysfunction in patients with preoperative cognitive impairment, which domains are most vulnerable? *Anesthesiology* 2007; **106**: 431–5.

19. Steimetz J, Christensen KB, Lund T *et al.* Long-term consequences of postoperative cognitive dysfunction. *Anesthesiology* 2009; **110**: 548–55.

20. Hanning CD. Postoperative cognitive dysfunction. *Br J Anaesth* 2005; **95**: 82–7.

21. Price CC, Garvan CW, Monk TG. Type and severity of cognitive decline in older adults after noncardiac surgery. *Anesthesiology* 2008; **108**: 8–17.

22. Xie Z, Dong Y, Maeda U *et al.* Isoflurane-induced apoptosis, a potential pathogenic link between delirium and dementia. *J Gerontology* 2006; **61A**: 1300–1306.

23. Philips H. Alzheimer's alert over anaesthetics. *New Sci* 2007; **192**(2575): 12.

24. Crosby G, Culley D, Xie Z, Eckenhoff R. Fear of anaesthesia. *New Sci* 2008; **193**(2594): 22.

25. Culley DJ, Xie Z, Crosby G. General anesthetic-induced neurotoxicity, an emerging problem for the young and old? *Curr Opin Anaesthesiol* 2007; **20**: 408–13.

26. Mandal PK, Pettegrew JW, McKeag DW, Mandal R. Alzheimer's disease, halothane induces Abeta peptide to oligomeric form – solution NMR Studies. *Neurochem Res* 2006; **31**: 883–90.

27. Fodale V, Quattrone D, Trecroci C, Caminiti V, Santamaria LB. Alzheimer's disease and anaesthesia: implications for the central cholinergic system. *Br J Anaesth* 2006; **97**: 445–52.

28. Sampson EL, Raven PR, Ndhlovu PN *et al.* A randomised, double-blind, placebo-controlled trial of donezepil (Aricept) for reducing the incidence of postoperative delirium after elective total hip replacement. *Int J Geriatr Psychiatry* 2007; **22**(4): 343–9.

29. Planel E, Richter KEG, Nolan CE *et al.* Anesthesia leads to tau hyperphosphorylation through inhibition of phosphatase activity by hypothermia. *J Neurosci* 2007; **27**: 3090–97.

30. Run X, Liang Z, Zhang L *et al.* Anesthesia induces phosphorylation of tau. *J Alzheimers Dis* 2009; **16**: 619–26.

132

Nutritional State

David N. Anderson[1] and Mohammed T. Abou-Saleh[2]

[1]*Mossley Hill Hospital, Liverpool, UK*
[2]*Division of Mental Health, St George's University of London, London, UK*

Dietary surveys of elderly people in several countries over the past three decades have shown that a substantial proportion of subjects had intake below recommended standards. Two US National Health and Nutrition surveys showed that 50% of the populations, especially the elderly, were deficient in one or more nutrients. In 1979, a Department of Health and Social Security survey in the UK suggested that 7% of those aged 65 years or more may be undernourished and twice this proportion of those aged 80 years or greater[1]. In Sidney, Australia deficiency in the intake of nutrients by older people was similar to that found in the UK at that time[2].

There is little evidence that the situation has improved. The National Dietary and Nutrition Survey in the UK has reported since 1992 and, while most older people seem to receive adequate nutritional intake, the most recent survey has drawn attention to greater risk in particular groups of older people, including those who have lost their own teeth, those in institutions, the older age groups and those with low socioeconomic status[3]. A study of people aged 65 years or greater, using a validated malnutrition screening tool, identified more than 10% at medium or high risk of malnutrition[4-7]. Single nutrient deficiency is much more common than malnutrition, and in people in this age group, 29% of those who were independent and 35% of those in institutions were found to be folate deficient and 14% and 40%, respectively, deficient in vitamin C[3].

Of great concern is clear and consistent evidence that the highest rates of malnutrition reported in developed countries are those older people in hospital or care homes. In these populations malnutrition has been reported in 10–60% depending on age and medical conditions[4-7]. These populations will have high proportions of people with physical and mental illness. Inevitably, malnutrition is a common cause and consequence of illness but the number of undernourished people leaving National Health Service hospitals in England rose by almost 85% in the 10 years up to 2006, reaching almost 140 000 in 2006–7[8]; and 70–80% of malnourished people enter and leave hospital without a diagnosis or treatment[9,10].

Those older people at most risk include the housebound, those with cognitive impairment, a history of depression or long-term conditions, and the oldest old. Poor dentition, swallowing difficulties and not having regular cooked meals are further factors placing people at risk of malnutrition (Table 132.1).

The prevalence of malnutrition is certainly higher in older people where countries report this data. Poor financial reserves, isolation, physical handicap, dental problems and mental disorder all contribute, and the effects of disease, disability and ageing can combine to change a marginally sufficient diet into a grossly deficient one. Higher proportions of older people in these circumstances live in relative poverty and have greater prevalence of disease. The diet of lower socioeconomic groups provides cheap energy and is lower in essential nutrients like calcium, iron, magnesium, folate and other vitamins[11].

Malnutrition is a state in which a deficiency of energy, protein and/or other nutrients causes measurable adverse effects on tissue/body form, composition, function or clinical outcome[6]. It has significant implications for people at risk, causing increased vulnerability to infection by compromising the immune system, delayed wound healing, impairing function of heart and lungs, muscle weakness and depression and, in the extreme, death[12].

It increases rates of medical attendance, admission to hospital, length of hospital admissions and mortality. People with malnutrition have two to three times more complications following surgery[13]. Furthermore, the consequences of malnutrition include depression, apathy, decline of social interaction and confusion, which will conspire to produce a spiralling decline of nutritional status[7]. Malnutrition is a significant predisposing factor for the development of delirium in older people admitted to hospital medical wards[14]. Finally, malnutrition will affect the way the body handles prescribed medications.

Despite this information 30–40% of malnourished people do not receive care according to present scientific evidence and 20–25% receive care that is not needed or is potentially harmful[15]. Though single nutritional deficiencies are more common than malnutrition they commonly co-exist[7].

But the most common nutritional problem in developed countries is obesity. This has direct relevance to mental health as it contributes significantly to vascular risk and the metabolic syndrome. It is now clear that vascular risk is not only important for the development of vascular brain disease, which may manifest as dementia, depression or psychosis in later life, but also as a risk factor for the development of Alzheimer's disease. Obesity can impair independent function and ambulation, add to the burden on arthritic joints or impaired cardiopulmonary function and exacerbate other long-term conditions, creating a situation where older people can then become depressed.

While ageing is usually accompanied by weight loss, some older people will become vulnerable to weight gain if their lives become more sedentary and their diet unbalanced. Of course, obesity may also be associated with single deficiencies and people who are obese can

Principles and Practice of Geriatric Psychiatry, 3rd edn. Edited by Mohammed T. Abou-Saleh, Cornelius Katona and Anand Kumar

Table 132.1 People at most risk of poor nutrition

Circumstances
* Increasing age
* Low socioeconomic status
* Care homes
* Hospitals
* Housebound
* Isolated

Clinical
* Dementia
* Depression
* Alcohol misuse
* Poor dentition
* Dysphagia
* Low body mass index
* Unintentional weight loss
* Poor absorptive capacity
* Increased nutrient loss
* Catabolic states

become malnourished. Drugs used for the treatment of mental illness often carry the risk of weight gain and the metabolic syndrome.

Those most at risk of malnutrition or who may need nutritional support are summarized in Table 132.1.

ASSESSMENT AND DIAGNOSIS

Part of the problem is difficulty diagnosing malnutrition and agreeing diagnostic criteria. The assessment of nutritional state is complex and any single measure seems inadequate. However, anthropometric measurements, including body mass index (BMI), are the foundation but this needs to be done by professionals with expertise who understand the clinical context. Biochemical markers are often unreliable, particularly with people who are ill, as these are affected by acute phase responses. People most at risk of being malnourished are those who are thin or with recent unintentional weight loss, including people who are obese[6,7,16]. Other clinical circumstances will further identify people at risk of becoming malnourished, for example, people with dysphagia or excessive nutrient loss[13].

Routine screening of people on admission to hospital or care homes is now recommended and identification of those likely to need nutritional support based on a combination of BMI, unintentional weight loss and clinical contexts placing people at risk[13]. Screening instruments like the Malnutrition Universal Screening Tool can be useful, easy to use and require little training[6]. Screening is considered cost effective for older people admitted to hospital[13]. While over 95% of malnutrition is in the community (including care homes), most malnutrition-related expenditure occurs in hospitals[17,18].

MENTAL HEALTH

Malnutrition and nutrient deficiencies are more likely to be a consequence rather than a cause of mental illness in older people. Classical single deficiency states as cause of mental illness are rare in developed countries though there is a strong suspicion that suboptimal nutrition often contributes to ill health in old age. The immediate significance of single deficiency states is confined to a few specific circumstances, for example, thiamine deficiency and the Wernicke–Korsakoff syndrome; B12 and folate with cognitive impairment, dementia and depressive states[19]. In most instances, the import of nutritional status on mental function is less direct and more subtle.

Certainly, the consequences of malnutrition will complicate treatment of mental illness and impair prospects for recovery. In addition, effects on physical strength, organ function and the immune system increase the risk of falls, fractures, pressure sores, infection, hospital admission and mortality. These risks will need to be addressed in care plans and will substantially increase the hazards associated with prescribing psychotropic drugs to older people.

Under-nutrition may arise from quantitative and qualitative dietary inadequacy, and a number of problems facing older people and the mentally ill place them at particular risk. Social isolation, loneliness, poor socioeconomic position, physical and sensory disability and co-morbid long-term conditions are common accompaniments of mental health problems in later life. Depression and dementia, in particular, are associated with reduced appetite, weight loss and poor attention to diet resulting from apathy, loss of interest and cognitive difficulties. Furthermore, effects of nutrient deficiency, including apathy, depression and cognitive impairment, will compound an already difficult situation and may lead to a spiral of decline.

PREVENTION

The overwhelming priority in the management of under-nutrition among elderly populations is prevention. A major impetus must ultimately come from changes in public policy that improve the older person's social, material and financial position in society, address inequalities and ensure the efficient provision of services to those in need.

The market-led approach to nutrition that operates in many food-rich countries has been found to increase the disparity between the nutrition and health of the rich and poor[20]. The provision of domiciliary care services is inequitably distributed, often inefficiently organized and frequently determined by demand rather than need[21]. In the UK a younger person with equivalent need to an older person has much greater access to social care and mental health services[22,23].

In the modern era food suppliers are often large impersonal stores sited some distance from communities, making shopping difficult for physically and mentally disabled people. Low income with disability not only restricts ability to afford a protective diet but also limits access to retailers where healthy food can be purchased more cheaply. Local shops in developed countries are less prevalent and can be significantly more expensive than distantly sited supermarkets[24].

Often the presentation and supervision of meals is poor. This is particularly evident in hospitals and care homes. A leading charity for older people in the UK[25] has drawn attention to the problem in hospitals and this report along with other national guidelines recommends a number of changes to practice that could address this need[13,26]. The National Diet and Nutrition Survey in the UK found the food supply in care homes to be sufficient but biochemical measures revealed poor vitamin and mineral status[3]. While the explanation of this is not clear it may be the result of poor intake and absorption due to poor presentation and timing of food, need for more assistance with eating or changes in absorption and the general medical condition.

Simple measures like providing meals in a form that is appealing and easily edible, at a time when appetite is greatest or when people are most motivated, providing assistance and allowing enough time for meals to be eaten are often all that is required yet all too often not part of the regimes of hospitals or care homes. Some people, particularly people with dementia, will take food from family or friends and not care staff or from certain care staff, and these institutions need to provide greater flexibility of approach and ensure that areas catering for older people and people with dementia have sufficient number of staff. The ready availability of fresh produce, particularly fruit and vegetables, is lacking. Modern catering is not always sensitive to the needs and preferences of older people.

Diet is a poor source of vitamin D, which depends on exposure to ultraviolet light for its formation. More exposure to natural sunlight is the most important preventive measure but for those older people at risk of little exposure, calcium and vitamin D supplements are recommended[27].

Easy access to health and dental care is important. People with long-term conditions and poor dentition are at particular risk of dietary deficiency. Dental care is especially overlooked yet a study of hospitalized people aged 61–99 years found 60% to have disease of the oral soft tissue[28]. For those living in the community, preventive dental and health care with early recognition and treatment of illness is needed.

The elderly population may benefit from greater education and advice about healthy and affordable eating, issues normally targeted at younger people. The judicious use of fruit juice, frozen foods and some convenience foods might ease the burden of food preparation in those at risk of neglecting their diet. Occupational therapy assessments can find practical solutions to problems arising from visual impairment, arthritic joints and disability or the need for someone to help with shopping and food preparation. The teaching of culinary skills may be particularly helpful to the older bereaved man who never cooked while his wife was alive.

Diet is connected with lifestyle and opportunity and so moderate alcohol consumption is associated with better health and less risk of developing depression but also with a more active and sociable lifestyle, better self-rated health status[29] and higher intake of various nutrients[30]. Whether these variables are independent is not clear but the evidence would suggest that older people who can remain active, exercise and remain socially connected seem to take a better diet and protect themselves from some of the mental health problems occurring in later life.

In a prospective study of relatively healthy and active European men aged 70–89 years, low cholesterol but not dietary factors was associated with increased risk of developing depression[31]. The relationship of cholesterol levels to mental health in later life remains confusing as, while raised levels might suggest increased vascular risk, high levels may reduce risk of dementia, with declining levels reported before incident dementia[32].

TREATMENT

Recommendations for the treatment of malnutrition and the maintenance of optimal nutrition are available[13]. But assessment and treatment require considerable expertise as there are dangers. If correction is too rapid there is the risk of precipitating re-feeding syndrome or Wernicke–Korsakoff syndrome. The former seems to arise from the body's adaptation to malnourishment when rapid change precipitates micronutrient deficiency and dangerous change in fluid and electrolyte balance. This may lead to cardiac failure, pulmonary oedema, cardiac dysthymia, fluid overload or depletion, low levels of phosphate, potassium and magnesium, and raised glucose. People with alcohol problems, in particular, are at risk of rapid re-feeding, causing increased thiamine demand and the Wernicke–Korsakoff syndrome.

The preferred approach is always to improve dietary intake by natural means. Guidance on the risk benefits and approaches to artificial nutrition are available though studies have rarely involved older people with mental illness[13].

Where single nutrient deficiencies are found it is usually better to replace them though there is little evidence to demonstrate that this has clinically detectable effects on mental health other than in exceptional circumstances. Thiamine replacement in Wernicke's encephalopathy is curative. Thiamine supplementation in people with serious alcohol misuse or undergoing detoxification and correction of B12 and folate deficiency in cognitive impairment or dementia may protect or enhance cognitive function. Because single deficiencies often co-exist with more general under-nutrition or the risk of developing malnutrition they should prompt a more detailed assessment of nutritional status. If it clearly arises as a consequence of mental disorder the imperative is to treat that and address the disability or need underlying dietary neglect.

There are a large number of heterogeneous randomized controlled trials of nutritional supplements of mixed quality and results that, in general, show benefits of producing weight gain with fewer complications and mortality and they are acceptable to patients[13]. Similarly, studies of vitamin and mineral supplements produce conflicting results and, although of uncertain benefit, are thought to be beneficial for older people where there is concern about their food intake[13]. These studies rarely consider the effects on mental state.

In extreme circumstances assisted enteral or parenteral methods, including surgical procedures like percutaneous endoscopic gastrostomy (PEG), are considered to sustain nutrition with clear evidence-based guidelines for their use[13].

DEMENTIA

Particular concerns arise about decisions on feeding for people with dementia. While all general principles apply, dementia raises issues rather different from the rest of mental health due to the combination of people who lack capacity to make decisions and who are also suffering a terminal illness.

There are a number of reasons why people with dementia have difficulty sustaining nutrition. Dietary intake may be reduced due to a natural decline of appetite and hunger, difficulty with the feeding process or food preparation due to cognitive deficits, and problems swallowing.

Furthermore, weight loss is a recognized consequence of dementia, regardless of diet, which may develop before the diagnosis is made. A 32-year prospective study showed increasing difference in BMI between people with and without dementia during the 6-year period before the diagnosis was made[33]. Though the reasons are not entirely clear, a number of possibilities are proposed, not least that this is part of the neurodegenerative process[34].

If people with dementia suddenly lose appetite or weight the possibility of other causes must be considered. New physical illness, pain, oral and dental problems, newly prescribed medication, constipation or impaction, and depression may present this way and can be difficult to recognize in more severe dementia when the person's ability to communicate symptoms is compromised. This situation requires a more detailed examination of physical and mental function followed by appropriate investigation.

Many of the essential approaches to facilitating dietary intake and maintaining nutrition have been covered and the prevailing view, when these begin to fail, is to continue with a conservative, palliative care approach rather than take recourse to more invasive and artificial procedures. In advanced disease there is no good evidence that tube feeding prevents aspiration pneumonia (paradoxically the most common adverse association), malnutrition, pressure ulcers or infection, or improves survival, function or comfort[35]. Similar lack of benefit and adverse consequences has been found with PEG[36].

However, this is a difficult situation because while the evidence for tube feeding or PEG fails to provide convincing evidence of benefit in people with dementia, and does demonstrate significant risks, these studies have been conducted on frail people with advanced disease and there is an absence of evidence for people with earlier disease at risk of nutritional deficiency[37].

All commentators emphasize the need for clarity about the purpose of artificial nutrition in this situation, recognizing that there are occasions when such procedures may be warranted; for example, when the problem is reversible and not a direct result of the dementia[38].

Ultimately, decisions will need to be made on an individual basis, acknowledging the evidence base and considering what is in the best interest of a particular individual should they be unable to express their own wishes or have not made that clear through an advance statement.

CONCLUSION

A great deal more needs to be known about the relationship between diet, nutrition and mental health in older people – not only understanding how nutritional deficiency might exert effects on mental function but also identifying people who may be predisposed to develop mental disorder where modification of diet and lifestyle could afford protection[39]. There is no doubt that lifestyle characteristics affect health; improving diet would be expected to improve general health and, thereby, reduce the risk of certain mental health problems in later life. For example, intake of fruit and vegetables is an independent risk factor for stroke[40], a physical health problem with significant psychiatric morbidity.

At present nutritional deficiencies and malnutrition are far more likely to be a consequence than a direct cause of mental illness though in less developed parts of the world they may have greater relevance to the causation of mental disturbance. What is very clear is that older people, people in isolation with long-term conditions and those who are socioeconomically disadvantaged are at greater risk of malnutrition and these are groups also at greater risk of mental illness.

Despite many countries having national policies on nutrition and there being many guidelines and recommendations from professional bodies, the problem of malnutrition continues to be significant. Public policy will also have to address the serious inequalities that exist for older people in many parts of the world. Training for doctors, nurses and medical students on nutrition will need to improve[8,41–43] and rates of malnutrition are highest in hospitals and care homes, where guidance does not seem to be changing practice. Stronger enforcement of this guidance, including routine screening, is probably necessary[8].

The evidence connecting nutrition and morbidity that impairs function, and increases risk and mortality makes this an essential area of knowledge for all professionals working with older people. There is a good case for a specialist practitioner able to provide nutritional assessment and advice to be available to mental health teams working with older people, and these assessments should now be routine for all people admitted to hospital and care homes. The consequences of malnutrition will have significant impact on the treatment of mental illness, risk and recovery.

Further exploration of the relationship between dietary constituents and the course of mental illness may yet yield significant information relevant to the management of mental illness in later life. The chicken and egg question is difficult to unravel, and large prospective studies that control for a substantial number of variables will be needed to address this intriguing association. What is certainly the case at present is that the fundamental need for a nutritious diet to maintain optimal health is still missing in the lives of many older people and its importance overlooked or ignored by health and social care services.

REFERENCES

1. Department of Health and Social Security. *A Nutrition Survey of the Elderly*. London: HMSO, 1979.
2. Stuckey SJ, Darnton-Hill I, Ash S *et al*. Dietary patterns of elderly people living in Sydney. *Hum Nutr Appl Nutr* 1984; **38A**: 255–64.
3. Finch S, Doyle W, Lowe C *et al*. *National Diet and Nutrition Survey: People Aged 65 Years and Over*, Vol 1: *Report of the Diet and Nutrition Survey*. London. The Stationery Office, 1998.
4. Elia M, Stratton RJ. How much undernutrition is there in hospitals? *Br J Nutr* 2000; **84**: 257–9.
5. Elia M, Stratton RJ. Geographical inequalities in nutrient status and risk of malnutrition among English people aged 65 years and over. *Nutrition* 2005; **21**(11). 1100–106
6. Elia M. *The 'MUST' Report: Nutritional Screening of Adults: a Multidisciplinary Responsibility. Development and Use of the Malnutrition Universal Screening Tool (MUST) for Adults*, a report by the Malnutrition Advisory Group of the British Association for Parenteral and Enteral Nutrition (BAPEN). Redditch: BAPEN, 2003.
7. Stratton RJ, Green CJ, Elia M. *Disease Related Malnutrition: An Evidence Based Approach to Treatment*. Walllingford: CABI, 2003.
8. Lean M, Wiseman M. Malnutrition in hospitals: still common because screening tools are underused and poorly enforced. *Br Med J* 2008; **336**: 290.
9. Kelly IE, Tessier S, Cahill A *et al*. Still hungry in hospital: identifying malnutrition in acute hospital admissions. *Q J Med* 2000; **93**: 93–8.
10. McWhirter JP, Pennington CR. Incidence and recognition of malnutrition in hospital. *Br Med J* 1994; **308**: 945–8.
11. Philip W, James T, Nelson M *et al*. The contribution of nutrition to inequalities in health. *Br Med J* 1997; **314**: 1545–9.
12. Todorovic V, Russell C, Stratton R *et al*. *The MUST Explanatory Booklet: A Guide to the Malnutrition Universal Screening Tool (MUST) for Adults*. Redditch: BAPEN, 2003.
13. National Collaborating Centre for Acute Care. *Nutrition support in Adults: Oral Nutrition Support, Enteral Tube Feeding and Parenteral Nutrition*. London: National Collaborating Centre for Acute Care, 2006.
14. Inouye SK, Viscoli CM, Horwitz RI *et al*. A predictive model for delirium in hospitalized elderly medical patients based on admission characteristics. *Ann Intern Med* 1993; **119**: 474–81.

15. Heyland DK, Dhaliwal R, Drover JW *et al*. Nutrition support in mechanically ventilated, critically ill adult patients: are we ready for evidence based clinical practice? *Nutr Clin Pract* 2004; **19**: 193–200.

16. Stratton RJ, Hackston A, Longmore D *et al*. Malnutrition in hospital outpatients and inpatients: prevalence, concurrent validity and ease of use of the 'malnutrition universal screening tool' (MUST) for adults. *Br J Nutr* 2004; **92**: 799–808.

17. Amand-Battandier F, Malvy D, Jeandel C *et al*. Use of oral supplements in elderly patients living in the community: a pharmoeconomic study. *Clin Nutr* 2004; **23**: 1096–103.

18. Edington J, Barnes R, Bryan F *et al*. A prospective randomized controlled trial of nutrient supplementation in malnourished elderly in the community: clinical and health economic outcomes. *Clin Nutr* 2004; **23**: 195–204.

19. Scott TM, Peter I, Tucker KL *et al*. The Nutrition, Ageing and Memory in Elders (NAME) study: design and methods for a study of micronutrients and cognitive function in a homebound elderly population. *Int J Geriatr Psychiatry* 2006; **21**: 519–28.

20. Milio N. Nutrition and health: patterns and policy perspectives in food rich countries. *Soc Sci Med* 1989; **29**(3): 413–23.

21. Sinclair I, Parker R, Leat D, Williams J. *The Kaleidoscope of Care: A Review of Research on Welfare Provision for Elderly People*. London: HMSO, 1990.

22. Forder J. *The Costs of Addressing Age Discrimination in Social Care*, PSSRU discussion paper 2538, 2008. At www.pssru.ac.uk/pdf/dp2538.pdf, accessed 12 Feb 2010.

23. Beecham J, Knapp M, Fernández J-L *et al*. *Age Discrimination in Mental Health Services*, PSSRU discussion paper 2536, 2008. At www.pssru.ac.uk/pdf/dp2536.pdf, accessed 12 Feb 2010.

24. Piachaud D, Webb J. *The Price of Food: Missing out on Mass Consumption*. London: Sticerd, 1996.

25. Age Concern. *Hungry to Be Heard: The Scandal of Malnourished Older People in Hospital*. London: Age Concern, 2006. At www.ageconcern.org.uk/AgeConcern/Documents/Hungry_to_be _Heard_August_2006.pdf, accessed 12 Feb 2010.

26. NHS Quality Improvement Scotland. *Food, Fluid and Nutritional Care in Hospitals*, 2003. At www.nhshealthquality.org/nhsqis/ controller?p_service=Content.show&p_applic=CCC&pContentID =3196, accessed 12 Feb 2010.

27. Committee on Medical Aspects of Food Policy. *Report of the Panel on Dietary Reference Values for Food, Energy and Nutrients for the United Kingdom*. London: HMSO, 1991.

28. Sweeney MP, Shaw A, Yip B, Bagg J. Oral health of elderly institutionalized patients. *Br J Nurs* 1995; **4**: 1204–8.

29. Hajat S, Haines A, Bulpitt C, Fletcher A. Patterns and determinants of alcohol consumption in people aged 75 years and over:

30. Walmsley CM, Bates CJ, Prentice A, Cole TJ. Relationship between alcohol and nutrient intake and blood status indices of older people living in the UK: further analysis of data from the National Diet and Nutrition Survey of people aged 65 years and over, 1994/5. *Public Health Nutr* 1998; **1**: 157–67.

results from the MRC trial of assessment and management of older people in the community. *Age Ageing* 2004; **33**: 170–77.

31. Bots S, Tijhuis M, Giampaoli S *et al*. Lifestyle and diet related factors in late life depression – a 5 year follow-up of elderly European men: the FINE study. *Int J Geriatr Psychiatry* 2008; **23**: 478–84.

32. Mielke MM, Zandi P, Sjogren M *et al*. High total cholesterol levels in late life associated with reduced risk of dementia. *Neurology* 2005; **64**: 1689–95.

33. Stewart R, Masaki K, Xu QL *et al*. A 32 year prospective study of change in body weight and incident dementia. *Arch Neurol* 2005; **62**: 20–22.

34. Turpenny B, Brown A. Feeding problems in dementia. *Geriatr Med* 2007; **37**: 15–19.

35. Finucane TE, Chirstmas C, Travis K. Tube feeding in patients with advanced dementia: a review of the evidence. *JAMA* 1999; **282**: 1365–70.

36. Sanders DS, Hurlestone DP, McAlindon ME. PEG placement in patients with dementia: a contentious ethical and clinical dilemma. *Gastrointest Endosc* 2004; **60**: 492–3.

37. Hughes JC, Jolley D, Jordan A, Sampson EL. Palliative care in dementia: issues and evidence. *Adv Psychiatr Treat* 2007; **13**(4): 251–60.

38. Gillick MR. Rethinking the role of tube feeding in patients. *New Engl J Med* 2000; **342**: 206–10.

39. Kim J-M, Stewart R, Kim S-W *et al*. Methylenetetrahydrofolate reductase gene and risk of Alzheimer's disease in Koreans. *Int J Geriatr Psychiatry* 2008; **23**: 454–9.

40. Myint, PK, Luben RN, Wareham NJ *et al*. Combined effect of health behaviours and risk of first ever stroke in 20,040 men and women over 11 years follow-up in Norfolk cohort of European Prospective Investigation of Cancer (EPIC Norfolk): prospective population study. *Br Med J* 2009; **338**: b349.

41. Lennard-Jones JE. *A Positive Approach to Nutrition as Treatment*. London: King's Fund, 1992.

42. Parker D, Emmett PM, Heaton KW. Final year medical students' knowledge of practical nutrition. *J R Soc Med* 1992; **85**: 338.

43. Royal College of Nursing. *Nutrition Standards and the Older Adult*. London: Royal College of Nursing, 1993.

133

Caregiver Support

Kathleen C. Buckwalter, Mary Ellen Stolder, Charlene S. Aaron and Catherine Messinger

University of Iowa College of Nursing, Iowa City, IA, USA

INTRODUCTION

Alzheimer's disease and related dementias (ADRD) are neurodegenerative, progressive, chronic illnesses with an unpredictable clinical course. Compounding this tragedy is that caregivers' mental and physical well-being suffers, and their activities and social relationships are disrupted, leading them to discontinue home care. This chapter highlights the vital caregiver role, and the costs to and support for home caregivers and those in the process of relocating a patient to an institutional setting. We review the positive and negative effects of caregiving, the psychosocial and physiological outcomes, and variables that mediate the stressors inherent in caregiving.

THE CAREGIVER ROLE

Of the estimated 5.3 million Americans with ADRD, over 80% are cared for by family members and friends, typically spouses[1-3]. Most families want to forestall or avert institutionalization of those with ADRD, so the aging US population presents a significant societal challenge.

Who are Family Caregivers?

Caregiving typically falls to women, who provide 72% of care: 29% are adult daughters and 43% are wives[4]. Nonetheless, both men and women caregivers of persons with dementia (PwDs) devote a similar amount of time to caregiving service and, more importantly, perceive similar levels of stress. Most stress arises from dealing with behavioural problems. This stress is a common precipitant of institutionalization[5,6].

Public Policy and Cost Implications of Caregiving

Policy makers recognize that families are the mainstay of caregiving and that such care comes at considerable cost (i.e. home modifications, assistive devices, special food, high utility costs and lost wages[7-9]). Conservative estimates indicate that family caregivers of PwDs saved the US health care system $350 billion in 2006[10]. With the population ageing, this estimate will increase. Although family caregiving greatly relieves costs to society, it concentrates financial burdens onto caregiving families. Moreover, monetary estimates in no way reflect the human costs of this devastating disease. Indeed, caregiving correlates with other adverse consequences, such as poor health[11-13].

CAREGIVER STRESS AND BURDEN AND ITS IMPACT ON CAREGIVER WELL-BEING

The concept of caregiver burden is used as an all-encompassing term referring to the financial, social, physical and emotional effects of caregiving. Numerous studies have examined the burden and stress of caring for a PwD, the effects on mental and physical health, and the use of a variety of interventions to relieve caregiving burden.

Family caregivers of persons with ADRD experience stressors that affect their health and well-being, and precipitate institutionalization of the care recipient. Hence, 'stress' has emerged as an important concept, with the words 'stress', 'burden', and 'distress' often used interchangeably. Spouses may be at greatest risk, as they are often elderly themselves[14]. In a common pattern, the distress and depression caregivers experience precipitates physiological changes and poor health habits, leading to illness[15].

Models of Caregiver Stress

Several theoretical frameworks have guided studies of PwDs, their family caregivers and how interventions affect both[16]. Stress models, in particular, have guided much of this research, showing that the care recipient's level of impairment is not a linear predictor of caregiver stress[17,18]; instead, caregiver stress is moderated by many factors, including the caregiver's physical health, social support, financial assets, coping abilities and personality. For example, Vitaliano et al.[19,20] stratified resources and vulnerability variables of both the caregiver and care recipient, to pinpoint relationships among stressors, resources and burden. Vitaliano considered both psychological and biological markers of distress, and expressed them in a mathematical formula in which the level of caregiver distress (burden) decreases with reduced undesirable variables or increased desirable variables:

$$\text{Distress} = \frac{\text{Exposure to stressors} + \text{Vulnerability}}{\text{Psychological resources} + \text{Social resources}}$$

Principles and Practice of Geriatric Psychiatry, 3rd edn. Edited by Mohammed T. Abou-Saleh, Cornelius Katona and Anand Kumar
© 2011 John Wiley & Sons, Ltd

Other studies, examining racial differences in caregivers of PwDs, found stress levels to be affected by overarching factors that reflect personal context (e.g. being able to financially provide for their family and getting leisure time away)[21].

Stressors Associated with Family Caregiving

The profound cognitive and behavioural changes of ADRD include progressive loss of memory, judgment, the ability to interpret abstraction, and language and motor skills, as well as personality changes. ADRD culminate in an inability to perform instrumental activities of daily living (IADLs), such as cooking and managing money and, as the disease progresses, more basic activities like bathing and toileting. Researchers disagree on whether the level of a care recipient's functional or cognitive impairment correlates with caregiver burden[22,23]. Notably, however, a recent study found caregivers' quality of life did correlate with the severity of the care recipient's behavioural disorders and duration of the disease process[24].

ADRD has an unpredictable course and pace of decline; the only certainty is that the disease is progressive. As dementia progresses, caregivers must be increasingly vigilant, since a PwD may unexpectedly leave home or injure themselves. In the final stages, patients are often completely dependent on their caregivers, making caring for a PwD eventually an all-consuming job.

Behavioural Impairments in Care Recipients

Most commonly, the reported behavioural changes of ADRD include lethargy, withdrawal, sleep disturbance, restlessness, wandering, aggression, destroying property and verbally disruptive or sexually inappropriate behaviour[25-27]. The stress of providing 24-hour care mounts when the PwD becomes agitated, stressed or disoriented. Behavioural abnormalities appear in up to 67% of care recipients upon diagnosis[28], in 65% of institutionalized persons[26], and in 70–90% of persons with advanced dementia[29,30]. They worsen with disease progression and may be related to fatigue, change, overstimulation, excessive demands or physical stressors[31]. Moreover, the care recipient's behavioural problems are the characteristic that overwhelmingly predicts caregiver distress[22,32], making this a strong predictor of institutionalization[33].

Other Factors that Influence Caregiver Stress

Caregiving for persons with ADRD entails years of constant demands. Over the disease trajectory, the intensity and/or frequency of a caregiver's level of distress may vary widely. To understand this variability, investigators try to identify factors associated with differing outcomes. Stress may be influenced by whether the caregiver and recipient reside together, the abruptness of the disease onset, the family relationship, and the caregiver's coping strategies[34,35]; also caregiver burden was reportedly more intense for spouses than for adult children[32]. Positive outcomes, however, are associated with a strong social network and satisfactory support[36].

In sum, the relationship between the caregiver's psychological distress and physical impairment depends on many variables, for instance the care recipient's behaviours and caregiver vulnerability (e.g. age, gender, neuroticism, pre-existing hypertension, and social support). Nonetheless, the factors contributing to caregiver distress have only recently been delineated well enough to effectively direct interventions or preventative strategies[37-40].

Dementia Versus Non-dementia Caregiving

The risk for health problems increases with the physical demands of caregiving, prolonged distress and the biological vulnerability of older caregivers. Research suggests that caring for a PwD is more demanding than caring for physically impaired older adults[41]. In a review of studies of caregiving in different types of illnesses, Biegel, Sales, and Schulz[42] observed different patterns of distress. Distress peaked after the initial diagnosis, but, as time passed, the level of distress fell. This pattern, however, was not observed in family caregivers of persons with a gradual onset, where no relief of distress was observed[43].

POSITIVE AND NEGATIVE OUTCOMES OF FAMILY CAREGIVING FOR PERSONS WITH DEMENTIA

It is notable that mounting evidence suggests that some caregivers find satisfaction in the caregiving role and report life satisfaction, emotional uplifts, enhanced self-esteem and self-efficacy, optimism, and growth and meaning[44-49]. Interviews of 50 caregivers of PwDs found 58% experienced 'self-fulfilling' experiences during caregiving, with the same percentage expressing 'losses and difficulties'[50]. Positive aspects of caregiving were related to the caregiver's competence. Brown and colleagues[51] found that caregivers who provided instrumental support to friends, relatives or neighbours, or who provided emotional support to their spouses, had lower five-year mortality rates.

IMPACT OF CAREGIVING ON HEALTH OF CAREGIVERS

Despite some inconsistent findings concerning how caring for PwDs affects mental and physical health, most but not all studies find increased psychiatric and physical morbidity[52-55]. This suggests that inconsistencies are attributed to differences in caregivers' coping strategies.

Mental Health Outcomes

Caring for an older person with ADRD puts one at risk for extreme psychological distress. A number of studies link stress to factors such as the strain of providing direct care, grief from witnessing the decline of their loved ones, social isolation and role changes. These effects occur with home care, following institutionalization, and during bereavement[37,56].

Depression

Depressive symptoms are among the mental health changes most frequently reported by family caregivers of PwDs. A complex interaction of cultural factors[57,58], caregiver and receiver characteristics come into play, predicting depression[59-61]. Moreover, depression among caregivers is associated with the intensity of their reactions to the patients' memory and behaviour problems[62] and to other outcomes such as increased physical and subjective burden[63,64], and the use of psychotropic medications[22,65].

Predictors of caregiver depression include a younger age of caregiver and care receiver, Caucasian race, Hispanic ethnicity compared to black ethnicity, higher education, activities of daily living dependence, and the recipient's behavioural abnormalities (particularly aggressive or angry behaviour). Other predictors include low income, spousal status, hours spent caregiving and functional dependence of the caregiver[61,66]. Depression is greater among females than males[6] and appears to increase over time among residential caregivers and decrease over time following institutionalization and bereavement[67]. Compared to non-caregiving men, male spouse caregivers have higher levels of depression, respiratory symptoms, and poorer health habits, although the groups did not differ on other measures of physical and mental health[68].

Anxiety

Several investigators incorporated self-reported measures of anxiety when examining depression among caregivers. Some found that caregivers who presented with symptoms of depression also often reported symptoms of anxiety[18,69]. Overall, strong evidence suggests caregivers are at risk for psychiatric symptomatology. Yet, caution must be exercised when interpreting the generalizability of these findings since many samples may be biased towards more distressed caregivers. For example, most caregivers are recruited from chapters of the Alzheimer's Association, support groups, or through referrals by health professionals; either individuals who have little difficulty with the caregiving role or are so distressed or constrained that they cannot participate in supportive programmes or visit health care professionals, may be under-represented. Additionally, transient psychiatric symptoms may be more common than diagnosable depression. Moreover, caregiver burden does not always predict depressive symptoms, suggesting that the relationship between caregiver burden and caregiver depression is complex[66].

Physical Health Outcomes

Most studies examining the physical effects of caregiving used one or more indicators of caregiver health: (i) self-reported health status; (ii) self-reported incidence of illness-related symptoms; (iii) self-reported utilization of health care services; (iv) self-reported medication use; and (v) disease susceptibility. Predictors of poor physical health outcomes for caregivers include being older, a spouse and female[22,70]. Interestingly, however, in some cases caregiving was also reported to improve physical health. Family caregivers with coronary heart disease (CHD), who experienced emotional uplifts, also showed less severe metabolic signs that predict CHD[20,71].

The psychoneurological and immunological effects of caregiving are receiving increased attention. One study indicated that long-term residential caregiving for PwDs decreased measures of cellular immunity and increased the duration of infection; most affected were caregivers who reported less social support and more stress[72]. Stress-induced changes in physiological function increase the probability of illness[73]. Caregiver wear and tear, from repeated arousal and inefficient control of the physiological responses of stress, can also lead to pathophysiology[74,75]. Stressors can cause impaired health habits, physiological responses, physical illness and even death[11,20,76,77].

Similarly, psychological stress can increase caregiver vulnerability to disease by compromising immune system integrity[20,78]. A well-controlled study examined caregiver depression and distress as immunological modifiers and linked the poorer immune response to lower levels of helper T-lymphocytes and natural killer (NK) cells[78]. Here, caregivers also reported nearly three-fold more stress-related symptoms and higher rates of psychotropic drug use, especially if they lived with the PwD. While some studies reported that caregivers use more psychotropic medications[22,72], most reports suggest use of somatic medication does not significantly increase[20,79].

In summary, the findings for the effects of caregiving on physical health are more equivocal than those for mental health; however, the evidence is still generally weak. This may be due to different definitions of health, health outcome measures, caregiving and control samples (varying levels of vulnerability and resources), care recipient samples (functional versus behavioural impairments), and that some self-report measures of physical health may primarily reflect life satisfaction. Moreover, caregivers who provide assistance with activities of daily living (ADLs) exhibit poor nutrition and poor decision-making regarding their own health care appointments[80].

Evaluating links between caregiver distress and health will ultimately require testing complex, multivariate models. Despite methodological challenges inherent in evaluating caregiving outcomes, data suggest chronic stressors do contribute to affective disorders and may alter caregivers' sympathetic, neuroendocrine and immunological function.

FAMILY CAREGIVING: RELOCATING THE CARE RECIPIENT

Placing a relative in a nursing home is stressful for both caregiver and patient. Yet PwDs are usually placed in nursing homes only when all other avenues and resources are exhausted[81,82]. Generally, the decision is postponed long past the time when more objective persons see it as appropriate[83]. One reason for this delay is that some caregivers, especially spouses, believe their role obliges them to sole caregiving responsibility and to reject institutionalization[84]. Although children are comparatively more likely to rely on formal services and place the PwD in institutional care, they nevertheless often delay placement decisions because of reluctance to reverse roles and take charge of a parent's life[85].

Overall, the literature indicates a care recipient's extent of cognitive impairment, loss of self-care abilities, and disruptive behaviours are predictive of institutionalization. Cohen et al.[81] described seven variables that affect a caregiver's decision to institutionalize a dependent elder with dementia: use of services, enjoyment of caregiving, caregiver burden and health, caregiver rating and reaction to care receiver behaviour and memory problems, and presence of troublesome behaviours. Six variables predicted actual institutionalization: caregiver health and burden, use of services, care receiver cognitive function and troublesome behaviours, and caregiver reaction to behaviours. Montgomery and Kosloski[85] compared predictors of placement for adult child caregivers and spouse caregivers. Higher income, eligibility for Medicaid, lower morale and age of the elder were associated with placement for both groups, but other predictors were different. Notably, the level of affection predicted placement for children, but not spouses, while sense of obligation was predictive for spouses, but not children, who were always more likely to institutionalize the PwD. The probability of placement declined with time for a while, levelled off, and then rose as caregiving exceeded 30 months, with the probability increasing more sharply for adult child caregivers than for spouses.

Increasingly, services are supporting family caregiving in the home, but the extent to which they are meeting needs is questionable[86,87]. Neither should it be assumed that family members know how to provide all of the needed care or have access to the resources to assist them with providing care in the home[87]. One study found that 40% of family caregivers who had placed their loved one in a nursing home reported that at least one additional community service would have delayed institutionalization[88].

Relocation raises the prospect of sharp role transition. For most spouses, relocation changes a long-standing pattern of living together and providing for the other. For children, it can restore a pattern in which the child is not living with and/or is not directly responsible for the care of the parent. PwDs placed in nursing homes may be highly resistant and fearful of the change. Given their diminished capacity for reasoning, it can be challenging to convince them they require institutionalization. This presents a stressful dilemma, and one that may be more difficult for child caregivers, because of the need to reverse roles. Constant requests to be taken home are especially stressful to families. Spouses may find it more difficult if their relationship has been loving. Family Involvement in Care (FIC) interviews[89] revealed the regret felt when placing the relative in a nursing home, but also often reflected ambivalence because a burden was lifted.

When caregivers cannot manage the care recipient's difficult behaviours, such behaviours often escalate[31,90]; this is often the primary reason for institutionalizing a family member with dementia[91,92]. Considering the psychological and financial expense associated with institutionalizing a PwD, interventions that help caregivers prevent or manage behaviours are significant. Appropriately, national recommendations emphasize research that focuses on reducing the burdens of care for family members of PwDs[1]. Indeed, the American Association of Geriatric Psychiatry, the Alzheimer's Association and the American Geriatrics Society agree, 'Interventions that reduce the risk of caregiver depression and improve tolerance and the capacity to care for patients in the home, including educational materials, counseling support groups, day care and respite care' are among the most urgent areas for research[93].

Dang et al.[94] recommend that clinicians use the American Medical Association's 'Caregiver Self-Assessment Questionnaire', which can be placed in waiting rooms, handed to caregivers of patients with dementia, or mailed to them prior to the scheduled appointment. The questionnaire could alert providers to problems (e.g. signs of potential abuse or caregiver 'burn out'), prompting them to suggest education or counselling interventions. Although providing educational materials alone does little to relieve caregiver burden, a meta-analysis of 34 studies concluded that it significantly benefits caregiver psychological distress, caregiver knowledge and patient mood[94]. Another study showed that counselling caregivers delayed nursing home placement for an average of six months, and was particularly effective for adult-daughter caregivers[69].

CONCLUSION

Caring for a PwD is a responsibility usually shouldered by family members, and can be chronically demanding and often overwhelming[1]. Informal caregiving of elders with chronic illnesses and disabilities has become commonplace, in part from demographic shifts. Although medical advances are increasing life expectancy, escalating health care costs shortens hospital stays and limits reimbursement for at-home professional care. Adverse outcomes depend upon the unique characteristics of both the caregiver and the care receiver. Accordingly, research suggests that combined interventions, tailored for both caregivers and care receivers, can significantly improve caregiver well-being and health and, in some instances, problematic care receiver behaviours[95].

REFERENCES

1. Alzheimer's Study Group. *A National Alzheimer's Strategic Plan: The Report of the Alzheimer's Study Group*, 2009. At www.alz.org/documents/national/report_ASG_alzplan.pdf, accessed 17 Mar 2010.
2. Zhu C, Scarmeas N, Torgan R et al. Clinical characteristics and longitudinal changes of informal cost of Alzheimer's disease in the community. *J Am Geriatr Soc* 2006; **54**(10): 1596–602.
3. Gaugler JE, Kane RL, Kane RA. Family care for older adults with disabilities: Toward more targeted and interpretable research. *Int J Aging Hum Dev* 2002; **54**(3): 205–31.
4. Horowitz A. Family caregiving to the frail elderly. In Eisdorfor C (ed.), *Annual Review of Gerontology and Geriatrics*. New York: Springer Press, 1985, 194–246.
5. Ford GR, Goode KT, Barrett JJ et al. Gender roles and caregiving stress: an examination of subjective appraisals of specific primary stressors in Alzheimer's caregivers. *Aging Ment Health* 1997; **1**: 158–65.
6. Pinquart M, Sorenson S. Gender differences in caregiver stressors, social resources, and health: an updated meta-analysis. *J Gerontol B Psychol Sci Soc Sci* 2006; **61**(1): 31–45.
7. Arno P, Levine C, Memmott M. The economic value of informal caregiving. *Health Aff* 1999; **18**(2): 182–8.
8. Bloom G, Pouvourville N, Straus W. Cost of illness of Alzheimer's disease: how useful are the current estimates? *Gerontologist* 2003; **43**: 158–64.
9. Covinsky K, Eng C, Liu L et al. Reduced employment in caregivers of frail elders: Impact of ethnicity, patient clinical characteristics and caregiver characteristics. *J Gerontol A Biol Sci Med Sci* 2001; **56**(11): M707–13.
10. United States Administration on Aging. *A Profile of Older Americans 2008*. At www.mowaa.org/Document.Doc?id=69, accessed 22 Feb 2009.
11. Pinquart M, Sorenson S. Correlates of physical health of informal caregivers: a meta-analysis. *J Gerontol B Psychol Sci Soc Sci* 2007; **62**(2): 126–37.
12. Schulz R, Newsom J, Mittelmark M et al. Health effects of caregiving: the caregiver health effects study: an ancillary study of the cardiovascular health study. *Ann Behav Med* 1997; **19**(2): 110–16.
13. Schulz R, Hebert R, Dew M et al. Patient suffering and caregiver compassion: new opportunities for research, practice and policy. *Gerontologist* 2007; **47**: 4–13.
14. Pushkar-Gold D, Reis MF, Markiewicz D et al. When home caregiving ends: a longitudinal study of outcomes for caregivers of relatives with dementia. *J Am Geriatr Soc* 1995; **43**: 10–16.
15. Schulz R, Sherwood P. Physical and mental health effects of family caregiving. *Am J Nurs* 2008; **108**(9): 23–7.
16. Pearlin LI, Mullan JT, Semple SJ et al. Caregiving and the stress process: an overview of concepts and their measures. *Gerontologist* 1990; **30**: 583–94.
17. Hadjistavropoulos T, Taylor S, Tuokko H et al. Neuropsychological deficits, caregivers' perceptions of deficits and caregiver burden. *J Am Geriatr Soc* 1994; **42**: 308–14.
18. Vitaliano PP, Russo J, Young HM et al. Predictors of burden in spouse caregivers of individuals with Alzheimer's disease. *Psychol Aging* 1991; **6**: 392–402.
19. Vitaliano PP, Maiuro RD, Ochs H et al. *A Model of Burden in Caregivers of DAT Patients*. DHHS Publication No. (ADM)89-1569. Bethesda: National Institute of Health, 1989.

20. Vitaliano P, Zhang J, Scanlan J. Is caregiving hazardous to one's physical health? A meta-analysis. *Psychol Bull* 2003; **129**: 946–72.

21. Williams I. Emotional health of black and white dementia caregivers: a contextual examination. *J Gerontol B Psychol Sci Soc Sci* 2005; **60**(6): P287–95.

22. Baumgarten M, Battista RN, Infante-Rivard C *et al.* The psychological and physical health of family members caring for an elderly person with dementia. *J Clin Epidemiol* 1992; **45**: 61–70.

23. Cattanach L, Tebes JK. The nature of elder impairment and its impact on family caregivers' health and psychosocial functioning. *Gerontologist* 1991; **31**: 246–55.

24. Ferrara M, Langiano E, Di Brango T *et al.* Prevalence of stress, anxiety and depression in with Alzheimer caregivers. *Health Qual Life Outcomes* 2008; **6**(6): 93.

25. Folstein MF, Bylsma FW. Noncognitive symptoms of Alzheimer's disease. In Terry RD, Katzman R, Bick KL (eds), *Alzheimer's Disease*. New York: Raven Press, 1994, 27–40.

26. Nasman B, Bucht G, Erikson S. Behavioral symptoms in the institutionalized elderly: relationship to dementia. *Int J Psychiatry* 1993; **8**: 67–73.

27. Teri L, Traux P, Logsdon R *et al.* Assessment of behavioral problems in dementia: the revised memory and behavior problems checklist. *Psychol Aging* 1992; **7**: 622–31.

28. Cacabelos R. Diagnosis of Alzheimer's disease: defining genetic profiles. *Acta Neurol Scand* 1996; **93**: 572–84.

29. Swearer JM, Drachman DA, O'Donell BF *et al.* Troublesome and disruptive behaviors in dementia: relationships to diagnosis and disease severity. *J Am Geriatr Soc* 1988; **36**: 784–90.

30. Teri L, Larson E, Reifler BV. Behavioral disturbance in dementia of the Alzheimer's type. *J Am Geriatr Soc* 1988; **36**: 1–6.

31. Hall GR, Buckwalter KC. Progressively lowered stress threshold: a conceptual model for care of adults with Alzheimer's disease. *Arch Psychiatr Nurs* 1987; **1**: 399–406.

32. Pinquart M, Sorensen S. Associations of stressors and uplifts of caregiving with caregiver burden and depressive mood: a meta-analysis. *J Gerontol B Psychol Sci Soc Sci* 2003; **58**(2): 112–28.

33. Zimmer J, Watson N, Treat A. Behavioral problems among patients in skilled nursing facilities. *Am J Public Health* 1984; **74**: 1118–21.

34. Quayhagen MP, Quayhagen M. Alzheimer's stress: Coping with the caregiving role. *Gerontologist* 1988; **28**: 391–6.

35. Zarit SH, Birkel RC, MaloneBeach E. Spouses as caregivers: stresses and interventions. In Goldstein MY (ed.), *Family Involvement in Treatment of the Frail Elderly*. Washington, DC: American Psychiatric Press, 1989, 26–62.

36. Seltzer MM, Li LW. The transitions of caregiving: subjective and objective definitions. *Gerontologist* 1996; **36**: 614–26.

37. Schulz R, Burgio L, Burns R *et al.* Resources for enhancing Alzheimer's caregiver health (REACH): overview, site-specific outcomes, and future directions. *Gerontologist* 2003; **43**(4): 514–20.

38. Mittelman M, Roth D, Haley W *et al.* Effects of caregiver intervention on negative caregiver appraisals of behavior problems in patients with Alzheimer's disease: results of a randomized trial. *J Gerontol J Gerontol B Psychol Sci Soc Sci* 2004; **59**: P27.

39. Schulz R, O'Brien A, Czaja S *et al.* Dementia caregiver intervention research: in search of clinical significance. *Gerontologist* 2002; **42**: 589–602.

40. Sorenson S, Pinquart M, Duberstein P. How effective are interventions with caregivers? An updated meta-analysis. *Gerontologist* 2002; **42**: 356–72.

41. Kim V, Schulz R. Family caregivers' strains: comparative analysis of cancer caregiving with dementia, diabetes, and frail elderly caregiving. *J Aging Health* 2008; **20**(5): 483–503.

42. Biegel DE, Sales E, Schulz R. *Family Caregiving in Chronic Illness: Alzheimer's Disease, Cancer, Heart Disease, Mental Illness, and Stroke*. Newbury Park: Sage, 1991.

43. Reese DR, Gross AM, Smalley DL *et al.* Caregivers of Alzheimer's disease and stroke patients: immunological and psychological characteristics. *Gerontologist* 1994; **34**: 534–40.

44. Cohen C, Colantino A, Vernich L. Positive aspects of caregiving: rounding out the caregiver experience. *Int J Geriatr Psychiatry* 2002; **17**(2): 184–8.

45. Butcher H, Holkup P, Buckwalter K. The experience of caring for a family member with Alzheimer's disease. *West J Nurs Res* 2001; **23**(1): 33–5.

46. Gonyea J, O'Connor M, Carruth A *et al.* Subjective appraisal of Alzheimer's disease caregiving: the role of self-efficacy and depressive symptoms in the experience of burden. *Am J Alzheimers Dis Other Demen* 2005; **20**: 273–80.

47. Kolanowski A, Fick D, Waller J *et al.* Spouses of persons with dementia: their healthcare problems, utilization and costs. *Res Nurs Health* 2004; **27**(5): 296–306.

48. Mausbach B, Aschbacher K, Patterson T *et al.* Avoidant coping partially mediates the relationship between patient problem behaviors and depressive symptoms in spousal caregivers. *Am J Geriatr Psychiatry* 2006; **14**: 299–306.

49. Tarlow B, Wisniewski S, Belle S *et al.* Positive aspects of caregiving: contributions of the REACH project to the development of new measures for Alzheimer's caregiving. *Res Aging* 2004; **26**(4): 429–80.

50. Narayan S, Lewis M, Tornatore J *et al.* Subjective responses to caregiving for a spouse with dementia. *J Gerontol Nurs* 2001; **27**(2): 19–28.

51. Brown SL, Nesse RM, Vinokur AD *et al.* Providing social support may be more beneficial than receiving it: results from a prospective study of mortality. *Psychol Sci* 2003; **14**(4): 320–7.

52. Gottlieb B, Rooney J. Coping effectiveness: determinants and relevance to the mental health and affect of family caregivers of persons with dementia. *Aging Ment Health* 2004; **8**: 364–73.

53. Clyburn L, Stones M, Hadjistavropoulos T *et al.* Predicting caregiver burden and depression in Alzheimer's disease. *J Gerontol B Psychol Sci Soc Sci* 2000; **55**(1): S2–13.

54. Bell C, Araki S, Neuman P. The association between caregiver burden and caregiver health-related quality of life in Alzheimer's disease. *Alzheimer Dis Assoc Disord* 2001; **15**(3): 129–36.

55. Connell C, Janevic M, Gallant M. The costs of caring: impact of dementia on family caregivers. *J Geriatr Psychiatry Neurol* 2001; **14**(4): 179–87.

56. Schulz R, Boerner K, Shear K *et al.* Predictors of complicated grief among dementia caregivers: a prospective study of bereavement. *Am J Geriatr Psychiatry* 2006; **14**(8): 650–8.

57. Janevick M, Connel C. Racial, ethnic, and cultural differences in the dementia caregiver experience: recent findings. *Gerontologist* 2001; **41**: 334–47.

58. Torti F, Gwyther L, Reed S *et al.* A multinational review of recent trends and reports in dementia caregiver burden. *Alzheimer Dis Assoc Disord* 2004; **18**(2): 99–109.

59. Adams B, Aranda M, Kemp B *et al.* Ethnic and gender differences in distress among Anglo American, African American, Japanese American and Mexican American spousal caregivers of persons with dementia. *J Clin Geropsychol* 2002; **8**: 279–301.

60. Coon D, Williams M, Moore R *et al.* The northern California chronic care network for dementia. *J Am Geriatr Soc* 2004; **52**(1): 150–6.

61. Covinsky K, Newcomer R, Fox P *et al.* Patient and caregiver characteristics associated with depression in caregivers of patients with dementia. *J Gen Intern Med* 2003; **18**(2): 1006–14.

62. Croog S, Burleson J, Sudilovski A *et al.* Spouse caregivers of Alzheimer's patients: problem responses to caregiver burdens. *Aging Ment Health* 2006; **10**(2): 87–100.

63. Gaynor SE. The long-haul: the effects of home care on caregivers. *Image J Nurs Sch* 1990; **22**: 208–14.

64. Neundorfer MM. Coping and health outcomes in spouse caregivers of persons with dementia. *Nurs Res* 1991; **40**: 260–5.

65. Clipp EC, George LK. Psychotropic drug use among caregivers of patients with dementia. *J Am Geriatr Soc* 1990; **38**: 227–35.

66. Sherwood P, Given C, Given B *et al.* Caregiver burden and depressive symptoms: analysis of common outcomes in caregivers of elderly patients. *J Aging Health* 2005; **17**(2): 125–47.

67. Gaugler J, Kane R, Newcomer R. Resilience and transitions from dementia caregiving. *J Gerontol B Psychol Sci Soc Sci* 2007; **62**(1): P38–44.

68. Fuller-Jonap F, Haley WE. Mental and physical health of male caregivers of a spouse with Alzheimer's disease. *J Aging Health* 1995; **7**: 99–118.

69. Andren S, Elmstahl S. Effective psychosocial intervention for family caregivers lengthens time elapsed before nursing home placement of individuals with dementia: a five-year follow-up study. *Int Psychogeriatr* 2008; **20**: 1177–92.

70. Young RF, Kahana E. Specifying caregiver outcomes: gender and relationship aspects of caregiving strain. *Gerontologist* 1989; **29**: 660–6.

71. Vitaliano PP, Scanlan JM, Siegler IC *et al.* Caregiving exacerbates the metabolic syndrome associated with coronary heart disease. Paper presented at the American Psychosomatic Medicine Society Annual Meeting, 1997, Santa Fe, New Mexico.

72. Kiecolt-Glaser JK, Dura JR, Speicher CE, Trask OJ, Glaser R. Spousal caregivers of dementia victims: longitudinal changes in immunity and health. *Psychosom Med* 1991; **53**: 345–62.

73. Brantley P, Garrett V. *Psychobiological Approaches to Health and Disease*. New York: Plenum Press, 1993, 647.

74. Chrousos G, Gold P. The concepts of stress and stress system disorders. *JAMA* 1992; **267**: 1244–52.

75. McEwen B. The neurobiology of stress: from serendipity to clinical relevance. *Brain Res* 2000; **886**: 172–89.

76. Schulz R, Visintainer P, Williamson GM. Psychiatric and physical morbidity effects of caregiving. *J Gerontol* 1990; **45**: 181–91.

77. Christakis NA, Allison PD. Mortality after the hospitalization of a spouse. *N Engl J Med* 2006; **354**(7): 719–30.

78. Kiecolt-Glaser J, Glaser R. Psychosocial moderators of immune function. *Ann Behav Med* 1987; **9**: 16.

79. Brodaty H, Hadzi-Pavlovic D. Psychosocial effects on carers of living with persons with dementia. *Aust N Z J Psychiatry* 1990; **24**: 351–60.

80. Burton L, Zdaniuk B, Schulz R *et al.* Transitions in spousal caregiving. *Gerontologist* 2003; **43**(2): 230–41.

81. Cohen C, Gold D, Shulman K *et al.* Factors determining the decision to institutionalize demented individuals: a prospective study. *Gerontologist* 1993; **33**: 714–20.

82. Tipton-Smith S, Tanner G. Coping with placement of a parent in a nursing home through preplacement education. *Geriatr Nurs* 1994; **15**: 322–6.

83. Ade-Ridder L, Kaplan L. Marriage, spousal caregiving, and a husband's move to a nursing home: a changing role for the wife. *J Gerontol Nurs* 1993; **19**: 13–23.

84. Dellasega C, Mastrian K. The process and consequences of institutionalizing an elder. *West J Nurs Res* 1995; **17**: 123–40.

85. Montgomery R, Kosloski K. A longitudinal analysis of nursing home placement for dependent elders cared for by spouses versus adult children. *J Gerontol* 1994; **49**: S62–74.

86. Applebaum R, Phillips P. Assuring the quality of in-home care: the "other" challenge for long term care. *Gerontologist* 1990; **30**: 444–50.

87. Kelley LS, Buckwalter KC, Maas ML. Access to health care resources for family caregivers of elderly persons with dementia. *Nurs Outlook* 1998; **47**: 8–14.

88. Collins C, Stommel M, Wang S *et al.* Caregiving transitions: changes in depression among family caregivers of relatives with dementia. *Nurs Res* 1994; **43**: 220–5.

89. Maas M, Swanson E. *Nursing Interventions for Alzheimer's: Family Role Trials*. Research Grant, National Institute of Nursing Research R01-NR01689. Rockville: National Institutes of Health, 1992.

90. Vitaliano PP, Young HM, Russo J *et al.* Does expressed emotion in spouses predict subsequent problems among care recipients with Alzheimer's disease? *J Gerontol* 1993; **48**: 202–9.

91. Teri L. Behavior and caregiver burden: behavioral problems in patients with Alzheimer's disease and its association with caregiver stress. *Alzheimer Dis Assoc Disord* 1997; **11**: S35–8.

92. Pruchno RA, Potashnik L. Caregiving spouses: physical and mental health in perspective. *J Am Geriatr Soc* 1989; **37**: 697–705.

93. Small GW, Rabins PV, Barry PP *et al.* Diagnosis and treatment of Alzheimer's disease and related disorders. Consensus statement of the American Association for Geriatric Psychiatry, the Alzheimer's Association, and the American Geriatrics Society. *JAMA* 1997; **278**: 1363–71.

94. Dang S, Badiye A, Kelkar G. The dementia caregiver-a primary care approach. *South Med J* 2008; **101**(12): 1246–51.

95. Pinquart M, Sorenson S. Helping caregivers with dementia: which interventions work and how large are their effects? *Int Psychogeriatr* 2006; **18**(4): 577–95.

134

Elder Abuse – Epidemiology, Recognition and Management

Alexander M. Thomson[1] and Martin J. Vernon[2]

[1]*Department of Elderly Care, Salford Royal Hospitals NHS Foundation Trust, UK*
[2]*Department of Elderly Medicine, University Hospitals of South Manchester NHS Foundation Trust, UK*

INTRODUCTION

During the 1980s elder abuse emerged as a health and social issue of international importance[1]. It is defined as 'a single or repeated act or lack of appropriate action occurring within any relationship where there is an expectation of trust which causes harm or distress to an older person'[2]. While most authorities include self-neglect within the broad definition, acts which threaten an elder's well-being as a consequence of their competently made decisions are specifically excluded.

Abuse may occur in one of two settings. Domestic abuse is perpetrated within the home of the victim or a caregiver by either a relative or other care provider. Institutional abuse occurs within a designated care facility (residential or nursing home or hospital) perpetrated by one or more individuals having an obligation to care for and protect the victim.

Five major categories of abuse have been identified[3,4]:

1. Physical: any activity involving force to generate bodily injury or pain, including striking or burning. This includes the use of physical or pharmacological restraint (e.g. by means of over-sedation or withholding medication to assist movement such as analgesics or medications for Parkinson's disease).
2. Sexual: any form of non-consensual sexual contact, including unwanted touching, rape, sodomy and coerced nudity.
3. Psychological: the infliction of emotional distress through verbal or non-verbal acts, including insults, threats, humiliation, infantilization and harassment.
4. Financial: the improper use of an elder's property or assets, including theft, deception, coercion and misuse of authority to act, such as power of attorney.
5. Neglect: the refusal or failure to fulfil basic care obligations including the provision of food, water, clothing, medication, comfort and protection.

PREVALENCE AND INCIDENCE

Variability in case definition obscures direct comparison, although the prevalence of elder abuse is broadly similar throughout Europe and North America. To date there are few data from developing countries. With the exception of the United States, a paucity of robust national incidence data reflects widespread absence of formal mechanisms for case reporting and validation.

Differing study populations and sampling techniques have also contributed to a range of prevalence and incidence estimates[5]. The work by Thomas[6] described a range of estimates across studies of between 2% and 10%. This suggests elder abuse is sufficiently prevalent to be regularly encountered by all health care workers looking after older adults. Lachs and Pillemer[5] estimate that for every 20–40 older adults seen, there is one victim of abuse.

VICTIM CHARACTERISTICS

Likelihood of abuse increases with age[7]. Older women are more likely than men to be victims[8] but this observation may be confounded by greater likelihood of longer life expectancy[3]. Poverty elevates the risk of abuse[7].

Shared living is considered a major risk factor, due to increased opportunities for contact. Living alone is associated with lower risk, except for financial abuse[9,10]. Social isolation from other family members and friends (apart from the perpetrator(s)) is an additional risk factor[11].

Dementia is associated with higher rates of abuse than in cognitively intact older adults[11,12]. Cooper *et al.*[13] described an abuse prevalence of 52% from carers among a population with dementia. They discussed the 'spectrum of behaviour' in patterns of abuse, with 34% reporting seemingly important levels of abuse and lower rates of more serious abuse or physical harm. Behaviour disturbance, agitation or aggression is likely to fuel caregiver abuse. Carers are themselves also at risk of physical abuse from those with challenging behaviours. In one series, a third of carers reported physical abuse by the patient, which in turn was associated with abuse of the patient by the carer[14].

Interestingly, neither the level of dependency of an older adult on a caregiver nor the severity of caregiver stress have been identified as risk factors in a variety of research studies[5]. Similarly there is no proven relationship between degree of physical impairment and abuse.

Principles and Practice of Geriatric Psychiatry, 3rd edn. Edited by Mohammed T. Abou-Saleh, Cornelius Katona and Anand Kumar
© 2011 John Wiley & Sons, Ltd

Abuse in institutional care settings has been associated with a number of factors: inadequate staffing levels, frequent use of non-permanent staff, poor staff training, development and supervision, and inadequate incident reporting systems.

Vulnerability to abuse has been associated with certain personality traits[15]. Victims of psychological abuse have less ability to control problem situations and tend to react aggressively when feeling anger or frustration. In contrast, physical abuse victims pursue passive or avoidant behaviour, while financial abuse victims possess negative beliefs of self-efficacy and turn aggression or frustration on themselves.

ABUSER CHARACTERISTICS

Greater understanding of abusive situations has focused attention on those perpetrating abuse. Nearly half of all abusers are related to the victim, but only a small minority are the primary carer[3]. Carers who do abuse suffer social isolation, feel unsupported and may be financially dependent on the person they are abusing.

The strongest associations with perpetrators of abuse are with mental health disorders and drug and alcohol misuse. In particular depression and anxiety among carers are associated with abusive behaviour[16,17].

Abusers identified as misusing substances are likely to be male children of the victim, less likely to provide care and more likely to cause physical or psychological abuse than financial abuse[18]. Alcohol misuse and dependency have been demonstrated to have a strong association with the abuser across a number of studies[19,20].

NATURAL HISTORY OF ABUSE

The inconsistencies in definitions, poor recognition and under-reporting of cases create difficulties in examining outcomes. Corroborated abuse is associated with greater risk of death for elderly victims (odds ratio 3.1; 95% confidence interval 1.4–6.7) after adjusting for co-morbid and demographic factors[21]. However abuse rarely leads to homicide: in one American study only 2% of elderly homicides could be attributed to abuse[22].

Association has also been established between abuse and adverse outcomes including depressive illness and entry to 24-hour care[23]. Victims are also more likely to use behavioural health services[24].

RECOGNITION

Diagnosis of elder abuse requires a high index of suspicion. Professionals should be alert to the presence of one or more risk factors for abuse (Table 134.1) and sensitive to principal abuse signals. Although advocated by some authorities, no good evidence exists to support the routine use of screening tools to detect abuse[5]. Some assessment instruments have had limited value, but are poorly validated and lack outcome improvements to support their regular employment. There is no replacement for the general vigilance of health care workers supported by high-quality training in recognition, assessment and management.

In cases of suspected abuse, a coordinated multi-agency approach must identify all care needs and deficiencies. Corroborated history must be obtained from all participants including victim, alleged

Table 134.1 Risk factors for abuse

Victim	Age >75
	Living alone (financial abuse)
	Living with spouse or child (physical, sexual or psychological abuse)
	Low income
	Cognitive impairment
	Poor premorbid relationship with carer
	Abusive, passive or avoidant behaviour
Abuser	Male (physical abuse)
	Female (psychological abuse)
	Social isolation
	Financial dependency
	Impaired physical or mental health
	Substance abuse
	History of receiving or perpetrating abuse

abuser and designated carers with careful verification of information obtained from cognitively impaired individuals.

Symptoms and signs of abuse must be elicited during a comprehensive clinical assessment to which the victim consents (Table 134.2). Accurate documentation including note keeping, radiology and photography will facilitate planning and may be vital for future prosecutions.

MANAGEMENT

Central to effective management is the establishment of a single co-ordinating agency providing education, advice and access to resources. Intervention models should be low cost, multidisciplinary, collaborative and capable of evaluating outcomes[25]. Denial, resistance to intervention, ignorance of intervention protocols, confidentiality and fear of reprisal have all been cited as professional barriers to the management of elder abuse[26].

Identification of incipient abuse should generate a brisk response to avoid escalation. Integral to management of cases is the aim to preserve autonomous choice for the victim and avoid paternalistic action which seeks to provide a speedy resolution, perhaps through institutionalization. Assessment of mental capacity is essential to determine the extent to which they can contribute to the assessment and management process. Accurate identification of unmet care needs should generate planned and effective care strategies which engender safety without intrusion. Given that abuse may be multidirectional, attention may need to be focused on both victim and abuser.

Overtly criminal activity such as theft or assault should be dealt with by prevailing criminal law. Most countries have eschewed a legislative approach to elder abuse, relying instead upon health and social service agencies to develop locally applicable policies and procedures. In the United States mandatory reporting laws have achieved only limited success and professionals remain unfamiliar with reporting procedures[27]. Of greater potential benefit for the future is the emergence of national organizations aiming to prevent the abuse of older people by disseminating research, informing public policy and providing specialist advice and training to both professionals and the general public[28].

Table 134.2 Symptoms and signs of abuse (National Center on Elder Abuse, 2000)

Physical abuse	Carer refusal to permit examination
	Reports of being hit, kicked or mistreated
	Unexplained behavioural disturbance
	Presence of unexplained bruises, lacerations, ligature marks, fractures
	Untreated injuries in various stages of healing
	Inappropriate use of prescribed medication
Sexual abuse	Reports of sexual assault or rape
	Bruising of breasts or genital area
	Torn, stained or bloody underclothing
	Unexplained genital infection or bleeding
Psychological abuse	Reports of verbal or emotional mistreatment
	Withdrawal, non-communication or non responsiveness
	Unexplained or unusual agitation or behavioural disturbance
Financial abuse	Reports of financial exploitation
	Unauthorized or unexplained changes in banking practice
	Abrupt, unauthorised or unexplained changes to financial documentation
	Unexplained disappearance of assets
	Unmet care needs in the presence of adequate financial resources
	Sudden appearance of individuals asserting their rights to an elder's assets
Neglect	Reports of mistreatment
	Failure to provide food and hydration
	Failure to meet clearly identified care needs
	Hazardous or unsanitary living conditions

REFERENCES

1. Bennett G, Kingston P. *Elder Abuse: Concepts, theories and interventions*. London: Chapman and Hall, 1993.
2. World Health Organization. *Missing Voices; Views of Older People on Elder Abuse*. Geneva: WHO, 2002.
3. Action on Elder Abuse. *Hidden Voices: Older People's Experience of Abuse*. London: Help the Aged, 2004.
4. National Center on Elder Abuse. Briefing Papers, National Aging Information Center, Washington, 2000.
5. Lachs MS, Pillemer K. Elder abuse. *Lancet* 2004; **364**: 1263–72.
6. Thomas C. First National Study of Elder Abuse and Neglect: contrast with results from other studies. *J Elder Abuse Neglect* 2002; **12**: 1–14.
7. Lachs MS, Williams C, O'Brien S, Hurst L, Horwitz R. Older adults: An 11-year longitudinal study of adult protective service use. *Arch Intern Med* 1996; **156**: 449–53.
8. Wilson G. Abuse of elderly men and women among clients of a community psychogeriatric service. *Br J Social Work* 1994; **42**: 681–700.
9. Lachs MS, Williams C, O'Brien S, Hurst L, Horwitz R. Risk factors for reported elder abuse and neglect: a nine year observational cohort study. *Gerontologist* 1997; **37**: 469–74.
10. Choi NG, Kulick DB, Mayer J. Financial exploitation of elders: analysis of risk factors based on county adult protective services data. *J Elder Abuse Neglect* 1999; **10**: 39–43.
11. Lachs MS, Berkman L, Fulmer T, Horowitz RI. A prospective community-based pilot study of risk factors for the investigation of elder mistreatment. *J Am Geriatr Soc* 1994; **42**: 169–73.
12. Dyer CB, Pavlik VN, Murphy KP, Hyman DJ. The high prevalence of depression and dementia in elder abuse or neglect. *J Am Geriatr Soc* 2000; **48**: 205–208.
13. Cooper C, Selwood A, Blanchard M, Walker Z, Blizard R, Livingston G. Abuse of people with dementia by family carers: representative cross-sectional survey. *BMJ* 2009; **338**: 583–86.
14. Coyne A, Reichman WE, Berbig LJ. The relationship between dementia and elder abuse. *Am J Psychiatry* 1993; **150**: 643–46.
15. Comijs HC, Jonker C, van Tilburg W, Smith JH. Hostility and coping capacity as risk factors of elder mistreatment. *Soc Psychiatry Psychiatr Epidemiol* 1999; **34**: 48–52.
16. Homer A, Gilleard CJ. Abuse of elderly people by their carers. *BMJ* 1990; **301**: 1359–62.
17. Paveza GJ, Cohen D, Eisdorfer C *et al.* Severe family violence and Alzheimer's disease: prevalence and risk factors. *Gerontologist* 1992; **32**: 493–97.
18. Hwalek MA, Neale AV, Goodrich CS, Quinn K. The association of elder abuse and substance abuse in the Illinois Elder Abuse System. *Gerontologist* 1996; **36**: 694–700.
19. Reay AM, Browne KD. Risk factor characteristics in carers who physically abuse or neglect their elderly dependants. *Aging Ment Health* 2001; **5**: 56–62.
20. Anetzberger GJ, Korbin JE, Austin C. Alcoholism and elder abuse. *J Interpers Violence* 1994; **9**: 184–93.
21. Lachs MS. Williams CS, O'Brien S, Pillemer KA, Charlson ME. The mortality of elder mistreatment. *JAMA* 1998; **280**: 428–32.
22. Falzon AL, Davis GG. A 15 year retrospective review of homicide in the elderly. *J Forensic Sci* 1998; **43**: 371–74.
23. Lachs MS, Williams CS, O'Brien S, Pillemer KA. Adult protective service use and nursing home placement. *Gerontologist* 2002; **42**: 734–39.
24. Schonfeld L, Larsen RG, Stiles PG. Behavioural health services utilisation among older adults identified within a state abuse hotline database. *Gerontologist* 2006; **46**: 193–99.
25. Reis M, Nahmiash D. When seniors are abused: an intervention model. *Gerontologist* 1995; **35**: 666–71.
26. Krueger P, Patterson C. Detecting and managing elder abuse: challenges in primary care. *Can Med Assoc J* 1997; **157**: 1095–100.
27. Jones JS, Veenstra TR, Seamon JP, Krohmer J. Elder mistreatment: national survey of emergency physicians. *Ann Emerg Med* 1997; **30**: 473–79.
28. Jenkins G, Asif Z, Bennett G. *Listening is not Enough*. London: Action on Elder Abuse, 2000.

135

Care of the Dying

Adrian Treloar, Monica Crugel and Waleed Fawzi

Oxleas NHS Foundation Trust, Memorial Hospital, London, UK

MENTAL ILLNESS AND DYING

It is well recognized that serious mental illnesses of all kinds are associated with higher morbidity and mortality[1,2].

In dementia, the average life expectancy after diagnosis is only 4.7 years[3]. A variety of reasons contribute to mortality from almost all medical conditions occurring during a dementia illness. Dementia itself makes patients prone to acquire pneumonia (due to swallowing difficulties), urine infections (due to poor fluid intake, incontinence) and fractures (due to mobility problems). Dementia will also lead to late diagnosis with consequent higher mortality from many conditions. It limits the treatment options for conditions such as cancer, where the dementia may make intensive and painful treatments too burdensome to consider. Poor compliance with treatment also causes mortality. When dementia occurs in people with Parkinson's disease or Huntington's disease, these increase mortality as well[4]. However, in practice, most death certificates for people who die with dementia make no mention of any contribution made to the death by the dementia[5].

Delirium, which has a high incidence in the elderly and especially in those with multiple physical pathologies, is also associated with a high mortality[6]. While the mortality of delirium is most often thought to be due to its medical causes, death is also undoubtedly more likely due to the poor compliance and reduced motivation to rehabilitate that will be seen in delirium. People with a hyperactive delirium may pull out their drips and resist treatment just when they really need it.

In delirium, the therapeutic aim would be, of course, to make people better and avoid the excess mortality. Much too can be done in schizophrenia to reduce mortality through optimizing treatment, risk management, advice on smoking, diet, exercise and treatment for the antipsychotic-associated diabetes, hyperlipidaemias etc. However, in conditions such as dementia and Parkinson's disease it becomes clear at a certain time that life is indeed drawing towards an end. At such time, care rightly becomes more palliative (with the aim of maximizing comfort and quality of life), ahead of curative treatment.

Palliative care is the active holistic care of patients with advanced progressive illness. Management of pain and other symptoms and provision of psychological, social and spiritual support is paramount. The goal of palliative care is achievement of the best quality of life for patients and their families. Many aspects of palliative care are also applicable earlier in the course of the illness in conjunction with other treatments. Palliative care should help people to live as well as possible until they die. It accepts natural death but seeks neither to prolong nor shorten life.

Clinicians, patients' families and nursing home staff need to recognize and treat advanced dementia as a terminal illness requiring palliative care[7,8].

INTERNATIONAL PERSPECTIVE

Internationally, practice is not uniform but there is a widespread interest and increasing understanding of the need to develop a good evidence base and improved palliative care for people with advanced dementia[7,9,10]. Although in the USA, people with advanced dementia do not need to have another serious illness to qualify for hospice care[7], access of people with advanced dementia to palliative care services is limited both in Europe and in the USA[11]. In the UK, despite the willingness to see non-cancer patients, people with dementia in acute hospitals are only a third as likely to be referred to palliative care as other patients[12], and few are admitted to inpatient hospices[13]. A recent US study has highlighted the low referral rate to palliative care services (22%) and high occurrence of burdensome interventions in people with advanced dementia (40.7% in their last three months of life)[8].

In Germany there is concern about the lack of clear clinical and ethical guidance for decision making in advanced dementia, including the appropriateness of using tube feeding[14]. In France there is increasing interest in developing adequate specific services which follow a palliative care model and a few studies are underway[9]. In some countries (e.g. USA, Germany) it is much commoner to use artificial nutrition and hydration in those dying with dementia[15]. The insertion of PEG tubes (as well as the use of mittens and restraints which are sometimes needed to enable this practice) may be seen as preserving life or, by some, as a burdensome medical intervention which may not be appropriate. UK practice is quite firmly against such methods[16]. But conversely, there is substantial concern in the UK about the underuse of hydration in those who are dying and there are clear reports of a harrowing death occurring without the use of any fluids[17]. We suspect that there is a need for balance here. European continental practice does include more use of parenteral fluids when these are well tolerated by the patient[9].

In other jurisdictions, where euthanasia is legal (e.g. Holland, Belgium, Switzerland, Oregon), euthanasia can also be applied without consent to people with dementia who lack capacity to decide for themselves. But many worry that the availability of euthanasia may make good palliative care less important, and training of lower quality[18]. Deep sedation has been seen as an alternative to euthanasia in Holland[19]. Concern has also been expressed in the UK about the use of some care pathways for those who are dying[20]. Perhaps the biggest worry is that if a diagnosis of dying is made in someone who is not actually imminently dying, the care consequent upon that diagnosis (such as administration of inappropriate sedatives and withdrawal of fluids) may sometimes assure a death that was not imminent. But in the end whichever the jurisdiction there is a very clear need for good and appropriate care for those who are dying. It is entirely unacceptable that those who are dying might not have access to good palliative care in whichever jurisdiction they live. After all, palliative care exists to help people live as well as they can until they die and that must, surely, be available to all.

WHAT ARE THE KEY AIMS OF GOOD PALLIATIVE CARE OF DEMENTIA?

1. Perhaps the greatest aim of good care of the dying is to enable people to live as well as possible until they die. Frail and demented elderly often contribute in many ways to their family and others during their last illness and many people with dementia live well.
2. When patients with dementia or other terminal illnesses are distressed, then that distress ought to be alleviated.
3. Discussion about dying, with a willingness to inform both patients and carers, is important. Discussions enable advance illness planning which can be of great help later on in enabling those with dementia to live as well as possible and also to die well. Last-minute trips to hospital via A&E are to be avoided, and this will most likely be through good discussion and planning.
4. Care of the dying should seek to ensure that treatments given are effective, appropriate and not burdensome, primarily focused on enabling the patient to live well until they die and to reduce suffering.

PRINCIPLES OF PALLIATIVE CARE AS THEY APPLY TO DEMENTIA

Upon its founding, the hospice movement saw symptom control and the alleviation of distress as priorities. Hospices moored this alongside high-quality care and good environments providing oases of quality that were originally mainly afforded to those dying with cancer.

Dame Cicely Saunders, who founded the hospice movement, identified the reality of 'total pain':

- Pain is not just physical, but mental and existential too. All forms of pain/distress must be addressed and treated. It should be said here that the notion that pain (distress) can be both mental and physical is hardly alien to dementia care. Such an understanding has always been a central part of old-age psychiatric care.
- She saw that the patient is a whole person, an interplay of physical, psychological, social and spiritual dimensions. These all have an effect in a single individual and interplay together. So doctors must recognize and respond to psychosocial and spiritual distress, and not just deal with physical disease.
- She saw that the family was the unit of care and that care had to become centred around the person by recognizing the broader family and community.

- She established that symptoms could be analysed scientifically in the same way as any other illness so as to enable best care[21].

The models of palliative care bring with them some useful ethical views. It has long been accepted that sometimes the importance of distress reduction may mean that side effects of treatment might shorten life (double effect). A comfortable death can often be achieved by the appropriate use of medicines, and this may be one reason (see below) why antipsychotics may be justified. The oft-quoted ethics of 'first do no harm' may work a little less well. If the only aim is to avoid harmful treatments, it may not be possible to adequately alleviate distress. The Hippocratic position of 'I will never intend harm' would apply better as all treatment may bring a risk of harm but the intention must always be to improve the patient's condition. So, in the end, the purpose of care is central. If in the care of the dying the primary purpose of care may well be to reduce suffering, while accepting some risk of harm, that is fine. But if the primary purpose is to shorten life, then of course that is not.

The other key concept here is burden of care. When we are mentally well we will accept burdensome treatments so as to become well again, but as frailty increases and death nears, it becomes increasingly wrong to apply burdensome treatments. This helps to define appropriate and inappropriate care.

WHEN IS A MOVE TOWARDS PALLIATIVE CARE INDICATED IN DEMENTIA AND SIMILAR ILLNESSES?

Palliative care may be provided from the onset of an illness if symptoms are distressing. But generally, early on in illness, attempts at a cure and active treatment have more prominence. In progressive, fatal conditions there will, however, be a switch towards a more palliative approach. Factors that indicate that a switch is appropriate are set out in Box 135.1[22].

Box 135.1

Indicators for a transition towards more palliative care
  Severe distress (mental or physical) which is not easily amenable to treatment
  Or
  Severe physical frailty which is not easily amenable to treatment
  Or
  Another condition (e.g. co-morbid cancer) which merits palliative care in its own right
  Occurring in someone with a diagnosis of moderate or severe dementia or other progressive and fatal mental illness.

Therefore, in a frail and weak person with dementia, who can barely walk and is unlikely to survive acute medical care, a gentler and more palliative approach is needed. Similarly, in someone who is suffering due to ongoing mental distress or physical pain a palliative approach is needed. Finally, if someone has cancer and the demands of chemotherapy would be too great (due to the dementia), the focus of treatment must be palliative.

The *Gold Standard Framework* also sets out two ways of identifying when end-of-life care is appropriate[23]. Firstly it asks whether or not the clinician would be surprised if the patient died in the next year. This is a simple question but it is clear that accurate prognosis is very hard in dementia. So, the question will often not be answered positively even in advanced dementia. Many who die would not have been identified by clinicians using the Surprise Question[24]. Moreover, those living happily with dementia may not need specific end-of-life care.

The Gold Standard Framework also suggests that the following indicate the need for end-of-life care:

- unable to walk without assistance; and
- urinary and faecal incontinence; and
- no consistently meaningful verbal communication; and
- unable to dress without assistance;
- Barthel score < 3;
- reduced ability to perform activities of daily living (ADL).

Plus any one of the following: 10% weight loss in previous six months without other causes; pyelonephritis or UTI; serum albumin <25 g/l; severe pressure scores, e.g. stage III/IV; recurrent fevers, reduced oral intake/weight loss; aspiration pneumonia.

However, these indicators are very physical in nature and there is a lack of consistency in the indicators of severity. Inability to communicate meaningfully sits awkwardly alongside reduced ADL skills as an indicator of severity. More importantly, these indicators do not recognize the importance of distress reduction in those with a difficult dementia complicated by behavioural challenge and psychological distress.

WHAT ARE THE FEATURES OF DISTRESS IN PEOPLE WITH ADVANCED DEMENTIA AND OTHER CONDITIONS WHERE IT IS HARD FOR THEM TO EXPRESS THEMSELVES?

Distress might be demonstrated by some or all of the following:

- anger/frustration
- aggression/agitation
- fear/anxiety
- tearfulness/misery
- pain when still
- discomfort on moving
- restlessness
- insomnia
- calling out/vocalization
- wandering and persistent challenging behaviours when these appear to be driven by distress or fear
- autonomic arousal, sweating, tachycardia, hypertension.

WHAT ARE THE CAUSES OF DISTRESS?

Distress may be caused by mental illness, other mental and psychological difficulties and physical difficulties/pain. Distress is in essence pain that is either mental or physical and no sort of distress is less worthy of palliation than any other. So the following causes of distress must be explored:

- depression
- psychosis
- pain

- poor understanding
- fear and anxiety
- insomnia
- hunger and diet
- boredom, isolation and lack of spiritual care
- poor environment including poor staff practices, etc.

In a chapter of this length we can but mention the causes and make a few comments. Physical pain is frequently missed and undertreated in dementia. Its treatment provides a real modality to reduce distress in patients dying with dementia and other mental illnesses. The prevalence of pain in US nursing homes has been estimated between 26% and 83%[25]. Pain is not reported by the elderly who are cognitively intact as it is often attributed to 'natural ageing' and those with dementia are often unable to express their pain[26]. However, studies have demonstrated that patients with a diagnosis of dementia are less likely to receive analgesia compared to those without this diagnosis[27].

Those who appear depressed may well respond to an antidepressant and those who show evidence of psychosis may respond to antipsychotics. Of course, given the harm that we know they do[28], a discussion about risk of harm must always be had whatever the indication or the use of antipsychotics. But if, in the end, antipsychotics represent the best way to reduce severe distress in someone with dementia, then their use may be justified[29].

ADVANCE CARE PLANNING

Receiving a diagnosis such as dementia will rightly lead to a desire to think about and make plans for the future. But the fear that dementia brings may be huge and it is important to give an opportunity to discuss and allay fears where possible. In truth, dementia is a distressing condition, but patients need reassurance that distress is usually managed with the right care, support and medications. Discussion of living well with dementia may be very reassuring. Understanding the palliative model of care may help considerably. A discussion on prognosis and advance care planning can start at diagnosis, and be developed further during the transition from restorative care towards more palliative care.

Of course, early on it is right to treat the memory impairment and to work out ways to delay or reduce disease progression. But, as the illness progresses, treatment is more focused on symptom control and reduction of distress. Various methods allow the planning of care as dementia advances:

Advance Patient Statements

These are broad statements of preference about future care and can be very useful. Patients may ask for specific care at specific times, or ask for assurance that fluids will be given[30]. Most often a simple statement such as "If I have an untreatable or terminal illness I ask for sensible treatments that have a reasonable chance of benefit and that avoid excessive burden" may be helpful. Such statements can enable the patient to guide others towards more appropriate care once capacity has been lost.

Preferred Priorities of Care

The preferred priorities of care protocols[31] enable people with any diagnosis to set out what their priorities are and where they would like to be cared for during their last illness. Of course most choose home, but other preferences too may be helpful. Some will wish a certain style of care, others to see the right people, some to have the right spiritual care etc. Of course such statements should preferably be advisory and not binding as it is hard to predict precisely what needs there will be. In dementia care it is not infrequent to find patients have an expressed desire not to go into nursing care, but that at the time, it turns out that this may be the best care and that they are demonstrably happier (see problems with advance refusals below).

Illness Contingency Planning

As illness progresses it is sensible to consider the scenarios that may lead to change of care. In the UK there is anxiety that death at home is uncommon and also that transfer to acute hospitals from nursing care at a time when patients are, in fact simply dying, occurs too often[32]. It is perfectly sensible to hope to avoid the chaos of acute hospital care at a time when death is inevitable, but with dementia there are special difficulties in achieving this and support for dementia at home until death (though highly effective and well regarded by carers[33]) is rarely available and there are very few specialist services that aim to support such care. This is in complete (and unjustifiable) contrast to the situation for cancer care and other illnesses.

Inevitably though, infections and pneumonias may, unless already thought through, trigger a referral to an emergency department. Several questions can be usefully asked and discussed with carers and advocates and may take into account the declining physical functions and increased risk of other illnesses, infections, falls and fractures associated with dementia, see Box 135.2. It is probably true that the most effective part of this is the discussion itself. A discussion with carers will often have a good effect and enable confidence around ongoing care and dying.

Box 135.2

Advance illness planning questions

Is cardiopulmonary resuscitation, ventilation or intensive care medicine appropriate?

Would treatments with severe side effects be appropriate?

Would complex surgical procedures (such as a major abdominal operation) be appropriate?

Would hospital admission be appropriate for injuries such as fractures?

Would hospital admission be appropriate for illness such as chest infections?

If dehydration occurs and is causing the patient to suffer then would hospital admission be appropriate to treat?

When dying is imminent and the patient is distressed *we would expect* that medication will be given to alleviate the distress that may occur during death.

For some problems the solution will still be hospital. The best treatment of a broken hip is to mend it. The best treatment of a urine infection is antibiotics. But with a pneumonia, oral antibiotics with care at home by usual carers may well be associated with a better outcome than a transfer to hospital. So any plan must always remain flexible to a degree so that contingency can be dealt with.

Advance Decisions to Refuse Treatment

Advance decisions to refuse treatment (ADRTs) may be more challenging in dementia care. In England, Wales[34] and Scotland they are binding but are, fortunately, subject to stringent tests of validity and applicability. As with advance statements, they may well be helpful and give good advice but must be specific and valid. They do enable those who lose capacity to continue to guide their care, but they also carry some risks, and a binding decision might cause unanticipated effects[35].

Case Example

A person with dementia has stated that he only wants symptomatic treatment once his dementia is moderate or severe. Restorative treatment is refused, in the hope that this will enable comfort and that he will not suffer unduly. He then develops a urine infection.

- Does the ADRT prohibit treatment of the infection or can the antibiotic be construed as symptomatic treatment? If it cannot, must the enhanced suffering of living without antibiotics be accepted even though the intention was to reduce distress?
- What if he develops a fractured hip? Is surgery the best analgesic and is it prohibited by the ADRT?
- What if, at the stage of dementia he has, he is happy, enjoying living with his family and all seems well?

The Mental Capacity Act gives some helpful clues here. The ADRT would be invalid if:

- the person withdrew the decision while they still had capacity to do so
- after making the ADRT the person made a lasting power of attorney (LPA) giving an attorney authority to make treatment decisions that are the same as those covered by the ADRT
- the person has done something, which is not in accordance with the ADRT remaining their fixed decision (i.e. they have changed their mind).

The ADRT would be inapplicable if:

- the proposed treatment is not the treatment specified in the ADRT
- the circumstances are different from any specified in the ADRT
- there are reasonable grounds for believing that circumstances have now arisen, which were not anticipated by the person when making the ADRT and which would have affected the ADRT had he anticipated them at the time.

In the case set out, there is a lack of specificity about treatment of a UTI or broken hip making the ADRT not applicable. There would also be reasonable grounds to think that the current circumstance was not anticipated. And, of course, questions about the level of understanding at the time of making the ADRT must be raised. Finally, note that ADRT's are not valid if they apply to life sustaining treatment and are not in witnessed and writing.

Given the complexity, possible benefits and also the possible harms of ADRTs, it is clearly appropriate that dementia specialists ought to advise those thinking of making an ADRT of the risks of making them as well as some of the possible benefits[35].

Lasting Power of Attorney (LPA)

The Mental Capacity Act in England and Wales and Adults with Incapacity Act in Scotland also allow people to appoint decision makers (such as a relative, friend or solicitor) to make decisions for them at a time when they lose capacity. Generally an LPA will trump an advance statement. Authority passes from the ADRT to the LPA if an LPA is appointed. The LPA, of course, must include a respect for the previous wishes and views of the patient in their decision-making process.

PARTNERSHIP WITH PALLIATIVE CARE

Specialist palliative care services do not have the capacity to provide the palliative care needs for those with dementia. Moreover, old-age psychiatry settings, including continuing care units can be seen as providing palliative care by virtue of the work they do in reducing the distress of severe and complex dementia. It is true that old-age psychiatry often underestimates physical pain in dementia, but, on the other hand, specialist palliative care services may struggle with patients who wander and present challenging behaviour. In each district therefore both old-age psychiatry and specialist palliative care can form useful partnerships and undertake mutual learning from each other. This is described in much fuller detail elsewhere[22].

CONCLUSION

The care of the dying is an integral part of good care of the elderly. Mental health services will do well to acknowledge this and develop their understanding of what they already do in terms of palliative care and to then learn more about what they do not do well.

REFERENCES

1. Miller BJ, Paschall CB, III, Svendsen DP. Mortality and medical comorbidity among patients with serious mental illness. *Focus* 2008; **6**: 239–45.
2. Treloar A. Mental health, palliative care for older people and end of life care. In Williamson T (ed.), *Older People's Mental Health Today: A Handbook*. Brighton: Pavilion, 2009.
3. Xie J, Brayne C, Matthews FE. Survival times in people with dementia: analysis from population based cohort study with 14-year follow-up. *BMJ* 2008; **336**: 258–62.
4. National Council of Palliative Care. *Focus on Neurology – Addressing Palliative Care for People with Neurological Conditions*. The National Council of Palliative Care, 2007.
5. NCPC and the Alzheimer's Society. *Exploring Palliative Care for People with Dementia – A Discussion Document*. NCPC and the Alzheimer's Society, 2006.
6. Treloar A. Delirium: prevalence, prognosis and management. Rev Clin Gerontol 1998; **8**: 241–9.
7. Sachs GA. Dying from dementia. *N Engl J Med* 2009; **361**: 1595–6.
8. Mitchell SL, Teno JM, Kiely DK, Shaffer ML, Jones RN, Prigerson HG *et al.* The clinical course of advanced dementia. *N Engl J Med* 2009; **361**: 1529–38.
9. Lopez-Tourres F, Lefebvre-Chapiro S, Fétéanu D, Trivalle C. Soins palliatifs et maladie d'Alzheimer. *La Revue de Médecine Interne* 2009; **30**: 501–7.
10. Kunz R. Palliative care for patients with advanced dementia: evidence-based practice replaced by values-based practice. *Z Gerontol Geriatr* 2003; **36**: 355–9.
11. Volicer L. *End-of-Life Care for People with Dementia in Residential Care Settings*. Alzheimer's Association, 2005.
12. Sampson EL, Gould V, Lee D *et al.* Differences in care received by patients with and without dementia who died during hospital admission: a retrospective case note study. *Age Ageing* 2006; **35**: 187–9.
13. Hughes JC, Robinson L, Volicer L. Specialist palliative care in dementia. Specialised units with outreach and liaison are needed. *BMJ* 2005; **330**: 57–8.
14. Synofzik M. Tube-feeding in advanced dementia. An evidence-based ethical analysis. *Nervenarzt* 2007; **78**: 418–28.
15. Mitchell SL, Teno JM, Roy J, Kabumoto G, Mor V. Clinical and organizational factors associated with feeding tube use among nursing home residents with advanced cognitive impairment. *JAMA* 2003; **290**: 73–80.
16. RCP/BSG Working Party. *Oral Feeding Difficulties and Dilemmas. A Guide to Practical Care, Particularly Towards the End of Life*. Report of a Joint RCP/BSG Working Party Royal College of Physicians and the British Society of Gastroenterology, 2010.
17. Craig G. Artificial hydration and nutrition. Medical treatment or basic human need? In Craig GM (ed.), *Patients in Danger: The Dark Side of Medical Ethics*. Northampton: Enterprise House, 2006, 6–14.
18. Zylicz Z. 'Death on Request' and Dutch euthanasia policy. *Prog Palliat Care* 1995; **3**: 43–4.
19. Reitjens J *et al.* Continuous deep sedation for patients nearing death in the Netherlands: descriptive study. *BMJ* 2008; **336**: 810–13.
20. Treloar AJ. Dutch research reflects problems with the Liverpool care pathway. *BMJ* 2008; **336**: 905–2017.
21. Richmond C. Dame Cicely Saunders. *BMJ* 2005; **331**: 238.
22. National Council for Palliative Care. *The Power of Partnership: Palliative Care in Dementia*. National Council for Palliative Care, 2009.
23. Gold Standards Framework. At http://www.goldstandardsframework.nhs.uk/, accessed 22 Jan 2010.
24. Mitchell SL, Kiely DK, Hamel MB. Dying with advanced dementia in the nursing home. *Arch Intern Med* 2004; **164**: 321–6.
25. Warden V, Hurley AC, Volicer L. Development and psychometric evaluation of the Pain Assessment in Advanced Dementia (PAINAD) scale. *J Am Med Dir Assoc* 2003; **4**: 9–15.
26. Herr KA, Mobily PR. Complexities of pain assessment in the elderly. Clinical considerations. *J Gerontol Nurs* 1991; **17**: 12–19.
27. Nygaard HA, Jarland M. Are nursing home patients with dementia diagnosis at increased risk for inadequate pain treatment? *Int J Geriatr Psychiatry* 2005; **20**: 730–7.
28. Ballard C, Hanney ML, Theodoulou M, Douglas S, McShane R, Kossakowski K *et al.* The dementia antipsychotic withdrawal trial (DART-AD): long-term follow-up of a randomised placebo-controlled trial. *Lancet Neurol* 2009; **8**: 151–7.

29. All-Party Parliamentary Group on Dementia. *Always a Last Resort. Inquiry into the Prescription of Antipsychotic Drugs to People with Dementia Living in Care Homes*, 2008.

30. *R (on the application of Burke) vs. GMC*. 3 WLR 1132; 2005.

31. NHS End of Life Care Publications. *Preferred Priorities for Care (PPC)*, 2008. At www.endoflifecareforadults.nhs.uk/eolc/eolcpub .htm, accessed 11 March 2009.

32. Department of Health. *End of Life Care Strategy – Promoting High Quality Care for All Adults at the End of Life*. London: Department of Health, 2008.

33. Treloar A, Crugel M, Adamis D. Palliative care of dementia at home is feasible and rewarding – results from the 'Hope for Home' study. *J Dementia Care* (Special Issue on Palliative Care. At www.careinfoorg/dementiacare/, accessed Aug 2009.

34. HMSO. *Mental Capacity Act 2005. Code of Practice*. London: HMSO, 2005.

35. NHS End of Life Care Programme and the National Council for Palliative Care. *Advance Decisions to Refuse Treatment. A Guide for Health and Social Care Professionals*, 2008. At www.endoflifecareforadults.nhs.uk/eolc/eolcpub.htm, accessed Aug 2009.

136

Prevention of Mental Disorders in Late Life

Pim Cuijpers[1], Filip Smit[2], Barry D. Lebowitz[3] and Aartjan T. F. Beekman[4]

[1]Department of Clinical Psychology and EMGO Institute for Health and Care Research, VU University and VU University Medical Centre, Amsterdam, The Netherlands
[2]Trimbos Institute (Netherlands Institute of Mental Health and Addiction), and EMGO Institute for Health and Health Care Research, VU University Medical Centre, Utrecht, The Netherlands
[3]University of California, San Diego School of Medicine, La Jolla, CA, USA
[4]Department of Psychiatry VU Medical Centre and GGZ inGeest and EMGO Institute for Health and Care Research, VU University and VU University Medical Centre, Amsterdam, The Netherlands

INTRODUCTION

Prevention in the mental health field has been seen, traditionally, as an area that has been implicitly restricted to issues in childhood and adolescence. If anything, prevention in geriatrics was seen as an oxymoron. Theory and research in prevention were, for a long time, restricted to issues of child development and intervention early in the life course. In an influential report, the Institute of Medicine (IoM) of the US National Academy of Sciences assessed the state of knowledge in prevention research in the 1990s, but could find hardly any studies aimed at prevention of mental disorders in older adults[1]. A more recent follow-up report on prevention of mental disorders by that same institute is aimed completely at children, youth and young adults, while prevention in older adults is not mentioned at all[2].

At the same time, however, prevention of mental disorders in older adults has been the focus of a new line of research. This research has resulted in a growing body of knowledge on how to identify those with the highest risk of developing a mental disorder, several preventive interventions, and some randomized controlled trials showing that prevention may be possible and effective in older adults. Furthermore, considerable progress has been achieved in the field of prevention of mental disorders for younger adults in recent years. The growing number of randomized controlled trials has shown that prevention of depressive and anxiety disorders in adults in general is probably effective, and there is no reason to assume that interventions which are effective in younger adults would not be effective in older adults.

Why be concerned with prevention in late life? As is well covered in other sections of this text, there is the demographic imperative brought about by the overall ageing of the world population and in particular by the ageing of the older population. As pointed out in the classic paper by Kramer (1980)[3], the same dynamics: public health measures, technological development and lifestyle changes, that created this growth in the overall population were also relevant to growth of the population of those with chronic illnesses and disabilities. They

conclude that, in the absence of cures or effective preventive strategies, we will see an explosion in the number of older persons with serious and persistent disabling illnesses, particularly mental disorders. The availability of more efficacious treatments and the accessibility of appropriate services in the community combined to produce huge gains in the life expectancy of those with mental disorders, who in earlier times would have died long before reaching old age. This demographic imperative leads to the conclusion that prevention must be an important part of the agenda of geriatric psychiatry.

For example, major depression currently affects about 3.6–4.8% of persons of 60 years or older, and many more report clinically relevant depressive symptoms[4,5]. At this moment, major depression in all age groups is the fourth disorder worldwide in terms of disease burden, and it is expected to be the disorder with the highest disease burden in high-income countries by the year 2030[6]. Furthermore, the prevalence of depressive disorders in older adults is projected to double from its present level by 2050[7]. Depression is not only a highly prevalent disorder, but it is also associated with a huge loss of quality of life in patients and their relatives[8,9], with increased mortality rates[10], with high levels of service use and with enormous economic costs. The economic costs of depression in the United States were estimated to be $83 billion in 2000[11].

Another reason why prevention is important is that current treatments can reduce the disease burden of depression only to a limited extent. A recent study in Australia estimated that about 16% of the disease burden of major depression is averted in the current health system[12]. Because many patients do not receive an evidence-based treatment, this percentage could rise to 23% if all patients received such an evidence-based treatment. Furthermore, about 40% of all people with a depressive disorder do not receive any treatment. If it would be possible to deliver treatment to all patients with a depressive disorder, 34% of the disease burden of depression could be averted. So, although current treatments are usually considered to be effective in treating depressive disorders, it is estimated that these treatments can reduce the disease burden of

Principles and Practice of Geriatric Psychiatry, 3rd edn. Edited by Mohammed T. Abou-Saleh, Cornelius Katona and Anand Kumar
© 2011 John Wiley & Sons, Ltd

depression by a maximum of 34%[12]. Prevention of the incidence of new cases of major depression has been suggested as an alternative for treatment which may reduce a part of the 66% of the disease burden which is not averted by current treatments[13,14].

In the current chapter we will give an overview of the field of prevention of mental disorders in older adults. First, we will give a definition of prevention in the mental health field. Then we will focus on recently developed methods of identifying the optimal high-risk groups for preventive interventions. Finally, we will describe the interventions that have been developed and the results of research examining the effects of these interventions.

WHAT IS PREVENTION?

The traditional public health view derives from infectious disease and is divided into primary, secondary and tertiary prevention. Primary prevention is directed towards maintaining health by isolating the causes of disease and eliminating or counteracting them. Secondary prevention is directed towards enhancing recovery by case identification and prompt intervention early in the course of illness. Tertiary prevention is directed towards those already ill and emphasizes treatment and rehabilitation.

There is a growing consensus that the traditional public health view is not optimal in mental health. The components of this approach including, for example, concepts such as pathogens, risk factors, disease vectors and definitions of caseness do not translate easily into psychopathology or chronic disease. In the definition of depression which is currently used by most researchers and practitioners in the mental health field, prevention comprises all interventions which are conducted before subjects meet the formal criteria of a mental disorder (according to the DSM-IV[1]). Curative interventions are given to persons who suffer from acute disorders, and maintenance treatments are given to patients with chronic disorders. In this spectrum of interventions, three types of prevention can be distinguished:

Universal prevention is aimed at the general population or parts of the general population, regardless of whether they have a higher than average risk of developing a disorder. The best-known examples of universal prevention include school programmes aimed at all students, whether they have an increased likelihood of developing a mental disorder or not; and mass media campaigns, aimed at the general population.

Selective prevention is aimed at high-risk groups, who have not yet developed a mental disorder. High-risk groups include people who have recently experienced a stressful life event or who experience a chronic stressor, such as divorce, losing a family member through death, caring for an ill family member, and unemployment.

Indicated prevention is aimed at individuals who have some symptoms of a mental disorder but do not meet diagnostic criteria.

In this chapter, we will give an overview of selective and indicated preventive interventions for older adults. Because universal interventions have not been developed systematically or examined in well-designed trials, we will not discuss these possibilities here. Then we will look at the research examining whether preventive interventions are actually capable of preventing the incidence of new cases of mental disorders, and we will describe new methods of identifying optimal target groups for prevention of mental disorders in older adults.

SELECTIVE PREVENTION

In the past decades, several indicated preventive interventions for older adults have been developed, including interventions aimed at widows and widowers, caregivers of frail older adults, older adults with a chronic general medical illness, and inhabitants of homes for the elderly and nursing homes. Several of these interventions are not specifically aimed at older adults, because there are also younger adults who lose their spouse or get a chronic general medical disorder, but the chance of belonging to such a high-risk group is much greater among older adults. Therefore, it seems reasonable to consider such interventions as prevention for older adults.

One important group of selective preventive interventions is aimed at widows and widowers. They are an important high-risk group for mental disorders[15], and several preventive interventions have been developed, including social support groups and widow-to-widow programmes. In social support groups, widows and widowers come together in small groups to exchange experiences and emotions, with a clear preventive focus. However, research examining the effects of these groups has not resulted in strong evidence for their effectiveness[16]. Another preventive intervention developed for widows and widowers are the so-called 'Widow-to-widow' programmes[17,18]. In these programmes, widows who have recently lost their spouse are visited by another widow who lost their spouse some time earlier. Early research showed promising effects of these programmes, but a larger recent trial did not find any beneficial health effects of such a programme[19].

Another group of selective preventive interventions is aimed at caregivers of frail older adults. Because of the stressful situation they live in and the burden of care, this is an important high-risk group for the development of mental disorders[20]. Several types of interventions have been developed for caregivers, many of which have a clear preventive goal in terms of preventing mental disorders or severe stress-related problems. Interventions for these caregivers include support groups and psycho-educational interventions[21], respite care[22], home visits[23], and multi-component interventions in which different interventions are combined and adapted to the need of the caregiver[24]. Research examining these interventions has typically resulted in small to moderate effect sizes on mental health outcomes in caregivers, with limited clinical impact[25,26], although multi-component interventions seem to be more effective[27].

Several multifaceted interventions have been developed for the prevention of late-life depression in residential care[28,29], where the prevalence of depressive disorders is very high[30]. Such interventions focus on the training of nurses and doctors, on consultation and on supportive interventions for the residents. A few trials have found encouraging effects of these interventions[28,29]. Another study found significant effects for screening and early intervention in residential homes for the elderly[31], although this should be considered as indicated prevention or even treatment.

Older adults with chronic general medical illnesses are another important target group for selective prevention. In this area, several well-designed studies have been conducted, and these studies have actually examined whether preventive interventions are capable of preventing the onset of new cases of mental disorders. Rovner and colleagues (2007)[32] screened older patients with neovascular macular degeneration, and found that problem-solving treatment resulted in a significantly lower incidence rate of new cases of depressive disorders at two and six months follow-up. Robinson and colleagues

(2008)[33] found that both problem-solving treatment and antidepressive medication resulted in a significantly lower incidence rate of major depressive disorders in stroke patients.

This overview of selective preventive interventions is not comprehensive, but it gives a good idea of the possibilities that are available for developing preventive interventions for older adults at risk of getting a mental disorder.

INDICATED PREVENTION

In the past decades, several indicated preventive interventions, aimed at older adults with sub-threshold symptoms but no mental disorder, have been developed. Until now, these interventions have focused mainly on depression. The first type of indicated prevention we want to present is the psycho-educational 'Coping with Depression' course (CWD). This intervention was originally developed as a group treatment for depression. However, because of its psycho-educational nature, it can also be applied relatively easy as a preventive intervention. As we will see later on, the CWD (for all age groups) has been used in 6 of the 19 randomized controlled trials which have examined the effects of prevention on the incidence of major depression in those who did not have a depressive disorder at baseline.

The CWD is a cognitive behavioural intervention which is usually conducted in group format with 8 to 12 participants. Because of the psycho-educational format, there is no therapist or patient, but only teachers and students. Therefore, older adults with depressive symptoms do not have to go into treatment, but only go to a course where they learn how to improve their mood. Apart from behavioural activation, the students also learn cognitive restructuring skills, and social skills. The CWD is not only used in older adults, but also in many other target groups, including adolescents, minority groups, primary care patients, and general medical patients. There is much research examining the effects of the CWD as treatment of existing depressive disorders and as prevention of new cases[34,35]. These studies show that the CWD is an effective treatment for depression, but is also effective in preventing new cases of depressive disorders. A recent randomized controlled trial in the Netherlands, where the CWD is offered as a preventive intervention to older adults in about 80% of the regions, showed that the CWD effectively reduces the level of depressive symptoms in participants in these courses[36]. However, this study also showed that about 40% of the participants in these courses in routine care did have an established major depressive disorder, and so it cannot be seen as a purely preventive intervention. However, because of the low threshold for participation, and the reluctance of many older adults to seek treatment for existing depressive disorders[37], this does not seem to be a problem from a public health point of view.

Another preventive intervention for depression in older adults is life review and reminiscence. In life review interventions, older adults discuss their life and the evaluation of each important period in their life with a trained professional. Several randomized controlled studies and meta-analyses have shown that these interventions are effective in reducing existing depressive symptoms[38], as well as increasing life-satisfaction and emotional well-being[39]. Although the effects have not yet been examined in target groups in which sub-threshold depression was established with a diagnostic interview, life review seems to be an excellent intervention for indicated prevention, because of its low threshold for participation, because the stigmatizing word 'depression' is not needed, and because no understanding of negative thoughts or other complex psychological issues is necessary for participating successfully in this intervention.

More recently, the internet has been found to offer promising new opportunities for the prevention of mental disorders in all age groups, including older adults. A considerable number of studies have found that internet-based cognitive behaviour therapy (CBT) is effective in the treatment of depression and anxiety disorders[40]. In one study, internet-based CBT has been found to be effective in the treatment of sub-threshold depression in older adults[41], which can be seen as indicated prevention. This study showed that internet-based CBT had large effects on depressive symptomatology in older adults, and was as effective as a preventive group intervention.

Another recent development is the use of stepped-care models for the prevention of depressive disorders in older adults with sub-threshold depression or anxiety[42,43]. In a large, randomized, controlled trial, older adults with sub-threshold depression or anxiety were recruited from primary care and assigned to a preventive stepped-care programme or usual care. Stepped-care participants sequentially received watchful waiting, CBT-based bibliotherapy, CBT-based Problem Solving Treatment, and finally referral to primary care for medication, if required. It was found that cumulative incidence of DSM-IV major depressive disorder or anxiety disorder after 12 months was reduced from 24% (20/84) in the usual care group to 12% (10/86) in the stepped-care group, which indicates a relative risk of 0.49 (95% confidence interval: 0.24–0.98). These results are better than those found in the meta-analysis of preventive interventions for depression[44], and may indicate that stepped care is an excellent method for the prevention of mental disorders in older adults.

IS IT POSSIBLE TO PREVENT THE INCIDENCE OF MAJOR DEPRESSION?

In the past decades, hundreds of controlled studies have examined the effects of mental health programmes aimed at preventing mental health problems in children, adolescents, adults and older adults[14,20]. This considerable body of research has shown that some prevention programmes in mental health are capable of strengthening protective factors, such as social skills, problem-solving skills, stress-management skills, pro-social behaviour and social support; that these programmes can reduce the consequences of risk factors, psychiatric symptoms and substance use; and that they may have positive economic effects. Despite this large body of research, however, relatively few studies have examined whether these prevention programmes are actually capable of reducing the incidence of new cases of mental disorders defined according to diagnostic criteria, although this research question can easily be regarded as one of the most important ones, both from a public health perspective and from a scientific point of view.

In the past 15 years, a growing number of studies has examined whether it is possible to prevent the incidence of mental disorders in persons who do not have an established disorder at the start of the preventive intervention. Most of these studies are aimed at the prevention of depression[44], and some are aimed at the prevention of anxiety disorders[45-48]. A recent meta-analysis of studies examining the effects of preventive interventions on the incidence of depressive disorders found that the incidence rate ratio of developing a depressive disorder was 0.78 (95% confidence interval: 0.65–0.93) for participants in the prevention conditions compared to control subjects, which indicates that participants in the preventive interventions have 22% less chance of developing a depressive disorder in the next year[44].

Only a few of the studies in this area have been conducted with older adults[32,33,43], but those that have been conducted find results which are comparable to the studies that have been conducted with younger adults. More research is clearly needed to establish the possibility of preventing the incidence of mental disorders in older adults, but research in younger adults suggests that this is a promising field of investigation.

IDENTIFYING TARGET GROUPS FOR PREVENTIVE INTERVENTIONS

As we have seen earlier in this chapter, several interventions have been developed for older adults who are at risk for developing a mental disorder, such as caregivers of frail elderly, those who have lost their spouse, people who have chronic general medical disorders, and people with sub-threshold depression. Although many of such risk indicators for mental disorders are known, their specificity is low. This means that most people in these high-risk groups will never develop a mental disorder[14,49]. Although much epidemiological research is available showing that such indicators are associated with an increased risk of developing a mental disorder, this research is not very useful in identifying the optimal high-risk groups for preventive interventions. The traditional indicators of the strength of a predictor for the incidence of such disorders, such as a relative risk or odds ratio, are not sufficient for identifying the best target populations for preventive interventions. Suppose, for example, that the risk of developing a major depressive disorder in the general population is 2.5% in one year[50,51]. If a high-risk group has a relative risk of developing a depressive disorder of 4.00, this will be highly significant (if the research population is large enough). But, this means that still only about 10% of the high-risk group will actually develop a depressive disorder, and 90% will not. A high-risk group will probably be difficult to motivate for participation in a preventive programme if only 10% eventually will develop the disorder, apart from the question of whether it is ethically acceptable to intervene in such a population. Furthermore, such an intervention is probably not very efficient and cost effective, because by far the majority will never develop a disorder and the intervention has no preventive effect in this majority.

Recently, more advanced methods have been developed to identify the optimal target groups for preventive interventions in at-risk older adults. After the identification of significant risk indicators, this method starts with calculating three other statistics that can help us in identifying the optimal target populations. First, the exposure rate (ER), which gives the percentage of the population exposed to the risk indicator. The second statistic is the population attributable fraction (AF), which indicates by how many percentage points the current incidence rate of depression in the population would be reduced if the adverse effect of the risk indicator is completely blocked[13,52]. This equals the maximum possible impact of a completely successful preventive intervention. Third, the number-needed-to-be-treated (NNT) can be interpreted as the number of people that should be targeted by a preventive intervention to avoid the onset of the disorder in one person (assuming that the preventive intervention is completely successful in containing the adverse effect of the risk factor).

When target populations for preventive interventions are selected, the ER and the NNT should be as small as possible, while the AF of the target population should be as high as possible. This allows us to identify small target populations with the largest possible proportion of new incident cases, while the number of subjects that have to be treated with the preventive intervention is as small as possible. There are several ways of finding the most optimal combinations of risk indicators (small ER and NNT, large AF), including a straightforward exploration of all possible combinations of significant risk indicators[13], but also more sophisticated methods such as CART analyses (classification and regression tree analysis), and bootstrap aggregation (bagging).

In one study, it was found that older adults with (subclinical) depressive symptoms, functional limitations, a small social network, and female gender comprised only 8% of the total older population (ER), while 24.2% of the new incident cases could be attributed to this group (AF)[53]. The number of subjects from this population that would have to receive a preventive intervention in order to prevent one incident case (NNT) was 4 (assuming that the intervention was 100% successful). In another prospective study among older adults, CART analyses were used to identify the optimal groups for indicated prevention (high-risk groups) and universal prevention (sub-threshold depression present)[54]. In the selective prevention model, spousal death showed the highest risk, becoming even higher if the subjects also had a chronic illness. In the indicated prevention model, sub-syndromal symptoms of depression were associated with a risk of almost 40% of developing depression and an NNT of 5.8, accounting for 24.6% of new cases. Adding more risk factors raised the absolute risk to 49.3%, with a lower NNT, but also lower AF values. Overall, the attributable fraction values in the indicated model were found to be higher, identifying more people at risk. A third prospective study was aimed at the identification of the optimal target groups for prevention of anxiety disorders among older adults[55]. In this study it was found that several factors were significantly associated with increased risk of developing anxiety, including sub-threshold anxiety, depression, two or more chronic illnesses, poor sense of mastery, poor self-rated health and low educational level.

Although this methodology of identifying the optimal target groups for preventive interventions in epidemiological research has been developed well, it has not yet been used in actual intervention studies. Designing such studies is certainly one of the most important challenges for interventions researchers in the years to come.

CONCLUSIONS

In this chapter, we have tried to illustrate why prevention of depression in older adults is important. Reasons for its importance include its very high prevalence, incidence, disease burden and the huge economic costs of depression. It is also important because current treatments can reduce the disease burden by about one-third, while two-thirds cannot be avoided, even when only evidence-based treatments are given and all depressed patients receive such an intervention.

We also showed that traditional epidemiological research cannot identify the best target populations for prevention. Relatively simple statistics, such as the exposure rate, the population attributable fraction, and the numbers-needed-to-be-treated can be used to select those high-risk groups which are as small as possible, but explain as many of the new incident cases as possible.

Research in the past decade has also shown that preventive interventions in all age groups are probably effective and can reduce the incidence by about one-quarter, and the few studies that have been conducted with older adults find comparable results. Psycho-educational cognitive behaviour therapy is the most used preventive intervention for depression and is already implemented in some countries. In the next few years, the internet will probably give new opportunities for the broad implementation of preventive interventions, because access is easy, scalable, economically affordable and effective. Another important development is stepped-care interventions with more intensive treatments when no reduction of depressive symptoms has been realized. It is expected that this type of intervention will be able to reduce the incidence of depression in older adults further.

There is a significant epidemiological transition towards older age and greater morbidity. This process is equally manifest in the workforce for health. After all, the average age of the health care professionals is increasing rapidly. To illustrate, over 50% of the nurses in the European Union are older than 45 years, and their mean age is still on the increase. Increasing demands for health care and restricted supply is one of the key problems in the near future. Therefore a health care system needs to be able to produce significant health gains in an acceptable, effective, scalable and economically affordable way. Empowering people to become the managers of their own good health via preventive self-help interventions offered over the internet is probably one of the most important steps that we need to take now for a better future.

REFERENCES

1. Mrazek PL, Haggerty RI (eds). *Reducing Risks for Mental Disorders: Frontiers for Preventive Intervention Research*. Washington, DC: National Academy Press, 1994.
2. O'Connell ME, Boat T, Warner KE (eds). *Preventing Mental, Emotional, and Behavioral Disorders among Young People: Progress and Possibilities*. Committee on the Prevention of Mental Disorders and Substance Abuse Among Children, Youth and Young Adults: Research Advances and Promising Interventions; Institute of Medicine; National Research Council. Washington, DC: The National Academies Press, 2009.
3. Kramer M. The rising pandemic of mental disorders and associated chronic diseases and disabilities. *Acta Psychiatr Scand* 1980; **62** (Suppl 285): 382–97.
4. Beekman A, Copeland J, Prince M. Review of community prevalence of depression in later life. *Br J Psychiatry* 1999; **174**: 307–11.
5. Steffens D, Skoog I, Norton M *et al*. Prevalence of depression and its treatment in an elderly population: The Cache County study. *Arch Gen Psychiatry* 2000; **57**: 601–7.
6. Mathers CD, Loncar D. Projections of global mortality and burden of disease from 2002 to 2030. *PLoS Med* 2006; **3**: e442.
7. Heo M, Murphy C, Fontaine K, Bruce M, Alexopoulos G. Population projection of US adults with lifetime experience of depressive disorder by age and sex from year 2005 to 2050. *Int J Geriatr Psychiatry* 2008; **23**: 1266–70.
8. Ustun TB, Ayuso-Mateos JL, Chatterji S, Mathers C, Murray CJL. Global burden of depressive disorders in the year 2000. *Br J Psychiatry* 2004; **184**: 386–92.
9. Saarni SI, Suvisaari J, Sintonen H *et al*. Impact of psychiatric disorders on health-related quality of life: general population survey. *Brit J Psychiat* 2007; **190**: 326–32.
10. Cuijpers P, Smit F. Excess mortality in depression: a meta-analysis of community studies. *J Affect Dis* 2002; **72**: 227–36.
11. Greenberg P, Kessler R, Birnbaum H *et al*. The economic burden of depression in the United States: how did it change between 1990 and 2000? *J Clin Psychiatry* 2003; **64**: 1465–75.
12. Andrews G, Issakidis C, Sanderson K, Corry J, Lapsley H. Utilising survey data to inform public policy: comparison of the cost-effectiveness of treatment of ten mental disorders. *Br J Psychiatry* 2004; **184**: 526–33.
13. Smit F, Ederveen A, Cuijpers P, Deeg D, Beekman A. Opportunities for cost-effective prevention of late-life depression: an epidemiological approach. *Arch Gen Psychiatry* 2006; **63**: 290–6.
14. Cuijpers P. Examining the effects of prevention programs on the incidence of new cases of mental disorders: The lack of statistical power. *Am J Psychiatry* 2003; **160**: 1385–91.
15. Onrust S, Cuijpers P. Mood and anxiety disorders in widowhood: a systematic review. *Aging Ment Health* 2006; **10**: 327–34.
16. Schut H, Stroebe MS, van den Bout J, Terheggen M. The efficacy of bereavement interventions: determining who benefits. In Stroebe MS, Hansson RO, Stroebe W, Schut H (eds), *Handbook of Bereavement Research. Consequences, Coping and Care*. Washington, DC: American Psychological Association, 2001, 705–37.
17. Silverman PR. Widow-to-widow: a mutual help program for the widowed. In Price R, Cowen E, Lorion RP, Ramos-McKay J (eds), *Fourteen Ounces of Prevention: A Casebook for Practitioners*. Washington, DC: American Psychological Association, 1988, 175–86.
18. Vachon ML, Lyall WA, Rogers J, Freedman Letofsky K, Freeman SJ. A controlled study of self-help intervention for widows. *Am J Psychiatry* 1980; **137**: 1380–4.
19. Onrust S, Smit F, Willemse G, van den Bout J, Cuijpers P. Cost-utility of a visiting service for older widowed individuals: randomised trial. *BMC Health Serv Res* 2008; **8**: 128.
20. Cuijpers P, van Straten A, Smit F. Preventing the incidence of new cases of mental disorders: a meta-analytic review. *J Nerv Ment Dis* 2005; **193**: 119–25.
21. Brodaty H, Green A, Koschera A. Meta-analysis of psychosocial interventions for caregivers of people with dementia. *J Am Geriatr Soc* 2003; **51**: 657–64.
22. Lee H, Cameron M. Respite care for people with dementia and their carers. *Cochrane Database Syst Rev* 2004; **2**: CD004396.
23. Stuck AE, Aronow HU, Steiner A *et al*. A trial of annual in-home comprehensive geriatric assessments for elderly people living in the community. *N Engl J Med* 1995; **333**: 1184–9.
24. Schulz R, Burgio L, Burns R *et al*. Resources for Enhancing Alzheimer's Caregiver Health (REACH): overview, site-specific outcomes, and future directions. *Gerontologist* 2003; **43**: 514–20.
25. Schulz R, O'Brien A, Czaja S *et al*. Dementia caregiver intervention research: in search of clinical significance. *Gerontologist* 2002; **42**: 589–602.
26. Pinquart M, Sörensen S. Helping caregivers of persons with dementia: which interventions work and how large are their effects? *Int Psychogeriatr* 2006; **18**: 577–95.
27. Gitlin LN, Belle SH, Burgio LD *et al*. Effect of multicomponent interventions on caregiver burden and depression: the REACH multisite initiative at 6-month follow-up. *Psychol Aging* 2003; **18**: 361–74.
28. Llewellyn-Jones RH, Baikie KA, Smithers H *et al*. Multifaceted shared care intervention for late life depression in residential care: randomised controlled trial. *BMJ* 1999; **319**: 676–82.
29. Cuijpers P, Van Lammeren P. Secondary prevention of depressive symptoms in elderly inhabitants of residential homes. *Int J Geriatr Psychiatry* 2001; **16**: 702–8.
30. Rovner BW, German PS, Brant LJ *et al*. Depression and mortality in nursing homes. *JAMA* 1991; **265**: 993–6.

31. Eisses AM, Kluiter H, Jongenelis K *et al.* Care staff training in detection of depression in residential homes for the elderly: randomised trial. *Br J Psychiatry* 2005; **186**: 404–9.

32. Rovner BW, Casten RJ, Hegel MT, Leiby BE, Tasman WS. Preventing depression in age-related macular degeneration. *Arch Gen Psychiatry* 2007; **64**: 886–92.

33. Robinson, RG, Jorge RE, Moser DJ *et al.* Escitalopram and problem-solving therapy for prevention of poststroke depression: a randomized controlled trial. *JAMA* 2008; **299**: 2391–2400.

34. Cuijpers P. A psycho-educational approach to the treatment of depression; a meta-analysis of Lewinsohn's 'Coping with Depression' course. *Behav Ther* 1998; **29**: 521–33.

35. Cuijpers P, Muñoz RF, Clarke GN, Lewinsohn PM. Psychoeducational treatment and prevention of depression: the "Coping with Depression" course thirty years later. *Clin Psychol Rev* 2009; **29**: 449–58.

36. Haringsma R, Engels GI, Cuijpers P, Spinhoven P. Effectiveness of the Coping With Depression (CWD) course for older adults provided by the community-based mental health care system in the Netherlands: a randomized controlled field trial. *Int Psychogeriatr* 2006; **18**: 307–25.

37. Friedhoff AJ. Barriers to care for older adults. In Schneider LS, Reynolds III CF, Lebowitz BD, Friedhoff AJ, *Diagnosis and Treatment of Depression in Late Life; Results of the NIH Consensus Development Conference*. Washington, DC: American Psychiatric Press, 1994, 377–96.

38. Bohlmeijer E, Smit F, Cuijpers P. Effects of reminiscence and life-review on late-life depression: a meta-analysis. *Int J Geriatr Psychiatry* 2003; **18**: 1088–94.

39. Bohlmeijer E, Roemer M, Cuijpers P, Smit F. The effects of reminiscence on psychological well-being in older adults: a meta-analysis. *Aging Ment Health* 2007; **11**: 291–300.

40. Spek V, Cuijpers P, Nyklíček I *et al.* Internet-based cognitive behavior therapy for mood and anxiety disorders: a meta-analysis. *Psychol Med* 2007; **37**: 319–28.

41. Spek V, Nyklíček I, Smits N *et al.* Internet-based cognitive behavioural therapy for sub-threshold depression in people over 50 years old: a randomized controlled clinical trial. *Psychol Med* 2007; **37**: 1797–1806.

42. Van 't Veer-Tazelaar PJ, van Marwijk HWJ, van Oppen P *et al.* Prevention of anxiety and depression in the age group of 75 years and over: a randomised controlled trial testing the feasibility and effectiveness of a generic stepped care programme among elderly community residents at high risk of developing anxiety and depression versus usual care. *BMC Publ Health* 2006; **6**: 186.

43. Van 't Veer-Tazelaar PJ, van Marwijk HWJ, van Oppen P *et al.* Stepped-care prevention of anxiety and depression in late life: a randomized controlled trial. *Arch Gen Psychiatry* 2009; **66**: 297–304.

44. Cuijpers P, van Straten A, Smit F, Beekman A. Preventing the onset of depressive disorders: a meta-analytic review of psychological interventions. *Am J Psychiatry* 2008; **165**: 1272–80.

45. Dadds MR, Spence SH, Holland DE, Barrett PM, Laurens KR. Prevention and early intervention for anxiety disorders: a controlled trial. *J Consult Clin Psychol* 1997; **65**: 627–35.

46. Schmidt NB, Eggleston AM, Woolaway-Bickel K *et al.* Anxiety Sensitivity Amelioration Training (ASAT): a longitudinal primary prevention program targeting cognitive vulnerability. *J Anx Dis* 2007; **21**: 302–19.

47. Gardenswartz CA, Craske MG. Prevention of panic disorder. *Behav Ther* 2001; **32**: 725–37.

48. Swinson RP, Soulios C, Cox BJ, Kuch K. Brief treatment of emergency room patients with panic attacks. *Am J Psychiatry* 1992; **149**: 944–6.

49. Maclure M. Refutation in epidemiology: why else not? In Rothman KJ (ed.), *Causal Inference*. Chestnut Hill, PA: Epidemiology Resources, 1988, 131–8.

50. Bijl RV, De Graaf R, Ravelli A, Smit F, Vollenbergh WAM. Gender and age specific first incidence of DSM-III-R psychiatric disorders in the general population. Results from the Netherlands Mental Health Survey and Incidence Study (Nemesis). *Soc Psychiatry Psychiatr Epid* 2002; **37**: 372–9.

51. Smit F, Beekman A, Cuijpers P, De Graaf R, Vollebergh W. Selecting key-variables for depression prevention: results from a population-based prospective epidemiological study. *J Affect Dis* 2004; **81**: 241–9.

52. Rothman KJ, Greenland S. *Modern Epidemiology*. Philadelphia: Lippincott-Raven, 1998.

53. Smit F, Cuijpers P, Oostenbrink J *et al.* Excess costs of common mental disorders: population-based cohort study. *J Ment Health Pol Econ* 2006; **9**: 193–200.

54. Schoevers RA, Smit F, Deeg DJH *et al.* Prevention of late-life depression in primary care; do we know where to begin? *Am J Psychiatry* 2006; **163**: 1611–21.

55. Smit F, Comijs HC, Schoevers R *et al.* Target groups for the prevention of late-life anxiety. *Br J Psychiatry* 2007; **190**: 428–34.

137

The Principles of UK Mental Health Law: A View from the Clinic

Julian C. Hughes

Northumbria Healthcare NHS Foundation Trust and Institute for Ageing and Health, Newcastle University, UK

INTRODUCTION

On 12 November 1962, in *The New York Times*, Earl Warren, the Chief Justice of the United States, wrote:

> In civilized life law floats in a sea of ethics. Without law, the least scrupulous might prevail, but without ethics, law itself could not exist... without ethical understanding, the law, as a ship of state, would be stranded on dry land.

Mental health is the branch of clinical practice where clinicians can deprive people of their liberty and enforce treatments on them against their wishes. Our clinical decisions are, at one and the same time, ethical; but our ethical decisions must also be, at one and the same time, legal. Our concepts – 'mental disorder', 'incapacity' – carry clinical, ethical and legal weight and show the links between law, ethics and practice.

In this chapter, I shall sketch the mental health legislation that governs England and Wales. For the sake of brevity and prudence, I shall mention other UK jurisdictions only in passing. (Fuller accounts of the laws governing England and Wales can be found in standard texts[1,2].) I shall attempt to raise some broader issues of principle. In this I want to take my lead from Earl Warren, because I want to point to the ways in which there is a necessary interaction between ethics, which in this context I take to imply practice, and law.

In the spirit of questioning, I shall first set the historical scene and gesture at areas of debate. I shall then briefly sketch the main provisions of the two laws now governing practice in England and Wales: the *Mental Capacity Act 2005* (MCA) and the *Mental Health Act* (MHA) *2007*.

SLOW BIRTHS AND CONTROVERSIES

Law is not static, but evolving. The MHA 1983, which was amended by the MHA 2007, had its roots in the 1959 Act, which incorporated the recommendations of the Percy Commission of 1957. That Commission had concluded:

> ...that the law should be altered so that whenever possible suitable care may be provided for mentally disordered patients with no more restriction of liberty or legal formality than is

applied to people who need care because of other types of illness, disability or social difficulty[3].

The Percy Commission recommended that compulsory detention should only be employed where necessary. They made it clear that they wished to see 'the need for care' and 'the justification for compulsion' as two quite separate questions[3]. The assumption, they suggested, that compulsory powers must be used unless the patient can express a positive desire for treatment should be abandoned and replaced by 'the offer of care without deprivation of liberty, to all who need it and are not unwilling to receive it'[3]. This seems very humane and it got rid of the previous situation in which incapacitated compliant patients had to be detained, because they could not agree to treatment. However, although the subsequent 1959 Act was,

> heralded as a great piece of liberalising legislation, ... its reputation became tarnished by concern about failures of services and abuses of professional power. The Act was seen as being deficient in safeguarding the rights of detained patients[4].

So the pendulum swung in favour of greater safeguards for patients. Now we are concerned that the pendulum has gone too far: beyond safeguarding patients to protecting the public from the risks of the potentially dangerous mentally ill[4]. The insistence on reform of the 1983 Act on the part of the government came about when Michael Stone, who had an antisocial personality disorder and had been under psychiatric care, killed a mother and daughter. This led to the home secretary, Jack Straw, offering the following condemnation of psychiatrists:

> Quite extraordinarily for a medical profession, they have said they will only take on those patients they regard as treatable. If that philosophy applied anywhere else in medicine there would be no progress whatsoever. It's time, frankly, that the psychiatric profession seriously examined their own practices and tried to modernize them in a way that they have so far failed to do[5].

The strength of feelings was shown by the response of Robert Kendell, then the President of the Royal College of Psychiatrists, in a radio interview:

Principles and Practice of Geriatric Psychiatry, 3rd edn. Edited by Mohammed T. Abou-Saleh, Cornelius Katona and Anand Kumar
© 2011 John Wiley & Sons, Ltd

There may be a place for some form of preventative detention for men like this. That is an issue for parliament. The home secretary cannot expect psychiatrists to do his dirty work for him when it is at present excluded by law[6].

On the grounds that the 1983 Act was intended for a time when community treatment was in its infancy, when detention in hospital was the main issue, the government set about modernizing mental health law in England and Wales[4]. The subsequent history is well documented: following an expert scoping report, a green paper, a white paper, two draft bills and eight years, in the face of 'vehement, sustained, and almost unanimous opposition from those with an interest in mental health care'[7], the government announced that it would simply amend the 1983 legislation rather than try to bring in a new Act. Nonetheless, as many feared[7], it is arguable that the government's agenda of public safety won the day.

There are certainly contradictory views of the MHA 2007. Writing just before it was passed, Lepping highlighted 'a clear shift away from liberal individualism towards utilitarian thinking'[8]. His complaint was that the government was focusing largely on risk. He felt that innovations such as community treatment orders and the broadening of the definition of mental disorder favoured 'public safety considerations over individual rights'[8]. Responding to this paper, just after the Bill became law, Maden retorted that, 'The best that professionals can do under the 1983 law is sometimes not enough to prevent foreseeable disaster'[9]. He was somewhat dismissive of medical ethics ('... much of medical ethics consists of coming to terms with scientific discoveries') and upbeat about the possibility of predicting violence. In his view, the new Act was a continuation of a process that started with the murder of Jonathan Zito by a psychotic patient in 1992. Since then, he argued, there had been,

a general increase in aversion to risk which is not confined to mental health or, indeed, to any one country. There is no ethical basis for arguing that mental health should remain exempt from this trend, which has swept through most democracies[9].

Maden then referred to changes to criminal justice legislation in England and Wales that 'resulted in judges imposing about 150 indeterminate sentences each month on the grounds of public protection'[9]. This reference was to the *Criminal Justice Act 2003*, which allows dangerous offenders to be given indeterminate sentences, even if their offences do not otherwise justify such detention. Maden presents this almost as a justification for the changes to mental health legislation, as if to say that psychiatrists should stop moaning about rights and get on with accepting their duty to protect the public. Other psychiatrists, however, have not been so happy with the *Criminal Justice Act 2003*, and specifically not with its ethical implications. For,

... under the 2003 Act, psychiatrists are required to give evidence about risk to the sentencing court in relation to a person's mental disorder, irrespective of the treatability of that disorder. This poses similar ethical dilemmas concerning the use of psychiatry solely for public protection, as well as for punishment of offenders, rather than for treatment[7].

Furthermore, the emphasis on public protection flies in the face of recommendations made by the government's own scoping committee – the Richardson Committee:

We are convinced that whatever the precise scope of a mental health act it must primarily be seen as a health measure and must be consistent with the professional ethics of the health services. This is not to deny the importance of public protection but to place it within the appropriate context within which it can best be promoted. The importance of respecting and enhancing patient autonomy is now gaining increased recognition within the health services generally ... and we are satisfied that it must acquire similar recognition within mental health services specifically[10].

If the MHA 2007 took almost 10 years to be born, the MCA took even longer. It emerged in response to high-profile cases in the late 1980s of people with learning disabilities and enforced sterilization[11]. Whereas reform of the MHA has been surrounded by controversy, the MCA developed from an exceptionally well-argued Law Commission Report[12], which led to a very cogent document from the government[13] and a good deal of agreement as subsequent documents emerged prior to its delivery. One largely groundless concern has been that the MCA might bring in euthanasia by the back door. The Act, however, contains a number of defences against this possibility. More alarming to the clinician, perhaps, is the amendment to the MCA – the Deprivation of Liberty Safeguards (DOLS) – brought in by the MHA 2007, to which we shall return.

Nevertheless, there was debate concerning whether, in fact, there should be two Acts (for capacity and for mental health) or just one. It has recently been announced that Northern Ireland will have a single Act, which many elsewhere in the UK will regard with envy. Meanwhile, in Scotland, capacity legislation was amongst the first Acts to be passed by the Scottish Parliament in the form of the *Adults with Incapacity (Scotland) Act 2000*. There is separate mental health legislation, but in the *Mental Health (Care and Treatment) (Scotland) Act 2003*, decision-making ability is a criterion for both emergency detention (36(4)(b)) and for short-term detention (44(4)(b)), where 'because of the mental disorder, the patient's ability to make decisions about the provision of medical treatment is significantly impaired'.

The argument about whether incapacity should be the criterion for compulsory detention and treatment harks back (in a sense) to the aspiration of the Percy Commission[3] that mental illness should be treated no differently from other illnesses. The suggestion is that the rationale for imposing treatment on someone should only be that the person lacks the capacity to make a decision him- or herself. Because this could be applied equally to people with mental illness and to those with other illnesses, it has been argued that this is a way to decrease discrimination and stigma.

The message is as follows, though ill, those with a mental disorder are somehow different. That is why they require separate legislation. They may be treated against their will irrespective of whether they have the capacity to consent to treatment. This suggests a pervasive and disturbing notion that 'mental' patients somehow are incapable of possessing a full degree of autonomy; mental disorder automatically diminishes the sufferer; he or she is not a complete 'person'[14].

Pursuing this point is beyond my present remit and, in the context of England and Wales, is purely academic. I shall turn to consider some of the details of the Acts, with the caveat that what follows is merely a sketch (see[1,2]).

MENTAL HEALTH ACT 2007

The MHA and the MCA both have accompanying Codes of Practice. Whilst the Codes merely provide guidance, it is clear that they cannot be ignored or deviated from without good reason. Box 137.1 contains the five guiding principles of the MHA Code of Practice.

Box 137.1

Summary of Guiding Principles in the MHA Code of Practice

Purpose Principle: Decisions under the Act must be taken with a view to minimizing the harm done by mental disorder, maximizing the safety and well-being of patients and protecting the public from harm.

Least Restriction Principle: People taking action without a patient's consent must attempt to keep to a minimum the restrictions they impose on the patient's liberty, having regard to the purpose for which the restrictions are imposed.

Respect Principle: Diverse needs, values and circumstances, including race, religion, culture, gender, age and sexual orientation must be respected.

Participation Principle: Patients must be involved as far as is possible in planning care. The involvement of carers and others with an interest in patients' welfare should be encouraged unless there are particular reasons to the contrary.

Effectiveness, Efficiency and Equity Principle: Resources are to be used in the most effective, efficient and equitable way.

Some of the changes to the MHA are less likely to affect the older patient. For instance, the MHA 2007 now defines mental disorder simply as 'any disorder or disability of the mind' (Section 1(2)). As in the past, dependence on alcohol or drugs is excluded from the definition of a disorder or disability of the mind, but promiscuity, other immoral conduct and sexual deviancy have been removed from the exclusions. The presumed reasoning behind this change and others is that they allow the detention of a broader range of people who can be subjected to a broader array of treatments. It is coupled with a change that broadens the professional groups that undertake particular roles, so that, instead of 'responsible medical officers', the MHA 2007 talks about 'responsible clinicians', who no longer need to be medical doctors. In addition, the treatability test has been replaced by an 'appropriate treatment test' (Section 4), where this means that the medical treatment is appropriate to the person's case and broadly conceived to alleviate or prevent a worsening of the person's disorder, or one or more of its symptoms or manifestations.

Of more relevance to older patients is the new right to apply to a county court to change the nearest relative (Section 23). This can be seen as a way for patients to maintain their autonomy. Similarly, the amendments in the MHA 2007 include the provision that patients have a right to an advocacy service when under compulsion (Section 30). Patients who are detained should be offered an Independent Mental Health Advocate (IMHA). Again, this could be potentially very helpful to older patients, although how this will work in practice is as yet unsure.

Perhaps the most significant change that could potentially affect older patients is the new provision of Supervised Community Treatment (SCT) (Sections 32–36). SCT provides a framework for the management of patient care in the community, following detention

under e.g. Section 3, and gives the responsible clinician the power to recall the patient to hospital for treatment if necessary. SCT is an alternative to Guardianship, concerning which the law has also been changed. It is now possible to convey the person to the place where he or she is required to reside, which is one of the powers given to the Guardian. The other two powers are: to require the patient to attend for treatment and to allow relevant professionals to have access to the place where the patient lives. In deciding between guardianship and SCT, the Code of Practice suggests that under SCT the focus is on ensuring that the patient continues to receive necessary medical treatment for mental disorder without having to be detained again and it allows compulsory recall, especially where speed is likely to be important (Chapter 28 MHA Code of Practice). On the other hand, the focus of Guardianship is on the patient's general welfare rather than being specifically on medical treatment. Guardianship should be considered where there is little risk of the patient needing to be admitted compulsorily and quickly to hospital. But Guardianship is required where there is a need for enforceable powers to require the patient to reside at a particular place. However, this does not allow the person to be deprived of their liberty and, if this is likely to be the case, then this must be authorized separately under the MCA. The Code also says that it will not always be best to use guardianship as the way to decide where patients who lack capacity must live, since it would be possible to, more simply, use Section 5 of the MCA, which allows that the person's liberty can be restricted. However, some legal experts suggest that Guardianship provides a greater degree of protection to all concerned.

MENTAL CAPACITY ACT 2005

The MCA is much more routinely applicable to older patients, being relevant whenever a person cannot make decisions for him- or herself. It has a dual function: it enables people to retain some control or influence over the decisions that are made on their behalf and it protects those who must provide care to people who cannot decide for themselves. Box 137.2 shows the principles that summarize the intent of the MCA.

Box 137.2

Principles of the MCA (Section 1)

- A person is assumed to have capacity.
- All practicable steps must be taken to help the person to make a decision.
- People are entitled to make unwise decisions.
- Any actions taken on behalf of a person who lacks capacity must be in the person's best interests.
- Before any action is taken it should be the least restrictive of the person's rights and freedom of action.

Section 2 of the MCA defines incapacity as follows:

. . . a person lacks capacity in relation to a matter if at the material time he is unable to make a decision for himself in relation to the matter because of an impairment of, or a disturbance in the functioning of, the mind or brain.

This leads to a two-stage test of incapacity: first, does the person have an impairment of, or a disturbance in the functioning of, their mind or brain? Secondly, does the impairment or disturbance mean the person is unable to make a specific decision when they need to? This is judged by asking whether the person is able to retain (at least for a short while), understand and weigh up the relevant information and communicate his or her decision.

If the person lacks capacity, the central plank of the MCA is that decisions must be made in the person's best interests (Section 4). The MCA Code of Practice explains that 'best interests' cannot be defined because it will be so particular in different circumstances for different people. But it sets out (in Chapter 4) a checklist to help judgements to be made. At the heart of the checklist is the idea that the person's past and present wishes and feelings, values and beliefs, should inform the decisions that are made on his or her behalf. In addition, the views of anyone else engaged in caring for the person or anyone who might have an interest in the person's welfare must be consulted if at all possible. Whilst the details of the MCA should be consulted, this brings into view two other important aspects of the Act. First, it confirms the legal standing of valid and applicable advance refusals of treatment (but they must be both valid and applicable). Secondly, it establishes the concept of a Lasting Power of Attorney (LPA), to make decisions about matters of welfare, which include decisions about healthcare and changes to the place of residence. A LPA, like the previous Enduring Power of Attorney, can also be made to cover property and finance. But a welfare LPA means that a doctor might be faced by a relative with the power to give or withhold consent to the patient's treatment. However, as with all decisions for people who lack capacity, the decisions made by the donee of the LPA must be in the person's best interests and they can be challenged in the Court of Protection if they are not.

Unlike the MHA, the MCA does not allow everyone to have an advocate, but where serious medical treatment decisions or changes to the place of residence are being contemplated, *if the person is not supported* other than by professionals, an Independent Mental Capacity Advocate (IMCA) must be appointed. This is yet another way in which the MCA seeks to protect and enhance the rights of people who lack capacity. This brings to mind Sabat writing:

The means by which we evaluate, and arrive at our conclusions about, the afflicted person's competency may well ultimately be a test of our own competency as thoughtful, judicious, humane human beings[15].

Sections 5 and 6 of the MCA allow that a person may be restrained as long as this is proportionate. However, by an amendment to the MCA brought in by the MHA 2007, it is made clear that, even if restrictions of liberty can be sanctioned under certain circumstances, a deprivation of liberty requires greater safeguards and must be avoided if at all possible. If, where the person lacks capacity and in his or her best interests, a deprivation of liberty is required, then appropriate authorization must be sought. These are the Deprivation of Liberty Safeguards (DOLS). The technicalities of DOLS are beyond the scope of this chapter (see[16]). The distinction between a *restriction* of liberty and a *deprivation* of liberty seems crucial in this connection, but it, too, like 'best interests', cannot be pinned down. This makes life difficult and uncertain at the coalface, but is of con-siderable conceptual interest. The issue is nonetheless clear: as a matter of human rights, vulnerable people must be protected by the law.

CONCLUSION

This brief foray into the law brings us back to Earl Warren: 'Without law, the least scrupulous might prevail, but without ethics, law itself could not exist'. We can see how the laws establish principles as guides to practice, but in the end it is practitioners who must put the law into effect. It is our patterns of practice – be they ethical or unethical – that shape our lives and thereby, collectively, the moral standing of our societies.

REFERENCES

1. Bowen P. *Blackstone's Guide to the Mental Health Act 2007*. Oxford: Oxford University Press, 2007.
2. Bartlett P. *Blackstone's Guide to the Mental Capacity Act 2005*. Oxford: Oxford University Press, 2008.
3. Percy Commission. *Report of the Royal Commission on the Law Relating to Mental Illness and Mental Deficiency 1954–1957* (Cmnd 169). London; HMSO, 1957.
4. Grounds A. Reforming the Mental Health Act. *Br J Psychiatry* 2001; **179**: 387–9.
5. Hansard. *The Parliamentary Debates. Official Report. Sixth Series, Vol. 318*; Column 9, 26 Oct 1998. At www.publications.parliament.uk/pa/cm199798/cmhansrd/vo981026/debtext/81026-02.htm, accessed 24 Jan 2010.
6. Warden J. Psychiatrists hit back at home secretary. *BMJ* 1998; **317**: 1270.
7. Eastman N. Reforming mental health law in England and Wales. *BMJ* 2006; **332**: 737–8.
8. Lepping P. Ethical analysis of the new proposed mental health legislation in England and Wales. *Philos Ethics Humanit Med* 2007; **2**: 5.
9. Maden A. England's new Mental Health Act represents law catching up with science: a commentary on Peter Lepping's ethical analysis of the new mental health legislation in England and Wales. *Philos Ethics Humanit Med* 2007; **2**: 16.
10. Report of the Expert Committee. *Review of the Mental Health Act 1983*. London: Department of Health, 1999.
11. Gillon R. On sterilising severely mentally handicapped people. *J Med Ethics* 1987; **13**: 59–61.
12. Law Commission. *Report No. 231, Mental Incapacity*. London: HMSO, 1995.
13. Lord Chancellor's Department. *Who Decides? Making Decisions on Behalf of Mentally Incapacitated Adults*. London: HMSO, 1997.
14. Szmuckler G, Holloway F. Mental health law is now a harmful anachronism. *Psychiatric Bull* 1998; **22**: 662–5.
15. Sabat SR. *The Experience of Alzheimer's Disease: Life Through a Tangled Veil*. Oxford: Blackwell, 2001.
16. Ministry of Justice. *Mental Capacity Act 2005 Deprivation of Liberty Safeguards: Code of Practice to supplement the main Mental Capacity Act 2005 Code of Practice*. London: The Stationery Office, 2008.

138

Training Requirements for Old Age Psychiatrists in the UK

Susan Mary Benbow[1] and Aparna Prasanna[2]

[1]Centre for Ageing and Mental Health, Staffordshire University, Stafford, UK
[2]Wolverhampton Primary Care Trust, Penn Hospital, Wolverhampton, UK

In the UK over the past 30 plus years increasing numbers of psychiatrists have specialized in working with older adults. Various terms are used to describe this area of work: psychogeriatrics, geriatric psychiatry, old age psychiatry and older people's mental health are probably the most common. In 1978 the Royal College of Psychiatrists formed a Section (which later became a Faculty) of Old Age Psychiatry and in 1989 the Department of Health recognized old age psychiatry as a specialty: this was regarded as a milestone in the specialty's development at the time. The Royal Colleges of Physicians and Psychiatrists produced a Joint Report in 1989, which devoted a chapter to education and training in the psychiatry of old age[1]. Prior to this there was no designated training programme for psychiatrists aiming to work with older people.

BACKGROUND: GROWTH OF THE SPECIALTY

In the early 1980s two surveys of old age psychiatry services reported considerable growth in the developing specialty[2,3], and over 200 consultants were identified by late 1983. The authors predicted continuing growth in the specialty and a need to expand training placements. At that time the Joint Committee on Higher Psychiatric Training at the Royal College of Psychiatrists required higher trainees to spend 12 to 18 months in posts where the majority of the work was in old age psychiatry, and 28 senior registrar placements were identified.

In 1990 there were 360 consultants working mainly in old age psychiatry and by 1993 the total had increased to 405[4]. Figures collected by the Faculty of Old Age Psychiatry showed a continuing gradual increase in consultant numbers, but with a high vacancy rate.

The first Joint Report[1] had recommended that each medical school should have a senior academic in old age psychiatry and that all medical undergraduates should receive training in the subject. Faire and Katona[5] surveyed undergraduate teaching in the UK and reported a considerable expansion in academic old age psychiatry posts. However, they also found a great variation in the amount of clinical experience on offer and the authors felt there was a strong case for all medical students having clinical experience in the specialty as recommended by the Joint Report. Gregson and Dening[6] surveyed teaching hospital psychiatrists and found that many teachers set no

learning objectives in old age psychiatry. Most respondents wanted their teaching to impart enthusiasm for the subject, a sense of hope in working with mentally ill older adults, and an awareness of issues specific to ageing and ageism.

The second Joint Report[7], published in 1998, recommended that the characteristics of mental disorders in older people and the principles of good quality care should be included in the core curricula of all schools of medicine and nursing, and by the time the second edition of this book was published, there were chairs or readerships at a number of medical schools in the UK, although some gaps remained. The twenty-first century brought with it the National Service Framework for Older People[8], which estimated that by 2009, extrapolating from the numbers of existing trainees, there would be 670 old age psychiatrists. It argued the case for increased staff numbers to improve the mental health of older people, and also noted that its recommendations had implications for education and training in undergraduate and postgraduate medicine.

Despite growth in the specialty of old age psychiatry, the long-term prospects continue to cause concern. The Dean of the Royal College of Psychiatrists wrote in his May 2009 newsletter[9] that recruitment into psychiatry as a medical specialty is 'in crisis' with only 6% of candidates for paper 2 of the Membership examination in summer 2008 having gained their primary medical qualification in the United Kingdom. One response to this has been initiatives to try to attract more UK medical students into the specialty, e.g. an official Royal College of Psychiatrists group has been set up on a popular social networking website.

Alongside these developments, postgraduate education has undergone considerable reorganization over recent years. *Modernising Medical Careers*[10] was published in 2004. It aimed to streamline training based on competency-based curricula, and also brought in the foundation programme for newly graduated doctors. In 2005 the Postgraduate Medical Education and Training Board (PMETB)[11] took over responsibility for standards and quality assurance of postgraduate education, training and assessment in medicine and dentistry. The foundation programme has introduced foundation posts in psychiatry to many areas, and with it an opportunity to attract new medical graduates into the psychiatric specialties.

Principles and Practice of Geriatric Psychiatry, 3rd edn. Edited by Mohammed T. Abou-Saleh, Cornelius Katona and Anand Kumar
© 2011 John Wiley & Sons, Ltd

SPECIALIST TRAINING IN OLD AGE PSYCHIATRY

The total minimum duration of specialist training in old age psychiatry is currently six years, of which three years is in core or generic training (core trainee CT1–3) and three years in advanced training (specialty registrar ST4–6). A new curriculum for specialty training in psychiatry and its specialties was approved by PMETB in April 2009 and was introduced in August 2009[12]. Figure 138.1 illustrates the structure of training.

Core Training

A newly qualified doctor intending to specialize in psychiatry will first spend two years on a foundation programme. Following this, competitive recruitment into psychiatry in England is by a standardized national recruitment programme through the Royal College of Psychiatrists. The trainee will undertake core training, which lasts three years and concentrates on providing a range of experience in the specialties and subspecialties of psychiatry. This part of training is common to the various psychiatric specialties. Core training aims to develop history taking, formulation and case presentation skills, therapeutic skills and clinical judgement, relationship with patients/carers and colleagues, and appropriate use of mental health legislation. Experience in old age psychiatry is regarded as an important part of core training because of the increasing elderly population and the high rates of mental illness in older people.

During this time the trainee is preparing to take his/her examination for membership of the Royal College of Psychiatrists. The minimum requirement to sit the Parts 1, 2 and 3 written papers for the Membership examination is 12 months' experience in psychiatry. This may include four or six months of experience of old age psychiatry. The Clinical Assessment of Skills and Competencies (CASC) exam can only be taken after 30 months of experience in psychiatry and is a requirement for entry into advanced training in the different specialties.

In addition, throughout their core and advanced training, trainees undergo a series of workplace-based assessments (WPBA). A number of assessment tools such as assessment of clinical expertise (the trainee's ability to assess a case), case-based discussion (discussion of a clinical case in which the trainee has made a significant contribution) and direct observation of procedural skills (assessment of a practical procedure) can be used[14]. Evidence of achieved competencies is collected using a combination of electronic and paper portfolios.

By the end of three years of approved supervised placements in core training, the trainee is ready to move onto advanced training and will hold the Membership of the Royal College of Psychiatrists (MRCPsych). They will have had sufficient exposure to the psychiatric specialties to decide on their career intentions.

Advanced Training

Higher training offers an educational programme that aims to prepare a trainee for independent practice in psychiatry. Following competitive entry into a specialty training programme, a National Training Number (NTN) is awarded by a Postgraduate deanery. The PMETB sets the standards for training and approves the curriculum, which is developed by the Royal College of Psychiatrists[15]. Trainees receive educational and clinical supervision by approved trainers. On successful completion of an advanced training programme, the Certificate of Completion of Training (CCT) is awarded by the PMETB on recommendation by the Royal College[16]. This gives entry to the General Medical Council's Specialist Register[17]. Since 1997, entry into the Specialist Register has been mandatory for specialists who wish to take up a consultant post in the National Health Service.

Currently, trainees can gain a single CCT in six psychiatric specialties: General Adult, Old Age, Forensic, Child and Adolescent, Learning Disabilities, and Psychotherapy. General Adult psychiatry trainees can gain further endorsements in Liaison, Substance Misuse and Rehabilitation psychiatry. Old Age psychiatry trainees spend three years in advanced training of which one year may be spent in General Adult psychiatry or one of its subspecialties. Academic Clinical Fellows and Clinical Lecturers can (with prior approval) count the time spent in such posts towards a CCT.

During their training, specialty registrars are expected to develop their professional attributes, core knowledge and skills, carry out audit, get involved in teaching and management, and develop research and/or special interests. Eight 'core' sessions are devoted to experience in old age psychiatry (or other specialty). This involves working with a multidisciplinary team to provide a service to a defined population. Two sessions are available to develop research and audit experience or other special interests. Trainees could opt to gain formal higher qualifications relevant to old age psychiatry during this time. Many trainees choose to gain further experience in psychological therapies[18]. They are also expected to gain experience of geriatric medicine at some stage of their training, and this is usually achieved either as a short-term attachment or using special interest sessions.

CONTINUING PROFESSIONAL DEVELOPMENT AS A CONSULTANT

Loane and Barker[19] surveyed newly appointed old age psychiatrists to investigate their views of their higher training experience. Overall their respondents felt that clinical experience was satisfactory, but management experience was lacking in a number of areas, and training was identified as insufficient in relation to experience in dealing with complaints, dealing with difficult professional relationships, recruitment and disciplinary proceedings. Higher trainees are

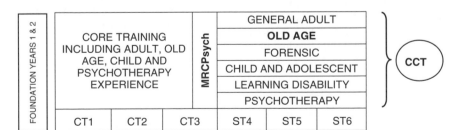

FOUNDATION YEARS 1 & 2	CORE TRAINING INCLUDING ADULT, OLD AGE, CHILD AND PSYCHOTHERAPY EXPERIENCE		MRCPsych	GENERAL ADULT			CCT
				OLD AGE			
				FORENSIC			
				CHILD AND ADOLESCENT			
				LEARNING DISABILITY			
				PSYCHOTHERAPY			
	CT1	CT2	CT3	ST4	ST5	ST6	

Figure 138.1 Training pathway in psychiatry (adapted from six-year psychiatry plan, Royal College of Psychiatrists[13])

expected to get training in management but it is difficult to pitch it at the right level, and constant changes in the health service are challenges to confidence and competencies.

Today lifelong learning is regarded as essential for all health care professionals[20]. Learning does not stop at the transition from trainee to consultant; indeed, some might say that this is the point at which learning really starts. In 2001 the Royal College of Psychiatrists introduced personal development plans (PDPs) as a way of planning continuing professional development prospectively and linked to clear objectives; together with this, participation in peer groups is required in order to review and assist in developing PDPs[21]. This means that consultant old age psychiatrists plan their CPD, although it needs to be flexible and to evolve with the specialty, the individual and the job, since increasingly consultants' interests, disciplines and posts evolve as their career progresses. This may be one way for people to re-energize and deal with the stresses of their multiple roles[22]. CPD is a positive opportunity for consultants to continue learning and developing throughout their working lives.

LIFELONG LEARNING

Learning starts in medical school and continues throughout the working life of the old age psychiatrist. As is true of the whole of medicine, the context within which the specialty operates is constantly evolving, and the specialty itself continues to develop and change[23]. There are always threats and opportunities on the horizon. Old age psychiatry and its practitioners cannot stand still. The enthusiasm which teaching hospital psychiatrists aim to impart to their medical undergraduates can be maintained throughout specialist training and boosted during the course of a consultant career by continuing professional development and the challenge of working in a constantly changing health and social services context.

REFERENCES

1. Royal College of Physicians of London and Royal College of Psychiatrists. *Care of Elderly People with Mental Illness: Specialist Services and Medical Training*. London: Royal College of Physicians, 1989.
2. Wattis JP, Wattis L, Arie T. Psychogeriatrics: a national survey of a new branch of psychiatry. *Br Med J* 1981; **282**: 1529–33.
3. Wattis J, Arie T. Further developments in psychogeriatrics in Britain. *Br Med J* 1984; **289**: 778.
4. Benbow SM, Jolley DJ. A specialty register: uses and limitations. *Psychiatr Bull* 1996; **20**: 459–60.
5. Faire GM, Katona CLE. Survey of undergraduate teaching of old age psychiatry in the United Kingdom. *Psychiatr Bull* 1993; **17**: 209–11.
6. Gregson CA, Dening T. Teaching old age psychiatry to medical schools in England. *Int J Geriatr Psychiatry* 1995; **10**: 883–6.
7. Working Party of the Royal College of Psychiatrists and Royal College of Physicians. *The Care of Older People with Mental Illness: Specialist Services and Medical Training*. London: Royal College of Psychiatrists, 1998.
8. Department of Health. *National Service Framework for Older People*. At www.dh.gov.uk/dr_consum_dh/groups/dh_digitalassets/@dh/@en/documents/digitalasset/dh_4071283.pdf, accessed 15 Feb 2010.
9. Howard R. The Dean's Newsletter, 2009. At www.rcpsych.ac.uk/pdf/May%202009%20Dean%20News.pdf, accessed 12 Jun 2009.
10. Department of Health. *Modernising Medical Careers: The Next Steps*, 2004. At www.dh.gov.uk/en/Publicationsandstatistics/Publications/PublicationsPolicyAndGuidance/DH_4079530, accessed 7 Jun 2009.
11. Postgraduate Medical Education and Training Board. (2003) *PMETB Order 2003*. At www.pmetb.org.uk/index.php?id=order, accessed 7 Jun 2009.
12. Royal College of Psychiatrists. (2009) *A Competency Based Curriculum for Specialist Training in Psychiatry, Specialist Module in Old Age Psychiatry*. At http://rcpsych.ac.uk/training/curriculum/curriculum2009.aspx, accessed 7 Jun 2009.
13. Royal College of Psychiatrists. Six-year psychiatry plan. At http://rcpsych.ac.uk/pdf/6%20year%20psychiatry%20plan.pdf, accessed 10 Jun 2009.
14. Royal College of Psychiatrists. *Trainees' Guide to Workplace Based Assessment*, 2007. At www.rcpsych.ac.uk/docs/Trainees%20guide%20to%20WPBA%2031%2010%2007.doc, accessed 12 Jun 2009.
15. PMETB (2008) *A Reference Guide for Postgraduate Specialty Training in the UK, The Gold Guide*, 2nd edn, June 2008. At http://rcpsych.ac.uk/pdf/Gold%20Guide%202008.pdf, accessed 7 Jun 2009.
16. Royal College of Psychiatrists. *How to Apply for Your CCT*. At www.rcpsych.ac.uk/training/routestospecialistregister/completionoftrainingcct.aspx#apply, accessed 7 Jun 2009.
17. General Medical Council. The Medical Register. At www.gmc-uk.org/register/index.asp, accessed 7 Jun 2009.
18. Stephenson M, Puffett A. Special interest sessions in psychiatry – survey of one higher training scheme. *Psychiatr Bull* 2000; **24**: 187–8.
19. Loane R, Barker A. Newly appointed consultants in old age psychiatry and the adequacy of higher training. *Psychiatr Bull* 1996; **20**: 388–90.
20. Department of Health (2001) *Working Together, Learning Together: A Framework for Lifelong Learning for the NHS*. At www.dh.gov.uk/en/Publicationsandstatistics/Publications/PublicationsPolicyAndGuidance/DH_4009558, accessed 7 Jun 2009.
21. Royal College of Psychiatrists. *CR90. Good Psychiatric Practice: CPD*, 2001. At www.rcpsych.ac.uk/publications/collegereports/cr/cr90.aspx, accessed 7 Jun 2009.
22. Benbow SM, Jolley DJ. Burnout and stress amongst old age psychiatrists. *Int J Geriatr Psychiatry* 2002; **17**: 710–14.
23. Pitt B, Arie T, Benbow SM, Garner J. The history of old age psychiatry in the UK. *Int Psychogeriatr Assoc Bull* 2006; **23**(2): 8–10.

139

Training Requirements in North America

Paul D. Kirwin[1] and Kirsten M. Wilkins[2]

[1]Associate Professor of Psychiatry, Geriatric Psychiatry Fellowship Director, Yale University School of Medicine, VA CT Healthcare System
[2]Assistant Professor of Psychiatry, University of Oklahoma College of Medicine-Tulsa, Tulsa, OK

The imperative for training specialists in geriatric psychiatry has never been greater. As the United States' 76 million baby boomers near retirement age, the number of Americans over age 65 will double to 70 million, one-fifth of the U.S. population. Americans older than 85 represent the fastest growing segment of this population and are projected to grow from five million today to an estimated 21 million by 2050. By the year 2010, there will be approximately 40 million people in the United States over the age of 65[1]. Almost 20 percent of those people will experience mental health problems[2].

Facing this exploding demographic imperative is a shrinking workforce of those with specialty training in the diagnosis and treatment of neuropsychiatric disorders in late life. In 2001, there were about 2,600 geriatric psychiatrists in the U.S. By 2007 there were only 1,596 geriatric psychiatrists–rather than the 5,000 needed to provide adequate care for the current population of older adults. The steep decline in the numbers of geriatric psychiatrists is accounted for by attrition and a failure of many who remain in active practice to recertify. Recruitment into the field is also waning, with less than half of geriatric psychiatry fellowship positions filled in 2006–2007. We are currently graduating approximately 80 new geriatric psychiatrists a year. By the year 2030 accounting for attrition, we are projected to have approximately 1,659 geriatric psychiatrists, or one geriatric psychiatrist per 20,195 older Americans. The field of geriatric medicine faces parallel workforce shortages with a 25% drop in geriatricians in the last five years. Over the next 20 years this disproportion is expected to worsen: from 1 geriatrician per 2,456 elderly currently to 1 per 4,254 older Americans by 2030. By 2030, it is projected that less than one third of the required geriatricians will be available for older Americans. Clearly there is a pressing need to train more experts in geriatric psychiatry and medicine, and to expand clinical training in geriatrics in both general psychiatry and medicine residency programs to adequately prepare a workforce ready to care for the expanding U.S. elder population[3].

The problem extends to other specialists in mental health and aging. In social work, only about 1,115 (3.6%) of Master's level social work students specialize in aging and only about 5% of practitioners at any level identify aging as their primary area of practice, even though the National Institute on Aging projected that by 2020, 60,000–70,000 gerontological social workers will be needed. Among psychologists, only about 3% view geriatrics as their primary area of practice and only 28% of all graduate psychologists have some graduate training in geriatrics[4].

Training in general psychiatry and then in the sub-specialty of geriatric psychiatry is extensive. The Accreditation Council for Graduate Medical Education (ACGME) in conjunction with the American Board of Psychiatry and Neurology stipulate that one must complete four years of post medical school graduate training in general psychiatry before being eligible to enter advanced training in geriatric psychiatry. One month of general psychiatry residency is dedicated to training in geriatric psychiatry. The quality of this geriatric psychiatry experience, in particular, the quality and attributes of the educators providing the training are associated with the development of interest in the field[5]. Following completion of the general psychiatry residency, the geriatric psychiatry fellowship is typically one year in length. Many programs offer additional training years for research, but these are optional and not required to sit for the advanced board exam in geriatric psychiatry.

The ACGME provides program requirements that specify the scope and content of training in general psychiatry and all psychiatry subspecialties. Programs undergo periodic "site visits" by the ACGME to ensure that the quality of the training program meets the expectations outlined in the program requirements. The twenty-plus page ACGME Geriatric Psychiatry Program Requirements necessitate that training experiences are rooted in six core competencies. The program must demonstrate that fellows have educational opportunities to gain knowledge, skills, behaviors and attitudes in these six domains: Patient Care, Medical Knowledge, Practice-Based Learning and Improvement, Interpersonal and Communication Skills, Professionalism, and Systems-Based Practice. These six core competencies have been adapted to fit the scope of training needs of a geriatric psychiatry fellow[6].

Ideally, training in geriatric psychiatry offers a rich combination of experiences designed to provide psychiatrists with expertise in the diagnosis and treatment of psychiatric and neuropsychiatric disorders in late life, to develop skills as educators, and to stimulate interest in research. A training program should provide opportunities to learn about the socio-cultural, legal, ethical and financial issues associated with the care of older adults. Supervised clinical training should occur in a broad array of settings, including outpatient and inpatient environments, nursing home and long term care

Principles and Practice of Geriatric Psychiatry, 3rd edn. Edited by Mohammed T. Abou-Saleh, Cornelius Katona and Anand Kumar

settings, cross disciplinary consultation opportunities, home-based services, community-based offices and clinics, and both inpatient and outpatient-based research programs.

A critical element in a successful geriatric psychiatry training program is mentorship. Unlike large residency training programs, fellows often work side-by-side with their program directors and senior attending psychiatrists. This day to day interaction is fundamental to a fellow's professional and personal development as a colleague. Imparting enthusiasm, attending to a fellow's interests, encouraging their abilities, and assisting with their limitations are essential for a fellow's growth. Successful mentorship relationships often last far beyond training and become an essential resource during the development of a career. They also serve as powerful models for developing one's own mentorship sensibilities. Mentorship is a deeply satisfying process and is vital to the overall success of the training program.

In 2008, the Institute of Medicine (IOM) released a study of the readiness of the nation's healthcare workforce to meet the needs of its aging population. *Re-tooling for an Aging America: Building the Health Care Workforce* called for immediate investments in preparing our health care system to care for older Americans and their families[7]. Yet the prescient and insightful report precluded in-depth consideration of the workforce needed for treating mental illness. The American Association for Geriatric Psychiatry (AAGP) formally requested that the study be followed by a complementary study focused on the specific challenges in the geriatric mental health field. The AAGP asserts that "virtually all healthcare providers need to be fully prepared to manage the common medical and mental health problems of old age. In addition, the number of geriatric health specialists, including mental health providers, needs to be increased both to provide care for those older adults with the most complex issues and to train the rest of the workforce in the common medical and mental health problems of old age. The small numbers of specialists in geriatric mental health, combined with increases in life expectancy and the growing population of the nation's elderly, foretell a crisis in health care that will impact older adults and their families nationwide. Unless changes are made now, older Americans will face long waits, decreased choice, and suboptimal care"[8]. Then, in December of 2009, after extensive efforts by the AAGP and other organizations, Congress passed legislation designating $900,000 for the Institute of Medicine (IOM) to conduct a study on the mental health workforce necessary for our nation's growing geriatric and ethnic populations, which promises to provide guidance on how to address geriatric mental health workforce inadequacies.

Multifaceted incentives to enter training in geriatric psychiatry are necessary. Initiatives in the public policy arena include legislation to provide loan forgiveness for health care professionals who enter geriatric specialties. The AAGP has promoted legislation to create a new program for loan repayment for specialists across disciplines that enter geriatric specialties. The AAGP also supports legislation to allow fellows in geriatric medicine and geriatric psychiatry to include fellowship training as part of their obligated service under the National Health Corps Loan Repayment Program, a program designed to encourage health professionals to provide clinical care to underserved populations. The AAGP has also requested that the ACGME review the current structure of fellowship training to allow for more flexibility and promote recruitment of psychiatrists into the field of geriatric psychiatry. Specifically, the AAGP has asked the ACGME to consider allowing residents to use their fourth year elective time in general residency training to specialize in geriatric psychiatry and then be eligible to sit for the general and subspecialty certification at the end of four years of training. The organization also supports a training model to integrate research training in geriatric mental health over a two year period, the fourth and fifth year of training, to stimulate and encourage academic research careers.

Recently, there have been promising developments which should promote easier access to skilled mental health care for the elderly. The U.S. Congress passed legislation (over President Bush's veto) on July 15th, 2008 that eliminated long standing discriminatory co-payment rates for Medicare outpatient psychiatric services. Cost sharing for outpatient mental health services will phase down from 50 percent to 20 percent by 2014. On the private insurance side, in 2008 Congress also passed legislation to ensure mental health parity which stipulates that for employers with greater than 50 employees, any limits on mental health treatments (including substance abuse) must be no greater than the limits placed on medical and surgical benefits.

The demographics of aging and mental illness clearly indicate a growing need for specialists trained in comprehensive psychiatric care of older adults. Despite the availability of geriatric psychiatry training and the growing population of older adults, current statistics suggest an alarming paucity of psychiatrists who are specialty trained in geriatrics. As such, it is essential to increase the geriatric psychiatry workforce. This includes increasing recruitment of general psychiatric trainees into the geriatric psychiatry sub-specialty, in order to both provide care for the growing population of older adults and to train general psychiatric and medical practitioners, who will likely be providing the bulk of the psychiatric care of older adults. Several strategies to increase the geriatric psychiatry workforce are currently being explored, including structural changes in sub-specialty training programs, financial incentives such as loan repayment programs, and earlier and broader experiences with geriatric psychiatrist educators during general psychiatry residency training. Equally important in ensuring that the elderly will receive optimal care are initiatives directed at improving their access to specialty mental health services.

In spite of an evolving economic landscape, a decision to enter the field of geriatric psychiatry has always been a decision of the heart, and not the pocket-book. It attracts those who love to hear stories from those who have lived the longest and acquired wisdom borne of life long experiences. For most elderly, the onset of mental illness is a new and horrifying experience. Their distress is profound, as is their gratitude for skilled intervention. One gets to make a difference in geriatric psychiatry, and this ability to intervene with patients and families in both curative and supportive ways brings the geriatric psychiatrist deep satisfaction. Working with the elderly attracts those with a sense of mission, a calling to take care of our most vulnerable citizens – those who face the double prejudice of old age and mental illness.

REFERENCES

1. Federal Interagency Forum on Aging-Related Statistics. Older Americans 2008: Key Indicators of Well-Being. Federal Interagency Forum on Aging-Related Statistics, Washington, DC: U.S. Government Printing Office. March 2008.
2. Mental Health: A Report of the Surgeon General 1999. U. S. Department of Health and Human Services, Office of the Surgeon General, SAMHSA.
3. Association of Directors of Geriatric Academic Programs (ADGAP). (2007) Fellows in geriatric medicine and geriatric psychiatry programs. *The Status of Geriatrics Workforce Study: Training and Practice Update* 5(2): 1–7.

4. Rosen, AL. Testimony on behalf of the National Coalition on Mental Health and Aging to the White House Conference on Aging Steering Committee. January 24, 2005.

5. Lieff SJ, Tolomiczenko GS, Dunn LB. (2003) Effect of training and other influences on the development of career interest in geriatric psychiatry. *Am J Geriatr Psychiatry* 11(3): 300–308.

6. Lieff SJ, Kirwin P, Colenda CC. (2005) Proposed geriatric psychiatry core competencies for specialty training. *Am J Geriatr Psychiatry* 13(9): 815–821.

7. Committee on the Future Healthcare Workforce for Older Americans. Retooling for an aging America: building the health care workforce. Institute of Medicine of the National Academy of Sciences Report. April 2008: 1–4.

8. Kirwin, Paul D. Testimony on behalf of the American Association for Geriatric Psychiatry to the United States House of Representatives, Appropriations Subcommittee on Labor, Health and Human Services, and Education. March 18, 2009.

140

Education in Old Age Psychiatry: Recent and Future Developments

Hugo de Waal

East of England Postgraduate School of Psychiatry, Fulbourn, Cambridge, UK

INTRODUCTION

Over the past few decades geriatric psychiatry has developed as a psychiatric subspecialty to varying degrees in different countries[1]: while in some it is recognized as such at governmental level (e.g. the UK[i]), elsewhere it developed a defined medical identity more within the medical profession (e.g. the USA, Australia, Canada), or it functions as a less well circumscribed area of special interest of medical practitioners, whose designation often lies in other specialties, such as general psychiatry, neurology or geriatric medicine (e.g. the Netherlands).

In 1998 the World Health Organization (WHO) in collaboration with the International Psychogeriatric Association (IPA) published three consensus statements on geriatric psychiatry, the third of which focused on education. Its aim was 'to propose wide guidelines favouring an education of good quality, taking into account the complexity of the subject to teach and of the public concerned'[2] – not a straightforward ambition, given the fact that worldwide geriatric psychiatric services and education range from non-existent to highly sophisticated and mature, well-embedded in health provision and educational accreditation systems.

The following presents the impact of various circumstances and factors upon the development of education in geriatric psychiatry and highlights some trends that may prove important for the future of training and education in this subspecialty.

THE LINKS BETWEEN EDUCATION, CAREER CHOICE, SERVICE PROVISION AND SUBSPECIALTY RECOGNITION

Career Choice

Training and education in geriatric psychiatry are influenced to a considerable extent by factors related to career choices made by medical graduates in general. In the United States, Bragg and Warshaw reported that problems persist in recruitment and retention of 'high-quality USMGs' (United States Medical Graduates) in both geriatric medicine and geriatric psychiatry. They identified early exposure to geriatrics as an important factor in selecting it as a career[3], as did Lieff et al., who investigated more fully which particular experiences showed a positive effect: they mention specific teacher attributes, training experiences, personal experiences with seniors, and the medical, neuropsychiatric and multifactorial nature of the field[4]. Similarly, in the United Kingdom, McParland et al. showed how undergraduate experience is essential in choosing the specialty and the more so if that experience is positive and of a high quality[5].

There are other, related factors at play with regard to career choice: Goldacre et al. report that in the United Kingdom non-white consultants who qualified abroad were at 18.4% significantly over-represented in geriatric psychiatry[6]. This pattern of skewed ethnic representation can be recognized in general in British psychiatric training: in his recent newsletter the Dean of the Royal College reported that at the last sitting of the final membership examination (the so-called Clinical Assessment of Skills and Competencies) only one out of eight candidates was a UK graduate[7]. It is therefore clear that the UK remains a net importer of doctors, and this pertains to geriatric psychiatry even more than to some of the other psychiatric subspecialties. He believes that two important explanatory factors can be found in 'the current dismal experience of many medical school clinical attachments' and 'the poor penetration of psychiatry into the Foundation years' (the British version of post-qualification, pre-registration training). One could therefore conclude that even in the UK there are major difficulties in recruitment and retention in psychiatry (and therefore in geriatric psychiatry), regardless of the fact that internationally the UK could be regarded as advanced in its development of geriatric psychiatric services and related training and education.

Service Provision

Surveying the international picture of education in old age psychiatry, it soon becomes clear that it appears mature and sophisticated in those countries where psychogeriatric services exist, which themselves are mature and established. On the contrary, education tends to be poorly structured, educationally isolated and occurring in an ad hoc fashion in those countries where psychogeriatric services are either non-existent, or are an 'afterthought' featuring in other medical specialties.

---

[i]Old Age Psychiatry is recognised in the UK by the Postgraduate Medical Education and Training Board as a subspecialty, carrying its own Certificate of Completion of Training.

Principles and Practice of Geriatric Psychiatry, 3rd edn. Edited by Mohammed T. Abou-Saleh, Cornelius Katona and Anand Kumar
© 2011 John Wiley & Sons, Ltd

In 2001 the World Psychiatric Association (WPA) section on old age psychiatry surveyed the level of development of medical education in geriatric psychiatry in 93 countries. A total of 48 countries responded, which in itself at 52% was a worryingly low response rate – even for a postal questionnaire – given that the survey was particularly aimed at those clinicians who were known to have a special interest in and affinity to the subspecialty. Of the responders, 40 countries reported the existence of old age psychiatric services and 44 formal teaching at undergraduate level, but only 13 full recognition of the discipline as a subspecialty. The member societies furthermore considered support for the development of postgraduate training as their most pressing need[8].

In those countries where there is a drive to develop both services and education, there is often the problem of how to tackle the 'chicken and egg' phenomenon: it is, perhaps predictably, quite difficult to get education going when clinically there is no defined basis for that to occur in, although it must be pointed out that in the case of geriatric psychiatry some lessons have been learned from geriatric medicine. The same survey found that chairs in geriatric medicine – as a reasonable indication of structured advanced educational activity – only exist in countries where geriatric medicine is recognized as a subspecialty. This appeared not to be the case for geriatric psychiatry; several countries reported chairs in geriatric psychiatry to be in existence, even when the discipline was not yet formally recognized.

Subspecialty Recognition

The process of developing services when there are only a few appropriately skilled and motivated medical specialists pushing the psychogeriatric agenda is understandably a laborious exercise. But even when there are such interested parties present, the response from the wider professional body may be felt to be less than supportive. For example, in Canada Herrmann[9] pointed out that there exists a very active geriatric psychiatric subspecialty. The Canadian Academy of Geriatric Psychiatry counted in 2004 more than 190 members and organizes annual academic meetings, residency training programmes, numerous undergraduate and postgraduate training programmes and fellowship awards. It developed the Canadian Coalition for Seniors' Mental Health (CCSMH), which – among many activities and initiatives – co-hosted and organized the 9th Congress of the International Psychogeriatric Association. Yet the Canadian Royal College of Physicians and Surgeons did not demand any particular clinical and training time requirement in geriatric psychiatry until 2008, when it incorporated a mandatory six months' placement in geriatric psychiatry into its junior residency training programme[10] and to this day it does not recognize geriatric psychiatry as a subspecialty, while it does list geriatric medicine as such[11]. Hermann points out that such subspecialty recognition is vitally important to 'strengthen the awareness and profile of geriatric psychiatry, increasing the likelihood of recruitment into the practice'. If such recognition is not forthcoming in a country such as Canada, then how difficult will it be in countries that do not feature highly regulated professional bodies and training accreditation processes?

With or without such support from regulatory bodies, there is no doubt that high-level insistence on guidelines and standards has a positive effect on further developments. The earlier mentioned WHO consensus statement has led to a number of initiatives with immediate impact. In Europe it led to a consensus curriculum on Skill-Based Objectives in Old Age Psychiatry in 2002 (the so-called Lausanne statement). Apart from formulating a comprehensive list of areas of competence and learning objectives, Gustafson et al. express the hope that implementation of the curriculum 'should help ensure that . . . each European country has a number of specialists who can provide leadership in clinical service development, training and research'[12]. In the USA Lieff et al. formulated core competencies for geriatric psychiatric training and certification; their list appears equally inspired by the WHO consensus statement[13].

Implicitly they may be considered to base such expectations on the experience in the UK, where geriatric psychiatry managed to become a fully-fledged, mature and sophisticated subspecialty on the back of the energetic advocacy from initially only a few 'pioneers', such as Sam Robinson, Felix Post, Klaus Bergmann, Tom Arie, David Jolley, Brice Pitt, Elaine Murphy, Gordon Langley and John Wattis, to name the most prominent ones. Their inspirational efforts span across close to three decades, and to gain some understanding of how such pioneers and champions went about creating a new subspecialty, the Guthrie Trust Witness Seminar, entitled *The Development of Old Age Psychiatry from the 1960s until 1989*, provides a unique account and an important insight into how enthusiasm on one hand and tenacity on the other proved to be essential cornerstones of the process of establishing and developing old age psychiatry in the UK[14].

FUTURE DEVELOPMENTS

Research

Apart from the obvious and regularly reported demographic projections, which in themselves are likely to lead to increased attention and professional interest in geriatric psychiatric services on one hand, and subspecialty medical education on the other, there are other – very interesting – factors that may lead to a more fertile appreciation of the subspecialty within the medical profession at large. While historically geriatric psychiatry was quite limited in its therapeutic arsenal with respect to its most prominent disease category, i.e. dementia, the relatively recent availability of cholinesterase inhibitors, particularly in the developed countries, has served to improve its perceived status within the younger generations in medicine. This is likely to be further enhanced by the accelerated production of other therapeutic medications coming out of a research establishment which until fairly recently would have found it difficult to spend much time and energy on an illness category it considered to be largely beyond therapy or profit. The International Conference on Alzheimer's Disease (ICAD) in July 2009 in Vienna featured no fewer than eight distinct therapeutic target areas. Progress appears to be being made, for instance, in pyroglutamate-related pathways, tau aggregation inhibition, protection against tau hyperphosphorylation via activity-dependent neuroprotective protein (ADNP), normalization of metal–protein interactions via so-called metal protein attenuating compounds (MPAC), β-secretase inhibition, prevention of neuronal re-entry into the cell cycle, and so on (see www.alz.org/icad/overview.asp). Although many of these projects are some considerable time away from leading to clinically relevant therapeutic agents, there is little doubt that over time a more varied therapeutic arsenal will lead to more interest from all sorts of corners, including budding specialists.

Service Development

The link between such therapeutic power on one hand, and the ongoing development of a speciality and related focus on training and education on the other, was recognized by Foucault, who described and analysed such links as cornerstones of a more or less mature specialist discourse, even if he then goes on to critique such discourse[15]. One unpredictable issue at this stage is the possibility that a super-specialty may develop within geriatric psychiatry, solely devoted to dementia: the inexorable and fast accelerating progress of therapeutic research into this area, combined with projections of an ageing population, would potentially lead to segregation between such a service and services for older patients with so-called functional illnesses. Such a path would follow Foucault's analyses of the medical discourse: whenever medicine is able to pinpoint causative pathophysiological processes it has a tendency to devote specialist attention to them, and this is further reinforced when therapeutic interventions become feasible and prove to be efficacious. Should this occur, then a new threat may be surfacing to the integrity and cohesion of geriatric psychiatry: one should be guarded if such a development leads to a decrease of specialist attention to the functional illnesses of old age, and it could be considered a negative and unintended consequence if the functional side of geriatric psychiatry winds up being reabsorbed into more generic psychiatric services.

Postgraduate Schools

From 2007 in the UK postgraduate training in all medical specialties is being commissioned and quality assured by newly established Postgraduate Schools, on behalf of the longer established Postgraduate Deaneries. Such Schools function through operational boards, which are almost exclusively manned by medical trainers and educationalists, with additional representation of senior management, Royal College officers, trainees, and patients and carers. These Schools are proving quite powerful in developing, driving and improving postgraduate training, and this is particularly important for those subspecialties that otherwise might wind up in a 'Cinderella position'. The British concept of the Postgraduate Schools may well prove an excellent mechanism through which other countries might try to foster such subspecialty developments. If so, it would be a rare example of a situation in which a high intensity of political interference with educational structures (as is the case in the United Kingdom) actually turns out to be beneficial to the profession and its training and education.

CONTENT OF TRAINING, ASSESSMENT AND APPRAISAL PROCESSES

With the establishment of Postgraduate Schools in the UK, the Royal College's role became more specifically focused on curricular development and the setting of standards for training and education. This gave the College the opportunity to formulate detailed, competency-based curricula, which directly link to assessment and appraisal processes, and these in turn form the core evidence on which specialist accreditation is based. The curricula undergo regular revision, and the latest version with respect to geriatric psychiatry can be accessed at www.rcpsych.ac.uk/PDF/Old_Age_Feb09.pdf.

Additionally the College took the lead role in developing workplace-based assessments particular to psychiatric training, which shifted the training experience from an apprentice model to a 'managed learning' model. These assessments replaced in part the traditional knowledge-testing function of the Royal College membership examination; workplace-based assessments specifically test clinical and professional competencies through direct observation and feedback, the latter being particularly important in providing a

learning tool to the trainee, with increased levels of self-reflection on performance.

Already in 2003 Gustafson et al. called for training programmes to:

- be rooted in evidence-based practice
- be clinically relevant
- have explicit evaluation criteria
- include feedback from trainees
- be reviewed regularly.

He also highlighted that 'training program participants should have both formative (constructive feedback) and summative assessments'[11]. The former is thus now a crucial component of specialist training in the UK (as it has been for some time in the USA and Canada), while the latter is particularly important if one is to expect such training programmes and assessment processes to be linked to accreditation of specialists. Gustafson calls for the setting up of geriatric psychiatric accreditation through national systems in all European countries. All of this flows directly from the Lausanne statement[11], in turn the result of the WHO/IPA consensus statement[2].

It is worth noting that in the UK, with the implementation of the new streamlined postgraduate curriculum and assessment processes in 2007, totally new workplace-based assessments have been developed. These were to some degree based on the tools already in use in the USA and Canada, but they underwent extensive adaptation and re-validation for the purposes of psychiatric training. More recently a further assessment tool has been developed, particularly aiming to test for higher, non-clinical skills (the so-called Direct Observation of non-Clinical Skills, or DOnCS); it tests and assesses the trainee's skills in competencies not directly related to the clinician–patient interaction, but more to do with higher, so-called 'meta-level', skills. The categories are taken from CanMEDS, the Canadian framework, which organizes core competencies around seven key physician roles:

- medical expert
- communicator
- collaborator
- manager
- health advocate
- scholar
- professional.

It aims to provide formative and summative learning opportunities to the trainee in their post-membership training, and is expected to aid in their preparation for their subsequent role as consultant old age psychiatrists. In the British National Health Service there is a strong appreciation that the consultant role must exceed the provision of clinical, patient-centred care, and should incorporate a variety of roles, such as team leader, service developer, inter-agency negotiator, strategic planner etc. Given that particularly in geriatric psychiatry there is a relatively strong emphasis on collaboration with other agencies and an ensuing interest in strategic service and educational development, the DOnCS could be particularly powerful in fostering such skills in specialists being educated and trained in geriatric psychiatry, were it to be adopted elsewhere. More information about this assessment tool can be found at https://training.rcpsych.ac.uk/doncs-assessor-guidance.

CONCLUSION

With the large variety of political, cultural and economic factors on one hand and the huge diversity of service configuration and related existence of medical education on the other, combined furthermore with the varying levels of governmental interest or disinterest in either, the way forward will at least have to be a two-pronged one: top-down with the involvement and guidance of institutions such as the World Health Organization and the International Psychogeriatric Association and bottom-up through 'champions and pioneers'.

The role of champions and pioneers should start with undergraduate training. One noteworthy initiative, recently started by the UK Royal College and led by its Psychiatric Trainees' Committee, is designed to engage with medical students: in medical schools up and down the country undergraduate Psychiatry Societies are starting up, linked into a network in which a new College grade of Student Associate of the Royal College features prominently. The UK Royal College website now has a dedicated section for medical students who are interested in psychiatry and who want to find out more about the specialty, the training and education, career options etc. (www.rcpsych.ac.uk/specialtytraining/students.aspx). It provides an opportunity for interested medical students to enrol as a Student Associate of the Royal College. Further information on the Old Age section of this website can be found at www.rcpsych.ac.uk/specialtytraining/students/subspecialties /oldagepsychiatry.aspx.

In short, one can discern a number of factors that should lead to a higher profile for geriatric psychiatry and its training and education:

1. continued efforts by international and national professional organizations
2. increased efforts to provide the relevant exposure to medical students
3. enthusiasm and active 'proselytizing' by clinicians and educators
4. the projected increase in the size of the older age groups
5. an expected increase in therapeutic options.

REFERENCES

1. Draper B, Melding P, Brodaty H (eds). *Psychogeriatric Service Delivery: An International Perspective*. Oxford: Oxford University Press, 2005.
2. World Health Organization, World Psychiatric Association. *Education in Psychiatry of the Elderly: A Technical Consensus Statement*. Geneva: WHO and WPA, 1998.
3. Bragg EJ, Warshaw GA. Evolution of geriatric medicine fellowship training in the United States. *Am J Geriatr Psychiatry* 2003; **11**(3): 280–90.
4. Lieff SJ, Tolomiczenko GS, Dunn LB. Effect of training and other influences on the development of career interest in geriatric psychiatry. *Am J Geriatr Psychiatry* 2003; **11**(3): 300–308.
5. McParland M, Noble LM, Livingston G *et al*. The effect of a psychiatric attachment on students' attitudes to and intention to pursue psychiatry as a career. *Med Educ* 2003; **37**: 447–54.
6. Goldacre MJ, Davidson JM, Lambert TW. Country of training and ethnic origin of UK doctors: database and survey studies. *Br Med J* 2004; **329**(7466): 597.
7. Royal College of Psychiatrists. The Dean, Professor Rob Howard, Celebrates His First Anniversary. At www.rcpsych.ac.uk /members/rcpsychnews/july2009.aspx#title2, accessed 4 Jul 2009.
8. Camus V, Katona C, de Mendonça Lima CA *et al*. Teaching and training in old age psychiatry: a general survey of the World Psychiatric Association member societies. *Int J Geriatr Psychiatry* 2003; **18**: 694–9.
9. Hermann N. Geriatric psychiatry: a subspecialty whose time has come. *Can J Psychiatry* 2004; **49**(7): 415–16.
10. Royal College of Physicians and Surgeons of Canada. *Specialty Training Requirements in Psychiatry* (rev), 2008. At http://rcpsc.medical.org/residency/certification/training /psychiatry_e.pdf, accessed 15 Feb 2010.
11. Royal College of Physicians and Surgeons of Canada. *Policies and Procedures for Certification and Fellowship*, 2009. At http://rcpsc.medical.org/residency/certification/policy-procedures_e.pdf, accessed 15 Feb 2010.
12. Gustafson L, Burns A, Katona C *et al*. Skill-based objectives for specialist training in old age psychiatry. *Int J Geriatr Psychiatry* 2003; **18**: 686–93.
13. Lieff SJ, Kirwin P, Colenda CC. Proposed geriatric psychiatry core competencies for subspecialty training. *Am J Geriatr Psychiatry* 2005; **13**(9): 815–21.
14. Hilton C (ed.). *The Development of Old Age Psychiatry, from the 1960s until 1989*, Guthrie Trust Witness Seminar, Centre for the History of Medicine, University of Glasgow, 9 May 2008. At www.gla.ac.uk/media/media_107314_en.pdf, accessed 15 Feb 2010.
15. Foucault M. *Naissance de la clinique: une archéologie du regard médical*. Paris: Presses Universitaires de France, 1973.

Subject Index

suspended-sediment-rich plumes and turbidity currents. On stable cratons, sediment fluxes from the deeply weathered regolith may be negligible, and runoff dominated by organic fluxes. In the seas and oceans, very high organic productivity gives a productive 'carbonate factory' away from areas of siliciclastic input.

2 Low-latitude Trade Wind belts over continents are arid with little vegetation, so chemical weathering is negligible, and physical breakdown predominates. Aeolian processes in great sand seas (ergs) are characteristic, with regionally steady Trade Winds. Evaporite mineral precipitation is widespread, from groundwaters, playas and coastal lagoons. Sabkha anhydrite is indicative of extreme aridity and very high summer temperatures. In shallow marine environments carbonate production is again high. Adjacent to oceans, offshore or shore-parallel wind regimes give strong upwelling, high primary productivity, with shelf anoxia encouraging 'black shale' type facies to form (Chapter 26).

3 Semiarid climates with scrub vegetation have low water tables but sufficient summer convective or weak monsoonal precipitation to develop characteristic calcisols, vertisols and *in situ* oxidative weathering of shallow buried sediment to produce 'red beds'.

River regimes are characteristically 'flashy', with a great propensity for delivery of hyperconcentrated and debris flows (but these are *not* climatically diagnostic in their own right).

4 Mid- to temperate-latitude maritime climates develop deciduous woodlands under which acidic surface waters cause development of strongly leached podzol-type soils.

5 Polar climates show negligible chemical weathering. Areas under ice and in the permafrost zone feature a wide range of glacial and periglacial facies and structures (Chapter 20).

Further reading

Lockwood (1979) is an excellent, though idiosyncratic, introduction to modern climatology. A more recent text is Linacre and Geerts (1997), with a refreshing antipodean bias. Scorer (1997) is more physical. Lamb (1995) is incomparable for historic climate change. Wright *et al.* (1993) is indispensable for post-18 ka climate change. Older palaeoclimate is comprehensively covered by Frakes *et al.* (1992). A host of good papers on the sedimentological consequences of orbital forcing are to be found in de Boer and Smith (1994).

14   Changing sea level and sedimentary sequences

Then come, come, come, let her spend her
Quivering momentum where I lie here,
Wedding words to her waves, and able to tend her
Every swirl and sound with eye and ear.

Hugh MacDiarmid, 'The Point of Honour', *Complete Poems*, Vol. 1, Carcanet

14.1 Introduction: sea level as datum

The instantaneous position of a shoreline is perhaps the most important datum that sedimentary geologists have in their inventory of tricks to interpret the sedimentary record. Leaving aside here the details of exactly how we use sediments to discover ancient shorelines (see Chapter 23), we may note that the position of a shoreline in time and space is determined by three competing variables (Fig. 14.1):

- subsidence rate, with deepening due to subsidence or shallowing due to uplift;
- sediment deposition rate, with shallowing due to deposition;
- absolute sea level.

The important lesson to be gained from Fig. 14.1 is that the concept of changing sea-level datum requires a consideration of both relative and absolute changes in sea level.

14.2 Sea-level changes

The confirmation of the Austrian geologist Suess's original idea from 1888 that global sea level has not been constant but has varied, sometimes periodically, by up to several hundred metres through geological time has been one of the major developments of 20th-century geology. Conditions of maximum and minimum sea level are referred to as highstands and lowstands respectively. Such global, or eustatic, changes must be distinguished from the myriad of local or regional changes induced by faulting, thermal subsidence, volcanism, intraplate stresses due to subduction, thermal uplift, sediment compaction and other causes (for examples and discussion see Burgess *et al.*, 1997; Dewey & Pitman, 1998). Whilst local

sea-level change may be very important, for example in estimating the relative movements along faults or folds, it is the elucidation of global sea-level change that represents the major breakthrough in stratigraphic and sedimentary studies. Just how may we estimate whether sea level has changed globally?

1 From evidence in the sedimentary and/or fossil record for shallowing or deepening or of shoreline shift to landward or seaward.

2 By the correlation in time of firmly established sea-level changes over significant parts of the global sedimentary record.

3 By oxygen isotopic evidence from oceanic calcareous plankton for the abstraction of seawater or return of fresh water into and out of the polar ice-caps.

The first two methodologies have been around for some time in the geological literature and constrain the older geological record (> 10 Ma), whilst the latter is a relatively new technique (since the mid-1970s) and has been applied with spectacular success to the younger record of Neogene 'icehouse Earth'. Needless to say, this latter oxygen isotope record is considerably the more accurate. The broad pattern of worldwide sea-level changes for Mesozoic to Cainozoic times is indicated in Fig. 14.2, with details of the relative rates and low frequencies of change determined for the greenhouse Jurassic period. By way of contrast, the high frequency of sea-level change for icehouse Neogene times is emphasized in Fig. 14.3. A major development in the past few years has been the integration of both oxygen isotope and sedimentological records of cyclicity during Neogene times (e.g. Hilgen, 1991, 1994; Lourens *et al.*, 1996; Naish, 1997; see Fig. 14.6).

Landward shoreline shifts are termed *transgressions* (marine floods by some) and seaward shifts

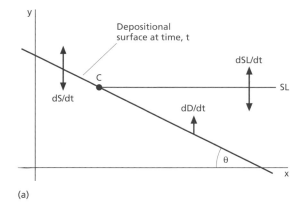

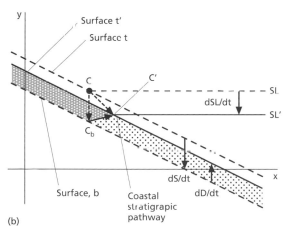

Fig. 14.1 Sketches to show controls on shoreline position. (a) Definition of terms: C = position of coastline on depositional surface sloping at angle θ; SL = sea level; dSL/dt = time rate of change in eustatic sea level; dS/dt = time rate of subsidence or uplift leading to a relative sea-level change; dD/dt = time rate of sediment deposition. (b) From time t to t', the position of the coastline migrates from C to C'. Concurrently, the original coastline C and the depositional surface on which it was located are buried, to C_b and surface b, respectively. C_b to C' thus defines the coastal pathway through the stratigraphic section and the facies boundary between continental (stipple) and marine (dash) sediments. (After Collier *et al*., 1990.)

regressions. If the mean gradient, θ, of the coastal lowlands is low, then the transgressing or regressing sea may travel far inland or on to the shelf, in fact for a distance δSL/tan θ (Fig. 14.1). If the sea-level change is very fast, then there will be a rapid changeover in sedimentary facies observed at any one point. Here we come to the first difficulty in assessing whether

eustatic changes have taken place, that is, the determination of the age of the first marine deposits (the initial transgressive or marine flooding surface), which will vary in space. It may be that such an age variation is impossible to estimate from the range of fossils or other evidence available to the stratigrapher; the further back we go in the geological record, the more difficult the task becomes.

Once it is established that a sea-level change has occurred, then we must check by fieldwork and by further study of the literature whether this change has happened the world over in deposits of equivalent age (we must look well outside a particular tectonic province in case the cause is a regional tectonic one; see Underhill, 1991 for a revealing example). The problem now becomes one of correlation, a process largely entrusted to palaeontological colleagues. Correlation to time levels of less than a few million years clearly becomes almost impossible in many Precambrian sedimentary rocks (see discussion of Miall, 1997), this despite remarkable technical advances in the past two decades concerning precision dating of single crystals of minerals like zircon and monazite in crystal tuffs and lava flows intercalated within such sequences.

14.3 Rates and magnitude of sea-level change

Once we are satisfied that particular sea-level changes may be correlated widely, from plate to plate, we can be more confident that a eustatic change has taken place. We next need to enquire as to the rate of recurrence of the sea-level change and its magnitude.

Mesozoic (greenhouse) sea-level changes appear as low-frequency ups and downs, typically of about 0.5–3 Myr duration, superimposed on a gross secular change at very low frequencies of the order 10^2 Myr (Fig. 14.2). Estimates of the magnitude of the higher of these frequencies (Hallam, 1997) are in the range of a few tens of metres. Estimates of the magnitude of the secular changes are very much more difficult to call (because of post-Mesozoic tectonics), but may range from 100 to 300 m above present-day sea level (Heller *et al*., 1996). From these data we infer that rates of absolute Mesozoic sea-level change were very low, in the range 0.001–0.05 mm/yr. Such rates are usually less than relative sea-level changes brought about by the slow thermal and flexural subsidence

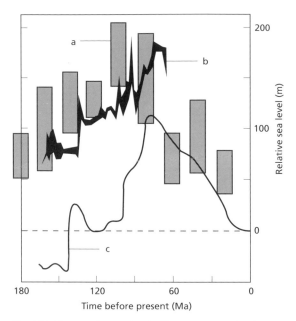

Fig. 14.2 Three estimates (a–c) of long-term sea-level change from the Mesozoic and Cainozoic stratigraphic record as compiled by Heller *et al.* (1996). Note that, despite the wide range of estimates for magnitude of sea-level variation, the broad trends to and from the late-Cretaceous highstand are comparable.

of rifted continental margins (see data in Fig. 15.3). Under such conditions the correlation of apparent sea-level changes from different continental margins must be done with very great care.

Upper Cainozoic (icehouse) sea-level changes revealed in the oxygen isotope record appear as high-frequency ups and downs of between 20 and 100 kyr duration reflecting the Milankovitch-band periodicities discussed in Chapter 13 (Fig. 14.3). Prior to the onset of major continental glaciations, at about 800 ka, back to about the Miocene, the predominant signal is of a 40 kyr periodic fluctuation of about 20–50 m magnitude. From about 800 ka to present the 40 kyr fluctuation is superimposed upon, and reinforces, a highly asymmetrical 100 kyr periodic fluctuation of about 125 m magnitude. The fluctuation is asymmetrical in that the rising limb is very much steeper than the falling limb. From these data, calculated rates of absolute upper Cainozoic sea-level change were very high, in the range 1–10 mm/yr. Such rates are very much greater than sea-level changes brought about by most tectonic mechanisms,

other than slip rates along particularly active faults (see examples in Gawthorpe *et al.*, 1994).

The situation regarding sea-level changes further back in geological time is much less clear. Speculations for the whole Phanerozoic record are presented by Vail *et al.* (1977). It seems reasonable to suppose that periods with 'icehouse Earth' conditions would have shown similar high-frequency signals to those seen more recently. Certainly that is the message from studies of cyclical deposits of Permo-Carboniferous age on the ancient Pangaean megaplate (e.g. Heckel, 1986; Maynard & Leeder, 1992). Although we can clearly apply the lessons of fast-acting eustasy to former 'icehouse' epochs like the Permo-Carboniferous, upper Ordovician and late Precambrian, the majority of the Earth history was probably enacted under conditions more akin to 'greenhouse Earth'. So, under such boundary conditions we expect 'slow eustasy' to dominate. But here the rates involved are very, very slow relative to most tectonic or sedimentary processes, hence the strong probability that noneustatic signatures will dominate the sedimentary record. All is not lost, however, for there is good evidence that, although major ice-caps were never present during what we call 'greenhouse Earth', smaller caps certainly were and it is these that probably waxed and waned at axial tilt frequencies through time. For example, such cycles have been widely recognized in the Triassic platform carbonates described in Chapter 24.

14.4 Origins of global sea-level change: slow vs. fast eustasy

The next question is 'Why should sea level change globally?' At first we may think that any such change is a paradox, since the total amount of water in the hydrosphere cannot vary much and we can probably rule out any major flux of juvenile water from the Earth's mantle. There seem to be two possible eustatic mechanisms, one extremely slow-acting and only detectable under 'greenhouse Earth' conditions, and the other rather fast and limited to 'icehouse Earth' conditions.

Slow-acting eustasy works on the 'bath-tub' principle in that the total amount of global seawater is conserved in the oceans but that the containing ocean basins may grow smaller or larger in volume, due basically to tectonic processes. Since we know that in

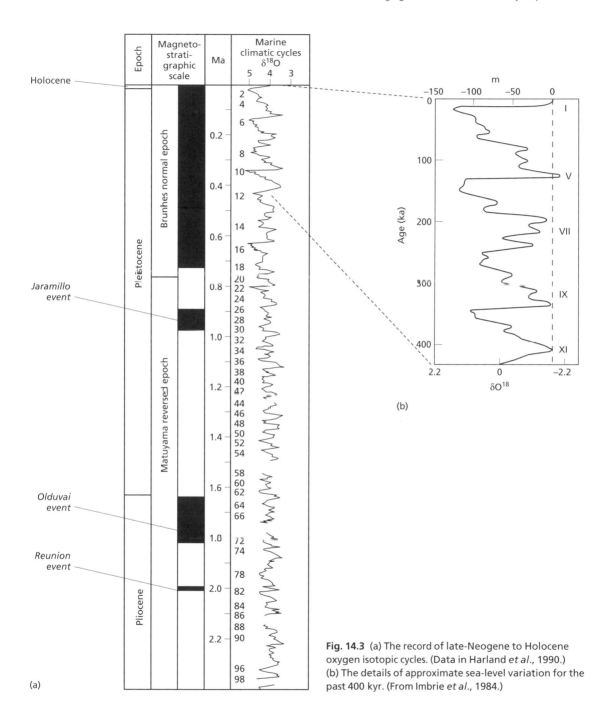

Fig. 14.3 (a) The record of late-Neogene to Holocene oxygen isotopic cycles. (Data in Harland *et al.*, 1990.) (b) The details of approximate sea-level variation for the past 400 kyr. (From Imbrie *et al.*, 1984.)

the long term the Earth is not increasing or decreasing in diameter, and the cycle of plate tectonic interactions must conserve lithospheric mass, the dilation or shrinkage of the ocean basins or the uplift and/or subsidence of the continents must involve a very complicated sequence of feedback mechanisms (for a nice review see Dewey & Pitman, 1998). How can this happen?

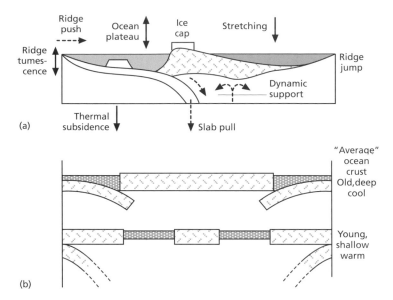

Fig. 14.4 (a) The main tectonic controls acting to determine mean oceanic and continental volume and (b) the relative oceanic shallowing induced by break-up of a former supercontinent between young, warm oceanic crust.

1 Traditionally, since the classic paper by Pitman (1978) at least, the effect has been ascribed to the swelling or shrinking of mid-ocean ridges as seen in the proxy evidence for faster or slower spreading rates apparently recorded in the Cretaceous ocean crust of the Pacific. Recent data make it unlikely that such changes in spreading rates actually occurred (Heller *et al.*, 1996; see Fig. 14.2). Also, this cause cannot be directly established for rocks other than the oldest ocean crust, about 180 Ma in the early Jurassic.

2 A second mechanism concerns the eruption of large volumes of basalts from mantle plumes into the ocean basins, so reducing their volume, during so-called megaplume episodes. Such bursts of plume activity are postulated for several intervals of Earth history, particularly the middle Cretaceous. They may be related to triggering events in the D″ region of the core–mantle boundary, the so-called 'slab graveyard'. Contrary to this view is the argument that such plume eruptions are essentially random, or even more sceptically, that plumes do not exist (Heller *et al.*, 1996).

3 A third mechanism notes the coincidence of rising global sea levels in the Jurassic and Cretaceous with the onset of the total break-up of the continental superplates and the destruction of Tethys (Heller *et al.*, 1996). This would have led to the replacement of very old, cool and dense oceanic lithosphere by young, warm and less dense oceanic lithosphere. Since

it is well known that ocean depth is a function of cooling age, then the younger Mesozoic oceans would have been shallower on average than older oceans. Hence global mean sea level would have increased during progressive rifting, reached a maximum and then declined as thermal cooling counteracted the shallowing tendency (Fig. 14.4).

4 A fourth mechanism appeals to the notion of dynamic topographical support of the continents by a combination of sublithospheric mantle convection and mantle advection inboard induced by oceanic lithosphere subduction (Gurnis, 1993; Burgess *et al.*, 1997). Direct tests of the idea are difficult to make, particularly in the light of Heller *et al.*'s criticisms of mechanism 2 above. Indirect tests (Burgess *et al.*, 1997) achieve some explanations of *c.* 100 Myr cratonic 'cycles' but require rather naive assumptions concerning palaeoplate tectonics and basin scale models.

Fast-acting eustasy results as ice is abstracted to form the major polar ice-caps or is melted to return fresh water to the oceans. Thus the global oceanic sea-water volume is not conserved and we are dealing with the continental ice-caps as sinks and sources for about 5% by volume of the oceans. As we have noted previously, the explanation for such changes in global ice volumes involves the effect of changing annual radiation balances at eccentricity, axial tilt and axial precession wavelengths. For the past eight 100 kyr cycles, the progression from conditions of highstand to lowstand is considerably longer, 'bumpier' and slower overall than is the relatively smooth and short passage from lowstand to highstand. Continental ice-caps clearly melted quicker than they took to form, not something that is easy to understand without very large-scale oceanic convective warming leading to polar sea-ice break-up.

14.5 Sequence stratigraphy: layers, cheesewires and bandwagons

Sedimentary deposits are layered, interleaved and generally arranged in 3-D patterns that reflect the history of their formation. Stratigraphy is the discipline that deals with the investigation of sedimentary layers —arranging, mapping and correlating them using a very wide range of techniques, from seismic reflection lines to fossils to palaeomagnetism. The readers of this book need not worry themselves with the details of stratigraphic practice, but a few basic remarks will serve to prevent confusion and help to facilitate inter-change of ideas with stratigraphers and palaeonto logists. Like the foundations, walls, floors and roofs of buildings, we may break down depositional mosaics into what have been called architectural 'elements' (Miall, 1997). When we can map such subdivisions around the surface or subsurface landscape, we can then define a basic lithostratigraphy or arrangement of distinctive layers. It should be stressed that such an arrangement of layers/strata exists absolutely inde-pendently of any time constraints. Lithostratigraphic units form a hierarchy of layers in 3D space based wholly on the ability of the geologist to map or trace them between exposures or wells. The situation faced by a subsurface mapper using seismic reflection traces is somewhat analogous. Here the layercake must be split up based on the succession of distinctive reflector horizons to define seismic stratigraphic units. Frequently, in this case, use is made of the nature of the top and bottom contacts between distinctive layers to shed light on the nature of processes respons-ible for deposition of the units in question (Fig. 14.5). At this stage the explorer has no knowledge of the nature of the rocks in question far below the surface (although he or she can make some inspired guesses based on the nature of the seismic response). Once a well or a number of wells have been drilled through

such seismic stratigraphic units, then the seismic units may be transferred into lithostratigraphic ones.

Local, regional or global changes in sea level enable sedimentary deposits to be subdivided according to the phase of the sea-level curve in which they were deposited or in which erosion occurred (Fig. 14.5). Those sediments laid down between successive low-stands are termed a *sequence*. Sequences are easiest to recognize where the sequence boundary is also a surface of erosion or nondeposition, made clear by a distinct mappable surface and/or on the basis of a time gap indicated by a mature palaeosol or from fossil evidence (Fig. 14.6). Erosion during lowstands is most obvious where the continental shelf is exposed to the atmosphere, giving the opportunity for the cut-ting of new drainage channels and the downcutting of pre-existing channels into the former marine sedi ments of the highstand shelf. More controversial is the situation at lowstand on the former coastal plain. For situations where the slope of the newly exposed continental shelf is significantly greater than that of the coastal plain, then it is to be expected that a 'wave' of channel incision and soil formation will work its way up the river channels at a rate determined by the slope difference and the erosive power of the river. It is also expected that the rate of the stream propaga-tion will decrease with time and the depth of erosion will decrease with distance upstream. As the channels incise, so the likelihood of floodplain accretion will decrease and soils will begin to develop on terraces (see Wright & Marriott, 1993; Aitkens & Flint, 1995; Gibling & Bird, 1994; Tandon & Gibling, 1997). For situations where the slopes of the coastal plain and shelf are similar or where the former is less than the latter, then it is less likely that incision will occur. Further discussion of river behaviour during cycles of sea-level change may be found in Chapter 17.

As sea level begins to rise from lowstand, then the formerly eroding shelf or coastal plain experiences a marine transgression and progressive water deepen-ing until highstand is reached (Fig. 14.6). The trans-gressive deposits of this stage of the cycle and those of the succeeding highstand and regressive phase overlie the lower sequence boundary and are in turn bounded by the next lowstand erosion surface. All the deposits between successive lowstand surfaces comprise a sequence. Each of the subdeposits has 'jargony' appel-lations (e.g. systems tracts) whose details need not concern us further.

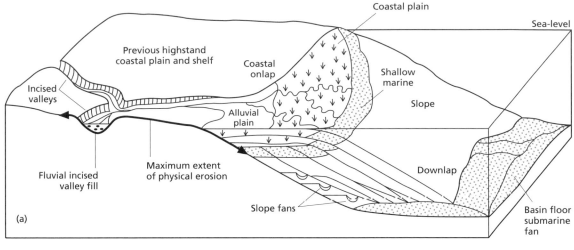

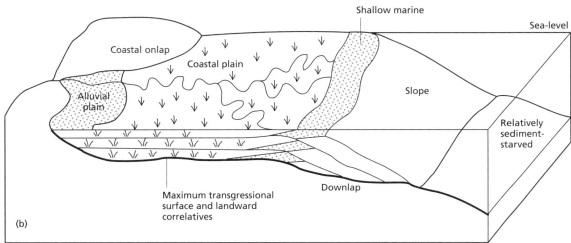

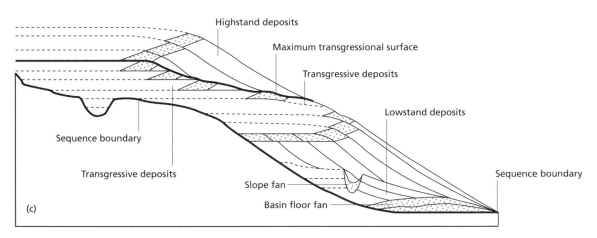

Fig. 14.5 Diagrams to illustrate stratal geometries, lowstand and highstand sequences. (a) Components of lowstand deposits on a subsiding continental margin with a wide coastal plain and a narrow shelf. (b) Components of highstand deposits on a similar shelf to (a). (c) Architectural summary scheme for a complete sequence on the same margin as (a) and (b). (Loosely after van Waggoner et al., 1988; mostly after Myers & Milton, 1996.)

(a)

(b)

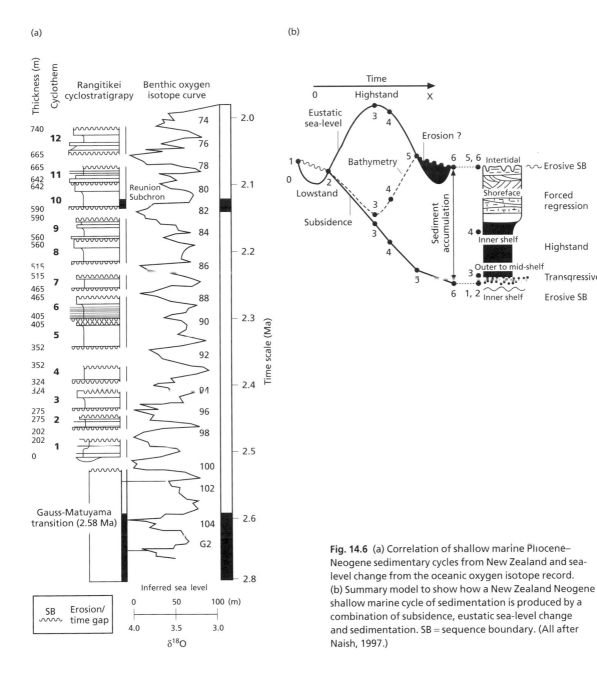

Fig. 14.6 (a) Correlation of shallow marine Pliocene–Neogene sedimentary cycles from New Zealand and sea-level change from the oceanic oxygen isotope record. (b) Summary model to show how a New Zealand Neogene shallow marine cycle of sedimentation is produced by a combination of subsidence, eustatic sea-level change and sedimentation. SB = sequence boundary. (All after Naish, 1997.)

It is in offshore and oceanic environments below the level of the lowstand that the concepts of sequence stratigraphy are most useful, and sometimes most difficult, to apply (for example, see Poulsen *et al.*, 1998). During lowstands (Fig. 14.5) rivers may debouch their sediment loads closer to the shelf edge, avoiding reworking by tide and wave with the likelihood that sediment density underflows and slumping of rapidly deposited materials to form surge-type turbidity flows will greatly increase in frequency. The idea is that, under such conditions, submarine fans and their feeder channels should show rapid growth until rising sea level to highstand brings the process to an end with the fan now draped by fine-grained sediments of hemipelagic types.

Although it is not the purpose of this account to offer a treatise on the lore of sequence stratigraphy, there are a few points upon which we must expand in order that the reader may more fully appreciate the context of sedimentology in relation to stratigraphy.

1 The term *regression* refers quite generally to a seaward shift in the position of a shoreline. Such seaward shifting may simply arise because sediment is being dumped at the shoreline causing the coastal plain to expand on to an adjacent lagoon or shelf. The outward movement of deltas or the human-assisted reclamation of coastal lands are examples that readily spring to mind. Now, in such cases no upward or downward movement of relative sea level is involved, and the process may be best called *progradational regression*. Should seaward movement of the shoreline occur in response to a relative sea-level fall, then the process is called *forced regression*. Clearly, regressions may involve combinations of both forced and progradational causes. The case of transgressions is similar, although the example of *erosional transgressions* in the absence of relative sea-level rise is rarely considered in stratigraphy. Much more common is the *forced transgression*. The term *parasequence* has been widely adopted by stratigraphers to describe the depositional products of a progradational regression that is terminated by a relatively abrupt relative sea-level rise.

2 Many stratigraphers and some sedimentologists have a compulsion for classifying sedimentary deposits according to 'orders'. Since orbital parameters may control sequence development over 20, 40 and 100 kyr, then such datum points may clearly have a use in dividing up cycles into bins at these levels. However, we have the problem that slow-acting eustasy and tectonic alterations to sea level may act on overlapping scales of anything in the range of 10^3–10^8 yr. There seems to be consensus in referring to cycle duration in terms of units of powers of 10, with 100 Myr cycles being first-order, 10 Myr cycles second-order, and so on.

3 The term *accommodation space* is much used by sequence stratigraphers—the author has even heard respected sedimentologists (who should know better) refer to 'negative accommodation space' as a synonym for environments where deposition is not possible! This pseudo-quantitative concept exactly equates to what normal geologists refer to as water depth of seas and lakes. It is simply the available volume within which sediment may be subaqueously deposited. Yet, it is a profoundly misleading concept since it must be applied not only to subaqueous but also to subaerial environments. How can we envisage accommodation space for environments open to the atmosphere?

Further reading

Miall (1997) is the most scholarly account of the whole business of sequences, eustasy and much else. Emery and Myers (1996) is more 'cookbookish'. Case histories and much to ponder over appear in the twin peaks of Weimer and Posamentier (1993) and Loucks and Sarg (1993). Poulsen *et al.* (1998) is a careful account of the 3-D complexities of 'real world' stratigraphy. The very important science of 'cyclostratigraphy' for Neogene times is presented in seminal papers by Hilgen (1991, 1994) and is reviewed by de Boer and Smith (1994).

15   Tectonics, denudation rates and sediment yields

And what are two thousand years? (asked Mrs Ramsay ironically, staring at the hedge). What, indeed, if you look from a mountaintop down the long wastes of the ages? The very stone one kicks with one's boots will outlast Shakespeare.

Virginia Woolf, *Mrs Dalloway*, p. 256, Penguin Omnibus Edition, 1992.

15.1 Basic geodynamics of uplift

We explore, in general terms, the relationship between denudation and the growth of relief due to tectonics. These control the elevation and gradient of any part of the Earth's surface. Some definitions of uplift, erosion and denudation are presented in Fig. 15.1.

The total tectonic displacement of any part of the solid Earth's surface may be described by a vector that is the sum of both local horizontal and local vertical changes in position and elevation. Relative plate motions are usually drawn as horizontal vectors on maps, but locally the vertical component of motion due to uplift, denudation or deposition may be a significant proportion of the horizontal displacement.

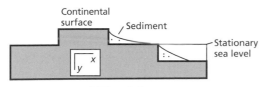

(a) Denudation
Deeper rock is exhumed due to removal of overlying material
(reference axes are fixed internally)

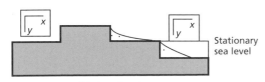

(b) Elevation change
Surface changes height due to denudation, uplift or subsidence
(reference axes are fixed externally or at fixed sea level)

Fig. 15.1 Coordinate systems for movement of the Earth's surface and of buried rock masses through denudation, uplift, subsidence and exhumation.

Sedimentary and geomorphological studies contribute much to the determination of the vertical component of motion, e.g. mapping and dating emergent marine terraces. Major mechanisms for surface uplift and subsidence are indicated in Fig. 15.2.

The rate of denudation is important in a number of diverse disciplines, from metamorphic geology, where pressure–temperature–time paths are critically controlled by the rate of denudation, to basin analysis, where the rate of sediment transfer from tectonic uplands down the regional gravity slope controls the rate of infill of sedimentary basins. Denudation rates are compared with uplift, subsidence and changing sea-level rates in Fig. 15.3.

15.2 Elevation and gradients

We have seen in previous chapters that surface gradient is a major control on rates of erosion and surface transport of solids. Observed gradients in any landscape, subaerial or submarine, are the result of a delicate balance between tectonic or volcanic construction and erosional or depositional modification. Zones of greatest submarine slope are usually relatively narrow features, reflecting the narrowness of most oceanic plate boundaries. They include those at the prominent system of subduction zones and associated island arcs (mean slope often > 3.4°), particularly on the inner trench slope (~ 5°), around volcanic chains and along oceanic transform faults. Among the diverging plate boundaries, slow-spreading ridges like the Mid-Atlantic Ridge form large areas of moderately steep slopes of high roughness, whilst fast-spreading ridges like the East Pacific Rise have very low slopes. Average ridge slopes decrease exponentially with increasing spreading rate. The slopes around

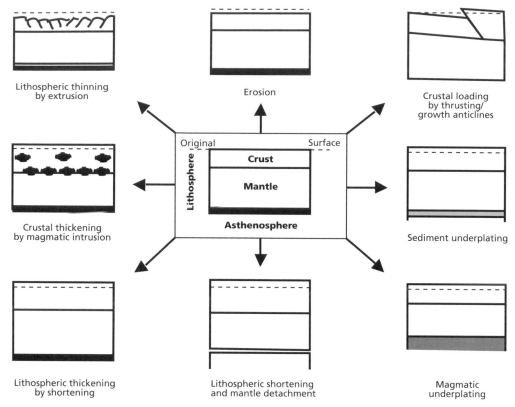

Fig. 15.2 The major tectonic processes responsible
for uplift and subsidence of the Earth's surface.

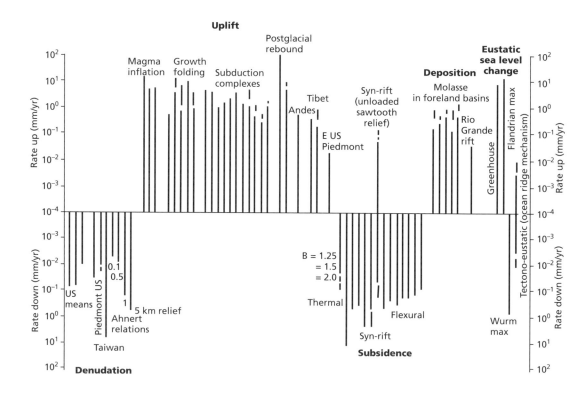

More information on isostasy and surface deformation

Imagine that the piece of lithosphere upon which you are now sitting is part of a reference volume such as that drawn as a 'streamtube' in Fig. B15.1. The base is fixed at some depth, y_0, in the asthenosphere. The top on which you are sitting is fixed at the mean elevation of the land surface, y, above y_0, and the density, ρ, of the whole volume is taken as an integrated mean $\int \rho \, dy$ over the whole depth y_0. Many geological processes may now affect the reference volume, including denudation, surface loading (by ice or by thrusting), extension, compression, magma intrusion, and heating or cooling. These processes may affect both the thickness and the density of the lithosphere. Let v_x, v_y, v_z be the components of material velocity, v, entering and leaving the volume. These will define the mass flux ρv of material moved into and out of the reference volume. Other density changes may be due to new metamorphic mineral growth, phase changes, or density changes, to *local* heating and to magma generation. These processes, arising within the reference volume, are termed sinks or sources and are represented by the symbol ψ. Using these various definitions we may write the

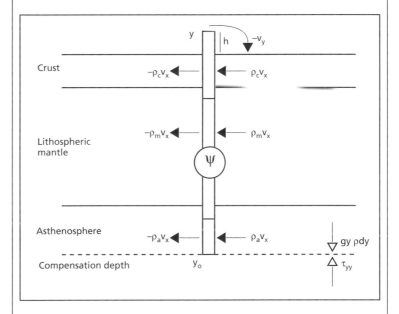

Fig. B15.1 Isostasy through a streamtube (see text for explanation).

continued on p. 270

Fig. 15.3 (*opposite*) The 12 orders of magnitude of the velocity of the Earth's surface caused by tectonic subsidence, uplift, denudation, deposition and eustatic sea-level changes. Note that subsidence and uplift are generally of greater magnitude than denudation, and that uplift is generally greater than deposition. Note the very high rates of eustatic sea-level change produced by glacial melting and the very rapid uplift rates produced by glacial rebound. By contrast, note the very low values of sea-level change produced by mid-ocean-ridge inflation/deflation mechanisms.

fundamental continuity equation for the changing density with time of a unit volume of lithosphere as:

$$\frac{\partial \rho}{\partial t} = \psi - \nabla \cdot \rho v \qquad \text{(B15.1)}$$

The geological theory of isostasy, an application of Archimedes' theory of buoyancy, demands that the vertical component of stress, τ_y, acting at the base of our reference volume must be equal to that in all adjacent volumes. So, from the continuity equation, any change in density or thickness due to the geological processes noted above will cause a corresponding change in elevation with time, $\partial y/\partial t$. Thus surface elevation change may be caused by the contributions and feedback from lithospheric thickening or thinning, metamorphic phase changes, denudation, loading and internal heating.

Let us briefly apply the above principles to surface uplift and subsidence. Consider a section through the lithosphere of unit area in the xy plane. Let h be the mean elevation above or below sea level, and let $v_{x,y}$ be the velocity of material of density ρ' into or out of lithosphere of density ρ over a time t. The new elevation h' is given by:

$$h' = h + v_{x,y} t \left(\frac{\rho - \rho'}{\rho} \right) \qquad \text{(B15.2)}$$

So in unit time the velocity of the Earth's surface u_y, in the absence of denudation or deposition, is given by:

$$u_y = v_{x,y} \left(\frac{\rho - \rho'}{\rho} \right) \qquad \text{(B15.3)}$$

The rate of surface uplift or subsidence thus depends upon the rate of material or thermal flux and on the density contrast.

More information on isostasy and surface deformation [*continued*]

passive continental margins that have been evolving for up to 10^2 Myr are often remarkably steep, except of course where they are blanketed by depositional features like large submarine fans. The global zone of maximum steepness (Fig. 15.4) is 1–2 km deep with a mean value of some 1.8°. Submarine slope evolution involves both progradational outbuilding and also periodic submarine landsliding to preserve the initial form of the shelf slope break. The largest areas of low submarine slopes occur on the abyssal plains, usually with slopes of < 0.3° at 5.8 km depth.

Although areas of high continental elevation tend, on average, to have the higher gradients (Plates 7 & 8), there are many exceptions, for example much of southern Africa, the interior of the Tibetan Plateau and the interior central Andes. Subaerial slopes are generally less than submarine slopes, reflecting the wider and more diffuse nature of continental plate boundaries, more active processes of deposition and erosion, and less spectacular volcanic constructions. All continental plates show a marked zone of low slopes close to sea level (Fig. 15.4), usually around 0.2°. This is a constructional feature, reflecting the deposition of sediments along coastal plains and on the coastal zone and the shallow shelf. The most prominent zones of steep subaerial slopes are associated with the thrusted margins of the Alpine–Himalayan and Andean mountain belts. The south Himalayas and northern Tibetan fronts are the only continental slopes comparable in magnitude and linear extent to those of the oceanic margins. Areas of continental extension such as the Basin and Range and central

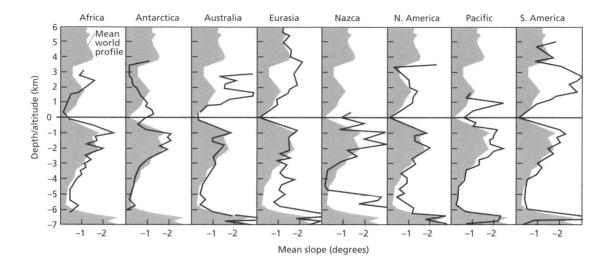

Fig. 15.4 The mean slope calculated for all points within 250 m increments of elevation for each of the major plates, together with the (shaded) grand mean world slope trend against elevation for comparison. Polar data are eliminated beyond 75° latitude because of distortion on the original digital image. (After Moore & Mark, 1986.)

Greece produce low-wavelength/high-frequency slope terrains of great complexity. By way of contrast, the great East African Rift system has longer-wavelength and lower-frequency slopes, reflecting regional-scale updoming and bending of the lithosphere.

15.3 Catchment processes

Weathering provides dissolved and solid materials for transport by moving fluids at the Earth's surface. It seems that in many cases the rate of weathering and the rate of removal in catchments are in long-term equilibrium (e.g. Reneau & Dietrich, 1991; McKean et al., 1993). Catchment transfer processes and rates of landscape denudation are relevant to the sedimentologist because the mass flux of sediment and dissolved materials out of a catchment and into a sedimentary basin are one of the chief controls on the extent and rate of basin infill. The stratigraphy of deposits results from the competition between sediment supply, tectonics and relative sea- or lake-level change. Denudation by weathering and erosion controls the exhumation of subsurface rock masses and, together with uplift, determines the elevation of

the crustal surface. During landscape erosion and denudation, three rates of change are involved:

- the rate of removal of surface soil particles by erosion, determining the rate of lowering of the surface (V_1 in Fig. 15.5);
- the rate, V_2, of descent of the soil front;
- the rate, V_3, of descent of the saprolitization front.

We have noted already the aphorism that the drainage basin is 'the fundamental unit of geomorphology'. We may relate water and sediment runoff to the surface area, relief, gradient, drainage density and vegetational state of a drainage basin. The highest relief ratios occur in smaller basins and these tend to have more peaked hydrographs with shorter lag between precipitation and flood peak. Thus for a given rock type and climate, smaller basins produce a higher sediment yield per unit area. Drainage density, the length of watercourses per unit area, usually reflects precipitation intensity, with the highest densities in semiarid areas and the lowest in humid temperate areas. The higher the drainage density, the higher the sediment yield. Although there is a general decrease in concentration of dissolved load with increased runoff, the amount of dissolved load transported generally increases. This is because the decrease in concentration is more than offset by the increase of volume (flux or load being a product of concentration times volume).

Precipitation and temperature, more precisely their yearly distribution, control the development of vegetation. Degree and type of natural vegetation

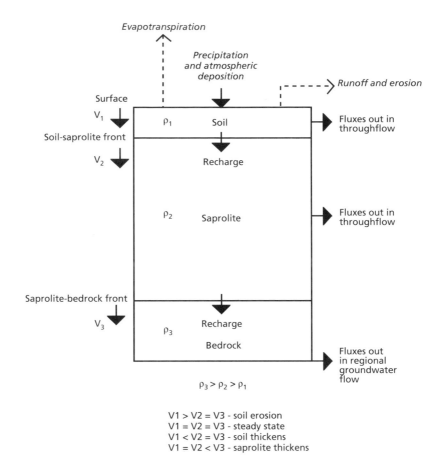

Fig. 15.5 Definition diagram to illustrate the various soil and weathering fronts, their velocities of descent and the fluxes out of the hillslope weathering system.

cover strongly control weathering rates through the influence of the soil ecosystem. Sediment yield is sensitive to degree of vegetation cover because of sheltering and binding effects that reduce rainsplash erosion and surface rilling. Vegetation also has a major role in the hydrological cycle, contributing major losses of water through evapotranspiration. As well as precipitation, rock type is an important independent variable, partly controlling runoff character, the location of springs, the rate of weathering, and the nature of solid and dissolved loads.

Sediment budgets may be calculated for catchments using an accounting system based upon mass conservation. Dissolved load is measured at the drainage

outlets. Solid sediment is derived from weathered surface layers, then transported as surface wash by overland flow or as colluvium by creep and mass flow down hillslope hollows into the stream system. Detailed studies in the unglaciated catchments of Oregon (Reneau & Dietrich, 1991) reveal an approximate long-term balance between rock provided by exfoliation on the hillslopes and sediment plus ions exported by streams from their catchments. But not all sediment that is eroded from the landscape (input) necessarily appears immediately at the drainage outlet (output) because of storage in internal sinks within the drainage or sedimentary basin. The erosion of stored sediment may act as an important marker during periods of environmental change, e.g. deforestation, leading to very high hinterland erosion rates and basinal deposition over relatively short periods of time. This is well illustrated by the late-Quaternary

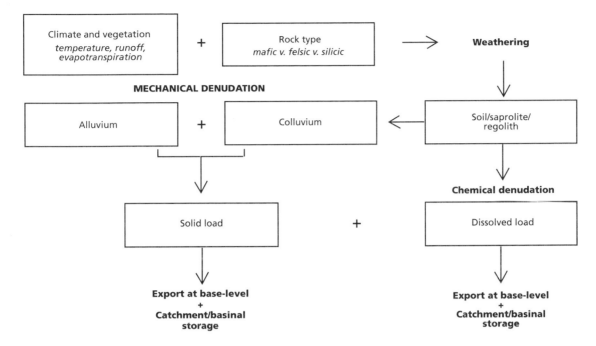

Fig. 15.6 Flow diagram to establish the relationship between mechanical and chemical denudation.

depositional record in many areas of the world (see Bull, 1991). *Homo sapiens* neatly imitates Nature when they clearcut forests—appallingly high sediment yields result.

15.4 Erosion and denudation

It is important to establish the essential difference between erosion and denudation:

Erosion is a removal of material from the Earth's surface and must be defined with reference to co-ordinates fixed beneath the surface, since the surface potential elevation may itself change because of tectonics. Erosion rates may refer to local measured absolute values or to regional values integrated over a catchment.

Denudation refers to the loss of material from both surface and subsurface parts of a drainage basin or regional landscape by all types of weathering, physical and chemical. It includes the important chemical mass flux through soil and saprolite zones (about equal in magnitude), measured ultimately as dissolved load in streams and moving groundwater. We can thus speak of mechanical and chemical denudation

(Fig. 15.6), their sum being the total denudation (see Carson & Kirkby, 1972, pp. 264–6). Like erosion, denudation is defined with reference to fixed internal coordinates.

So, the important difference between erosion and denudation is that erosion may be directly and locally measured but that denudation is not always accompanied by erosion. Saprolite formation by chemical denudation may be accompanied by substantial export of ions (in certain climates) and a decrease of density, but not necessarily by noticeable erosion at the surface. Since chemical denudation leads to a loss of mass, changes in surface elevation due to isostatic recovery will result.

Rates of chemical denudation are usually correlated positively with runoff. Under some climatic conditions, this rate may exceed the mechanical denudation rate, but it is usually lower. The positive correlation arises because of the chemistry of the weathering process discussed previously (Chapter 2). Thus increased runoff and infiltration enable new, more acidic pore-water to displace *in situ* porewater. Rock type exerts a very strong control over the magnitude and nature of the dissolved load. Several studies have shown that porous and permeable immature sandstones give much higher dissolved yields than acid plutonics or supermature quartzites.

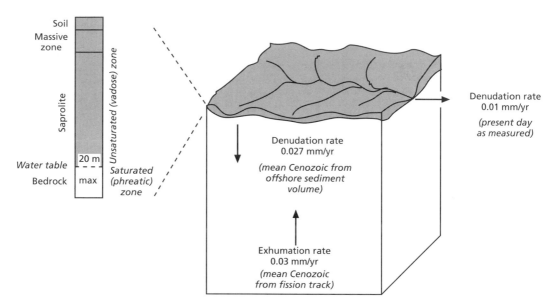

Cenozoic Appalachian Piedmont–a landscape in steady state

Fig. 15.7 Schematic indicating that there is an approximate long-term equivalence between estimates of surface denudation (lowering) and the exhumation rate of bedrock. (After Pavich, 1985, 1986.)

Estimates of historic rates of total denudation are usually made over a whole catchment or part of a catchment by measuring the mass fluxes of suspended load, bedload and dissolved load at suitably placed gauging stations on rivers. Such techniques were pioneered in the USA in the early part of the 20th century. Many of these records show us more about how human interference has changed the fluxes involved. Longer-term erosion estimates must be made with reference to dated geomorphic surfaces such as river terraces, raised beaches, pediment levels, etc. Local rates of surface erosion may be determined by direct measurement, either mechanical measurements or proxy measurements by cosmically derived isotopes such as [10]Be—see review in Morris (1991) and for applications to deposition and erosion rates see, respectively, Lee *et al.* (1993) and McKean *et al.* (1993). Mean exhumation rates integrated over several million years may be deduced from apatite fission track lengths and their statistical distributions (Gleadow *et al.*, 1986). The technique depends upon the accurate estimation of geothermal gradient over the time

interval in question. Apatite fission track analysis (AFTA) has revolutionized studies of exhumation and vertical motions of the denuding crust in the past 10 years or so (e.g. van der Beek *et al.*, 1994).

The simplest field example of mass conservation to consider is that of the isostatic or flexural response to denudation, with no other imposed vertical or horizontal tectonic motions. Mass-balance studies by Pavich (1985, 1986; Fig. 15.7) in the Piedmont zone of the Appalachian orogenic belt support an approximate long-term balance there between denudation and exhumation determined by apatite fission track studies (Boettcher & Milliken, 1994). The mean exhumation rate for the post-early Cretaceous is 0.028 mm/yr, with clear indication of a Miocene acceleration of unroofing due to a warm-to-cool climate change. The implications of erosion to Appalachian landscape evolution and sediment delivery rates are discussed by Pazzaglia and Brandon (1996).

15.5 Large-scale studies of denudation rates

As we discussed in Chapter 1, denudation makes a major contribution to global plate recycling. The major loci of deposition are shown in Fig. 15.8. The estimated observed sediment delivery rate to the

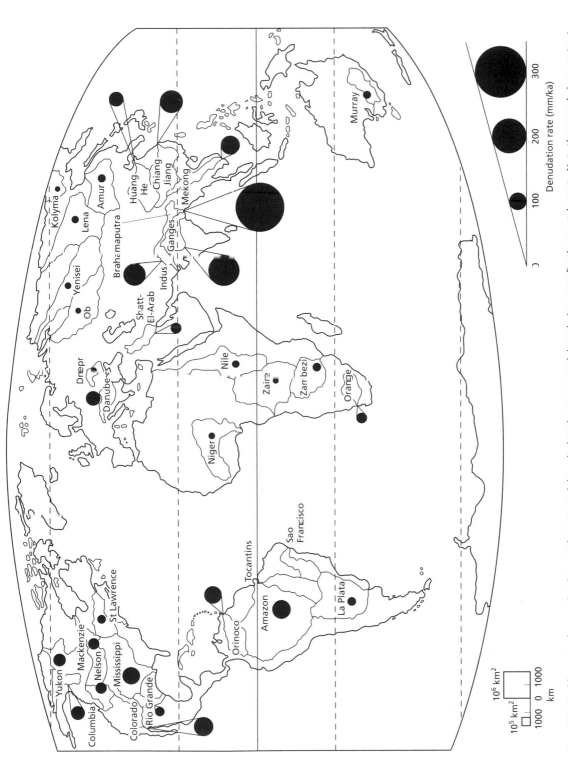

Fig. 15.8 World map to show major river catchments and the calculated mean annual denudation rates for these catchments. Note the very obvious contrast between the high rates from the continent–continent collision zone of the Himalayas compared to, say, the low rates from the relatively tectonically stable African continental plate. (Data of Summerfield & Hulton, 1994.)

oceans gives a sediment yield of some 150 t/km^2 yr (Milliman & Meade, 1983). Some of the difference between measured oceanic delivery and estimated upland denudation is due to temporary storage of sediment in catchment interfluves, floodplains and deltas. More important to the geologist is the sediment stored by subsidence of sedimentary basins. It is likely that 'natural' early-Holocene sediment yields were much reduced compared to those presently measured, perhaps by 50%. Calculations (Milliman & Syvitski, 1992) suggest that the pre-forest-clearance total sediment discharge to the oceans may have been about 10 billion tonnes per year, only about half present (pre-dam era) estimates.

The effects of mean annual precipitation on erosion rates in drainage basins from the North American Mid-West are discussed in a classic and much-quoted paper by Langbein and Schumm (1958). Schumm's (1968a) graph is shown in Fig. 15.9. Yields are low from arid drainage basins because runoff is low. They are high in semiarid basins because highly peaked runoff occurs with sparse vegetation. Yields were thought to be relatively lower in temperate and tropical basins where vegetation is abundant. The Langbein and Schumm results have not been duplicated on geographically wider data sets (Jansson, 1988; Milliman & Syvitski, 1992; Summerfield & Hulton, 1994; Ludwig & Probst, 1996; Hovius, 1997), which include the influence of catchment area, gradient, relief and rainfall regime.

In his classic study, Fournier (1960) used measurements of suspended sediment yield from 78 drainage basins ranging in size from 2.5×10^3 to 1.0×10^6 km^2. Sediment yield E (t/km^2 yr) was correlated with mean drainage basin elevation h, slope α and a precipitation peakedness parameter p^2/P, where p is the highest monthly rainfall and P is the mean annual rainfall. By multiple regression

$$\log E = 2.65 \log \left(\frac{p^2}{P} \right) + 0.46 \log h \tan \alpha - 1.56$$

$$(15.1)$$

This equation may be used to predict yield when climate and relief are known. High yields are thus to be expected in the high-gradient, seasonally humid tropics, with lower rates in equatorial zones where seasonal effects are lacking. Fournier used climatic records for p^2/P to give a world map of erosion, but it is likely that the absence of data on dissolved loads

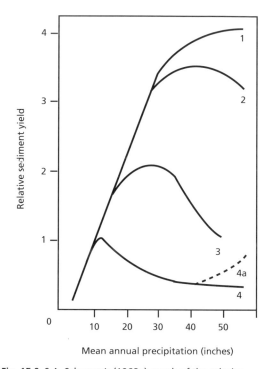

Fig. 15.9 S.A. Schumm's (1968a) graph of the relative trend of predicted sediment yield for different times in the geological past (curves 1–3) compared to that of the present (curve 4; after Langbein & Schumm, 1958). Curve 1 described the pre-Silurian, prior to the appearance of land vegetation. Curve 2 follows the appearance of primitive land vegetation in the Siluro-Devonian. Curve 3 follows the appearance of post-Cretaceous grasses.

has led to some underestimation of the denudation rate in certain basins. A more serious criticism is that sediment yields more properly reflect local basin relief rather than basin elevation. Also, the yields from smaller drainage basins, particularly those in steep mountainous terrains subject to abundant landsliding (Hovius et al., 1997), are well known to be much higher per unit area than in larger basins (Scott & Williams, 1978; Milliman & Syvitski, 1992). This effect, together with the increased influence of local rock properties such as erodibility, make the Fournier equation (and others) unsuitable for small-scale basin modelling. Nevertheless, data from mountainous terrains with across-range changes in precipitation bear out the basic message of Fournier's approach (Fig. 15.10).

In an attempt to overcome some of the above problems, Ahnert (1970), in an influential study,

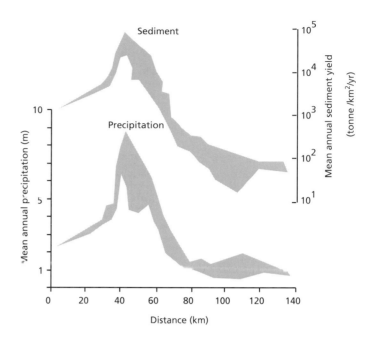

Fig. 15.10 (a) Variation of sediment yield with precipitation in a west–east transect across the New Zealand Alps. The data are presented here as an envelope of curves from local maxima to minima. The data are spectacularly consistent and show the close positive relationship between precipitation and sediment yield in this uplifting and orogenically active area. The rate of change of precipitation is itself controlled by topography, since the New Zealand rains are orographic in nature. (b) Comparison of denudation vs. uplift rates in a west–east transect across central South Island, New Zealand. Note that the denudation along the transect always exceeds the measured rates of uplift. Note, too, that the denudation rate (due, perhaps in large part, to landsliding and subsequent transport-limited streamflow) is very, very high. (After Selby, 1993, figs 19.5 & 19.6, and sources cited therein; see also Hovius *et al.*, 1997.)

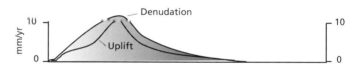

choose 20 mid-latitude, northern-hemisphere drainage basins ranging in area from 1.0×10^2 to 1.0×10^3 km² with mean annual precipitation of 250–2500 mm/yr. Although large enough to show no influence of particular rock types, none of these basins have pronounced seasonality of precipitation, eliminating any peakedness influence of the kind recognized in Fournier's approach. Denudation rates D (mm/yr) were calculated from data on both dissolved and suspended loads, and the data were regressed against mean drainage basin relief (h) as determined from numerous 20 × 20 km² grids. The following linear relationship was derived (Fig. 15.11):

$$D = (1.54 \times 10^{-4})h - 1.09 \times 10^{-2} \qquad (15.2)$$

Ahnert's result has an exponential form since the rate of change of relief, D, is proportional to the relief itself. In symbols:

$$D = -\frac{dh}{dt} = kh \qquad (15.3)$$

Integrating, we have:

$$h = -k \int h \; dt = h_0 e^{-tk} \qquad (15.4)$$

or

$$h = h_0 e^{-t/\tau} \qquad (15.5)$$

where h_0 is relief at $t = 0$ and $\tau = 1/k$ is the denudational time constant, calculated as 6.5 Myr from Ahnert's relationship. A criticism of the approach is that it neglects to take account of isostatic recovery, which always acts regionally to restore a proportion of the surface relief removed by denudation. The Ahnert denudation time constants are thus considerable underestimates.

More recent worldwide studies (Pinet & Souriau, 1988; Milliman & Syvitski, 1992; Summerfield & Hulton, 1994; Ludwig & Probst, 1996; Hovius, 1997) have clearly shown the importance of Ahnert's basic point concerning the importance of drainage basin relief upon denudation rates. Despite the relief–yield correlation, the tremendous variations in the

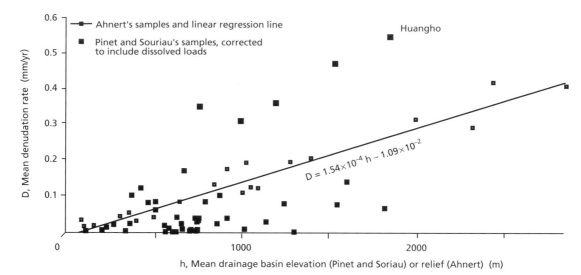

Fig. 15.11 The relationship between mean drainage basin relief (Ahnert, 1970) or elevation (Pinet & Souriau, 1988) plotted against mean total denudation rate for large catchments worldwide. Note the well-constrained Ahnert linear relationship but the very large scatter (shotgun effect) when all the data points are considered. There does seem to be a very generalized positive correlation, but clearly there are additional variables affecting total denudation rate.

other variables (Fig. 15.12) suggest that a great deal of caution should be used when assessing the parametrization of erosion rates in basin modelling studies.

Although it is obvious that many areas of active tectonics have been or are being uplifted, the isostatic response to denudation causes elevation to decline only gently. This is well seen in the uplifting accretionary prism of Taiwan (Li, 1976) and in South Island, New Zealand (Selby, 1993). It should be noted that in such areas rates of denudation are extraordinarily high because of the dominance of landsliding in young easily erodible rocks (Hovius *et al.*, 1998) and the effects of orographic precipitation. In certain cases where major downcutting by rivers or glaciers has occurred, it may be that mountain elevation actually increases due to valley erosion (Molnar & England, 1990).

15.6 Basinal studies of denudation and sediment flux: the inverse approach

Methods for determining longer-term (10^2–10^7 yr) sediment fluxes out of catchments are based upon estimations of eroded or deposited volumes, assessed with respect to bounding surfaces of known age (Ibbeken & Schleyer, 1991; Collier *et al.*, 1995;

Pazzaglia & Brandon, 1996; Fig. 15.13). Usually in such cases a correction has to be made for dispersion of the dissolved contribution and for the increased volume (decreased density) of the sediment over and above that of the eroded bedrock. Sometimes the estimates may be checked against independent indicators of exhumation or sediment yields.

The simplest case is that of river discharge into a lake or reservoir. Take the example of Lake Mead on the Colorado river in Arizona. The Hoover Dam was constructed in 1929. Over the 14 years to 1943, an estimated volume accumulated on the reservoir floor corresponding to an annual flux of 144×10^6 t/yr. Direct measurements indicate an annual dissolved load of some 10×10^6 t/yr. These fluxes sum to yield a mean erosion rate of about 0.144 mm/yr over the 392 118 km² drainage basin of the Colorado river and tributaries.

A very useful methodology makes use of deposition from a catchment on to a datable surface. Consider the Milner Creek alluvial fan, which is sourced in the White Mountains of east-central California (Beaty, 1970). The Pleistocene fan sediments were deposited upon the 700 kyr Bishops Tuff, whose subsurface extent may be extrapolated from surface mapping.

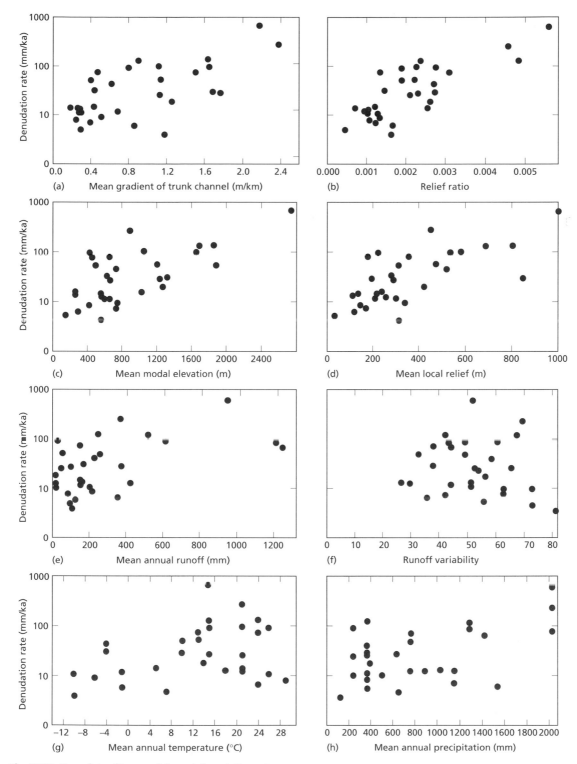

Fig. 15.12 Crossplots of large-catchment denudation rates against several catchment variables. (From Summerfield & Hulton, 1994.)

As noted previously, the change of position of a fixed rock volume with respect to some earth-surface datum (such as fixed sea level) records the exhumation of that volume. This is the so-called 'uplift rate' recorded by fission track dating (see Molnar & England, 1990). The rate of change of mean surface elevation, $\partial h/\partial t$, is the sum of the denudation $(-u_d)$, isostatic recovery (u_i) and tectonic (u_t) velocities:

$$\frac{\partial h}{\partial t} = u_t - u_d + u_i \tag{B15.4}$$

This equation must be solved iteratively to yield the changing continental elevation over successive small time increments, δ_t. Thus:

$$h_{(\delta t)} = h_0 + \frac{\rho_c}{\rho_m}(u_t\delta t)e^{-\delta t/\tau} \tag{B15.5}$$

where h_0 is the original elevation, τ is the denudational time constant and ρ_c and ρ_m are mean crustal and mantle densities respectively ($\rho_c/\rho_m = 0.83$). An example of this expression is graphed in Fig. B15.2.

A note on denudation rates, elevation changes and the isostatic response

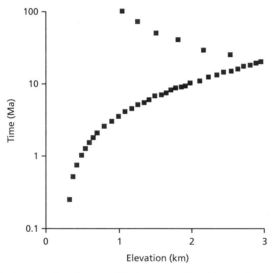

Fig. B15.2 The elevation change with time as predicted by eqn (B15.5) with a typical crust/mantle density ratio of 0.83, $\tau = 2.5$ Myr, $u_t = 0.25$ km/Myr for 20 Myr, then $u_t = 0$ for 80 Myr; $h_0 = 0.25$ km.

The 1.733 km² volume of the fan represents a mean erosion rate of some 0.06 mm/yr from the 35.5 km² area of the Milner Creek catchment. This estimate is uncorrected for any export of dissolved ions, the magnitude of which is unknown in the area but which is unlikely to exceed 10%. Using similar techniques a number of other basin fills from Nevada yield mean erosion rates for the last 15 million years or so of around 0.06 mm/yr.

The usefulness of the inverse catchment method is best illustrated by stepping up a scale. Consider the Ganges–Brahmaputra catchment, which drains the eastern Himalayas and part of southern Tibet. Sediment from this drainage area of 6.1×10^5 km² has

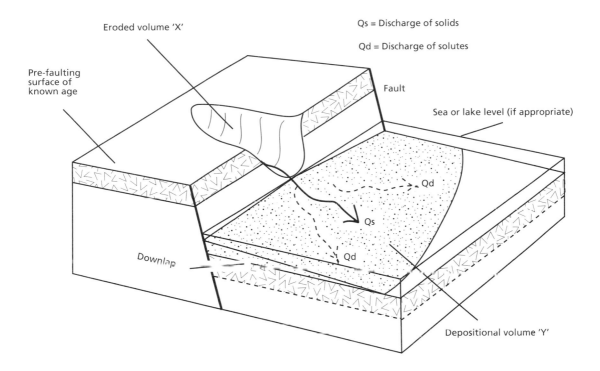

Fig. 15.13 Sketch to show the basic methodology for estimating eroded rock volumes from observed sediment volumes present above a dated datum plane. (After Collier et al., 1995.)

accumulated in marginal fans, in the Ganges–Brahmaputra foreland basin and on the vast Bengal submarine fan over the last 40 Myr since the collision of the Indian plate with Asia. An estimated 1.4×10^7 km³ of sediment solids (corrected for density differences from bedrock) is preserved onshore and offshore. Today, the catchment exports an additional 20% of dissolved contributions (Milliman & Mead, 1983). Assuming that this has remained constant over time, we arrive at a grand total exported volume of 1.54×10^7 km³ in 40 Myr. This translates into a mean eroded thickness of 23 km over the catchment at a mean rate of some 0.58 mm/yr. It should be stressed that this result is a mean estimate integrated over the whole catchment and does not take into account shorter-term changes in erosion rates consequent upon the uplifting of the Tibetan Plateau in the last 5 Myr or so. This has led to estimates of > 1 mm/yr erosion rates from geochronological studies of Tibetan basement (Copeland & Harrison, 1990).

15.7 Sediment supply, vegetation and climate change: implications for basin stratigraphy

In the past few years geologists have tended to concentrate on exploring tectonic controls on relief, slope and sediment supply. At the same time the occurrence of climate change during Quaternary times has been well established, together with increasing appreciation of its effects on the sedimentary record during earlier geological epochs (e.g. Perlmutter & Mathews, 1989; Frakes et al., 1992). In particular, with the advent of sequence stratigraphic concepts, it is a matter of great importance to explore whether ups and downs of sea or lake level are accompanied by more or less sediment supply from continental catchments. That is, do sea level and sediment supply change in phase or out of phase? The rate of sediment supply to a sedimentary basin depends upon the rate of surface soil and rock erosion in the basin-bordering catchments, minus any sediment stored or otherwise exported, e.g. by wind. As we have seen, it is determined, in complex ways, by catchment geology, relief and slope and by the role of climate in determining vegetation and runoff. The lack of success of

where β is the rate of decomposition at temperature T (°C) and $β_0$ is the rate at 0 °C. Having established GPP and plant losses, the net primary productivity (NPP) is calculated following standard International Biological Programme methodologies (Newbould, 1967; Milner & Hughes, 1968), which underlie the entire vegetation growth model. The vegetation and soil are allowed to develop until vegetation equilibrium is achieved. Equilibrium is presently defined as existing when the monthly levels of vegetation and soil are replicated year on year. It is for this equilibrium condition that the erosion potential values are calculated, although the model may also be used in a transient mode.

Overland flow generation is controlled by a soil-water storage threshold. This threshold is controlled by the equilibrium vegetation–soil complex in four ways:

1 The soil organic matter acts as a dynamic store of soil water.
2 Above-ground biomass intercepts and evaporates raindrops from leaf surfaces, modifying groundwater and local water balances.
3 A large, but less dynamic, soil-water store is provided by the degree of mineral soil present.
4 By reducing raindrop impact on the soil, the vegetation cover also prevents soil crusting, which further modifies the threshold value.

Until the soil storage threshold has been reached (based on the interaction between the above-ground input and the subsurface store drainage), overland flow will not occur. Once it does occur, it is assumed that a proportion of the excess generates overland flow, and the resulting discharge will accumulate linearly downslope. The sediment yield resulting from this discharge is modelled as a power law with exponent 2:

$$S = q^2 \Lambda = k[(r-h)a]^2 \Lambda \qquad (B15.7)$$

where S is sediment transport, q is water discharge, Λ is hillslope gradient, k is the erodibility coefficient, r is a single rainfall event, h is soil-moisture storage threshold and a is the area drained per unit flow width. Equation (B15.7) is combined with a standard mass-balance equation. The CSEP is written as the nonspatial part of eqn (B15.7):

$$CSEP = \Sigma(r-h)^2 \qquad (B15.8)$$

where the summation is over the distribution of daily rainfalls for each month. With N_0 and r_0 as empirical parameters of the rainfall distribution for a given month and R as the total monthly precipitation, the annual CSEP is obtained by summing over each month of the year:

$$CSEP = 2N_0 r_0^2 \exp(-h/r_0) = 2r_0 R \exp(-h/r_0) \qquad (B15.9)$$

A full derivation of eqn (B15.9) is given in Kirkby and Cox (1995). The value of the CSEP obtained is a *relative* erosion potential based on the integrated effects of climate and the developing vegetation–soil system at the centre of the grid cell.

Further information on CSEP
[*continued*]

estimates will vary according to the nature of the investigation proposed. For example, the determination of erosion rates relevant to geophysical models for basin margin deformation requires data on a long timescale, perhaps over 10^6–10^7 yr, such as those provided from Australia by Nott and Roberts (1996). Students of fluvial architecture, on the other hand, require data on changing rates of sediment delivery over timespans of the order 5–100 kyr so that they can try to distinguish between climatic, sea-level and tectonic origins for fluvial cycles (e.g. Blum, 1993). Finally, archaeological, geomorphological and environmental studies often require information on timescales of 10–1000 yr.

We may illustrate the effects of climate on sediment yields with reference to the Mediterranean area, where there is pollen evidence for periodic major changes in later Quaternary vegetation at eccentricity and, to a lesser extent, precessional timescales (Tzedakis, 1993). Glacial maxima were characterized by widespread development of treeless steppe, and the interglacials by Mediterranean forest. The direct evidence of the glacial vegetation, water-balance models (Prentice et al., 1992) and evidence for higher lake levels suggest cooler temperatures with similar yearly rainfall to the present day for glacial maximum times, but with an increase in winter runoff. CSEP computational experiments (Figs 15.15 & 15.16) indicate that the vegetation cover of each month under the 18 ka climate was lower than that of today. Total runoff was

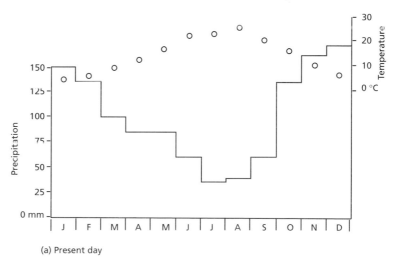

(a) Present day

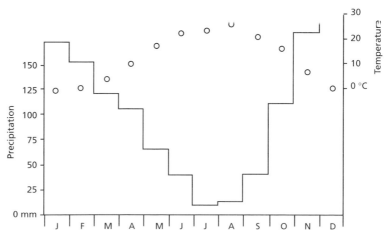

Fig. 15.15 Climatic data (from Prentice et al., 1992) used in CSEP experiments (Leeder et al., 1998): (a) present-day monthly climatic data for northern Greece; (b) glacial maximum (18 ka) data.

(b) Glacial maximum, 18 kyr

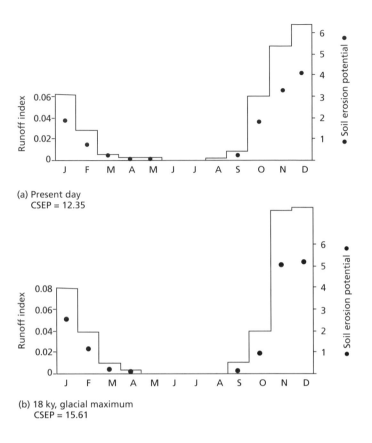

(a) Present day
CSEP = 12.35

(b) 18 ky, glacial maximum
CSEP = 15.61

Fig. 15.16 Results of CSEP experiments (Leeder *et al.*, 1998) for present-day and glacial climate scenarios. The vegetation cover (not shown here) of each month under the 18 ka climate is lower than that of today. Total runoff was higher at 18 ka ago than today, with high winter runoff a major feature. In terms of monthly potential erosion levels, there is a major difference between the two times, with higher levels of potential erosion in the cool wet winters of 18 ka. Overall the total annual erosion at 18 ka is about 25% higher, with a CSEP index of 15.6, compared with today's value of 12.4.

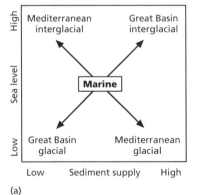

(a)

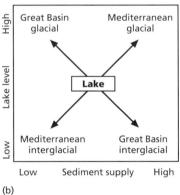

(b)

Fig. 15.17 Relative rates of sediment supply in relation to (a) sea and (b) lake level for Mediterranean (high sediment yields in glacial epochs) and Great Basin (high sediment yields in interglacial epochs) Quaternary climatic regimes. (See Leeder *et al.*, 1998.) For the marine scenario, the Great Basin case is indicative and generalized, in the sense that much of the drainage here is internal—the response of the Colorado catchment and delta to climate change would be a direct and interesting test of the thesis.

higher at 18 ka than today, with increased winter runoff a major feature. In terms of monthly erosion levels, there is a major difference in the distribution of erosion between the two times, with higher levels in the cool wet winters of the glacial maximum. Overall the annual erosion at 18 ka is higher, with a CSEP index of 15.6, compared with today's value of 12.4.

Although we have stressed the role of major glacial to interglacial climatic changes in altering the balance of sediment and water discharges in rivers, we stress that channels are sensitive to shorter-term climatic fluctuations. The cases of the San Pedro, Paria and Gila rivers in the southwestern USA (Burkham, 1972; Graf *et al.*, 1991; Hereford, 1993; Huckleberry, 1994) are instructive. Here the coincidence of the onset of channel degradation and widening with the onset of large winter floods above the base discharge suggests that seasonal distribution of floods controls

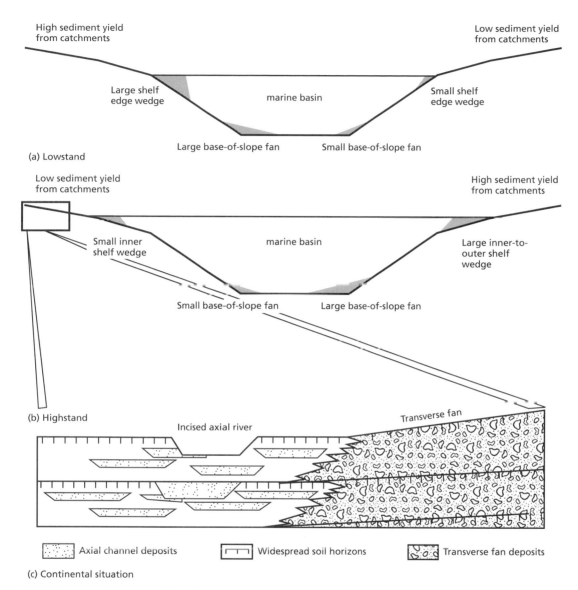

High sediment yield
from catchments

Low sediment yield
from catchments

Large shelf
edge wedge

marine basin

Small shelf
edge wedge

Large base-of-slope fan   Small base-of-slope fan

(a) Lowstand

Low sediment yield
from catchments

High sediment yield
from catchments

Small inner
shelf wedge

marine basin

Large inner-to-
outer shelf
wedge

Small base-of-slope fan   Large base-of-slope fan

(b) Highstand

Incised axial river   Transverse fan

Axial channel deposits   Widespread soil horizons   Transverse fan deposits

(c) Continental situation

Fig. 15.18 Cartoons to illustrate effects of variations in sediment supply to the development of marine coarse-grained clastic wedges during (a) lowstand and (b) highstand conditions. The inset (c) tries to show the development of fluviatile cycles in relation to climate change (in the spirit of Blum, 1993). These may occur independently of sea- or lake-level changes. Incision, fan retreat and soil formation are shown occurring during periods of low sediment supply from catchments to fans and axial rivers. Aggradation and fan growth (progradation) occur during periods of high sediment yield.

the channel aggradation–degradation process. Winter floods due to frontal rains, although smaller and less frequent than summer and autumn floods, carry very little sediment and have a greater ability to erode the channel than do summer and autumn floods due to storms. These latter may also be insufficient to increase the main channel's discharge, so that accumulation of the introduced sediment results (Blum, 1993).

Turning briefly to marine and lake environments within sedimentary basins, we return to the sediment supply scenarios sketched out previously and summarized in Figs 15.17 and 15.18.

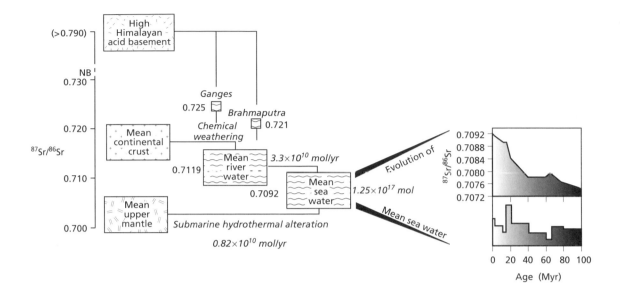

Fig. 15.19 The major ^{87}Sr and ^{86}Sr fluxes and sources, and the change and rate of change of mean oceanic ^{87}Sr/^{86}Sr ratio over the last 100 Myr. The oceanic mean composition is very strongly modulated by input from the high ^{87}Sr/^{86}Sr acid leucogranites of the High Himalayas. (Various data from Richter *et al.*, 1992; Krishnaswami *et al.*, 1992.)

For catchments feeding marine environments with low sediment discharges during full-glacial climate and sea-level lowstand, the production of incised valleys due to the gradient changes accompanying sea-level fall at the shelf–coastal break will be accentuated by lack of sediment availability. Although lowstand conditions enable shelf bypass and shelf erosion to occur, the lack of sediment availability from the hinterlands will limit the development of lowstand turbidite fans. For lake environments the situation is different, with cool, wetter glacial maxima and lowered sediment yields coinciding with high lake levels due to a combination of increased runoff and/or decreased evaporation. We thus expect the development of upstream fluvial incision to coincide with the production of highstand deltas whose lack of sediment supply will cause low rates of highstand lake-margin delta progradation.

In environments with greater sediment discharges during glacial climates, marine lowstands coincided with aggradational conditions in river basins away from the influence of the shelf–coastal break. The high sediment supply causes rapid lowstand progradation and the development of prominent submarine fans. During highstands sediment supply is much reduced and river incision is likely to occur. Highstand deltas will migrate slowly seawards due to low sediment supply. For lakes, increased winter runoff during glacial times led to high lake levels at the same time as enhanced sediment supply.

A fascinating but little developed area of study is the likely changes in sediment yield through geological time brought about by the evolution of vegetation. Little has been done on this problem since Schumm's penetrating analysis of 30 years ago (Schumm, 1968a; Fig. 15.9). Major changes in vegetation cover since the advent of *Homo sapiens*, chiefly the replacement of forest cover by arable farmlands, has had a sometimes drastic effect upon sediment yields.

15.8 Marine strontium isotope ratio and continental erosion rates

Remarkable insight into time and spatial variation of erosion rates is provided by geochemical markers in the world's oceans. The strontium isotope ratio ^{87}Sr/^{86}Sr is of particular interest (Palmer & Elderfield, 1985). That of modern seawater is 0.709 (Fig. 15.19)

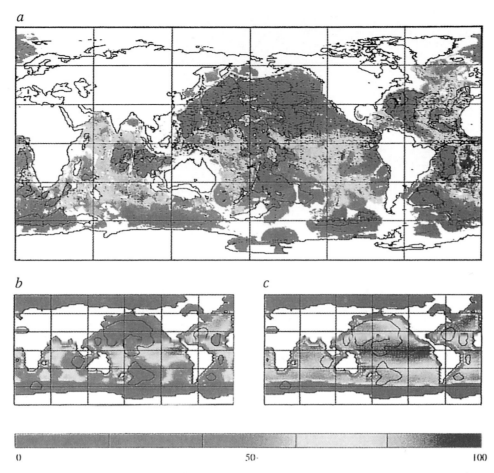

Plate 1 (a) Distribution of sedimentary calcite (dry weight per cent) in seafloor sediments. (b) Modelled distribution using present day CaCO₃ fluxes and a coupled ocean-sediment C-cycle model. (c) Modelled distribution resulting from an increased deep-sea CaCO₃ flux (×2.6 present day level) such as might have drawn down the CO_2 content of the atmosphere into the glacial ocean. The fact that such abundances of $CaCO_3$ are not seen in glacial-age ocean sediments indicates that another mechanism for drawdown must exist. Contour is the 5 km isobath (Figures and discussion after Archer and Maier-Reimer 1994.)

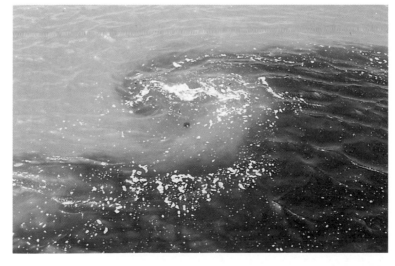

Plate 2 Spectacular vertical axis Kelvin-Helmholtz wave eddy at the interface between the Solimos and Negro tributaries to the Amazon. Solimos is loaded with suspended sediment and is brown. Negro water is organic-rich and black. View about 10 m across. (Photo by and courtesy of M. Pèrez-Arlucea.)

[facing page 288]

(a)

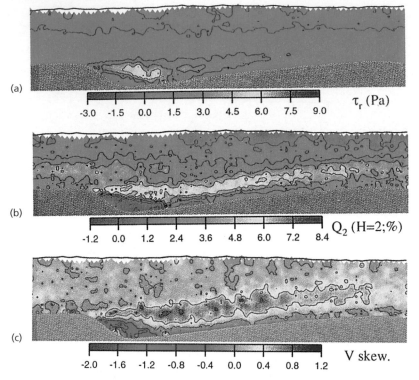

τ_r (Pa)

-3.0   -1.5   0.0   1.5   3.0   4.5   6.0   7.5   9.0

(b)

Q_2 (H=2;%)

-1.2   0.0   1.2   2.4   3.6   4.8   6.0   7.2   8.4

(c)

V skew.

-2.0   -1.6   -1.2   -0.8   -0.4   0.0   0.4   0.8   1.2

Plate 3 Contour maps (Bennett and Best 1995) of flow and turbulence parameters measured by Laser-Doppler anemometry over fixed experimental dune-like bedforms (colourscale forms at base of each image). Flow is from left to right in each case. (a) Distribution of Reynolds stress $\rho \overline{u'v'} = \tau_r$. Note the high stresses extending to the bed associated with the free shear layer of the leeside roller of separated flow and their persistence but gradual decay downstream. (b) Percentage distribution of Quadrant 2 bursting events. Note the persistence of bursting intensity along the downstream extension of the free-shear layer associated with eddies arising from Kelvin–Helmholtz instability (c) Distribution of skewness of the vertical velocity, reinforcing the plot of (b).

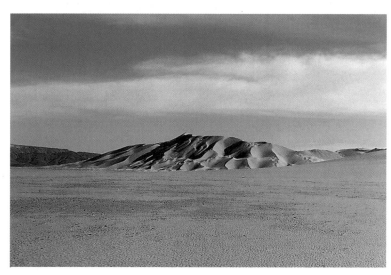

Plate 4 Ground view of large star-shaped dune from the Erg Mehedjibat, 100 km south of In Saleh, Algeria. Dune is approximately 300 m high. (Photo courtesy of R. Dixon.)

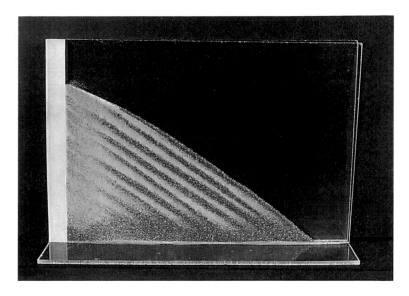

Plate 5 Experimental (Makse *et al.* 1997) segregation and stratification produced when a mixture of grains is poured into the left hand side of a perspex gate of width 5 mm. Typical result showing the formation of successive layers (about 1.2 cm wide) of fine and coarse grains where the white grains are glass beads of average diameter 0.27 mm, while the larger red grains are sugar crystals of typical size 0.8 mm. (Photo courtesy of H. Makse.)

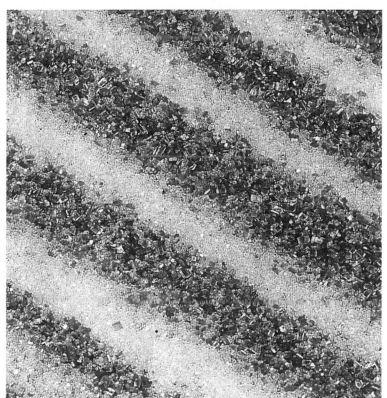

Plate 6 Close-up of laminations in Plate 5 showing the coarse/fine couplets. (Photo courtesy of H. Makse.)

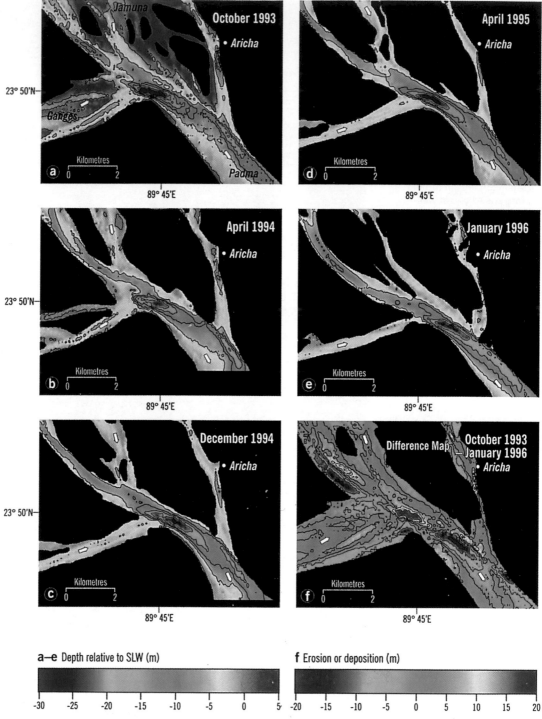

Plate 11 Bathymetry of the Jamuna–Ganges confluence region, Bangladesh, over a 28-month period, for five surveys between October 1993 and January 1996. Bed heights are expressed relative to a standard low water datum (SLW) at Aricha. Parts (a)–(e) show bed morphology for each survey period; part (f) shows the change in bed level over the total survey period. Note the large fluvial conference scours, which erode up to 27m below present sea level and are highly mobile in the lateral sense. These features mean that apparent ancient incision due to sea level fall must be treated with caution. (After Best & Ashworth, 1997; images courtesy of Jim Best and Phil Ashworth.)

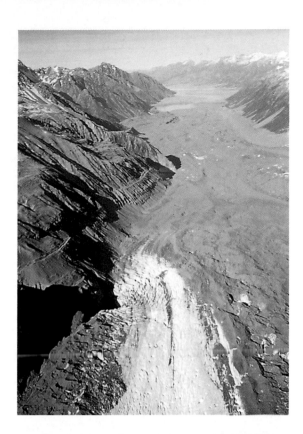

Plate 12 Near snout of the Glacier, South Island, New Zealand. Note extreme dirtiness of the glacier ice surface which is largely covered with debris from surrounding slopes. (Photograph courtesy of Bruce Yardley.)

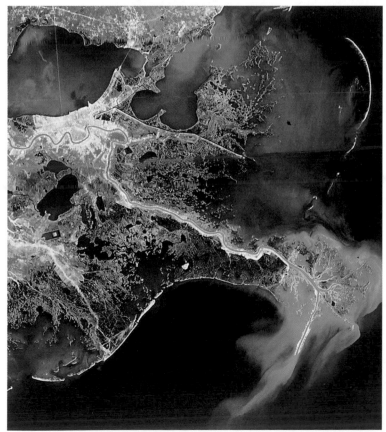

Plate 13 Infrared colour composite of the Mississippi delta as photographed by the Landsat satellite on 9 April 1976. Vegetation appears red, clear water dark blue and suspended sediment light blue. Note the south-westerly deflection of the sediment plumes by the prevailing shelf currents as they enter the Gulf of Mexico from the modern birdsfoot distributary mouths. This westward transport includes massive introduction of farmland-runoff with nutrients; leading to widespread annual hypoxia all along the Louisiana–Texas Shelf (see Malakoff, 1998) (Landsat images 2443–15 and 2443–15 462 as assembled and discussed by G. T. Moore (1979).)

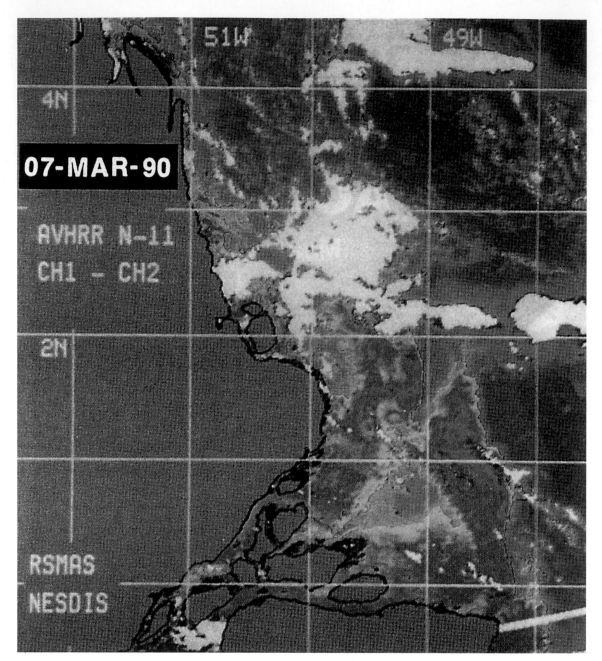

Plate 14 Satellite image of the turbid plume emanating from the mouth of the Amazon River in March 1990. This image was obtained with the Advanced-Very-High-Resolution-Radiometer (AVHRR) on the NOAA 9 satellite, using a composite image created from channel 1 (visible) and channel 2 (near infrared). The most turbid water is located on the continental shelf along the frontal zone, where tidal resuspension and convergence of the estuarine circulation create extremely high concentrations of suspended sediment. The plume of turbid water extending seaward and northward from the river mouth shows considerable variability in structure, reflecting temporal fluctuations on the order of days to weeks. Note also turbid surface water extending northwards along the coast. (Image used courtesy of C. Nittrouer.)

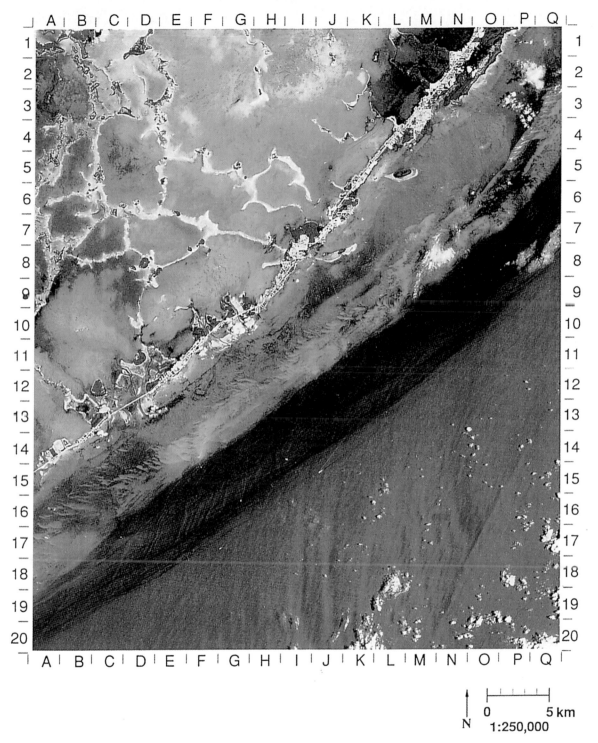

0   5 km

N   1:250,000

Plate 15 Landsat TM image of the south-central part of the Florida barrier/lagoon carbonate complex (from Harris and Kowalik 1994). Note: Florida Bay mudbanks and islands; the Keys (barriers) with their ebb and flood tidal deltas; The inner reef with muddy carbonate and local buildups. The outer reef with prominent dunes in skeletal sands. (See Fig. 24.15.)

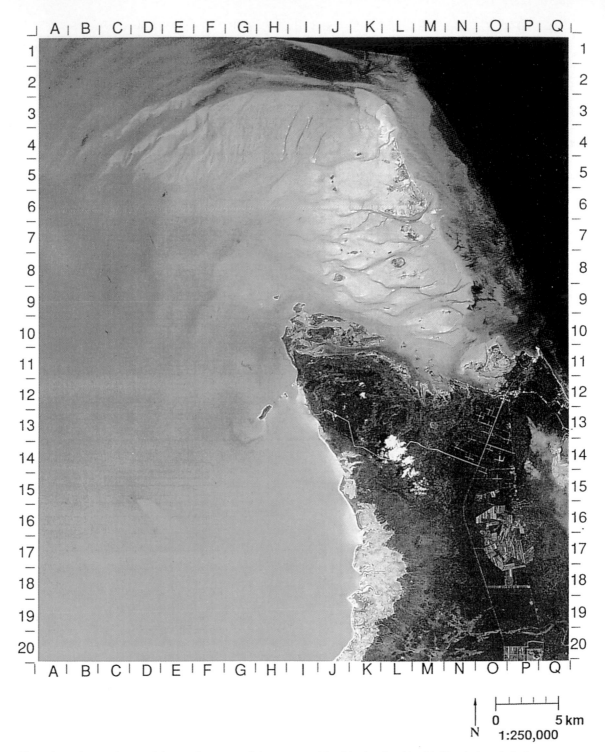

Plate 16 Landsat TM image of the northern part of the Great Bahama Bank with the northern tip of the Island of Andros, the deepwater tongue of the ocean to the north-west (from Harris and Kowalik 1994). Image shows coastal mudflats and drainage channels of the leeward side of Andros (see Fig. 24.12); windward platform bordering the tongue of the ocean; the prominent tidal channels and oolite sand shoals to the leeward of Joulters Cay. (See Fig. 24.16.)

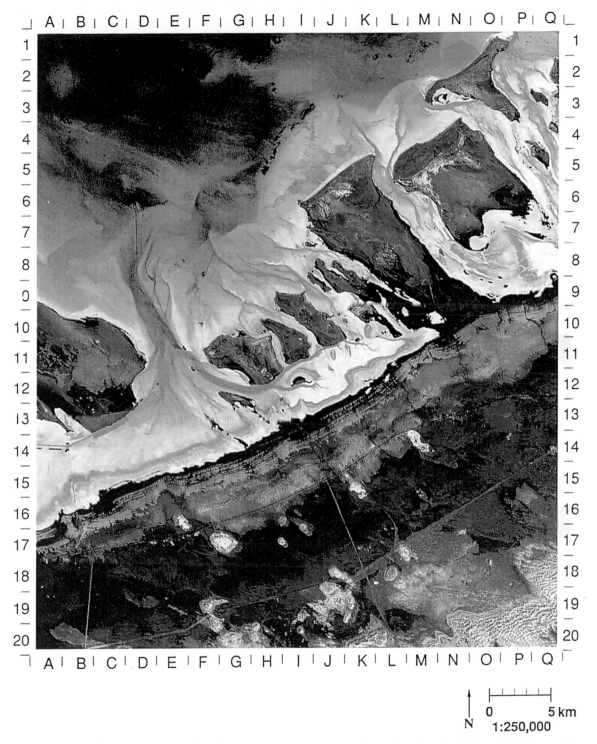

Plate 17 Landsat TM image of eastern Abu Dhabi area, Trucial Coast (from Harris and Kowalik 1994). Note barrier islands; intervening tidal inlets and ebb tidal deltas; ooid and skeletal sand tidal chanels; dark intertidal stromatolite flats; sabkha with numerous beach ridges; fringe of desert dunes to the SW. (See Section 24.2.)

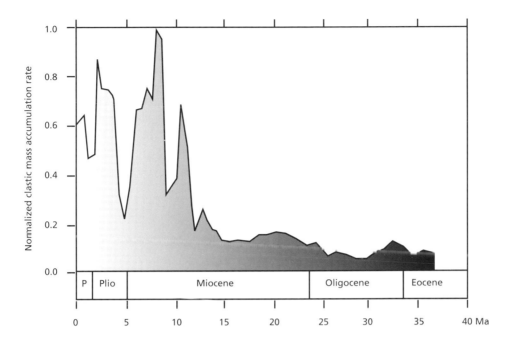

Fig. 15.20 The mean normalized clastic mass accumulation rates for the north-east Indian ocean over the past 40 Myr. The large peaks between about 8 and 12 Ma are approximately coincident with the uplift of the Tibetan Plateau and a presumed increase in the effectiveness of the Indian–Asian monsoon. (After Rea, 1993.)

and is identical, within measurement errors, from ocean to ocean and from the surface to great depths. The ratio is the result of thorough mixing in the ocean (10^3 yr timescale), a long residence time for strontium (about 10^7 yr) and a balance between two main sources of strontium, continental crust and mid-ocean-ridge basalt. The continental crust has a high ratio of rubidium (Rb) to strontium (Sr), and thus the process of chemical weathering generates a lot more radiogenic [87]Sr (provided by the decay of the abundant isotope [87]Rb to [87]Sr) than does the hydrothermal alteration of seafloor basalts of the ocean crust, which are low in radiogenic Sr. Thus the average [87]Sr/[86]Sr ratio of river-water is some 0.712, whilst that of seafloor hydrothermal vents is 0.703. So to keep the oceanic [87]Sr/[86]Sr ratio at its current level requires a mixture of about two-thirds river-water and one-third water from hydrothermal vents. These proportions

are confirmed by observed current river flux and by estimates of heat flux and hydrothermal emission rates from the ocean ridges.

A proxy record of the evolving [87]Sr/[86]Sr ratio in oceanic waters of the past may be gained by analysis of marine skeletal calcites precipitated by organisms in contact with seawater. This calcite may be shown to be in exact isotopic equilibrium with seawater. Provided that the samples are unaltered by diagenesis and no extra mineral phases are present, they may be analysed by mass spectrometry to yield [87]Sr/[86]Sr. Analyses show that the ratio has increased gradually, but spectacularly, over the past 40 Myr (Palmer & Elderfield, 1985; Fig. 15.19). The increase is not thought to be the result of isotopic or flux changes involving the seafloor basalt hydrothermal system, since this is thought to be highly conservative. Rather, it must reflect either regional or global changes in the continental isotopic ratio and/or the flux of continental weathering products into the oceans. One popular solution (Richter *et al.*, 1992) is the coincidental observation that around 40 Ma the Himalayas were formed by plate collision. At that time a huge mass of highly radiogenic gneisses and granitoids were uplifted into the High Himalayas by thrusting and unroofed by intense chemical and physical weathering.

Part 6
Sediment Deposition, Environments and Facies in Continental Environments

16   Aeolian sediments in low-latitude deserts

The bulk of the grains flowed as a dense fog, rising no higher than five feet from the ground. Over it we could see each other quite clearly, head and shoulders only, as in a swimming bath. Up above the great fine-grained crests of the dunes were on the move. Cornices dissolved as we looked, swaying along the curving surfaces in heavy dark folds, as if the mane of some huge animal was being ruffled and reset in a new direction by a gale.

R.A. Bagnold, *Libyan Sands*, Hodder and Stoughton

16.1 Introduction

A desert is generally defined by limited available precipitation and a general deficiency of water for weathering, runoff and accumulation. The technical definition depends on the ratio between actual precipitation (P) and the ability of solar energy and vegetation to return moisture to the atmosphere by evaporation and evapotranspiration (ET_p). Thus a desert is an arid zone that has a P/ET_p ratio of < 0.2. There is no sharp boundary defining a desert, rather a gradation of conditions from extremely arid to semiarid and subhumid (Fig. 16.1). A desert is a provider, accumulator and exporter of sediment. It may contain marginal rivers, fans, lakes and deltas, and may lie immediately adjacent to a coastline. Low-latitude deserts have only about 20% of their surface area covered by sand dunes. The following narrative concentrates on wind-blown processes in modern deserts. But it should be remembered that aeolian reworking also widely affects beaches, sabkhas, exposed river channel bars and fluvioglacial deposits.

The major deserts of the world with active sand flow occur in the central and southern parts of the subtropical high-pressure cells where descending dry warm air forms the Trade Wind belts (see Chapter 13). A further category of desert occurs in the continental lee or 'rain-shadow' of uplifted mountain belts such as the western USA, Central Asia and Patagonia. In many of these semiarid and arid zones, sedimentary grains are liberated from upland areas by weathering and transferred by ephemeral stream flow along wadis. Here the sediment undergoes sorting processes and is moulded into various aeolian bedforms (see Chapter 8), which may coalesce to form sand seas, or ergs (an Arabic name) as they are widely known. Loess sheets result in adjacent areas after deposition of wind-blown dust. The Namib sand sea is noteworthy for its sediment source, which includes major high-energy coastal areas to the south, the erg being fed by narrow deflation corridors that stretch from the coast through over 100 km of intervening bedrock (Corbett, 1993). In all ergs, sand-grade sediment and finer is very selectively taken into the local or regional wind system.

Figure 16.2 also shows areas of 'fixed' or inactive ergs that border the active ergs. These 'fixed' ergs attest to much-expanded Trade Wind belts of the Pleistocene glacial maxima. Vast areas of Pleistocene loess in temperate, Mediterranean and subtropical latitudes underline the vigorous nature of full-glacial planetary winds. The North African Trade Winds, for example, were active much further south during the last glaciation. The 'fixed' ergs, now stranded and stabilized by vegetation in the northern savannah fringes (Talbot & Williams, 1979; Talbot, 1980, 1985), attest to the long time interval needed to destroy an erg and lead to the expectation that erg facies ought to be preserved in the geological record.

16.2 Physical processes and erg formation

In Chapter 8 we discussed the various aeolian bedforms. Here we consider ergs and their relations to continental wind systems. In the great Trade Wind deserts, such as the North African Sahara and central Australia, there is a close correspondence between dominant wind flow and sand transport.

Meteorological observations, bedform orientations and the trend of erosional lineations (yardangs) enable sand-flow distributions to be mapped out regionally (Wilson, 1971; Mainguet & Canon, 1976; McKee,

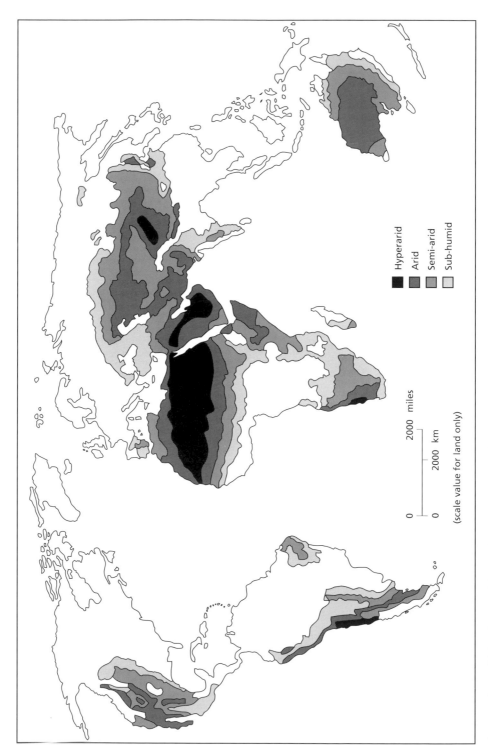

Fig. 16.1 The world distribution of deserts. (From UNESCO, 1977.) Hyperarid zones have $P/ET_p < 0.03$; arid zones $0.03 < P/ET_p < 0.20$; semiarid zones $0.20 < P/ET_p < 0.5$; subhumid zones $0.50 < P/ET_p < 0.75$. P/ET_p is the Thornthwaite index of aridity (see text). There are Trade Wind deserts (North Africa, Arabia and south-central Australia), continental deserts (Central Asia), rain-shadow/continental deserts (western North America and sub-Andean South America), and Trade Wind/cool offshore current deserts (Atacama and Namib).

Hyperarid

Arid

Semi-arid

Sub-humid

0   2000   km

0   2000   miles

(scale value for land only)

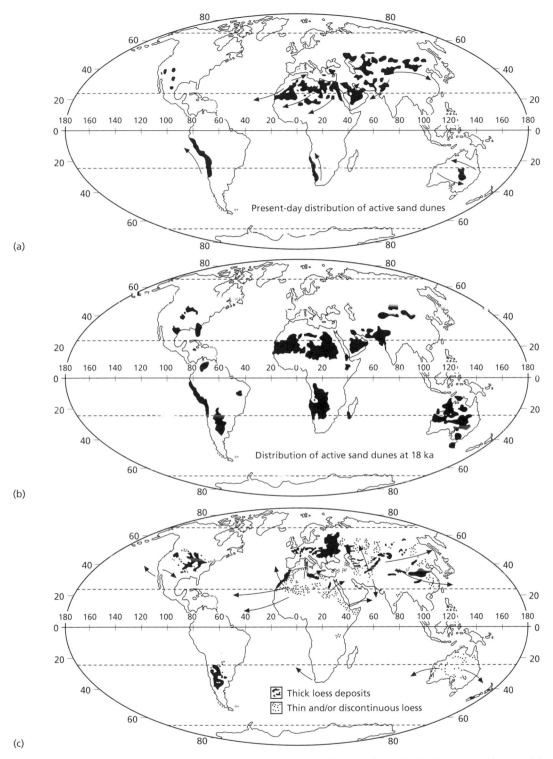

Fig. 16.2 Distribution of: (a) present-day active sand dunes and mean dune-forming wind regimes; (b) glacial-maximum active sand dunes; and (c) present-day distribution of mostly glacial-maximum loess and the mean trajectories of modern aerosol dust tracks. (Mostly after Williams *et al.*, 1993, and sources cited therein.)

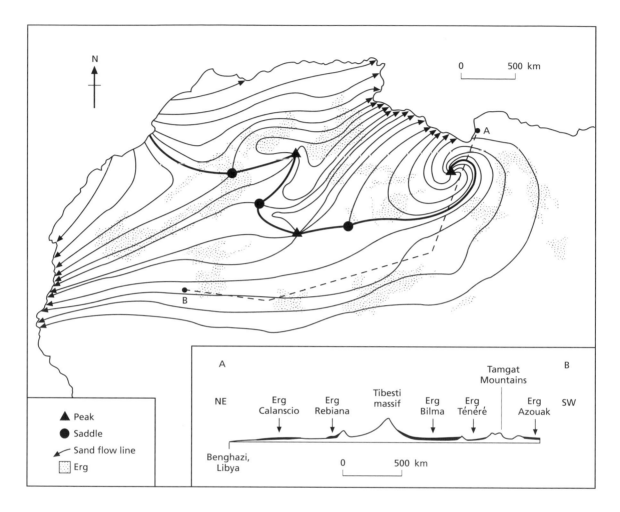

Fig. 16.3 Wilson's (1971) classic mean resultant sand-flow map for Saharan ergs, together with an approximate topographic section from Benghazi to Niger.

1978; Mainguet, 1978, 1983). Ideally, a sand-flow map should show resultant directions as flowlines *and* resultant magnitudes as contours, analogous to a combined wind direction and pressure map. Information currently available is generally inadequate to achieve this aim. Sand-flow maps are also analogous to drainage maps in that they show divides separating distinct 'drainage' basins: peaks in fixed high-pressure areas and saddles in between them. Unlike water drainage, there is little direct relation between sand flow and topography since winds and their sandy bedload may blow uphill.

The flowlines for North Africa (Fig. 16.3) extend from erg to erg, implying very long transport distances downwind, giving ample time for aeolian abrasion and transport processes to work. Evidence for this erg-to-erg transport is provided by satellite photographs showing linear traces (yardangs) of aeolian corrosion in between erg areas along sand-flow lines (Mainguet, 1978, 1983; for ancient yardangs see Tewes & Loope, 1992). All the sand-flow lines arise within the desert itself, with the main clockwise circulatory cell roughly corresponding to the subtropical high-pressure zone. The lines eventually lead to the sea, giving rise to a great plume of Saharan dust extending out for thousands of kilometres into the Atlantic ocean. A significant part reaches as far as the Lesser Antilles, providing a steady rain of fine silt- to clay-grade particles into the deep ocean (Fig. 16.4).

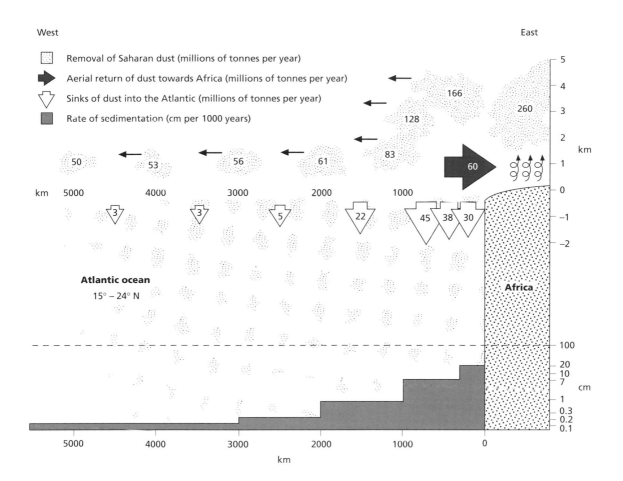

Fig 16.4 Modern annual aerosol dust budgets for Sahara and adjacent Atlantic ocean. (After sources and data in Middleton et al., 1986.)

Mineral dust in the size range 0.1–1 μm is a potent light-scattering aerosol and may have an important cooling role to play in climate change (Li *et al.*, 1996; Tegen *et al.*, 1996). It has been estimated that some 2.6×10^8 tonnes of Saharan mineral dust per year is removed in this way (Coudé-Gaussen, 1984). The magnitude of this sediment flux varied throughout the Quaternary in response to cycles of climate change causing Trade Winds to fluctuate greatly in strength. Present-day fluxes are likely to be low compared to those at the last glacial maximum. The evidence comes from deep-sea cores, which enable dust deposition rates to be calculated as far back as the late Cretaceous (Lever & McCave, 1983).

The other spectacular example of Trade Wind-orientated desert dunes occurs in the great ergs of central Australia, where the migrating high-pressure cell provides the dominant control of anticlockwise sand movement along longitudinal dune systems (Brookfield, 1970). The pattern of sand flow here is much simpler than in North Africa, since the sand flow circulation is largely undisturbed by topographic obstacles.

Individual desert ergs are confined to basins, whatever their absolute height. They terminate at any pronounced slope break. Ergs can form only when the wind is both fully charged with bedload and decelerating in either time or space according to the sediment mass continuity equation (Chapter 6). They can form at sand-flow centres, at saddles and in local areas controlled by topography. Some possible basinal configurations for erg formation are shown in Fig. 16.5.

Reduction of total
sandflow energy

Reduction of resultant
sandflow energy

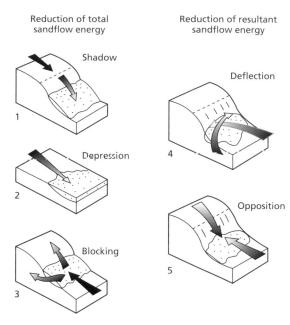

Fig. 16.5 Ergs, topography and sand deposition. As sand-bearing winds decelerate in time and/or space (according to the sediment continuity equation), they deposit their sand load. Sketches show various situations leading to deposition. (After Fryberger & Ahlbrandt, 1979.)

Deposition and deflation are controlled not only by the regional wind system, but also in a complex manner by more local bedform hierarchies present on the erg (see Wilson, 1971). Despite the continental scale of low-latitude desert sand flow, major local influences upon wind flow are exerted by topography and by mesoscale circulation at wavelengths of 10–100 km (Atkinson & Zhang, 1996). Winds have to flow around as well as over some high-relief areas, much as turbidity currents interact with submarine topography (Chapter 11). The resulting accelerations, decelerations, lee waves and helical flow paths create much interesting complexity whose effects have rarely been appreciated in the geological record (for a simple introduction see Greeley & Iverson, 1985). For example, it is likely that smaller-scale ergs not linked to a regional Trade Wind system and hence to extra-erg sand supply will be much more prone to climatic or base-level induced interruptions to sedimentation and the production of bounding surfaces (Section 16.4).

16.3 Modern desert bedform associations and facies

The margins of many ergs are marked by relatively thin sand accumulations, so-called sand sheets (Fryberger *et al.*, 1979; Kocurek & Nielsen, 1986; Lancaster, 1995; Fig. 16.6). There is insufficient fine sand supply here, and maybe other unfavourable conditions (such as high water table, surface stabilization), for significant dunes to form. Sand sheets form a transitional facies between aeolian dunes and nonaeolian deposits. They originate by gentle wind deceleration in the lee of small surface irregularities, and exhibit small dunes, aeolian ripple remnants, granule ridges, surface lag deposits and internal low-angle erosion surfaces and climbing ripple laminae (Fig. 16.6).

In many ergs, areas of inter-dune or inter-draa deposition occur that have many similarities to the deposits of sand sheets. The exact nature of such areas depends upon the availability of sand, and the moisture content of the depression floor brought about by changing water table, freshwater flooding, saline groundwater invasion or marine intrusion in coastal ergs. Sparse sand availability under 'dry' conditions leads to dune or draa migration over the areas of immobile sediments and the nonpreservation of inter-bedform sediment. In this case the inter-bedform areas are merely transport paths for sand between adjacent dunes.

The careful analysis of true inter-bedform deposits, analysed in the manner of Kocurek (1981) or Crabaugh and Kocurek (1993), may provide valuable evidence for the general palaeogeographic and palaeoclimatic conditions that existed during erg evolution. Periodic, albeit rare, wet conditions arise when runoff down dune surfaces and between adjacent depressions of varying depth causes subaqueous current ripple and even small subaqueous dunes to form. These may be covered with thin mud drapes as ponding occurs and thereafter cracked up by desiccation, sometimes to be incorporated in the wind-blown sands of the next arid period. Sabkhas occur where a saline water table intersects the inter-dune troughs (Glennie, 1970). Blown sand driving across moist areas causes build-up of highly porous adhesion-accreted sands. Evaporation leads to evaporite precipitation as crusts and subsurface nodules. Crusty surfaces do not trap sand along transport paths; rather the hard

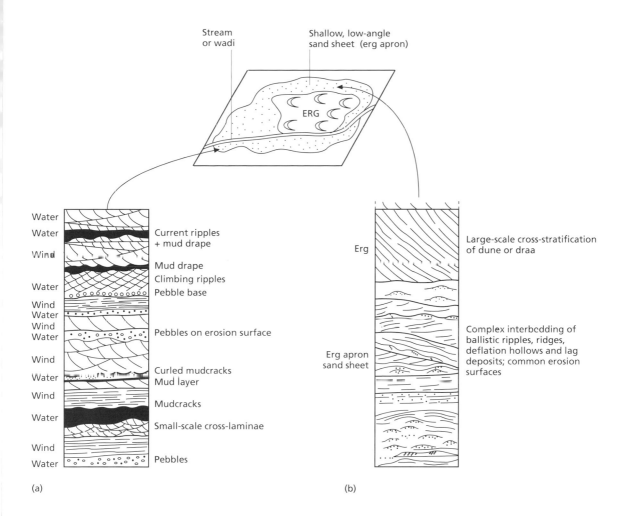

Fig. 16.6 Vertical sequences liable to be generated at the margin of ergs. (After Fryberger et al., 1979.) (a) Facies produced by alternations of water and air flow such as might be found close to a stream or wadi system. (See for example Langford, 1989; Langford & Chan, 1989.) (b) Facies produced by air flow alone on the erg apron margin.

surfaces accelerate transport on to the next dune, draa or erg (Mainguet, 1983). In some areas temporary playa lakes may form in inter-dune depressions following extensive rainfall. Spectacular examples of inter-dune playas between stabilized dunes occur around Lake Chad near Timbuktoo (Talbot, 1980). Oscillation ripples and algal carbonates may develop when such lakes remain for appreciable periods of time. Dry inter-dune depressions develop soil horizons, aeolian ripple remnants and other features similar to those of sand sheets. The generally poorly sorted and fine-grained character of inter-dune deposits contrasts markedly with those of the main erg bedforms. They form important permeability barriers in both aquifers and hydrocarbon reservoirs, and have thus received much recent study.

16.4 Aeolian architecture

The detailed architecture of an erg cannot be directly imaged. So it has been through the invention of conceptual models based upon modern desert surface processes and the testing of these on very extensive outcrops of ancient aeolian deposits, particularly in

once-active bedforms are subject to soil development and sediment redistribution into inter-dune troughs by runoff and mass flow (Talbot & Williams, 1979). They are eloquent testimony to the ability of climate change to form regional bounding surfaces (Talbot, 1985), termed 'supersurfaces' by later authors (e.g. Kocurek *et al.*, 1991; Lancaster, 1992). Such surfaces are of much greater extent than those within individual draas or dunes discussed in the previous section; they bound *all* elements of the once-active erg. If the aeolian system becomes operative once more and a sand flux into the area is provided, then such regional surfaces will become preserved, bounding a new sequence of aeolian sediments. This process of episodic stratigraphic accumulation is very well illustrated in the Gran Desierto of northern Mexico (Blount & Lancaster, 1990; Lancaster, 1992), where several generations of dunes separated by regional bounding surfaces may be seen. The dunes have formed, been abandoned and then re-formed due probably to cycles of late Quaternary climatic change and changes in sediment supply from the adjacent Colorado River delta. This area is particularly interesting as an analogue for ancient deposits because it is located in an area of strong subsidence associated with the transtensional regime of the San Andreas Fault and associated faults. Another highly relevant study in the southwestern Saharan fringes (Kocurek *et al.*, 1991) also reveals cycles of draa development, abandonment and inter-draa lake, wetland and sabkha formation during the late Pleistocene and Holocene.

Many dried-up, formerly freshwater, lake beds occur within the Trade Wind deserts (Williams *et al.*, 1993; Williams, 1994; see Chapter 19). For example, the lakes of central Australia became progressively more saline about 25 000 yr ago due to climatic aridity when gypsum was deposited together with clays. Complete desiccation of the lakes led to wind reworking of the finely powdered gypsum and clay into elliptical 'lunette' and parabolic dunes now seen on the downwind lake margins. Longitudinal dunes then migrated across the lake floors (Bowler, 1977).

16.6 Ancient desert facies

Permian Rotliegendes of north-west Europe

One of the best-known deposits is the Permian Rotliegendes Sandstones of the southern and northern North Sea basin (Fig. 16.9), which form an important regional natural gas reservoir in the British and Dutch sectors (Glennie, 1986; George & Berry, 1993). The two ergs were separated by the Mid North Sea High, an area of presumed wind deflation. Detailed well-log studies (e.g. Heward, 1994) and studies of onshore outcrops in north-east England reveal a series of complex fossilized erg sand bodies up to 500 m thick with marginal facies of fluvial wadi sediments and a basin centre facies of lacustrine clays and playa evaporites. The onshore exposures around the erg margins give convincing evidence for the existence of compound longitudinal draas separated by inter-dune areas (Glennie, 1982; Steele, 1983; Clemmensen, 1989; Chrintz & Clemmensen, 1993). The latter authors give impressive draa reconstructions.

Regional palaeocurrent studies reveal that the Rotliegendes was deposited by a clockwise-rotating air cell. Cored intervals, production and dipmeter data cannot establish dune type with any certainty because of correlation problems, but dry and wet inter-dune horizons have been clearly identified. It is not clear whether regional stabilization (super)surfaces occur. Drying-upwards cycles have been recognized from many wells and these have been used, somewhat imaginatively, to infer numerous (five or more) periods of large-scale erg contraction and expansion (George & Berry, 1993). It is possible that these cycles may reflect Milankovitch-driven responses to mid–late Permian climatic changes, since this was a major icehouse period of Earth history. The final extinction of the great Rotliegendes erg occurred as the global Permian sea level rose upon final melting of the Gondwanan glaciers. A distinctive water-reworked horizon, the Weissliegend, with soft sediment deformation in underlying dunes, marks the event in onshore exposures (Glennie & Buller, 1983).

Ancient ergs of the western USA

Owing to the Tertiary downcutting activities of the Colorado and other rivers, no area has such breathtaking exposures of aeolian sediments as the Colorado Plateau of the western USA. Noteworthy pioneer studies by Kocurek (1981) and more recent work by Crabaugh & Kocurek (1993), Herries (1993), Havholm *et al.* (1993) and Blakey *et al.* (1996) have set out to test conceptual models for erg evolution and architecture. In his classic work on the

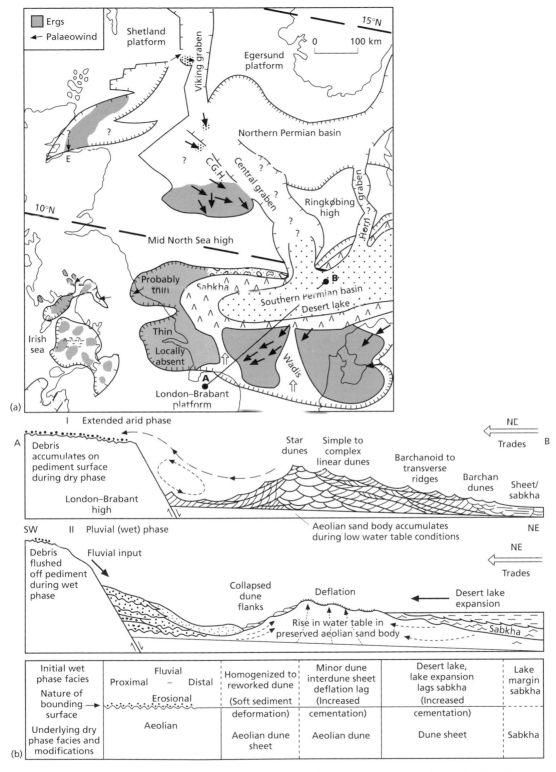

Fig. 16.9 The extent of Permian ergs in the North Sea basin (after Glennie, 1982) together with an interesting climatic hypothesis for the formation of repeated bounding supersurfaces (after George & Berry, 1993).

Upper Jurassic Entrada Sandstone, Kocurek (1981) demonstrated the occurrence of inter-dune deposits (Fig. 16.8) and climbing dune sets whose geometry did not support regional water-table influences on their development. More recent work (Crabaugh & Kocurek, 1993) has swung full circle with the recognition of additional regional unconformable surfaces within the deposit that *do* attest to periods of widespread erg stabilization. Havholm *et al.* (1993) and Blakey *et al.* (1996) have also established that regional bounding surfaces may be identified and traced out over hundreds of kilometres in the Middle Jurassic Page Sandstone of Utah and Arizona. It is possible that age dating of zircons from associated bentonites may aid chronostratigraphic correlation of these surfaces in future. Clemmenson *et al.* (1989) and Herries (1993) have both documented the facies architecture developed in zones of intertonguing between ergs and adjacent river systems, in the Lower Jurassic Moenave/Wingate and Kayenta/Navajo Formations respectively. In both cases the position of the river/erg boundary appears to have suffered repeated major lateral translations, on a scale of 1–100 km, perhaps in response to climate change affecting sand flow and river sediment dynamics. The result is a series of 'drying-upwards' and 'wettening-upwards' cycles passing from fluviatile to erg facies and back again.

The palaeoclimatic (and economic) implications of these discoveries are profound. If the Jurassic was indeed a hothouse era (see Frakes *et al.*, 1992), then the major changes in erg dynamics implied by environmental analysis are difficult to explain, particularly since palaeocurrent data and climate modelling (Peterson, 1988; Parrish & Peterson, 1988) indicate quite stable or slowly rotating wind regimes during the periods in question. The timing of the climatic cyclicity is low frequency and not immediately explicable other than by perhaps the long-term eccentricity contribution (*c.* 400 Kyr) from Milankovitch-type orbital forcing mechanisms (Clemmenson, 1989). It may be that a major long-term cyclical switch between Trade Winds (arid) and monsoonal winds (seasonally moist) is being recorded, tracked by motions of the contemporary equatorial zone of convergence. Comparisons with the icehouse Permian erg cycles of north-west Europe might reveal some fundamental truths about the longer-term behaviour of planetary Trade Wind belts and their dynamic ergs. On the other hand, it seems clear that at least some regional supersurfaces, notably those of the Middle Jurassic Page Sandstone (Blakey *et al.*, 1996), correlate with basinwards marine transgressions whose effect was to cut off sand supply and raise the regional water table, causing erg stabilization and abandonment.

Ancient ergs of Pangaea and palaeoplate reconstructions

Knowledge that modern ergs of continental scale are adjusted to the motions of the Trade Wind system encourages the hope that ancient erg deposits may be used in conjunction with continental reassemblies to reconstruct ancient wind systems. Much progress has been made in this field in recent years since the early synthesis by Bigarella (1973). In a wide-ranging study, Parrish & Peterson (1988) present a stimulating comparison between measured palaeocurrents and computed model Trade Winds for the late Palaeozoic to Mesozoic of the western USA. The area lay in the northern hemisphere and on the western side of the Pangaean supercontinent. Both summer monsoonal and summer subtropical high-pressure circulations are thought to have had a particular influence during Triassic and Jurassic times.

Further reading

Cooke *et al.* (1993), Thomas (1989), Abrahams and Parsons (1994) and Kocurek (1996) are readable summaries of many features of desert geomorphology and sedimentology. McKee (1978) contains superb satellite photographs of erg features, many in colour. Ancient desert deposits are featured in North and Prosser (1993a) and Pye and Lancaster (1993).

17   Rivers

I do not know much about gods; but I think that the river
Is a strong brown god—sullen, untamed and intractable, . . .

T.S. Eliot, 'The Dry Salvages', *Four Quartets*, Faber

17.1 Introduction

Some part of the precipitation that falls on to the Earth's surface eventually finds itself flowing as channelized runoff: river channels are conduits for the dispersal of weathering products derived from their catchments. River deposits are thus highly sensitive indicators of tectonic slope changes, sourceland geology and climate. The supply of sediment to all other sedimentary systems is controlled by rivers they tell us more about more geological and geomorphological evolution than any other sedimentary system.

17.2 Channel magnitude and gradient

River channels in sedimentary basins vary greatly in size, over more than four orders of magnitude, from mere ditches to the > 20 km wide lower reaches of the Brahmaputra and Ganges (Fig. 17.1). The magnitude of any channel may be described in terms of its width, w, and depth, h, for bankfull flow. These basic measures of channel size help to determine the extent of coarse-grained channel deposits. The bigger the channel, the more water it can carry through itself, so we must also characterize channels according to the magnitude of the mean annual discharge. Since the mean flow velocity, u, in any channel is Q/wh, we have $Q = whu$. Expressing width, depth and mean velocity of flow as functions of the mean discharge, we can derive the basic expressions of hydraulic geometry:

$$w = aQ^d \qquad h = bQ^e \qquad u = cQ^f \qquad (17.1)$$

where $abc = 1$ and $d + e + f = 1$. The magnitudes of the exponents and constants vary according to different stream types and climatic conditions. The ratio w/h is a particularly key relationship for it appears quite generally that high w/h ratios are characteristic of low-sinuosity channels (Fig. 17.1).

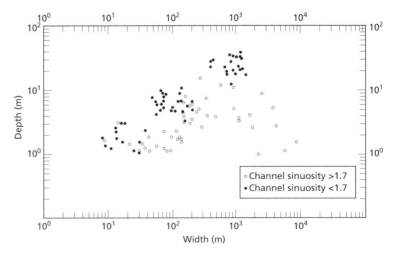

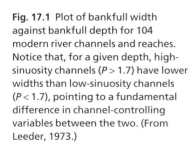

Fig. 17.1 Plot of bankfull width against bankfull depth for 104 modern river channels and reaches. Notice that, for a given depth, high-sinuosity channels ($P > 1.7$) have lower widths than low-sinuosity channels ($P < 1.7$), pointing to a fundamental difference in channel-controlling variables between the two. (From Leeder, 1973.)

307

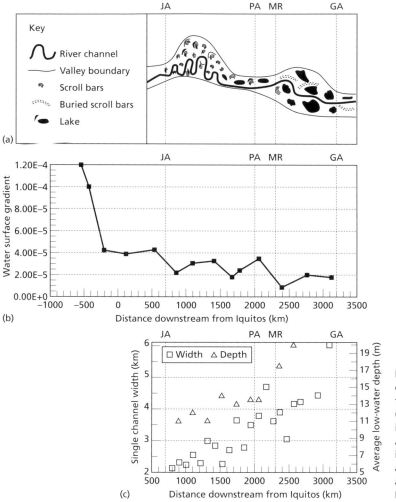

Fig. 17.2 (a) Indicative planform changes in Amazon river downstream from Iquitos bends—not to scale. (b) The general downstream decrease in water surface gradient along the Amazon river. (c) The downstream increase of mean low-water depth and single-channel low-water width along the Amazon river. (All after Mertes *et al.*, 1996.)

The remarkably smooth longitudinal profiles of most channels once they emerge from their bedrock valleys reflect a long-term ability to overcome original, and subsequently imposed, irregularities in topography by the combined effects of erosion and deposition. River profiles are usually concave (Fig. 17.2); all initial or imposed convexities have to decay to concave slopes with time. This can be readily understood by noting that the downstream increase in discharge associated with all stream networks (Fig. 17.2) must be accompanied by a downstream decrease in slope if equilibrium, i.e. neither erosion nor deposition, is to be maintained. If slope stayed constant or increased, then erosion would result in a lowering of

the bed and the production of a concavity. Profile concavity may be described by an equation of the form

$$H = H_0\, e^{-kL}$$

where H is local profile height with respect to an initial height H_0, k is an erosional or depositional constant and L is distance downstream.

Major changes in the gradients of channel networks may arise in highly active tectonic areas, such as when a river crosses particularly large thrust faults. The Himalayan examples in Fig. 17.3 reinforce the observation that the production of a smooth profile requires massive redistribution of materials, something that may take many millions of years to achieve *once the*

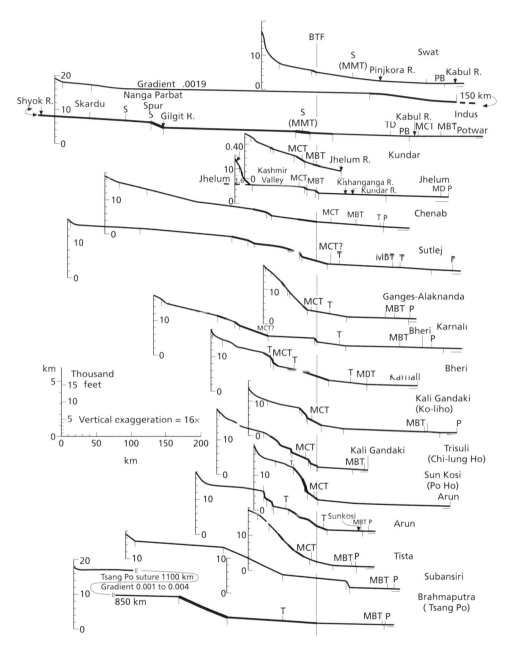

Fig. 17.3 Longitudinal profiles of the major Himalayan rivers (arranged west to east, top to bottom) to show common zones of high gradients (thickened lines) and curvature convexities associated with great thrust fronts like the Main Central Thrust (MCT) that separate the Greater and Lesser Himalayas. The existence of such curvatures shows that river disequilibrium is common across actively uplifting geological structures. The trans-Himalayan Indus river in the west shows no such development. The Main Boundary Thrust (MBT) separates Front Ranges from foreland basin. (After Seeber & Gornitz, 1983.)

tectonic activity stops. The rate at which a particular channel can make adjustments to its profile will clearly depend on the magnitude of the system in question.

The downstream concavity of profile in most aggrading rivers (ignoring the effects of tributaries) leads to a diminution of bed shear stress and hence to a general downstream fining of grain size, although abrasion due to transport undoubtedly also contributes. Downstream fining is particularly marked in mixed gravel–sand systems (e.g. Ferguson *et al.*, 1996) where there are marked changes in river curvature (Sambrook-Smith & Ferguson, 1995). Such gradient changes are most marked in tectonically active basins at faulted mountain fronts (Fig. 17.3) where gravel 'trapping' is commonly observed. Gravel trapping generally is a complicated result of the attainment or otherwise of 'equal mobility' of gravel–sand mixtures (see Chapter 7). Since equal mobility depends upon bed shear stresses attaining more than about twice the value to transport the median grain size of the mixture (Wilcock & McArdell, 1993), then downstream decrease of bed shear stress will inevitably result in gravel deposition and selective sand transport (Ferguson *et al.*, 1996). However, the situation cannot apply universally since most rivers increase their discharge and depth downstream as tributaries join them. The sign of downstream changes in flow strength will then depend upon the exact nature of the slope–discharge parameters for a particular river.

17.3 Channel form

Channels possess form as well as magnitude and are best described (Fig. 17.4) by a combination of:
- a planform description of channel deviation from a straight path (*sinuosity*, P);

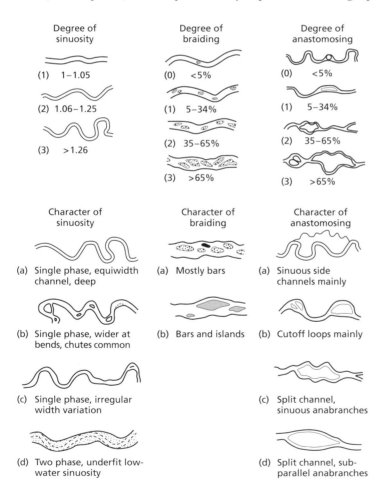

Fig. 17.4 Sketches to show the range of river channel types. (Adapted after Brice, 1984.)

- the degree of channel subdivision by large migrating bedforms and accreting islands around which channel reaches diverge and converge (*braiding*);
- more permanent distributive channel subdivision into stationary smaller channels (separated by floodplain) that each contain their own channel and point bars (*anastomosing*).

No rigid classification of any single channel on anything longer than a reach level (a few channel widths) is universally practicable since many rivers show combinations of sinuosity and braiding. We noted previously the tendency for high w/h ratios to occur in low-sinuosity channels, and vice versa for high-sinuosity channels. As discharge and therefore channel cross-sectional size increase, so does the planform wavelength, λ, of any meanders involved. Measurements of many natural bends reveal that $\lambda = 10.9w^{1.01}$, with a standard error of about 0.3 log units. This approximates to $\lambda \propto 11w$. A second useful scaling relationship is that between meander wavelength and mean annual discharge, $\lambda = 106Q^{0.46}$, with a standard error of about 0.05 log units. This approximates to $\lambda \propto \sqrt{Q}$.

Much of the literature on ancient river deposits seeks too rigid a classification of ancient rivers and too narrow interpretations of the reasons for particular channel form; the tectonic and palaeohydrological inferences thus made are frequently in error. Thus braided rivers do not *have* to occur on steeper slopes, in coarser sediments and in catchments with 'flashy' discharge regimes. They may be made experimentally with invariant discharges. Neither do they comb their floodplains constantly, thus leaving no floodbasin fines for preservation in the river's own stratigraphic record. Gravel-bed meandering rivers are not uncommon. Further, there is no one single cause as to channel sinuosity or braiding index. The causes of braiding or meandering behaviour remain obscure (see the reviews by Ferguson, 1987; Bridge, 1993). The much-quoted slope dependence of braiding (discriminators of the kind $S = aQ^{-b}$) cannot be the whole story since sediment supply characteristics clearly play an important role in determining whether or not a reach will meander or be of low sinuosity. Ferguson has suggested that a discriminant function between braiding and nonbraiding should include a grain-size term, thus $S = aQ^{-b}D^{c}$, whilst van den Berg (1995) suggests a combined stream power : grain size criterion.

Another variable that influences channel form is bank stability: unerodible banks will contain a perfectly straight channel, whilst totally cohesionless banks will be free to widen indefinitely until the decrease of depth and applied bed shear stress at the bank margins can no longer do any eroding (Parker, 1976). The main point is that braided rivers must be able to let their flows converge and diverge around barforms; indeed, simple but powerful cellular models of braiding achieve exactly this form with these boundary conditions (Murray & Paola, 1994). Stable banks will clearly contain more cohesive sediment, such as peat, clay or silty clay, than sand. If the river is transporting an appreciable volume of suspended fines, then the floodplain should contain dominantly fine-grained sediment. By defining a parameter M that expresses the amount of silt–clay in the channel perimeter, Schumm (1960, 1963a) was able to show a high degree of correlation in Great Plains rivers (but this is *not* generally applicable) between M and both w/h and sinuosity (P). Thus $w/h = 225M^{-1.08}$, with a standard error of 0.2 log units, and $P = 0.94M^{-0.25}$, with a standard error of 0.06 log units.

Anastomosing channel patterns, in which the spanwise position of individual channel branches and adjacent vegetated islands are stable, have been suggested to reflect the combination of ultrastable banks and substrates and very low gradients in areas of rapid rise of base level (Smith & Smith, 1980; Smith, 1983; Törnqvist, 1993). Since the channel branches are often quite sinuous, and the channels do not migrate significantly laterally, it appears that they must evolve by vertical accretion from sinuous crevasses issuing from an original channel that was not anastomosing (Smith & Smith, 1980).

17.4 Channel sediment transport processes, bedforms and internal structures

The largest river bedforms have dimensions that bear some constant relationship with the dimensions of the containing channel. The bedforms, henceforth referred to as 'bars', are said to *scale with* the channel size, usually expressed as total active channel width, and are frequently referred to as 'macroforms'. These include point, lateral and in-channel bars. Helical flow is the common denominator to each; downstream bar migration is thus accompanied by bar lateral accretion. The former positions of barforms

The flow of water and sediment around bends (Fig. B17.1) occurs in all manner of channels: river, delta, tidal and submarine fan. It is a universal principle that any steady, curved movement of a body, be it stirred coffee in a cup or a motor vehicle around a bend of radius r, results in a net force being set up. This follows directly from Newton's second law, since, although the speed of motion, u, is steady, the direction of the motion has changed. Since velocity is a vector, the result is a radial acceleration of magnitude u^2/r acting inwards from the bend, causing an inward-acting (centripetal) force of magnitude $\rho u^2/r$ per unit volume. Note that the centripetal force increases with the square of the velocity, but decreases with increasing radius of curvature (as every motorist knows). This centripetal force is opposed by an equal and opposite centrifugal force that tends to force the water outwards from the centre of the radius of bend curvature. As in our stirred coffee (but not in the case of the car because the wheels, hopefully, grip the road and restrain the outward force by friction) a water surface slope develops downwards from the outer to the inner bank. We now have an interesting situation in that the water surface slope induced by the centrifugal tendencies must give rise to a hydrostatic lateral pressure

Further information on flow in bends

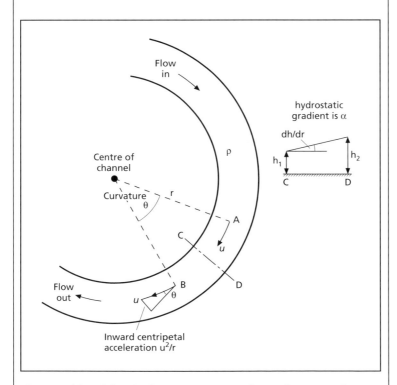

Fig. B17.1 (a) To define the forces acting in curved water flows around channel bends.

continued on p. 313

Further information on flow in bends [*continued*]

gradient, positive from outer to inner bank. This lateral gradient will *not* change with water depth and is $\rho g \, \mathrm{d}h/\mathrm{d}r$ per unit volume. At equilibrium the centrifugal and hydrostatic forces are equal:

$$\rho g \frac{\mathrm{d}h}{\mathrm{d}r} = \rho \frac{u^2}{r} \tag{B17.1}$$

or

$$\frac{\mathrm{d}h}{\mathrm{d}r} = \frac{u^2}{gr} \tag{B17.2}$$

The force set up by the gradient will try to oppose the centrifugal force set up by the curved flow. This may be impossible in the upper part of the flow, in the outer boundary layer; but as the velocity of flow decreases towards the bed, the centrifugal force will rapidly decay (remember the square function). Since the hydrostatic pressure force is unchanged with depth, it becomes possible there for it to oppose the

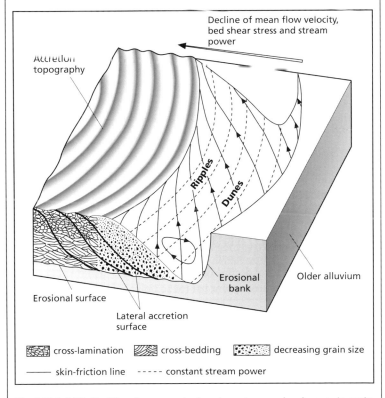

Fig. B17.1 (b) Helical flow in a meander bend causing regular changes in grain size, bedforms and sedimentary structures in the deposits of the accretionary point bar. (After several authors.)

continued on p. 314

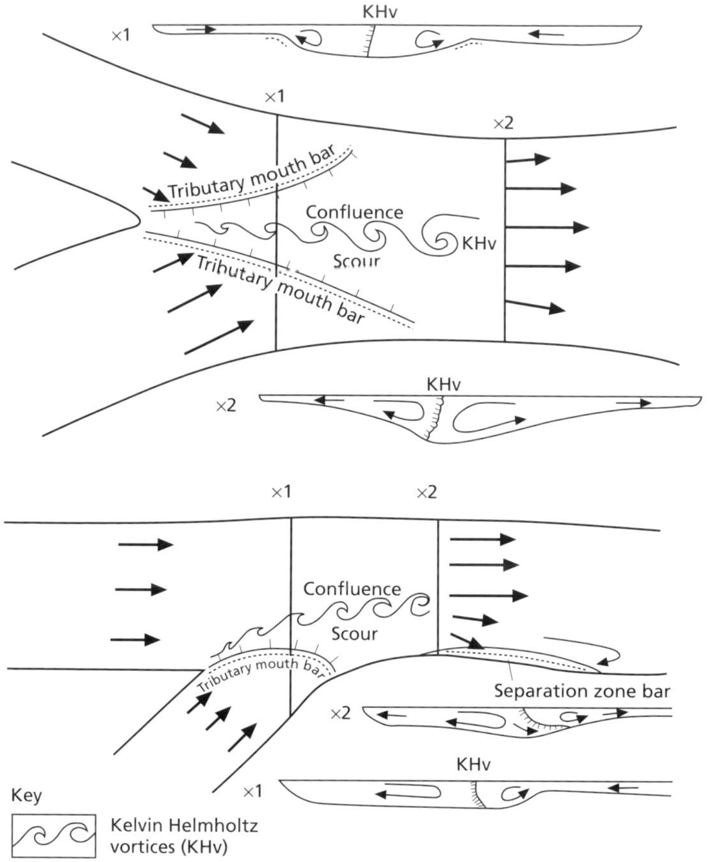

Fig. 17.6 Flow, scour and bedform patterns at river confluences. Arrows are vectorial indicators of mean flow velocity. (After Best, 1987; Best & Roy, 1991.)

Point bars and meander bends

The basic dynamics of meanders leads to erosion on the outside parts of bends and deposition of a point bar on the inside. Decreasing bed shear stress from the deep toe to the shallow top of the point bar also leads to the development of distinct bedform suites on the point bar surface, and, in sections of the bend where the flow is fully developed, an upwards fining of grain size (Figs B17.1 & 17.7). Current ripples, dunes and upper plane beds are the commonest bedforms observed, their occurrence and distribution over the bar surface depending upon the particular hydraulics of the river in question. It is common to find a general downstream fining around point bars, related to the decay of the next upstream helical flow cell (Jackson, 1975; Bridge & Jarvis, 1982).

Erosion of the cut bank depends upon the structure of the bank and the properties of its constituents—whether they are noncohesive, cohesive or composite. Bank undercutting by the river leads to collapse along planes formed by soil shrinkage. Clay banks may fail along rotational slides. In both cases, failure and collapse occur preferentially during falling river stage in response to changing porewater levels and pore pressures.

The combined processes of outer bank erosion and inner bank accretion over the surface of the point bar lead to whole-channel migration. Channel bends may grow, migrate and rotate with time, frequently leading to the formation of meander cutoffs as the channels take short-cut routes across meander necks during high discharges. Periodic bend migration and point bar accretion in response to major floods lead to

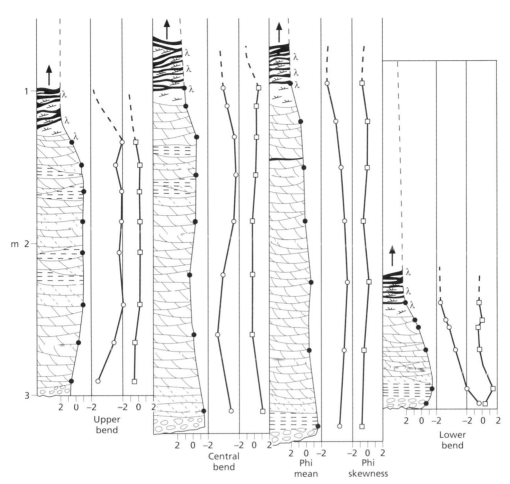

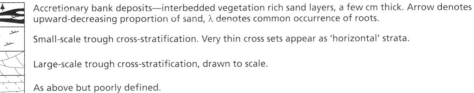

Accretionary bank deposits—interbedded vegetation rich sand layers, a few cm thick. Arrow denotes upward-decreasing proportion of sand, λ denotes common occurrence of roots.

Small-scale trough cross-stratification. Very thin cross sets appear as 'horizontal' strata.

Large-scale trough cross-stratification, drawn to scale.

As above but poorly defined.

Poorly defined 'horizontal' stratification, transitional with above.

Gravel and slumped bank material on erosion surface.

— grain sizes in φ units ($\phi = -\log_2$ mm)

Fig. 17.7 Logs from vibracores to illustrate sedimentary successions developed at various positions around a meander bend. (From Bridge & Jarvis, 1982.)

vertical mud accretion also characterizes the arid-zone and stomosing river plains of the Channel Country, central Australia, where again the channel positions remain fixed (Gibling *et al.*, 1998).

17.5 The floodplain

Adjacent to river channels are swathes of periodically flooded wetlands whose ecological well-being has often been neglected in the cause of floodplain cultivation and habitation. Events in the recent past in the mid-west of the USA (Gomez *et al.*, 1995) and many other regions have brought these hard facts home to roost in no uncertain terms. Floodplain sediments have a special interest since they are the sites of upward accretion and thus preservation of soils, habitats,

habitations and organic remains. The alternation of channel and floodplain sediments in stratigraphic sections emphasizes that the processes of alluvial architecture depend on a dynamic interaction in time and space between the two environments. In recent years there have been abundant new data on this interaction, particularly on avulsive depositional sequences (Smith *et al.*, 1989; Smith & Pérez-Arlucea, 1994; Pérez-Arlucea & Smith, 1999; Figs 17.12–17.15) and the role of floodplains as sequesterers of downstream-moving sediment (Mertes *et al.*, 1996; Allison *et al.*, 1998).

Perhaps the least-understood aspect of river sedimentation dynamics is the out-of-channel vertical accretion process that occurs on levees, on crevasse splays and in the marshy wetlands and shallow lakes of flood basins. Levee sediment strength is reduced by increased internal pore pressures as the river stage rises. Initial floodwater may break through a levee via a channel or a levee slope-failure scar leading to a crevasse splay (Fig. 17.13) or spill into the floodbasin

Fig. 17.12 Map to show the spectacular break-out zone of the Cumberland Marshes avulsion on the Saskatchewan River. Box shows detailed study area of Fig. 17.15. (From Pérez-Arlucea & Smith, 1999.)

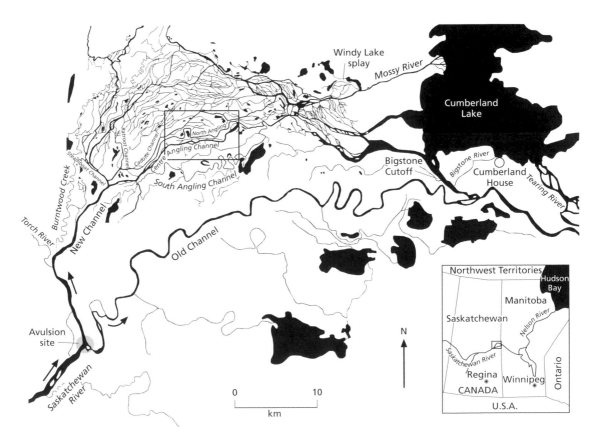

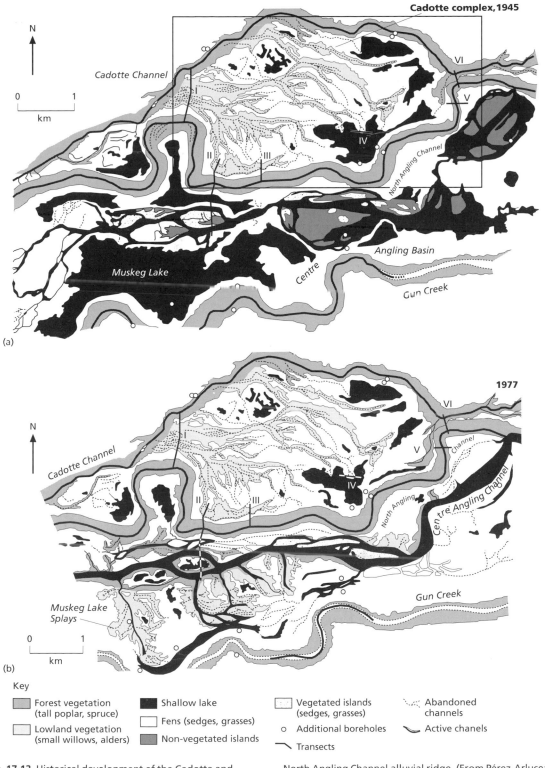

Fig. 17.13 Historical development of the Cadotte and Muskeg Lake splay complexes developing against the North Angling Channel alluvial ridge. (From Pérez-Arlucea & Smith, 1999.)

over the levee as a sheet flood. The deceleration of floodwater leads to a gradual deposition of progressively smaller amounts of finer sediment further from the channel margin. Floodbasin infill will be followed by downvalley flow of the shallow sheet of floodwaters, again with deposition rates decreasing away from the channel (Mertes, 1994). Continued flood discharges from the channel will deepen and speed up the floodbasin flow so that widespread deposition on levees results due to deposition from periodic flow vortices at the channel margins (Sellin, 1964). Pizzuto (1987) suggested that suspended sediment 'diffuses' down concentration gradients out into a floodplain from the channel, but the physics of this concept seem wrong and predictions of the idea (Marriott, 1996) have proven negative. Data on the magnitude of deposition during flooding events are sparse, but careful trapping experiments, comparisons of upstream and downstream gauging station records, and radiometric dating of floodplain cores reveal that a surprisingly high (30–70%) proportion of upstream suspended load may be deposited on the floodplain reach during flooding (Allison *et al.*, 1998). Most sand is dumped on the levees very close to the channel margins (Gretener & Stromquist, 1987; Asselmann & Middelkoop, 1995; Gomez *et al.*, 1995; Marriott, 1996).

The net effect of repeated flooding is the production of an alluvial ridge, whose topography of levees and active and abandoned meander loops stands above the general floodplain level. The observed fall-off in mean net deposition rate r at any distance z from the edge of the channel over the levee to the floodplain margin is most simply given by power-law expressions like:

$$r = a(z + 1)^{-b} \qquad (17.2)$$

where a is the maximum net deposition rate at the edge of the channel belt, and b is an exponent that describes the rapidity with which the rate of deposition decreases with distance from the meander belt (Bridge & Leeder, 1979; Allison *et al.*, 1998). The constants vary according to factors such as climate, river size, timing of flood and sediment load (see Asselmann & Middelkoop, 1995; Gomez *et al.*, 1995). Such expressions fail to predict the observed impact of abandoned channels and other depressions on the floodplain, which very markedly increase deposition rates (Gretener & Stromquist, 1987; Asselmann & Middelkoop, 1995) since they tend to trap and route floodwaters once they have left the levee flanks.

Flood deposits themselves may be dated using various techniques and the time distribution of flooding established—an important exercise in developing hazard analysis in floodplains via 'palaeoflood analysis' (for a polemic against statistical flood analysis, see Baker, 1994). The link between channel change, climate and flooding levels then enables conclusions to be made concerning the causes of palaeofloods, like climate change vs. land-use change, etc. (Macklin *et al.*, 1992; O'Connor *et al.*, 1994; Ely *et al.*, 1996). Cycles of flooding and discharge variations occur on an approximately decadal timescale in the west of North America due to the oscillating El Niño Southern Ocean (ENSO) effect, causing variations in Pacific-sourced winter storm frequency and magnitude (Graf *et al.*, 1991).

Since river floods are periodic, newly deposited sediment is at once acted upon by processes leading to soil formation. Rapid vegetation growth in humid climates leads to the formation of peat beds separated by thin partings of flood-derived muds and silts. Both soil formation and peat formation will be encouraged by slow sedimentation. Well-marked horizonated soils are generally poorly developed in areas of active floodplains because of the rapidity of sediment deposition (Leeder, 1975; Kraus & Aslan, 1993). Simple models for soil development are possible because there must always be an inverse relationship between the extent of pedogenesis and the rate of sedimentation. The concept of a 'residence interval' is a useful one in this respect. This is the time during which pedogenesis can act upon a volume of alluvium initially at the floodplain surface. Residence intervals are generally low in upstream areas of alluvial basins because of high sedimentation rates, whereas downstream (particularly in terminal fans) soil formation may be inhibited by high water tables and development of shallow lakes and ponds with carbonate precipitation (Sanz *et al.*, 1995; McCarthy *et al.*, 1997). In the latter case, interesting cycles of soil, lake and floodplain sediment result (Sanz *et al.*, 1995).

17.6 Channel belts, alluvial ridges, combing and avulsion

Prolonged occupation of an area by a river leads to the production of a channel belt occupied by active and abandoned reaches. The relatively sudden movement of a whole channel belt (not just a single reach or bend cutoff) to another position on the floodplain is

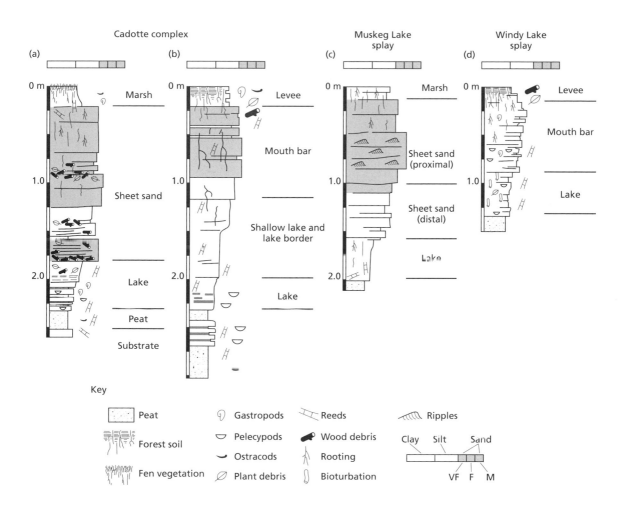

Key

Peat

Forest soil

Fen vegetation

Gastropods

Pelecypods

Ostracods

Plant debris

Reeds

Wood debris

Rooting

Bioturbation

Ripples

Clay   Silt   Sand

VF F   M

Fig. 17.14 Logs from vibracores through the Cadotte and Muskeg Lake splay complexes to show various coarsening-upwards sequences. (From Pérez-Arlucea & Smith, 1999.)

termed *avulsion*. The process occurs in meandering *and* braided rivers and is recorded by abandoned channel belts preserved on floodplains or buried partly or wholly beneath them. The frequency of avulsion appears to vary very widely indeed (10–6000 yr), with no clear underlying control, although Törnqvist (1993) has clear evidence for increased avulsion frequency in the lower Rhine–Meuse at a time of rapidly changing sea level (pre-4.5 ka) and during the Iron Age (2.8–1.4 ka).

Avulsion leaves very characteristic deposits in the stratigraphic record of a floodplain. This is best seen in the lower Saskatchewan River, Canada (Figs 17.12

& 17.13), where an avulsion in the 1870s has led to the production of a vast complex of splays, wetlands and channels in the Cumberland Marshes (Smith *et al.*, 1989; Smith & Pérez-Arlucea, 1994; Pérez-Arlucea & Smith, 1999). The diversions are actually gradual and ongoing, with a general progradational aspect well seen in the coarsening-upwards sequences produced by splay-infill of lakes and floodplains (Figs 17.14 & 17.15). A possible ancient analogue is documented by Kraus (1996).

There is some evidence from other rivers that discharge may be split between older and younger courses for considerable time periods (Autin *et al.*, 1991), but in yet others (Mack & Leeder, 1998) the process can be very rapid (weeks or months) and frequent. Perhaps the term 'combing' is more appropriate for these frequent avulsions. Some authors consider that avulsion is more likely to occur from

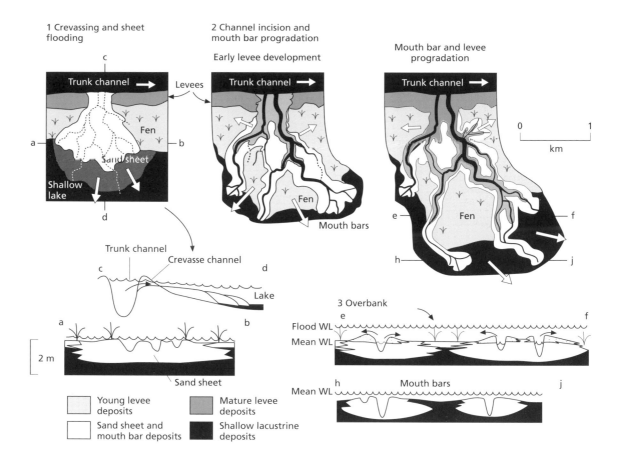

Fig. 17.15 Sketches to show model for crevasse splay development, Cumberland Marshes. (From Pérez-Arlucea & Smith, 1999.)

higher, older, alluvial ridges since the process involves floodwater seeking a gradient advantage over the old course (Bryant *et al.*, 1995; Heller & Paola, 1996). On the other hand, the process must be *easier* when the levees are low. In the present author's opinion, avulsion is generally more likely to be related to large-magnitude floods. It is also known from tectonically active areas that vertical crustal movements play an important role in both initiating and controlling avulsion. Thus diversions may be established along floodplain lows because of fault subsidence (Alexander & Leeder, 1987; Blair & McPherson, 1994a, b; Peakall, 1998). But we still have a lot to learn about channel avulsion. Data from the River Kosi (Wells & Dore,

1987) indicate that major shifts here seem stochastic and autocyclic, with no correlation between them and either severe earthquakes *or* major floods.

17.7 River channel changes, adjustable variables and equilibrium

A river may adjust the following variables in response to independently imposed climatic or tectonic changes (i.e. changes to runoff/discharge and slope over which the river itself has absolutely no control): cross-sectional size (wd), cross-sectional ratio (w/d), bed configuration, bed material grain size, planform shape (sinuosity) and size (meander wavelength), and channel bed slope. If equilibrium forms truly exist in Nature, then they will include that Holy Grail of equilibrium geomorphology, the graded stream. A graded stream has been defined (Leopold & Bull, 1979) as '. . . one in which, over a period of years,

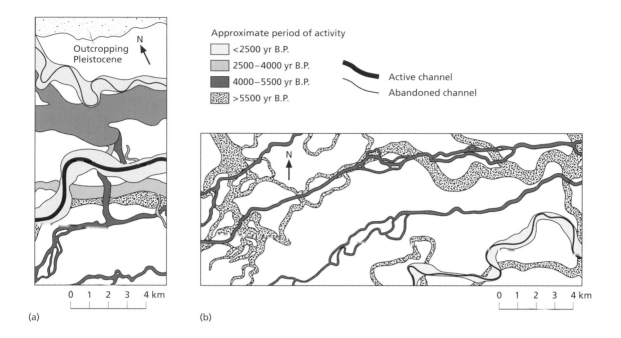

(a)

(b)

Fig. 17.16 Palaeochannel patterns (flow east to west) of the Holocene Rhine–Meuse in the region of Utrecht as revealed by extremely high density of shallow boreholes. Note the anastomosed and meandering channel styles and the tendency for westward channel diminution. (From Törnqvist et al., 1993, and data sources cited therein.)

slope, velocity, depth, width, roughness and channel morphology mutually adjust to provide the power and efficiency necessary to transport the load supplied from the drainage basin *without aggradation or degradation of the channels*' [my italics]. It is the view of the present author that the italicized passage is unnecessarily restrictive, since by the main part of the definition, equilibrium applies only to the sediment load, i.e. to a condition of (sediment in) = (sediment out), or $\nabla \cdot Q_\mathrm{s} = 0$.

As we have seen, a river channel of a particular type has several attributes like depth, width and slope that are related in a complex way to imposed sediment load and water discharge. Clues as to the origins of channel type come from changes over time—channels are extremely sensitive to perturbations in slope, sediment load and water discharge. These perturbations may be imposed by climate change, base-level change and tectonics. For example, the hydraulic geometry

equations imply that the magnitude of water discharge and the nature of sediment load should radically affect channel sinuosity. Many river systems around the world record major changes in channel magnitude and geometry since the last glacial maximum, commonly exhibiting a trend from large, braided, aggrading channels to large and then smaller, meandering, incised channels (Northern and Central Europe: Starkel, 1983; Vanderburghe, 1995; North America: Knox, 1983; Schumm & Brackenridge, 1987; South Australia: Schumm, 1968b; Page & Nanson, 1996; North Africa: Adamson et al., 1980). These changes have occurred due to large decreases in sediment supply in response to a general decrease in runoff and increase in vegetation in the past 15 000 yr. Increased temperature and humidity after the last Ice Age caused vegetation growth and substantially reduced the amount of coarse sediment liberated from drainage basins (see Chapter 13).

Downstream and vertical (time) channel changes from meandering to anastomosing have been carefully documented from tens of thousands of boreholes in the Rhine–Meuse delta, where the cause has been ascribed to a period of rapid sea-level rise about 4–5 ka reaching the depositional area (Fig. 17.16; Törnqvist, 1993; Törnqvist et al., 1993). An interesting thing about Fig. 17.16 is the downstream distributive nature of the channel change from meandering to anastomosing, with many blind crevasses and the trunk channel decreasing in magnitude also. These bear some resemblance to the Cumberland Marshes avulsion sequences described previously and are even reminiscent of Friends' (1978) 'terminal fans'.

17.8 The many causes of channel incision–aggradation cycles

The advent of sequence stratigraphy has focused attention on single cause effects, like relative base-level change, to explain incision/aggradation of river and delta channels. The fluvial system, however, is complex (in the chaotic sense) since many possible causes for incision exist and there is much nonlinearity due to feedbacks of one sort or another. The state of any river system may thus be seen as the interplay between an 'intrinsic' set of variables (like discharge of water and sediment) controlled by the climate and characteristics of its whole catchment, set against external variables like tectonic and eustatic changes in sea level (Schumm, 1977; Bull, 1991).

Base-level change does not affect river channel behaviour in a simple linear fashion, since it takes some time for the wave of incision initiated by base level falling below a previous shoreline and on to a gentle continental slope to pass upstream, which it does at a declining rate proportional to $\sqrt{t}$ (Fig. 17.17). The rate of upstream progression of the modified gradient change (the 'knickpoint') and the distance of travel of the upstream limit to incision will vary according to the initial difference in gradients between river/delta plain (Miall, 1991) and shelf, and the transport capacity of the river channel in question, more specifically its ability to erode and transport away the sediment at the migrating point of maximum gradient change. In symbols, a simple linear diffusional approach (Begin, 1988) yields:

$$\frac{\partial y}{\partial t} = \kappa \frac{\partial y^2}{\partial^2 x} \tag{17.3}$$

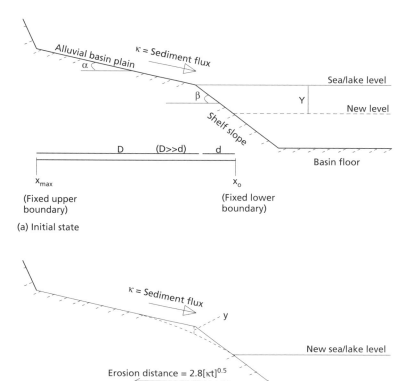

(a) Initial state

(b) With deposition unable to compensate for sea level change

Fig. 17.17 Definition sketches to show the upstream migration of a gradient curvature between shelf and alluvial plain following a fall in sea level. (From Leeder & Stewart, 1996.)

where x and y are the horizontal and vertical coordinates respectively, t is time and κ is the sediment transport coefficient with dimensions LT^{-1}. The position of the knickpoint is defined as where the term on the RHS of eqn. (17.3) is at a maximum. Some solutions

Fig. 17.18 The rate of upstream migration (x) of a gradient curvature between shelf and alluvial plain following a fall in sea level for various values of the sediment transport coefficient, κ. (From Leeder & Stewart, 1996.)

to this equation for various initial values of alluvial and shelf slope are shown in Fig. 17.18.

Another factor concerns the river's own ability to alter its planform rather than necessarily incising or aggrading in response to imposed gradient changes (Schumm, 1993). Thus sinuous river channels have an extra degree of freedom with which to respond to gradient changes: they can change their sinuosity to counteract the imposed gradient change. This is because a high-sinuosity channel has a lower mean

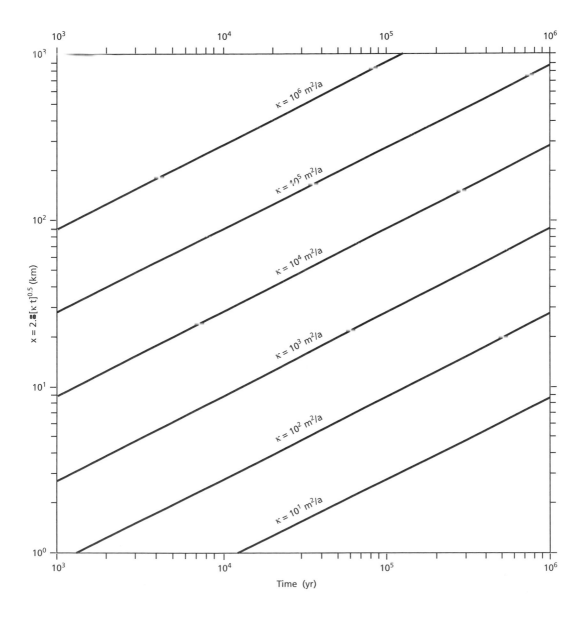

channel gradient than a low-sinuosity channel flowing down the same valley floor.

Channel aggradation–incision cycles may also have a climatic origin, in that weathering/erosion changes in the drainage catchment cause greater or lesser amounts of sediment and/or water to discharge into the alluvial and deltaic plains (Autin *et al.*, 1991; Blum, 1990). Cycles of aggradation or degradation thus result independently of or out of phase with sea-level change. For example, in the Colorado River there is a Holocene cycle of alluviation and incision unrelated to sea-level change since both post-date the last great transgression (Blum, 1990). Similarly in the Mississippi delta the maximum phase of incision only affects the river up to Baton Rouge; and in the alluvial valleys to the north, aggradation occurs at the glacial peak and beginning of waning stages due to the massive amounts of sediment and meltwater coming down the river from the north (Autin *et al.*, 1991).

Regional cycles of stream incision, followed by aggradation (of 40–50 yr duration) seem to have occurred in the American south-west over the past 100 yr or more. Channel incision occurred during periods of high winter storm activity. These winter storms cause much channel discharge but they do not cause so much surface erosion from interfluves as high-intensity summer thunderstorms. The winter discharges are therefore dilute and undersaturated, capable of picking up more sediment from stream beds and therefore causing incision. Aggradation occurred when winter storms were less common and floodplain construction could proceed following overbank deposition caused by the high sediment yield produced during runoff following dominant summer thunderstorms (Burkham, 1972; Hereford, 1993; Graf *et al.*, 1991).

17.9 Fluvial architecture: scale, controls and time

Figure 17.19 illustrates the continuum of scales in fluvial architecture with which the sedimentologist must work. Basin type is established by tectonics (see Part 8) and provides the large-scale framework for fluvial deposition. Timescales are in the range 10^5–10^8 yr, with horizontal length scales of 10–10^3 km and vertical length scales of 1–10 km. River systems in fault-bounded asymmetric basins such as

rifts, pull-aparts or thrust top basins are likely to be strongly influenced by tectonic effects. In other larger sedimentary basins, river sedimentation patterns are unlikely to be primarily controlled by active tectonics, either because subsidence is steady and slow (e.g. thermal sagging) and/or because the magnitude of periodic tectonic deformation is too slow to influence channel behaviour.

On a medium scale, fluviatile sand bodies within their 'matrix' of floodplain fines and palaeosol horizons record the occurrence of a significant number of channel avulsions over timescales in the range 10^3–10^6 yr and vertical length scales of 1–10 km. The architectural pattern is controlled by the two-dimensional migratory response of channels to tectonic gradient changes, climatic fluctuations causing discharge changes, base-level changes causing incision and aggradation, and the effects of compaction and pedogenesis upon channel stability and migration.

The small-scale features of fluvial deposits reflect the form of the channels themselves and their bedforms, and in particular the discontinuities within and between individual channel sand bodies. These characteristics are dominated by the changing fluvial hydrograph on timescales of 10^{-2}–10^2 yr and may typically be seen in sand bodies at length scales of 10^{-4}–10^{-1} km. Such features include sand-body thickness and stratification type, clay abandonment plugs in channels or reaches, clay drapes and palaeosols over bar surfaces. They record the effects of channel type, sediment load and channel changes due to bankfull discharge, reach/bend cutoff and migration, flood scour, slack water settling and the local effects of gradient changes due to tectonics and other base-level changes.

We may identify our macro-architectural scale with the concept of *cyclic time* (the length of an erosion cycle, *c.* 10^6 yr or more); meso-architectural scale with *graded time* (a short span of cyclic time in which a graded or dynamic equilibrium exists, *c.* 10^2 yr); and micro-architectural scale with *steady or unsteady time* (steady or unsteady discharge, 10^{-2}–1 yr).

17.10 Fluvial deposits in the geological record

Analysis of ancient point bar deposits, with economic and palaeontological implications, may be found in Wood (1989), Willis (1993), Diaz-Molina (1993) and

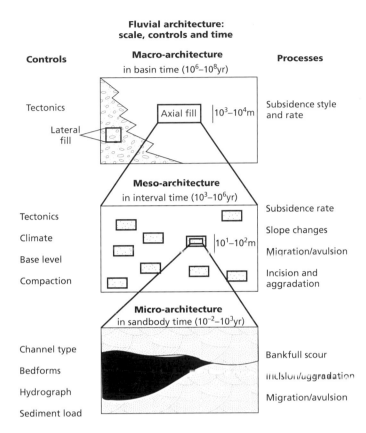

Fig. 17.19 Sketches to illustrate contrasting scale, controls and time in studies of alluvial architecture. (From Leeder, 1993.)

Daams *et al.* (1996). Miall (1994) is good on 3D reconstructions of in-channel bars (from the famous Castlegate Sandstone of Utah). Marzo *et al.* (1988) document an impressive valley-fill sequence in the Castissent Sandstone of the Spanish Pyrenees. The alluvial history of the great north-west European rivers (Thames, Rhine, Meuse) over the last 3 Myr is impressively documented by Gibbard (1988). Outstanding studies of fluvial sediments within the sub-Himalayan Siwalik foreland basin are provided by Willis and Behrensmeyer (1994), Khan *et al.* (1997) and Zaleha (1997a, b). Mack and Leeder (1999) provide an account of the interaction between lateral alluvial fans and the axial ancestral Rio Grande in the Rio Grande rift. Particularly careful analyses of alluvial architecture via detailed facies analysis are to be found in Ramos *et al.* (1986) and Clemente and Pérez-Arlucea (1993).

Further reading

Miall (1996) is massive, informative but sometimes rather uncritical. Best and Bristow (1993) is excellent on braided rivers. Ashworth *et al.* (1996) is more technical, but none the worse for that, on channel flow structures. Knighton (1998) is a nice geomorphological account of fluvial forms and process whilst Anderson *et al.* (1996) has much of relevance to floodplain processes. Purseglove (1989) is delightful.

18.1 Introduction

Alluvial fans and fan deltas are fan-shaped accumulations of sediment traversed by stream flow or debris flow channels (Fig. 18.1). They are point-sourced by streams issuing from a drainage catchment. In radial section the fan profile is straight to concave, in cross-section invariably convex upwards. The fan toe grades gently into a basin floor environment like a flood-plain, lake or marine shoreline. Toe-trimmed fans result when axial-fluvial or beachface erosion of the lower fan occurs and a cliff profile is formed. It is common to find linear zones of adjacent coalesced fans, particularly along faulted mountain fronts; these are called *bajada*.

18.2 Controls on the size (area) of fans

No scale has yet been implied for fans, yet fan size has numerous implications for basin-margin architecture. The chief controls upon fan area have been investigated by many field studies, chiefly in the American south-west, Appalachia and southern Spain. All other things being equal, drainage area is the major influence, through its control of runoff and hence sediment discharge (Fig. 18.2). This is expressed in relations of the kind:

$$A_f = cA_d{}^b \qquad\qquad (18.1)$$

where A_f is fan area, b and c are coefficients gained from regression analysis and A_d is drainage catchment area. But there are no universal values of the coefficients, although b approximates to 0.9 in many cases. This is because other factors, such as climate and catchment geology, intervene and cause considerable scatter when data from different areas are plotted together. In general, mean fan slope also decreases with increasing fan size.

Some authors, notably Blair and McPherson (1994a, b), regard alluvial fans as essentially small-scale features dominated by hyperconcentrated flow deposition, and as somehow separate from the sorts of large alluvial fans with well-defined fluvial channels such as the Kosi and Okavango that issue from very large catchments. In reality there is a complete gradation of catchment area, fan size and transport mechanism. A good account of the spectrum of fan scales and types may be found in Stanistreet and McCarthy (1993). In the present author's opinion, too much reliance has been placed in the literature on the small-scale, often debris-flow-dominated, fans of the Basin and Range extensional province of the western USA.

A final point concerns the evolutionary aspects of fan growth in relation to tectonic processes acting in or adjacent to the drainage catchment. Fault and fold propagation has a major effect here, being capable of fan uplift, tilting, channel incision and the focusing of catchment outlets (Leeder & Jackson, 1993; Jackson & Leeder, 1994; Jackson et al., 1996; Gupta, 1997). The focusing effects are spectacularly seen in the Nepalese Himalayas (Gupta, 1997), where formerly (prior to c. 10 Ma) a dozen or so fans emerged from outlets along the mountain front. Subsequent propagation of the Main Frontal Thrust has focused the entire drainage of the 750 km long sector into just three outlets as megafans, including the well-known Kosi Fan (Fig. 18.3). Such major changes in basin-margin fan size are likely to dominate the stratigraphic architecture of foreland basins.

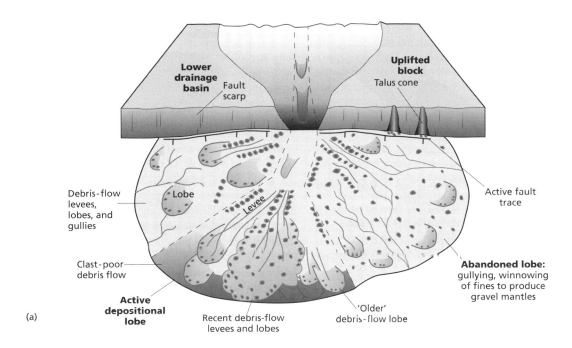

(a)

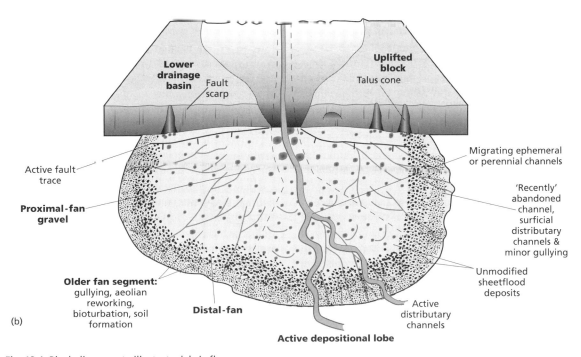

(b)

Fig. 18.1 Block diagrams to illustrate debris-flow-
and stream-flow-dominated alluvial fans adjacent
to active normal faults. (Modified after Blair & McPherson,
1994a.)

18.4 Debris-flow-dominated alluvial fans

Debris-flow-dominated fans occur in both humid and semiarid climates and in some high mountain locations where flow over the fan surface may be regarded as ephemeral and where transport by debris flows is predominant. In some areas, e.g. Betic Range of southern Spain (Harvey, 1990), it may be demonstrated that smaller, steeper catchments tend to encourage debris flow dominance, although source-rock characteristics (e.g. matrix-rich saprolite, mudrocks) play an important role. Smaller-scale debris fans may occur *within* many catchments. These are due to the runout and spreading of individual debris flows generated after high-rainfall events on hillslopes—for good examples of humid debris fans from within Appalachian catchments see Kochel (1990). Morphologically, debris-flow-dominated alluvial fans comprise a main rockhead valley, which may pass, but not always, into a fanhead channel, canyon or trench and hence into a distributive network of fan channels and mid-fan lobes. These fan channels may have been cut by previous fluvial processes but reoccupied by successive generations of debris flows (Whipple & Dunne, 1992). The active lobes are separated by interlobe and interchannel areas and the whole mid-fan area passes gradationally into a distal fan apron. Each of these areas gives rise to characteristic sedimentary facies.

A number of down-fan changes in the general nature of sedimentary deposits are apparent from studies of recent fans. There is usually a down-fan decrease in mean grain size, bed thickness and channel depth, and a down-fan increase in sediment sorting. Because of the short transport distances involved in dry fans, there is usually little discernible down-fan change of grain shape. Important changes in flow mechanism are responsible for some of these trends; thus there may be a down-fan change in dry fans from thick debris flow lobes with levees to more fluid mudflows and sheet floods on the lower fan apron. In the coarse deposits of the upper fan, much of the runoff may percolate through the subsurface, causing the rapid deposition of a gravel lobe as a sieve deposit (Hooke, 1967). The infiltration may deposit detrital clays in the interstices of the open gravel framework beneath.

Catchment valley and fanhead trench subenvironments contain localized accumulations of poorly sorted, angular and coarse gravels, with the clasts being grain- or matrix-supported. Internal stratification is poorly developed. Deposition occurs by scree fall, colluvial mass flow and in-channel debris flow. Fanhead trenches range in depth from a few metres up to tens of metres. At the intersection point of the fan trench with the general alluvial fan surface (Hooke, 1967), the confined flow changes into a distributive network of shallow channels. The major locus of deposition on the fan occurs downstream of this intersection point. Both debris flow deposits and water-lain deposits occur over the mid-fan area. The former comprise interdigitated sheets with nonerosive basal contacts, or occupy prior channels cut by water flow action (Beaty, 1990; Whipple & Dunne, 1992). The detailed morphology of 'dry' fan surface depends critically upon the effective viscosity of the debris flows themselves (Whipple & Dunne, 1992). Low-viscosity flows tend to move further down-fan where they spread and radiate, thus smoothing prior topographic regularities and filling in channel traces. High-viscosity flows by way of contrast are unable to move from the upper fan, where they remain as rough, leveed landscape features, each flow influencing the paths of its predecessors. It is thus clear that whatever controls debris flow viscosity (sediment type, weathering, precipitation) will also control fan steepness and size (Whipple & Dunne, 1992).

Stratigraphic models for the sedimentary sequences built up over time by alluvial fans are largely based upon the hypothetical behaviour of a prograding or retrograding fan system (Heward, 1978). A prograding fan is expected to give rise to large-scale coarsening-upwards sequences as the depositional processes become increasingly proximal. Progradation may be caused by increasing intensity of basin-margin faulting or by increasingly humid climate giving higher runoff and sediment transport rates. A retrograding fan system should give rise to a fining-upwards sequence by the reverse of the above. Initial fan growth along a new scarp or fault scarp should also give rise to a coarsening-upwards sequence, as will advance of active subsidiary fans after deep fanhead trenching.

18.5 Stream-flow-dominated alluvial fans

Stream-flow-dominated ('wet') fans (Gole & Chitale, 1966; Gohain & Parkash, 1990; Kochel, 1990; Maizels, 1990) receive perennial or seasonal stream flow. The avulsion and migration of stream channels dominate the sequences produced on such fans. Some wet fans are very large, with low gradients, an example being the Kosi and other fans noted previously issuing from the Nepal Himalaya fan in northern India. 'Wet' fans often show a proximal–distal change from coarse alluvium deposited in rapidly shifting braided channels to finer sediment of meandering channel and overbank flood deposits (see Amorosi *et al.*, 1996). They, too, may often show entrenched fanhead channels. Such fans often originate from high ranges or mountains subject to very high seasonal rainfall. In the largest of these fans, coalescence and fluvial invasion by adjacent stream systems is common (Mukerji, 1990). Additionally the fans may be so large and gently sloping that they source their own drainage systems on the temporarily inactive fan surfaces. All these features add considerable complexity to 'wet' fan sequences.

Notable examples of 'wet' fans occur on a large scale adjacent to many thrust belts such as the Himalayas (Fig. 18.3; Gupta, 1997) and Alps (Guzzetti *et al.*, 1997) where they feed trunk axial rivers. Many semiarid rift basin fans (e.g. Rio Grande rift) are also of this type (Mack & Leeder, 1998). Fans that have no outlet and which lose their entire discharge to percolation, evaporation, etc., are termed *terminal fans* (Friend, 1978). As noted previously, the fans are dominated by the migratory behaviour of river channel courses. Indeed, the capricious behaviour of the Kosi channels led to its being named after the heroine of a Hindi legend concerning an abused low-caste flirt (see Gohain & Parkash, 1990). The active channel belt of the Kosi today lies to the extreme west of the fan accumulation. It has migrated there in successive avulsions over the past several hundred years (Gole & Chitale, 1966; Wells & Dorr, 1987). Slopes decrease markedly from proximal to distal, accompanied by a braided to meandering change over the 160 km or so of the fan length. Groundwater-fed streams that rework abandoned fan surface deposits become increasingly common distally (Singh *et al.*, 1993). Similar trends are evident in the subsurface deposits of the Bologna alluvial fan bajada that extends 15–20 km basinwards of the Appennine Thrust Front in northern Italy (Fig. 18.4; Amorosi *et al.*, 1996). This area is noteworthy for the influence of both climatic and tectonic controls on fan archtiecture. It is also one of very few examples

where correlations have been made between catchment valley processes of downcutting and terrace formation and the deposition of fan sediment. Avulsive behaviour, but not of a sweeping migratory kind, is also recorded on the Assiniboine Fan (with its spectacular channel levees) of Manitoba, Canada (Rannie, 1990) and on the spectacular abandoned Pleistocene fans of northern Oman (Maizels, 1990).

The Okavango Fan of north-west Botswana is extraordinary (McCarthy *et al.*, 1991; Stanistreet *et al.*, 1993). Rivers rising in the humid Mozambique Highlands feed discharge down to the hyperarid Kalahari desert. The main discharge enters a tectonic rift through a 'panhandle'-like gorge, whereupon periodic combing motions of the initially sinuous streams have created a vast wetland fan traversed by channels. The very low proportions of suspended load do not prevent the occurrence of meandering or straight channel forms since the channel margins are encased in thick cohesive peat levees of the papyrus plant community, which stabilize the channels. Periodic abandonment in the distal fan is accompanied by natural peat burnings, which cause the levees to crumble and the abandoned channel sands to stand out in relief.

18.6 Recognition of ancient alluvial fans

The majority of ancient fan deposits are located at basin-margin positions adjacent to once-active normal (e.g. Leeder & Jackson, 1993), reverse (e.g. Gupta, 1997) or strike-slip faults (e.g. Ridgway & DeCelles, 1993). Individual fans or coalesced bajada may be recognized by a combination of palaeocurrent, grain-size and facies trends. The purist will insist that the radiating form of any contemporary fan-shaped body be established *a priori* from palaeocurrent or channel trend mapping. The nature of the fan should be established by a consideration of the predominance of stream flow vs. hyperconcentrated flow features. Upward changes in grain size and facies in the basin-margin stratigraphy should reflect cycles of fan growth and shrinkage. The influence of tectonics upon fan cycles should be carefully investigated with reference to field and theoretical models of the effects of subsidence rate upon fan dynamics. Climatic and eustatic base-level effects will be at least as severe as, if not more than, tectonics. But they should be investigated with a clear knowledge of local and

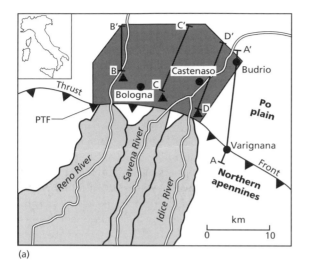

(a)

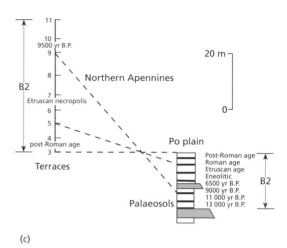

(c)

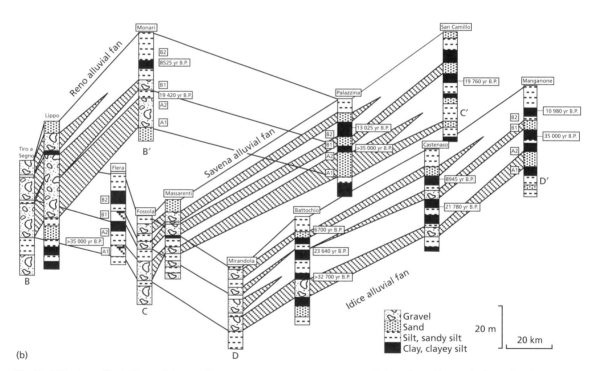

(b)

Fig. 18.4 The large fluvial fans of the northern Appennines. (a) Location, catchments and fans investigated. (b) A 3D reconstruction of facies correlations in the subsurface indicating northward fining and thinning common to all three fans. (c) Correlations of Holocene erosive terrace intervals with fan depositional and palaeosol intervals. (After Amorosi et al., 1996.)

regional climatic evidence, and from a general appreciation of the climatic dynamics of the geological period in question, namely whether greenhouse or icehouse conditions prevailed worldwide.

A well-documented study of Quaternary stacked fan complexes by Nemec & Postma (1993) revealed cycles of entrenchment and backfilling reflecting climatic change as well as regional upwarp of Crete and sea-level changes. Yoshida (1994) describes the growth of a system of mixed stream-flow/debris-flow fans related to Pleistocene thrusting in south-west Japan. Of particular interest is the lateral expulsion and disruption of a prior axial-fluvial system by the growing fans and by an upward change from stream flow to debris flow mechanisms with time as the thrust-related mountains grew. We have already drawn attention to the revealing studies of the Bologna bajada by Amorosi *et al.* (1996).

Crews and Ethridge (1993) ascribe a humid fan origin to a 750 m thick package of interbedded sandstones and conglomerates, which form a marginal facies to the lower Eocene Wasatch Formation bounded by the thrust-related Uinta uplift. They record a grossly coarsening-upwards and then fining-upwards sequence thought to have resulted from the growth and abandonment of a syntectonic fan on whose surface braided stream channels migrated to and fro. Other good accounts of large-scale fluvially dominated fans are by Galloway (1980), Nichols (1987) and Daams *et al.* (1996).

18.7 Fan deltas

A fan delta is an alluvial fan whose active front is an interface with standing water, marine or lacustrine, into which the fan delta is prograding and with which it interacts (Fig. 18.5; Nemec & Steel, 1988). Marine fan deltas in lower latitudes may exhibit significant biogenic carbonate sedimentation from fringing reefs and patch reefs (Hayward, 1982). Although these coral–algal communities may be periodically disturbed or overwhelmed by flood sediment discharges, the overall sedimentation rate is too low and the rate of biological production too high to prevent colonization. Particularly fine examples of such mixed siliciclastic and carbonate environments occur along the modern faulted coastline of the Gulf of Aqaba (Hayward, 1985). Interesting ancient analogues feature

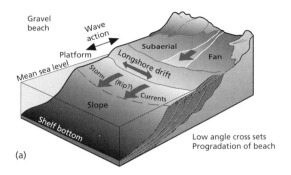

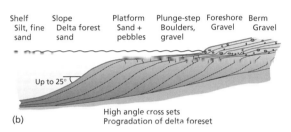

Fig. 18.5 Sketch to illustrate a wave-dominated fan delta with characteristic low-angle beachface foresets overlying steeper delta-front foresets of 'Gilbert' type. (After Dabrio *et al.*, 1991b.)

in the late Neogene of south-east Spain (Dabrio & Polo, 1988).

The nature of the beachface to offshore transition (Fig. 18.5) is clearly of primary importance in any investigation of variability amongst fan deltas (Ethridge & Westcott, 1984; Colella, 1988; Massari & Colella, 1988; Postma, 1990; Dabrio *et al.*, 1991b). Ramp-type fan deltas have relatively gentle offshore slope with a degree of wave and tide reworking. Little sediment bypasses the gently offshore gradients. The internal structure of individual fan delta complexes is thus dominated by relatively low-angle accretion surfaces recording periodic changes in progradation rate. Ramp-type fan deltas are common where tectonic subsidence is low, along inactive faults and particularly on the subsiding hanging walls of extensional basins or the footwall ramps of thrust-related basins. Certainly the most spectacular and instructive ancient example of a shelf-type fan delta complex is that of the historic Eocene Montserrat fan delta of Catalonia (Marzo & Anadon, 1988). A great pile of alluvial fan conglomerates coarsens upwards over 1300 m. Within this sequence, eight individual units (75–250 m thick) that fine and thin outwards into the basin can be distinguished. Each of these passes from proximal alluvial fan debris- and stream-flow conglomerates to distal fan sandy channel and overbank fines, to beachface, shoreface and mouthbar sands and gravels, and finally to offshore fines. Five of the fan units are separated by thin transgressive marine and overlying fan delta progradational coarsening-upwards sequences. The complex represents the vertical stacking of wave-reworked fan delta complexes periodically swept landwards by subsidence-induced transgressions followed by renewed progradation. Subtle changes in the character of the fan delta front during transgression (wave-dominated) and progradation (fluvial-dominated, with coarse mouthbars, even debris flows!) may reflect preservation potential and very marked variations in sediment supply.

Gilbert-type fan deltas have an abrupt discontinuity of slope at or near the shoreface such that the subsequent depositional submarine gradient may reach 25° or more. Although the shoreface of the fan delta may be reworked by wave and tide to form significant beachface and shoreface units (Massari & Collela, 1988; Dabrio *et al.*, 1991b; Horton & Schmitt, 1996), a significant sediment flux bypasses the zone during flood events. This sediment is deposited at the top of the delta slope and, together with material provided by frequent submarine failures, is transported down the steep delta front as debris/grain flow avalanches or density currents in broad shallow chute channels (Fig. 18.6; Ferentinos *et al.*, 1988; Prior & Bornhold, 1988, 1990). Lower down the slope the avalanche deposits cease their motion as frictional forces overcome internal driving forces. They accrete on to the pre-existing slope and stand at the angle of repose for the sediment flow in question. At the foot of the delta slope there may be an abrupt hydraulic jump or gradational change to deposits of the basin floor, which may feature resedimented coarse sediment lobes (Figs 18.7 & 18.8; Postma & Roep, 1985; Postma *et al.*, 1988). Sediment entrained into density currents on the delta slope chutes or generated at the hydraulic jump carries on down across the basin floor where eventual radial spreading and deceleration will cause deposition of sand and gravel in subaqueous fan lobes interdigitated with basinal fine sediments (Surlyk, 1978; Postma & Roep, 1985; Ferentinos *et al.*, 1988; Prior & Bornhold, 1988; Syvitski &

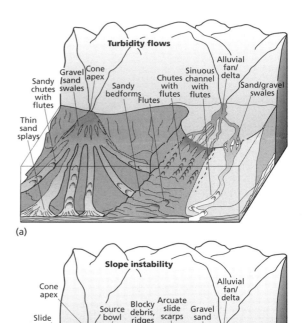

(a)

(b)

Fig. 18.6 Schematic 3D views of avalanche, inertia flow, turbidity flow and slope instability features of Gilbert-type fan deltas. In each case the left-hand fan delta has little subaerial surface expression, typical of very young fan deltas or those on very steep slopes such as fjord sides. (After Prior & Bornhold, 1990.)

Farrow, 1989; Chough *et al.*, 1990; Falk & Dorsey, 1998). Narrow basin floors will encourage long runout distances and perhaps the attainment of very high current velocities (Prior & Bornhold, 1988).

Recognition of Gilbert-type fan deltas is aided by the mapping of the low-angle so-called topsets of the alluvial fan channel complex, the connection of these topsets with curvilinear plan foresets and their connection in turn with bottomset and basinal resedimented fan lobes. The thickness of individual Gilbert complexes will thus depend upon local basin water depths, ranging from a few to many hundreds of

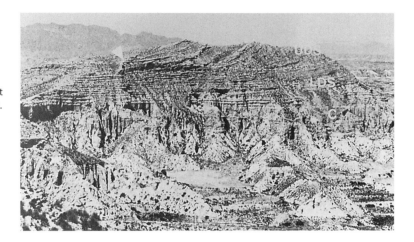

Fig. 18.7 View of El Hacho (south-east Spain) Gilbert-type fan delta deposits. The foreset beds are clearly visible dipping at high angles to the left. These grade out into low-angle bottomsets with thickened gravel beds deposited at the position of a hydraulic jump by high-density turbidity currents sourced from the foresets (see also Fig. 18.8). (From Postma & Roep, 1985.)

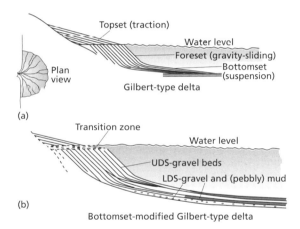

Fig. 18.8 An illustration of low-angle bottomsets with thickened gravel beds deposited at the position of a hydraulic jump by high-density turbidity currents sourced from the foresets (see also Fig. 18.7). (From Postma & Roep, 1985.)

metres. The detailed shapes of the foresets are a response to variations in sediment supply, water depth and relative sea-level change (Postma, 1990). Because fan delta foresets are clearly imaged in shallow seismic profiles, they are of great use in elucidating the relationship between relative sea-level change and sedimentary response, particularly in the great Flandrian sea-level rise of the Holocene (e.g. Somoza

& Rey, 1991). Successive cycles of Gilbert-type fan delta, fluvial and marine transgressive facies reflect changing relative sea level and sediment supply (Dart *et al.*, 1994; Hardy *et al.*, 1994). Convincing evidence for a tectonic subsidence control on repeated high-frequency (~10 kyr) cycles adjacent to the Loreto Fault, Baja California, is given by Dorsey *et al.* (1997)

In deep water and where the subaerial feeder fan channel gradients are very high, there may be only a very small area of subaerial delta exposed, as well seen in some fjords (Fig. 18.6; Prior & Bornhold, 1988; Syvitski & Farrow, 1989). Spectacular examples of Gilbert fan delta complexes have been mapped out in the uplifted southern portions of the Corinth graben, central Greece, where foreset complexes of coarse gravels occupy whole mountainsides up to 600 m high (Ori, 1989; Dart *et al.*, 1994). Other outstanding exposures (and descriptions) of ancient Gilbert-type fan deltas and associated submarine slope facies are to be found in the pioneering paper of Surlyk (1978) and, more recently, by Falk and Dorsey (1998).

Further reading

Useful conference volumes on alluvial fans and fan deltas are Colella and Prior (1990), Nemec and Steel (1988) and Dabrio *et al.* (1991a).

19   Lakes

A lake allows an average father, walking slowly,
To circumvent it in an afternoon,
And any healthy mother to halloo the children
Back to her bedtime from their games across:
(Anything bigger than that, like Michigan or Baikal,
Though potable, is an 'estranging sea').

W.H. Auden, 'Lakes', *Selected Poems*, Penguin Books

19.1 Introduction

Lakes are sinks for both water and sediment. They form on the continental surface when runoff or river flow is interrupted, usually because a depression causes water build-up. The commonest causes of large, deep and steeply shelving lake basins are tectonic (particularly extensional tectonics) and glacial erosion. Large shallow lakes occur in crustal sags (Lake Chad) or have been reconstructed from thrust-loaded foreland basins (Eocene Lakes Gosuite and Uinta). Smaller examples occur widely in coastal, deltaic and fluvial wetlands. Lakes contain about 0.02% by volume of the biosphere's water, and cover about 2% of the Earth's surface. Despite these small percentages, lakes have great ecological and economic importance: their sink-like properties make them highly important repositories of evidence for climate change (Talbot, 1990).

Looking at the surface of a lake in the landscape, one is unaware of the complex processes that go on in the apparently tranquil waters (Fig. 19.1). The length

Fig. 19.1 Aspects of the whole lake system. The sedimentology of lakes is a balance between clastic input by rivers and deltas, longshore and offshore redistribution by waves and wave-produced currents, downslope mass movements and turbidity current generation, and *in situ* biological and chemical production. These processes are all modulated by changes in lake level, which cause transgressive and regressive sequences to form.

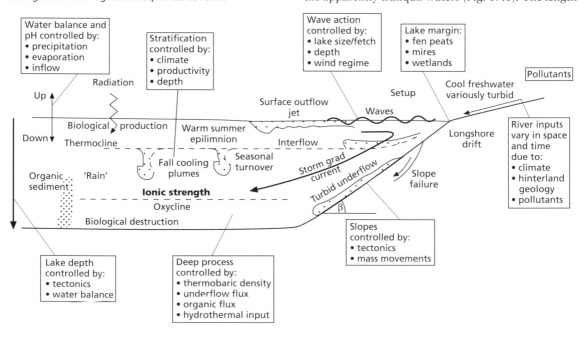

scales and gradients of the water body may be immediately identified as independent variables controlling many aspects of lake dynamics. Depth, lake bottom slopes and surface area represent balances between the basin-forming processes and the hydrological variables of outward flow, evaporation and inward flow. Climate thus appears as the chief modulator of lake dynamics. Solar radiation provides one means of energy transfer through its control of surface water temperature and hence density. Sunlight provides photosynthetic opportunities at the base of the food chain upon which all else in the biomass depends. Clastic sediment particles and dissolved ions enter the water body mostly at point sources such as river deltas, although wind-blown detritus may be important locally. Plumes of sediment then interact with basin floor slopes. Wind shear on the lake surface provides kinetic energy, the more important as surface area increases, to erode and transport bottom sediment introduced by rivers or provided by organic cycling.

There are thus a great variety of lakes, ranging from large, deep and permanent freshwater lakes such as the North American Great Lakes, the deeper East African Rift Valley lakes and Russian Lake Baikal to shallow, ephemeral, saline lakes such as those in the Basin and Range of the western USA and central Iran. Spectacular ephemeral lakes may form in continental interior basins after abnormal rainfall events—witness the astonishing Lake Eyre, South Australia. Chemical classifications of lakes such as those in East Africa (Talling & Talling, 1965) and Amazonia (Rai & Hill, 1980) are based upon the ionic concentrations through measurable conductivity, a feature closely related to alkalinity. It is sometimes useful to distinguish closed lakes (perfect sinks), which lose no water or sediment supplied to them, from open lakes (imperfect sinks), which may either have a surface outlet controlling maximum lake level or lose water and dissolved ions through vadose groundwater flow.

19.2 Lake stratification

Not only are lake-waters subject to the influence of surface waves, currents and turbidity currents, they also develop distinct layers (stratification) that differ in their density, chemical composition and biochemical processes. Thermal density stratification is caused by the production of density gradients due to surface heating (Fig. 19.2). Chemical density stratification

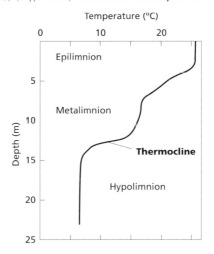

Fig. 19.2 Schematic section to illustrate summer lake stratification, thermocline, epilimnion, metalimnion and hypolimnion. (After Wetzel, 1983.)

More information on stratification

Let us examine the process of thermal density stratification in more detail. Take the case of a temperate lake in summertime. This will show well-marked thermal stratification, with an upper, warm layer called the *epilimnion* separated from deeper, cold water that makes up the *hypolimnion* by a layer of water exhibiting a changing temperature, the *metalimnion*. The *thermocline* is a term used to define an imaginary planar surface of maximum temperature gradient (Fig. B19.1). Most heat is trapped in the surface epilimnion until, in autumn, cooling from the water surface downwards causes density inversions and mixing of the epilimnion with the deep hypolimnion. Melting of winter ice causes wholesale sinking of cold surface water, giving rise to the spring

continued on p. 342

**More information on
stratification** [*continued*]

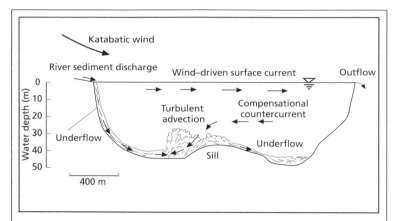

Fig. B19.1 The steady underflow of cold, sediment-rich meltwater and interaction with a deep countercurrent produce an intensely turbulent bottom current that ponds against and then spills over an intrabasinal sill. Based on evidence from Peyto Lake, Alberta, Canada. (After Chikita *et al.*, 1996; see also Plate 9.)

overturn. In early spring the water of a moderately deep lake will all be at a temperature of about 4 °C. The topmost waters will be gradually warmed by solar radiation and mixed downwards by wind action. As heating continues, the isothermal, warm surface water will become buoyant enough to resist wholesale mixing and will remain above the cold deep water. In deep tropical lakes the water stratification into epilimnion and hypolimnion is permanent. The process of overturn in thermally stratified lakes causes the production of alternating sediment- and organic-rich laminae of a varve-like nature. Lake stratification may also be disrupted by currents travelling along the density interface. These may be sufficiently strong to cause entrainment and mixing at the interface.

There are a large number of variations in lake circulation and stratification recognized by limnologists. Some of these, applied to lakes deep enough to form a hypolimnion, are summarized below:

- *Amictic*—lakes permanently isolated from the atmosphere by ice cover.
- *Cold monomictic*—lake-water never rises above 4 °C, with one period of circulation in the summer.
- *Cool dimictic*—lake-water freely circulates twice yearly in spring and autumn (process described previously).
- *Warm monomictic*—lake-water temperatures never drop below 4 °C, freely circulating in the winter and stratifying directly in the summer.
- *Oligomictic*—lake-water rarely circulates, temperatures always well above 4 °C (i.e. tropical), and stable stratification with small temperature vs. depth variations.
- *Polymictic*—lakes with frequent or continuous circulation due to strong winds and/or strong short-term temperature variations.
- *Meromictic*—lakes with a chemocline separating a near-permanent bottom layer that never mixes with the main water mass.

occurs when a layer of salty water is stable beneath upper layers of less-saline fluid, the two separated by a pycnocline of salinity gradient. Such conditions occur in some coastal lakes fed by marine seepage and in solar ponds. Another kind of chemical stratification is the separation of an upper oxygenated layer from a lower deoxygenated layer along a chemocline.

19.3 Clastic input by rivers and the effect of turbidity currents

Water and sediment inputs to lakes come as point sources via fan and river deltas. Only a small proportion of surface runoff enters a lake as a surface plume because of the generally higher density of the cool inflowing water with respect to the warm lake-surface water. Proximity to source is a fundamental control on the nature of lake sedimentary facies. Successively finer sediment will be deposited outwards from the point source, although this regular pattern is affected by surface currents due to direct wind shear. Channelized runoff from steep tectonic or glacial slopes encourages formation of Gilbert-type fan deltas whose steep slopes are prone to sediment failure and downslope mass movement. Indeed, the formation, runout and mixing of these flows with lake-water dominates many lake sediment distribution patterns. Lake turbidites commonly interrupt the more-or-less regular seasonal varves formed by intrinsic lake processes (Sturm & Matter, 1978; Pickrill & Irwin, 1983). Base-of-slope fans are preferentially formed during lowstands when subaerial fan deltas become incised and bypassed (Oviatt et al., 1994).

Turbidity currents in lakes are caused by inflow of sediment-laden, generally cool, river-waters of greater density than the lake (Fig. B19.1; Plate 9). There is a very delicate balance between the density of the inflow and that of the lake itself. Density current development is hindered by turbulent dissipation in very shallow, well-mixed lakes with gently sloping margins. The density contrasts that drive subaqueous currents vary with temperature and sediment concentration. Detailed monitoring provides evidence of the variability of density underflows on a daily basis (Weirich, 1986) and their interactions with wind-forced currents (Chikita et al., 1996). In thermally stratified lakes the density of the inflowing water may be greater than that of the lake epilimnion but less than that of the hypolimnion, so that the density

current moves along the top of the metalimnion as an interflow (Wunderlich, 1971; Sturm & Matter, 1978). Thus, high concentrations of suspended sediment occur at this level, which may then be dispersed over the lake by wind-driven circulation. Other inflows are denser than the hypolimnion and flow along the lake floor as underflows. The underflows bring oxygenated water into the deep hypolimnion and prevent permanent stagnation in deep lakes. It is possible that the phenomenon of turbidity current 'lofting' (see Chapter 11) might also occur once the sediment load has been largely dissipated.

19.4 Wind-forced physical processes

Away from the effects of point-sourced river influxes, water movement in lakes is controlled entirely by wind-driven progressive waves and gradient currents. Even the world's largest lakes are too small to exhibit more than minute (< 2 cm) tidal oscillations. Wind-driven surface waves effectively mix the upper levels of lake-water and give rise to wave currents along shallow lake margins (Csanady, 1978). These processes are accompanied by the seasonal density overturns described previously. The size and effectiveness of lake waves depend upon the square root of the fetch of the lake winds and therefore on the physical size of the lake itself. The energy associated with travelling waves is dissipated along the shoreline as the waves break, the nearshore sediment distribution being largely controlled by these effects. Progressive waves may also form at the epilimnion–metalimnion interface.

A steady wind causes a mass transport of surface water by wind shear (Fig. 19.3), the direction of water movement being oblique to the direction of wind flow due to Coriolis effects. In very large and deep lakes, this deviation can reach a maximum at the surface of 45°, decreasing down from the surface and thus defining the so-called *Ekman spiral* (see Chapter 26). The Ekman effect becomes progressively less as the the lake decreases in area and depth. A measurable tilting of the lake-water surface results from wind shear, the downwind part being higher than the upwind part (similar effects in very large lakes may arise due to differences in barometric pressure). It can be shown (e.g. Csanady, 1978) that a static equilibrium is possible if the wind stress is balanced by a surface elevation gradient of magnitude u^*/gh, where u^*

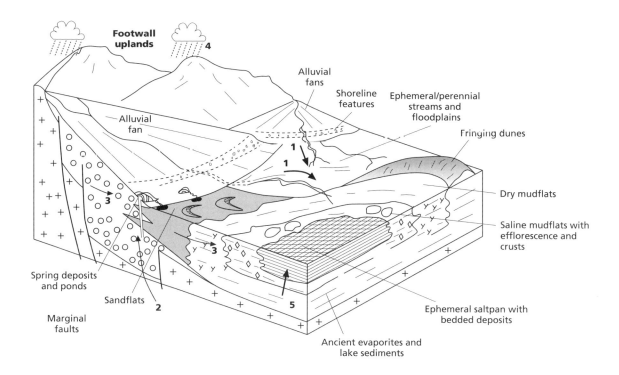

Fig. 19.5 Diagrams to illustrate depositional environments and sources of groundwater in typical playa basins: 1, surface runoff; 2, hydrothermal outflows; 3, groundwater; 4, direct rain recharge; 5, connate water. (After Hardie *et al.*, 1978; Rosen, 1994.)

most typical example. Such playas collect runoff from surrounding footwall and hangingwall uplands, but precipitation is often minimal and a negative water balance exists for most of the year. Clastic detritus is trapped on alluvial fans that fringe such basins so that only solute-laden waters and springs issue into the saline lake. Replenishment flow into the playa may be mainly subsurface via springs, charged by the topographic relief of surrounding uplands, or from ephemeral stream flow with evaporation causing evaporite crusts to appear at the surface. A concentric arrangement of evaporite precipitates is usually seen, with the mineral phases present being controlled by the nature of the weathering reactions in the surrounding hinterlands. Subsurface growth of both evaporite salts in the basin centre and dolomite (as dolocrete—see Colson & Cojan, 1996) in the flanking highs may occur. In some tectonically active rifts associated with volcanism, there may be a significant input of salts (containing Na, Ca and Cl) from juvenile

magmatic sources. Some enclosed playas are still open hydrologically because they may still lose subsurface water and ions to adjacent basins (see review by Rosen, 1994). Saline waters are usually dominated by Na–Ca–Cl–SO_4, although great variety can occur. Many present-day saline playas of the western USA were once deep perennial lakes during glacial maximum times. Death Valley, for example (Li *et al.*, 1997), was up to 90 m deep between 10 and 35 ka, precipitating calcite, some halite and with significant clastic mud deposition. This contrasts with the playa-like state of the past 10 kyr dominated by Na–Ca–SO_4 precipitates. Other lakes show well-developed laminated black shale facies of algal origins during lake highstands (e.g. Newton, 1994, for Mono lake, California).

Deep permanent saline lakes such as the Dead Sea (Neev & Emery, 1967) show appreciable river-water influx, which balances net evaporation. Most of the solute influx, however, comes from small marginal saline springs around the periphery rather than from the River Jordan itself since diversion and training in the past 30 years. The lake-waters are very saline (> 300 000 ppm) and of an unusual Na–Mg–(Ca)–Cl type, with low sulphate and bicarbonate. The deep (~300 m) main basin has historically been density-stratified because of salinity differences, both ara-gonite and gypsum precipitating from surface waters. Natural halite precipitation also occurred in the deep lake about 1500 yr ago when the evaporation/inflow ratio reached into the halite supersaturation field. The Dead Sea is now well mixed and its level dropping since an overturn in 1979, and coarsely crystalline halite, aragonite and gypsum deposits are being precipitated and preserved on the lake floor (Neev, 1978). Seismic sections (Csato et al., 1997) reveal evidence for many phases of climatically driven lake-level rises and falls in the past 5 Myr (see Yechieli et al., 1998).

19.6 Biological processes and cycles

Nutrients brought into lakes by runoff are utilized by a variety of biological communities. Photosynthetic phytoplankton thrive in the well-lit epilimnion and provide the basic rung of the lake food chain. Diatoms are often highly important in nutrient-poor (oligo-trophic) lakes like Baikal (Colman et al., 1995). Below a certain depth, freshwater lakes with low degrees of vertical mixing (for various reasons) are prone to chemical stratification. Thus most dissolved oxygen is used up in the bacterially mediated oxida-tion of detrital organic matter, phytoplankton, zoo-plankton and higher members of the food chain that have settled out after death on to the lake floor from the productive upper waters. It can be appreciated that the abundant fertility of upper lake levels may cause the 'death' of the lower lake—witness the explo-sion of productivity felt in many lakes polluted by abundant phosphates and nitrogenous compounds. Permanently chemically stratified (meromictic) lakes are thus able to preserve almost all incoming organic debris, causing the formation of black, laminated organic-rich muds. However, seasonal fluctuations in the depth of oxygenation may cause the production of distinctive organic-rich and organic-poor laminae to be preserved below a certain depth (Kelts & Hsu, 1978; Dickman, 1985). Dickman has described how early-winter mixing of the upper lake-waters of meromictic Lake Crawford caused oxygenation and mass mortality of anaerobic bacteria, which sedi-mented to form an organic-rich layer on the deep lake floor (Fig. 19.6). These thin (~1 mm) layers be-come enriched in iron monosulphides after reactions between dissolved or particulate Fe^{2+} and the sulphur-rich bacterial carcasses (the photosynthetic bacteria themselves oxidize sulphides to elemental sulphur

during life). This illustrates the great importance of bacteria in the biogeochemical cycling of lakes.

19.7 Modern temperate lakes and their sedimentary facies

The facies pattern of a cool dimictic lake is well illus-trated by Lake Brienz, Switzerland (Sturm & Matter, 1978), a 14 km long and 261 m deep lake in the Swiss Alps. Sediment deposition is entirely clastic, the detritus being introduced by rivers that enter the lake from opposite ends. As noted above, the fluvial sediment is transported and deposited in the seasonally stratified lake by overflows, interflows and under-flows, depending on the density difference between the river- and lake-waters. High-density turbidity currents form underflows and deposit thick (< 1.5 m) graded sand layers. These deposits occur only once or twice per century in response to catastrophic flooding. The underflows formed by low-density turbidity currents occur annually during periods of high river discharge and deposit centimetre-thick, faintly graded sand layers. Fine sediment introduced by overflows and interflows is mixed over the whole lake surface by circulation and it settles continuously during the summer thermal stratification to form the summer half of a varve couplet. At turnover in the autumn the remaining sediment trapped in the thermocline settles out and forms the winter half of the varve couplet. Turbidites grade laterally into thin dark laminae similar to the summer part of the varve noted above. The mechanisms of turbidite deposition and clastic summer varve formation are thus related, the two layers having a common sediment source but a differ-ing level of introduction during periods of thermal stratification. The light-coloured winter layer is of uniform thickness over the whole basin and it forms when the lake is wholly mixed.

In contrast to the clastic facies of Lake Brienz, the sediments currently being laid down in Lake Zurich, Switzerland, are mostly biogenic and chemical, since flood-control dams have almost stopped fluvial sedi-ment input into the lake since about 1900. The varved sediments laid down here form in response to an annual chemical and biological cycle. The varves are present below 50 m depth but are destroyed on slopes by slow creep. Close analogies may be made between the chalky varved sediments of Lake Zurich and the Neogene lacustrine chalks penetrated by deep-sea drilling in the Black Sea (Kelts & Hsu, 1978).

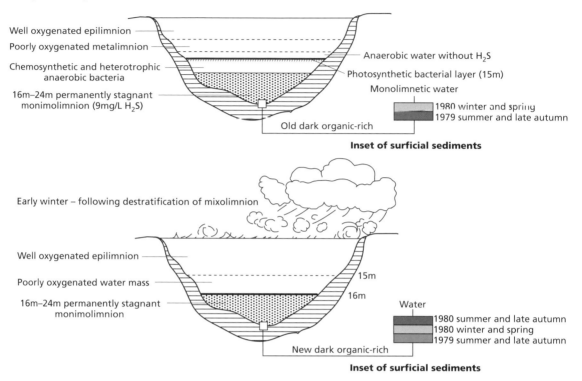

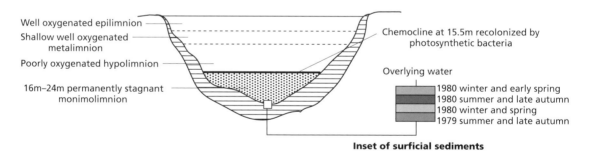

Fig. 19.6 Sketches to illustrate the seasonal changes in a meromictic lake, specifically the mortality of photosynthetic bacteria at the chemocline and their impact on dark organic-rich varve laminations. (After Dickman, 1985.)

19.8 Lakes in the East African rifts

Lakes Malawi (Nyasa) and Tanganyika typify the large stratified freshwater lakes developed in half-grabens of the East African rift system (Fig. 19.7). In Lake Malawi (area 45 000 km², maximum depth 730 m) up to 4.5 km of sediment has accumulated in the lake basin in the past 5 Myr or so. In Lake Tanganyika (area 23 000 km², maximum depth 1470 m) more than 4 km has accumulated in the past 1 Myr. In each half-graben the bathymetric framework is dominated by the asymmetric basin form and the effects of fault segmentation (Fig. 19.7; Ebinger *et al.*, 1987; Scholz *et al.*, 1990; Scholz & Finney, 1994; Johnson *et al.*, 1995; Lezzar *et al.*, 1996). Lakewards of active faults, the steep subaqueous slopes are predominantly bypass

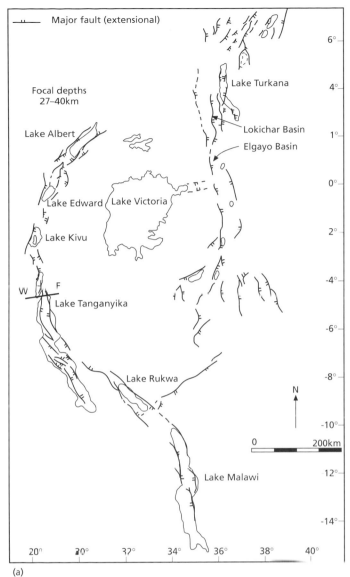

(a)

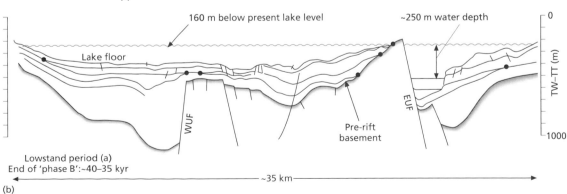

(b)

Fig. 19.7 (a) Regional tectonic map of the East African rift system and (b) a west–east cross-section across northern Lake Tanganyika rift to illustrate typical asymmetrical lake floor slopes produced by intrabasinal footwall uplift and hangingwall subsidence. Drawn for a −160 m lake lowstand at about 35 ka. EUF, WUF—Eastern and Western Ubwar Faults. Lake floor sediments are maximum 300 m thick, going back about 1 Myr. (After Lezzar *et al.*, 1996.)

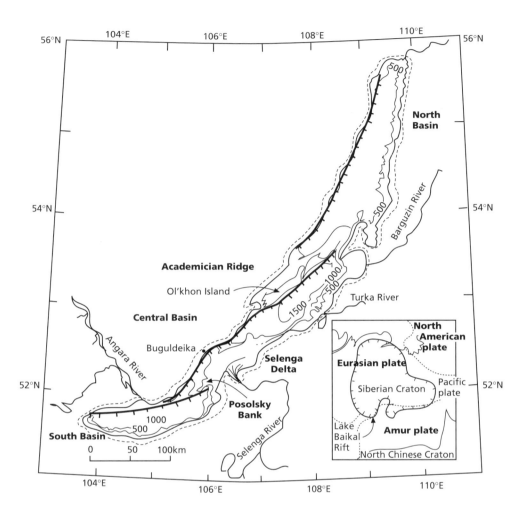

Fig. 19.9 Bathymetry, inflowing rivers and the three major right-stepping normal faults that border Lake Baikal. Note ridges and highs located on stepover zones and major river inflow from the southern hangingwall uplands. (After Scholz et al., 1993.)

data on continental evaporites are given in Chapters 24 and 26.

19.11 The succession of facies as lakes evolve

To the student of modern lakes (e.g. Wetzel, 1983) it seems inevitable that lakes should evolve through time (lake 'ontogeny') as they infill from their margins. Such changes might involve the succession of facies laid down in stratified freshwater lakes, from the products of the lake hypolimnion to the epilimnion, and hence to the clastic input sites at the lake margins, and finally to the products of wetlands and bogs around the lake margins. At its crudest, we might expect a coarsening-upwards trend in grain size and a trend from algal-dominant to higher-plant-dominated organic facies. This sedimentary trend might also record the geochemical change from relatively high-pH to low-pH conditions as the alkaline hypolimnion gives way to the acidic groundwater conditions afforded by encroaching freshwater *Sphagnum* peats (Wetzel, 1983). Saline lakes will show a characteristic infill pattern, with subaqueous evaporites passing upwards into particulate forms with wind reworking and dissolution surfaces (Warren, 1982).

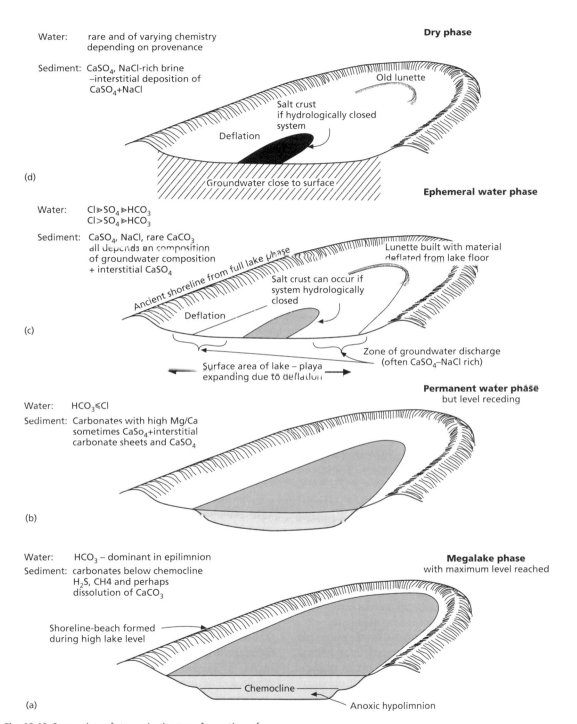

Water: rare and of varying chemistry
           depending on provenance

Sediment: $CaSO_4$, NaCl-rich brine
           –interstitial deposition of
           $CaSO_4$+NaCl

Dry phase

Old lunette

Salt crust
if hydrologically closed
system

Deflation

(d)

Groundwater close to surface

Ephemeral water phase

Water: $Cl \gg SO_4 \gg HCO_3$
           $Cl > SO_4 \gg HCO_3$

Sediment: $CaSO_4$, NaCl, rare $CaCO_3$
           all depends on composition
           of groundwater composition
           + interstitial $CaSO_4$

Ancient shoreline from full lake phase

Lunette built with material
deflated from lake floor

Salt crust can occur if
system hydrologically
closed

Deflation

(c)

Surface area of lake – playa
expanding due to deflation

Zone of groundwater discharge
(often $CaSO_4$–NaCl rich)

Permanent water phase
but level receding

Water: $HCO_3 \leqslant Cl$

Sediment: Carbonates with high Mg/Ca
           sometimes $CaSo_4$+interstitial
           carbonate sheets and $CaSO_4$

(b)

Megalake phase
with maximum level reached

Water: HCO_3 – dominant in epilimnion
Sediment: carbonates below chemocline
           H_2S, CH4 and perhaps
           dissolution of $CaCO_3$

Shoreline-beach formed
during high lake level

Chemocline

Anoxic hypolimnion

(a)

Fig. 19.10 Succession of stages in the transformation of a
pluvial-period permanent lake to a dry-period salina or
playa. (After DeDekker, 1988.)

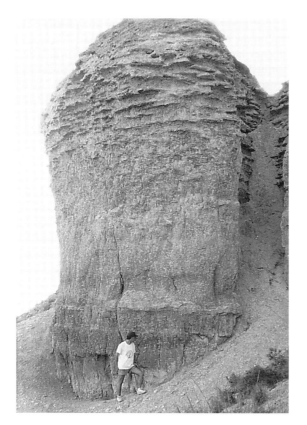

Fig. 19.12 Close-up view of the transition from palaeosols to pond facies in the tertiary of the Madrid Basin. The lower part of the exposure shows pedified mudrock with dolomitized calcisols. The upper part reveals ledges of gypsum crusts. (Photo courtesy of J.P. Calvo.)

thin partings of dolomitic mudstone interpreted to result from increased evaporative concentration of the playa lake that gave rise to the oil shale facies. Bioturbated calcareous mudstones present in the Laney member contain freshwater molluscs and ostracods. There is an upward trend in the Laney member cycles from playa to shallow freshwater lake environments. Cross-stratified sandstones with frequent channel forms are indicative of alluvial fan and braidplain environments with Gilbert delta facies recorded occasionally in the Laney member. The clastic facies intertongue with lacustrine facies and are sourced from syntectonic highs within and adjacent to the lake basins.

Tertiary Lake Madrid

The tertiary deposits of the Madrid Basin, Spain, have well-developed lacustrine facies. In particular, spectacular upward transitions occur from well-drained lake margin alluvial plains, with dolomitized calcisols, to shallow evaporating carbonate pond (paludal) deposits with gypsum crests (Fig. 19.12; Sanz *et al.*, 1995).

Further reading

Many papers of interest for both modern and ancient lake studies are to be found in the volumes edited by Matter and Tucker (1978), Lerman (1978), Fleet *et al.* (1988), Renaut and Last (1994) and Rosen (1994). Talbot and Allen (1996) is a well-balanced review of lake processes and sedimentary products. A fundamental reference on the physics and chemistry of lakes is Hutchinson (1957), and an excellent general text on limnology is Wetzel (1983).

periodically exposed lake floor. High rates of organic productivity are inferred, with the playa flats acting as efficient sediment traps preventing the introduction of much clastic material. Bedded trona deposits contain

20   Ice

. . . and then the earth namely the air and then the earth in the great cold the great dark the air and the earth abode of stones in the great cold alas alas in the year of their Lord six hundred and something the air the earth the sea the earth abode of stones in the great deeps the great cold on sea on land and in the air . . .

Samuel Beckett, [from Lucky's soliloquy], 'Waiting for Godot', *Complete Dramatic Works*, Faber

20.1 Introduction

Some 10% of the Earth's surface area is covered by ice, representing about 80% of surface fresh water. A further area of 20% is affected by permafrost. This total 30% of the frigid land surface is our cryosphere (Williams *et al.*, 1993), an environment quite unlike any other. Of the ice-lands, the Antarctic ice-cap has about 86% by area, Greenland has about 11% and the many other valley and piedmont glaciers make up the remaining tiny fraction. Yet earlier in Quaternary times a staggering 30% of the Earth's surface was ice-covered, with vast areas of North America and Europe subjected to glacial erosion and deposition and even larger areas in the permafrost zone. At least 11 epochs during Earth history had very extensive and long-lasting 'icehouse-mode' climates, the longest

and best-documented being the Gondwanan Permo-Carboniferous glaciation (Fig. 20.1).

As discussed in Chapter 13, periodicity in glaciation is best explained by the Milankovitch mechanism (Hays *et al.*, 1976)—but for an antidote read the sceptical, and sometimes outrageous, Hoyle (1981). However, the Milankovitch effect is small and cannot trigger an Ice Age. Even in our present interglacial conditions, the Earth's oceanic heat engine is thoroughly dominated by the exchange of heat from deep, cold, polar water masses to warm surface currents that feed air masses with latent heat from condensation. It is these warm winds, not subtle radiation changes, that prevent temperate latitudes from developing permanent ice cover. The presence of continents over the polar regions and a deep oceanic meridional circulation (see Chapter 26) are obviously a major prerequisite for glaciation, variations in solar energy input and reflection/trapping efficiency being secondary controls.

Fig. 20.1 Time series for glaciations and their approximate magnitude during Earth's history. (After Hambrey, 1994.)

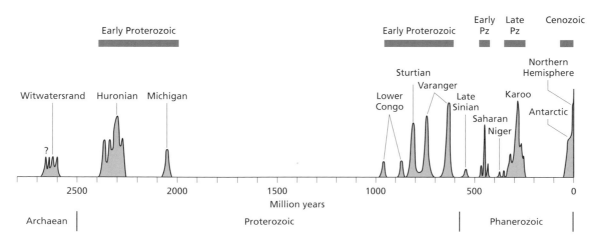

The major environments of glacier ice are:
- ice-sheets and their associated fast-moving outlet ice streams and coastal ice shelves;
- valley glaciers (Plate 12) and their marine outlets called tidewater glaciers;
- piedmont glaciers—divergent, fan-like ice masses formed after a valley glacier becomes unconfined.

In all glaciers, a dynamic equilibrium exists between snow input, ice formation, ice motion and terminal melting. Depositional products are dominated by a variety of subglacial facies and by meltout facies of glacial outwash plains on land and glacimarine and glacilacustrine environments under water. The preservation potential of glacial environments will generally be low unless the depositional and erosional features are produced in areas of subsidence. For this reason the depositional products of the glacimarine environments on rifting or thermally subsiding margins, with their wide ring of ice shelves and calving icebergs, are probably the most likely to be preserved.

20.2 Physical processes of ice flow

Ice as a sediment transporting system is poorly understood and so radically different from any other we have hitherto encountered in this book (it is difficult to do flume experiments with ice) that a short discussion of the basic principles seems necessary. We are dealing with the bulk sliding and/or gravitational deformation of a crystalline solid phase due to its own body force under the influence of gravity. The direction of movement is set in response to regional pressure gradients caused by the 3D distribution of ice mass and/or a bedrock slope. The radial flow of a mound-like ice-sheet will pay little attention to local or even regional bedrock relief, i.e. ice commonly moves uphill. Valley glaciers, on the other hand, move downvalley in response to the downslope component of gravitational force acting on the ice mass. The slow mean surface laminar flow of glacier ice is usually measured in metres per year, with values between 10 and 200 m/yr for valley glaciers and 200–1400 m/yr for ice streams. Corresponding strain rates are also small. Although usually slow and steady, spectacular glacier surges occur periodically when ice velocity increases by an order of magnitude and more.

Ice is composed of an aggregate of roughly equigranular crystals whose crystal size increases with time and/or depth. When stressed, by burial in a glacier or insertion in a test rig in the laboratory, each crystal deforms easiest internally along glide planes parallel to the basal planes of the hexagonal crystal lattice. Since crystals in ice are not usually aligned along common axes, the polycrystalline aggregate rearranges, and recrystallization takes place during strain or flow. Natural ice crystals in the actively deforming layer of a glacier also contain a myriad of gaseous, liquid and solid impurities and inclusions (Sharp *et al.*, 1994). It is not surprising therefore that natural ice deformation is rather complex, with time-dependent behaviour seen during the application of continued stress. Primary, secondary and tertiary creep regimes may be identified, with secondary creep (a sort of steady state) dominant in glaciers, which are usually responding to load- and slope-induced stresses in the range 50–200 kPa (0.5–2 bar). For applied stresses of this magnitude in the laboratory, the shear strain rate of secondarily creeping glacier ice is given by Glen's law:

$$\frac{\mathrm{d}u}{\mathrm{d}y} = k\tau^n \qquad (20.1)$$

where n is an exponent ranging between 1.5 and 4.2, k is an experimental constant and τ is the shear stress. (Compare this to the Newtonian law for fluids when $n = 1$ and $1/k$ is the molecular viscosity.) It has been stated that n is most reliably estimated as 3 (see Paterson, 1994), whilst k is partly a temperature-dependent (Arrhenius) function controlled by the energy required to activate creep. It is also a function of crystal size, shape and inclusion content. It ranges in value from 5.3×10^{-15}/s kPa at 0 °C to 5.4×10^{17}/s kPa at −30 °C. In view of all this complexity, the reader should note the dissenting evidence from Antarctic studies by Doake and Wolff (1985) who found that a linear flow law for the strain rate, of the form $\dot{e} = k\tau$, with $k = 10^{-15}$/s Pa best fitted their deformation studies from borehole data.

The shear stress arising from valley glacier ice sliding over a plane inclined bed may be approximately given by the familiar tractive stress equation:

$$\tau = \rho g h \sin \alpha \qquad (20.2)$$

where ρ is the density of ice, h is the thickness of ice and α is the mean valley floor (or ice surface) slope.

20.3 Glacier flow and surges

Our previous discussion of the mechanical flow of ice left out the most vital part of the whole process, namely that of the interaction of the basal ice layer in

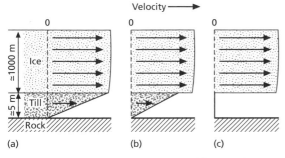

Fig. 20.2 Schematic velocity profiles possible for sliding glacier ice in contact with a basal till overlying solid bedrock. (a) Predominant till deformation, as proposed for Antarctic ice streams. (b) Till deformation plus basal sliding, appropriate for near-polar glacial termini. (c) Basal ice sliding only, probably rare in Nature. (After Alley *et al.*, 1986.)

a real glacier with a solid and sediment substrate and with glacial waters. It is the coupling of the three materials (see Boulton & Hindmarsh, 1987) that is really the key to the whole process. Two fundamental types of flowing glacial ice (Fig. 20.2) may be identified:

1 'Cold' and dry ice beds are an uncommon (and largely hypothetical) state when ice lies well below its pressure melting point at depth. A condition of 'no slip' exists at the ice–bed interface, and there is a general absence of englacial or subglacial drainage. Forward motion of such ice is therefore by internal creep alone. Glacial debris is transported within the ice, with substrate erosion due to plucking and grinding effective only at the summits of protuberances on the bed.

2 'Warm' and wet ice beds lie close to the pressure melting point at the glacier sole (ignoring the conditions throughout the rest of the ice column), and the glacier slides over its bed on a *décollement* plane on fluid-rich and highly porous sediment. Most glaciers, including both polar ice streams (Blankenship *et al.*, 1986; Alley *et al.*, 1986; Smith, 1997) and valley glaciers, seem to exist in this state. It is quite instructive to remember that the weight of over 1000 m of Antarctic ice is held up by pore fluid pressure in a thin (5–6 m) basal deforming layer of till. It seems that up to 90% of total glacier movement may occur by basal sliding, the rest by internal deformation. The concept of effective stress (Chapter 12) is relevant again here, for the shear strength, τ_s, of subglacial sediment must be exceeded by that of the driving bed shear stress, τ_0, for ice flow if deformation is to occur at all. Ignoring cohesive strength, assuming that resistance is due to solid friction (ϕ) and that strength is much reduced by high porewater pressures, we may write:

$$\tau_0 \geq \tau_s \tag{20.3}$$

or

$$\rho g h \sin \alpha \geq \Delta P \tan \phi \tag{20.4}$$

where ΔP is the excess of lithostatic pressure above porewater pressure. The reduced strength allows the driving force provided by the tractive force of the glacier—actually quite small for most glaciers due to the low slopes involved, and about 20 kPa for the Antarctic ice-cap (Alley *et al.*, 1986)—to cause deformation and steady forward motion. Direct subglacial measurements of rates of till deformation (Fischer & Clarke, 1994) indicate values of 'viscosity' for deforming till of between 3×10^9 and 3×10^{10} Pa s, with yield stresses of about 50–60 kPa. But we know little about the *in situ* properties of deforming till; it may even be unlikely that normal concepts of yield stress and flow law behaviour apply. In any case, it seems clear that both the glacier ice *and* the deforming subglacial till must move along.

The process of basal sliding (Weertmann, 1957; see Glen's law above) must also involve enhanced creep around drag-creating obstacles, pressure melting around obstacles and direct lubrication by abundant basal meltwater (Murray & Clarke, 1995). The latter comes from surface meltwaters let into the sole by crevasses and ice tunnels, ice melted by geothermal heat (e.g. spectacular Lake Vostok under the Antarctic ice cap; see Kapitsa *et al.*, 1996), and ice melted by pressure at the glacier sole (see Fountain & Walder, 1998 for a review of water in temperate glaciers). The water under ice streams is often modelled as a thin (few centimetres) film but is more realistically thought to occur in a network of very shallow sub-ice channels cut into the deforming till (Walder & Fowler, 1994; Fig. 20.3). It may be possible to characterize a glacier bed by some roughness coefficient or friction factor, analogous to the flow of water over sediment beds and bedforms.

Glacier flow is unsteady and nonuniform on a variety of timescales (e.g. Harbor *et al.*, 1997; Fig. 20.4) due mainly to variations in the rate of basal sliding vs. internal ice deformation caused by variation of water content. Slow winter flow occurs because meltwater is in short supply and subglacial drainage is minimal. Flow accelerates in spring and summer as more water becomes available. Glaciers may also suddenly surge

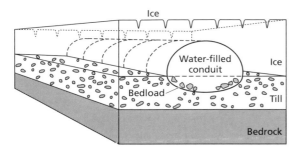

Fig. 20.3 Sketch to show an idealized subglacial tunnel conduit moving at an ice–till interface. (From Walder & Fowler, 1994.)

after years of steady slow flow and over a few months move orders of magnitude faster than in preceding and subsequent months. The process suggests that some deformation threshold is crossed—maybe the onset of high shear strain as the ice accumulation increases, a consequence of the Glen third-power law of deformation. Given the roles that basal fluid pressure and deforming sediment have upon glacier behaviour, it seems more likely that changing near-bed conditions play a crucial role.

The Bering glacier of Alaska is a well-known example in which surges occur quite regularly, every 20 yr or so, the most recent initiated in 1993. As in flooding rivers, surging reflects an imbalance between supply from the gathering area upstream and the geometry of the channel downstream. In addition, resistance to flow is strongly dependent upon water content at the glacier sole. The icy kinematic floodwave that quickly travels through the system causes tectonic thickening, intense crevassing, extreme local velocity gradients, abundant discharges of meltwater and the intense mixing of lateral and medial moraines. As the surge dissipates and the glacier resumes its sluggish phase once more, the advanced snout (but note that surges do not *always* reach the snout) decays back to its equilibrium position. Distinctive surge moraines then mark the previous maximum position of the glacier front.

20.4 Sediment transport, erosion and deposition by flowing ice

The debris found within glacial ice may come from the glacier top, sides (Plate 12) or sole. In the former cases a variety of angular particles are supplied by the very effective freeze–thaw mechanisms acting on surrounding bedrock slopes. It is supplied to the

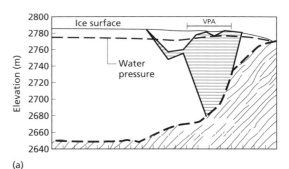

(a)

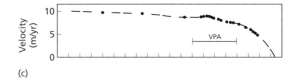

(b)

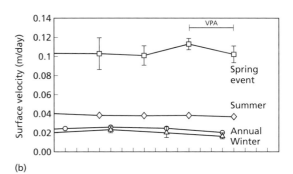

(c)

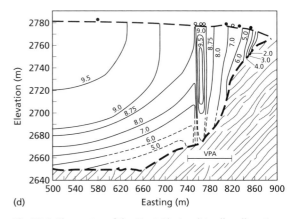

(d)

Fig. 20.4 Flow rates of the Haut Glacier d'Arolla; all sections are half-sections normal to flow. (a) Half cross-section to show ranges of water pressure and local ice overburden pressure and a variable pressure axis (VPA) zone. (b) Seasonal surface velocity variations. (c) Mean annual surface velocities and the glacial boundary layer. (d) The cross-sectional mean annual velocities (note the high gradients in the region of the VPA. (After Harbor *et al.*, 1997.)

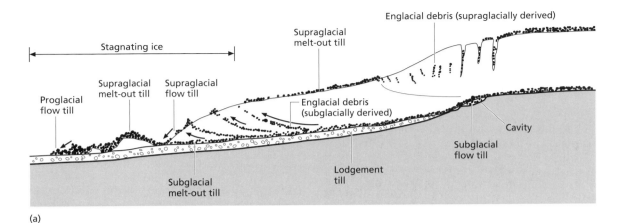

(a)

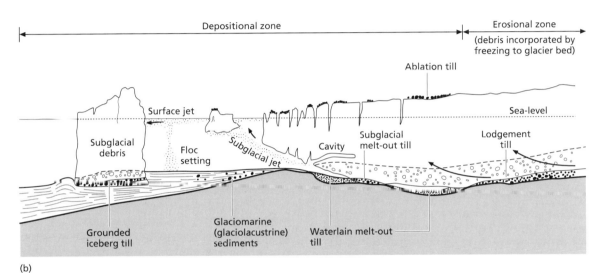

(b)

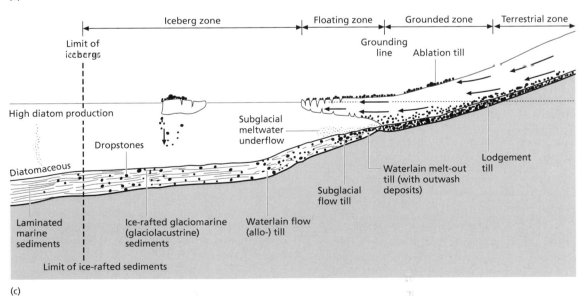

(c)

Fig. 20.5 Longitudinal (flow-parallel) sections of glacier termini (not to scale) to show modes of till, outwash and subaqueous proglacial deposition: (a) terrestrial glacial deposition; (b) grounded glacier deposition; (c) floating glacier deposition. (After Hambrey & Harland, 1981, and the many sources cited therein, with some modifications.)

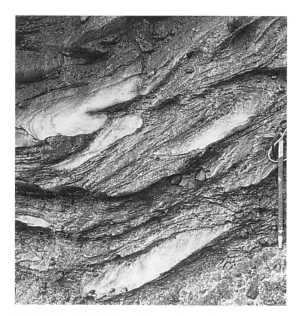

Fig. 20.6 Basal glacier ice of the Variegated Glacier, Alaska, to show intensely sheared and folded pure ice (white) and debris-rich (≈10%) ice (grey). Foliation planes are about parallel to glacier bed. Ice axe is 85 cm long. (From Sharp et al., 1994. Photo courtesy of M. Sharp.)

glacier margin by scree build-up and subsequent rock-fall avalanches and debris flows. Successive bands of debris within temperate glaciers record seasonal cycles of snow accumulation and debris fall from rock outcrops. Some proportion of the supraglacial debris finds its way to the sole via crevasses (Fig. 20.5) and intraglacial tunnels, where it is modified in shape and size during ice motion. Polar ice characteristically contains a thick basal zone of layered regelation ice, heavily charged with debris caused by upstream pressure melting and downstream refreezing around obstacles such as gravel and boulders. Thin regelation layers also occur in warm glaciers but these are lost downflow as the basal sliding process takes over. Subglacial erosion is effected by both sediment-charged subglacial water and by plucking, abrasion, crushing and fracturing. Subglacial transport processes cause frequent grain-to-grain interactions resulting in abrasion and a degree of rounding. Also formed are striated facets (Boulton, 1978) and the formation of the abundant rock 'flour' that dominates the suspended load of glacial outwash streams. Thrust planes may arise at the glacier snout (Fig. 20.5a) in response to compressional stresses between the slow-moving or stationary snout and the fast-moving

upstream ice, particularly during surges. These thrusts carry subglacial debris to high positions in the ice front, where it can both melt out and flow.

Deposition (lodgement) of glacial debris at the active ice sole will occur in response to the cohesive smearing of clay-rich sediment on to bedrock or pre-existing sediments. The process is aided by melting around the upstream parts of bed roughness elements and the deposition of the released materials downstream. Thick layers of lodgement till with shear fabric thus gradually build up (Fig. 20.5a). Clast orientation within lodgement till and spectacular shear foliation of the ice itself (Fig. 20.6) point to the effectiveness of the shearing–smearing process. Clasts may be orientated with their long a-axis parallel to flow, as observed in many grain flows and debris flows, but with a varying proportion of imbricate intermediate b-axis orientations, as seen in sediments deposited by bedload rolling mechanisms (for a discussion of active till fabrics see Benn, 1995).

20.5 Glacigenic sediment: nomenclature and classification

Much care is needed in the description, nomenclature and interpretation of glacigenic sediments, particularly those that are coarse, poorly sorted and matrix-rich. Such muddy, sandy and gravelly deposits are given the quite general and nongenetic term *diamict(ite)*, the suffix for lithified examples in the geological record. This is not for pedantic or semantic reasons, but because of the great controversy (and difficulty!) often associated with the identification of ancient glacial deposits. Thus a diamictite could have an origin as a true subglacial primary lodgement till (see below) or it could have been redeposited by a debris flow related (Eyles & Eyles, 1989) or quite unrelated to any glacier ice. Many extra observations of both the deposit and its relationships with adjacent deposits are needed before a glacigenic origin can be confidently stated.

The following terms are in general modern use and increasingly accepted as standard by workers in the glacial field—see Dreimanis (1989) for an exhaustive account and Hambrey (1994) for a mercifully concise summary:

- *Primary till* is unmodified diamictite deposited directly from glacier ice on land or under the sea. The latter is also known as waterlain till. Deposition is most commonly due to meltout from stationary ice or lodgement from the moving glacier or iceberg base.

- *Secondary till* is diamictite that is modified after deposition (but not by significant addition of melt-water), most commonly by gravity flow, slumping or debris flow.

An important point concerns the physical state of lodgement tills, which are frequently quite dense and overcompacted. This was not their condition during glacial flow (at least away from the terminus) since we have seen above that most ice flows on a highly porous and overpressured water-rich sediment base. The till fabric and physical state must evolve rapidly as the snout is approached, with *massive* dewatering and compaction.

20.6 Quaternary and modern glacial environments and facies

A broad spectrum of depositional environments and facies exists in association with the movement and melting of glacier ice. We may usefully divide the depositional environments and products (see summary in Fig. 20.5) into:

- ice-produced, by direct lodgement from subglacial flow or by passive meltout;
- ice-produced by subsequent gravity flows from the glacial terminus;
- water-produced, within the ice or at the subaerial ice contact zone: confined or unconfined stream, tunnel flow and delta deposits;
- glacimarine, after ice or meltwater comes into contact with marine waters: a great variety of till, density current (plumes and jets) and meltout deposits;
- glacilacustrine, after ice or meltwater comes into contact with lacustrine waters: a great variety of till, density current (plumes and jets) and meltout deposits.

In terms of geological preservation potential, the last two are most favoured because the products, particularly those on the shelves and in the oceans, may be spread over vast areas. Picking up this glacigenic signal amongst the deposits of 'normal' shelf and oceanic deposits is obviously highly important for reconstructions of pre-Holocene ice dynamics and distributions (see Chapter 26 for Heinrich events). Not a little skill is needed to do this, and the following sections are designed to provide a brief introductory background to the topic.

20.7 Ice-produced glacigenic facies and the periglacial realm

These are dominated by poorly sorted, often matrix-rich, gravelly tills (an older term is boulder clay). As noted previously a number of distinct genetic varieties of till are known. Lodgement tills result from deposition at the base of temperate ice by a plastering effect. There is often evidence of an upper, more porous, deformed layer with a good development of shear fabric overlying a more massive, denser layer with spaced shear planes (Boulton, 1979; Boulton & Hindmarsh, 1987; Dowdeswell & Sharp, 1986; Benn, 1994). Larger clasts may resist the shear stress of the glacier ice by their greater stability if they 'keel down' into the lower nonshearing layer. Such lodged boulders may resist the shearing stress set up by the glacier bed and act as nuclei for the downstream accretion of finer sediment to form ridge-like mounds a few metres or tens of metres long (these are sometimes called flutes, but because the same name is in widespread usage for quite different erosive structures the term *ridge* seems preferable). Accretion has been postulated to have been brought about by a spanwise component of motion of till into the zone of changed pressure gradients in the lee of the obstructing pebble (Boulton, 1976). The spanwise motion has recently been confirmed by analysis of pebble orientations (Benn, 1994). On a larger scale, but possibly in a similar way to these ridges, till deposited from ice-sheets or streams may be moulded into streamlined drumlin bedforms over pre-existing topographic nuclei that resist internal shear (for a recent compilation see Menzies & Rose, 1989).

Meltout or ablation tills (Fig. 20.5a) result from the seasonal melting of debris-laden ice in temperate glaciers. Such tills should show no development of internal structures or fabrics and may locally overlie lodgement tills. Flow tills are extremely common at the glacier front and result from thick supraglacial accumulations of debris derived from the meltout of debris bands (Boulton, 1968). These poorly sorted deposits then move down the local gravity slope at the glacier snout or lateral margins as coherent slumps or as debris flows. Flow tills may come to overlie meltout and lodgement tills to form a characteristic tripartite subdivision (Boulton, 1972b). Spectacular, valley-wide diamicts of debris flow origin are sometimes produced during deglaciations (Eyles *et al.*, 1988).

Moraines are essentially glacitectonic ridges produced by glacial dumping of both ice-deposited tills and water-deposited outwash. High, laterally extensive terminal moraines mark periods when forward motion is exactly balanced by melting over a long period of time. Spectacular glacitectonics is recorded in many outwash deposits, moraines, diamictons and interglacial fluvial terraces that are overrun by later glacial advances. Fine examples are to be seen in the Pleistocene of the East Anglian coast (Hart & Boulton, 1991), in central Holland (Ruegg, 1991) and in the Karakorum Mountains (Owen, 1988) to name but a few examples.

We must finally briefly mention the widespread periglacial realm in which frozen ground conditions may reach hundreds of metres below the surface. Diagnostic near-surface features are produced by brief summer thaws and deep winter freezes above a permanently frozen substrate. Ice wedge casts and various forms of patterned ground are particularly characteristic of periglacial conditions. Rock glacier flows and deposits are ice-cored remnants (an example in Antarctica has the oldest known ice, at about 8 Ma; see Sugden *et al.*, 1995) covered with an often thick layer of avalanche, debris flow or collapse talus. They may slowly creep downslope from cirques or ice fronts.

20.8 Glaciofluvial processes at and within the ice front

Subglacial drainage usually occurs along distinct channels or tunnels that may be alongside or within the ice or at its base. Deep tunnel valleys may be cut below ice-sheets overlying relatively easily erodible sediments. Fluvial depositional facies at the base or sides of glaciers or in the ice contact zone include *esker* ridges and *kame* terraces. An esker is a linear accumulation of stratified sands or gravels that was deposited by a stream wholly or partly confined by glacier ice resting usually directly on bedrock. They are commonly a few metres to tens of metres high, tens to hundreds of metres wide and kilometres to tens of kilometres long. Kames form by subaqueous deposition adjacent to ice masses in contact with bedrock surfaces. They commonly have relatively flat-topped surfaces with slumped margins marking the former position of the melting ice boundary. Deposits of cnglacial streams are 'let down' to the local bedrock surface during ice melting and, as a result, may show marginal slump and fault structures related to this movement. Certain eskers are thought to have formed subaqueously as subglacial streams debouched into lake bodies. Most eskers are associated with temperate glaciers and are thought to have formed at or fairly close to a retreating glacier terminus. The deposits of eskers are dominated by current-produced sedimentary structures. Climbing ripple cross-laminations with a high angle of climb attest to the rapidity of sediment deposition. Esker beads are thought to be caused by flow acceleration and deceleration at the front of subaqueous subglacial streams, giving rise to characteristic down-bead fining (Bannerjee & McDonald, 1975). Subaqueous esker facies intertongue with marine or lacustrine facies.

Summer meltwater discharged from the glacier front is free to erode, transport and deposit sediment as in any other fluvial system. Although outwash discharges are often heavily charged with suspended rock flour, the abundance of gravel- to boulder-grade debris in the bedload determines the intensely braided form of most outwash plains (see Plate 9). Outwash plains (known by the Icelandic term *sandur*) may exhibit single or coalesced fan-like forms. Downstream trends include decreasing grain size and increasing predominance of point and lateral bars (Boothroyd & Ashley, 1975). Peculiar effects caused both by seasonal freezing of the fan channel beds and by melting of buried ice masses occur on outwash plains and valley flats. In the latter case, large-scale cross-beds and coarsening-upwards sequences are thought to result from the transport of outwash, as deltas prograde into local depressions (kettleholes) formed by the melting of buried ice masses. Most sandurs do not exhibit large-scale foresets because of the very shallow water depths. Imbricate gravels are much more common in proximal areas, with particles transported and deposited in layers parallel to the surface of the bar–channel network (Rust, 1975).

We cannot leave the subject of glacier-front fluvial processes without briefly mentioning two kinds of mass flooding events: proglacial lake breakout and Jökulhlaups. Detailed investigation (Baker, 1973, 1990, 1994) of the enormous late Pleistocene/early Holocene Lake Missoula breakout floods have significantly affected our attitude towards extreme events and catastrophism in the geological record. Jökulhlaups are also major floods but this time due to the bursting of subglacial meltwater reservoirs produced by subglacial volcanic activity. Their *locus typicus* is Iceland and the last spectacular example occurred in 1996 (Einarsson *et al.*, 1997). They contribute significantly to the architecture and build-up of sandur outwash plains (see Maizels, 1989).

20.9 Glacimarine environments

Proximal glacimarine environments (Figs 20.5b,c) include ice shelves and ice stream and valley glacier termini at fjord and valley heads in both temperate and polar climates. Here, in these ground-line environments, deposition rates may be very high, up to several millimetres per year. These proximal environments grade out into the more distal shelf and shelf edge, where deposition rates decline exponentially as glacial debris forms less and less of the local sediment flux. A floating ice mass is produced when a mass of glacier ice (sheet, stream or valley ice) reaches the coastline and interacts with the marine environment at the limit of ice–bed contact, the ground-line (Molnia, 1983b; Anderson *et al.*, 1991). The freezing point of average seawater is −1.8 °C and the temperature of the ambient seawater is clearly always going to be higher than that of the ice terminus. The complicated dynamics of an ice shelf may be approximated by considering a wedge-shaped tongue of moving ice that tapers seawards. A mass balance is set up between ice and sediment delivered to the front, contact melting at the ice–seawater interface, ice wedge flotation and ice taken away by iceberg calving. Lodgement till may continue to be delivered to the ice terminus where, under stable conditions of sea level, it may oversteepen and be resedimented down the local marine basinal slope as debris flows (Blankenship, 1993). Above any *in situ* lodgement till deposited by a former glacier surge or during a period of lowered sea level there will occur a thickness of subaqueous stratified till with dropstones derived from meltout of the ice roof of the tapering wedge of the ice shelf (e.g. Gibbard, 1980). But this facies should thin seawards as the layer of basal debris itself dies out due to the ice shelf taper (Anderson *et al.*, 1991).

Along the subaerial ice front, flow tills will form in the usual way (Fig. 20.5c), but then become subaqueous bodies (Hicock *et al.*, 1981) with the possibility of remobilization into turbidity currents should conditions be right. Delivery of copious silt and mud at the shelf edge during glacial sea-level lowstands leads to the generation of long-runout glacigenic mudflows (Vogt *et al.*, 1993). The discrete exit of meltwaters from subglacial tunnels occurs as jets and evolves into plumes; underflows are rare because of the high sediment concentrations needed to form them (Syvitski, 1989), but interflows are commonly observed (Domack & Ishman, 1993). The meltwaters may have cut deep tunnel valleys or deposited eskers in the forward part of the glacier: their deposits are characteristically coarse (Eyles & McCabe, 1989). At the ice terminus bedload sediment from the meltwater is rapidly deposited as mound-shaped fans, termed grounding-line fans (Powell, 1990). The fans may exhibit imbricated gravel bedforms in their proximal parts, fining downcurrent and exhibiting well-defined delta-front foresets. Should conditions allow, the subaqueous grounding-line fans may grow to sea level and produce subaerial ice-contact deltas. Very energetic jet flow at high discharge stages is postulated to cause sets of avalanche faces rather in the style of Gilbert-type subaqueous fan deltas. After flow expansion and deceleration the jets then provide surface or stratified plume-like extrusions of buoyant meltwater laden with suspended sediment (Domack & Ishman, 1993). Fine examples of late-Pleistocene ice-contact deltas, now uplifted above sea level by postglacial rebound and dissected, are described in a classic paper by Rust and Romanelli (1975) and more recently by McCabe and Eyles (1988).

Temperate valley glaciers will obviously liberate much more sediment from their copious meltwaters into buoyant brackish overflows than will polar ice-sheets: higher deposition rates ensue from temperate glaciers than from polar ones (Eyles *et al.*, 1985; Syvitski *et al.*, 1987). Concentrations as high as 800 mg/L have been recorded from Alaskan glacially sourced plumes (Cowan & Powell, 1990). The suspended load settles out rapidly, fining seawards as the plume decelerates, cooled from below by mixing and conduction. Deposition rates decrease markedly due to plume dissipation. Finely laminated sedimentary couplets of coarse and fine grains (not varves) may form in the zone due to the interaction of the buoyant outflow and the cycle of local tidal processes, should these be significant (Cowan & Powell, 1990; Phillips *et al.*, 1991). Seawards, this zone, dominated by buoyant outflows, is also affected by iceberg calving, which may cause basal scour and the addition of extra sediment from meltout.

Sediment rafted along by icebergs may become widely dispersed over the adjacent shelf. Dowdeswell *et al.* (1994) describe how the style of sedimentation depends on the nature of the calved ice masses. For example, very thick bergs (> 600 m) are produced by calving from the fast-moving outlet glaciers fed from the Greenland ice-cap. Not only do these produce copious sediment as their debris-rich basal layers melt, but their deep keels extensively scour and mix up existing shelf sediment. Sediment coring reveals thick sequences of massive diamicton over wide areas of the East Greenland Shelf, whilst seafloor imaging reveals ample evidence of iceberg scours. Many examples of Pleistocene glacial-epoch iceberg scours and deposits may be found on temperate shelves (Heinrich, 1988; Bond *et al.*, 1992, 1993; Hesse & Khodabakhsh, 1998). By way of contrast, abundant icebergs calved from the great floating ice shelfs of the Antarctic tend to be much thinner and less rich in debris, reflecting the seaward-tapering nature of the ice apron and the extensive *in situ* meltout that takes place below the shelf prior to calving. In one fairly recent major calving event, in 1986, the calved mass was a staggering 13 000 km² in area and fragments may have reached 38°S, the latitude of Buenos Aires. It should be said that polar mountain glaciers will deliver more sediment-rich bergs than the ice-sheets themselves, but these are in a minority volumetrically in Antarctic conditions (Anderson *et al.*, 1991).

The distinction between sequences of iceberg meltout diamictons on a continental shelf, as distinct from diamictons formed by nearshore meltout adjacent to the grounding-line, is an important one (Dowdeswell *et al.*, 1994). Shelf diamictons will be widespread, intercalated within 'normal' shelf sequences as distance from the shoreline increases and should contain a very wide variety of debris sourced from various calving ice streams. These features, together with the occurrence of seabed scours, might lead to the identification of Greenland-type grounded ice outlets rather than the presence of an Antarctic-type ice shelf.

The three-dimensional distribution of facies in glacimarine environments is dependent upon the dual control of local relative base level by glacioeustasy and by the regional crustal response to glacial loading and unloading (Boulton, 1990). The response time of ice-sheets to global warming is rapid compared to the response of the asthenosphere to glacial unloading. The two effects are thus out of phase, with maximum subsidence occurring after ice-sheet retreat. At first this causes marine transgression over former shoreline and land glacial facies, but as the crust responds to unloading the late-glacial and transgressive facies are uplifted and incised.

20.10 Glacilacustrine environments

Many of the processes outlined above in the glacimarine environment are present in the glacilacustrine, much simplified by the lack of tides and the lower effectiveness of waves and absence of other ocean currents. The other difference is the greater density of cold suspended-sediment-rich meltwater over the (often) stratified lake-waters. Jet- or plume-like underflows are therefore much commoner in glacilacustrine environments.

Proglacial lakes are fed by calving icebergs and by seasonal outwash, which may debouch into the lake to form a steeply dipping delta front of Gilbert type. Finer-grained material finds its way out into the lake body proper by processes of overflow (rare), interflow or underflow, depending upon the relative density of the incoming suspended-sediment-rich water and the ambient lake-waters. The seasonal melt–freeze process gives rise to varved deposits, which may show complex internal rhythms (Ashley, 1975) caused by interference between sediment supplied by overlapping density currents.

20.11 Glacial facies in the pre-Quaternary geological record

The identification of glacial deposits in the geological record should be attempted using all available local and regional evidence for glacier advance, retreat, meltout and general climatic frigidity. Deposits thought to be tills are best termed diamictites so as to emphasize their characteristics at the expense of a finalized genetic description. This point is best illustrated by the attribution by Eyles and Eyles (1989) of thick late Precambrian diamictites not to a direct origin as tillites, but as resedimented till deposited as debris flows. The very broad range of modern till types and sedimentary processes discussed above should be remembered when criteria for establishing ancient tills are being searched for. A major source and a fundamental record of the Earth's glacial sedimentary record is the impressive book by Hambrey and

Harland (1981), workers who combine knowledge of both recent and ancient glacial environments.

Detailed studies of particular ancient glaciations include the Permo-Carboniferous glaciations of Gondwanaland (Crowell, 1983; Eyles *et al.*, 1998), which played such a key role in the 1940s and 1950s in determining that continental drift had occurred. Notable in this respect is an account of tectonic control upon the glaciers that sourced the rapidly subsiding extensional graben of the Parana Basin (Eyles *et al.*, 1993). Glaciers (from southern Africa) delivered their loads right to the margins of the faulted footwall uplands of these basins where most of it was subsequently resedimented as turbidity or debris flow deposits over the fault lines, probably from fan deltas of fjord type (see Chapter 18). Analogous situations may be seen today, though from remnant valley glaciers into a subaerial basin, in the footwall uplands of the magnificent Grand Tetons half-graben of Wyoming. Another fascinating account with a Gondwanan theme involves the various subglacial and proglacial deposits found in the Omani Mountains, whose subsurface equivalents contain vast reserves of oil and gas (Levell *et al.*, 1988). Highly recommended and well-illustrated accounts of ancient glacigenic deposits are provided for the Huronian of Ontario by Miall (1985).

Further reading

Good, concise and up-to-date accounts of glacial environments, with many fine illustrations, are given by Hambrey (1994). Longer tomes are by Benn and Evans (1998) and Menzies (1995). Hooke (1998) gives an accessible account of ice and glacier mechanics. The Quaternary context of glacial processes is well discussed by Williams *et al.* (1993) and by Dawson (1992). Many important papers are to be found in the volumes edited by Jopling and McDonald (1975), Dreimanis (1989), Molnia (1983a), Dowdeswell and Scourse (1990) and Anderson and Ashley (1991). Paterson (1994) is good on physical aspects of ice behaviour; see also the volume edited by Colbeck (1980). The 'bible' for studies of how Quaternary glacier studies may be applied to ancient deposits is the massive Hambrey and Harland (1981), whilst numerous papers of interest occur in Anderson and Ashley (1991). A good review of waterflow through temperate glaciers is by Fountain and Walder (1998).

Part 7
Sediment Deposition, Environments and Facies in Marine Environments

21 Estuaries

'These, I take it, are sandbanks,' said Stephen.
'Just so. And the little figures show the depth at high water and at low: the red is where they are above the surface.'
'A perilous maze. I did not know that so much sand could congregate in one place.'

Patrick O'Brien, [Stephen Maturin and Jack Aubrey consulting charts], *Post Captain*, Harper Collins

21.1 Introduction

Estuaries are funnel-shaped embayments, narrowing upstream, the site of constant interaction between unsteady and nonuniform freshwater river and marine tidal currents and waves (Fig. 21.1). An estuary is not a delta (which has distributaries) or a tidal inlet along a linear clastic shoreline (with no attached river). We can take a biological, ecological or chemical view and define an estuary as 'a semi-enclosed coastal body of water which has a free connection with the open sea and within which sea water is measurably diluted with fresh water of river origin' with Pritchard (1967). The definition restricts the term to the dynamic interface between river-water and sea-water as measured by salinity. Many delta distributary outlets show estuarine characters by this definition, but that need not worry us. A more sedimentologically appropriate definition (shortened and modified after Dalrymple *et al.*, 1992) goes as 'the seaward termination of a single river channel which receives a fluvial and marine sediment flux that is acted upon by tidal, wave and fluvial fluid forces to produce an

Fig. 21.1 Sketch to illustrate the major processes affecting estuarine sedimentation. (Mostly after Dyer, 1989.)

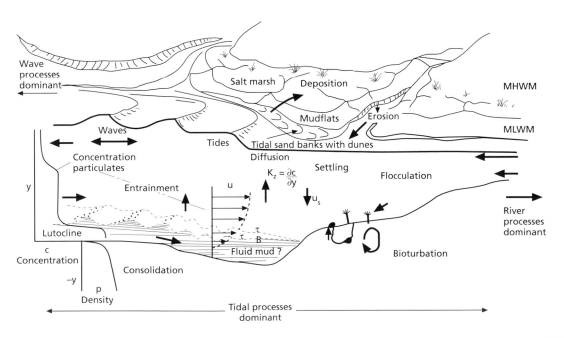

Water and sediment dynamics in estuaries are closely dependent upon the relative magnitude of tidal, river and wave processes. The incoming progressive tidal wave is modified as it travels along a funnel-shaped estuary whose width and depth steadily decrease upstream. The following derivations are from Pond and Pickard (1983). For a 2D wave that suffers little energy loss due to friction or reflection (a severe simplification), the wave energy flux will remain constant, causing the wave to amplify and shorten as it passes upstream into narrower reaches. This is the *convergence* effect. Thus for wave energy, E, per unit length of an estuary, Eb is the energy per unit length, where b is total estuary width. Multiplying by the wave speed, c, gives the energy flux up the estuary as Ebc = constant. Writing $E = (\rho g A^2)/2$ and the long-wave equation for shallow water waves as $c = (gh)^{0.5}$ we have:

$$0.5(\rho g A^2)b\sqrt{gh} = \text{constant} \tag{B21.1}$$

or

$$A \propto b^{-0.5}h^{-0.25} \tag{B21.2}$$

We can see that narrowing has more effect on changing wave amplitude than shallowing. Shallowing also causes the wave speed to decrease and, since wave frequency is constant, the wavelength must decrease by the argument $c = f\lambda$. Since:

$$\lambda = \frac{c}{f} = \frac{\sqrt{gh}}{f} \tag{B21.3}$$

we have

$$\lambda \propto h^{0.5} \tag{B21.4}$$

Thus tidal waves increase in amplitude and decrease in wavelength up many estuaries, the so-called *hypsosynchronous* effect. But we cannot ignore frictional retardation of the tidal wave in this discussion; frictional energy losses are greatest when channel depth decreases rapidly upstream. Frictional retardation causes a reduction in amplitude of the tide upstream, the *hyposynchronous* mode. Estuaries where the tidal wave changes little in amplitude, where the convergence effect is exactly balanced by the frictional retardation, are termed *synchronous*. Good examples of such modes are provided by Borrego *et al.* (1995). Resonant effects with tide or wave may also affect currents in estuaries of gulfs and straits—these are discussed further in Chapter 25.

Further information on estuarine dynamics

Type A, well-stratified, estuaries are those river-dominated estuaries where tidal and wave mixing processes are permanently or temporarily at a minimum. The stratified system is dominated by river discharge, with the tidal : river discharge ratio being low, about < 20 (Fig. 21.4). An upstream tapering salt wedge occurs, over which the fresh river-water flows as a buoyant plume. The picture is exactly the same as in river-dominated delta distributaries such as the modern Mississippi delta (section 22.5) and is further exemplified by the estuarine-like behaviour of the distributaries of the Fraser River delta, Canada,

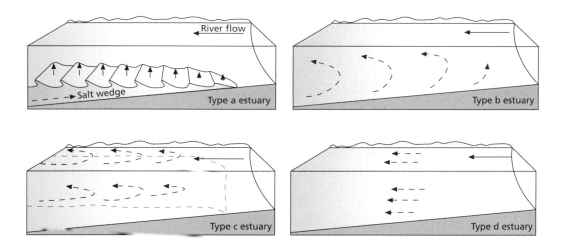

Fig. 21.3 Schematic diagrams to show the four major types of estuarine circulation defined by Pritchard and Carter (1971).

during periods of high river flow ('freshet') discharge (Kostaschuk *et al.*, 1992; see Fig. 21.5). Internal waves are thought to form at the sharp salt-wedge/river-water interface and these cause limited upward mixing of salt water with fresh water (advection), but not vice versa. A prominent zone of shoaling at the tip of the salt wedge arises when sediment deposition from bedload occurs in both fresh water and seawater. This zone of deposition shifts upstream and downstream in response to changes in river discharge and, to a much lesser extent, to tidal

oscillation. Thus, deposited fine bedload sediment and flocculated suspended load are periodically flushed out of the system by turbulent shear during high river stage.

Some river-dominated estuaries do not necessarily fit easily into the above classification, as exemplified by the estuaries of the wave dominated and micro-tidal coastline of southern Africa (Cooper, 1993). These are often characterized by beach barrier cusps and spits partially shielding their approaches and thus preventing simple salt-wedge intrusion. These beach barriers are periodically destroyed during periodic high-magnitude river discharges, the resulting Gilbert-type delta being itself subsequently destroyed by wave action and the barriers re-formed during long periods of normal river discharge.

Fig. 21.4 The division of estuaries into types A (stratified), B (partially stratified) and C (well stratified) according to the ratio of tidal discharge to that of fluvial discharge, with data for spring (S), mean (M) and neap (N) tides for the Guadiana and Odiel estuaries, southern Spain. (After Borrego *et al.*, 1995.)

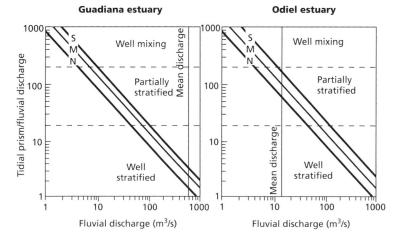

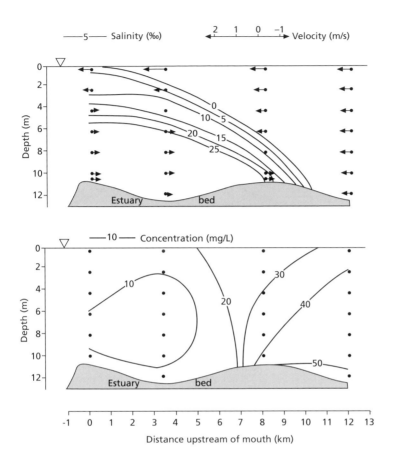

Fig. 21.5 Salinity, velocity and suspended sediment profiles taken during high tide along a transect of the well-stratified (salt wedge) type A estuary of the Fraser River, Canada. (After Kostaschuk *et al.*, 1992.)

Type B, partially stratified, estuaries are those in which tidal turbulence destroys the upper salt-wedge interface, producing a more gradual salinity gradient from bed to surface water by both advectional and diffusional mechanisms. The tidal : river discharge ratio is between about 20 and 200. Down-estuary changes in the salinity gradient at the mixing zone occur so that the zone moves upwards towards higher salinities. Earth rotational effects cause the mixing surface to be slightly tilted so that in the northern hemisphere the tidal flow up the estuary is nearer the surface and strongest to the left. Sediment dynamics will be strongly influenced by the upstream and downstream movement of salt water over the various phases of the tidal cycle (Allen *et al.*, 1976, 1980; Uncles & Stephens, 1989). The resulting turbidity maximum (Fig. 21.6) is particularly prominent in the upper estuary (around 1–5‰ salinity) on spring and large neap ebb and flood tidal phases, and less prominent at slackwater periods due to settling and deposition. Turbidity maxima are affected by the magnitude of freshwater runoff. A seasonal cycle of dry-season upstream migration of the turbidity maximum and locus of maximum deposition is followed by wet-season downstream migration and resuspension by erosion (Uncles & Stephens, 1989). The turbidity maximum is also acted on by gravity-induced circulations arising from its own excess density.

Type C, well-mixed, estuaries are those in which strong tidal currents completely destroy the salt-wedge/fresh-water interface over the entire estuarine cross-section. The ratio of tide : river discharge is > 200. Longitudinal and lateral advection and lateral diffusion processes dominate. Vertical salinity gradients no longer exist but there does exist a steady downstream increase in overall salinity. In addition, the rotational effect of the Earth may still cause a pronounced lateral salinity gradient, as in type B estuaries. Sediment dynamics are dominated by strong tidal flow, with estuarine circulation gyres produced by the

Fig. 21.6 Typical longitudinal distributions of depth-averaged concentration (ppm) of suspended particulate matter in a typical macrotidal, partially mixed estuary: (a) large neap tide, low runoff; (b) small neap tide, low runoff. Note well-marked turbidity maxima, particularly during the large neap tide. (Data from Tamar estuary, England; data of Uncles & Stephens, 1989.)

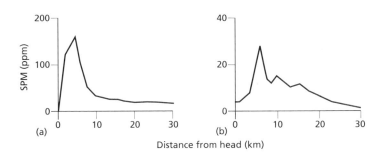

Fig. 21.7 A remarkable graph (after Grabemann & Krause, 1989) to illustrate the repeatable hysteresis (over three tidal cycles, but details not shown) of suspended matter concentration (C) with mean tidal current velocity at a measuring station in the well-mixed and macrotidal Weser estuary, Germany. Velocities are negative for flood, positive for ebb. Results indicate local advection from downstream at the height of the flood, then deposition during the slack, then resuspension during the ebb, and finally redeposition during the slack. Some net deposition at the site is the end-result.

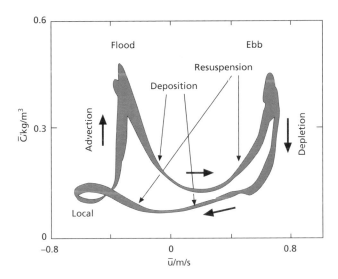

lateral salinity gradient. Extremely high suspended sediment concentrations may occur close to the bed in the inner reaches of some tidally dominated estuaries. Sediment particles of river origin, some flocculated, will undergo various transport paths, usually of a 'closed loop' kind (Fig. 21.7), in response to settling into the salt layer and subsequent transport by the net upstream tidal flow. Settling of bound aggregates of silt- and sand-sized particles creates large areas of stationary and moving mud suspensions that characterize the outer estuarine reaches of tide-dominant estuaries like the Severn of England (Kirby & Parker, 1983) and the Gironde of France (Allen *et al.*, 1975). Major areas of high-density suspensions (up to > 200 g/l) are a major feature in the outer Severn estuary. These suspensions may be mobile or fixed, the latter grading into areas of more-or-less settled mud. Stationary suspensions up to 3 m thick may be deposited very quickly (in seconds according to Kirby & Parker, 1983), cores through such deposits revealing structureless muddy silts with occasional thin sandy laminae. Stationary suspensions show sharp upper surfaces on sonar records. They form during slackwater periods, progressively thickening during the spring-to-neap transition. They are easily eroded by the accelerating phases of spring tidal cycles, to be taken up in suspension once more.

Type D estuaries are theoretical end-members of the estuarine continuum in that they show both lateral and vertical homogeneity of salinity. Such conditions apply only in the outer parts of many type B and C estuaries; they are clearly transitional to open shelf conditions. Under equilibrium conditions, saline water is diffused upstream to replace that lost by advective mixing. Sediment movement is dominated entirely by tidal motions, again with no internal sediment trap.

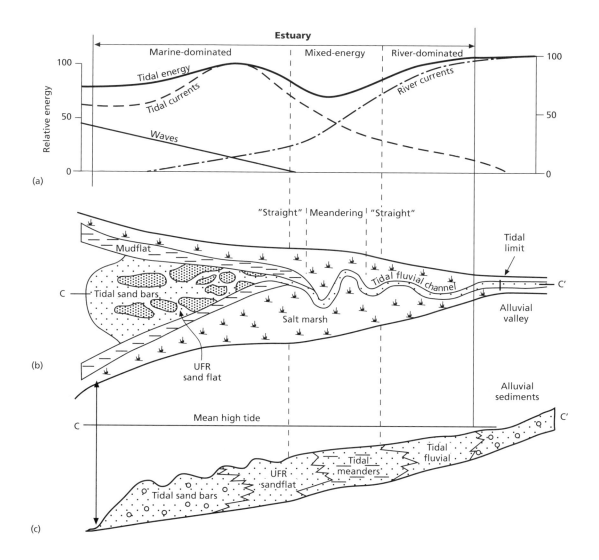

Fig. 21.8 Sketch map and section to illustrate the salient characteristics of well-mixed tide-dominated estuaries. (After Dalrymple *et al.*, 1992.)

Our brief review of estuarine dynamics has stressed the interplay between river and tide. Most estuaries are those with type B characters and hence tend to act as trappers of sediment, particularly of fine grades. Whilst recognizing the efficiency of such estuaries as sediment traps, it should also be pointed out that advective plumes of seaward-directed fine sediment may be driven by both residual tidal and wave currents far out on to the shelf (see Chapter 25). We stress again that, although estuary classification is of some

use, their behaviour varies according to season and climate. This is best exemplified by estuaries along the macrotidal coastline of northern Australia (Woodroffe *et al.*, 1985). These are usually tide-dominated (tidal ranges up to 10 m) type C or D, but during the monsoonal season the tremendous freshwater efflux causes lengthy periods of type B behaviour.

21.3 Modern estuarine facies

For sedimentological purposes we may broadly divide estuaries into tide- and wave-dominated end-members, recognizing that a complete gradation exists between them (Figs 21.8 & 21.9).

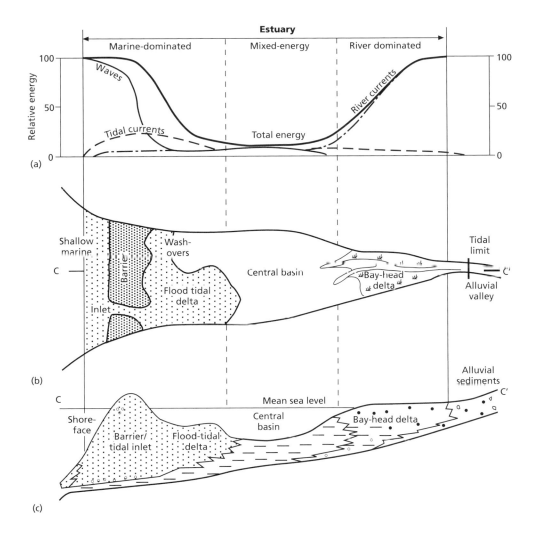

Fig. 21.9 Sketch map and section to illustrate the salient characteristics of partially barred, wave-dominated estuaries. (After Dalrymple *et al.*, 1992.)

Estuaries with appreciable tidal ranges are bordered by coastal tidal flats with saltmarsh (mangrove swamps in tropical estuaries—see Woodroffe *et al.*, 1985) and minor drainage channels. Seaward progradation of funnel-shaped estuarine complexes on a coastal plain will cause the deeper-channel estuarine environments to become progressively overlain by fining-upwards tidal-flat facies. Studies of main estuarine channels such as the Parker estuary, New England (Hayes, 1971), and of the outer estuary of the Bay of Fundy (Dalrymple *et al.*, 1990) show well-developed ebb and flood tidal channels and associated shoals with extensive bordering dunefields. Frequently the flood tide dominates in the upstream estuary and the ebb tide dominates in the downstream, as in the Gironde estuary, France (Berné *et al.*, 1993), where the orientation of dunes is adjusted to this spatial variation in net tidal vector. At the point of equal influence, a suite of symmetrical dunes have developed. The magnitude, type, migration rates and orientation of estuarine tidal shoal dunes depend strongly on timing with respect to the neap/spring cycle, quasi-equilibrium forms evolving at and shortly after the spring tidal phase (Langhorne & Read, 1986; Larcombe & Jago, 1996). Large (> 2 m high) dunes cannot be so

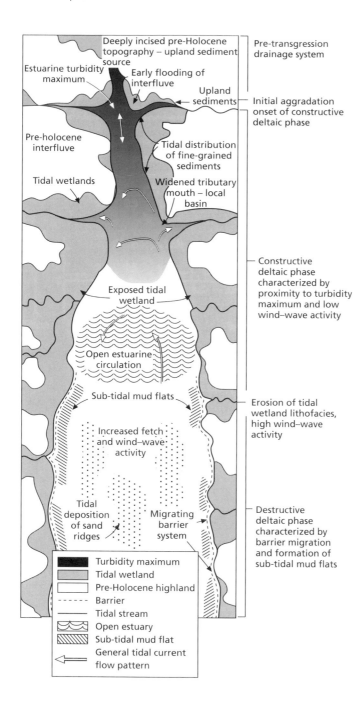

Fig. 21.10 Sketch to illustrate the morphology of a modern estuary (Delaware) whose outer estuary was once tidally dominant during the early Holocene sea-level rise (turbidity maxima moving upstream) but which now is wave-dominated. Meanwhile the modern turbidity maxima and the locus of fine-grained tidal wetland deposition have moved well up the estuary. (After Fletcher *et al.*, 1990.)

altered by the fortnightly tidal variation (Berné et al., 1993) but must reflect longer-term changes in estuarine dynamics and river floods. Sediment particles are dominantly derived from offshore in many outer well-mixed estuaries. Thus in the Thames estuary, England, fully marine ostracods are found up to 20 km inland from their life habitats and the sediment shows a decreasing mean grain size upstream (Prentice et al., 1968). Vertical sequences through such sediments would reveal alternating packets of ebb- and flood-orientated cross beds with clay interbeds resting on channel-floor erosion planes.

21.4 Estuaries and sequence stratigraphy

The identification of incised lowstand alluvial valleys is a key element in the steps of logic that lead to the reconstruction of ancient episodes of relative sea-level change. But as we noted previously (Chapter 17) their identification (and causes) may be far from simple and obvious. The association between incised valleys and estuarine environments thus provides an important link in the sequence stratigraphic argument. The high-frequency changes of relative sea level in late-Pleistocene to Recent times have enabled estuarine workers to make a decisive and important contribution here. For example, one prominent feature of Holocene estuarine systems in microtidal regimes is the development of bay-head deltas that prograde seawards to infill the estuarine valley (see, for example, the studies of Nichol et al., 1997; Sondi et al., 1995). Changing sea level in a seaward-deepening and -widening estuary is accompanied by very significant changes in tidal resonance and hence tidal range. Lowstand estuaries may be significantly different in terms of the relative strengths of wave, tide and river currents. This is exemplified by the Holocene evolution of the Delaware Bay estuary complex (Fig. 21.10; Fletcher et al., 1990). Here, as relative sea level rose, the developing locus of turbidity maximum, and hence site of maximum mud deposition, migrated steadily upstream. Changes in wave power due to variations in climate or to the effects of estuarine channel migration on offshore water depth and tidal currents led to local episodes of tidal-flat erosion and deposition at highstand. The sediment infill of an estuarine complex is thus time- and space-dependent, as illustrated by the Cobequid/Salmon River estuary in the Bay of Fundy (Dalrymple & Zaitlin, 1994).

21.5 Ancient estuarine facies

In a prograding nondeltaic coastal plain, estuarine facies should overlie and partly cut out a variety of marine nearshore facies. They, in their turn, will be overlain and partly cut out by fluvial facies. Within these broad limits the identification of estuarine facies will depend upon the recognition of channelized tidal depositional facies, marginal tidal-flat facies overlying the channelized estuarine complex and evidence for salinities intermediate between fresh and fully marine. Tidal processes are relatively easy to recognize in rock products (for a detailed discussion see Shanley et al., 1992). Recognition of a salinity spectrum will, of necessity, depend entirely upon biological inferences (e.g. Hudson, 1963). It may therefore be impossible to recognize pre-Phanerozoic estuarine facies.

The reader is referred to the papers of Bosence (1973), Campbell and Oakes (1973) and Richards (1994) for detailed discussions of the possible estuarine attributes of Tertiary, Cretaceous and Triassic successions, respectively. Time and space variations in estuarine dynamics are neatly reconstructed by Willis (1997) in his study of Cretaceous estuarine valley-fill complexes from South Dakota, USA. The study of Porebski (1995) has already been noted above, and his reconstruction of a palaeoestuary architectural fill is shown in Fig. 21.11. This paper along with several in the volume edited by Dalrymple et al. (1994) explore the important links between sea-level change, incised fluvial valley formation and estuarine infill sequences. The importance of the identification of estuarine channel complexes in a sequence stratigraphic framework (see Shanley et al., 1992; Willis, 1997) should do much to resurrect interest amongst geologists in the attributes of modern estuaries.

Further reading

Many papers on aspects of estuarine sediment transport may be found in Burt et al. (1997). Black et al. (1998) also contains much of relevance to estuarine tidal flat processes of erosion and sedimentation. Dyer (1989) provides a useful review of estuarine sediment transport. As noted above, sequence stratigraphic aspects of estuarine sediments are found in Dalrymple et al. (1994).

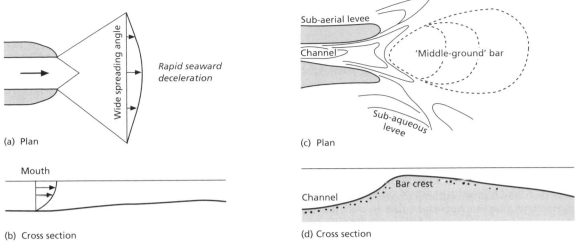

Fig. 22.3 Plan and section views of friction-dominated jets and their 'middle-ground' distributary mouth bars. (After Wright, 1977.)

(a) Plan

Wide spreading angle

Rapid seaward deceleration

(b) Cross section

Mouth

(c) Plan

Sub-aerial levee

Channel

'Middle-ground' bar

Sub-aqueous levee

(d) Cross section

Channel

Bar crest

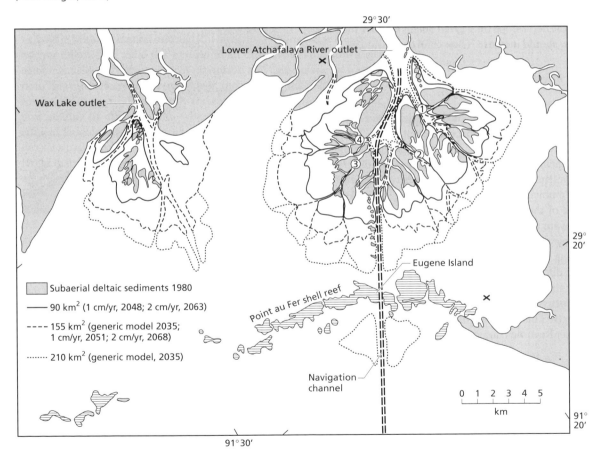

29° 30′

Lower Atchafalaya River outlet

Wax Lake outlet

Eugene Island

Point au Fer shell reef

Navigation channel

29° 20′

91° 20′

Subaerial deltaic sediments 1980

90 km² (1 cm/yr, 2048; 2 cm/yr, 2063)

155 km² (generic model 2035; 1 cm/yr, 2051; 2 cm/yr, 2068)

210 km² (generic model, 2035)

0 1 2 3 4 5
km

91° 30′

Fig. 22.4 The shoal-water Atchafalaya delta (formed by a partial avulsion of the Mississippi river) is the result of the fused growth of numerous 'middle-ground' bars. The growth of the delta is modelled by curves for the next 100 or so years (from 1980) for a 'slow' (1 cm/yr) and a rapid (2 cm/yr) relative sea-level rise (Wells, 1987). This is a good example of continued deltaic progradation *despite* a sea-level rise (somewhat disquieting for sedimentologically challenged proponents of sequence stratigraphy).

effects arising from bottom drag on the plume become very important. Such plumes experience rapid seaward spreading, deceleration and hence deposition of bedload sediment (Figs 22.3 & 22.4). Such friction-dominated jets quickly deposit a 'mid-ground' distributary mouth bar bordered on its margins by a Y-shaped channel bifurcation. Bars of this type are particularly characteristic of subdelta growth in the Mississippi interdistributary bays (see Section 22.5) and of the Atchafalaya (Fig. 22.4). They are analogous in some ways to crevasse splay lobes described previously from the River South Saskatchewan (Chapter 17).

Low values of *Fr'* (< 1) suggest dominance by buoyant forces whereby the outflow spreads as a narrow expanding plume above a salt wedge that may extend for a considerable distance up the distributary channel (Figs 22.5–22.7). Such jets are termed *hypopycnal*. As we discussed in the context of estuary behaviour in Chapter 21, salt wedges are best developed in deep channels with low tidal ranges. Internal waves that are generated at the salt-wedge/effluent boundary cause vertical mixing, rapid deceleration and deposition of coarse sediment as a simple mouth bar. During periods of high river flow the salt wedge is expelled from the distributary channel to a position just seaward of the bar crest where bedload deposition occurs as the effluent separates from the salt water. Continuing deposition of successively finer sediment occurs on the seaward bar slope. Good examples of such seaward-fining distributary mouth bars occur at the front of the major Mississippi outfalls, but nothing is known of the bedforms and resulting internal structures due to the salt wedging and flushing. The effluent jets remain dominant far on to the shelf (Plates 13 & 14).

When the combined density of the effluent plume water and its suspended solids exceeds that of the basin ambient fluid ($\rho_e/\rho_a > 1$), the conditions are set for the plume to underflow. The plume is then in a state known as *hyperpycnal*. This is obviously more likely to occur in lake-waters since a suspended load of at least > 28 kg/m³ must be present just to counteract the density of normal seawater. Perhaps the most spectacular underflowing delta system is that of the Huanghue, whose colossal suspended load picked up on its passage through the central China loess belt (see Van Gelder *et al.*, 1994) enables it to sink without trace in the offshore region.

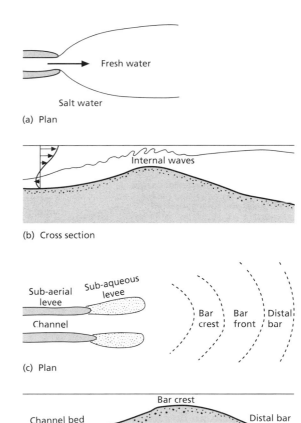

(a) Plan

(b) Cross section

(c) Plan

(d) Cross section

Fig. 22.5 Plan and section views of buoyancy-dominated jets and their distributary mouth bars. (After Wright, 1977.)

Let us now turn to the modifying effects that waves and tides have on these simple jet models of delta front dynamics (Wright & Coleman, 1973). Wave power is substantially reduced as waves pass from offshore areas over very gently sloping offshore–nearshore zones; indeed some extremely gentle offshore slopes may cause complete dissipation of wave energy. In coastal areas of high wave power relative to river discharge, effluent jets may be completely disrupted by wave reworking. The coastlines of such deltas tend to be very much more linear in plan view than those of more moderate wave power. The effects of wave reworking include shoreward

local position and may travel kilometres offshore, the stratigraphic arrangements within the slide blocks remaining more-or-less intact, although dipping at a high angle to the local horizontal, above the basal slide planes. Continued 'normal' deposition leaves these shallow-water 'orphans' completely surrounded and entombed within the offshore deposits—providing interesting stratigraphic hydrocarbon traps, not to say great puzzles, for interpretation should they be preserved in the geological record.

22.4 Organic deposition in deltas

The formation of wetland mires and peat is the eventual fate of the majority of the lakes, lagoons, abandoned channels and crevasses in a prograding and avulsing delta system. Mires comprise large portions of the on-delta area but, as Kosters (1989) forcefully reminds us, they have been neglected by organically-challenged sedimentologists. Tropical delta backswamps are particularly widespread and have an incredibly high rate of primary plant production, reaching several tens of centimetres per year in some areas. For example, peat mires cover 50–80% of the surface area of the Rajang river delta in Sarawak (Staub & Esterle 1993). Even in the high-flux sediment regime of the Holocene Mississippi, thick peats developed periodically behind reworked shorelines that sheltered abandoned delta lobes (see further below; Kosters, 1989). To gain an understanding of the importance of deltaic organic facies, it is important to understand that thick peats do not form featureless sheets. They actually accumulate as extensive raised mires (peat domes) several metres higher than even the raised levees of the distributary channels that pass through them (Anderson, 1964; Coleman et al., 1970; McCabe, 1984). In common with raised mires in temperate wet upland areas, the living vegetation gets its supply of water and nutrients largely from rainfall. In lowland tropical deltas the raised mires therefore act as important barriers to channel migration, floodwater runoff and avulsion (a similar role is played by papyrus peats in the Okavango fan delta—see Chapter 18). It has been postulated (McCabe & Shanley, 1992) that the stabilizing effect of raised coastal mires enables them to resist high rates of sea-level rise. Not only that, the largest mires actually act as local hinterlands, exporting intercepted rainfall into the 'normal' delta distributaries as low-suspended-load humic runoff (Staub & Esterle, 1993). This low-density discharge often overlies the denser suspended-rich runoff, causing sediment bypass to the delta front rather than loss to levees and floodplain.

22.5 Delta case histories

Mississippi delta

River-dominated deltaic environments, with well-developed buoyant forces dominant during jet discharge, are exemplified by the well-studied Mississippi delta (Fig. 22.9; Plate 13; Fisk, 1944; Fisk et al., 1954; Coleman & Gagliano, 1964; Coleman et al., 1964; Wright & Coleman, 1973; Penland et al., 1988; Kosters, 1989). The Mississippi delta front has low tidal range (about 0.3 m), moderately high all-round water discharge (approximately 10–30 m³/s from low to high stage), a fine-grained sediment load and moderate degrees of incident wave energy. The latter attenuate markedly, typically to around 0.034×10^7 erg/s in the nearshore area. This attenuation is a direct consequence of the fine-grained nature of the Mississippi sediment load, creating a gently sloping apron to the nearshore zone. It is upon this apron that deep-water wave energy is expended.

The 'exposed' delta plain is dominated by a small number of large distributaries and a host of minor ones (Fig. 22.9). Because of the very low slopes involved, these channels tend to be straight. Frequent avulsion occurs as the delta progrades, the channels periodically seeking new routes to the sea with gradient advantages. The 'birdsfoot' morphology of the delta results from these avulsions, with the 'claws' marked by channels and the 'webbed' connections marked by interdistributary bays. The bays are shallow, brackish to marine, and are gradually infilled by minor crevasse deltas. Frictional effects dominate in these shallow water bodies and Y-shaped mid-ground-type mouth bars form as the crevasse channels debouch their discharge. Gradually, by crevasse progradation and overbank flooding, the bays become part of the subaerial marsh of the delta plain. Cores through the prograding marshes and minor channels of the interdistributary bays reveal a variety of coarsening-upwards successions, capped by vegetation colonization surfaces, wetland peats of various kinds (Kosters, 1989) and sharp-based fining-upwards successions resulting from deposition in minor channels.

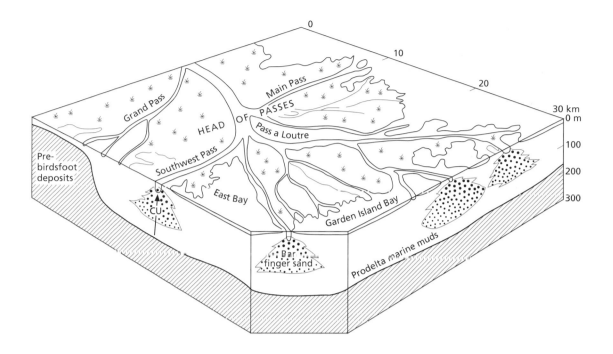

Fig. 22.9 Block diagram to show the morphology and major facies present around the front of the modern Mississippi birdsfoot delta. CU indicates coarsening upwards. Elongate bar finger sands form after continued progradation of distributary mouth bar sands. (After the classic work by Fisk *et al.*, 1954.)

At the delta front the major distributaries widen and pass into well-developed lunate distributary mouth bars. Shoaling from the distributary channel to the mouth bar crest results from the dynamics of salt-wedge intrusion discussed previously. During progradation the channel erodes a portion of the bar crest that is directly downstream from it, causing the thick (50–150 m) coarsening-upwards mud-to-sand succession of the mouth bar to be cut by an erosive-based, fining-upwards distributary channel sand. Deposition of thick successions of muds in the delta front area encourages the development of a wide range of soft sediment deformation, slump and growth fault features.

Over the past few thousand years the active parts of the Mississippi delta have undergone periodic avulsive shifts along the coast of Louisiana as successive channels have searched for gradient advantages over their precursors (Figs 22.10 & 22.11). Transfer of the river to a new location causes abandonment of the previously active delta constructional system (Frazier, 1967; Törnqvist *et al.*, 1996). The latest delta lobe is that created by the Atchafalaya avulsion (Roberts *et al.*, 1980)—Steinberg (1995) has an interesting slant on the history and economic consequences of the Atchafalaya avulsion.

Wetland expansion and peat accumulation in the coast-protected environment are followed by eventual marine or bay/lake expansion as very early compactional subsidence (see Nadon 1998) causes local submergence and transgression (Kosters, 1989). This process thereby leads to the production of a characteristic abandonment facies at the top of a delta-lobe facies association. Renewed clastic input from further avulsions of the trunk channel may subsequently terminate the shallow bays and lakes. A mechanism thus exists within a switching delta for producing complex deltaic 'cycles', so long as the coastal plain is located in an area of net tectonic subsidence (as is indeed the case in the Gulf of Mexico). Wetland loss is now a serious matter for concern in the Mississippi area (as in most delta complexes world-wide). A good discussion is to be found in Walker *et al.* (1987).

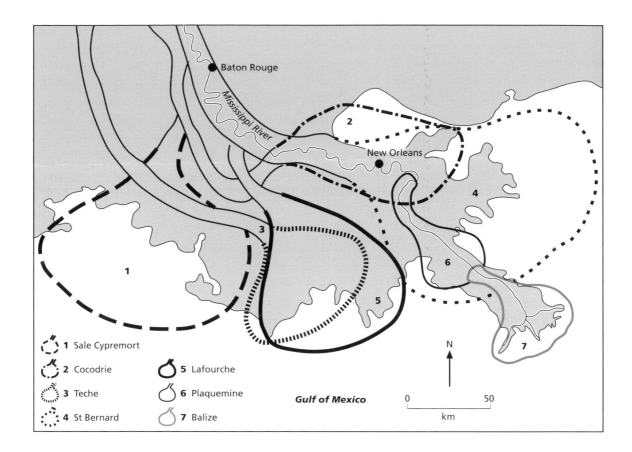

1 Sale Cypremort

2 Cocodrie

3 Teche

4 St Bernard

5 Lafourche

6 Plaquemine

7 Balize

N

Gulf of Mexico

0   50

km

Fig. 22.10 The seven Holocene delta lobes of the Mississippi delta plain. (After Kolb & Van Lopik, 1958; Colman, 1976; for a revised chronology see Törnqvist *et al.*, 1996.)

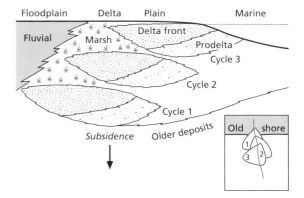

Fig. 22.11 How successive delta cycles may be produced by delta lobe switching in a subsiding and prograding coastal plain. (After Coleman & Gagliano, 1964.)

The birdsfoot phase of the Holocene evolution of the Mississippi coastal plain is quite atypical of the numerous previous delta lobes that have shifted around the coastal plain due to periodic avulsions. Most of the five or so pre-Recent deltas prograded into much shallower water than the modern birds-foot, whose effluent plumes nowadays almost reach the shelf break. These shoal water deltas now exist as eroded and partial remnants whose coarser sand deposits of abandoned mouth bar and channel have been reworked by waves by a sequence of events comprising: (1) flanking barrier/spits. (2) transgressive barrier island arcs with migrating tidal channels, and

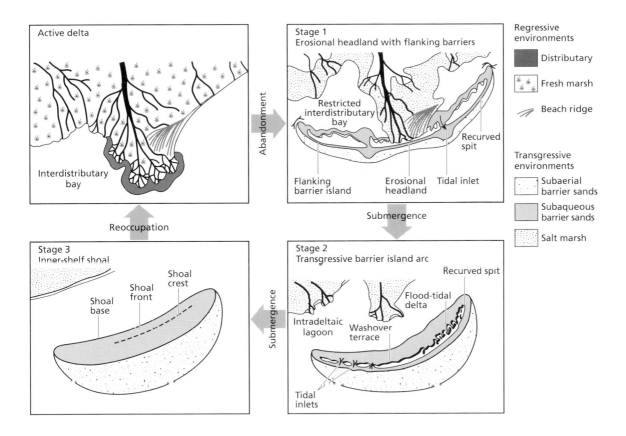

Fig. 22.12 The evolution of delta lobe abandonment sequences, appropriate to Mississippi-type shoal water deltas. (After Penland *et al.*, 1988.)

(3) remnant inner shelf shoals (Fig. 22.12; Penland *et al.*, 1988).

Niger delta

By way of contrast to the Mississippi delta, the mixed regime (tide/wave-dominated) Niger delta (Oomkens, 1974) has coastal environments dominated by the occurrence of major coastal barrier islands separated by tidal inlets (Fig. 22.13). The great trunk stream of the braided River Niger breaks up into a host of smaller channels, each of which is tide-dominated. Sandy bedload deposited in ebb tidal deltas is redistributed alongshore by severe wave action. Delta-front facies are thus dominated by tidal inlet channel fills and coastal barrier sands. Continued delta pro-

gradation results in reworking and destruction of these facies at the expense of the upper delta-plain facies. Investigations of thick (9–12 km!) Tertiary proto-Niger delta deposits in the subsurface indicate the overwhelming importance of delta slope failure in understanding facies distributions. Seismic and well penetration indicates that the whole thick sequence is broken by a myriad of growth faults, slide blocks and slumps, many of which have a tectonic control by basement structures.

Nile delta

This, the type delta since the nomination of Herodotus, has been somewhat neglected in the more recent past since attention was shifted to the Mississippi and Niger, both oil-rich. By contrast the Nile (Fig. 22.14) has few hydrocarbon reservoirs in its subsurface, but has dominated the rise, fall and rebirth of Egyptian civilization for 7000 yr. It is just

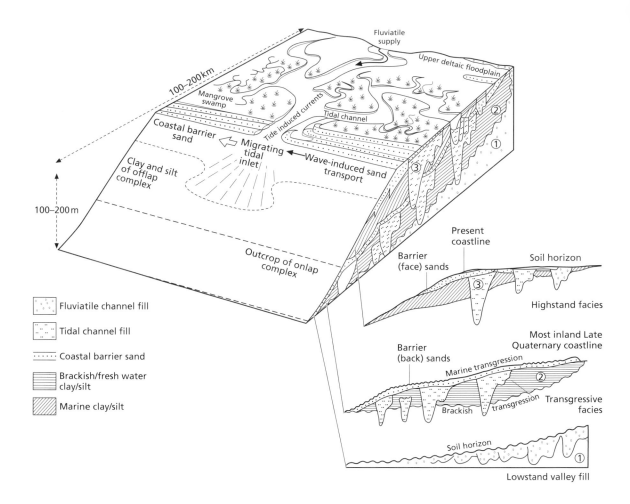

Fig. 22.13 Lithofacies relations in the mixed-regime late-Quaternary Niger delta. (After Oomkens, 1974.)

because of its enormous richness in archaeological remains, and its great importance in the understanding of the rise of ancient civilizations, that modern archaeosedimentologists have returned to this fascinating area (Stanley & Warne, 1993). A further reason lies in the construction of the Aswan High Dam in 1964, which, although assuring Lower Egypt of a steady supply of water for irrigation and power, has led to a vast impoundment of sediment that would otherwise have been added to the floodplains and to the delta front. Very serious coastal erosion is now threatening much of the Nile coastline as a con-

sequence. Sestini (1989) summarizes much information gathered during successive UNESCO studies of the effects of dam construction on the delta.

The Nile delta is a wave-dominated system on a microtidal coastline with important east-flowing offshore currents that deflect the effluent plumes. The delta itself is unusual for its site in an arid climate, the river collecting its waters mainly from the summer monsoons that drench the Ethiopian Plateau and feed the Blue Nile, rich in suspended sediment. The delta front is dominated by a 500 km long barrier–beach complex, which formerly sheltered extensive back-barrier lakes and lagoons. These are now mostly drained and reclaimed. The coastal barriers are broken by the promontory-like outlets of the two modern subdeltas of the Rosetta and Damietta branches

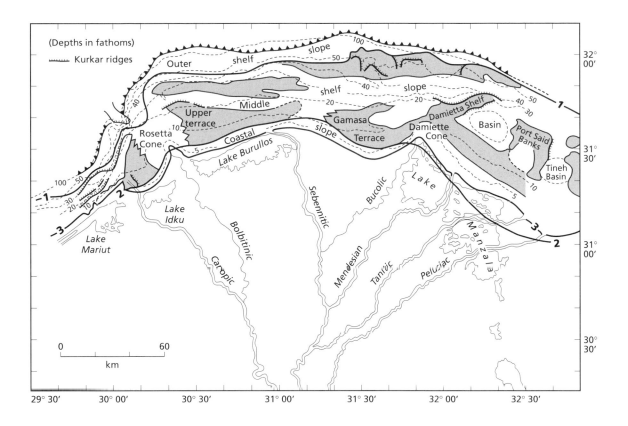

Fig. 22.14 Map of the Nile delta and shelf showing major morphological features, isobaths and successive (1) early Holocene, (2) historical and (3) modern shorelines. Of the numerous Holocene distributaries, only the Bolbitinic (Rosetta) and Bucolic (Damietta) are presently active. (After Said, 1981; Scheihing & Gaynor, 1991.)

(a total of perhaps six major prehistoric abandoned distributary courses have been recognized; Fig. 22.14). The modern channels are fringed by prominent beach ridges, particularly on their eastern sides, leeward of the prevailing northwesterlies. Post-1964 erosion of several kilometres has occurred in response to lack of sand-grade sediment input to compensate wave erosion and longshore transport.

Great insights into the late-Pleistocene to Holocene history of the delta have been gained in recent years from extensive archaeosedimentary studies (Stanley & Warne, 1993). It appears that during the glacial maximum (20–18 ka) the Nile ran out to the shelf edge as a sand-dominated incised braidplain. Rapid sea-

level rise to 8 ka led to a lowering of river gradients over the present delta and the eventual establishment around 7 ka BC of stable floodplains that received abundant silts and clays from the flooding river, which was no longer in a state of sediment bypass. Thus deposition formed the broadening fertile floodplains that were to provide the springboard for establishment of pre-Dynastic agriculture.

Tiber delta

This is another 'classical' Mediterranean delta, this time intimately tied up with the history of Roman civilization. Detailed studies (Bellotti *et al.*, 1994) reveal that the modern delta evolved from a bay-head delta infilling lagoons during the immediate postglacial sea-level rise to the wave-dominated highstand feature with reclaimed lagoons that we see today (Fig. 22.15). Progradation has accelerated in the past 500 yr, so much so that the Imperial city's main port for the import of North African wheat, Ostia Antica now lies 5 km or so inland.

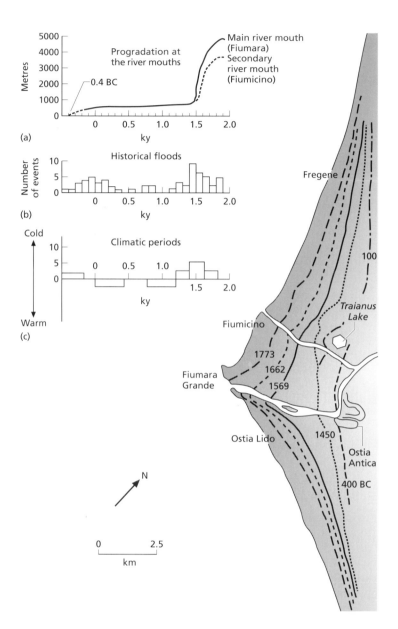

Fig. 22.15 Map and inset graphs to show the growth of the Tiber delta. (From Bellotti *et al.*, 1994.) Despite obscure records from Rome's Dark Ages, note the surge of growth from the late Renaissance onwards, presumably reflecting careless human developments in the catchment.

Some tidally dominated deltas

Deltas are common on macrotidal coasts where wave action is limited, such as the Ganges–Brahmaputra (Coleman, 1969) and Mahakam, Indonesia (Gastaldo *et al.*, 1995), and where onshore monsoonal wave-creating winds are strong, as in the Fly River delta of the Gulf of Papua (Baker *et al.*, 1995). They show a very distinctive delta-front facies dominated by

a dense network of tidal channels and islands, which pass offshore into a network of coast-normal linear tidal current ridges. Delta progradation has caused gradual emergence of the tidal current ridges so that they become coated with a sequence of intertidal and supratidal fine-grained sediments. The areas between the tidal current ridges eventually become tidal channels and ultimately fluvial channels as progradation continues. In the Fly River delta, for example, the predominant facies in the channels are finely laminated well-sorted sands and silts thought to be deposited during neap tides when wave-induced oscillatory currents are weak. Bioturbation levels are low because of the very high tidal current velocities (up to 2.4 m/s) and high suspended loads (up to 40 g/1).

Further reading

Aspects of modern and ancient deltas are dealt with in the collections of papers edited by Whateley and Pickering (1989), Lyons and Alpern (1989) and Rahmani and Flores (1984).

23   'Linear' clastic shorelines

. . . When the chalk wall falls to the foam and its tall ledges
Oppose the pluck
And knock of the tide,
And the shingle scrambles after the suck-
ing surf, . . .

W.H. Auden, 'Seascape', *Selected Poems*, Penguin Books

23.1 Introduction

Hayes (1975, 1979) was the first to show the variation of coastal morphology as a function of both tidal
range and wave energy (Figs 23.1 & 23.2). When tidal
currents are strong and a plentiful supply of sediment
is available, particularly muds and silt, a low-gradient
wedge of tidal-flat sediment builds out seawards. Not
only is incoming swell wave power greatly reduced
by the low-gradient flat but also waves cannot break
on any one part of the tidal flat for any length of
time. The effectiveness of waves on such macrotidal
coasts is thus greatly reduced. The opposite conclusions apply to microtidal coasts dominated by high
wave power.

Depositional coastlines away from estuary mouths
or deltas may be subdivided according to whether the
coastline is 'attached' or 'detached'. In the latter case
there exist offshore barrier islands, which physically
protect an inner, more sheltered, coastline that surrounds a bay or lagoon. The major environments of
coastal deposition (Fig. 23.3) comprise (i) attached
beaches and intertidal flats, (ii) partly attached spits,
(iii) detached barriers, tidal inlets and lagoon complexes, and (iv) the shoreface slope and shoreface-
to-shelf transition. In all these environments we may
usually speak of a single, well-mixed and friction-
dominated boundary layer, usually fully turbulent.
At the shallow depths of most such shorefaces (from
about 4 m down to about 20 m or so) the Coriolis

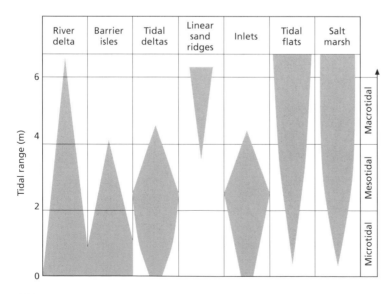

Fig. 23.1 Variation of coastal
morphology with tidal range.
(After Hayes, 1975.)

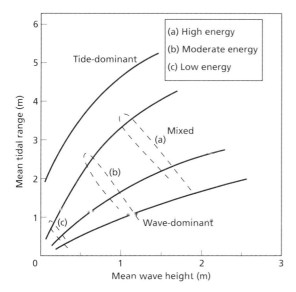

Fig. 23.2 Characterization of shorelines on a mean tidal range vs. mean local wave height plot. High-energy area (a) approximates to the German Bight; moderate-energy area (b) to the Georgia Bight; low-energy area (c) to the west Florida Bight. (After Hayes, 1979.)

Fig. 23.3 Morphological sketches of various coastlines, all with moderate wave energy. (a) Macrotidal coast; note absence of barrier islands and occurrence of tidal current ridges. (b) Mesotidal coast; note barriers with tidal inlets and ebb tidal deltas. (c) Microtidal coast; note abundant washovers, rare tidal inlets and flood tidal deltas. (After Hayes, 1979.)

force may usually be neglected in fluid force balances. This serves to distinguish the shoreface zone physically from the inner shelf, where stratified boundary layers are commoner and where Coriolis effects leading to Ekman transport become increasingly important in turning geostrophic currents and buoyant plume discharges.

The distinction between beach and tidal flat can never be sharply defined, but generally beaches occur as narrow intertidal to supratidal features dominated by wave action in which the sediment coarsens from offshore to onshore. In direct contrast, tidal flats are wider areas dominated by to-and-fro and rotary tidal motions in which the sediment fines from offshore to onshore. Tidal flats tend to be best developed on open, macrotidal coasts or as part of back-barrier complexes on mesotidal coasts. Chenier plains are particular coastal marsh and tidal mudflat environments, broken by very extensive lateral shell ridges up to 50 km long and 3 m high.

Coastal barriers (Fig. 23.3) are commonest on meso- and microtidal coasts; they require some steady riverine or longshore supply of sand for their sustained development. Those on microtidal coasts are long and linear with sedimentary processes in the back barrier lagoons dominated by storm washover effects. Barriers on meso- and macrotidal coasts are broken by frequent tidal inlets with flood tidal deltas in lagoons and bays on the back-barrier side and ebb tidal deltas on the seaward side. Fringing tidal flats

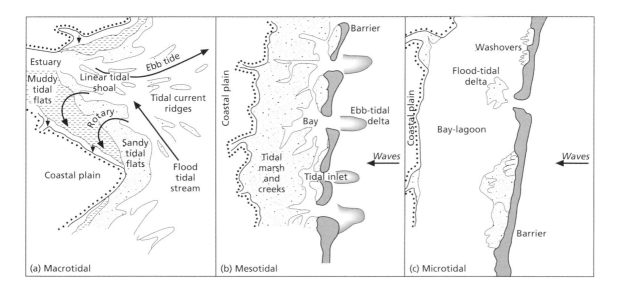

occur in the back-barrier environment, sheltered by the barrier from most wave action.

23.2 Physical processes on linear coasts

Controversy still exists concerning the physics of wave generation, though pressure fluctuations in the wind boundary layer and wave sheltering effects upon wind flows play an important role. Storms generate a spectrum of waves in a generating area. As these waves propagate outwards with the wind, the dispersive effect operates, longer waves travelling faster (Section 9.2). Even so, the generation of waves occurs at different times in different areas, so that all wave-recording stations record a range of wave sizes over any period of time. Statistics such as significant wave height and period refer to the mean height of the highest one-third of waves measured over some time interval. Apropos of our previous discussion on wave energy, it should be realized that the total energy accumulated over a portion of coast is obtained by integration of the wave spectrum over the entire frequency range. As in several other modes of wave motion, superposition of waveforms leads to positive or negative amplification or neutralization depending upon the wavelengths involved. Groups of gravity waves (defined by the beat frequency) in deep water are separated by low-amplitude neutralization areas, which travel with only half the velocity of the waves themselves. Small-amplitude waves passing from neutralization areas grow in amplitude as they pass through a group. After passing through the midpoint of the group, they decrease in amplitude away from it. The energy transported by waves thus travels with the group velocity appropriate to the beat rather than the wave velocity; simple wave theory gives this group velocity as half the wave velocity.

The simple linear (Airy) wave theory that we used previously (Chapter 9) to understand wave dynamics in the context of bedform development neglects terms of wave height to the second and higher orders. These terms are included in Stokes' theory (for an accessible derivation see Lighthill, 1978) and they serve to enhance wave crest amplitude and decrease the trough amplitude. In fact the wave profile has become more similar to that of natural waves. Trochoidal waves approximate best to many natural wave profiles but the theory of trochoidal waves need not detain us here. Concerning Stokes waves, one interesting

departure from linear (Airy) theory is that the wave orbitals are not closed, so that a steady mass transport of water must occur, i.e. a drift velocity exists, which is the mean velocity of a fluid particle averaged over a wave period (see Chapter 9). Such drifting determines a net sediment transport vector for shallow waves approaching a shoreline. It is interesting to note that Stokes waves transporting net water mass in the direction of the wave propagation must have a compensatory near-bed *seaward* flow of water. But this is quite the opposite to that detected by experiments and field measurements (Bagnold, 1940). This disagreement between theory and practice was caused by the noninclusion of viscous terms in the derivation. Once such terms are included (Longuet-Higgins, 1953), good agreement between theory and experiment occurs. Recent measurements indicate that the shoreward flux of momentum (radiation stress—see box below) at the seafloor due to asymmetric orbital velocities in steepening Stokes waves outside the surf zone may actually be reversed in the presence of wave ripples (Krause & Horikawa, 1990; Nielsen, 1992).

As the typical sinusoidal 'swell' of the deep ocean passes over the continental shelf towards coastlines, the waves undergo a transformation as they react to the bottom at values of between about 0.5 and 0.25 of their deep-water wavelength. Wave speed and wavelength decrease whilst wave height increases. Peaked crests and flat troughs develop as the waves become more solitary in behaviour until oversteepening causes wave breakage. Stokes' theory can also be used to shed light on the wave-breaking phenomenon. Waves will break when the water velocity at the crest is equal to the wave speed. This occurs as the apical angle of the wave reaches a value of about 120°. In deep water the tendency towards breaking may be expressed in terms of a limiting wave steepness given by:

$$\frac{H}{\lambda} \cong \frac{1}{7} \qquad (23.1)$$

Breaking waves may be divided into spilling, plunging and surging types (Fig. 23.4). Wave refraction effects occur in response to bottom topography or incidence of wave attack (Fig. 23.5). The behaviour of waves on beaches varies according to the steepness of the beach face (Huntley & Bowen, 1975a). Steep beaches possess a narrow surf zone in which the waves steepen rapidly and show high orbital velocities. Wave collapse is dominated by the plunging

More information on wave energy and radiation stresses

Concerning wave energy, it is the rhythmic conversion of potential to kinetic energy and back again that maintains the wave motion; our previous derivations of simple wave theory in Chapter 9 were dependent upon this approach. The displacement of the wave surface from the horizontal provides potential energy that is converted into kinetic energy by the orbital motion of the water. The total wave energy per unit area is given by:

$$E = \tfrac{1}{2}\rho g a^2 = \tfrac{1}{8}\rho g H^2 \tag{B23.1}$$

where a is wave amplitude and H is wave height $(=2a)$. The energy flux (or wave power) is the rate of energy transmitted in the direction of wave propagation and is given by:

$$\omega - Ecn - \tfrac{1}{8}\rho g H^2 cn \tag{B23.2}$$

where c is the local wave velocity, and $n = 0.5$ in deep water and $n = 1$ in shallow water. In deep water the energy flux is related to the wave group velocity rather than to the wave velocity, and it can be shown that this group velocity is about half the wave velocity (see Acheson, 1993).

Because of the forward energy flux, Ec, associated with waves approaching the shore, there exists also a shoreward-directed momentum flux or stress (radiation stress) outside the zone of breaking waves (Longuet-Higgins & Stewart, 1964). This may be regarded as the excess shoreward flux of momentum due to the presence of groups of water waves, the waves outside the breaker zone exerting a thrust on the water inside the breaker zone. This thrust arises because the net forward velocity associated with the arrival of groups of shallow-water and Stokes waves gives rise to a net flux of wave momentum. The two nonzero components of the momentum flux tensor, τ_{ij}, are:

$$\tau_{xx} - E(2n - \tfrac{1}{2}) = E/2 \tag{B23.3}$$

for deep water or $3E/2$ for shallow water, and

$$\tau_{yy} = E(n - \tfrac{1}{2}) = 0 \tag{B23.4}$$

for deep water or $E/2$ for shallow water. (The x-axis is in the direction of wave advance and the y-axis is parallel to the wave crest.) Radiation stress plays an important role in the origin of a number of coastal processes, including wave set-up and set-down, generation of longshore currents and the origin of rip currents amongst others. We shall examine a number of these aspects below.

mechanism and there is much interaction on the breaking waves by backwash from a previous wave-collapse cycle. A rip cell circulation (Fig. 23.6) may also be present. Gently sloping beaches show a wide surf zone in which the waves steepen slowly, show low orbital velocities, and surge up the beach with very minor backwash effects. Rip cells are not associated with such beaches; steady longshore currents exist instead.

The nearshore current system may include a remarkable cellular system of circulation comprising rip and longshore currents (Shepard & Inman, 1950)

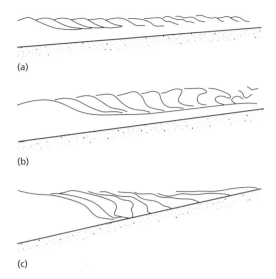

(a)

(b)

(c)

Fig. 23.4 Three types of breaking waves. Note that every gradation occurs between these types. (a) In *spilling* waves the crest steepens and the wave becomes asymmetric until the unstable crest cascades down as bubbles and foam. (b) In *plunging* waves the shoreward wave face curls over and impacts its whole momentum upon the beach. (c) In *surging* waves the shoreward wave face steepens as if to plunge, but the wave then moves as a surge (rather like a bore) up the beach, causing the wave face to disappear. (After Galvin, 1968.)

Fig. 23.5 Definition sketches for wave refraction on sloping coastlines. (After Collins, 1976.)

(Fig. 23.6). The narrow zones of rip currents make up the powerful 'undertow' on many steep beaches and are potentially hazardous to swimmers because of their high velocities (several metres per second). Rip currents arise because of variations in wave set-up (Longuet-Higgins & Stewart, 1964; Huntley & Bowen, 1975a) along steep beaches. Wave set-up is the small (centimetre to metre) rise of mean water level above still water level caused by the presence of shallow-water waves (Fig. 23.7; for field measurements see Hequette & Hill, 1993). It originates from that portion of the radiation stress τ_{xx} remaining after wave reflection and bottom drag and is balanced close inshore by a pressure gradient due to the sloping water surface. Now, in the breaker zone the set-up is greater shoreward of large breaking waves than smaller waves, so that a longshore pressure gradient causes longshore currents to move from areas of high to low breaking waves (Bowen, 1969; Bowen & Inman, 1969). These currents turn seawards where set-up is lowest and where adjacent currents converge.

What mechanism(s) can produce variations in wave height parallel to the shore in the breaker zone? Wave refraction is one such (Fig. 23.5), and some rip current cells are closely related to offshore variations in topography. Since rip cells also exist on long straight beaches with little variation in offshore topography, another mechanism must also act to provide lateral variations in wave height. This is thought to be that of standing edge waves (Huntley & Bowen, 1975b),

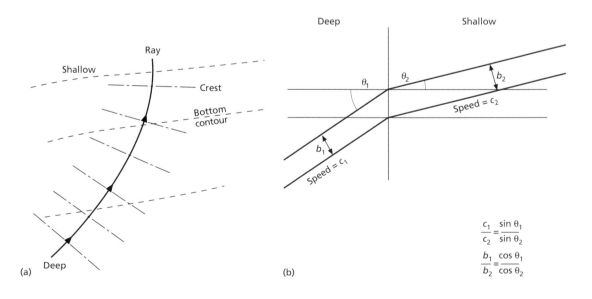

(a)

(b)

$$\frac{c_1}{c_2} = \frac{\sin \theta_1}{\sin \theta_2}$$

$$\frac{b_1}{b_2} = \frac{\cos \theta_1}{\cos \theta_2}$$

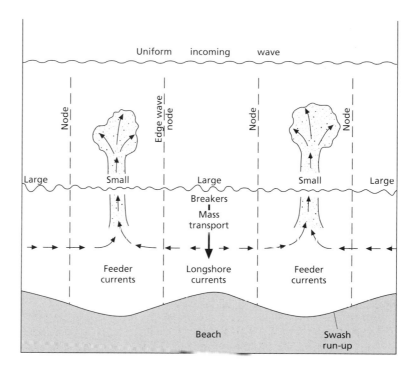

Fig. 23.6 Rip current cells located in areas of small breakers where incoming waves and standing edge waves are out of phase. (After Shepard & Inman, 1950; Komar 1975.)

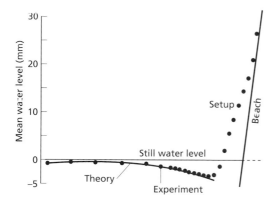

Fig. 23.7 Wave set-up and set-down produced by the radiation stress (momentum flux) of incoming waves in a laboratory wave tank and artificial beach. (From Bowen et al., 1968.)

which form as trapped waveforms due to refracting wave interactions with strong backflowing wave swash on relatively steep beaches. Edge waves were first detected on natural beaches (Huntley & Bowen, 1975b) as short-period waves acting at the first subharmonic of the incident wave frequency, decaying rapidly in amplitude offshore. The addition of incoming waves to edge waves is expected to give marked longshore variations in breaker height, the summed height being greatest where the two wave systems are in phase (Fig. 23.6). It is thought that trapped edge waves may be connected with the formation of the common cuspate form of many beaches; these have wavelengths of a few to tens of metres, approximately equal to the known wavelengths of measured edge waves (see Huntley & Bowen, 1975b). More recent results concerning the effects of edge waves and 'leaky' mode standing waves (where some proportion of energy is reflected seawards as long waves at infragravity frequency, 0.03–0.003 Hz) indicate that both shoreward and seaward transport of suspended sediment may result depending on conditions (Wright et al., 1991). Usually, sediment entrainment under groups of large waves in arriving wavepackets is preferentially transported seawards under the trough of the bound long-period group wave.

The second group of nearshore currents are those produced by oblique wave attack upon the shoreline. (It should be noted that such currents may be superimposed upon the rip cells described previously.) Such currents, which give a lateral thrust to the water and sediment in the surf zone, are caused by τ_{xy}, the flux towards the shoreline (x direction) of momentum directed parallel to the shoreline (y direction). Longuet-Higgins (1970) gives:

$$\tau_{xy} = \tfrac{1}{4} E \sin 2\alpha \qquad (23.2)$$

where α is the angle between wave crest and shore (shore-parallel crests = 0°; shore-normal = 90°). The τ_{xy} value reaches a maximum when $\sin 2\alpha = 1$, or when the angle of wave incidence is 45°. The longshore velocity component, u_L, is:

$$u_L = \left(\frac{5\pi \tan \beta}{8C_f}\right) u_{max} \sin \alpha \qquad (23.3)$$

where $\tan \beta$ is the beach slope, C_f is the drag coefficient, and u_{max} is the maximum orbital velocity at the breaker zone. However, Komar and Inman (1970) found no dependence of u_L on slope, and Komar (1971, 1975) suggests that $(\tan \beta)/C_f$ is approximately constant so that:

$$\bar{u}_L = 2.7 u_{max} \sin \alpha \cos \alpha \qquad (23.4)$$

in good agreement with field measurements at mid-surf. Concerning sediment transport in the nearshore zone, Bagnold (1963) has related sand transport by immersed weight i_b to the wave energy flux (power ω), such that $i_b = k\omega$, where k is a constant that approximates to 0.28 from empirical data. Under purely to-and-fro water motion, the wave power simply acts to suspend sediment grains with no net transport. Net transport occurs only in the presence of a shoreward-directed residual current, u', caused by shoaling waves or a longshore current, u_L (or combinations thereof). In such cases the net transport rate, i, is given by:

$$i = k\omega \frac{u'}{u_{max}} \qquad (23.5)$$

which for longshore transport yields:

$$i_L = kECn \cos \alpha \; \frac{\bar{u}_L}{u_{max}} \qquad (23.6)$$

where n = 0.5 in deep water and 1 in shallow water (see p. 401) in good agreement with field measurements (Komar & Inman, 1970).

It must be stressed that the long-term longshore transport of sediment depends upon the summed effects of all wave systems that impact upon a coastline. Such long-term transport vectors cancel out seasonal effects and are visually impressed upon the mind of the casual coastal visitor by piling-up of sediment against groynes, jetties and breakwaters around coastlines and by the migration directions of coastal spits.

A final point concerns wave-produced bedforms. We have already discussed the moulding effect that purely oscillatory and combined oscillatory–current flows have upon loose beds of sediment grains (Chapter 9). All gradations exist between purely oscillatory and combined oscillatory–current flows in the nearshore and beach environments, but in general we might expect an increasing degree of flow asymmetry, and hence bedform asymmetry, as the water depth decreases towards the shoreline. In fact, large seasonal variations in the degree of asymmetry are to be expected, causing complex interrelations to be preserved in the sedimentary structures of the nearshore and beach zone.

23.3 Beach dynamics and sedimentation

Comparison of summer and winter beach profiles reveals major changes. In *summer*, swell waves with low steepness values transport sediment onshore, forming narrow linear ridges called *beach berms*. In *winter*, storm waves with high steepness values transport sediment offshore forming *offshore bars*. Rip current cells are commoner in winter on steeper beaches. The beachface slope is governed by the asymmetry of offshore and onshore transport vectors discussed previously. The seaward backwash is generally weaker and longer-lasting than the rapid shoreward movement of water from collapsing waves because of percolation and frictional drag on the swash (see Hughes *et al.*, 1997). Sediment is thus continually moved up the beach slope until an equilibrium is established (Hardisty, 1986). Maximum percolation occurs on the most permeable gravel beaches and these usually have the highest slopes. Assuming that gravity opposes the net shoreward drift of sediment, Inman and Bagnold (1963) obtain the following relationship for local beach slope $\tan \beta$:

$$\tan \beta = \tan \phi \left(\frac{1-c}{1+c}\right) \qquad (23.7)$$

where ϕ is the coefficient of internal friction, and c is the asymmetry term for offshore vs. onshore wave energy. When $c = 1$ no asymmetry occurs and $\tan \beta = 0$. If the asymmetry is large then $c \to 0$ and $\tan \beta \to \tan \phi$, the beach slope approaching the angle of repose. The coarsening-onshore trend found in almost all beach and nearshore systems (from about surf line inwards) is explained by the fact that the forward orbital motion under shallow-water wave crests is short-lived but powerful compared to the seaward return flow (Bagnold, 1940; Kemp, 1975). This leads to the concept of a net landward flux of wave-induced momentum (also called radiation stress), resulting in coarse particles being preferentially transported onshore.

As noted previously, beaches show a general offshore to onshore increase in sediment grain size and a great sensitivity to storm intensity (for a well-illustrated review see Massari & Parea, 1988). The majority of beachface accretion takes place after storm events and during fair-weather periods when low-angle accretion laminae exhibit characteristic open framework sorting, and seaward dipping imbrication of common discoid pebbles (Orford, 1975). Storms themselves leave evidence of their occurrence in the form of erosional and truncation surfaces in the beachface and berm washovers. Along the shoreface and offshore it is a different matter since net offshore transport by rip and gradient currents occurs during storms, giving rise to sharp-based and sheet-like poorly sorted gravels and sands exhibiting hummocky cross-stratification. Shoreface and foreshore topography reflects the presence of various 'bars', ridges and troughs as well as wave-formed current ripples and dunes (Fig. 23.8). Scuba observations (Hart & Plint, 1989) of high-gradient upper shoreface environments, down to depths of 6 m or so below a prominent plunge-pool step at low water mark, indicate large-wavelength (up to 2 m) asymmetrical (shore-facing) gravel bedforms up to 0.25 m or so in height.

Larger offshore bars occur on all but the steepest high-energy beaches and are controlled in a complex way by the position of spilling waves during storm conditions. Successive coast-parallel or crescentic bars with wavelengths of tens to hundreds of metres occur on low-gradient shorefaces. The bars tend to increase in height (up to 1.5 m) away from the shore, perhaps individually reflecting the average spilling position of waves of a certain height. The bars (Fig. 23.8) show variably dipping internal sets of tabular cross-stratification directed landwards, and the troughs show small-scale cross-laminations produced by landward-migrating wave–current ripples (Davidson-Arnott & Greenwood, 1974, 1976; Davidson-Arnott & Pember, 1980; Gruszczynski *et al.*, 1993). Measurements taken during storm conditions indicate that sediment accumulates on bar

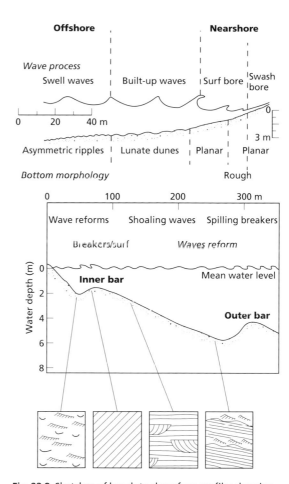

Fig. 23.8 Sketches of beach to shoreface profiles showing the relations of bedforms to waveforms. (After Clifton *et al.*, 1971; Davidson-Arnott & Greenwood, 1974.)

crests and is eroded from troughs, and that the latter are the site of significant shore-parallel flows (Greenwood & Sherman, 1993). When bars occur in the foreshore area, they are termed ridge and runnel topography (Wunderlich, 1972). During rising and falling tides the runnels come under the influence of slope-controlled flows as they alternately fill up and drain: current-produced bedforms including dunes and upper plane beds result whose orientation is shore-parallel (Moore *et al.*, 1984).

Osborne and Greenwood (1992) analyse the problem of the across-shoreface transport of suspended sediment and assembled field data that suggested both time-averaged (mean) cross-shore currents and oscillatory currents are critical in determining net transport. In the surf zone of bars there is onshore transport at low wave frequencies (seasonal storm conditions). Outside the surf zone the linkage between the effects of a steady seaward mean current and the energy and suspended sediment transport in long-frequency, bounded, wave groups leads to offshore transport. Rip current processes are a distinctive physical mechanism for across-shoreface transport. They have been largely neglected by students of ancient coastal facies. The very characteristic rip current cells that occur on many steeper beaches, particularly during storms, produce spaced channels that may dissect offshore bars (Gruszczynski *et al.*, 1993) and contain sharp-based shelly sands and pebbly sands with shell lags. The fan-like terminations to rip current channels deposit seaward-dipping cross-sets.

23.4 Barrier–inlet systems and their deposits

The origin of barrier systems has become clearer since the advent of multidisciplinary studies involving shallow geophysics, vibracoring and carbon dating (e.g. Siringan & Anderson, 1993; Wellner *et al.*, 1993; Aubrey & Geise, 1993). Early theories suggested that barriers resulted from the upbuilding of submerged offshore bars into emergent islands. The absence of offshore facies beneath modern lagoons discredits the theory. We have already seen (Chapter 22) that barriers like those of the Chandeleur Islands overlie marsh and delta-front deposits and mark the reworked rim of abandoned subdeltas of the Mississippi. Periodically, portions of these islands are destroyed by hurricanes, but they may re-form again by emergence of the remnant submerged sand bars if sand supply is provided. Other barrier islands formed over abandoned deltas isolated from a continuing sand supply may be vulnerable to the washover of sand into the lagoons and bays on the landward side during storms. For example, large-scale destruction of the Isles Dernieres off coastal Louisiana occurred after Hurricane Andrew in 1992 (Fig. 23.9).

Inherited coastal topography generated during low sea-level stands plays a key role in barrier evolution

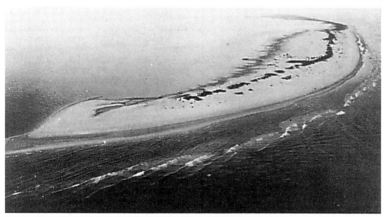

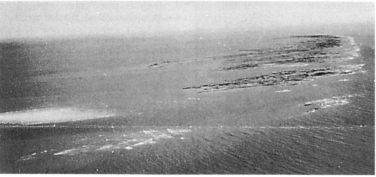

Fig. 23.9 Raccoon Island, Louisiana, before (top) and after (bottom) the passage of Hurricane Andrew in August 1992. The detached barrier island was originally 3 miles long but was heavily scoured, shortened and flattened by washover erosion. (From EOS, 1992.)

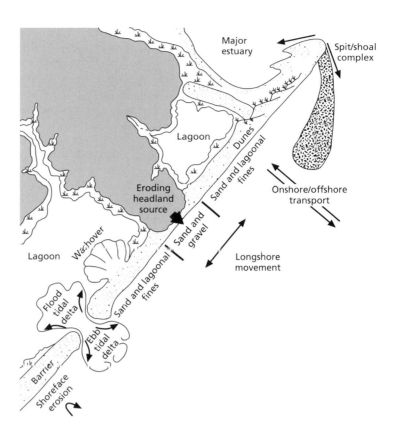

Fig. 23.10 Sketch of barrier/spit/ lagoon/tidal inlet complex to indicate various sediment sources and sinks. Many tidal inlets are now known to overlie partly buried lowstand fluvial channels, whilst eroding headlands, formerly incised valley slopes, supply clastic sediment to the coastal system. (After Kraft *et al.*, 1987.)

(Halsey, 1979; Oertel, 1979; Fitzgerald, 1993). Lowstand palaeochannel networks are separated by higher interfluve areas. During transgression, beaches formed against the eroding interfluves and estuaries formed along the river channel outlets (Fig. 23.10). A variety of barrier, spit, lagoon and tidal-flat environments evolve as transgression continued. Of great importance is a ready supply of sand or fine gravel sediment. One such source may be lowstand sub-aerial deltas, delta fronts (particularly glacial outwash deltas) or older barriers and their ebb tidal delta shoals now stranded offshore. On a relatively tectonically stable coastline such as the eastern USA, these might represent Isotope stage 3 or 4 lowstand deposits, now well within modern storm wave base at depths of 30–50 m. A good example is the Merrimack delta off Cape Cod, whose sands are thought to have supplied the Holocene Cape Cod barrier system (Fitzgerald, 1993).

Tidal inlets are present along barriers in macrotidal, mesotidal and, to a lesser extent, microtidal areas. They play an important role, transferring oceanic waters into and out of the back-barrier lagoon or bay. Tidal currents and range are usually enhanced in the inlet compared to the adjacent shelf. They are the main flushing arteries, or orifices in Oertel's (1988) metaphor, vital to the ecological well-being of highly prized and productive lagoonal ecosystems. The flow passing along the inlet in response to tidal and storm forcing issues as an expanding jet behind and in front of the barrier. In both cases predominantly sandy sediment bodies form as flood and ebb tidal deltas respectively (Figs 23.10 & 23.11). Inlets are often dynamic items, migrating, rotating, opening and closing—see Sha and de Boer (1991) for a long-term historical view of Dutch tidal inlets—or they may remain stationary for thousands of years. Inlet behaviour depends upon local conditions of sediment supply, tidal and wave characteristics, and the changing nature of the tidal prism supplied by the back-barrier catchment (see Oertel, 1988; Biegel & Hoekstra, 1995; Oost & de Boer, 1994). It also depends upon the inherited topography of the seafloor, for, as noted previously, many prominent

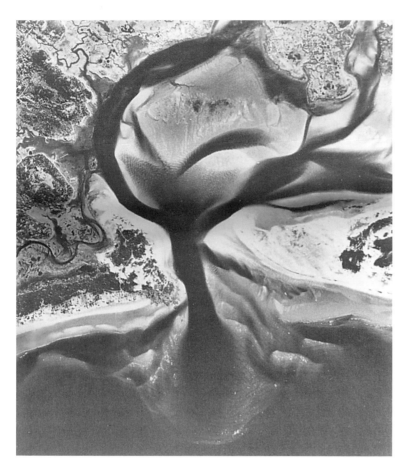

Fig. 23.11 A 1976 vertical aerial photograph of the Essex River tidal inlet, Ipswich Bay, Massachusetts, showing ebb and flood tidal deltas, attached and detached barrier ridges, barrier tip accretion surfaces and coastal tidal wetlands. Local longshore drift is right to left, approximately NW to SE. Mean local wave height is ≈0.2 m, with a mean tidal range of about 2.7 m. (Data and photograph from Fitzgerald, 1993.)

stationary modern inlets are found to be coincident with drowned lowstand river and estuary valleys (Fitzgerald, 1993; Siringan & Anderson, 1993; Levin, 1995). Coriolis effects are important in larger tidal inlets at higher latitudes, causing the position of the maximum flood and ebb tides to alternate in opposite directions so that one side of inlet channels are flood-dominant whilst the other is ebb-dominant (e.g. see Vilas *et al.*, 1991). Inlets play a vital role in the nourishment or starvation of adjacent portions of a barrier. This depends on the degree of bypassing of sediment across the inlet channel. Periodic growth, accretion and then cutoff of ebb tidal deltas control the accretion rate of the barrier itself (Fitzgerald, 1988).

A particularly well-studied example of inlet initiation is in the Cape Cod area of Massachusetts where a major spring tide coincided with a succession of great NE storms in the winter of 1987. A storm surge overwhelmed the existing barrier opposite Chatham

estuary and eroded sufficient sediment that over a period of days a rapidly widening channel began to transfer water through it. Over a few months a major inlet up to 700 m wide had been cut across the once-continuous barrier, now with tidal currents flowing at over 1 m/s. In this and other equilibrium tidal inlets it is the strong tidal currents that maintain the channel in face of opposition from the deposition of sand by longshore wave-induced currents. It is the delicate balance between longshore supply and tidal currents that determines inlet behaviour (e.g. Fitzgerald, 1993), channels migrating in the direction of longshore supply (see Levin, 1995). The net transport of sediment in an inlet (onshore vs. offshore) depends upon the residual current regime caused primarily by the mean sea-level difference between onshore and the open ocean during the course of the tidal cycle. Tidal amplitude and the phase difference between the two ends of the channel also play a role. In general, the bigger the tidal

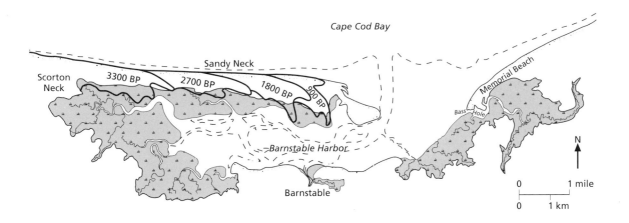

Fig. 23.12 Map to show the growth and development of the attached barrier–spit of Sandy Neck, Barnstable, northern shoreline of Cape Cod, Massachusetts. Sediments are derived from erosion of Pleistocene cliffs to the north. (After Fitzgerald, 1993.)

range, the deeper, larger and more powerful is the channel flow in inlets.

Seaward-prograding barrier islands will produce coarsening-upwards successions similar to those of attached beaches but with the major addition of tidal inlet and back-barrier lagoon or bay facies. Back-barrier lagoons vary tremendously, depending upon climate, degree of tidal flushing by inlets, river inflow and extent of storm washover events. Lagoons in microtidal areas are dominated by storm washovers so that the bioturbated lagoonal silts and muds are intercalated with sheets up to 1.5 m thick of parallel-laminated sands derived from storm breaching of the exposed barrier profile. Washover fans produced in this way may show delta-like landward terminations with internal sets of landward-dipping planar cross-stratification (Schwartz, 1975). Microtidal lagoons in semiarid climates such as the Texan Laguna Madre show evaporite growth of sabkha types, carbonate precipitation as ooliths, and growth of algal mats (Fisk, 1959; Rusnak, 1960). Flood tidal deltas in mesotidal lagoons occur on the inner sides of tidal inlets in response to flow expansion and decelera-tion (Hayes, 1979). The subaqueous delta surface is covered by landward-directed tidal dune bedforms. Some sandflat platforms are wave-dominated but the tidal drainage channels are current-dominated (Davis & Flemming, 1995). The remainder of the lagoon in

such cases approximates to the physiography of a tidal flat as discussed below. Ebb tidal deltas have a morphology and symmetry that strongly reflect the relative strength of tidal and longshore currents and their ability to transport away sediment (Oertel, 1979; Nummedal & Penland, 1981). Strongly asymmetric deltas tend to develop when longshore currents are strong.

The growth of coast-attached spit systems (Fig. 23.12) is of some interest. Along most of their length the seaward-facing spit might show only lim-ited seaward progradation, since the predominant sediment transport vector is shoreface-parallel. At the tip of the spit, below a beach platform and a series of subtidal sand bars, gravel and sand are periodically supplied to the deeper water of the estuarine inlet by avalanching. This process gives rise to a very char-acteristic sequence of giant, steeply dipping, foreset beds overlain by beach and shoreface deposits (Johannessen & Nielsen, 1986).

In summary, as barriers migrate seawards under conditions of net sediment supply and sea-level high-stand, an upward-coarsening sequence is produced that may be broken by fining-upwards tidal-inlet channel facies and the complex facies of ebb tidal deltas. The inlet association may comprise up to 50% of the total along-barrier sediment volume, the exact amount depending upon rates of inlet migration. It is to be expected that, in examples formed after preced-ing lowstands, the tidal inlet may become stabilized in position above a lowstand valley and its deposits (see Siringan & Anderson, 1993). The barrier may eventu-ally be overlain by lagoonal, tidal-flat or flood tidal delta facies, which reverse the coarsening-upwards trend.

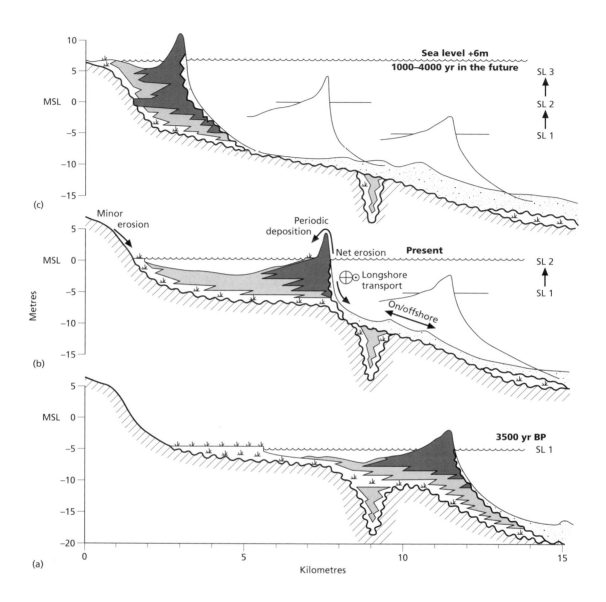

Fig. 23.13 A series of sketch profiles to illustrate the morphology and lateral relationships of sedimentary environments in response to changing sea level, from 3.5 kyr BP (bottom), now (middle) and perhaps 1–4 kyr in the future should sea level continue to rise (top). (After Kraft et al., 1987.)

It is less evident how barrier–lagoon systems maintain an equilibrium morphology during transgressions. Early studies (Rampino & Sanders, 1981) proposed that regions subject to rapid sea-level rise with low sand supply would favour stepwise retreat of barriers. Areas with slow sea-level rise and high sand influx (Bourgeois, 1980) might show continuous

shoreface retreat and the production of a gently sloping erosional or 'ravinement' surface overlying a truncated shoreface sequence. Barriers would then be free to prograde once more at sea-level highstand (Ashley et al., 1991; Wellner et al., 1993).

The behaviour of regressive barrier systems during periods of stable sea level should be contrasted with that of transgressing barriers (see Kraft & John, 1979; Kraft et al., 1987; Pilkey & Davis, 1987; Everts, 1987). In the latter case little of the barrier facies themselves may be preserved offshore if transgression is slow and sediment supply low. The whole barrier system simply translates onshore (Fig. 23.13), erosional action at the shoreface zone during storms producing a 'ravinement' erosion surface over the original ramp slope, with an overlying thin reworked offshore sand body that may eventually overlie the lagoon facies directly as transgression continues (Kraft, 1971; Kraft et al., 1987; Ashley et al., 1991). Lagoonal environments themselves may narrow and infill as they are forced against higher-gradient land surfaces during transgression and barrier retreat (Finkelstein & Ferland, 1987). Older subsurface lagoonal deposits onlapped by the barrier may also be removed by the action of migrating tidal inlets (Kumar & Sanders, 1974). It is possible that high rates of sediment supply combined with rapid transgression may cause barrier preservation (Bourgeois, 1980). The behaviour of coastal barrier–beach systems in the context of present-day sea-level rise is a fascinating topic (Fig. 23.13); the beach-hut-owning reader is referred to the stimulating papers by Everts (1987) and Pilkey and Davis (1987) for reviews of possible scenarios.

23.5 Tidal flats and chenier ridges

Tidal flats are generally sinks for fine-grained sediment, whether originating from estuary outlets and tidal inlets or in larger-scale coastal embayments, like the Wash, England, or Jade, Germany. In the Wash, for example (Ke et al., 1996), a net supply of fine-grained sediment arrives from offshore North Sea, mostly at spring tides, because of a net residual flood tidal current. Fining onshore across tidal flats has generally been attributed to two related processes that encourage silt- and mud-grade sediment to accumulate on the upper tidal flats. First there is the tendency for maximum fine sediment deposition from suspension to occur at spring tidal high water mark. This deposits fine sediment in a position where subsequent lower tidal levels cannot resuspend it. Secondly, once deposited during the high flood tide, fine sediment is more difficult to erode at the equivalent point in the ebb because of cohesive forces at the bed, early compaction and algal binding.

Limited percolation of tidal waters occurs on muddy tidal flats because of low permeability. This encourages surface runoff and the establishment of meandering tidal channel networks. Careful measurements of tidal flows both in channels and on adjacent flats (Carling, 1981; Collins et al., 1981) reveal a broad rotary pattern as a coast-parallel tide swings

on to the tidal flats during the course of the flood tide to become shore-normal. Tidal creeks split the alongshore tidal prism into a number of cells. It is commonly found that there exists a strong residual sediment transport towards the shoreline over the tidal flats, with weaker residual transport seawards in the channels (Fig. 23.14). The overall result is a net shoreward transport of sediment and vertical accretion of the tidal-flat surface. Sediment concentrations in the water peak strongly at the beginning of the flood tide and the end of the ebb, reflecting substrate erosion by the shallow, fast gravity-controlled tidal residual and gravity runoff. The latter is a neglected but important seaward transporting process when copious rainwater falls on to exposed tidal flats (Bridges & Leeder, 1976).

The facies of tidal flats (e.g. Evans, 1965; Reineck, 1967; Collins et al., 1981) are dominated by the nearshore-to-offshore coarsening trend noted previously (Fig. 23.15). Seaward progradation produces an upward-fining sequence, broken by intertidal and subtidal channels and capped by a rootlet bed or peat accumulation of the saltmarsh. The supratidal salt-marsh zone with halophytic (salt-loving) plants passes gradationally outwards at a very low slope (1 : 100 to 1 : 800) into a mudflat with a rich infauna. Seaward coarsening gives rise to a mixed sand/mudflat with a variety of laminations including flasers. Again, bioturbation by the abundant infauna is intense. Tidal channels rework much of the tidal-flat deposits and give rise to inclined lateral accretion deposits of interlaminated silts and muds (Reineck, 1958; Bridges & Leeder, 1976). Rapid deposition on the point bars discourages infaunas, and hence these deposits are relatively free of bioturbation. The sandflats that occur at mean low water mark show a great variety of wave- and current-formed ripple bedforms with complex interference forms caused by gravity runoff effects. Local dunes may result if tidal flows are strong enough. In many areas intertidal channels pass offshore into a subtidal zone of deep channels with major dune bedforms whose migration and accretion are dominated by the periodic ebb and flow of the tidal wave (e.g. Reineck, 1967, 1972). Frequently ebb and flood channels (like the tidal inlet channels already discussed) are separate, so that resulting cross-stratified sand deposits tend to show either ebb or flood dominance. More rarely, evidence for a mixture of the two vectors may be seen in the occurrence of reactivation surfaces cut into the lee-side deposits

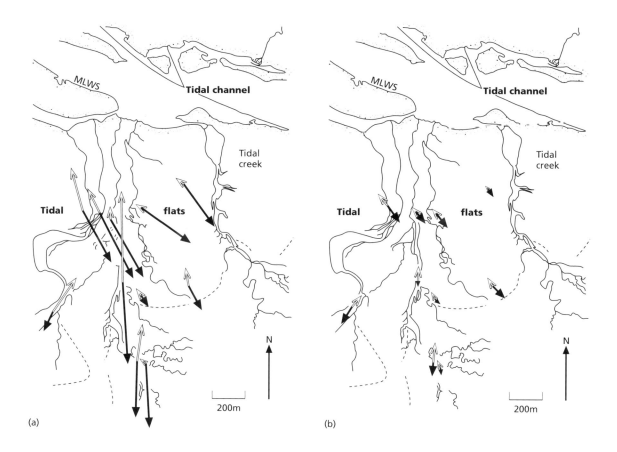

(a)   (b)

Fig. 23.14 Maps to show the sediment transport pattern for (a) spring and (b) neap tides across tidal flats. Black vectors are flood tide transport residuals, and white vectors are ebb tide residuals. Note the strong onshore asymmetry in sediment flux. MLWS, mean low-water spring-tide level. (After Carling, 1981.)

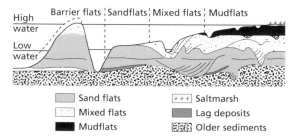

Fig. 23.15 Section through a tidal-flat complex to show the various subdivisions and the sort of sequence produced after tidal-flat progradation. (After Reineck & Singh, 1973.)

of the dominant dune bedform (de Mowbray & Visser, 1984).

The classic cheniers occur in Louisiana, westwards of the modern lobe of the Mississippi delta. Periods of mudflat outbuilding appear to coincide with abundant longshore mud supply from the Mississippi. Periods of mudflat erosion occur when mud supply is sparse (perhaps following a lobe avulsion) and waves rework the nearshore mudflats and concentrate shell material as chenier storm ridges bordering the mudflats. Chenier sand or shell facies are dominated by storm washover effects that produce landward-dipping, low-angle to planar cross-sets on the landward (washover) side of the biconvex ridge. The nature of the base of the chenier succession varies from a sharp contact with marsh facies on the landward side of the ridge to a gradational contact with shallow-water or mudflat facies on the seaward side.

23.6 Ancient clastic shoreline facies

Identification of true shoreline and nearshore facies is of the utmost importance in palaeogeographic reconstructions, since firm limits may then be put on the extent of sea during a particular time interval. Additionally, identification of shoreline facies enables deductions to be made according to the magnitude of the tides, the relative importance of waves vs. tides and the absolute bathymetry of the shoreline facies for palaeoecological studies. Now-classic accounts of storm-generated sequences of the shoreface and inner shelf with hummocky cross-stratification are provided by Dott and Bourgeois (1982) and by Hunter and Clifton (1982). Prave *et al.* (1996), in a study of Devonian shoreline deposits, establish shallowing-upwards sequences in which offshore storm-dominated deposits give way to nearshore tidally dominated sequences. Okazaki and Masuda (1995) reconstruct the coastal dynamics of palaeo-Tokyo Bay in terms of a barrier–inlet coast. DeCelles' (1987) analysis of a coarse-grained wave-generated deposit in the mid-Tertiary of southern California postulates storm wave reworking of introduced fluvial deposits and the rip current transport of sand and gravel obliquely offshore.

Further reading

Useful accounts of the physical and geomorphological processes that affect clastic shoreline sedimentation appear in the text by Komar (1998) and in the volumes edited by Hails and Carr (1975), K. S. Davis and Ethington (1976), R. A. Davis (1985), Leatherman (1979), Aubrey and Geise (1993), Carter and Woodruffe (1994), Flemming and Bartholema (1995) and Black *et al.* (1998). Coastal sediment transport and water wave dynamics are nicely discussed (but you will need to brush up your mathematics) by Nielsen (1992) and Fredsoe and Deigaard (1992).

24 Carbonate-evaporite shorelines, shelves and basins

*They fell with a regular thud. They fell with the concussion of horses' hooves on the turf . . .
They drew in and out with the energy, the muscularity, of an engine which sweeps its force out
and in again.*

Virginia Woolf, *The Waves*, p. 92, Penguin, 1964.

24.1 Introduction: carbonate 'factories' and their consequences

Despite the physical aspects (i.e. wave and tidal processes) of coastal and shelf carbonate environments being comparable to those of siliciclastic environments, carbonate sediments are distinctive because of:

- their local or *in situ* biogenic or chemical origins;
- spatial and time gradients in grain type and production rates;
- altered hydrodynamic properties of queer-shaped carbonate grains;
- rapid accretion of wave-resistant subtidal to deep shelf 'build-ups';
- their tendency to become lithified during exposure;
- steep lithified/accreted carbonate platform margin slopes.

Nothing in sedimentology is simple, however, for it is common in the stratigraphic record to find carbonate and clastic sediments superimposed vertically or juxtaposed horizontally. Investigation of such sequences has undoubtedly been hampered by artificial separation of many sedimentological research schools into 'carbonate' or 'clastic'.

As sketched in Fig. 24.1, the greatest source for carbonate grains is the warm shallow photic zone of the subtidal environment, the *carbonate 'factory'*, from whence storms and mass flows transfer detritus at declining rates onshore and offshore. The highest organic productivity of the 'factory' on Recent subtropical and tropical shallow shelves occurs in coral reefs at platform margins, leading to the production of rimmed shelves with abrupt, steep seaward margins and landward lagoons (Fig. 24.2; Plates 15 & 16). This is essentially Darwin's 1842 coral growth model for atolls. Major rimmed offshore banks completely

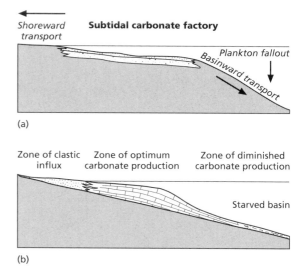

Fig. 24.1 The shallow subtidal carbonate factory, with its import : export fluxes and the control upon offshore slope by *in situ* and redistributive (diffusional, advective) processes.

isolated from terrigenous clastic input occur as fragmented continental crustal 'microcontinents' bordered by abyssal plains and deep channels. Such an example is seen in the Bahamas Banks, one of the largest and most studied modern carbonate platforms. Here the distribution of environments reflects both distribution of *in situ* producers and wave/tide energy levels (Hine *et al.*, 1981b). Steep reefal platform margins owe their origins to basement structural controls; deep seismic profiles (Eberli & Ginsburg, 1987; Fig. 24.2; Plate 16) reveal the banks formed by coalescence of smaller nuclei, probably originally fault-controlled, combined with significant lateral progradation to the leeward (westerly in this case).

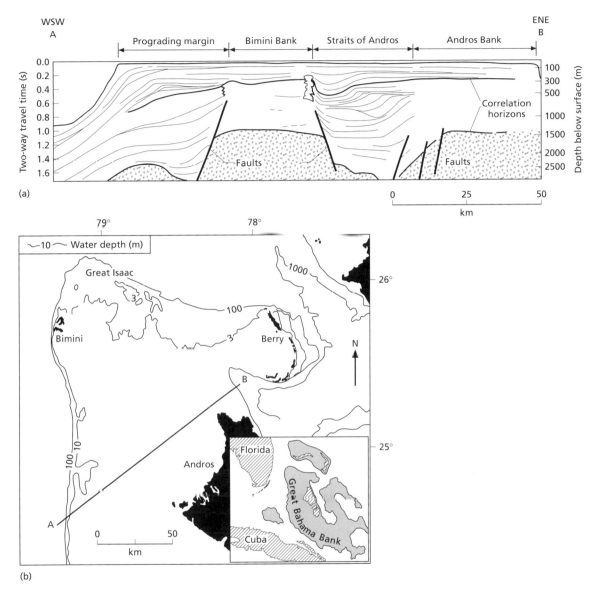

Fig. 24.2 SW–NE (a) cross-section (after Eberli & Ginsburg, 1987) and (b) location map of Great Bahama Bank to illustrate (1) modern rimmed platform of wide main bank (the Bahamas 'carbonate factory') bounded by steep (15–30°) western rimmed margin, (2) growth of western margin through time from ramp to rimmed bank and (3) the fused, composite nature of the modern bank, witnessed by the infill of the Straits of Andros by a prograding ramp to steep (25–30°) rimmed shelf through time.

On the other hand, carbonate *ramp* shorelines and shelves (Fig. 24.3) are, as their name implies, mostly depicted as uniformly and gently sloping (a degree or so) depositional surfaces (Ahr, 1973; Read, 1984) that decline away from a prograding shoreline into deeper water with no *pronounced* (< 5°) platform margin break of slope. They have been much investigated in ancient (where of course their form can only be *inferred*) carbonate sediments thought to have developed in regionally subsiding shelf basins without

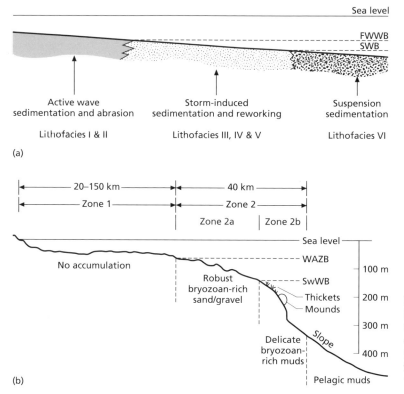

Fig. 24.3 Ramp models in practice. (a) Simple model for the Deschambault Formation, Ordovician of Quebec, Canada (Lavoie, 1995). (b) Modern situation on the Lacepede Shelf, southern Australia (James *et al.*, 1992).

fault control. In order to maintain such a ramp profile, as distinct from a steep, reef-rimmed shelf break with a landward more-or-less protected interior, the rate of *in situ* carbonate production and/or seaward redistribution by storms must decrease from shoreline to offshore (Aurell *et al.*, 1995). The effects of nearshore sediment production maxima eventually lead to the formation of a gentle gradient change offshore, a feature simulated from given carbonate production rates by superimposing a spatially varying sediment supply on a uniform linear subsidence rate under conditions of rising sea levels (Fig. 24.4; Bosence & Waltham, 1990; Bosence *et al.*, 1994; Aurell *et al.*, 1995; Whitaker *et al.*, 1997).

In reality, non-Bahamian platform-type shelves *are* often seen to be *combinations* of rimmed shelves and ramps, and the distinction may be scholastic. Take the case of the Queensland shelf, for example. Here the southern and northern shelfward margins are marked by disconnected linear fragments of wall reefs that mark the abrupt shelf edge (see the classic account of Maxwell & Swinchatt, 1970). Yet all across this

sometimes very wide gently sloping shelf there is a high degree of tidal mixing, such that to all intents and purposes the wide reef-rimmed shelf may be regarded as a carbonate ramp–seaway with no discernible chemical or physical barriers across it. The Torres Strait peripheral foreland basin of NE Australia/ Papua New Guinea, at the northernmost extremity of the Great Barrier Reef, is another fine example of such a reef-strewn seaway, with strong tidal currents between the reefs leading to spectacular dunefields (Keene & Harris, 1995). An older example of a ramp–seaway geometry is deduced by Anastasa *et al.* (1997) for the tidally swept temperate carbonate dunefields of the Te Kuiti Group, North Island of New Zealand.

It seems evident from the stratigraphic record (Read, 1984; Burchette & Wright, 1992) that ramps have sometimes been commoner on pre-Cainozoic carbonate shelves (for detailed examples and modelling runs see Aurell *et al.*, 1995). To *avoid* production of a rimmed shelf margin, shallow-water reefs or build-ups must be limited somehow: mechanisms are

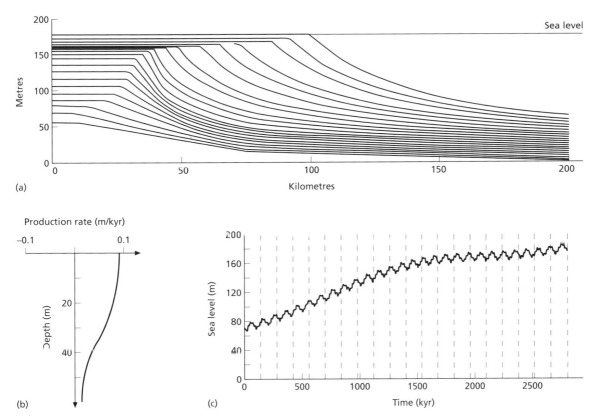

(a)

(b)   (c)

Fig. 24.4 Modelling ramp evolution on the computer. Simplified version of output from the model of Aurell *et al.* (1995). (a) Evolution of an equilibrium offshore slope (nonlinear 'ramp') from an initial linear ramp via a carbonate production rate function (b), a gradually varying sea level (c), a linear subsidence rate and a 'redistribution' function representing onshore lowstand erosion and offshore sediment transport during storms. Lines in (a) represent 140 kyr time increments.

discussed in a later section. In contrast to the 'rimmed' northern and southern Great Barrier Reef, the central part of the Queensland shelf has no rimmed margin (Maxwell & Swinchatt, 1970), gently sloping offshore as a ramp. Ramp conditions also pertain today in the Arabian Gulf and the West Florida shelf, for example, and the West Florida ramp (Roof *et al.*, 1991) passes from shoreface to deep water with no pronounced shelf-slope break, although in common with most examples the oceanward ramp slope increases somewhat. It may sometimes be useful to distinguish inner, mid and outer ramps according to the decreasing degree of wave–current reworking. However, the variation of this and the neglected importance of tidal currents and storm surges within the general hydrodynamic setting of carbonate basins make any generalities as to the absolute water depths appropriate to these zones impossible.

Although carbonate production reaches greatest levels in low latitudes, we must not neglect the often important and distinctive production in the cooler waters of mid-latitude shelves. All shelf sediments contain some proportion of organic-sourced carbonates, but in some areas where siliciclastic supply is limited these may become dominant. Such environments are exemplified by the Cainozoic to Recent deposits of the New Zealand shelf (Nelson *et al.*, 1988; Anastasa *et al.*, 1997) and particularly the southern Australian shelf, the world's largest modern cool-water carbonate province (James *et al.*, 1992).

24.2 Arid carbonate tidal flats and evaporite sabkhas

Arid tidal flats and sabkhas along the southern shores of the Arabian (Persian) Gulf (Fig. 24.5) were intensely studied in the 1960s, in a series of classic papers (Wells & Illing, 1964; Illing *et al.*, 1965; Kinsman, 1966; Evans *et al.*, 1969). Similar, though less extremely arid, environments around the deeply indented margins of Shark Bay, Western Australia (Fig. 24.6), have also been documented by painstaking fieldwork (Logan *et al.*, 1970, 1974). Both areas are dominated by evaporation resulting from a combination of extreme aridity and high annual temperatures. Thus rainfall in Shark Bay is a variable 230 mm/yr with evaporation at 2200 mm/yr. Rainfall in the Gulf is a sporadic 40–60 mm/yr with evaporation 1500 mm/yr. The major effect of such aridity on the supratidal and high intertidal sediments is greatly increased sediment porewater salinity, which leads to evaporite precipitation (minor at Shark Bay itself) and dolomitization.

In both areas, intertidal sedimentation is dominated by the growth of stromatolitic algal mats, which show well-defined lateral zonation of growth forms due to variations in exposure. Around the Trucial Coast the intertidal algal mat zone, up to 2 km wide (Figs 24.5, 24.7–24.9; Plate 17), is broken up by an irregular network of channels and covered by discontinuous shallow ponds. Storm processes drive subtidal lagoonal sediments on to the intertidal flats and provide a major proportion of the pelletal sediment bound by the algal mats. Buried algal mat sections reached through pits in the prograding sabkha reveal that few of the detailed surface mat forms survive. This low preservation potential is caused by a combination of gypsum precipitation within the buried mat, and compaction and bacterial destruction of the organic-rich algal laminae (Park, 1976, 1977).

Low-energy environments in Shark Bay (e.g. Nilemah embayment; Woods & Brown, 1975) are dominated by continuous algal mats (Fig. 24.6). Well-laminated sediments with narrow cavities (fenestrae) occur beneath areas of smooth mat in the lower intertidal zone, whilst poorly laminated sediments with irregular fenestrae occur beneath areas of pustular mat in the middle to upper intertidal zone. Dominant grain types in the tidal flats are pellets, altered skeletal grains and intraclasts, the last named being derived as storm rip-up clasts from areas of partially lithified sediment below algal mats in the high intertidal zone. Higher-energy environments in Shark Bay are typified by the northwestern margin of the Hutchison embayment (Hagan & Logan, 1974). Here lithified algal columns and ridges (Figs 24.9 & 24.10) form a stromatolitic reef that thickens seawards. The 'reef' is associated with a beach–ridge barrier comprising large-scale, cross-stratified molluscan coquinas.

The Trucial Coast sabkhas (Figs 24.5 & 24.8) slope gently seawards at about 0.4 m/km and may be up to 16 km wide. Dolomite and a characteristic suite of evaporitic minerals occur in the shallow subsurface, the most distinctive feature being anhydrite and gypsum with nodular (chicken-mesh) and enterolithic (twisted, gut-like) textures indicative of growth of the evaporite in a carbonate matrix (Shearman, 1966) provided by the seaward-prograding carbonate

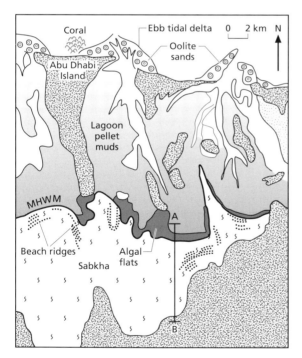

Fig. 24.5 Map to show the distribution of lithofacies in the Abu Dhabi area of the southern Arabian Gulf. A–B is the indicative location of the cross-section in Fig. 24.7. See also satellite image, Plate 17. (After Butler, 1970.)

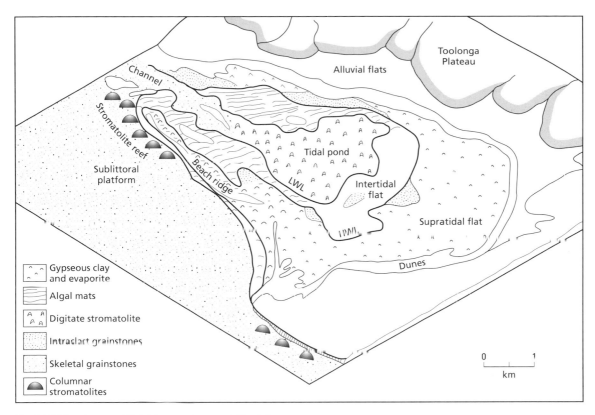

Fig. 24.6 Sketch map of Hutchison embayment, Shark Bay, Western Australia, to show intertidal flat, lagoon and stromatolite facies. LWL, low water level; HWL, high water level. (After Hagan & Logan, 1974.)

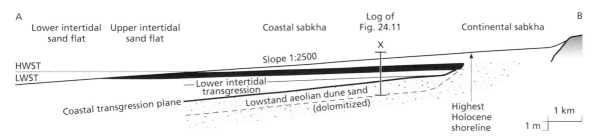

Fig. 24.7 Generalized north–south cross-section (A–B of Fig. 24.5) of the Abu Dhabi sabkha to show slope of sabkha surface and shallow subsurface Holocene progradational sediment wedge above the 7 ka transgressional plane. LWST, low water spring tide; HWST, high water spring tide. (After Evans *et al.*, 1969.)

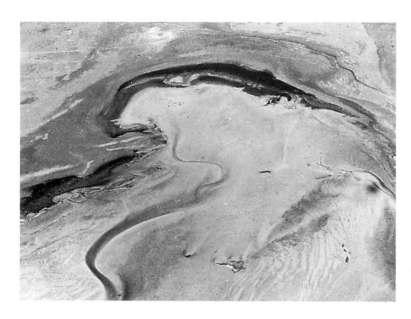

Fig. 24.8 Aerial view of lagoon/intertidal pellet sandflats, tidal channel, intertidal algal belt (black) and sabkha (S), Abu Dhabi. (Photo courtesy of R. Till.)

lagoons. The Quaternary sediments below the sabkha surface (Fig. 24.11) reveal Pleistocene lowstand dolomitized sequences (Chafetz & Rush, 1994) and evidence for a major transgressive event that modified a sandy coastal desert zone at about 7000 yr BP (Evans *et al.*, 1969). The open coastal embayment so formed was changed into a lagoon/tidal-flat complex when a small (perhaps 1 m) relative sea-level fall caused the emergence of barrier islands and restricted circulation at about 3750 yr BP. Subsequent tidal-flat progradation caused the modern sabkha flats to develop. These are now subject to storm and storm tidal processes, which periodically renew the interstitial porewaters.

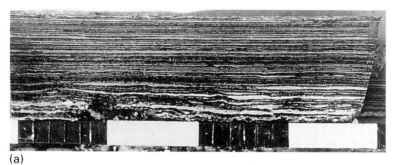

(a)

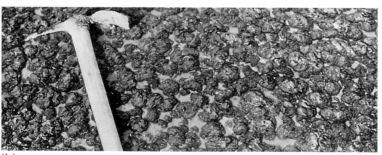

(b)

Fig. 24.9 (a) Smooth, regularly laminated algal stromatolite from the lower intertidal zone of the Trucial Coast. Note dark (algal-rich) and light (sediment-rich) interlaminations; white scale bar = 10 cm. (b) View of blister algal stromatolites from the mid-upper intertidal zone of the Trucial Coast. *Continued opposite.*

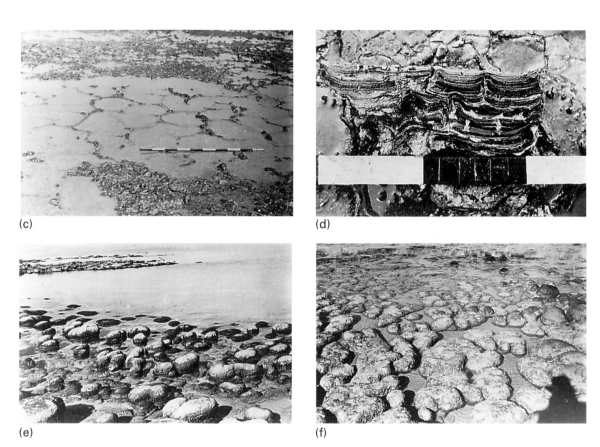

(c)
(d)
(e)
(f)

Fig. 24.9 (*continued*) (c) View of large-scale polygonal algal mat with raised rims and areas of blister mat growth, Trucial Coast. (d) Section through smooth algal mat disrupted by polygonal shrinkage cracks. Note raised rims to polygons and periodic 'healing' (e) Lithified stromatolite columns showing seaward asymmetry, Shark Bay, Western Australia. (f) Lithified stromatolitic ridges in exposed, high-energy intertidal zone of Shark Bay, Western Australia. Ridges are separated by skeletal carbonate sands and show elongation parallel with the direction of wave propagation. (Photos (a)–(d) courtesy of R. Till. Photos (e) and (f) courtesy of P.G. Harris.)

The Shark Bay tidal flats record a similar history of initial transgression (4000–5000 yr BP), sea-level fall and coastal progradation. As the supratidal surface expanded, porewater concentrations reached aragonite and gypsum precipitation levels. Gypsum is the major component in the upper intertidal and supratidal zones. A profile of the Hutchison embayment tidal-flat area is shown in Fig. 24.6.

Ancient sabkha facies have been described from many areas. Well-illustrated accounts are given by Wood and Wolfe (1969), Shearman and Fuller (1969), Fuller and Porter (1969), Holliday and Shepard-Thorne (1974) and West (1975).

24.3 Humid carbonate tidal flats and marshes

The extensive tidal flats and supratidal marshes on the west, leeward, side of Andros Island, Bahamas (Shinn *et al.*, 1969; Hardie, 1977), serve as type examples of nonevaporitic flats (Figs 24.12–24.14; Plate 16). Similar examples occur around other smaller carbonate platforms (e.g. Wanless *et al.*, 1988a,b) and the Florida Coast. A tropical maritime climate with winter storms and occasional hurricanes prevails in the area with mean annual rainfall of about 130 cm/yr (range 65–230 cm/yr). This abundant rainwater freshens the

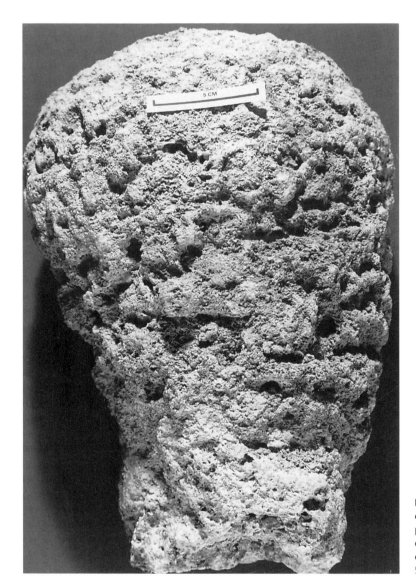

Fig. 24.10 Single lithified Shark Bay columnar stromatolite head with pustulose mat growth forms. Head comprises algal-bound and aragonite-cemented skeletal debris. Scale bar is 5 cm.

supratidal marsh during summer months and prevents development of sabkha-type evaporites. Salinities of the tidal waters usually fall in the range 39–42‰ but may fall as low as 5‰ after heavy rainfall. This periodic freshwater 'flushing' creates a 'high-stress' environment and is responsible for a restricted biota on the flats. The semidiurnal tides have a mean maximum range of 0.5 m, but the tidal range is much affected by periodic storm surges. Wave action is not usually important because of the sheltered nature of Great

Bahama Bank lagoon. The tidal-flat sediments are dominantly pelleted carbonate muds, with < 10% of skeletal material, dominantly foraminifera, and extensive algal mats. Three major subenvironments may be defined (Shinn *et al.*, 1969; Hardie, 1977; Fig. 24.12): (a) nearshore marine belt, (b) tidal-flat complex of channels with levees and tidal ponds, and (c) supratidal algal marsh.

The nearshore marine belt comprises thoroughly bioturbated, muddy pelletal sands loosely bound by

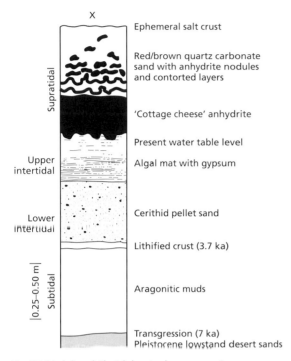

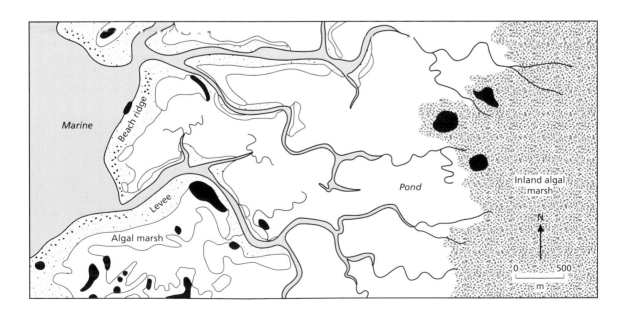

Fig. 24.11 (*above*) Sketch log to show regressive highstand sabkha–lagoon sequence overlying lowstand aeolian sands produced at position X in Fig. 24.7. (After Till, 1978.)

a surface 'scum' of algae. Callianassid (crustacean) burrows are particularly common. The exposed shorelines between channel openings are beach ridges with terraces and washover fans. The latter comprise intraclast gravels and rippled sands showing well-developed internal laminations. Similar facies, with lithified intertidal beachrocks, make up much of the eastern, windward, coastline of Andros Island.

The intertidal flats, partly protected by the beach ridges, are cut by a dense tidal channel network (Fig. 24.12). The channels are 1–100 m wide and 0.2–3 m deep. They meander but show little evidence of lateral migration, in contrast to channels on temperate siliciclastic tidal flats. The channels contain lag gravels of skeletal debris, intraclasts and fragments of Pleistocene bedrock. The channel banks and stationary point bars are heavily bioturbated by crabs and overgrown by mangroves, and are covered by complex hemispherical stromatolite heads. Sections through these heads reveal well-preserved domal laminae with abundant uncalcified filaments of the

Fig. 24.12 (*below*) Map to show the environments of deposition in the Three Creeks area, leeward shore of Andros Island, Bahamas (see also Plate 16). Dark patches indicate the occurrence of cemented surface crusts. (After Hardie & Garrett, 1977.)

Inland algal marsh
Channelled belt
Offshore marine
Pinelands
Periodic hurricane layers
Buried channel
Channel
X
Pond
Levee
Beach ridge
+1
Sea level
0
−1
−2 m
X
Pleistocene bedrock
Thin-bedded to thick laminated
Thinly laminated
Bioturbated

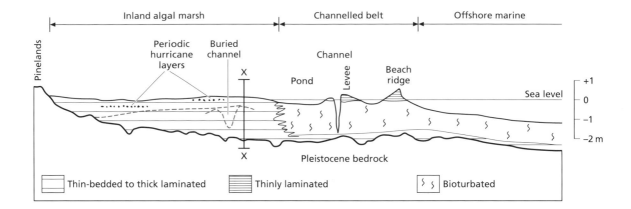

Fig. 24.13 Schematic section through the Three Creeks tidal flats shown in Fig. 24.12. Section assumes that Holocene progradation of the shoreline has occurred since highstand. (Modified after Hardie & Ginsburg, 1977.)

Fig. 24.14 Schematic log at position X, adjacent to an earlier Holocene beach–channel complex, of Fig. 24.13 to illustrate general nature of the progradational sequence.

sediment-binding alga *Schizothrix calcicola*. The channel levees are only rarely covered by tidal waters and are coated by a thin algal mat. Sections reveal a fine millimetre-scale lamination without disruptions. The levee toes show small desiccation cracks.

In between adjacent channels lie extensive tidal ponds bounded by algal marshes. The ponds are frequently covered by tidal waters and the muddy sediment has a thin surface algal mat that is grazed by

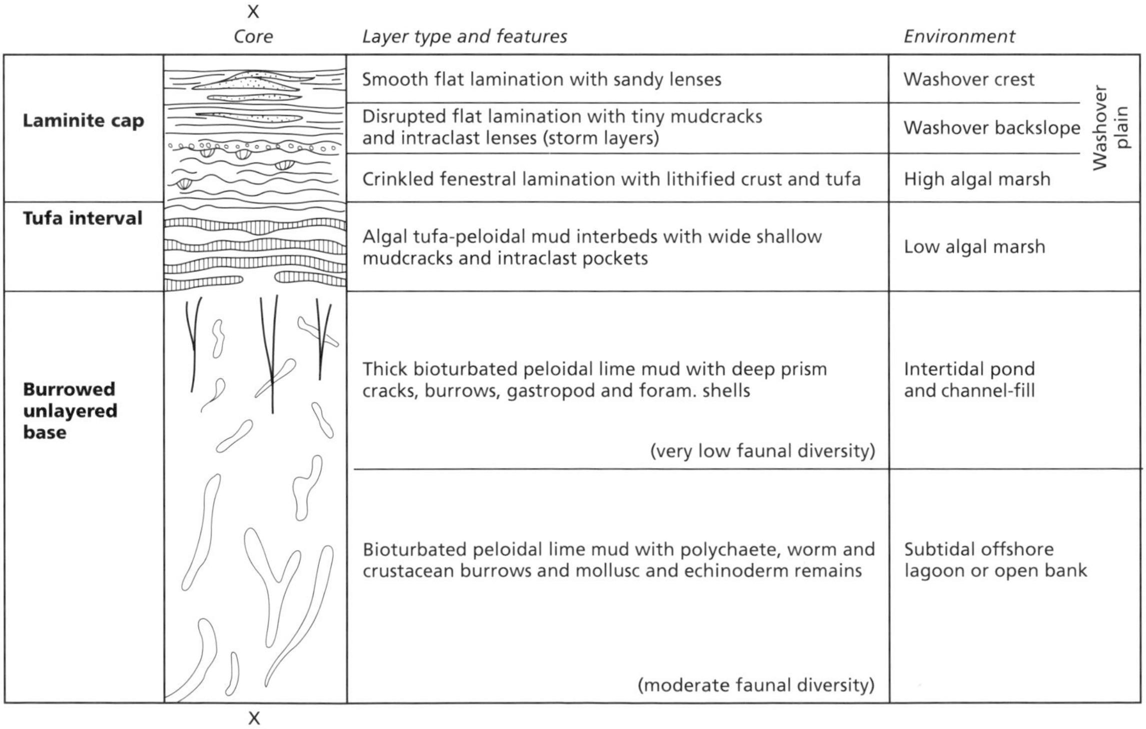

X
Core
Layer type and features
Environment
Laminite cap
Smooth flat lamination with sandy lenses
Washover crest
Disrupted flat lamination with tiny mudcracks and intraclast lenses (storm layers)
Washover backslope
Washover plain
Crinkled fenestral lamination with lithified crust and tufa
High algal marsh
Tufa interval
Algal tufa-peloidal mud interbeds with wide shallow mudcracks and intraclast pockets
Low algal marsh
Burrowed unlayered base
Thick bioturbated peloidal lime mud with deep prism cracks, burrows, gastropod and foram. shells
(very low faunal diversity)
Intertidal pond and channel-fill
Bioturbated peloidal lime mud with polychaete, worm and crustacean burrows and mollusc and echinoderm remains
(moderate faunal diversity)
Subtidal offshore lagoon or open bank
X

cerithid gastropods and polychaete worms. Sections reveal unlayered, bioturbated pelletal muds cut by deep (up to 30 cm) desiccation cracks that form during winter and spring low-water periods. The fringing algal marshes comprise a high marsh with continuous algal mats of the freshwater genus *Scytonema* and a low marsh with 'pincushion' growths of *Scytonema*. Patchy cementation by high-magnesian calcite and aragonite occurs, sections through the mats revealing a well developed crinkly lamination with fenestrae (see Fig. 24.14). The laminations seen in tidal-flat sediments are thought to be due to sporadic onshore winter storms (generated by southward-pushing cold fronts), which suspend and transport lagoonal sediments onshore.

The inland algal marsh lies about 20 cm above the mean high-water level of the channelled tidal flats. A similar zonation of low 'pincushion' marsh to high 'carpet' marsh occurs as noted above from around the tidal ponds. No invertebrates live in this marsh, which may be up to 8 km wide. The *Scytonema* algal mats are frequently lithified by high-magnesian calcite, forming a discontinuous algal tufa. Desiccated mats give rise to characteristic polygon heads as the algae attempt to heal over the upturned polygon rims. Sections through the inland marsh reveal up to 1.7 m of laminated sediment with abundant fenestrae (see below). These marsh laminae (1–10 mm thick) are tropical storm layers, the result of periodic hurricane-driven sheet floods, which carry lagoonal pelletal sediments on to and over the entire tidal flat and marsh—see data of Wanless *et al.* (1988a, b) for Hurricane Kate on the Caicos platform. The initially cross-laminated sediment is then bound by renewed *Scytonema* growth and the laminae preserved. The fenestrae are predominantly horizontal sheet cracks with subordinate vertical 'palisade' cracks. They form as primary voids from air pockets and as secondary voids from bacterial breakdown of algal filaments in vertical and horizontal layers and clusters. Lithification of the mats obviously enhances the preservation potential of the fenestrae. Indeed, spar-filled fenestrae ('birds-eye' fabric) in ancient carbonate sediments can (but see Shinn, 1983) provide good evidence of high intertidal to supratidal origin in ancient carbonate sediments.

Lateral and vertical sections through the entire Bahamian tidal-flat complex are shown in Figs 24.13 and 24.14. Note that the supratidal zone contrasts markedly with arid tropical sabkhas. It is evaporite-free and it contains lithified algal tufa of freshwater-dominated marsh origin. The calcified *Scytonema* filaments and fenestrae in the latter serve to distinguish the stromatolites from the unlithified algal peats found in the intertidal zone of the Arabian Gulf.

Ancient analogues of Bahamian-type tidal-flat and marsh deposits, sometimes with good evidence for wildly fluctuating fresh to saline conditions (schizohaline state), are to be found in the Triassic Lofer Cycles of Austria (Fischer, 1964, 1975; Hardie, 1977), the Devonian Manlius facies of the central Appalachians (Laporte, 1971), the Precambrian of South Africa (Eriksson, 1977) and, widely, in the Purbeckian of Tethyan to southern Boreal Europe (Francis, 1984; Strasser, 1988).

24.4 Shorefaces, lagoons and bays

Subtropical carbonate lagoons and bays are relatively quiet-water environments periodically traversed by storms and hurricanes. They typify 'detached' shorelines, being partially separated from open marine environments by low offshore islands of lithified Pleistocene limestones (Arabian Gulf), reefs (Honduras, Great Barrier), or a combination of the two (Florida, Bahamas). These fringing 'rims' (like siliciclastic barriers or spits) protect the lagoons and bays to a greater or lesser extent from onshore winds and hence the effects of waves. Tidal currents are forced to enter the lagoons via narrow inlets. Efficient tidal exchange may keep lagoons close to oceanic salinity, but in arid tropical areas high evaporation of the shallow water bodies may cause salinity to rise as high as 67‰ (Abu Dhabi). In humid tropical areas lagoonal and bay water may be considerably freshened by freshwater runoff from the tidal flats and hinterland (West Coast of Andros Island, Florida Bay). Thus, for the most part, shallow coastal lagoons and bays tend to be 'high-stress' environments and a restricted biota occurs.

Lagoonal sediments usually comprise pelleted lime muds, with decreasing amounts of mud as wave action increases in importance. The wave-stirred Trucial Coast lagoons, for example, are floored by pellet sands. The current-scoured outer Florida lagoon (Fig. 24.15) is floored by a winnowed lag of skeletal debris. Pellets are excreted by crabs, cerithid gastropods and polychaete worms. Aragonite mud

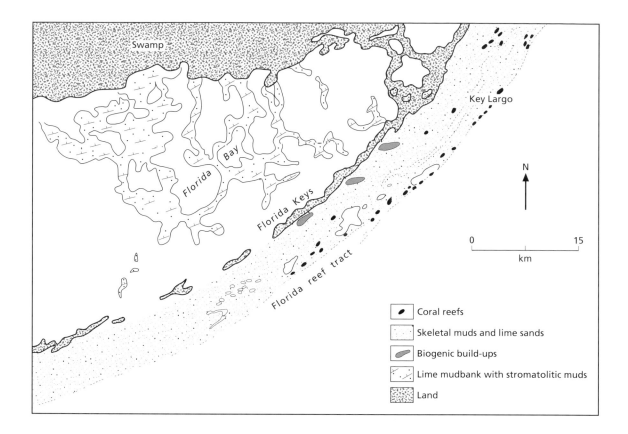

Fig. 24.15 Recent sedimentary facies of south Florida. See also Plate 15. (After Griffith *et al.*, 1969.)

is predominantly of algal origin in the inner Florida and Honduras lagoons, coccoliths being an important contributor in the latter area (Matthews, 1966). Controversy still rages as to the origin of Bahamian bank-top lagoonal aragonite muds, but the very detailed exploration of aragonite whitings by Shinn *et al.* (1989), and chemical (Milliman *et al.*, 1993) and morphological evidence (Loreau, 1982) on the Great Bahamas Bank, indicate that most is probably chemical in origin and not resuspended algal material (see Chapter 3). Minor skeletal debris usually comprises foraminifera and molluscs. Most lagoons support a thriving infauna, particularly crabs, which effectively destroy any primary laminations. *Thalassia* (seagrass) stands occur in Florida Bay and the Bahamas and Arabian lagoons. In the inner part of Florida Bay the *Thalassia* banks act as sediment baffles and have

built up numerous winding mud mounds and islands that show vertical and lateral accretion trends with time (Enos & Perkins, 1979). Patch reefs occur in many lagoons and are surrounded by a halo of coarse, reef-derived bioclastic grains. Variations in Holocene lagoonal sediment thickness are caused by differential topography of the lithified Pleistocene bedrock surfaces that underlie the lagoons. Some of this topography reflects the relief of buried karst (Purdy, 1974). Hurricanes may have temporary smoothing effects on depositional topography of bays and lagoons and lead to the infill and abandonment of open burrows like those of callianassid shrimps (Wanless *et al.*, 1988b). The long-term trend in bays/lagoons like those of Florida is for coastal progradation to occur behind the barrier reef as islands coalesce and are replaced by coastal mangrove swamps and a supratidal zone with shallow lakes (see Enos & Perkins, 1979). Carbonate sediment budget studies in Bahamian lagoons reveal a substantial overproduction compared with accurately dated deposition rates

(Neumann & Land, 1975; Boardman & Neumann, 1984). This is accounted for by storm and tidal current export of bank-top lagoonal sediment, mostly chemically precipitated aragonite (Shinn *et al.*, 1989; Milliman *et al.*, 1993), to periplatform areas.

Strandline carbonate sequences of Holocene age facing high-energy, open marine environments are rare, probably because of the predominance of offshore reef build-ups. An interesting example of a late-Pleistocene wave-dominated beach–ridge plain has been documented from the Yucatan Peninsula of Mexico by Ward and Brady (1979). Here a 7 m sequence of shoreface to beachface grainstones, including common ooids in the upper shoreface, accumulated in a seaward-prograding coastal plain that was up to 4 km wide and 150 km long at its maximum extent. The interesting, and perplexing, thing about this occurrence is the fact that the entire high-energy coastal-plain sequence prograded behind a contemporary offshore barrier reef that obviously had no discernible 'protective' influence further inshore (see previous comments on the Great Barrier Reef).

In the ancient carbonate record, Francis (1984), Strasser (1988) and Joachimski (1994) give accounts of shoaling-upwards sequences produced by the seaward progradation of ramp peritidal (often schizohaline) environments.

24.5 Enhanced-salinity bays and embayments

Carbonate sedimentation in the bays of unrimmed, indented coastlines is best illustrated by further brief reference to Shark Bay, Western Australia. The general absence of freshwater input and imperfect tidal flushing causes a general landward increase of salinity up to 70‰. The hypersaline portions of the bay are dominated by a monotypic coquina of the small bivalve *Fragum hamelini*, which is salinity-tolerant. These subtidal coquinas fringe the arid tidal flats discussed previously. The metahaline and oceanic parts of the bay are dominated by spectacular sea-grass-bound carbonate build-ups. These have topographic relief on the seafloor, lack an internal skeletal frame, and are composed of *in situ* and locally derived skeletal carbonate from the grass epibiota and sheltered benthos (Davies, 1970; Hagan & Logan, 1974). Skeletal breakdown causes much silt- and mud-grade material to be admixed with the coarser debris of molluscan, algal and foraminiferal origins. The build-ups occur as fringing, patch and barrier types. There is a vertical trend as the sea-grass meadows accrete upwards towards mean tide level from matrix-rich skeletal packstones and wackestones to well-washed skeletal grainstones.

24.6 Tidal delta and margin-spillover carbonate tidal sands

There is close correlation between strong tidal currents and oolite formation, although the presence of the former is not always accompanied by the latter. Tidal currents are amplified as they pass on to the rimmed Bahamian shelf or into the Trucial Coast lagoons through constrictions in reefal barriers tidal inlets. Active oolite and skeletal carbonate sand shoals result as ebb and flood tidal deltas. By way of contrast, the high-energy carbonate sand belt of the southwestern Florida Keys (around and to the west of Marquesas Keys) lacks ooliths (Shinn *et al.*, 1990). Here skeletal (algal/coral) sands are moulded into dune-like bedforms, which laterally accrete westwards under the influence of strong north–south directed tidal currents.

On the Bahamas Bank, active oolite shoals form at many localities around the perimeter (Illing, 1954; Purdy, 1963; Ball, 1967; Harris, 1979; Hine *et al.*, 1981b). The shoals take the form of flood tidal deltas and storm spillover lobes. The lobes have an axial channel and may be up to 1 km long and 0.5 km wide. The lobes terminate at steeply dipping 'noses' and show internal large-scale foresets up to 1.75 m high. Smaller lobes superimposed on the larger forms show variable ebb and flood orientations. Lobes are covered by current ripple and dune bedforms, which travel parallel to the lobe long axes. The larger spillover lobes may be active only when onshore storms or hurricanes assist the normal flood tidal currents. The active oolite shoals disappear bankwards, replaced by a stabilized oolite and grapestone sands covered with a thin subtidal algal mat and *Thalassia* stands. In other areas, notably the inter-shoal channels of southern Exuma Islands, giant (up to 2 m high) variously shaped stromatolites, some analogous (in external form at least) to the well-known Shark's Bay examples, exist *within* active dunefields (see Dill *et al.*, 1986; Shapiro *et al.*, 1995). They nucleated on to highs on underlying Pleistocene lowstand karst.

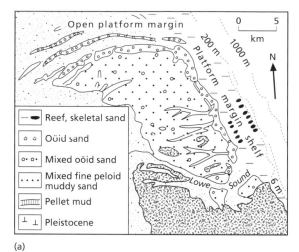

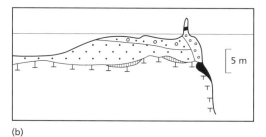

(a)

(b)

Fig. 24.16 (a) Environments around Joulters Oolite Shoal, Bahamas. The shoal is a shallow sandflat (fine stipple), cut by tidal channels and fringed on the ocean side by mobile sands (coarse stipple). (b) Section to show the vertical and lateral distributions of facies: note oceanwards and vertical coarsening-upwards pattern.

The growths are periodically constructed by sediment-binding activities of filamentous green algae, cyanobacteria and diatoms, destruction occurring by the activities of boring sponges and molluscs, endolithic algae and grazing fish. Growth and decay alternate in a complex series of events as the stromatolites are alternately exposed and buried by dune migration.

Lateral facies changes from bank edge to lagoon are well illustrated by the Joulters Cay Shoal (Harris, 1979; Fig. 24.16). Here the site of active ooid sands is located as a windward fringe, 4 m thick, with an extensive bankward spread of altered ooids mixed with skeletal grains and aragonitic muds. The muds are stabilized by grasses and algal films, are extensively bioturbated and are up to 10 m thick. There is an

upward trend towards less mud within the inactive interior shoal. Numerous horizons within the interior shoal show penecontemporaneous cementation in areas of stabilized bottom covered by algal scum.

Distinctive oolite shoals occur in the Schooners Cay area at the north end of Exuma Sound (Ball, 1967). Here the shoals take the form of linear tidal ridges whose long axes are parallel to the dominant flood tidal currents. Individual ridges are up to 8 km long and 750 m wide with amplitudes of about 5 m. Spillover lobes occur with their long axes orientated subparallel to the ridge long axes. They indicate a component of on-bank flow that is reflected in the asymmetry of the ridges, whose steeper sides are directed bankwards. Ripples and dunes superimposed upon the ridges are also orientated bankwards. Flow in the channels separating ridges is dominantly parallel to the ridge long axes. These linear ridges are very similar to those described from clastic tidally influenced shelves (Chapter 25) and are expected to show the same internal structures, i.e. cross-sets dipping obliquely to perpendicularly with respect to the ridge long axis. The ridges overlie burrowed muddy pelletal sands. Penecontemporaneous cementation may occur in the channel floors between the active oolite ridges.

Ancient oolitic complexes are well described from the Pleistocene of Florida (Halley *et al.*, 1977) and the Middle Jurassic of northwest Europe (e.g. Sellwood & McKerrow, 1973; Purser, 1979).

24.7 Open carbonate shelf ramps

As noted previously, the majority of Holocene carbonate sediments are being formed on rimmed platform margins, and thus few studies of modern open carbonate shelves or ramps may be found in the literature. Since Mesozoic to Recent hexacoral reef development is hindered by the production of excess nutrients (see Section 24.8), we might expect that ancient and modern ramps are preferentially located in seas close to the sites of oceanic upwelling. This is certainly the case with the Arabian Gulf inshore of the Arabian Sea upwelling. Over most of its area (Pilkey & Noble, 1967) the shelf waters show salinities between normal seawater values and 42%. In shallow coastal areas (5–30 m deep) skeletal grainstones comprising well-rounded and well-sorted molluscan, foraminiferal, algal and (localized) coral debris are accumulating. In deeper offshore areas (> 30 m) sorting becomes poorer and skeletal fragments are more angular, their sharp fracture surfaces perhaps being caused by *in situ* mechanical breakdown. Increasing admixtures of silt- and mud-grade low-magnesian calcite occur in deeper areas, giving rise to packstone and wackestone fabrics and, ultimately, marls. The fines are thought to be derived from wind-blown carbonate dusts. Although 'whitings' of precipitated aragonite mud occur periodically in the Gulf, no trace of this aragonite has been recorded in the offshore sediments. Much of the Gulf shelf is covered by a thin, lithified subtidal hardground (Shinn, 1969) that supports a specialized epifauna adapted to hard substrate life. This cemented horizon indicates low offshore productivity and sedimentation rates.

The Yucatan shelf (Ginsburg & James, 1974) is a ramp with an inner zone 130–190 km wide extending down to depths of 60 m where a zone of relict Quaternary build-ups occurs along the shelf break. The modern sedimentary cover comprises a thin layer of molluscan debris, everywhere less than 1 m thick. At the shelf break there are build-ups associated with relict Quaternary lime sands with ooids, peloids and lithoclasts. At greater depths these nonskeletal sands are increasingly diluted with the tests of winnowed pelagic foraminifera. This pattern of relict outer-shelf facies and contemporary inner-shelf molluscan debris occurs on most tropical or subtropical clastic-free shelves, emphasizing the extreme importance of the shallow subtidal carbonate 'factory' as a sediment producer.

Cool-water carbonate ramp deposits occur widely on the New Zealand (Nelson *et al.*, 1988) and Southern Australia shelves. The Lacepede Shelf, South Australia (James *et al.*, 1992), for example, is a gently sloping, ramp-like feature (Fig. 24.3b) that extends from the siliciclastic beach ridges bordering the Coorong Lagoons, of which more later, down to a shelf break at about 200 m. Although the NW margins of the Coorong Lagoons mark the site of the large Murray River, little clastic sediment reaches the shelf from the now-restricted lower reaches of this sluggish system. The outer shelf from about 100 m depth slopes more steeply oceanwards into the canyoned slope and hence into the adjacent abyssal plain. The wide shallow shelf is mostly at depths of 40–60 m and is dominated by a swell wave regime of high (> 2.5 m), long-period (> 12 s) modal waves. During the summer

the shelf water mass is stratified with surface waters of temperature 18 °C overlying a thermocline at 30–80 m and bottom waters of about 13 °C. The shelf waters are well mixed during the winter, with mean temperatures of around 18 °C down to depths of 100 m. The distribution of facies contrasts markedly in several ways with those on low-latitude warm carbonate shelf ramps and platforms. Sediment types include various proportions of terrigenous clastic sands and silts, relict skeletal carbonates of pre-Holocene strandlines and 'modern' skeletal carbonate materials, chiefly bryozoan and mollusc sands and gravels. These latter are never dominant in shallow-water areas, usually representing at most 45% of the total and mainly comprising abraded mollusc debris sourced from storm-wave-reworked infaunal bivalves. The main carbonate production comes from an outer-shelf 'bryozoan factory' at depths greater than about 80 m, below the depth of high abrasive stresses on animal and plant communities but well above the swell wave base. Here the bryozoan-rich carbonates are coarse detritus sourced from production (including calcareous algae) on harder substrates lithified by lowstand carbonate precipitation. The deposits are frequently moved by winter swell waves and sorted into rippled patches. Below about 150 m the sediment becomes muddier and generally finer, reflecting the growth of more fragile bryozoan species. The location of the main carbonate factory on the outer shelf has important implications for ancient cool-water facies models for wave-dominated regimes. Also important is the close proximity of this factory to the edge of the slope and thus the expectation that significant losses of carbonate occur downslope.

Many examples of ancient open carbonate ramp/ shelf facies have been described, including Wilson's (1975) pioneering work and Kerans *et al.*'s (1994) more recent work on the Smackover Formation of Texas. Lavoie (1995) presents a brave attempt at analysing an Ordovician carbonate unit in terms of a temperate-water ramp environment.

24.8 Platform margin reefs and carbonate build-ups generally

Modern carbonate platforms are frequently rimmed by reefal (predominantly coral) carbonate build-ups, which control, to a greater (Bahamas) or lesser (Queensland) extent, the resultant distribution of carbonate facies on the platform itself because of their influence on the physical processes of wind, wave and tide. But as we go back into the geological record, the composition, depth distribution and influence of build-ups have changed. Embrey and Klovan (1971), Wilson (1975) and James and Gravestock (1990) define the following terms, which are used, somewhat variably, by authorities on build-ups and reefs:

- *Calcimicrobes*—calcified microbial fossils (a 'dust-bin' term for a large group of ancient problematica, including suspected cyanobacteria, etc.) with a very long geological history that are increasingly seen to play an important role in strengthening the basic coral framework of modern and ancient reefs (Camoin & Montaggioni, 1994) and also in cementing non-framework build-ups such as the Miocene *Halimeda* mounds described by Braga *et al.* (1996).
- *Carbonate* boundstone—a reefal fabric in a limestone characterized by few metazoan fossil remains but with features indicative of 'antigravitational' carbonate trapping, cementation or binding often associated with calcimicrobes.
- *Carbonate build-up*—mostly organic bodies of locally formed and laterally restricted carbonate sediment that possesses topographic relief.
- *Carbonate mound*—equidimensional or ellipsoidal build-up.
- *Carbonate pinnacle*—conical or steep-sided upward-tapering mound.
- *Patch reef*—small isolated subaqueous circular build-up in shallow water.
- *Knoll reef*—small isolated subaqueous circular build-up in deeper water.
- *Atoll*—ring-like organic accumulation projecting to surface, surrounding a lagoon.
- *Barrier island reef*—curvilinear belt projecting to sea level (often made up of individual wall reefs) of organic accumulation, steep to seawards, situated somewhat offshore and separated from the coast by a lagoon or broad shelf.
- *Shelf-edge reef*—submerged in 15–60 m water, relict or actively growing sometimes deeper-water corals, often buttressed and grooved to windward (see Blanchon & Jones, 1997).
- *Fringe reef*—belt of organic accumulation built out directly from the shoreline.

The very existence of a carbonate build-up depends upon a local carbonate production rate that exceeds that of surrounding areas in which excess production

is conserved. Some surplus production may be locally or regionally exported. The higher production measured over the Holocene mounds off the Florida Keys for example (Bosence *et al.*, 1985) is due to the localized growth of standing crops of the green algae *Neogoniolithon* and *Halimeda* and the coral *Porites*. Coring reveals that the gravel-grade sediments of the modern mound are derived from *in situ* breakdown at a rate of about 2 mm/yr. Early microbially mediated cementation just below the sediment–water interface must also play a role in preventing sediment export by tide and wave and in stabilizing nonframework build-ups such as Palaeozoic phylloid algae and the Cretaceous-to-modern green alga *Halimeda* (Braga *et al.*, 1996).

Relatively low-energy ramp margins of the geological record (Fig. 24.17) contain a remarkable variety of (predominantly) downslope build-ups of microbiologically precipitated carbonate mud, *in situ* skeletons and organic detritus. The finer-grained build-ups evidently formed below storm wave base (depths > 100 m). The build-ups take the form of mounds, linear fringes, ridges or barriers, perhaps best seen in the spectacularly exhumed Middle Devonian of the Algerian Sahara (Wendt *et al.*, 1993, 1997; Figs 24.18 & 24.19), where contemporary water depths are thought to have been of the order of 100–200 m. The cementing, binding, trapping and/or baffling organisms may be calcimicrobes, as in many Proterozoic and Palaeozoic reefs (Turner *et al.*, 1993; Narbonne & James, 1996; Wendt *et al.*, 1997), calcified sponges and primitive coral-like ancestors in the earliest (Lower Cambrian) shallow-water metazoan reefs (Savarese *et al.*, 1993; Wood *et al.*, 1993), bryozoans (Ordovician–Permian), platy algae (upper Carboniferous), crinoids (Silurian–Carboniferous), rudist bivalves (Cretaceous), the green alga *Halimeda* (Cretaceous–Recent) and marine grasses (Tertiary–Recent). Proof of topographic relief on ancient build-ups revolves around recognition of contemporary, nontectonic dips using boundstone markers, internal sediment, sparry calcite spirit levels and talus spreads tonguing out from the build-up flanks. Sea-level fluctuations may impress karstic phenomena upon the build-up framework (see Narbonne & James, 1996), sometimes accentuating evidence for build-up slopes. Recent studies (Harris, 1993) of the famous Triassic Latemar platform margin in the Dolomites (see also section 24.9) reveals that a narrow reefal build-up here comprised

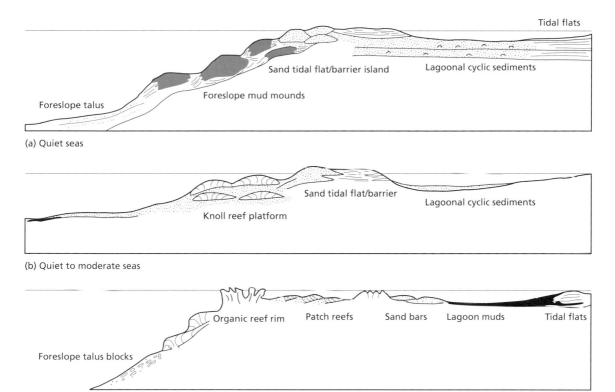

(a) Quiet seas

(b) Quiet to moderate seas

(c) Rough seas

Fig. 24.17 The three types of build-ups at ancient and modern carbonate platform/shelf margins defined by Wilson (1975). (a) Downslope mud mound accumulations of relatively quiet-water seas (common as Waulsortian facies of the upper Palaeozoic). (b) Knoll reef platforms of moderate-energy (periodic hurricane-swept) margins like those of Florida. (c) Robust hexacoral reef-rimmed platform of high-energy seas (Great Barrier Reef and many others). In each case the energy levels in the back-build-up lagoons and bays may be highly variable depending on the efficacy of the wave damping exerted by the coastal zone.

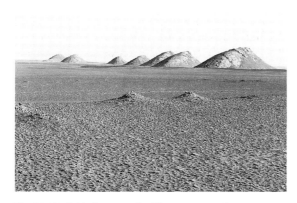

Fig. 24.18 Field photograph of linear group of seven spectacular exhumed Devonian build-ups of the Algerian Sahara, each 25–30 m high. (Photo courtesy of A.J. Wendt.)

wave-resistant boundstones involving the microscopic problematica *Tubiphytes* and a variety of organic crustal carbonate growths and cements, but very little skeletal framework support.

No subtidal ramp is *dominated* by framework-poor build-ups at the present day, but mounds of *Halimeda* are common in waters 20–50 m deep on many carbonate platform margins (e.g. Queensland; Orme *et al.*, 1978). The *Thalassia*-bound build-ups of Shark Bay (see Section 24.2) and Florida Bay represent modern examples in 'lagoonal' environments. Deep-water build-ups on the flanks of the Bahamas platform (Neumann *et al.*, 1977; Mullins & Neumann, 1979) provide important modern analogues to ancient lime mud mounds (Lees & Miller, 1985).

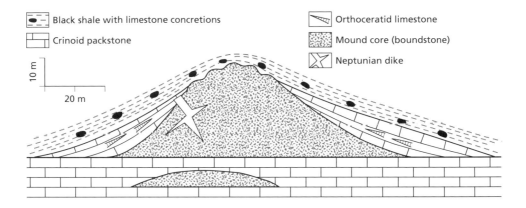

Black shale with limestone concretions

Crinoid packstone

Orthoceratid limestone

Mound core (boundstone)

Neptunian dike

10 m

20 m

Fig. 24.19 Schematic restored section of the Algerian Devonian mud mounds featured in Fig. 24.18. Note overlying black shales suggesting nutrient-induced termination of build-up. (From Wendt *et al.*, 1997.)

Intermediate- to high-energy shoalwater margins (Fig. 24.17) comprise framebuilt reef rims that grow up to or close to mean sea level (but prolifically from 15 m to as deep as 60 m). Mesozoic to Holocene examples are dominantly scleractinian coral associations and occur where sunlight radiation levels that benefit the coral–algal symbionts are at maximum; hence they grow into the zone of greatest storm or hurricane wave energy. They form barrier, fringing or shelf-edge reefs (preferentially on the windward coastlines of carbonate platforms) and are zoned ecologically in parallel belts, with their hexacoral growth forms (platy, domal or branching—see Blanchon & Jones, 1997) precisely reflecting light intensity, sediment concentration, exposure level and energy levels (James & Ginsburg, 1979; Chappell, 1980; Hallock & Schlager, 1986; Hallock, 1988). It is likely that microbial crusts play an important role in protecting and strengthening the primary coral framework in some examples (Camoin & Montaggioni, 1994). The reefs usually show steep seaward slopes with abundant reef talus and the majority show, or are expected to show, seawards lateral accretion with time as the reef spurs and ridges move uncertainly seawards (interrupted by hurricane disruptions) over their substrate of talus. Recent data from the Grand Cayman shelf-edge reef (Blanchon & Jones, 1997) reveal that the seaward reef wall at depths of 15 to 60 m is variably buttressed and channelled according to the

degree of exposure to hurricane-induced storm wave (and presumably gradient) currents (Fig. 24.20). The Great Barrier Reef of the Queensland coast of Australia (Maxwell & Swinchatt, 1970) has well-developed linear wall reefs at the steep gradient shelf edges in the northern and southern sectors (where tidal currents are also at maximum) and a variety of fringing, ring and concentric platform reefs scattered across the gently sloping shelf (really a ramp, see previous discussions) to the landwards until a coastal zone of siliciclastics is reached. Framebuilt reefs support not only a highly diverse coral community but also a flourishing reefal epifauna and infauna (often destructive) of molluscs, echinoids, coralline algae, microbial crusts and foraminifera.

Sand fringes in the backreef and forereef areas of Queensland, Florida and the Bahamas are often dominated by calcareous algal fragments, particularly *Halimeda*, coral not being a good sand-former. In the Floridan reef tract the extensive backreef environment, with its patch reefs and sublittoral coral/algal sand spreads, grades into the backreef lagoon. The seaward margins to the Belize barrier and atoll reefs (James & Ginsburg, 1979) comprise four facies belts passing seawards from the reef front. The reef front down to 70 m depth comprises coarse coral and *Halimeda* sands and conglomerates with grainstone fabrics. The reef wall (65–120 m) is made up of well-cemented coral-rich limestones, which yield ages in the range 8000–15 000 yr BP. The forereef talus fans comprise muddy *Halimeda* sands showing packstone and wackestone fabrics. Cements in the reef wall include common high-magnesian calcite and subordinate aragonite. Isotopic and trace-element analyses

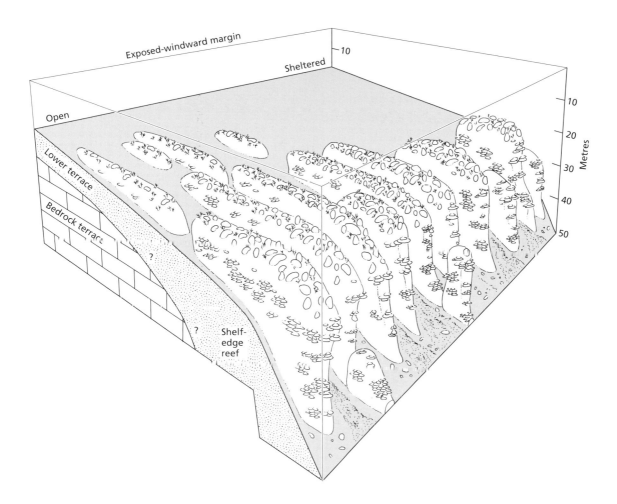

Fig. 24.20 Drawing to show the highly elongated buttressed spurs and embayed talus spreads typical of domed growths of *Acropora palmata* corals situated on exposed high-energy reef margins. The trend to more sheltered conditions is also shown, with the elongated spurs being replaced by more equidimensional 'crowned' growths at depths > 20 m. (Drawing courtesy of P. Blanchon; see Blanchon & Jones, 1997.)

prove the marine origins of these cements. James and Ginsburg (1979) propose an accretionary model for the seaward margin to the Belize platform, with erosion during lowstand, and rapid coral growth 'plastering' the reef wall during sea-level rise. Reef wall growth is thus envisaged as a discontinuous lateral accretion process, with submarine cementation occurring after each period of accretion.

A similar pattern of offshore 'stranded' shallow-water reefs formed by rapid accretion accompanying the Holocene sea-level rise is found off the Florida shelf margin. These relict reefs are now colonized by deeper-water communities and form a characteristic stepped profile offshore. The reason for their demise (see Macintyre, 1988) is not simply 'drowning', since *Acropora palmata*, the main shallow-water reef-building species, is capable of growth rates of 10–15 mm/yr, easily matching the rate of sea-level rise. Increased mid-Holocene turbidity, higher nutrient levels (see below) and the invasion of cold water masses during wintertime may have all contributed.

In important contributions to our understanding of the controls upon Mesozoic to Recent hexacoral reef development (Fig. 24.21), Hallock and Schlager (1986) and Hallock (1988) point out that all reef

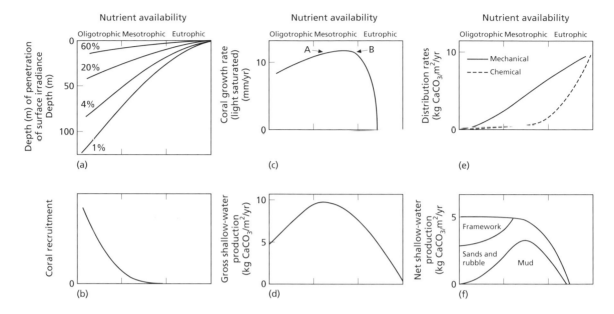

Fig. 24.21 Hallock's (1988) attempt to illustrate how several parameters associated with reef development change as nutrient availability increases from oligotrophic (phosphate levels often < 0.1 μM), through mesotrophic to oligotrophic (often > 1 μM).

development hinges upon the ability of the framework-building corals to achieve growth rates that exceed the local bio-erosion rate. Now, high nutrient availability affects bio-erosion, competition and coral growth, the former two by encouraging the growth of coral predators and competing 'fleshy' algae and the latter by making the corals excrete excess mucus, which encourages bacterial attack on the coral–algal community, so killing them. Since coastal upwelling often controls the amount of nutrient supplied, it follows that coral reefs should be largely absent amongst the carbonate platform margins of upwelling coastlines, a prediction that concurs with observation.

A second control on reef development is rate of sea-level rise. Even the fast-growing *Acropora palmata* may be overwhelmed by extremely high short-term glacial meltout rates attributable to catastrophic ice-sheet reorganization (Blanchon & Shaw, 1995). The result is a series of drowned reef crests at depths of about 80, 50 and 15 m in the Caribbean area, each correlated with rates of sea-level rise of > 45 mm/yr.

Long before the days of sequence stratigraphy, Purdy (1974) drew attention to the effects that Quaternary

sea-level oscillations have had upon reef development. He amplified MacNeil's (1954) hypothesis of karst-induced effects upon atoll and barrier reef morphology. His antecedent karst theory envisages lowstand sub-aerial exposure of a limestone platform surrounded by a relatively steep structural or depositional slope. $CaCO_3$ dissolution is concentrated in the middle of atoll-like offshore banks and on the landward flanks of barrier-like ramps. Karstic rims and tower karsts acted as nuclei for coral growth during rising sea level to produce the present-day atoll rims, barrier reefs and lagoonal pinnacle reefs. This idea has been developed by Schlager and is discussed by Ginsburg *et al.* (1991; see next section). [It should be noted that Purdy's examples taken from Belize/Honduras lagoons have been shown to be incorrect—the karstic foundations here have in fact turned out to be the undulating remains of a lowstand siliciclastic coastal plain (Choi & Ginsburg, 1982; see also below).] More recently there has been great interest in the behaviour of reef complexes during periods of sea-level change, epitomized by the detailed architectural studies of well-exposed Miocene Mallorcan reefs by Pomar and Ward (1994). These remarkable rocks give evidence for prograding lowstand reef growth with erosion landwards, aggradational growth during sea-level rise, progradation once more at highstand, followed finally by off- and downlapping with landward erosion at the forced regression of falling stage (Fig. 24.22).

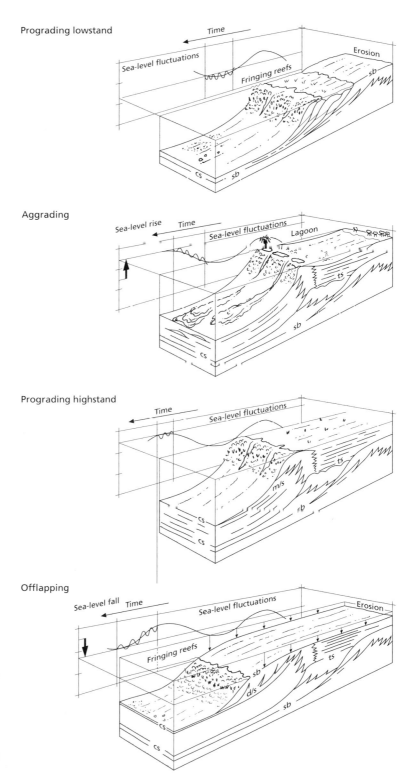

Fig. 24.22 The response of Mallorcan late-Miocene hexacoral reefs to sea-level changes and the types of sedimentary architecture produced. d/s, downlap surface; cs, condensed section; sb, sequence boundary; ts, transgressive surface. (After Pomar & Ward, 1994.)

24.9 Platform margin slopes and basins

Relatively little is known about the characteristically steep (compared with siliciclastic margins—see Schlager & Camber, 1986) modern slopes to carbonate platform margins and their associated basins compared with what we know about shelf and nearshore deposits. The majority of our knowledge comes from integrated studies of the Bahamian platform margins, in particular the results of deep seismic profiles (see Fig. 24.2; Eberli & Ginsburg, 1987). Much has also been inferred from ancient carbonate platform complexes subject to varying sea level, in particular the insightful studies of the magnificent exposures of Triassic carbonate platform margins in the Italian Dolomites (Bosellini, 1984; Harris, 1993; Fig. 24.23), the Permian Capitan reef front of Texas (Melim &

Scholle, 1995) and the Devonian reefs of the Canning Basin margin (George *et al.*, 1997). These have shed much light on previous inferences concerning platform growth (Kendall & Schlager, 1981; Schlager & Camber, 1986) and form important tests for the computational depositional models of Bosence and Waltham (1990) and Bosence *et al.* (1994).

In their early study of Bahamian slopes and basins, Mullins and Neumann (1979) recognized the following controls upon sedimentation at bank margins: (i) presence or absence of bank margin faults; (ii) direction and magnitude of off-bank sediment transport; (iii) amount of mass flows and pelagic deposits; (iv) nature of the oceanographic circulation; (v) degree of submarine cementation; and (vi) presence of deepwater organic build-ups. Subsequent work highlights item (ii) as the major of these controls, with the max-

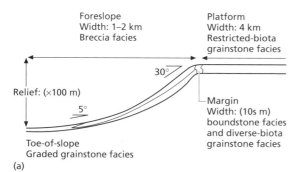

(a)

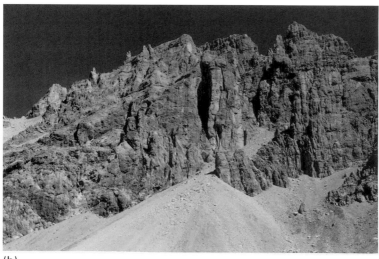

(b)

Fig. 24.23 View of mountainside exposure of the transition from steeply dipping foreslope to horizontally bedded platform deposits of the Triassic Latemar build-up, northern Italy. (From Harris, 1993.)

imum export of bank-top carbonate sediment occurring during highstands when shallow-water lagoonal production was greatest (Droxler & Schlager, 1985).

Seismic reflection imaging of platform margins (e.g. Hine *et al.*, 1981a,b; Eberli & Ginsburg, 1987, 1989; Mullins & Hine, 1989; Wilber *et al.*, 1990) and daring submersible dives (e.g. Ginsburg *et al.*, 1991) have begun to bridge the gap between ancient, modern and computational models. It has become evident that the rates of leeward lateral growth (to the west in the case of the Bahamas, see Fig. 24.2) of platform margins during stable sea level is very much greater than vertical growth, windward growth being negligible. This implies that there exists an efficient leeward transport system, probably storm-induced currents, to take *in situ* produced materials from the platform top—where both green algal production rates (Neumann & Land, 1975; Hine *et al.*, 1981a; Boardman & Neumann, 1984) and chemical precipitation rates (Shinn *et al.*, 1989) are known to vastly exceed deposition rates—to the platform margin (Hine *et al.*, 1981a,b; Wilber *et al.*, 1990).

The extensive scalloped margins of the smaller platforms of the southeast Bahamas suggested to Mullins and Hine (1989) that periodic gravity collapse due to undercutting or faulting may have disrupted a once more extensive marginal platform. Certainly the extensive dives undertaken by Grammer *et al.* (1993) bear out the dominant role of lowstand collapse in forming periplatform breccias (Fig. 24.24). However, despite these observations, seismic data make clear that lateral bank growth and the infilling of original structural depressions like Bimini embayment and the Straits of Andros by lee-side accretion during highstands of sea level were predominant over the long term (Eberli & Ginsburg, 1987). The submersible observations of Ginsburg *et al.* (1991) bear out the role of highstand lateral accretion of upper bank margins by outgrowing coral ledges, their periodic collapse down very steep (50°) bypass walls to the limit

Fig. 24.24 (right) Diagrams to illustrate how platform margins and their foreslopes respond to sea-level changes. Based on Holocene evolution of the Tongue of the Ocean margins, Bahamas Bank. (After Grammer *et al.*, 1993.)

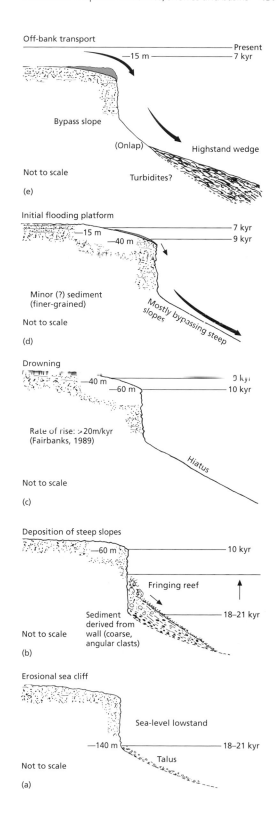

of Pleistocene sea-level lowstands, and the cementation of a residual forereef slope below about 150 m water depth. On leeward platform margins, exported bank-top aragonite sediment predominates during highstands (Droxler & Schlager, 1985), draping the lowstand breccia wedge (Grammer *et al.*, 1993).

Hemipelagic and gravity-flow processes dominate bank margin sedimentation. Suspension during storms of fine- to sand-grade sediment is the main export process (Neumann & Land, 1975; Hine *et al.*, 1981a, b; Boardman & Neumann, 1984; Mullins *et al.*, 1984; Droxler & Schlager, 1985; Shinn *et al.*, 1989). Wilson and Roberts (1992) envision sediment and water stirred up by cold winter storms to sink laterally on to the margins as 'cold water cascades' or density plumes. Pelagic carbonates are important on slopes only when not winnowed by bottom currents, diluted by gravity flows or dissolved below the carbonate compensation depth. Gravity flows are important where slopes are steep. Thick graded carbonate turbidites occur on the lower slopes around the Little Bahamas Bank and as thinner beds in the basins, where they are interbedded with pelagic oozes. Slope breccias of debris flow origin occur on the gentle muddy slopes, whilst grain flows occur at the base of very steep (~18°) slopes around the marginal escarpment. Very extensive slump, debris flow and turbidity flow deposits occur in Exuma Sound basin, Bahamas (Crevello & Schlager, 1981). Ancient analogues to these gravity flows are described and discussed by Mountjoy *et al.* (1972), James (1981) and Spence and Tucker (1997).

Extensive areas of submarine cementation occur west of the northern Bahamas and in the Tongue of the Ocean down to depths > 500 m. These lithified slopes are very stable and the cementation combined with strong current scour undoubtedly help to maintain the steep gradients observed in all the deep embayments separating the Bahamian platforms (Schlager *et al.*, 1976). In general the degree of cementation decreases downslope from well-lithified hardgrounds at depths < 375 m, to lithified nodules in a soft muddy matrix at depths from 375 to 500 m, and to soft oozes at depths greater than 500 m (Mullins *et al.*, 1980a). The nodules are multigeneration intramicrites to intramicrudites cemented by high-magnesian calcite in layers up to 1.5 m thick. The cementation is greatest along slopes where the Florida Current flows.

There are also spectacular sediment drifts in the Straits of Florida between Florida and the Bahamas Banks to the east (Mullins *et al.*, 1980b). These are very large (thousands of square kilometres), thick (> 600 m) accumulations of mostly shallow-water-derived carbonate sand-grade sediment reworked by energetic ocean floor (depths up to 800 m) contour currents with velocities up to 0.6 m/s. Most of the sediment is that exported from the prolific 'carbonate factory' of the Great Bahama Bank. Cementation and bottom currents also play a role in localizing the spectacular 'ribbon' of deep-sea build-ups, which extends over 200 km from the Blake Plateau along the western margin of the Little Bahama Bank to Bimini (Neumann *et al.*, 1977; Mullins & Neumann, 1979). These build-ups occupy a zone some 15 km wide in water depths of 600–700 m. They show up to 50 m relief and may be hundreds of metres long, orientated parallel to the northerly deep current flow. Observations from submersibles confirm their contemporary origin and reveal a dense and diverse benthic community of crinoids, ahermatypic corals and sponges, which must baffle and trap sediment provided by the bottom currents. The build-ups are constructed *in situ* by lithification of successive layers of trapped sediment by micritic high-magnesian calcite.

Particular insights into the evolution of carbonate margins with time have come from the magnificent exposures across exhumed margins in the Triassic of the Italian Dolomites (Bosellini, 1984; Harris, 1993; Fig. 24.23). Here, episodic progradation recorded by clinoforms might suggest lee-side accretion during highstands (as noted above for the Bahamas Bank). However, petrographic compositions suggested to Blendinger (1994) that the majority of steeply dipping clinoform sediment is more-or-less *in situ* (and boundstone-like): it seems that the clinoforms were their own carbonate 'factory'. Regardless of their origins, the nature of the lower and upper boundaries to the slope clinoforms yields important information on the processes and rates of aggradation and progradation.

In recent years it has been discovered that platform margin deposits are important sources of information about sea-level changes and platform-top carbonate production (Bosellini, 1984; Melim & Scholle, 1995; George *et al.*, 1997). Highstands were often periods of high forereef production alternating with periods of relative sediment starvation (despite the influx of karstic detritus) and algal encrustation on the lower forereef slopes during lowstands.

24.10 Carbonate sediments, cycles, sequences and sea-level changes

The effects of sea-level change causing landward and seaward migration of facies belts and the standard concepts of sequence stratigraphy work well with carbonate/evaporite sediments. This is because the effects of regressions and lowstands are pronounced (especially on very low-gradient, shallow platform tops), and therefore easy to recognize, owing to the drastic effects that exposure to fresh water and the atmosphere has on carbonate sediments:

1 Dissolution and reprecipitation of aragonitic and high-magnesian calcite carbonate as low-magnesian calcite causes distinctive cement fabrics, vugs, cavities and solution pits. A useful attempt to simulate the resulting complicated and overlapping diagenetic patterns during cycles of glacioeustatic sea-level change acting on a uniformly subsiding platform is reported by Whitaker et al. (1997).

2 Larger-scale karstification occurs as meteoric/phreatic water tables descend through highstand sequences. The lower limit to karstification, cave dissolution and stalagmite formation is a valuable palaeo-sea-level marker and is found at the base of the freshwater lens that overlies saline phreatic seawater (Mylroie & Carew, 1988, 1990). Karst is expected to be better developed and more extensive on flat-topped rimmed shelves than on sloping ramps. Such features and deposits figure prominently in the stratigraphic record of carbonate platforms like those of Bermuda (Vollbrecht & Meischner, 1996).

3 Distinctive supratidal soils develop in humid carbonate environments like terra rossa whose origins owe much to both in situ dissolution and also import of wind-blown dust (Boardman et al., 1995).

4 Development of significant spreads of wind-reworked carbonate sands occurs as aeolianites, given onshore winds and an adequate supply of carbonate sediment. Meteoric cementation and soil development on these gives them high preservation potential (Carew & Mylroie, 1995).

5 There is seaward spread of distinctive supratidal sabkha and salina evaporites during regression and lowstand in arid climates. The reader should also note the common occurrence of evidence for mixed saline and fresh conditions (the schizohaline environment of Folk, 1974) in the supratidal zone of more humid carbonate environments like those widely developed in the Purbeckian of western Europe (Francis, 1984; Strasser, 1988; Joachimski, 1994).

6 Seaward spread of distinctive fluviodeltaic and coastal siliciclastic sediments occurs adjacent to coastal plains with freshwater runoff. There is evidence for incision by channel systems.

7 Successive levels of solution notches are produced at platform margins at the marine phreatic–meteoric interface (Grammer et al., 1993).

8 Important jointing and cracking of karstified and partly lithified build-up carbonates occurs along steep lowstand margins due to wave action (Grammer et al., 1993).

9 There is lowstand collapse of cracked and jointed blocks to form distinctive talus cones at the foot of periplatform slopes (Grammer et al., 1993).

All these features may be used to track the course of significant sea-level falls or lows, either in core samples, seismic work or at outcrop. The lowstand features are draped by often quite contrasting transgressive and highstand sedimentary facies with a record of 'switching-on' any bank-top carbonate factory and the rapid burial of lowstand wedges by highstand finer-grained drapes resulting from renewed export of bank-top carbonate in response to prevailing wind directions.

It is common to observe sedimentary cycles developed in carbonate sediments. Some are of shallow-water origins witness those a few metres thick of peritidal origins deposited on extensive ramp-type margins—and are useful in determining the pattern of sedimentary cyclicity due to ancient sea-level changes (e.g. Fischer, 1964; Grotzinger, 1986; Hardie et al., 1986; Read et al., 1986; Strasser, 1988; Kerans et al., 1994). Spectral analysis of deposits like the famous Triassic Latemar Limestone (Schwarzacher & Fischer, 1982; Goldhammer et al., 1990; Hinnov & Goldhammer, 1991) have led to the proposal of precession- and eccentricity-driven shoaling-upwards cycles deposited during periods of sea-level change. However, precise dating and correlation of the Latemar sequence (Brack et al., 1996) reveal that depositional time was too short (by about 50%) to allow such an interpretation of all 600 or so cycles. There is clearly a big problem to be resolved here (see Drummond & Wilkinson, 1993)!

Another type of small-scale cyclic sequence of great interest comprises relatively thin alternations a few decimetres to metres thick of carbonates (> 60% $CaCO_3$) and more marly (around 40% $CaCO_3$) intervals richer in siliciclastic clays. These are common in the Mesozoic (DeBoer & Wonders, 1984) and Cainozoic record. The Pliocene examples of southern Italy have been ascribed to climatic fluctuations at the 20 kyr Milankovitch time band (e.g. DeVisser et al., 1989). The sedimentary origins of the cycles are somewhat controversial. They are clearly of shelfal to basinal origins, mostly well below storm wave base. Some workers ascribe the marly layers to periods of increased freshwater runoff and higher clastic sediment yield; comparable cycles on the West Florida ramp (Roof et al., 1991) result from periodic Mississippi-induced changes in shelf sediment plume activity. The carbonate units were deposited during more arid climates (DeVisser et al., 1989). Evidence that the two components of the cycles have quite distinctive microfaunas and floras (Thunnell et al., 1991), with the carbonates richer in foraminiferae indicative of highly productive cool upwelling conditions, leads to an alternative explanation that the cycles represent alternation between high- (limestones) and low-intensity (marls) upwelling conditions related to the precession-dependent strength of the Pliocene wind (monsoon?) system.

24.11 Destruction of carbonate environments: siliciclastic input and eutrophication

One of the problems in using the isolated carbonate platforms of the Bahamas and Florida as analogues for the stratigraphic record is the very common occurrence in that record of alternating carbonate and siliciclastic facies. These cycles imply that periodically the relatively shallow-water (< 200 m) carbonate depositional environments were displaced by the introduction of siliciclastic sediment (and then vice versa), perhaps due to relative sea-level or climatic changes. This implies that the two contrasting environments, of carbonate and siliciclastic sediment, are laterally situated relative to one another at any one time, ready either to expand or contract in area in response to external forcing. Such situations today have been little studied, probably because of the

regrettable and artificial schism that seems to exist between 'carbonate' and 'clastic' sedimentologists. Early attention was drawn to the potential of the Queensland coast for such studies (Maxwell & Swinchatt, 1970), for here the coastal plain and shallow shelf are dominated by the siliciclastic detritus brought in by ferocious, monsoon-fed rivers like the Burdekin. Only 15 km or so offshore lies the Great Barrier Reef complex (up to 100 km wide) in waters of 15–150 m depth. With such an example, it is easy to imagine the seaward or landward shift in clastic and carbonate facies belts during periods of sea-level change. A similar situation pertains in the Arabian Gulf where the Tigris–Euphrates delta and its extensive organic-rich wetlands are present adjacent to coastal sabkhas and shallow-water carbonate deposits (see Aqrawi & Evans, 1994; Evans, 1995). Further light is shed on the problem from shallow seismic and coring explorations in the Belize lagoons of Honduras (Choi & Ginsburg, 1982), where it is evident that the modern highstand lagoonal reefs and carbonates behind the fringing barrier platform overlie lowstand clastic sediments deposited in fluvial and deltaic distributary channel complexes. The palaeomorphology (levees, etc.) and compactional relief over this siliciclastic foundation has strongly influenced the locus of subsequent reef formation. Interesting accounts of alternating carbonate and clastic facies in the stratigraphic record and various theories to explain that alternation may be found in Rankey (1997) and Soreghan (1994).

A second reason for the demise of carbonate producers involves the phenomenon of eutrophication (see Brasier, 1995), whereby an increase in the abundance of nutrients in the seawater (perhaps induced by upwelling) causes replacement of carbonate deposits by organic-rich black shales. In fact, there is a distinct absence of modern carbonate platforms along all eastern oceanic basin margins, precisely those that tend to be affected by upwelling (Ziegler et al., 1984). We have already noted the controls upon coral reefs provided by nutrient availability and, as pointed out by Caplan et al. (1996), many examples of carbonate successions succeeded by black shales are known in the sedimentary record. The occurrence of ancient eastern ocean carbonate platforms in the western USA has been ascribed to the development of structural barred basins along back-arcs and forelands (Whalen, 1995).

24.12 Subaqueous evaporites

Until the sabkha evaporite model was outlined in the mid-1960s, it was almost universally assumed that evaporitic salts in the geological record were 'straight' chemical precipitates from bodies of standing brines as outlined in Chapter 3.

The crux of the modern dilemma regarding subaqueous evaporites hinges around: (i) the extremely large area over which some ancient evaporites may be traced, (ii) the scarcity of modern examples of such large evaporite basins, and (iii) the lack of knowledge concerning the evolution of sabkha plains with time. It is possible that continued sabkha progradation over periods of > 10^5 yr, combined with locally high subsidence rates, might produce standing evaporitic brine bodies in local basins above the sites of the old sabkhas—see Peryt (1994) on the Werra Anhydrite for a possible example.

Some light is shed on the matter of scale by reference to the early evaporite phase that many opening and closing oceans seem to pass through. As we shall discuss in Chapter 28, marine transgression into an incipient oceanic rift often seems to have been followed by a period of massive evaporite precipitation from shallow to deep brine bodies. Continued seafloor spreading ultimately encourages better exchange with the parent oceanic mass, evaporite precipitation ceases and the thick halite-dominated evaporite succession is overlain by 'normal' oceanic sediments.

Leaving aside these examples of oceanic evaporite sequences, it is apparent that recognition of ancient subaqueous evaporites must be made on as broad a basis as possible. Brine bodies may form in a multitude of settings, including on-sabkha depressions, abandoned coastal intra-dune depressions (Warren, 1982; Warren & Kendall, 1985), desert rift basin playas, barred lagoons, intra-platform basins (Peryt, 1994) and intra-build-up basins. Cathro et al., (1992), in their study of the vast lower Palaeozoic Canning evaporite basin of north-west Australia, propose the term 'saltern' for all dominantly subaqueous evaporite water bodies. Consideration of local and regional facies should serve to delimit such settings. Lateral facies changes may allow basinal subaqueous evaporitic units to be traced into contemporary nearshore and saltern margin facies with evidence of shallow-water or continental deposition. In such

cases a *prima facie* case for basin topography may emerge. Subaqueous nonevaporitic facies that overlie and underlie an evaporite unit may also be helpful in this respect, although these will not necessarily prove that the evaporite unit is subaqueously deposited. In the last resort it is the features of the evaporites themselves that may prove decisive. Let us, with Warren and Kendall (1985) and Lowenstein and Hardie (1985), briefly examine features that might indicate subaqueous, as distinct from subaerial, evaporite deposition:

1 Shallow brine bodies should be affected by wave-driven and, perhaps, tidal currents. Primary bedforms and sedimentary structures should therefore result. Clastic textures within the evaporite will also be formed, but these, together with some of the current-produced laminations, may be completely destroyed during burial diagenesis, particularly if the gypsum-to-anhydrite change is involved. Gradual infill of the brine bodies should lead to production of a shoaling-upwards sequence. Lateral gradations in brine salinity from basin centre to margin should lead to concentric (bulls-eye in plan view) or at least shore-parallel changes in evaporite mineralogy. Modern salinas are dominated by gypsum, and less commonly halite (Fig. 24.25; Orti-Cabo et al., 1984), precipitation, in marked contrast to the anhydrites of the Arabian sabkhas. It should be noted, however, that gypsum will always recrystallize to anhydrite with burial below about 500 m of overburden.

2 Should evaporite successions be subject to pene-contemporaneous differential applied stresses, then secondary structures will be formed, ranging from sedimentary deformation (load casts) to slump-like mass flows and beds resedimented into deeper water. Should rapidly moving mass flows be subject to mixing with the ambient brine, then redeposited evaporite beds with internal clastic turbidite-like characteristics will be produced (Schreiber et al., 1976). Some redeposited deep-water evaporites may have been derived from pre-existing poorly lithified shallow-water to supratidal evaporites that have been disrupted and uplifted by fault motions (e.g. Rouchy et al., 1995).

3 Subaqueous evaporite deposition favours the production of widely traceable (tens to hundreds of kilometres) varve-like laminations (Chapter 3).

4 Subaqueous evaporites should show evidence of crystal growth either at the brine–air interface or at the brine–sediment interface (using a term borrowed

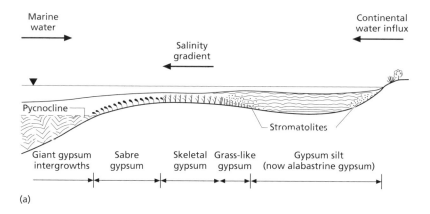

(a)

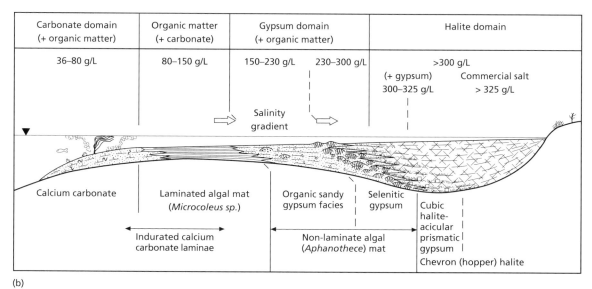

(b)

Fig. 24.25 (a) Subaqueous evaporite facies reconstruction for the gypsiferous successions of the Badenian of Western Ukraine. (From Peryt, 1996.) (b) Subaqueous halite–gypsum facies of modern Spanish coastal salinas. (From Orti-Cabo *et al.*, 1984.)

from igneous petrology, Lowenstein and Hardie (1985) call such precipitates, *cumulates*). Delicate rafts of hopper halite crystals form at the brine–air interface whilst upward-growing chevron halite and other growth forms occur at the brine–sediment interface as epitaxial growths from capsized hopper rafts (Shearman, 1970; Arthurton, 1973). Layers of large, vertically standing, elongate to curved gypsum crystals (swallow-tail crystals) with internal horizontal

inclusion trails and dissolution surfaces are also thought to indicate growth upwards from the sediment surface into brine (e.g. Schreiber *et al.*, 1976; Peryt, 1996). Intriguing and analogous features occur as halite growths in the industrial Dead Sea salterns (Talbot *et al.*, 1996). All such growth fabrics may be subject to recrystallization during evaporite burial.

5 The distinctive salt-pan evaporites that occupy many playas of the semiarid western USA and the magnificent Lake Eyre salt-pan of Australia show distinctive repeated cycles. The brackish lake phase occurs after flooding due to high runoff, followed by evaporative concentration in saline lakes and, finally, desiccation of the layered evaporites to give surface polygons and subsurface precipitation due to

concentration of groundwater brine. The two most distinctive features are laterally extensive dissolution surfaces and thin clastic laminae, formed as the under-saturated brackish waters initially flood the dry pan. A variety of other more subtle features are discussed by Lowenstein and Hardie (1985). Examples of ancient 'saltern' cycles with somewhat variable mineralogy according to local conditions are given by Hovorka (1987), Lowenstein (1988) and Cathro *et al.* (1992).

Further reading

Tucker and Wright (1990) is a major source for all things carbonate. Kendall and Harwood (1996) and Wright and Burchette (1996) provide good summaries. The reader is implored to read, mark and inwardly digest the sedimentological im-plications of the magnificent collection of satellite images and their discussion by Harris and Kowalik (1994); three of these are reproduced by permission in the present text (Plates 15–17). Logan (1987) is the most impressive single study of an evaporite environment and repays close study.

25 Shelves

Once, with my boy's body little I knew
But her furious thresh on my flesh;
But now I can know her through and through
And, light like, her tide enmesh

Hugh MacDiarmid, 'The Point of Honour', *Complete Poems*, Vol. 1, Carcanet

25.1 Introduction

The continental shelves are half-way houses for sediment on its journey from continent to deep ocean. They also act as final resting places (*sinks*) for sediment, being sites of active subsidence. In order for clastic sediment to arrive on to the shelf, it must previously have bypassed various nearshore traps such as estuaries, bays, lagoons, deltas and tidal flats. Once on the shelf, a complicated fluid dynamical mixture of tidal, wave, wind, oceanic and density currents disperse the sediment, allowing some proportion to 'escape' over the shelf edge into the deep ocean basins. *In situ* production (*sources*) of calcareous shelly debris may be important, $CaCO_3$ concentrations approaching 40% in significant areas of the NW European temperate shelf, for example (Wilson, 1982).

Some 18 000 yr ago, during the last glacial maximum, sea level stood closer to most modern shelf edges. This led to shelf-edge deltas (e.g. Suter *et al.*, 1987; Winn *et al.*, 1995) and shelf sand ridge features (e.g. Stride *et al.*, 1982), now stranded and defunct in water depths of 150–200 m. Shoreline retreat features enable a continuum to be traced on the shelf from lowstand to present day (we have already discussed examples on barrier-fronted coasts in Chapter 23). Thus modern shelves are, to a greater or lesser extent, relict in the sense that pre-Holocene sediment is exposed and is being current-reworked. Despite this, the majority of shelf sediment seems to be in hydrodynamic equilibrium with present-day flows. Shelf architecture, revealed by high-resolution marine seismic surveys, presents a universal picture (extending back well into the middle Tertiary) of lowstand erosion and outbuilding, alternating with transgressive erosion and highstand coastal sediment trapping (Fig. 25.1).

Shelves extend from the limits of the shoreface (say in the region 4–20 m water depth) out to a prominent shelf-edge break, at the top of the continental slope. The depth of the shelf edge (20–550 m) and the shelf width (2–1500 km) are tremendously variable, depending largely upon tectonic setting. Shelves on Atlantic-type ('passive') continental margins tend to be much wider than those on Andean-type or Pacific margins. The relatively smooth, gentle offshore slope to most shelves is basically a constructional feature moulded by shelf currents and deposited sediment. Shelf subsidence is another factor, since most shelves are underlain by extremely thick sedimentary successions that lie in fault-bounded linear basins and/or in broader downsags superimposed on these relicts of continental break-up. These successions were deposited in relatively shallow water (< 100 m water depth), implying that shelves are prone to continued, gentle subsidence, with rates of sediment supply and production usually able to keep pace with that subsidence.

Simple shelves outboard a continent and inboard a passive continental margin are the most common type. They show an oceanward-dipping prism of sediments (Fig. 25.1) and have been referred to as *pericontinental* shelves. By way of contrast, some very wide modern shelves like the North Sea, Yellow Sea and Timor–Arafura Seas lie well inboard of the continental margin, in the former case because of its status as a failed arm or rift dating back to Mesozoic times. Such *epicontinental*, or epeiric, shelves covered much larger areas in past geological epochs of continental plate evolution, especially in the Mesozoic of NW Europe, Tethys and the Western Interior Seaway,

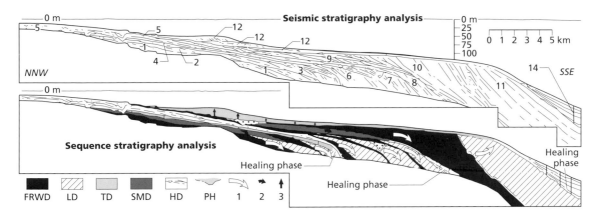

Fig. 25.1 High-resolution seismic reflection profile across the Gulf of Cadiz shelf, SW Spain, to illustrate the episodic progradation of the shelf edge in response to high-frequency Pleistocene sea-level changes over the period since about 3000 kyr BP. 1–12, depositional sequences and subsequences; FRWD, forced regressive wedge deposits (sea level falling); LD, lowstand deposits; TD, transgressive deposits; SMD, shelf-margin deposits; HD, highstand deposits; PH, incised palaeochannel and infills. Arrow 1, major progradation; arrow 2, minor progradation; arrow 3, aggradation. (Simplified after Somoza et al., 1997.)

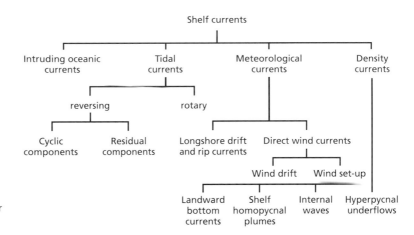

Fig. 25.2 Components of the shelf current velocity field. (Modified after Swift, 1972.)

but also in the upper Palaeozoic of North America and NW Europe. Narrower shelves exist on destructive or collisional plate margins because shelf sediment 'damming' has occurred behind outboard positive relief features formed by faulting and accretionary prism growth (e.g. Pacific coast of the Americas, Miocene of the Central European Paratethys).

25.2 Shelf water dynamics: general

The dynamics of water and sediment movement on shelves is complicated because of the several influences at work, from land-based to ocean-sourced currents (Figs 25.2, 25.3). The components of the shelf velocity field are summarized in Fig. 25.2. The most important of these are tide, wave and wind, the latter including net mass transport of water by direct wind shear. These all act on incident water and sediment density plumes from river estuaries and delta distributary mouths. Coriolis force is important as a dynamical consideration on the shelf.

Shelves have been classified into tide- and weather-dominated, but most shelves show a mixture of processes in both time and space. The majority of

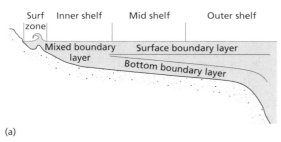

(a)

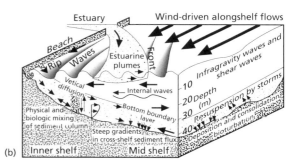

(b)

Fig. 25.3 (a) Simple division of shelf waters into mixed, surface and bottom boundary layers. Inner shelf has tide and wave mixing and is said to be frictionally dominated. Outer shelf is often stratified into an upper layer dominated by geostrophic flow and a bottom boundary layer of low friction. (b) Simple diagram to show the major physical processes responsible for cross-shelf flow and sediment transport. (Both after Nittrouer & Wright, 1994.)

pericontinental shelves are meso- to macrotidal only around their shallower margins; most have a tidal range < 2 m. Even the epicontinental North Sea shelf, with its powerful rotary tidal gyres, is macrotidal only over about 50% if its area. It is thus important for geologists to remember that the tidal regime of a whole basin cannot be inferred from evidence gathered from just a small area. Despite all these warnings about complexity, it is considered useful in the context of shelf physical processes to consider a generalized model for shelf physiography and water characteristics that involves an inner shelf mixed layer where frictional effects of wave and tide are dominant. Then the deepening mid- to outer shelf exhibits increasing differentiation into surface and bottom boundary layers separated by a 'core' zone (Fig. 25.3).

25.3 Shelf tides

In the oceans the twice-daily tidal wave is still of shallow-water (long-wave) type since the tidal wavelength is very large (about 10 000 km) compared with the depth of the oceans (say 5 km). The maximum tidal velocity in the open oceans is given approximately by $u = \zeta(g/h)^{0.5}$, where h is water depth and ζ is tidal wave amplitude, about 50 cm. Substituting realistic values we find that typical open oceanic tidal currents (from the M_2 tide, i.e. the principal lunar tide component) are only of a few centimetres

per second magnitude. So why does the tidal wave cause so much stronger tidal currents on some shelves and in some seas, but not others?

The open ocean tidal wave (Fig. 25.4) decelerates as it crosses the shallowing waters at the shelf edge. This causes wave refraction of obliquely incident waves into parallelism with the shelf break and partial reflection of normally incident waves. At the same time the wave amplitude of the transmitted tidal wave will be enhanced and so will the resulting tidal currents. This is because the energy of a wave must be conserved (we neglect bottom frictional losses here), and from the energy equation for gravity waves (Chapter 9) we have:

$$E = 0.5\rho gH^2(gh)^{0.5} \tag{25.1}$$

So if water depth, h, is decreased then H, wave height, must increase in due proportion. The tidal currents increase because they are dependent on the instantaneous amplitude of the wave. Tidal strength may also vary because of the nature of the connection between the shelf or sea and the open ocean. In the case of the Mediterranean Sea, for example, the connection with the Atlantic has become so narrow and restricted that the tide cannot reach any significant range in most of the sea. Locally, in the Straits of Gibraltar, the Straits of Messina and the Venetian Adriatic, for example, the tidal currents (but not necessarily the tidal range) may be very much amplified when water levels between unrelated tidal gyres or standing waves interrelate.

Another cause of spatially varying tidal strength concerns the resonant effects of the shelf acting upon the open oceanic tide. Resonant effects may very greatly increase the oceanic tidal range in nearshore environments and lead to the establishment of dynamic tidal currents and processes. In a *closed*

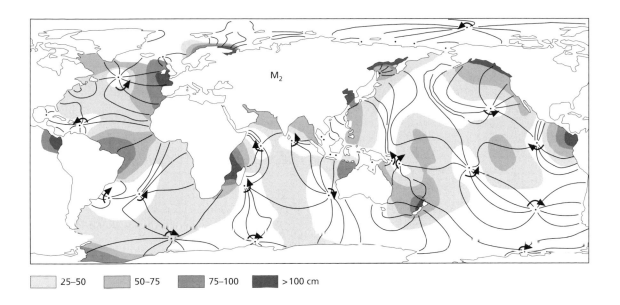

M_2

Fig. 25.4 Map to show computed M_2 high-water tidal ranges for the open oceans, with lines joining places where the time of high water is coincident. (From Schwiderski, 1979.)

25–50   50–75   75–100   >100 cm

basin a standing wave of resonant period, T, with a node in the middle and antinodes at the ends, has a wavelength, λ, twice the length, L, of the basin. The speed of the wave is thus $2L/T$ and, treating the tidal wave as a shallow-water wave ($h/\lambda < 0.1$), we may write *Merian's formula* as:

$$\frac{2L}{T} = \sqrt{gh} \qquad (25.2)$$

or

$$T = \frac{2L}{\sqrt{gh}} \qquad (25.3)$$

T is now the characteristic resonant period of the basin, dependent upon basin length and inversely dependent upon the square root of water depth. When the period of incoming waves equals this resonant period, then amplification occurs.

Now, *open* coastal basins like estuaries, bays and lagoons must receive the 12-hourly oceanic tidal wave and a standing wave (of period 12 h) may be set up, with a node at the mouth and an antinode at the end (by no means the only resonant possibility). In this scenario L is only 0.25λ and thus we have:

$$T = \frac{4L}{\sqrt{gh}} \qquad (25.4)$$

Should the shelf or embayment width, y, be odd numbers (1/4, 3/4, 5/4, etc.) of the tidal wavelength, then resonance will also occur and the tidal wave amplified, but with the effects of friction dampening the resonant amplification as distance from the shelf edge increases (Fig. 25.5). Most modern shelf widths are too narrow to show significant resonance across them (i.e. $y < 1/4$ tidal wavelength) and in most cases, for example the shelf of the eastern USA, a simple slow linear increase of tidal amplitude and currents occurs across the shelf.

It is possible to use the expressions above also to deduce the magnitude of the ancient tidal wavelength, since rearrangement of eqn (25.4) gives:

$$L = \frac{T(gh)^{0.5}}{4} \qquad (25.5)$$

where T is the period of the semidiurnal M_2 tide. The Bay of Fundy, maritime Canada, is the world's most spectacular example of a gulf that resonates with the period of the ocean's tides. The gulf has a length of about 270 km (calculated from the gulf head to the major change of slope at the shelf edge) and is about 70 m deep on average, giving the required 12 h characteristic resonant period. The standing resonant oscillation has a node at its entrance, which causes

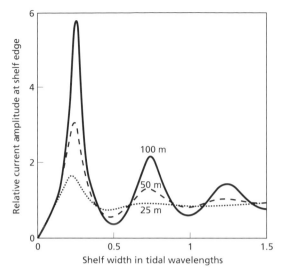

Fig. 25.5 Relative tidal wave amplitude at a shelf edge vs. shelf width in tidal wavelengths for depths of 100, 50 and 25 m. (After Haworth, 1982.)

the tidal range to increase from 3 m to a spring maximum of some 15.6 m along its length. Since h may be estimated from sedimentological evidence (e.g. by measuring the thickness of sediment from mean high-water mark (MHWM) saltmarsh to mean low-water mark (MLWM) sandflat facies, see Figs 23.14, 24.15),

it is then possible to solve for L, as the minimum length of an ancient basin that can resonate a tide (Sztano & DeBoer, 1995).

The Coriolis force acts as a moderating influence on tidal streams in semi-enclosed large shelves, like the NW European shelf, the Yellow Sea and the Gulf of St Lawrence. In the former, the progressive anticlockwise tidal wave of the North Atlantic enters first into the Irish Sea and the English Channel, then several hours later it veers down into the North Sea proper through the Norway–Shetland gap in a great anticlockwise rotary wave (whose passage north to south was noted by the monk Bede in the eighth century). Why should such rotary motions occur? The answer is that the tidal gravity wave has a sufficiently long period that it must be affected by the Coriolis force. Since the water on continental shelves is bounded by solid coastlines, often on two or three sides on the inner shelf, the tide rotates. Such waves of rotation against solid boundaries are termed *Kelvin waves* (Fig. 25.6; after the enobled William Thompson, the 19th-century Scottish physicist), the propagating wave being forced against the solid boundaries by the effects of the Coriolis parameter, f. The water builds up as a wave whose radial slope exerts a pressure gradient that exactly balances the Coriolis effect at equilibrium. The elevation, ε, of the wave is given by:

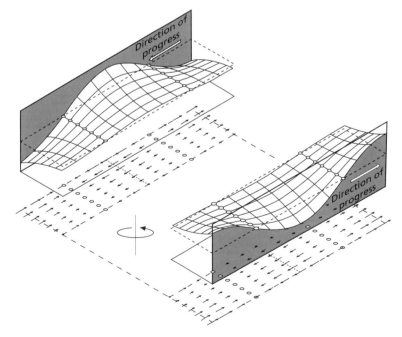

Fig. 25.6 Topography and bottom flow associated with a rotating northern hemisphere Kelvin tidal wave in a wide 'channel'. (After Wells, 1986.)

$$\varepsilon = \varepsilon_0 \exp(-y/L) \cos(\sigma t - kx) \qquad (25.6)$$

where $L = \sigma/fk = \sqrt{gh}/f$, σ is the wave frequency, k is the wavenumber and y is horizontal distance from the solid boundary. The tidal wave has maximum amplitude at $y = 0$, decaying exponentially towards the amphidromic point of no displacement. The wave has the properties of a shallow-water wave with the water velocity positive where associated with the high elevation and vice versa. The resonant period in the North Sea is around 40 h, a figure large enough to support three multinodal standing waves. The Coriolis force causes the stationary waves to become rotary, advancing anticlockwise about a nodal point of no displacement with maximum tidal displacements around the margins adjacent to the coastlines (Fig. 25.7).

The crest of the tidal Kelvin wave is a radius of the (roughly) circular basin and is also a cotidal line along which tidal minima and maxima coincide. Concentric circles drawn about the node are co-range lines of equal tidal displacement. Tidal range is thus increased outwards from the amphidromic node by the rotary action, and further resonant and funnelling amplification may of course take place at the coastline. Pingree and Griffiths (1979) and Harris et al. (1995) make the point that the apices of the amphidromic cells in shallow waters are also sites of maximum bed shear stress. This has relevance to the distribution of sediment grain size and bedforms, points discussed further below in connection with 'bedload partings' on shelves.

But not all basins can develop the rotary tidal wave: there must be sufficient width, since as we have seen

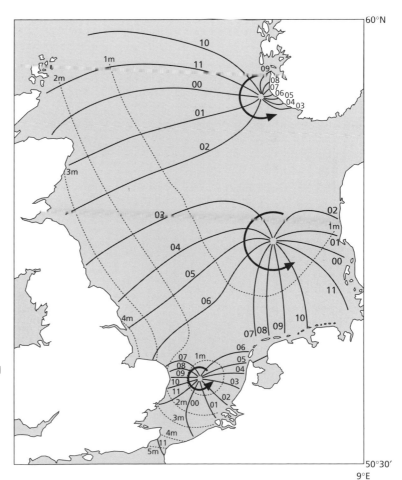

Fig. 25.7 The three subordinate Kelvin waves of the southern North Sea, defining amphidromic (Greek, literally 'running around') tidal systems. Continuous curves are cotidal lines joining up places of similar high water given in lunar hours (62 min) after the Moon's meridional passage at 0° longitude. The pecked curves give shelf average tidal ranges. (Note that these may be considerably amplified close to shore; not shown here in detail.) (From Harvey, 1976.)

the wave decays away exponentially with distance (see Pugh, 1987). The critical width is termed the *Rossby radius* of deformation, given by the ratio of the velocity of a shallow-water wave to the magnitude of the Coriolis parameter:

$$R = \left(\sqrt{gh}\right)/f \tag{25.7}$$

At this distance the amplitude of any Kelvin wave has reduced to 1/e, or 0.37, of its initial value.

We discussed previously (Chapter 9) the vector variation of tidal currents by means of a tidal current ellipse whose ellipticity is a direct function of tidal current type and vector asymmetry. For example, the inequality between ebb and flood on the NW European continental shelf is largely determined by the M_4 harmonic of the main lunar tide (Pingree & Griffiths, 1979). Since sediment transport is a cubic function of current velocity (Chapter 6) it can be appreciated that quite small residual tidal currents can cause appreciable net sediment transport in the direction of the residual current (Belderson *et al.*, 1978). The turbulent stresses of the residual currents will be further enhanced should there be a superimposed wave oscillatory flow close to the bed. A further important consideration arises from the fact that turbulence intensities are higher during decelerating tidal flow than during accelerating tidal flow. This arises from the greater intensity of the burst/sweep process in the unfavourable pressure gradients of nonuniform and unsteady flows. Increased bed shear stress during deceleration thus causes increased sediment transport compared to that during acceleration, so that the net transport direction of sediment will lie at an angle to the long axis of the tidal ellipse (McCave, 1979; Johnson *et al.*, 1981).

A final point concerns the importance of internal tides and other internal waves, particularly upon the outer shelf region (Cacchione & Southard, 1974; Heathershaw, 1985). These are common in the summer (fair-weather) months when the outer-shelf water body is at its most density-stratified, with a stable, warm, surface layer of density ρ_1 overlying a denser layer ρ_2. They are also common in fjords. Now, if a wave motion is set up at the stable density interface (due to a storm or the spring tide), the restoring force of gravity is $(\rho_2 - \rho_1)g$ and, because ρ_1 is a large fraction of ρ_2 (unlike in surface waves when $\rho_1 \ll \rho_2$), the waves cannot be damped quickly. Internal waves are thus of longer period than surface waves. For short

internal waves (very deep, lower, denser layers) the forward speed is given by:

$$c = \sqrt{gh'\frac{(\rho_2 - \rho_1)}{\rho_2}} \tag{25.8}$$

where h' is the depth of the less dense fluid. Thus a 20 m deep layer of fresh water overlying seawater will propagate internal waves of speed about 2 m/s, a significant speed for sediment erosion and transport. For long internal waves (wavelengths $\gg$ total flow depth), wave speed is given by:

$$c = \sqrt{g\frac{h_1 h_2}{h_1 + h_2}\frac{(\rho_2 - \rho_1)}{\rho_2}} \tag{25.9}$$

where h_2 is the depth of the lower layer.

25.4 Wind drift currents

Although all continental shelves suffer the action of storms, weather-dominated shelves are those that usually show low tidal ranges (< 1 m) and correspondingly weak tidal currents (< 0.3 m/s). Also it is not uncommon for the inner shelf to shoreface to be tide-dominated during the summer months but wave-dominated during the winter. In any case, tidal currents and wave currents are progressively less important offshore, so that at the outer shelf margin it is only the largest storms that affect the sediment bottom. In these areas of the outer shelf it is common to find a multilayer water system (Fig. 25.1), with a surface boundary layer dominated by wind shear effects, a middle 'core' layer, and a basal boundary layer dominated by upwelling, downwelling or intruding ocean currents. Winter wind systems assume an overriding dominance on most shelves, causing net residual currents arising from wind drift, wind set-up and storm surge. Wind shear causes water and sediment mass transport at an angle to the dominant wind direction because of the Ekman effect arising from the influence of the Coriolis force (see box below). For example, northward-blowing, coast-parallel winds with the coast to the left in the northern hemisphere will cause net offshore transport of surface waters and the occurrence of compensatory upwelling. The reader can thus appreciate that outer-shelf sediment dynamics and budgets are extremely sensitive to the vector magnitude of shelf wind systems. Depending upon dominant wind regime, either import or export is possible.

More information on Coriolis force and Ekman transport

External forces acting on seas and oceans are caused by direct wind shear on surface water layers and by the Coriolis force. The latter arises when there is velocity relative to the rotating Earth's surface. It is an apparent force in the sense that it is seen only by observers in the fixed frame of reference that is the solid Earth. The magnitude of the horizontal component of the Coriolis force, f, is given by

$$f = 2\omega \sin \phi u$$

Where ω is the angular velocity of the Earth, ϕ is latitude, and u is the horizontal velocity of an object or flow. The horizontal component of the Coriolis force increases with latitude; at the equator it is zero, since here $\sin \phi = 0$. The Coriolis force is directed normal to the object velocity, to the right in the northern hemisphere and to the left in the southern hemisphere. The Coriolis force thus deflects every physical object that moves horizontally over the Earth's surface. Slowly moving air and water masses are particularly subject to deflection. The main motivators for surface ocean currents are wind stress, giving rise to drift currents, and horizontal pressure gradients, giving rise to gradient currents. The Coriolis force and internal friction act as a result of movements set up by wind and pressure. They cannot cause the water masses to move, but they have a strong effect on the resultant motion.

But the movement of surface waters by direct wind stress is more complicated than appears at first sight (Fig. B25.1). Comparisons between the velocity paths of icebergs and the prevailing wind in Arctic seas showed an angular difference of 20–40° to the right of the wind for iceberg (and hence near-surface water) travel. The physicist Ekman established a quantitative solution to this problem by a consideration of

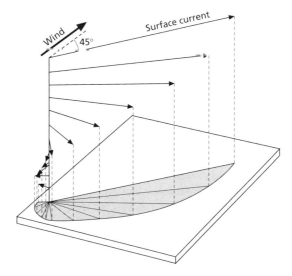

Fig. B25.1 The Ekman spiral produced by wind action upon a deep water mass.

continued on p. 452

viscous accelerations and Coriolis acceleration. His solution requires that the surface water velocity is directed at 45° to the right of the surface wind stress, the angular difference increasing with depth until a small reverse flow occurs; the velocity vector of a wind drift current with depth is thus in the form of a spiral. The magnitude of the current falls off exponentially with depth, and below a certain depth the effects of surface winds upon water motion ceases. Because of the Coriolis effect, this depth is latitude-dependent as well as velocity-dependent; at intermediate latitudes the effective depth limit is around 100 m. Ekman's drift-current theory assumes no horizontal pressure gradients to be present in the ocean. Should such gradients be present because of variations in density or due to driving up of water by Ekman transport (drift currents causing pressure differences), then gradient currents can result. These are discussed further in Chapter 26.

More information on Coriolis force and Ekman transport [*continued*]

25.5 Storm set-up and wind-forced geostrophic currents

Let us examine the effects of storm winds in more detail, for, as we shall see below, major shelf erosion and deposition result during such episodes. As we saw in lakes, wind shear drift causes set-up of coastal waters; should this coincide with a spring high tide, then major coastal flooding results. The effects are well known, for example, in the southern North Sea (where the Thames Barrage now protects low-lying London), in the Bay of Bengal and in the Venetian Adriatic (where in both places the people are not so lucky). Coastal tornadoes hitting the southeastern and southern USA are particularly effective at raising the set-up of coastal waters, sometimes up to 4 m or more above mean high-water level, as in Hurricane Carla on Padre Island, Gulf of Mexico, 1961 (Morton, 1981). The magnitude of the set-up for the 1953 storm surge in the southern North Sea can be roughly estimated (Wells, 1986) by assuming that the shearing stress, τ, due to the wind balances the pressure gradient due to the sloping sea surface, $\partial \xi / \partial x$. That is:

$$g\frac{\partial \xi}{\partial x} = \frac{\tau}{\rho h} \tag{25.10}$$

where h is water depth and ρ is water density. Solving for the slope term for storm winds of 30 m/s acting on 40 m water depth yields about 2.2×10^{-6} for the 600 km long North Sea, leading to a southern

superelevation of about 1.3 m. This is 50% or so less than the observed surge height because we have neglected important effects due to the Coriolis force, which forces the current against the shoreline where it is further amplified by resonance and funnelling. In the case of the southern North Sea in 1953, the southerly directed wind drift was first forced westwards on to the Scottish coast with the southward travelling (anticlockwise) Kelvin tidal wave, where it ultimately gave rise, some 18 h later to a ~3.0 m superelevated surge along the Dutch and Belgian coasts (Fig. 25.8). The Kelvin wave nature of storm surges enables them to be predicted for vulnerable areas like the North Sea and the Adriatic by reference to upcurrent changes in sea level during storm development. In addition to dynamic effects resulting from wind shear, the very low barometric pressures during storms cause a sea-level rise under the storm pressure minimum. The magnitude of this effect is about 1 cm rise per millibar decrease of pressure. So passage of the eye of a storm of pressure 960 mbar might cause a few tens of centimetres of sea-level rise.

Offshore, the importance of wave set-up during storms is that there must exist a compensatory bottom flow out to sea, driven by the pressure gradient (Fig. 25.9). Such geostrophic or gradient currents (which may be turned by Coriolis forcing) have been proven by measurements during storms to reach over 1 m/s, running for several hours (Murray, 1970; Gienapp, 1973; Forristal *et al.*, 1977; Hequette & Hill, 1993). Such flows are a major means by which

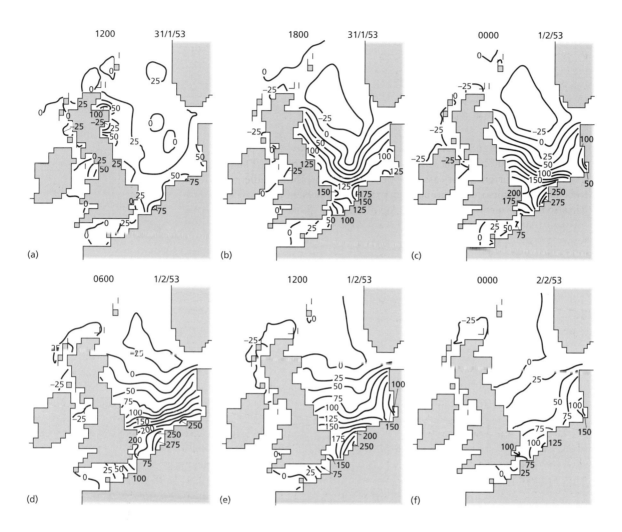

Fig. 25.8 Snapshots of storm surge elevations (25 cm contour interval) computed from a numerical model for the 1953 floods of the southern North Sea. Note some anticlockwise translation of the surge maxima and gradual amplification to almost 3 m at the Dutch coast. (After Flather, 1984.)

sediment is transferred from coast to shelf (Gadow & Reineck, 1969; Morton, 1981; Aigner & Reineck, 1982).

25.6 Shelf density currents

Density currents are very important in distributing and transferring mud-, silt- and sand-grade sediments across the shelf. Hypopycnal (positively buoyant) jets of fresh to brackish water with some suspended sediment (but not more than about 20 kg/m³) issue from most estuaries and delta distributary mouths. In higher latitudes, small to moderate buoyancy fluxes are soon turned by the Coriolis force, and they may be trapped along-source in the mid- to inner shelf where they form coastal currents or linear fronts. Particularly splendid vortices have developed along the free shear layer between a coastal front and off-shore circulating shelf waters in southern Turkey, for example (Evans *et al.*, 1995). Plumes are very sensitive to the effects of coastal upwelling or downwelling currents caused by winds. They may reach some way out into the mid-shelf or right across the shelf break,

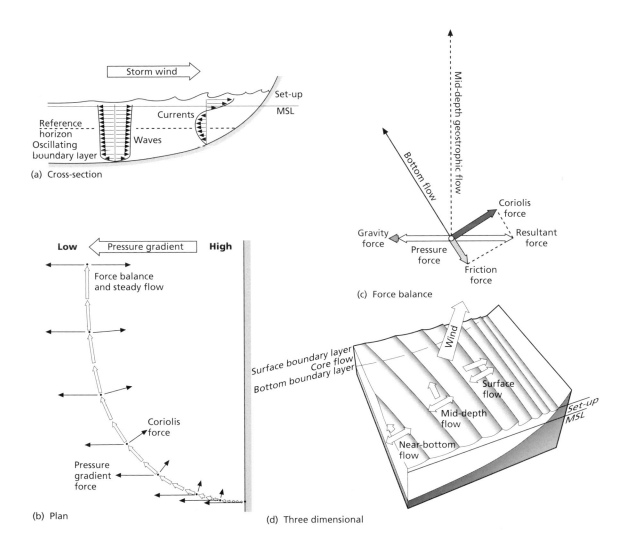

Fig. 25.9 Simple sketches to illustrate the basic pattern of storm-driven geostrophic circulation due to surface storm waves driven on to a shoreface in the northern hemisphere. MSL, mean sea level. (After Duke, 1990.)

depending upon their dynamic characteristics, those of the shelf winds and currents, and the slope of the shelves. Low slopes encourage long passage, whilst the development of vorticity on steeper slopes encourages turning and termination. The large buoyancy flux of many late spring and summer Arctic rivers (Becker, 1994) causes plumes to extend for up to 500 km offshore, well into the Arctic ocean basin.

During periods of high river discharge, the huge Amazon brackish plume (Plate 14) overrides a salt-wedge front at about 100 km from the shoreline (see papers in Nittrouer & Kuehl, 1995). The jet reaches mid-shelf, a distance of up to 200 km from the coast, before it is turned NW, parallel to the shelf contours, by the strong offshore North Brazilian Current (the Coriolis force is negligible at these low latitudes). The shelfward extent of the plume, at about 70 m water depth, forms a well-defined front due to tidal resuspension at the line of convergence with the plume head. The fast-moving (~1 m/s) jet fluid is laden with suspended mud and silt kept aloft by intense internal and externally forced tide- and wave-driven turbulence.

In inshore regions (< 12 m) sediment concentrations are 1–5 g/l and the water column is well mixed. A noteworthy feature between 12 and 30 m depth is the presence of 'fluid mud', with very high concentrations recorded indeed, up to 100 g/l, but generally around 10 g/l close to the shelf bottom. The fact that these high concentrations are recorded seawards of a well-mixed zone might suggest that the flow has not evolved into a hyperconcentrated underflow, but that some sort of 'turbidity maximum' has occurred due to settling and resuspension. Further out, surface concentrations are generally < 10 g/l, with bottom concentrations < 3 g/l.

Negatively buoyant jets form hyperpycnal underflows that issue from the mouths of rivers and distributaries able to provide the excess of suspended sediment needed to maintain negative bouyancy ($\gtrsim$ 30 kg/m³). Perhaps the most noteworthy example is that of the Huanghe (Yellow River), which dominates transport across the Yellow Sea (Wright et al., 1986). But the abundance of such hyperpycnal flows is strongly underestimated, as casual observations during flights over tropical areas indicate. Little is known about the deposits due to hyperpycnal underflows: it is an interesting question as to whether such flows lead to the formation of outer-shelf or deeper 'fluid-mud' deposits. Plumes of suspended-sediment-rich waters also result from the oscillatory effects of strong surface storm waves upon the bottom sediments, which suspend fine sediment into the water column. This suspension is then available for transport by the residual drift currents noted above, or by powerful onshore-to-offshore currents.

25.7 Across-shelf transport

It was pointed out some years ago (McCave, 1972; Schubel & Okabo, 1972) that, since most fine-grained inorganic deep-sea sediment is derived from the continents, it must have crossed the shelves to reach the oceans. Yet the routes and mechanisms of this escape remain obscure. As we have seen, much fine sediment is deposited well before the shelf break by the advection and turbulent decay of turbid plumes issuing from coastal tidal inlets, estuaries and deltas. These usually flow obliquely across the shelf (Ridge & Carson, 1987) under the combined influence of buoyancy, shelf current and Coriolis forces. Many such plumes end in mid-shelf as a well-defined front,

contributing to what we may call the *mid-shelf sink*. Even very extreme flood runoff may be of insufficient concentration to allow advection over and out of the shelf (Drake et al., 1972). On the other hand, sediment budget studies from a variety of river source indicate that some proportion (10–50% according to local dynamic conditions) always escapes to the continental slope (see review in Nittrouer & Wright, 1994).

Trans-shelf water and sediment fluxes are well demonstrated for the Arctic (Becker, 1994) and Oregon shelves (Komar et al., 1972; Baker & Hickey, 1986). In the latter case, long-period southwesterly storm waves stir the bottom to water depths of 200 m. The resuspension is then transported as plumes of sediment, which bypass the shelf in surface and mid-water eventually to deposit sediment on the continental slope up to 100 km offshore. Net southward transport on and across the South Texas shelf (Shideler, 1978) is attributed mainly to advection by residual drift currents, which reflect a winter-dominated hydraulic regime. Frequent winter storms characterized by the relatively strong northerly winds that accompany the passage of cold fronts appear to be the dominant regional dispersal agents acting on the buoyant plumes issuing from the Mississippi delta outlets (Plate 13).

25.8 Recent shelf facies

The distribution of sediment of differing grain sizes on highstand shelves depends on a variety of factors, e.g. point vs. line coastal sources, magnitude of freshwater and suspended sediment discharge, existence of advected buoyant plumes, wind/wave/tidal current vectors and regime, and a variety of others, including the general shape of the coastline produced by tectonics. It must be stressed that there is no general pattern of offshore fining with increasing water depth, for muds may accumulate almost anywhere across a shelf, dependent upon the nature of the current and source regime. A further important consideration is historical, being the influence of lowstand processes, particularly old river valleys, moraines and so on. These provide environments sheltered from tide and wave for muds to accumulate, for example. Many shelves have embayments and gulfs; these are important because generally the flooding, bore-like, tidal wave is less dissipated than that of the ebb, and so net up-embayment transport is maintained.

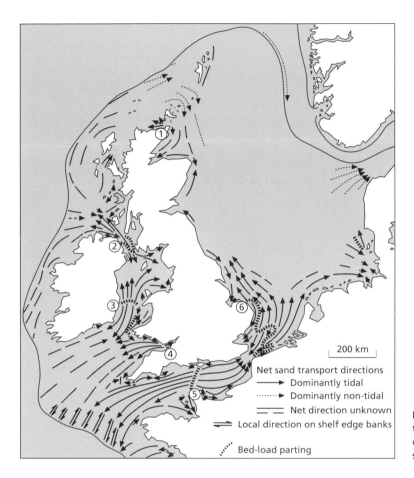

Fig. 25.10 Map to show generalized tidal current transport paths on part of the NW European continental shelf. (After Johnson *et al.*, 1981.)

On tide-dominated shelves the distribution of grain size, bedforms and facies depends to a great extent upon position with respect to tidal current transport paths. These are computed from combined M_2 and M_4 tidal current predictions, and show the direction and relative magnitude of *net* bedload transport (Pingree & Griffiths, 1979; Johnson *et al.*, 1981). Detailed studies on the northwest European tide-dominated shelf, for example (Fig. 25.10; Stride, 1963; Kenyon & Stride, 1970; Belderson *et al.*, 1978), have defined tidal current transport paths by a combination of observations on (i) surface tidal velocities, (ii) elongation and asymmetry of tidal current ellipses, (iii) facing direction of sandwaves, and (iv) trends of sand ribbons (see Fig. 25.12) and grain size. (The reader should compare the methodology of this approach with the principles used to construct sand flow paths in the great Saharan desert ergs, as discussed in Chapter 16.) Note the position of irregular 'bedload

partings' that separate opposing sand and gravel pathways. These are associated either with the centres of amphidromic cells or with local acceleration of the tidal streams in coastline constrictions (Harris *et al.*, 1995). There is always a general trend towards decreasing grain size down the tidal current paths, perhaps from coarse sand to mud depending upon the availability of sediment. This trend is due to decreasing net current strength. The concept of bedload partings seems to fall down when residual currents and the nonuniform 3D flows of outer estuaries, embayments and firths are considered (Harris & Collins, 1991). Here the ebb and flood tidal currents separate into distinct pathways in space, leading to the situation of nonuniformity across the whole tidal prism.

The upstream parts of tidal current paths, with velocities in excess of 1 m/s, may show sand ribbon bedforms up to 20 km long, 0.2 km wide and about 0.1 m thick (Fig. 25.11). These features occur in

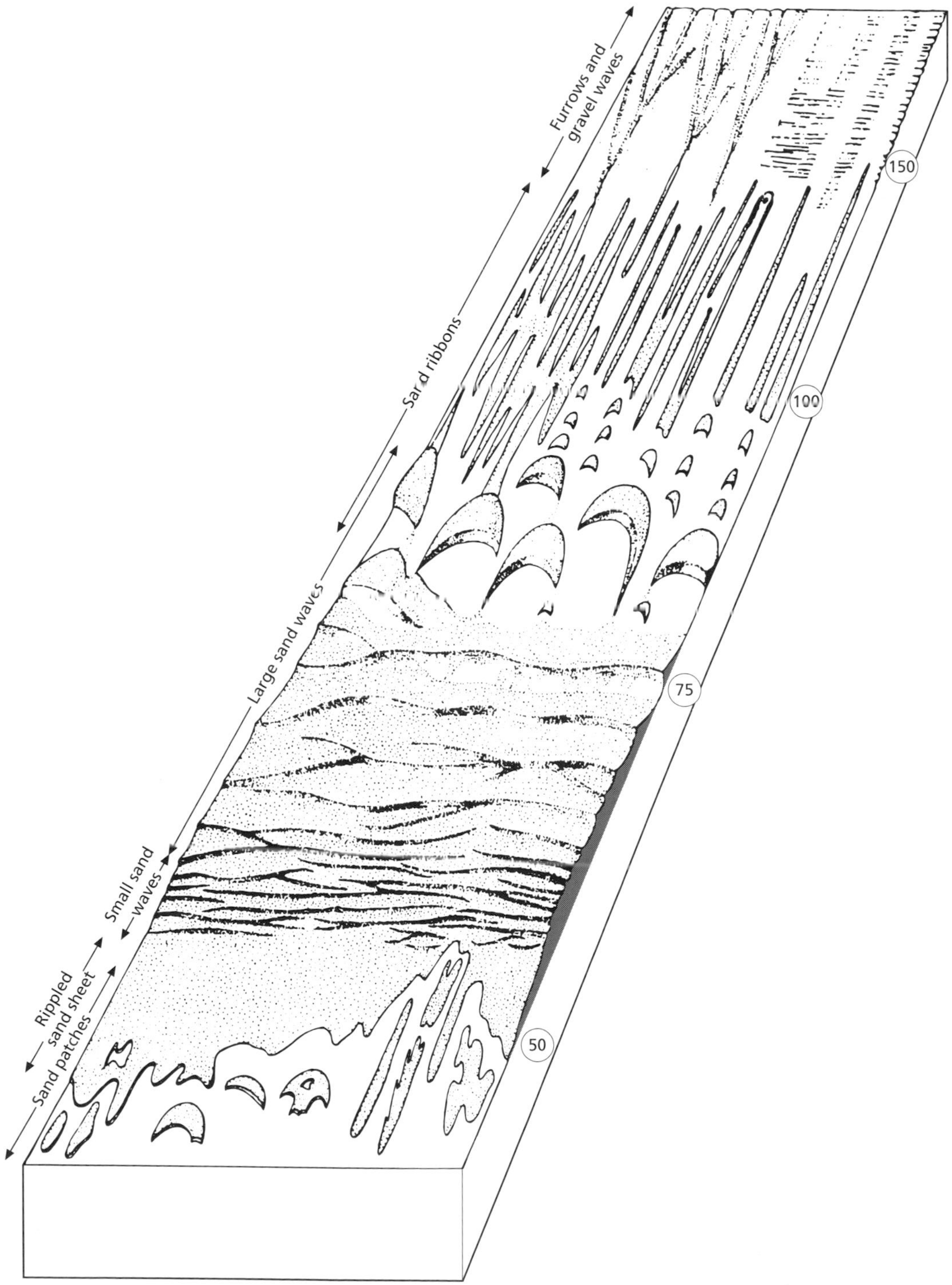

Fig. 25.11 Block diagram to show the lateral sequence of bedforms and sediment types observed down a typical tidal current transport path, with mean spring tide peak near-surface tidal currents in centimetres per second. (After Belderson *et al.*, 1981)

water depths of 20–100 m on gravel substrates that
have a sparse cover of coarse sands. Simple parallel
sand ribbons may owe their existence to secondary
flows involving pairs of counter-rotating helical vortices, but there are several different candidates for the
origin of such features (Pantin & Hamilton, 1987).

Another characteristic sheet-like shelf depositional
facies comprises dunes (Johnson *et al.*, 1981; Stride
et al., 1982). These cover large areas (> 100 km²)
along the higher-energy parts of tidal transport paths.
The dunes are 3–15 m high with wavelengths of up to
0.6 km. Given a sufficient supply of sand these bedforms will develop as asymmetric forms in areas of
marked tidal ellipse asymmetry and as symmetric
forms at bedload partings where ellipse asymmetry
is absent (McCave, 1971; Johnson *et al.*, 1981).
During storms, dune heights and wavelengths are
significantly reduced, whilst the forms are absent in
nearshore areas where wave activity is persistently
high. They die out down tidal transport paths, as bed
shear stresses decline, offering limited opportunities
for dunes to develop. Little is known concerning the
internal structures of the dunes, but it may be inferred
that they comprise dominantly unimodal large-scale
cross-stratification with perhaps smaller-scale sets with
opposed orientations. Sandwaves with low-angle lee
slopes tend to occur in areas of weaker mean tidal currents and may be expected to show numerous internal
sets of cross-stratification separated by downcurrent
dipping set boundaries (Reineck, 1963).

A very prominent feature of tide-dominated
shelves, like those of the southern North Sea
(Figs 25.12 & 25.13), Celtic, Yellow and White Seas,
is numerous parallel, large-scale linear tidal *ridges*
(sometimes called *banks*). These are the most spectacular bedforms of the continental shelves (Kenyon
et al., 1981; Belderson *et al.*, 1982; Stride *et al.*, 1982),
reminding us in their scale and persistence of the
linear seif dunes and draa of Trade Wind deserts. The
ridges in the North Sea comprise shelly, well-sorted,
medium sands up to 40 m high, 2 km wide, 60 km
long with spacings of 3–12 km and covered by active
dunes. In between the ridges the substrate is usually
coarser, sometimes gravelly. The ridge systems are in
clear equilibrium with the present tidal regime. They
have their crest lines oriented slightly obliquely (up to
20°, usually clockwise) to the direction of the maximum peak tidal current velocity. They are usually
asymmetric, with the steep face inclined at a *maximum*

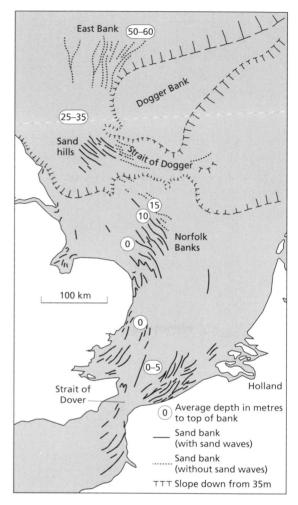

Fig. 25.12 Areas of tidal sand ridges in the southern and
central North Sea. The East Bank, Sand Hills and outermost
Norfolk Banks are largely relict features. (After Houboult,
1968; Kenyon *et al.*, 1981.)

of about 6° to the horizontal and *in the direction* of
the net regional sand transport. The superimposed
dunes migrate over the backs of the ridges until they
reach the crests, where they turn clockwise to begin
their orthogonal descent down the slightly steeper
face (Fig. 25.13). Internal structure is revealed by
shallow seismic surveys (Houboult, 1968; Laban &
Schüttenhelm, 1981; Fig. 25.14), which show evidence
for ridge build-up growth and preferential migration.
It is clear that the ridges did not develop over pre-
Holocene positive or negative relief features developed on the tills and glacial outwash that underlie the

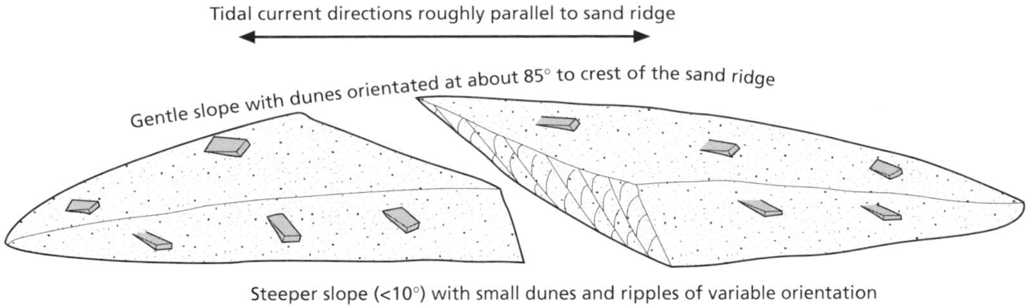

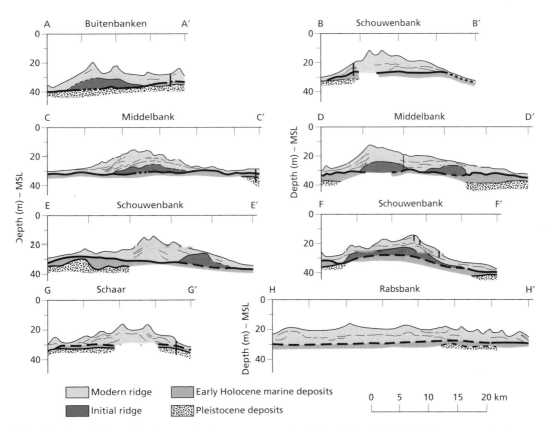

Tidal current directions roughly parallel to sand ridge

Gentle slope with dunes orientated at about 85° to crest of the sand ridge

Steeper slope (<10°) with small dunes and ripples of variable orientation

Fig. 25.13 Morphology, currents and likely internal structure of an asymmetric tidal sand ridge.   (Modified from Houboult's, 1968, account of Wells Bank.)

Fig. 25.14 Seismic profiling and coring reveals the internal structure of these tidal current sand ridges from   the Zeeland (Flemish) Banks. MSL, mean sea level. (From Laban & Schüttenhelm, 1981.)

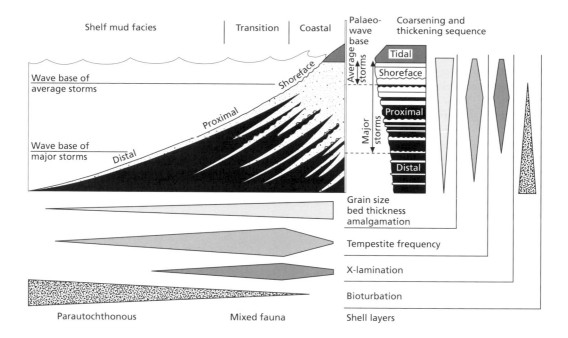

Fig. 25.15 Summary of the coastal to offshore trends observed in coring transects off the storm-dominated Helgoland Bight of the southern North Sea and their use in constructing an idealized vertical facies sequence resulting from coastal progradation. (After Aigner & Reineck, 1982.)

area. Asymmetric ridges show internal inclined low-angle foresets parallel to the steeper face, indicative of ridge migration in this seawards direction. Symmetrical ridges show only build-up surfaces internally (Laban & Schüttenhelm, 1981). Large fields of apparently inactive ridges occur in deeper waters (> 130 m) adjacent to the modern shelf break, perhaps most spectacularly developed in the Celtic Sea. These are thought to represent 'fossil' ridges dating back to lowstand times.

The distal ends of tidal transport paths comprise isolated sand patches and small sandwaves with numerous ripple bedforms and bioturbation features, the paths finally ending in areas of mud deposition. Bioturbated offshore mud deposits with rich infauna can occur only in relatively deep areas of low wave activity, the high deposition rates (3–5 mm/yr) indicating continuous mud fallout from suspension with important storm-produced suspensions contributing significantly (Reineck, 1963; Gadow & Reineck,

1969). Studies of the mud belt developed in the Helgoland (German) Bight of the North Sea (see Aigner & Reineck, 1982) reveal frequent, thin, graded sand and shell layers attributed to storm gradient (geostrophic) currents, which have transported intertidal sands and fauna up to 40 km out into the deep offshore (Figs 25.15 & 25.16). Measured storm underflow currents (e.g. during the winter storms of 1965—see Gienapp, 1973) reach well over 1 m/s. A well-developed proximal to distal trend is found in these 'tempestite' deposits: from amalgamated, parallel, laminated and hummocky(?) sands with shelly lags in up to 5 m water depth, via interbedded, thinner, sharp-based sands and silts with thin, wave-rippled zones and bioturbated mud caps in 5–15 m water depth, to very thin silts and sands set in thick muds in > 15 m depth, some 60 km or so from the shoreline. Thin graded sands are also common off those parts of the Gulf of Mexico coast that are both rich in a sand source (Siringan & Anderson, 1994) and traversed by hurricanes that set up gradient currents. For example, the aforementioned Hurricane Carla of 1961 has left its legacy as a prominent, laterally extensive, graded storm bed up to 0.25 m thick (Morton, 1981). There is evidence that shore-normal gradient currents may be significantly turned parallel

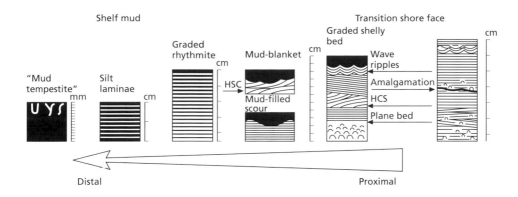

Fig. 25.16 Simple representation of the sedimentary structures in distal and proximal storm layers. (After Aigner & Reineck, 1982.)

to bathymetric contours by regional wind drift currents (Siringan & Anderson, 1994, their figure 12).

On shelves dominated by the advection of sediment-laden, but positively buoyant, plumes, maximum deposition tends to occur at or about mid-shelf where the plume front is halted as it is redistributed by tidal, wave or offshore vorticity. At higher latitudes the turning effect of the Coriolis force on the predominant offshore wind regime is crucial. The destination of the plume depends upon the orientation of the effective shelf wind regime. That of the Washington coast of northwest USA encourages oblique passage of river-borne plumes to the mid- to outer shelf (Baker & Hickey, 1986), presumably with declining deposition rates all the way. This pattern of dispersal should give rise to lobate mud/silt lobes that fine and thin towards the shelf break. The Amazon buoyant plume has deposited a subaqueous mud-delta wedge over 100 km out from the shoreline into water depths of 70 m or so (Nittrouer & Kuehl, 1995). In shallow inshore areas, interlaminated and interbedded sediments on a millimetre to centimetre scale represent diurnal and spring–neap tidal current variations. The topset wedge ends at a slope break in about 25 m water depth, fluid mud facies occurring landward of this point. On the upper foresets, short-term deposition rates of up to 100 mm/yr have been recorded; not surprisingly there are abundant signs of slope instability in these areas.

Little is known about the distribution of shelf facies in areas dominated by negatively buoyant flows, save for the widespread deposition of muds and silts mapped out in the Gulf of Bohai and along the axis of the Yellow Sea shelf (Lee & Chough, 1989). These may mark the course of the River Huanghe (Yellow River) turbid underflow but also coincide with the surface advection of dilute suspensions in the Bohai current up to a concentration of 5 mg/l. Other areas of fine-grained sediments are relict, recording former positions of the Huanghe, or are the advected plumes of active riverine input from the great Changjiang (Yangtze) translated southwards along the coastal shelf by strong shelf currents. Very large areas of shelf sands are thought to be relict tidal sand ridges that formed as lowstand deposits and during the post-glacial transgression.

Overall, weather-dominated shelves tend to show a general offshore decrease in grain size and Holocene sediment thickness in response to attenuating wave power. This trend is well shown by the Bering, Oregon and southwestern Gulf of Mexico shelves (Sharma *et al.*, 1972; Kulm *et al.*, 1975; Shideler, 1978). Mud-grade sediments settling out close to the shelf-edge break are often intermixed with partly reworked transgressive relict sands on the outer shelf. As already noted, wave-formed ripples can occur at depths up to 200 m on the Oregon shelf, indicating that rippled sand laminae may be expected to be common in many offshore areas. But fair-weather reworking by burrowing organisms may destroy these storm laminae.

The Middle Atlantic Bight, the wide (75–180 km) shelf off the eastern USA (Fig. 25.17) between latitudes

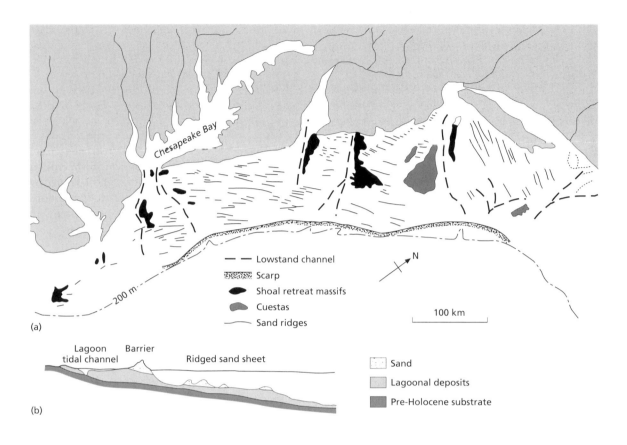

(a)

(b)

Lowstand channel
Scarp
Shoal retreat massifs
Cuestas
Sand ridges

N

100 km

Lagoon
tidal channel Barrier Ridged sand sheet

Sand
Lagoonal deposits
Pre-Holocene substrate

Fig. 25.17 (a) Morphology of the Middle Atlantic Bight
of the eastern USA to show features of relict and
transgressive origins. (b) Section across shelf to show
transgressive barrier and progressively abandoned shelf
sand ridges. (After Swift *et al.*, 1973; Swift, 1974.)

35 and 41°N, stands as a particularly well-investigated
weather-dominated shelf of complex morphology
(data from Swift *et al.*, 1973, 1981; Field, 1980).
The shelf slopes gently eastwards from the lower
shoreface (at a somewhat arbitrary 20 m depth) with
the shelf break at between 50 and 150 m water depth.
Tides are generally insignificant (apart from in some
estuaries and the Nantucket Shoals area around 41°N)
and sediment transport is dominated by the passage
of storms. The highest-wave months are September
and January–March, with the former bearing the
brunt of subtropical-sourced long-period waves and
the latter the shorter-period northeasterlies. On the
inner shelf and lower shoreface there is an upper
water regime of asymmetric oscillatory flow landwards, with an important time-mean lower water
flow (of geostrophic origins) seawards, the latter
enhanced for sediment transport as a combined flow
by storm wave orbital motions. All-in-all the surface
sediment of the modern Bight is remarkably coarse,
with muds and silts being restricted largely to estuaries and back-barrier lagoons. This reflects the paucity
of modern sediment flux on to the shelf (compare
the Amazon shelf discussed above) and the efficiency
of the storm wave transport process acting on sands
made available from the pre-Holocene lowstand. The
surface of the modern shelf shows abundant evidence
that precursor, lowstand and rising sea-level relief
features influence and control modern sedimentary
processes. This control has been increasingly obvious
in recent years with the advent of high-resolution

shallow geophysical surveys and extensive coring programmes (e.g. Ashley *et al.*, 1991, 1993; Wellner *et al.*, 1993; Levin, 1995). Thus traces of incised pre-Holocene river and estuarine channels date from the last glacial lowstand; the landward extension of the smaller of these has already been shown to influence the position of barrier island inlets. Larger channels, such as those of the palaeo-Chesapeake, Hudson and Delaware, may often be traced out as prominent bathymetric valleys all the way to the shelf edge. The pattern of sand distribution on the shelf tracks in a remarkable way the successive positions of the cape and headland high-energy beaches and barriers off New Jersey, Maryland/Delaware and North Carolina that separate the major coastal estuaries. It is envisaged that the predominantly onshore to offshore transport of sand seen in shoreface environments has occurred continuously during transgression, causing the observed modern sand sheet down to depths of 50 m or more to remain under the influence of storm wave processes.

In detail, much of the eastern USA shelf sheet sand (10 m or so mean thickness) is dominated by fields of linear, northeast-trending, ridges up to 10 m high with slopes of a few degrees (usually < 3° nearshore). Shoals are separated by linear hollows bearing gravel over the Pleistocene lowstand surface. Clusters of shoals merge with the modern shoreface in water only 3 m deep. The ridges make small angles (< 35°) with the modern coastline. Seismic profiles through the more offshore ridges reveal low-angle surfaces that dip to the southeast, the direction of ridge asymmetry. The active shoreface shoals are forming at the present time in response to storm-generated currents running approximately parallel to the shoal crests. Shoal detachment from the shoreface is thought to have occurred periodically during the Flandrian transgression, the detached shoals continuing to evolve at the present day in response to the storm wave surge and water drift currents. This idea is supported by the onshore to inner-shelf transition of ridge morphology observed off the Maryland coast. Here, nearshore ridges are 'attached' to the shoreface as shown by their contours. They are steeper, of lower cross-sectional area and less asymmetric seawards than those detached ridges that lie progressively offshore. Regarding grain size, it is found that the coarsest grain sizes occur in the landward flanks, not on the

ridge crests. Long-term studies indicate that the ridges migrate in response to sediment transport aligned south and slightly offshore relative to the ridge crests. It is likely that the ridges owe their origins to the shelf-parallel time-mean geostrophic flows discussed previously. The reasons why such ridges should begin to form as attached spurs on the shoreface is unknown. Also, little is known about the internal structure of the ridges, but it is likely that inclined internal surfaces seen on geophysical records represent storm erosion planes. Successive internal planes may be separated by fine sediment showing small-scale cross-laminations in the wave troughs produced by wave oscillations in normal weather conditions. The reader should note that the Middle Atlantic Bight linear ridges produced by time-mean wave–current flows are quite similar in broad morphology to the tide-dominated ridges noted previously. It is left to the ingenuity of the reader to distinguish between the two in terms of tell-tale internal structures.

25.9 Ancient clastic shelf facies

Anderton (1976) is a classic account of an ancient (Dalradian, Scotland) tidally swept shelf environment. Perhaps the best accounts of ancient shelf deposits (detailed work on magnificent exposures) are those of the Cretaceous western North American seaway, from Colorado to Alberta (e.g. Plint *et al.*, 1986; Plint, 1988; Pozzobon & Walker, 1990; Pattinson & Walker, 1992). Bridges (1982) made the first reconstruction of any ancient rotary tidal system based upon this Cretaceous seaway. He deduced the presence of several amphidromic cells acting in the narrow seaway. More recently these ideas have been extended by Slingerland *et al.* (1996). Another excellent physical reconstruction of an ancient resonating tidal gulf (discussed already above) was undertaken by Sztano and DeBoer (1995) for the Miocene of the North Hungarian Bay. Boyles and Scott (1982) discussed migrating sandy shelf bars in the Mancos Shale of NW Colorado, which they compared with those of the wave-dominated Holocene Middle Atlantic Bight. A more recent account of equivalent facies in Wyoming (Mellere & Steel, 1995) concentrates on sea-level influences on detailed sand body geometries. Leckie and Krystink (1989), Duke (1990) and Midtgaard (1996) contribute to the debate on

Coriolis-induced turning of gradient storm currents. Brenchley *et al.* (1993) describe coarsening-upwards and thickening-upwards cycles of Ordovician age, which they attribute to cycles of outer- and inner-shelf adjustment to changing sea levels. Sinclair (1993) discusses the Tertiary Gres d'Annot shelf storm sequences as part of regressive/transgressive cycles involving a barrier shoreline with inlets and also extruding hypopycnal plumes.

Further reading

Despite the explosion of research on shelf flows and sedimentology there is no up-to-date introductory account that explains processes and sedimentary products. Batist and Jacobs (1996) and Swift *et al.* (1991) contain many papers of interest, the latter including a long series of reviews. Nittrouer and Wright (1994) is a more precise and advanced review. For a single case-study of great interest the reader is advised to browse through the collection of papers on the Amazon shelf in Nittrouer and Kuehl (1995).

26   Oceanic processes and sediments

We must be humble. We are so easily baffled by appearances
And do not realise that these stones are one with the stars.
It makes no difference to them whether they are high or low,
Mountain peak or ocean floor, palace, or pigsty.

Hugh MacDiarmid, 'On a Raised Beach', *Complete Poems*, Vol. 1, Carcanet

26.1 Introduction

Since the *Magellan* mission to Venus it is often quipped that we know more about the surface of that distant planet, from radar range-finding probes, than we do about the two-thirds of Earth that is the ocean floor. The relative opacity of seawater to electromagnetic waves and the slowness of ocean-going survey vessels are both responsible for this. But things are rapidly changing with the advent of satellite altimetry, remote sensing and deep towed sonar devices of great range and accuracy. We may especially mention GLORIA (Geological Long Range Inclined ASDIC, where ASDIC is a sonar system) and its successor TOBI (Towed Bottom Water Instrument). Major advances in our understanding of ocean water dynamics, biological productivity and sedimentation have also occurred as a result of the development of automated sediment traps (Honjo & Doherty, 1988). We now know from moored subsurface recorders that ocean surface currents coexist with deep currents of some strength, and that any section through the ocean reveals distinct water masses with often sharp vertical and horizontal discontinuities in temperature, salinity, turbidity and velocity. Analysis of the thousands of cores taken during the many research cruises (over 160) of the Deep Sea Drilling Project (DSDP) and the Ocean Drilling Project (ODP) has revolutionized our understanding of the effects on ocean currents and sediments of both climatic change and changing oceanic configurations. Perhaps the major advance here was the ability to determine the O_2 isotopic composition of minute quantities of calcareous foraminifera.

The nature and preservation of pelagic deep-sea sediments are closely controlled (Fig. 26.1) by input of particulates and nutrients, by variations in the depth of the oxygen minimum layer, and by the carbonate compensation depth. Maximum accumulation of planktonic remains corresponds closely to areas of high organic primary productivity in the productive surface layer of the oceans, especially where mixing of water masses occurs. Since the 1950s it has been postulated that the fringe of thick clastic sediments around the continental slopes and inner abyssal plains was mostly deposited by turbidity current flows. More recent (1970s) recognition of the depositional and erosional importance of deep ocean currents, and of debris flows and sediment slumps, has blurred the issue a little. Sedimentation around the ocean margins is closely related to the type of plate-tectonic boundary, in addition to the sediment dispersal system of coastal plain and continental shelf. We shall consider the detailed physiography of the ocean basins and the major tectonic controls on oceanic sediment distributions in Chapter 28.

26.2 Physical oceanic processes: general

The ocean waters form one part of the coupled ocean–atmosphere heat engine that redistributes the latitudinally (zonal) unequal radiant heat energy received from the Sun (Fig. 26.2). Solar heating drives atmospheric flows that cause direct wind drag of the surface waters. It also produces density differences during heating, cooling, evaporation and precipitation. Before we consider the broad pattern of oceanic circulation, it is necessary to note the nature of the forces acting upon the ocean reservoirs:
1 *External* forces are caused by direct wind shear on the surface oceanic layers and by the Coriolis force. We have seen previously that the oceanic tides are generally weak.

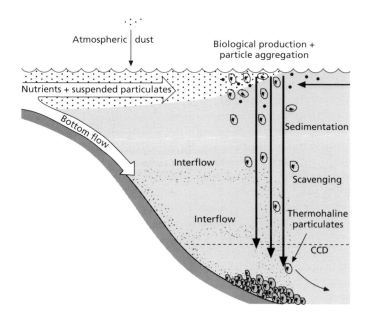

Fig. 26.1 Particle fluxes to the oceans; CCD, carbonate compensation depth. (Mostly after Ittikot *et al.*, 1991.)

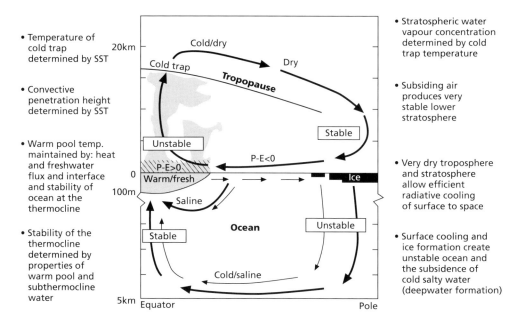

Fig. 26.2 Components of the coupled ocean–atmosphere system: SST, sea surface, temperature (After Webster, 1994.)

2 *Internal* forces are caused by horizontal pressure gradients arising from variations in the height of the oceanic surface, by horizontal and vertical gradients arising from variations in density due to temperature, suspended particles and salinity, and by friction at the ocean boundaries.

The main causes of surface and deep ocean currents are thus wind stress, giving rise to drift currents, and horizontal pressure gradients, giving rise to gradient currents. The Coriolis force and internal friction act as a result of movements set up by wind and pressure.

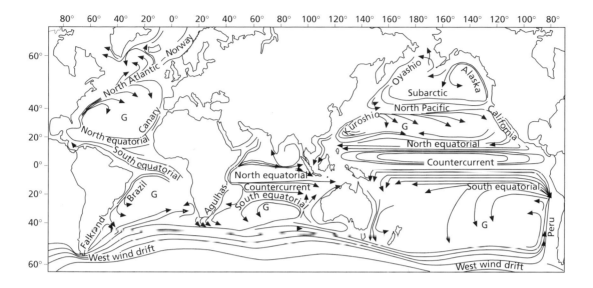

Fig. 26.3 Global average of surface ocean currents drawn as streamlines so that streamline spacing is inversely proportional to flow magnitude. G are subtropical gyres. (After Charnock, 1996, and sources cited therein.)

They cannot cause the water masses to move, but they have a strong effect on the resultant motion.

26.3 Surface oceanic currents and circulation

We may view the upper part of the oceans (the top 100 m or so) as a boundary layer in which strong gradients of temperature, salinity, turbulence, photic energy and oxygen content occur. The zone is one of active interaction between the moving atmosphere and the ocean waters (Fig. 26.2). It is also a layer that is differentially heated by solar radiation from equator to pole. The dynamics of ocean surface mixing are thus rather complicated, involving convection due to heating and cooling, convectional stability induced by freshwater precipitation and glacial meltout waters, and, most importantly, deep mixing caused by periodic strong wind shear (e.g. Moum & Caldwell, 1994). The drift currents associated with direct wind shear are considerably modified by surface gravity waves, the two setting up the remarkably regular pattern of wind-parallel vortex motions known as 'Langmuir circulation'. These are seen to good effect on any lake or sea surface as wind-parallel rows of

foam bubbles or surface debris during a brisk wind on choppy water. Persistence of the bubble windrows at depths up to tens of metres shows that the circulation is important in the mixing process carried on in the upper ocean boundary layer. Less obvious to the observer, but probably much more important volumetrically, is the mixing produced by the breaking of internal waves generated by tidal or surface gravity waves along marked density gradients.

The major surface currents of the ocean (Fig. 26.3) are closely related to the planetary wind system, whose major features were discussed in Chapter 16. Starting with the omnipresent Trade Winds, these begin the process of wind shear in low latitudes, creating the North and South Equatorial Currents whose warm waters journey westwards and northwards into higher latitudes on the western margins of the oceans. Between 25 and 30° latitudes they are further urged on by coupling with the strong westerly winds. In high latitudes a return flow of cool waters is initiated along the eastern sides of the oceans. Thus in each ocean we may identify a very basic circulatory pattern centred on the tropics. These very large-scale motions are termed the 'subtropical gyres', characterized over much of their centres by a generally low biological productivity because of nutrient depletion. The physics of atmosphere–ocean 'coupling' are hidden in the term *wind shear*, for subtle forces are set up during shear which govern the course of surface currents. Thus wind movement around these great anticyclonic 'highs'

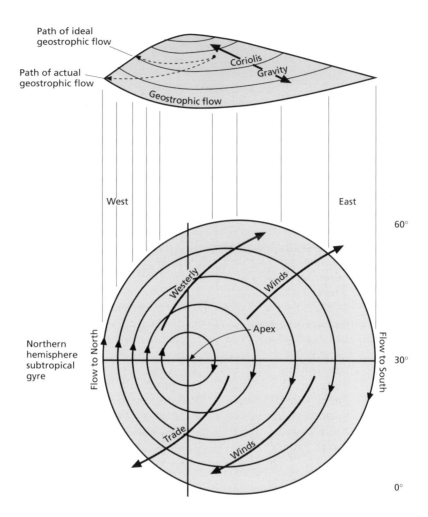

Fig. 26.4 Streamline sketches to illustrate the balance of Coriolis-driven Ekman transport and restoring gravity forces about oceanic gyre vortical circulations. The westerly intensification of transport is indicated by the closer spacing of the closed streamlines. (After Thurman, 1991.)

causes Ekman transport of surface waters in towards their centres. This transport causes a downward slope of the ocean surface to develop outwards from the centre of the high, causing gravitational flow in opposition. Thus the ocean surface flow is set up as gradient currents that run mostly oblique to the dominant winds (Fig. 26.4). The existence of positive topography (about 1.4 m maximum) over the subtropical gyres has been vividly confirmed by satellite altimetry in recent years.

Along the intertropical zone of convergent Trade Winds north and south of the equator, Ekman transport polewards (at about 0.1 m/s) by the westward-flowing equatorial currents causes steady equatorial upwelling of about 1 m per day. The North and South Equatorial Currents are bisected by a prominent narrow eastwards-flowing surface counter-current and a spectacular shallow subsurface counter-counter-current towards the west at up to 1 m/s. Shear interactions in these near-equatorial zones cause powerful convergences and divergences, upwelling of cold nutrient-rich waters and marked eddy mixing (Flament *et al.*, 1996). Seasonal variations in eddy strength control the degree of nutrient-rich upwelling and the amount of phytoplankton subsequently delivered to the seafloor as 'marine snow' (see

Section 26.7). Other very important near-surface current boundaries occur around the Arctic and, particularly strikingly, Antarctica between 50 and 70° latitude. These are the subpolar gyres of the Norwegian and Weddell seas, the Arctic and Antarctic Convergences respectively. The Antarctic Convergence, or Polar Front, marks the boundary between converging cold Antarctic surface waters and much warmer sub-Antarctic waters. The descent of the former as Antarctic Intermediate Water is accompanied by upwelling of nutrient-rich warm waters and massive planktonic productivity (see Section 26.7).

In the past 20 years periodicity in the linked west-directed tropical and oceanic circulations has been explained by the action of an oscillation termed ENSO, the El Niño–Southern Oscillation. The effects of this were particularly prominent in the 1982–83 event, the strongest of the century. ENSO is due to major reduction in the strength of the tropical Trade Winds causing periodic (approximately decadic) outflows of warm tropical waters as rotating Kelvin waves from the western to the eastern Pacific. This is because the normal Trade Winds 'hold up' the warm waters of the western Pacific higher, by about 0.5 m, than those of the cooler eastern Pacific. Once it reaches the coasts of Central America, the wave is reflected polewards into the North Pacific as Rossby waves. These seriously affect ocean currents such as the Kuro Shio Current up to 10 years later (Jacobs *et al.*, 1994). The main ENSO event decreases the magnitude of precipitation over northern Australia and Indonesia, and reduces the degree of upwelling off the coast of NW South America. The upwelling cycle causes major fluctuations in the whole food chain of the upper oceans, in the lean years of which the South American fisheries industry is the major loser. The periodic ENSO-motivated delivery of organic mass to the bottom sediment and the linked development of ocean-water anoxic conditions are expected to give rise to marked cyclicity of shelf and ocean-floor sediments. The effects of ENSO events are also felt widely over the globe, since the workings of the tropical 'heat engine' have knock-on effects on world climate.

One of the most striking features of the general oceanic wind-driven circulation described above is the intensification of surface flow on the western borders of the oceans (Figs 26.3 & 26.4). These are manifest as the great warm western boundary currents such as the North Atlantic Gulf Stream, South Atlantic Brazil Current, Pacific Kuro Shio Current and Indian Ocean Agulhas Current. It is common to measure speeds of over 1.4 m/s (about 5 km/h) in these currents. The asymmetry of the subtropical gyres is explicable in terms of vortex theory (Stommel, 1948; for an introduction see Harvey, 1976). The effect adds to the existing vorticity (equal to the Coriolis force) of the symmetrical wind-driven motions on the western sides of oceans and opposes it on the eastern sides. To establish a steady state, the total vorticity cannot rise without some limiting effect. The braking action is provided by frictional effects (proportional to velocity squared), which cause the warm western currents to be extremely strong, up to 10 times the strength of the cool eastern currents. Major erosive events on the Blake Plateau (see Fig. 28.8) have been attributed to Gulf Stream flow during glacial epochs when the current was thought to be at its strongest (Kaneps, 1979).

Satellite images of western boundary currents reveal spectacular eddy motions, meanders and cutoffs of cooler waters to form 'cold core' eddies. Direct current measurements and bottom scour features (Gross *et al.*, 1988) indicate that these strong vortex motions are able to propagate turbulent energy all the way (i.e. > 4 km) down to the ocean floor, where they cause unsteadiness in the deep thermohaline current flow (so-called deep-sea 'storms'), enhanced resuspension of bottom sediment (Hollister & McCave, 1984) and nutrient mixing (McGillicuddy *et al.*, 1998).

An important consequence of Ekman transport (Chapter 25) is the phenomenon of upwelling. Convergent winds or coast-parallel winds cause strong surface water flow divergence away from the line of wind convergence and the coastline respectively. This forcing away of surface waters is accompanied by the upwelling of deeper waters to take their place. Upwelling is particularly important, for example, off the coasts of Peru, northwest and southwest Africa, and California. Upwelling waters bring with them nutrients such as phosphorus and nitrogen, which cause a greatly increased plankton biomass to be supported in the surface waters. Distinctive sedimentological 'signatures' of upwelling include well-preserved diatom and radiolarian assemblages, increased amount of fish debris and the occurrence of phosphorite grains. Seasonal or decadal variations in upwelling flux (such as those noted previously for

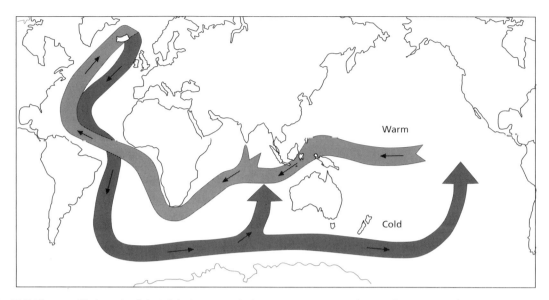

Fig. 26.5 The most likely path of the 'global conveyor belt' of heat via warm Pacific Upper Water moving west (in a highly complex way) through the Indonesian archipelago and Indian ocean into the North Atlantic, where it is cooled to form North Atlantic Deep Water that forms the Western Boundary Undercurrent and a Circum-Antarctic Undercurrent before finally dissipating back in the Pacific. (After Wells *et al.*, 1996, as gleaned from many sources; for a long discussion see Schmitz, 1995.)

ENSO) cause strong signatures in the bottom sediments, such as laminations of varying thickness and organic content.

26.4 Oceanic deep currents and circulation

The surface oceanic circulation described above is merely the most obvious visible sign of a deeper, more thoroughgoing, circulation system that affects the whole ocean mass (Fig. 26.5). Radioisotope tracers indicate that all deep waters must re-establish contact with the atmosphere on a 500 yr timescale. The first evidence for such large-scale recycling was collected by the German 'Meteor' expedition in the 1920s. Following the pioneering theoretical treatment of Stommel (1957), detailed temperature, density and isotopic studies worldwide have revealed a system of deep, dense waters that dominate ocean-floor processes (see review by Schmitz, 1995). These dense currents are termed *thermohaline currents*, from the dual role that temperature and salinity have in producing them. At low latitudes the upper ocean is heated by solar radiation (density decreases), but loses water by evaporation (density increases). At high latitudes the upper ocean is cooled by contact with a colder lower atmosphere (density increases), but freshened by precipitation, river runoff and inflows of polar glacial meltwater (density decreases); also the production of sea ice leads to a saltier residual seawater (density increases). Thermohaline circulation can thus have several causes, favoured by the destabilizing processes that lead to density inversions due to increased surface water density. Today these are prominent in the northern North Atlantic and the Southern oceans (Fig. 26.6). The thermohaline currents are linked to compensatory intermediate and shallow warmer currents in a complicated pattern of downwelling and upwelling whose detailed paths in the Pacific and Indian oceans are still uncertain. The amount of water discharged by the currents is staggering, one estimate for deep water being some 50×10^6 m³/s. This is about 50 times the flow of the world's rivers; about half of the total ocean volume is sourced from the cooled sinking waters of the polar oceans. The nature of the oceanic circulation, with its links from surface to depth, and its role in heat transport and redistribution, has led to its description as a 'global conveyor belt' of both heat and kinetic energy. The

Fig. 26.6 Diagram to show thermohaline circulations (chiefly of the variation in North Atlantic Deep Water (NADW) in an Atlantic meridional cross-section from north (NP) to south (SP) poles with the factors likely to influence this circulation. Apart from any change in shape of the basins due to tectonics, we have: $R_{in} - R_{out}$, radiation balance; V, extent of snow and ice cover; T, global mean temperature; $P_{rain} - P_{ev}$, changes in precipitation and evaporation over oceans; $P_{snow} - P_{abl}$, changes in snow and ice cover; ABW, Atlantic bottom water. (After sources cited in Moum & Caldwell, 1994.)

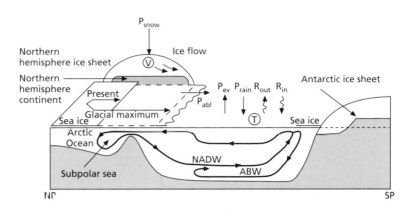

sedimentological consequences of this deep circulation are profound, since steady current velocities of up to 0.25 m/s have been recorded in some areas where the normally slow (~0.05 m/s) thermohaline currents are accelerated on the western sides of oceans and in topographic 'constrictions'.

The basic reasons for the existence of active deep oceanic currents are to be found in the extreme temperature variations that exist today from the equator polewards. Warm subtropical Atlantic waters are driven northwards as surface currents by westerly winds. Closure of the current system occurs by sinking of cooled and denser waters at high latitudes. Thus dense water masses from the Antarctic and Arctic seas sink to become the Antarctic Bottom Water (ABW) and North Atlantic Deep Water (NADW) respectively. ABW forms the majority of the bottom flow around the Antarctic as a circumpolar current, receiving NADW from the western South Atlantic and leaking large discharges northwards from the Weddell sea and other sources into the South Atlantic (under and alongside the NADW), Indian and Pacific oceans. Much is currently being learnt about the paths of these deep-water thermohaline currents during oceanic exploration. Recent results (e.g. Polzin et al., 1996) confirm earlier observations that indicate movement of deep water through fracture zones and across mid-ocean ridges. Thus transfer of ABW from the western to the eastern side of the South Atlantic occurs through the larger silled fracture zones of the Mid-Atlantic Ridge, with intense turbulent mixing along the upper interface. We may ask whether such results are typical for thermohaline

currents in general, given their astonishingly widespread and constant properties. Tracer studies at the interface of other shallow water masses reveal a low value of the mixing rate, about 10^{-5} m²/s. This implies a low rate of turbulent mixing along density interfaces relative to lateral spread, a conclusion also established by turbulent stress calculations. However, it is likely that other mixing mechanisms exist, for example internal waves, which will lead to much larger turbulent dissipation.

Despite expectations to the contrary, there is little evidence from radioisotope studies that the oceanic conveyor belt between the North Atlantic and Southern ocean was more active during the longer glacial intervals (Yu et al., 1996). Yet in the North Atlantic there are clear signals in the quartz silt content of continental-rise sediments (McCave, 1995) and from oxygen and carbon isotopes in benthic forams (Charles & Fairbanks, 1992; Cortijo et al., 1994) that periodic unsteadiness in the generation of NADW has occurred in both the last glacial and interglacial. This seems sensible given the enormous effect in these latitudes of the production of surface, fresh, cold waters and deep, cold, saline waters from the southern front of the Northern Hemisphere Ice-Sheet. Similarly, during the last deglaciation and Holocene there is evidence from sediment cores of very rapid deep water fluctuations which may be due to rapid changes in the thermohaline conveyor belt in its northern generative area (Bianchi & McCave, 1999). There is, in fact, a growing consensus that the linked pattern of surface and thermohaline circulation plays a major role in climate change in northern latitudes.

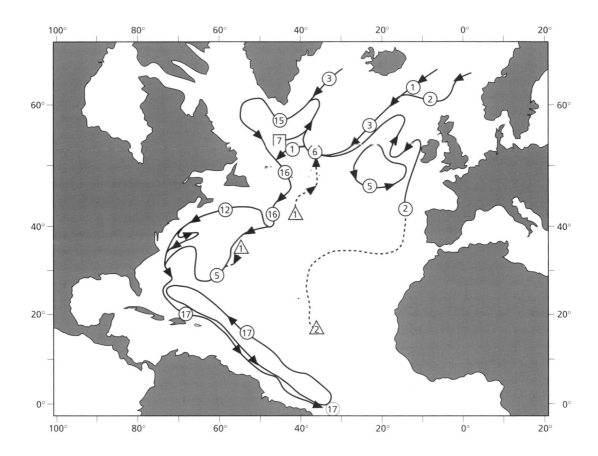

Fig. 26.7 Maps to show the generalized paths and transport rates of North Atlantic Deep Water (1.8–4 °C) circulation. Curved paths indicate that flows are following submarine topography, thus the older term for thermohaline flows used by geologists—contour currents. Rates are in sverdrups (10⁶ m³/s), squares represent sinking, and triangles upwelling. (After Schmitz & McCartney, 1993.)

The NADW is particularly important on the western margin of the North Atlantic ocean where the current is termed the Western Boundary Undercurrent. It flows parallel to and southwards over the continental rise at velocities of up to 0.25 m/s (Fig. 26.7). Seismic studies and coring reveal a thick (kilometre scale) sediment 'drift' comprising alternations of thin, very fine sands, silts and bioturbated muds. The sands and silts are thinly bedded, ungraded, well sorted, and may contain heavy mineral placers in small-scale cross-laminations (Heezen & Hollister, 1963; Hollister

& Heezen, 1972; Bouma & Hollister, 1973). Small ripple-like forms, other tractional features and current scour features are recorded during periodic intensification of the near-bottom flow during deep-sea 'storms' (McCave, 1985; Gross et al., 1988).

The silty and fine sandy deposits of boundary undercurrents in general are termed *contourites*; their good sorting, due to winnowing, distinguishes them from thin distal turbidites, but it is difficult to tell the two deposits apart in the geological record (see discussion in Stow & Lovell, 1979; McCave et al., 1981; Shanmugam et al., 1993). Stow and Piper (1984) catalogue the various attributes of contourites (but see the criticisms of Shanmugam et al., 1993), and Hollister (1993) gives a useful contourite retrospective. The erosional effects of cold undercurrents are also important; many stratigraphic gaps in deep-sea sediment cores from Oligocene times onwards have been attributed to contour-current erosion. Whether drifts form generally or not, and their distribution

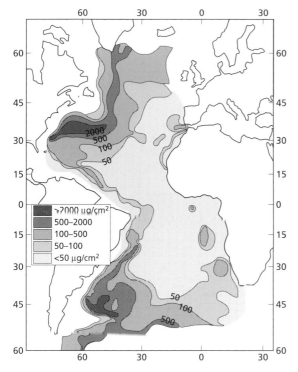

Fig. 26.8 Biscaye and Eittreim's (1977) classic map to show the excess of suspended sediment in the Atlantic Deep Water defining a turbid nepheloid layer. Note that the existence of spatial gradients in concentration (∇c) along such transport paths as indicated in Fig. 26.7 indicates substantial local deposition (on sediment drifts) and erosion (from glacigenic and turbidite fans).

in space, involves a complex interaction between thermohaline flow acceleration, seafloor lithology and submarine-fan sediment supply—see Carter and McCave (1997) for a south Pacific example, and Shanmugan *et al.* (1993) for a Gulf of Mexico example.

A final feature of deep ocean waters is attributed in part to the action of thermohaline currents and in part to the occurrence of deep-sea 'storms', i.e. deep downward transfer of ocean surface eddy energy. This is the phenomenon of increased suspended material in nearbottom water, revealed by light-scattering techniques. The source of the suspended sediment in these bottom nepheloid layers (Fig. 26.8) is variable: distant sourcing (from polar regions especially), local erosional resuspension of ocean-floor muds by 'storms' and

enhanced thermohaline currents, and dilute distal turbidity current flows probably all may have a role. Some nepheloid layers may be up to 2 km thick, although 1–200 m is a more usual figure (Eittreim *et al.*, 1975; Biscaye & Eittreim, 1977). Sediment in nepheloid layers is usually < 2 μm although fine silt up to 12 μm may be suspended, normally at concentrations of up to 500 mg/l rising to 5000 mg/l a few metres off the bottom during deep-sea 'storms' (Gross *et al.*, 1988). Nepheloid layers are also known in many areas from intermediate depths (e.g. Drake & Gorsline, 1973; Pak *et al.*, 1980; Dickson & McCave, 1986), often at the junction between different water masses. These are thought to arise through the erosion of bottom sediments by internal waves and tides amplified on certain critical bottom slopes (Huthnance, 1981). The layers, once formed, intrude laterally into the adjacent open ocean as tongues many tens of metres thick (Fig. 26.9).

26.5 Sculpturing and resedimentation: canyons, slides, slumps and debris flows

The major environments where appreciable volumes of terrigenous clastic sediment occur are the continental rise and inner abyssal plains. We consider these environments of deposition generically, leaving the details of particular types of oceanic basins to Chapter 28. Chief amongst these generic depositional environments are submarine fans, fed by canyons and valleys cutting the continental slope and often extending on to, and sometimes across, the continental shelf. The continental slope, or more precisely the slope break, marks a fundamental division between shallow shelf and the deep marine environment. Unfaulted slopes around passive ocean margins are best seen as (relatively) steep (up to 6°) portions of logistic curves that flatten shelfwards and oceanwards. Large deltas such as the Niger and Mississippi may prograde right out to such slope margins (even at sea-level highstands), where they accentuate the slope by rapid deposition and define wide and distinctive features cut by myriad normal growth faults. The simple form of some slopes may be severely disrupted by the effects of salt intrusion (originating during early rifting), with chaotic salt diapiric topography. Faulted slopes with gradients up to 30° dominate young ocean rifted margins, many subducting margins and coastal extensional basins; they have been referred to as *slope*

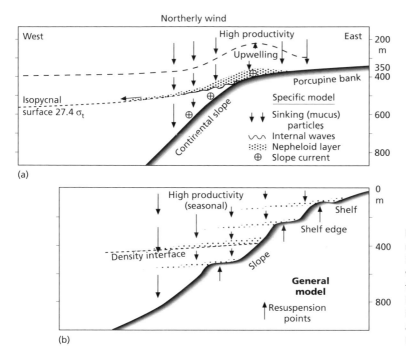

Fig. 26.9 The origin of internal nepheloid layers at isopycnal surfaces is encouraged at their intersection with shelf or slope ramps. The excess turbidity is due to a variety of factors, including bottom resuspension by internal waves, high local productivity and slope currents. (After Dickson & McCave, 1986.)

aprons. Characteristic base-of-slope-apron deposits include talus collapse breccias, slump mounds, debris flow masses and steep-sided gully fills (for very distinctive examples see Surlyk, 1987). Periodic small submarine fans are located at canyon exits through fault scarps.

Continental slopes are dynamic surfaces (see Ross *et al.*, 1994), encouraged to prograde seawards by deposition, smoothed by slow downslope diffusional creep but at the same time ravaged by gullies and slide scars due to downslope mass movements on scales of a few cubic metres to thousands of cubic kilometres (Fig. 26.10). Our modern continental slopes at depths > 100 m have been dominated by the effects of the past 1 Myr of high-amplitude sea-level fluctuations. During sea-level lowstands, much coarse sediment is delivered by rivers, those in high latitudes gorged by glacial meltwaters, in incised canyons almost to the shelf edge. During highstands, deposition is from shelf-edge fine-sediment plumes. A fundamental point concerns the instability of such alternations of coarse- and fine-grained outer-shelf and continental-slope sediment. Generally high water contents (Keller *et al.*, 1979) and the development of gas hydrates (Bugge *et al.*, 1988) encourage periodic mass failure after shocks and abnormal pressures produced by earthquakes (seismic and seismo-volcanic), tsunamis and internal waves. Lower values of shear strength in the

vicinity of submarine canyons are related to a combination of increased concentrations of organic matter and fine-grained sediment. Some idea of the effects of passing surface waves on bottom sediment may be gained from the calculations of Watkins and Kraft (1978) that large storm waves, particularly during hurricanes, may induce pressure anomalies with wavelengths of 300 m and amplitudes of 70 kN/m² in water depths of 60 m. Although the amplitude of these wave-induced pressure anomalies should decrease in deeper water, the effect is considered important on shelf-edge sediments always liable to failure.

Submarine canyons occur on shelves, submarine slopes and submarine fans. They are important conduits for transfer of sediment from shelf to deep marine basin, particularly during sea-level lowstands. Canyons may originate by some or all of the following processes:

• shelfward enlargement (*retrogressive slope failure*) of slope slump scars (see Farre *et al.*, 1983; Piper *et al.*, 1998) by internal waves, tides and surges;
• direct river cutting during sea-level lowstands;
• erosive action of turbidity underflows.

The major canyons of the world's continental margins usually occur seawards of major rivers, usually cutting across the shelf and deepening downwards before flaring wider and shallowing on the continental rise. They commonly have dimensions of hundreds

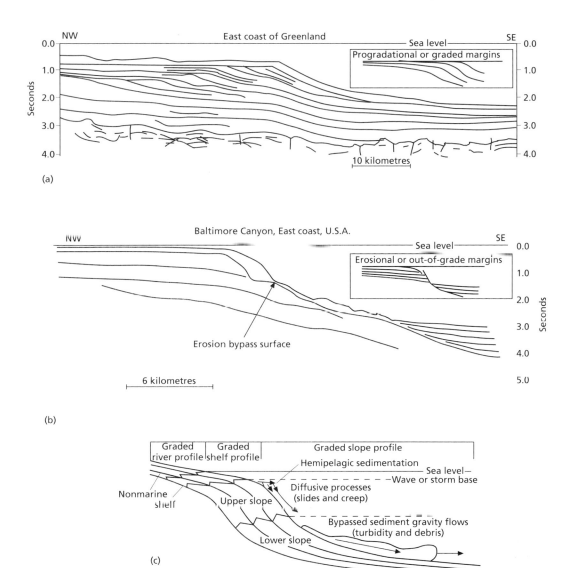

Fig. 26.10 Progradational and erosional continental margins. (a) Progradational (outbuilding and periodically upbuilding) margin of East Greenland. (b) Erosional margin of Baltimore Canyon, east coast, USA. (c) Cartoon of prograding slope to show processes affecting 'graded' slope profile. (From Ross *et al.*, 1994, and sources cited therein.)

of metres deep and kilometres wide, and have a V-shaped cross-sectional form in their upper parts. They are the great bypass conduits for oceanwards sediment transfer and the majority owe their origins to current erosion by rivers and/or associated river-derived turbidity underflows, mostly during low-stands. Their precise courses on the continental slope are governed by local topographic funnelling due to major ocean margin and submarine topography, slide enlargement, slump scars, faulting and the reoccupation of shallow buried antecedent lowstand canyons (Pratson *et al.*, 1994). Some canyons were cut mostly by glacial meltwater discharges, like the great Northwest Atlantic Mid-Ocean Channel (NAMOC) that connected streams of the North American Laurentide ice-cap with the Labrador slope and

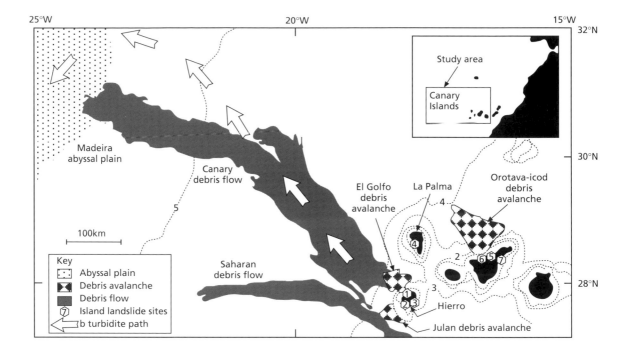

Fig. 26.11 Location of debris flows and debris avalanches around the western Canary Islands, a group of plume-related volcanic edifices rising from the Atlantic floor to the west of the Sahara. (After Masson, 1996.)

abyssal plains as distant as the Sohm to the south (Hesse *et al.*, 1987, 1996; Hesse & Rakofsky, 1992). NAMOC is up to 4000 km long and shows spectacular depositional features like meanders, channel bars and giant levees. Klaucke *et al.* (1997) present interesting palaeohydraulic reconstructions of this remarkable feature.

The majority of canyons are 'headless' in the sense that they do not extend on to the shelf and owe their origins to slump scar enlargement, forming prominent scalloped enclaves into the upper continental slope. The process of competitive growth of these scars leads to a fairly regular canyon spacing of a few kilometres or so (Orange *et al.*, 1994). The orientation of the canyons and gullies is sometimes strongly structurally controlled by faults, by joints and by sedimentary layering in the slope basement. Headless canyons are still conduits, serving to funnel ocean and internal tides, storm waves and shelf plumes into and out of the shelf margins.

Currents in submarine canyons (Shepard *et al.*, 1979) show a strong ocean tidal signature, with up and down water motions strongly modified by current reflections and refractions, the tendency for denser suspensions to move downslope, wave currents, storm surge (gradient) currents and internal waves. More persistent and strong downcanyon flows (over 1 m/s, sometimes over several days, but usually a few hours) record the onset of turbidity current events triggered by any of the previously mentioned currents or by direct river underflows.

Detailed exploration of the ocean margins with GLORIA (e.g. Bugge *et al.*, 1988; Moore *et al.*, 1989; Masson *et al.*, 1992) confirms that large-volume submarine slides, avalanches and debris flows are very important depositional processes in a variety of deep marine environments (for early discoveries see Embley, 1976; Flood *et al.*, 1979). Such mass flows (a mixed igneous–sedimentary *mélange*) are perhaps most commonly and easily derived by failure from the steep (5–10°) slopes associated with intra-oceanic plate volcanic edifices like those of the Hawaian chain in the Pacific (Moore *et al.*, 1989) and the Canary Islands in the central eastern Atlantic (Fig. 26.11; Masson *et al.*, 1992; Masson, 1996). Volumes of individual events involved in the former area may exceed 5000 km³ and occur as a halo of dispersed blocks (some of which are kilometres in extent) around the volcanic centres. It seems that gravity is the main destructive agent of the igneous islands built up slowly over millions of years of plume-induced melting. Major slides and debris flows have been discovered in recent years derived from nonvolcanic continental slopes. Embley (1976) first identified debris flow deposits of enormous extent that were generated by large sediment slides off the Spanish Sahara on the northwest African continental margin (Fig. 26.11). The debris flow travelled on slopes as low as 0.1° for a distance of several hundred kilometres. The deposits cover an area of about 30 000 km² and originated from a massive slump of volume 600 km³ on the upper continental rise where a prominent slide scar several tens of metres deep now exists. Recognition of the debris flow deposits is based on a characteristic geometry, a distinctive acoustic character, a pebbly mudstone fabric and sharp angular contacts in cores, and an undulating surface morphology revealed by bottom photographs. Recent GLORIA and TOBI surveys (Masson *et al.*, 1992; Masson, 1996) identified numerous large volcanic avalanches and slides from the Canary Islands with downslope debris flow deposits and finally turbidity current deposition on the Madeira abyssal plain. It appears from detailed core and GLORIA studies (Masson, 1994) that the turbidity current and the debris flow parted company close to the source area and followed separate paths. Eventually the slower debris flow caught up with the slowly depositing turbidity current on the abyssal plain, burying the lower deposits and then becoming buried itself by the

later flow deposits. It is well known that the Grand Banks earthquake of 1926 in the NW North Atlantic produced a major debris flow that ran out into the Sohm abyssal plain. The stupendous 5500 km³ Storrega slide and debris flow ran out some 800 km into the Norwegian sea, giving rise to a basinwide megaturbidite and triggering a spectacular tsunami whose effects are widely recorded in Scotland and coastal Norway (see Dawson *et al.*, 1993). Today the slide scar actually defines the continental margin and is some 300 km wide and 300 m deep.

26.6 Submarine fans

Submarine fans (Fig. 26.12) abut against feeder submarine channels on the continental slope, the larger ones extending across the continental rise into the abyssal plain. As in many marine environments, fans are very sensitive to sea-level change (Posamentier *et al.*, 1991; Posamentier & Erskine, 1991; Armentrout *et al.*, 1991). In the past million years or so, fan activity has been at maximum during lowstands, with high deposition rates and the formation of lowstand 'wedges' (Fig. 26.13). This trend was accentuated in fans like the Mississippi where huge quantities of glacial meltwater and associated sediment were discharged to the shelf edge, subsequently to descend as underflows to the Mississippi submarine fan. Many fans have become inactive during the Holocene highstand with very low deposition rates of fine-grained pelagic or hemipelagic sediment as their valley heads became far removed from direct riverine input of sediment, with the shelf acting as a sediment 'trap' (for the Amazon fan see Damuth *et al.*, 1988; Cramp *et al.*,

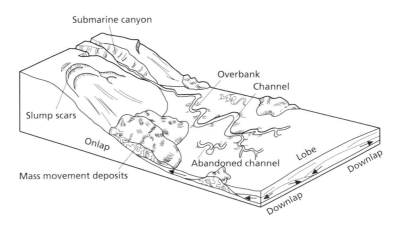

Fig. 26.12 Diagram to show features of submarine fans and adjacent basin margins. (After Normark *et al.*, 1993.)

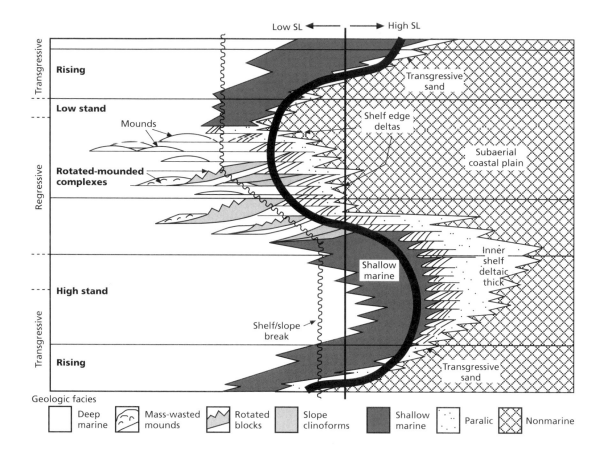

Fig. 26.13 The distribution of coastal plain, shelf and basinal sedimentary facies in time and space through a cycle of sea-level change. Note the lowstand shelf-edge deltas feeding directly downslope into submarine fans and the highstand entrapment. (After Armentrout, 1991.)

1995). High-resolution stratigraphic studies in older sediments pre-dating the 'eccentricity-driven' cycles of the upper Pleistocene also point to a periodic control on turbidity current activity, driven perhaps in Mediterranean areas by precession-induced (~23 kyr) changes in continental runoff rather than by direct sea-level controls (Postma *et al.*, 1993a; Weltje & DeBoer, 1993). Also, the surface of fans and of travelling turbidity currents on western oceanic boundaries must be strongly affected both by ocean 'storms' descending from energetic upper ocean eddies and by thermohaline current activity, yet we know little about such influences.

Our ideas on the nature and morphology (if not the processes) of submarine fans have had to undergo a radical shift in the past several years as a result of the increased resolution provided by new generations of high-resolution seismic reflection profiling, imaging from GLORIA and TOBI, and drilling by DSDP/ODP legs. These have revealed an astonishing variety of details concerning fan morphology and evolution. Even before these new data, it was well appreciated that submarine fans are rarely regularly fan-shaped (or even fan-shaped at all!) since their growth is often closely controlled by submarine topography, with which intruding turbidity currents and debris flows must interact. Thus not only is there a great range in fan area, reflecting sediment and water discharge from feeder canyons and slopes, but also great variability in shape. Yet only a pedant would argue against established usage since the term *fan* serves as a useful unifying concept, linking as it does all point-sourced submarine sediment bodies. Thus submarine

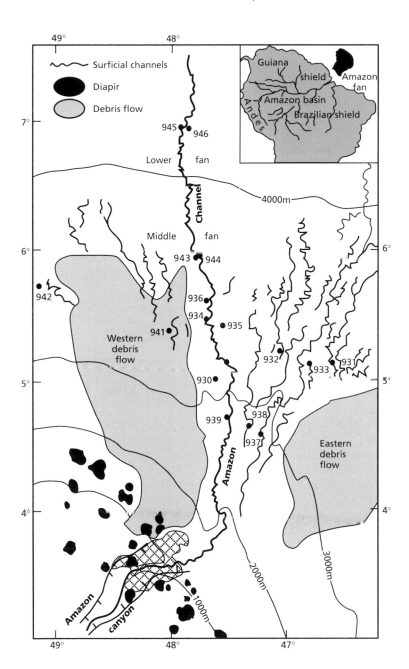

Fig. 26.14 Map of Amazon fan to show active Amazon channel and numerous abandoned channels. Numbered sites refer to core locations. (After Cramp *et al.*, 1995.)

fans are directly analogous to the more regularly and perfectly fan-shaped alluvial fans (where topographic constraints are often absent in fault-bounded basins) in that dispersal of sediment across the fan is controlled by a migrating and avulsive distributive channel system separated by levees and interchannel areas (see various examples by: Normark & Piper, 1972, 1984; Colella & Normark, 1984; Colella & di Geronimo, 1987; Damuth *et al.*, 1988; Flood *et al.*, 1991; Twichell *et al.*, 1991; Weimer, 1991; O'Connell, 1991; McHargue, 1991). Basically the majority of a submarine fan deposit is made up of an amalgam of stacked and leveed channels (Figs 26.14 & 26.15).

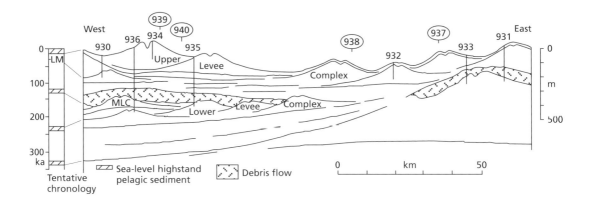

Fig. 26.15 Schematic cross-section of the Amazon fan. Numbers are sites in Fig. 26.14. Note the stacked and offset lowstand channel–levee complexes formed in response to channel switching, and the burial and onlap of the debris flow deposits by fan sediment. MLC, middle levee complex; LM, 30 ka Lake Mungo event. (After Cramp *et al.*, 1995.)

Despite the variability noted above, it is still useful to admire the prescience of pioneering facies models for submarine fans such as those proposed by Walker and Mutti (1973) and Walker (1976, 1978). We may subdivide fans into the following sectors:

1 *Upper fan*. This contains the main feeder channel issuing from a submarine canyon (rarely, as in the Crati fan, from a tributary network) and usually bordered by major levees. Debris flow lobes may occur on this portion, spreading down on to the middle fan.

2 *Middle fan*. Here the main channel splits into leveed distributaries of different ages (usually only one channel is active at any time). These show meandering patterns or braid between interchannel areas bounded by levees. Some channels terminate in the mid-fan to pass into 'supra-fan' lobes (noteworthy examples occur on Delgada and Navy fans).

3 *Lower or outer fan*. This is often smooth, or with a myriad of smaller channels (a few metres in depth), sometimes (noteworthy examples occur on Navy and Mississippi fans) ending in well-defined (to GLORIA II anyway) terminal fan lobes.

Fan channels are closely analogous to river channels. High-resolution GLORIA images, shallow seismic profiles and deep drilling results from the Amazon (Damuth *et al.*, 1988; Leg 155 Shipboard

Scientific Party, 1994), Mississippi (Twichell *et al.*, 1991; Weimer, 1991) and Indus (McHargue, 1991) fans reveal convincing evidence for channel meandering, meander migration, lateral accretion, meander loop cutoff and avulsion of entire channels (Figs 26.14 & 26.16). Many channels end with a distributive nature at well-defined terminal lobes (for a fine example from Delgada fan see Drake *et al.*, 1989; Fig. 26.17), which mark the onset of rapid radial deceleration and turbidity current dissipation (Fig. 26.18). Avulsive nodes and terminal lobe development are exceptionally clearly described from the fan valley of the Petit-Rhône, NW Mediterranean sea (Torres *et al.*, 1997). It is possible that, for submarine fans dominated by underflow, terminal lobe sites mark the occurrence of flow lofting (Sparks *et al.*, 1993) and rapid deposition of fines on the lower fan to form what have been christened 'hemiturbidites' (Stow & Wetzel, 1990).

Since submarine fans are dominated by the dynamics of channels, let us take a closer look at the processes that might occur in and around such features. The first point to make concerns timing of channel cutting, occupation and migration (Fig. 26.19). It seems that the majority of channels seen on or near the surface of modern fans were cut during lowstand or in the transition to highstand times, since Holocene highstand draping by fine hemipelagic sediment is almost universal. The very existence of fan channels means that at some point turbidity currents issuing from the feeder canyons must have had the excess power available to cut such channels, otherwise the turbidity current would have spread radially at the canyon exit, depositing uniformly as it did so. The fact that channels are still seen hundreds of kilometres

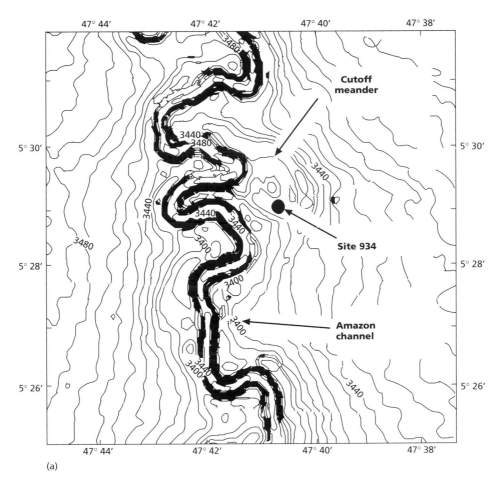

(a)

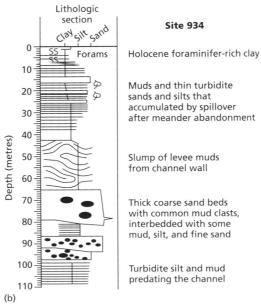

(b)

Fig. 26.16 (a) Bathymetric map showing the spectacular Amazon channel meanders and the cutoff meander sampled at Site 934. (b) Log of core through meander cutoff. (After Cramp et al., 1995.)

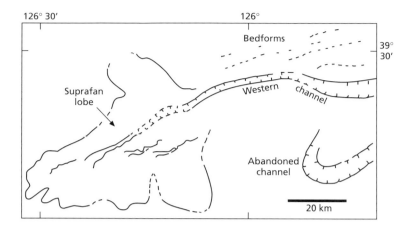

Fig. 26.17 Interpretation of a sonograph mosaic from Delgada fan to show the well-developed supra-fan lobe at the end of the downstream-tapering fan channel. (After Drake *et al.*, 1989, where the original sonograph image may also be seen.)

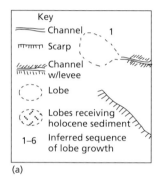

(a)

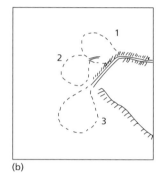

(b)

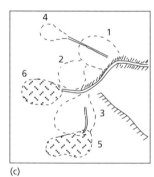

(c)

Fig. 26.18 Sketches to show how fan channel frontal lobes construct a larger area of lobate form (cut by later channels) by a combined process of progradation and periodic lobe switching. (After Normark *et al.*, 1979.)

downfan from the main feeder canyon (e.g. for the Mississippi fan see Twichell *et al.*, 1991) means that this power was almost always available—perhaps because the heads of travelling currents are *always* erosive, no matter how dilute the flow? Once cutting has begun, the channel then serves to guide subsequent currents, which may in turn enlarge the channel by erosion or infill the channel incrementally depending upon the state of the current locally. At the same time the channel-bordering levees are being constructed as currents overtop the channel margins (Hay *et al.*, 1982) and interact with the surrounding fan surface. Levee growth is preferentially to the right in the northern hemisphere (vice versa for the southern)

because of the Coriolis effect (see Komar, 1969; Klaucke *et al.*, 1997). The rates of growth of levees and of the deepening or shallowing of channels then control the dynamics of the whole fan system. In many upper and middle fan sectors it seems that some sort of depositional (aggradational) equilibrium between channel and levee was attained, since leveed channels now perch with their talwegs (deepest parts) high above the surface of the surrounding fan. We know from evidence of modern rivers and modelling studies of rivers (Mackey & Bridge, 1995) that such a topography leads to a system of offset stacking of successive channel–levee complexes as channel avulsion occurs with time. Such offset stacks have been nicely imaged by high-resolution seismic reflection studies on the Mississippi (Weimer, 1991; Twichell *et al.*, 1991), Indus (McHargue, 1991) and Amazon (Damuth *et al.*, 1988; Leg 155 Shipboard Scientific Party, 1994; Cramp *et al.*, 1995) fans (Fig. 26.15). Another process that may have great importance in

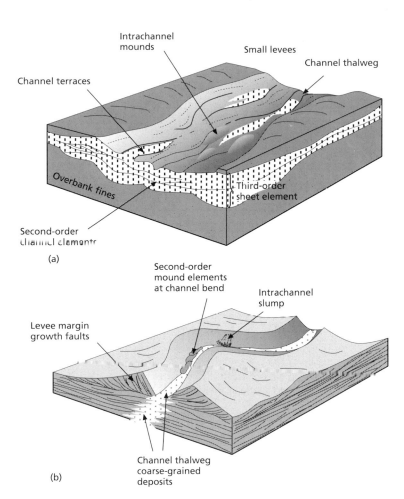

Fig. 26.19 Schematic block diagrams to illustrate contrasting low-sinuosity fan channels producing sheet sands by lateral migration, with high-sinuosity channels with abundant spillover producing ribbon sands in an aggrading package of levee deposits. (After Clark & Pickering, 1996.)

controlling levee deposition, terminal lobe formation and avulsion is that of flow stripping, first deduced from the well-studied Navy fan off the California borderlands (Piper & Normark, 1983; Bowen *et al.*, 1984). Here, large-magnitude flows negotiating a meander bend or other sharp bend split into two, with the denser, sandier, lower portion carrying on round the bend and the upper portion leaving the channel confines to erode the levee and escape on to the surrounding fan surface, where it may lay down a lobe-shaped deposit during its radial deceleration. Under some circumstances of major flow and levee failure, the process may lead to complete channel avulsion. Many levees are covered with regular wavy dune-like bedforms.

On a large scale the architecture of fans is a response to both changing sea level, producing the fan lobe sequences of Twichell *et al.* (1991) and Weimer (1991), and the shifting locus of sediment input at the continental shelf break. The Mississippi fan shows this latter effect *par excellence* as the changing Quaternary position of the Mississippi river has influenced the sites of successive shelf and slope canyons (Weimer, 1991). The resulting spaghetti-like arrangement of about 17 Plio-Pleistocene channel–levee complexes in a lateral wedge-shaped amalgamation of fans is impressive. A similar sequence of lobe shifting following movement of feeder river channels is documented in the smaller elongate Crati fan (Colella & Normark, 1984; Colella & di Geronimo, 1987). Major new data on fan stacking was provided by Leg 155 drilling into the Amazon fan (Leg 155 Shipboard Scientific Party, 1994; Cramp *et al.*, 1995), with spectacular offset stacking within individual prograding lowstand fan lobe sequences and abandonment highstand pelagic drapes separating successive sequences (Fig. 26.15).

Our all-too-brief synthesis of submarine fans must end with some attempt to guide geologists in their difficult attempts to make sense of ancient deposits thought to be of fan origins—for an excellent account in much more detail see Mutti and Normark (1991). Channel deposits are believed to fine downstream from source and to contain aggraded or laterally accreted sequences of sand- and/or gravel-grade sediments depending on available sediment supply. Hydraulic considerations lead to the expectation of channel and point bars covered with dune bedforms and thus the production of laterally accreted cross-stratified deposits with frequent erosion surfaces. The magnitude of modern channels should prepare the geologist for major, kilometre-wide, hundreds of metres deep complexes of great internal complexity (Fig. 26.19). Clark *et al.* (1992) and Clark and Pickering (1996) divide channel deposits into two end-members, *erosional* and *aggradational*. The former tend to occur on smaller fans and are usually low-sinuosity channels with low levees transporting coarse sediment down relatively steep slopes; avulsions are frequent and a high degree of channel deposit density is achieved locally. The latter are usually highly sinuous channels with large levees on gentler slopes; avulsions are infrequent and depositional sequences are dominated by the vertical aggradation of the channel deposits. Cores from modern fan levees are dominated by thin-bedded fine sand beds with internal small-scale cross-laminations. The form of levees indicates that over kilometres or tens of kilometres all units should fine and thin away from the channels. Complete levee sequences might reach hundreds of metres thick for the largest submarine fans. Interchannel flats between channel levee complexes comprise bioturbated muds and thin silts. Terminal lobes like those of Navy and Delgada fans might be mapped out as such in an area of good exposure, showing downlobe diminution of channels, fining and thinning of thin turbidite laminae and beds.

The overall depositional pattern of a fan involves a downfan fining from thick coarse sand- or gravel-grade turbidites and debris flows in the upper fan channels to thin, very fine sand- or silt-grade turbidites on the lower fan apron. Sections normal to the fan axis on the mid-fan show channelized turbidites

separated by fine interchannel areas. Fan progradation is postulated to cause a gross coarsening-upwards succession (Walker & Mutti, 1973) as progressively more proximal fan facies overlie the fan apron.

26.7 Biological and chemical oceanic processes

The biological productivity of the surface layer of the oceans is due to the abundance of light, enabling the primary producers, *phytoplankton*, to thrive and photosynthesize, forming the basis of the oceanic food chain. The major phytoplanktonic groups are the siliceous diatoms, the calcareous nanoplanktonic coccoliths and the organic-walled dinoflagellates. *Primary production* is the term given to the daily amount of carbon fixed by photosynthetic reactions in the surface layers of the oceans. This varies over two orders of magnitude, the amount of carbon fixed ranging up to about 200 g/m² yr (only *c.* 25% of the highest values for equatorial rainforest environments). About 1% of this carbon reaches the ocean floor as organic sediment, defining the mass sink from the surface layer 'organic carbon pump'. Combined with the loss of carbon through $CaCO_3$ precipitation, the result is an unsteady and nonuniform rain of inorganic detritus from coastal plumes, organic tissue, siliceous opal and calcium carbonate to the ocean floor (Fig. 26.20). Unsteadiness is a seasonal, annual, decadal or longer-term response to water mass characteristics, including elemental supply, inorganic input, nutrient content, temperature, light levels and so on. Variation in these factors is responsible for near-surface planktonic 'blooms', increased probability of organic/inorganic aggregation and the production of sediment interlaminations. Low productivity occurs in the surface waters of the subtropical gyres. The highest production comes from areas within the influence of large-scale river-derived nutrient input and where forced coastal upwelling of deep, cool, nutrient-rich waters occurs due to Ekman transport. In low-surface-productivity areas, vertical transport of nutrients by rising and descending diatom mats has been established as a dynamic process whereby some surface productivity still occurs in the absence of *in situ* nutrients (Villareal *et al.*, 1993). An interesting theory (Martin *et al.*, 1994; de Baar *et al.*, 1995) points out that in the Southern ocean, even though upwelling waters occur associated with the Circum-

Fig. 26.20 The fundamental controls upon the transformation of organic matter, pelagic sediment and organisms into the aggregated and sedimenting particles known as marine 'snow'. The principal processes are: A. metabolic release of respiration products, excretion and desorption; B. assimilation by microorganisms, adsorption; C. grazing on fine particles; D. fine particle production via grazing; E. aggregation (low turbulent shear); F. fragmentation, disaggregation (high turbulent shear); G. faecal packaging; H. grazing on large particles; I. assimilation of dissolved substances by microbes associated with large particles; J. excretion and metabolic release of dissolved substances by microbes associated with large particles; K. assimilation of dissolved substances by zooplankton; L. excretion by zooplankton. (After Bruland *et al.*, 1989; Jahnke, 1990.)

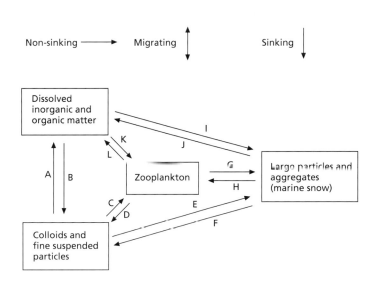

Antarctic Current, primary productivity here is very low and characteristic high-nutrient/low-chlorophyll waters exist. These all coincide with very low available iron contents due to the paucity of wind-blown dusts with their iron oxide coatings. Iron thus turns out to be a limiting element in primary productivity, a feature illustrated by experiments involving seeding the upper ocean waters of such areas with iron compounds and by observations of water mass characteristics at the great convergences of the Antarctic Polar Front. Additionally there is evidence for markedly increased primary productivity in glacial times when wind-blown dust supplies from Patagonia to the Southern ocean were much increased (Kumar *et al.*, 1995), general oceanic upwelling increased and nitrate loss by denitrification much reduced (see Ganeshram *et al.*, 1995). It has been calculated that this increased glacial productivity and the return of the sequestered carbon into sediments was more than ample to cause the reduced CO_2 content of the glacial atmosphere.

Our purpose here with chemical processes is to focus on two important 'fences' that exist in ocean water, the junctions between carbonate saturation and undersaturation (CCD; see Chapter 3) and between oxygen enrichment and depletion. Variation

of the CCD with time is beautifully illustrated by events at the Eocene–Oligocene boundary revealed in deep-sea cores (Kennett & Shackleton, 1976). Oxygen isotope measurements on deep benthic forams revealed a rapid temperature fall caused by the initiation of the deep Antarctic Bottom Current at this time. Onset deep oceanic circulation (see below) caused increased oceanic turnover, which in turn caused increased calcareous biogenic production in the central Pacific. This was closely followed by a major and apparently rapid deepening of the carbonate compensation depth. The regions of the ocean that show particular productivity, and hence high sedimentation rates, are along the eastern ocean margins where cold nutrient-rich waters upwell (see below) and at the convergence of major oceanic gyres in equatorial and polar regions.

The second important chemical 'fence' marks the junction between the upper oxygenated levels of the ocean and lower, oxygen-deficient, levels. Oxygen in seawater is derived from the atmosphere and as a byproduct of photosynthesis. Saturation is usually achieved in near-surface levels, but oxygen contents generally fall with increasing depth (50–100 m). Below the photosynthetic zone, processes such as the oxidation of organic material reduce the oxygen content. In deeper water the oxygen content may rise again if cold, oxygen-rich thermohaline currents are present. A major development in the past 20 years has been the location of vast areas of open ocean that show marked oxygen deficiency at depths of 1000–2000 m (see reviews in Demaison & Moore, 1980; Wignall, 1994). It is no coincidence that such areas are close to regions of upwelling and therefore of high organic productivity. The absence of anoxic waters in the open Atlantic ocean is attributed to more efficient flushing by ocean currents and to the general paucity of phosphate, which limits primary production levels. The large area of anoxic ocean water found in the Arabian sea is noteworthy because it is accompanied by abundant hydrogen sulphide in the bottom sediments.

Anoxic water masses also exist in basins that have a narrow connection with the open ocean across a shallow sill. Intermittent anoxic conditions occur in many fjords and small bays, whilst permanent anoxic conditions occur in the Black sea. In all cases anoxism is caused by the development of mid-water stratification produced by salinity or temperature gradients, often a result of saline density currents intruding into the basin over the entrance sill. Oceanographic research has identified periodic anoxic events in many oceans; examples from the Santa Barbara and Cariaco basins will be discussed further later (see Section 26.10).

Sediment below anoxic water is rich in organic material and provides a broad modern analogue to some black shales, which are a frequent occurrence in the geological record (Wignall, 1994). Such organic-rich sediments are important potential oil source rocks. The high organic content is a consequence of the enhanced organic productivity that produced the anoxic conditions in the first place. Significant occurrences of light hydrocarbon produced by bacteria occur in sediment below the anoxic waters. Many marine black shales are enriched in uranium, a feature that eases their recognition in exploration and production wells, since their production of gamma-rays is readily recorded. The reason for this enrichment is that, in the porewaters of reducing sediments, dissolved uranium complexes are reduced to insoluble U_4O_2, the rate of accumulation being inversely proportional to the depth of the uranium redox boundary from the sediment–water interface (Lovely *et al.*, 1991).

26.8 Pelagic oceanic sediments

In oceanic environments below the carbonate compensation depth (CCD) and in areas of low surface water productivity for siliceous plankton, the chief sediment type is red clays (actually chocolate to red-brown silty clays). These accumulate at very slow rates of between 0.0001 and 0.001 mm/yr and are predominantly of clay minerals whose compositions reflect continental climatic regimes (illite, chlorite, kaolinite) or intra-oceanic basic igneous source rocks (montmorillonite). Slow-growing manganese nodules are common in certain areas of red clay deposition. Adjacent to Trade Wind deserts such as the Sahara, appreciable amounts of wind-blown silt occur in red clay facies, much of it 'wüstenquartz' with its characteristic iron oxide coating. As discussed previously, this wind-blown dust supplies biologically available iron to the surface ocean waters. Studies of aeolian dust in North Atlantic cores (Chapter 16) has proved of great help in elucidating desert expansion and contraction during the Quaternary.

On the ocean floor above the CCD, biogenic calcareous oozes dominate, with the main culprits being the coccolithophores (see Honjo, 1976), foraminiferae and pteropods, which fall through the ocean column as part of 'marine snow' (Fig. 26.20) or in faecal pellets from predators higher in the food chain. Mapping the distribution and thickness of calcareous oozes in subsurface oceanic sediments provides critical evidence for the chemical dynamics of the ocean with time. Other estimates of palaeoproductivity are the ratio of benthic to planktonic foraminiferae, the abundance of the former reflecting the amount of suitable organic matter supplied to the ocean floor.

Calcareous oozes predominate over the crests and flanks of the mid-ocean ridges where the resultant deposits may be strongly modified by bio-irrigation, local gravity flowage, density currents and bottom currents.

The components of silicic oozes are the opaline skeletons of the planktonic diatoms, silicoflagellates and the predatory protozoan radiolarians. Preservation of opal is largely independent of water depth, i.e. there is no silica compensation depth. Hence siliceous biogenic sediments may be a good indicator of ocean surface productivity *if* postdepositional dissolution can be estimated. Diatom oozes are typical high-latitude deposits at the present day, Antarctic waters accounting for over 50% of the world's opaline silica production. This has not always been the case in the past and they are abundant in certain lower-latitude areas today (e.g. Gulf of California; see Pike & Kemp, 1997). Radiolarians are more common in low latitudes. The overall distribution of opaliferous deposits reflects high-fertility areas of the ocean marked by either coastal upwelling, surface water divergence, as in equatorial regions like the eastern Pacific, or convergence, as at the Antarctic Polar Front. In such areas high phosphate and nitrate contents arise from annual thermocline breakdown and deep-water mixing processes. Pike and Kemp (1997) have documented the production of delicately varved diatomaceous laminites produced in this way, with important records of decadal to half-century cyclicity in the ocean current systems responsible in the eastern Pacific/Gulf of California. As noted previously, siliceous planktonic productivity is severely iron-limited in areas away from the influx of wind-blown dust.

26.9 Palaeo-oceanography of modern oceans

It is the ocean sediments and their contained fauna and flora that provide the memory bank that can be used to trace the physical and chemical evolution of oceanic water masses. Oceanic sediments are thus a record of the ocean's productivity (see review by Berger & Herguera, 1992) but by their very nature only proxy records, through the use of organic carbon content, for example. The fact that oceanic circulation patterns have a major effect on world climate through their role as the major 'conveyor belt' of thermal energy transfer from atmosphere to ocean means that palaeo-oceanography must also address and reconstruct this aspect. A prerequisite for oceanic reconstruction is some knowledge of the evolution of oceanic shape, size and depth. Linear ocean-crust magnetic anomalies enable shape and size to be reconstructed, while models for ocean-crust cooling and subsidence enable palaeodepths to be estimated. Data from offshore deep-water exploration wells and multichannel seismic reflection profiles enable stratigraphic and sedimentary successions to be defined and delimited, and the nature of the sedimentary record to be related to ocean basin evolution. Typically a Mesozoic-aged opening ocean involved initial accumulation of evaporites followed by carbonate

platforms and ramps and the subsequent development of submarine fans as continental-scale drainage systems developed. The onset of deep thermohaline circulation in the Cainozoic and the onset of rapid and high-magnitude sea-level variations in the Quaternary compete the major controls.

Estimates of the carbonate compensation depth (CCD) in ancient oceans depend upon plots of $CaCO_3$ accumulation rates against palaeodepth. The position of the CCD can then be computed from a regression equation, being the intercept of depth as the accumulation rate tends to zero (see van Andel et al., 1977). Curves relating CCD to time show strong similarities between all oceans, implying control by circulation of deep oceanic waters. Evidence for ocean anoxic events comes from widespread black shale horizons (sapropels), whilst upwelling is recorded by cherts, phosphorite and fish debris. Very extensive cherts record high equatorial productivity of radiolarian species. Studies of biogenic silica in Pacific cores, for example, reveal that the maximum accumulation rates have occurred at the equator for the past 50 Myr, indicating the persistence of equatorial upwelling caused by divergence (Leinen, 1979). However, once deposited, the opaline skeletons of plankton are vulnerable to early diagenetic dissolution by porewaters, with much silica diffusion back into the ocean water. Studies in the Southern ocean (Kumar et al., 1995) reveal a greatly increased diatom production, as seen in opal accumulation rates, but decreased carbonate accumulation rates (due to increased dissolution) in glacial times as compared with today. Generally it is found that the glacial equatorial oceans were characterized by a higher surface productivity and increases in the rate of burial of organic carbon ('carbon events'), probably due to an increase in rates of coastal upwelling. However, this increase in organic carbon burial does not seem to have given rise to more widespread oceanic anoxia even in more physically isolated basins such as the Panama basin (Yang et al., 1995). Contour-current activity is indicated by thick continental-rise 'contourites', whilst submarine fans of turbiditic origin witness the growth of terrestrial drainage systems on continental areas adjacent to the opening ocean.

As noted previously, two perturbations are responsible for changes in ocean water dynamics—polar cooling to create cool dense waters, and equatorial heating to give warm saline waters. Both have the

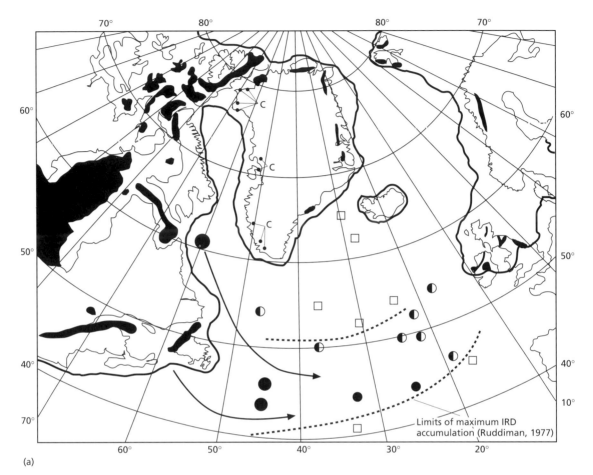

(a)

Fig. 26.21 (a) Map to show the distribution of oceanic ice-rafted debris (IRD) sourced from carbonate-rich rocks (outcrops shaded; mainly North America) of the last glacial catchments. Maximum limits of the last glacial ice are shown. The sizes of the filled circles indicate the relative abundance of limestone-sourced IRD. Half-filled circles indicate IRD not present in all Heinrich layers. Squares are localities with no limestone-rich IRD. Arrows indicate possible iceberg paths from the major calving area of Greenland–Labrador and St Lawrence icestreams. (After Bond *et al.*, 1992)

potential to give rise to thermohaline currents, but the local oceanic topography must be capable of letting the water masses 'feed' into and circulate around the world's oceans. Kennett (1977) was the first to point out that oceanic circulation depends upon the particular topographic evolution of the ocean basins, the zonal position of the continents *and* the world climate. The present-day circulation results from thermohaline deep currents due to a strong zonal temperature gradient and the development of a circum-Antarctic seaway after seafloor spreading

had opened up Drake's Passage. The former process provided the necessary dense water, whilst the latter allowed deep dispersal of this water into the world's oceans. Thus increased flux of warm equatorial water polewards causes a tendency for 'greenhouse' interglacial conditions, whilst increases in cool polar water equatorwards gives glacial conditions. Oxygen isotope studies reveal that the warmest Cainozoic ocean temperatures occurred at the Palaeocene–Eocene boundary, when a major reorganization of oceanic circulation must have taken place. It is probable that

Atlantic Ocean (O'Connell *et al.*, 1996). Subsequent to this warm interval, Antarctic ice began to accumulate. The onset of ADW in the Cainozoic (Kennett *et al.*, 1974; Kennett & Shackleton, 1976) is documented in the isotopic composition of deep-dwelling benthonic forams, which give evidence for a 5 °C decline in bottom-water temperature over about 100 000 yr at the Eocene–Oligocene boundary. There is plentiful evidence (see Hodell *et al.*, 1986) from oxygen isotopes that a major uptake of ocean water into ice occurred in the upper Miocene to the Miocene–Pliocene boundary. This marks a global sea-level fall, which coincidentally made a major contribution to the subsequent isolation and desiccation of the entire Mediterranean sea (see Section 26.11). Data from ODP drilling in the Arctic ocean indicates that the outflow of NADW into the Atlantic did not occur before that late Miocene. Prior to this, poorly ventilated bottom conditions dominated, with preservation of sapropels and a siliceous diatom record of high surface productivity. Abundant dropstones in lower Pliocene sediments attest to the development of ice, with a marked increase in their frequency at about 2.5 Ma.

Detailed isotopic and grain-size studies of ocean sediment (see McManus *et al.*, 1999) and of ice-sheet cores reveal that, super-imposed upon the shortest-term Milankovitch band timescale of 20 kyr, there are short-duration (~1–5 kyr) rapid climatic switches termed 'Dansgaard–Oeschger' events. They give rise to cyclical variations in sediment type in high-latitude oceans (50–60°) because of the periodic increase in discharge of icebergs produced in glacial surges during cold periods. They result in widespread dissemination of meltout sediments (Heinrich layers), both to seafloor and to deep thermohaline currents as the nepheloid layer intensifies (Heinrich, 1988; Bond *et al.*, 1992; Fig. 26.21). The actual effects of massive iceberg discharge on thermohaline circulation are unknown, though theoretical studies (Paillard & Labeyrie, 1994) suggest that the resultant freshening of the ocean surface waters (confirmed by oxygen data on planktonic forams) may temporarily stop the deeper circulation due to surface buoyancy increase. In this way the occurrence of climatic fluctuations has a major effect upon oceanic circulation and sedimentation patterns.

Spectacular results from DSDP and ODP cores in the equatorial Pacific ocean include the discovery

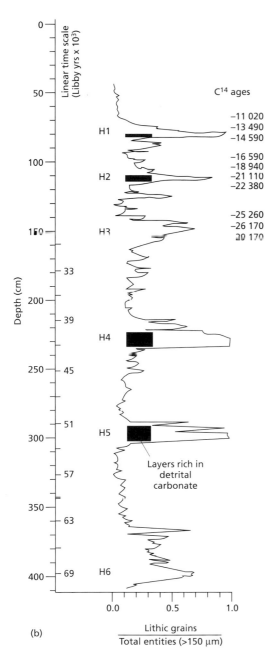

Fig. 26.21 (b) Log of DSDP Site 609 to show Heinrich layers and those rich in carbonate IRD. (After Bond *et al.*, 1992.)

strong latitudinal gradients in sea surface temperatures caused evaporation to exceed precipitation greatly in low-latitude semi-restricted areas of the old and closing Tethys Ocean or the new, opening South

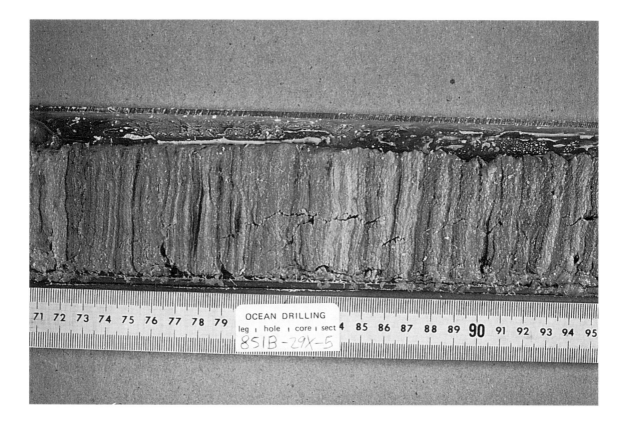

Fig. 26.22 Core photo to show diatom-laminated ooze, Site 851, eastern Pacific. (From Kemp & Baldauf, 1993; photo courtesy of A. Kemp.)

(Kemp & Baldauf, 1993) of repeated episodes of increased equatorial primary production in the Neogene between 15 and 4 Ma (middle Miocene to lower Pliocene). These are represented by laminated deposits rich in the strand-like diatom *Thalassiothrix* (Fig. 26.22) and interpreted to be the foundered remains of surface 'mats' (see Villareal *et al.*, 1999). The laminated intervals, centimetres to decimetres in thickness, are distinctive and unusual in the sense that 'normal' oceanic sediment in the areas is bioturbated and unlaminated. The laminations are not due to development of open-ocean anoxia because the benthic foraminifera associated with the laminations are normal open-ocean forms. It is thought that the rapid descent of vast volumes of tough diatomaceous mat simply overwhelmed the local benthic organisms' ability to bioturbate the sediment. It may be that other intervals of laminated sediment may also be due to diatomaceous mat growth, rather than to the development of oxygen deficiency. The discoveries shed new light on variations in carbonate and silica production in ancient oceans, for the abundance of silica in this case is not due to preferential dissolution of carbonate. The periodic nature of the smaller-scale laminations, probably reflecting decadal timescales, suggests a mechanism such as the ENSO phenomenon. The decimetre-scale interbedding of the siliceous oozes and the 'normal' nanoplankton-rich sediment must be due to longer-scale processes. It is thought that the major phases of surface mat production coincide with major periods of cooling and reorganization of oceanic element supplies. For example, an interval from 10.5 to 9.5 Ma is coeval with a major shift in silica production from the Atlantic to the Pacific, whilst the absence of mats in the upper Pliocene to Recent correlates with the global shift of major silica production to the Southern ocean.

26.10 Anoxic events of seas and oceans

Anoxic oceanic pelagic sediments are typically black, laminated, organic-rich shales called *sapropels*. As noted previously, oceans may experience anoxic events caused by the development of oxygen minimum layers. These develop at the intersection point of the oxygen minimum layer either with the ocean margin (Thiede & van Andel, 1977) or with oceanic plateaux or continental shelves (Schlanger & Jenkyns, 1976). It is the *origin* of ocean anoxism that has proven controversial.

The Black Sea (Degens & Ross, 1974) is perhaps the largest and best-known example of a sea that has periodically been anoxic. This silled basin is up to 2200 m deep, with an O_2/H_2S interface at a mean depth of about 200 m. Surface salinities are 17.5–19‰, whilst the remainder is at about 22‰. Early Quaternary shallow-water deposits comprise 'megavarves' (10–100 mm thick), evaporites, chalky oozes (*seekreide*) and oil shales formed in a stratified water body fluctuating between fresh and saline (Degens & Stoffers, 1980). The upper Pleistocene to Recent deposits are successively: terrigenous turbidites and fines deposited in oxic freshwater lake lowstand environments (pre-7.5 ka), a sapropel representing marine transgressive anoxic conditions (2.7–7.5 ka), and chalky pelagic oozes marking modern-day 'marine' oxic conditions (for details of chronology see Jones & Gagnon, 1994). The Holocene sapropel is a few centimetres to decimetres thick with ~10% organic matter. Well-developed varves are present, with dark microlaminae originating from seasonal mass mortality of planktonic bacteria. Associated pyrite evidently precipitated within the water column (Lyons, 1997). The sapropel formed over short time intervals (thousands of years) during times of warm climate when successive saline spills from the Mediterranean sea intruded as density currents over the Bosphorus sill on to the megalake bed to form a rising front that gradually moved through the water mass. Termination of sapropel deposition occurred when the O_2/H_2S interface was constant, so that the permanent density stratification produced a planktonic community adjusted to the new stable habitat (Degens & Stoffers, 1980). Thus the present stable conditions in the Black Sea have lasted for about 1000 yr, the youngest sapropel being overlain by annually varved coccolith oozes (with low organic contents, see Calvert & Karlin, 1998) that continue to form today.

Periodic Quaternary anoxic events in the eastern Mediterranean (Thunell *et al.*, 1977) provide an interesting link with those described from the Black Sea above. Periodic sapropel layers here (see review by Cramp and O'Sullivan 1999) are marked by absence of benthic microfossils and by the presence of an abnormal planktonic foraminifera containing a high proportion of a particular salinity-sensitive form. The deposition of sapropels was synchronous in the eastern Mediterranean and correlates with a precessional periodicity (Hilgen 1991; Lourens *et al.*, 1996). One reason for the onset of anoxic conditions may have been increased runoff. The low-salinity overspill would have formed a surface layer that prevented oxygenation of the basin at depth. Whether the freshwater overspill *out* of the Black Sea was coincident with and compensation for the salt-water underspill *into* the Black Sea from the Mediterranean noted above is an intriguing but unanswered question. Recently, the role of migrating diatom mats in sapropel formation has been stressed (Sancetta, 1994; Kemp *et al.*, 1999).

Instructive examples of the periodic onset of anoxic conditions are provided by the silled basins of the California Borderland (Fig. 26.23; Behl & Kennett, 1996) and of the Caraico basin, Venezuela (Hughen *et al.*, 1996). In these basins O_2-deficient waters occur below sill depths at the present day. The low O_2 concentrations and high surface productivity encourage the rapid deposition of unbioturbated, laminated, organic-rich silts and clays with forams of O_2-tolerant types. However, sediment cores reveal that such anoxic conditions have alternated with periods when well-ventilated bottom waters occurred, producing bioturbated sediments with new suites of more oxygen-loving forams. The resultant cycles (Fig. 26.23) seem to correlate well with rapid climate excursions in Greenland ice cores, giving evidence that changes in the outflow of thermohaline currents and related changes in Trade Wind strength and upwelling can alter the pattern of productivity and oxygenation worldwide in certain restricted basins in quite short timespans. This is not to say that any majority of the world's oceans become anoxic; we have already stated evidence from the Panama basin (Yang *et al.*, 1995) that, despite generally higher glacial organic production, anoxic waters did not develop.

Part 8
Sedimentology in Sedimentary Basins

27   Tectonic subsidence and deposition

To speak of knowledge is futile. All is experiment and adventure. We are forever mixing ourselves with unknown quantities.

Virginia Woolf, *The Waves* (Bernard speaking), p. 100, Penguin, 1964.

27.1 Introduction: basins and basin analysis

The large-scale pattern of sediment distribution and the partitioning of the Earth's surface into areas of erosion and deposition depend largely upon tectonics. We must therefore attempt to understand these basic tectonic controls—they are too important to be left to tectonicists. It is particularly important for the geologically orientated sedimentologist to understand the mechanisms of subsidence in particular sedimentary basins (and the patterns of accompanying uplift) so that the nature and extent of ancient basins can be reconstructed. Here we make broad subdivisions of sedimentary basins according to the processes of tectonic subsidence.

Sedimentary basins come in all shapes and sizes with a variety of tectonic origins. Rather than attempting an artificially narrow or wide definition, we may note a number of common features:
- basins are repositories for sediment;
- basins owe their origins to crustal subsidence relative to surrounding, often uplifted, areas.

Basins may be active for hundreds of millions of years, yet within a few million become sourcelands themselves through structural deformation and uplift: a process known as *inversion*. The sediments that accumulated in the basin are now at the mercy of weathering and erosion processes as they are recycled into some adjacent or distant structure.

The sedimentary fill of a basin can provide unique evidence for the environmental conditions that pertained during the basin's lifetime: evidence such as water depth, rate of subsidence, contemporary climate, source of sediment, etc. The sedimentologist has a vital role here, for it is largely the evidence written in the rocks that provides data for geochemists and geophysicists to construct their grand theories of Earth evolution. The general arrangement of rock types and their structural relationships comprise what has been called *basin architecture*; it is the sedimentologist who must disentangle this. It is important therefore that the contents of a basin are, metaphorically speaking, carefully sieved, just as an archaeologist would in an important 'dig'. In fact, basin analysis means much more than just the examination of this basin fill, for this can rarely be understood without careful consideration of tectonics and structural evolution. The concept of a basin as a repository finds full meaning when the origin of economically important byproducts of the sedimentary process is considered. It is virtually impossible nowadays to explore for, and produce, oil, gas, water and metals without a very detailed idea of basin evolution built up from outcrop, well and geophysical viewpoints. This is because the way a basin evolves determines the spatial relationships of sourcerock, migration, seal and reservoir.

The nature of a basin's sedimentary infill depends upon a number of sometimes interrelated variables, including local climatic regime, hinterland geology, continentality, prebasinal elevation, topography, sediment flux, subsidence and uplift history, eustasy and volcanism. Thus any particular basin, whether active or deceased, will possess its own unique sedimentary architecture. Models for whole-basin architecture are presented in the final chapter of this book.

27.2 Preservation of sediment in basins

In previous sections we have discussed the origin of sediment and the various ways that it is transported over the surface of the Earth, part of the vast recycling system that accompanies the conveyor belt of plate

occurs by faulting. Below it, deformation is of pure-shear type, taken up by some form of slow, possibly continuous, plastic creep (see Bourne *et al.*, 1998) at a rate determined by imposed tectonic stresses and mineralogical composition of the lower crust. Olivine-dominated mantle rocks are initially more resistant to deformation than the lower crust, but become progressively less so towards the base of the lithosphere. It should be noted that the depth of the brittle-to-ductile transition is extremely sensitive to thermal gradient: increased gradients cause the transition to migrate upwards.

Actively extending rift basins

Here 'active' refers to displacement along normal faults during syn-rift lithospheric extension. The result is rotation of rigid crustal blocks about horizontal axes (Fig. 27.3; Jackson *et al.*, 1988). Relative uplift of the immediate foot walls to the faults is subordinate (about 10–20%) to the subsidence of the hanging walls. The characteristic basins and ranges produced are individual, linear, rift-like structures, often of half-graben form, or broad zones of such structures, such as found in continental rift valleys, broad Great Basin type rift provinces, back-arc and intra-arc basins and along mid-ocean ridges (Fig. 27.4).

1 *Closed-system or passive rifting.* In such rifting, magma results from decompressive partial melting of the asthenosphere. Local or regional flank uplifts result from fault-block rotation, the inherent asymmetry of nonuniform extension, flexure, lateral heat flow from the narrow rift and local magma production.

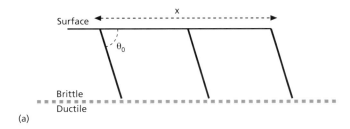

(a)

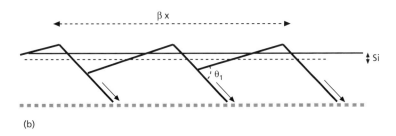

(b)

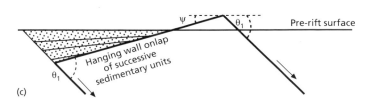

(c)

Fig. 27.3 Sketches of typical extensional tectonic blocks. Horizontal-axis rotation of the crustal blocks bounded by normal faults occurs in domino fashion. (After Jackson *et al.*, 1988.) The depth to brittle–ductile transition in the crust and hence the maximum depth of major normal faulting varies according to temperature gradient and strain rate (see Fig. 27.2). In many areas of active extension it lies between 10 and 20 km deep. Here x is initial crustal length; βx is the length after extension over time t by a factor β; θ_0 is the initial fault dip; θ_1 is the dip after extension β; y is the total tilt after extension β; S_i is the initial (nonthermal) subsidence produced by the extension β.

1 Closed, uniform, pure

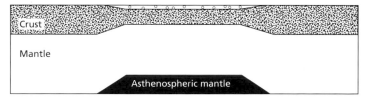

Crust

Mantle

Asthenospheric mantle

2 Closed, non-uniform, pure

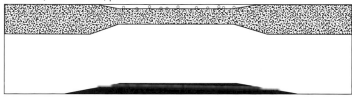

3 Closed, uniform, pure with *in-situ* magma production

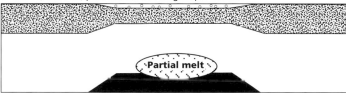

Partial melt

4 Closed, non-uniform, pure with *in-situ* magma production

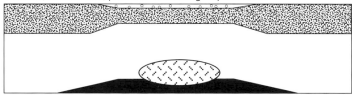

5 Closed, simple

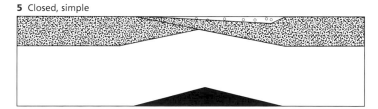

Fig. 27.4 Schematic diagrams to illustrate possible combinations of pure and simple shear, uniform or nonuniform stretching, and magma production. Local (Airy-type) isostatic compensation is assumed throughout (i.e. lithosphere has small elastic thickness). Surface and upper-crustal deformation by faulting is not shown.

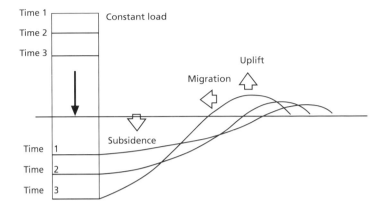

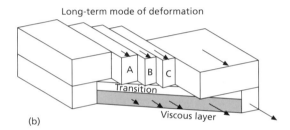

Fig. 27.9 How a viscoelastic plate (i.e. one that is free to flow by viscous creep in response to loading) loaded instantaneously by a constant load responds through time to that load. The zone of subsidence narrows as creep takes place and the forebulge migrates loadwards and amplifies at the same time. Of course, in Nature, loads are neither applied instantaneously nor constant, being subject to erosion. (From Quinlan & Beaumont, 1984.)

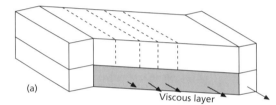

Fig. 27.10 How strike-slip faults work in a zone of lithosphere subjected to simple shear. Between earthquakes, the blocks bounded by faults remain locked, as they are subject to basal stress and they accumulate elastic strain. During earthquakes, the blocks move relative to each other—in practice, bends in the faults (not shown here, but see Chapter 28) create uplifts and depressions. The total long-term velocity of the rigid blocks is the same as that of the underlying flowing lithosphere/asthenosphere. (From Bourne et al., 1998.)

Tilt blocks

Owing to isostatic adjustments, uniform extension of stretch β over time t leads to an initial mean subsidence rate (Fig. 27.3) of *all* portions of the tilt blocks of:

$$S_i = 2.5(1 - 1/\beta)/t \qquad (B27.1)$$

the value of the constant depending upon the initial thermal structure, the density and the length scales of the crust, mantle and asthenosphere (McKenzie, 1978). This is superimposed on differential footwall uplift and subsidence due to the horizontal-axis rotation of the fault with time, $\delta\theta/t$, resulting in the growth of a sawtooth topography of amplitude:

$$y = d \sin (\delta\theta/t) \qquad (B27.2)$$

where d is the block width.

More information about mechanisms and rates of subsidence

continued on p. 505

More information about mechanisms and rates of subsidence [*continued*]

Thermal subsidence

Cooling of any solid volume, and rocks are no exception, leads to contraction as atomic lattice vibrations decrease in mean amplitude. The flow rate of heat energy, Q, depends on the thermal conductivity, κ, of the solid and the gradient of temperature, dT/dy, across the solid's boundary. For the simplest possible 1D case of Fourier's law we have:

$$Q = -\kappa \frac{dT}{dy} \tag{B27.3}$$

where y is direction of cooling. Now, this does not necessarily imply that T must change with time. Any rate of change of T with time (dT/dt) depends on the *net* flow of heat outwards or inwards, plus any heat generated within the solid (say, by radioactive decay or metamorphic reactions, etc.) and, of course, the thermal capacity (specific heat) of the material. In the simplest possible statement of this, we find that the rate of change of temperature with time is proportional to the rate of change of the gradient of the temperature with distance (a typical 'diffusive' relationship similar to one that holds in discussions of river incision). We can write this as:

$$\frac{dT}{dt} \propto \frac{d^2T}{dy^2} \tag{B27.4}$$

Solutions to the full form of this expression are rather frightening (to a geologist, at any rate), but their essence is captured by the simple relationship that the cooling rate of subsidence and therefore the cumulative subsidence due to cooling of previously heated crust or lithosphere declines proportionately according to $\sqrt{t}$ (Fig. 27.6).

Load-induced bending subsidence

A lithospheric plate has the strength to bear surface loads up to a certain magnitude and generally supports short-wavelength topographic loads without undergoing bending or flexure. A herd of elephants presents no problems, but the topographic mass of an ice-sheet or a large thrust slice of upper crust most certainly does so. The exact size of load to bend the lithosphere depends on a number of factors, but chiefly on a temperature-sensitive parameter of lithospheric rigidity termed the *flexural rigidity*, D (see Fig. 27.8):

$$D = \frac{Eh^3}{12(1 - \nu^2)} \tag{B27.5}$$

where E and ν are elastic material properties known as Young's modulus and Poisson's ratio, respectively, and h is the lithospheric thickness. Once bent or flexed, we may describe the subsidence (deflection)

continued on p. 506

due to the load mathematically. The details of this need not bother us here, suffice to say that for the bending of an infinitely long plate normal to its long axis, the lateral rate of change of the gradient (the curvature) of the lateral bending moment, M, in the plane normal to the length must be found, i.e. d^2M/dx^2. At equilibrium, this is equal to the sum of the downward acting force per unit area, q, and the horizontal force per unit length, P, times the vertical curvature of deflection, d^2w/dx^2, where w is the deflection. Finally, M is also given by dividing the plate's flexural rigidity by d^2w/dx^2. We arrive at the rather formidable-looking expression for the deflection of any elastic plate:

$$D\frac{d^4w}{dx^4} + P\frac{d^2w}{dx^2} = q \qquad (B27.6)$$

This expression ignores isostatic effects since any bent lithosphere will experience a reactive force due to gradients of stress resulting from the replacement of mantle-density rocks by either lower-density water (oceanic case) or thickened lower-density continental crust. So, for real-world oceanic and continental lithosphere, the downward load, q, is effectively reduced by a density contrast $\Delta\rho$, giving rise to a net hydrostatic reactive force $\Delta\rho gw$, where w is the deflection produced by loading. The final expression for bending is therefore:

$$D\frac{d^4w}{dx^4} + P\frac{d^2w}{dx^2} + \Delta\rho gw = q \qquad (B27.7)$$

which can be solved for w in various ways to determine the nature of bending in time and space.

More information about mechanisms and rates of subsidence [*continued*]

Cratonic basins

Major breakthroughs have been made recently in our understanding of the dynamic processes responsible for large-scale (up to 10^4 km^2) subsidence of the continental interiors, and the origins of so-called 'cratonic' basins, although many problems remain. Briefly, the process of deep subduction, and even penetration of subducted lithospheric slab material through the 650 km phase-change boundary (see Fig. 1.5), causes transient patterns of mantle flow and density changes that induce subsidence or uplift over 10^7 My or so (see Gurnis, 1992; Burgess & Gurnis, 1995; Pysklywec & Mitrovica, 1998).

Further reading

The reader is pointed to Allen and Allen (1990) for a thorough introduction to mechanisms of basin subsidence and for details of the treatment of sediment compaction, loading and lithospheric flexure. Turcotte and Schubert (1982) is *the* fundamental source, though not for the mathematically challenged.

28 Sedimentology in sedimentary basins: a user's guide

The word 'time' split its husk; poured its riches over him; and from his lips fell like shells, like shavings from a plane, without his making them, hard, white, imperishable, words, and flew to attach themselves to their places in an ode to Time; an immortal ode to Time.

Virginia Woolf, *Mrs Dalloway*, p. 78, Penguin, 1992.

28.1 Introduction

We conclude this book with brief accounts of the major tectonic basin environments in which sediment is deposited. This is meant to be no more than a 'sampler' to a vast (and still-growing) literature on basin analysis, including the tailor-made journal *Basin Analysis* itself. Suggestions for further reading are presented at the end of sections, with one or two illuminating case histories. Two books, *Tectonics of Sedimentary Basins* (Busby & Ingersoll, 1995) and *Sedimentary Basins* (Einsele, 1992), present much interesting material, the former more tectonic, the latter more sedimentary in approach. Allen and Allen (1990) is the soundest account of basin subsidence mechanisms. The reader should remember that the tectonic 'templates' described here are nothing more than that; the bare tectonic bones described must be fleshed out with regard for climate, vegetation and sea-level controls on sediment fluxes and sequence development. These aspects were discussed earlier in this book (Chapters 13–15).

28.2 Continental rifts

Stretching of continental lithosphere causes the formation of elongate fault-bounded rifts. The oldest preserved sedimentary basins on Earth (c.3.55 Gy) are thought to have been extensional rift-like structures in greenstone belts (Nijman *et al.*, 1998). Rift basins and flank uplifts become depositional sinks and erosional sources, respectively, for sediment. The broad history of rift flank uplift may be elucidated using fission-track techniques, the information being used for large-scale models of rift evolution (see van der

Beek *et al.*, 1994). The structural and sedimentary architecture of rift basin infills is often referred to as the *syn-rift* phase of lithospheric extension. Classic rift valleys are narrow (50–100 km), long (up to 1000 km) features, much segmented in detail, atop major regional surface upwarps or domes covering many thousands of square kilometres. They are typified by the East Africa, Baikal, Rhine and Rio Grande rifts. By way of contrast, wide (> 1000 km) rift provinces like the Basin and Range of the western USA and the Greek and Turkish Aegean include a plethora of individual, narrow (15–30 km) rift basins separated by range uplifts.

The length of normal fault segments (10–50 km) approximately equals the thickness of the local brittle crustal layer. Segments may be offset by stepover or separated by more extensive transfer or accommodation zones where fault polarity reverses. The extension is taken up across numerous small normal faults, causing the offset zones to stand at higher elevations than the intervening basins and thus to be barriers to sediment transport. Crossover accommodation zones are frequently the site of abundant volcanism in the East African rift system and in extensional back-arc basins. Multiple basin-margin faults are known where initially wide tiltblocks are fragmented into smaller blocks by new faults in the old hanging wall. Cessation of activity on the old bounding fault is followed by footwall uplift, erosional dissection and transport of the old basin fill into the newly subsiding basin.

Over time a crudely wedge-shaped accumulation develops in rift basins, with the characteristic structural asymmetry exerting a fundamental control on the distribution of sedimentary environments and lithofacies. Footwall uplands adjacent to main basin-

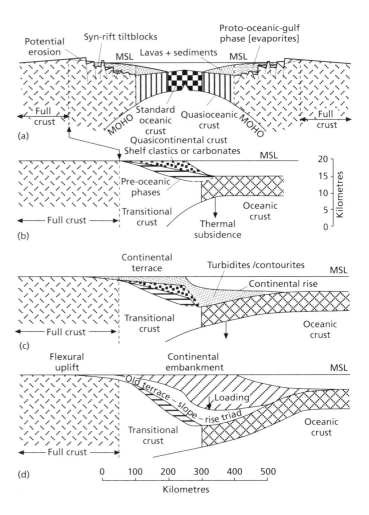

Fig. 28.5 Sketches to show the sequential development of a passive continental margin. MSL, mean sea level. (Modified after Ingersoll's, 1988, modification of Dickinson, 1976.)

magma including dyke swarms equivalent in age to those commonly found intruded on land along both sides of the Red Sea. To the south, the western tip of the slow-spreading (16 mm/yr) Gulf of Aden rift comes onshore in Djibouti as the Asal rift. The Red Sea rift is also propagating westwards into the Afar depression towards Asal. The forces required to stretch the slowly NE-drifting Afro-Arabian plate were presumably provided by slab-pull edge forces on the subducting plate descending beneath the Zagros Mountains of Iran and Iraq to the northeast. These forces had the effect of slightly accelerating the NE-drifting Arabian area of the plate, causing regional tensional stresses in the crust.

Prior to formation of the initial rift, the Red Sea area had low relief and was part of a northward-deepening epicontinental area from the late Cretaceous to the early Oligocene. The widespread presence of marine conditions at many localities along the Red Sea and Gulf of Suez margins prior to and shortly after the first evidence for extensional faulting implies that pre-rift doming was not important and that closed-system rifting conditions with decompressive mantle melting were operative. Fission-track dating of flank uplift indicates basement exhumation of up to 2.5–5 km since the middle Miocene. Syn-rift sedimentation was typified by marginal alluvial fans and fan deltas together with a variety of nearshore carbonate and clastic environments. The Gulf of Suez rift is noteworthy for its evidence for syn-rift fault growth. During Miocene times, enormous thicknesses of evaporites formed in the periodically isolated proto-oceanic trough. Normal marine salinities resumed during Pliocene to Recent times. Holocene sedimentation in the central Red Sea has been dominated by pelagic foram–pteropod oozes with high sedimentation rates. A highly stratified water column developed during early deglaciation times (14–8 ka) with low productivity in the upper mixed layer, very high bottom salinities and accumulation of sapropels. Today the situation is much changed, with generally good mixing and well-oxygenated conditions, though deep brine pools exist along the axial ridge.

28.4 Coastal plains, shelf terraces and continental rises

After active rifting has given way to seafloor spreading, the continental mosaic of crustal-scale faults that define tilted blocks and graben becomes inactive (Fig. 28.5) and the long, slow(ing) process of thermal subsidence and continental margin construction begins (Figs 28.6 & 28.7), the rate being greatest in the thinnest continental crust as β tends to infinity. At the same time, the strongly modified continental crust,

particularly in areas underplated by lower-crustal basic intrusives, and the oldest oceanic crust carry on their own cooling, shrinkage and subsidence. Once the rift basins are filled, the construction begins of the coastal plain, shelf terrace and rise (Fig. 28.6). The net result is a bathymetric profile that slowly increases in slope from the continent across the hinge line to the stretched continental crust, rapidly increases across the (underplated) transition to ocean crust, and finally slowly decreases once more across the ocean basin proper. The profile is a sigmoid, approximating in form to the logistic growth function. Construction of the shelf terrace is achieved by deposition from and moulding by tides, waves and ocean currents, modified across the more steeply sloping shelf rise by mass failure and gravity flows. It is important to realize that the form of the mature continental margin is largely a constructional feature formed by the interplay between differential subsidence, deposition and resedimentation. The continued deposition of sediment over the terrace and on the rise takes the form

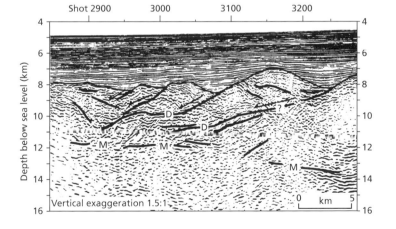

Fig. 28.6 Deep seismic reflection image (prestack, depth-migrated) from the Iberian Atlantic passive continental margin to show highly extended continental crust. Note synrift/proto-oceanic tiltblocks capped by syn-rift (Mesozoic) sediments and bounded by low-angle detachments (D); note also draping by postrift gently oceanward-dipping sediments. (From Pickup *et al.*, 1996.)

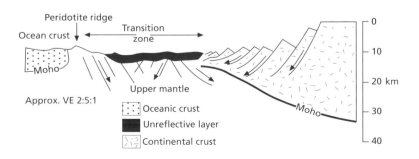

Fig. 28.7 Summary sketch of the highly extended Iberia abyssal plain continental margin; postextension sediments not shown. (From Pickup *et al.*, 1996.)

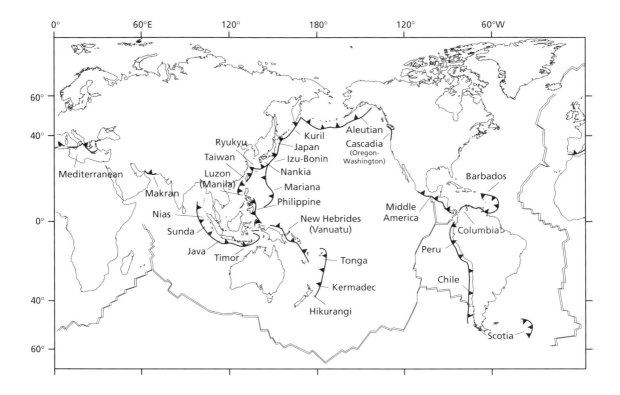

Fig. 28.9 Global distribution of active oceanic subduction zones. (After Underwood & Moore, 1995.)

from (admittedly crude) mass-balance calculations that there has been a small net growth of continental crust due to these two processes. Although consumption of oceanic lithosphere is a common feature, there are important differences in the nature of convergence that cause the morphology of convergent margins to differ markedly. These arise because of differences in relative plate motions and the degree of coupling between the subducting and the overriding plates as expressed in the angle of subduction determined from earthquake mechanisms. The paradoxical feature is that convergent margins may be (or have been) at least for some time in their history the site of significant extension, leading to preservation of characteristic back-arc extensional volcanic and sedimentary associations.

Compressional arc–trench systems have strongly coupled descending and overriding plates with the whole overriding plate advancing faster and in the opposite or strongly oblique direction relative to the descending plate. The majority of the overriding plate is in strong compression with many great earthquake epicentres in a broad band parallel to the shallow-dipping subduction zone. Compressional margins tend to occur when the rate of plate convergence and the negative buoyancy of the subducting slab are high and the angle of plate descent is low. Morphologically, compressional margins are characterized by relatively shallow trenches, voluminous calc-alkaline plutonism and volcanism, and high relief. The effects of compresssion are felt widely across the overriding plate to the extent that crustal-scale thrust tectonics may occur thousands of kilometres away from the trench behind the arc. This causes the formation of retro-arc foreland basins as seen in the eastern Andean foreland province and deduced for the early Tertiary history of the Rocky Mountains. The amount of sediment input depends strongly upon climate and drainage controls, typified by along-strike variations in the Andean chain.

Extensional arc–trench systems have weakly coupled descending and overriding plates with the whole

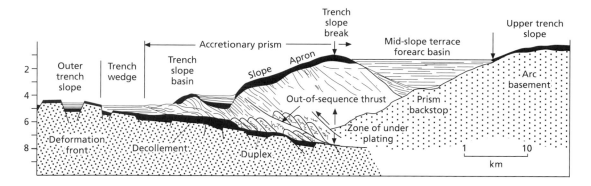

Fig. 28.10 Section to show the major bathymetric features, structural deformation and depositional sites associated with subduction zones. (After Underwood & Moore, 1995.)

overriding plate advancing slowly and/or in the same direction as or strongly oblique relative to the descending plate. The majority of the overriding plate is in extension with few strong earthquakes along a narrow seismic zone atop a steeply dipping subduction zone. Extensional margins tend to occur when the rate of plate convergence and the negative buoyancy of the subducting plate are both low and the angle of plate descent is high. They are common along destructive intra-oceanic convergent margins in the Pacific ocean. Evidence from within the Rocky Mountain cordillera and Andes indicates that such margins were very typical of the early stages of convergence of the Pacific margins in Mesozoic times. Morphologically, extensional margins are characterized by deep trenches, voluminous calc-alkaline and basaltic volcanism. The effects of extension are felt widely across the overriding plate to the extent that crustal-scale extensional tectonics may occur thousands of kilometres away from the trench behind the arc. This results in the formation of a plethora of intra-arc and back-arc extensional basins with their characteristic block-faulted and tilted morphologies, as seen to perfection in the Aegean or Marianas.

In conclusion it seems that the majority of destructive margins are expected to show, perhaps in both time *and* space, some combination of compressional, extensional or obliquely convergent features. This makes the detailed and careful basin analysis of ancient convergent-margin sediments both difficult and interesting.

28.6 Subduction zones: trenches and trench-slope basins

During its journey in time and space from ocean ridge to subduction zone, oceanic lithosphere cools and slowly subsides to equilibrium isostatic depths. Some but not all of the ocean-floor relief is obscured by a layer-cake of sediment. Still in evidence are a myriad of seamounts, remnant fracture zones and associated features. As oceanic plate moves progressively closer to a subduction zone, it comes under the influence of immense flexural forces caused by bending and by loading due to the weight of the overriding plate as the subducting plate turns into the subduction zone (Fig. 28.11). These forces cause the production up to 150 km oceanwards of a peripheral bulge 300–500 m high above the oceanic depths. The ocean floor then slopes gently in towards the locus of maximum depth along the trench itself. The passage of ocean floor from abyssal plain to bulge and then to trench is marked by the shallowing, then deepening, and the onset of extensional stresses, which act upon basement weaknesses such as old fractures and normal faults once active closer to the mid-ocean ridge. Renewed subsidence along normal faults occurs as the surface of the outer trench slope moves towards the trench, the perched basins receiving sediment from local submarine fans or turbidity flows sourced axially or on the inner trench slope. Bounded on its oceanward side by the outer trench slope, the trench rises more steeply up the inner trench slope, the surface expression of a wedge of offscraped sediment known as an *accretionary complex* or *prism*. Restricting our attention for the moment to the trench, its bathymetry and shape are determined by:

- *style and rate of subduction*, i.e. shallow vs. steep angle of lithosphere descent, slow or fast plate

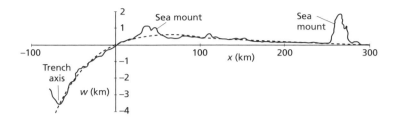

Fig. 28.11 The bending of the Pacific plate (solid line) as it enters into the Mariana Trench. (From Turcotte & Schubert, 1982.) Pecked line shows profile according to flexural theory (Chapter 27; eqn 3.159 of Turcotte & Schubert).

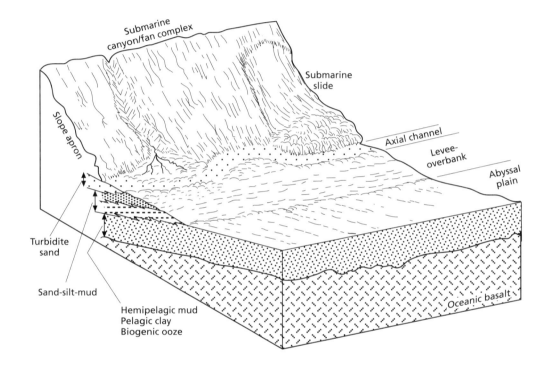

Fig. 28.12 Simplest possible relationships for lateral submarine fan input to a subduction margin; a coarsening-upwards sequence is produced. (From Piper et al., 1973.) In practice, inner slope basins, axial deflections and runout/reversal behaviour complicate the picture (see Chapter 26).

sinking, giving rise to shallow and deep trenches respectively;
- *bathymetry of descending plate*, particularly the occurrence of seamounts, aseismic ridges, active ridges and fracture zones, which cause the trench to be segmented axially;
- *flux of detrital sediment* into the trench, with large fluxes causing trench infill, flat floors, gentle gradients and marginal onlap on to trench walls and

axial segment boundaries, and low-flux trenches being deep, bathymetrically irregular and with steep local gradients;
- *flux of ocean-floor sediment* sequences into the trench and the efficiency and magnitude of the 'scrape-off' process as witnessed by the lateral and vertical extent of the accretionary prism.

The junction between trench floor and inner trench slope approximates to the beginning of the active thrust front (or *décollement*) bounding the accretionary prism. The position of this frontal thrust relative to height above the oceanic crustal basement determines the preservation potential of the total oceanic and trench sedimentary sequence (Fig. 28.12): the higher the *décollement*, the more sequence is subducted and is available for underplating. The

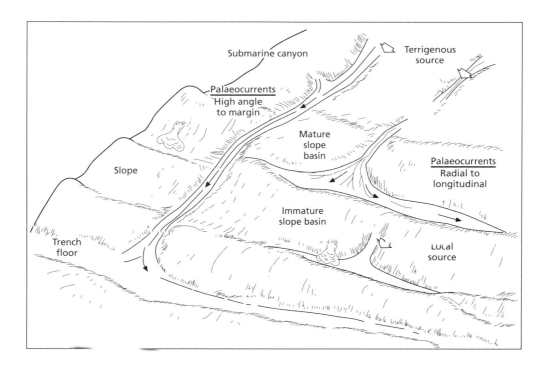

Fig. 28.13 Sketch to show the nature of an inner trench slope on an accretionary prism, with the many slope basins formed by the intersection of thrust faults with the prism surface. (After Underwood & Bachman, 1982.)

position of the *décollement* depends upon a number of factors, chiefly the internal shear resistance profile of the sedimentary sequence. However, it is usual for most of the terrigenous clastic sediments supplied to the trench floor to be scraped off and accreted, but both oceanic pelagic sediment and ocean crust itself may be scaped off into the prism as ophiolite slivers. Underplated material finds its way down the subduction zone, perhaps eventually to be partly recycled as part of an arc-derived volcanic or plutonic rock.

The inner trench slope developed upon the ever-uplifting and seaward-expanding accretionary prism may range from a relatively smooth surface with a drape of hemipelagic clays and silts to a very intricate bathymetric profile dependent upon intersections of various generations of thrust and normal fault planes with the seafloor surface (Fig. 28.13). Many trench slopes have small to very large smooth-floored basins formed in depressions between active or once-active

thrust surfaces. These act as efficient sediment traps for local turbidity currents. In general the major offscraping thrust faults become older towards the volcanic arc, though backthrusts, out-of-sequence thrusts, normal faults developed on the trench slope, and shallow extensional slides, slumps and debris-flow channels all complicate the picture in detail. The innermost part of an accretionary prism (usually the oldest) marks the trench-slope break, arcwards of which is usually developed a prominent flat or gently sloping feature known as a *fore-arc basin* (see below). Perhaps in no other environment on the Earth's surface do sedimentation and tectonics interact more closely and on such a variety of scales. It can be appreciated that the interpretation of ancient accretionary prisms may be an extremely complicated and painstaking task.

Further reading

The tectonics and sedimentation of trenches and trench-slope basins is thoroughly and clearly reviewed by Underwood and Moore (1995). A useful quantitative modelling approach to trench wedge accretion is provided by Mountney and Westbrook (1996).

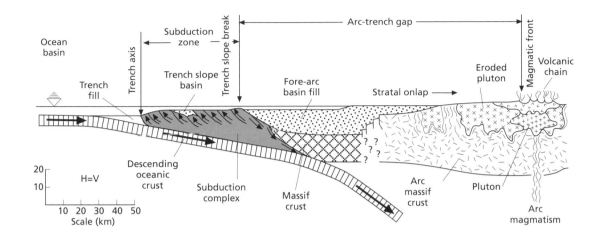

Fig. 28.14 Dickinson's (1995) sketch section to show the tectonic setting of fore-arc basins. (From Dickinson, 1995.)

28.7 Fore-arc basins

Along destructive margins, fore-arc refers to linear areas seawards of continental or oceanic volcanic arcs and landwards of any accretionary prism or trench (Fig. 28.14). A subsiding fore-arc is referred to as a fore-arc basin, rooted in either modified continental or oceanic crust. Bathymetrically, fore-arcs are rather variable. Most are shelf-like, with gentle slopes up to

Fig. 28.15 Facies and environments of the Sunda fore-arc. (From sources cited in Dickinson, 1995.)

100 km or more wide (Sunda arc; Fig. 28.15). Some are much more complex (Cretan fore-arc), with a plethora of sub-basins and local uplifted highs associated with both thrust and normal faulting. They act as sediment traps for the often prodigious sediment fluxes issuing from adjacent volcanic arcs. Volcanic airfalls, submarine slumps and eruption-driven turbidity currents transfer sediment downslope. Floating pumice rafts disperse more widely over the destructive margin. The efficiency of the fore-arc trap increases as ridge-like barriers form by accretionary offscraping at the trench-slope break. The tendency with time is for the initially shallow fore-arc, with its coarse-grained basal deposits, to deepen quickly and then to infill gradually with a coarsening-upwards, predominantly turbiditic facies of arc volcanic provenance (Fig. 28.16).

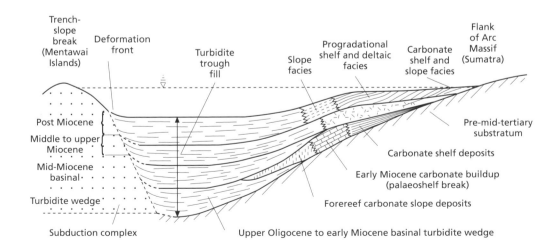

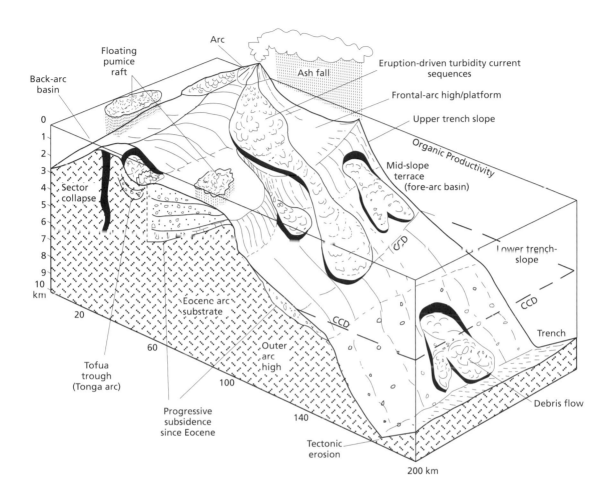

Fig. 28.16 Facies and environments of a typical volcanigenic oceanic fore-arc. CCD, carbonate compensation depth. (Based mainly on Tonga; after Underwood *et al.*, 1995.)

With time, the fore-arc broadens and shallows by sediment onlap both oceanwards and landwards. The end-result is an increasingly inefficient trap configuration. Basin fills from Cainozoic and Mesozoic examples may reach up to 10 km in thickness. The Great Basin of California is perhaps the best-exposed and investigated example of an ancient fore-arc, whilst amongst active examples the Sumatra–Java fore-arc shows many classic features.

In order to understand how many fore-arc basins originate as residual features superimposed upon older oceanic or continental-margin basement, it is necessary to conduct a thought experiment by imagining the likely sequence of events when subduction is initiated along a passive continental margin. During such a process, oceanic slab failure and reversely buoyant descent will occur oceanwards of the last thinned or modified continental crust. Fore-arcs are thus underlain by oceanic, modified oceanic or thinned continental crust, and bounded oceanwards by the first offscraped sediment of the nascent accretionary prism. Water depths are initially deep, liable to rapid infill by copious sediment flux from the adjacent arc. Sediment loading induces extra flexural subsidence around the basin margins, causing forebulges, then waves of subsidence to migrate outwards towards both the trench-slope break and the volcanic arc, causing progressive onlap on to these features. Fore-arc terrains along periodically extensional destructional margins undergo alternating uplift due to shortening and subsidence as the area of the whole trench–arc gap episodically increases due to stretching.

Further reading

The best general account of fore-arc basins is that by Dickinson (1995). A useful account of western Pacific fore-arc basins penetrated by deep ocean drilling is given by Underwood *et al.* (1995). The Great Basin of California is discussed by Ingersoll (1979), amongst many others. The intricacies of the Cretan fore-arc are discussed by Postma *et al.* (1993b).

28.8 Intra-arc basins

Volcanic arcs are major constructional features along zones of plate destruction. They share a constructional nature, albeit of a different kind, with the off-scraped accretionary complexes discussed previously. Ample opportunities exist for the preservation of pyroclastic flows, ashfalls and volcanically derived sediments adjacent to volcanic centres in the often deep-water areas that separate individiual volcanic centres. Also, many volcanic arcs are (or were) in a state of extension, with basin margins bounded by major normal faults allowing preservation of thick volcaniclastic sequences. In addition, the rise and collapse of magmatic domes and caldera formation also allow for shallow normal faulting and preservation of portions of the volcanic superstructure. Not all volcanically derived material finds its resting place in the inter-arc, for significant amounts may be erupted or flow laterally into adjacent fore-arc or back-arc basins. Intra-arc basins may develop from back-arc or fore-arc basins as the style or polarity of subduction changes. Moreover, larger-scale forces are also at work in the arc environment for long-wavelength subsidence results when low-angle subduction changes to high-angle. Also, rising diapirs of calc-alkaline or alkaline magma may force themselves upwards to change a previously depositional submarine site into an uplifted one.

Further reading

Intra-arc basins are reviewed by Smith and Landis (1995), with a valuable extra perspective provided by Underwood *et al.* (1995).

28.9 Back-arc basins

The vast majority (> 70%) of back-arc basins occur associated with the destructive plate margins of the Pacific ocean (Fig. 28.17). Other notable examples occur in the Scotia Sea and Mediterranean Sea (Tyrrhenian, Aegean). We have already noted how destructional plate margins may, for a variety of reasons, be brought under a state of extensional stress. The result is that a formerly active volcanic arc or an area of continental crust may be split by active rifting, first into a series of tilted blocks, accompanied perhaps by basaltic or calc-alkaline volcanism, and finally, once the extension has reached a certain limit, the site of new ocean crust formation. Such back-arc basins are, or were, active in the sense that they owe their presence to active plate-margin processes. A second group of back-arc basins owes its origin to a reorganization of subduction whereby an oceanward shift in the site of subduction leaves stranded an abandoned volcanic arc and an area of pre-existing ocean floor behind the new arc. Such 'passive' or 'residual' back-arc basins are typified by the Bering Sea and West Philippine basins.

Early stages of active back-arc rifting in oceanic settings are exemplified by the young (< 5 Ma) Izu–Bonin arc, northern Owo Jima ridge, Phillipine–Japan Sea (Carey & Sigurdsson, 1984; Taylor *et al.*, 1991; Klaus *et al.*, 1992). This comprises half-grabens arranged in long (700 km) chains up to 40 km wide behind or sometimes between a line of arc volcanoes. The grabens, separated by volcanically active transfer zones, are bounded by active normal faults with up to 2.5 km throw. Fault development follows closely the pattern of major continental half-grabens, whereby a large half-graben develops against a master normal fault on one side and an antithetic fault on the other side. Sediment fluxes are dominated by pyroclastic flows and by resedimented volcanically derived material in gravity flows down the slopes formed by tectonics (see Fig. 28.18 for the Tonga back-arc situation). Further development of back-arc rifts into the seafloor spreading phase is accompanied by localization of rifting and the onset of spreading along a narrower axial zone. Subsidence over much of the now inactive syn-rift remnant volcanic arc and earlier spreading centres is due to thermal subsidence, as in the post-rift phase of young oceanic rifts.

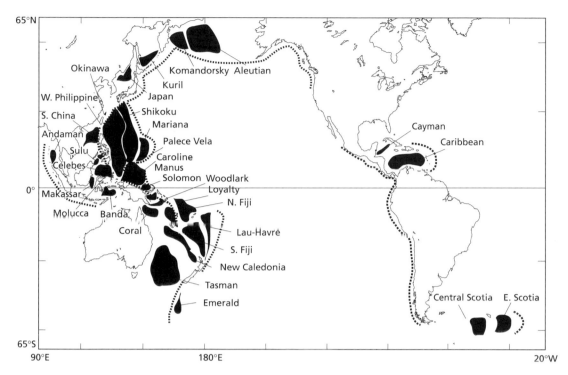

Fig. 28.17 Distribution of trenches and back-arcs in the circum-Pacific region. (After Tamaki & Honza, 1991.)

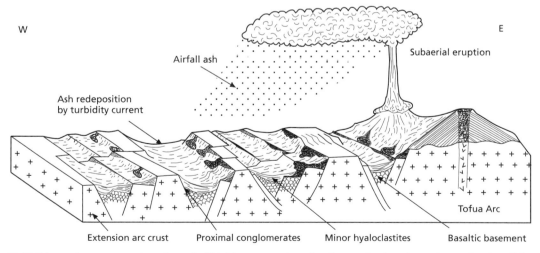

Fig. 28.18 Schematic representation of a typical highly extended oceanic back-arc basin. Note the plethora of extensional tiltblocks in ocean crust and their role in trapping the proximal products of arc volcanism. (After Marsaglia *et al.*, 1995.)

Back-arc basins forming in continental crust are typified by the largely submarine Okinawa Trough and the Aegean sea where, in the latter case, well-defined half-grabens have horst flanks extending well above sea level, providing clastic sediment to the deep-water rift basins. There is a trend from lacustrine conditions early on in the extensional process to marine conditions with abundant influx of detrital sediment. Steep, fault-controlled continental and submarine slopes result in spectacular examples of sediment dispersal by gravity flows.

Further reading

Marsaglia's (1995) review is a good starting point, followed by the seminal work of Carey and Sigurdsson (1984) and the more tectonically correct summaries of recent western Pacific back-arcs by Marsaglia *et al.* (1995) and Clift (1995). Taylor *et al.* (1991) and Klaus *et al.* (1992) present a mass of fascinating and detailed data on the extensional tectonics of Philippine back-arcs.

28.10 Foreland basins

Foreland basins (Fig. 28.19) develop on continental crust along the length of collisional plate margins or along compressional destructive margins. They are certainly the most-studied type of sedimentary basin, because they lie adjacent to Earth's major mountain chains and contain the only real geological data with which the evolution of these orogenic belts and their time–temperature–pressure paths (gained from fission-track and mineral closure temperature ages) can be reconstructed. 'Foreland' refers to the relatively undeformed (in the shortening sense) continental crust or continental margin over which major thrust faults transfer great wedges of crust from an orogenic belt. It is these thrust wedges that play a

dual role in the evolution of a foreland basin and its sedimentary infill:
- they load the foreland plate, which in turn responds by flexural bending;
- they form the uplifted source areas for river catchments to develop and provide a sediment source for the developing basin.

There are two major types of foreland basin, differentiated on the basis of position relative to the orogenic belt:

1 *Collisional (peripheral) foreland basins* lie on the continental crust of the subducting plate at collision zones. They are typified by the active Indo-Gangetic foreland basins south of the Himalayan frontal thrusts, the inactive Molasse basins of the Alps and Pyrenees, and the active Tigris–Euphrates–Arabian Gulf basins west of the Zagros Mountains in Iraq.

2 *Retro-arc foreland basins* (Fig. 28.20) lie on the continental crust of the overriding plate at destructive margins on the continental side of the orogenic belt away from (behind) the subducting plate. They are typified by the mosaic of active basins to the east of the Andes and by the inactive basins in the eastern forelands of the Rocky Mountains.

The two types are quite distinctive in respect of tectonic position but share the common feature of flexure-induced subsidence caused by thrust loading. Active thrusting produces geologically instantaneous subsidence in the foot wall of the thrust around the periphery of the load. The magnitude and extent of the subsequent flexural subsidence depend upon those of the load and upon the elastic properties of the over-ridden plate. Loading is obviously a time-dependent feature since the total extent of thrusting is accumulative (but not necessarily steady). Not only will the loading mass increase with time, but the rate of removal of the load by erosion will also increase, giving an increase in sediment flux into the developing basin with time. Further out into the overthrust plate

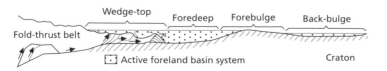

Fig. 28.19 Schematic cross-section of a composite foreland basin system, based on the central Andean foreland basin. (After Horton & DeCelles, 1997.) The origin of the thin saucer-shaped back-bulge depression is poorly known. For wedge-top basins, see Horton (1998).

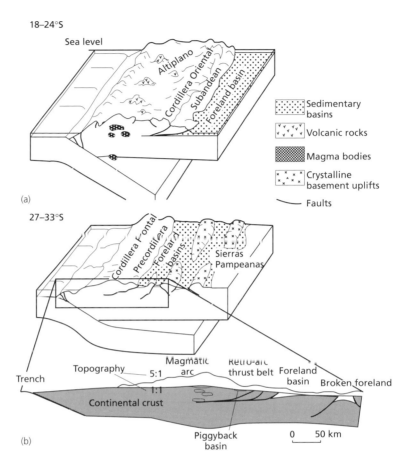

18–24°S

Sea level

Altiplano

Cordillera Oriental

Subandean

Foreland basin

Sedimentary basins

Volcanic rocks

Magma bodies

Crystalline basement uplifts

Faults

(a)

27–33°S

Cordillera Frontal

Precordillera

Foreland basins

Sierras Pampeanas

Trench

Topography   5:1

1:1

Continental crust

Magmatic arc

Retro-arc thrust belt

Foreland basin

Broken foreland

Piggyback basin

0   50 km

(b)

Fig. 28.20 Schematic diagrams of the zonal variation in subduction geometry and foreland basin development in the Andes. (a) Northern section with steep subduction and thin-skinned sub-Andean foreland basin. (b) Central section has flat subduction with shortening deformation on deep thrusts far out into the sub-Andean (broken) foreland. (After Jordan, 1995, and sources cited therein.)

from the point of application of the thrusted load, subsidence and uplift reflect the development of peripheral bulging, whose height and distance from the load closely depend upon the elastic properties of the underlying lithosphere. If we first consider the case of a stationary noneroding load increasing only in mass with time, then it is clear that a complete wave of subsidence and uplift will migrate across the loaded plate with time, increasing in magnitude as it migrates. We can thus characterize given points in space according to their movement vectors. Superimposed on these will be the modifying effects of deposition. It seems that, in the majority of cases, after an initial acceleration of subsidence as the load grows and advances from the far-field, high subsidence rates result in rapid water deepening close to the thrust front, with uplift of the peripheral bulge causing shallowing-upwards trends in any pre-existing deposits of the overridden plate. Deposition subsequently

causes infill of the bathymetry and the production of coarsening-upwards sequences. The nature of any foreland basin thus depends critically upon the ability of the sediment depositional systems feeding the basin to fill it with sediment so that all slopes are changed from tectonic to depositional. Such considerations lead to concepts of underfilled vs. overfilled sedimentary basins (Figs 28.21 & 28.22).

Local and regional tectonic and drainage factors play an extremely important role in the evolution of foreland basins:
1 Because of their role in providing orographic rainfall, drainage sourcelands are prone to the effects of climatic change on runoff, vegetation and sediment supply (de Boer *et al.*, 1991).
2 Thrust faults propagate and the locus of faulting migrates with time, causing unsteadiness and nonuniformity in tectonic slopes produced by growth folding (Anadon *et al.*, 1986). Thrust-parallel fault

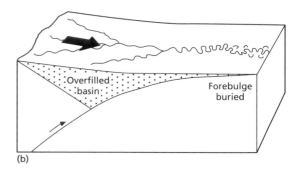

Fig. 28.21 Cartoons to show contrasts between (a) underfilled (water-filled in this case) and (b) overfilled foreland basins. (After Crampton & Allen, 1995.)

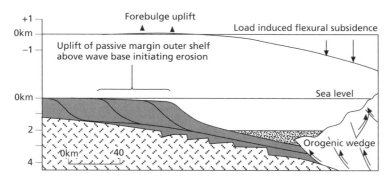

Stage 1 Initial loading of outer passive margin, e.g., present day Taiwan, Timor and Papua New Guinea. Palaeocene in the Alps.

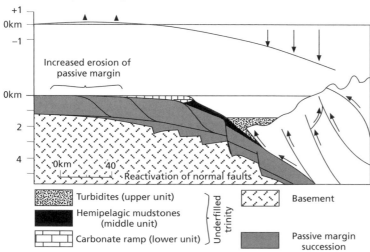

Stage 2 Development of underfilled trinity as flexural profile passes over passive margin

Fig. 28.22 Sketches to show the sequential evolution of an initially marine foreland basin as it narrows and is affected by forebulge migration in response to advance of the orogenic wedge along a thrust front. (After Sinclair, 1997.)

Stage 3 Steady state migration of the underfilled trinity over the craton i.e., rate of thrust front advance equals rate of cratonic onlap

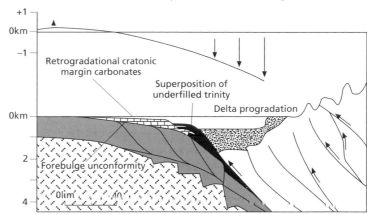

Stage 4 Transition of foreland basin from an underfilled to a filled depositional state. Siliciclastics from orogen fill the basin, smothering the underfilled stratigraphy.

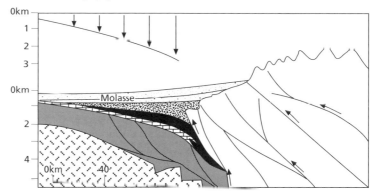

Fig. 28.22 (*continued*)

and fold propagation may cause marked basinwards shifts in the locus of sediment outfall due to drainage coalescence (Gupta, 1997), whilst basinward propagation causes the uplift of portions of previously level proximal basins into so-called piggyback basins (Ori & Friend, 1984).

3 Thrusting itself may be fixed in space but episodic over timespans very appreciably longer (> 500 kyr) than the recurrence intervals between major thrust earthquakes. This longer-term unsteadiness may allow alternating periods of quiescence and activity during which basin-transverse fans and axial rivers must adjust to the imposition or removal of tectonic slopes (see Nyman, 1998 for an outstandingly documented example). Although frequently used as the basis for models of sedimentation in active foreland basins, independent evidence for longer-term un-

steadiness in faulting is difficult to come by. In fact, major problems in the exact interpretation of foreland basins arise because of general inability to date phases of structural deformation independently.

4 The development of axial drainage from the coalescence of transverse drainages leads to a massive increase in throughflux of sediment. Peripheral foreland basins are usually characterized by axial drainage, whilst much-segmented retro-arc basins exhibit local drainage or major cross-basin drainage normal to basin strike.

5 The uplift and erosion of the sedimentary fill to piggyback and wedge top basins may cause large-scale drainage reorganization and the rapid production of major alluvial fans. Other basin fills have higher preservation potential (Horton, 1998).

Retro-arc foreland basins are characteristic of

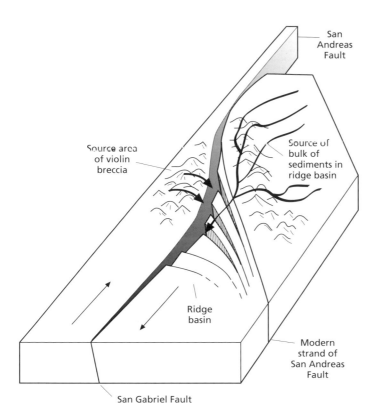

Fig. 28.23 Crowell's classic notion of slide-apart basin formation along a bend in a major strike-slip fault as gleaned from the famous Ridge Basin along the now-defunct San Gabriel Fault, California. Drainages are indicative only. (From Crowell, 1974a.)

modern convergent plate boundaries under states of compression brought about by the various factors discussed previously, e.g. shallow subduction angle, net plate convergence, etc. One of their most characteristic features is the occurrence of combined zones of thin-skinned tectonics and scattered basement uplifts originating along much deeper and steeper thrusts, which bring crystalline crustal basement to the surface in the foot wall of thrusts. Such forelands with their isolated uplifts and subsiding basins are termed 'broken' forelands, as distinct from the more continuous foreland basin plains brought about by thin-skinned thrusts. The broken forelands of the eastern Andes, the Sierras Pampeanas of Argentina, have propagated far eastwards in an area coincident with the shallowest angle of the subducting plate (Fig. 28.20). Broken forelands are characterized by both local basement uplift sediment sources and more regional sourcing from the Andes thin-skinned thrust belt to the west. The identification of these sources is vital in the elucidation of the history of ancient broken foreland basins like those of the Rocky Mountains formed during Mesozoic and early Tertiary Sevier and Laramide subduction to the west.

Further reading

Peripheral foreland basins are generally reviewed by Miall (1995) and retro-arc (broken) forelands by Jordan (1995). DeCelles and Giles (1996) is a thought-provoking analysis of the latter, with interesting comments on the development of a 'backbulge' behind the sub-Andean forebulge provided by Horton and DeCelles (1997). Allen and Homewood (1986) and Allen *et al.* (1992) contain useful collections of foreland basin studies. The dynamics of forebulges are revealed in neat integrative tectono-sedimentary studies by Allen *et al.* (1991), Crampton and Allen (1995) and Sinclair (1997). Ori and Friend (1984) originated the piggyback concept. The use of closely dated foreland basin sediments to elucidate thrust evolution in orogens is illustrated in the Rocky Mountain broken foreland by Lawton (1986) and Talling *et al.* (1994), in the Pyrenean foreland basin by Burbank *et al.* (1992), in the Himalayan foreland basin by Burbank and Raynolds (1988), and in the Swiss Alpine foreland basin by Schlunegger *et al.* (1997). Interesting reconstructions of the drainage systems of the latter area are provided by Schlunegger

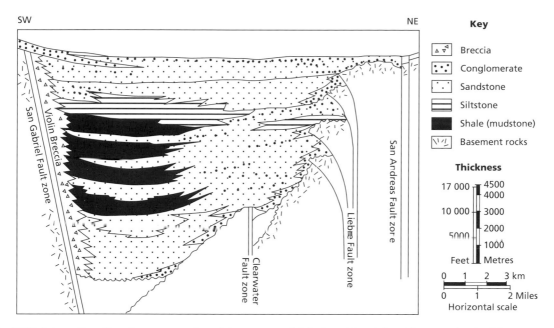

Fig. 28.24 Schematic sedimentary cross-section of the Ridge Basin to show central lacustrine 'fines' and coarse alluvial fan/fan-delta clastic tongues sourced from the narrow catchments in the San Gabriel Fault to the SW (Violin Breccia) and the wider sourcelands of the fragmented 'slide-apart' uplands to the NE. (After Crowell & Link, 1982.)

et al. (1998). Drainage and unconformity development around growth folds are discussed by Anadon *et al.* (1986), DeCelles (1988), Jackson *et al.* (1996) and Gupta (1997).

28.11 Strike-slip basins

Major strike-slip faults (see review by Woodcock, 1986) are broadly linear features. Some penetrate the whole lithosphere as plate-bounding transform faults like the San Andreas Fault of California. Others, the majority, penetrate the brittle crust as transcurrent boundaries to sliding and rotating crustal blocks driven by basal traction against a uniformly deforming lower lithosphere. These latter are common within impacting continental terrains, as in the North Anatolian Fault of Turkey (Mann, 1997) or the Pannonian Basin margin to the Vienna Basin (Royden, 1988). Strike-slip faults are often echelon-segmented and may show marked departures from linearity along-strike. It is the along-strike interaction between different parts of the fault that results in a vertical component of slip leading to the production of sedimentary basins. Major basins usually result from two 'pull-apart' mechanisms:

- lateral echelon stepping or jogging, creating rhomboid-shaped areas of subsidence between the steps (dilational jogs of Sibson, 1985) as in the Dead Sea basin of Jordan and Israel;
- 'calving' tendencies along normal to oblique-slip antithetic faults at major fault bends (Fig. 28.23), as first proposed in the classic work by Crowell (1974a,b) on the Ridge Basin of California.

Strike-slip basins of all sorts show rapid (several millimetres per year) asymmetric subsidence against the major strike-slip segment, rapidly rotating antithetic faults, infill by transverse fans feeding lakes or axial, fault-parallel rivers and submarine fans (Figs 28.24 & 28.25). The strike-slip movement itself creates along-strike offset of source areas, changing sediment provenance with time at a point and the occurrence of laterally migrating centres of deposition along the length of the elongating basin.

Further reading

Strike-slip basins are reviewed by Nilsen and Sylvester (1995). Everyone should read Crowell's (1974a, b) classic papers.

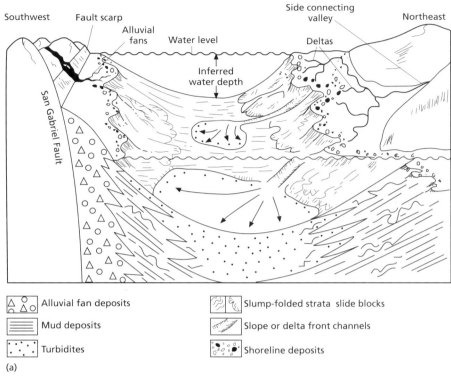

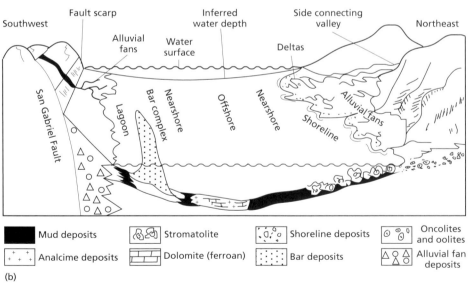

Fig. 28.25 Sketches to show the depositional environments in the Ridge Basin during (a) lake highstand and (b) lake lowstand. (After Link & Osborne, 1982.)

References

Abbott, J.E. & Francis, J.R.D. (1977) Saltation and suspension trajectories of solid grains in a water stream. *Philosophical Transactions of the Royal Society, London (A)*, **284**, 225–54.

Abers, G.A., Mutter, C.Z. & Fang, J. (1977) Shallow dips of normal faults during rapid extension: earthquakes in the Woodlark–D'Entrescasteaux rift system, Papua New Guinea. *Journal of Geophysical Research*, **102**, 15301–17.

Abrahams, A.D. & Parsons, A.J. (eds) (1994) *Geomorphology of Desert Environments*. Chapman and Hall, London.

Acarlar, M.S. & Smith, C.R. (1987) A study of hairpin vortices in a laminar boundary layer. Part 1. Hairpin vortices generated by a hemispherical protuberance. *Journal of Fluid Mechanics*, **175**, 1–41.

Acheson, D.J. (1990) *Elementary Fluid Dynamics*. Oxford University Press, Oxford.

Adamson, D.A., Gasse, F., Street, F.A. & Williams, M.A.J. (1980) Late Quaternary history of the Nile. *Nature*, **288**, 50–5.

Ahnert, F. (1970) Functional relationships between denudation, relief and uplift in large mid-latitude drainage basins. *American Journal of Science*, **268**, 243–63.

Aigner, T. & Reineck, H.-E. (1982) Proximality trends in modern storm sands from the Helgoland Bight (North Sea) and their implications for basin analysis. *Senckenbergiana Maritima*, **14**, 183–215.

Aitken, J.F. & Flint, S.S. (1995) The application of high-resolution sequence stratigraphy to fluvial systems: a case study from the Upper Carboniferous Breathitt Group, eastern Kentucky. *Sedimentology*, **42**, 3–30.

Alexander, J. & Fielding, C. (1997) Gravel antidunes in the tropical Burdekin River, Queensland, Australia. *Sedimentology*, **44**, 327–37.

Alexander, J.A. & Leeder, M.R. (1987) Active tectonic control of alluvial architecture. In: *Recent Developments in Fluvial Sedimentology* (eds F.G. Ethridge, R.M. Flores & M.D. Harvey), pp. 243–52. Special Publication no. 39, Society of Economic Palaeontologists and Mineralogists.

Alexander, J.A. & Morris, S. (1994) Observations on experimental, nonchannelised, high-concentration turbidity currents and variations in deposits around obstacles. *Journal of Sedimentary Research (A)*, **64**, 899–909.

Allen, G.P., Sauzay, G., Castaing, P. & Jouanneau, J.M. (1975) Transport and deposition of suspended sediment in the Gironde estuary, France. *Estuarine Processes 2*, Academic Press, New York, 63–79.

Allen, G.P., Salomon, J.C., Bassoulet, P., Du Penhoat, Y. & De Gandpre, C. (1980) Effects of tides on mixing and suspended sediment transport in macrotidal estuaries. *Sedimentary Geology*, **26**, 69–90.

Allen, J.R.L. (1964) Primary current lioneation in the Lower Old Red Sandstone (Devonian), Anglo-Welsh Basin. *Sedimentology*, **3**, 89–108.

Allen, J.R.L. (1969) Some recent advances in the physics of sedimentation. *Proceedings of the Geologists Association*, **80**, 1–42.

Allen, J.R.L. (1970) *Physical Processes of Sedimentation*. George Allen and Unwin, London.

Allen, J.R.L. (1972) A theoretical and experimental study of climbing-ripple cross-lamination, with a field application to the Uppsala esker. *Geografiska Annaler*, **53A**, 157–87.

Allen, J.R.L. (1973) Phase differences between bed configuration and flow in natural environments, and their geological relevance. *Sedimentology*, **20**, 323–9.

Allen, J.R.L. (1982) *Sedimentary Structures: Their Character and Physical Basis*. Elsevier, Amsterdam.

Allen, J.R.L. (1985) *Principles of Physical Sedimentology*. Allen and Unwin, London.

Allen, J.R.L. & Banks, N.L. (1972) An interpretation and analysis of recumbent-folded deformed cross-bedding. *Sedimentology*, **19**, 257–83.

Allen, P.A. (1984). Reconstruction of ancient sea conditions with an example from the Swiss Molasse. *Marine Geology*, **60**, 455–73.

Allen, P.A. (1997) *Earth Surface Processes*. Blackwell Science, Oxford.

Allen, P.A. & Allen, J.R. (1990) *Basin Analysis*. Blackwell Scientific Publications, Oxford.

Allen, P.A. & Homewood, P. (eds) (1986) *Foreland Basins*. Special Publication no. 8, International Association of Sedimentologists.

Allen, P.A., Crampton, S.L. & Sinclair, H.D. (1991) The inception and early evolution of the North Alpine foreland basin, Switzerland. *Basin Research*, **3**, 143–63.

Allen, P.A., England, P.C., Grotzinger, J. & Sinclair, H. (eds) (1992) Thematic set on foreland basins. *Basin Research*, **4**, 169–352.

Alley, R.B., Blankenship, D.D., Bentley, C.R. & Rooney, S.T. (1986) Deformation of till beneath ice stream, West Antarctica. *Nature*, **322**, 57–9.

Allison, M.A., Kuehl, S.A., Martin, T.C. & Hassan, A. (1998) Importance of flood-plain sedimentation for river sediment budgets and terrigenous input to the oceans: insights from the Brahmaputra–Jamuna River. *Geology*, **26**, 175–8.

Alonso-Zarza, A.M., Wright, V.P., Calvo, J.P. & Garcia del Cura, M.A. (1992) Soil–landscape and climatic relationships in the middle Miocene of the Madrid basin. *Sedimentology*, **39**, 17–35.

Amiotte Suchet, P. & Probst, J.L. (1993) Flux de CO_2 consomme par alteration chimique continentale: influences du drainage et de la lithologie. *Comptes Rendus, Academie des Sciences, Paris (II)*, **317**, 615–22.

Amorosi, A., *et al.* (1996) Genetically related alluvial deposits across active fault zones: an example of alluvial fan-terrace correlation from the upper Quaternary of the southern Po Basin, Italy. *Sedimentary Geology*, **102**, 275–95.

Anadon, P., *et al.* (1986) Syntectonic intraformational unconformities in alluvial fan deposits, eastern Ebro Basin margins (NE Spain). In: *Foreland Basins* (eds P.A. Allen & P. Homewood), pp. 259–71. Special Publication no. 8, International Association of Sedimentologists.

Anastasa, A.S., Dalrymple, R.W., James, N.P. & Campbell, S.N. (1997) Cross-stratified calarenites from New Zealand: subaqueous dunes in a cool-water Oligo-Miocene seaway. *Sedimentology*, **44**, 869–91.

van Andel, T.H. (1975) Mesozoic/Cenozoic calcite compensation depth and the global distribution of calcareous sediments. *Earth and Planetary Science Letters*, **26**, 187–94.

van Andel, T.H. & Komar, P.D. (1969) Ponded sediments of the Mid-Atlantic Ridge between 22° and 23° north latitude. *Bulletin of the Geological Society of America*, **80**, 1163–90.

van Andel, T.H., Thiede, J., Sclater, J.G. & Hay, W.W. (1977) Depositional history of the S. Atlantic Ocean during the last 125 million years. *Journal of Geology*, **85**, 651–98.

Anderson J.A.R. (1964) The structure and development of the peat swamps of Sarawak and Brunei. *Journal of Tropical Geography*, **18**, 7–16.

Anderson, J.B. & Ashley, G.M. (eds) (1991) *Glacial Marine Sedimentation: Palaeoclimatic Significance*. Special Publication no. 261, Geological Society of America.

Anderson, J.B., Kennedy, D.S., Smith, M.J. & Domack, E.W. (1991) Sedimentary facies associated with Antarctica's floating ice masses. In: *Glacial Marine Sedimentation: Palaeoclimatic Significance* (eds J.B. Anderson & G.M. Ashley), pp. 1–26. Special Publication no. 261, Geological Society of America.

Anderson, M.G., Walling, D.E. & Bates, P.D. (eds) (1996) *Floodplain Processes*. Wiley, Chichester.

Anderson, R.S. & Bunas, K.L. (1993) Grain size segregation and stratigraphy in aeolian ripples modelled with a cellular automaton. *Nature*, **365**, 740–3.

Anderton, R. (1976) Tidal shelf sedimentation: an example from the Scottish Dalradian. *Sedimentology*, **23**, 429–58.

Andrews, J.E., Singhvi, A.K. & Kailath, A.J. (1998) Do stable isotope data from calcrete record Late Pleistocene monsoonal climate variation in the Thar Desert of India? *Quaternary Research*, **50**, 240–51.

Andrews, J.E., Brimblecombe, P., Jickells, T.D. & Liss, P.S. (1996) *An Introduction to Environmental Chemistry*. Blackwell Science, Oxford.

Aqrawi, A.A.M. & Evans, G. (1994) Sedimentation in the lakes and marshes (Ahwar) of the Tigris–Euphrates delta, southern Arabia. *Sedimentology*, **41**, 755–76.

Archer, D. (1991) Modeling the calcite lysocline. *Journal of Geophysical Research*, **96**, 17037–50.

Archer, D. & Maier-Reimer, E. (1994) Effect of deep-sea sedimentary calcite preservation on atmospheric CO_2 concentration. *Nature*, **367**, 260–3.

Armentrout, J.M. (1991) Paleontologic constraints on depositional modelling: examples of integration of biostratigraphy and seismic stratigraphy, Pliocene-Pleistocene, Gulf of Mexico. In: *Seismic Facies and Sedimentary Processes of Submarine Fans and Turbidite Systems* (eds P. Weimer & M.H. Link), pp. 137–70. Springer, Berlin.

Armentrout, J.M., Malaceck, S.J., Braithwaite, P. & Beeman, C.R. (1991) Seismic facies of slope-basin turbidite-reservoirs, East Breaks 160–161 Field: Pliocene-Pleistocene, Northwest Gulf of Mexico. In: *Seismic Facies and Sedimentary Processes of Submarine Fans and Turbidite Systems* (eds P. Weimer & M.H. Link), pp. 223–40. Springer, Berlin.

Arnott, R.W.C. & Hand, B.M. (1989) Bedforms, primary structures and grain fabric in the presence of sediment rain. *Journal of Sedimentary Petrology*, **59**, 1062–9.

Arthurton, R.S. (1973) Experimentally produced halite compared with Triassic layered halite-rock from Cheshire, England. *Sedimentology*, **20**, 145–60.

Ashley, G.M. (1975) Rhythmic sedimentation in glacial Lake Hitchcock, Massachusetts–Connecticut. In: *Glaciofluvial and Gaciolacustrine Sediments* (eds A.V. Jopling & B.C. McDonald), pp. 304–20 Special Publication no. 23, Society of Economic Palaeontologists and Mineralogists.

Ashley, G.M. (1990) Classification of large scale subaqueous bedforms: a new look at an old problem. *Journal of Sedimentary Petrology*, **60**, 160–72.

Ashley, G.M., Wellner, R.W., Esker, D. & Sheridan, R.E. (1991) Clastic sequences developed during late Quaternary glacio-eustatic sea-level fluctuations on a passive margin: example from the inner continental shelf near Barnegat Inlet, New Jersey. *Bulletin of the Geological Society of America*, 103, 1607–21.

Ashworth, P.J., Bennett, S.J., Best, J.L. & McClelland, S.J. (1996) Wiley, Chichester.

Asselman, N.E.M. & Middelkoop, H. (1995) Floodplain sedimentation: quantities, patterns and processes. *Earth Surface Processes and Landforms*, 20, 481–99.

Atkins, P.W. (1992) *The Elements of Physical Chemistry*. Oxford University Press, Oxford.

Atkinson, B.W. & Zhang, J.Wu. (1996) Mesoscale shallow convection in the atmosphere. *Reviews of Geophysics*, 34, 403–31.

Aubrey, J. & Geise, F.J. (eds) (1993) *Formation and Evolution of Multiple Tidal Inlets*, Monograph, American Geophysical Union.

Aurell, M., Bosence, D. & Waltham, D. (1995) Carbonate ramp depositional systems from a late Jurassic epeiric platform (Iberian Basin, Spain): a combined computer modelling and outcrop analysis. *Sedimentology*, 42, 75–94.

Autin, W.A., Burns, S.F., Miller, B.J., Saucier, R.T. & Snead, J.I. (1991) Quaternary geology of the Lower Mississippi Valley. In: *The Geology of North America*; Vol. K2, *Quaternary Nonglacial Geology; Conterminous US* (ed. R.B. Morrison). Geological Society of America, Boulder, CO.

de Baar, H.J.W., *et al.* (1995) Importance of iron for plankton blooms and carbon dioxide drawdown in the Southern Ocean. *Nature*, 373, 412–15.

Baas, J.H. (1994) A flume study on the development and equilibrium morphology of small-scale bedforms in very fine sand. *Sedimentology*, 41, 185–209.

Baas, J.H., *et al.* (1993) Time as an independent variable for current ripples developing towards linguoid equilibrium morphology. *Terra Nova*, 5, 29–35.

Bagnold, R.A. (1936) The movement of desert sand. *Proceedings of the Royal Society of London*, A157, 594–620.

Bagnold, R.A. (1940) Beach formation by waves: some model experiments in a wave tank. *Journal of the Institute of Civil Engineers*, 15, 27–52.

Bagnold, R.A. (1946) Motion of waves in shallow water: interactions between waves and shallow bottoms. *Philosophical Transactions of the Royal Society, London (A)*, 187, 1–18.

Bagnold, R.A. (1954a) Experiments on a gravity-free dispersion of large solid spheres in a Newtonian fluid under shear. *Philosophical Transactions of the Royal Society, London (A)*, 225, 49–63.

Bagnold, R.A. (1954b) *The Physics of Blown Sand and Desert Dunes*, 2nd edn. Chapman and Hall, London.

Bagnold, R.A. (1955) Some flume experiments on grains but little denser than the transporting fluid, and their implications. *Proceedings of the Institute of Civil Engineers*, 4, 174–205.

Bagnold, R.A. (1956) The flow of cohesionless grains in fluids. *Philosophical Transactions of the Royal Society, London (A)*, 249, 335–97.

Bagnold, R.A. (1962) Auto-suspension of transported sediment: turbidity currents. *Philosophical Transactions of the Royal Society, London (A)*, 265, 315–19.

Bagnold, R.A. (1963) Mechanics of marine sedimentation. In: *The Sea* (ed. M.N. Hill), pp. 507–23. Wiley, New York.

Bagnold, R.A. (1966a) The shearing and dilation of dry sand and the 'singing' mechanism. *Philosophical Transactions of the Royal Society, London (A)*, 295, 219–32.

Bagnold, R.A. (1966b) *An Approach to the Sediment Transport Problem from General Physics* Professional Paper no. 422-I, United States Geological Survey.

Bagnold, R.A. (1973) The nature of saltation and of 'bed-load' transport in water. *Philosophical Transactions of the Royal Society, London (A)*, 332, 473–504.

Bagnold, R.A. (1991) *Sand, Wind and War: Memoirs of a Desert Explorer*. University of Arizona Press, Tucson.

Baikal Drilling Project Members (1997) Project-96 (Leg 2). Continuous paleoclimate record recovered for last 5 million years. *EOS, December*, 597–604.

Baker, E.K., Harris, P.T., Keene, J.B. & Short, S.A. (1995) Patterns of sedimentation in the macrotidal Fly River delta, Papua New Guinea. In: *Tidal Signatures in Modern and Ancient Sediments*, pp. 193–211. Special Publication no. 24, International Association of Sedimentologists.

Baker, E.T. & Hickey, B.M. (1986) Contemporary sedimentation processes in and around an active west coast submarine canyon. *Marine Geology*, 71, 15–34.

Baker, V.R. (1973) *Palaeohydrology and Sedimentology of Lake Missoula Flooding in Eastern Washington*. Special Paper 144, Geological Society of America.

Baker, V.R. (1990) Geological fluvial geomorphology. *Bulletin of the Geological Society of America*, 100, 1157–67.

Baker, V.R. (1994) Geomorphological understanding of floods. *Geomorphology*, 10, 139–56.

Ball, M.M. (1967) Carbonate sand bodies of Florida and the Bahamas. *Journal of Sedimentary Petrology*, 37, 556–91.

Banerjee, I. & McDonald, B.C. (1975) Nature of esker sedimentation. In: *Glaciofluvial and Glaciolacustrine Sediments* (ed A.V. Jopling & B.C. McDonald), pp. 132–54 Special Publication no. 23, Society of Economic Palaeontologists and Mineralogists.

Banks, N.L. (1973) The origin and significance of some downcurrent-dipping cross-stratified sets. *Journal of Sedimentary Petrology*, 43, 423–7.

Barker, G. & Grimson, M. (1990) The physics of muesli. *New Scientist*, May.

Barros, A.P. & Lettenmaier, D.P. (1994) Dynamic modeling of orographically induced precipitation. *Reviews of Geophysics*, 32, 265–84.

Barshad, I. (1966) The effect of variation in precipitation on the nature of clay mineral formation in soils from acid and basic igneous rocks. In: *Proceedings of the 1st International Clay Conference*, Jerusalem, pp. 167–73.

Bates, C.C. (1953) Rational theory of delta formation. *Bulletin of the American Association of Petroleum Geologists*, 37, 2119–62.

Bathurst, R.G.C. (1966) Boring algae, micrite envelopes and lithification of molluscan biosparites. *Geological Journal*, 5, 15–32.

Bathurst, R.G.C. (1968) Precipitation of ooids and other aragonitic fabrics in warm seas. In: *Recent Developments in Carbonate Sedimentology in Central Europe* (eds G. Muller & G.M. Friedman), pp. 1–10. Springer, Berlin.

Bathurst, R.G.C. (1975) *Carbonate Sediments and their Diagenesis*. Elsevier, Amsterdam.

de Batist, M. & Jacobs, P. (eds) (1996) *Geology of Siliciclastic Shelf Seas*. Geological Society of London Special Publication 117.

Bazylinski, D.A., Heywood, B.R. Mann, S. & Frankel, R.B. (1993) Fe$_3$O$_4$ and Fe$_3$S$_4$ in a bacterium. *Nature*, 366, 218.

Beard, D.C. & Weyl, P.K. (1973) Influence of texture on porosity and permeability of unconsolidated sand. *Bulletin of the American Association of Petroleum Geologists*, 51, 349–69.

Beaty 1967

Beaty, C.B. (1970) Age and estimated rate of accumulation of an alluvial fan, White Mountains, California, USA. *American Journal of Science*, 268, 50–77.

Beaty, C.B. (1990) Anatomy of a White Mountains debris-flow—the making of an alluvial fan. In: *Alluvial Fans: A Field Approach* (eds A.H. Rachocki & M. Church), pp. 69–89. Wiley, New York.

Beaumont, C. (1981) Foreland basins. *Geophysical Journal of the Royal Astronomical Society*, 65, 291–329.

Becker, P. (1994) Density plumes of the Ob, Yenisei and Mackenzie Rivers. In: *AGU Fall Meeting Abstract Volume*, p. 317.

van der Beek, P., Cloetingh, S. & Andriessen, P. (1994) Mechanisms of extensional basin formation and vertical motions at rift flanks: constraints from tectonic modelling and fission track thermochronology. *Earth and Planetary Science Letters*, 121, 417–33.

Beghin, P., Hopfinger, E.J. & Britter, R.E. (1981) Gravitational convection from instantaneous sources on inclined boundaries. *Journal of Fluid Mechanics*, 107, 407–22.

Begin, Z.B. (1988) Application of a diffusion–erosion model to alluvial channels which degrade due to base level lowering. *Earth Surface Processes and Landforms*, 13, 487–500.

Behl, R.J. & Kennett, J.P. (1996) Brief interstadial events in the Santa Barbara basin, NE Pacific, during the past 60 ky. *Nature*, 379, 243–6.

Belderson, R.H., Johnson, M.A. & Stride, A.H. (1978) Bedload partings and convergences at the entrance to the White Sea, USSR and between Cape Cod and Georges Bank, USA. *Marine Geology*, 28, 65–75.

Belderson, R.H., Johnson, M.A. & Kenyon, N.H. (1982) Bedforms. In: *Offshore Tidal Sands: Processes and Deposits* (ed. A.H. Stride), pp. 27–57. Chapman and Hall, London.

Bellotti, P., et al. (1994) Sequence stratigraphy and depositional setting of the Tiber delta: integration of high-resolution seismics, well logs, and archeological data. *Journal of Sedimentary Research*, 64, 416–32.

Benn, D.I. (1994) Fluted moraine and till genesis below a temperate valley glacier: Slettmarkbreen, Jotunheimen, southern Norway. *Sedimentology*, 41, 279–92.

Benn, D.I. (1995) Fabric signature of subglacial till deformation, Breidamerkurjokull, Iceland. *Sedimentology*, 42, 735–47.

Benn, D.I. & Evans, D.J.A. (1998) *Glaciers and Glaciation*. Arnold, London.

Bennett, S.J. & Best, J.L. (1995) Mean flow and turbulence structure over fixed, two-dimensional dunes: implications for sediment transport and dune stability. *Sedimentology*, 42, 491–514.

Bennett, S.J. & Best, J.L. (1996) Mean flow and turbulence structure over fixed ripples and the ripple–dune transition. In: *Coherent Flow Structures in Open Channels* (eds P.J. Ashworth et al.). pp. 281–304, Wiley, Chichester.

Bennett, S.J. & Bridge, J.S. (1995) The geometry and dynamics of low-relief bedforms in heterogenous sediment in a laboratory channel, and their relationship to water flow and sediment transport. *Journal of Sedimentary Research (A)*, 65, 29–39.

Benson, L. & Thompson, R.S. (1987) The physical record of lakes in the Great Basin. In: *The Geology of North America*, Vol. K3, *North America and Adjacent Oceans During the Last Deglaciation* (eds W.F. Ruddiman & H.E. Wright), pp. 241–60. Geological Society of America, Boulder, CO.

van den Berg, J.H. & van Gelder, A. (1993) A new bedform stability diagram, with emphasis on the transition of ripples to plane bed in flows over fine sand and silt. In: *Alluvial Sedimentation* (eds M. Marzo & C. Puigdefabregas), pp. 11–21. Special Publication no. 17, International Association of Sedimentologists.

Berger, W.H. (1982) Increase of carbon dioxide during deglaciation: the coral reef hypothesis. *Naturwissenschaften*, 69, 87–8.

Berger, W.H. & Herquera, J.C. (1992) Reading the sedimentary record of the ocean's productivity. In: *Primary Productivity and Biogeochemical Cycles in the Sea* (eds P.G. Falkowski & A.D. Woodhead), pp. 455–86. Plenum, New York.

Berné, S., Castaing, P., LeDrezen, E. & Lericolais, G. (1993) Morphology, internal structure and reversal of asymmetry of large subtidal dunes in the entrance to Gironde estuary (France). *Journal of Sedimentary Petrology*, 63, 780–93.

Berner, R.A. (1969) Goethite stability and the origin of red beds. *Geochimica et Cosmochimica Acta*, **33**, 267–73.

Berner, R.A. (1970) Sedimentary pyrite formation. *American Journal of Science*, **208**, 1–23.

Berner, R.A. (1971) *Principles of Chemical Sedimentology*. McGraw-Hill, New York.

Berner, R.A. (1975) The role of magnesium in the crystal growth of calcite and aragonite from sea water. *Geochimica et Cosmochimica Acta*, **39**, 489–504.

Berner, R.A. (1976) The solubility of calcite and aragonite in seawater at atmospheric pressure and 34.5‰ salinity. *American Journal of Science*, **276**, 713–30.

Berner, R.A. (1992) Weathering, plants and the long-term carbon cycle. *Geochimica et Cosmochimica Acta*, **56**, 3225–32.

Berner, R.A. (1995) Chemical weathering and its effect on atmospheric CO_2 and climate. In: *Chemical Weathering Rates of Silicate Minerals* (eds A.F. White & S.L. Branfield) American Mineralogical Society, Washington, DC.

Berner, R.A. & Lasaga, A.C. (1989) Modelling the geochemical carbon cycle. *Scientific American*, **260**, 54–61.

Berner, R.A., Westrich, J.T., Graber, R., Smith, J. & Martens, C.S. (1978) Inhibition of aragonite precipitation from supersaturated seawater. A laboratory and field study. *American Journal of Science*, **278**, 816–37.

Berner, R.A., Lasaga, A.C. & Garrels, R.M. (1983) The carbonate–silicate geochemical cycle and its effect on atmospheric carbon dioxide over the past two million years. *American Journal of Science*, **283**, 641–83.

Best, J.L. (1987) Flow dynamics at river channel confluences: implications for sediment transport and bed morphology. In: *Recent Developments in Fluvial Sedimentology* (eds F.G. Ethridge, R.M. Flores & M.D. Harvey), pp. 27–35. Special Publication no. 39, Society of Economic Palaeontologists and Mineralogists.

Best, J.L. (1988) Sediment transport and bed morphology at river channel confluences. *Sedimentology*, **35**, 481–98.

Best, J.L. (1992a) On the entrainment of sediment and initiation of bed defects from recent developments within turbulent boundary research. *Sedimentology*, **39**, 797–811.

Best, J.L. (1992b) Sedimentology and event timing of a catastrophic volcaniclastic mass flow, Volcan Hudson, Southern Chile. *Bulletin of Volcanology*, **54**, 299–318.

Best, J.L. (1993) On the interactions between turbulent flow structure, sediment transport and bedform development: some considerations from recent experimental research. In: *Turbulence: Perspectives on Flow and Sediment Transport* (eds Clifford *et al.*), pp. 62–91. Wiley, London.

Best, J.L. & Ashworth, P.J. (1997) Scour in large braided rivers and the recognition of sequence stratigraphic boundaries. *Nature*, **387**, 275–7.

Best, J.L. & Bridge, J.S. (1992) The morphology and dynamics of low amplitude bedwaves upon upper-stage plane beds and the preservation of planar laminae. *Sedimentology*, **39**, 737–52.

Best J.L. & Bristow, C.S. (1993) (eds) *Braided Rivers*. Geological Society of London Special Publication 75.

Best, J.L. & Leeder, M.R. (1993) Drag reduction in turbulent muddy seawater flows and some sedimentary consequences. *Sedimentology*, **40**, 1129–37.

Best, J.L. & Roy, A.G. (1991) Mixing-layer distortion at the confluence of channels of different depths. *Nature*, **350**, 411–13.

Bianchi, G.G. & McCave, I.N. (1999) Holocene periodicity in North Atlantic climate and deep-ocean flow south of Iceland. *Nature*, **397**, 515–17.

Bidle, K.D. & Azam, F. (1999) Accelerated dissolution of diatom silica by marine bacterial assemblages. *Nature*, **397**, 508–12.

Biegel, E. & Hoekstra, P. (1995) Morphological response characteristics of the Zoutkamperlaag, Frisian inlet (The Netherlands), to a sudden reduction in basin area. In: *Tidal Signatures in Modern and Ancient Sediments*, pp. 85–99. Special Publication no. 24, International Association of Sedimentologists.

Bigarella, J.J. (1973) Paleocurrents and the problem of continental drift. *Geologische Rundschau*, **62**, 447–77.

Biscaye, P.E. & Eittreim, S.L. (1977) Suspended particulate loads and transports in the nepheloid layer of the abyssal Atlantic Ocean. *Marine Geology*, **23**, 155–72.

Black, K.S., Paterson, D.M. & Cramp, A. (eds) (1998) *Sedimentary Processes in the Intertidal Zone*. Geological Society of London Special Publication **139**.

Blair, T.C. & McPherson, J.G. (1994a) Alluvial fans and their natural distinction from rivers based on morphology, hydraulic processes, sedimentary processes, and facies assemblages. *Journal of Sedimentary Research*, **64**, 450–89.

Blair, T.C. & McPherson, J.G. (1994b) Alluvial fan processes and forms. In: *Geomorphology of Desert Environments* (eds A.D. Abrahams & A.J. Parsons), pp. 354–402. Chapman and Hall, London.

Blakey, R.C., Havholm, K.G. & Jones, L.S. (1996) Stratigraphic analysis of eolian interactions with marine and fluvial deposits, Middle Jurassic Page Sandstone and Carmel Formation, Colorado Plateau, USA. *Journal of Sedimentary Research*, **66**, 324–42.

Blanchon, P. & Jones, B. (1997) Hurricane control on shelf-edge-reef architecture around Grand Cayman. *Sedimentology*, **44**, 479–506.

Blanchon, P. & Shaw, J. (1995) Reef drowning during the last deglaciation: evidence for catastrophic sea-level rise and ice-sheet collapse. *Geology*, **23**, 4–8.

Blankenship, D.D. (1993) The depositional environment at the grounding zone of a contemporary Antarctic ice stream. *EOS Abstracts Spring Meeting*, p. 309.

Blankenship, D.D., Bentley, C.R., Rooney, S.T. & Alley, R.B. (1986) Seismic measurements reveal a saturated porous layer beneath an active Antarctic ice stream. *Nature*, **322**, 54–7.

Blatt, H., Middleton, G.V. & Murray, R. (1980). *Origin of Sedimentary Rocks*, 2nd edn. Prentice Hall, New Jersey.

Blendinger, W. (1994) The carbonate factory of Middle Triassic buildups in the Dolomites, Italy: a quantitative analysis. *Sedimentology*, **41**, 1147–59.

Blount, G. & Lancaster, N. (1990) Development of the Gran Desierto sand sea, northwestern Mexico. *Geology*, **18**, 724–8.

Blum, A.E. & Stillings, L.L. (1995) Feldspar dissolution kinetics. In: *Chemical Weathering Rates of Silicate Minerals* (eds A.F. White & S.L. Branfield). American Mineralogical Society, Washington, DC.

Blum, M.D. (1990) Climatic and eustatic controls on Gulf Coastal plain fluvial sedimentation: an example from the late Quaternary of the Colorado River, Texas. *GCSSEPM Foundation 11th Annual Research Conference*, pp. 71–83.

Blum, M.D. (1993) Genesis and architecture of incised valley-fill sequences: a late Quaternary example from the Colorado River, Gulf coastal plain of Texas. In: *Siliciclastic Sequence Stratigraphy: Recent Developments and Applications* (eds P. Weimer & H.W. Posamentier), pp. 259–83. Memoir 58, American Association of Petroleum Geologists.

Boardman, M.R. & Neuman, A.C. (1984) Sources of periplatform carbonates: Northwest Providence Channel, Bahamas. *Journal of Sedimentary Petrology*, **54**, 1110–23.

Boardman, M.R., McCartney, R.F. & Eaton, M.R. (1995) Bahamian paleosols: origin, relation to palaeoclimate and stratigraphic significance. In: *Terrestrial and Shallow Marine Geology of the Bahamas and Bermuda* (eds A.A. Curran & B. White), pp. 33–51. Special Paper 300, Geological Society of America.

Boersma, J.R. (1967) Remarkable types of mega cross-stratification in the fluviatile sequence of a sub-Recent distributary of the Rhine, Amerongen, the Netherlands. *Geologie Mijnbouw*, **46**, 217–35.

Boettcher, S.S. & Milliken, K.L. (1994) Mesozoic–Cenozoic unroofing of the Southern Appalachian Basin: apatite fission track evidence from Middle Pennsylvanian sandstones. *Journal of Geology*, **102**, 655–63.

Bond, G., *et al*. (1992) Evidence for massive discharges of icebergs into the north Atlantic ocean during the last glacial period. *Nature*, **360**, 245–9.

Bond, G., Kominz, M.A. & Sheridan, R.E. (1995) Continental terraces and rises. In: *Tectonics of Sedimentary Basins* (eds C. Busby & R. Ingersoll), pp. 149–78, Blackwell Science, Oxford.

Boothroyd, J.C. & Ashley, G.M. (1975) Processes, bar morphology and sedimentary structures on braided outwash fans, northeastern Gulf of Alaska. In: *Glaciofluvial and Glaciolacustrine Sediments* (eds A.V. Jopling & B.C. McDonald), pp. 193–222, Special Publication no. 23, Society of Economic Palaeontologists and Mineralogists.

Borchert, H. & Muir, R.O. (1964) *Salt Deposits*. Van Nostrand Reinhold, London.

Borrego, J., Morales, J.A. & Pendon, J.G. (1995) Holocene estuarine facies along the mesotidal coast of Huelva, south-western Spain. In: *Tidal Signatures in Modern and Ancient Sediments*, pp. 151–70. Special Publication no. 24, International Association of Sedimentologists.

Bosellini, A. (1984) Progradation geometries of carbonate platforms: examples from the Triassic of the Dolomites, northern Italy. *Sedimentology*, **31**, 1–24.

Bosence, D.W.J. (1973) Facies relationships in a tidally influenced environment: a study from the Eocene of the London Basin. *Geologie Mijnbouw*, **52**, 63–7.

Bosence, D.W.J. (1983a) Description and classification of rhodoliths (rhodoids, rhodolites). In: *Coated Grains* (ed. T.M. Peryt), pp. 217–24. Springer, Berlin.

Bosence, D.W.J. (1983b) The occurrence and ecology of recent rhodoliths—a review. In: *Coated Grains* (ed. T.M. Peryt), pp. 225–42. Springer, Berlin.

Bosence, D.W.J. & Waltham, D.A. (1990) Computer modelling the internal architecture of carbonate platforms. *Geology*, **18**, 26–30.

Bosence, D.W.J., Rowlands, R.J. & Quine, M.L. (1985) Sedimentology and budget of a Recent carbonate mound, Florida Keys. *Sedimentology*, **32**, 317–43.

Bosence, D.W.J., Pomar, L.P., Waltham, D.A. & Lankester, T.H.G. (1994) Computer modelling a Miocene carbonate platform, Mallorca, Spain. *Bulletin of the American Association of Petroleum Geologists*, **78**, 247–66.

Boulton, G.S. (1972) Modern Arctic glaciers as depositional models for former ice sheets. *Quarterly Journal of the Geological Society of London*, **128**, 361–93.

Boulton, G.S. (1976) The origin of glacially-fluted surfaces—observations and theory. *Journal of Glaciology*, **17**, 287–309.

Boulton, G.S. (1978) Boulder shapes and grain size distributions of debris as indicators of transport paths through a glacier and till genesis. *Sedimentology*, **25**, 773–99.

Boulton, G.S. (1979) Processes of glacier erosion on different substrates. *Journal of Glaciology*, **23**, 15–38.

Boulton, G.S. (1990) Sedimentary and sea level changes during glacial cycles and their control on glacimarine facies architecture. In: *Glacimarine Environments* (eds J.A. Dowdeswell & J.D. Scourse) pp. 15–52. Special Publication no. 53, Geological Society of London.

Boulton, G.S. & Hindmarsh, R.C.A. (1987) Sediment deformation beneath glaciers: rheology and geological consequences. *Journal of Geophysical Research*, **92B**, 9059–82.

Bouma, A.H. (1962) *Sedimentology of Some Flysch Deposits: A Graphic Approach to Facies Interpretations*. Elsevier, Amsterdam.

Bouma, A.H. & Hollister, C.D. (1973) Deep ocean basin sedimentation. In: *Turbidites and Deep Water*

Sedimentation, pp. 79–118. Society of Economic Palaeontologists and Mineralogists Short Course, Anaheim.

Bourgeois, J. (1980) A transgressive shelf sequence exhibiting hummocky stratification: the Cape Sebastion Sandstone (U. Cretaceous), SW Oregon. *Journal of Sedimentary Petrology*, **50**, 681–702.

Bourne, S.J., England, P.C. & Parsons, B. (1998) The motion of crustal blocks driven by flow of the lower lithosphere: implications for slip rates of faults in the South Island of New Zealand and Southern California. *Nature*, **391**, 655–9.

Bowen, A.J. (1969) Rip currents, 1: Theoretical investigations. *Journal of Geophysical Research*, **74**, 5467–78.

Bowen, A.J. & Inman, D.L. (1969) Rip currents, 2: Laboratory and field observations. *Journal of Geophysical Research*, **74**, 5479–90.

Bowen, A.J., Inman, D.L. & Simmon, V.P. (1968) Wave 'set down' and 'set up'. *Journal of Geophysical Research*, **73**, 256–77.

Bowen, A.J., Normark, W.R. & Piper, D.J.W. (1984) Modelling of turbidity currents on Navy Submarine Fan, California Continental Borderland. *Sedimentology*, **31**, 169–85.

Bowler, J.M. (1977) Aridity in Australia: age, origins and expression in aeolian landforms and sediments. *Earth Science Reviews*, **12**, 279–310.

Boyles, J.M. & Scott, A.J. (1982) A model for migrating shelf-bar sandstones in Upper Mancos Shale (Campanian), northwest Colorado. *Bulletin of the American Association of Petroleum Geologists*, **66**, 491–508.

Brack, P., Mundil, R., Oberli, F., Meier, M. & Rieber, H. (1996) Biostratigraphic and radiometric age data question the Milankovitch characteristics of the Latemar cycles (Southern Alps, Italy). *Geology*, **24**, 371–5.

Bradshaw, M.J., James, S.J. & Turner, P. (1980) Origin of oolitic ironstones discussion. *Journal of Sedimentary Petrology*, **50**, 295–9.

Braga, J.C., Martin, J.M. & Riding, R. (1996) Internal structure of segment reefs: *Halimeda* algal mounds in the Mediterranean Miocene. *Geology*, **24**, 35–8.

Brantley, S.L. & Chen, Y. (1995) Chemical weathering rates of pyroxenes and amphiboles. In: *Chemical Weathering Rates of Silicate Minerals* (eds A.F. White & S.L. Branfield), American Society of Mineralogy, Washington, DC.

Brasier, M.D. (1995) Fossil indicators of nutrient levels. 1: Eutrophication and climate change. In: *Marine Palaeoenvironmental Analysis from Fossils* (eds D.J.W. Bosence & P.A. Allison), pp. 113–32. Special Publication no. 83, Geological Society of London.

Brayshaw, A.C., Frostick, L.E. & Reid, I. (1983) The hydrodynamics of particle clusters and sediment entrainment in coarse alluvial channels. *Sedimentology*, **30**, 137–43.

Breed, C.S. (1977) Terrestrial analogs of the Hellespontus dunes, Mars. *Icarus*, **30**, 326–40.

Brenchley, P.J., Pickerill, R.K. & Stromberg, S.G. (1993) The role of wave reworking on the architecture of storm sandstone facies, Bell Island Group (Lower Ordovician), eastern Newfoundland. *Sedimentology*, **40**, 359–82.

Brice, J.C. (1984) Planform properties of meandering rivers. In: *River Meandering, Proceedings Rivers '83 Conference* pp. 1–15. American Society of Civil Engineers, New York.

Bridge, J.S. (1976) Bed topography and grain size in open channel bends. *Sedimentology*, **23**, 407–14.

Bridge, J.S. (1977) Flow, bed topography, grain size and sedimentary structures in open channel bends: a three dimensional model. *Earth Surface Processes*, **2**, 401–16.

Bridge, J.S. (1985) Palaeochannel patterns inferred from alluvial deposits: a critical evaluation. *Journal of Sedimentary Petrology*, **55**, 579–89.

Bridge, J.S. (1993) The interaction between channel geometry, water flow, sediment transport and deposition in braided rivers. In: *Braided Rivers* (eds J.L. Best & C.S. Bristow), pp. 13–71. Special Publication no. 75, Geological Society of London.

Bridge, J.S. & Bennett, S.J. (1992) A model for the entrainment and transport of sediment grains of mixed sizes, shapes and densities. *Water Resources Research*, **28**, 337–63.

Bridge, J.S. & Best, J.L. (1997) Preservation of planar laminae due to migration of low-relief bed waves over aggrading upper-stage plane beds: comparison of experimental data with theory. *Sedimentology*, **44**, 253–62.

Bridge, J.S. & Gabel, S.L. (1992) Flow and sediment dynamics in a low-sinuosity, braided river: Calamus River, Nebraska Sandhills. *Sedimentology*, **39**, 125–42.

Bridge, J.S. & Jarvis, J. (1982) The dynamics of a river bend: a study in flow and sedimentary processes *Sedimentology*, **29**, 499–541.

Bridge, J.S. & Leeder, M.R. (1979) A simulation model of alluvial stratigraphy. *Sedimentology*, **26**, 617–44.

Bridge, J.S., *et al.* (1986) Sedimentology and morphology of a low-sinuosity river: Calamus River, Nebraska Sand Hills. *Sedimentology*, **33**, 851–70.

Bridge, J.S., *et al.* (1995) Ground-penetrating radar and coring used to study the large-scale structure of point-bar deposits in three dimensions. *Sedimentology*, **42**, 839–52.

Bridges, P.H. & Leeder, M.R. (1976) Sedimentary model for intertidal mudflat channels with examples from the Solway Firth, Scotland. *Sedimentology*, **23**, 533–52.

Bridges, P.H. (1982) Ancient offshore tidal deposits. In: *Offshore Tidal Sands* (ed A.H. Stride), 172–92. Chapman & Hall, London.

Bridgman, P.W. (1911) Water, in the liquid and five solid forms, under pressure. *Proceedings of the American Academy of Arts and Sciences*, **47**, 439–558.

Brimblecombe, P. & Davies, T.D. (1982) The Earth's atmosphere. In: *The Cambridge Encyclopaedia of Earth Sciences* (ed. D.G. Smith). Cambridge University Press, Cambridge.

Bristow, C.S. (1993) Sedimentary structures exposed in bar tops in the Brahmaputra River, Bangladesh. In: *Braided Rivers* (eds J.L. Best & C.S. Bristow), pp. 277–90. Special Publication no. 75, Geological Society of London.

Bristow, C.S., Best, J.L. & Roy, A.G. (1993) Morphology and facies models of channel confluences. In: *Alluvial Sedimentation* (eds M. Marzo & C. Puigdefabregas), pp. 91–100. Special Publication no. 17, International Association of Sedimentologists.

Bristow, C.S., Pugh, J. & Goodall, T. (1996) Internal structure of aeolian dunes in Abu Dhabi determined using ground-penetrating radar. *Sedimentology*, **43**, 995–1003.

Britter, R.E. & Linden, P.F. (1980) The motion of the front of a gravity current travelling down an incline. *Journal of Fluid Mechanics*, **99**, 531–43.

Broecker, W.S. (1974) *Chemical Oceanography*. Harcourt Brace Jovanovich, New York.

Broecker, W.S. & Takahashi, T. (1966) Calcium carbonate precipitation on the Bahama Banks. *Journal of Geophysical Research*, **71**, 1575–602.

Brookfield, M. (1970) Dune trends and wind regime in Central Australia. *Zeitschrift fur Geomorphologie, Suppl.*, **10**, 121–53.

Brookfield, M.E. (1977) The origin of bounding surfaces in ancient aeolian sandstones. *Sedimentology*, **24**, 303–30.

Brown, D.A., Sherriff, B.L. & Sawicki, J.A. (1997) Microbial transformation of magnetite to haematite. *Geochimica et Cosmochimica Acta*, **61**, 3341–8.

Bruland, K.W., *et al.* (1989) Flux to the seafloor. In: *Productivity of the Oceans: Present and Past* (eds W.H. Berger *et al.*), pp. 193–216. Wiley, New York.

Bryant, M., Falk, P. & Paola, C. (1995) Experimental study of avulsion frequency and rate of deposition. *Geology*, **23**, 365–8.

Bugge, T., Belderson, R.H. & Kenyon, N.H. (1988) The Storegga slide. *Philosophical Transactions of the Royal Society, London (A)*, **325**, 357–88.

Bull, W.B. (1979) Threshold of critical power in streams. *Bulletin of the Geological Society of America*, **90**, 453–64.

Bull, W.B. (1991) *Eomorphic Response to Climate Change*. Oxford University Press, New York.

Burbank, D.W. & Raynolds, R.G.H. (1988) Stratigraphic keys to the timing of thrusting in terrestrial foreland basins: applications to the NW Himalaya. In: *New Perspectives in Basin Analysis* (eds K.L. Kleinspehn & C. Paola), pp. 331–51. Springer, New York.

Burbank, D.W., Puigdefabregas, C. & Muños, J.A. (1992) The chronology of the Eocene tectonic and stratigraphic development of the eastern Pyrenean foreland basin, northeast Spain. *Bulletin of the Geological Society of America*, **104**, 1101–20.

Burchette, T.P. & Wright, V.P. (1992) Carbonate ramp depositional systems. *Sedimentary Geology*, **79**, 3–57.

Burchfiel, B.C. (1966) Tin Mountain landslide, southeastern California, and the origin of megabreccia. *Bulletin of the Geological Society of America*, **77**, 95–100.

Burgess, P.M. & Gurnis, M. (1995) Mechanisms for the formation of cratonic sequences. *Earth and Planetary Science Letters*, **136**, 647–63.

Burgess, P.M., Gurnis, M. & Moresi, L. (1997) Formation of sequences in the cratonic interior of North America by interaction between mantle, eustatic and stratigraphic processes. *Bulletin of the Geological Society of America*, **108**, 1515–35.

Burkham, D.E. (1972) *Channel Changes of the Gila River in Safford Valley, Arizona, 1846–1970*. Professional Paper no. 655-G, United States Geological Survey.

Burt, N., Parker, R. & Watts, J. (eds) (1997) *Cohesive Sediments*. Wiley, Chichester.

Burton, E.A. & Walter, L.M. (1987) Relative precipitation rates of aragonite and Mg calcite from seawater— temperature or carbonate ion control? *Geology*, **15**, 111–14.

Burton, E.A. & Walter, L.M. (1990) The role of pH in phosphate inhibition of calcite and aragonite precipitation in seawater. *Geochimica et Cosmochimica Acta*, **54**, 797–808.

Busby, C.J. & Ingersoll, R.V. (eds) (1995) *Tectonics of Sedimentary Basins*. Blackwell Science, Oxford.

Cacchione, D.A. & Southard, J.B. (1974) Incipient sediment movement by shoaling internal gravity waves. *Journal of Geophysical Research*, **79**, 2237–42.

Calvert, S.E. & Karlin, R.E. (1998) Organic carbon accumulation in the Holocene sapropel of the Black Sea. *Geology*, **26**, 107–10.

Calvo, J.P., Alonso-Zarza, A.M. & Garcia del Cura, M.A. (1989) Models of Miocene marginal lacustrine sedimentation in response to varied depositional regimes and source areas in the Madrid basin (central Spain). *Palaeogeography, Palaeoclimatology, Palaeoecology*, **70**, 199–214.

Camoin, G.F. & Montaggioni, L.F. (1994) High energy coralgal–stromatolite frameworks from Holocene reefs (Tahiti, French Polynesia). *Sedimentology*, **41**, 655–76.

Campbell, C.S. (1989) Self-lubrication for long runout landslides. *Journal of Geology*, **97**, 653–65.

Campbell, C.S., Cleary, W. & Hopkins, M. (1995) Large-scale landslide simulations: global deformation, velocities and basal friction. *Journal of Geophysical Research*, **100**, 8267–83.

Campbell, C.V. & Oakes, R.Q. (1973) Estuarine sandstone filling tidal scours, Lower Cretaceous Fall River Formation, Wyoming, *Journal of Sedimentary Petrology*, **43**, 765–78.

Campbell, S.E. (1979) Soil stabilisation by a prokaryotic desert crust: implications for PreCambrian land biota. *Origins of Life*, **9**, 335–48.

Caplan, M.L., Bustin, R.M. & Grimm, K.A. (1996) Demise of a Devonian–Carboniferous carbonate ramp by eutrophication. *Geology*, 24, 715–18.

Carew, J.L. & Mylroie, J.E. (1995) Depositional model and stratigraphy for the Quaternary geology of the Bahamas Islands. In: *Terrestrial and Shallow Marine Geology of the Bahamas and Bermuda* (eds A.A. Curran & B. White), pp. 5–32. Special Paper 300, Geological Society of America.

Carey, S.N. & Sigurdsson, H. (1984) A model of volcanogenic sedimentation in marginal basins. In: *Marginal Basin Geology* (eds B.P. Kokelaar & M.F. Howell), pp. 37–58. Special Publication no. 16, Geological Society of London.

Carling, P.A. (1981) Sediment transport by tidal currents and waves: observations from a sandy intertidal zone (Burry Inlet, South Wales). In: *Holocene Marine Sedimentation in the North Sea Basin.* (eds S.D. Nio, et al.) International Association of Sedimentologists Special Publication 5, 65–80.

Carroll, D. (1958) Role of clay minerals in the transportation of iron. *Geochimica et Cosmochima Acta*, 14, 1–27.

Carson, M.A. (1971) *The Mechanics of Erosion*. Pion, London.

Carson, M.A. & Kirkby, M.J. (1972) *Hillslope Form and Process*. Cambridge University Press, Cambridge.

Carter, L. & McCave, I.N. (1997) The sedimentary regime beneath the deep Western Boundary Current inflow to the Southwest Pacific Ocean. *Journal of Sedimentary Research*, 67, 1005–17.

Carter, R.W.G. & Woodroffe, C.D. (eds) (1994) *Coastal Evolution: Late Quaternary Shoreline Morphodynamics*. Cambridge University Press, Cambridge.

Casey, W.H. & Bunker, B. (1991) The leaching of mineral and glass surfaces during dissolution, in mineral–water interface geochemistry. *Reviews of Mineralogy*, 23, 397–426.

Casey, W.H., Westrich, H.R., Banfield, J.F., Ferruzzi, G. & Arnold, G.W. (1993) Leaching and reconstruction at the surfaces of dissolving chain-silicate minerals. *Nature*, 366, 253–5.

Cathro, D.L., Warren, J.K. & Williams, G.E. (1992) Halite saltern in the Canning Basin, Western Australia: a sedimentological analysis of drill core from the Ordovician–Silurian Mallowa Salt. *Sedimentology*, 39, 983–1002.

Causse, C., Coque, R., Fontes, J.Ch., Gasse, F., Gibert, E., Ben Ouezdou, H. & Zouari, K. (1989) Two high levels of continental waters in the southern Tunisian chotts at about 90 and 150 ka. *Geology*, 17, 922–5.

Chadwick, O.A., et al. (1999) Changing sources of nutrients during four million years of ecosystem development. *Nature*, 397, 491–7.

Chafetz, H.S. & Rush, P.F. (1994) Diagenetically altered sabkha-type Pleistocene dolomite from the Arabian Gulf. *Sedimentology*, 41, 409–21.

Chahine, M.T. (1992) The hydrological cycle and its influence on climate. *Nature*, 359, 373–80.

Chappell, J. (1980) Coral morphology, diversity and reef growth. *Nature*, 286, 249–52.

Charles, C.D. & Fairbanks, R.G. (1992) Evidence from Southern Ocean sediments for the effect of North Atlantic deep-water flux on climate. *Nature*, 355, 416–19.

Charnock, H. (1996) The atmosphere and the ocean. In: *Oceanography, An Illustrated Guide* (eds C.P. Summerhayes & S.A. Thorpe), ch. 2, Manson Press, London.

Chave, K.E. & Suess, E. (1970) Calcium carbonate saturation in seawater: effects of organic matter. *Limnology and Oceanography*, 15, 633–7.

Chepil, W.S. (1961) The use of spheres to measure lift and drag on wind eroded soils. *Proceedings of the Soil Science Society of America*, 25, 343–5.

Chesworth, W. (1992) Weathering systems. In: *Weathering, Soils and Palaeosols* (eds I.P. Martini & W. Chesworth). Elsevier, Amsterdam.

Chikita, K.A., Smith, N.D., Yonemitsu, N. & Pérez-Arlucea, M. (1996) Dynamics of sediment-laden underflows passing over a subaqueous sill: glacier-fed Peyto Lake, Alberta, Canada. *Sedimentology*, 43, 865–75.

Choi, D.R. & Ginsburg, R.N. (1982) Siliciclastic foundations of Quaternary reefs in the southernmost Belize Lagoon, British Honduras. *Bulletin of the Geological Society of America*, 93, 116–26.

Chough, S.K., Hwang, I.G. & Choe, M.Y. (1990) The Miocene Doumsan fan-delta, southeast Korea: a composite fan-delta system in back-arc margin. *Journal of Sedimentary Petrology*, 60, 445–55.

Chrintz, T. & Clemmenson, L.B. (1993) Draa reconstruction, the Permian Yellow Sands, northeast England. In: *Aeolian Sediments Ancient and Modern* (ed. K. Pye), pp. 151–61. Special Publication no. 16, International Association of Sedimentologists.

Clark, J.D. & Pickering, K.T. (1996) Architectural elements and growth patterns of submarine channels: application to hydrocarbon exploration. *Bulletin of the American Association of Petroleum Geologists*, 80, 194–221.

Clark, J.D., Kenyon, N.H. & Pickering, K.T. (1992) Quantitative analysis of the geometry of submarine channels: implications for the classification of submarine fans. *Geology*, 20, 633–6.

Cleary, P.W. & Campbell, C.S. (1993) Self-lubrication for long runout landslides: examination by computer simulation. *Journal of Geophysical Research*, 98, 21911–24.

Clemente, P. & Pérez-Arlucea, M. (1993) Depositional architecture of the Cuerda Del Pozo Formation, Lower Cretaceous of the Extensional Cameros Basin, North-Central Spain. *Journal of Sedimentary Petrology*, 63, 437–52.

Clemmenson, L.B. (1987) Complex star dunes and associated aeolian bedforms, Hopeman Sandstone (Permo-Triassic), Moray Firth basin, Scotland. In: *Desert Sediments: Ancient and Modern* (eds L. Frostick & I. Reid), pp. 213–31. Special Publication no. 35, Geological Society of London.

Clemmenson, L.B. (1989) Preservation of interdraa and draa plinth deposits by the lateral migration of large linear draas (Lower Permian Yellow Sands, northeast England) *Sedimentary Geology*, **65**, 139–51.

Clemmenson, L.B., Olsen, H. & Blakey, R.C. (1989) Erg-margin deposits in the Lower Jurassic Moenave Formation and Wingate Sandstone, southern Utah. *Bulletin of the Geological Society of America*, **101**, 759–73.

Clifford, N.J., French, J.R. & Hardisty, J. (eds) (1993) *Turbulence: Perspectives on Flow and Sediment Transport*. Wiley, Chichester.

Clift, P.D. (1995) Volcaniclastic sedimentation and volcanism during the rifting of Western Pacific Backarc basins. In: *Active Margins and Marginal Basins of the Western Pacific*, pp. 67–96. Geophysical Monograph no. 88, American Geophysical Union.

Clifton, H.E. & Dingler, J.R. (1984). Wave-formed structures and palaeoenvironmental reconstruction. *Marine Geology*, **60**, 165–98.

Clifton, H.E., Hunter, R.E. & Phillips, R.L. (1971) Depositional structures and processes in the non-barred, high energy nearshore. *Journal of Sedimentary Petrology*, **41**, 651–70.

Cloud, P.E. (1962) *Environment of Calcium Carbonate Deposition West of Andros Island, Bahamas*. Professional Paper 350, United States Geological Survey.

Cody, R.D. & Hull, A.B. (1980) Experimental growth of primary anhydrite at low temperatures and water salinities. *Geology*, 505–9.

Cohen, A.S., *et al.* (1997) Lake level and palaeoenvironmental history of Lake Tanganyika, Africa, as inferred from late Holocene and modern stromatolites. *Bulletin of the Geological Society of America*, **109**, 444–60.

Colbeck, S.C. (1980) (ed) *Dynamics of Snow and Ice Masses*. Academic Press, New York.

Colella, A. (1988) Pliocene–Holocene fan deltas and braid deltas in the Crati Basin, southern Italy: a consequence of varying tectonic conditions. In: *Fan Deltas: Sedimentology and Tectonic Settings* (eds W. Nemec & R.J. Steel), pp. 50–74. Blackie, London.

Colella, A. & di Geronimo, I. (1987) Surface sediments and macrofaunas of the Crati submarine fan (Ionian Sea, Italy). *Sedimentary Geology*, **51**, 257–77.

Colella, A. & Normark, W.R. (1984) High-resolution side-scanning sonar survey of delta slope and inner fan channels of Crati submarine fan (Ionian Sea). *Memoir of the Geological Society of Italy*, **27**, 381–90.

Colella, A. & Prior, D.B. (1990) (eds) *Coarse-Grained Deltas*. International Association of Sedimentologists Special Publication **10**.

Coleman, J.M. (1969) Brahmaputra River: channel processes and sedimentation. *Sedimentary Geology*, 3, 129–239.

Coleman, J.M. (1976) *Deltas: Processes of Deposition and Models for Exploration*. Continuing Education Publishing, Champaign, IL.

Coleman, J.M. & Gagliano, S.M. (1964) Cyclic sedimentation in the Mississippi river delta plain. *Transactions of the Gulf Coast Association of Geological Societies*, **14**, 67–80.

Coleman, J.M., Gagliano, S.M. & Webb, J.E. (1964) Minor sedimentary structures in a prograding distributary. *Marine Geology*, 1, 240–58.

Coleman, J.M., Gagliano, S.M. & Smith, W.G. (1970) Sedimentation in a Malaysian high tide tropical delta, pp. 185–97. Special Publication no. 15, Society of Economic Palaeontologists and Sedimentologists.

Coleman, N.L. (1981) Velocity profiles with suspended sediment. *Journal of Hydraulic Research*, **19**, 211–29.

Collier, R.E.Ll. & Thompson, J. (1991) Transverse and linear dunes in an Upper Pleistocene marine sequence, Corinth basin, Greece. *Sedimentology*, **38**, 1021–40.

Collier, R.E.Ll., Leeder, M.R. & Maynard, J.R. (1990) Transgressions and regressions: a model for the influence of tectonic subsidence, deposition and eustasy, with application to Quaternary and Carboniferous examples. *Geological Magazine*, **127**, 117–28.

Collier, R.E.Ll., Jackson, J.A. & Leeder, M.R. (1995) Quaternary drainage development, sediment fluxes and extensional tectonics in Greece. In: *Mediterranean Quaternary River Environments* (eds J. Lewin, M.G. Macklin & J.C. Woodward), pp. 31–44. Balkema, Rotterdam.

Collins, J.I. (1976) Approaches to wave modelling. In: *Beach and Nearshore Sedimentation* (eds K.S. Davis & R.L. Ethington), pp. 54–68. Special Publication no. 24, Society of Economic Palaeontologists and Mineralogists, Tulsa.

Collins, M.B., Amos, C.L. & Evans, G. (1981) Observations of some sediment-transport processes over intertidal flats, The Wash, UK. In: *Holocene Marine Sedimentation in the North Sea Basin* (eds S.-D. Nio, R.T.E. Schüttenhelm & T.C.E. van Weering), pp. 81–98. Special Publication no. 5, International Association of Sedimentologists.

Collinson, J.D. (1970) Bedforms of the Tana River, Norway. *Geografiska Annaler*, **52A**, 31–56.

Collinson, J.D. & Thompson, D.B. (1982) *Sedimentary Structures*. Allen and Unwin, London.

Colman, S.M. (1981) Rock-weathering rates as functions of time. *Quaternary Research*, **15**, 250–64.

Colman, S.M. & Pierce, K.L. (1981) *Weathering Rinds on Andesitic and Basaltic Stones as a Quaternary Age*

Indicator, Western United States. Professional Paper 1210, US Geological Survey.

Colman, S.M., *et al.* (1995) Continental climate response to orbital forcing from biogenic silica records in Lake Baikal. *Nature*, 378, 769–71.

Colson, J. & Cojan, I. (1996) Groundwater dolocretes in a lake-marginal environment: an alternative model for dolocrete formation in continental settings (Danian of the Provence basin, France). *Sedimentology*, 43, 175–88.

Cook, P.J., Colwell, J.B., Firman, J.B., Lindsay, J.M., Scwebel, D.A. & Von der Borch, C.C. (1977) The late Cenozoic sequence of southeast South Australia and Pleistocene sealevel changes. *Bulletin of the Bureau of Mineral Resources of Australia*, 2, 81–8.

Cooke, R.U. (1979) Laboratory simulation of salt weathering processes in arid environments. *Earth Surface Processes*, 4, 347–59.

Cooke, R.U. & Warren, A. (1973) *Geomorphology in Deserts*. Batsford, London.

Cooke, R.U., Warren, A. & Goudie, A.S. (1993) *Desert Geomorphology*. UCL Press, London.

Cooper, J.A.G. (1993) Sedimentation in a river-dominated estuary. *Sedimentology*, 40, 979–1017.

Copeland, P. & Harrison, T.M. (1990) Episodic rapid uplift in the Himalaya revealed by 40Ar/39Ar analysis of detrital K-feldspar and muscovite, Bengal fan. *Geology*, 18, 354–7.

Corbett, I. (1993) The modern and ancient pattern of sandflow through the southern Namib deflation basin. In: *Aeolian Sediments Ancient and Modern* (ed. K. Pye), pp. 45–60. Special Publication no. 16, International Association of Sedimentologists.

Cortijo, E., *et al.* (1994) Eemian cooling in the Norwegian Sea and North Atlantic Ocean preceding continental ice-sheet growth. *Nature*, 372, 446–8.

Coudé-Gaussen, G. (1984) Le cycle des poussieres eoliennes desertiques actuelles et la sedimentation des loess peridesertiques quaternaires. *Bulletin du Centre Recherches et Exploration-Production Elf-Aquitaine*, 8, 167–82.

Coussot, P. & Proust, S. (1996) Slow, unconfined spreading of a mudflow. *Journal of Geophysical Research*, 101, 25217–29.

Cowan, E.A. & Powell, R.D. (1990) Suspended sediment transport and deposition of cyclically interlaminated sediment in a temperate glacial fjord, Alaska, USA, pp. 75–89. In: *Glacimarine Environments* (eds J.A. Dowdeswell & J.D. Scourse) Special Publication no. 53, Geological Society of London.

Cowan, E.A. & Powell, R.D. (1991) Ice-proximal sediment accumulation rates in a temperate glacial fjord, southeastern Alaska. In: *Glacial Marine Sedimentation: Palaeoclimatic Significance* (eds J.B. Anderson & G.M. Ashley), pp. 61–73. Special Publication no. 261, Geological Society of America.

Crabaugh, M. & Kocurek, G. (1993) Entrada Sandstone: an example of a wet aeolian system. In: *The Dynamics and Environmental Context of Aeolian Sedimentary Systems* (ed. K. Pye), pp. 103–26. Special Publication no. 72, Geological Society of London.

Craig, H. (1994) Vertical mixing in Lake Baikal: an 'ocean in reverse'. *AGU Fall Meeting Abstracts*, p. 388.

Cramp, A. & O'Sullivan, G. (1999) Neogene sapropels in the Mediterranean: a review. *Marine Geology*, 153, 11–28.

Cramp, A., Maslin, M., Long, D. & the Shipboard Scientific Party Leg 155 (1995) The Amazon submarine fan: sedimentary processes and climate change: initial results from ODP Leg 155. *Geoscientist*, 5, 23–5.

Crampton, S.L. & Allen, P.A. (1995) Recognition of forebulge unconformities associated with early stage foreland basin development: example from the North Alpine foreland basin. *Bulletin of the American Association of Petroleum Geologists*, 79, 1495–514.

Crane, K., Hecker, B. & Golubev, V. (1991) Heat flow and hydrothermal vents in Lake Baikal, USSR. *EOS*, 72, 585.

Crans, W., Mandl, G. & Harembource, J. (1980) On the theory of growth faulting: a geomechanical delta model based on gravity sliding. *Journal of Petroleum Geology*, 2, 265–307.

Crevello, P.D. & Schlager, W. (1980) Carbonate debris sheets and turbidites, Exhuma Sound, Bahamas. *Journal of Sedimentary Petrology*, 50, 1121–48.

Crews, S.G. & Ethridge, F.G. (1993) Laramide tectonics and humid fan sedimentation, NE Uinta uplift, Utah and Wyoming. *Journal of Sedimentary Petrology*, 63, 420–36.

Cronin, T.M. and Raymo, M.E. (1997) Orbital forcing of deep-sea benthic species diversity. *Nature*, 385, 624–27.

Cronin, S.J., Neall, V.E., Lecointre, J.A. & Palmer, A.S. (1996) Unusual 'snow slurry' lahars from Ruapehu volcano, New Zealand, September 1995. *Geology*, 24, 1107–10.

Crowell, J.C. (1974a) Sedimentation along the San Andreas Fault, California, pp. 292–303. In: *Modern and Ancient Geosynclinal Sedimentation* (eds R.H. Dott & R.H. Shaver) Special Publication no. 19, Society of Economic Palaeontologists and Mineralogists.

Crowell, J.C. (1974b) Origin of late Cenozoic basins in southern California, pp. 190–204. Special Publication no. 22, Society of Economic Palaeontologists and Mineralogists.

Crowell, J.C. (1983) Ice ages on Gondwanan continents. *Transactions of the Geological Society of South Africa*, 86, 230–61.

Crowell, J.C. & Link, M.H. (1982) *Geological History of the Ridge Basin, Southern California (Book 22)*. Pacific Section of the SEPM, Los Angeles.

Csanady, G.T. (1978) Water circulation and dispersal mechanisms. In Lerman (1978), 21–64.

Csato, I., Kendall, C.G.St.J., Nairn, A.E.M. & Baum, G.R. (1997) Sequence stratigraphic interpretations in the southern Dead Sea basin, Israel. *Bulletin of the Geological Society of America*, **108**, 1485–501.

Curtis, C.D. (1976) Stability of minerals in surface weathering reactions: a general thermochemical approach. *Earth Surface Processes*, **1**, 63–70.

Curtis, C.D. & Spears, D.A. (1968) The formation of sedimentary iron minerals. *Economic Geology*, **63**, 257–70.

Daams, R., Diaz-Molina, M. & Mas, R. (1996) Uncertainties in the stratigraphic analysis of fluvial deposits from the Loranca Basin, central Spain. *Sedimentary Geology*, **102**, 187–209.

Dabrio, C.J. & Polo, M.D. (1988) Late Neogene fan deltas and associated coral reefs in the Almanzora Basin, Almeria Province, southeastern Spain. In: *Fan Deltas: Sedimentology and Tectonic Settings* (eds W. Nemec & R.J. Steel), pp. 354–67. Blackie, London.

Dabrio, C.J., Zazo, C. & Goy, J.L. (eds) (1991a) *The Dynamics of Coarse-Grained Deltas*. Cuadernos de Geologia Iberica no. 15, Universidad Complutense, Madrid.

Dabrio, C.J., Barbaji, T., Zazo, C. & Goy, J.L. (1991b) Effects of sea-level changes on a wave-worked Gilbert-type delta (Late Pliocene, Aguilas Basin, SE Spain). In: *The Dynamics of Coarse-Grained Deltas* (eds C.J. Dabrio, C. Zazo & J.L. Goy), pp. 103–137. Cuadernos de Geologia Iberica no. 15, Universidad Complutense, Madrid.

Dade, W.B., Lister, J.R. & Huppert, H.E. (1994) Fine-sediment deposition from gravity surges on uniform slopes. *Journal of Sedimentary Research*, **64**, 423–32.

Dalrymple, R.W. & Zaitlin, B.A. (1994) High-resolution sequence sratigraphy of a complex, incised valley succession, Cobequid Bay–Salmon River estuary, Bay of Fundy, Canada. *Sedimentology*, **41**, 1069–91.

Dalrymple, R.W., Knight, R.J., Zaitlin, B.A. & Middleton, G.V. (1990) Dynamics and facies model of a macrotidal sand-bar complex, Cobequid Bay–Salmon River Estuary (Bay of Fundy). *Sedimentology*, **37**, 577–612.

Dalrymple, R.W., Zaitlin, B.A. & Boyd, R. (1992) Estuarine facies models: conceptual basis and stratigraphic implications. *Journal of Sedimentary Petrology*, **62**, 1130–46.

Dalrymple, R.W., Boyd, R. & Zaitlin, B.A. (eds) (1994) *Incised-Valley Systems: Origin and Sedimentary Sequences*. Special Publication no. 51, Society for Sedimentary Geology.

Damuth, J.E., *et al.* (1988) Anatomy and growth pattern of Amazon deep sea fan as revealed by long-range sidescan sonar (GLORIA) and high resolution seismic studies. *Bulletin of the American Association of Petroleum Geologists*, **72**, 885–911.

Dart, C., *et al.* (1994) Sequence stratigraphy of Pliocene–Quaternary synrift, Gilbert-type fan deltas, northern Peloponnesos, Greece. *Marine and Petroleum Geology*, **11**, 545–60.

Davidson, J.F., Harrison, D. & Guedes de Carvalho, J.R.F. (1977) On the liquidlike behaviour of fluidised beds. *Annual Reviews of Fluid Mechanics*, **9**, 55–86.

Davidson-Arnott, R.G.D. & Greenwood, B. (1974) Bedforms and structures associated with bar topography in the shallow water wave environment, Kouchibougvac Bay, New Brunswick, Canada. *Journal of Sedimentary Petrology*, **44**, 698–704.

Davidson-Arnott, R.G.D. & Greenwood, B. (1976) Facies relationships on a barred coast, Kouchibougvac Bay, New Brunswick, Canada. In: *Beach and Nearshore Sedimentation* (eds K.S. Davis & R.L. Ethington), pp. 149–68. Special Publication no. 24, Society of Economic Palaeontologists and Mineralogists, Tulsa.

Davidson-Arnott, R.G.D. & Pember, G.F. (1980) Morphology and sedimentology of multiple parallel bar systems, southern Georgian Bay, Ontario. In: *The Coastline of Canada* (ed. S.B. McCann), pp. 417–28. Paper 80–10, Geological Society of Canada.

Davies, G.R. (1970) Algal-laminated sediments, Gladstone embayment, Shark Bay, Western Australia. *Memoir of the American Association of Petroleum Geologists*, **13**, 169–205.

Davies, P.J., Bubela, B. & Ferguson, J. (1978) The formation of ooids. *Sedimentology*, **25**, 703–30.

Davis, K.S. & Ethington, R.L. (eds) (1976) *Beach and Nearshore Sedimentation*. Special Publication no. 24, Society of Economic Palaeontologists and Mineralogists, Tulsa.

Davis, R.A. (ed.) (1985) *Coastal Sedimentary Environments*, 2nd edn. Springer, New York.

Davis, R.A. & Flemming, B.W. (1995) Stratigraphy of a combined wave- and tide-dominated intertidal sand body: Martens Plate, East Friesian Wadden Sea, Germany. In: *Tidal Signatures in Modern and Ancient Sediments*, pp. 121–32. Special Publication no. 24, International Association of Sedimentologists.

Dawson, A.G. (1992) *Ice Age Earth*. Routledge, London.

Dawson, A.G., *et al.* (1993) Tsunamis in the Norwegian Sea and North Sea caused by the Stoegga submarine landslide. In: *Tsunamis in the World* (ed. S. Tinti), pp. 31–42. Kluwer, Dordrecht.

De Boer, P.L. & Smith, D.G. (eds) (1994) *Orbital Forcing and Cyclic Sequences*. Special Publication no. 19, International Association of Sedimentologists. Blackwell Science, Oxford.

De Boer, P.L. & Smith, D.G. (1994) Orbital forcing and cyclic sequences. In: *Orbital Forcing and Cyclic Sequences* (eds P.L. De Boer & D.G. Smith), pp. 1–14. Special Publication no. 19. International Association of Sedimentologists. Blackwell Science, Oxford.

De Boer, P.L. & Wonders, A.A.H. (1984) Astronomically induced rhythmic bedding in Cretaceous pelagic sediments near Moria (Italy). In: *Milankovich and Climate* (eds Berger *et al.*), Part 1, pp. 177–90. Reidel, Dordrecht.

De Boer, P.L., Oost, A.P. & Visser, M.J. (1989) The diurnal inequality of the tide as a parameter for recognizing tidal influences. *Journal of Sedimentary Petrology*, **59**, 912–21.

De Boer, P.L., Pragt, J.S.J. & Oost, A.P. (1991) Vertically persistent sedimentary facies boundaries along growth anticlines and climate-controlled sedimentation in the thrust-sheet-top South Pyrenean Tremp-Graus foreland Basin. *Basin Research*, **3**, 623–78.

DeCelles, P.G. (1987) Variable preservation of Middle Tertiary, coarse-grained, nearshore to outer-shelf storm deposits in southern California. *Journal of Sedimentary Petrology*, **57**, 250–64.

DeCelles, P.G. (1988) Lithologic provenance modeling applied to the Late Cretaceous synorogenic Echo Canyon Conglomerate, Utah: a case of multiple source areas. *Geology*, **16**, 1039–43.

DeCelles, P.G. & Giles, K.A. (1996) Foreland basin systems. *Basin Research*, **8**, 105–23.

DeCelles, P.G., Langford, R.P. & Schwartz, R.K. (1983) Two new methods of paleocurrent determination from trough cross-stratification. *Journal of Sedimentary Petrology*, **53**, 629–42.

DeDekker, P. (1988) Large Australian lakes during the last 20 million years: sites for petroleum source rocks or metal ore deposition or both? In: *Lacustrine Petroleum Source Rocks* (eds A.J. Fleet, K. Kelts & M.J. Talbot), pp. 45–58. Special Publication no. 40, Geological Society of London.

Deelman, J.C. (1978) Experimental ooids and grapestones: carbonate aggregates and their origin. *Journal of Sedimentary Petrology*, **48**, 471–2.

Degens, E.T. & Ross, D.A. (eds) (1974) *The Black Sea Geology, Chemistry and Biology*. Memoir no. 20, American Association of Petroleum Geologists.

Degens, E.T. & Stoffers, P. (1980) Environmental events recorded in Quaternary sediments of the Black Sea. *Journal of the Geological Society of London*, **137**, 131–8.

Demaison, G.J. & Moore, G.T. (1980) Anoxic environments and oil source bed genesis. *Bulletin of the American Association of Petroleum Geologists*, **64**, 1179–209.

Denny, M.W. (1993) *Air and Water: The Biology and Physics of Life's Media*. Princeton University Press, Princeton, NJ.

DePloey, J., Kirkby, M.J. & Ahnert, F. (1991) Hillslope erosion by rainstorms—a magnitude–frequency analysis. *Earth Surface Processes and Landforms*, **16**, 339–409.

Derbyshire, E. & Owen, L.A. (1990) Quaternary alluvial fans in the Karakorum Mountains. In *Alluvial Fans: A Field Approach* (eds A.H. Rachocki & M. Church), pp. 27–53. Wiley, Chichester.

DeVisser, J.P., *et al*. (1989) The origin of rhythmic bedding in the Pliocene Trubi Formation of Sicily, southern Italy. *Palaeogeography, Palaeoclimatology, Palaeoecology*, **69**, 45–66.

Dewey, J.F. (1982) Plate tectonics and the evolution of the British Isles. *Journal of the Geological Society of London*, **139**, 371–414.

Dewey, J.F. & Pitman, W.C. (1998) Sea-level changes: mechanisms, magnitudes and rates. In: *Eustasy and the Tectonostratigraphic Evolution of Northern South America*. Special Publication no. 58, Society of Economic Palaeontologists and Mineralogists.

Diaz-Molina, M. (1993) Geometry and lateral accretion patterns in meander loops: examples from the Upper Oligocene–Lower Miocene, Loranca basin, Spain. In: *Alluvial Sedimentation* (eds M. Marzo & C. Puigdefabregas), pp. 115–31. Special Publication no. 17, International Association of Sedimentologists.

Dickinson, W.R. (1976) *Plate Tectonic Evolution of Sedimentary Basins*. Continuing Education Course Notes Series 1, American Association of Petroleum Geologists.

Dickinson, W.R. (1995) Forearc basins. In: *Tectonics of Sedimentary Basins* (eds C. Busby & R. Ingersoll), pp. 221–62. Blackwell Science, Oxford.

Dickman, M. (1985) Seasonal succession and microlamina formation in a meromictic lake displaying varved sediments. *Sedimentology*, **32**, 109–18.

Dickson, J.A.D. (1995) Palaeozoic Mg Calcite preserved: implications for the Carboniferous ocean. *Geology*, **23**, 535–8.

Dickson, R.R. & McCave, I.N. (1986) Nepheloid layers on the continental slope west of Porcupine Bank. *Deep Sea Research*, **33**, 791–818.

Diem, B. (1985) Analytical method for estimating palaeowave climate and water depth from wave ripple marks. *Sedimentology*, **32**, 685–704.

Dill, R.F., Shinn, E.A., Jones, A.T., Kelly, K. & Steinen, R.P. (1986) Giant subtidal stromatolites forming in normal salinity waters. *Nature*, **324**, 55–8.

Doake, C.S.M. & Wolff, E.W. (1985) Flow law for ice in polar ice sheets. *Nature*, **314**, 255–7.

Domack, E.W. & Ishman, S. (1993) Oceanographic and physiographic controls on modern sedimentation within Antarctic fjords. *Bulletin of the Geological Society of America*, **105**, 1175–89.

Donovan, R.N. & Foster, R.J. (1972) Subaqueous shrinkage cracks from the Caithness Flagstone series (Middle Devonian) of NE Scotland. *Journal of Sedimentary Petrology*, **42**, 309–17.

Dorsey, R.J., Umhoefer, P.J. & Falk, P.D. (1997) Earthquake clustering inferred from Pliocene Gilbert-type fan deltas in the Loreto basin, Baja California Sur, Mexico. *Geology*, **25**, 679–82.

Dott, R. & Bourgeois, J. (1982) Hummocky cross-stratification: significance of its variable bedding sequences. *Bulletin of the Geological Society of America*, **93**, 663–80.

Dove, P.M. (1995) Kinetic and thermodynamic controls on silica reactivity in weathering environments. In: *Chemical Weathering Rates of Silicate Minerals* (eds A.F. White & S.L. Branfield), ch. 6. American Mineralogical Society, Washington, DC.

Dove, P.M. & Elston, S.F. (1992) Dissolution kinetics of quartz in sodium chloride solutions: analysis of existing data and a rate model for 25°. *Geochimica et Cosmochimica Acta*, **56**, 4147–56.

Dove, P.M. & Hochella, M.F. (1993) Calcite precipitation mechanisms and inhibition by orthophosphate: in situ observations by scanning force microscopy. *Geochimica et Cosmochimica Acta*, **57**, 705–14.

Dowdeswell, J.A. & Scourse, J.D. (1990) *Glacimarine Environments*. Special Publication no. 53, Geological Society of London.

Dowdeswell, J.A. & Scourse, J.D. (1990) On the description and modelling of glacimarine sediments and sedimentation, pp. 1–13. Special Publication no. 53, Geological Society of London.

Dowdeswell, J.A. & Sharp, M.J. (1986) Characterization of pebble fabrics in modern terrestrial glacigenic sediments. *Sedimentology*, **33**, 699–710.

Dowdeswell, J.A., Whittinton, R.J. & Marienfeld, P. (1994) The origin of massive diamicton facies by iceberg rafting and scouring, Scoresby Sund, East Greenland. *Sedimentology*, **41**, 21–35.

Drake, D.E. & Gorsline, D.S. (1973) Distribution and transport of suspended particulate matter in submarine Hueneme, Redondo, Newport and La Jolla submarine canyons, California. *Bulletin of the Geological Society of America*, **84**, 3949–68.

Drake, D.E., Kolpack, R.L. & Fischer, P.J. (1972) Sediment transport on the Santa Barbara–Oxnard shelf, Santa Barbara Channel, California. In: *Shelf Sediment Transport* (eds D.J.P. Swift, D.B. Duane & O.H. Pilkey), pp. 307–31. Stroudsberg, PA: Dowden, Hutchinson and Ross.

Drake, D.E., *et al.* (1989) Morphology and growth history of Delgada fan: implications for the Neogene evolution of Point Arena basin and the Mendocino triple junction. *Journal of Geophysical Research*, **94**, 3139–58.

Dreimanis, A. (1989) Tills: their genetic terminology and classification. In: *Genetic Classification of Glacigenic Deposits* (eds R.P. Goldthwait & C.L. Matsch), pp. 17–83. Balkema, Rotterdam.

Drever, J.I. (1988) *The Geochemistry of Natural Waters*. Prentice Hall, New Jersey.

Drever, J.I. & Clow, D.W. (1995) Weathering rates in catchments. In: *Chemical Weathering Rates of Silicate Minerals* (eds A.F. White & S.L. Branfield), ch. 10. American Mineralogical Society, Washington, DC.

Drever, J.I., Li, Y.-H. & Maynard, J.B. (1988) Geochemical cycles: the continental crust and the oceans. In: *Chemical Cycles in the Evolution of the Earth* (eds C.B. Gregor *et al.*), pp. 17–54. Wiley, New York.

Droxler, A.W. & Schlager, W. (1985) Glacial versus interglacial sedimentation rates and turbidite frequency in the Bahamas. *Geology*, **13**, 799–802.

Drummond, C.N. & Wilkinson, B.H. (1993) Carbonate cycle stacking patterns and hierarchies of orbitally-forced eustatic sea level change. *Journal of Sedimentary Petrology*, **63**, 369–77.

Drummond, C.N., Wilkinson, B.H. & Lohmann, K.C. (1996) Climatic control of fluvial-lacustrine cyclicity in the Cretaceous Cordilleran Foreland Basin, western United States. *Sedimentology*, **43**, 677–89.

Duke, W.L. (1990) Geostrophic circulation of shallow marine turbidity currents? The dilemma of palaeoflow patterns in storm-influenced prograding shoreline systems. *Journal of Sedimentary Petrology*, **60**, 870–83.

Dyer, K.R. (1989) Sediment processes in estuaries: future research requirements. *Journal of Geophysical Research*, **94C**, 14327–39.

van Dyke, M. (1982) *An Album of Fluid Motion*. Parabolic Press, Stanford, CA.

Eberli, G.P. & Ginsburg, R.N. (1987) Segmentation and coalescence of Cenozoic carbonate platforms, northwestern Bahamas Bank. *Geology*, **15**, 75–9.

Eberli, G.P. & Ginsburg, R.N. (1989) Cenozoic progradation of northwestern Great Bahamas Bank, a record of lateral platform growth and sealevel fluctuations. In: *Controls on Carbonate Platform and Basin Development* (eds P.D. Crevello *et al.*), pp. 339–51. Special Publication no. 44, Society of Economic Palaeontologists and Mineralogists.

Ebinger, C.J., Rosendahl, B.R. & Reynolds, D.J. (1987) Tectonic model of the Malawi rift, Africa. *Tectonophysics*, **141**, 215–35.

Edwards, D.A., *et al.* (1994) On experimental reflected density currents and the interpretation of certain turbidites. *Sedimentology*, **41**, 437–61.

Eggleton, R.A. (1986) The relations between crystal structure and silicate weathering rates. In: *Rates of Chemical Weathering of Rocks and Minerals* (eds S.M. Colman & D.P. Dethier), pp. 21–40. Academic Press, New York.

Einarsson, P., *et al.* (1997) Center of the Icelandic Hotspot experiences volcanic unrest. *EOS*, **78**, 369–75.

Einsele, G. (1992) *Sedimentary Basins: Evolution, Facies and Sediment Budget*. Springer, Berlin.

Eisma, D., Dyer, K.R. & van Leussen, W. (1997) The in situ determination of the settling velocities of suspended fine-grained sediment—a review. In: *Cohesive Sediments* (eds N. Burt, R. Parker & J. Watts), pp. 17–44. Wiley, New York.

Eittreim, S., Biscaye, P.E. & Amos, A.F. (1975) Benthic nepheloid layers and the Ekman thermal pump. *Journal of Geophysical Research*, **80**, 5061–7.

El-Tabakh, M., Riccione, R. & Schreiber, B.C. (1997) Evolution of late Triassic rift basin evaporites (Passaic Formation): Newark Basin, Eastern North America. *Sedimentology*, **44**, 767–90.

Ely, L.L., *et al.* (1996) Changes in the magnitude and frequency of late Holocene monsoon floods on the

Narmada River, central India. *Bulletin of the Geological Society of America*, **108**, 1134–48.

Embley, R.W. (1976) New evidence for occurrence of debris flow deposits in the deep sea. *Geology*, **4**, 371–4.

Embrey, A.F. & Klovan, (1971) A late Devonian reef tract on the northeastern banks island NWT. *Bulletin of Canadian Petroleum Geology*, **19**, 730–81.

Emery, D. & Myers, K.J. (1996) *Sequence Stratigraphy*. Blackwell Science, Oxford.

Enos, P. & Perkins, R.D. (1979) Evolution of Florida Bay from island stratigraphy. *Bulletin of the Geological Society of America*, **90**, 59–83.

EOS (1992) Andrew shortens lifetime of Louisiana barrier islands. *EOS*, **73/47**, 505.

Eriksson, K.A. (1977) Tidal flat and subtidal sedimentation in the 2250 Ma Malmani Dolomite, Transvaal, South Africa. *Sedimentary Geology*, **18**, 223–44.

Ethridge, F.G. & Westcott, W.A. (1984) Tectonic setting, recognition and hydrocarbon reservoir potential of fan-delta deposits. In: *Sedimentology of Gravels and Conglomerates* (eds E.H. Koster & R.J. Steel), pp. 217–35. Memoir no. 10, Canadian Society of Petroleum Geologists.

Eugster, H.P. & Hardie, L.A. (1975) Sedimentation in an ancient playa-lake complex: The Wilkins Peak member of the Green River Formation of Wyoming. *Bulletin of the Geological Society of America*, **86**, 319–34.

Eugster, H.P. & Hardie, L.A. (1978) Saline lakes: In: *Lakes: Chemistry, Geology, Physics* (ed. A. Lerman), pp. 237–334. Springer, New York.

Evans, G. (1965) Intertidal flat sediments and their environments of deposition in the Wash. *Quarterly Journal of the Geological Society of London*, **121**, 209–45.

Evans, G. (1995) The Arabian Gulf: a modern carbonate–evaporite factory; a review. *Cuadernos de Geologia Iberica*, **19**, 61–96.

Evans, G., Schmidt, V., Bush, P. & Nelson, H. (1969) Stratigraphy and geologic history of the sabkha, Abu Dhabi, Persian Gulf. *Sedimentology*, **12**, 145–59.

Evans, G., Lane-Serf, F., Collins, M.B., Ediger, V. & Pattiaratchi, C.B. (1995) Frontal instabilities and suspended sediment dispersal over the shelf of the Cilician Basin, southern Turkey. *Marine Geology*, **128**, 127–36.

Everts, C.H. (1987) Continental shelf evolution in response to a rise in sea level. In: *Sea Level Fluctuation and Coastal Evolution* (eds D. Nummedal, O.H. Pilkey & J.D. Howard), pp. 49–57. Special Publication no. 41, Society of Economic Palaeontologists and Mineralogists.

Eyles, C.H., Eyles, N. & Franca, A.B. (1993) Glaciation and tectonics in an active intracratonic basin: the Late Palaeozoic Itararé Group, Parana Basin, Brazil. *Sedimentology*, **40**, 1–25.

Eyles, C.H., Eyles, N. & Gostin, V.A. (1998) Facies and allostratigraphy of high-latitude, glacially-influenced marine strata of the Early Permian southern Sydney Basin, Australia. *Sedimentology*, **45**, 121–61.

Eyles, N. & Eyles, C.H. (1989) Glacially-influenced deep-marine sedimentation of the Late Precambrian Gaskiers Formation, Newfoundland, Canada. *Sedimentology*, **36**, 601–20.

Eyles, N. & McCabe, A.M. (1989) Glaciomarine facies within subglacial tunnel valleys: the sedimentary record of glacio-isostatic downwarping in the Irish Sea basin. *Sedimentology*, **36**, 431–48.

Eyles, N., Eyles, C.H. & Miall, A.D. (1985) Models of glaciomarine sedimentation and their application to the interpretation of ancient glacial sequences. *Palaeogeography, Palaeoclimatology, Palaeoecology*, **51**, 15–84.

Eyles, N., Eyles, C.H. & McCabe, A.M. (1988) Late Pleistocene subaerial debris-flow facies of the Bow Valley, near Banff, Canadian Rocky Mountains. *Sedimentology*, **35**, 465–80.

Faber, T.E. (1995) *Fluid Dynamics for Physicists*. Cambridge University Press, Cambridge.

Falco, R.E. (1977) Coherent motions in the outer regions of turbulent boundary layers. *Physics of Fluids*, **20**, 124–32.

Falk, P.D. & Dorsey, R.J. (1998) Rapid development of gravelly high-density turbidity currents in marine Gilbert-type deltas, Loreto Basin, Baja California Sur, Mexico. *Sedimentology*, **45**, 331–49.

Farre, J.A., McGregor, B.A., Ryan, W.B.F. & Robb, J.M. (1983) Breaching the shelfbreak: passage from youthful to mature phase in submarine canyon evolution. In: *The Shelfbreak: Critical Interface on Continental Margin* (eds D.J. Stanley & G.T. Moore), pp. 25–39. Special Publication no. 33, Society of Economic Palaeontologists and Mineralogists.

Ferentinos, G., Papatheodourou, G. & Collins, M.B. (1988) Sediment transport processes on an active submarine fault escarpment: Gulf of Corinth, Greece. *Marine Geology*, **83**, 43–61.

Ferguson, J., Bubela, B. & Davies, P.J. (1978) Synthesis and possible mechanism of formation of radial carbonate ooids. *Chemical Geology*, **22**, 285–308.

Ferguson, R. (1987) Hydraulic and sedimentary controls of channel pattern. In: *River Channels: Environments and Process* (ed. K.S. Richards), pp. 125–58. Blackwell Scientific, Oxford.

Ferguson, R., Hoey, T., Wathen, S. & Werrity, A. (1996) Field evidence for rapid downstream fining of river gravels through selective transport. *Geology*, **24**, 179–82.

Field, M.E. (1980) Sand bodies on coastal plain shelves: Holocene record of the US Atlantic inner shelf off Maryland. *Journal of Sedimentary Petrology*, **50**, 505–28.

Fineberg, J. (1996) Physics in a jumping sandbox. *Nature*, **382**, 763–4.

Finkelstein, K. & Ferland, M.A. (1987) Back-barrier response to sea-level rise, eastern shore of Virginia.

In: *Sea Level Fluctuation and Coastal Evolution* (eds D. Nummedal, O.H. Pilkey & J.D. Howard), pp. 145–55. Special Publication no. 41, Society of Economic Palaeontologists and Mineralogists.

Fischer, A.G. (1964) The Lofer cyclothems of the Alpine Triassic. In: *Symposium on Cyclic Sedimentation* (ed. D.F. Merriam), pp. 107–49. Bulletin no. 169, Geological Survey of Kansas.

Fischer, A.G. (1975) Tidal deposits, Dachstein Limestone of the North Alpine Triassic. In: *Tidal Deposits* (ed R.N. Ginsburg), 235–42. Springer, New York.

Fischer, U.H. & Clarke, G.K.C. (1994) Ploughing of subglacial sediment. *Journal of Glaciology*, **40**, 97–106.

Fisk, H.N. (1944) *Geological Investigations of the Alluvial Valley of the Lower Mississippi River*. Mississippi River Commission, Vicksberg, MS.

Fisk, H.N. (1959) Padre Island and the Laguna Madre flats, coastal South Texas. *National Academy of Science-National Research Council 2nd Coastal Geography Conference* 103-SI.

Fisk, H.N., McFarlan, E., Kolband, C.R. & Wilbert, L.J. (1954) Sedimentary framework of the modern Mississippi delta. *Journal of Sedimentary Petrology*, **24**, 76–99.

Fitzgerald, D.M. (1988) Shoreline erosional–depositional processes associated with tidal inlets. In: *Hydrodynamics and Sediment Dynamics of Tidal Inlets* (eds D.G. Aubrey & L. Weishar), pp. 186–225. Springer, Berlin.

Fitzgerald, D.M. (1993) Origin and stability of tidal inlets in Massachusetts. In: *Formation and Evolution of Multiple Tidal Inlets* (eds Aubrey, J. & Geise, F.J.), pp. 1–61. Monograph, American Geophysical Union.

Flament, P.J., *et al.* (1996) The 3D structure of an upper ocean vortex in the tropical Pacific Ocean. *Nature*, **383**, 610–13.

Flather, R.A. (1984) A numerical model investigation of the storm surge of 31 January and 1 February 1953 in the North Sea. *Quarterly Journal of the Royal Meteoreological Society*, **110**, 591–612.

Fleet, A.J., Kelts, K. & Talbot, M.J. (eds) (1988) *Lacustrine Petroleum Source Rocks*. Special Publication no. 40, Geological Society of London.

Flemings, P.B. & Jordan, T.E. (1990) Stratigraphic modelling of foreland basins: interpreting thrust deformation and lithospheric rheology. *Geology*, **18**, 430–5.

Flemming, B.W. & Bartholema (eds) (1995) *Tidal Signatures in Modern and Ancient Sediments*. Special Publication 24, International Association of Sedimentologists.

Fletcher, C.H., Knebel, H.J. & Kraft, J.C. (1990) Holocene evolution of an estuarine coast and tidal wetlands. *Bulletin of the Geological Society of America*, **102**, 283–97.

Flood, R.D., Hollister, C.D. & Lonsdale, P. (1979) Disruption of the Feni sediment drift by debris flows from Rockall Bank. *Marine Geology*, **32**, 311–34.

Flood, R.D., *et al.* (1991) Seismic facies and late-Quaternary growth of Amazon submarine fan. In: *Seismic Facies and Sedimentary Processes of Submarine Fans and Turbidite Systems* (eds P. Weimer & M.H. Link), pp. 415–34. Springer, Berlin.

Folk, R.L. (1955) Note on the significance of 'turbid' feldspars. *American Mineralogist*, **40**, 356–7.

Folk, R.L. (1962) Spectral division of limestone types. In: *Classification of Carbonate Rocks* (ed W.E. Ham), 62–84, Memoirs of the American Association of Petroleum Geologists, Tulsa, Oklahoma.

Folk, R.L. (1971) Longitudinal dunes of the northwestern edge of the Simpson Desert, Northern Territory, Australia. 1: Geomorphology and grain size relationships. *Sedimentology*, **16**, 5–54.

Folk, R.L. (1974) The natural history of crystalline calcium carbonate: effect of magnesium content and salinity. *Journal of Sedimentary Petrology*, **44**, 40–53.

Folk, R.L. & Patton, E.B. (1982) Buttressed expansion of granite and development of grus in central Texas. *Zeitschrift für Geomorphologie*, **26**, 17–32.

Follmi, K.B. (1995) 160 my record of marine sedimentary phosphorus burial: coupling of climate and continental weathering under greenhouse and icehouse conditions. *Geology*, **23**, 859–62.

Forristall, G.Z., Hamilton, R.C. & Cardone, V.J. (1977) Continental shelf currents in Tropical Storm Delia: observations and theory. *Journal of Physical Oceanography*, **7**, 532–46.

Fountain, A.G. & Walder, J.S. (1998) Water flow through temperate glaciers. *Reviews of Geophysics*, **36**, 299–328.

Fournier, F. (1960) *Climat et Erosion: la Relation entre l'Erosion du Sol par l'Eau et les Precipitations Atmospheriques*. Presses Universitaire de France, Paris.

Frakes, L.A., Francis, J.E. & Sykes, J.I. (1992) *Climate Modes of the Phanerozoic*. Cambridge University Press, Cambridge.

Francis, J.E. (1984) The seasonal environment of the Purbeck (Upper Jurassic) fossil forests. *Palaeogeography, Palaeoclimatology, Palaeoecology*, **48**, 285–307.

Francis, J.R.D. (1969) *A Textbook of Fluid Mechanics*. Edward Arnold, London.

Francis, J.R.D. (1973) Experiments on the motion of solitary grains along the bed of a water stream. *Philosophical Transactions of the Royal Society, London (A)*, **332**, 443–71.

Frazier, D.E. (1967) Recent deltaic deposits of the Mississippi delta: their development and chronology. *Transactions of the Gulf Coast Association of Geological Societies*, **17**, 287–315.

Fredsoe, J. & Deigaard, R. (1992) *Mechanics of Coastal Sediment Transport*. World Scientific, Singapore.

Friedman, S.J. (1998) Rock-avalanche elements of the Shadow Valley Basin, Eastern Mojave Desert, California: processes and problems. *Journal of Sedimentary Research*, **67**, 792–804.

Friend, P.F. (1978) Distinctive features of some ancient river systems. In: *Fluvial Sedimentology* (ed A.D. Miall), pp. 531–42, Memoirs of the Canadian Society of Petroleum Geologists 5.

Frostick, L.E. & McCave, I.N. (1979) Seasonal shifts of sediment within an estuary mediated by algal growth. *Estuarine and Coastal Marine Science*, 9, 569–76.

Frostick, L.E. & Reid, I. (1986) Evolution and sedimentary character of lake deltas fed by ephemeral rivers in the Turkana basin, northern Kenya. In: *Sedimentation in the African Rifts* (ed. L. Frostick), pp. 113–25. Special Publication no. 25, Geological Society of London.

Fryberger, S.G. (1993) A review of aeolian bounding surfaces, with examples from the Permian Minnelusa Formation, USA. In: *Characterisation of Fluvial and Aeolian Reservoirs* (eds C.P. North & D.J. Prosser), pp. 167–97. Special Publication no. 73, Geological Society of London.

Fryberger, S.G. & Ahlbrandt, T.S. (1979) Mechanism for the formation of aeolian sand seas. *Zeitschrift fur Geomorphologie*, 23, 440–50.

Fryberger, S.G. & Schenk, C.J. (1988) Pinstripe lamination: a distinctive feature of modern and ancient eolian sediments. *Sedimentary Geology*, 55, 1–15.

Fryberger, S.G., Ahlbrandt, T.S. & Andrews, S. (1979) Origin, sedimentary features and significance of low-angle eolian 'sand sheet' deposits. Great Sand Dunes National Monument and vicinity, Colorado. *Journal of Sedimentary Petrology*, 49, 733–46.

Fuller, J.G.C.M. & Porter, J.W. (1969) Evaporite formations with petroleum reservoirs in Devonian and Mississippian of Alberta, Saskatchewan and N. Dakota. *Bulletin of the American Association of Petroleum Geologists*, 53, 909–26.

Furrer, G. & Stumm, W. (1986) The coordination chemistry of weathering, 1. Dissolution kinetics of δ-Al₂O₃ and BeO. *Geochimica et Cosmochimica Acta*, 50, 1847–60.

Gabel, S.L. (1993) Geometry and kinematics of dunes during steady and unsteady flows in the Calamus River, Nebraska. *Sedimentology*, 40, 237–69.

Gadow, S. & Reineck, H.E. (1969) Ablandiger sand transport bei Sturmfluten. *Senckenbergiana Maritima*, 3, 103–33.

Galloway, W.E. (1980) Deposition and early hydrological evolution of Westwater Canyon wet alluvial-fan system, pp. 59–69. Memoir no. 38, New Mexico Bureau of Mines and Mineral Resources.

Galvin, C.J. (1968) Breaker type classification on three laboratory beaches. *Journal of Geophysical Research*, 73, 3651–9.

Ganeshram, R.S., Pederson, T.F., Calvert, S.E. & Murray, J.W. (1995) Large changes in oceanic nutrient inventories from glacial to interglacial periods. *Nature*, 376, 755–8.

Gardulski, A.F., Mullins, H.T. & Weiterman, S. (1990) Carbonate mineral cycles generated by foraminiferal and

pteropod response to Pleistocene climate: west Florida ramp slope. *Sedimentology*, 37, 727–43.

Garrels, R.M. & Christ, C.L. (1965) *Solutions, Minerals and Equilibrium*. Harper and Row, New York.

Gasse, F., Tehet, R., Durand, A., Gibert, E. & Fontes, J.-C. (1990) The arid–humid transition in the Sahara and the Sahel during the last deglaciation. *Nature*, 346, 141–6.

Gastaldo, R.A., Allen, G.P. & Huc, A.-Y. (1995) The tidal character of fluvial sediments of the modern Mahakam River delta, Kalimantan, Indonesia. In: *Coarse-Grained Deltas* (eds A. Colella & D.B. Prior), pp. 193–211. Special Publication no. 10, International Association of Sedimentologists.

Gawthorpe, R.L. & Colella, A. (1990) Tectonic controls on coarse-grained delta depositional systems in rift basins. In: *Coarse-Grained Deltas* (eds A. Colella & D.B. Prior), pp. 113–28. Special Publication no. 10, International Association of Sedimentologists.

Gawthorpe, R.L., Fraser, A.J. & Collier, R.E.Ll. (1994) Sequence stratigraphy in active extensional basins: implications for the interpretation of ancient basin-fills. *Marine and Petroleum Geology*, 11, 642–58.

Gawthorpe, R.L., Sharp, I., Underhill, J.R. & Gupta, S. (1997) Linked sequence stratigraphic and structural evolution of propagating normal faults. *Geology*, 25, 795–8.

George, A.D., Playford, P.E., Powell, C.McA. & Tornator, P.M. (1997) Lithofacies and sequence development on an Upper Devonian mixed carbonate–siliciclastic fore-reef slope, Canning Basin, Western Australia. *Sedimentology*, 44, 843–67.

George, G. & Berry, J.K. (1993) A new lithostratigraphy and depositional model for the Upper Rotliegend of the UK sector of the southern North Sea, In: *Characterisation of Fluvial and Aeolian Reservoirs* (eds C.P. North & D.J. Prosser), pp. 291–320. Special Publication no. 73, Geological Society of London.

Gibbard, P. (1980) The origin of stratified Catfish Creek Till by basal melting. *Boreas*, 9, 71–85.

Gibbard, P.L. (1988) The history of the great northwest European rivers during the past three million years. *Philosophical Transactions of the Royal Society, London*, 318, 559–602.

Gibbs, R.J., Mathews, M.D. & Link, D.A. (1971) The relationship between sphere size and settling velocity. *Journal of Sedimentary Petrology*, 41, 7–18.

Gibling, M.R., Nanson, G.C. & Maroulis, J.C. (1998) Anastomosing river sedimentation in the Channel Country of central Australia. *Sedimentology*, 45, 595–619.

Gibling, M.R. & Bird, D.J. (1994) Late Carboniferous cyclothems and alluvial palaeovalleys in the Sydney basin, Nova Scotia. *Bulletin of the Geological Society of America*, 106, 105–17.

Gienapp, H. (1973) Strömingen während der Stormflut vom 2 November 1965 in der Deutschen Bucht und ihre

Bedeutung für den Sedimenttransport. *Senckenbergiana Maritima*, **5**, 135–51.

Gile, L.H., Hawley, J.W. & Grossman, R.B. (1981) *Soils and Geomorphology in the Basin and Range Area of Southern New Mexico—Guidebook to the Desert Project*. Memoir no. 39, New Mexico Bureau of Mines and Mineral Resources, Socorro, NM.

Gill, R. (1989) *Chemical Fundamentals of Geology*. Chapman and Hall, London.

Gill, W.D. & Keunen, P.H. (1958) Sand volcanoes on slumps in the Carboniferous of County Clare, Ireland. *Quarterly Journal of the Geological Society of London*, **113**, 441–60.

Ginsburg, R.N., Harris, P.M., Eberli, G.P. & Swart, P.K. (1991) The growth potential of a bypass margin, Great Bahama Bank. *Journal of Sedimentary Petrology*, **61**, 976–87.

Gleadow, A.J.W., Green, P.F. & Lovering, J.F. (1986) Confined track lengths in apatite—a diagnostic tool for thermal history analysis. *Contributions to Mineralogy and Petrology*, **94**, 405–15.

Glennie, K.W. (1970) *Desert Sedimentary Environments*. Elsevier, Amsterdam.

Glennie, K.W. (1982) Early Permian (Rotliegendes) palaeowinds of the North Sea. *Sedimentary Geology*, **34**, 245–65.

Glennie, K.W. (1986) Early Permian Rotliegend. In: *Introduction to the Petroleum Geology of the North Sea*. (ed K.W. Glennie), pp. 63–86, Blackwell Science, Oxford.

Glennie, K.W. & Buller, A.T. (1983) The Permian Weissliegend of NW Europe: the partial deformation of aeolian dune sands caused by the Zechstein transgression. *Sedimentary Geology*, **35**, 43–81.

Gohain, K. & Parkash, B. (1990) Morphology of the Kosi Megafan. In: *Alluvial Fans: A Field Approach* (eds A.H. Rachocki & M. Church), pp. 151–78. Wiley, New York.

Goldhammer, R.K., Dunn, P.A. & Hardie, L.A. (1990) Depositional cycles, composite sea-level changes, cycle stacking patterns, and the hierarchy of stratigraphic forcing: examples from Alpine Triassic platform carbonates. *Bulletin of the Geological Society of America*, **102**, 535–62.

Gole, C.V. & Chitale, S.V. (1966) Inland delta building activity of Kosi River. *Journal of the Hydraulics Division, American Society of Civil Engineers*, **92**, 111–26.

Gomez, B., *et al.* (1995) Sediment characteristics of an extreme flood: 1993 upper Mississippi River valley. *Geology*, **23**, 963–6.

Goudie, A.S. (1985) *Salt Weathering*. Research Paper no. 33, School of Geography, University of Oxford.

Goudie, A.S., Cooke, R.U. & Evans, I.S. (1970) Experimental investigation of rock weathering by salts. *Area*, **4**, 42–8.

Grabemann, I. & Krause, G. (1989) Transport processes of suspended matter derived from time series in a tidal estuary. *Journal of Geophysical Research*, **94C**, 14373–9.

Graf, J.B., Webb, R.H. & Hereford, R. (1991) Relation of sediment load and floodplain formation to climatic variability, Paria River drainage basin, Utah and Arizona. *Bulletin of the Geological Society of America*, **103**, 1405–15.

Grammer, G.M., Ginsburg, R.N. & Harris, P.M. (1993) Timing of deposition, diagenesis, and failure of steep carbonate slopes in response to a high-amplitude/high-frequency fluctuation in sea level, Tongue of the Ocean, Bahamas. In: *Carbonate Sequence Stratigraphy* (eds R.G. Loucks & J.F. Sarg), pp. 107–32. Memoir no. 57, American Association of Petroleum Geologists.

Grant, W.D. & Williams, A.J. (1984) Bottom stress estimates and their prediction on the northern California continental shelf during CODE-1: the importance of wave–current interaction. *Journal of Physical Oceanography*, **14**, 506–27.

Grass, A.J. (1970) Initial instability of fine bed sand. *Journal of the Hydraulics Division, American Society of Civil Engineers*, **96**, 619–32.

Grass, A.J (1971) Structural features of turbulent flow over smooth and rough boundaries. *Journal of Fluid Mechanics*, **50**, 233–55.

Gratz, A.J., Hillner, P.E. & Hansma, P.K. (1993) Step dynamics and spiral growth rate on calcite. *Geochimica et Cosmochimica Acta*, **57**, 491–5.

Gray, W.A. (1968) *The Packing of Solid Particles*. Chapman and Hall, London.

Greeley, R. & Iverson, J.D. (1985) *Wind as a geological process: on Earth, Mars, Venus and Titan*. Cambridge University Press, Cambridge.

Green, M.O., Rees, J.M. & Pearson, N.D. (1990) Evidence for the influence of wave–current interactions in a tidal boundary layer. *Journal of Geophysical Research*, **C95**, 9629–44.

Greenwood, B. & Sherman, D.J. (1993) Waves, currents, sediment flux and morphological response in a barred nearshore system. *Marine Geology*, **60**, 31–61.

Gregory, K.J. & Walling, D.E. (1973) *Drainage Basin Form and Process*. Edward Arnold, London.

Gretener, B. & Stromquist, L. (1987) Overbank sedimentation rates of fine grained sediments. A study of the recent deposition in the lower River Fyrisan. *Geografiska Annaler*, **69A**, 139–46.

Griffin, R.A. & Jurinak, J.J. (1973) The interaction of phosphate with calcite. *Proceedings of the Soil Science Society of America*, **37**, 847–50.

Griffith, L.S., Pitcher, M.G. & Rice, G.W. (1969) Quantitative environmental analysis of a lower cretaceous reef complex. In: *Depositional Environments in Carbonate Rocks* (ed. G.H. Friedman), pp. 120–37. SEPM, Tulsa.

Gross, T.F., Williams, A.J. & Nowell, A.R.M. (1988) A deep-sea sediment transport storm. *Nature*, **331**, 518–20.

Grotzinger, J.P. (1986) Cyclicity and palaeoenvironmental dynamics, Rocknest platform, northwest Canada.

Bulletin of the Geological Society of America, **97**, 1208–31.

Gruszczynski, M., Rudowski, S., Semil, J., Slominski, J. & Zrobek, J. (1993) Rip currents as a geological tool. *Sedimentology*, **40**, 217–36.

Gunatilaka, A. (1976) Thallophyte boring and micritisation within skeletal sands from Connemara, W. Ireland. *Journal of Sedimentary Petrology*, **46**, 548–54.

Gupta, S. (1997) Himalayan drainage patterns and the origin of fluvial megafans in the Ganges foreland basin. *Geology*, **25**, 11–14.

Gurnis, M. (1992) Rapid continental subsidence following the initiation and evolution of subduction. *Science*, **255**, 1556–8.

Gurnis, M. (1993) Phanerozoic marine inundation of continents driven by dynamic topography above subducting slabs. *Nature*, **364**, 589–93.

Gust, G. (1976) Observations on turbulent drag reduction in a dilute suspension of clay in sea water. *Journal of Fluid Mechanics*, **75**, 29–47.

Guzzetti, F., Marchetti, M. & Reichenbach, P. (1997) Large alluvial fans in the north-central Po Plain (Northern Italy). *Geomorphology*, **18**, 119–36.

Hagan, G.M. & Logan, B.W. (1974) Development of carbonate banks and hypersaline basins, Shark Bay, Western Australia. In: *Evolution and Diagenesis of Quaternary Carbonate Sequences, Shark Bay, W. Australia* (eds B.W. Logan et al.), pp. 61–139. Memoir no. 22, American Association of Petroleum Geologists.

Hails, J. & Carr, A. (eds) (1975) *Nearshore Sediment Dynamics and Sedimentation*. Wiley, London.

Hallam, A. (1997) Estimates of the amount and rate of sea-level change across the Rhaetian–Hettangian and Pliensbachian–Toarcian boundaries (latest Triassic to early Jurassic). *Journal of the Geological Society of London*, **154**, 773–9.

Halley, R.B. (1977) Ooid fabric and fracture in the Great Salt Lake and the geologic record. *Journal of Sedimentary Petrology*, **47**, 1099–120.

Halley, R.B., Shinn, E.A., Hudson, J.H. & Lidz, B.H. (1977) Pleistocene barrier bar seaward of ooid shoal complex near Miami, Florida. *Bulletin of the American Association of Petroleum Geologists*, **61**, 519–26.

Hallock, P. (1988) The role of nutrient availability in bioerosion: consequences to carbonate buildups. *Palaeogeography, Palaeoclimatology, Palaeoecology*, **63**, 275–91.

Hallock, P. & Schlager, W. (1985) Nutrient excess and the demise of coral reefs and carbonate platforms. *Palios*, **1**, 389–98.

Halsey, S.D. (1979) Nexus: new model of barrier island development. In: *Barrier Islands* (ed. S.P. Leatherman), pp. 185–210. Academic Press, New York.

Hambrey, M. (1994) *Glacial Environments*. UCL Press, London.

Hambrey, M. & Harland, W.B. (eds) (1981) *Earth's pre-Pleistocene Glacial Record*. Cambridge University Press, Cambridge.

Hampton, M.A. (1972) The role of subaqueous debris flow in generating turbidity currents. *Journal of Sedimentary Petrology*, **42**, 775–93.

Hanna, S.R. (1969) The formation of longitudinal sand dunes by large helical eddies in the atmosphere. *Journal of Applied Meteorology*, **8**, 874–83.

Harbor, J., et al. (1997) Influence of subglacial drainage conditions within a glacier cross section. *Geology*, **25**, 739–42.

Hardie, L.A. (1967) The gypsum-anhydrite equilibrium at one atmosphere pressure. In: Special Publication 5, International Association of Sedimentologists, 187–210.

Hardie, L.A. (ed.) (1977) *Sedimentation on the Modern Carbonate Tidal Flats of NW Andros Island, Bahamas*. Johns Hopkins Press, Baltimore.

Hardie, L.A. (1996) Secular variation in seawater chemistry: an explanation for the coupled secular variation in the mineralogies of marine limestones and potash evaporites over the past 600 my. *Geology*, **24**, 279–83.

Hardie, L.A. & Garrett, P. (1977) General environmental setting. In: *Sedimentation on the Modern Carbonate Tidal Flats of NW Andros Island, Bahamas* (ed. L.A. Hardie), pp. 12–49. John Hopkins Press, Baltimore.

Hardie, L.A. & Ginsburg, R.N. (1977) Layering: the origin and environmental significance of lamination and thin bedding. In: *Sedimentation on the Modern Carbonate Tidal Flats of NW Andros Island, Bahamas* (ed. L.A. Hardie), pp. 50–123. John Hopkins Press, Baltimore.

Hardie, L.A., Smoot, J.P. & Eugster, H.P. (1978) Saline lakes and their deposits: a sedimentological approach. In: *Modern and Ancient Lake Sediments* (eds A. Matter & M.E. Tucker), 7–42. Special Publication no. 2, International Association of Sedimentologists. Blackwell Scientific Publications, Oxford.

Hardie, L.A., Bosellini, A. & Goldhammer, R.K. (1986) Repeated subaerial exposure of subtidal carbonate platforms, Triassic, northern Italy: evidence for high frequency sea level oscillations on a 10^4 year scale. *Palaeooceanography*, **1**, 447–57.

Hardisty, J. (1986) A morphodynamic model for beach gradients. *Earth Surface Processes and Landforms*, **11**, 327–33.

Hardisty, J. & Whitehouse, R.J.S. (1988) Evidence for a new sand transport process from experiments on Saharan dunes. *Nature*, **332**, 532–4.

Hardy, S., Dart, C.J. & Waltham, D. (1994) Computer modelling of the influence of tectonics on sequence architecture of coarse-grained fan deltas. *Marine and Petroleum Geology*, **11**, 561–74.

Harland, W.B., et al. (1990) *A Geological Time Scale*. Cambridge University Press, Cambridge.

Harms, J.C., Southard, J.B., Spearing, D.R. & Walker, R.G. (1975) *Depositional Environments as Interpreted from Primary Sedimentary Structures and Stratification Sequences*. Short Course Notes 2.

Harris, M.T. (1993) Reef fabrics, biotic crusts and syndepositional cements of the Latemar reef margin (Middle Triassic), northern Italy. *Sedimentology*, 40, 383–401.

Harris, P.M. (1979) *Facies Anatomy and Diagenesis of a Bahamian Ooid Shoal*. Sedimenta 7, Comparative Sedimentology Laboratory, University of Miami, Florida.

Harris, P.M. & Kowalik, W.S. (1994) *Satellite Images of Carbonate Depositional Settings. Examples of Reservoir and Exploration Scale Geological Facies Variation*. American Association of Petroleum Geologists, Methods in Exploration Series, 11. Tulsa, OK.

Harris, P.T. & Collins, M.B. (1991) Sand transport in the Bristol Channel: bedload parting zone or mutually evasive transport pathways? *Marine Geology*, 101, 209–16.

Harris, P.T., Pattiaratchi, C.B., Collins, M.B. & Dalrymple, R.W. (1995) What is a bedload parting? In: *Tidal Signatures in Modern and Ancient Sediments*, pp. 3–18. Special Publication no. 24, International Association of Sedimentologists.

Hart, B.S. & Plint, A.G. (1989) Gravelly shoreface deposits: a comparison of modern and ancient facies sequences. *Sedimentology*, 36, 551–7.

Hart, J.K. & Boulton, G.S. (1991) The glacial geology of north east Norfolk. In: *The Glacial Deposits of Britain* (eds J. Rose *et al.*), pp. 233–44. Balkema, Rotterdam.

Harvey, A.M. (1990) Factors influencing Quaternary alluvial fan development in SE Spain. In: *Alluvial Fans: A Field Approach* (eds A.H. Rachocki & M. Church), pp. 247–69. Wiley, Chichester.

Harvey, J.G. (1976) *Atmosphere and Ocean: Our Fluid Environments*. Artemis Press, Sussex.

Harvie, C.E., Eugster, H.P. & Weare, J.H. (1982) Mineral equilibria in the six-component seawater system, Na–K–Mg–Ca–SO$_4$–Cl–H$_2$O at 25 °C. 2. Composition of the saturated solutions. *Geochimica et Cosmochimica Acta*, 46, 1603–18.

Harvie, C.E., Møller, N. & Weare, J.H. (1984) The prediction of mineral solubilities in natural waters: the Na–K–Mg–Ca–HSO$_4$–Cl–H$_2$O–SO$_4$–OH–HCO$_3$–CO$_3$–CO$_2$ system to high ionic strengths at 25 °C: composition of the saturated solutions. *Geochimica et Cosmochimica Acta*, 48, 723–51.

Haughton, P.D.W. (1994) Deposits of deflected and ponded turbidity currents, Sorbas basin, SE Spain. *Journal of Sedimentary Research*, A64, 233–46.

Havholm, K.G., Blakey, R.C., Capps, M., Jones, L.S., King, D.D. & Kocurek, G. (1993) Aeolian genetic stratigraphy: an example from the Middle Jurassic Page sandstone, Colorado Plateau. In: *Aeolian Sediments Ancient and Modern* (ed. K. Pye), pp. 87–107. Special Publication no. 16, International Association of Sedimentologists.

Haworth, M. (1982) Tidal currents. In: *Offshore Tidal Sands: Processes and Deposits* (ed. A.H. Stride), pp. 8–40. Chapman and Hall, London.

Hay, A.E., Burling, R.W. & Murray, J.W. (1982) Remote acoustic detection of a turbidity current surge. *Science*, 217, 833–5.

Hayes, M.O. (1971) Geomorphology and sedimentation of some New England estuaries. In: *The Estuarine Environment* (ed. J.R. Schubel), pp. 1–71. American Geological Institute, Washington, DC.

Hayes, M.O. (1975) Morphology of sand accumulations in estuaries. In: *Estuarine Research* (ed. L.E. Cronin), pp. 3–22. Academic Press, New York.

Hayes, M.O. (1979) Barrier island morphology as a function of tidal and wave regime. In: *Barrier Islands* (ed. S.P. Leatherman), pp. 1–27. Academic Press, New York.

Haynes, C.V. (1989) Bagnold's barchan: a 57-year record of dune movement in the eastern Sahara and implications for dune origin and palaeoclimate since Neolithic times. *Quaternary Research*, 32, 153–67.

Hays, J.D., Imbrie, J. & Shackleton, N.J. (1976) Variations in the Earth's orbit: pacemaker of the ice ages. *Science*, 194, 1121–32.

Hayward, A.B. (1982) Coral reefs in a clastic sedimentary environment: fossil (Miocene, SW Turkey) and modern (Recent, Red Sea) analogues. *Coral Reefs*, 1, 109–14.

Hayward, A.B. (1985) Coastal alluvial fans (fan deltas) of the Gulf of Aqaba (Gulf of Eilat), Red Sea. *Sedimentary Geology*, 53, 241–60.

Head, M.R. & Bandyopadhyay, P. (1981) New aspects of turbulent boundary layer structure. *Journal of Fluid Mechanics*, 107, 297–338.

Heath, G.R. (1974) Dissolved silica and deep-sea sediments. In: *Studies in Paleo-oceanography* (ed. W.W. Hay), pp. 77–93. SEPM, Tulsa.

Heathershaw, A.D. (1985) Some observations of internal wave current fluctuations at the shelf edge and their implications for sediment transport. *Continental Shelf Research*, 4, 485–93.

Heckel, P.H. (1986) Sea level curve for Pennsylvanian eustatic marine transgressive depositional cycles along Midcontinent outcrop belt, North America. *Geology*, 14, 330–4.

Heezen, B.C. & Hollister, C.D. (1963) Evidence of deep sea bottom currents from abyssal sediments. International Union Geodesy and Geophysics 6, 111.

Heinrich, H. (1988) Origin and consequences of cyclic ice-rafting in the northeast Atlantic Ocean during the past 130 000 years. *Quaternary Research*, 29, 143–52.

Heller, P.L. & Paola, C. (1996) Downstream changes in alluvial architecture: an exploration of controls on channel-stacking patterns. *Journal of Sedimentary Research*, 66, 297–306.

Heller, P.L., Anderson, D.L. & Angevine, C.L. (1996) Is the middle Cretaceous pulse of rapid sea-floor spreading real or necessary? *Geology*, **24**, 491–4.

Hequette, A. & Hill, P.R. (1993) Storm-generated currents and offshore sediment transport on a sandy shoreface, Tibjak Beach, Canadian Beaufort Sea. *Marine Geology*, **113**, 283–304.

Herd, D.G. (1986) The 1985 Ruiz volcano disaster. *EOS*, 13 May, 457–60.

Hereford, R. (1993) *Entrenchment and Widening of the Upper San Pedro River, Arizona*. Special Paper no. 282, Geological Society of America.

Herries, R.D. (1993) Contrasting styles of fluvial–aeolian bounding surfaces, with examples from the Permian Minnelusa Formation, USA. In: *Characterisation of Fluvial and Aeolian Reservoirs* (eds C,P, North & D.J. Prosser), pp. 199–218. Special Publication no. 73, Geological Society of London.

Hesse, R. & Khodabakhsh, S. (1998) Depositional facies of late Pleistocene Heinrich events in the Labrador Sea. *Geology*, **26**, 103–6.

Hesse, R. & Rakofsky, A. (1992) Deep sea channel/submarine yazoo system of the Labrador Sea: a new deep water facies model. *Bulletin of the American Association of Petroleum Geologists*, **104**, 680–707.

Hesse, R., Chough, S.K. & Rakofsky, A. (1987) The Northwest Mid-Ocean Channel of the Labrador Sea. V. Sedimentology of a giant deep sea channel. *Canadian Journal of Earth Sciences*, **24**, 1595–624.

Hesse, R., *et al.* (1996) Imaging Laurentide ice sheet drainage into the deep sea: impact on sediments and bottom water. *GSA Today*, September, 3–8.

von Heune, R. & Scholl, D.W. (1991) Observations at convergent margins concerning sediment subduction, and the growth of continental crust. *Reviews of Geophysics*, **29**, 279–316.

von Heune, R., Bourgois, J., Miller, J. & Pautot, G. (1989) A large tsunamogenic landslide and debris flow along the Peru trench. *Journal of Geophysical Research*, **94**, 1703–14.

Heward, A.P. (1978) Alluvial fan sequence and megasequence models: with examples from Westphalian D–Stephanian B coalfields, northern Spain. In Miall (1978), 669–702.

Hickin, E. (1974) The development of meanders in natural river channels. *American Journal of Science*, **274**, 414–42.

Hicock, S.R., Dreimanis, A. & Broster, B.E. (1981) Submarine flow tills at Victoria, British Colombia. *Canadian Journal of Earth Sciences*, **18**, 71–80.

Hilgen, F.J. (1991) Astronomical calibration of Gauss to Matuyama sapropels in the Mediterranean and implication for the geomagnetic polarity timescale. *Earth Planetary Science Letters*, **104**, 226–44.

Hilgen, F.J. (1994) An astronomically calibrated (polarity) time scale for the Pliocene–Pleistocene: a brief review. In: *Orbital Forcing and Cyclic Sequences* (eds P.L. De Boer & D.G. Smith), 109–116. Special Publication no. 19, International Association of Sedimentologists. Blackwell Science, Oxford.

Hine, A.C., Wilber, R.J., Bane, J.M., Neumann, A.C. & Lorenson, K.R. (1981a) Offbank transport of carbonate sands along open leeward carbonate margins: Northern Bahamas. *Marine Geology*, **42**, 327–48.

Hine, A.C., Wilber, R.J. & Neumann, A.C. (1981b) Carbonate sand bodies along contrasting shallow bank margins facing open seaways in the northern Bahamas. *Bulletin of the American Association of Petroleum Geologists*, **64**, 261–90.

Hinnov, L.A. & Goldhammer, R.K. (1991) Spectral analysis of the Middle Triassic Latemar Limestone. *Journal of Sedimentary Petrology*, **61**, 1173–93.

Hiscott, R.N. (1994) Traction-carpet stratification in turbidites—fact or fiction? *Journal of Sedimentary Research*, **A64**, 204–8.

Hochella, M.F. & Banfield, J.F. (1995) Chemical weathering of silicates in nature: a microscopic perspective with theoretical considerations. In: *Chemical Weathering Rates of Silicate Minerals* (eds A.F. White & S.L. Branfield), ch. 8. American Mineralogical Society, Washington, DC.

Hodell, D.A., Elstrom, K.M. & Kennett, J.P. (1986) Latest Miocene benthic $\delta^{18}O$ changes, global ice volume, sea level and the 'Messinian salinity crisis'. *Nature*, **320**, 411–14.

Holdren, G.R. & Speyer, P.M. (1985) Reaction rate-surface area relationships during the early stages of weathering, 1, Initial observations. *Geochimica et Cosmochimica Acta*, **49**, 675–81.

Holland, H.D. (1978) *The Chemistry of the Atmospheres and Oceans*. Wiley, New York.

Holliday, D.W. & Shephard-Thorne, E.R. (1974) *Basal Purbeck Evaporites of the Fairlight Borehole, Sussex*. Report no. 74/4, Institute of Geological Sciences.

Hollister, C.D. (1993) The concept of deep-sea contourites. *Sedimentary Geology*, **82**, 5–15.

Hollister, C.D. & Heezen, B.C. (1972) Geological effects of ocean bottom currents: western North Atlantic. In: *Studies in Physical Oceanography* (ed. A.L. Gordon), pp. 37–66. Gordon and Breach, New York.

Hollister, C.D. & McCave, I.N. (1984) Sedimentation under deep-sea storms. *Nature*, **309**, 220–5.

Holzhausen, G.R. (1989) Origin of sheet structure, 1. Morphology and boundary conditions. *Engineering Geology*, **27**, 225–78.

Honji, H., Kaneko, A. & Matsunaga, N. (1980) Flows above oscillatory ripples. *Sedimentology*, **27**, 225–9.

Honjo, S. (1976) Coccoliths: production, transportation and sedimentation. *Marine Micropalaeontology*, **1**, 65.

Honjo, S. & Doherty, K.W. (1988) Large aperture time-series sediment trap: design, objectives, construction and application. *Deep Sea Research*, **35**, 133–49.

Hooke, R.LeB. (1967) Processes on arid-region alluvial fans. *Journal of Geology*, **75**, 438–60.

Hooke, R.LeB. (1972) Geomorphic evidence for Late Wisconsin and Holocene tectonic deformation, Death Valley, California. *Bulletin of the Geological Society of America*, **83**, 2073–98.

Hooke, R.LeB. (1998) *Principles of Glacier Mechanics*. Prentice Hall, Englewood Cliffs, NJ.

Hopfinger, E.J. (1983) Snow avalanche motion and related phenomena. *Annual Review of Fluid Mechanics*, **15**, 47–76.

Horton, B.K. (1998) Sediment accumulation on top of the Andean orogenic wedge: Oligocene to late Miocene basins of the Eastern Cordillera, southern Bolivia. *Bulletin of the Geological Society America*, **110**, 1174–92.

Horton, B.K. & DeCelles, P.G. (1997) The modern foreland basin system adjacent to the central Andes. *Geology*, **25**, 895–8.

Horton, B.K. & Schmitt, J.G. (1996) Sedimentology of a lacustrine fan-delta system, Miocene Horse Camp Formation, Nevada, USA. *Sedimentology*, **43**, 133–55.

Horvorka, S.D. (1987) Depositional environments of marine-dominated halite, Permian San Andres Formation, Texas. *Sedimentology*, **34**, 1029–54.

Houboult, J.J.H.C. (1968) Recent sediments in the southern Bight of the North Sea. *Geologie en Mijnbouw*, **47**, 245–73.

Hovius, N. (1997) Controls on sediment supply by large rivers. In: *Relative Role of Eustasy, Climate and Tectonics in Continental Rocks* (eds K.W. Shanley & P.J. McCabe). Special Publication, Society of Economic Palaeontologists and Mineralogists.

Hovius, N. & Leeder, M.R. (eds.) (1998) Thematic Set on Sediment Supply to Basins. *Basin Research*, **10/1**, 1–174.

Hovius, N., Stark, C.P. & Allen, P.A. (1997) Sediment flux from a mountain belt derived by landslide mapping. *Geology*, **25**, 231–4.

Hovius, N., Stark, C.P., Tutton, M.A. & Abbott, L.D. (1998) Landslide-driven drainage network evolution in a presteady-state mountain belt: Finisterre Mountains, Papua New Guinea. *Geology*, **26**, 1071–74.

Hoyle, F. (1981) *Ice*. Hutchinson, London.

Hsu, K.J. (1966) Origin of dolomite in sedimentary sequences: a critical analysis. *Mineralum Depositum*, **2**, 133–8.

Hsu, K.J. (1972) Origin of saline giants: a critical review after the discovery of the Mediterranean evaporite. *Earth Science Reviews*, **8**, 371–96.

Hsu, K.J. (1975) On Sturzoms—catastrophic debris streams generated by rockfalls. *Bulletin of the Geological Society of America*, **80**, 129–40.

Hsu, K.J., Montadert, L., Bernoulli, D. *et al.* (1977) History of the Mediterranean salinity crisis. *Nature*, **267**, 399–403.

Huckleberry, G. (1994) Contrasting channel response to floods on the middle Gila River, Arizona. *Geology*, **22**, 1083–6.

Hudson, J.D. (1963) The recognition of salinity-controlled mollusc assemblages in the Great Estuarine Series (Middle Jurassic) of the Inner Hebrides. *Palaeontology*, **6**, 318–26.

Hughan, K.A., Overpeck, J.T., Peterson, L.C. & Trumbore, S. (1996) Rapid climatic changes in the tropical Atlantic region during the last deglaciation. *Nature*, **380**, 51–4.

Hughes, M.G., Masselink, G. & Brander, R.W. (1997) Flow velocity and sediment transport in the swash zone of a steep beach. *Marine Geology*, **138**, 91–103.

Hunter, R.E. (1977) Basic types of stratification in small eolian dunes. *Sedimentology*, **24**, 361–87.

Hunter, R.E. & Clifton, H.E. (1982) Cyclic deposits and hummocky cross-stratification of probable storm origin in Upper Cretaceous rocks of the Cape Sebastian area, southwest Oregon. *Journal of Sedimentary Petrology*, **52**, 127–43.

Huntley, D.A. & Bowen, A.J. (1975a) Comparison of the hydrodynamics of steep and shallow beaches. In: *Nearshore Sediment Dynamics and Sedimentation* (eds J. Hails & A. Carr). Wiley, New York.

Huntley, D.A. & Bowen, A.J. (1975b) Field observations of edge waves and their effects on beach material. *Journal of the Geological Society of London*, **131**, 69–81.

Hutchinson, G.E. (1957) *A Treatize on Limnology, 1: Geography, Physics and Chemsitry*. Wiley, New York.

Hutchinson, D.R., Golmshtok, A.J., Zonenshain, T.C., Moore, T.C., Scholz, C.A. & Klitgord, K.D. (1992) Depositional and tectonic framework of the rift basins of Lake Baikal from multichannel seismic data. *Geology*, **20**, 589–93.

Huthnance, J.M. (1981) Waves and currents near the continental shelf edge. *Progress in Oceanography*, **10**, 193–226.

Ibbeken, H. & Schleyer, R. (1991) *Source and Sediment: A Case Study of Provenance and Mass Balance at an Active Plate Margin (Calabri, Southern Italy)*. Springer, Berlin.

Illing, L.V. (1954) Bahamian calcareous sands. *Bulletin of the American Association of Petroleum Geologists*, **38**, 1–95.

Illing, L.V., Wells, A.J. & Taylor, J.C.M. (1965) Penecontemporaneous dolomite in the Persian Gulf. In: *Dolomitisation and Limestone Diagenesis: A Symposium* (eds L.C. Pray & R.C. Murray), pp. 89–111. Special Publication no. 13, Society of Economic Palaeontologists and Mineralogists, Tulsa.

Imbrie, J. & Imbrie, K.P. (1979) *Ice Ages: Solving the Mystery*. Macmillan, New York.

Imbrie, J., *et al.* (1984) The orbital theory of Pleistocene climate: support from a revised chronology of the marine $\delta^{18}O$ record. In: *Milankovitch and Climate*, Part 1 (eds Berger *et al.*), pp. 269–305. Reidel, Dordrecht.

Ingersoll, R.V. (1979) Evolution of the Late Cretaceous forearc basin, northern and central California, USA. *Bulletin of the Geological Society of America*, 90, 813–26.

Inman, D.L. & Bagnold, R.A. (1963) Littoral processes. In: *The Sea*, Vol. 3 (ed. M.N. Hill), pp. 529–83. Wiley, New York.

Inman, D.L. & Bowen, A.J. (1963) Flume experiments on sand transport by waves and currents. *Proceedings of the 8th Conference on Coast Engineering*, pp. 137–50.

Ittekot, V., *et al.* (1991) Enhanced particle fluxes in Bay of Bengal induced by injection of freshwater. *Nature*, 351, 385.

Iverson, R.M. (1997) The physics of debris flows. *Reviews of Geophysics*, 35, 245–96.

Jackson, J.A. & Leeder, M.R. (1994) Drainage systems and the development of normal faults: an example from Pleasant Valley, Nevada. *Journal of Structural Geology*, 16, 1041–59.

Jackson, J.A., White, N.J., Garfunkel, Z. & Anderson, H. (1988) Relations between normal-fault geometry, tilting and vertical motions in extensional terrains: an example from the southern Gulf of Suez. *Journal of Structural Geology*, 10, 155–70.

Jackson, J.A., Norris, R. & Youngson, J. (1996) The structural evolution of active fault and fold systems in central Otago, New Zealand: evidence revealed by drainage patterns. *Journal of Structural Geology*, 18, 217–34.

Jackson, R.G. (1975) Velocity–bedform texture patterns of meander bends in the lower Wabash River of Illinois and Indiana. *Bulletin of the Geological Society of America*, 86, 1511–22.

Jackson, R.G. (1976b) Depositional model of point bars in the lower Wabash River. *Journal of Sedimentary Petrology*, 46, 579–94.

Jackson, T.A. & Keller, W.D. (1970) Comparative study of the role of lichens and inorganic processes in the chemical weathering of recent Hawaiian lava flows. *American Journal of Science*, 269, 446–66.

Jacobs, G.A., *et al.* (1994) Decade scale trans-Pacific propagation and warming effects of an El Niño anomaly. *Nature*, 370, 360–3.

Jaeger, H.M., Nagel, S.R. & Behringer, R.P. (1996) The physics of granular materials. *Physics Today*, 49, 32–6.

Jahnke, R.A. (1990) Ocean flux studies: a status report. *Reviews of Geophysics*, 28, 381–98.

James, N.P. (1978a) Introduction to carbonate facies models. In: Walker (1978b), 105–8.

James, N.P. (1978b) Reefs. In: Walker(1978b), 121–32.

James, N.P. & Ginsburg, R.N. (1979) The seaward margin of Belize barrier and reefs. *The Seaward Margin of Belize Barrier and Atoll Reefs* (eds N.P. James & R.N. Ginsberg) Special Publication no. 3, International Association of Sedimentologists.

James, N.P. & Gravestock, D.I. (1990) Lower Cambrian shelf and shelf margin buildups, Flinders Ranges, South Australia. *Sedimentology*, 37, 455–89.

James, N.P., Bone, Y., Von der Borch, C.C. & Gostin, V.A. (1992) Modern carbonate and terrigenous clastic sediments on a cool water, high energy, mid-latitude shelf: Lacepede, southern Australia. *Sedimentology*, 39, 877–903.

Jansson, M.B. (1988) A global survey of sediment yield. *Geografiska Annaler*, 70A, 81–98.

Jeffreys, D.J. (1982) Aggregation and break-up of clay flocs in turbulent flow. *Advances in Colloid and Interface Science*, 17, 213–18.

Joachimski, M.M. (1994) Subaerial exposure and deposition of shallowing upward sequences: evidence from stable isotopes of Purbeckian peritidal carbonates (basal Cretaceous), Swiss and French Jura Mountains, *Sedimentology*, 41, 805–24.

Johannessen, P.N. & Nielsen, L.H. (1986) A sedimentological model for spit systems prograding into deep water. *IAS 7th Regional Meeting Abstracts Volume*, Cracow. International Association of Sedimentologists.

Johansen, C., Larsen, T. & Peterson, O. (1997) Experiments on erosion of mud from the Danish Wadden Sea. In: *Cohesive Sediments* (eds N. Burt, R. Parker & J. Watts), pp. 305–14. Wiley, New York.

Johnson, A.M. (1970) *Physical Processes in Geology*. Freeman, Cooper, San Francisco.

Johnson, M.A., Stride, A.H., Belderson, R.H. & Kenyon, N.H. (1981) Predicted sand-wave formation and decay on a large offshore tidal-current sand sheet. In: *Holocene Marine Sedimentation in the North Sea Basin* (eds S.-D. Nio, R.T.E. Shuttenhelm & T.C.E. van Weering), pp. 247–56. Special Publication no. 5, International Association of Sedimentologists.

Johnson, T.C., Halfman, J.D., Rosendahl, B.R. & Lister, G.S. (1987) Climatic and tectonic effects on sedimentation in a rift-valley lake: evidence from high-resolution seismic profiles, Lake Turkana, Kenya. *Bulletin of the Geological Society of America*, 98, 439–47.

Johnson, T.C., Wells, J.D. & Scholz, C.A. (1995) Deltaic sedimentation in a modern rift lake. *Bulletins of the Geological Society of America*, 107, 812–29.

Jones, C.M. & McCabe, P.J. (1980) Erosion surfaces within giant fluvial cross-beds of the Carboniferous in N. England. *Journal of Sedimentary Petrology*, 50, 613–20.

Jones, G.A. & Gagnon, A.R. (1994) Radiocarbon chronology of Black Sea sediments. *Deep-Sea Research*, 41, 531–57.

Jones, K.P.N., McCave, I.N. & Weaver, P.P.E (1992) Textural and dispersal patterns of thick mud turbidites from the Madeira Abyssal Plain. *Marine Geology*, 107, 149–73.

Jongmans, A.G., *et al.* (1997) Rock-eating fungi. *Nature*, 389, 682–3.

Jopling, A.V. & McDonald, B.C. (eds) (1975) Glaciofluvial and Glaciolacustrine Sediments. Special Publication 23, Society of Economic Palaeontologists and Mineralogists.

Jordan, T.E. (1995) Retroarc foreland and related basins. In: *Tectonics of Sedimentary Basins* (eds C.J. Busby & R.V. Ingersoll), pp. 331–62. Blackwell Science, Boston.

Jullien, R., Meakin, P. & Pavlovitch, A. (1992) Three-dimensional model for particle-size segregation by shaking. *Physical Review Letters*, 69, 640–3.

Kahle, C.F. (1974) Ooids from Great Salt Lake, Utah, as an analogue for the genesis and diagenesis of ooids in marine limestones. *Journal of Sedimentary Petrology*, 44, 30–39.

Kaneps, A.G. (1979) Gulf Stream: velocity fluctuations during the late Cenozoic. *Science*, 204, 297–301.

Kapdasli, M.S. (1991) Threshold conditions of sand particles under codirectional combined wave and current flow. In: *Sand Transport in Rivers, Estuaries and the Sea*, Eromecht 262 (eds R.L. Soulsby & R. Bettess), pp. 31–6. Balkema, Rotterdam.

Kapitsa, A.P., *et al.* (1996) A large deep freshwater lake beneath the ice of the central East Antarctic. *Nature*, 381, 684–6.

Ke, X., Evans, G. & Collins, M.B. (1996) Hydrodynamics and sediment dynamics of The Wash embayment, eastern England. *Sedimentology*, 43, 157–74.

Keene, J.B. & Harris, P.T. (1995) Submarine cementation in tide-generated bioclastic sand dunes: epicontinental seaway, Torres Straits, north-east Australia. In: *Tidal Signatures in Modern and Ancient Sediments*, pp. 225–36. Special Publication no. 24, International Association of Sedimentologists.

Keller, C.K. & Wood, B.D. (1993) Possibility of chemical weathering before the advent of vascular land plants. *Nature*, 364, 223–5.

Keller, G.H., Lambert, D.N. & Bennett, R.H. (1979) Geotechnical properties of continental slope deposits— Cape Hatteras to Hydrographer Canyon. In: *Geology of Continental Slopes* (eds L.J. Doyle & O.H. Pilkey), pp. 131–51. Special Publication no. 27, Society of Economic Palaeontologists and Mineralogists.

Kelts, K. & Hsu, K.J. (1978) Freshwater carbonate sedimentation. In: *Lakes: Physics, Chemistry and Geology* (ed A. Lerman), pp. 295–321. Springer, New York.

Kemp, A.E.S. & Baldauf, J.G. (1993) Vast Neogene laminated diatom mat deposits from the eastern Equatorial Pacific Ocean. *Nature*, 362, 141–4.

Kemp, P.H. (1975) Wave asymmetry in the nearshore zone and breaker area. In: *Nearshore Sediment Dynamics and Sedimentation* (eds J. Hails & A. Carr), pp. 47–68. Wiley, New York.

Kemp, P.H. & Simons, R.R. (1982) The interaction between waves and a turbulent current: waves propagating with the current. *Journal of Fluid Mechanics*, 116, 227–50.

Kemp, A.E.S. *et al.* (1999) The role of mat-forming diatoms in the formation of Mediterranean sapropels. *Nature*, 398, 57–61.

Kendall, A.C. & Harwood, G.M. (1996) Marine evaporites: arid shorelines and basins. In: *Sedimentary Environments: Processes, Facies and Stratigraphy* (ed H.G. Reading), pp. 281–324. Blackwell Science, Oxford.

Kendall, G.S.C. & Schlager, W. (1981) Carbonates and relative changes in sea level. *Marine Geology*, 44, 180–212.

Kennedy, J.F. (1963) The mechanics of dunes and antidunes on crodible-bed channels. *Journal of Fluid Mechanics*, 16, 521–44.

Kennett, J.P. (1977) Cenozoic evolution of Antarctic glaciation, the circum-Antarctic ocean, and their impact on global palaeo-oceanography. *Journal of Geophysical Research*, 82, 3843–60.

Kennett, J.P. & Shackleton, N.J. (1976) Oxygen isotope evidence for the development of the psychrosphere 38 Ma ago. *Nature*, 260, 513–15.

Kennett, J.P., *et al.* (1974) Development of the circum-Antarctic current. *Science*, 186, 144–7.

Kent, P.E. (1966) The transport mechanism in catastrophic rockfalls. *Journal of Geology*, 74, 79–83.

Kenyon, N.H. & Stride, A.H. (1970) The tide-swept continental shelf sediments between the Shetland Isles and France. *Sedimentology*, 14, 159–73.

Kenyon, N.H., Belderson, R.H., Stride, A.H. & Johnson, M.A. (1981) Offshore tidal sand banks as indicators of net sand transport and as potential deposits. In: *Holocene Marine Sedimentation in the North Sea Basin*, (eds S.-D. Nio, R.T.E. Schüttenhelm & T.C.E. van Weering), pp. 257–68. Special Publication no. 5, International Association of Sedimentologists.

Kenyon, R.M. & Turcotte, D.L. (1985) Morphology of a delta prograding by bulk sediment transport. *Bulletin of the Geological Society of America*, 96, 1457–65.

Kerans, C., Lucia, F.J. & Senger, R.K. (1994) Integrated characterisation of carbonate ramp reservoirs using Permian San Andres Formation outcrop analogues. *Bulletin of the American Association of Petroleum Geologists*, 78, 181–216.

Kersey, D.G. & Hsu, K.J. (1976) Energy relations and density current flows: an experimental investigation. *Sedimentology*, 23, 761–90.

Keulegan, G.H. (1957) *Thirteenth Progress Report on Model Laws for Density Currents: An Experimental Study of the Motion of Saline Water from Locks into Freshwater Channels*. Report no. 5168, US National Bureau of Standards.

Khan, I.A., Bridge, J.S., Kappelman, J. & Wilson, R. (1997) Evolution of Miocene fluvial environments, eastern Potwar plateau, northern Pakistan. *Sedimentology*, 44, 221–51.

Kiehl, J.T. (1994) Clouds and their effects on the climate system. *Physics Today*, November, 36–42.

Kimberley, M.M. (1979) Origin of oolitic iron formations. *Journal of Sedimentary Petrology*, 49, 111–32.

Kinsman, D.J.J. (1966) Gypsum and anhydrite of Recent age, Trucial Coast, Persian Gulf. In: *Second Symposium on Salt* (ed. J.L. Rau), pp. 302–26. Northern Ohio Geological Society, Cleveland, OH.

Kinsman, D.J.J. (1975a) Salt floors to geosynclines. *Nature*, 255, 375–8.

Kinsman, D.J.J. (1975b) Rift valley basins and sedimentary history of trailing continental margins. In: *Petroleum and Global Tectonics* (eds A.G. Fischer & S. Judson), pp. 83–126. Princeton University Press, Princeton, NJ.

Kinsman, D.J.J. (1976) Evaporites: relative humidity control of primary mineral facies. *Journal of Sedimentary Petrology*, 46, 273–9.

Kirby, R. & Parker, W.R. (1983) Distribution and behavior of fine sediment in the Severn Estuary and Inner Bristol Channel, UK. *Canadian Journal of Fisheries and Aquatic Sciences*, 40, 83–95.

Kirkbride, A. (1993) Observations of the influence of bed roughness on turbulence structure in depth-limited flows over gravel beds. In: *Turbulence: Perspectives on Flow and Sediment Transport* (eds N.J. Clifford, J.R. French & J. Hardisty), pp. 185–96. Wiley, Chichester.

Kirkby, M.J. (1995) Modelling the links between vegetation and landforms. *Geomorphology*, 13, 319–35.

Kirkby, M.J. & Cox, N.J. (1995) A climatic index for soil erosion potential (CSEP) including seasonal and vegetation factors. *Catena*, 25, 333–52.

Kirkby, M.J. & Neale, R.H. (1987) A soil erosion model incorporating seasonal factors. In: *International Geomorphology 1986*, Part 2 (ed. V. Gardiner), pp. 189–210. Wiley, New York.

Klaucke, I., Hesse, R. & Ryan, W.B.F. (1997) Flow properties of turbidity currents in a low-sinuosity giant deep-sea channel. *Sedimentology*, 44, 1093–102.

Klaus, A., *et al.* (1992) Structural and stratigraphic evolution of the Sumisu Rift, Izu–Bonin Arc. *Proceedings of the Ocean Drilling Program, Scientific Results*, 126, 555–74.

Kline, S.J., Reynolds, W.C., Schraub, F.A. & Runstadler, P.W. (1967) The structure of turbulent boundary layers. *Journal of Fluid Mechanics*, 30, 741–73.

Kneller, B.C. (1996) Beyond the turbidite paradigm: physical models for deposition of turbidites and their implication for reservoir prediction. In: *Characterisation of Deep Marine Clastic Systems* (eds A. Hartley & D.J. Prosser), pp. 29–46. Special Publication no. 94, Geological Society of London.

Kneller, B.C. & Branney, M.J. (1995) Sustained high density turbidity currents and the deposition of massive sands. *Sedimentology*, 42, 607–16.

Kneller, B.C., *et al.* (1991) Oblique reflection of turbidity currents. *Geology*, 19, 250–2.

Knighton, D. (1998) *Fluvial Forms and Processes: a New Perspective*. Arnold, London.

Knight, J.B., Jaeger, H.M. & Nagel, S.R. (1993) Vibration-induced size separation in granular media: the convection connection. *Physical Review Letters*, 70, 3728–31.

Knox, J.C. (1983) Response of river systems to Holocene climates. In: *Late Quaternary Environments of the United States*, Vol. 2, *The Holocene* (ed. H.E. Wright Jr), pp. 26–41. University of Minnesota Press, Minneapolis.

Knuepfer, P.L.K. (1988) Estimating ages of late Quaternary stream terraces from analysis of weathering rinds and soils. *Bulletin of the Geological Society of America*, 100, 1224–36.

Kobluk, D.R. & Risk, M.J. (1977) Calcification of exposed filaments of endolithic algae, micrite envelope formation and sediment production. *Journal of Sedimentary Petrology*, 47, 517–28.

Kochel, R.C. (1990) Humid fans of the Appalachian Mountains. In: *Alluvial Fans: A Field Approach* (eds A.H. Rachocki & M. Church), pp. 109–30. Wiley, New York.

Kocurek, G. (1981) Significance of interdune deposits and bounding surfaces in eolian dune sands. *Sedimentology*, 28, 753–80.

Kocurek, G. (1988) First-order and super bounding surfaces in eolian sequences—bounding surfaces revisited. *Sedimentary Geology*, 56, 193–206.

Kocurek, G. (1996) Desert aeolian systems. In: *Sedimentary Environments: Processes, Facies and Stratigraphy* (ed H.G. Reading), pp. 125–55. Blackwell Science, Oxford.

Kocurek, G. & Nielson, J. (1986) Conditions favourable for the formation of warm-climate aeolian sand sheets. *Sedimentology*, 33, 795–816.

Kocurek, G., Havholm, K.G., Deynoux, M. & Blakey, R.C. (1991) Amalgamated accumulations resulting from climatic and eustatic changes, Akchar Erg, Mauritania. *Sedimentology*, 38, 751–72.

Kocurek, G., *et al.* (1992) Dune and dunefield development on Padre Island, Texas, with implications for interdune deposition and water-table-controlled accumulation. *Journal of Sedimentary Petrology*, 62, 622–35.

Kolb, C.R. & Van Lopik, J.R. (1958) *Geology of the Mississippi River Deltaic Plain*. Technical Reports nos. 3483 and 3484, US Corps of Engineers Waterways Experimental Station.

Komar, P.D. (1969) The channelized flow of turbidity currents with applications to Monterey deep-sea fan channel. *Journal of Geophysical Research*, 74, 4544–58.

Komar, P.D. (1971) The mechanics of sand transport on beaches. *Journal of Geophysical Research*, 76, 713–21.

Komar, P.D. (1974) Oscillatory ripple marks and the evaluation of ancient wave conditions and environments. *Journal of Sedimentary Petrology*, 44, 169–80.

Komar, P.D. (1975) Nearshore currents: generation by obliquely incident waves and longshore variations in breaker height. In: *Nearshore Sediment Dynamics and Sedimentation* (eds J. Hails & A. Carr), pp. 17–46. Wiley, New York.

Komar, P.D. (1998) *Beach processes and sedimentation*. Prentice Hall, Englewood Cliffs, NJ.

Komar, P.D. & Inman, D.L. (1970) Longshore sand transport on beaches. *Journal of Geophysical Research*, 75, 5914–27.

Komar, P.D., Neudeck, R.H. & Kulm, L.D. (1972)

Observations and significance of deep water oscillatory ripple marks on the Oregon continental shelf. In: *Shelf Sediment Transport: Process and Pattern* (eds D.J.P. Swift, D.B. Duane & O.H. Pilkey), pp. 601–19. Dowden, Hutchinson and Ross, Stroudsberg, PA.

Konhauser, K.O., Mann, H. & Fyfe, W.S. (1992) Prolific organic SiO_2 precipitation in a solute-deficient river: Rio Negro, Brazil. *Geology*, **20**, 227–30.

Koons, P.O. (1989) The topographic evolution of collisional mountain belts: a numerical look at the Southern Alps, New Zealand. *Annual Review of Earth and Planetary Sciences*, **23**, 375–408.

Kostaschuk, R.A. & Church, M.A. (1993) Macroturbulence generated by dunes: Fraser River, Canada. *Sedimentary Geology*, **85**, 25–37.

Kostaschuk, R.A. & Villard, P. (1996) Flow and sediment transport over large subaqueous dunes: Fraser River, Canada. *Sedimentology*, **43**, 849–63.

Kostaschuk, R.A., Church, M.A. & Luternauer, J.L. (1992) Sediment transport over salt-wedge intrusions: Fraser River estuary, Canada. *Sedimentology*, **39**, 305–17.

Koster, E.H. (1978) Transverse ribs: their characteristics, origin and palaeohydraulic significance. In: *Fluvial Sedimentology* (ed. A.D. Miall), pp. 161–86. Memoir no. 5, Canadian Society of Petroleum Geologists.

Kosters, E.C. (1989) Organic–clastic facies relationships and chronostratigraphy of the Barataria interlobe basin, Mississippi delta plain. *Journal of Sedimentary Petrology*, **59**, 98–113.

Kraft, J.C. (1971) Sedimentary facies patterns and geologic history of a Holocene marine transgression. *Bulletin of the Geological Society of America*, **82**, 2131–58.

Kraft, J.C. & John, C.J. (1979) Lateral and vertical facies relations of transgressive barrier. *Bulletin of the American Association of Petroleum Geologists*, **63**, 2145–63.

Kraft, J.C., Chrzastowski, M.J., Belknap, D.F., Toscano, M.A. & Fletcher, C.H. (1987) The transgressive barrier–lagoon coast of Delaware: morphostratigraphy, sedimentary sequences and responses to relative rises in sea level. In: *Sea Level Fluctuation and Coastal Evolution* (eds D. Nummedal, O.H. Pilkey & J.D. Howard), pp. 129–44. Special Publication no. 41, Society of Economic Palaeontologists and Mineralogists.

Kranck, K. (1975) Sediment deposition from flocculated suspensions. *Sedimentology*, **22**, 111–23.

Kranck, K. (1981) Particulate matter grain-size characteristics and flocculation in a partially mixed estuary. *Sedimentology*, **28**, 107–14.

Kraus, M.J. (1996) Avulsion deposits in Lower Eocene alluvial rocks, Bighorn Basin, Wyoming. *Journal of Sedimentary Research*, **66**, 354–63.

Kraus, M.J. & Aslan, A. (1993) Eocene hydromorphic paleosols: significance for interpreting ancient floodplain processes. *Journal of Sedimentary Petrology*, **63**, 453–63.

Krause, N.C. & Horikawa, K. (1990) Nearshore sediment

transport. In: *The Sea*, Vol. 9, *Ocean Engineering Science* (eds B. LeMehaute & D.M. Hanes), pp. 775–814. Wiley, New York.

Krauskopf, K.B. (1979) *Introduction to Geochemistry*, 2nd edn. McGraw-Hill, New York.

Krishnaswami, S., *et al.* (1992) Strontium isotopes and rubidium in the Ganga–Brahmaputra river system: weathering in the Himalaya, fluxes to the Bay of Bengal and contributions to the evolution of oceanic $^{87}Sr/^{86}Sr$. *Earth and Planetary Science Letters*, **109**, 243–53.

Kulm, L.D. *et al.* (1975) Oregon continental shelf sedimentation: interrelationships of facies distribution and sedimentary processes. *Journal of Geology*, **83**, 145–76.

Kumar, N. & Sanders, J.E. (1974) Inlet sequences: a vertical succession of sedimentary structures and textures created by the lateral migration of tidal inlets. *Sedimentology*, **21**, 491–532.

Kumar, N., *et al.* (1995) Increased biological productivity and export production in the glacial Southern Ocean. *Nature*, **378**, 675–80.

Kutzbach, J.E. & Street-Perrott, F.A. (1985) Milankovich forcing of fluctuations in the level of tropical lakes from 18 to 0 kyr BP. *Nature*, **317**, 130–4.

Laban, C. & Schüttenhelm, R.T.E. (1981) Some new evidence on the origin of the Zeeland ridges. In: *Holocene Marine Sedimentation in the North Sea Basin* (eds S.-D. Nio, R.T.E. Schüttenhelm & T.C.E. van Weering), pp. 239–45. Special Publication no. 5, International Association of Sedimentologists.

Lamb, H. (1945) *Hydrodynamics*, 6th edn. Cambridge University Press, Cambridge.

Lamb, H.H. (1948) *Hydrodynamics*. Cambridge University Press, Cambridge.

Lamb, H.H. (1995) *Climate, History and the Modern World*, 2nd edn. Routledge, London.

Lambe, T.W. & Whitman, R.V. (1969) *Soil Mechanics*. Wiley, New York.

Lancaster, N. (1989) The dynamics of star dunes: an example from Gran Desierto, Mexico. *Sedimentology*, **36**, 273–89.

Lancaster, N. (1992) Relations between dune generations in the Gran Desierto of Mexico. *Sedimentology*, **39**, 631–44.

Lancaster, N. (1995) *Geomorphology of Desert Dunes*. Routledge, London.

Langbein, W.B. & Schumm, S.A. (1958) Yield of sediment in relation to mean annual precipitation. *Transactions of the American Geophysical Union*, **39**, 1076–84.

Langford, R.P. (1989) Fluvial–aeolian interactions: Part 1, Modern systems. *Sedimentology*, **36**, 1023–35.

Langford, R.P. & Chan, M.A. (1989) Fluvial–aeolian interactions: Part 2, Ancient systems. *Sedimentology*, **36**, 1037–51.

Langford, R.P. & Chan, M.A. (1993) Downwind changes within an ancient dune sea, Permian Cedar Mesa

Sandstone, southeast Utah. In: *Aeolian Sediments Ancient and Modern* (ed. K. Pye), pp. 109–26. Special Publication no. 16, International Association of Sedimentologists.

Langhorne, D.N. & Read, A.A. (1986) The evolution and mechanics of modern intertidal and subtidal bedforms: their relevance to geological structures. *Journal of the Geological Society of London*, **143**, 957–62.

Laporte, L.F. (1971) Palaeozoic carbonate facies of the Central Appalachian Shelf. *Journal of Sedimentary Petrology*, **41**, 724–40.

Larcombe, P. & Jago, C.F. (1996) The morphological dynamics of intertidal megaripples in the Mawddach Estuary, North Wales, and the implications for palaeoflow reconstructions. *Sedimentology*, **43**, 541–59.

Larronne, J.B. & Reid, I. (1993) Very high rates of bedload sediment transport by ephemeral desert rivers. *Nature*, **366**, 148–50.

Lasaga, A.C. (1995) Fundamental approaches in describing mineral dissolution and precipitation rates. In: *Chemical Weathering Rates of Silicate Minerals* (eds A.F. White & S.L. Branfield), ch. 2. American Mineralogical Society, Washington, DC.

Lautridou, J.-P. & Ozouf, J.C. (1982) Experimental frost shattering: 15 years of research at the Centre de Géomorphologie du CNRS. *Progress in Physical Geography*, **6**, 215–32.

Lautridou, J.-P. & Scppala, M. (1986) Experimental frost shattering of some PreCambrian rocks, Finland. *Geografiska Annaler*, **68A**, 89–100.

Lavoie, D. (1995) A Late Ordovician high energy temperate-water carbonate ramp, southern Quebec, Canada: implications for Late Ordovician oceanography. *Sedimentology*, **42**, 95–116.

Lawton, T.F. (1986) Fluvial systems of the Upper Cretaceous Mesaverde Group and Paleocene North Horn Formation, central Utah: a record of transition from thin-skinned to thick-skinned deformation in the foreland region, pp. 423–42. Memoir no. 41, American Association of Petroleum Geologists.

Leatherman, S.P. (ed.) (1979) *Barrier Islands*. Academic Press, New York.

Leckie, D.A. & Krystink, L.F. (1989) Is there evidence for geostrophic currents preserved in the sedimentary record of inner to middle shelf deposits? *Journal of Sedimentary Petrology*, **59**, 862–70.

Leddy, J.O., Ashworth, P.J. & Best, J.L. (1993) Mechanism of anabranch avulsion within gravel-bed braided rivers: observation from a scaled physical model. In: *Braided Rivers* (eds J.L. Best & C.S. Bristow), pp. 119–27. Special Publication no. 75, Geological Society of London.

Ledwell, J.R., Watson, A.J. & Law, C.S. (1993) Evidence for slow mixing across the pycnocline from an open-ocean tracer release experiment. *Nature*, **364**, 701–3.

Lee, H.J. & Chough, S.K. (1989) Sediment distribution, dispersal and budget in the Yellow Sea. *Marine Geology*, **87**, 195–205.

Lee, M.R. & Parsons, I. (1995) Microtextural controls of weathering of perthitic alkali feldspars. *Geochimica et Cosmochimica Acta*, **59**, 4465–88.

Lee, M.R. & Parsons, I. (1998) Microtextural controls of diagenetic alteration of detrital alkali feldspars: a case study of the Shap Conglomerate (Lower Carboniferous), NW England. *Journal of Sedimentary Research*, **68**, 198–211.

Lee, T., You, C.-F. & Liu, T.-K. (1993) Model-dependent [10]Be sedimentation rates for the Taiwan Strait and their tectonic significance. *Geology*, 423–6.

Leeder, M.R. (1973) Fining-upwards cycles and the magnitude of palaeochannels. *Geological Magazine*, **110**, 265–76.

Leeder, M.R. (1975) Pedogenic carbonates and flood sediment accretion rates: a quantitative model for alluvial arid-zone lithofacies. *Geological Magazine*, **112**, 257–70.

Leeder, M.R. (1983) On the dynamics of sediment suspension by residual Reynolds stresses—confirmation of Bagnold's theory. *Sedimentology*, **30**, 485–91.

Leeder, M.R. (1993) Tectonic controls upon drainage basin development, river channel migration and alluvial architecture: implications for hydrocarbon reservoir development and characterization. Special Publication of the Geological Society of London **73**, 7–22.

Leeder, M.R. (1995) Continental rifts and proto-oceanic rift troughs. In: *Tectonics of Sedimentary Basins* (eds C. Busby & R. Ingersoll), pp. 119–48, Blackwell Science, Boston.

Leeder, M.R. (1996) Sedimentary basins: tectonic recorders of sediment discharge from drainage catchments. *Earth Surface Processes and Landforms*, **22**, 229–37.

Leeder, M.R. & Gawthorpe, R.L. (1987) Sedimentary models for extensional tiltblock/half graben basins. In: *Continental Extensional Tectonics* (eds M.P. Coward, J.F. Dewey & P.L. Hancock), pp. 139–52. Special Publication no. 28, Geological Society of London.

Leeder, M.R. & Jackson, J.A. (1993) The interaction between normal faulting and drainage in active extensional basins with examples from the Western United States and Greece. *Basin Research*, **5**, 79–102.

Leeder, M.R. & Stewart, M.D. (1996) Fluvial incision and sequence stratigraphy: alluvial responses to relative sea-level fall and their detection in the geologic record. In: *Sequence Stratigraphy in British Geology* (eds S.P. Hesselbo & D.N. Parkinson), pp. 25–39. Special Publication no. 103, Geological Society of London.

Leeder, M.R., Harris, T. & Kirkby, M.J. (1998) Sediment supply and climate change: implications for basin stratigraphy. *Basin Research*, **10**, 7–18.

Lees, A. (1975) Possible influences of salinity and temperature on modern shelf carbonate sedimentation. *Marine Geology*, **19**, 159–98.

Lees, A. & Miller, J. (1985) Facies variation in Waulsortian buildups, 2. Mid-Dinantian buildups from Europe and

North America. *Geological Journal*, **20**, 159–80.

Leg 155 Shipboard Scientific Party (1994) Drilled cores divulge history of continental and oceanic palaeoclimate. *EOS*, September, 435–7.

Leinen, M. (1979) Biogenic silica accumulation in the Central Equatorial Pacific and its implications for Cenozoic palaeo-oceanography. *Bulletin Geological Society America*, **90**, 801–3.

Leopold, A. (1991) *The River of the Mother of God and Other Essays* (eds S.L. Flader & J.B. Callicott). University of Wisconsin Press, Madison.

Leopold, L.B. & Bull, W.B. (1979) Base level, aggradation and grade. *Proceedings of the American Philosophical Society*, **123**, 168–202.

Lerman, A. (ed) (1978) *Lakes: physics, chemistry and geology.* Springer, New York.

van Leussen, W. (1997) The Kolmogorov microscale as a limiting value for the floc sizes of suspended fine-grained sediments in estuaries. In: *Cohesive Sediments* (eds N. Burt, R. Parker & J. Watts), pp. 45–62. Wiley, New York.

Levell, B.K., Braakman, J.H. & Rutlen, K.W. (1988) Oil-bearing sediments of Gondwana glaciation in Oman. *Bulletin of the American Association of Petroleum Geologists*, **72**, 775–96.

Lever, A. & McCave, I.N. (1983) Eolian components in Cretaceous and Tertiary North Atlantic sediments. *Journal of Sedimentary Petrology*, **53**, 811–32.

Levin, D.R. (1995) Occupation of a relict distributary system by a new tidal inlet, Quatre Bayou Pass, Louisiana. In: *Tidal Signatures in Modern and Ancient Sediments*, pp. 71–84. Special Publication no. 24, International Association of Sedimentologists.

Lezzar, K.E., *et al.* (1996) New seismic stratigraphy and Late Tertiary history of the North Tanganyika Basin, East African Rift system, deduced from multichannel and high resolution reflection seismic data and piston core evidence. *Basin Research*, **8**, 1–28.

Li, J., Lowenstein, T.K. & Blackburn, I.R. (1997) Responses of evaporite mineralogy to inflow water sources and climate during the past 100 ky in Death Valley, California. *Bulletin of the Geological Society of America*, **109**, 1361–71.

Li, X., *et al.* (1996) Dominance of mineral dust in aerosol light-scattering in the North Atlantic trade winds. *Nature*, **380**, 416–19.

Li, Y.-H. (1976) Denudation of Taiwan Island since the Pliocene Epoch. *Geology*, **4**, 105–7.

Lighthill, J. (1978) *Waves in Fluids.* Cambridge University Press, Cambridge.

Ligrani, P.M. & Moffat, R.J. (1986) Structure of transitionally rough and fully rough turbulent boundary layers. *Journal of Fluid Mechanics*, **162**, 69–98.

Linacre, E. & Geerts, B. (1997) *Climates and Weather Explained.* Routledge, London.

Link, M.H. & Osborne, R.H. (1982) Sedimentary facies of Ridge Basin, southern California. In: *Geologic History of Ridge Basin, Southern California* (eds J.C. Crowell & M.H. Link), pp. 63–78. Pacific Section, Society of Economic Palaeontologists and Mineralogists.

Lippmann, F. (1973) *Sedimentary Carbonate Minerals.* Springer, New York.

Lisitzin, A.P. (1996) *Oceanic Sedimentation.* American Geophysical Union, Washington, DC.

Livingstone, D.A. (1963) *Chemical Composition of Rivers and Lakes.* Professional Paper no. 440G, US Geological Survey.

Livingstone, I. & Thomas, D.S.G. (1993) Modes of linear dune activity and their paleoenvironmental significance: an evaluation with reference to southern African examples. In: *The Dynamics and Environmental Context of Aeolian Sedimentary Systems* (ed. K. Pye), pp. 91–101. Special Publication no. 72, Geological Society of London.

Lockwood, J.G. (1979) *Causes of Climate.* Edward Arnold, London.

Logan, B.W., *et al.* (eds) (1970) *Carbonate Sedimentation and Environments, Shark Bay, Western Australia.* Memoir no. 13, American Association of Petroleum Geologists.

Logan, B.W., *et al.* (eds) (1974) *Evolution and Diagenesis of Quaternary Carbonate Sequences, Shark Bay, W. Australia.* Memoir no. 22, American Association of Petroleum Geologists.

Logan, B.W. (1987) *The MacLeod Evaporite basin, Western Australia.* Memoir 44, American Association of Petroleum Geologists.

Longuet-Higgins, M.S. (1953) Mass transport in water waves. *Philosophical Transactions of the Royal Society, London (A)*, **245**, 535–81.

Longuet-Higgins, M.S. (1970) Longshore currents generated by obliquely incident sea waves. *Journal of Geophysical Research*, **75**, 6778–801.

Longuet-Higgins, M.S. & Stewart, R.W. (1964) Radiation stress in water waves; a physical discussion with applications. *Deep-Sea Research*, **11**, 529–63.

Loope, D.B. (1984) Origin of extensive bedding planes in aeolian sandstones: a defence of Stokes' hypothesis. *Sedimentology*, **31**, 123–32.

Loreau, J.-P. (1982) *Sédiments Aragonitique et leur Genese.* Memoires, Serie C, no. 47, Museum d'Histoire Naturelle, Paris.

Loreau, J.-P. & Purser, B.H. (1973) Distribution and ultrastructure of Holocene ooids in the Persian Gulf. In: *The Persian Gulf Holocene Carbonate Sedimentation and Diagenesis in a Shallow Epicontinental Sea* (ed. B.H. Purser), pp. 279–328. Springer, Heidelberg.

Loucks, R.G. & Sarg, J.F. (1993) *Carbonate Sequence Stratigraphy*, Memoir no. 57, American Association of Petroleum Geologists, Tulsa.

Lourens, L.J.A. *et al.* (1996) Evaluation of the Plio-Pleistocene astronomical timescale. *Palaeoceanography*, **11**, 391–431.

Lovelock, J.E. (1979) *Gaia: A New Look at Life on Earth.* Oxford University Press, Oxford.

Lovely, D.R., Stolz, J.F., Nord, G.L. & Phillips, E.J.P. (1987) Anaerobic production of magnetite by a dissimilatory iron-reducing microorganism. *Nature*, 330, 252–4.

Lovely, D.R., Phillips, E.J.P., Gorby, Y.A. & Landa, E.R. (1991) Microbial reduction of uranium. *Nature*, 350, 413–15.

Lowe, D.R. (1975) Water escape structures in coarse-grained sediments. *Sedimentology*, 22, 157–204.

Lowe, D.R. (1976) Grain flow and grain flow deposits. *Journal of Sedimentary Petrology*, 46, 188–99.

Lowe, D.R. (1982) Sediment gravity flows: 2. Depositional models with special reference to the deposits of high density turbidity currents. *Journal of Sedimentary Petrology*, 52, 279–97.

Lowe, D.R. & Lopiccolo, R.D. (1974) The characteristics and origins of dish and pillar structures. *Journal of Sedimentary Petrology*, 44, 484–501.

Lowenstam, H.A. (1963) Biologic problems relating to the composition and diagenesis of sediments. In: *The Earth Sciences—Problems and Progress in Current Research* (ed. T.W. Donnelly) 137–95. University of Chicago Press, Chicago.

Lowenstein, T.K. (1988) Origin of depositional cycles in a Permian 'saline giant': the Salado (McNutt Zone) evaporites of New Mexico and Texas. *Bulletin of the Geological Society of America*, 100, 592–608.

Lowenstein, T.K. & Hardie, L.A. (1985) Criteria for the recognition of salt-pan evaporites. *Sedimentology*, 32, 627–44.

Lucchi, R. & Camerlenghi, A. (1993) Upslope turbiditic sedimentation on the south eastern flank of the Mediterranean Ridge. *Bollettino di Oceanologia Teorica ed Applicata*, 11, 3–25.

Ludwig, W. & Probst, P. (1996) Predicting the oceanic input of organic carbon by continental erosion. *Global BioGeoChemical Cycles*, 10(1), 23–41.

Lustig, L.K. (1965) Clastic sedimentation in Deep Springs Valley, California. pp. 131–92. Professional Paper no. 352F, US Geological Survey.

Lynch, H.D. & Morgan, P. (1987) The tensile strength of the lithosphere and action of extension. In: *Continental Extensional Tectonics* (eds M.P. Coward, et al.), pp. 53–65. Special Publication no. 28, Geological Society of London.

Lyons, P.C. & Alpern, B. (eds) (1989) Peat and coal: origin, facies, and depositional models. *International Journal of Coal Geology*, 12, 1–4.

Lyons, T.W. (1997) Sulphur isotope trends and pathways of iron sulphide formation in upper Holocene sediments of the anoxic Black Sea. *Geochimica et Cosmochimica Acta*, 61, 3367–82.

McCabe, M. & Eyles, N. (1988) Sedimentology of an ice-contact glaciomarine delta, Carey Valley, Northern Ireland. *Sedimentary Geology*, 59, 1–14.

McCabe, P.J. (1984) Depositional environments of coal and coal bearing strata. In: *Sedimentology of Coal and Coal-bearing Sequences* (eds R.A. Rahmani & R.M. Flores), pp. 13–42. Special Publication no. 7, International Association of Sedimentologists.

McCabe, P.J. & Shanley, K.W. (1992) Organic control on shoreface stacking patterns: bogged down in the mire. *Geology*, 20, 741–4.

McCarthy, P.J., Martini, I.P. & Leckie, D.A. (1997) Anatomy and evolution of a Lower Cretaceous alluvial plain: sedimentology and palaeosols in the upper Blairmore Group, south-western Alberta, Canada. *Sedimentology*, 44, 197–220.

McCarthy, T.S., Stanistreet, I.G. & Cairncross, B. (1991) The sedimentary dynamics of active fluvial channels on the Okavango fan, Botswana. *Sedimentology*, 38, 471–87.

McCave, I.N. (1971) Sand waves in the North Sea off the coast of Holland. *Marine Geology*, 10, 199–225.

McCave, I.N. (1972) Transport and escape of fine-grained sediment from shelf areas. In: *Shelf Sediment Transport: Process and Pattern* (eds D.P. Swift, D.B. Doane & O.H. Pilkey), pp. 225–48. Dowden, Hutchinson and Ross, Stroudsberg, PA.

McCave, I.N. (1979) Tidal currents at the North Hinder lightship, southern North Sea: flow directions and turbulence in relation to maintenance of sand bars. *Marine Geology*, 31, 101–14.

McCave, I.N. (1995) Sedimentary processes and the creation of the stratigraphic record in the Late Quaternary North Atlantic Ocean. *Philosophical Transactions of the Royal Society of London*, B348, 229–41.

McCave, I.N. (1985) *Marine Geology*, 66, 169–88.

McCave, I.N. & Jones, K.P.N. (1988) Deposition of ungraded muds from high-density non-turbulent turbidity currents. *Nature*, 333, 250–2.

McCave, I.N., Lonsdale, P.F., Hollister, C.D. & Gardner, W.D. (1981) Sediment transport over the Halton and Gardar contourite drifts. *Journal of Sedimentary Petrology*, 50, 1049–62.

McClennan, S.M. (1993) Weathering and global denudation. *Journal of Geology*, 101, 295–303.

McEwan, I.K. & Willetts, B.B. (1993) Adaption of near-surface wind to the development of sand transport. *Journal of Fluid Mechanics*, 252, 99–115.

McEwan, I.K. & Willetts, B.B. (1994) On the prediction of bed-load sand transport rate in air. *Sedimentology*, 41, 1241–51.

McGillycuddy, D.J. et al. (1998) Influence of mesoscale eddies on new production in the Sargasso Sea. *Nature*, 394, 263–66.

McHargue, T.R. (1991) Seismic facies, processes and evolution of Miocene Inner Fan Channels, Indus submarine fan. In: *Seismic Facies and Sedimentary*

Processes of Submarine Fans and Turbidite Systems (eds P. Weimer & M.H. Link), pp. 403–14. Springer, Berlin.

Macintyre, I.G. (1988) Modern coral reefs of Western Atlantic: new geological perspective. *Bulletin of the American Association of Petroleum Geologists*, **72**, 1360–9.

Mack, G.H. & James, W.C. (1994) Paleoclimate and the global distribution of paleosols. *Journal of Geology*, **102**, 360–6.

Mack, G.H. & Leeder, M.R. (1998) Channel shifting of the Rio Grande, southern Rio Grande Rift: implications to alluvial stratigraphic models. *Sedimentary Geology*, **117**, 207–19.

Mack, G.H. & Leeder, M.R. (1999) Footwall-derived alluvial-fan and axial-fluvial lithofacies in the Plio-Pleistocene Palomas Half Graben, southern Rio Grande Rift, USA. *Journal of Sedimentary Research*, (in press).

Mack, G.H. & Seager, W.R. (1990) Tectonic control on facies distribution of the Camp Rice and Palomas Formations (Pliocene–Pleistocene) in the southern Rio Grande rift. *Bulletin of the Geological Society of America*, **102**, 45–53.

Mack, G.H., James, W.C. & Monger, H.C. (1993) Classification of paleosols. *Bulletin of the Geological Society of America*, **105**, 129–36.

Mack, G.H., *et al.* (1994) Stable oxygen and carbon isotopes of pedogenic carbonate as indicators of Plio-Pleistocene paleoclimate in the southern Rio Grande rift, south-central New Mexico. *American Journal of Science*, **294**, 621–40.

McKean, J.A., Dietrich, W.E., Finkel, R.C., Southon, J.R. & Caffee, M.W. (1993) Quantification of soil production and downslope creep rates from cosmogenic [10]Be accumulations on a hillslope profile. *Geology*, **21**, 343–6.

McKee, E.D. (1966) Structure of dunes at White Sands National Monument, New Mexico. *Sedimentology*, **7**, 1–61.

McKee, E.D. (ed.) (1978) *A Study of Global Sand Seas*. Professional Paper no. 1052, US Geological Survey.

McKenzie, D.P. (1978) Some remarks on the development of sedimentary basins. *Earth and Planetary Science Letters*, **40**, 25–32.

Mackenzie, F.T. & Morse, J.W. (1992) Sedimentary carbonates through Phanerozoic time. *Geochimica et Cosmochimica Acta*, **56**, 3281–95.

Mackey, S.D. & Bridge, J.S. (1995) Three-dimensional model of alluvial stratigraphy: theory and application. *Journal of Sedimentary Research*, **65**, 7–31.

Macklin, M.G., Rumsby, B.T. & Heap, T. (1992) Flood alluviation and entrenchment: Holocene valley-floor development and transformation in the British uplands. *Bulletin of the Geological Society of America*, **104**, 631–43.

McLellan, H. (1965) *Elements of Physical Oceanography*. Pergamon, Oxford.

McManus, J.F., Oppo, D.W. & Cullen, J.L. (1999) A 0.5–million-year record of millenial-scale climate variability in the North Atlantic. *Science*, **283**, 971–75.

MacNeil, F.S. (1954) Organic reefs and banks and associated detrital sediments. *American Journal of Science*, **252**, 385–401.

McTigue, D.F. (1981) Mixture theory for suspended sediment transport. *Journal of the Hydraulics Division, American Society of Civil Engineers*, **107**, HY6, 659–73.

Maddox, J. (1990) Sandpiles as paradigms of noise. *Nature*, **347**, 225.

Mainguet, M. (1978) The influence of trade winds, local airmasses and topographic obstacles on the aeolian movement of sand particles and the origin and distribution of dunes and ergs in the Sahara and Australia. *Geoforum*, **9**, 17–28.

Mainguet, M. (1983) Tentative mega-morphological study of the Sahara. In: *Mega-geomorphology* (eds R. Gardner & H. Scoging), pp. 113–33. Clarendon Press, Oxford.

Mainguet, M. & Canon, L. (1976) Vents et paleovents du Sahara. Tentative d'approche paleoclimatique. *Revue Geographie Physique et de Geologie Dynamique*, **18**, 241–50.

Maizels, J. (1989) Sedimentology, paleoflow dynamics and flood history of Jökulhlaup deposits: palaeohydrology of Holocene sediment sequences in southern Iceland Sandur deposits. *Journal of Sedimentary Petrology*, **59**, 204–23.

Maizels, J. (1990) Long-term palaeochannel evolution during episodic growth of an exhumed Plio-Pleistocene alluvial fan, Oman. In: *Alluvial Fans: A Field Approach* (eds A.H. Rachocki & M. Church), pp. 271–304. Wiley, New York.

Major, J.J. (1997) Depositional processes in large-scale debris-flow experiments. *Journal of Geology*, **105**, 345–66.

Makse, H.A., Havlin, S., King, P.R. & Stanley, H.E. (1997) Spontaneous stratification in granular mixtures. *Nature*, **386**, 379–82.

Makse, H.A., *et al.* (1998) Experimental studies of stratification in a granular Hele–Shaw cell. *Philosophical Magazine*, **77B**, 1341–51.

Malakoff, D. (1998) Death by suffocation in the Gulf of Mexico. *Science*, **281**, 190–92.

Mann, P. (1997) Model for the formation of large, transtensional basins in zones of tectonic escape. *Geology*, **25**, 211–14.

Marriott, S.B. (1996) Analysis and modelling of overbank deposits. In: Floodplain Processes (eds M.G. Anderson *et al.*), pp. 63–93. Wiley, New York.

Marsaglia, K.M. (1995) Interarc and backarc basins. In: *Tectonics of Sedimentary Basins* (eds C. Busby & R. Ingersoll), pp. 299–330, Blackwell Science, Oxford.

Marsaglia, K.M., *et al.* (1995) Sedimentation in Western Pacific backarc basins: new insights from recent ODP drilling. In: *Active Margins and Marginal Basins of the Western Pacific*, pp. 291–314. Geophysical Monograph no. 88, American Geophysical Union.

Martin, J.H., Gordon, R.M. & Fitzwater, S.E. (1990) Iron in Antarctic waters. *Nature*, **345**, 156–8.

Martin, J.H. *et al.* (1994) Testing the iron hypothesis in ecosystems of the Equatorial Pacific, *Nature*, **371**, 123–9.

Marzo, M. & Anadon, P. (1988) Anatomy of a conglomeratic fan-delta complex: the Eocene Montserrat Conglomerate, Ebro Basin, northeastern Spain. In: *Fan Deltas: Sedimentology and Tectonic Settings* (eds W. Nemec & R.J. Steel), pp. 318–41. Blackie, London.

Marzo, M., Nijman, W. & Puigdefabregas, C. (1988) Architecture of the Castissent fluvial sheet sandstones, Eocene, South Pyrenees, Spain. *Sedimentology*, **35**, 719–38.

Massari, F. & Colella, A. (1988) Evolution and types of fan-delta systems in some major tectonic settings. In: *Fan Deltas. Sedimentology and Tectonic Settings* (eds W. Nemec & R.J. Steel), pp. 103–22. Blackie, London.

Massari, F. & Parea, G.C. (1988) Progradational gravel beach sequences in a moderate- to high-energy, microtidal marine environment. *Sedimentology*, **35**, 881–913.

Massey, B.S. (1979) *Mechanics of Fluids*, 4th edn. Van Nostrand Reinhold, New York.

Masson, D.G. (1994) Late Quaternary turbidity current pathways to the Madeira abyssal plain and some constraints on turbidity current mechanisms. *Basin Research*, **6**, 17–33.

Masson, D.G. (1996) Catastrophic collapse of the volcanic island of Hierro 15 ka ago and the history of landslides in the Canary Islands. *Geology*, **24**, 231–4.

Masson, D.G., Kidd, R.B., Gardner, J.V., Huggett, Q.J. & Weaver, P.P.E. (1992) Saharan continental rise: facies distribution and sediment slides. In: *Geologic Evolution of Atlantic Continental Rises* (eds C.W. Poag & P.C. de Graciansky), pp. 327–43. Van Nostrand Reinhold, New York.

Matter, A. & Tucker, M.E. (eds) (1978) *Modern and Ancient Lake Sediments*. International Association of Sedimentologists, Special Publication **2**.

Mathews, R.K. (1966) Genesis of recent lime mud in British Honduras. *Journal of Sedimentary Petrology*, **36**, 428–54.

Matyas, E.L. (1984) Profiles of modern prograding deltas. *Canadian Journal of Earth Sciences*, **21**, 1156–60.

Maxwell, W.G.H. & Swinchatt, J.P. (1970) Great Barrier Reef: regional variation in a terrigenous-carbonate province. *Bulletin of the Geological Society of America*, **81**, 691–724.

Mayer, L., Gerson, R. & Bull, W.B. (1984) Alluvial gravel production and deposition: a useful indicator of Quaternary climatic change in deserts. *Catena Supplement*, **5**, 137–51.

Maynard, J.R. & Leeder, M.R. (1992) On the periodicity and magnitude of Late Carboniferous glacio-eustatic sea-level changes. *Journal of the Geological Society of London*, **149**, 303–11.

Mazullo, S.J., Bischoff, W.D. & Teal, C.S. (1995) Holocene shallow subtidal dolomitization by near-normal seawater, northern Belize. *Geology*, **23**, 341–4.

Medwedeff, D.A. & Wilkinson, B.H. (1983) Cortical fabrics in calcite and aragonite ooids. In: *Coated Grains* (ed. T.M. Peryt), pp. 109–15. Springer, Berlin.

Meehl, G.A. (1992) Effect of tropical topography on global climate. *Annual Review of Earth and Planetary Sciences*, **20**, 85–112.

Mehta, A.J. (1989) On estuarine cohesive sediment suspension behaviour. *Journal of Geophysical Research*, **94**, 14303–14.

Mehta, A. & Barker, G.C. (1991) Vibrated powders: a macroscopic approach. *Physical Review Letters*, **67**, 394–7.

Melim, L.A. & Scholle, P.A. (1995) The forereef facies of the Permian Capitan Formation: the role of sediment supply vs sea-level changes. *Journal of Sedimentary Research*, **B65** 107–18.

Mellere, D. & Steel, R.J. (1995) Facies architecture and sequentiality of nearshore and 'shelf' sandbodies: Haystack Mountains Formation, Wyoming, USA. *Sedimentology*, **42**, 551–74.

Melosh, H.J. (1979) Accoustic fluidisation: a new geological process? *Journal of Geophysical Research*, **84**, 7513–20.

Melosh, H.J. (1987) The mechanics of large rock avalanches. In: *Debris Flows/Avalanches: Processes, Recognition, and Mitigation* (eds J.E. Costa & G.F. Wieczorek), pp. 41–9. Reviews in Engineering geology no. 7, Geological Society of America.

Melton, M.A. (1965) The geomorphic and palaeoclimatic significance of alluvial deposits in southern Arizona. *Journal of Geology*, **73**, 1–38.

Menzies, J. (1995) *Modern Glacial Environments*. Butterworth Heinemann, Oxford.

Menzies, J. & Rose, J. (eds) (1989) Subglacial bedforms—drumlins, Rogen moraine and associated subglacial bedforms. *Sedimentary Geology*, **62**, 2–4.

Mertes, L.A.K. (1994) Rates of flood-plain sedimentation on the central Amazon River. *Geology*, **22**, 171–4.

Mertes, L.A.K., Dunne, T. & Martinelli, L.A. (1996) Channel–floodplain geomorphology along the Solimões–Amazon River, Brazil. *Bulletin of the Geological Society of America*, **108**, 1089–107.

Meyer, G.A., Wells, S.G., Balling, R.C. & Jull, A.J.T. (1992) Response of alluvial systems to fire and climate change in Yellowstone National Park. *Nature*, **357**, 147–50.

Meyer, H.J. (1984) The influence of impurities on the growth rate of calcite. *Journal of Crystal Growth*, **66**, 639–46.

Miall, A.D. (1985) Sedimentation on an early Proterozoic continental margin under glacial influence: the Gowganda Formation (Huronian), Elliott Lake area, Ontario, Canada. *Sedimentology*, **32**, 763–88.

Miall, A.D. (1991) Stratigraphic sequences and their chronostratigraphic correlation. *Journal of Sedimentary Petrology*, **61**, 497–505.

Miall, A.D. (1994) Reconstructing fluvial macroform architecture from two-dimensional outcrops: examples from the Castlegate Sandstone, Book Cliffs, Utah. *Journal of Sedimentary Research*, **64**, 146–58.

Miall, A.D. (1995) Collision-related foreland basins. In: *Tectonics of Sedimentary Basins* (eds C. Busby & R. Ingersoll), pp. 393–424, Blackwell Science, Oxford.

Miall, A.D. (1996) *The Geology of Fluvial Deposits*. Springer, Berlin.

Miall, A.D. (1997) *The Geology of Stratigraphic Sequences*. Springer, Berlin.

Middleton, G.V. (1965) Antidune cross-bedding in a large flume. *Journal of Sedimentary Petrology*, **35**, 922–7.

Middleton, G.V. (1966a) Experiments on density and turbidity currents. 1: Motion of the head. *Canadian Journal of Earth Sciences*, **3**, 523–46.

Middleton, G.V. (1966b) Experiments on density and turbidity currents. 2: Uniform flow of density currents. *Canadian Journal of Earth Sciences*, 3, 627–37.

Middleton, G.V. (1966c) Experiments on density and turbidity currents. 3: Deposition of sediment. *Canadian Journal of Earth Sciences*, 4, 475–505.

Middleton, G.V. (1970) Experimental studies related to problems of flysch sedimentation. In: *Flysch Sedimentology in N. America* (ed. J. Lajoie), pp. 253–72. Report no. 7, Geological Association of Canada.

Middleton, G.V. & Wilcock, P.R. (1994) *Mechanics in the Earth and Environmental Sciences*. Cambridge University Press, Cambridge.

Middleton, N.J., Goudie, A.S. & Wells, G.L. (1986) The frequency and source areas of dust storms. In: *Aeolian Geomorphology* (ed. W.G. Nickling), pp. 237–60. Allen and Unwin, Boston.

Midtgaard, H.H. (1996) Inner-shelf to lower-shoreface hummocky sandstone bodies with evidence for geostrophic influenced combined flow, Lower Cretaceous, West Greenland. *Journal of Sedimentary Research*, **66**, 343–53.

Miller, E.K., Blum, J.D. & Friedland, A.J. (1993) Determination of soil exchangeable-cation loss and weathering rates using Sr isotopes. *Nature*, **362**, 438–41.

Miller, M.C., McCave, I.N. & Komar, P.D. (1977) Threshold of sediment motion under unidirectional currents. *Sedimentology*, **24**, 507–28.

Milliman, J.D. & Mead, R.H. (1983) World-wide delivery of river sediment to the oceans. *Journal of Geology*, **91**, 1–21.

Milliman, J.D. & Syvitski, J.P.M. (1992) Geomorphic/tectonic control of sediment discharge to the ocean: the importance of small mountainous rivers. *Journal of Geology*, **100**, 525–44.

Milliman, J.D., Freile, D., Steinen, R.P. & Wilber, R.J. (1993) Great Bahama Bank aragonite muds: mostly inorganically precipitated, mostly exported. *Journal of Sedimentary Petrology*, **63**, 589–95.

Milner, C. & Hughes, R.E. (1968) *Methods for Estimating the Primary Production of Grasslands*, IBP Handbook no. 6. Blackwell Scientific Publications, Oxford.

Molnar, P. & England, P.C. (1990) Late Cenozoic uplift of

mountain ranges and global climate change: chicken or egg? *Nature*, **346**, 29–34.

Molnar, P., England, P. & Martinod, J. (1993) Mantle dynamics, uplift of the Tibetan Plateau, and the Indian monsoon. *Reviews of Geophysics*, **31**, 357–96.

Molnia, B.F. (ed.) (1983a) *Glacial-Marine Sedimentation*. Plenum, New York.

Molnia, B.F. (1983b) Subarctic glacial-marine sedimentation: a model. In: *Glacial-Marine Sedimentation* (ed. B.F. Molnia), pp. 95–144. Plenum, New York.

Moore, G.T. (1979) Mississippi river delta—April 9, 1976—from Landsat 2. *Bulletin of the American Association of Petroleum Geologists*, **63**, 660–7.

Moore, J.G. & Mark, R.K. (1986) World slope map. *EOS*, 2 December, 1353–62.

Moore, J.G., *et al.* (1989) Prodigious submarine landslides on the Hawaiian Ridge. *Journal of Geophysical Research*, **94**, 17465–84.

Moore, J.N., Fritz, W.J. & Futch, R.S. (1984) Occurrence of megaripples in a ridge and runnel system. Sapelo Island, Georgia: morphology and processes. *Journal of Sedimentary Petrology*, **54**, 615–25.

Morris, J.D. (1991) Applications of cosmogenic [10]Be to problems in the earth sciences. *Annual Review of Earth and Planetary Sciences*, **19**, 313–50.

Morse, J.W. (1974) Dissolution kinetics of calcium carbonate in sea water. III. A new method for the study of carbonate reaction kinetics. *American Journal of Science*, **274**, 97–107.

Morse, J.W. & Berner, R.A. (1972) Dissolution kinetics of calcium carbonate in seawater. 11: A kinetic origin for the lysocline. *American Journal of Science*, **272**, 840–51.

Morse, J.W., *et al.* (1984) The carbonate chemistry of Grand Bahama Bank waters: after 18 years, another look. *Journal of Geophysical Research*, **89**, 3604–14.

Morse, J.W., Wang, Q. & Tsio, M.Y. (1997) Influences of temperature and Mg:Ca ratio on $CaCO_3$ precipitates from seawater. *Geology*, **25**, 85–7.

Morton, R.A. (1981) Formation of storm deposits by wind-forced currents in the Gulf of Mexico and the North Sea. In: *Holocene Marine Sedimentation in the North Sea Basin* (eds S.-D. Nio, R.T.E. Schüttenhelm & T.C.E. van Weering), pp. 385–96. Special Publication no. 5, International Association of Sedimentologists.

Moum, J.N. & Caldwell, D.R. (1994) Experiment explores the dynamics of ocean mixing. *EOS*, **75**, 489–90.

Mountjoy, E.W., Cook, H.E. & Pray, L.C. (1972) Allochthonous carbonate debris flows—worldwide indicators of reef complexes, banks or shelf margins. *Proceedings of the 24th International Geological Congress*, Vol. 6, pp. 172–89.

Mountney, N.P. & Westbrook, G.K. (1996) Modelling sedimentation in ocean trenches: the Nankai Trough from 1 Ma to present. *Basin Research*, **8**, 85–101.

de Mowbray, T. & Visser, M.J. (1984) Reactivation surfaces in subtidal channel deposits, Oosterchelde, southwest Netherlands. *Journal of Sedimentary Petrology*, **54**, 811–24.

Muck, M.T. & Underwood, M.B. (1990) Upslope flow of turbidity currents: a comparison among field observations, theory, and laboratory models. *Geology*, **18**, 54–7.

Muir, I.J., Bancroft, G.M., Shotyk, W. & Nesbitt, H.W. (1990) A SIMS and XPS study of dissolving plagioclase. *Geochimica et Cosmochimica Acta*, **54**, 2247–56.

Mukerji, A.B. (1990) The Chandigarth Dun alluvial fans: an analysis of the process–form relationship. In: *Alluvial Fans: A Field Approach* (eds A.H. Rachocki & M. Church), pp. 131–49. Wiley, New York.

Mulder, T. & Syvitski, J.P.M. (1995) Turbidity currents generated at river mouths during exceptional discharges to the world's oceans. *Journal of Geology*, **103**, 285–99.

Mulder, T., Savoye, B. & Syvitski, J.P.M. (1997) Numerical modelling of a mid-sized gravity flow: the 1979 Nice turbidity current (dynamics, processes, sediment budget and seafloor impact). *Sedimentology*, **44**, 305–26.

Muller, A. & Gyr, A. (1982) Visualisation of the mixing layer behind dunes. In: *Mechanics of Sediment Transport*, Euromech 156 (eds B. Mutlu Sumer & A. Muller), pp. 41–5. Balkema, Rotterdam.

Muller, A. & Gyr, A. (1986) On the vortex formation in the mixing layer behind dunes. *Journal of Hydraulic Research*, **24**, 359–75.

Mullins, H.T. & Hine, A.C. (1989) Scalloped bank margins: beginning of the end for carbonate platforms? *Geology*, **17**, 30–3.

Mullins, H.T. & Neumann, A.C. (1979) Deep carbonate bank margin structure and sedimentation in the northern Bahamas. In: (eds L. Doyle & D.H. Pilkey) Special Publication **27**, Society of Economic Palaeontologists and Mineralogists.

Mullins, H.T., Neumann, A.C., Wilber, R.J. & Boardman, M.R. (1980a) Nodular carbonate sediment on Bahamian slopes: possible precursors to nodular limestones. *Journal of Sedimentary Petrology*, **50**, 117–31.

Mullins, H.T., Neumann, A.C., Wilber, R.J., Hine, A.C. & Chinburg, S.J. (1980b) Carbonate sediment drifts in Northern Straits of Florida. *Bulletin of the American Association of Petroleum Geologists*, **64**, 1701–17.

Mullins, H.T., Heath, K.C., Van Buren, M. & Newton, C.R. (1984) Anatomy of a modern open ocean carbonate slope: Northern Little Bahama bank. *Sedimentology*, **31**, 141–68.

Murray, A.B. & Paola, C. (1994) A cellular model of braided rivers. *Nature*, **371**, 54–7.

Murray, P.B., Davies, A.G. & Soulsby, R.L. (1991) Sediment pick-up in wave and current flows. In: *Sand Transport in Rivers, Estuaries and the Sea*, Euromech 262 (eds R.L. Soulsby & R. Bettess), pp. 37–44. Balkema, Rotterdam.

Murray, S.P. (1970) Bottom currents near the coast during hurricane Camille. *Journal of Geophysical Research*, **75**, 4579–82.

Murray, T. & Clarke, G.K.C. (1995) Black-box modelling of the subglacial water system. *Journal of Geophysical Research*, **100**, 10 231–45.

Muto, T. (1989) A method of detecting tectonic tilting events from geologic records of coastal alluvial fans. *Journal of Geology*, **97**, 640–5.

Mutti, E. & Normark, W.R. (1991) An integrated approach to the study of turbidite systems. In: *Seismic Facies and Sedimentary Processes of Submarine Fans and Turbidite Systems* (eds P. Weimer & M.H. Link), pp. 75–106. Springer, Berlin.

Myers, K.J. & Milton, N.J. (1996) Concepts and principles of sequence stratigraphy. In: *Sequence Stratigraphy* (eds D. Emery & K.J. Myers), pp. 11–44. Blackwell Science, Oxford.

Mylroie, J.E. & Carew, J.L. (1988) Solution conduits as indicators of late Quaternary sea level position. *Quaternary Science Reviews*, **7**, 55–64.

Mylroie, J.E. & Carew, J.L. (1990) The flank margin model for dissolution cave development in carbonate platforms. *Earth Surface Processes and Landforms*, **15**, 413–24.

Myrow, P.M. & Southard, J.B. (1991) Combined-flow model for vertical stratification sequences in shallow marine storm-deposited beds. *Journal of Sedimentary Petrology*, **61**, 202–10.

Nadon, G.C. (1998) Magnitude and timing of peat-to-coal compaction. *Geology*, **26**, 727–30.

Nagy, K.L. (1995) Dissolution and precipitation kinetics of sheet silicates. In: *Chemical Weathering Rates of Silicate Minerals* (eds A.F. White & S.L. Branfield), ch. 5. American Mineralogical Society, Washington, DC.

Naish, T. (1997) Constraints on the amplitude of late Pliocene eustatic sea-level fluctuations: new evidence from the New Zealand shallow marine sediment record. *Geology*, **25**, 1139–42.

Nanson, G.C. (1980) Point bar and floodplain formation of the meandering Beatton River, northeastern British Columbia, Canada. *Sedimentology*, **27**, 3–29.

Narbonne, G.M. & James, N.P. (1996) Mesoproterozoic deep-water reefs from Borden Peninsula, Arctic Canada. *Sedimentology*, **43**, 827–48.

Needham, R.S. (1978) Giant-scale hydroplastic deformation structures formed by the loading of basalt on to water-saturated sand, Middle Proterozoic, Northern Territory, Australia. *Sedimentology*, **25**, 285–96.

Neev, D. (1978) Messinian and Holocene gypsum deposits of relatively deep water. *Abstracts Volume 10th International Association of Sedimentologists Meeting*, Jerusalem, Vol. 2, p. 459.

Neev, D. & Emery, K.O. (1967) The Dead Sea: depositional processes and environments of evaporites, *Israel Geological Survey Bulletin*, **41**, 1–147.

Nelson, C.S., Keane, S.L. & Head, P.S. (1988) Non-tropical carbonate deposits on the modern New Zealand shelf. *Sedimentary Geology*, **60**, 71–94.

Nemec, W. & Postma, G. (1993) Quaternary alluvial fans

in southwestern Crete: sedimentation processes and geomorphic evolution. In: *Alluvial Sedimentation* (eds M. Marzo & C. Puigdefabregas), pp. 235–76. Special Publication no. 17, International Association of Sedimentologists.

Nemec, W. & Steel, R.J. (eds) (1988) *Fan Deltas: Sedimentology and Tectonic Settings*. Blackie, London.

Nesbitt, H.W. & Young, G.M. (1982) Early Proterozoic climates and plate motions inferred from major element chemistry of lutites. *Nature*, **299**, 715–17.

Nesbitt, H.W. & Young, G.M. (1989) Formation and diagenesis of weathering profiles. *Journal of Geology*, **97**, 129–47.

Nesbitt, H.W., Fedo, C.M. & Young, G.M. (1997) Quartz and feldspar stability. Steady and non-steady state weathering, and petrogenesis of siliciclastic sands and muds. *Journal of Geology*, **105**, 173–91.

Neumann, A.C. & Land, L.S. (1975) Lime mud deposition and calcareous algae in the Bight of Anaco, Bahamas: a budget. *Journal of Sedimentary Petrology*, **45**, 763–86.

Neumann, A.C., Kofoed, J.W. & Keller, G.H. (1977) Lithoherms in the Straits of Florida. *Geology*, **5**, 4–10.

Newbould, P.J. (1967) *Methods for Estimating the Primary Production of Forests*. IBP Handbook no. 2. Blackwell Scientific Publications, Oxford.

Newton, M.S. (1994) Holocene fluctuations of Mono Lake, California: the sedimentary record. In: *Sedimentology and Geochemistry of Modern and Ancient Saline Lakes* (eds R.W. Renaut & W.M. Last), pp. 143–57. Special Publication no. 50, Society of Economic Palaeontologists and Mineralogists.

Nguyen, Q.D. & Boger, D.V. (1992) Measuring the flow properties of yield stress fluids. *Annual Review of Fluid Mechanics*, **24**, 47–88.

Nichol, S.L., Zaitlin, B.A. & Thom, B.G. (1997) The upper Hawkesbury River, New South Wales, Australia: a Holocene example of an estuarine bayhead delta. *Sedimentology*, **44**, 263–86.

Nichols, G.J. (1987) Structural controls on fluvial distributary systems—the Luna System, northern Spain. In: *Recent Developments in Fluvial Sedimentology* (eds F.G. Ethridge, R.M. Flores & M.D. Harvey), pp. 269–78. Special Publication no. 39, Society of Economic Paleontologists and Mineralogists.

Nichols, R.J. (1995) The liquification and remobilisation of sandy sediments. In: *Characterisation of Deep Marine Clastic Systems* (eds A.J. Hartley & D.J. Prosser), pp. 63–76. Special Publication no. 94, Geological Society of London.

Nichols, R.J., Sparks, R.S.J. & Wilson, C.J.N. (1994) Experimental studies of the fluidisation of layered sediments and the formation of fluid escape structures. *Sedimentology*, **41**, 233–53.

Nielsen, P. (1992) *Coastal Bottom Boundary Layers and Sediment Transport*. World Scientific, Singapore.

Nijman, W. (1998) Cyclicity and basin axis shift in a piggyback basin: towards modelling of the Eocene Tremp-Ager Basin, South Pyrenees, Spain. In: (eds Mascle *et al.*) Cenozoic Foreland Basins of Western Europe. Geological Society of London, Special Publication **134**, 135–62.

Nijman, W., Willigers, B.J.A. & Krikke, A. (1998) Tensile and compressive growth structures: relationships between sedimentation, deformation and granite intrusion in the Archaean Coppin Gap greenstone belt, Eastern Pilbara, Western Australia. *PreCambrian Research*, **88**, 83–108.

Nilsen, T.H. & Sylvester, A.G. (1995) Strike-slip basins. In: *Tectonics of Sedimentary Basins* (eds C. Busby & R. Ingersoll), pp. 425–58. Blackwell Science, Oxford.

Nittrouer, C.A. & Kuehl, S.A. (eds) (1995) Geological significance of sediment transport and accumulation on the Amazon continental shelf. *Marine Geology*, **125**, 175–399.

Nittrouer, C.A. & Wright, L.D. (1994) Transport of particles across continental shelves. *Reviews of Geophysics*, **32**, 85–113.

Normark, W.R. & Piper, D.J.W. (1972) Sediments and growth pattern of Navy deep-sea fan, San Clemente Basin, California Borderland. *Journal of Geology*, **80**, 198–223.

Normark, W.R. & Piper, D.J.W. (1984) Navy Fan, California Borderland: growth pattern and depositional processes. *Geo-Marine Letters*, **3**, 101–8.

Normark, W.R., Piper, D.J.W. & Hess, G.R. (1979) Distributary channels, sand lobes, and mesotopography of Navy submarine fan, California Borderland, with applications to ancient fan sediments. *Sedimentology*, **26**, 749–74.

Normark, W.R., Posamentier, H. & Mutti, E. (1993) Turbidite systems: state of the art and future directions. *Reviews of Geophysics*, **31**, 91–116.

North, C.P. & Prosser, D.J. (eds) (1993a) *Characterisation of Fluvial and Aeolian Reservoirs*. Special Publication no. 73, Geological Society of London.

Nott, J. & Roberts, R.G. (1996) Time and process rates over the past 100 my: a case for dramatically increased landscape denudation rates during the late Quaternary in northern Australia. *Geology*, **24**, 883–7.

Nummedal, D. & Penland, S. (1981) Sediment dispersal in Norderneyer Seegate, West Germany. In: (eds S.D. Nio, *et al.*) Special Publication 5, International Association of Sedimentologists, 187–210.

O'Connell, S., Ryan, W.B.F. & Normark, W.R. (1991) Evolution of a fan-channel on the surface of the outer Mississippi fan: evidence from side-looking sonar. In: *Seismic Facies and Sedimentary Processes of Submarine Fans and Turbidite Systems* (eds P. Weimer & M.H. Link), pp. 365–382. Springer, Berlin.

O'Connell, S., Chandler, M.A. & Ruedy, R. (1996) Implications for the creation of warm saline deep water: Late Palaeocene reconstructions and global climate model simulations. *Bulletin Geological Society America*, **108**, 270–84.

O'Connor, J.E., *et al.* (1994) A 4500 year record of large

floods on the Colorado River in the Grand Canyon, Arizona. *Journal of Geology*, 102, 1–9.

Oertel, G.F. (1979) Barrier island development during the Holocene recession, SE United States. In: *Barrier Islands* (ed. S.P. Leatherman), pp. 273–90. Academic Press, New York.

Oertel, G.F. (1988) Processes of sediment exchange between tidal inlets, ebb deltas and barrier islands. In: *Hydrodynamics and Sediment Dynamics of Tidal Inlets* (eds D.G. Aubrey & L. Weishar), pp. 297–318. Springer, Berlin.

Okazaki, H. & Masuda, F. (1995) Sequence stratigraphy of Palaeo–Tokyo Bay. In: *Tidal Signatures in Modern and Ancient Sediments*. pp. 85–99. Special Publication no. 24, International Association of Sedimentologists.

Olsen, P.E. (1986) A 40-million-year record of early Mesozoic climatic forcing. *Science*, 234, 842–8.

Ono, Y. (1990) Alluvial fans in Japan and South Korea. In: *Alluvial Fans: A Field Approach* (eds A.H. Rachocki & M. Church), pp. 91–107. Wiley, New York.

Oomkens, E. (1974) Lithofacies relations in the Late Quaternary Niger delta complex. *Sedimentology*, 21, 195–222.

Oost, A.P. & de Boer, P.L. (1994) Sedimentology and development of barrier islands, ebb-tidal deltas, inlets and backbarrier areas of the Dutch Wadden Sea. *Senckenbergiana Maritima*, 24, 65–115.

Opdyke, B.N. & Walker, J.C.G. (1992) Return of the coral reef hypothesis: basin to shelf partitioning of $CaCO_3$ and its effect on atmospheric CO_2. *Geology*, 20, 733–6.

Opdyke, B.N. & Wilkinson, B.H. (1993) Carbonate mineral saturation state and cratonic limestone accumulation. *American Journal of Science*, 293, 217–34.

Orange, D.L., Anderson, R.S. & Breen, N.A. (1994) Regular canyon spacing in the submarine environment: the link between hydrology and geomorphology. *GSA Today*, 4, 36–9.

Orford, J.D. (1975) Discrimination of particle zonation on a pebble beach. *Sedimentology*, 22, 441–63.

Ori, G.-G. (1989) Geologic history of the extensional basin of the Gulf of Corinth (Pliocene–Pleistocene), Greece. *Geology*, 17, 918–21.

Ori, G.-G. & Friend, P.F. (1984) Sedimentary basins formed and carried piggyback on active thrust sheets. *Geology*, 12, 475–8.

Orme, G.R., Flood, P.G. & Sargent, G.E.G. (1978) Sedimentation trends in the lee of outer (ribbon) reefs, northern region of the Great Barrier Reef province. *Philosophical Transactions of the Royal Society, London (A)*, 291, 85–99.

Orti-Cabo, F., Pueyo Mur, J.J., Geisler-Cuseey, D. & Dulau, N. (1984) Evaporitic sedimentation in the coastal salinas of Santa Pola (Alicante, Spain). *Rev. Inst. Inv. geol.*, 38/39, 169–220.

Orton, G.J. & Reading, H.G. (1993) Variability of deltaic processes in terms of sediment supply, with particular emphasis on grain size. *Sedimentology*, 40, 475–512.

Osborne, P.D. & Greenwood, B. (1992) Frequency dependent cross-shore suspended sediment transport. 2. A barred shoreface. *Marine Geology*, 106, 25–51.

Osborne, P.D. & Greenwood, B. (1993) Sediment suspension under waves and currents: time scales and vertical structure. *Sedimentology*, 40, 599–622.

Ovviatt, C.G., McCoy, W.D. & Nash, W.P. (1994) Sequence stratigraphy of lacustrine deposits: a Quaternary example from the Bonneville basin, Utah. *Bulletin of the Geological Society of America*, 106, 133–44.

Owen, G. (1996) Experimental soft-sediment deformation: structures formed by the liquefaction of unconsolidated sands and some ancient examples. *Sedimentology*, 43, 279–93.

Owen, L.A. (1988) Wet-sediment deformation of Quaternary and recent sediments in the Skardu Basin, Karakoram Mountains, Pakistan. In: *Glaciotectonics: Forms and Process* (ed. D.G. Croot), pp. 123–47.

Owen, R.B., Bartelme, J.W., Renant, R.W. & Vincens, A. (1982) Palaeolimnology and archaeology of Holocene deposits NE of Lake Turkana, Kenya. *Nature*, 298, 523–9.

Page, K.J. & Nanson, G.C. (1996) Stratigraphic architecture resulting from Late Quaternary evolution of the Riverine Plain, south-eastern Australia. *Sedimentology*, 43, 927–45

Paillard, D. & Labeyrie, L. (1994) Role of the thermohaline circulation in the abrupt warming after Heinrich events. *Nature*, 372, 162–4.

Pak, H., Zaeveld, J.R.V. & Kitchen, J. (1980) Intermediate nepheloid layers observed off Oregon and Washington. *Journal of Geophysical Research*, 85, 6697–708.

Palmer, M.R. & Elderfield, H. (1985) Sr isotope composition of seawater over the past 75 my. *Nature*, 314, 526–8.

Panagiotopoulos, I., Sylaios, G. & Collins, M.B. (1994) Threshold studies of gravel size particles under the co-linear combined action of waves and currents. *Sedimentology*, 41, 951–62.

Pantin, H.M.P. (1979) Interaction between velocity and effective density in turbidity flow: phase plane analysis, with criteria for autosuspension. *Marine Geology*, 31, 59–99.

Pantin, H.M.P. & Leeder, M.R. (1987) Reverse flow in turbidity currents: the role of internal solitons. *Sedimentology*, 34, 1143–55.

Pantin, H.M.P., Hamilton, D. & Evans, C.D.R. (1987) Theoretical modelling of deep ocean sediment transport—comment. *Marine Geology*, 76, 163–7.

Paola, C. & Borgman, L. (1991) Reconstructing random topography from preserved stratification. *Sedimentology*, 38, 553–65.

Paola, C., *et al.* (1992) Downstream fining by selective deposition in a laboratory flume. *Science*, 258, 1757–60.

Park, R.K. (1976) A note on the significance of lamination in stromatolites. *Sedimentology*, 23, 379–93.

Park, R.K. (1977) The preservation potential of some recent

stromatolites. *Sedimentology*, **24**, 485–506.

Parker, G. (1976) On the causes and characteristic scales of meandering and braiding in rivers. *Journal of Fluid Mechanics*, **76**, 457–80.

Parker, G., Klingeman, P.C. & McLean, D.C. (1982) Bedload and size distribution in paved gravel-bed streams. Journal of the Hydraulics Division. *American Society of Civil Engineers*, **108**, 544–71.

Parker, G., Fukushima, Y. & Pantin, H.M. (1986) Self-accelerating turbidity currents. *Journal of Fluid Mechanics*, **171**, 145–81.

Parrish, J.T. & Peterson, F. (1988) Wind directions predicted from global circulation models and wind directions determined from eolian sandstones of the western United States—a comparison. *Sedimentary Geology*, **56**, 261–82.

Parsons, B. & Sclater, J.G. (1977) An analysis of the variation of ocean floor bathymetry and heat flow with age. *Journal of Geophysical Research*, **82**, 803–27.

Paterson, D.M. (1997) Biological mediation of sediment erodibility: ecology and physical dynamics. In: *Cohesive Sediments* (eds N. Burt, R. Parker & J. Watts), pp. 215–29. Wiley, New York.

Paterson, W.S.B. (1994) *The Physics of Glaciers*, 3rd edn. Pergamon, Oxford.

Pattinson, S.A.J. & Walker, R.G. (1992) Deposition and interpretation of long, narrow sandbodies underlain by a basinwide erosion surface: Cardium Formation, Cretaceous Western Interior Seaway. *Journal of Sedimentary Petrology*, **62**, 292–309.

Pavich, M.J. (1985) Appalachian piedmont morphogenesis: weathering, erosion and Cenozoic uplift. In: *Tectonic Geomorphology* (eds M. Morisawa & J.T. Hack), pp. 299–320. Allen and Unwin, Boston.

Pavich, M.J. (1986) Processes and rates of saprolite production and erosion on a foliated granitic rock of the Vuginia Piedmont. In: *Rates of Chemical Weathering of Rocks and Minerals* (eds S.M. Colman & D.P. Dethier), pp. 552–90. Academic Press, Orlando.

Pazzaglia, F.J. & Brandon, M.T. (1996) Macrogeomorphic evolution of the post-Triassic Appalachian mountains determined by deconvolution of the offshore basin sedimentary record. *Basin Research*, **8**, 255–78.

Peakall, J. (1998) Axial river evolution in response to half-graben faulting: Carson River, Nevada. *Journal of Sedimentary Research*.

Peakall, J., Ashworth, P. & Best, J. (1996) Physical modelling in fluvial geomorphology: principles, applications and unresolved issues. In: *The Scientific Nature of Geomorphology* (eds B.L. Rhoads & C.R. Thorn), pp. 221–53. Wiley, New York.

Peng, T.-H. & Broecker, W.S. (1991) Dynamical limitations on the Antarctic iron fertilisation strategy. *Nature*, **349**, 227–9.

Penland, S., Boyd, R. & Suter, J.R. (1988) Transgressive depositional systems of the Mississippi delta plain: a model for barrier shoreline and shelf sand development.

Journal of Sedimentary Research, **58**, 932–49.

Pérez-Arlucea, M. & Smith, N.D. (1999) Depositional patterns following the 1870's avulsion of the Saskatchewan River (Cumberland Marshes, Saskatchewan). *Journal of Sedimentary Research*, **69**, 62–73.

Perlmutter, M.A. & Mathews, M.D. (1989) Global cyclostratigraphy—a model. In: *Quantitative Dynamic Stratigraphy* (ed. T.A. Cross), pp. 233–60. Prentice Hall, Englewood Cliffs, NJ.

Pernetta, J. (1994) *Atlas of the Oceans*. Mitchell Beazly, London.

Peryt, T.M. (1994) The anatomy of a sulphate platform and adjacent basin system in the Leba sub-basin of the Lower Werra Anhydrite (Zechstein, Upper Permian), northern Poland. *Sedimentology*, **41**, 83–113.

Peryt, T.M. (1996) Sedimentology of Badeneian (middle Miocene) gypsum in eastern Galicia, Podolia and Bukowina (West Ukraine). *Sedimentology*, **43**, 571–88.

Peterson, F. (1988) Pennsylvanian to Jurassic eolian transportation systems in the western United States. *Sedimentary Geology*, **56**, 207–60.

Phillips, A.C., Smith, N.D. & Powell, R.D. (1991) Laminated sediments in prodeltaic deposits, Glacier Bay, Alaska. In: *Glacial Marine Sedimentation: Palaeoclimatic Significance* (eds J.B. Anderson & G.M. Ashley), pp. 1–26. Special Publication no. 261, Geological Society of America.

Pickering, K.T. & Hiscott, R.N. (1985) Contained (reflected) turbidity currents from the Middle Ordovician Cloridorme Formation, Quebec, Canada: an alternative to the antidune hypothesis. *Sedimentology*, **34**, 1143–55.

Pickering, K.T., Hiscott, R.N. & Hein, F.J. (1989) *Deep Marine Clastic Environments: Clastic Sedimentation and Tectonics*. Unwin Hyman, London.

Pickering, K.T., Underwood, M.B. & Taira, A. (1992) Open-ocean to trench turbidity-current flow in the Nankai Trough: flow collapse and reflection. *Geology*, **20**, 1099–102.

Pickrill, R.A. & Irwin, J. (1983) Sedimentation in a deep glacier-fed lake—Lake Tekapo, New Zealand. *Sedimentology*, **30**, 63–75.

Pickup, S.L.B., Whitmarsh, R.B., Fowler, C.M.R. & Reston, T.J. (1996) Insight into the nature of the ocean–continent transition off West Iberia from a deep multichannel seismic reflection profile. *Geology*, **24**, 1079–82.

Pierson, T.C. (1981) Dominant particle support mechanisms in debris flows at Mt Thomas, New Zealand, and implications for flow mobility. *Sedimentology*, **28**, 49–60.

Pierson, T.C. (1985) Initiation and flow behaviour of the 1980 Pine Creek and Muddy River lahars, Mt St Helens, Washington. *Bulletin of the Geological Society of America*, **96**, 1056–69.

Pierson, T.C. (1995) Flow characteristics of large eruption-triggered debris flows at snow-clad volcanoes: constraints for debris-flow models. *Journal of Volcanology and Geothermal Research*, **66**, 283–94.

Pierson, T.C. & Scott, K.M. (1985) Downstream dilution of a lahar: transition from debris flow to hyperconcentrated streamflow. *Water Resources Research*, **21**, 1511–24.

Pigott, J.D. & Mackenzie, F.T. (1979) Phanerozoic oöld diagenesis: a signature of paleo-ocean and -atmospheric chemistry. *Geological Society of America Abstracts*, **11**, 495–6.

Pike, J. & Kemp, A.E.S. (1997) Early Holocene decadal-scale ocean variability recorded in Gulf of California laminated sediments. *Paleooceanography*, **12**, 227–38.

Pilkey, O.H. & Davis, T.W. (1987) An analysis of coastal recession models: North Carolina coast. In: *Sea Level Fluctuation and Coastal Evolution* (eds D. Nummedal, O.H. Pilkey & J.D. Howard), pp. 59–70. Special Publication no. 41, Society of Economic Palaeontologists and Mineralogists.

Pilkey, O.H. & Noble, D. (1967) Carbonate and clay mineralogy of the Persian Gulf. *Deep Sea Research*, **13**, 1–16.

Pinet, P. & Souriau, M. (1988) Continental erosion and large-scale relief. *Tectonics*, **7**, 563–82.

Pingree, R.D. & Griffiths, D.K. (1979) Sand transport paths around the British Isles resulting from M_2 and M_4 tidal interactions. *Journal of the Marine and Biological Association, UK*, **59**, 497–513.

Piper, D.J.W., Cochonate, P. & Morrison, M.L. (1999) The sequence of events around the epicentre of the 1929 Grand Banks earthquake: initiation of debris flows and turbidity current inferred from sidescan sonar. *Sedimentology*, **46**, 79–97.

Piper, D.J.W., von Heune, R. & Duncan, J.R. (1973) Late Quaternary sedimentation in the active eastern Aleutian Trench. *Geology*, **1**, 19–22.

Piper, D.J.W., *et al.* (1985) Sediment slides and turbidity currents on the Laurentian fan: sidescan sonar investigations near the epicentre of the 1929 Grand Banks earthquake. *Geology*, **13**, 538–41.

Pitman, W.C. (1978) Relationship between eustasy and stratigraphic sequences of passive margins. *Bulletin of the Geological Society of America*, **89**, 1389–403.

Pizzuto, J.E. (1987) Sediment diffusion during overbank flows. *Sedimentology*, **34**, 301–17.

Plafker, G. & Ericksen, G.E. (1978) Nevados Huascarán avalanches, Peru. In: *Rockslides and Avalanches*, Vol. 1, *Natural Phenomena* (ed. B. Voight), pp. 277–314. Developments in Geotechnical Engineering no. 14A.

Platt, N.H. (1989) Lacustrine carbonates and pedogenesis: sedimentology and origin of palustrine deposits from the Early Cretaceous Rupelo Formation, W. Cameros Basin, N. Spain. *Sedimentology*, **36**, 665–84.

Plint, A.G. (1988) Sharp-based shoreface sequences and 'offshore bars' in the Cardium Formation of Alberta: their relationship to relative changes in sea level. In: *Sea Level Changes: An Integrated Approach* (eds C.K. Wilgus *et al.*), pp. 357–70. Special Publication no. 42, Society of

Economic Palaeontologists and Mineralogists.

Plint, A.G., Walker, R.G. & Bergman, K.M. (1986) Cardium Formation 6. Stratigraphic framework of the cardium in the subsurface. *Bulletin of Canadian Petroleum Geologists*, **34**, 313–25.

Plummer, L.N. (1977) Defining reactions and mass transfer in part of the Floridan aquifer. *Water Resources Research*, **13**, 801–12.

Polzin, K.L., Speer, K.G., Toole, J.M. & Schmitt, R.W. (1996) Intense mixing of Antarctic Bottom Water in the equatorial Atlantic Ocean. *Nature*, **380**, 54–7.

Pomar, L. & Ward, W.C. (1994) Response of a late Miocene Mediterranean reef platform to high-frequency eustasy. *Geology*, **22**, 131–4.

Pond, S. & Pickard, G.L. (1983) *Introductory Dynamical Oceanography*, 2nd edn. Pergamon, London.

Porebski, S.J. (1995) Facies architecture in a tectonically-controlled incised-valley estuary: La Meseat Formation (Eocene) of Seymour Island, Antarctic Peninsula. *Studia Geologica Polonica*, **107**, 7–97.

Porebski, S.J., Meischner, D. & Gorlich, K. (1991) Quaternary mud turbidites from the South Shetland Trench (West Antarctica): recognition and implications for turbidites facies modelling. *Sedimentology*, **38**, 691–715.

Posamentier, H.W. & Erskine, R.D. (1991) Seismic expression and recognition criteria of ancient submarine fans. In: *Seismic Facies and Sedimentary Processes of Submarine Fans and Turbidite Systems* (eds P. Weimer & M.H. Link), pp. 197–222. Springer, Berlin.

Posamentier, H.W., Erskine, R.D. & Mitchum, R.M. (1991) Models for submarine fan deposition within a sequence stratigraphic framework. In: *Seismic Facies and Sedimentary Processes of Submarine Fans and Turbidite Systems* (eds P. Weimer & M.H. Link), pp. 127–36. Springer, Berlin.

Postma, G. (1990) An analysis of the variation in delta architecture. *Terra Nova*, **2**, 124–30.

Postma, G. & Roep, T.B. (1985) Resedimented conglomerates in the bottomsets of Gilbert-type gravel deltas. *Journal of Sedimentary Petrology*, **55**, 874–85.

Postma, G., Babic, L., Zupanic, J. & Roe, S.-L. (1988) Delta-front failure and associated bottomset deformation in a marine, gravelly Gilbert-type fan delta. In: *Fan Deltas: Sedimentology and Tectonic Settings* (eds W. Nemec & R.J. Steel), pp. 91–102. Blackie, London.

Postma, G., Hilgen, F.J. & Zachariasse, W.J. (1993a) Precession-punctuated growth of a late-Miocene submarine-fan lobe on Gavdos (Greece). *Terra Nova*, **5**, 438–44.

Postma, G., Fortuin, A.R. & Van Wamell, W.A. (1993b) Basin-fill patterns controlled by tectonics and climate: the Neogene 'fore-arc' basins of eastern Crete as a case history. pp. 335–62. Special Publication no. 20, International Association of Sedimentologists.

Pouliquen, O., Delour, J. & Savage, S.B. (1997) Fingering

in granular flows. *Nature*, **386**, 816–17.

Poulsen, C.J., Flemings, P.B., Robinson, R.A.J. & Metzger, J.M. (1998) Three-dimensional stratigraphic evolution of the Miocene Baltimore Canyon region: Implications for eustatic interpretations and the systems tract model. *Bulletin Geological Society of America*, **110**, 1105–22.

Powell, R.D. (1990) Glacimarine processes at grounding-line fans and their growth to ice-contact deltas. In: (eds J.A. Dowdeswell & J.D. Scourse) *Glacimarine Environments*, pp. 53–73. Special Publication no. 53, Geological Society of London.

Pozzobon, J.G. & Walker, R.G. (1990) Viking Formation (albion) at Eureka, Saskatchewan: a transgressed and degraded shelf sand ridge. *Bulletin of the American Association of Petroleum Geologists*, **74**, 1212–27.

Pratson, L.F., Ryan, W.B.F., Mountain, G.S. & Twichell, D.C. (1994) Submarine canyon initiation by downslope-eroding sediment flows: evidence in late Cenozoic strata on the New Jersey continental slope. *Bulletin of the Geological Society of America*, **106**, 395–412.

Prave, A.R. (1990) Clarification of some misconceptions about antidune geometry and flow character. *Sedimentology*, **37**, 1049–52.

Prave, A.R., Duke, W.L. & Slattery, W. (1996) A depositional model for storm- and tide-influenced prograding siliciclastic shorelines from the Middle Devonian of the central Appalachian foreland basin, USA. *Sedimentology*, **43**, 611–29.

Prentice, I.C., Guiot, J. & Harrison, S.P. (1992) Mediterranean vegetation, lake levels and palaeoclimate at the Late Glacial Maximum. *Nature*, **360**, 658–60.

Prentice, J.E., *et al.* (1968) Sediment transport in estuarine areas. *Nature*, **218**, 1207–10.

Priestley, C.H.B. & Taylor, R.J. (1972) On the assessment of surface heat flux and evaporation using large-scale parameters. *Monthly Weather Review*, **100**(2), 81–92.

Prior, D.B. & Bornhold, B.D. (1988) Submarine morphology and processes of fjord fan deltas and related high-gradient systems: modern examples from British Columbia. In: *Fan Deltas: Sedimentology and Tectonic Settings* (eds W. Nemec & R.J. Steel), pp. 125–43. Blackie, London.

Prior, D.B. & Bornhold, B.D. (1990) The underwater development of Holocene fan deltas. In: *Coarse-Grained Deltas* (eds A. Colella & D.B. Prior), pp. 75–90. Special Publication no. 10, International Association of Sedimentologists.

Prior, D.B., Bornhold, B.D., Wiseman, W.J. & Lowe, D.R. (1987) Turbidity current activity in a British Columbia fjord. *Science*, **237**, 1330–3.

Pritchard, D.W. (1955) Estuarine circulation patterns. *Proceedings, American Society of Civil Engineers*, **81**, 1–11.

Pritchard, D.W. (1967) What is an estuary: physical viewpoint. In: *Estuaries* (ed. G.H. Lauff), pp. 1–10. American Association for the Advancement of Science, Washington, DC.

Pritchard, D.W. & Carter, H.H. (1971) Estuarine circulation patterns. In: *The Estuarine Environment* (ed. J.R. Schubel), pp. 1–17. American Geological Institute, Washington, DC.

Pugh, D.T. (1987) *Tides, Surges and Mean Sea Level*. Wiley, London.

Purdy, E.G. (1963) Recent calcium carbonate facies of the Great Bahama Bank. 2: Sedimentary facies. *Journal of Geology*, **71**, 472–97.

Purdy, E.G. (1974) Reef configurations: cause and effect. In: *Reefs in Time and Space* (ed. L.F. Laporte), pp. 9–76. Special Publication no. 18, Society of Economic Palaeontologists and Mineralogists.

Purseglove, J. (1989) *Taming the Flood: A History and Natural History of Rivers and Wetlands*. Oxford University Press, Oxford.

Purser, B.H. (1979) Middle Jurassic sedimentation on the Burgundy Platform. *Symp. Sed. Jurass. W. Europe*, pp. 75–84. Publication no. 1,

Pye, K. (1982) Morphological development of coastal dunes in a humid tropical environment, Cape Bedford and Cape Flattery, North Queensland. *Geografiska Annaler*, **A64**, 213–27.

Pye, K. (1993) Late Quaternary development of coastal parabolic megadune complexes in northeastern Australia. In: *Aeolian Sediments: Ancient and Modern* (eds K. Pye & N. Lancaster), pp. 23–44. Special Publication no. 16, International Association of Sedimentologists. Blackwell Scientific Publications, Oxford.

Pye, K. & Lancaster, N. (eds) (1993) *Aeolian Sediments: Ancient and Modern*. Special Publication no. 16, International Association of Sedimentologists.

Pye, K. & Tsoar, H. (1990) *Aeolian Sand and Sand Dunes*. Chapman and Hall, London.

Pysklywec, R.N. & Mitrovica, J.X. (1998) Mantle flow mechanisms for the large-scale subsidence of continental interiors. *Geology*, **26**, 687–90.

Pytkowicz, R.M. (1965) Rates of inorganic calcium carbonate nucleation. *Journal of Geology*, **73**, 196–9.

Quinlan, G.M. & Beaumont, C. (1984) Appalachian thrusting, lithospheric flexure and the Palaeozoic stratigraphy of the eastern interior of North America. *Canadian Journal of Earth Sciences*, **21**, 973–96.

de Raaf, J.F.M. Boersma, J.R. & van Gelder, A. (1977) Wave-generated structures and sequences from a shallow marine succession. Lower Carboniferous, County Cork, Ireland. *Sedimentology*, **24**, 451–83.

Rahmani, R.A. & Flores, R.M. (eds) (1984) *Sedimentology of Coal and Coal-bearing Sequences*, Special Publication no. 7, International Association of Sedimentologists.

Rai, H. & Hill, G. (1980) Classification of central Amazon lakes on the basis of their microbiological and physico-chemical characteristics. *Hydrobiologia*, **72**, 85–99.

Ramos, A., Sopeña, A. & Pérez-Arlucea, M. (1986) Evolution of Buntsandstein fluvial sedimentation in North-West Iberian Ranges (Central Spain). *Journal of Sedimentary Petrology*, **56**, 862–75.

Rampino, M.R. & Sanders, J.E. (1981) Evolution of the barrier islands of Southern Long Island, New York. *Sedimentology*, **28**, 37–48.

Rankey, E.C. (1997) Relations between relative changes in sea level and climate shifts: Pennsylvanian–Permian mixed carbonate–siliciclastic strata, western United States. *Bulletin of the Geological Society of America*, **109**, 1089–100.

Rannie, W.F. (1990) The Portage La Prarie 'floodplain fan'. In: *Alluvial Fans: A Field Approach* (eds A.H. Rachocki & M. Church), pp. 179–93, Wiley, New York.

Raudkivi, A.J. (1976) *Loose Boundary Hydraulics*. Pergamon, Oxford.

Raudkivi, A.J. & Hutchinson, D.L. (1974) Erosion of kaolinite clay by flowing water. *Proceedings of the Royal Society of London*, **A337**, 537–54.

Rea, D.K. (1993) Geologic records in deep sea muds. *GSA Today*, **3**(8), 205–10.

Read, J.F. (1982) Carbonate platforms of passive (extensional) continental margins: types, characteristics and evolution. *Tectonophysics*, **81**, 195–212.

Read, J.F. (1984) Carbonate platform facies models. *Bulletin of the American Association of Petroleum Geologists*, **69**, 1–21.

Read, J.F., Grotzinger, J.P., Bova, J.A. & Koershner, W.F. (1986) Models for generation of carbonate cycles. *Geology*, **14**, 107–10.

Reddy, M.M. (1977) Crystallisation of calcium carbonate in the presence of trace concentrations of phosphorus-containing anions. *Journal of Crystal Growth*, **41**, 287–95.

Reineck, H.E. (1958) Longitudinale schragschit im Watt. *Geologische Rundschau*, **47**, 73–82.

Reineck, H.E. (1963) *Sedimentgefuge in Bereich der Sudlichen Nordsee*. Gesellschaft Nr. 505, Abteilung Senckenbergiana Naturforschung.

Reineck, H.E. (1967) Layered sediments of tidal flats, beaches and shelf bottoms of the North Sea. In: *Estuaries* (ed. G.D. Louff), pp. 191–206. American Association for the Advancement of Science, Washington, DC.

Reineck, H.E. (1972) Tidal flats. In: *Recognition of Ancient Sedimentary Environments* (eds J.K. Rigby & W.K. Hamblin), pp. 146–59. Special Publication no. 16, Society of Economic Palaeontologists and Mineralogists.

Reineck, H.E. & Singh, I.B. (1973) Genesis of laminated sand and graded rhythmites in storm-sand layers of shelf mud. *Sedimentology*, **18**, 123–8.

Reineck, H.E. & Singh, I.B. (1980) *Depositional Sedimentary Environments*, 2nd edn. Springer, Berlin.

Reineck, H.E. & Wunderlich, F. (1968) Zur unter scheidung von asymmetrischen oszillationrippen und Stromungsrippeln. *Senckenbergiana Lethaia*, **49**, 321–45.

Renaut, R.W. & Last, W.M. (eds) (1994) *Sedimentology and Geochemistry of Modern and Ancient Saline Lakes*. Special Publication no. 50, Society of Economic Palaeontologists and Mineralogists.

Renaut, R.W. & Tiercelin, J.-J. (1994) Lake Bogoria, Kenya rift valley—a sedimentological overview. In: *Sedimentology and Geochemistry of Modern and Ancient Saline Lakes* (eds R.W. Renaut & W.M. Last), pp. 101–23. Special Publication no. 50, Society of Economic Palaeontologists and Mineralogists.

Reneau, S.L. & Dietrich, W.E. (1991) Erosion rates in the southern Oregon Coast Range: evidence for an equilibrium between hillslope erosion and sediment yield. *Earth Surface Processes and Landforms*, **16**, 307–22.

Retallack, G.J. (1990) *Soils of the Past: An Introduction to Palaeopedology*. Unwin Hyman, London.

Reymer, A. & Schubert, G. (1984) Phanerozoic addition rates to the continental crust and crustal growth. *Tectonics*, **3**, 63–77.

Richards, M.T. (1994) Transgression of an estuarine channel and tidal flat complex: the Lower Triassic of Barles, Alpes de Haute Provence, France. *Sedimentology*, **41**, 55–82.

Richardson, J.F. & Zaki, W.N. (1958) Sedimentation and fluidization. *Transactions Institute of Chemical Engineers*, **32**, 35–53.

Richter, D.K. (1983) Calcareous ooids: a synopsis. In: *Coated Grains* (ed. T.M. Peryt), pp. 71–99. Springer, Berlin.

Richter, F.M., Rowley, D.B. & DePaolo, D.J. (1992) Sr isotope evolution of seawater: the role of tectonics. *Earth and Planetary Science Letters*, **109**, 11–23.

Richter-Bernberg, G. (1955) Uber salinaire sedimentation 2. *Deutsche Geologische Gesellschaft*, **105**, 593–6.

Ridge, M.J.H. & Carson, B. (1987) Sediment transport on the Washington continental shelf: estimates of dispersal rates from Mount St Helens ash. *Continental Shelf Research*, **7**, 759–72.

Ridgeway, K.D. & DeCelles, P.G. (1993) Stream-dominated alluvial fan and lacustrine depositional systems in Cenozoic strike-slip basins, Denali fault system, Yukon territory, Canada. *Sedimentology*, **40**, 645–66.

Riding R. (1983) Cyanoliths (cyanoids): oncoids formed by calcified cyanophytes. In: *Coated Grains* (ed. T.M. Peryt), pp. 277–83. Springer, Berlin.

Riech, V. & von Rad, U. (1979) Silica diagenesis in the Atlantic Ocean: diagenetic potential and transformations. In (ed M. Ewing). American.

Roberts, H.H., Adams, R.D. & Cunningham, R.H.W. (1980) Evolution of the sand-dominant subaerial phase, Atchafalaya Delta, Louisiana. *Bulletin of the American Association of Petroleum Geologists*, **64**, 264–79.

Roof, S.R., *et al.* (1991) Climatic forcing of cyclic carbonate sedimentation during the last 5.4 million years along the West Florida continental margin. *Journal of Sedimentary Petrology*, **61**, 1070–88.

Rosato, A., *et al.* (1987) Why the Brazil nuts are on top: size segregation of particulate matter by shaking. *Physical Review Letters*, **58**, 1038–40.

Rosen, M.R. (1994) The importance of groundwater in playas: a review of playa classifications and the sedimentology and hydrology of playas. In: *Paleoclimate and Basin Evolution of Playa Systems* (ed. M.R. Rosen). Special Paper no. 289, Geological Society of America.

Ross, W.C., *et al.* (1994) Slope readjustment: a new model for the development of submarine fans and aprons. *Geology*, **22**, 511–14.

Rothwell, R.G., Pearce, T.J. & Weaver, P.P.E. (1992) Late Quaternary evolution of the Madeira Abyssal Plain, Canary Basin, NE Atlantic. *Basin Research*, **4**, 103–31.

Rothwell, R.G., Thomson, J. & Kahler, G. (1998) Low sea-level emplacement of a very large Late Pleistocene 'megaturbidite' in the western Mediterranean Sea. *Nature*, **392**, 377–80.

Rottman, J.W. & Simpson, J.E. (1989) The formation of internal bores in the atmosphere: a laboratory model. *Quarterly Journal of the Royal Meteorological Society*, **115**, 941–63.

Rouchy, J.-M., Pierre, C. & Sommer, F. (1995) Deep-water resedimentation of anhydrite and gypsum deposits in the Middle Miocene (Belayim Formation) of the Red Sea, Egypt. *Sedimentology*, **42**, 267–82.

Rowe, P.W. (1962) The stress-dilatancy relation for static equilibrium of an assembly of particles in contact. *Proceedings of the Royal Society, London(A)*, **269**, 500–27.

Roy, A.G. & Bergeson, N. (1988) Hydraulic geometry and changes in flow velocity at a river confluence with coarse bed material. *Earth Surface Processes and Landforms*, **13**, 583–98.

Royden, L. (1988) Late Cenozoic tectonics of the Pannonian Basin system. In: pp. 27–48. Memoir no. 45, American Association of Petroleum Geologists.

Rozovskii, I.L. (1961) *Flow of Water in Bends of Open Channels*. Israel Programme for Scientific Translations, Jerusalem, p. 233.

Ruddiman, W.F. & Kutzbach, J.E. (1991) Plateau uplift and climatic change. *Scientific American*, March.

Ruegg, G.H.J. (1991) Pleistocene fluviatile deposits in ice-pushed position, Wageningen, The Netherlands. *Mededelingen Rijks Geologische Dienst*, **46**, 3–25.

Rusnak, G.A. (1960) Sediments of Laguna Madra, Texas. In: *Recent Sediments of the NW Gulf of Mexico* (eds F.P. Shepard, F.B. Phleger & T.H. van Andel), pp. 153–96. American Association of Petroleum Geologists, Tulsa, OK.

Rust, B.R. (1975) Fabric and structure in glaciofluvial gravels. In (eds A.V. Jopling & B.G. McDonald) *Glaciofluvial and Glaciolacustrine Sediments*, pp. 238–48. Special Publication **23**, Society of Economic Palaeotologists and Mineralogists.

Rust, B.R. & Romanelli, R. (1975) Late Quaternary subaqueous outwash deposits near Ottawa, Canada. In: pp. 177–92. Special Publication no. 23, Society of Economic Paleontologists and Mineralogists.

Sack, D. (1994) Geomorphic evidence of climate change from desert-basin paleolakes. In: *Geomorphology of Desert Environments* (eds A.D. Abrahams & A.J.

Parsons), pp. 616–30. Chapman and Hall, London.

Said, R. (1981) *The Geological Evolution of the River Nile*. Springer, New York.

Sallenger, A.H. (1979) Inverse grading and hydraulic equivalence in grain-flow deposits. *Journal of Sedimentary Petrology*, **49**, 553–62.

Sambrook-Smith, G. & Ferguson, R.I. (1995) The gravel–sand transition along alluvial river channels. *Journal of Sedimentary Research*, **A65**, 423–30.

Sancetta, C. Mediterranean sapropels: seasonal stratification yields high production and carbon flux. *Palaeoceanography*, **9**, 195–6.

Sandberg, P.A. (1975) New interpretations of Great Salt Lake ooids and of ancient nonskeletal carbonate mineralogy. *Sedimentology*, **22**, 497–537.

Sandberg, P.A. (1983) An oscillating trend in Phanerozoic non-skeletal carbonate mineralogy. *Nature*, **305**, 19–22.

Santantonio, M. (1993) Facies associations and evolution of pelagic carbonate platform/basin systems: examples from the Italian Jurassic. *Sedimentology*, **40**, 1039–67.

Sanz, M.E., Alonso-Zarza, A.M. & Calvo, J.P. (1995) Carbonate pond deposits related to semi-arid alluvial systems: examples from the Tertiary Madrid Basin, Spain. *Sedimentology*, **42**, 437–52.

Saunderson, H.C. & Lockett, F.P. (1983) Flume experiments on bedforms and structures at the dune–plane bed transition. In: *Modern and Ancient Fluvial Sediments* (eds J.D. Collinson & J. Lewin), pp. 49–58. Special Publication no. 6, International Association of Sedimentologists.

Savage, S.B. (1979) Gravity flow of cohesionless granular materials in chutes and channels. *Journal of Fluid Mechanics*, **92**, 53–96.

Savarese, M., Mount, J.F., Sorauf, J.E. & Bucklin, L. (1993) Paleobiologic and paleoenvironmental context of coral-bearing Early Cambrian reefs: implications for Phanerozoic reef development. *Geology*, **21**, 917–20.

Scheihing, M.H. & Gaynor, G.C. (1991) The shelf sand-plume model: a critique. *Sedimentology*, **38**, 433–44.

Schlager, W. & Camber, O. (1986) Submarine slope angles, drowning unconformities, and self-erosion of limestone escarpments. *Geology*, **14**, 762–5.

Schlager, W., Hooke, R.L. & James, N.P. (1976) Episodic erosion and deposition in the Tongue of the Ocean (Bahamas). *Bulletin of the Geological Society of America*, **87**, 1115–18.

Schlanger, S.O. & Jenkyns, H.C. (1976) Cretaceous oceanic anoxic events: causes and consequences. *Geologieen Mijnbouw*, **55**, 79–84.

Schilsche, R.W. (1992) Structural and stratigraphic development of the Newark extensional basin, eastern North America: evidence for the growth of the basin and its bounding structures. *Bulletin of the Geological Society of America*, **104**, 1246–63.

Schlische, R.W. & Olsen, P.E. (1990) Quantitative filling model for continental extensional basins with applications to early Mesozoic rifts of eastern North

America. *Journal of Geology*, **98**, 135–55.

Schlunegger, F., Leu, W. & Matter, A. (1997) Sedimentary sequences, seismic facies, subsidence analysis, and evolution of the Burdiglian Upper Marine Molasse Group, central Switzerland. *Bulletin of the American Association of Petroleum Geologists*, **81**, 1185–207.

Schlunegger, F., Slingerland, R. & Matter, A. (1998) Crustal thickening and crustal extension as controls on the evolution of the drainage network of the central Swiss Alps between 30 Ma and the present: constraints from the stratigraphy of the North Alpine Foreland Basin and the structural evolution of the Alps. *Basin Research*, **10**, 197–212.

Schminke, H.V., Fisher, R.V. & Waters, A.C. (1975) Antidune and chute-and-pool structures in the base surge deposits of the Laacher See area, Germany. *Sedimentology*, **20**, 553–74.

Schmitz, W.J. (1995) On the interbasin-scale thermohaline circulation. *Reviews of Geophysics*, **33**, 151–74.

Schmitz, W.J. & McCartney, M.S. (1993) On the North Atlantic circulation. *Reviews of Geophysics*, **31**, 29–49.

Scholz, C.A. & Finney, B.P. (1994) Late Quaternary sequence stratigraphy of Lake Malawi (Nyasa), Africa. *Sedimentology*, **41**, 163–79.

Scholz, C.A., Rosendahl, B.R. & Scott, D.L. (1990) Development of coarse-grained facies in lacustrine rift basins: examples from East Africa. *Geology*, **18**, 140–4.

Scholz, C.A., Klitgord, K.D., *et al.* (1993) Results of 1992 seismic reflection experiment in Lake Baikal. *EOS*, **74**, 465.

Schott, J. & Berner, R.A. (1985) Dissolution mechanism of pyroxenes and olivines during weathering. In: *The Chemistry of Weathering* (ed. J.I. Drever), pp. 35–53. Reidel, Hingham, MA.

Schreiber, B.C., Friedman, G.M., Decima, A. & Schreiber, E. (1976) Depositional environments of Upper Miocene (Messinian) evaporite deposits of the Sicilian basin. *Sedimentology*, **23**, 729–60.

Schubel, J.R. (1971b) A few notes on the agglomeration of suspended sediment in estuaries. In: *The Estuarine Environment* (ed. J.R. Schubel). American Geological Institute, Washington, DC.

Schubel, J.R. (1971c) Estuarine circulation and sedimentation. In: *The Estuarine Environment* (ed. J.R. Schubel). American Geological Institute, Washington, DC.

Schubel, J.R. & Okabo, A. (1972) Comments on the dispersal of suspended sediment across the continental shelves. In: *Shelf Sediment Transport: Process and Pattern* (eds D.J.P. Swift, D.B. Duane & O.H. Pilkey), pp. 333–46. Dowden, Hutchinson & Ross, Stroudsberg, PA.

Schumm, S.A. (1968a) Speculations concerning paleohydrologic controls of terrestrial sedimentation. *Bulletin of the Geological Society of America*, **79**, 1573–88.

Schumm, S.A. (1968b) *River Adjustment to Altered Hydrologic Regimen—Murrumbidgee River and paleochannels, Australia*. Professional Paper no. 598, US Geological Survey.

Schumm, S.A. (1977) *The Fluvial System*. Wiley, New York.

Schumm, S.A. (1993) River response to baselevel change: implications for sequence stratigraphy. *Journal of Geology*, **101**, 279–94.

Schumm, S.A. & Brackenridge, G.R. (1987) River response. In: *The Geology of North America*, Vol. K3, *North America and Adjacent Oceans during the Last Deglaciation* (eds W.F. Ruddimann & H.E. Wright Jr), pp. 221–40. Geological Society of America, Boulder, CO.

Schwartz, R.K. (1975) *Nature and Genesis of Some Washover Deposits*. Technical Memo no. 61, US Army Corps of Engineers, Coastal Engineering Research Centre.

Schwartzman, D.W. (1993) Comment on 'Weathering, plants, and the long-term carbon cycle' by Robert A. Berner. *Geochimica et Cosmochimica Acta*, **57**, 2145–6.

Schwartzman, D.W. & Volk, T. (1989) Biotic enhancement of weathering and the habitability of Earth. *Nature*, **340**, 457–60.

Schwarz, T. (1996) High latitude laterite as palaeoclimatic indicator of Middle Miocene greenhouse conditions. In: *Proceedings of the 4th International Symposium on the Geochemistry of the Earth's Surface* (ed. S.H. Bottrell), pp. 216–20. University of Leeds.

Schwarzacher, W. & Fischer, A.G. (1982) Limestone–shale bedding and perturbations of the Earth's orbit. In: *Cyclic and Event Stratification* (eds G. Einsele & A. Seilacher), pp. 72–95. Springer, Berlin.

Scoffin, T.P. (1970) The trapping and binding of subtidal carbonate sediments by marine vegetation in Bimini Lagoon, Bahamas. *Journal of Sedimentary Petrology*, **40**, 249–73.

Scoffin, T.P. (1987) *An Introduction to Carbonate Sediments and Rocks*. Blackie, London.

Scorer, R.S. (1997) *Dynamics of Meteorology and Climate*. Wiley, New York.

Scott, K.M. & Williams, R.P. (1978) *Erosion and Sediment Yields in the Transverse Ranges, Southern California*. Professional Paper no. 1030, US Geological Survey.

Seeber, L. & Gornitz, V. (1983) River profiles along the Himalayan arc as indicators of active tectonics. *Tectonophysics*, **92**, 335–67.

Selby, M.J. (1993) *Hillslope Materials and Processes*. Oxford University Press, Oxford.

Sellin, R.H.J. (1964) A laboratory investigation into the interaction between the flow in the channel of a river and that over its floodplain. *Houille Blanche*, **19**, 793–801.

Sellwood, B.W. (1968) The genesis of some sideritic beds in the Yorkshire Lias (England). *Journal of Sedimentary Petrology*, **38**, 854–8.

Sellwood, B.W. & McKerrow, W.S. (1973) Depositional environments in the lower part of the Great Oolite Group of Oxfordshire and North Gloucestershire. *Proceedings of the Geologists Association*, **85**, 189–210.

Seltzer, G.O., *et al.* (1998) High-resolution seismic reflection profiles from Lake Titicaca, Per-Bolivia: evidence for Holocene aridity in the tropical Andes. *Geology*, **26**, 167–70.

Seppälä, M. & Linde, K. (1978) Wind tunnel studies of ripple formation. *Geografiska Annaler*, **60**, 29–42.

Sestini, G. (1989) Nile Delta: a review of depositional environments and geological history. In: *Deltas: Sites and Traps for Fossil Fuels* (eds M.K.G. Whateley & K.T. Pickering), pp. 99–128. Special Publication no. 41, Geological Society of London.

Sha, L.P. & de Boer, P.L. (1991) Ebb-tidal delta deposits along the west Friesian Islands (The Netherlands): processes, facies architecture and preservation. In: *Clastic Tidal Sedimentology* (eds D.G. Smith *et al.*), pp. 199–218. Memoir no. 16, Canadian Society of Petroleum Geologists.

Shanley, K.W., McCabe, P.J. & Hettinger, R.D. (1992) Tidal influence in Cretaceous fluvial strata from Utah, USA: a key to sequence stratigraphic interpretation. *Sedimentology*, **39**, 905–30.

Shanmugam, G., Spalding, T.D. & Rofheart, D.H. (1993) Traction structures in deep-marine, bottom-current-reworked sands in the Pliocene and Pleistocene, Gulf of Mexico. *Geology*, **21**, 929–32.

Shapiro, A.H. (1961) *Shape and Flow: The Fluid Dynamics of Drag*. Doubleday, New York; Heinemann, London.

Shapiro, R.S., Aalto, K.R., Dill, R.F. & Kenny, R. (1995) Stratigraphic setting of a subtidal stromatolite field, Iguana Cay, Exumas, Bahamas. In: *Terrestrial and Shallow Marine Geology of the Bahamas and Bermuda* (eds A.A. Curran & B. White), pp. 139–55. Special Paper no. 300, Geological Society of America.

Sharma, G.D., Naidu, A.S. & Hood, D.W. (1972) Bristol Bay: a model contemporary graded shelf. *Bulletin of the American Association of Petroleum Geologists*, **56**, 2000–12.

Sharp, M., Jouzel, J., Hubbard, B. & Lawson, W. (1994) The character, structure and origin of the basal ice layer of a surge-type glacier. *Journal of Glaciology*, **40**, 327–40.

Shearman, D.J. (1966) Origin of marine evaporites by diagenesis. *Transactions of the Institute of Mining and Metallurgy*, **75B**, 208–15.

Shearman, D.J. (1970) Recent halite rock, Baja California, Mexico. *Transactions of the Institute of Mining and Metallurgy*, **79B**, 155–62.

Shearman, D.J. & Fuller, J.G.C.M. (1969) Anhydrite diagenesis, calcitisation and organic laminites, Winnipegosis Formation, M Devonian, Saskatchewan. *Bulletin of the Canadian Society of Petroleum Geologists*, **17**, 496–525.

Shearman, D.J., Twyman, J. & Karimi, M.Z. (1970) The genesis and diagenesis of oolites. *Proceedings of the Geologists Association*, **81**, 561–75.

Shepard, F.P. & Inman, D.L. (1950) Nearshore circulation. In: *Proceedings of the 1st Conference on Coastal Engineering*, pp. 50–9. Council on Wave Research, Berkeley, CA.

Shepard, F.P., Marshall, P.A., McLoughlin, P.A. & Sullivan, G.G. (1979) *Currents in Submarine Canyons and Other Sea Valleys*. Studies in Geology no. 8, American Association of Petroleum Geologists.

Sheridan, R.E. & Grow, J.A. (eds) (1988) *The Geology of North America*, Vol. I2, *The Atlantic Margin: US*. Geological Society of America, Boulder, CO.

Shideler, G.L. (1978) A sediment-dispersal model for the South Texas continental shelf, NW Gulf of Mexico. *Marine Geology*, **26**, 284–313.

Shinn, E.A. (1969) Submarine lithification of Holocene carbonate sediments in the Persian Gulf. *Sedimentology*, **12**, 109–44.

Shinn, E.A. (1983) Birdseyes, fenestrae, shrinkage pores, and loferites: a reevaluation. *Journal of Sedimentary Petrology*, **53**, 619–28.

Shinn, E.A., Lloyd, R.M. & Ginsburg, R.N. (1969) Anatomy of a modern carbonate tidal mat, Andros Island, Bahamas. *Journal of Sedimentary Petrology*, **39**, 1202–28.

Shinn, E.A., Steinen, R.P., Lidz, B.H. & Swart, P.K. (1989) Whitings: a sedimentological dilemma. *Journal of Sedimentary Petrology*, **59**, 147–61.

Shinn, E.A., Lidz, B.H. & Holmes, C.W. (1990) High-energy carbonate sand accumulation, the Quicksands, southwest Florida Keys. *Journal of Sedimentary Petrology*, **60**, 952–67.

Shotyk, W. & Metson, J.B. (1994) Secondary ion mass spectrometry (SIMS) and its application to chemical weathering. *Reviews of Geophysics*, **32**, 197–220.

Shreve, R.L. (1968) *The Blackhawk Landslide*. Special Paper no. 108, Geological Society of America.

Sibson, R.H. (1985) Stopping of earthquake ruptures at dilational fault jogs. *Nature*, **316**, 248–51.

Siegenthaler, U. & Sarmiento, J.L. (1993) Atmospheric carbon dioxide and the ocean. *Nature*, **365**, 119–25.

Siever, R. (1992) The silica cycle in the PreCambrian. *Geochimica et Cosmochimica Acta*, **56**, 3265–72.

Simkiss, K. (1964) Phosphates as crystal poisons of calcification. *Biological Review*, **39**, 487–505.

Simons, D.B., Richardson, E.V. & Nordin, C.F. (1965) Sedimentary structures generated by flow in alluvial channels. In: *Primary Sedimentary Structures and Their Hydrodynamic Interpretation* (ed. G.V. Middleton), pp. 34–52. Special Publication, Society of Economic Palaeontologists and Mineralogists.

Simpson, J.E. (1972) Effects of the lower boundary on the head of a gravity current. *Journal of Fluid Mechanics*, **53**, 759–68.

Simpson, J.E. (1987) *Gravity Currents: In the Environment and the Laboratory*. Ellis Horwood/Wiley, Chichester.

Simpson, J.E. & Britter, R.E. (1979) The dynamics of the head of a gravity current advancing over a horizontal surface. *Journal of Fluid Mechanics*, **94**, 477–95.

Sinclair, H.D. (1993) High resolution stratigraphy and facies differentiation of the shallow marine Annot Sandstones, south-east France. *Sedimentology*, **40**, 955–78.

Sinclair, H.D. (1994) The influence of lateral basin slopes on turbidite sedimentation in the Annot Sandstone of SE France. *Journal of Sedimentary Research*, **64**, 42–54.

Sinclair, H.D. (1997) Tectonostratigraphic model for underfilled peripheral foreland basins: an Alpine perspective. *Bulletin of the Geological Society of America*, **109**, 324–46.

Singh, H., Parkash, B. & Gohain, K. (1993) Facies analysis of the Kosi megafan deposits. *Sedimentary Geology*, **85**, 87–113.

Siringan, F.P. & Anderson, J.B. (1993) Seismic facies architecture and evolution of the Bolivar Roads tidal inlet/delta complex, east Texas Gulf Coast. *Journal of Sedimentary Petrology*, **63**, 794–808.

Siringan, F.P. & Anderson, J.B. (1994) Modern shoreface and inner-shelf storm deposits off the East Texas coast, Gulf of Mexico. *Journal of Sedimentary Research*, **64**, 99–110.

Sleath, J.F.A. (1984) *Sea Bed Mechanics*. Wiley, New York.

Slingerland, R.L., et al. (1996) Estuarine circulation in the Turonian Western Interior seaway of North America. *Bulletin Geological Society America*, **108**, 941–52.

Smith, A.M. (1997) Basal conditions on Rutford Ice Stream, West Antarctica, from seismic observations. *Journal of Geophysical Research*, **102**, 543–52.

Smith, C.R. & Walker, J.D.A. (1990) A conceptual model of wall turbulence. In: *Proceedings of the NASA Langley Boundary Layer Workshop* (ed. S. Robinson).

Smith, D.G. (1983) Anastomosed fluvial deposits: modern examples from Western Canada. In: *Modern and Ancient Fluvial Systems* (eds J.D. Collinson & J. Lewin), pp. 155–68. Special Publication no. 6, International Association of Sedimentologists.

Smith, D.G. & Smith, N.D. (1980) Sedimentation in anastomosed river systems: examples from alluvial valleys near Banff, Alberta. *Journal of Sedimentary Petrology*, **50**, 157–64.

Smith, G.A. & Landis, C.A. (1995) Intra-arc basins. In: *Tectonics of Sedimentary Basins* (eds C. Busby & R. Ingersoll), pp. 263–98, Blackwell Science, Oxford.

Smith, J.D. & McLean, S.R. (1977) Spatially averaged flow over a wavy surface. *Journal of Geophysical Research*, **82**, 1735–46.

Smith, N.D. & Pérez-Arlucea, M. (1994) Fine-grained splay deposition in the avulsion belt of the lower Saskatchewan River, Canada. *Journal of Sedimentary Research*, **B64**, 159–68.

Smith, N.D., Cross, T.A., Dufficy, J.P. & Clough, S.R. (1989) Anatomy of an avulsion. *Sedimentology*, **36**, 1–23.

Somoza, L. & Rey, J. (1991) Holocene fan deltas in a 'Ria' morphology: prograding clinoform types and sea level control. In: *The Dynamics of Coarse-Grained Deltas* (eds C.J. Dabrio, C. Zazo & J.L. Goy), pp. 37–48. Cuadernos de Geologia Iberica no. 15, Universidad Complutense, Madrid.

Somoza, L., Hernandez-Molina, F.J., De Andres, J.R. & Rey, J. (1997) Continental shelf architecture and sea level cycles: Late Quaternary high-resolution stratigraphy of the Gulf of Cadiz, Spain. *Geo-Marine Letters*, **17**, 133–9.

Sondi, I., Juracic, M. & Pravdic, V. (1995) Sedimentation in a disequilibrium river-dominated estuary, the Rasa River estuary (Adriatic Sea, Croatia). *Sedimentology*, **42**, 769–82.

Soreghan, G.S. (1994) The impact of glacioclimatic change on Pennsylvanian cyclostratigraphy. In: (eds A.F. Embry, B. Beauchamp & D.J. Glass), pp. 523–43. Memoir no. 17, Canadian Society of Petroleum Geologists.

Southard, J.B. (1971) Representation of bed configurations in depth–velocity–size diagrams. *Journal of Sedimentary Petrology*, **41**, 903–15.

Southard, J.B. (1991) Experimental determination of bed-form stability. *Annual Review of Earth and Planetary Sciences*, **19**, 423–55.

Southard, J.B. & Boguchwal, L.A. (1990a) Bed configurations in steady unidirectional water flows, Part 1. Synthesis of flume data. *Journal of Sedimentary Petrology*, **60**, 658–79.

Southard, J.B. & Boguchwal, L.A. (1990b) Bed configurations in steady unidirectional water flows, Part 2. Effects of temperature and gravity. *Journal of Sedimentary Petrology*, **60**, 680–6.

Southard, J.B., et al. (1990) Experiments on bed configurations in fine sands under bidirectional purely oscillatory flow, and the origin of hummocky cross-stratification. *Journal of Sedimentary Petrology*, **60**, 1–17.

Sparks, R.S.J., Bonnecaze, R.T., Huppert, H.E., et al. (1993) Sediment-laden gravity currents with reversing buoyancy. *Earth and Planetary Science Letters*, **114**, 243–57.

Spence, G.H. & Tucker, M.E. (1997) Genesis of limestone megabreccias and their significance in carbonate sequence stratigraphic models: a review. *Sedimentary Geology*, **112**, 163–93.

Spencer, R.J., et al. (1984) Great Salt Lake, and precursors, Utah: the last 30 000 years. *Contributions to Mineralogy and Petrology*, **86**, 321–34.

Sperling, C.H.B. & Cooke, R.U. (1985) Laboratory simulation of rock weathering by salt crystallisation and hydration processes in hot, arid environments. *Earth Surface Processes and Landforms*, **10**, 541–55.

Stanistreet, I.G. & McCarthy, T.S. (1993) The Okavango Fan and the classification of subaerial fan systems. *Sedimentary Geology*, **85**, 115–33.

Stanistreet, I.G., Cairncross, B. & McCarthy, T.S. (1993) Low sinuosity and meandering bedload rivers of the Okavango Fan: channel confinement by vegetated levees without fine sediment. *Sedimentary Geology*, **85**, 135–56.

Stanley, D.J. & Warne, A.G. (1993) Sealevel and initiation of Predynastic culture in the Nile delta. *Nature*, **363**, 435–8.

Starkel, L. (1983) The reflection of hydrologic change in the fluvial environment of the temperate zone during the last 15 ky. In: *Background to Paleohydrology* (ed. K.J. Gregory), pp. 213–35. Wiley, New York.

Staub, J.R. & Esterle, J.S. (1993) Provenance and sediment dispersal in the Rajang River delta/coastal plain system, Sarawak, East Malaysia. *Sedimentary Geology*, **85**, 191–201.

Steele, R.P. (1983) Longitudinal draa in the Permian Yellow Sands of NE England. In: *Eolian Sediments and Processes* (eds M.E. Brookfield & T.S. Ahlbrandt), pp. 543–50. Developments in Sedimentology no. 38. Elsevier, Amsterdam

Steinberg, T. (1995) *Slide Mountain, or the Folly of Owning Nature*. University of California Press, Berkeley, CA.

Stockman, K.W., Ginsburg, R.N. & Shinn, E.A. (1967) The production of lime mud by algae in South Florida. *Journal of Sedimentary Petrology*, **37**, 633–48.

Stokes, W.L. (1968) Multiple parallel-truncation bedding planes—a feature of wind deposited sandstone formations. *Journal of Sedimentary Petrology*, **38**, 510–15.

Stommel, H. (1948) The westward intensification of wind-driven ocean currents. *Transactions of the American Geophysical Union*, **29**, 202–6.

Stommel, H. (1957) The abyssal circulation. *Deep-Sea Research*, **41**, 49–84.

Stow, D.A.V. & Bowen, A.J. (1980) A physical model for the transport and sorting of fine-grained sediment by turbidity currents. *Sedimentology*, **27**, 31–46.

Stow, D.A.V. & Faugeres, J.C. (1998) Special issue: Contourites, turbidites and process interaction. *Sedimentary Geology*, **115**, 1–386.

Stow, D.A.V. & Lovell, J.P.B. (1979) Contourites: their recognition in modern and ancient sediments. *Earth Science Reviews*, **14**, 251–91.

Stow, D.A.V. & Piper, D.J.W. (1984) Deep-water fine-grained sediments: facies models. In: *Fine-Grained Sediments: Deep-Water Processes and Facies* (eds D.A.V. Stow & D.J.W. Piper), pp. 611–46. Special Publication no. 15, Geological Society of London.

Stow, D.A.V. & Shanmugam, G. (1980) Sequences of structures in fine-grained turbidites: comparison of recent deep sea and ancient flysch sediments. *Sedimentary Geology*, **25**, 23–42.

Stow, D.A.V. & Wetzel, A. (1990) Hemiturbidite: a new type of deep-water sediment. *Proceedings of the Ocean Drilling Program Scientific Results*, **116**, 25–34.

Strasser, A. (1988) Shallowing-upward sequences in Purbeckian peritidal carbonates (lowermost Cretaceous, Swiss and French Jura Mountains). *Sedimentology*, **35**, 369–83.

Stride, A.H. (1963) Current swept floors near the southern half of Great Britain. *Quarterly Journal of the Geological Society of London*, **119**, 175–99.

Stride, A.H., Belderson, R.H., Kenyon, N.H. & Johnson, M.A. (1982) Offshore tidal deposits: sand sheet and sand bank facies. In: *Offshore Tidal Sands: Processes and Deposits* (ed. A.H. Stride), pp. 95–125. Chapman and Hall, London.

Stumm, W. (1992) *Chemistry of the Solid–Water Interface*. Wiley, New York.

Stumm, W. & Wollast, R. (1990) Coordination chemistry of weathering. *Reviews of Geophysics*, **28**, 153–69.

Sturm, M. & Matter, A. (1978) Turbidites and varves in Lake Brienz (Switzerland): deposition of clastic detritus by density currents. In (eds A. Matter & M.E. Tucker), *Modern and Ancient Lake Sediments*, pp. 145–66. International Association of Sedimentologists, Special Publication **2**.

Suess, E. & Futterer, D. (1972) Aragonitic ooids: experimental precipitation from seawater in the presence of humic acid. *Sedimentology*, **19**, 129–39.

Sugden, D.E., *et al.* (1995) Preservation of Miocene glacier ice in East Antarctica. *Nature*, **376**, 412–14.

Sumer, B.M. & Deigaard, R. (1979) *Experimental Investigation of Motion of Suspended Heavy Particles and the Bursting Process*. Series Publication no. 23, Institute of Hydrodynamics and Hydraulic Engineering, Technical University of Denmark.

Sumer, B.M. & Oguz, B. (1978) Particle motions near the bottom in turbulent flow in an open channel. *Journal of Fluid Mechanics*, **86**, 109–27.

Summerfield, M.A. & Hulton, N.J. (1994) Natural controls of fluvial denudation rates in major world drainage basins. *Journal of Geophysical Research*, **99B**, 13871–85.

Summerhayes, C.P. & Thorpe, S.A. (1996) *Oceanography: an illustrated guide*. Manson Publishing, London.

Summerhayes, C.P., *et al.* (eds) (1995) Upwelling in the Ocean. Wiley, Chichester.

Sumner, D.Y. & Grotzinger, J.P. (1996) Were kinetics of Archean calcium carbonate precipitation related to oxygen concentration? *Geology*, **24**, 119–22.

Surdam, R.C. & Stanley, K.O. (1979) Lacustrine sedimentation during the culminating phase of Eocene Lake Gosuite, Wyoming (Green River Formation). *Bulletin of the Geological Society of America*, **90**, 93–110.

Surlyk, F. (1978) *Submarine Fan Sedimentation Along Fault Scarps on Tilted Fault Blocks (Jurassic–Cretaceous Boundary, East Greenland)*. Bulletin no. 128, Gronlands Geologiske Undersogelse.

Surlyk, F. (1987) Slope and deep shelf gully sandstones, Upper Jurassic, East Greenland. *Bulletin of the American Association of Petroleum Geologists*, **71**, 464–75.

Surlyk, F. (1990) Mid-Mesozoic synrift turbidite systems: controls and predictions. In: (ed. J.D. Collinson) *Correlation in Hydrocarbon Production*, pp. 231–41. Graham and Trotman, London.

Suter, J.R., Berryhill, H.L. & Penland, S. (1987) Late Quaternary sea-level fluctuations and depositional sequences, southwest Louisiana continental shelf. In: *Siliciclastic Shelf Sediments* (eds R.W. Tillman & C.T. Siemans), pp. 199–219. Special Publication no. 34, Society of Economic Palaeontologists and Mineralogists.

Suttner, L.J., Basu, A. & Mack, G.H. (1981) Climate and the origin of quartz arenites. *Journal of Sedimentary Petrology*, 51, 1235–46.

Sverdrup, H. & Warfinge, P. (1995) Estimating field weathering rates using laboratory kinetics. In: *Chemical Weathering Rates of Silicate Minerals* (eds A.F. White & S.L. Branfield), ch. 11. American Mineralogical Society, Washington, DC.

Swift, D.J.P. (1972) Implications of sediment dispersal from bottom current measurements; some specific problems in understanding bottom sediment distribution and dispersal on the continental shelf: a discussion of two papers. In: *Shelf Sediment Transport: Process and Pattern* (eds D.J.P. Swift, D.B. Duane & O.H. Pilkey), pp. 363–71. Dowden, Hutchinson & Ross, Stroudsberg, PA.

Swift, D.J.P. (1974) Continental shelf sedimentation. In: *The Geology of Continental Margins* (eds C.A. Burk & C.L. Drake), pp. 117–35. Springer, Berlin.

Swift, D.J.P., Duane, D.B. & McKinney, T.F. (1973) Ridge and swale topography of the Middle Atlantic Bight, North America: secular response to the Holocene hydraulic regime. *Marine Geology*, 15, 227–47.

Swift, D.J.P., Oertel, G.F., Tillman, R.W. & Thorne, J.A. (eds) (1991) Shelf Sand and Sandstone Bodies. Special Publication 14, International Association of Sedimentologists.

Swift, D.J.P., Young, R.A., Clarke, T.L., Vincent, C.E., Niedoroda, A. & Lesht, B. (1981) Sediment transport in the Middle Atlantic Bight of North America: synopsis of recent observations. In: *Holocene Marine Sedimentation in the North Sea Basin* (eds S.-D. Nio, R.T.E. Schüttenhelm & T.C.E. van Weering), pp. 361–83. Special Publication no. 5, International Association of Sedimentologists.

Syvitski, J.P.M. (1989) On the deposition of sediment within glacier-influenced fjords: oceanographic controls. *Marine Geology*, 85, 301–29.

Syvitski, J.P.M. & Farrow, G.E. (1989) Fjord sedimentation as an analogue for small hydrocarbon-bearing fan deltas. pp. 21–43. Special Publication no. 41, Geological Society of London.

Syvitski, J.P.M., Burrell, D.C. & Skei, J.M. (1987) *Fjords: Processes and Products*.

Sztano, O. & DeBoer, P.L. (1995) Basin dimensions and morphology as controls on amplification of tidal motions (the early Miocene North Hungarian Bay). *Sedimentology*, 42, 6665–82.

Takahashi, T. (1975) Carbonate chemistry of seawater and the calcite compensation depth in the oceans pp. 11–26. Special Publication no. 13, Cushman Foundation for Foraminiferal Research.

Takahashi, T. (1978) Mechanical characteristics of debris flow. *Journal of the Hydraulics Division, American Society of Civil Engineers*, 104, HY8, 1153–69.

Talbot, C.J., Stanley, W., Soub, R. & Al-Sadoun, N. (1996) Epitaxial salt reefs and mushrooms in the southern Dead Sea. *Sedimentology*, 43, 1025–47.

Talbot, M.R. (1973) Major sedimentary cycles in the Corallian Beds. *Palaeogeography, Palaeoclimatology, Palaeoecology*, 14, 293–317.

Talbot, M.R. (1980) Environmental responses to climatic change in the West African Sahel over the past 20 000 years. In: *The Sahara and the Nile* (eds M.A.J. Williams & H. Faure), pp. 37–62. Balkema, Rotterdam.

Talbot, M.R. (1985) Major bounding surfaces in aeolian sandstones—a climatic model. *Sedimentology*, 32, 257–65.

Talbot, M.R. (1990) A review of the palaeohydrological interpretation of carbon and oxygen isotopic ratios in primary lacustrine carbonates. *Chemical Geology*, 80, 261–79.

Talbot, M.R. & Williams, M.A.J. (1979) Cyclic alluvial fan sedimentation on the flanks of fixed dunes, Janjari, Central Niger. *Catena*, 6, 43–62.

Talbot, M.R. & Allen, P.A. (1996) Lakes. In: *Sedimentary Environments: Processes, Facies and Stratigraphy* (ed H.G. Reading), pp. 83–124. Blackwell Science, Oxford.

Talling, J.F. & Talling, I.B. (1965) The chemical composition of African lake waters. *International Review of Hydrobiology*, 50, 421–63.

Talling, P.J., *et al.* (1994) Magnetostratigraphic chronology of Cretaceous-to-Eocene thrust belt evolution, Central Utah, USA. *Journal of Geology*, 102, 181–96.

Tamaki, K. & Honza, E. (1991) Global tectonics and formation of marginal basins: role of the Western Pacific. *Episodes*, 14, 224–30.

Tandon, S.K. & Gibling, M.R. (1997) Calcretes at sequence boundaries in Upper Carboniferous cyclothems of the Sydney Basin, Atlantic Canada. *Sedimentary Geology*, 112, 43–67.

Taylor, A. & Blum, J.D. (1995) Relation between soil age and silicate weathering rates determined from the chemical evolution of a glacial chronosequence. *Geology*, 23, 979–82.

Taylor, B., Klaus, A., Brown, G.R. & Moore, G.F. (1991) Structural development of the Sumusi Rift, Izu–Bonin Arc. *Journal of Geophysical Research*, 96, 16113–29.

Taylor, S.R. & McLennan, S.M. (1995) The geochemical evolution of the continental crust. *Reviews of Geophysics*, 33, 241–65.

Tegen, I., Lacis, A.A. & Fung, I. (1996) The influence on climate forcing of mineral aerosols from disturbed soils. *Nature*, 380, 419–21.

Tewes, D.W. & Loope, D.B. (1992) Palaeo-yardangs: wind-scoured desert landforms at the Permo-Triassic unconformity. *Sedimentology*, 39, 251–61.

Tharp, T.M. (1987) Conditions for crack propagation by frost weathering. *Bulletin of the Geological Society of America*, 99, 94–102.

Thiede, J. & van Andel, T.H. (1977) The paleoenvironment of anaerobic sediments in the late Mesozoic South Atlantic Ocean. *Earth and Planetary Science Letters*, **33**, 301–9.

Thomas, D.S.G. (ed.) (1989) *Arid Zone Geomorphology*. Belhaven Halsted, New York.

Thorne, C.R., Bathurst, J.C. & Hey, R.D. (1987) *Sediment Transport in Gravel Bed Rivers*. Wiley, Chichester.

Thorne, C.R., MacArthur, R.C. & Bradley, J.B. (1988) *The Physics of Sediment Transport by Wind and Water: a collection of hallmark papers by R.A. Bagnold*. American Society of Civil Engineers, New York.

Thunell, R.C., Williams, D.F. & Kennett, J.P. (1977) Late Quaternary palaeoclimatology, stratigraphy and sapropel history in eastern Mediterranean deep-sea sediments. *Marine Micropalaeontology*, **2**, 371–88.

Thunnell, R., Rio, D., Sprovieri, R. & Raff, I. (1991) Limestone–marl couplets: origin of the early Pliocene Trubi marls in Calabria, southern Italy. *Journal of Sedimentary Petrology*, **61**, 1109–22.

Thurman, H.V. (1991) *Introductory Oceanography*, 7th edn. Macmillan, New York.

Tiedermann, W.G., Luchik, T.S. & Bogard, D.G. (1985) Wall-layer structure and drag reduction. *Journal of Fluid Mechanics*, **156**, 419–37.

Till, R. (1978) Arid Shorelines and Evaporites. In: (ed. H.G. Reading) *Sedimentary Environments and Facies*, 1st edn. Blackwell Science Ltd., Oxford.

Törnqvist, T.E. (1993) Holocene alternation of meandering and anastomosing fluvial systems in the Rhine–Meuse delta (Central Netherlands) controlled by sea-level rise and subsoil erodibility. *Journal of Sedimentary Petrology*, **63**, 683–93.

Törnqvist, T.E., van Ree, M.H.M. & Faessen, E.L.J.H. (1993) Longitudinal facies architectural changes of a Middle Holocene anastomosing distributary system (Rhine–Meuse delta, central Netherlands). *Sedimentary Geology*, **85**, 203–19.

Törnqvist, T.E., et al. (1996) A revised chronology for Mississippi River subdeltas. *Science*, **273**, 1693–6.

Torres, J., et al. (1997) Deep-sea avulsion and morphosedimentary evolution of the Rhône Fan Valley and Neofan during the Late Quaternary (north-western Mediterranean Sea). *Sedimentology*, **44**, 457–77.

Trewin, N.H. (1986) Palaeoecology and sedimentology of the Achanarras fish bed of the Middle Old Red Sandstone, Scotland. *Transactions of the Royal Society of Edinburgh, Earth Sciences*, **77**, 21–46.

Tricker, R.A.R. (1964) *Bores, Breakers, Waves and Wakes*. Mills and Boon, London; Elsevier, New York.

Tritton, D.J. (1988) *Physical Fluid Dynamics*. Oxford University Press, Oxford.

Tsoar, H. (1978) *The dynamics of longitudinal dunes*. Final technical report, European Research Office, US Army, London.

Tsoar, H. (1982) Internal structure and surface geometry of longitudinal (seif) dunes. *Journal of Sedimentary Petrology*, **52**, 823–31.

Tsoar, H. (1983) Dynamic processes acting on a longitudinal (seif) sand dune. *Sedimentology*, **30**, 567–78.

Tucker, M.E. (1982) Precambrian dolomites: petrographic and isotopic evidence that they differ from Phanerozoic dolomites. *Geology*, **10**, 7–12.

Tucker, M.E. & Wright, V.P. (1990) *Carbonate Sedimentology*. Blackwell Scientific Publications, Oxford.

Tucker, R.M. & Cann, J.R. (1986) A model to estimate the depositional brine depths of ancient halite rocks: implications for ancient subaqueous evaporite depositional environments. *Sedimentology*, **33**, 401–12.

Turcotte, D.L. & Schubert, G. (1982) *Geodynamics: Applications of Continuum Physics to Geological Problems*. Wiley, New York.

Turner, E.C., Narbonne, G.M. & James, N.P. (1993) Neoproterozoic reef microstructures from the Little Dal Group, northwest Canada. *Geology*, **21**, 259–62.

Tuschall, J.R. & Brezonik, P.L. (1980) Characterisation of organic nitrogen in natural waters: its molecular size, protein content and interactions with heavy metals. *Limnology and Oceanography*, **25**, 495–504.

Twichell, D.C., Kenyon, N.H., Parson, L.M. & McGregor, B.A. (1991) Depositional patterns of the Mississippi fan surface: evidence from GLORIA II and high-resolution seismic profiles. In: *Seismic Facies and Sedimentary Processes of Submarine Fans and Turbidite Systems* (eds P. Weimer & M.H. Link), pp. 349–64. Springer, Berlin.

Tzedakis, P.C. (1993) Long-term tree populations in northwest Greece through multiple Quaternary climatic cycles. *Nature*, **364**, 437–40.

Umbanhowar, P.B., Melo, F. & Swinney, H.L. (1996) Localised excitations in a vertically vibrated granular layer. *Nature*, **382**, 793–6.

Uncles, R.J. & Stephens, J.A. (1989) Distributions of suspended sediment at high water in a macrotidal estuary. *Journal of Geophysical Research*, **94**, 14395–405.

Underhill, J.R. (1991) Controls on late-Jurassic seismic sequences, Inner Moray Forth, UK North Sea: a critical test of a key segment of Exxon's original global cycle chart. *Basin Research*, **3**, 79–98.

Underwood, M.B. & Bachman, S.B. (1982) Sedimentary facies associations within subduction zones, pp. 537–50. Special Publication no. 10, Geological Society of London.

Underwood, M.B. & Moore, G.F. (1995) Trenches and trench slope basins. In: *Tectonics of Sedimentary Basins* (eds C. Busby & R. Ingersoll), pp. 179–220. Blackwell Science, Oxford.

Underwood, M.B., et al. (1995) Sedimentation in forearc basins, trenches, and collision zones of the Western Pacific: a summary of results from the Ocean Drilling Program. In: *Active Margins and Marginal Basins of the Western Pacific*, pp. 315–53. Geophysical Monograph no. 88, American Geophysical Union.

UNESCO (1977) *World Distribution of Arid Regions*. CNRS, Paris.

Vago, R., Gill, E. & Collingwood, J.C. (1997) Laser measurements of coral growth. *Nature*, **386**, 30–1.

Vail, P.R., *et al*. (1977) Seismic stratigraphy and global changes of sea level. In: *Seismic Statigraphy* (ed. C.E. Payton), pp. 49–205. Memoir no. 26, American Association of Petroleum Geologists.

Valeton, I. (1996) Tectono-morphogenetic evolution of late Mesozoic–early Tertiary palaeosurfaces and extension of saprolite–bauxite deposits. In: *Proceedings of the 4th International Symposium on the Geochemistry of the Earth's Surface* (ed. S.H. Bottrell), pp. 234–40. University of Leeds.

Vallance, J.W. & Scott, K.M. (1997) The Osceola Mudflow from Mount Rainier: sedimentology and hazard implications of a huge clay-rich debris flow. *Bulletin of the Geological Society of America*, **109**, 143–63.

Valyashko, M.G. (1972) Playa lakes—a necessary stage in the development of a salt-bearing basin. In: *Geology of Saline deposits* (ed. G. Richter-Bernberg), pp. 41–51. UNESCO, Paris.

Vanderburghe, J. (1995) Timescales, climate and river development. *Quaternary Science Reviews*, **14**, 631–8.

Van den Berg, J.H. (1995) Prediction of alluvial channel pattern of perennial rivers. *Geomorphology*, **12**, 259–79.

Van Gelder *et al*. (1994) Overbank and channelfill deposits of the modern Yellow River delta. *Sedimentary Geology*, **90**, 293–305.

Van Houten, F.B. (1962) Cyclic-sedimentation and the origin of analcime-rich Upper Triassic Lockatong Formation, west central New Jersey and adjacent Pennsylvania. *American Journal of Science*, **260**, 561–76.

Van Houten, F.B. (1964) Cyclic lacustrine sedimentation, Upper Triassic Lockatong Formation, central New Jersey and adjacent Pennsylvania. *Bulletin of the Geological Survey of Kansas*, **169**, 497–531.

Vardy, A. (1990) *Fluid Principles*. McGraw-Hill, New York.

Vasconcelos, C. & McKenzie, J.A. (1997) Microbial mediation of modern dolomite precipitation and diagenesis under anoxic conditions (Lagoa Vermelha, Rio de Janeiro, Brazil). *Journal of Sedimentary Research*, **67**, 378–90.

Vasconcelos, C., *et al*. (1995) Microbial mediation as a possible mechanism for natural dolomite formation at low temperature. *Nature*, **377**, 220–2.

Villareal, T.A., Altabet, M.A. & Culver-Rymsza, K. (1993) Nitrogen transport by vertically migrating diatom mats in the North Pacific Ocean. *Nature*, **363**, 709–12.

Villareal, T.A., *et al*. (1999) Upward transport of oceanic nitrate by migrating diatom mats. *Nature*, **397**, 423–5.

Vilas, F., *et al*. (1991) The Corrubedo beach–lagoon complex, Galicia, Spain: dynamics, sediments and recent evolution of a mesotidal coastal embayment. *Marine Geology*, **97**, 391–404.

Vincent, C.E. & Green, M.O. (1990) Field measurements of the suspended sand concentration profiles and fluxes and of the resuspension coefficient over a rippled bed. *Journal of Geophysical Research*, **95**, 11 591–601.

Visser, M.J. (1980) Neap-spring cycles reflected in Holocene subtidal large-scale bedform deposits: a preliminary note. *Geology*, **8**, 543–6.

Vitousek, P.M., *et al*. (1997) Soil and ecosystem development across the Hawaiian Islands. *GSA Today*, **7**, 1–8.

Vogel, S. (1994) *Life in Moving Fluids*. Princeton University Press, Princeton, NJ.

Vogt, P.R., Crane, K. & Sundvor, E. (1993) Glacigenic mudflows on the Bear Island submarine fan. *EOS*, October 5.

Vollbrecht, R. & Meischner, D. (1996) Diagenesis in coastal carbonates related to Pleistocene sea level, Bermuda Platform. *Journal of Sedimentary Research*, **66**, 243–58.

van Waggoner, J.C., *et al*. (1988) An overview of the fundamentals of sequence stratigraphy. In: *Sea Level Changes—An Integrated Approach* (eds Wilgus *et al*.), pp. 71–108. Special Publication no. 42, Society of Economic Palaeontologists and Mineralogists.

Wahlstrom, E.E. (1948) Pre-Fountain and Recent weathering on Flagstaff Mountain near Boulder, Colorado. *Bulletin of the Geological Society of America*, **59**, 1173–90.

Walder, J.S. & Fowler, A. (1991) Channelized subglacial drainage over a deformable bed. *Journal of Glaciology*, **40**, 3–15.

Walder, J. & Hallet, B. (1985) A theoretical model of the fracture of rock during freezing. *Bulletin of the Geological Society of America*, **96**, 336–46.

Walker, F.D.L., Parsons, I. & Lee, M.R. (1995) Micropores and micropermeable texture in alkali feldspars: geochemical and geophysical implications. *Mineralogical Magazine*, **59**, 507–36.

Walker, H.J., Coleman, J.M., Roberts, H.H. & Tye, R.S. (1987) Wetland loss in Louisiana. *Geografiska Annaler*, **69A**, 189–200.

Walker, J.C.G. (1977) *Evolution of the Atmosphere*. Macmillan, New York.

Walker, J.C.G. (1980) Biogeochemical cycles: oxygen. In: *Handbook of Environmental Chemistry* (ed. O. Hutzinger), pp. 87–104. Springer, Heidelberg.

Walker, J.C.G. & Drever, J.I. (1988) Geochemical cycles of atmospheric gases. In: *Chemical Cycles in the Evolution of the Earth* (eds C.B. Gregor *et al*.), pp. 55–76. Wiley, New York.

Walker, J.G.C., Hays, P.B. & Kasting, J.F. (1981) A negative feedback mechanism for the long-term stabilization of Earth's surface temperature. *Journal of Geophysical Research*, **86**, 9776–82.

Walker, R.G. (1965) The origin and significance of the internal structures of turbidites. *Proceedings of the Yorkshire Geological Society*, **35**, 1–32.

Walker, R.G. (1976) Facies models. 2, Turbidites and

associated coarse clastic deposits. *Geosciences Canada*, 3, 25–36.

Walker, R.G. (1978) Deep water sandstone facies and ancient submarine fans: models for exploration for stratigraphic traps. *Bulletin of the American Association of Petroleum Geologists*, 62, 932–66.

Walker, R.G. & Mutti, E. (1973) Turbidite facies and facies associations. In: *Turbidites and Deep Water Sedimentation* (eds G.V. Middleton & A.H. Bouma), pp. 119–57. Pacific Section Short Course, Society of Economic Palaeontologists and Mineralogists.

Wallmann, K., *et al.* (1997) Salty brines on the Mediterranean sea floor. *Nature*, 387, 31–2.

Wan, Z. (1982) *Bed Material Movement in Hyperconcentrated Flows*. Series paper no. 31, Institute of Hydrodynamics and Hydraulic Engineering, Technical University of Denmark.

Wan, Z. & Wang, Z. (1994) *Hyperconcentrated Flow*. Balkema, Rotterdam.

Wanless, H.R., Tyrrell, K.M., Tedesco, L.P. & Dravis, J.J. (1988a) Tidal-flat sedimentation from Hurricane Kate, Caicos Platform, British West Indies. *Journal of Sedimentary Petrology*, 58, 724–38.

Wanless, H.R., Tedesco, L.P. & Tyrrell, K.M. (1988b) Production of subtidal tubular and surficial tempestites by Hurricane Kate, Caicos Platform, British West Indies. *Journal of Sedimentary Petrology*, 58, 739–50.

Ward, W.C. & Brady, M.J. (1979) Strandline sedimentation of carbonate grainstones, Upper Pleistocene, Yucatan Peninsula, Mexico. *Bulletin of the American Association of Petroleum Geologists*, 63, 362–9.

Warren, J.K. (1982) The hydrological setting, occurrence and significance of gypsum in late Quaternary salt lakes in South Australia. *Journal of Sedimentary Petrology*, 52, 1171–201.

Warren, J.K. & Kendall, C.G.S.C. (1985) Comparison of sequences formed in marine sabkha (subaerial) and salina (subaqueous) settings—modern and ancient. *Bulletin of the American Association of Petroleum Geologists*, 69, 1013–23.

Wasson, R.J. & Hyde, R. (1983) Factors determining desert dune type. *Nature*, 304, 337–9.

Watkins, D.J. & Kraft, L.M. (1978) Stability of continental shelf and slope off Louisiana and Texas: geotechnical aspects. In: *Framework Facies and Oil-Trapping Characteristics of the Upper Continental Margin* (eds A.H. Bouma, G.T. Moore & J.M. Coleman), pp. 267–86. Studies in Geology no. 7, American Association of Petroleum Geologists, Tulsa, OK.

Weaver, P.P.E. & Thomson, J. (1993) Calculating erosion by deep-sea turbidity currents during initiation and flow. *Nature*, 364, 136–8.

Weber, K.J. & Daukoru, E. (1975) Petroleum geology of the Niger delta. *Proceedings of the 9th World Petroleum Congress*, Tokyo, Vol. 2, pp. 209–21. Applied Science, London.

Webster, P.J. (1994) The role of hydrological processes in ocean–atmosphere interactions. *Reviews of Geophysics*, 32, 427–76.

Weertman, J. (1957) On the sliding of glaciers. *Journal of Glaciology*, 3, 33–8.

Wei, T. & Willmarth, W.W. (1991) Examination of velocity fluctuations in a turbulent channel flow in the context of sediment transport. *Journal of Fluid Mechanics*, 223, 241–52.

Weimer, P. (1991) Seismic facies, characteristics, and variations in channel evolution, Mississippi fan (Plio-Pleistocene), Gulf of Mexico. In: *Seismic Facies and Sedimentary Processes of Submarine Fans and Turbidite Systems* (eds P. Weimer & M.H. Link), pp. 323–48. Springer, Berlin.

Weimer, P. & Posamentier, H.W. (1993) *Siliciclastic Sequence Stratigraphy*. Memoir no. 58, American Association of Petroleum Geologists, Tulsa, OK.

Weirich, F.H. (1986) The record of density-induced underflows in a glacial lake. *Sedimentology*, 33, 261–77.

Wellner, R.W., Ashley, G.M. & Sheridan, R.E. (1993) Seismic stratigraphic evidence for a submerged middle Wisconsin barrier: implications for sea-level history. *Geology*, 21, 109–12.

Wells, A.J. & Illing, L.V. (1964) Present day precipitation of calcium carbonate in the Persian Gulf. In: *Deltaic and Shallow Marine Deposits* (ed. L.M.J.U. Van Straten), pp. 429–35. Elsevier, Amsterdam.

Wells, J.T. (1987) *Effects of Sea-Level Rise on Deltaic Sedimentation in South-Central Louisiana*. Special Publication, Society of Economic Palaeontologists and Mineralogists.

Wells, N. (1986) *The Atmosphere and Ocean: A Physical Introduction*. Taylor and Francis, London.

Wells, N.A. & Dore, J.A. (1987) Shifting of the Kosi River, northern India. *Geology*, 15, 204–7.

Wells, N.C., Gould, W.J. & Kemp, A.E.S. (1996) The role of ocean circulation in the changing climate. In: (eds C.P. Summerhayes & S.A. Thorpe), ch. 3. Manson Press, London.

Weltje, G.J. & DeBoer, P.L. (1993) Astronomically induced paleoclimatic oscillations reflected in Pliocene turbidite deposits on Corfu (Greece): implications for the interpretation of higher order cyclicity in ancient turbidite systems. *Geology*, 21, 307–10.

Wendt, J., Belka, Z. & Moussine-Pouchkine, A. (1993) New architectures of deep-water carbonate buildups: evolution of mud mounds into mud ridges (Middle Devonian, Algerian Sahara). *Geology*, 21, 723–6.

Wendt, J., Belka, Z., Kaufman, B., Kostrewa, R. & Hayer, J. (1997) The world's most spectacular carbonate mud mounds (Middle Devonian, Algerian Sahara). *Journal of Sedimentary Research*, 67, 424–36.

Werner, B.T. (1995) Eolian dunes: computer simulations and attractor interpretation. *Geology*, 23, 1107–10.

West, I.M. (1975) Evaporites and associated sediments of

the basal Purbeck Formation (U. Jurassic) of Dorset. *Proceedings of the Geological Association*, **86**, 205–25.

Westbroek, P. (1991) *Life as a Geological Force*. Norton, New York.

Wetzel, R.G. (1983) *Limnology*, 2nd edn. Saunders College Publishing, Philadelphia.

Whalen, M.T. (1995) Barred basins: a model for eastern ocean basin carbonate platforms. *Geology*, **23**, 625–8.

Whateley, M.K.G. & Pickering, K.T. (eds) (1989) *Deltas: Sites and Traps for Fossil Fuels*. Special Publication no. 41, Geological Society of London.

Whipple, K.L. (1997) Open-channel flow of Bingham fluids: applications in debris-flow research. *Journal of Geology*, **105**, 243–62.

Whipple, K.L. & Dunne, T. (1992) The influence of debris flow rheology on fan morphology, Owens Valley, California. *Bulletin of the Geological Society of America*, **104**, 887–900.

Whitaker, F., Smart, P., Hague, Y., Waltham, D. & Bosence, D. (1997) Coupled two-dimensional diagenetic and sedimentological modeling of carbonate platform evolution. *Geology*, **25**, 175–8.

Whitaker, J.H. McD. (1973) Gutter casts. *Norsk Geologisk Tidsskrift*, **53**, 403–17.

White, A.F. (1995) Chemical weathering rates of silicate minerals in soils. In: *Chemical Weathering Rates of Silicate Minerals* (eds A.F. White & S.L. Brantley), ch. 9. American Mineralogical Society, Washington, DC.

White, A.F. & Brantley, S.L. (1995) Chemical weathering rates of silicate minerals: an overview. In: (eds A.F. White & S.L. Brantley) *Chemical Weathering Rates of Silicate Minerals*, Ch. 1. American Mineralogical Society, Washington DC.

White, A.F. & Brantley, S.L. (1995) *Chemical Weathering Rates of Silicate Minerals*. American Mineralogical Society, Washington DC.

Whiting, P.J., Dietrich, W.E., Leopold, L.B., Drake, T,G. & Shreve, R.L. (1988) Bedload sheets in heterogenous sediment. *Geology*, **16**, 105–8.

Widdel, F., Schnell, S., Heising, S., Ehrenreich, A., Assmus, B. & Schink, B. (1993) Ferrous iron oxidation by anoxygenic phototrophic bacteria. *Nature*, **362**, 834–6.

Wignall, P.B. (1994) *Black Shales*. Oxford University Press, Oxford.

Wilber, R.J., Milliman, J.D. & Halley, R.B. (1990) Accumulation of bank-top sediment on the western slope of Great bahama bank: rapid progradation of a carbonate megabank. *Geology*, **18**, 970–4.

Wilcock, P.R. & McArdell, B.W. (1993) Surface-based fractional transport rates: mobilisation thresholds and partial transport of a sand–gravel sediment. *Water Resources Research*, **29**, 1297–312.

Wilcock, P.R. & Southard, J.B. (1989) Bedload transport of mixed size sediment: fractional transport rates, bed forms, and the development of a coarse bed surface layer. *Water Resources Research*, **25**, 1629–41.

Wilkinson, B.H., Owen, R.M. & Carroll, A.R. (1985) Submarine hydrothermal weathering, global eustasy and carbonate polymorphism in Phanerozoic marine oolites. *Journal of Sedimentary Petrology*, **55**, 171–83.

Williams, M.A.J. (1994) Cenozoic climatic changes in deserts: a synthesis. In: *Geomorphology of Desert Environments* (eds A.D. Abrahams & A.J. Parsons), pp. 644–70. Chapman and Hall, London.

Williams, M.A.J., et al. (1993) *Quaternary Environments*. Arnold, London.

Williams, P.B. & Kemp, P.H. (1971) Initiation of ripples on mat sediment beds. *Journal of the Hydraulics Division, American Society of Civil Engineers*, **97**, 505–22.

Willis, B.J. (1993) Interpretation of bedding geometry within ancient point-bar deposits. In: *Alluvial Sedimentation* (eds M. Marzo & C. Puigdefabregas), pp. 101–14. Special Publication no. 17, International Association of Sedimentologists.

Willis, B.J. (1997) Architecture of fluvial-dominated valley-fill deposits in the Cretaceous Fall River Formation. *Sedimentology*, **44**, 735–57.

Willis, B.J. & Behrensmeyer, A.K. (1994) Architecture of Miocene overbank deposits in northern Pakistan. *Journal of Sedimentary Research*, **64**, 60–7.

Wilson, A.G. & Kirkby, M.J. (1975) *Mathematics for Geographers and Planners*. Oxford University Press, Oxford.

Wilson, I.G. (1971) Desert sandflow basins and a model for the development of ergs. *Geographical Journal*, **137**, 180–99.

Wilson, I.G. (1972a) Aeolian bedforms—their development and origins. *Sedimentology*, **19**, 173–210.

Wilson, I.G. (1972b) Universal discontinuities in bedforms produced by the wind. *Journal of Sedimentary Petrology*, **42**, 667–9.

Wilson, I.G. (1973) Ergs. *Sedimentary Geology*, **10**, 77–106.

Wilson, J.B. (1982) Shelly faunas associated with temperate offshore tidal deposits. In: *Offshore Tidal Sands: Processes and Deposits* (ed. A.H. Stride), pp. 126–71. Chapman and Hall, London.

Wilson, J.L. (1975) *Carbonate Facies in Geologic History*. Springer, Berlin.

Wilson, P.A. & Roberts, H.H. (1992) Carbonate-periplatform sedimentation by density flows: a mechanism for rapid off-bank and vertical transport of shallow-water fines. *Geology*, **20**, 713–16.

Winn, R.D., Roberts, H.H., Kohl, B., Fillon, R.H., Bouma, A.H. & Constans, R.E. (1995) Latest Quaternary deposition on the outer shelf, northern Gulf of Mexico: facies and sequence stratigraphy from Main Pass Block 303 core. *Bulletin of the Geological Society of America*, **107**, 851–66.

Witten, T.A. (1990) Structured fluids. *Physics Today*, July, 21–8.

Wollast, R. & Mackenzie, F.T. (1983) The global cycle of

silica. In: *Silicon Geochemistry and Biochemistry* (ed. S.R. Ashton), pp. 39–76. Academic Press, San Diego.

Wollast, R., Garrels, R.M. & Mackenzie, F.T. (1980) Calcite–seawater reactions in ocean surface waters. *American Journal of Science*, **280**, 831–48.

Wood, G.V. & Wolfe, M.J. (1969) Sabkha cycles in the Arab/Darb Formation off the Trucial Coast of Arabia. *Sedimentology*, **12**, 165–91.

Wood, J.M. (1989) Alluvial architecture of the Upper Cretaceous Judith River Formation, Dinosaur Provincial Park, Alberta, Canada. *Bulletin of the Canadian Society of Petroleum Geologists*, **37**, 169–81.

Wood, R., Zhuravlev, A.Y. & Anaaz, C.T. (1993) The ecology of Lower Cambrian buildups from Zuune Arts, Mongolia: implications for early metazoan reef evolution. *Sedimentology*, **40**, 829–58.

Woodcock, N.H. (1986) The role of strike-slip fault systems at plate boundaries. *Philosophical Transactions of the Royal Society, London (A)*, **317**, 13–29.

Woodroffe, C.D., Thom, B.G. & Chappell, J. (1985) Development of widespread mangrove swamps in mid-Holocene times in northern Australia. *Nature*, **317**, 711–13.

Woods, P.J. & Brown, R.G. (1975) Carbonate sedimentation in an arid zone tidal flat, nilemash Embayment, Shark Bay, Western Australia. In: (ed. R.N. Ginsburg) *Tidal Deposits*, pp. 223–33. Springer, New York.

Wopfner, H. & Twidale, C.R. (1988) Formation and age of desert dunes in the Lake Eyre depocentres in central Australia. *Geologische Rundschau*, **77**, 815–34.

Worden, R.H., Walker, F.D.L., Parsons, I. & Brown, W.L. (1990) Development of microporosity, diffusion channels and deuteric coarsening in perthitic alkali feldspars. *Contributions to Mineralogy and Petrology*, **104**, 507–15.

Wright, H.E., *et al.* (eds) (1993) *Global Climates Since the Last Glacial Maximum*. University of Minnesota Press, Minneapolis.

Wright, L.D. (1977) Sediment transport and deposition at river mouths: a synthesis. *Bulletin of the Geological Society of America*, **88**, 857–68.

Wright, L.D. (1985) River deltas. In: *Coastal Sedimentary Environments* (ed. R.A. Davis), pp. 1–76. Springer, New York.

Wright, L.D. & Coleman, J.M. (1973) Variations in morphology of major river deltas as functions of ocean wave and river discharge regimes. *Bulletin of the American Association of Petroleum Geologists*, **57**, 370–98.

Wright, L.D., Boon, J.D., Kim, S.C. & List, J.H. (1991) Modes of cross shore sediment transport on the shoreface of the Middle Atlantic Bight. *Marine Geology*, **96**, 19–51.

Wright, L.D., *et al.* (1986) Hyperpycnal plumes and plume fronts over the Huanghe (Yellow River) delta front. *Geo-Marine Letters*, **6**, 97–105.

Wright, V.P. & Marriott, S.B. (1993) The sequence stratigraphy of fluvial depositional systems: the role of floodplain sediment storage. *Sedimentary Geology*, **86**, 203–10.

Wright, V.P. & Burchette, T.P. (1996) Shallow-water carbonate environments. In: *Sedimentary Environments: Processes, Facies and Stratigraphy* (ed H.G. Reading), pp. 325–94. Blackwell Science, Oxford.

Wunderlich, F. (1972) Georgia coastal region, Sapelo Island, USA: sedimentology and biology, 3, Beach dynamics and beach development. *Senckenbergiana Maritima*, **4**, 15–45.

Wunderlich, W.O. (1971) The dynamics of density-stratified reservoirs. In: *Reservoir Fisheries and Limnology* (ed. G.E. Hall), pp. 219–31. Special Publication no. 8, American Fisheries Society, Washington, DC.

Wyngaard, J.C. (1992) Atmospheric turbulence. *Annual Reviews of Fluid Mechanics*, **24**, 205–33.

Yang, Y.-L., Elderfield, H., Pederson, T.F. & Ivanovich, M. (1995) Geochemical record of the Panama basin during the last glacial maximum carbon event shows that the glacial ocean was not suboxic. *Geology*, **23**, 1115–18.

Yarnold, J.C. (1993) Rock-avalanche characteristics in dry climates and the effects of flow into lakes: insights from mid-Tertiary sedimentary breccias near Artillery Peak Arizona. *Bulletin of the Geological Society of America*, **105**, 345–60.

Yechieli, Y., Gavrieli, I., Berkowitz, B. & Ronen, D. (1998) Will the Dead Sea die? *Geology*, **26**, 755–8.

Yoshida, F. (1994) Interaction between alluvial fan sedimentation, thrusting, and sea level changes: an example from the Komeno Formation (Early Pleistocene), southwest Japan. *Sedimentary Geology*, **92**, 97–115.

Yu, E.-F., Francois, R. & Bacon, M.P. (1996) Similar rates of modern and last-glacial ocean thermohaline circulation inferred from radiochemical data. *Nature*, **379**, 689–94.

Yuretich, R.F. (1979) Modern sediments and sedimentary processes in Lake Rudolf (Lake Turkana), eastern Rift Valley, Kenya. *Sedimentology*, **26**, 313–32.

Yuretich, R.F. & Cerling, T.E. (1983) Hydrogeochemistry of Lake Turkana, Kenya: mass balance and mineral reactions in an alkaline lake. *Geochimica et Cosmochimica Acta*, **47**, 1099–109.

Zaleha, M. (1997a) Intra- and extra-basinal controls on fluvial deposition in the Miocene Indo-Gangetic foreland basin, northern Pakistan. *Sedimentology*, **44**, 369–90.

Zaleha, M. (1997b) Fluvial and lacustrine palaeoenvironments of the Miocene Siwalik Group, Khaur area, northern Pakistan. *Sedimentology*, **44**, 349–68.

Ziegler, A.M., Hulver, M.L., Lottes, A.L. & Schmachtenberg, W.F. (1984) Uniformitarianism and paleoclimates: inferences from the distribution of carbonate rocks. In: *Fossils and Climate* (ed. P.J. Brenchley), pp. 3–25. Wiley, New York.

Index

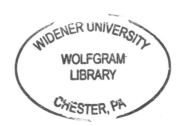